CURRENT THERAPY IN

AVIAN MEDICINE
AND SURGERY

CURRENT THERAPY IN

AVIAN MEDICINE AND SURGERY

FIRST EDITION

Editor-in-Chief

BRIAN L. SPEER, DVM, DABVP (Avian Practice), DECZM (Avian)

The Medical Center for Birds
Oakley, California

ELSEVIER

ELSEVIER

3251 Riverport Lane
St. Louis, Missouri 63043

Content Strategy Director: Penny Rudolph
Content Development Manager: Jolynn Gower
Publishing Services Manager: Julie Eddy
Design Direction: Ashley Miner

Printed in China

Last digit is the print number: 9 8 7 6 5 4 3 2

Contributors

Mélanie Ammersbach, DVM
Department of Pathobiology
Ontario Veterinary College
University of Guelph
Guelph, Ontario, Canada
Variability and Limitations in Clinical Avian Hematology
Clinical Biochemistry

Natalie Antinoff, DVM, DABVP (Avian Practice)
Gulf Coast Avian & Exotics
Gulf Coast Veterinary Specialists
Houston, Texas
Clinical Avian Neurology and Neuroanatomy

Heather Barron, BSA, DVM, DABVP (Avian Practice)
Hospital Director
Clinic for the Rehabilitation of Wildlife
Sanibel, Florida
Table of Common Drugs and Approximate Doses

Hugues Beaufrère, DVM, PhD, DABVP (Avian Practice), DECZM (Avian Practice), DACZM
Service Chief, Avian and Exotic Service
Health Sciences Centre, Ontario Veterinary College
University of Guelph
Guelph, Ontario, Canada
Cardiology
Variability and Limitations in Clinical Avian Hematology
Clinical Biochemistry
Medicine of Strigiformes

R. Avery Bennett, DVM, MS, DACVS
Zorro Veterinary Surgery
Fort Lauderdale, Florida
Approaches to the Coelom and Selected Procedures
Selected Coelomic Surgical Procedures

Laurie Bergman, VMD, DACVB
Keystone Veterinary Behavior Services
Villanova, Pennsylvania
Behavior

Jeleen A. Briscoe, VMD, DABVP (Avian Practice)
Avian Specialist
Chief of Staff, Animal Care
Chair, AC Civil Rights and Diversity Advisory Committee
USDA APHIS Animal Care
Washington, DC
Animal Welfare Legislation and Its Influence on Avian Welfare

James W. Carpenter, MS, DVM, DACZM
Professor
Department of Clinical Sciences
Kansas State University
Manhattan, Kansas
Table of Common Drugs and Approximate Doses
Normal Biological Data

Thomas E. Catanzaro, DVM, MHA, LFACHE
CEO
Veterinary Consulting International
Boondall, Queensland, Australia
Practice Management

Crissa Cooey, MS
Graduate Student
Division Forestry and Natural Resources
West Virginia University
Morgantown, West Virginia
Diagnostic Testing of Age of Birds and Its Applications

Lorenzo Crosta, Med Vet, PhD
Co-owner
Clinica Veterinaria Valcurone
Missaglia, Italy
Chlamydiosis (Psittacosis)
The Conservation Project of the Rarest Parrot: The Spix's Macaw (Cyanopsitta spixii)

Ricardo de Matos, LMV, MSc, DABVP (Avian), DECZM (Avian, Small Mammal)
Lecturer
Department of Clinical Sciences
Cornell University College of Veterinary Medicine
Ithaca, New York
Diseases of the Endocrine System—Protein Hormones

Robert Doneley, BVSc, FANZCVS
Associate Professor, Avian and Exotic Pet Medicine
School of Veterinary Science
University of Queensland
Gatton, Queensland, Australia
Common Conditions of Commonly Held Companion Birds in Multiple Parts of the World

Michael Scott Echols, DVM, DABVP (Avian Practice)
Associate Veterinarian, Co-Founder
Mobile Avian Surgical Services
The Medical Center for Birds
Oakley, California
Navigating the Nutraceutical Industry: A Guide to Help Veterinarians Make Informed Clinical Decisions
Approaches to the Coelom and Selected Procedures
Selected Coelomic Surgical Procedures

Dorianne Elliott, DVN, BVSc
Head Veterinarian
Bird and Exotic Animal Hospital
Onderstepoort
Pretoria, Gauteng, South Africa
  Common Conditions of Commonly Held Companion Birds in Multiple Parts of the World

Nienke Endenburg, PhD
Assistant Professor
Department of Animals in Science and Society
Faculty of Veterinary Sciences
Utrecht, Netherlands
  The Human–Avian Bond

Brenna Colleen Fitzgerald, DVM, DABVP (Avian Practice)
Associate Veterinarian
Medical Center for Birds
Oakley, California
  Cardiology

Susan G. Friedman, PhD
Department of Psychology
Utah State University
Logan, Utah
  Behavior

Alan M. Fudge, DVM, DABVP (Avian Practice)
Clinical Veterinarian/Photographer
Mobile Veterinary Services: Birds & Fish
Alan Fudge Photography
Greenville, South Carolina
Former Director
Bird Doctor
California Avian Laboratory
El Dorado Hills, California
  Normal Clinical Pathologic Data

Brett D. Gartrell, BVSc, PhD, MANZCVS (Avian Health)
Associate Professor
Wildbase, Institute of Veterinary Animal and Biomedical Sciences
Massey University
Palmerston North, New Zealand
  Veterinary Involvement in the Takahe Recovery Program

Stacey Gelis, BSc, BVSc (Hons), MACVSc (Avian Health)
Senior Veterinarian
Melbourne Bird Veterinary Clinic
Scoresby, Victoria, Australia
  Advancements in Nutrition of Loridae

Jennifer Graham, DVM, DABVP (Avian and Exotic Companion Mammal Practice), DACZM
Assistant Professor of Zoological Companion Animal Medicine
Department of Clinical Sciences
Cummings School of Veterinary School at Tufts University
North Grafton, Massachusetts
  Neoplastic Diseases in Avian Species

Cheryl B. Greenacre, DVM
Professor
Small Animal Clinical Sciences, CVM
University of Tennessee
Knoxville, Tennessee
  Euthanasia

James M. Harris, BS, DVM
Mayfair Veterinary Clinic
Sandy Bay, Tasmania, Australia
  Foreword

Michelle G. Hawkins, VMD, DABVP (Avian Practice)
Director, California Raptor Center
Associate Professor, Companion Avian and Exotic Pets
Department of Medicine and Epidemiology
School of Veterinary Medicine
University of California, Davis
Davis, California
  Recognition, Assessment, and Management of Pain in Birds
  Table of Common Drugs and Approximate Doses

Darryl Heard, BSc, BVMS, PhD, DACZM
Associate Professor Zoological Medicine
Small Animal Clinical Sciences
University of Florida
Gainesville, Florida
  Anesthesia

Edward W. Hsu, PhD
Associate Professor
Department of Bioengineering
University of Utah
Salt Lake City, Utah
  Advances in Diagnostic Imaging

Hillar Klandorf, PhD
Professor
Division of Animal and Nutritional Science
College of Agriculture, Natural Resources and Design
West Virginia University
Morgantown, West Virginia
  Diagnostic Testing of Age of Birds and Its Applications

Eric Klaphake, DVM, DACZM, DABVP (Avian Practice)
Associate Veterinarian
Cheyenne Mountain Zoo
Colorado Springs, Colorado
  Specialization in Avian Medicine and Surgery

V. Wensley Koch, DVM
Assistant Staff Officer
USDA, APHIS, Animal Care
Fort Collins, Colorado
Animal Welfare Legislation and Its Influence on Avian Welfare

Elizabeth Koutsos, PhD
Director
Mazuri Exotic Animal Nutrition
PMI Nutrition Intl LLC
Gray Summit, Missouri
Foundations in Avian Nutrition

Charlotte Lacroix, DVM, JD
Owner and CEO
Veterinary Business Advisors, Inc.
Managing Risk in Avian Practice

Nathaniel K.Y. Lam, DVM, DACVS
Chief of Surgery
VCA Oahu Veterinary Specialists
Pearl City, Hawaii
Approaches to the Coelom and Selected Procedures
Selected Coelomic Surgical Procedures

Delphine Laniesse, DMV, IPSAV
Resident in Avian Medicine
Health Sciences Centre
Ontario Veterinary College
University of Guelph
Guelph, Ontario, Canada
Medicine of Strigiformes

Angela Lennox, DVM, DABVP (Avian Practice),
ECM, ECZM-SA
Avian and Exotic Animal Clinic
Indianapolis, Indiana
Mycobacteriosis
Critical Care

Anna Le Souef, BSc (Hons), BVMS, PhD
Research Fellow
Black Cockatoo Health and Demographics Project
Murdoch University
Veterinarian
Perth Zoo
Perth, Western Australia, Australia
Diagnostic Testing of Age of Birds and Its Applications

Marla Lichtenberger, DVM, DACVECC
Owner and Critical Care Specialist
Milwaukee Emergency Center for Animals
Milwaukee, Wisconsin
Critical Care

Michael Lierz, Prof Dr Med Vet, DZooMed, DECZM,
DECPVS
Professor
Faculty of Veterinary Medicine
Clinic for Birds, Reptiles, Amphibians and Fish
Justus Liebeig University Giessen
Giessen, Germany
Avian Bornavirus and Proventricular Dilation Disease
Advancements in Methods for Improving Reproductive Success
Advancements in Methods for Decreasing Reproductive Success

Johannes Thomas (Sjeng) Lumeij, DVM, PhD,
DECZM (Avian Practice)
Associate Professor
Division of Zoological Medicine
Department of Clinical Sciences of Companion Animals
Faculty of Veterinary Medicine
Utrecht University
Utrecht, Netherlands
Usutu Virus

Philip M. Marsh
Takahē Liaison
Department of Conservation
Te Papa Atawhai
New Zealand
Veterinary Involvement in the Takahe Recovery Program

An Martel, DVM, MSc, PhD, DECZM (Wildlife
Population Health)
Professor
Faculty of Veterinary Medicine
Department of Pathology, Bacteriology and Avian Diseases
Division of Poultry, Exotic Animals, Wildlife and Laboratory
    Animals
Ghent University
Merelbeke, Belgium
Aspergillosis

Anne McDonald, DVM
Night Owl Bird Hospital
Vancouver, British Columbia, Canada
*Common Conditions of Commonly Held Companion Birds in
    Multiple Parts of the World*

Alicia McLaughlin, DVM, BS
Associate Veterinarian
Center for Bird and Exotic Animal Medicine
Bothell, Washington
Neoplastic Diseases in Avian Species

Steve Mehler, DVM, DACVS
Chief of Surgery
Hope Veterinary Specialists
Malvern, Pennsylvania
Approaches to the Coelom and Selected Procedures
Selected Coelomic Surgical Procedures

Franck L.B. Meijboom, MA, PhD
Assistant Professor
Ethics Institute
Department of Animals in Science & Society
Faculty of Veterinary Medicine
Utrecht University
Utrecht, Netherlands
*As Free as a Bird on the Wing: Some Welfare and Ethical
Considerations on Flight Restraint Methods in Birds*

Alessandro Melillo, DVM
OMNIAVET Vet Clinic
Rome, Italy
Chlamydiosis (Psittacosis)

Michael Mison, DVM, DACVS
Surgeon
Seattle Veterinary Specialists
Kirkland, Washington
Affiliate Assistant Professor
Department of Comparative Medicine
University of Washington
Seattle, Washington
*Approaches to the Coelom and Selected Procedures
Selected Coelomic Surgical Procedures*

**Deborah Monks, BVSc (Hons), CertZooMed, DECZM
(Avian Practice), FANZCVSc (Avian Medicine)**
Principal
Brisbane Bird and Exotics Veterinary Service
Macgregor, Queensland, Australia
*Diseases of the Endocrine System—Protein Hormones
Common Conditions of Commonly Held Companion Birds in
Multiple Parts of the World*

Geoffrey P. Olsen, DVM, DABVP (Avian Practice)
Medical Center for Birds
Oakley, California
*Common Conditions of Commonly Held Companion Birds in
Multiple Parts of the World*

Glenn H. Olsen, DVM, MS, PhD
Veterinary Medical Officer
USGS Patuxent Wildlife Research Center
Laurel, Maryland
*Conservation Medicine
The Whooping Crane Recovery Project*

**Susan E. Orosz, PhD, DVM, DABVP (Avian Practice),
DECZM (Avian)**
Owner
Bird and Exotic Pet Wellness Center
Toledo, Ohio
*Clinical Avian Neurology and Neuroanatomy
Anatomy and Physiology of the Endocrine System—Protein
Hormones*

Joanne Paul-Murphy, DVM
Diplomate American College of Zoological Medicine
Diplomate American College of Animal Welfare
Professor
Veterinary Medicine & Epidemiology
University of California, Davis
Davis, California
*Recognition, Assessment, and Management of Pain in Birds
Foundations in Avian Welfare*

Helene Pendl, DrMedVet
PendlLab
Zug, Switzerland
*Immunology
Cytology*

Olivia A. Petritz, DVM, DACZM
Avian & Exotics Division
ACCESS Specialty Animal Hospital
Los Angeles, California
*Advancements in Methods for Decreasing Reproductive Success
Clinical Applications and Considerations for the use of GnRH
Agonists*

David Phalen, DVM, PhD, DABVP (Avian Practice)
Associate Professor
Faculty of Veterinary Science
University of Sydney
Camden, New South Wales, Australia
*Psittacid Herpesviruses and Associated Diseases
Macrorhabdosis*

Christal Pollock, DVM, DABVP (Avian Practice)
Veterinary Consultant
Lafeber Company
Cornell, Illinois
*A Historical View of Avian Medicine
Normal Biological Data*

Julia B. Ponder, DVM
Executive Director
The Raptor Center, College of Veterinary Medicine
University of Minnesota
St. Paul, Minnesota
Orthopedics

Shane Raidal, BVSc, PhD, FACVSc, DECZM
Professor
Veterinary Pathobiology
Charles Sturt University
Wagga Wagga, New South Wales, Australia
Psittacine Beak and Feather Disease

**Drury R. Reavill, DVM, DABVP (Avian and Reptile
& Amphibian Practice), DACVP**
Zoo/Exotic Pathology Service
Carmichael, California
Neoplastic Diseases in Avian Species

Patrick Redig, DVM, PhD
Professor
Veterinary Clinical Sciences
College of Veterinary Medicine
Co-Founder and Director Emeritus
The Raptor Center
University of Minnesota
St. Paul, Minnesota
    Orthopedics

Jorge Rivero, DVM
Sierra Vista, Arizona
    Common Conditions of Commonly Held Companion Birds in
        Multiple Parts of the World
    The Perspective on Avian Medicine in South America

Jacob A. Rubin, DVM
Assistant Professor
Department of Clinical Sciences
Michigan State University
East Lansing, Michigan
    Principles of Microsurgery

Jeffrey J. Runge, DVM, DACVS
Assistant Professor of Minimally Invasive Surgery
Department of Clinical Studies, Section of Surgery
University of Pennsylvania, School of Veterinary Medicine
Philadelphia, Pennsylvania
    Principles of Microsurgery

Elizabeth Marie Rush, DVM, DACZM
Staff Specialist – Antech Imaging Services
Associate Professor, Pathobiology Academic Program
Coordinator, Wildlife and Zoological Research
School of Veterinary Medicine
St. George's University
Grenada, West Indies
    Foundations in Clinical Pathology

Jaime Samour, MVZ, PhD, DECZM (Avian)
Director of Wildlife
Wildlife Division
Wrsan
Abu Dhabi, United Arab Emirates
    Advancements in Methods for Decreasing Reproductive Success

David Sanchez-Migallon Guzman, LV, MS, DECZM
(Avian), DACZM
Veterinary Teaching Hospital
School of Veterinary Medicine
University of California, Davis
Davis, California
    Recognition, Assessment, and Management of Pain in Birds

Robert E. Schmidt, DVM, PhD, DACVP
Zoo/Exotic Pathology Service
Anthem, Arizona
    Forensic Necropsy

Petra Schnitzer, DVM, Resident ECZM (Avian)
Resident
Avian Specialty
Veterinari Montevecchia
Montevecchia, Italy
    Chlamydiosis (Psittacosis)

Nico J. Schoemaker, DVM, PhD, DECZM (Small
Mammal and Avian Practice), DABVP (Avian
Practice)
Associate Professor
Division of Zoological Medicine
Department of Clinical Sciences of Companion Animals
Faculty of Veterinary Medicine
Utrecht University
Utrecht, Netherlands
    Advances in Diagnostic Imaging
    As Free as a Bird on the Wing: Some Welfare and Ethical
        Considerations on Flight Restraint Methods in Birds

Brian L. Speer, DVM, DABVP (Avian Practice),
DECZM (Avian)
The Medical Center for Birds
Oakley, California
    Approaches to the Coelom and Selected Procedures
    Selected Coelomic Surgical Procedures
    Practice Management
    Common Conditions of Commonly Held Companion Birds in
        Multiple Parts of the World
    Normal Clinical Pathologic Data

Nicole Stacy, DVM, DrMedVet, DACVP (Clinical
Pathology)
University of Florida
Large Animal Clinical Sciences
College of Veterinary Medicine
Gainesville, Florida
    Cytology

Cynthia E. Stringfield, DVM
Faculty and Veterinarian
Exotic Animal Training and Management
Moorpark College
Moorpark, California
    Veterinary Contributions to the Recovery of the California
        Condor

Darrel K. Styles, DVM, PhD
Senior Staff Veterinarian
Surveillance, Preparedness, and Response Division
National Preparedness and Incident Coordination Staff
USDA APHIS Veterinary Services
Riverdale, Maryland
    An Overview of Avian Influenza in Domestic and Nondomestic
        Avian Species

W. Michael Taylor, DVM
Clinician Consultant
Taylor Avian and Exotics
Port Perry, Ontario, Canada
Clinical Significance of the Avian Cloaca: Interrelationships with the Kidneys and the Hindgut
Pleura, Pericardium, and Peritoneum: The Coelomic Cavities of Birds and their Relationship to the Lung–Air Sac System

Ian Tizard, BVMS, PhD, AVCM, DSc
University Distinguished Professor of Immunology
Veterinary Pathobiology
Texas A&M University
College Station, Texas
Immunology

Yvonne R.A. van Zeeland, DVM, MVR, PhD, DECZM (Avian, Small Mammal)
Associate Professor
Division of Zoological Medicine
Department of Clinical Sciences of Companion Animals
Faculty of Veterinary Medicine
Utrecht University
Utrecht, Netherlands
Behavior
Advances in Diagnostic Imaging
As Free as a Bird on the Wing: Some Welfare and Ethical Considerations on Flight Restraint Methods in Birds

Claire Vergneau-Grosset, DVM, IPSAV, DACZM
Staff Veterinarian
Companion Avian and Exotic Pet Medicine
University of California, Davis
Davis, California
Clinical Biochemistry

Frank Verstappen, DVM, DECZM (Avian)
Avian & Exotic Veterinarian
Dierenkliniek Hoofdstraat
Driebergen, Netherlands
Common Conditions of Commonly Held Companion Birds in Multiple Parts of the World

Claudia M. Vinke, PhD
Associate Professor
Department of Animal in Science & Society
Faculty of Veterinary Medicine
Utrecht University
Utrecht, Netherlands
As Free as a Bird on the Wing: Some Welfare and Ethical Considerations on Flight Restraint Methods in Birds

Patricia Wakenell, DVM, PhD, DACVP
Head of Avian Diagnostics
Associate Professor of Comparative Pathobiology
Animal Disease Diagnostic Laboratory
Purdue University
West Lafayette, Indiana
Management and Medicine of Backyard Poultry

Kristin Warren, BSc, Hons, BVMS, PhD, Dipl ECZM (Wildlife Population Health)
Associate Professor
Conservation Medicine Program
College of Veterinary Medicine, Murdoch University
Murdoch, Western Australia
Diagnostic Testing of Age of Birds and Its Applications

James F.X. Wellehan Jr., DVM, MS, PhD, DACZM, DACVM (Virology, Bacteriology/Mycology), DECZM (Herpetology)
Zoological Medical Service
College of Veterinary Medicine
University of Florida
Gainesville, Florida
Critical Thinking and Practical Application of Evidence-Based Medicine in Avian Practice
The Pathogenesis of Infectious Diseases
Coccidial Diseases of Birds
Molecular Diagnostic Testing

Morena Wernick, DrMedVet, DECZM (Avian)
ExoticVet GmbH
Jona, St. Gallen, Switzerland
Foundations in Clinical Pathology

Maggie Weston, DVM
New Frontier Animal Medical Center
Sierra Vista, Arizona
Common Conditions of Commonly Held Companion Birds in Multiple Parts of the World
The Perspective on Avian Medicine in South America

Tina Wismer, DVM, DABVT, DABT
Medical Director
ASPCA Animal Poison Control Center
Urbana, Illinois
Advancements in Diagnosis and Management of Toxicologic Problems

Enrique Yarto-Jaramillo, DVM, MSc
Clinical Advisor—ZooLeon
Leon, Guanajuato, Mexico
President of Instituto Mexicano de Fauna Silvestre y Animales de Compañía
Adjunct Veterinarian—Exotic Pets and Wildlife
Centro Veterinario Mexico
Distrito Federal, Mexico
Common Conditions of Commonly Held Companion Birds in Multiple Parts of the World
Additional Perspectives from Mexico and Central America

Ashley Zehnder, DVM, DABVP (Avian Practice)
Postdoctoral Scholar
Department of Dermatology
Stanford University
Stanford, California
Neoplastic Diseases in Avian Species

To my immediate and extended family,
every one of you.
At the end of the day,
it is all of you that are the real deal.

And to the birds themselves,
who continue to inspire us to soar to new heights.

Foreword

My first nonhuman companion was a 6-week-old Budgie that my father bought on a business trip to Scotland. For the 500-mile drive returning to our home in London, the bird in a box on the front seat of the car heard its name, "Joey," every 10 seconds. When it arrived home it was put in a cage located behind my seat at the dining table where it could look out the window into our yard. The next morning when I came downstairs for breakfast it said "Joey." From there the vocabulary expanded to some 500 words; Joey displayed an amazing cognitive understanding of language. When he was asked, "Where do you live," "16 Litchfield Way Hampstead Garden Suburb" was the clear reply. As a young boy I always left my meat for last as it was my favorite food. Mum would say, "Jimmy, eat your meat." If all was consumed on my plate except for the protein, Joey would remind me to eat my meat, saving my mum from having to remind me. Family members were greeted each morning by name. Years later, working with my late dear friend Dr. Louis Baptista, I would learn much more about the vocalization and the language of birds. At the age of 6, I announced to my father that I was going to be a veterinary surgeon and I was off to the greatest adventure of my life.

After graduating from Michigan State University, College of Veterinary Medicine in 1958, I relocated to Oakland, California. In 1961 at one of our monthly veterinary association dinner meetings, I announced that I was starting my own practice. I was going to lease a space in a shopping center, have an appointment book, and see birds.

A colleague across the room was laughing so hard he fell off his chair as he shouted, "You won't last 3 months." A lot of water has passed under the veterinary bridge since that time, and needless to say, my passion for healthcare delivery for birds has only grown.

Robert Stroud's book was pretty much all there was to read on avian medicine. I think I still have a copy somewhere, collecting dust on one of my shelves. Now my medical library has three full shelves of Avian Medicine and Surgery texts, ranging from poultry to parrots, birds of prey, and more. And the colleague that came to me as a young mixed-animal practitioner in 1985 and asked me to mentor him as he was interested in Avian Medicine and Surgery is now editing this volume. It did not take long for him to surpass me in his knowledge and skill as an avian specialist. He is not alone at this time in our development of the field of Avian Medicine and Surgery. The list of contributors to this volume speaks highly of how the field has progressed and advanced as a specialty within our profession.

Predominantly an American interest a little over 30 years ago, Avian Medicine and Surgery is now a worldwide entity, with avian veterinary organizations in Australasia, Europe, and other parts of the world. Interest internationally is growing among our colleagues, benefitting birds kept by humans as well as the 10,000 or so avian species that inhabit every corner of our planet from the Arctic to the Antarctic and every geographical habitat between.

In addition to the interest and dedication we in the profession have toward avian species, the wealth of literature now available, and those in teaching positions at veterinary training institutions, those involved with research have contributed to our knowledge and allowed avian diagnosis and treatment to progress to the current advanced state. We have made good progress but have just scratched the surface. There is so much more we need to understand and apply for the benefit of our patients and clients in clinical practice, as well as of the wildlife we treat.

Finally, I must give thanks to the industries that we are dependent on for our pharmaceuticals and the specialized equipment needed in our daily work. Their contribution to avian medicine cannot be overstated.

I for one look forward to adding this volume to my medical library. I hope it is the first of a continuous series of volumes that periodically present *Current Therapy in Avian Medicine and Surgery*.

My sincere thanks to Brian Speer for his eager interest in this project, to the contributors of each section, and to the publishers for making this material available.

James M. Harris, OAM, BS, DVM, FRSPH
Mayfair Veterinary Clinic
Sandy Bay, Tasmania, Australia
16 April, 2014

Preface

This, the first edition of our text, originated over a series of conversations and meetings with Penny Rudolph spanning a handful of years, prior to my acceptance of the offer to undertake the project. There was a need for a newer avian medicine text, one with a newer format that was representative of the breadth and scope that avian medicine and surgery had grown to be and would become in the future. The format of *Current Therapy in Avian Medicine and Surgery* offers a more appropriate means with which to introduce up-to-date, cutting-edge material that is more broadly relevant to this continually evolving species discipline. The vast opportunity to incorporate evidence-based principles in a way that best demonstrates advancements and to fortify clinical knowledge in a manner that is clinically relevant was clear. Furthermore, this delivery system offered the chance to open doors to new thought processes within avian medicine and surgery, new clinical techniques and paradigms of healthcare, and myriad other areas to explore and develop for future editions. Excited by this promise and honored to have been asked to take on the challenge, I accepted the offer. This text has been written with two audiences in mind: those colleagues who are beginning their careers and those who are continuing to broaden their understanding and expertise.

The first outline was written in January 2013, and after 47 collaborative modifications to the table of contents, the layout of this text finally emerged; needless to say, it went well beyond my original vision. Excited contributors and friends offered their thoughts, suggestions, and energy to the project and in turn helped bring it to its final form. Potential contributors were contacted as early as September 2013, and the editing process soon began for each and every written portion. An impressive total of 87 contributors, recognized experts and authors all, were able to bring their work forward. As this first edition approaches completion, information and ideas are already being gathered for the second!

This book contains four sections: (1) *Advances in Avian Medicine*, (2) *Advances in Anesthesia, Analgesia, and Surgery*, (3) *Advances in Welfare, Conservation, and Practice Management*, and (4) *Pattern Recognition*. Throughout the 25 chapters of this edition, tables, boxes, figures, artwork, and algorithms are used to provide readers with streamlined overviews and aids to clinical thought processes and concepts. The interconnections between topics should be apparent to readers. Each of these chapters provides important pieces of the whole, but also relies on the others to help build a more complete picture of the delivery of avian healthcare.

The first section, *Advances in Avian Medicine*, is also the largest and includes 18 chapters. Chapter 1 reviews the past history of avian medicine, helping readers understand how we have arrived at where we are today. It outlines in detail the means by which veterinarians may pursue specialization in the field, which aids in empowering colleagues to fortify their passion for birds and to turn that passion toward the service of avian healthcare and conservation. The foundation for the art of delivery of optimal healthcare lies in critical thought

processes, our ability to use the best evidence possible, which is explored in the final portion. Chapter 2 focuses on select infectious diseases. Most of the topics included are not simple and pose a challenge to understand, diagnose, or manage. A foundational, unifying, and introductory view into the complexity of pathogenesis of infectious disease is provided at the beginning; infectious disease is dependent on far more than merely the pathogen alone. Readers will find a mixture of well-published diseases such as aspergillosis, chlamydiosis, mycobacteriosis, psittacine beak and feather disease, and psittacid herpesvirus and its associated diseases. Information is current, relevant, and clinically applicable. Relatively newer diseases such as macrorhabdosis, Usutu virus, and some of the coccidial diseases of birds are included as well, bringing light to their associated pathogens, pathogenesis, diagnosis, and treatment options. In particular, avian bornavirus and proventricular dilation disease are discussed from a current, complete, and critical viewpoint, with practical and clinically relevant recommendations for testing, diagnosis, and preventative management. Finally, the timely and ever-important topic, avian influenza virus, is reviewed. Chapter 3 brings forward an in-depth and current review of neoplastic diseases of birds. It offers clinicians an innovative view of clinically relevant options for diagnosis, staging, and treatment. Chapter 4 explores some of the current aspects of nutrition and nutritional therapy, first by reviewing foundations in nutrition and then by providing an in-depth review of our current understanding of nutrition of the Loridae family. Finally, a critical look at what veterinarians need to know to best use nutraceuticals in the care and treatment of their patients is included. Chapter 5 brings behavioral medicine to the forefront, its proper position as an important component of *Advances in Avian Medicine*. The days of simplistically separating a bird's behavioral health from its physical health are becoming a thing of the past. This chapter provides readers with current, well-delivered foundations with which clinicians can integrate sound behavioral medical principles into the care that they provide for avian patients. Chapter 6 addresses cardiology in a complete, dynamic, well-researched, and applicable manner. It is an excellent go-to reference site for those who seek to improve their understanding of this increasingly prevalent category of disease in avian species. Chapters 7 and 8 explore the anatomy, form, and function of the cloaca and the coelomic cavities of birds; through a careful and detailed review of foundational literature, these chapters highlight the complexity of their relevant anatomy and function, providing an opportunity to understand the manifestations of disease, means of diagnosis, and treatment options. Clinical neurology is presented in Chapter 9 in a refreshed manner, with new, reimagined artwork and a clinical eye on applicability through improved understanding. The protein hormones of birds and their endocrinology are discussed in Chapter 10 in a current and clinically relevant manner, placing this material in a single location that clinicians can quickly reference for helpful information. Chapter 11 tackles the complexities of the immune system, bringing forward a current review and discussion of relevant immune mechanisms, diseases, syndromes, and diagnostic and therapeutic considerations. Reproduction, the subject of Chapter 12, is approached in a different manner, with the focus on ways to increase or decrease reproductive success. Current topics, including artificial insemination, external and internal vasectomy, and GnRH agonists, are offered in a critical, in-depth, and applicable manner that should function as an excellent means for forming the framework for decision making in clinical settings. Chapter 13 includes a broad window to the breadth of clinical pathology for avian species, ranging from its foundational principles to the diagnostic testing of age in birds. Hematology and serum biochemistry are explored in a different light, seeking to identify their strengths and potential limitations and the means with which diagnosticians can best use these important tools. Advanced imaging modalities, discussed in Chapter 14, clarify the indications, equipment, materials, and methods for these to be considered and applied in clinical settings. Backyard poultry and owls are the two individual species groups that are included in Chapters 15 and 16, bringing new and practical information in a readily available manner for those who see these species in practice. Critical care and toxicology are reviewed, updated, and presented in an informative, practical, and useful manner in Chapters 17 and 18.

In the second section, anesthesia, analgesia, and surgery are addressed. Anesthesia is discussed first, bringing readers a current literature review and practical applications and recommendations. Then pain management is brought forward in a comprehensive and current, as well as practical, manner, with tables to facilitate quick reference. Surgery is then approached by first reviewing the principles of microsurgery, which is an essential aspect of most procedures in small bird species. Surgical procedures of the coelom and orthopedics are presented in the second portion of the surgery section. Anatomic detail and procedural detail are brought together to facilitate improved surgical success.

The third section presents topics that are less commonly included in an avian medical text: welfare, conservation, and practice management. Welfare is an immensely important component of every facet of avian healthcare, and the subject is thoughtfully and factually written for readers in a manner that provides points that can be put into action for change. Welfare-associated legislation can directly and indirectly influence what veterinarians do for birds, and this relevant information is presented to both inform and empower veterinarians, now and in the future. Important, timely, and individual welfare topics are further discussed with an ethical perspective, including deflighting or flight-limiting procedures and the human–avian bond. Conservation topics are foundationally introduced in a broad manner and then are brought to life through the tales of four different endangered species' conservation efforts and the veterinary involvements with each. Finally, without effective practice management, the ability to deliver avian medicine is inhibited, leading to unfulfilled dreams, curtailed practice growth, and limitations to the quality of healthcare that is ultimately received. The subject material is presented in practical wording in a manner that practitioners can use and apply to the art of what they do every day.

The final section of this text is an innovative effort to look at patterns of disease and problems that are seen in common pet bird species. Although evidence-based medical thought is essential in medical care, so is pattern recognition. A familiarity with the species that are more commonly held as pets in various parts of the world and what should be commonly expected has value for all. The discussion, as well as the tables in this section, offers a different window with which veterinarians can view disease patterns and some means with which a larger change in these patterns may be able to be effected, one practitioner at a time.

The three appendices are designed to provide a current drug formulary, normal clinical pathologic data, and normal biological data. The drug formulary regroups medications as compactly and usefully as possible. Not intended to replace the *Exotic Animal Formulary*, these compacted versions are included as an initial and immediate single-source reference for veterinarians.

All of us, contributors, editors, and collaborators, who have worked to bring this edition forward thank you for your interest, as well as for your dedication to remain current in the multiple facets of avian healthcare. It is true that as a whole, what we can do for birds as a profession is a powerful, ever-changing, and exciting thing. Thanks for being a part of the journey! As my father always told me, "Seems that the more you know, the more you know you need to know more." With that said, we'll be seeing you again soon.

Brian L. Speer

Acknowledgments

There are a large number of colleagues to whom I am grateful for their influence in the development, guidance, and maturation of my current view of avian medicine and surgery. Greg Harrison, who authored the first text on Clinical Avian Medicine and Surgery in 1986 and who was, in so many ways, a visionary and considerably ahead of his time in helping meet the need to unify medical knowledge and surgery. Walter Rosskopf, who helped pave the way so many years ago for me to see how much could be medically considered and done for birds, and James Harris, who also shared his excitement and passion for learning and shared his knowledge of science and birds, empowering me with those qualities. Nico Schoemaker and Yvonne van Zeeland, who considerably helped shape the vision of this text, contributed, and made efforts truly above and beyond the call of duty to help it become a reality. Scott Echols, Geoff Olsen, and Brenna Fitzgerald, who unfailingly supported me, tolerated my immense distractions from daily practice duties, and helped keep the practice healthy and growing throughout. The entire staff of the Medical Center for Birds must be acknowledged and thanked, as it was through their support that time could be preserved to enable my pursuit of this and other projects in the past. Other friends and colleagues should be named, who have had formative roles and influence including but not limited to David Phalen, Jamie Samour, Tom Tully, Joanne Paul-Murphy, Murray Fowler, Michelle Hawkins, Neil Forbes, Susan Orosz, Bob Doneley, Nigel Harcourt-Brown, Branson Ritchie, Helene Pendl, Keven Flammer, Helga Gerlach, and Susan Friedman. To all, I sincerely thank you for all that you have done and for what you continue to do.

And, family always remains the foundation of what our professional lives help support. Without the strength of family, life is not complete. My wife, Denise, has been unfailingly supportive and deserves my heartfelt thanks and appreciation. Thank you for being yourself and for seeing to it that this bird veterinarian, your husband, remains whole. Our children, Robin and Cody, also have tolerated their dad in a similar manner and have helped (with mom) to keep me on the straight and narrow, reminding me constantly of what really is important in life. My parents, Verl and Lucille, who raised me to be passionate about what I do and to always do the right thing, even if it means that decision will not be the easy road to travel. And finally, Taylor Richerson, who unfailingly supported me from childhood during good times and bad, through thick and thin, and showed me what it is to really, truly, be a friend. Thanks, man. We all miss you and know that you are still with us and seeing that we stay on schedule.

Brian L. Speer

Contents

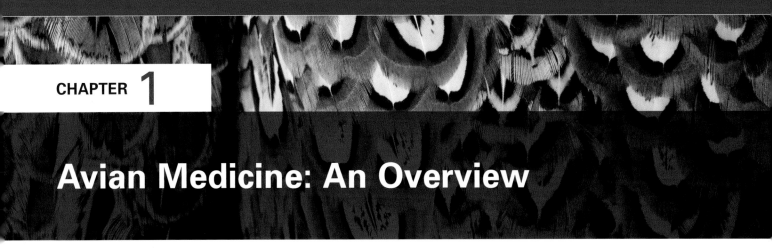

CHAPTER 1

Avian Medicine: An Overview

Christal Pollock • Eric Klaphake • James F.X. Wellehan Jr.

A HISTORICAL VIEW OF AVIAN MEDICINE

Christal Pollock

Although modern veterinary medicine has evolved over centuries, avian medicine is a relatively new field. Avian veterinarians today may manage commercial poultry flocks, treat companion birds, care for wildlife, and manage zoo specimens or even falconry birds; however, the path leading to such a wide range of opportunities has not been straightforward or easy.

> [T]he orderly contemplation of its own history is a proper and profitable pursuit for any profession—which takes pride in its ancestry and entertains some hope for posterity.[1]

ANCIENT BIRD CARE

Ancient Chinese writings dating back to 4000 BC record the use of herbs for curative purposes in humans and animals.[2] These early writings focus on horses but also include information on the care of other animals important to agriculture, such as ducks, geese, and chickens. The first mention of surgery in the bird comes from the Eastern Zhou dynasty (770 BC–221 BC) when castration of food animals, including cocks, was widely employed.[3]

Egyptian hieroglyphics from around 3500 BC show the presence of numerous types of domesticated animals.[2] The first written record of veterinary medicine from Egypt is provided by the Kahun Veterinary Papyrus (1800 BC), which discusses the diagnosis and treatment of diseases of domestic animals and fish (Figure 1-1).[4]

The first records of information on animal care and disease in Europe come from the Greco-Roman period. Information from this period primarily focuses on the horse and other hoofstock. Although there were many contributors to this knowledge base, Aristotle (384-322 BC) is considered by many to be the father of comparative anatomy and pathology.

Aristotle's *Historia Animalium* (Story of Animals) provides information on almost 500 animal species, including birds.[3]

FALCONRY

The origin of falconry is unclear, and it may be impossible to ever know exactly where and when the practice arose.[5] Nevertheless, one fact is certain: The origins of falconry go back much further than the origins of writing because the earliest records describe a highly complex and intricate form of hunting that must have taken many hundreds, if not thousands, of years to develop.[5,6] The sport of falconry was already well established in both Asia and the Middle East by 2000 BC, and gradually migrated westward to Greece, Italy, and the rest of Europe.[5]

In Western Europe, the sport of hawking or falconry attained most widespread popularity during the Middle Ages, and a number of treatises on falconry were published during this time. The most famous, *De Arte Venandi cum Avibus* (On the Art of Hunting with Birds), was written by Emperor Frederick II (1194-1250 AD). Lying between the Middle Ages and the Renaissance, this work is considered a hallmark of medieval science due to its systematic and scientific approach.[7-10] Albert the Great's section on falconry from *De Animalibus* in the thirteenth century includes an extensive list of treatments for diseases in falcons. These treatments included herbal concoctions (typically infused into the falcon's meat), special diets, theriacs (an ointment or other medicinal compound used as an antidote to snake venom or other poisons), plasters, bleeding, and cauterization.[8]

Other medieval treatises on falconry diseases describe aggrestyne (itch), agrum (rheum), anguellis (worms), booches (mouth ulcers), fallera (liver dx), filanders (worms), frounce (mouth sores), gleth (phlegm), poose (cough), and general debility or "unlustynesse."[11] Most of the medications are based on herbs or spices and a few minerals, including saffron, shepherd's purse, canell (cinnamon), gelofre (gillyflower), kersis (watercress), maryall (black nightshade), neppe (catmint),

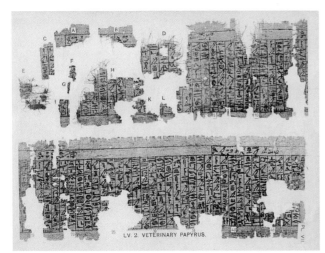

FIGURE 1-1 Rediscovered in 1889, the Kahun Veterinary Papyrus is the first written record of veterinary medicine from Egypt. (Photo courtesy Francis Llewellyn Griffith via Wikimedia Commons.)

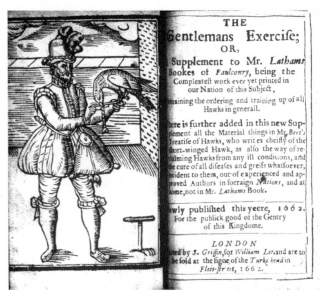

FIGURE 1-2 *Latham's Faulconry* or *The Faulcons Lure and Cure: In Two Books* describes ailments and medications for a variety of conditions in the falconry bird.

puliall (pennyroyal), venecreke (fenugreek), quicksilver, coral, ashes, urine, heron fat, pigeon, or even human feces.[11] A treasured ingredient in ointments and pills was also mummy, purchased from apothecaries.[8]

> [T]he most precious medicine for falcons' wounds; it is prepared from the flesh of dead men, and the finest is made from the head.[8]

In another treatise, *Libro de la caza de las aves* by the Chancellor of Castile López de Ayala (1332–1407), almost 60 ingredients are listed, and the falconer should always be equipped with these ingredients.[11,12]

Toward the end of the Middle Ages, the growing popularity of falconry as a recreational sport is indicated by the emergence of practical manuals or how-to guides (Figure 1-2). *The Boke of St. Alban* (1486) was the first work on falconry published in English.[8,13] *The Boke* contains references to many conditions, some of them still recognizable today.[13] For instance, great attention was paid to maintaining the condition of the plumage as a period of poor feeding could result in a visible hunger trace, a weak spot where feathers might break, called a "taynt."[11]

> [A] thing that gooth overwarte the federis of the wynges and of the tayll, lyke as and it were eetyn with wormys; and it begynyth first to breded at the body in the penne, and that same penne shall frete asunder and falle away thurrow the ssame taynte, and then is the hawke disparaged for all that yere.[11]

Another famous falconry tome is the *Baz-Nama-Yi Nasiri: A Persian Treatise on Falconry*. Published in 1868, the treatise summarizes much of the ancient knowledge on health conditions, including bumblefoot (Arabic: *saddah* or *seddah*), poxvirus (Arabic: *jeddrah* or *jidri*), and frounce (Arabic: *glah* or *jidri*). The text has been translated to English, French, and German.[14,15]

Chapter LXIII: Expedient If Meat Fail
Should you be caught in the snow far from your stage and have no means of procuring food for your hawks—a deadly cold wind springing up in your teeth, your hawks will certainly perish, unless fed. Remedy: at once dismount and bind the forearm of your horse. With the point of your pen-knife open the vein (1); hold a cup underneath so that the blood may collect and congeal in it, then give this blood to your hawk that she escape death.[15]

Chapter LXIV: Restoration After Drowning
Should your hawk fall into a stream and be swept away (2), and when recovered be lifeless, the treatment, even though the hawk has been apparently dead for half an hour, is as follows. Treatment: light a fire and lay the hawk down by the side of it. Collect the hot ashes under the wings and heap ashes on the back, and as soon as the ashes cool, pile on other ashes, fresh and warm. The ashes must not be so hot as to burn the feathers. In a short time, by God's decree, the dead hawk will come to life. This remedy is suitable for a man also, or indeed, for any beast that has been drowned. It is efficacious even up to half or three quarters of an hour after insensibility. I have several times successfully tried this remedy on man, beast, and bird.[15]

Chapter LIX: Operation of Opening the Stomach
…Item: if [recommendations for medical management of obstruction] also fail, then cast her and tie her up firmly in some quiet spot protected from wind and draughts. Have by ready a needle and silk, and yellow aloes powdered and mixed with antimony. Have the hawk's legs separated wide apart. Now, the hawk being on her back with her head away from you and raised, you will find at the root of the thigh and at the end of the sternum a fine skin (1): pluck out the small feathers from this, so as to lay bare the skin. Then with a sharp pen-knife make a slit lengthways in the skin, two fingers' breadth in length. After the "skin," you will find a second a third "fine-skin," which also slit. Now, with the greatest care, insert two fingers, and lift up and expose the guts to view. Quickly and dexterously open the stomach, replace it in its proper position, and after that sew up, one by one, the three "fine-skins" and lastly the outer "skin." On the outside wound sprinkle the powdered aloes and antimony, and then free the hawk and let her rest.
Feed her every day on the yolks of eggs: if she will not eat them, pound a little meat, about half a sparrow in quantity, and

mix it with the yolks of two eggs (1) and give it to her in the morning, and again at noon, and in the afternoon. If she eats this meat and "puts it over," again give her the yolks of two eggs with pounded meat. Feed her thus for two days. On the third day give her minced meat with the yolk of egg, and feed her thus for three days. Then for three days more give her meat, cut up into bits the size of filbert and mixed with the yolk of an egg. During this period you must on no account let her pull or tear at her food; for the exertion of pulling will burst the stitches, either inside or out, and if the stitches of even one of the skins give way, she is destroyed. Anyone accustomed to caponize cocks will have no difficulty in performing this operation: the two operations are practically the same.[15]

EVOLUTION OF THE VETERINARIAN
From Leech or Farrier to Scientist

During the Dark Ages, the medical care of hoofstock fell into the hands of self-proclaimed professionals such as the farrier, blacksmith, herdsman, or leech.[2,16,17] Leeches were uneducated individuals, and their practices (or "leechdom") were based on superstition.[18]

> To remove away eye pain, take a wolfs right eye, and prick it to pieces, and bind it to the suffering eye; it maketh the sore to wane, if it frequently be smeared therewith.[18]

The need for science-based animal doctors was not recognized until devastating epizootics of contagious animal diseases such as rinderpest swept through Western Europe during the eighteenth century. Claude Bourgelat, a horseman and attorney, established the first veterinary college at Lyon, France, in 1761. Other schools were soon established in the 1770s in Sweden, Germany, Denmark, and Austria. In 1844, the Royal College of Veterinary Surgeons was founded in Great Britain.[2,3]

Veterinary medical education in the United States began as a private enterprise, with the Veterinary College of Philadelphia opening in 1852.[3] These private schools were plagued with problems, and the trend of private veterinary schools was relatively short-lived. Even the veterinary program at Harvard University had lower standards for admission compared with other programs at the institution. The Ontario Veterinary College opened in Toronto in 1862. Iowa State University, the first state-run school, opened in 1879.[3,19]

Not surprisingly, the curriculum of these early veterinary colleges focused on the horse. Other species generally received little attention; however, there are exceptions to this rule. The veterinary anatomists Wilhelm Ellenberger (1848-1929) and Hermann Baum (1864-1932) published *Handbuch der Vergleichenden Anatomie der Haustierie* in 1898, and this tome includes a detailed chapter on birds (Figure 1-3).[3,20]

SCIENTIFIC INQUIRY AND THE GROWTH OF AVIAN MEDICINE

Although modern avian medicine came quite late to the veterinary stage, by the time individuals who called themselves "avian veterinarians" came to be, there was already a tremendous

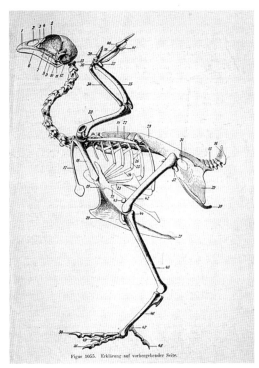

FIGURE 1-3 German veterinary anatomists Ellenberger and Baum worked with the artist, Hermann Dittrich, to create beautiful and accurate illustrations of animal anatomy, which were published in the *Handbuch der Vergleichenden Anatomie der Haustierie.*

amount of information available. This growing knowledge base was part of a surge in scientific inquiry led by interested individuals from a variety of fields.

Physicians

A new type of practitioner known as the surgeon-farrier appeared in the 1700s. These men were often physicians, surgeons, or apothecaries with a strong interest in animals.[2] An excellent example of the surgeon-farrier is John Hunter (1728-1793), a prominent physician and surgeon in London. Hunter was also a leading scholar of comparative anatomy, and his lectures stressed the relationship between structure and function in all living creatures.[2,3] Hunter's studies covered avian species as diverse as ostriches and sparrows.[21] The following is a description of Hunter's experimental work studying "air-cells" (air sacs) in a bird of prey[22]:

> I next cut the wing through the os humeri, in another fowl, and tying up the trachea, as in the cock, found that the air passed to and from the lungs by the canal in this bone. The same experiment was made with os femoris of a young hawk, and was attended with a similar result. But the passage of air through the divided parts, in both these experiments, especially in the last, was attended with more difficulty than in the former one; it was indeed so great as to render it impossible for the animal to live longer than evidently to prove that it breathed through the cut bone.[22]

The study of the gapeworm *(Syngamus trachea)* is another example of the physician's contribution to veterinary medicine. In 1797, Baltimore physician and anatomy professor

Dr. Andrew Wiesenthall wrote a letter to the *Medical and Physical Journal* reporting worms in the trachea of chickens and turkeys that displayed difficulty breathing and might have died gasping for breath. Dr. Wiesenthall reported success in removing parasites by twisting a feather, stripped of its barbs almost to the tip, into the trachea and withdrawing the feather shaft slowly, with the worms adhering to the implement. This method remained a means of treatment for affected birds for well over a century. In 1883, Dr. D.H. Walker, a busy small-town physician in Franklinville, New York, instituted a series of experiments that identified the earthworm as the gapeworm's intermediate host.[23]

Biologists and Ornithologists

In 1910, a massive die-off of hundreds of thousands of ducks in Utah and California was attributed to "western duck disease." The die-off recurred in 1912, and a young biologist with the U.S. Biology Survey was assigned to study the problem in 1913. Alexander Wetmore (1886-1978) noted that losses were almost always associated with declining water levels during late summer and fall when water temperatures were highest. Wetmore theorized that "duck sickness" was caused by the toxic action of certain soluble salts found in alkali around the western lakes, hence the historical term "alkali poisoning." Although Wetmore defined a piece of the puzzle, it was biologist Edwin R. Kalmbach (1884-1972) who confirmed that western duck disease was attributable to *Clostridium botulinum* type C in 1930.[24,25]

Physicians, Veterinarians, and Microbiologists

The zoonotic disease, psittacosis, is an excellent example of knowledge gained through the contributions of a variety of professionals. In 1879, the Swiss physician Dr. Jakob Ritter published the first detailed description of a disease resembling psittacosis, in which seven patients were affected and three individuals died. Ritter recognized that newly imported caged birds were the source of the infection he called "pneumotyphus." The French physician Morange first coined the term "psittacosis" in 1895 after *psittakos*, the Greek word for parrot.[26-28]

Sporadic cases and outbreaks of psittacosis were reported until the pandemic of 1929-1930. In the summer and fall of 1929, over 100 cases of an unusual and serious pneumonia were reported in Argentina.[26] All patients had been exposed to a large shipment of birds. Many of those birds were ill and dying, and the owners, wishing to minimize their losses, sold the birds quickly at a series of auctions. As the birds and auctions moved from city to city, human cases of psittacosis followed.[29] Cases eventually appeared in North America, England, Europe, North Africa, Japan, and Australia. The final worldwide count of cases was estimated to be between 750 and 800, with a mortality rate of approximately 15%. Germany was the most severely affected, with 215 cases and 45 deaths. England, the United States, and Argentina were the only countries with more than 100 human infections. Amazon parrots (*Amazona* spp.) were responsible for 43 of the 74 infection foci. Other species incriminated in the pandemic included "talking parrots," lovebirds (*Agapornis* spp.), canaries (*Serinus canaria*), "parakeets," and shell parakeets (*Melopsittacus undulatus*).[28]

Working independently in 1930, bacteriologists and virologists Levinthal, Coles, and Lillie all described small, filterable bodies in infectious material, now called Levinthal-Coles-Lillie (LCL) bodies. By the mid-1930s, work in England, Germany, France, and the United States established that psittacosis was not caused by a bacterium but by a filterable agent, which was presumed to be a virus.[27]

Also in the 1930s, research conducted by Dr. Karl Friedrich Meyer (1884-1974) of the Hooper Institute, in cooperation with the California State Public Health Department, led to the recognition of endemic psittacosis in psittacine aviaries in California and of latent infections in parakeets.[28,30] Meyer, who was born in Switzerland, earned his Doctorate of Veterinary medicine from the University of Zurich in 1909 and moved to the United States in 1910. Dr. Meyer coined the term "ornithosis" for chlamydophilosis in nonpsittacine birds, and he remained an authority on this disease until well after his retirement. During the 1960s, research led by Dr. Meyer established the efficacy of oral tetracycline therapy for psittacosis in birds.[28]

POULTRY MEDICINE

Although all branches of avian medicine have grown tremendously, there is probably no segment that has undergone more dramatic change than poultry medicine. The last quarter of the nineteenth century saw the height of the small farm flock, a time when each American farmer felt obliged to keep a flock of chickens as well as a few turkeys, ducks, geese, and/or guinea fowl. The day-to-day care of poultry was typically relegated to children.[23]

> The diseases of poultry have seldom received attention in this country, from persons qualified to treat them judiciously. The management of this…farm stock, both in sickness and health, is entrusted to children, or persons who are incapacitated for other business. The consequence is a general ignorance of their peculiar habits, as well as their diseases.[1]

As late as 1900, poultry diseases were poorly classified and little understood.[31,32] Published in 1897, *Diseases and Enemies of Poultry* by Leonard Pearson (1868-1909) and Benjamin H. Warren (1858-1926) described "catarrh of the nasal passages (pip) as a discharge from the nose, mouth, swelling of eyelids, depression of spirits, head drawn down and feathers ruffled." This mention of "pip" is an illustration of how little was known about the chicken in the late 1800s. In *Aldrovandi on Chickens*, written in 1598, the Italian naturalist, Ulisse Aldrovandi (1522-1605) described "pip" as a "flow of liquid or humor from the brain to the nostrils" . . . "Pip" was a widely used term, usually referring to a common sequel to a catarrhal affliction of the head and nostrils causing the bird to breathe through its mouth. The tongue would dry and harden on its tip, like a horny growth. This was the "pip," and the "horn" was commonly removed with the point of a penknife.[23]

Lack of knowledge did not prevent—and perhaps even spurred—the development of many home remedies for poultry. Milk, buttermilk, and sour milk were used extensively as "flushes" to treat digestive upsets and coccidiosis up until the advent of sulfa drugs in the 1940s. Epsom salts and sodium bicarbonate were also used as "flushes" to control a wide variety of diseases. Copper sulfate was frequently recommended for intestinal disorders.[23]

During the 1920s through the 1940s, there was rapid growth in the poultry industry and a significant trend toward intensification in management. Rising population density resulted in increased losses from infectious diseases and created a tremendous demand for remedies to reduce mortality rates. Family formulas were passed on to entrepreneurs, who used national advertising campaigns and effective sales techniques to sell a variety of products to poultrymen, who had no better source to turn for help (Figure 1-4).[3,23]

The need for science-based answers to poultry problems eventually led to research directed toward practical control of infectious diseases. This research was primarily conducted at U.S. land-grant universities and the Bureau of Animal Industry (BAI) of the U.S. Department of Agriculture. One of the most influential teachers in the first generation of American avian veterinary microbiologists was L. D. Bushnell of the Kansas State College of Agriculture. Dr. Bushnell was the head of the College's department of bacteriology, which even included a division of poultry bacteriology. It is of interest to note that Dr. Bushnell started his work on poultry diseases because the veterinary college at Kansas State would have nothing to do with chickens.[23]

Clearly, it took a while for veterinarians to become concerned with poultry disease problems. In writing on "What Veterinarians Should Know About Diseases of Poultry" B. F. Kaupp stated in 1914[1]:

> The poultry industry is being heralded as a billion dollar business.... It is high time the veterinarian was awakening to the possibilities of poultry practice. It is charged that the average poultryman is a "tight wad." But the fact remains that he is no tighter than many of us can remember he was in being "chary" about employing a veterinarian to treat his ill horse or cow twenty years ago. If the veterinarian really becomes proficient and shows his proficiency he will be in demand.[1]

Poultry veterinarians began to appear in the 1930s, and the field continued to make extraordinary progress in breeding,

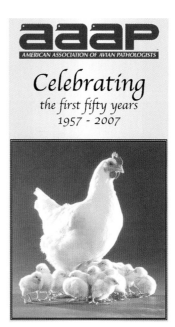

FIGURE 1-5 The American Association of Avian Pathologists has been diligent in chronicling its history. (Courtesy American Association of Avian Pathologists.)

nutrition, and understanding and managing diseases. In 1943, the first edition of *Diseases of Poultry* was published. This comprehensive reference on all aspects of poultry health and diseases is now in its 13th edition. The American Association of Avian Pathologists (AAAP) was founded in 1957 (Figure 1-5), and today all veterinary schools require courses in poultry diseases.[23]

PET BIRD CARE

When Europeans immigrated to North America in the seventeenth century, they brought with them the practice of bird keeping. By the nineteenth and early twentieth centuries, the bird was the most popular indoor pet in the United States. Solitary caged birds were common in working-class households, but more well-to-do families often cared for a variety of birds in aviaries. Native songbirds such as the goldfinch, mockingbird, and cardinal were initially very common but were eventually supplanted by imported birds such as the canary. The canary eventually became known as the "universal parlor bird," and it was considered the most popular caged bird through the 1930s. Parrots were relatively more expensive and far less common than songbirds in early American homes (Figure 1-6).[16,33]

In the event of injury or illness, most bird owners attempted nursing care at home because few veterinarians were interested in animal problems outside of an agricultural setting.[34,35] Bird dealers and pet store owners were a logical resource because of their practical experience with small animals and animal diseases.[33] Pet shops distributed proprietary bottled medications, dispensed written advice, and even performed procedures on sick or injured pets when the need arose.[16,33] Bird dealers also published "how-to" books on bird care.[16,36,37] The Nature Friend, Inc., in its popular booklet, recommended a 7-day feeding schedule for the family canary.

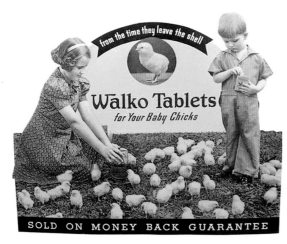

FIGURE 1-4 Walko tablets, consisting mostly of potassium permanganate, were added to poultry drinking water, and the attractive purple color convinced many owners that flock health hinged on faithful application of this treatment. (Used with permission from http://www.avianaquamiser.com.)

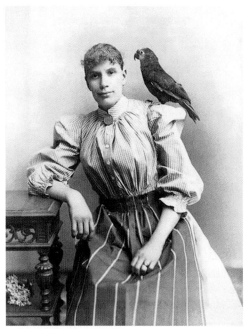

FIGURE 1-6 Songbirds were the most popular indoor pets in early America; parrots were relatively expensive and far less common. (Photo courtesy Julie Murad.)

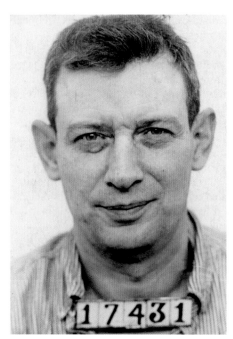

FIGURE 1-7 Robert Stroud, the "Birdman of Alcatraz," owned up to 300 birds and was even provided with two additional cells to house them.

The regime included *Magic Song Restorer*, and the booklet closed with "An Imprisoned Bird's Daily Prayer"[38]:

Oh Captor, consider that I am your little prisoner,
Give me daily food,
consisting of pure and wholesome rape and canary seed,
and pray do not omit to give me a separate small dish of
MAGIC SONG RESTORER and GENERAL HEALTH FOOD
...
Lead me not into temptation
by offering me some cheap imitation of the
so-called song restorer
If you deliver me from such evils
I will promise to sing my song of gratitude
for the rest of my imprisoned life.[38]

Robert Stroud (1890-1963), the infamous "Birdman of Alcatraz," marketed a line of extremely popular bird treatments, including Stroud's Effervescent Bird Salts, Stroud's Special Prescription, Stroud's Avian Antiseptic, and Stroud's Salts No. 1 (Figure 1-7).[39]

One of the world's leading authorities on birds and avian disease of his time, Robert Stroud was sentenced to 12 years in prison for murdering a bartender in 1909. He was then transferred to Leavenworth penitentiary after attacking an orderly in 1912. Stroud was later condemned to life in prison without the possibility of parole after fatally stabbing a prison guard. Although it was not unusual for prisoners to keep a single pet bird, Stroud owned up to 300 birds and was even provided with two additional cells in which to house them (see Figure 1-7).[40]

In an effort to understand avian anatomy and disease transmission, Stroud conducted research, and when his birds fell ill, he struggled to nurse them back to health. When this failed, he also performed necropsies, at first with no more than his fingernails. The government handbooks Stroud turned to did not explain the problems he was seeing, so in an effort to educate himself, Stroud devoured as many books as possible on pharmacology, chemistry, medicine, and bacteriology.[39]

Stroud wrote numerous articles for canary journals while corresponding with thousands of private bird owners and breeders desperate for advice and guidance. He wrote two detailed accounts of his findings: *Diseases of Canaries*, originally published in 1933, and *Digest on the Diseases of Birds* (1943). Both texts are still in print today. Stroud's *Digest* is a comprehensive treatise on avian medicine geared to the breeders of canaries and other pet birds; however, it also contains information for the ". . . poultryman . . . the zoologist (and) the pet dealer." Stroud also hoped his work would ". . . be acceptable to veterinarians and veterinary schools for Heaven knows they need it."[39-41]

Some sections of the *Digest* clearly illustrate Stroud's ruthlessness that had led to his incarceration.

Bird blood has great clotting power. Cut a man's leg off and without the application of methods for stopping the bleeding he will be pretty certain to bleed to death. Under the same circumstances, a bird will not bleed enough to weaken it noticeably.[41]

Although Stroud did not state that he actually removed any appendages, this passage does create a disturbing mental image of Stroud performing his research without the benefit of anesthesia or analgesia. Nevertheless, this passage also accurately describes avian physiology. Humane studies performed in the pigeon, domestic fowl, and quail all confirm that birds can, indeed, tolerate blood loss to a much greater extent than mammals.[40]

A particularly interesting entry is found under "Egg Binding." Today's avian veterinarians know that an increase in humidity may assist in delayed oviposition. This practice is based on an old aviculturist technique, which Stroud describes:[40]

> The bird is held over the open mouth of a large-mouth bottle or jar that has been filled two-third full with hot water. The abdomen is steeped in the rising vapor. This method will sometimes cause the tissues to relax and the eggs to pass.[41]

ZOO MEDICINE

Zoos and museums have long played a role in contributing to our understanding of the bird. The Zoological Society of London, along with similar organizations in Germany and France, vigorously pursued the study of avian anatomy in the early part of the nineteenth century. The incentive for many of these early comparative anatomy studies was to substantiate or disprove various taxonomic proposals.[42]

A great deal of general information on bird anatomy and pathology can also be found in a variety of zoo texts. For instance, the physician Herbert Fox authored *Diseases in Captive Wild Mammals and Birds* in 1923. Dr. Fox described both normal and abnormal findings in his work as pathologist for the Zoological Society of Philadelphia, where he performed more than 3500 necropsies on birds over a 20-year period.[43]

> In the class Aves the pancreas consist of two or three distinct lobes lying one in front and two behind the cleft between the limbs of the duodenal loop and it discharges its secretion into the duodenum by two or three ducts separately and almost invariably above the bile duct openings . . . .
> Passerine birds have two pancreatic ducts usually on the ascending loop of the duodenum, or there may be one ahead of the pyloric biliary duct . . .
> The picarian varieties possess three ducts as a rule, one near the beginning of the pylorus, one near its end and a third of inconstant location. Owls have a system like Passerines, but the relation between the organ and the intestinal loop is looser and the ducts are wider . . . .
> The amount of pancreas to be found in birds is greater than that in mammals. According to our figures the organ represents 1/400th of the body weight in the former and 1/600th in the latter . . .[43]

It is of interest to note that a detailed description of Dr. Fox's book was included in the "Book Notes" section of the May 24, 1924, issue of the *Journal of the American Medical Association*. This would never happen in today's world but was apparently of potential interest to the physician of that day.[44]

The American Association of Zoo Veterinarians (AAZV) was founded in 1946, and early avian veterinarians often attended the Annual Conference.[45] One pioneer in companion bird medicine, Dr. Greg Harrison, presented a talk on surgical sexing at the 1976 Annual Conference (Spink R, Personal Communication, May 24, 2013).

MODERN AVIAN MEDICINE

After World War I, utilitarian use of the horse began to decline and automated agriculture increased.[2] Subsequently,

veterinary medicine gradually turned to the care of dogs and cats. Once the care of companion animals became more commonplace, veterinarians were eventually called upon to see a variety of other companion species, including birds.

Veterinary Record, one of the oldest veterinary journals in existence, was founded in 1888. The first *Veterinary Record* article on caged birds, "Common ailments of canaries," was published in 1947. This article was actually a reproduction of a piece written by Dr. G.V. Narusu from the *Indian Veterinary Journal*.[46]

The Association of Avian Veterinarians (AAV), briefly called the American Association of Avian Practitioners, was founded in 1980 (Figure 1-8). The Association's first Board of Directors consisted of private practitioners, entrepreneurs, and academics and included some of the best-known avian veterinarians in the United States at that time (Box 1-1).[45]

The AAV was born out of discontent among avian practitioners attending the AAZV meetings. Avian medicine was only a small portion of the AAZV's focus, and, of course, topics in caged bird medicine were not generally addressed. The AAV was designed to meet the practitioner's crucial need for connection and dissemination of information.[45]

When the AAV was formed, the curriculum at veterinary medical schools barely touched on avian medicine, except as it applied to birds raised for production, such as turkeys and chickens. Educational resources available in the early 1980s included: *Caged Bird Medicine: Selected Topics* by Drs. Charles V. Steiner and Richard B. Davis, *Stroud's Digest* and *Diseases of Canaries*, and *Diseases of Cage and Aviary Birds* by Dr. Margaret Petrak.[45] First published in 1969, Dr. Petrak's book was the first veterinary textbook published on caged bird medicine, and veterinary medical students used her textbook for many years.[42] In her preface, Dr. Petrak explained:

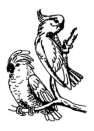

Attend the

American Association of

Avian Practitioners

1st Seminar & Workshop

on

"Avian Medicine"

June 21-22, 1980
SHERATON INN
Kalamazoo, Michigan

FIGURE 1-8 The first meeting of the Association of Avian Veterinarians, for a brief time called the American Association of Avian Practitioners, was held in Kalamazoo, Michigan, in June 1980. (Used with permission from the AAV.)

In early 1963, Mr. Theodore Phillips, then on the editorial staff at Lea & Febiger, asked me to edit a book on diseases of cage birds. The interest in the subject shown by veterinarians throughout the US and his own knowledge of veterinary literature had convinced him of the need for such a book. My developing concern in both medical and surgical treatment of cage birds and my frustration at the unavailability of pertinent literature influenced my decision to acquiesce . . .

We received some early criticism for presuming to write a book on a field of medicine still in its infancy. However in the five years since the book's conception all criticism has disappeared, to be replaced by encouragement and gratifyingly by impatience for publication of the work . . .[42]

Many segments of *Diseases of Cage and Aviary Birds* focus on the budgerigar parakeet, since this species was deemed the most numerous among those kept as pets.[42] The chapter on "Surgical techniques and anesthesia" by Dr. Charles P. Gandal, a veterinarian associated with the New York Zoological Society, stated, "Equi-Thesin is the drug of choice for most procedures . . ." Produced by Jensen-Salsbery Laboratories, a 500-mL vial of Equi-Thesin contained 328 g chloral hydrate, 75 g pentobarbital, and 164 g magnesium sulfate in aqueous solution of 35% propylene glycol with 9.5% alcohol. For inhalant anesthesia, Dr. Gandal reported[42]:

> . . . methoxyflurane and ether are quite satisfactory if properly administered . . . Small birds may be satisfactorily anesthetized with ether by placing them in a 1-quart glass jar, spraying 1 mL ether through a 25-gauge needle, capping the jar, and waiting approximately 30 seconds. When the bird stops struggling, it is immediately removed, and depending on the level reached, anesthesia may last 1 to 4 minutes. Further ether may be given intermittently by holding a cotton pledget moistened with ether close to the bird's nostrils, but great care must be exercised as a dangerous overconcentration may be rapidly attained . . . .
>
> . . . Methoxyflurane may also be used on larger birds by holding the bird's head in a 1-quart jar into which 0.2-0.4 mL of the drug has been sprayed and sealing the opening off with a towel. It may also be administered on a pledget of cotton held over the nostrils. Once a satisfactory stage of anesthesia has been reached an ET tube may be inserted and attached to a gas anesthetic machine . . . [42]

Today, most veterinary medical schools offer some form of didactic coursework in companion bird medicine. Most lectures introducing students to avian medicine are elective and are generally offered during the third year of veterinary school.[47]

THE TREND TO SPECIALIZATION

Specialty veterinary groups with advanced professional training began to appear after World War II. The American Veterinary Medical Association recognized both the American College of Poultry Veterinarians and the American College of Zoological Medicine in 1991, and the American Board of Veterinary Practitioners (ABVP) began avian board certification in 1993.[3] Today, the Avian Practice category is the second largest group within the ABVP, with approximately 135 active Diplomates.[48] The European College of Avian Medicine and Surgery (ECAMS) was also founded in 1993 and became recognized as a fully functional College in 2005.[49] ECAMS was expanded in 2007 to the European College of Zoological Medicine, which includes the avian specialty. In Australia and New Zealand, the equivalent specialty category is the Avian Chapter of the Australian and New Zealand College of Veterinary Scientists with fellowships in Caged and Aviary Birds or Poultry.[50]

CONCLUSION

The earliest references to medical care of birds refer to the castration of cockerels to produce capons and the nursing care of falconry birds. Modern avian medicine is a relatively new specialty; however, much of the information we hold as the foundation of our field is based on the work of a variety of pioneering scientists. As every veterinarian knows, there is no sharp line of demarcation between animal and human diseases, and therefore it should not be surprising that these scientific inquiries were answered by a variety of professionals: physicians, microbiologists, virologists, immunologists, zoologists, pathologists, ornithologists, aviculturists—and even veterinarians—although most of these early veterinarians would never have called themselves *avian* veterinarians. These exceptional individuals were often gifted with broad interests, great curiosity, creativity, and a keen intellect that they used to answer specific questions. In the case of poultry medicine, there were often immediate, practical applications for their research, but earlier workers often explored a topic merely to satisfy their own curiosity—in other words for the love of pure science.

> The history of avian medicine should evoke pride in today's achievements and appreciation of the pioneers who, with limited knowledge and inferior tools, paved the way for succeeding generations. . . . History is a compass bearing that gives a sense of direction for a continuing journey over winding roads. A look at the past is not a backward turn; it can lay the foundation of future progress.[23]

Modern avian medicine has grown tremendously since the founding of the AAV in 1980, and the advances made, in a relatively brief period, have been nothing short of amazing. There are many challenges facing avian medicine today, but the potential for growth is strong.

REFERENCES

1. Smithcors JF: *The American veterinary profession*, Ames, IA, 1963, Iowa State University Press.
2. Ho J: *Information resources on veterinary history at the National Agricultural Library: AWIC Resource Series No. 29. U.S. Department of Agriculture* (website). February 2005. http://www.nal.usda.gov/awic/pubs/VetHistory/vethistory.htm. Accessed September 9, 2014.
3. Dunlop RH, Williams DJ: *Veterinary medicine: an illustrated history*, St. Louis, MO, 1996, Mosby.
4. Schwabe W: *Veterinary medicine and human health*, ed 2, Baltimore, MD, 1969, Williams & Wilkins.
5. Epstein HJ: The origin and earliest history of falconry, *ISIS* 34: 497–509, 1943.
6. International Association of Falconry: *History of falconry* (website). http://www.iaf.org/HistoryFalconry.php. Accessed September 3, 2014.
7. Hohenstaufen, Frederick II: *De arte venandi cum avibus*, Wood CA, Fyfe FM, (translated and edited), Stanford, CA, 1943, Stanford University Press.
8. Aberth J: *An environmental history of the Middle Ages: the crucible of nature*, New York, 2013, Routledge Taylor & Francis Group.
9. Haskins CH: *Studies in the history of mediaeval science*, Cambridge, MA, 1924, Harvard University Press.
10. Grant E: *Medieval History in America*: Charles Homer Haskins, Indiana University Scholar Works (website), December 28, 1984. https://scholarworks.iu.edu/index.php. Accessed September 20, 2014.
11. Cummins J: *The hound and the hawk: the art of medieval hunting*, New York, 1988, St. Martin's Press.
12. López de Ayala P: *Libro de la caça de la saves*, London, U.K., 1986, JG Cummins.
13. Berners J: *The boke of St. Albans, facsimile edition in Rachel Hands. English Hawking and Hunting in 'The Boke of St. Albans,'* Oxford, U.K., 1975.
14. Upton R: *Arab falconry: history of a way of life*, Blaine, WA, 2002, Hancock House Publishers.
15. Mirza Husam 'd-Dawlah Taymur: *The Baz-nama-yi Nasiri: a Persian treatise on falconry*. https://archive.org/details/baznamayinasirip00husarich. Accessed Sep 20, 2014.
16. Grier KC: *Pets in America: a history*. Chapel Hill, NC, 2006, University of North Carolina Press.
17. Smithcors JF: Some early veterinary therapies, *Vet Heritage* 18:48–54, 1995.
18. Cockayne O, Cantab MA: *Leechdom, wortcunning, and starcraft of early England: being a collection of documents, for the most part never before printed illustrating the history of science in this country before the Norman conquest*, London, U.K., 1866, Longmans, Green, Reader and Dyer.
19. Smithcors JF: *The veterinarian in America 1625-1975*, Santa Barbara, CA, 1975, American Veterinary Publications, Inc.
20. Ellenberger W, Baum H: *Handbuch der vergleichenden Anatomie der Haustiere*, Berlin, 1912, Verlag Von August Hirschwald. https://archive.org/stream/handbuchdervergl00elle#page/n7/mode/2up. Accessed September 30, 2014.
21. Cooper JE: Some aspects of John Hunter's work on the diseases of birds of prey, *Ann R Coll Surg Engl* 64:345–347, 1982.
22. Hunter J: An account of certain receptacles of air in birds, which communicate with the lungs and Eustachian tube. In Palmer JF, editor: *The works of John Hunter*, FRS with notes, Vol 4, London, U.K., 1837, Longman.
23. Dunn J: *American association of avian pathologists celebrating the first fifty years: 1957–2007*, Athens, GA, 2007, Omnipress.
24. Garone P: The fall and rise of the wetlands of California's great central valley, Berkeley, CA, 2011, University of California Press, pp 146.
25. Kalmbach ER: *Western duck sickness: a form of botulism. USDA Technical Bulletin 411*, United States Department of Agriculture National Agricultural Library (website), May 1934. http://naldc.nal.usda.gov/download/CAT86200405/PDF. Accessed September 28, 2014.
26. Hull TG: *Diseases transmitted from animals to man*, Springfield, IL, 1947, CC Thomas, pp 212–230.
27. Pospischil A: From disease to etiology: historical aspects of *Chlamydia*-related diseases in animals and humans, *Drugs Today* 45(Suppl B): 141–146, 2009.
28. Ramsay EC: The psittacosis outbreak of 1929-1930, *J Avian Med Surg* 17:235–237, 2003.
29. Meyer KF: Psittacosis/ornithosis. In Biester HE, DeVries L, editors: *Diseases of poultry*, Ames, IA, 1943, Iowa State College Press, pp 433–465.
30. Meyer KF, Eddie B: Latent psittacosis infection in shell parakeets, *Proc Soc Exp Biol Med* 30:484–485, 1933.
31. Craig RA: *Common diseases of farm animals*, Philadelphia, PA, 1915, JP Lippincott Company.
32. Lewis HR: *Lippincott's farm manuals*, Philadelphia, PA, 1915, JP Lippincott Company.
33. Pollock CG: Companion birds in early America, *J Avian Med Surg* 27:148–151, 2013.
34. Drenan DM: The growth and development of small-animal practice in the United States, *J Am Vet Med Assoc* 169:42–49, 1976.
35. Jones SD: Pricing the priceless pet. In Jones SD, editor: *Valuing animals: veterinarians and their patients in modern America*, Baltimore, MD, 2003, Johns Hopkins University Press, pp 115–140.
36. Munroe J: *The bird keeper's guide and companion: containing plain directions for keeping and breeding canaries and all other song birds*, Cambridge, U.K., 1854, John Ford.
37. Nash JA: *Practical treatise on British song birds; in which is given every information relative to their natural history, incubation, &c. together with the method of rearing and managing both old and young birds*, London, U.K., 1824, Sherwood, Jones, and Co.
38. The Nature Friend Inc: *How to take care of your canary*, New York, 1935, Nature Friend.
39. O'Neil P: Prodigious intellect in solitary: impenitent killer Robert Stroud, who is famed for his treatise on birds, has a new hope for freedom, *Life* 48:147–149, 1960.
40. Pollock CG: The Birdman of Alcatraz, *J Avian Med Surg* 15:131–132, 2001.
41. Stroud R: *Stroud's digest on the diseases of birds*, Surrey, U.K., 1964, TFH Publications, Inc.
42. Petrak ML: *Diseases of cage and aviary birds*, Philadelphia, PA, 1969, Lea & Febiger.
43. Fox H: *Diseases in captive wild mammals and birds*, Philadelphia, PA, 1923, JB Lippincott.
44. Journal of the American Medical Association: Book notices, *J Am Med Assoc* 82:1717–1718, 1924.
45. Pollock CG: The "original" AAV: the founding of the Association of Avian Veterinarians, *J Avian Med Surg* 28:151–160, 2014.
46. Narusu GV: Common ailments of canaries, *Vet Rec* 59:53, 1947.
47. Pollock CG: Survey on avian medical education in US Veterinary Colleges: 2002–2004, *J Avian Med Surg* 18:183–188, 2004.
48. American Board of Veterinary Practitioners website: *Recognized veterinary specialties*, American Board of Veterinary Practitioners. http://www.abvp.com/veterinary-specialties. Accessed Sep 28, 2014.
49. European College of Zoological Medicine website: *Avian specialty*, European College of Zoological Medicine. https://www.eczm.eu/Avian%20Specialty.asp. Accessed November 18, 2014.
50. The Australian & New Zealand College of Veterinary Scientists. Chapters. *The Australian & New Zealand College of Veterinary Scientists*. http://www.anzcvs.org.au/info/chapters/. Accessed November 18, 2014.

SPECIALIZATION IN AVIAN MEDICINE AND SURGERY

Eric Klaphake

SPECIALIZATION

Receiving a veterinary degree in and of itself is an incredible achievement. However, there is always a push within any profession to "take things to another level," that is, to develop a higher level of expertise. At an initial level, this usually is addressed by reading journals, belonging to veterinary organizations, and attending conferences for continuing education. Over time, there can be a great drive to develop a niche within the profession, whether for the veterinary practice or an individual employed there. Part of this drive is for personal growth; in other cases, it may be more financially driven to develop a "product" that allows the practice to offer a service not otherwise available within the community. Legally and ethically, there are guidelines as to how one may advertise such a product. While beyond the scope of this chapter, the American Veterinary Medical Association's website (www.avma.org) provides such guidelines for the United States, and communicating directly with one's state veterinary board can also provide guidance as to how to advertise such skills. Ultimately, however, in both the United States and Europe, the term *specialist* is considered the gold standard for indicating the highest level of expertise. A veterinary graduate is legally able to treat any animal species, except human beings. However, most new graduates have developed a comfort level with a small subset of species, usually dogs and cats, horses, or food animals. A relatively new area of veterinary focus involves exotic animals as pets, wildlife, or part of a larger public or private collection. In many ways, the irony of working with such a diverse collection of animals truly challenges an individual to be able to become a specialist; in some cases, the phrase "jack-of-all-trades, master of none" is more applicable. These veterinarians know a little about a lot of species. Because this chapter resides within an avian textbook, the discussion will be directed toward four different opportunities for specialization in avian medicine and surgery: becoming a Diplomate of the American Board of Veterinary Practitioners (Avian Practice) (ABVP Avian Practice), a Diplomate of the American College of Zoological Medicine (ACZM), a Diplomate of the European College of Zoological Medicine (Avian) (ECZM) or either a Member or Fellow (two separate levels) of the Australian and New Zealand College of Veterinary Scientists (ANZCVS). Primary emphasis will be placed upon the former two routes.

COSTS OF SPECIALIZING

The efforts of getting accepted to and graduating from veterinary school can make one avoid considering further sacrifice. Some people immediately transition from veterinary school to an internship and then perhaps a residency. This can be one pathway for becoming a specialist and is often the fastest one, although by no means is it the only option available. So why become a specialist? In some fields, it can lead to a higher level of financial reward—either as a short-term bonus or reflected over the long term in the form of greater overall production revenue, which hopefully translates into a higher base salary or greater compensation in a commission-style contract. One should be aware that at this time, within the fields of zoological medicine, there is not always a direct correlation between specialization and salary increases. In academia, specialization is a requirement for promotion and tenure, and salary increases are often guaranteed. In referral centers, and even in some primary care practices, salary increases can be achieved by being able to charge higher fees and to offer a greater range of specialized services.

A specialist is also more likely to be sought locally, nationally, or even internationally for guidance by general practitioners or by other specialists. This may also translate into modest financial opportunities from speaking at veterinary conferences or from writing articles or book chapters. Specialists may become recognized in their community as the "go to" person for the media, local schools, and nonprofit organizations seeking that expertise. Although this may be viewed as either a perk or a burden, it is part of the mantle of being a specialist. Specializing also opens new doors of opportunity professionally. Most academic positions require some level of specialization, as do many secondary or tertiary private practices. Zoos have been slower to recognize the need for and benefit of specialists, but that has begun to change rapidly within the past few years.

Nonetheless, specializing does not come without costs, some of which are tangible and others intangible. The first route of pursuing specialization is through an approved residency.

The ACZM, ABVP, ECZM, and ANZCVS websites can direct an interested individual to the location of approved residencies if they exist for the particular organization. Approval can change rapidly based on changes of those in charge of such programs or an inability to meet the requirements of approved residencies. Likewise, new programs can be created just as quickly. Most of these residencies are quite competitive, so often an interested individual must begin the process by serving an internship or sometimes even two! This is an important cost consideration.

First, examine the loss of financial earning power. Most internships (1-year duration) pay approximately US $25,000 per year with some benefits, as of 2013. Some internships pay more, but one should evaluate the cost of living in the area, and usually the higher salary reflects this. Most residencies offer US $25,000 to $30,000 per year plus benefits and last 2 (ABVP) to 3 years (ACZM and ECZM). Compare this with the average starting salary for a private practitioner, approximately US $67,000 per year (2013 data). Doing the math, one sacrifices from US $50,000 to $120,000 or more, depending on the length of training. With U.S. veterinary student debt at ever-increasing levels, this should give individuals pause when considering this route to specialization. With some specialties such as surgery, one may quickly begin to recoup these financial losses, but this may not be so with ABVP (Avian Practice), ACZM, ECZM or ANZCVS.

Second, internships and residencies often necessitate continued movement across the country—veterinary school to internship, to second internship, to residency location. Some residencies even require living at different locations each year. The costs of moving and locating new housing may be compounded by significant others or spouses finding new employment at each location, creating the necessity of a long-distance relationship, or even leading to the fracturing of relationships. Ancillary to this financial cost can be the emotional cost on relationships with significant others or spouses and children. As with veterinary school, hours are often long, with emergency shifts, "free time" spent writing papers, and the need to come in on "off days" to see unique cases.

With approved residencies, a resident should be in a stronger position to qualify to successfully sit on specialty boards. In some cases, mentorship can be a benefit, but one is advised not to have high expectations. Some programs may espouse these virtues, but the reality may be that there is little supervision, and residents are left to figure things out for themselves, serving as cheap labor. One wishes this were not so, but I would be remiss if I did not acknowledge that many residents who have completed their programs are quite bitter about this aspect. However, if a resident goes into a residency recognizing that this opportunity will expedite the process, improve one's resume, and allow access to diagnostics, therapeutics, and unusual cases to which other practitioners will not be exposed, then it is unlikely the resident will become disillusioned or disappointed. Anything gained over and above that from a residency is simply a bonus. The reader should not feel that all approved residencies misrepresent what they offer, but it behooves an individual to diligently access the strengths and weaknesses of any program and not to be overly influenced by a program's reputation. Prospective applicants are strongly encouraged to talk to current or previous residents, and one should consider it a red flag if any program resists that open dialogue.

In theory, most approved residencies should allow for time to study for the specialty examination, prepare case reports or first author publications, and systematically review over the time of the entire residencies all of the didactic information to which one needs to be exposed. For example, the ACZM mandates a minimum of 5 hours of scholarly time away from clinical duties per week (approximately 30 days per year). In some cases, the opportunity to perform research may manifest itself, and, of course, completing a residency does enhance one's chance of employment in the academic sphere.

For either specialty, new employment opportunities may present themselves outside general practice, such as working in a zoo, for a nongovernmental organization often in field settings, as a federal or state wildlife veterinarian, as a teaching or research-only academician, or as a referral specialist.

A *board* is of equal standing to a *college* with regard to specialization, according to the American Board of Veterinary Specialties (ABVS). The role of this type of organization is simply to maintain the standards established by each specialty, and they make no effort or claim that one board or college is equal to another regarding difficulty.

For all of the following organizations, check regularly with their websites to access the most current information regarding timelines, credentialing and re-credentialing requirements, and examination structure and content.

Procrastinating is common among many residency candidates, both those pursuing the practitioner routes and those in residencies. Mentors often have the job of motivating residents to receive their credentials and pass their examinations, but mentors and their programs also benefit in membership size by having more of their residents take and eventually pass

boards. It is important for every individual to ascertain whether passing one of these examinations is a personal or career goal or whether they are only doing it for someone else. If potential applicants have no real interest in taking the examination, then they should forgo it so that someone who is dedicated can take that valuable place. One may never feel ready for such an examination, but a good course of action is to work on and complete the credentialing process and then focus on studying. Once one has committed to the field by becoming credentialed, the incentive to study and pass the examination becomes an intense motivator compared with studying for an examination sometime in the future. For credentialing, some may prefer to work through one case report or submit one publication at a time, whereas others may find it more efficient to work on several simultaneously. Having an online study group or a group to review case reports can be extremely helpful.

The ABVP does provide study and credentialing support groups, and further information is available on its website. Likewise, the ACZM offers dedicated short courses to aid candidates in examination preparation. Remember, both the ABVP and the ACZM examinations only require a score of 65% to 70%, which is the usual pass/fail line. This type of score may feel like failure to many veterinarians, but this is the level at which most veterinarians score in the examination process.

In the near future, all organizations should be completely paperless.

SPECIALTY BOARDS

The American Board of Veterinary Practitioners

The ABVP website is www.abvp.com (not .org). Their mission statement is: "To advance the quality of veterinary medicine through certification of veterinarians who demonstrate excellence in species-oriented clinical practice." This specialty is focused more on the private practitioner, although ABVP Diplomates are found in academia and other facets of veterinary medicine. ABVP Diplomates have demonstrated excellence in the care of the total patient. Certification provides professional and public recognition of advanced knowledge, skills, and competency in a species category. Diplomate status is granted with approval of the ABVS. The organization began in 1978, and the first examination was given in 1981. In 1993, the avian specialty was added. As of January 2014, approximately 968 Diplomates were in good standing across all species specialties, 121 of which were specialists in avian medicine, the second highest number of specialists within ABVP.

Two paths qualify an individual to submit credentials. One must either have practiced a minimum of 5 years in any combination of practice that allowed the minimal amount of professional exposure and caseload of birds as required or have completed an ABVP Avian-approved residency program. The applicant should contact the current ABVP Avian Regent for current requirements at the time of application. As of 2014, the credentialing process timeline is a short, simple first-time online application form and a fee—both due by September 1 of each year; this allows the candidate to take the examination no sooner than November of the following year if all requirements are met. The more complex credentials packet, which is described later, is due January 15 of the earliest year a candidate hopes to sit for the examination. The final evaluation of the credentials packet is completed and notification of acceptance or rejection (complete or partial) of that packet is provided to the candidate by June 1 of the earliest year a candidate hopes to sit. Studying then commences, and accepted candidates determine by September 1 if they will register for that year's examination or wait an additional year. Basic information regarding the contents of the 2014 Application and Credentials Packets can be found in Boxes 1-2 and 1-3; however, always refer to the website for changes in the process, form, and requirements. Both of these applications are now completely paperless and online.

One of the most challenging components of the credentials packet is the case report. As noted in Box 1-3, an applicant may submit one case report and a publication or two case reports. The process of one's selection of a particular case to report requires careful consideration. To demonstrate excellence in avian medicine and surgery, it behooves the candidate to show some breadth of expertise. Each case report's species and topic should be different. The topic of each case should generally avoid obscure, new, or uncommon diseases; instead, show expertise at thoroughly working up a standard case. Case reports must have been personally seen and worked up by the applicant within the past 5 years. Each case report must have adequate literature review and demonstrate a logical thought process and well-defended decisions and diagnostic interpretations. Applicants should demonstrate their thought processes and what they know in the case report: significant presenting signs, diagnostic characteristics, problem lists, pathophysiology, differential diagnoses, treatments, and management options. Other directions that could have been taken in hindsight for the aforementioned components should also be discussed for a complete case report.

More specific guidelines and example case reports are available on the website. Formatting is significantly different from most professional journals. The most common reason for failing to credential for examination is inadequate case reports! *Both* case reports, or *both* the single case report and the publication, must pass to qualify for the board certifying examinations.

BOX 1-2 AMERICAN BOARD OF VETERINARY PRACTITIONERS APPLICATION FORM

- ◆ Due September 1
- ◆ Requirements
  - ◆ Contact information
  - ◆ Listing of current position(s)
  - ◆ Graduation year and school
  - ◆ Listing of state license(s)
  - ◆ Designation of specialty category to which you are applying
  - ◆ Fee

Important: Once the first-time application and fee are received, applicants have 3 years to complete the credentialing process. If not successfully completed in the allotted 3 years, the process starts over from the beginning with submission of a new application and fee.

BOX 1-3 AMERICAN BOARD OF VETERINARY PRACTITIONERS CREDENTIALS PACKET

- ◆ Due January 15
- ◆ Veterinary diploma photocopy
- ◆ Curriculum vitae
- ◆ Synopsis of veterinary practice
- ◆ Self-reported job experience
- ◆ Continuing education documentation
- ◆ Applicant evaluation forms (3)
- ◆ Case reports (2)
  OR
- ◆ Case report (1) and publication (1)

It is highly advisable that applicants begin writing their case reports *before* submitting the application and application fee. Study groups are available from the ABVP and can help with the process of compiling a case report; taking advantage of this expertise and assistance is recommended. An outside review of the case report is also encouraged, but one must make sure that the individual is aware of the needed components of an ABVP case report. Correct grammar and syntax are important. Remember, this work represents the applicant's ability to function clinically at the level of a Diplomate.

For the refereed (peer-reviewed) publication, the applicant must be the first author. The topic of publication must make a meaningful contribution to the literature of the species specialty and must be different than that of the case report. The publication must be published no more than 5 years before the January 15 deadline, in a refereed, English-language, scientific journal. Conference proceedings, online publications, clinical vignettes, short/brief communications, serial features (e.g., ECG of the Month, Drug Topic of the Month, What's Your Diagnosis), and narrative review articles will *not* be accepted. If uncertain, one is advised to communicate directly with the executive director of the ABVP, well before any deadlines, to determine clarification of a publication on this issue. Acceptance for publication in a refereed scientific journal does not guarantee that the manuscript will be admissible in lieu of an ABVP-style case report.

Once an individual is credentialed to take the examination, preparation for the examination becomes critical. The ABVP examination has two components. One is an all-day two-part (morning and afternoon) general multiple-choice examination, in which each question has one correct answer and two distracters. The second component is a practical examination with slide images to be identified or to be used to answer the associated question. Generally, this second component may be the night before the all-day examination or the morning after. This is clarified by the ABVP once one has been accepted for the examination. The ABVP examination takes place in the fall, and examinees are informed of their own score and of the pass score within 45 days of the examination.

The American College of Zoological Medicine

The ACZM website is www.aczm.org. Work began in 1977 to create the ACZM. Established in 1983 by eight charter members, the ACZM is an international specialty organization for certification of veterinarians with special expertise in zoological medicine. Of note, zoological medicine includes all exotic species, so a Diplomate is not restricted to being just an avian specialist. Six individuals sat for the first examination in 1984. The ACZM became a stand-alone College in 1988. As of the completion of the 2014 examination cycle, there were more than 170 Diplomates in the College. ACZM is responsible for establishing training requirements, evaluating and accrediting training programs, and examining and certifying veterinarians in the veterinary specialty of zoological medicine.

ACZM Diplomates foster high-quality medical care for nondomestic animals and are actively involved in the discovery of new knowledge in the discipline and the dissemination of this knowledge to the veterinary profession and public. Eligibility for examination can occur either by practicing in 100% exotic or zoologic animal practices for at least 6 years, 50% for 12 years, or some combination thereof. Participation in an ACZM-approved residency program (3 years) can reduce the number of practice years needed to qualify to sit for the examination to a minimum of 4 years after graduation. Many residents find it difficult and daunting to take the examination that soon and may choose to wait an additional year or two. Unlike the ABVP, there is no case report component for qualifying; instead, the applicant for credentialing must have five, senior-authored (first author) peer-reviewed publications, and at least one must be original research, either prospective or retrospective. Papers must be fully accepted before the application deadline—a letter from the editor indicating this may be sufficient proof. Papers must make a meaningful contribution to the literature. Book chapters, review papers, and proceedings papers are *not* acceptable. See Box 1-4 for more general information regarding the credentialing application; however, always refer to the website for changes in the process, form, and requirements.

The ACZM examination also occurs over 2 days; however, it differs significantly from the ABVP examination. The examination takes 2 full days, and the total point allocation is 675 points. On Day 1, all candidates take five sections of the test: Avian, Herpetofauna, Mammal, Wildlife, and Aquatic. Box 1-5 shows the breakdown of the four components of the Day 1 sections. Continuation to Day 2 is contingent on passing all five Day 1 sections with a score of 65% or higher for each section. There are 75 multiple-choice questions for each of the five Day 1 components, and each question has one right answer and four distracters. Thus, 49 of 75 questions must be answered correctly in each section. On both the ACZM and the ABVP examinations, questions may be disqualified for various reasons during the grading process; thus, the actual number of correct answers needed to pass a Day 1 ACZM section can have some variation, but 49 is a starting point. There are still some encouraging rewards if three or four of the sections are passed. On returning the next year, examinees only need to pass the remaining one or two sections to continue on to ACZM Day 2. However, failure to pass those final one or two components in that second try will cause the examinees to have to repeat all five sections of the Day 1 examination the next year if they so desire to continue with the attempts.

The Day 2 examination for ACZM is based on one of four options of a subspecialty—General Zoo, Zoological Companion Animal, Aquatics, or Wildlife. See Box 1-6 for more

details of each. Obviously, birds are a component of each of these four options; however, many examinees choose one of the first two options. Each option has four sections—a practical examination, an essay examination, a slide examination, and an advanced multiple-choice examination (75 questions). One must pass with 65% or greater, but for Day 2, the score is cumulative. If examinees do not pass Day 2 on the first try (irrespective of whether first or second try for Day 1), they return the following year for one last try. Failure on the second try for Day 2 requires the examinee to start completely over with passing Day 1, all sections, again.

The European College of Zoological Medicine

The ECZM is a European Veterinary Specialist College formed under the auspices of the European Board of Specialisation (www.eczm.eu). The ECZM evolved from the European College of Avian Medicine and Surgery (ECAMS),

BOX 1-6 ZOOLOGICAL MEDICINE DAY 2 EXAMINATION OPTIONS

Aquatic Animal Medicine
- Fish, marine, and aquatic mammals, aquatic invertebrates, aquatic birds, and aquatic herpetofauna; either free-ranging or captive (including zoologic and aquaculture institutions)

General Zoo
- Captive mammals, birds, reptiles, amphibians, and fish, with an emphasis on species kept in standard zoologic institutions

Wildlife
- Free-ranging wildlife, including mammals, birds, and herpetofauna

Zoological Companion Animal Medicine
- Major emphasis on companion birds, herpetofauna, and mammals, some fish

itself a veterinary specialist organization founded in 1993. The ECAMS was an initiative of the European Committee of the Association of Avian Veterinarians, in response to a growing demand for better avian medical and surgical services for birds through specialization and a need to harmonize certification in this area. ECAMS became recognized as a fully functional College in 2005. In 2007, an initiative was commenced to broaden the membership and areas of specialty of the ECAMS. The aims were to strengthen the College by increasing membership, provide the opportunity for those working at a specialist level within allied zoologic fields to gain recognition, and facilitate greater recognition of the clinical area by the profession within veterinary academia, by governments, and by the public. The result was that the ECAMS changed to the ECZM. The ECZM website provides detailed information about the ECZM, including the constitution, bylaws, and information brochures on all specialties, including avian medicine. The latter contains information about requirements for admission to the College, a profile of the specialties, and application and examination procedures. As of October 2013, there were 33 ECZM Avian specialty Diplomates, including several in North America.

Diplomates in avian medicine and surgery work primarily as clinicians who are concerned with all aspects of diagnosis and management of diseases of birds other than poultry (companion birds, ornamental birds, zoo birds, racing pigeons, birds kept for falconry, free-range birds, and ratites). The primary objectives of the specialty are to advance avian medicine in Europe and increase the competency of those who practice in the field. However, non-Europeans may apply and become certified if they meet the same criteria as European applicants. In 2014, there were seven ECZM-approved avian residencies, with two of those in North America.

Currently, a specialist is only required to be active in the field for a minimum of 50% to 60% of the time. The current ECZM examination structure comprises a 1-day examination for a total of 370 points.

The Australian and New Zealand College of Veterinary Scientists—Avian Chapter

The Australian and New Zealand College of Veterinary Scientists (ANZCVS) seeks to serve the veterinary profession and reward excellence (www.anzcvs.org.au). *College Membership* signifies that a veterinarian has expertise and competence in a nominated subject area. To become a member of the College a candidate must have at least four years postgraduate experience as a veterinarian and have successfully completed both written and oral or practical examinations in one of the diverse range of subjects on offer. *College Fellowship* is associated with scholarly and technical excellence in a particular subject. Standards required for training and examination in Fellowship subjects meet or exceed the prerequisites for registration as a Veterinary Specialist in Australia, New Zealand, or both. Based on these descriptions, a Fellow is most analogous to a Diplomate in the other three systems previously mentioned. As of 2014, 64 individuals were listed as Members of the Avian Chapter and 9 of those individuals listed as Fellows. There are two separate Avian Health Chapters—a Caged and Aviary Birds Chapter and a Poultry Chapter, with the former more analogous to those of the other three groups.

The objectives of the Avian Chapter are:
- To provide the means of entry to the college for those specializing in avian health
- To provide a means of accreditation for avian health veterinarians
- To advance the science and art of avian health
- To facilitate the exchange of knowledge between avian health veterinarians
- To encourage exchange of knowledge with and collaborative work with other biological scientists in the field of avian health
- To encourage publication in the sphere of avian health
- To acquire, maintain, employ, and dispose of such real and personal property and to organize such services as will further the above aims

Candidates for Membership of the College should be eligible for registration as a veterinarian in an Australian State or in New Zealand. Council may at its discretion approve a candidate who has veterinary qualifications recognized as being equivalent to Australasian qualifications. Candidates must have spent at least 4 years in a full-time veterinary activity between graduation and taking the examination. Candidates who have not had the opportunity of working intensively in a limited field of activity and in a situation where an opportunity for learning from other veterinarians is available would well be advised to prolong their preparation period to 6 or even 8 years. Applicants will be assessed on their knowledge and skills at the Membership examination. Performance in the Membership examination is assessed on the basis that the candidate shall achieve a pass mark of 70% or above.

ANNOTATED SUGGESTED READING LISTS

For ABVP, ACZM, ECZM, and ANZCVS, lists are provided to guide veterinarians studying for the examination. They are *not* a comprehensive listing of all available material but rather a guide to facilitate finding information in areas in which the candidate does not have extensive experience. Questions are taken from the extant literature and are not confined only to information from the work on the list. Not all chapters in listed textbooks are necessarily of significance for the examination. Questions based on journal articles emphasize literature from the past 5 years, although older references may also be included. It is recommended that candidates prioritize study material within the references suggested.

EXAMINATION PREPARATION

No perfect method exists for studying for these examinations: different systems work for different people. Some basic recommendations include the following: Spend time reading (one of the main reasons for taking this examination is to give you the opportunity to, at least once, do a thorough review of the literature), start early (8 to 12 months before the examination), have a study plan, and have an examination-taking plan.

Beyond these steps, what follows are some of the strategies that may help some individuals better direct their energies. For ACZM credentialing, in most cases, candidates likely have a good idea of whether they meet the requirements. However, with credentials submitted by March 31, that only leaves about 5 months until the examination. Thus, some individuals indicate that they will take the examination the following year, giving themselves an 18-month time frame to study. For ABVP credentialing, notification of acceptance of credentials usually occurs in early summer, giving about 5 months until the next examination. As previously mentioned, no matter how much time one has to study, one will likely never feel prepared enough. Some examinees go into an examination with little or no preparation, using this strategy to see what they know and to analyze the question style to help preparation for the next year. Many current Diplomates frown on this strategy; however, it has worked for some individuals. This can be an expensive endeavor for many individuals because the examination fee, plane ticket, hotel expenses, and even the stress of waiting another year before trying again adds up. Using this strategy, one would need a multiyear examination plan from the beginning.

Another strategy often employed, particularly for the ACZM examination, is to try to pass the Day l examination in a multiyear approach. Again, while this strategy is not encouraged, it can be successful, particularly for those on the practitioner track, because these individuals often cannot devote large amounts of time to studying the enormous amount of information; however, if they perhaps focus on birds, herpetofauna, and aquatics, then a component of Day 1 might be passed. Disadvantages to this method include the cost of multiple examination site visits, as already mentioned; the stress of not being done after the first attempt; and the possibility that the sections with increased focus are actually failed. Nonetheless, given the huge breadth of ever-increasing knowledge required for passing the ACZM examination, this technique has worked well or occurred for a growing number of examinees. The technique does not work well for the ABVP examination because the only partial one can get is either passing only the practical or only the multiple-choice component, so partial passage is more incidental in most cases.

For those attempting to pass one of the examinations completely in one try, the first step is developing a technique to organize the information. Organizing by taxonomic groups or populations is one technique used, and another is to skim through core topics and recent research and organize by information source.

Working with a good mentor can be helpful; however, mentors not familiar with the current examination can sometimes be extremely detrimental because they may direct the examinee to study topics on the examination that are no longer relevant. Some mentors also put too much emphasis on the core topics, leaving the candidate blindsided by the examination question coverage. Speaking candidly with individuals previously mentored by that person can be extremely helpful in evaluating whether that particular mentor will be a benefit.

Practice examination questions from within a study group or that are completely self-created can help one to start thinking like a question writer and thus can help determine whether a particular paper may have value from an examination standpoint. Reading papers and references from the standpoint of taking an examination versus evaluating those same sources for clinical information usually requires an individual to look at those sources very differently. For either examination, assume that the results of a paper are valid, even if one personally disagrees. An exception to this is when another paper contradicts the other's findings; this controversy often leads to avoidance of that aspect of the topic for an examination question, although essay questions may touch on those controversies in the ACZM examination. Likewise, if findings are ambiguous or questionable, the results are not likely to be the focus of a question from that source.

For the ACZM Day 2 essay and practical portions, try to focus on the major topics in each area. For example, a question on brown kiwi reproductive surgery would be less likely than one on chlamydophilosis in a Columbiform species. Comparing and contrasting similar diseases are often a good way to cover such topics. Real-life scenarios (e.g., "You note a die-off of African penguins. How would you work it up? Then compare and contrast two major diseases that might be involved here.") are always helpful. Essay questions may be of ancillary benefit to ABVP examinees, but the learning format is not often helpful. Day 2 essays of the ACZM examination are used by many candidates as a significant portion of their combined Day 2 points because these questions focus more on showing what you know (usually a lot) versus what you do not know. However, points will be deducted for wrong information, so writing down everything possible hoping that some part of it is correct is not a good strategy.

Develop a pacing strategy for the examination. Remember, even if only guessing, one will be "correct" 33% of the time for the ABVP and 20% of the time for ACZM/ECZM examinations. Examinees then just need to combine what they already know and what they still need to learn in the area for the additional 37% to 45% to score in the 65% to 70% range. This perspective can help keep a candidate calm when feeling overwhelmed by the amount of information. For essays, examinees should quickly read through all of them, skipping those on which they have little or no information; the more well-known questions (and therefore the greater sources of points) should be completely answered first. Time should be allotted at the end of each section for writing down something for those questions that one does not have much to add.

For the practical and the slide portion of Day 2 ACZM, one often cannot return to certain stations or images, or, if the latter is allowed, only a brief reassessment may be performed. For the ABVP practical, the current practice is to print out images on to individual booklets for each examinee; however, video may still be shown in a manner described for the ACZM practical. Be careful about changing answers—sometimes first impressions are the best. However, also be careful about "easy question-answer combinations"; these are often screened from the question pools by examination committees, so quick associations of terms may not be the correct answer.

Having a study group for either examination does seem to improve the success of examinees. Some partner with a single other person, others with a larger group. Communication can be weekly, monthly, or even just once. Some try to form study groups with individuals of different backgrounds professionally so that each person brings something different to the group. Others prefer groups of like-minded people, who study and organize their summarized information similarly. Again, there is no single solution; it is different for everyone.

Images for the practical in both examinations and the slide portion of the Day 2 component of the ACZM examination should be reviewed in atlases, textbooks, journal articles, and on the Web. Most actual images on the examinations are rarely in the public domain, but similar ones have often been contributed to the examination.

Some people like to take time off 1 to 4 weeks before the examination for review of all topics. Many practitioners do not have the luxury of such an option. It is also important to realize that at this late stage of examination preparation, such reviews may help more by keeping a person focused and busy rather than allowing more time to gather novel information. Nonetheless, such reviews at the end or periodically throughout the study process may be helpful. It is very important to set a schedule so that one does not spend too much time on a particular topic or area and to also recognize that some topics of unfamiliarity may require greater energy and focus. Study groups often help keep one on schedule.

Do not panic during the studying process or during the examination, and try to stay positive. Everyone hits highs and, more commonly, lows during the process. Study group members can be helpful again in this regard. Also, do not forget that these examinations are not a matter of life and death: failure is not the end of the world (I passed the ACZM examination on the second try and am aware of some extremely well-respected zoo veterinarians and private practitioners who took the examination more than once). Make sure to dedicate time for family, pets, and a life outside of the examination process—no extra letter after one's name is worth that sacrifice or loss!

RE-CREDENTIALING

Currently, ABVP Diplomates are required to either retake the examination or re-credential via a point process every 10 years. Notification occurs in Year 8 to allow adequate time for this lengthy process and for the second or third attempt if early failure occurs so that Diplomate status is not lost. The ABVS is mandating such a process in the near future for all specialties, including the ACZM starting in 2016. Current Diplomates would be grandfathered in, although they would be encouraged to engage in the process. Re-credentialing, other than retaking the examination, requires a significant amount of documentation of appropriate specialty continuing education in the previous 5 years, publications, appropriate lectures, writing examination questions, and doing topic summaries, among other options. Re-credentialing should not be left until the last minute; some ABVP Diplomates have lost their Diplomate status because they lacked enough points. Interestingly, the ABVP offers recredentialing points if one has taken the ACZM examination and passed since the Diplomate last credentialed. The ECZM also has a compulsory re-credentialing system, which requires active Diplomates to re-credential every 5 years.

ACKNOWLEDGMENTS

I would like to specially thank the Executive Director of the ABVP, Marisa Hackemann, for the development of much of this information. Other members of the ABVP Core of Regents over the years also helped develop the Policies and Procedures, the Applicant Handbook, and the PowerPoint used to promote the ABVP that were a prominent source for this chapter. I would also like to give special thanks to the ABVP Credentialing and Examination Committees and, likewise, to the ACZM, its officers, and members of the Examination and Credentialing Committees, who contributed to earlier versions of this chapter, and, finally, Dr. Nico Shoemaker, who reviewed an earlier version of the material for the ECZM.

CRITICAL THINKING AND PRACTICAL APPLICATION OF EVIDENCE-BASED MEDICINE IN AVIAN PRACTICE

James F.X. Wellehan Jr.

The term "evidence-based medicine" is often misunderstood. A false dichotomy is often painted between "Western medicine" and "Eastern medicine," and claims are made that evidence-based medicine is not feasible, since we lack double-blinded controlled trials for everything. The reality is that the true division is between evidence-based medicine and doctrine-based medicine. Doctrine-based medicine involves acceptance of a set of teachings as truth, whether the doctrine is traditional Chinese medicine, information from a professor in a veterinary school, or from the book of the flying spaghetti monster. Evidence-based medicine works from the best information available, such as use of hypergravity for avian fracture repair,[1] but recognizes that further evidence may prove current theories incorrect. While the truth is approached, it is an ongoing and constantly revised process. When examined from this perspective, "Western medicine" is also riddled with doctrine, and the term denigrates the many excellent clinical scientists in Eastern countries; evidence transcends culture. Willow bark was used as an analgesic in traditional European medicine; accepting the controlled studies that have demonstrated this does not involve acceptance of the doctrine as a whole or letting bad blood out of patients because of imbalanced humors.[2] To hypothesize that placement of a needle in a specific site induces a neurophysiologic response causing analgesia is reasonable and merits further testing. To accept that this is caused by chi flow despite lack of supporting evidence of the existence of chi is doctrine-based medicine, and in this case, is acceptance of a doctrine that is leading to extinction of a significant number of species.[3]

A state of uncertainty and self-doubt is inherently less comfortable. It is a natural human tendency to seek clean black-or-white answers, and this is often the way information is taught in veterinary schools. Clients prefer their veterinarians to state answers with certainty. The problem with this was perhaps best stated by Mark Twain, "It ain't what you don't know that gets you into trouble. It's what you know for sure that just ain't so." While acting with surety is certainly easier, it occasionally leads to disastrous results. In the real world, everything is various shades of gray, and many factors play roles contributing to disease processes. It is important for the clinician to recognize uncertainty without letting it paralyze them into inaction, and to act on the apparent best path without forgetting other options. Evidence-based practitioners seek to identify, interpret, and apply the best and most relevant available evidence, while recognizing the limitations of said evidence.

IDENTIFYING EVIDENCE

The first step in evidence-based medicine is identification of evidence. Before searching for evidence, it is important to understand the choices for the presentation of evidence. The highest-quality evidence is original research found in peer-reviewed journals. When an author submits a manuscript to a journal, the standard process is that it is screened by an editor of the journal, and then sent to an associate editor on the subtopic of the journal relevant to the manuscript. If the manuscript is considered to merit further evaluation, the associate editor then identifies reviewers (typically two) who are experts on the topic, and these reviewers then read through the manuscript in detail, assessing the validity of the data and interpretation and clarity of presentation and noting any omissions or errors in the manuscript. The reviews are then returned to the associate editor, who decides whether the manuscript is rejected, accepted, or requires revision followed by re-evaluation. If revision is required, the manuscript is sent back to the authors, who must address all the concerns of the reviewers. If the revisions are addressed to the satisfaction of the reviewers and the editors, the manuscript then advances to publication. This peer review process is the most rigorous method of dissemination of data available and is the gold standard for modern science. It is not perfect, however, and depends on selection of appropriate reviewers by editors, as well as being vulnerable to reviewers who have their own biases and limitations on time available for reviews. Winston Churchill once said of democracy, "No one pretends that democracy is perfect or all-wise. Indeed, it has been said that democracy is the worst form of government except all those other forms that have been tried." Similarly, although peer-reviewed journals are flawed, they are not as flawed as other forms of evidence.

Lower-quality evidence includes review articles and textbooks. Many review articles are peer reviewed, but the original data on which statements are based is not directly available for the reader to assess. Textbooks are generally written by invited chapter authors and then reviewed primarily by the editor. Textbooks undergo a much less rigorous review process, and many textbooks do not even adequately cite the original data so that the reader can assess them, if needed. Brian Speer, as editor of this text, may very well let me get away with the statement on hypergravity therapy for avian fractures in the first paragraph of this section to illustrate the point. The reader should be especially cautious when a reference cited is another review or textbook; especially in avian medicine, many statements are repeated in various reviews and textbooks until they become gospel, but the original data on which the statement is based may be deeply flawed or absent.

Lower still in quality are conference proceedings. Conference proceedings are generally not peer reviewed and are often incomplete. Conference proceedings provide the opportunity to disseminate preliminary findings before publication but should be followed up by proper publication of a manuscript in a peer-reviewed journal. If a proceedings abstract is not followed in the next couple of years with a peer-reviewed manuscript, it should not be weighted heavily. One study in the field of human orthopedics found that 30% of published manuscript results differed from the conference proceedings where they were first presented,[4] and it is plausible that the accuracy rate of conference proceedings that never made it into publication may have been lower.

The least reliable sources of information are anecdotal. Of anecdotal information, the most reliable is personal experience, but it is very important to realize that there is a huge recollection bias. Good or bad outcomes from an insignificant number of cases without controls for comparison may significantly alter a veterinarian's behavior to an inappropriate extent. Bias from personal experience plays a larger role when data are uncertain, leading to incorrect clinical assessments.[5] It is important for the avian veterinarian to be aware of this and not overemphasize single case results when making clinical decisions. Objective interpretation of one's own biases is difficult and requires a very conscious effort.

Additional anecdotal sources of information include testimonials from avian medicine experts and product literature. While avian medicine experts may have seen larger caseloads and be more familiar with the literature, the same potentials for recollection bias exist, and this is essentially personal experience that is more challenging to assess bias because you were not present for this experience. Testimonials from product literature are even less reliable because the company producing the product has a vested interest in supporting the product and screening for positive testimonials.

When searching for evidence in avian medicine, there are two routes to take: reactive and proactive searching. Reactive searching is searching for data to best answer specific questions regarding a patient presented to the veterinarian. Proactive searching is screening the avian medical literature for information that may be useful with future cases that have not presented yet.

The most rapid way of reactive searching for high-quality evidence is through the use of literature databases. There are a number of literature database options available. The National Center for Biotechnology Information makes the PubMed (www.pubmed.gov) medical literature database available for free. Another free literature database is BioOne (www.bioone.org). This includes a number of natural history journals not present in PubMed that may be useful for determining appropriate husbandry conditions for captive birds. Google has produced the Scholar database (scholar.google.com), which is also free of charge. Although this database is currently less consistent than others discussed here, it has the advantage of linking to manuscripts citing the article of interest, potentially providing updates on the status of a topic since the original publication.

There are also several subscriber databases available. The largest and most extensive is ISI Web of Knowledge (wokinfo.com). This is an umbrella database covering several smaller databases, which cover a broad range of literature going back more than a century. Like Google Scholar, there are also links to manuscripts citing the article of interest, as well as backward links to manuscripts cited by the article of interest. Individual subscriptions are available, although most people access it through an academic library. It is worth investigating the possibility of alumni access to university libraries, or local colleges may also provide some public access. Another subscriber database is the Veterinary Information Network (VIN; www.vin.com).* The literature database covers a number of veterinary journals not on PubMed, although it is not as extensive as the Web of Knowledge. The VIN also has a number of experts in given areas who can offer opinions and more importantly point toward specific literature. It is important to remember that although an opinion may be given by an expert, it is still important to assess the data leading to that opinion.

When searching literature databases, it is important to narrow your search to exclude irrelevant items, as much as is feasible, but not to exclude relevant ones. Use of Boolean terms such as AND, OR, and NOT, can be very useful to help target your search appropriately. For example, if you are looking for information on fungal infection in house finches, which were moved from the genus *Carpodacus* to the genus *Haemorhous*, you might search for (Carpodacus OR Haemorhous) AND (fungal OR fungus). Many databases will also allow wildcard searches (often marked by an asterisk), meaning all words that start with a set of letters are included. For example, fung* would retrieve articles containing "fungal," "fungus," and "fungi."

The other approach to finding evidence is proactive evidence gathering. Proactive evidence gathering builds a knowledge base, reducing the amount of reactive searching needed when presented with a problem. There are a number of different common routes of proactive searching for evidence. One that all veterinarians share is attending veterinary school and attending continuing education following graduation. For proactive searching of the highest quality evidence, peer-reviewed journals, there are a number of options. The avian veterinarian can obtain journals through membership in societies that publish journals relevant to avian medicine, such as the Association of Avian Veterinarians, the Wildlife Disease Association, the American Association of Zoo Veterinarians, or the American Association of Avian Pathologists. However, relevant manuscripts for the avian veterinarian are spread across literally hundreds of journals, and it is not economically feasible to subscribe to all of them. Access to a library at a university with a veterinary school provides the opportunity to access a large number of veterinary journals. One practical option for remaining current with many journals is to have electronic table of contents (ETOCs) sent. Most journals provide emailing of ETOCs as a free service, even to non–journal subscribers. It is typically possible to sign up for this at a journal's web page. The reader can then rapidly browse titles, click to look at abstracts of interest, and decide whether the article is of sufficient interest to obtain and read in full. This is a very time efficient way of keeping up with the current literature.

OBTAINING EVIDENCE

The second step in evidence-based medicine is obtaining evidence that has been identified. More journals are becoming free online, and this is a rapid and easy way to obtain articles. For those with either online or physical access, an academic library is also a quick and easy route. Another route is to email an author to ask for an electronic reprint. Authors have put significant effort into creating scientific publications, and most authors are glad to know that their publication is of interest. Contact information for corresponding authors at the time of publication should be available with the abstract, and provision of reprints is considered basic scientific etiquette. Authors may also be able to help with directing the clinician toward other relevant evidence. Finally, most non–open access journals offer electronic reprints for a fee.

ASSESSING EVIDENCE

The third step in evidence-based medicine is assessing validity and relevance to your patient. With peer-reviewed journal articles, it is important to look at study design. The most easily misleading journal articles are case reports. These are primarily useful for determining whether a disease process exists in a given species. Treatment of the disease process in a case report means nothing about treatment safety or efficacy unless there is already known expected outcome without treatment. Even if there is an expected outcome, results of treatment of a single case may be an outlier, and not predictive of efficacy of treatment. If the talons of a falcon with enteritis are painted purple and the falcon recovers, that should not be taken as good evidence that painting the talons purple is a good treatment for enteritis in falcons.

Retrospective studies are studies that review past cases meeting diagnostic criteria and making associations with other factors and outcome. These also require caution when being interpreted—there may be significant selection bias involved in these cases. If, when treating cockatoos with renal disease, only the sickest animals are hospitalized and placed on intravenous fluids, then a retrospective study may find that cockatoos treated with intravenous fluids do not do as well.

Prospective studies are studies where diagnostic criteria for a case are defined in advance, and then patients are given one of two or more treatment protocols. These studies are the most reliable way of assessing comparative treatment efficacy. These studies may be clinical studies, or they may be experimental. Clinical studies use actual cases as they present to a clinic. One challenge, when dealing with uncommon conditions in uncommon species, is that it may be challenging to get sufficient numbers of cases to show statistical significance

---

*Disclosure: Jim Wellehan and Brian Speer are paid consultants for VIN.

for smaller differences. Another challenge is that when dealing with actual clinical cases, there are going to be a number of confounding factors causing variation. Diets may differ between toucanets in two different households. One household may have small children that cause significant stress to a bird. These factors will result in more variation in treatment groups and a need for larger sample sizes. Experimental studies use animals under controlled experimental conditions to reduce confounding factors, which should result in smaller sample sizes needed to find statistically significant differences. The main disadvantages of experimental studies are the large cost, and the need to induce the condition of concern in the animal. Some conditions such as rare tumors or infections with agents that have not been successfully cultured may be difficult to reproduce.

Finally, descriptive studies can be very important in avian medicine. Many descriptive natural history studies are crucial for proper husbandry. For determination of appropriate diets, stomach content studies of wild birds may provide the most useful data (and often differ dramatically from what is commonly fed in captivity). Morphology studies are useful for determining surgical approaches.

When assessing articles, the reader should first assess the methods to determine whether the approach is reasonable to answer the questions asked. Determining whether the methods result in an experiment that answers the question of concern is a significant issue. It is unfortunately not uncommon in avian medicine to see the use of unvalidated assays. The method of measuring albumin utilized by commercially available chemistry machines is very inaccurate for avian albumin.[6] Another common problem, given our lack of basic knowledge of the diversity of infectious agents of birds, is the use of serologic testing for an agent that has not been demonstrated in a given host species and may cross-react with yet unidentified related agents.

Statistical errors are common, including lack of presentation of confidence intervals, treatment of non-normal data using statistics that are only appropriate for data fitting a normal curve, and lack of correction for multiple comparisons. With a standard cutoff for statistical significance of 0.05, that means that there is only a 1 in 20 chance that the data are as divergent as they are by chance. However, if you are making a large number of comparisons, eventually you will find one that falsely appears divergent. There are a number of methods of correcting for this, the most common of which is the Bonferroni method.

A significant flaw of many manuscripts is to draw conclusions that are not supported by data. Some authors approach a study as an attempt to validate a theory, rather than an attempt to test it, and this bias may result in erroneous conclusions. This error may not be obvious from reading an abstract, and the reader generally needs to examine methods and results sections to identify these errors. Another common mistake is misinterpretation of an association as causality. There is probably a higher rate of lung cancer among humans who carry lighters. This does not mean that lighters cause lung cancer.

When assessing textbooks or review articles, it is important to ensure that adequate references are given to enable the reader to track down and assess the original data, if needed. Poor referencing is particularly a problem with textbooks, and some textbooks in avian medicine are poorly referenced. One example of a well-referenced text is the *Exotic Animal Formulary*.[7] When the references are examined more closely, it becomes very apparent that the data vary markedly in quality, ranging from peer-reviewed pharmacokinetic, safety, and efficacy studies to empirical doses based on personal communications. It is important for the reader to be aware of this and weigh information appropriately.

When assessing conference proceedings, the literature should be examined for articles resulting from the study initially presented in the proceedings. If it has resulted in a peer-reviewed publication, the reader should read and assess that instead of the proceedings. If it has been more than a couple of years since the proceedings presentation and no peer-reviewed publication has resulted, the data should be used with caution.

Once validity of data has been assessed, relevance to the case at hand needs to be determined. Hypergravity may improve avian fracture healing,[1] but given that the current practice of avian medicine is limited to one rather small planet, increasing gravity is not a practical option for therapy. The study population needs to be compared with the patient; while data on pharmacokinetics of azithromycin in healthy young blue and gold macaws may be available, this may differ in a 70-year-old macaw patient with hepatocellular carcinoma. In avian medicine, we often lack information in a given species, including anatomy, physiology, microbiology, and pharmacology. When information is lacking in a given species, the best model to use is typically the closest relative from which data are available. This requires knowledge of species relationships. Since humans are not commonly used for experimentation due to ethical concerns, common and appropriate laboratory models used are other primates, or the closest relatives of the primates, rabbits, and rodents. However, the understanding of animal classification that most current adults have been taught in grade school is fundamentally erroneous.

A definition is first necessary. The word *monophyletic* is an adjective used to describe a group that contains a common ancestor and all descendants. In comparative medicine, understanding what constitutes a monophyletic group is needed to understand relationships and to choose appropriate models. A group that is not monophyletic is called *paraphyletic*. Paraphyletic groups may not share a common ancestor or may exclude some descendants of the common ancestor. It is illogical to predict that paraphyletic groups would share characters that are not in nonmembers. Primates constitute a monophyletic group; when the primates except for humans are referred to, the term *nonhuman primates* is generally used. This qualification in the term helps the reader understand that a paraphyletic group is being referred to.

When the evolution of the tetrapods (terrestrial vertebrates) is examined, both the fossil record and the even stronger evidence from nucleic acid sequence phylogeny analyses are in agreement on relationships.[8] The earliest divergence among terrestrial vertebrates (tetrapods) is between amphibians and amniotes (Figure 1-9). The amniotes consist of reptiles (including birds) and mammals. The amnion was a major evolutionary advance, enabling amniotes to have a completely terrestrial life cycle without the need to return to water for reproduction.

Amniotes are then further divided into mammals and sauropsids (sauropsids are in green in Figure 1-9). Within the sauropsids, the first group to diverge is the squamate (lizards and snakes) or sphenodontid (tuatara) clade. Following this, Testudines (turtles) diverged, and the last two major sauropsid groups to diverge were crocodilians and dinosaurs, collectively known as Archosaurs. The recognition of dinosaurs as reptiles is widespread in our culture. However, what is not generally recognized is that dinosaurs are not extinct, and birds are the only surviving group of dinosaurs. This is supported both by fossil records and by sequence data.[9] Part of this failure may be due to an erroneous picture of nonavian dinosaurs—they shared a number of traits with birds, including feathers,[10] and there is evidence that they were warm-blooded.[11] Nevertheless, although birds themselves constitute a monophyletic group, if birds are not considered part of the reptiles, then reptiles are not a monophyletic group. What we really mean by reptiles is sauropsids, and birds are a group of reptiles. The term *nonavian reptile* should be used if excluding birds from the reptiles, an awkward term indicating a logically awkward paraphyletic group.

Birds and crocodilians share a number of medically relevant similarities. In a mammal, a persistent right aortic arch is a developmental problem that obstructs the esophagus, and the left aortic arch is the main outflow for oxygenated blood from the heart. In archosaurs, the right aortic arch is the major outflow.[12] Both birds and crocodilians have four-chambered hearts. They also both have a respiratory system with unidirectional, rather than tidal, air flow, a much more efficient design than the mammalian lung.[13] There are also similarities in susceptibility to infectious diseases.[14] Birds occupy a position in the middle of the reptile family tree. While information on birds would obviously be preferable when dealing with an avian patient, if the information is lacking, crocodilians are a better model than mammals. The obvious differences between a sparrow and a caiman underscore the more cryptic but greater differences between a sparrow and a big brown bat.

Within the birds, it is important to be familiar with relationships of taxa for model choice as well. The earliest divergence within the extant birds is the Palaeognathae–Neognathae divergence, occurring approximately 102 million years ago[15] (Figure 1-10). Palaeognathae comprises ostriches, rheas, emus, cassowaries, kiwis, and tinamous. Within Neognathae, the first divergence is between Galloanseres and Neoaves, approximately 88 million years ago.[15] Galloanseres include Galliformes (fowl, turkeys, quail, pheasants, cracids, and megapodids) and Anseriformes (ducks, geese, swans, and screamers). By far,

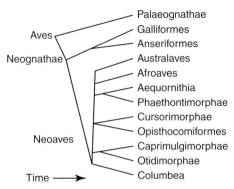

FIGURE 1-10 The relationships of the major avian clades. Descriptions of clades may be found in the text.

the most physiologic, microbiologic, and pathologic studies specific to birds involve the chicken, a member of Galliformes. Neoaves contain most of the living avian taxa, and resolution of their relationships has been complicated by the fact that nearly all families in this group (as well as the Galliformes–Anseriformes split) diverged shortly after the end-Cretaceous extinction, approximately 66 million years ago.[15] The loss of approximately 65% of species from the fossil record, associated with the Chicxulub crater asteroid impact, left many ecologic niches open, leading to an explosion in avian diversity within a short period. As a result, it is only with the recent advances in whole genome sequencing technology that we have gained sufficient resolution to understand these relationships, and several important clades for model choice have become clear as a result. Australaves (Passerines, Psittacines, Falcons, and Seriemas) contain the most commonly kept companion birds, with Passerines and Psittacines forming a subclade within Australaves, known as the Psittacopasserae or Passerimorphae, depending on the author.[15] Psittacopasserae share brain adaptations for vocal learning, a trait that has evolved independently in hummingbirds.[16] Afroaves contain several other taxa that are commonly seen in captivity, including hawks and eagles, new world vultures, owls, mousebirds, trogons, hornbills, woodpeckers, and bee eaters.[15] It should be noted that falcons are included in Australaves, while hawks and eagles are included in Afroaves; their similarity is convergent evolution. Aequornithia contains a variety of primarily aquatic birds, including loons, albatrosses, petrels, penguins, storks, cormorants, gannets, boobies, ibises, spoonbills, herons, and pelicans, and the sister group to Aequornithia is Phaethontimorphae, containing tropicbirds, sunbitterns, and the kagu. Cursorimophae are plovers and cranes, and the hoatzin is unique in Opisthocomiformes. Caprimulgimorphae (hummingbirds, swifts and nightjars) are the sister group of Otidimorphae (bustards, turacos, and cuckoos). The earliest divergence of Neoaves, the Columbea, is composed of Columbimorphae (doves, sandgrouse, and mesites) and Phoenicopterimorphae (flamingos and grebes). When working with poorly studied species, it is important to understand what the closest relative is with available data.

It is also important to consider environments in which birds have evolved. Eons of selective pressure have resulted in birds that have adapted to specific diets, habitats, and threats, and disease may result when captive conditions differ. Vitamin A deficiency is a common concern in parrots in the genus

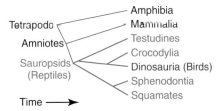

FIGURE 1-9 The relationships of the major vertebrate clades. It can be seen that the birds (Dinosauria) are in the middle of the reptiles and are a group of reptiles.

Amazona, native to tropical new world forests.[17] In contrast, induction of hypovitaminosis A in adult cockatiels is very difficult, and vitamin A toxicosis is comparatively easy to induce.[18] Cockatiels evolved in very xeric environments, where vitamin A may be expected to be relatively scarcer; treating all psittacine species identically from a nutritional standpoint can lead to significant clinical problems. Xanthomas can be a significant problem in birds fed levels of cholesterol beyond those to which they have adapted.[19] Some avian species may have adapted to toxins that may be fatal for other birds.[20,21]

Use of an evidence-based approach requires a conscious effort to keep an open mind about possibilities as cases progress and to avoid falling into routine assumptions. Especially in areas lacking data, such as avian medicine, the uncertainty can be initially discomforting, and most data need to be extrapolated from other model species. However, an evidence-based approach will enable clinicians to provide the best care possible for their avian patients and to improve approaches with the advent of new data.

REFERENCES

1. Negulesco JA: Effects of increased earth gravity and estrone treatment on intact and healing avian radii, *Calcified Tissue Res* 23:291–296, 1977.
2. Fuster V, Sweeny JM: Aspirin: a historical and contemporary therapeutic overview, *Circulation* 123:768–778, 2011.
3. Yiming L, Wilcove DS: Threats to vertebrate species in China and the United States, *Bioscience* 55:147–153, 2005.
4. Zelle BA, Zlowodzki M, Bhandari M: Discrepancies between proceedings abstracts and posters at a scientific meeting, *Clin Orthopaedics Related Res* 435:245–249, 2005.
5. Alexander M: Bias and asymmetric loss in expert forecasts: a study of physician prognostic behavior with respect to patient survival, *J Health Econ* 27:1095–1108, 2008.
6. Lumeij JT, de Bruijne JJ, Kwant MM: Comparison of different methods of measuring protein and albumin in pigeon sera, *Avian Pathol* 19:255–261, 1990.
7. Carpenter JW: *Exotic animal formulary*, ed 4, St. Louis, MO, 2012, W.B. Saunders.
8. Hugall AF, Foster R, Lee MS: Calibration choice, rate smoothing, and the pattern of tetrapod diversification according to the long nuclear gene RAG-1, *Syst Biol* 56:543–563, 2007.
9. Schweitzer MH, Zheng W, Organ CL, et al: Biomolecular characterization and protein sequences of the Campanian hadrosaur *B. canadensis*, *Science* 324:626–631, 2009.
10. Xu X, Wang K, Zhang K, et al: A gigantic feathered dinosaur from the lower cretaceous of China, *Nature* 484:92–95, 2012.
11. Eagle RA, Tütken T, Martin TS, et al: Dinosaur body temperatures determined from isotopic (^{13}C-^{18}O) ordering in fossil biominerals, *Science* 333:443–445, 2011.
12. Eme J, Gwalthney J, Owerkowicz T, et al: 2010. Turning crocodilian hearts into bird hearts: growth rates are similar for alligators with and without right-to-left cardiac shunt, *J Exp Biol* 213:2673–2680, 2011.
13. Farmer CG, Sanders K: Unidirectional airflow in the lungs of alligators, *Science* 327:338–340, 2010.
14. Temple BL, Finger JW Jr, Jones CA, et al: In ovo and in vitro susceptibility of American alligators (*Alligator mississippiensis*) to avian influenza virus infection, *J Wildl Dis* 51:187–198, 2015.
15. Jarvis ED, Mirarab S, Aberer AJ, et al: Whole-genome analyses resolve early branches in the tree of life of modern birds, *Science* 346:1320–1331, 2014.
16. Zhang G, Li C, Li Q, et al: Comparative genomics reveals insights into avian genome evolution and adaptation, *Science* 346:1312–1320, 2014.
17. Birgel EH, De Carvalho Periera P, et al: Hipovitaminose A em papagaios (*Amazonas aestiva aestiva*), *Revista da Faculdade de Medicina Veterinaria*, Universidade de Sao Paulo, 7:299–314, 1963.
18. Koutsos EA, Tell LA, Woods LW, et al: Adult cockatiels (*Nymphicus hollandicus*) at maintenance are more sensitive to diets containing excess vitamin A than to vitamin A-deficient diets, *J Nutr* 133:1898–1902, 2003.
19. Hoekstra KA, Nichols CR, Garnett ME, et al: Dietary cholesterol-induced xanthomatosis in atherosclerosis-susceptible Japanese quail (*Cotunix japonica*), *J Comp Pathol* 119:419–427, 1998.
20. Eriksson K, Nummi H: Alcohol accumulation from ingested berries and alcohol metabolism in passerine birds, *Ornis Fennica* 60:2–9, 1982.
21. Hewitt DG, Kirkpatrick RL: Ruffed grouse consumption and detoxification of evergreen leaves, *J Wildlife Manage* 61:129–139, 1997.

CHAPTER 2

Infectious Disease

James F. X. Wellehan Jr. • *Michael Lierz* • *David Phalen* • *Shane Raidal*
• *Darrel K. Styles* • *Lorenzo Crosta* • *Alessandro Melillo* • *Petra Schnitzer*
• *Angela Lennox* • *Johannes Thomas Lumeij*

THE PATHOGENESIS OF INFECTIOUS DISEASES

James F. X. Wellehan Jr.

Infectious disease is often thought of as a war against microbes. Koch's postulates, established in 1844, stipulated that a pathogen must be found in diseased but not healthy hosts, that it must be isolated in culture from a diseased host, that it should cause disease when introduced into a healthy host, and that the same organism should be isolated from the experimentally infected host after causing disease. While Koch's postulates have their use, they frequently result in a false dichotomous understanding of microbes as either pathogenic or nonpathogenic. Microbes are essential for all vertebrate life, for functions including digestion, nutrition, and defense, and disease is dependent on context. There is no such thing as a microbe that is always either a pathogen or a nonpathogen. There have been many asymptomatic human Ebola virus infections, and people have died of *Lactobacillus acidophilus* septicemia.[1,2]

Evolution and ecology are central to infectious disease. Evolution is an essential concept in biology. Indeed, when one considers definitions for life, perhaps the simplest and most elegant definition is that life consists of things that evolve. A microbe does not "want" to cause disease or not cause disease. All life on earth has been selected for billions of years to reproduce successfully, and this is all that matters from an evolutionary standpoint. If pathogenic traits provide an evolutionary advantage in a given situation, they will be selected for. If they provide a disadvantage, they will be selected against.

Multiple factors influence evolutionary rates, including generation times, fidelity of copying genes, and selective pressures. Microbes often have very short generation times. Ribonucleic acid (RNA) viruses, typically lacking proofreading, have high error rates when they make copies. As a result, evolution rates in microbes tend to be rapid, and RNA viruses are the most rapidly evolving organisms. This is useful for rapid adaptation to novel selective pressures such as immune selection and antimicrobial drug use. To compensate, the most rapidly evolving genes in vertebrates are immune related.

There are a number of important selective pressures impacting microbes in an avian host, including nutrient availability, temperature, competition with other microbes, the need to transfer to a new host, and the host immune system. A vertebrate host is a nutrient-rich environment. However, some nutrients may be sequestered; one example is iron, which is a limiting factor for the growth of many bacteria. Significant resources are spent by the host synthesizing transferrin, lactoferrin, and ferritin to make iron unavailable. Many bacterial virulence pathways have evolved to access this sequestered iron.[3,4]

Homeothermic vertebrates also provide a highly temperature-controlled environment, whereas poikilothermic hosts require the ability to survive at different temperatures. Infectious disease manifestation may be highly temperature dependent in poikilotherms.[5] In nonavian reptiles, temperature manipulation is often the most significant therapeutic approach. West Nile virus infection in alligators at avian-like body temperatures presents as hepatitis and encephalitis, as it does in a bird.[6] At cooler temperatures, alligators present with lymphohistiocytic foci in skin, known as *pix disease*, which is not life-threatening.[7] Significant temperature manipulation is not a reasonable therapeutic option in birds, unlike their closest relatives, although a fever response is clinically useful. Further investigation of the role of temperature in disease manifestation in birds is strongly indicated, especially with populations of many avian species critically declining and likely to be impacted by anthropogenic climate change.[8,9]

Fortunately for birds, they do not appear to be the most susceptible taxa to climate change. Many are familiar with the K-T extinction 66 million years ago as a result of a meteor impact at the end of the Cretaceous era. Approximately 65% of species disappeared from the fossil record at this time, including the nonavian dinosaurs. This is not the largest extinction in the fossil record; at the end of the Permian era, about 252 million years ago, approximately 95% of species went extinct as a result of the eruption of the volcanoes forming the Siberian steppes, burning extensive coal beds and releasing large quantities of carbon dioxide. This led to a global warming event that was unparalleled until now.[10,11] The dominant species in the late Permian era—carnivorous gorgonopsids and herbivorous dicynodonts—were in the lineage containing mammals, Therapsida. With highly soluble urea as nitrogenous waste requiring expensive loops of Henle, lack of a renal portal system to conserve water, and lack of an efficient unidirectional air flow respiratory system, the mammal lineage was hardest hit and nearly went extinct when Pangaea became a hot desert. The dinosaurs, more fit to deal with this, arose out of the ashes of this extinction and dominated the planet for the next 185 million years.

Microbial competition is also a major selective pressure in a bird; many organisms want to live in such a nutrient-rich environment. The majority of antimicrobials are derived from products secreted by other microbes that help them compete for ecologic niches. Animal guts are some of the most diverse and rich ecosystems to be found anywhere. Many organisms that have evolved in such a competitive environment have resistance to many antimicrobials, the *Enterococcus* sp. being a classic example.

The need to transfer to a new host creates significant selective pressure. This often involves secretion of large amounts of microbes via respiratory discharge or diarrhea, but other routes occur, such as the simultaneous behavioral changes and salivary gland shedding of rabies, or the use of insect vectors. There are three fundamental strategies that can be taken to deal with limited host lifespans. First, a microbe may survive well in the environment. Second, a microbe may adapt to a balance with the host environment. Finally, a microbe may move quickly to a new host.

Parasites often adapt to a balance with their host. Many parasites tend to have slower generation times compared with viruses or bacteria, making rapid reproduction and moving on to a new host less of a viable strategy. Many parasites bring relatively minimal costs to their definitive hosts, as it is advantageous to preserve their habitat. Bullfrog tadpoles carrying the pinworm *Gyrinicola batrachiensis* have better feed conversion and metamorphose earlier than uninfested controls, rendering the relationship mutualistic rather than parasitic.[12] However, for parasites with indirect life cycles, causing disease in an intermediate host may be advantageous. If a dove carrying *Sarcocystis calchasi* is debilitated, it is more likely to be eaten by a hawk, which would complete the life cycle. This may also result in greater disease in accidental hosts.[13] Some parasites do survive well in the environment; this reduces the selective pressure to not harm the host. Parasites that survive well in the environment are much more likely to cause significant disease.

Most fungi survive well in the environment, resulting in little selective pressure to keep their hosts alive. They compete significantly with bacteria for the same niches; this has resulted in the production of antibacterial compounds by fungi and antifungal agents by bacteria. The fungi are some of the closest relatives of animals; fungi, choanoflagellates, and metazoa (multicelled animals) form a clade known as the Opisthokonta.[14] A bird is much more closely related to a mushroom than it is to an oak tree. Antimicrobial drugs generally exploit differences in chemistry and metabolism between pathogen and host. Because fungi and avian hosts diverged more recently, there are fewer differences to exploit, and antifungal drugs tend to have narrower therapeutic indices and use a smaller subset of mechanisms.

Bacteria constitute a large portion of the avian ecosystem. There are far more bacterial cells in a normal bird than there are bird cells. Traditional approaches to examining bacterial diversity have depended on culture; this is a poor way of assaying diversity. Culture-independent methods such as 16S polymerase chain reaction (PCR) and cloning or high-throughput sequencing methods have revealed that standard culture-based methods will detect between 1% and 10% of bacterial species present in most ecologic niches. As an understanding of further diversity has arisen, it becomes clearer that a vertebrate is a complex ecosystem.[15] This system may be very dynamic. The gut flora of chickens changes significantly in response to antibiotic and anticoccidial use. After treatment with monensin and tylosin, bacteria in the phylum Firmicutes (the "classic" gram-positives, containing organisms such as *Clostridium*, *Staphylococcus*, and *Streptococcus*) shift away from the genus *Lactobacillus* and toward the genus *Clostridium*.[16]

Ecologic disturbance may have significant negative impacts on many aspects of health. Damage to healthy gut flora by antibiotic use provides opportunity for invasive species; recent treatment with antibiotics markedly increases host susceptibility to *Salmonella*.[17] A 5-day course of ciprofloxacin will change human gut flora diversity and composition for several weeks, and the original composition may never be reestablished.[18] In many ways, the use of broad-spectrum antibiotics for a bacterial infection in a vertebrate is analogous to starting a forest fire to get rid of coyotes. The ideal treatment for a bacterial pathogen would be as narrow spectrum as possible, minimally disturbing the rest of the host ecosystem. Fidaxomicin, which targets only *Clostridium difficile* and a few very closely related species and does not even significantly impact many other *Clostridium* spp., is an excellent example. Unfortunately, current market forces have resulted in pharmaceutical companies developing antibiotics with as broad a spectrum as possible, and narrow-spectrum antibiotics are often not put through further development and clinical trials.

Antibiotic use without consideration of microbial ecology and evolution rapidly leads to failure. Back in the 1990s, fluoroquinolones were used in poultry. Over the next few years, human *Campylobacter jejuni* isolates from humans acquired a high rate of ciprofloxacin resistance, which had previously been rare[19] and therefore posed a greater risk to human health than previously. Use of modern farming practices, including high stocking densities and use of antibiotics as growth promoters, leads to higher antibiotic resistance rates.[20] Wild birds typically have lower *Salmonella* carriage rates and less antibiotic resistance compared with farmed poultry.[21] The only realistic way to reduce the risk of *Salmonella* in farmed birds over the long term is to alter the ecology that the organism inhabits, including facilities engaged in companion bird breeding. Keeping farmed animals in high population densities increases contact rates, pathogen loads, and stress and lowers barriers to transmission. Increased ease of transmission reduces the selective pressure to keep the host alive and healthy.

Viruses are strictly dependent on host cells for replication. Therefore, living free in the environment as a strategy for dealing with limited host lifespans is not a viable option. There are a number of important properties that impact viral evolution and ecology. Enveloped viruses are surrounded by a lipid envelope. This envelope is usually essential for invading a host cell. Nonenveloped viruses use other mechanisms to invade a cell. The lipid envelope is easily damaged, making disinfection easier when dealing with an enveloped virus.

Segmentation of viral genomes, which allows reassortment, provides a hybrid advantage for crossing host species;

this has been best studied with influenza.[22] Random genetic mutations are much more likely to be deleterious than advantageous. Acquiring functional genes that are from a related organism is significantly more likely to be advantageous. Throughout biology, hybridization is a factor that allows for rapid nondetrimental change and for species to invade novel habitats.[23] New sites of infection or host species are novel virus habitats. Animals and plants invest significant resources into sex; it would be much easier to sit on the couch and bud, rather than having to take a shower and go on a date, but the advantage of more rapid evolution is worth the cost. Viral recombination is the equivalent of sex. Influenza, a negative stranded RNA virus in the family Orthomyxoviridae, is a segmented virus, and it changes so rapidly that a new vaccine is needed every year. Measles and its nearest avian relative, Newcastle disease, are caused by negatively stranded RNA viruses in the family Paramyxoviridae, which are biologically similar but are not segmented. Vaccination for paramyxoviruses typically results in lifelong protection because the virus does not do the viral equivalent of sex and therefore does not change rapidly. Another example of a segmented virus leading to rapid adaptation to divergent hosts is in the genus *Orthoreovirus*; a virus identified in parrots by one institution was nearly identical to one found by another institution in a case of abortion in a Steller sea lion in Alaska, representing an avian–mammal host jump.[24]

Nucleic acid type is another property with a major impact on viral evolution and ecology. Many large deoxyribonucleic acid (DNA) viruses adapt to a balance with their hosts, especially those with intranuclear replication. This is seen with latency or chronic infection, requiring a delicate balance with the host immune system, and a larger number of genes is often needed to maintain this balance. Because they are larger and more complicated, they require more accurate replication to avoid accumulating lethal mutations. DNA viruses usually have much more accurate replication, with either host or viral proofreading mechanisms in place. Many DNA viruses evolve at rates comparable with their hosts, enabling larger viral genomes with greater numbers of genes. Viruses reproducing in the nucleus often utilize the host replication machinery there, unlike viruses replicating in the cytoplasm which must supply their own replication proteins. This results in greater dependence on a given host, and large DNA viruses with intranuclear replication are the most host-specific viruses.[25] Adenoviruses and herpesviruses, both large intranuclear DNA viruses, have co-diverged evolutionarily along with their hosts. In Figure 2-1, a herpesviral phylogenetic tree is shown. The earliest amniote divergence is between mammals and reptiles, as seen in Chapter 1. All known β-herpesviruses and γ-herpesviruses use mammal hosts, and the longer branch lengths in this area indicate that these viruses have diverged over a longer period. In the α-herpesviruses, the first agents to diverge infect squamates; the squamates are the earliest divergence within the reptiles. The next group to diverge are the herpesviruses infecting turtle or tortoise hosts; this is also consistent with host divergence patterns. *Mardivirus* and *Iltovirus* infect avian hosts. However, the mammalian α-herpesviruses nest with the clade infecting avian hosts, closest to *Mardivirus*. The branch lengths within the mammalian α-herpesviruses are relatively short, indicating that these viruses have not diverged from each other to the same extent that mammalian

herpesviruses in the other subfamilies have. One plausible explanation for this is that the mammalian α-herpesviruses represent a host jump to mammals from the Dinosauria. Chicken pox, caused by the α-herpesvirus *Human herpesvirus 3*, may be a descendant of an avian virus and more aptly named than had been realized.

The host adaptation of some large DNA viruses provides selective advantage to causing minimal pathology in their hosts. A long-lived host may provide suitable habitat for decades. However, this balance in a definitive host may not apply to other hosts. Hosts that are similar enough for a virus to infect but dissimilar enough for the intricate balance of latency or chronic infection to not work often results in overwhelming and often fatal infection. The most significant pathology associated with herpesviruses is in aberrant hosts. A well-balanced host–virus relationship may actually be beneficial to the host. *Columbid herpesvirus 1*, endemic in rock doves, causes disease in squabs kept in stressful conditions, but the overall pathology is relatively minimal. However, in raptors, which prey on rock doves, *Columbid herpesvirus 1* causes an overwhelming infection that is rapidly fatal.[26] The advantage to the pigeon populations of killing off predators likely outweighs the disadvantage of minor disease in neonates.

RNA viruses reproduce less accurately. They usually lack proofreading and have the highest mutation rates of any organisms on Earth. These mutation rates mean that a large complex genome is not possible because their high error rates would cause offspring requiring a large gene set to be nonfunctional. RNA viruses therefore have small genomes and fewer genes. The advantage of such a high error rate is that RNA viruses are capable of rapidly outmaneuvering the host immune system. The strategy of RNA viruses is typically rapid reproduction and moving on to a new host. Because they have less complex relationships with their hosts, RNA viruses are much more capable of moving to new host species. The ability to move to new hosts reduces the selective pressure to not harm the host, and many RNA viruses are more pathogenic. One meta-analysis found that of the 20 virus families infecting the best-studied vertebrate species, humans, four RNA virus families, Reoviridae, Bunyaviridae, Flaviviridae, and Togaviridae, accounted for more than half of emerging and re-emerging viruses.[27] Most of the high-profile human viral diseases that have recently emerged are RNA viruses, including Ebola (Filoviridae), severe acute respiratory syndrome (SARS) and Middle East respiratory syndrome (MERS) (Coronaviridae), Chikungunya (Togaviridae), West Nile (Flaviviridae), influenza (Orthomyxoviridae), and Hendra (Paramyxoviridae) viruses.

Retroviruses have RNA genomes, and when actively replicating, they have very high mutation rates similar to other RNA viruses. However, retroviruses are unusual in that they reverse transcribe from RNA to DNA, and the DNA copy of their genome is then incorporated into the host genome. This has happened a lot over the course of evolution; approximately 1% of the typical vertebrate genome encodes for vertebrate proteins, whereas 8% to 9% of the typical mammal genome is retroviral in origin. The avian genome is much less burdened with retroviruses, at approximately 1.1% of the genome, but this is still formidable.[28] Numbers of identified endogenous retroviruses range from 132 endogenous retroviruses in the ostrich genome to 1032 in the American crow

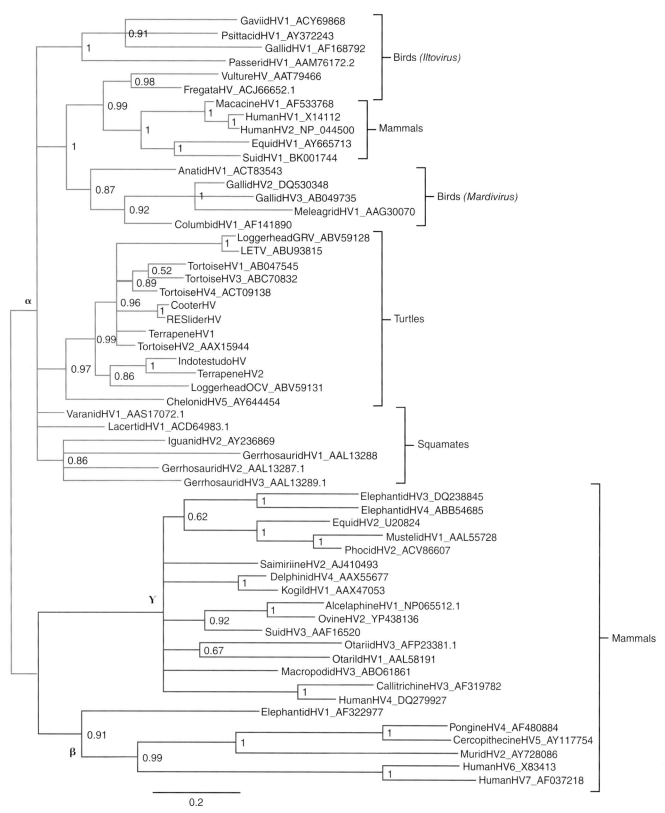

FIGURE 2-1 Phylogenetic tree of the herpesviruses suggestive of coevolution. The β-herpesviruses and γ-herpesviruses are all found in mammal hosts, whereas the α-herpesviruses are mostly reptile viruses and short by host class, with the exception of the α-herpesviruses of mammals, which have shorter branch lengths and cluster with avian herpesviruses, suggesting they may be of avian origin.

genome.[28] This makes retroviral discovery and diagnosis very challenging, not because they are hard to find but because they are widespread and present in such large numbers that it is difficult to sort out disease-associated viruses from clinically irrelevant endogenous viruses. Because of the prevalence of retroviruses in avian genomes, reverse transcriptase, the enzyme that converts viral RNA back to DNA, is commonly expressed in bird cells. This has also resulted in the incorporation of other viruses into host genomes, especially those that replicate in the nucleus, albeit less frequently. Bornaviruses, which have the uncommon trait for RNA viruses of nuclear replication, have been found to be incorporated into the genomes of many vertebrates, including avian species.[28] Incorporation of inactive bornavirus into host genomes complicates the interpretation of nucleic acid–based diagnostics for bornaviruses, some of which have been demonstrated to be causes of proventricular dilation disease in birds.[29,30] Circoviruses, small circular DNA viruses of which the best-studied member in birds is Beak and feather disease virus, are also incorporated into several avian genomes.[28] Interestingly, after retroviruses, the second most common endogenous viruses are the Hepadnaviridae, best known as the cause of hepatitis B in humans; there are 38 copies in the budgerigar genome and 68 in the great cormorant genome.[28] This is not seen in mammals, and this suggests a longer avian–hepadnavirus relationship. Although significant human pathogens, the clinical implications of hepadnaviruses in birds are not yet well understood, and they have only been described relatively recently in companion birds.[31] The chronic nature and lack of pathognomonic histologic lesions in humans make hepadnaviral disease more likely to avoid detection, and these lesions may be a significant unrecognized problem in birds. Endogenous parvoviruses have also been incorporated into avian genomes.[28]

Several routine husbandry practices in the avian pet trade create strong evolutionary selective pressures toward pathogenicity. First, overcrowding is common. The stress of close confinement has significant negative impacts on numerous health parameters.[32] High population densities lower transmission barriers, reducing pressure to keep the hosts alive and selecting toward virulence.[33] It is also common in the bird trade to select for color phases. This usually involves some degree of inbreeding to select for what are often recessive traits. A major driving force for the evolution of sex is the acquisition of genetic diversity for immune function. Inbreeding results in selection for greater disease.[34] Finally, variably stressed birds of species originating from all over the world are brought to breeders or distributors, often in the same facility. This is an ideal situation for pathogens to jump to new host species, which is where the most dramatic disease is seen.[35] The mixing of species by the exotic animal trade has already proved disastrous, with the transfer of monkey pox from Gambian pouched rats to prairie dogs to humans.[36]

Koch's postulates have led to another common erroneous conclusion—that most infectious diseases are caused by a single agent. When infectious disease is more properly considered as ecology, it seems obvious that a more typical scenario is several infectious agents in concert with other environmental factors. Chicken anemia virus and Fowl adenovirus 341 together cause hydropericardium syndrome in chickens, whereas this was not seen with either agent by itself.[37] Avian pneumovirus is much more significant when there is a co-infection with *Escherichia coli*, *Bordetella avium*, or *Ornithobacterium rhinotracheale*.[38] Co-infection does not always result in greater pathogenicity; avian influenza and Newcastle disease interfere with each other, resulting in lower pathogenicity[39].

With the development of next-generation sequencing tools, it has become possible to use nucleotide sequences to truly understand the diversity of flora present, whereas only a small fraction were previously identified by culture methods. Deeper investigation of enteritis in chickens revealed that while no single agent was a sole cause, exposure of specific pathogen-free chickens to flocks with chronic enteritis resulted in colonization with astroviruses, rotaviruses, picobirnaviruses, picornaviruses, and coronaviruses and also had significant shifts in bacterial gut flora.[40] Further work is needed to understand the microbial ecology of pathogen interactions, but the important thing for the clinician to understand at this point is that most infectious diseases involve the interaction of multiple microbes, and a frank single-pathogen disease is atypical.

To reduce the significant selective pressures toward highly pathogenic diseases, major changes in the associated avian industries are indicated. Genetic diversity in populations needs to be valued and monitored through appropriate use of studbooks and cooperative, rather than competitive, interactions with breeders. Breeding for color mutations needs to be discouraged. Housing needs to be entirely revised, with larger enclosures for individual animals or pairs designed such that feeding and cleaning can be done without cross-contamination to other animals. Facilities need to focus on single species and have smaller numbers of animals at lower densities. In conclusion, evolution is central to avian medicine and occurs in a clinically relevant time frame in avian infectious diseases. It is critical for the avian practitioner to take this into account, especially when dealing with the dynamics of interactions with population health (herd health), individual bird health, and infectious diseases.

REFERENCES

1. Leroy EM, Baize S, Volchkov VE, et al: Human asymptomatic Ebola infection and strong inflammatory response, *Lancet* 355:2210–2215, 2000.
2. Cannon JP, Lee TA, Bolanos JT, et al: Pathogenic relevance of Lactobacillus: a retrospective review of over 200 cases, *Eur J Clin Microbiol Infect Dis* 24:31–40, 2005.
3. Haley KP, Skaar EP: A battle for iron: host sequestration and Staphylococcus aureus acquisition, *Microbes Infect* 14:217–227, 2012.
4. Perry RD, Fetherston JD: Yersiniabactin iron uptake: mechanisms and role in Yersinia pestis pathogenesis, *Microbes Infect* 13:808–817, 2011.
5. Rojas S, Richards K, Jancovich JK, Davidson EW: Influence of temperature on Ranavirus infection in larval salamanders Ambystoma tigrinum, *Dis Aquat Organ* 63:95–100, 2005.
6. Klenk K, Snow J, Morgan K, et al: Alligators as West Nile virus amplifiers, *Emerg Infect Dis* 10:2150–2155, 2004.
7. Nevarez JG, Mitchell MA, Morgan T, et al: Association of West Nile virus with lymphohistiocytic proliferative cutaneous lesions in American alligators (Alligator mississippiensis) detected by RT-PCR, *J Zoo Wildl Med* 39:562–566, 2008.
8. Slenning BD: Global climate change and implications for disease emergence, *Vet Pathol* 47:28–33, 2010.

9. Hoberg EP, Brooks DR: Evolution in action: climate change, biodiversity dynamics and emerging infectious disease, *Philos Trans R Soc Lond B Biol Sci* 370(pii):20130553, 2015.

10. Sun Y, Joachimski MM, Wignall PB, et al: Lethally hot temperatures during the early Triassic greenhouse, *Science* 338:366–370, 2012.

11. Brand U, Posenato R, Came R, et al: The end-Permian mass extinction: a rapid volcanic CO_2 and CH_4-climatic catastrophe, *Chem Geol* 322-323:121–144, 2012.

12. Pryor GS, Bjorndal KA: Effects of the nematode Gyrinicola batrachiensis on development, gut morphology, and fermentation in bullfrog tadpoles (Rana catesbeiana): a novel mutualism, *J Exp Zool A Comp Exp Biol* 303:704–712, 2005.

13. Rimoldi G, Speer B, Wellehan JFX, et al: An outbreak of Sarcocystis calchasi encephalitis in multiple psittacine species within an enclosed zoological aviary, *J Vet Diagn Invest* 25:775–781, 2013.

14. Torruella G, Derelle R, Paps J, et al: Phylogenetic relationships within the Opisthokonta based on phylogenomic analyses of conserved single copy protein domains, *Mol Biol Evol* 29:531–544, 2012.

15. Robinson CJ, Bohannan BJ, Young VB: From structure to function: the ecology of host-associated microbial communities, *Microbiol Mol Biol Rev* 74:453–476, 2010.

16. Danzeisen JL, Kim HB, Isaacson RE, et al: Modulations of the chicken cecal microbiome and metagenome in response to anticoccidial and growth promoter treatment, *PLoS One* 6:e27949, 2011.

17. Croswell A, Amir E, Teggatz P, et al: Prolonged impact of antibiotics on intestinal microbial ecology and susceptibility to enteric Salmonella infection, *Infect Immun* 77:2741–2753, 2009.

18. Dethlefsen L, Relman DA: Incomplete recovery and individualized responses of the human distal gut microbiota to repeated antibiotic perturbation, *Proc Natl Acad Sci U S A* 108:4554–4561, 2011.

19. Smith KE, Besser JM, Hedberg CW, et al: Quinolone-resistant Campylobacter jejuni infections in Minnesota, 1992-1998. Investigation Team, *N Engl J Med* 340:1525–1532, 1999.

20. Schwaiger K, Schmied EM, Bauer J: Comparative analysis of antibiotic resistance characteristics of Gram-negative bacteria isolated from laying hens and eggs in conventional and organic keeping systems in Bavaria, Germany, *Zoonoses Public Health* 55:331–341, 2008.

21. Dobbin G, Hariharan H, Daoust PY, et al: Bacterial flora of free-living double-crested cormorant (Phalacrocorax auritus) chicks on Prince Edward Island, Canada, with reference to enteric bacteria and antibiotic resistance, *Comp Immunol Microbiol Infect Dis* 28:71–82, 2005.

22. Macken CA, Webby RJ, Bruno WJ: Genotype turnover by reassortment of replication complex genes from avian influenza A virus, *J Gen Virol* 87:2803–2815, 2006.

23. Rieseberg LH, Kim SC, Randell RA, et al: Hybridization and the colonization of novel habitats by annual sunflowers, *Genetica* 129:149–165, 2007.

24. Palacios G, Wellehan JF Jr, Raverty S, et al: Discovery of an orthoreovirus in the aborted fetus of a Steller sea lion (Eumetopias jubatus), *J Gen Virol* 92:2558–2565, 2011.

25. Pulliam JR, Dushoff J: Ability to replicate in the cytoplasm predicts zoonotic transmission of livestock viruses, *J Infect Dis* 199:565–568, 2009.

26. Pinkerton ME, Wellehan JF Jr, Johnson AJ, et al: Columbid herpesvirus-1 in two Cooper's hawks (Accipiter cooperii) with fatal inclusion body disease, *J Wildl Dis* 44(3):622–628, 2008.

27. Woolhouse ME, Gowtage-Sequeria S: Host range and emerging and reemerging pathogens, *Emerg Infect Dis* 11:1842–1847, 2005.

28. Cui J, Zhao W, Huang Z, et al: Low frequency of paleoviral infiltration across the avian phylogeny, *Genome Biol* 15:539, 2014.

29. Gancz AY, Kistler AL, Greninger AL, et al: Experimental induction of proventricular dilatation disease in cockatiels (Nymphicus hollandicus) inoculated with brain homogenates containing avian bornavirus 4, *Virol J* 6:100, 2009.

30. Mirhosseini N, Gray PL, Hoppes S, et al: Proventricular dilatation disease in cockatiels (Nymphicus hollandicus) after infection with a genotype 2 avian bornavirus, *J Avian Med Surg* 25:199–204, 2011.

31. Piasecki T, Harkins GW, Chrząstek K, et al: Avihepadnavirus diversity in parrots is comparable to that found amongst all other avian species, *Virology* 438:98–105, 2013.

32. Buijs S, Keeling L, Rettenbacher S, et al: Stocking density effects on broiler welfare: identifying sensitive ranges for different indicators, *Poult Sci* 88:1536–1543, 2009.

33. Borovkov K, Day R, Rice T: High host density favors greater virulence: a model of parasite-host dynamics based on multi-type branching processes, *J Math Biol* 66:1123–1153, 2013.

34. Morran LT, Schmidt OG, Gelarden IA, et al: Running with the Red Queen: host-parasite coevolution selects for biparental sex, *Science* 333:216–218, 2011.

35. Pulliam JR: Viral host jumps: moving toward a predictive framework, *Ecohealth* 5:80–91, 2008.

36. Bernard SM, Anderson SA: Qualitative assessment of risk for monkeypox associated with domestic trade in certain animal species, United States, *Emerg Infect Dis* 12:1827–1833, 2006.

37. Toro H, Gonzalez C, Cerda L, et al: Chicken anemia virus and fowl adenoviruses: association to induce the inclusion body hepatitis/hydropericardium syndrome, *Avian Dis* 44:51–58, 2000.

38. Jirjis FF, Noll SL, Halvorson DA, et al: Effects of bacterial coinfection on the pathogenesis of avian pneumovirus infection in turkeys, *Avian Dis* 48:34–49, 2004.

39. Ge S, Zheng D, Zhao Y, et al: Evaluating viral interference between Influenza virus and Newcastle disease virus using real-time reverse transcription-polymerase chain reaction in chicken eggs, *Virol J* 9:128, 2012.

40. Day JM, Oakley BB, Seal BS, et al: Comparative analysis of the intestinal bacterial and RNA viral communities from sentinel birds placed on selected broiler chicken farms, *PLoS One* 10:e0117210, 2015.

AVIAN BORNAVIRUS AND PROVENTRICULAR DILATION DISEASE

Michael Lierz

Proventricular dilation disease (PDD) is a common and fatal disease in birds and affects mainly psittacines. Only anecdotal reports describe the disease in other avian taxa. The disease was first described in the 1970s and named "Macaw wasting disease." The disease was always thought to be transferrable between birds, but the pathogen remained obscured for decades despite various speculations of potential candidates. Only recently, a novel virus, avian bornavirus (ABV) was proven to be the causative agent of this disease. It is now also known that this agent causes digestive tract disorders as well as other clinical signs in birds. Since its discovery, considerable research has been done on the disease and ABV, and knowledge has increased dramatically in the last 5 years. Many questions, however, are still unanswered or not clearly understood, in particular the clinical interpretation of test results in affected birds. This chapter will provide an overview of PDD, focusing on ABV and its clinical significance in the disease and diagnosis.

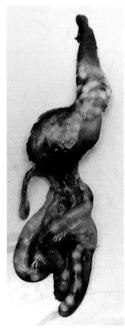

FIGURE 2-2 Gastrointestinal tract of a cockatiel with proventricular dilation disease (PDD). Note the thin proventricular wall, allowing the undigested seed to be seen. The same occurs even in the intestine, which is a rare event.

PROVENTRICULAR DILATION DISEASE

The first reports about PDD originated from the end of the 1970s, where a disease originally named "Macaw wasting disease" was described. Synonyms that have been used to describe the disease since then have included proventricular dilation syndrome (PDS), neuropathic dilation of the proventriculus, and myenteric ganglioneuritis.[1-7] It still remains unclear where the disease originated from, but there are speculations that it was first brought to the United States from Bolivia via imported parrots, followed by a further distribution to Europe.[8]

PDD is typically a disease of psittacines and has been described in more than 60 species.[9] Anecdotally, birds from other taxonomic orders, including Passeriformes, Anseriformes, and Piciformes, have been diagnosed with PDD.[10-12]

PDD is characterized by a nonpurulent inflammation of the peripheral nerves, in particular of the autonomic nervous system of the gastrointestinal tract (GI; esophagus, crop, proventriculus, and ventriculus).[6] As a result, neurologic function is impaired, and the smooth muscles of the GI tract atrophies.[5,13-15] This is followed by a functional impairment of peristaltic function, and food accumulates in the proventriculus and crop.[11] Food is maldigested, and the birds lose weight despite the frequent presence of a normal appetite. Dilation of the proventriculus can be extreme, leaving only a very thin proventricular wall (Figure 2-2), which can even rupture.[16] Nonpurulent inflammation can also be found in the central nervous system (CNS; brain, spinal cord), autonomic nerves of the heart, and adrenal glands.[5,6,17,18]

Clinical signs of PDD are usually nonspecific and detected relatively late in the progression of disease. They usually involve lethargy, weakness, and ruffled feathers but frequently a normal appetite. Owners then detect a loss of weight of the birds. Sudden death, without premonitory signs are described.[14,19] However, maldigestion is typically noted in birds that show a normal appetite, and in the later stages of the disease, undigested seed in feces and vomiting may be seen. Birds often die as a result of cachexia and functional starvation. Cardiac conduction disorders may also be reasons for death in some individuals afflicted with PDD.[20] Parallel to the affected digestive tract, CNS signs are described, mostly ataxia, lameness, tremor, and epileptic convulsions.[19-24] CNS signs and even blindness have also been linked to PDD without digestive disorders.[24,25]

PDD occurs in all ages, with no recognized age predilection. In a study involving 127 birds, the average age of the affected birds was 3.8 years, with a range of 10 weeks to 17 years;[6] therefore, long latent periods before the appearance of clinical signs were presumed, as single-housed birds also became affected after years of no known other outside exposure.[26]

PDD is often suspected if birds lose weight and have undigested seed in feces, although the differential diagnosis for that particular sign certainly includes other disease concerns. Importantly, a dilated proventriculus may occur because of reasons other than PDD. In particular, mycotic infections with *Candida* spp. and *Macrorhabdus ornithogaster* should be considered. Bacterial or parasitic infections, neoplasia, or foreign bodies are additional potential causes.[8,11] Intoxications, particularly with lead or zinc may be other considerations, especially if CNS symptoms additionally occur.

Conversely, CNS signs often are not part of typically suspected clinical signs, but PDD should almost always be one consideration in the differential diagnosis list for susceptible species and CNS signs. Radiography, including contrast imaging, may demonstrate the presence of a dilated proventriculus in typical cases. This does not have to be the case, however, if the myenteric ganglia of the proventriculus are not affected.

Often, when the proventriculus is enlarged as a result of PDD, the walls of the organ are appreciably much thinner than normal. In cases of a dilated proventriculus caused by other reasons (see above), the organ wall is usually thickened or unaltered. Additionally, the passage time of the contrast medium is prolonged in PDD.[8] Using contrast fluoroscopy, typically there is an absence of normal ventricular contractility that is visible and measurable.[27]

Endoscopic evaluation of a potentially dilated proventriculus has been described,[25] but it is usually difficult to judge the size of the organ and is of less value than radiography. In postmortem examinations, with the classic form of the disease, the proventriculus is highly dilated with a paper thin wall (see Figure 2-2) and filled with undigested food. The diagnosis of PDD is confirmed by demonstration of the typical inflammatory lesions of lymphoplasmacytic infiltrations in the ganglia of the nerves and therefore is often demonstrated post mortem only. In live birds, proventricular biopsies can be difficult to achieve, and may be contraindicated where there is considerable smooth muscle atrophy present. For this reason, crop biopsies have been used.[28] False-negative results of crop biopsy are not uncommon. In a study comparing 29 birds confirmed with PDD, only 22 birds had typical lesions in the crop, whereas 25 birds were positive in the proventriculus and 27 in the ventriculus.[29] These authors concluded that 24% of crop biopsy specimens seemed to have false-negative results, especially as those lesions were not distributed equally through the organ. This and other similar observations led to the recommendations to take proventricular and ventricular biopsy samples in cases where the crop biopsy was negative but the disease was suspected. The possibility of false-positive crop biopsy results should also be considered. Signs of inflammation may be seen in the ganglia but may only be temporary, not necessarily diagnostic for PDD. Evidence for this might be provided by the observation that birds that had positive results in the crop biopsy had repeat biopsy performed, had never been positive again, and did not show clinical signs for years. When these single-biopsy-positive birds ultimately died of unrelated causes, PDD was also not confirmed at postmortem examination. In the past, prior to the discovery of the causal role of ABV, crop biopsy represented the only tool to achieve at least a tentative diagnosis, in a minimally intrusive manner, compared with proventricular or ventricular biopsy. Today, crop biopsy is no longer viewed as a valuable tool, considering its comparative insensitivity and other diagnostic options being available (see below).

In cases where PDD has been diagnosed, therapy is difficult. Although some birds may clinically recover with treatment, many will not, and euthanasia may be appropriate when quality of life is poor. A first component of treatment is the provision of highly digestible, high-energy foodstuffs, preferably a formulated product. Metaclopramide has been symptomatically used to aid in promoting GI motility and cimetidine to reduce gastric acid secretion and for its histamine-blocking effects. Antibacterial medications and antimycotic treatment at the beginning of the therapy can be beneficial to treat secondary infection, if present. The use of cyclo-oxygenase-2 (COX-2) inhibitors and partial inhibitors (e.g., celecoxib (Celebrex, Pfizer; Meloxicam) seems to have the most beneficial effects in treatment, reducing the speed of progression of the disease.[13]

One of the major questions during the last 4 decades in avian medicine was the identification of the causative agent of PDD, although an infectious etiology has always been suspected because the disease seemed to be transferrable between birds. Gough et al[30] isolated cytopathogenic, 83-nm-large, enveloped virus particles from macaws with PDD but were unable to identify them. Gregory et al[31] were the first to prove the transmissible character of PDD, as they were able to reproduce the disease in healthy parrots after subcutaneous and intramuscular inoculation of homogenized tissue from birds with PDD. The inoculates contained 80-nm-large virus particles but could not be further characterized. During the last decades, many other viruses, especially neurotropic viruses, were speculated to be causative agents. This included adenoviruses, herpesviruses, coronaviruses, polyomaviruses, eastern equine encephalomyelitis virus, western equine encephalomyelitisvirus, and the latest avian paramyxovirus serotype 1 and 3.[a] However, none of these potential candidates was regularly demonstrated in birds with PDD, and Henle-Koch's postulates were not fulfilled. Therefore, those candidates always failed to be the proven cause. The latest candidate was identified in 2008 by two independent research groups, both demonstrating the same virus in PDD-affected birds.[35,36] Both groups characterized the virus as part of the bornavirus family and named it "avian bornavirus."

AVIAN BORNAVIRUS

Avian bornavirus (ABV) was first detected in 2008 from PDD-affected birds in Israel and the United States by microarray analysis[36] and pyrosequence analysis.[35] In nonaffected control birds, sequences of this virus were not found. The virus demonstrated a sequence homology to mammalian bornavirus by less than 70% but showed important features of the family Bornaviridae and was therefore named avian bornavirus. More detailed characteristics about the viral structure of ABV can be found in the literature.[37,38]

Until the discovery of ABV, the family Bornaviridae within the order of Mononegavirales contained only one genus (bornavirus) with all strains originating from mammals. The order Mononegavirales also includes Paramyxoviridae, Rhabdoviridae, and Filoviridae. The order is characterized as a relatively large enveloped virus with a monopartile single-stranded RNA genome of negative polarity.[38] In contrast to the other families within this order, bornaviruses use a cellular gene-splicing machinery for protein expression and replicate in the nucleus of the cell.[39-42] Bornaviruses are approximately 90 (70 to 130) nm in size and are neurotropic. In the 1920s, the viral etiology of borna disease in mammals was identified.[3] The virus was described in more detail in the 1970s[44] but since then, only two different genotypes of borna disease virus (BDV) have been described—that is, the genome of BDV is highly conserved.[45,46] BDV was distinguished into the classic BDV-1, where all the isolates shared a genomic nucleotide sequence level of more than 95%,[38] and BDV-2, the only variant so far (No/98) that is 85% similar to the other isolates in the genomic sequence. Only recently a novel mammalian bornavirus was isolated from squirrels that seems to have a zoonotic potential.[46a] This picture changed dramatically with the discovery of ABV. So far, eight ABV genotypes have been described from psittacines (ABV 1-8)[35,36,47-49] and seven from nonpsittacine birds, including strains isolated from Canada geese and trumpeter swans,[50,51] canaries,[12,52] and estrildid finches.[53] Within the group of ABV, the different strains share a 91% to 100% genomic similarity within their genotype, 68% to 85% between genotypes, and 60% to 69% with BDV.[36,38,51] The obvious difference between ABV and BDV is also supported by the fact that ABV replicates in cells of avian origin and only poorly, if at all, in mammalian cells compared with BDV, which replicates well in both.[38] This diversity within the genus *Bornavirus* required a novel taxonomy. Therefore, Kuhn et al[38] suggested naming at least five different species within the genus *Bornavirus*: Species 1 (mammalian 1 bornavirus), including the classic BDV-1 and BDV-2; species 2 (psittaciform 1 bornavirus), including ABV 1, 2, 3, 4, and 7; species 3 (passeriform 1 bornavirus), including the strains originating from canary birds (C1,C2, and C3) and from a Bengalese finch (LS); species 4 (waterbird 1 bornavirus), including the strains from waterfowl (062$_{CG}$); and species 5 (passeriform 2 bornavirus), including the isolate from an estrildid finch. ABV 5 and 6, MALL (originating from wild ducks[54]), and reptile bornaviruses described so far have remained unassigned, as the available sequences and the absence of isolates from those genotypes have not allowed classification so far.[38] The authors further suggested that the different bornavirus "variants" be named more descriptively. Therefore, in the future, ABV 1-7 should be named parrot bornavirus 1-7 (PaBV 1-7); C1-3 and LS as canary bornavirus 1-3 (CnBV 1-3) and munia bornavirus 1 (MuBV-1); ABV 062$_{CG}$ as aquatic bird bornavirus 1 (ABBV-1); EF as estrildid finch bornavirus 1 (EsBV-1), and the mammalian BDV 1-2 as borna disease virus 1 and 2 (BoDV 1-2). The variant of the Loveridge's garter snake belongs to a novel species (elapid 1 bornavirus) named Loveridge's garter snake virus 1 (LGSV-1), which is currently placed in the family Bornaviridae but not included in the genus *Bornavirus* so far because of insufficient characterization.[38] Only recently, a distinct ABV has been detected in captive psittacines in Brazil and has been named parrot bornavirus 8 (PaBV-8), forming a separate branch within psittaciform 1 bornavirus species.[49] As these nomenclature changes are not yet internationally accepted, the old nomenclature is used in this chapter. However, in the future, it is fair to assume that the new nomenclature will likely be used.

Interestingly, the avian bornavirus genome was also detected embedded in avian genomes in a low copy number.[55] This may point to the long coexistence of birds and viruses. The author in that report stated that birds obviously seem to be less susceptible to viral genome invasions or prevent them more efficiently compared with other taxonomic groups such as reptiles. So far, it is speculated that ABV represents a rather old virus with the same ancestor as BDV and that BDV evolved later (about 300 years ago).[56] The relationship of the separate lineages from waterfowl, songbirds, and psittacines remains speculative, especially if one evolved from another.[56] Further studies are needed for more detailed conclusions.

ABV as the Cause of PDD

The discovery of ABV in PDD-affected birds was surprising, as up until that discovery, only two mammalian bornavirus strains were known. Borna disease in mammals shows similar lesions to those typically of PDD in birds. BDV is difficult to isolate, however, as it does not show cytopathogenic effects in cell cultures and can easily be overlooked. At that point in time, a high possibility that ABV is the cause of PDD was presumed. However, in part as a result of the remaining large variety of different viruses that were also presumed to potentially have a causative role in the disease, doubts have remained if the cause of PDD was really discovered. First, studies indicated the causative role by demonstrating ABV-antigen in specific PDD lesions.[57,58]. These findings were followed by infection trials, where efforts were undertaken to induce the disease by artificial infection methods.

As a first trial, three cockatiels were inoculated intranasally, orally, and intramuscularly with the homogenized brain of a Grey parrot with PDD that was positive for ABV-4. Two birds demonstrated PDD-like symptoms 21 and 31 days after infection and ABV-RNA was demonstrated in tissue. Postmortem examinations showed histologic lesion typical for PDD.[59] The homogenized tissue, however, contained retrovirus and astroviruses as well, so a conclusive demonstration of ABV as the cause of PDD was not possible. In another trial, two Patagonian conures were inoculated intramuscularly with 8×10^4 international units (IU) of an ABV-4 isolate originating from a PDD-affected macaw. Both birds demonstrated PDD-like symptoms by 66 days after infection and seroconverted; ABV-RNA was found in both birds, and typical PDD lesions were detected at postmortem examination.[60] This experiment supported the hypothesis of ABV as the cause of PDD, but both conures were also known to be infected with a herpesvirus. Mirhosseini et al[61] infected (orally and intramuscularly) two cockatiels with an ABV-2 isolate originating from a cockatiel, PDD-like symptoms occurred 33 and 41 days after infection, and typical histologic lesions were demonstrated at postmortem examination. None of the birds shed ABV-RNA, but ABV-2 was demonstrated in the brain, spinal cord, and intestine. As both birds were known to be infected with ABV-4, the authors concluded that a superinfection with two different strains may cause PDD. Again, this study provided further evidence but still failed to prove ABV as the cause of PDD, particularly because of the low number of birds used and the questioned role of the other viruses found in those previous studies. Piepenbring et al[62] performed a larger infection trial involving 19 healthy cockatiels from a closely monitored research flock, which were known to be free of ABV, paramyxovirus-1, *Salmonella* spp., and *Chlamydia* spp. The birds were divided in two groups of nine birds each and a sentinel bird. One group was infected intracerebrally, the other intravenously with an ABV-4 isolate originating from a macaw. The birds were placed in an incubator, and the sentinel bird was added to the intracerebral group. The birds were closely monitored and sampled every other day for ABV RNA shedding and weekly for the production of ABV antibodies. The trial ended after 230 days, and all surviving birds were euthanized. During the trial, five birds demonstrated PDD-associated clinical signs. At histopathology, all inoculated birds demonstrated nerve lesions typical for PDD. Immunohistochemistry revealed ABV associated with the lesions, and reisolation of the inoculated ABV strain was successful, proving Henle-Koch's Postulates for the first time. All birds shed ABV-RNA in their feces, starting between day

18 and 71 after infection. All birds seroconverted, with titers constantly rising, up to as high as 1:20480. The first detectable antibodies were noted between day 7 and day 63 after infection. The findings of this study resembled the picture seen in daily practice, where infected birds do not always demonstrate clinical signs. This study clearly demonstrated that ABV is the cause of PDD and that it causes GI symptoms as well as neurologic signs, in combination or individually. Therefore, it has been suggested that PDD should be renamed avian bornavirus disease (ABVD), particularly because many more clinical signs beyond a dilation of the proventriculus can be seen. At present, it is becoming more important to understand ABV infection and its pathogenesis of disease in order to determine the route of transmission and to identify effective prophylactic measures. Knowing the pathogen opens new possibilities in fighting the disease. However, ABV infections are currently not completely understood, which is not surprising, as the virus has only been known for a few years.

Occurrence of Avian Bornavirus

Avian Bornavirus was first discovered in psittacines in single cases of PDD-affected birds in Israel and the United States.[35,36] Additionally, ABV has been demonstrated in Australia, several European countries,[47,63,64] Brazil,[49,65,66] Japan,[67] South Africa,[68] and Canada,[69] indicating a worldwide occurrence. Prevalence studies are rare, as most research has focused on the examination of diseased birds. Within Europe, a prevalence of 22.8% was detected, involving 1442 live and 73 dead parrots from 215 different flocks, including 33 genera of birds.[64] The study demonstrates that in all dead birds with histologically proven PDD, 100% were infected with ABV, whereas only 19% of the birds dying from other causes were ABV positive. In the live birds, 67% of birds showing PDD-like signs were infected compared with 19% of healthy birds investigated during a routine control examination.[64] This study not only supports the link between ABV and PDD, but it also demonstrates that the prevalence of ABV is considerably high in captive parrots and that clinically healthy, ABV-positive birds are common. A similar prevalence in a single flock was detected in 59 birds examined after two birds died from PDD with confirmed ABV infection. In 32.2% of the investigated clinically healthy birds, ABV-RNA was demonstrated in cloacal swabs.[63] In contrast, a study in Japan revealed only 4.3% of 93 investigated psittacines as ABV positive.[70] In the meantime, many breeders and veterinarians began to test and screen psittacine flocks, and it is not surprising that many asymptomatic individuals and flocks have been tested positive. It can realistically be assumed that nearly all larger breeding flocks of psittacines are infected, except those which are specifically making diligent efforts to clear the presence of the pathogen. Within a clinically healthy flock, about 10% to 45% of the birds are ABV positive, but exceptions to this general trend might occur. So far, all reports involved captive psittacines, but Encinas et al[65] detected ABV-4 in free-ranging birds in Brazil for the first time. This provides clear evidence that ABV is a pathogen that is not restricted to captive settings. In canaries, 12 of 30 investigated flocks (40%) were ABV positive, and both clinically healthy birds and diseased birds were seen. In waterbirds, ABV-RNA shedding prevalence in free-ranging asymptomatic birds varied according to species and sampling size between 0% and 13%, whereas antibodies were detected in all groups examined. This also clearly shows a wide distribution of ABV in waterfowl populations.[71] In addition, if waterfowl cases are selected by the presence of PDD-like histologic lesions, the prevalence of ABV-RNA detection in tissue samples of those birds increased up to 88.2%.[69]

In psittacines, predominantly ABV-2 and 4 are detected, with ABV-4 being the most common genotype.[72,73] This seems to be independent of the geographic origin, as those genotypes are reported on the various continents. Despite the reports of ABV-4 in psittacines in Brazil,[65,66] a novel type (PaBV-8) was reported in various birds in one study performed in Brazil.[49] Further studies are necessary to see if this strain is endemic to Brazil or if this will be reported more frequently in future. For now, ABV-2 and ABV-4 need to be considered as the most likely genotypes to be recovered, but seeing the high diversity of different strains, it seems likely that further genotypes will be described. The other psittacine genotypes described so far are only reported in single cases. It seems that other avian taxa do have distinctive specific strains, as waterbirds have consistently other genotypes than songbirds. Also within the family of songbirds distinctive genotypes are reported (canary bornavirus, estrildid bornavirus, munia bornavirus). So far, there is no evidence that the different ABV genotypes are able to cross family borders.

Avian Bornavirus Transmission

Because ABV-RNA is regularly detected in feces and urine as well as in cloacal–crop swabs, a fecal–oral route of transmission has been presumed.[37,72-75] Additionally, it was demonstrated that ABV spreads in a flock after infected birds are introduced into a collection.[76] Contact birds as well as noncontact birds became infected, but as seen in most flocks, not all birds became ABV positive. However, in this case, the prevalence of ABV in the affected flock prior to the first case was unknown, so it remains unclear how many birds were infected after introduction of the PDD case into the flock. By showing the occurrence of more clinically affected birds, the study underlines that transmission within a flock is possible. This is supported by an infection trial using canaries, where five healthy, noninfected birds were placed with 14 experimentally infected birds. Two of those contact birds developed a persistent infection, supporting the obvious conclusion that direct horizontal transmission between birds took place,[52] but three birds remained negative. Interestingly, those findings were questioned by the same researchers when they were able to infect cockatiels and canaries by inoculation and none of the contact birds of either species were shown to seroconvert or shed ABV-RNA.[53] The authors then concluded that horizontal transmission of ABV by direct contact is insufficient in immunocompetent fully fledged birds of the tested species. This finding was already presumed after a sentinel cockatiel, placed together with other experimentally infected birds, tested positive in feather and skin samples after contact, but never in one of the organs at necropsy; nor did they seroconvert. Exposure, therefore, most likely did not achieve persistent infection.[62] Further doubts of an easy transmission of ABV by fecal–oral route were raised when birds remained uninfected after being in contact with positive birds for years.[63] It is also a common finding, when investigating flocks, that infected and uninfected birds have had direct contact and that even in successful breeding pairs only one partner is ABV positive. The first experimental trials all used more than one infection route (oral, intramuscular, and intravenous)[59-61] or single routes that are artificial and do not represent the natural way of transmission (intracerebral and intravenous).[62] In the first infection trials mimicking more natural routes of transmission, birds could not be infected. In a study, two groups with nine cockatiels each were infected with an ABV-4 isolate orally and intranasally, respectively. The birds were monitored for several months and euthanized at the end of trial. None of the birds seroconverted, and ABV-RNA could not be demonstrated in any of the organs.[77,78] As it was possible to infect cockatiels with the same isolate under the same experimental conditions,[62] it is fair to presume that nasal or oral transmission in healthy cockatiels does not represent the common route of transmission, or at least other co-factors are needed for successful infection. Here the authors discussed the necessity of mucosal or skin lesions for the first time and other factors such as immune deficiency or incompetence in juvenile birds. These assumptions are supported by further trials involving Grey parrots. In a first study, Grey parrots could not be infected by oculonasal ABV gavage but were successfully infected when the same isolate was administered by the subcutaneous route.[79] The difficulties in transmission of the ABV between birds might be related to the viral nature. ABV, similar to BDV, persistently infects cells but those cells only release a very few infectious particles.[37,73,80,81] Potentially only certain cell types might be able to release an efficient amount of virus for transmission, as speculated for kidney cells.[74,81]

Another potential route of transmission that has been intensively discussed is vertical transmission. The first evidence to support the presence of vertical transmission was found in 2011, when the embryos of ABV-positive psittacine parents were tested positive for ABV-RNA in the brain.[82] Similarly, 10 eggs out of 61 eggs obtained from a psittacine flock with PDD-affected birds within it contained ABV-RNA either in the yolk or in the brain of two embryos.[83] This was further supported by a study demonstrating that embryos of ABV-positive sun conures contained not only ABV-RNA but also ABV-specific antibodies.[84] The authors also demonstrated the eggs and embryos of ABV-positive parents to be free of ABV-RNA and concluded that ABV can be vertically transmitted but that it is also possible to get negative offspring from infected parents by hand rearing or foster rearing. Embryonated eggs laid by experimentally infected canaries contained ABV-RNA, but the virus could not be reisolated.[52] However, there is still some doubt regarding vertical transmission of ABV, as all the studies demonstrated ABV-RNA only, and not viable virus. Both Lierz et al[82] and Monaco et al[83] stated that viable virus in a chick hatched from an infected egg needs to be proven before vertical transmission can be assumed. This is supported by findings of Wüst et al[84a] in 2015 investigating the survival of ABV after inoculation in embryonated cockatiel eggs. Of 32 embryos infected at day 3 to day 5 of incubation in the yolk sac, only nine demonstrated ABV-RNA in the brain at day 17 of incubation. All these embryos developed uneventfully, and no inflammation typical for PDD was seen. Reisolation of the virus was still ongoing during the preparation of this text, but these results again demonstrated that

vertical transmission is also not common and, if at all, only occurs when certain co-factors that are currently unknown are present. This is additionally supported by a study that failed to demonstrate ABV-RNA in the brain of newly hatched chicks or embryos from Canada geese originating from a known ABV-positive population. Only in the yolk of one unembryonated egg was ABV-RNA detected.[71]

Therefore, from clinical observation, the route of transmission, at least the circumstances of a successful transmission, is currently not fully understood, including vertical and horizontal means. The abilities and means by which ABV can overcome skin or mucosal barriers are unknown, viral factors (different genotypes and pathogenicities) are not fully understood, and host factors such as immunosuppression, incompetency in juvenile birds, or other immunologic variables might still play a role in the development of disease. However, both the irregular horizontal transmission as well as the uncommon vertical transmission of ABV opens large potential opportunities in preventing further spread of the virus and clearing flocks of ABV (see below).

Potential Pathogenesis

Today, there should remain no doubt that ABV is the causative agent of PDD and additional clinical signs, especially CNS abnormalities. However, it is also known that a considerable number of birds are infected but remain clinically healthy for long periods.[63,64,85-87] The circumstances leading an infection to clinical disease are presently not fully understood. ABV demonstrates a clear tissue tropism toward neural tissue,[63] especially in infected but clinically healthy birds. The highest virus load is always found in the brain, retina, or spinal cord.[88] In clinically diseased birds, the virus can be detected in a wider range of tissues, not exclusive to those of neural origin.[37,57,71] On the one hand, this is in part similar to BDV, as the mammalian virus also demonstrates neural tropism, but in contrast, BDV is not detected in various other tissues. Additionally, intravenous inoculation of BDV failed to infect rats,[89] whereas in cockatiels, those infection routes were successful.[62] Therefore, it is fair to assume that the pathogenesis of ABV has certain parallels to BDV but that differences might be present, so further work is needed to clarify the pathogenesis of ABV. However, BDV causes an immune-mediated disease (see also Chapter 11). Immunoincompetent or neonatal rats demonstrate a persistent infection with high virus load in CNS tissue compared with adult rats, which demonstrated an encephalitis 20 to 35 days after infection. Transmission of T lymphocytes from BDV-affected rats to infected but immunoincompetent (symptomless) rats induced clinical signs, clearly indicating a T cell–mediated disease at least in rats.[90] Here a neural invasion of CD8 T lymphocytes seems to cause the cellular damage and not the virus itself.[81,90-93] Obviously, a similar pathogenesis is presumed in ABV, and Payne et al[51] speculated a delayed-type hypersensitivity effect in inducing the clinical disease. It was also shown that ABV uses similar strategies in escaping the host immune system, by removing the 5' termini of the viral genome.[94] The authors further demonstrated that ABV infection of cell cultures is reduced by adding type 1 interferon (IFN) but that quail cells with a high load of viral ABV-RNA did not produce detectable levels of type 1 IFN as a sign of reducing the host response. The same was supported in a study comparing the type 1 IFN–reducing capacity of the X-protein of BDV and ABV, demonstrating similar capabilities.[95] The authors further detected that the level of depression of IFN-production was dose dependent with the amount of X-protein.

Prior to the detection of ABV, an immune-mediated pathogenicity of PDD was presumed, similar to Guillain-Barré syndrome in humans.[96] The study described antiganglioside antibodies as the cause of the nonpurulent inflammation typical of PDD and provided evidence, as the detection of those antibodies in PDD-confirmed cases were significantly higher than in healthy birds. The authors also concluded later[97] that the trigger for this could be ABV but also any other viral infection. However, this needs to be questioned, as it was not possible to find antiganglioside antibodies in confirmed PDD cases after experimental ABV infection and a very poor connection between ABV positivity and occurrence of antiganglioside antibodies in clinical cases has been shown.[97] A more detailed view of potential immune-mediated pathogenesis of ABV is provided in Chapter 11. It should also be kept in mind that the role of viral factors in the pathogenesis is not yet determined. It is known that different ABV strains act differently within the same host by terms of viral replication and pathogenicity. The first trial comparing the experimental infection of cockatiels with two different ABV genotypes under identical conditions, demonstrated that one strain (ABV-2) was more pathogenic to cockatiels than the other strain (ABV-4) and that viral RNA shedding occurred significantly earlier in ABV-4–infected birds compared with ABV-2–infected birds but that seroconversion occurred significantly earlier in the ABV-2 group.[98] More interestingly, the viral load of ABV-RNA in the different organs was significantly higher in the ABV-4–infected group despite the presence of fewer clinical signs. Additionally, in ABV-4–infected birds the tissue virus load findings were comparable in all birds, independently from the time point of death after infection or the route of inoculation (intracerebral versus intravenous). In the ABV-2–infected birds, the viral load in the different organs after infection depended on the route of infection (intracerebral-infected birds higher compared with intravenous-infected birds) and the time point of death after infection (early death birds had a lower load compared with late death birds). Last but not least, ABV-4 antigen was more often detected in the CNS of infected birds compared with that of birds infected with ABV-2, where antigen was found to be increased in the GI tract.[98] Most interestingly, reisolation was easily possible from ABV-4–infected birds from nearly all tissues within a couple of days, whereas re-isolation of ABV-2 depended on the time point of death or the identifiable disease of the host. Reisolation of virus from the birds that died earlier after experimental infection was successful only after several passages in cell culture compared with what was seen in infected birds that died later, where reisolation was typically possible in the first passage. These results indicated additionally that the amount of virus (and viral replication) is not correlated with the severity and speed of the disease and its progress. In addition, it is apparent that the virus induces the disease through mechanisms (e.g., earlier activation of the immune system) independently of the viral load or even that earlier activation of the immune system causes more severe disease but does not allow the virus to replicate quickly. This seems to be supported by

the fact that viral shedding was also noted significantly later compared with the ABV-4 group with a far higher viral replication and less severe symptoms. The infection patterns of ABV-2 demonstrates many parallels to BDV infection in mammals, as it is known that minimal viral replications can trigger the onset of clinical symptoms and that disease progression depends on host immune response.[99]

It needs to be considered, as clearly stated by Lierz et al,[98] that the differences found between ABV-2 and ABV-4 must not only be related to the different genotype, but they could also present strain specific variations and can theoretically also occur in different variants within a genotype. Additionally, the ABV-4 isolate used originated from a macaw compared with the ABV-2 isolate originating from a cockatiel and might therefore be differently adapted to the trial animals (cockatiels). However, they demonstrated varying viral factors influencing the viral kinetics and host–virus interactions. Further studies should focus on the interaction of ABV with the host to better understand the viral and host factors involved in triggering clinical disease after infection.

DIAGNOSIS

The diagnosis of the presence of an ABV infection basically follows the common rules of infectious medicine. It is focused on the demonstration of the pathogen in samples of the birds (direct proof) or the detection of specific antibodies against the pathogen (indirect proof). Both of these basic methods are possible in diagnosis of ABV infection in birds. However, for a straightforward diagnosis, knowledge regarding ABV kinetics in the host and its interaction with the immune system (circumstances of antibody production) must be known, but this knowledge is incomplete. As a result, interpretation of diagnostic test results is challenging. The first problem is when and how to judge a bird to be ABV positive; second, a bird owner or veterinarian will often request a prognosis about the clinical outcome for the bird. The first problem will be discussed below; the second problem has a very clear answer—a clinical prognosis is not possible in infected but clinically healthy birds.

The demonstration of the presence of ABV in samples from birds (e.g., cloacal swabs, tissue samples) is made by the detection of viral-RNA by reverse transcription polymerase chain reaction (RT-PCR). Conservative ABV-consensus PCR-protocols focus on the detection of the M-, N-, P-, or L- Gen,[35-37] with the M- and N- protocols appearing to have a higher sensitivity.[57,100] For an additional quantitative analysis of viral amount real-time RT-Taqman-PCR were initially developed for the detection of ABV-4 (Primer 1034-1322) and ABV-2 (Primer 1367).[35] As with all PCR protocols, the primers are able to detect specific gene sequences. As a result of the high variability of ABV, it should be kept in mind that those primers might fail to detect a specific ABV genome despite its presence because alterations in the specific gene sequence occurred. Therefore, negative PCR results should be interpreted in the context of the kind of PCR that has been used and, balanced with serologic results, the clinical picture in the patient or the potential occurrence of novel genomic variants. Enderlein et al[88] demonstrated that commonly used real-time RT-PCR protocols were not able to detect all known ABV genotypes. Similarly, an ABV-2 variant from cockatiels was not detected in the previously described real-time RT-PCR protocols[35] but by a conventional consensus RT-PCR,[98] making it necessary to alter the real-time RT-PCR protocol for detection. As ABV-4 and ABV-2 are the most common genotypes in psittacines, it seems fair to use those protocols in an initial diagnostic step. However, as stated earlier, in negative but suggestive cases, or to increase the confidence in the interpretive meaning of the results, further protocols should be applied. If focusing on the detection of ABV from other bird families (e.g., waterbirds, songbirds), specific PCR protocols need to be used.[52,69] Therefore, the laboratory receiving the samples should be able to handle the different PCR protocols that may be required and will need to know the origin of the sample. Additionally, laboratories need to be very experienced in handling samples for ABV or BDV investigation, as it is known that cross-contamination with Bornaviridae-RNA occurs more easily compared with other viruses. It cannot be overstated that ABV detection is a specific task that requires experience and that it is not easy to establish compared with other diagnostic PCR systems as commonly thought by veterinarians or commercial laboratories. Additionally, the details of sample selection, collection, storage, and transport to the laboratory surely can affect the results obtained. Commonly used samples are crop and cloacal swabs, feces, feather calamus, and blood. Feces carry certain disadvantages when used in PCRs, as inhibitors are commonly found in those samples. In a comparison of samples from 55 known ABV-positive psittacines, in 36 birds crop and cloacal swabs were positive for ABV-RNA, whereas in 11 cases only the crop and in 8 cases only the cloacal swab were positive. None of the whole blood samples of those birds were positive by PCR.[88] As a conclusion, a combined sample, including crop and cloacal swabs from one bird, merged in one tube for testing seemed superior for ABV detection in live birds. Interestingly, a recent study identified a high ABV-RNA content in urine,[74] potentially explaining the good results with cloacal swabs. Some authors suggest the feather calamus as a good sample,[101] but this view is not supported by the experience of some laboratories or by experimental studies, demonstrating other tissues more often positive.[62] Additionally, feathers always contain a higher risk of being contaminated by other birds or the environment, leading to false-positive results. In dead birds, brain or retinal tissue is the most superior sample for the detection of ABV-RNA.[62] Additional postmortem samples for viral detection might be the adrenal gland, proventriculus, and ventriculus. After collection, the samples should be stored in a cool environment or ideally placed in a special transport media (RNAlater, Quiagen) to be sent to the laboratory, as RNA within samples are sensitive to degradation, and false-negative results might occur because of poor transport conditions. The samples should reach the laboratory within a few days. In case samples need to be stored longer or are frozen, they should not be thawed and should reach the laboratory in the frozen state. Repeated thawing and freezing cycles degrade the RNA very quickly. The veterinarian should always keep in mind that a negative result of the sample might not automatically mean an ABV-negative bird. Apart from a false-negative result (e.g., sampling issues, loss of detectable viral genome as a result of transport), the sample might just not contain ABV-RNA because at the time of sampling the virus was not present in that location. This is a common problem, especially in live birds, as ABV is shed intermittently in some birds.[56] In tissue samples, the virus might not be in that particular tissue and may be found elsewhere (e.g., the brain). Especially in live birds, repeated testing might be recommended (see below).

ABV antigen can further be demonstrated in tissue by immunohistologic staining. This is commonly used in research settings but is of limited use in daily practice for diagnosis. Viral antigen is stained within the tissue by using polyclonal antiserum against nucleocapsid proteins[102] as well as against phosphoproteins[37,47,103] There seems to be high cross-reactivity between the antigens of the different ABV genotypes as well as between ABV and BDV, but this seems to depend on the target antigen.[104,105] It should also be kept in mind that used primary antibodies might cross-react with tissue antigens, complicating the interpretation of the results.[57]

Last but not least, the isolation of ABV from samples is another method for direct proof of the presence of the pathogen. As this is also not easy, susceptible to false-negative results (as a result of challenges in keeping the virus live during transport and cultivation), costly, and time-consuming, isolation is not a routine method in daily veterinary practice for the diagnosis of ABV infection. However, virus cultivation represents the only method to prove the viability of a virus known to be present, whereas a PCR only demonstrates the presence of a certain RNA sequence. Therefore, virus isolation is essential to answer certain questions and to understand the infection itself. As an example, the proof of vertical transmission requires the cultivation of a viable virus from embryos or newly hatched chicks, similar to the way that detection of means of shedding viable virus and infection trials can only be made if one is working with a live virus in hand. There are difficulties in cultivation of ABV in cell culture. During the search for the causative agent of PDD, several attempts to isolate the potential pathogen failed.[10,106] However, now it is known that ABV does not cause a cytopathic effect and therefore may have been overlooked when using cell cultures. Only Gough et al[30] demonstrated a cytopathic effect when he thought that the pathogen causing PDD was found, but so far it remains unproven if he did find ABV. ABV, independently of its origin (psittacine, canary bird, waterbirds), grows in cell cultures of avian origin such as in duck embryo fibroblasts[48,60,72] or quail cell lines (CEC32, or QM7).[37,48,52,105] ABV does not grow in cells of mammalian origin, and so far, only one study has reported a minimal growth of ABV in VERO cells.[52] The best virus cultivation results were achieved in CEC32 cells.[48,52] It should be kept in mind that different ABV isolates differ in their growth characteristics, especially in speed of replication and ability to infect cells,[98] making several passages necessary in some cases before a negative result can be assumed. As there is no cytopathogenic effect, additional tests such as real-time RT-PCR, immunofluorescence testing, or Western blot testing need to be applied to prove an increase in the amount of viral antigen to confirm a growing virus (Table 2-1).

The detection of ABV-specific antibodies in serologic assays is a very important diagnostic tool. So far, it is not fully understood under which circumstances detectable antibodies are present. In experimental setups, all infected birds developed antibodies independently of the genotype that the birds were infected with[52,62,98] following common rules of infections.

TABLE 2-1

Selected Tests for Detection of Avian Bornavirus Infection in Birds Commonly Offered by Commercial Laboratories*

Test	Use in Practice	Sample	Meaning	Interpretation	Remarks
Direct test to demonstrate the presence of virus particles. Minimum 18 days after infection shedding is detectable according to infection trials[62]; under natural circumstances this might be longer.					
Reverse transcriptase polymerase chain reaction (RT-PCR)	Good, sample easy to take, use transport media, cross contamination possible	Swabs, tissue, secretions	Detection of avian bornavirus ribonucleic acid (ABV-RNA)	Viral RNA demonstrated, does not imply the presence of viable virus	Could be caused by contamination, repeat if serology is negative, excellent for screening (see Figures 2-2 and 2-3)
Virus isolation	Less practical. Takes a longer time. Virus is sensitive to transport issues, and false-negative results can be seen	Swabs, tissue, secretions	Detection of viable virus	Complete viable virus, unlikely result of cross contamination	Takes long, expensive, more for research setups
Immunohistochemistry	Less practical, expensive, takes long, usually not commercially offered	Tissues	Detection of viral antigen in cells	In positive cases infection is clearly demonstrated	Sensitivity questionable, especially in latent cases usually not many cells infected; therefore not applicable in testing live birds
Indirect test (serology) to demonstrate the immunologic reaction of host against the presence of virus particles. Unclear if virus is still present, or even being likely in the case of ABV. Minimum 7 days after infection, seroconversion occurred according to infection trials[62]; under natural circumstances this might be longer.					
Immunofluorescence test – ABV-infected cell culture	Excellent; result takes 3–5 days	Serum, plasma	Detection of anti-ABV-specific antibodies	Bird's immune system had contact with virus. Persistent infection is presumed. Low titers may become negative, demonstrating non-infection of bird. Low titers (up to 1:80) should be rechecked if polymerase chain reaction (PCR) of bird is negative	ABV-infected cell cultures present various ABV antibodies, therefore higher chance of cross-reactivity between different antibodies. Antibodies cannot be distinguished against which protein they are directed

Continued

TABLE 2-1

Selected Tests for Detection of Avian Bornavirus Infection in Birds Commonly Offered by Commercial Laboratories*—cont'd

Test	Use in Practice	Sample	Meaning	Interpretation	Remarks
Multiple protein enzyme-linked immunosorbent assay (ELISA)	Excellent, results may take only 2 days	Serum, plasma	Detection of anti-ABV-specific antibodies	See Immunofluorescence, except that low and high titers should be interpreted by the laboratory using the test	Several proteins act as Antigen. Cross-reactivity likely, but less than as in immunofluorescence test. Depending on ELISA, antibodies, may be distinguishable against which protein they are directed. Low experience at present but may become a very valuable tool for research and clinical prognostication
Single-protein ELISA	Excellent, results may take only 2 days	Serum, plasma	Detection of anti-ABV-specific antibodies	See Immunofluorescence, except that low and high titers should be interpreted by the laboratory using the test	Titers should be rechecked, as huge variations between tests occur. Especially low titers in immunofluorescence test (IFT) sometimes not detected. Comparison trials between the various diagnostic test with large amount of samples necessary
Western blot	Good, result may be quick, only a few laboratories use this test	Serum, plasma	Detection of anti-ABV-specific antibodies	Interpretation of titers difficult	See Single-protein ELISA

*Refer to the text for more details.

In contrast, after natural infection, some birds are detected as shedders without seroconversion.[64,86] Additionally, the titer depends obviously on the time point of infection, the ABV genotype and other unknown factors, making interpretation of serologic test results challenging in spite of the apparent value that serology offers as a tool in flock management (see below). There are also hints that the titer correlates with the potential possibility of developing clinical signs[107] (see clinical interpretations below) and could be used for the interpretation of clinical cases. There are different assays available to detect anti-ABV-specific antibodies. These are indirect enzyme-linked immunosorbent assay (ELISA)[101,108] and Western blot[63] tests, using certain proteins as antigen. Those proteins are recombinant N-,[63,108,109] P-,[63,101] M-,[101] or X-[84] proteins from either BDV or ABV. Usually, single proteins in those tests are used, with expectations of cross-reactivity between BDV, ABV, and different ABV genotypes. However, as this cross-reactivity is not ensured between the different ABV genotypes, the sensitivity of those tests focusing on one protein only needs to be questioned until otherwise proven. At present, this is challenging, since gold standards for those tests for ABV-specific antibodies have not been set, as the disease and definition of ABV positive cases is poorly understood. However, sera from experimentally infected birds are available and should serve as samples for establishing those standards. The first published results of such tests had a sensitivity of 90% and a specificity of 82% in a Western blot test[72,104] and in an ELISA using the N-protein of 75% sensitivity and 75% specificity,[101] both unsatisfying results for use in clinical setups, especially in flock management and flock pathogen elimination strategies. It is presumed that in case of low titers, those tests might present false-negative results, and this presumption was supported by the first comparison tests performed. Tests based on ABV-infected cell cultures (e.g., indirect immunofluorescence test (IFT),[105] which present a wide range of different ABV antigens, seem to be superior in the detection of anti-ABV-specific antibodies in clinical case and flock management. However, those tests are more complicated to perform compared with ELISA. Additionally, in the indirect IFT, a complete antibody titer is measured, not distinguishing against which specific protein those antibodies are directed. For a clinical situation, this seems to be adequate. For research purposes, especially to obtain a better understanding of pathogenesis and disease development, it might be advantageous to know against which proteins the antibodies are directed in the different phases of infection.[101,110,111] Here, Dorrestein et al[112] made very interesting observations by developing an ELISA using different proteins as antigen. They detected that antibody titers against certain proteins (especially P16 and P24) increased when birds developed disease, whereas in infected but healthy birds only antibodies directed against the recombinant ABV protein P40 were detectable in the beginning.

Clinical Disease of Avian Bornavirus and Disease patterns

Clinically, ABV infections have the largest impact in psittacine birds. There are reports of clinical disease related to ABV infection in canaries, geese, and other species, but those are seen rarely, are usually anecdotal descriptions and the significance is still unclear. In psittacines, infection can lead to a deadly outcome. In psittacine species conservation projects, ABV can have a major impact. As an example, during the early 2000s, about 10% of Spix's macaws in the breeding program, one of the most endangered birds in the world and currently extinct in the wild, died from PDD, the major clinical outcome of an ABV infection.

ABV causes nonpurulent inflammation in nervous tissues with ensuing loss of function. Mainly lymphoplasmacytic infiltrations in ganglia are seen in histopathology. The most known clinical outcome of an ABV infection is PDD, as described above. However, other neurologic disorders should also be considered.[87] Especially, CNS signs seem to be more common than previously thought. CNS signs can range in severity from relatively minor signs, including slight tremor (e.g., of one toe), to epileptic convulsions and incoordination, loss of equilibrium, head shaking, opisthotonus, and so on. Fluck et al[107] examined CNS cases presented to avian practice and could clearly demonstrate a link to ABV infection, with more than half of those cases being ABV positive, by exclusion of other common potential causes. In the past, behavioral problems[70] and feather-damaging behaviors in psittacines had been associated with ABV,[113] but scientific proof for clear causality is still lacking. Fluck et al[107] included birds with feather-damaging behaviors in a study and found that about 50% of the examined birds were positive for ABV, but the amount of antibodies and viral RNA shed was comparable

with those of ABV-positive birds in a control group, whereas it was significantly lower compared with a group of CNS-diseased birds. A link between ABV and feather-damaging behaviors cannot be ruled out, but current evidence suggests that it is not likely. This stands out in contrast when compared with what is seen with clinical signs of CNS disease in a considerable number of those birds very likely caused by ABV. This is also supported by experimental infection trials, where cockatiels developed a classic manifestation of PDD after experimental infection (GI tract signs), but some birds also developed clear CNS signs either on their own or in combination with PDD.[62,98] Interestingly, some birds demonstrated only nonspecific clinical signs of ruffled feathers and diarrhea, and a few died suddenly without demonstrating any clinical signs prior to death.

It seems that the quality and quantity of clinical signs depend not only on host factors but also on the ABV variant. In a comparison trial, more birds developed clinical signs after infection with an ABV-2 variant compared with an ABV-4 variant. The incubation time can obviously be relatively short but can also be several months at least. The first signs occurred in experimental trial as soon as 22 days after infection with an ABV-2 variant and 33 days after infection with the ABV-4 variant.[62,98] In this same study, however, some birds developed clinical signs after as much as 20 weeks. It is repeatedly observed that single-housed birds died from PDD (with then-confirmed ABV infection) years after arrival, therefore making it likely that the incubation period of ABV might be as long as several years and the triggering factors might occur any time independent of the duration of existing ABV infection. These types of repeated clinical observations support the hypothesis that there is a delayed pathogenesis after infection in some birds; however, scientific challenge has not yet confirmed these observations to be true. Experimental trials have suggested that the clinical course of the disease in a single bird is unpredictable. After ABV-2 infection, three different types of courses were seen. There are (1) birds with a severe and acute onset of symptoms shortly after infection; (2) birds with a mild course of the disease developing first signs from approximately 80 days after infection, which might then develop to severe signs; and (3) birds with demonstrated signs late after infection (172 days after infection) with a mild progression of clinical disease or even remaining clinically healthy during the complete infection trial.[98] This array of clinical presentations is also seen in daily practice or when observing flocks. After introduction of ABV-positive birds into a collection, some contact birds died quickly with severe clinical signs, whereas others had a slow but progressive onset, and some remained infected but clinically healthy.[101] Additionally, it seems that it is not only the introduction of newly infected birds but other factors such as stress that may also aid in the induction of clinical disease in some birds in a flock. ABV-infected birds were followed up for years after being donated from owners who wished to exclude ABV-positive birds from their flocks. Repeatedly, it was observed that after translocation of those clinically healthy-appearing but ABV-infected birds, an initial die-off period was seen, with some of the translocated birds developing PDD or CNS signs shortly after translocation. Birds that survived this initial period of several months and did not demonstrate clinical signs during this time remained clinically healthy for at least

3.5 years despite being ABV positive. This observation is supported by a study monitoring ABV-infected birds for a year and demonstrating that some birds developed clinical signs, whereas others stayed clinically healthy for long periods.[86] Therefore, the prognosis for ABV-positive birds is nearly impossible to predict, as long as no directly attributable clinical signs of infection are noted.

In bird species other than psittacines, the clinical significance of an ABV infection seems to be low or unknown. The first description of a canary with enteric ganglioneuritis and encephalitis was linked to ABV infection.[47] In naturally ABV-infected canaries, GI and neurologic signs comparable with those observed in psittacines were discovered, but in contrast to the experimental trials in psittacines, these same clinical signs could not be reproduced in canaries experimentally infected with the ABV virus isolated from those diseased birds.[52] Histopathologic lesions, including lymphoplasmacytic perivascular cuffing in nervous tissue, similar to those of PDD in psittacines, were also discovered in Canada geese and trumpeter swans that were positive for ABV infection[69] but could not be linked to clinical signs, as only tissue was examined in that study without clinical history of those affected birds.

Clinical Diagnosis of Avian Bornavirus Infection

The most difficult question at present concerns the clinical interpretation of test results obtained from individual birds. Here, there is a considerable gap between the knowledge gained from experimental infection trials and what is seen in practice.

In two large experimental infection trials involving ABV-negative cockatiels, all inoculated birds seroconverted and started shedding ABV-RNA eventually. There was a difference between those trials in the maximum antibody titer reached, as ABV-4 caused significantly higher titers than an ABV-2 variant infection with lower and more varying titers,[62,98] but in the end, diagnosis of a successful ABV infection was made as all birds seroconverted and shed detectable levels of ABV-RNA. If those birds had been presented in a practice setup, they would easily have been detected as ABV-positive birds. Interestingly, it was also shown that 11 birds first tested positive for RNA shedding before seroconversion occurred, in 6 birds seroconversion was noted prior ABV-RNA shedding, and in 2 birds both occurred at the same time. These observations underline clearly the need for both direct and indirect tests when attempting to diagnose ABV infection. However, in those trials, birds were inoculated by the intravenous or intracerebral route, which might have affected the host response to infection.

In contrast, Heffels-Redmann et al[86] investigated naturally infected psittacines from different flocks repeatedly over a year. In this study, different infection patterns were observed. As in the experimental trials, there were birds with a high anti-ABV-antibody titer and shedding of ABV-RNA during the entire study, some of which developed clinical signs during the observation period, whereas others remained clinically healthy. However, those birds were clearly ABV infected. Another group of birds had a permanent but low anti-ABV-antibody titer and variable detection of ABV-RNA in crop and cloacal swabs. Those birds should also be interpreted as being

infected, as shedding of ABV seemed to be intermittent. However, the authors also observed two other groups of birds that are not easy to categorize, and those observations are also regularly seen in daily laboratory practice. There are birds demonstrating an intermittent low anti-ABV-antibody titer, meaning that sometimes they are serologically negative and at other times they have a low but measurable titer. Those birds never were noted to shed viral RNA during the observation period. In comparison, other birds shed viral-RNA in a low amount intermittently but never had a detectable antibody titer.[86] The last group may be explained as persistently infected birds, in which ABV was functionally hidden from the immune system, but the other group is much more difficult to explain. Those individuals may be persistently infected, with irregular contact of the virus to the immune system. However, both these hypotheses are at present very speculative, and the cause of those infection and host response patterns remains obscure. The route of transmission, as well as unclear host factors, might play a role in this. Veterinarians often have difficulties in explaining to bird owners if those birds should be considered ABV positive or not. As long as the details of infection remain incompletely understood, birds that have had positive signs for ABV should be considered potential carriers (see flock management) and tested repeatedly to get a clearer picture. Importantly, those observations very clearly underline the need that the investigation of birds for ABV positivity must include direct and indirect tests, that is, demonstration of viral presence (e.g., through PCR) as well as serology. With the use of only one laboratory test (e.g., PCR), the results are understandably incomplete and often inconclusive. Particularly in daily practice, cross-contamination of one sample with ABV-RNA from the environment cannot be excluded during sampling in places where several birds are kept or pass through.

In clinical settings, the following is suggested as long as the ABV infection is not better understood. Birds positive for the presence of virus (e.g., RT-PCR positive) and that are also positive by serology can be considered clearly ABV positive. Those being shown to be positive by PCR only should be retested to confirm this result and to exclude cross-contamination of the sample as a reason. At best, those tests should be repeated not earlier than 4 to 6 weeks after the first sample to see if seroconversion has occurred. During this time, the tested birds should be kept separate from others. If they seroconvert or are repeatedly positive for viral presence, they should be considered positive. Birds positive by serology only are a more difficult interpretive challenge. Usually, they are presumed to be carriers,[72] but clear evidence for this is lacking. However, birds with a high titer should be considered positive, as it is known that bornavirus in mammals causes persistent infections.[73] As described above, birds with a low titer are seen to be negative in additional tests, and therefore persistent infection in those remains unproven. There seems to be evidence that some birds are able to clear the ABV infection,[108] which could explain the varying titers seen in some birds, usually not seen in birds with a high ABV titer. This, however, needs to be scientifically proven. Additionally, false-positive reactions in serologic tests by cross-reaction with antibodies directed against other antigens cannot fully be excluded, even if unlikely. Therefore, low-titer birds should be kept separate and repeatedly tested by direct virus test (e.g., PCR) and serology approximately 4 to 6 weeks later. If the titer remains or increases, if virus is detected, or both, the birds should be considered positive. Decreasing titers or sero-negativity, together with negative virus detection (PCR negative), should lead to another retest 4 to 6 weeks later. Only if the seronegativity remains for both tests, and there is a repeated failure of virus demonstration by PCR, should the birds be considered ABV negative. Figure 2-3 provides an overview of suggested interpretation of test results to categorize tested birds.

An interesting question is the interpretation of what the meaning of a low or a high antibody titer is. This is not easy to answer, as this depends on the test used. Therefore, the laboratory should be contacted for interpretation. The greatest advantage is with laboratories that are experienced with ABV investigations, as they should have the experience to interpret those questionable results. Ideally, those laboratories have affiliations with clinical practice settings to provide the needed experience to compare with laboratory results obtained. By using the indirect IFT on infected cell cultures (see above) titers ranging up to 1:80 should be retested if viral detection by PCR failed.

As previously stated, PCR and serology laboratory results do not allow an individual prognosis for prediction of the onset of clinical disease in birds. These test results also do not necessarily indicate the cause of the clinical signs seen. Birds with a high titer and a high amount of shed virus remained clinically healthy for at least 3.5 years. It repeatedly is seen that clinically ill birds have a considerably high anti-ABV-antibody titers and do shed a considerable amount of virus or viral RNA. This was also seen by Fluck et al,[107] who detected significantly higher anti-ABV antibody titers and amount of ABV-RNA being shed in a group of neurologically diseased parrots, compared with a control or a feather-damaging group, despite the fact that the total number of ABV-positive birds was comparable between the feather-damaging and the neurologic group. This underlines the fact that laboratory results point to clinical diagnosis. However, there are cases when the antibody titers rise quickly shortly before the onset of clinical disease, but this point in time is not predictable, and birds cannot be monitored permanently in clinical setups. In experimental infection trials, it was also described that some birds developed the clinical signs very quickly after infection without developing high antibody titers or even shedding viral RNA. Therefore it must be summarized that in clinically sick birds, high titers or large amount of shed virus might be used carefully for interpretation of the cause. Conversely, those same results in clinically healthy birds cannot be used for a prognosis of clinical disease.

The question remains if diagnosis of ABV status is helpful for a PDD diagnosis. This question can be answered both No and Yes. In PDD cases, a single test (PCR or serology) for ABV alone is not helpful. An ABV test (PCR, serology, or both) can tell if a bird is infected with ABV, but it does not tell if the clinical signs of concern are caused by this infection. As described earlier, a considerable number of ABV-positive birds remain clinically healthy. If a bird is symptomatic with compatible signs of PDD, the factual cause of those signs can still be unrelated to ABV. Exclusion of other potential differential diagnoses such as toxicoses, gastric foreign bodies, or concurrent infections still is required to aid in the inductive

strength of a PDD diagnosis. Therefore, an ABV test—serology, PCR, or a combination—should not be taken as a PDD test. The typical PDD lesions can only be seen in histopathology. However, here comes the "Yes" that ABV investigation is helpful. In the situation where typical clinical signs of PDD or CNS signs are observed, ABV testing (serology and PCR) should be included in the diagnostic workup, and other common causes should be investigated. If those reasons cannot be confirmed, and ABV combined test results are positive, it is very likely that those signs are caused by ABV. This is particularly true if the ABV-titer or amount of shed ABV-RNA is high. For flock management, the combined ABV tests are essential (see below). Therefore it can be summarized that a combined antibody– PCR ABV test may be included in the examination panel in an avian practice but should not be taken as a "PDD test" and that single PCR or serologic assays are considerably less reliable for the purpose of screening and diagnosis of ABV status or the presence of PDD.

THERAPY

While several reports indicate partial success of therapy against PDD (see above), only a few studies have focused on the treatment of ABV infection itself. Antiviral treatment of ABV has not been successful to date.[73] Some authors[100,114] reported that amantadine hydrochloride reduced clinical symptoms in birds, but others[72] could not see an effect in reducing the viral shedding. It remains, therefore, unclear what the mode of action could have been in reducing the symptoms in the described studies. Ribavirin was reported to reduce ABV infection in cells in tissue cultures but also did not demonstrate an effect in reducing viral shedding in birds.[115] As long as no direct antiviral drug is available to reduce ABV infection, a treatment focus might be to interrupt the pathogenesis, thus not allowing the virus to trigger clinical disease. To achieve this, immunosuppressive drugs might be promising, as an increasing survival time of experimentally infected rats with BDV has been described.[91] This therapy focuses on selective T cell suppression, for example, accomplished with cyclosporine, and has been described as beneficial in single case reports in birds treated with cyclosporine-A.[116] Controlled studies in infected and clinically ill birds are necessary to prove the benefits. Additionally, it needs to be discussed how practical it is to immunosuppress a bird and reduce ABV-related symptoms, which would potentially then make the bird more susceptible to other infections. Those birds must then definitely be monitored very closely and may also return to clinical states of disease with PDD when immunosuppressive treatment is stopped. However, studies into this direction will be necessary to evaluate the pros and cons of this type of treatment. Recently, a study suggesting an immunomodulating approach using robenacoxib (anti-COX-2 nonsteroidal antiinflammatory drug) in combination with mycobacterial extracts was reported as being promising. The complete mixture applied remained proprietary, but it was reported that the T cell response was somehow redirected.[117] However, those studies had certain drawbacks, as proper case controls were lacking, and therefore the results should be considered carefully and need further confirmation.

As in the treatment of PDD, antiinflammatory drugs were suggested to reduce the ABV-induced signs of inflammation

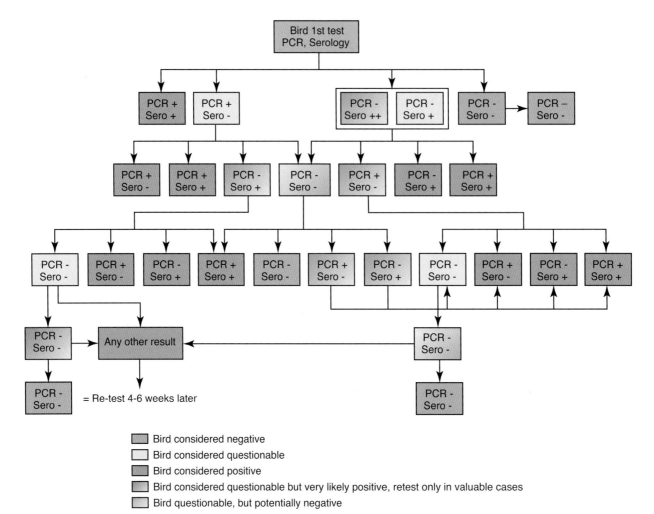

FIGURE 2-3 Suggested interpretation of laboratory test results to categorize birds as positive or negative for avian bornavirus (ABV). Polymerase chain reaction (PCR) should be made from a pooled cloacal and crop swabs of each bird, serology with a multiprotein enzyme-linked immunosorbent assay (ELISA) or preferably Immunofluorescence test based on ABV persistently infected cell culture (Herzog, et al, 2010). − = negative test result, + = positive test result, ++ high anti-ABV-antibody titer. Each box represents an individual bird, and so all the potential test results can be seen by following a box through the complete diagnosing process. Each arrow represents a retest 4 to 6 weeks apart with combined PCR and serology. Usually, most of the birds tested are assigned to a final result in the second row (after two tests) or third row (three tests). Only in very rare cases are more tests necessary, or the birds should be considered positive. First of all, the individual bird is tested and then assigned a positive, negative, or questionable status. Red means that those birds should be taken as positive. Yellow indicates that there is a questionable interpretive status and that from those birds all possibilities may arise; a retest is necessary. Green birds are negative, but it is advised to have at least two negative tests of one individual bird to ensure negativity. In the circumstance that a bird is considered positive, no retest is necessary. Often in clinical circumstances, a negative bird is considered as such in a single test. In the case where the bird is planned to be sold or integrated into a known negative flock, the test should be repeated, and only with a second negative result is the bird considered negative. In case a bird has a high antibody titer with a negative PCR, it should be considered positive. However, in the case of a bird that is deemed very rare or valuable species or individual, the test may be repeated. These birds are depicted as (red/yellow). Questionable birds are retested and usually will be assigned positive or potentially negative status. As described above, only in very rare events birds being positive in one of the test again may still be considered questionable and tested again. The vast majority of these previously positive cases, when retested, will remain positive. Potentially negative birds that were questionable status before are tested a third time and are only considered negative if they are deemed negative again, providing two consecutive negative tests. The odds that from a red/yellow box a result other than a positive can occur are very low, according to the experience of this author, but can theoretically happen.

and thus improve the observed clinical signs. For this, meloxicam was used in experimentally infected cockatiels[115] but demonstrated an adverse effect, with more severe lesions in ABV-infected birds that were treated compared with the control group that was ABV positive and not treated. It is fair to conclude that meloxicam had no observed beneficial effect in reducing clinical signs in experimentally infected cockatiels, but it remains unclear if the treatment had a role in increasing the severity of lesions observed in the treated group.

All in all, immune-modulating or symptomatic treatment might be beneficial in clinical circumstances for individual birds, but it should not be forgotten that those birds will likely remain ABV positive and are a potential risk of infecting other birds and spreading the virus.

FLOCK MANAGEMENT

The loss of a complete flock to ABV (or PDD) is a very rare event, if this has ever occurred. It seems that an initial period of PDD and CNS signs is reported more commonly in an infected flock, followed by longer periods of patency where no or only single birds become diseased. Usually, over years, only single birds die from ABV-related signs in these infected flocks. In some collections, even those single birds might have great value for financial, personal, or genetic reasons, and therefore this loss cannot be tolerated. However, some owners might decide to live with those losses and not to clear the flock from the virus. As ABV is very intensively discussed in the avian community, negative ABV test results are more often requested with a pre-purchase examination, in particular when large parrots are sold. Additionally, more and more boarding facilities request negative ABV test results on record prior to entry. Therefore, there is an increased pressure on breeding flocks to clear their flock from ABV, especially as ABV-positive or untested birds will be more and more impossible to sell. Unfortunately, the specifics of how these birds are being tested may be incomplete, leading to inconclusive findings or erroneous conclusions.

Viewing the common occurrence of ABV-positive birds and the high prevalence in different collections of psittacines, it is rational in some settings to initiate a proper flock health management strategy to exclude the virus from collections, particularly in psittacines. This complex task should only be supervised and planned by a veterinarian familiar with the particular details of the flock's particular management and goals and who understands what is most currently known about ABV and PDD. As with many complex disease processes, effective flock management strategy is far more than a series of test results alone. Informed consent prior to initiating the process to establish an ABV-free population is required.

The clearance of a flock from ABV is a long, expensive, and frustrating task and can only be accomplished with strict compliance of the owners. Many of them are enthusiastic at the start and want their flocks be examined. When they recognize that a considerable amount of birds are ABV positive, conflict often arises, especially if expensive and successfully breeding birds may need to be separated. It is not uncommon for aviculturists to stop further testing and abandon the effort to establish an ABV-free flock. Therefore, owners should be counseled as to exactly what is involved and expected at the onset of the effort to establish an ABV pathogen-free collection. If they accept this, a flock clearance and establishment of an ABV-negative flock is possible. This is particularly true as horizontal transmission of ABV seems to be not that easy (see above).

All birds of the flock need to be tested in a bimodal manner, by direct (virus demonstration, preferably RT-PCR of crop and cloacal swab) *and* indirect (serology) tests. Careful thought should be given to the specific choice of the serologic assay being used. This also applies in all further tests during the clearance process. After the first round of tests, three groups will be established and need to be maintained epidemiologically separate. This implies different logistical setups of compartments away from each other. One group contains the positive birds, the next the questionable birds, and the last the ABV-negative birds according to the diagnostic interpretation mentioned above (see clinical diagnosis and Figure 2-3). The assignment of the birds to one group is purely based on the laboratory results, not on the owners' preference or pairing status of the birds. If an owner does not want to split a pair when one partner is positive and the other negative, both birds must be included in the positive group. The compartments the different groups are located in are treated as separate units. These units are supplied and serviced by different caretakers or by the same caretakers who change their clothes, shoes, and so on, and disinfection is implemented when leaving one compartment. The negative compartment should be supplied (food, water, cleaning) first, followed by the questionable compartment and then the positive compartment. Owners might decide to give the positive birds away, which is a difficult task and might only be reached by rehoming them to private owners to be kept as pets. Euthanasia of positive birds is sometimes also requested but should only be considered in clinically affected birds. Ethically, euthanasia of ABV-positive but clinically healthy birds is very difficult and not recommended. It should also be considered that it seems possible to produce ABV-negative offspring from ABV-positive parents, and therefore those birds, as long as not clinically affected, do have their value as breeding birds (see below). In the end, it is the owners' informed decision, based on the advice of the veterinarian, whether the benefits outweigh the higher workload involved in keeping the ABV-positive birds and the risk of infecting the ABV-negative birds. In many cases of valuable breeding flocks, this is the case, and logistic plans should be made to keep the ABV-positive birds.

This first step is not the end of the way to clear a flock of ABV. In the second step, both groups (questionable and negative), are retested 4 to 6 weeks later. In the questionable group, some birds will now be treated as positives and transferred into this group, and some now potentially negative will remain here, but separated from other questionable birds (Figure 2-4). From the negative group, some birds will be transferred to one of the other groups and some remain still negative. The negative group can be taken as cleared when two consecutive combined tests performed 4 to 6 weeks apart reveal negative results in *all* birds of this group. Birds from the questionable group should be retested as often as only negative birds remains here, with two consecutive combined tests 4 to 6 weeks apart being negative. Those birds then can be placed back in the negative group. Whenever a bird shows

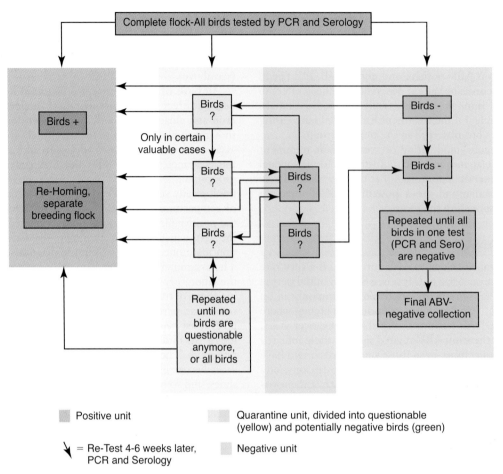

FIGURE 2-4 Suggested diagnostic workup plan to clear a flock from avian bornavirus (ABV) infection. The large box represents the epidemiologic units (populations), which should be clearly separated and treated as independent populations. The smaller boxes represent the group of birds which demonstrated the same results (positive, questionable, negative). Each arrow represents a retest 4 to 6 weeks later of *all* birds in that group at the same time. It is important that all birds within these groups are sampled on the same day and that always polymerase chain reaction (PCR) and serology are performed on an individual bird. First, the complete flock is tested, and three major groups are established (positive, questionable, and negative). A retest 4 to 6 weeks later places additional birds from the negative group into the positive and questionable groups and from the questionable group to the positive group and establishes a potentially negative group within the quarantine section. The negative group is only ultimately considered ABV-negative if ALL birds in that group are tested at the same time and are found to be negative in two consecutive tests. Questionable birds within the questionable groups are only placed in the negative group after two negative tests but are housed separately within the isolation area from the others after their first negative test result. Birds that are retested questionable (very rare; see Figure 2-3) should be considered positive for the purpose of clearing a flock of ABV; however, in very rare or valuable species, the risk might be taken to keep them in quarantine in the questionable group. However, should those birds test questionable again, they should definitely be considered positive. The isolation population is tested as long as all the birds are assigned to one of the other groups (positive or negative) or the owner decides that the remaining birds here should not be retested, and at that time, all remaining birds in isolation will be assigned to the positive group. Once a bird is assigned to the positive group, it will remain here.

up positive in one of those groups, the risk remains that virus was transferred from this bird to another, so the complete group should be retested. As stated above, a "test" means both direct (e.g., PCR) and indirect (serology) investigation (see Figure 2-4). Using this method, flocks were successfully cleared of ABV, with an observation period of approximately 3 years after exclusion of the last ABV-positive bird. This method was also utilized and effective in a flock of Spix's macaws. After separation of ABV-positive birds and strict hygiene measures, no further infections of previously negative birds were recorded over an observation period of 2 years in that flock.[118]

To keep a flock negative, strict measures must be applied to not include new birds in the flock. Only quarantined birds (at least 3 months or, even better, 6 months) that are repeatedly tested, as described above, and are negative should be included. Additionally, the flock should be retested on a regular schedule (yearly, biannually) to ensure the negative status. Also, the acceptance of other bird owners as visitors should be limited and shoe covers and coats should be supplied to them before entering the flock. This also will be beneficial to prevent various other infectious diseases.

As stated above, positive birds might still be used as breeding birds as vertical transmission of ABV seems to be rare, if occurring at all. Examination of eggs from ABV-positive parents has demonstrated that ABV-negative eggs are regularly found. Therefore eggs of positive parents should be taken away and the shell disinfected. It was shown that the shells of cockatiel eggs were effectively disinfected from ABV-RNA after cleaning with 3% hydrogen peroxide.[119] Following disinfection, those eggs should be artificially incubated, and the chicks should hatch separately from each other. Those chicks should then be kept singly housed, hand raised, and tested repeatedly using paired serology and PCR methods. In newly hatched chicks of small species, blood sampling for serology might not be possible, and only in this rare event PCR test for ABV-RNA detection by crop and cloacal swab should be used. It should be kept in mind that an anti-ABV-antibody titer in chicks could represent maternal antibodies transferred through the egg, as previously described.[101] This means that those birds should be retested 4, 6, and 8 weeks after hatch to see if the titer decreases, which is the case with maternal antibodies. If this is not the case and/or ABV-genome is detected, the birds are treated as positive. Chicks repeatedly testing negative can be grouped to avoid human imprints or can be transferred to ABV-negative foster parents. The last seems only to be possible in parrots when the birds are proven negative early enough for this procedure to be accepted by the parents. Transfer of newly hatched chicks to ABV-negative foster parents can be considered, and those chicks can be regularly tested there, although this maneuver poses a risk of the foster parents being infected. This is usually only done in setups where very valuable birds are bred and less valuable pairs are established as negative foster parents.

ABV-positive birds may remain clinically healthy for years. Therefore there may be a demand to rehome those birds as pets when breeders want to exclude them from their flocks. More and more owners also are starting to test their birds for ABV to try to determine their ABV status. This is particularly done if single birds are planned to be paired, even if breeding is not intended. Owners of ABV-negative birds usually request that the potential partner birds also be ABV negative. Conversely, owners of ABV-positive birds might plan to accept ABV-positive partners. Therefore rehoming of ABV-positive birds from flocks that are seeking to become ABV free is possible. Basically, this is a way that may be considered by the supervising veterinarian, if the right information about what is involved is relayed to the owner of the new home to which these birds are being transferred. However, it should be mentioned that ABV-positive birds might potentially carry different ABV genotypes. As a previous study has demonstrated, the infection of ABV-4-positive birds with ABV-2[61] triggered clinical disease; therefore, it

might be recommended that the genotype be evaluated first before paring those birds. On the other hand, it remains unclear at present if this observation and the potential different pathogenicity observed is really related to the genotype itself or to the single strain involved.[98] Compared with genotyping, strain differentiation within one genotype is very difficult, and therefore matching of the different ABV strains carried by potential partners is a task that can derail the plan to pair ABV-positive birds. The risk of triggering a clinical disease by pairing two ABV-positive birds remains, for practical extents and purposes, as anyway every ABV-positive bird carries the risk of getting a clinical disease at any time. This recommendation may be abandoned, changed, or supported when the factors triggering clinical disease are better understood.

VACCINATION

Whenever a novel pathogen is discovered as a cause of an important disease, the demand to produce a vaccine as a prophylactic measure and to protect the birds arises. In the case of ABV, this seems to be a very difficult task. As described above, high anti-ABV-antibody titers are detected in clinically diseased birds, and in many cases, there seem to be a correlation between the increase of the titer and onset of clinical symptoms. Therefore it is fair to state that the antibodies that have been detected so far specifically against ABV are not protective.[87] It seems also likely that the pathogenesis of the symptoms caused by ABV are immune mediated and that ABV has developed mechanisms to escape the recognition of the immune system.[94] All these facts do not make steps toward a vaccine production very promising. To the contrary, it might even be that vaccine could in some circumstances induce the clinical disease or at least increase the severity of clinical signs.[72] However, when the pathogenesis and the details of the host immune response and the nature of different anti-ABV-specific antibodies are better understood, the window for the development of specific vaccines might open, especially based on recombinant vaccines.

TAKE-HOME MESSAGE

Avian bornavirus has clearly been identified as the causative agent of PDD and other clinical symptoms such as CNS signs or sudden death. Despite being commonly observed in other avian taxonomic groups, its main clinical importance is seen in psittacines. So far, the triggering factors causing clinical disease out of an ABV infection are unknown, and the pathogenesis of the infection is poorly understood. However, for the clinician, it is important to know that ABV is widely distributed. The means of transmission or the circumstances under which the virus is successfully transmitted between birds are not completely understood, but viral transmission overall does not seem to be easily reproduced. Therefore, psittacine flocks can be managed to clear the virus from the flocks, which is possible by regular testing of birds using direct virus demonstration (e.g., PCR) and indirect (serologic) testing. Positive birds need to be separated from negative birds, and as long as they are clinically healthy, those positive birds should not be euthanized. In summary, ABV is a very important viral infection with a large impact, especially in psittacine management, but it seems to be controllable.

REFERENCES

1. Ridgway RA, Gallerstein GA: Proventricular dilatation in psittacines. In: *Proceedings of the Annual Conference of the Association of Avian Veterinarians*, 1983, pp 228–230.

2. Graham DL: An update on selected pet bird virus infections. In: Groskin R, editor: *Proceedings of the Annual Conference of the Association of Avian Veterinarians*, 1954, pp 267–280.

3. Busche RKF, Weingarten M: Zur Pathologie des macaw wasting-syndrome, Verhandlungsbericht 27. Symposium über Erkrankungen der Zootiere, St. Vincent/Toronto, 1985.

4. Clark FD: Proventricular dilatation syndrome in large psittacine birds, *Avian Dis* 28(3):813–815, 1984.

5. Hughes PE: The pathology of myenteric ganglioneuritis, psittacine encephalomyelitis, proventricular dilatation of psittacines, and macaw wasting syndrome. In: *Proceedings of the 33rd Western Poultry Disease Conference*, 1984, pp 85–87.

6. Graham DL: Wasting/proventricular dilatation disease: a pathologist's view. In: *Proceedings of the Annual Conference of the Association of Avian Veterinarians*, 1991, pp 43–44.

7. Grimm F: Der klinische Fall. *Tierärztliche Praxis* 19(21): 111–112, 1991.

8. Woerpel RJ, Rosskopf WJ, Hugues E: Proventricular dilatation and wasting syndrome: myenteric ganglioneuritis and encephalomyelitis of psittacines: an update. In: Groskin R, editor: *Proceedings of the Annual Conference of the Association of Avian Veterinarians*, 1984, pp 25–28.

9. Gregory CR, Latimer KS, Niagro FD, et al: A review of proventricular dilatation syndrome, *J Avian Med Surg* 8:69–75, 1994.

10. Daoust PY, Julian RJ, Yason CV, et al: Proventricular impaction associated with nonsuppurative encephalomyelitis and ganglioneuritis in two Canada geese. *J Wildlife Dis* 27(3):513–517, 1991.

11. Gregory CR: Proventricular dilatation disease. In: Ritchie BW, editor: *Avian viruses: function and control*, Lake Worth, FL, 1997, Wingers, pp 439–448.

12. Weissenböck H, Sekulin K, Bakonyi T, et al: Novel avian bornavirus in a nonpsittacine species (Canary; *Serinus canaria*) with enteric ganglioneuritis and encephalitis, *J Virol* 83(21):11367–11371, 2009.

13. Dahlhausen B, Aldred S: Resolution of clinical proventricular dilatation disease by cyclooxygenase 2 inhibition, *Proc Annu Conf Assoc Avian Vet* 9–12, 2002.

14. Grund CH, Ritter H: *Retrospektive feingewebliche Untersuchung von Psittaziden mit der Verdachtsdiagnose Neuropathische Magendilatation.* 14. Tagung über Vogelkrankheiten, München, 2004.

15. Lierz M: Proventricular dilatation disease. In: Harcourt-Brown N, Chitty J, editors: *BSAVA manual of psittacine birds*, Gloucester, U.K., 2005, British Small Animal Veterinary Association, pp 161–163.

16. Shivaprasad HL, Barr BC, Woods LW, et al: *Spectrum of Lesions (Pathology) of Proventricular Dilatation Syndrome Conference of the Association of Avian Veterinarians*, Philadelphia, Pennsylvania, 1995, Association of Avian Veterinarians.

17. Woerpel RW, Rosskopf WJ: *Clinical and pathologic features of macaw wasting disease*, 33rd Western Poultry Disease Conference, Davis, CA, 1984.

18. Vice CA: Myocarditis as a component of psittacine proventricular dilatation syndrome in a Patagonian conure, *Avian Dis* 36(4):1117–1119, 1992.

19. Lublin A, Mechani S, Farnoushi Y, et al: An outbreak of proventricular dilatation disease in psittacine breeding farm in Israel, *Israel J Vet Med* 61(1):16–18, 2006.

20. Berhane Y, Smith D-A, Newman S, et al: Peripheral neuritis in psittacine birds with proventricular dilatation disease, *Avian Pathol* 30(5):563–570, 2001.

21. Turner R: Macaw fading or wasting syndrome. 33rd Western Poultry Disease Conference, Davis, CA, 1984.

22. Phalen DN: An outbreak of proventricular dilatation syndrome (PPDS) in a private collection of birds and an atypical form of PPDS in a nanday conure. Conference of the Association of Avian Veterinarians, Miami, FL, 1986.

23. Mannl A, Gerlach H, Leipold R: Neuropathic gastric dilatation in psittaciformes, *Avian Dis* 31(1):214–221, 1987.

24. Steinmetz A, Pees M, Schmidt V, et al: Blindness as a sign of proventricular dilatation disease in a grey parrot (*Psittacus erithacus erithacus*), *J Sm Anim Pract* 49(12):660–662, 2008.

25. Boutette JB, Taylor M: Proventricular dilatation disease: a review of research, literature, species differences, diagnostics, prognosis, and treatment, Conference of the Association of Avian Veterinarians, New Orleans, LA, 2004.

26. Suedmeyer WK: Diagnosis and clinical progression of three cases of proventricular dilatation syndrome, *J Assoc Avian Vet* 6(3):159–163, 1992.

27. Beaufrère H, Nevarez J, Taylor WM, et al: Fluoroscopic study of the normal gastrointestinal motility and measurements in the Hispaniolan Amazon parrot (*Amazona ventralis*), *Vet Radiol Ultrasound* 51(4):441–446, 2010.

28. Doolen M: Crop biopsy—a low risk diagnosis for neuropathic gastric dilatation. Conference of the Association of Avian Veterinarians, Reno, NV, 1994.

29. Gregory CR, Latimer K, Campagnoli R, et al: Histologic evaluation of the crop for diagnosis of proventricular dilatation syndrome in psittacine birds, *J Vet Diagn Invest* 8(1):76–80, 1996.

30. Gough RE, Drury SE, Harcourt-Brown NA, et al: Virus like particles associated with macaw wasting disease, *Vet Rec* 139(1):24, 1996.

31. Gregory CRR, Latimer KS, SteffensWL, et al: Experimental transmission of psittacine proventricluar dilatation disease (PDD) and preliminary characterization of a virus recovered from birds with naturally occurring and experimentally induced PDD. Proceedings of International Virtual Conferences in Veterinary Medicine: diseases of psittacine birds, http://www.worldcat.org/title/proceedings-of-international-virtual-conferences-in-veterinary-medicine-diseases-of-psittacine-birds-may-15-june-30-1998/oclc/434494339

32. Gregory CR, Latimer KS, Niagro FD, et al: Investigations of eastern equine encephalomyelitis virus as the causative agent of psittacine proventricular dilatation syndrome, *J Avian Med Surg* 11(3):187–193, 1997.

33. Grund CH, Werner O, Gelderblom HR, et al: Avian paramyxovirus serotype 1 isolates from the spinal cord of parrots display a very low virulence, *J Vet Med B Infect Dis Vet Public Health* 49(9):445–451, 2002.

34. Gough RE, Drury SE, Culver F, et al: Isolation of a coronavirus from a green-cheeked Amazon parrot (*Amazon viridigenalis Cassin*), *Avian Pathol* 35(2):122–126, 2006.

35. Honkavuori KS, Shivaprasad HL, Williams BL, et al: Novel borna virus in psittacine birds with proventricular dilatation disease, *Emerg Infect Dis* 14(12):1883-1886, 2008.

36. Kistler AL, Gancz A, Cubb S, et al: Recovery of divergent avian bornaviruses from cases of proventricular dilatation disease: identification of a candidate etiologic agent, *Virol J* 5(1):88, 2008.

37. Rinder M, Ackermann A, Kempf H, et al: Broad tissue and cell tropism of avian bornavirus in parrots with proventricular dilatation disease, *J Virol* 83:5401–5407, 2009.

38. Kuhn JH, Duerwald R, Bao Y, et al: Taxonomic reorganization of the family Bornaviridae, *Arch Virol* 150(2):621–632, 2015.

39. Briese T, Schneemann A, Lewis AJ, et al: Genomic organization of Borna disease virus, *Proc Nat Acad Sci U S A* 91(10):4362–4366, 1994.

40. Cubitt B, Oldstone C, De La Torre JC: Sequence and genome organization of Borna disease virus, *J Virol* 68(3):1382–1396, 1994.

41. De La Torre JC: Molecular biology of borna disease virus: prototype of a new group of animal viruses, *J Virol* 68(12):7669–7675, 1994.

42. Schneemann A, Schneider PA, Lamb RA, et al: The remarkable coding strategy of borna disease virus: a new member of the nonsegmented negative strand RNA viruses, *Virology* 210(1):1–8, 1995.

43. Zwick W, Seifried O, Witte J: Experimentelle Untersuchungen über die seuchenhafte Gehirn–und Rückenmarksentzündung der Pferde (*Bornasche Kranheit*), *Z Inf Krkh Haustiere* 30:42–136, 1927.

44. Ludwig H, Becht H, Groh L: Borna disease (BD), a slow virus infection biological properties of the virus, *Med Microbiol Immunol* 158:275–289, 1973.

45. Nowotny N, Kolodziejek J, Jehle CO, et al: Isolation and characterization of a new subtype of Borna disease virus, *J Virol* 74(12):5655–5658, 2000.

46. Schwemmle M, Carbone KM, Tomonaga K, et al: *Virus taxonomy*, St. Louis, MO, 2012, Elsevier.

46a. http://ecdc.europa.eu/en/press/news/_layouts/forms/News_DispForm.aspx?List=8db7286c-fe2d-476c-9133-18ff4cb1b568&ID=1178

47. Weissenböck H, Bakonyi T, Sekulin K, et al: Avian bornaviruses in psittacine birds from Europe and Australia with proventricular dilatation disease, *Emerg Infect Dis* 15(9):1453–1459, 2009.

48. Rubbenstroth D, Rinder M, Kaspers B, et al: Efficient isolation of avian bornaviruses (ABV) from naturally infected psittacine birds and identification of a new ABV genotype from a salmon-crested cockatoo *(Cacatua moluccensis)*, *Vet Microbiol* 161(1-2):36-42, 2012.

49. Philadelpho NA, Rubbenstroth D, Guimaraes MB, et al: Survey of bornavirus in pet psittacines in Brazil reveals a novel parrot bornavirus, *Vet Microbiol* 174:584–590, 2014.

50. Delnatte P, Berkvens C, Kummrow M, et al: New genotype of avian bornavirus in wild geese and trumpeter swans in Canada, *Vet Rec* 169(4):108, 2011.

51. Payne S, Shivaprasad HL, Mirhosseini N, et al: Unusual and severe lesions of proventricular dilatation disease in cockatiels *(Nymphicus hollandicus)* acting as healthy carriers of avian bornavirus (ABV) and subsequently infected with a virulent strain of ABV, *Avian Pathol* 40(1):15–22, 2011.

52. Rubbenstroth D, Rinder M, Stein M, et al: Avian bornaviruses are widely distributed in canary birds *(Serinus canaria f. domestica)*, *Vet Microbiol* 165(3-4):287–295, 2013.

53. Rubbenstroth D, Schmidt V, Rinder M, et al: Discovery of a new avian bornavirus genotype in estrildid finches (Estrildidae) in Germany, *Vet Microbiol* 168(2-4):318–323, 2014.

54. Guo J, Shivaprasad HL, Rech RR, et al: Characterization of a new genotype of avian bornavirus from wild ducks, *Virol J* 19:11(1):197, 2014.

55. Cui J, Zhao W, Huang Z, et al: Low frequency of paleoviral infiltration across the avian phylogeny, *Genome Biol* 15(12):539, 2014.

56. He M, An TZ, Teng CB: Evolution of mammalian and avian bornaviruses, *Mol Phylogenet Evol* 79:385–391, 2014.

57. Raghav R, Taylor M, DeLay J, et al: Avian bornavirus is present in many tissues of psittacine birds with histopathologic evidence of proventricular dilatation disease, *J Vet Diagn Invest* 22:495–508, 2010.

58. Weissenböck H, Fragner K, Nedorost N, et al: Localization of avian bornavirus RNA by in situ hybridization in tissues of psittacine birds with proventricular dilatation disease, *Vet Microbiol* 145:9–16, 2010.

59. Gancz AY, Kistler AL, Greninger AL, et al: Experimental induction of proventricular dilatation disease in cockatiels *(Nymphicus hollandicus)* inoculated with brain homogenates containing avian bornavirus 4, *Virol J* 6:100, 2009.

60. Gray P, Hoppes S, Suchodolski P, et al: Use of avian bornavirus isolates to induce proventricular dilatation disease in conures, *Emerg Infect Dis* 16(3):473–479, 2010.

61. Mirhosseini N, Gray PL, Hoppes S, et al: Proventricular dilatation disease in cockatiels *(Nymphicus hollandicus)* after infection with a genotype 2 avian bornavirus, *J Avian Med Surg* 25(3):199–204, 2011.

62. Piepenbring AK, Enderlein D, Herzog S, et al: Pathogenesis of avian bornavirus in experimentally infected cockatiels, *Emerg Infect Dis* 18(2):234–241, 2012.

63. Lierz M, Hafez HM, Honkavuori KS, et al: Anatomical distribution of avian bornavirus in parrots, its occurrence in clinically healthy birds and ABV-antibody detection, *Avian Pathol* 38(6):491–496, 2009.

64. Heffels-Redmann U, Enderlein D, Herzog S, et al: Occurrence of avian bornavirus infection in captive psittacines in various European countries and its association with proventricular dilatation disease, *Avian Pathol* 40(4):419–426, 2011.

65. Encinas-Nagel N, Enderlein D, Piepenbring A, et al: Avian Bornavirus in free-ranging psittacine birds, Brazil, *Emerg Infect Dis* 20(12):2103–2106, 2014.

66. Donatti RV, Resende M, Ferreira, FC, et al: Fatal proventricular dilatation disease in captive native psittacines in Brazil, *Avian Dis* 58(1):187–193, 2014.

67. Ogawa H, Sanada Y, Sanada N, et al: Proventricular dilatation disease associated with avian bornavirus infection in a citron-crested cockatoo that was born and hand-reared in Japan, *J Vet Med Sci* 73:837–840, 2011.

68. Last RD, Weissenböck H, Nedorost N, et al: Avian bornavirus genotype 4 recovered from naturally infected psittacine birds with proventricular dilatation disease in South Africa, *J S Afr Vet Assoc* 83(1):Art. #938, 2012.

69. Delnatte P, Ojkic D, Delay J, et al: Pathology and diagnosis of avian bornavirus in Canada geese *(Branta canadensis)*, trumpeter swans *(Cygnus buccinator)* and mute swans *(Cygnus olor)* in Canada: a retrospective study, *Avian Pathol* 42(2):114–128, 2013.

70. Sassa Y, Horie M, Fujino K, et al: Molecular epidemiology of avian bornavirus from pet birds in Japan, *Virus Genes* 47(1):173–177, 2013.

71. Delnatte P, Nagy E, Ojkic D, et al: Avian bornavirus in free-ranging waterfowl: prevalence of antibodies and cloacal shedding of viral RNA, *J Wild Dis* 50(3):512–523, 2014.

72. Hoppes S, Gray PL, Payne S, et al: The isolation, pathogenesis, diagnosis, transmission, and control of avian bornavirus and proventricular dilatation disease, *Vet Clin North Am Exot Anim Pract* 13(3):495–508, 2010.

73. Staeheli P, Rinder M, Kaspers B: Avian bornavirus associated with fatal disease in psittacine birds, *J Virol* 84(13):6269–6275, 2010.

74. Heatley JJ, Villalobos AR: Avian bornavirus in the urine of infected birds, *Vet Med Res Rep* 3:19–23, 2012.

75. Enderlein DH, Herden C, Neumann D, et al: *Antikörper und Genomnachweis in PDD-positiven*, Vögeln. 1,DVG-Tagung über Vogel- und Reptilienkrankheiten, Leipzig, Germany, 2009.

76. Kistler AL, Smith JM, Greninger AL, et al: Analysis of naturally occurring avian bornavirus infection and transmission during an outbreak of proventricular dilatation disease among captive psittacine birds, *J Virol* 84(4):2176–2179, 2010.

77. Lierz M, Heckmann J, Piepenbring A, et al: *Investigations into different infection routes of avian bornavirus in psittacine birds*, Proceedings of the Annual AAV-Conference, New Orleans, LA, pp 19–20.

78. Heckmann J, Enderlein D, Piepenbring A, et al: Investigations on different infection routes of avian Bornavirus infection in cockatiels. Proceedings of the 2nd ICARE conference, Paris, France, 2015, p 258.

79. Rinder M, Högemann C, Hufen H, et al: Experimentelle Infektion von Kongo-Graupapageien (Psittacus erithacus erithacus) mit aviären Bornaviren: Klinische und pathologische Veränderungen. 1. Jahrestagung der DVG-Fachgruppe "Zier-, Zoo- und Wildvögel, Reptilien und Amphibien", München, 2014.

80. Sauder C, Staeheli P: Rat model of Borna disease virus transmission: epidemiological implications, *J Virol* 77:12886–12890, 2003.

81. Delnatte P: Avian bornavirus infection in waterfowl [Thesis], Guelph, Ontario, 2013, University of Guelph.

82. Lierz M, Piepenbring A, Herden C, et al:. Vertical transmission of avian bornavirus in psittacines, *Emerg Infect Dis* 17(12):2390–2391, 2011.

83. Monaco E, Hoppes S, Guo J, et al: The detection of avian bornavirus within psittacine eggs, *J Avian Med Surg* 26(3):144–148, 2012.

84. Kerski A, de Kloet AH, de Kloet SR: Vertical transmission of avian bornavirus in psittaciformes: avian bornavirus RNA and anti-avian bornavirus antibodies in eggs, embryos, and hatchlings obtained from infected Sun Conures *(Aratinga solstitialis)*, *Avian Dis* 56:471–478, 2012.

84a. Wust E, Malberg S, Enderlein D, et al: Experimental infection of cockatiel (*Nymphycus hollandicus*) eggs with avian ornavirus, *Proc ICARE* 258, 2015.

85. De Kloet SR, Dorrestein GM: Presence of avian bornavirus RNA and anti-avian bornavirus antibodies in apparently healthy macaws, *Avian Dis* 53(4):568–573, 2009.

86. Heffels-Redmann U, Enderlein D, Herzog S, et al: Follow-up investigations on different courses of natural avian bornavirus infections in psittacines, *Avian Dis* 56(1):153–159, 2012.

87. Lierz M, Herden C, Herzog S, et al: [Proventricular dilatation disease and Avian Bornavirus as a possible cause], *Tierarztl Prax Ausg K Kleintiere Heimtiere* 38(2):87–94, 2010.

88. Enderlein DH, Kaleta EF, Müller H, et al: Neue Erkenntnisse zur Rolle des aviären Bornavirus bei der Drüsenmagenerweiterung der Psittaziden. 16. DVG-Tagung über Vogelkrankheiten, München, München, Germany, 2010.

89. Narayan O, Herzog S, Frese K, et al: Pathogenesis of borna disease in rats: immune-mediated viral ophthalmoencephalopathy causing blindness and behavioral abnormalities, *J Infect Dis* 148(2):305–315, 1983.

90. Rott R, Herzog S, Richt J, et al: Immune-mediated pathogenesis of borna disease, *Zentralbl Bakteriol Mikrobiol Hyg A* 270(1–2):295–301, 1988.

91. Stitz L, Soeder D, Deschl U, et al: Inhibition of immune-mediated encephalitis in persistently borna disease virus-infected rats, *J Immunol* 143:4250–4256, 1989.

92. Hallensleben W, Schwemmle M, Hausmann J, et al: Borna disease virus-induced neurological disorder in mice: infection of neonates results in immunopathology, *J Virol* 72:4379–4386, 1998.

93. Matsumoto Y, Hayashi Y, Omori H, et al: Bornavirus closely associates and segregates with host chromosomes to ensure persistent intranuclear infection, *Cell Host Microbe* 11:492–503, 2012.

94. Reuter A, Ackermann A, Kothlow S, et al: Avian bornaviruses escape recognition by the innate immune system, *Viruses* 2:927–938, 2010.

95. Wensman JJ, Munir M, Thaduri S, et al: The X protein of bornaviruses interfere with type I interferon signaling, *J Gen Virol* 94:263–269, 2013.

96. Rossi G, Crosta L, Pesaro S: Parrot proventricular dilation disease, *Vet Rec* 163:310, 2008.

97. Rossi G, Enderlein D, Herzog S, et al: Comparison of anti-ganglioside antibodies and anti-ABV antibodies in psittacines, 11th European AAV Conference 2011, Madrid, Spain.

98. Lierz M, Piepenbring A, Heffels-Redmann U, et al: Experimental infection of cockatiels with different avian bornavirus genotypes. In: Bergman E, editor: *Proceedings of the 33rd Annual Conference of the Association of Avian Veterinarians*, Louisville, KY, Association of Avian Veterinarians, pp 9–10.

99. Carbone KM, Duchala CS, Griffin JW, et al: Pathogenesis of borna disease in rats: evidence that intra-axonal spread is the major route for virus dissemination and the determinant for disease incubation, *J Virol* 61:3431–3440, 1987.

100. Gancz AY, Clubb S, Shivaprasad HL: Advanced diagnostic approaches and current management of proventricular dilatation disease, *Vet Clin North Am Exot Anim Pract* 13(3):471–494, 2010.

101. De Kloet AH, Kerski A, De Kloet SR: Diagnosis of avian bornavirus infection in psittaciformes by serum antibody detection and reverse transcription polymerase chain reaction assay using feather calami, *J Vet Diagn Invest* 23(3):421–429, 2011.

102. Wünschmann A, Honkavuori K, Briese T, et al: Antigen tissue distribution of avian bornavirus (ABV) in psittacine birds with natural spontaneous proventricular dilatation disease and ABV genotype 1 infection, *J Vet Diagn Invest* 23:716–726, 2011.

103. Rebmeyer S, Herzog S, Enderlein D, et al: Distribution patterns of avian bornavirus in psittacine birds suffering from proventricular dilatation disease. In: *Proceedings of the Annual Conference of the European College of Veterinary Pathology*, 2010, pp 324.

104. Villanueva I, Gray P, Mirhosseini N, et al: The diagnosis of proventricular dilatation disease: use of a Western blot assay to detect antibodies against avian borna virus, *Vet Microbiol* 143(2-4):196–201, 2010.

105. Herzog S, Enderlein D, Heffels-Redmann U, et al: Indirect immunofluorescence assay for intra vitam diagnosis of avian bornavirus infection in psittacine birds, *J Clin Microbiol* 48(6):2282–2284, 2010.

106. Berhane Y: Studies on the etiology and pathology of proventricular dilatation disease [DVSc thesis], Guelph, Ontario, 2004, University of Guelph.

107. Fluck A, Enderlein D, Piepenbring A, et al: Avian bornavirus infection in psittacine birds with neurological signs and feather plucking. In: Proceedings of the 1st ICARE Conference, Wiesbaden, Germany, 2013.

108. Dorrestein GM, Honkavuori KS, Briese T, et al.; Overview of the role and diagnosis of avian bornavirus related to PDD in psittacines. In: Proceedings of the 7th International Congress on Wild and Exotic Animals, Paris, France, 2010.

109. Rinder M, Adrian K, Kaspers B, et al: Development of various diagnostic tests for avian bornavirus in psittacine birds. In: Samour J, editor: *Proceedings of the 11th European Association of Avian Veterinarians Conference*, 2011, pp 185–186.

110. De Kloet SR, Dorrestein GM: Presence of avian bornavirus RNA and antiavian bornavirus antibodies in apparently healthy macaws, *Avian Dis* 53:568–573, 2009.

111. McHugh JM, Kloet SR: Discrepancy in the diagnosis of avian bornavirus infection of psittacines by protein analysis of feather calami and enzyme-linked immunosorbent assay of plasma antibodies, *J Vet Diagn Invest* 27(2):150–158, 2015.

112. Dorrestein GM: Personal communication, New Orleans, LA, 2014.

113. Horie M, Ueda K, Ueda A, et al: Detection of avian bornavirus 5 RNA in *Eclectus roratus* with feather picking disorder, *Microbiol Immunol* 56:346–349, 2012.

114. Clubb SL: Proventricular dilation disease. In: Proceedings of the 81st Western Veterinary Conference, 2009, pp 707–711.

115. Hoppes S, Tizard I, Shivaprasad HL, et al: Treatment of avian bornavirus-infected cockatiels (*Nymphicus hollandicus*) with oral meloxicam and cyclosporine. In: Bergman E, editor: *Proceedings of the 33rd Annual Conference of the Association of Avian Veterinarians*, Louisville, KY, 2012, Association of Avian Veterinarians, p 27.

116. Gancz A, Elbaz D, Farnoushi Y, et al:. Clinical recovery from proventricular dilatation disease following treatment with cyclosporine-a in an African grey parrot (*Psittacus erithacus*). 17. DVG-Tagung über Vogelkrankheiten, Munich, Germany, 2012.

117. Rossi G, Crosta L, Ceccherelli R, et al: PDD: our point of view after 7 years of research. In: Bergman E, editor: *Proceedings of the 33rd Annual Conference of the Association of Avian Veterinarians*, Louisville, KY, 2012, Association of Avian Veterinarians, pp 79.

118. Enderlein DP, Herzog S, Herden C, et al: The situation of ABV in endangered psittacines like the Spix's macaw, 11th European AAV Conference, Madrid, Spain, 2011.

119. Wuest E, Malberg S, Herzog S, et al: Experimental infection of cockatiel eggs (*Nymphicus hollandicus*) with avian bornavirus. Proceedings of the 2nd ICARE Conference, Paris, France, 2015.

PSITTACID HERPESVIRUSES AND ASSOCIATED DISEASES

David Phalen

PSITTACID HERPESVIRUS 1

History and Description of the Virus

Psittacid herpesvirus 1 (PsHV-1) belongs to the subfamily (*Alphaherpesvirinae*) and genus (*Iltovirus*). It has four major genotypes and at least three serotypes (Table 2-2 and Table 2-3).[1] It is the cause of Pacheco disease, which is an acute rapidly fatal disease of parrots and, rarely, passerine species, as well as mucosal papillomas and associated neoplasms of parrots.[1,2]

Outbreaks of Pacheco disease were first recognized in Brazil in the late 1920s in captive parrots and were not seen again until the late 1970s when large numbers of parrots were exported from South America into Europe and North America.[1,2] As of this time, the frequency of outbreaks has diminished to the point where they are relatively rare, but they still occur in mixed collections of parrots originating from multiple sources. The prevalence of mucosal papillomatosis in parrots has also diminished, but to a lesser extent.

Species Affected and Geographic Distribution

Pacheco disease occurs in parrots of either sex and of any age, originating from all of their distributions, so potentially all species are susceptible to infection with PsHV-1 and the development of disease (see Table 2-3).[3] There is no age or sex predilection. Mucosal papillomas have the greatest prevalence in Amazon parrots (*Amazona* spp.), macaws (*Ara* spp.), Hawk-headed parrots (*Deroptyus accipitrinus*), and conures (*Aratinga* spp.) but have also been infrequently reported in other species. Mucosal papillomas and related neoplasms are found in birds of both sexes. They can also occur in parrots as young as 6 months of age. Pacheco disease outbreaks and or mucosal papillomatosis have been documented in North America, Europe, the Middle East, Japan, New Zealand (in quarantine birds), and Australia.[2,4]

Clinical Manifestations

Pacheco disease

Pacheco disease should be suspected when a parrot in a collection dies unexpectedly and when multiple deaths occur over a short period. Signs are rare and generally nonspecific; however, some birds will have biliverdin-stained (yellow or green) urates immediately prior to death.[2]

Mucosal papillomatosis

Mucosal papillomas can occur most frequently in the cloaca and the oral cavity. Signs may be lacking and the lesions only observed on physical examination. When the lesions are advanced, birds may exhibit upper respiratory signs, strain to defecate, and have blood in their droppings, and the papillomatous lesions from the cloaca may protrude. A more generalized form of the disease can also occur where the papillomatous lesions extend into the esophagus, crop, and, rarely, to the level of the proventriculus and ventriculus. These birds may experience a chronic wasting disease. Regurgitation is uncommon but may occur. Mucosal papillomas are typically raised and pink and have a cauliflower-like surface. More diffuse lesions that involve the entire cloaca may have a cobblestone appearance. Oral papillomatous lesions are most commonly found along the margins of the choanae and at the base of the tongue. They can be very subtle, resulting in an asymmetric thickening of the choana or a blunting of the papillae. In many instances, the first indication of oral mucosal papillomas is a loss of pigment at the site of the lesion. Lesions can wax and wane, disappear completely, or become progressive.[2,4,5]

Bile duct and pancreatic duct carcinomas are fairly common sequelae to mucosal papillomatosis. Birds with these lesions do not show evidence of disease until the lesions are severe. When they do show signs, they are typically signs of chronic liver disease, including weight loss, an overgrown beak, and poor feather quality. Bile and pancreatic duct carcinomas develop in the months and years following the onset of mucosal papillomas.[5]

TABLE 2-2

Psittacid Herpesviruses and Their Associated Diseases

Virus	Pacheco Disease	Respiratory Disease	Mucosal Papillomas
Psittacid herpesvirus 1	Yes	No	Yes
Psittacid herpesvirus 2	No	No	Grey parrots only
Psittacid herpesvirus 3	No	Yes	No

TABLE 2-3

Serotype and Disease Potential for the Four Genotypes of Psittacid Herpesvirus 1

Genotype	Serotype	Pacheco Disease	Mucosal Papillomas	Bile Duct Carcinomas
1	1	Amazons, Australian species	Uncommon	No
2	2	Amazons, Grey parrots	Uncommon	No
3	3	Predominately Amazons, less commonly other species	Very common	Yes
4	1	Most species	No	No

From Tomaszewski EK, Gravendyck M, Kaleta EF, et al: Isolation of psittacid herpesvirus genotype 1 from a superb starling (*Lamprotornis superbus*), *Avian Dis* 48:212–214, 2004.

Diagnosis

Pacheco disease

It is rare that a bird with Pacheco disease survives long enough to have blood collected and tested, and as a result, the diagnosis of Pacheco disease is usually made at necropsy. If a bird survived long enough to be seen by a veterinarian, experimental infections would indicate that they likely have a leukopenia and marked elevations in their plasma aspartate aminotransferase concentrations.[2] The hematologic picture, however, might change if the birds do not die immediately, which is uncommon.

Gross lesions in birds with Pacheco disease are variable. Some birds will only show very subtle changes in the liver that resemble a diffuse lipidosis. Others will have prominent swelling of the liver and spleen. Multifocal areas of discoloration, representing areas of necrosis, and gross evidence of pancreatitis and enteritis are seen less frequently. Most birds will be in good to excellent body condition. Microscopically, hepatic and splenic necroses, varying from moderate to massive, are characteristic lesions. The pattern of necrosis in the liver may appear to be random, but generally the periportal hepatocytes are spared. Pan-nuclear eosinophilic inclusions are generally present in the liver but, in some instances, can be difficult to find; they are often abundant in the spleen. Pancreatic necrosis and necrosis of the intestinal and crop mucosa with intralesional inclusion bodies occur with infection with certain genotypes. There is a single report of a cockatiel with chronic active pancreatitis secondary to PsHV-1 infection. This bird exhibited both endocrine and exocrine pancreatic insufficiency.[2]

Mucosal papillomatosis and associated neoplasms

Mucosal papillomas are diagnosed through careful examination of the oral cavity and eversion of the cloacal mucosa with a lubricated swab (Figure 2-5). Anesthesia may be required to observe subtle mucosal changes. If there are diffuse lesions, crop thickening may be detected with palpa-tion. The gross papillary changes are characteristic, and biopsy is generally not necessary to make a diagnosis. In the author's experience, PCR assays will reveal all of these birds to be positive for PsHV-1, so testing for PsHV-1 is not necessary.[2]

Despite extensive liver involvement, it is rare that the liver of birds with bile duct carcinomas is sufficiently enlarged that the edge of the liver can be palpated. Radiographically, the liver may have rounded margins. Bile duct carcinomas are readily visualized with ultrasonography as multifocal to coalescing hyperechoic regions of the liver that are replacing the adjacent normal areas of the liver. Increases in the γ-glutamyl transferase (GGT) have been reported in birds with bile duct carcinomas. It has been the author's experience that the GGT will increase in older parrots in a range of species, so changes in the GGT are not specific for bile duct carcinomas. Diagnosis can be confirmed by liver biopsy. Pancreatic duct carcinomas are very difficult to diagnose, but ultrasonography may reveal lesions, and biopsy can also lead to antemortem confirmation of diagnosis.[2]

Grossly, mucosal papillomas can be difficult to recognize in the dead bird, but if the animal is fresh, these mucosal papillomas will retain the same characteristics as those seen in the live bird. Microscopically, mucosal papillomas are made up of multiple fimbriae with a variably wide to narrow base. Each fimbria is composed of a fibrovascular core surrounded by a pseudostratified or stratified cuboidal to columnar epithelium. The lesions may be ulcerated. Lymphoplasmacytic infiltrations of the fibrovascular cores occur intermittently.[4]

Bile duct carcinomas are pale tan to gray colored, confluent to slightly raised, and multifocal to coalescing. Only small amounts of normal liver may remain. Similarly, pancreatic duct carcinomas are gray and nodular, and, in some instances, may be coalescing. Neither the bile duct carcinoma nor the pancreatic duct carcinoma metastasizes.[2]

The author has rarely seen cloacal carcinomas (Figure 2-6) in psittacine birds. However, in the three cases that have been seen, all contained PsHV-1 DNA, and all three metastasized to other organs in the body. Whether these tumors were caused by the virus or not is not known.

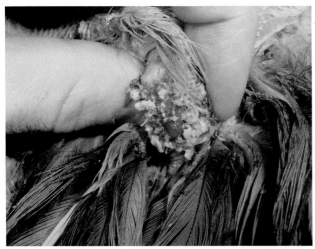

FIGURE 2-5 Everted mucosal papilloma of the cloaca of a blue and gold macaw. Persistent soiling of the mucocutaneous junction around the vent has resulted in infection and ulceration.

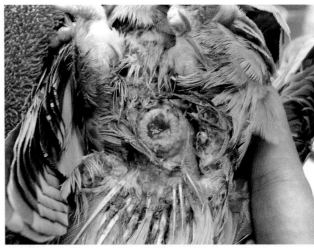

FIGURE 2-6 Cloacal carcinoma in an Amazon parrot.

Treatment

Acyclovir has been used to treat individual birds and entire aviaries during outbreaks of Pacheco disease. Published reports and anecdotal evidence suggest that treatment is highly effective in preventing mortality in these outbreaks. A range of routes of administration and drug dosages have been used. The author has used acyclovir orally by gavage at 80 to 100 milligrams per kilograms (mg/kg) three times a day for 10 days with apparent success. While treated birds may survive, they are not cured of infection and will become carriers of the virus. Carriers and those with overt mucosal papillomas are not impacted by treatment with acyclovir.[2]

Mucosal papillomas should be left alone unless they are clearly causing the bird discomfort or interfering with breathing or defecation. These lesions are rarely static and may spontaneously regress or may worsen. In many cases, they will shrink only to return again in the weeks or months to follow. If surgical intervention is required, the papillary lesions can be debulked with sharp dissection, laser surgery, radiosurgery, and treatment with topical silver nitrate. It is the author's impression that surgical remove of part of the diseased tissue can result in regression of the surrounding lesion in some instances. Repeated surgical intervention can result in cloacal scarring. To prevent cloacal scarring, the author uses sharp dissection to remove the diseased mucosa and sutures the margins. There is minimal evidence of successful treatments for bile duct carcinomas.[2] There is a case report of treatment of a pancreatic duct carcinoma in a green-winged macaw (*Ara chloroptera*) with carboplatin. In that case, the lesions resolved but ultimately returned.[6]

Epizootiology and Preventive Measures

It has been hypothesized that the four genotypes of PsHV-1 have coevolved with some South American species of parrot.[1] Infected birds shed the virus in oral secretions and droppings. Infection is thought to be the result of ingestion of contaminated material. The incubation period is 5 to 7 days. In the adapted host, infection is unlikely to cause disease, and these birds develop lifelong infections and are potential sources for future outbreaks if housed with other parrots that have not been exposed to the virus. When nonadapted parrots are exposed to certain PsHV-1 genotypes, Pacheco disease occurs. Which parrots in an aviary will develop Pacheco disease will depend on the species of the exposed bird and the genotype of the virus, as well as husbandry and other undefined factors.[1] For example, densely housed indoor collections are more prone to outbreaks of Pacheco disease. Many infections are subclinical, and the affected birds become carriers. Subclinically infected birds and those that have survived Pacheco disease are at high risk for developing mucosal papillomas if they are infected with genotype 3 and have a lower risk if infected with genotypes 1 and 2. To date, all birds that developed bile duct and pancreatic duct carcinomas and were tested were found to be infected with genotype 3.[4]

Keeping the birds infected with PsHV-1 out of a virus-free collection can be achieved by performing routine testing. PCR-based assays that can detect all four genotypes of PsHV-1 have been developed. In one study, the virus was consistently found in birds that were repeatedly tested over the course of a year by a PCR assay of combined oral and cloacal swabs. PsHV-1 DNA could also be detected in heparinized blood, but blood samples proved to be less sensitive than mucosal swabs. Serology may also be a useful tool for detecting subclinically infected birds, but sera would have to be tested against all three serotypes.[7]

Vaccines have been developed from PsHV-1 isolates and may prove to be useful tools in high-risk flocks.[2] It is not known, however, if vaccination with one serotype of PsHV-1 will protect against infection with other serotypes. In at least one instance, two different serotypes have been detected in the same bird, which indicates that a polyvalent vaccine may be required to protect against all three serotypes of PsHV-1.[7]

PSITTACID HERPESVIRUS-2

History and Description of the Virus

Psittacid herpesvirus 2 (PsHV-2) is of the genus *Iltovirus* of the subfamily Alphaherpesvirinae. It is most closely related to PsHV-1 but has never been associated with a Pacheco-like disease.[8]

Species Affected and Geographic Distribution

PsHV-2 has only been detected in Congo African Grey parrots (*Psittacus erithacus erithacus*) in the United States and Germany. Infections have been found in both wild-caught and domestically raised birds. In the only extensive survey done, even in mixed aviaries, infection was confined to Grey parrots and was not even detected in the closely related Timneh parrot (*Psittacus timneh*).[8,9] The only other bird known to be infected with PsHV-1 was a blue-and-gold macaw in a collection in the United States.[7] Widespread testing for this virus has not been done, so it is expected that it may have a wider geographic range than is currently known.

Clinical Manifestations

PsHV-2 infections can either be subclinical or result in the development of mucosal and, less commonly, mucocutaneous papillomas of the oral cavity and eye. The papillomas are benign but can be fairly extensive. Differential diagnoses for PsHV-2-induced papillomas include cutaneous papillomas caused by parrot papillomavirus-1 (PePV-1) and other neoplastic diseases of the oral cavity. PePV-1 is rare, causes extensive lesions of the skin of the face, and has only been reported in wild-caught birds.[8,9]

Diagnosis

Gross lesions are characteristic but can be confirmed by biopsy where the characteristic fibropapillomatous lesions will be demonstrated. Virus inclusions have not been reported in these lesions. Primers that detect PsHV-1 DNA can be used in PCR assays to detect PsHV-2 DNA in the papillomatous tissue or combined oral and cloacal swabs from clinically and subclinically infected Congo African Grey parrots.[2]

Treatment

There are no reports of treatment attempts. Surgical removal would be indicated if the lesions were interfering with air flow. Given that these lesions are not thought to be associated with replicating virus, acyclovir will not be effective against them.

Epizootiology and Preventive Measures

Current data suggest that this virus is host-adapted to Grey parrots and entered Europe and the United States by the movement of wild-caught Grey parrots. Twenty percent of aviaries in Germany were found to have infected birds.[9] Individual birds could be screened for infection by using PCR assays of oral and cloacal swabs designed to detect PsHV-2. The sensitivity of this assay is not known.

PSITTACID HERPESVIRUS 3

History and Description of the Virus

For several decades, an uncharacterized herpesvirus that predominately targets the trachea of parrots has been reported to occur sporadically in a range of parrots in North America and Europe. Recent work has shown this virus to belong to the subfamily Alphaherpesvirinae and the genus *Iltovirus*. It has been named psittacid herpesvirus-3 (PsHV-3) and is most closely related to the passerid herpesvirus-1, another respiratory herpesvirus.[10]

Species Affected and Geographic Distribution

PsHV-3 infection has only been confirmed by sequencing of the virus in an outbreak of disease in Bourke's parrots (*Neopsephotus bourkii*) in the United States and in two eclectus parrots (*Eclectus roratus*) in Australia.[10,11] It is likely that PsHV-3 has a more widespread geographic and species range because a similar disease has been described in Amazon parrots (*Amazona* spp.), Indian ring-necked parrots (*Psittacula krameri*), a cockatiel (*Nymphicus hollandicus*), and a princess parrot (*Polytelis alexandrae*) in Europe and Japan and other locations in Australia and the United States.[10]

Clinical Manifestations

The outbreak in the two Bourke's parrots lasted several months. Infected birds coughed, had difficulty breathing, and exhibited ocular and nasal discharge. The birds died within 3 to 7 days after signs were first noticed. Other species of parrots in the collection did not develop the disease.[10] Both eclectus parrots were in poor body condition and appeared to have been ill for some time. Respiratory signs were observed in one of the eclectus parrots, but the majority of the signs exhibited by these birds was nonspecific and may have been the result of concurrent infectious diseases.[11]

Diagnosis

Diagnosis in the live bird

No work has been done on the diagnosis of PsHV-3 in the live bird. It should be considered a potential differential diagnosis in any psittacine bird that is exhibiting signs of tracheal or pulmonary disease, especially if these signs are accompanied by ocular and nasal discharge. Cytology of the conjunctiva and trachea has the potential to detect syncytial cells as well as cells with characteristic eosinophilic intranuclear inclusion bodies. The partial sequence of PsHV-3 is known, and virus-specific primers could be developed for use in a PCR

assay. It is also possible to detect PsHV-3 by using pan-herpesvirus primers.[11]

Postmortem diagnosis

Potential gross lesions include conjunctivitis, tracheitis, and changes in the lungs suggestive of diffuse or locally extensive pneumonia and air sacculitis.[10] One of the eclectus parrots exhibited multiple pale foci in the pancreas caused by pancreatic necrosis. Both eclectus parrots also had concurrent aspergillosis.[11] Microscopically, diagnosis of PsHV-3 infection is presumptively made by detecting syncytial cells containing pan-nuclear eosinophilic inclusion bodies in the bronchi and parabronchi and to a lesser extent in the trachea, conjunctiva, air sac, and respiratory epithelium of the turbinates. Similar lesions were also seen in numerous other tissues, including the spleen, pancreas, inner ear, meninges, kidney, thymus, bursa, and gonads. Lymphoplasmacytic inflammation of varying degrees was often present, and hyperplasia of the respiratory epithelium was a common finding. In contrast to the acute form of the disease caused by PsHV-1, the liver is not a primary target.[10,11] Both eclectus parrots also had severe mycotic bronchopneumonia.[11]

Treatment

The outbreak in the Bourke's parrot collection stopped with the onset of acyclovir treatment. However, multiple other management changes were made at the same time, and whether acyclovir treatment was the reason the outbreak was stopped is not known.[10] Given the apparent success and safety of acyclovir treatment in birds with acute PsHV-1 infections, it would seem reasonable to use acyclovir to treat PsHV-3 infections if an antemortem diagnosis were made.

Epizootiology and Preventive Measures

If this virus behaves like many other avian herpesviruses, then it is likely that it is host adapted and does not cause disease in its host or hosts but does cause a persistent infection. If so, persistently infected birds are likely to intermittently or continuously shed the virus and would be the source of outbreaks when they do occur. It is possible that subclinically infected birds could be detected with PCR-based assays of oral swabs, cloacal swabs, or blood samples.

Both eclectus parrots described here were concurrently infected with the psittacine beak and disease virus (PBFDV).[11] It is therefore likely that these birds were immunosuppressed, which resulted in their *Aspergillus* infections. It is possible that immunosuppression may have also resulted in the PsHV-3 infection causing disease, whereas it would not have in an immune competent bird. Testing of birds with confirmed PsHV-3 infection for PBFDV will be necessary to prove this hypothesis.

REFERENCES

1. Tomaszewski EK, Kaleta EF, Phalen DN: Molecular phylogeny of the psittacid herpesviruses causing Pacheco's disease: correlation of genotype and phenotypic expression, *J Virol* 77:11260–11267, 2003.
2. Phalen DN: Implications of viruses in clinical disorders. In: Harrison GJ, Lightfoot T, editors: *Clinical avian medicine*, Vol 2, Palm Beach, FL, 2008, Spix Publishing, pp 721–746.

3. Tomaszewski EK, Gravendyck M, Kaleta EF, et al: Isolation of psittacid herpesvirus genotype 1 from a superb starling *(Lamprotornis superbus)*, *Avian Dis* 48:212–214, 2004.

4. Styles DK, Tomaszewski EK, Phalen DN: Psittacid herpesviruses associated with mucosal papillomas of neotropical parrots, *Virology* 235:24–35, 2004.

5. Styles DK: Psittacid herpesviruses associated with internal papillomatous disease and other tumors of psittacine birds [dissertation], College Station, TX, 2005, Department of Veterinary Pathology, Texas A&M University. Available from: http://repository.tamu.edu/bitstream/handle/1969.1/2646/etd-tamu-2005B-VTMI-Styles.pdf?sequence=1, 2005 (Accessed July 2014).

6. Speer BL, Eckermann-Ross C: Diagnosis and clinical management of pancreatic duct adenocarcinoma in a green-winged macaw *(Ara chloroptera)*. In: *2001 Proc EAAV ECAMS*, pp 20–21.

7. Tomaszewski EK, Wigle W, Phalen DN: Tissue distribution of psittacid herpesviruses in latently infected parrots, repeated sampling of latently infected parrots and prevalence of latency in parrots submitted for necropsy, *J Vet Diagn Invest* 18:536–544, 2006.

8. Styles DK, Tomaszewski EK, Phalen DN: A novel psittacid herpesvirus in African gray parrots *(Psittacus erithacus erithacus)*, *Avian Path* 34:150–154, 2005.

9. Legler M, Kothe R, Wohlsein P, et al: First detection of psittacid herpesvirus 2 in Congo African grey parrots *(Psittacus erithacus erithacus)* associated with pharyngeal papillomas and cloacal inflammation in Germany, *Berl Munch Tierarztl Wochenschr* 127:222–226, 2014.

10. Shivaprasad HL, Phalen DN: A novel herpesvirus associated with respiratory disease in Bourke's parrots *(Neopsephotus bourkii)*, *Avian Pathol* 41:531–539, 2012.

11. Gabor ML, Gabor J, Peacock L, et al: Psittacid herpesvirus 3 infection in the *Eclectus* parrot *(Eclectus roratus)* in Australia, *Vet Pathol* 50:1053–1057, 2013.

PSITTACINE BEAK AND FEATHER DISEASE

Shane Raidal

PSITTACINE BEAK AND FEATHER DISEASE

Psittacine beak and feather disease (PBFD) is a well-recognized disease that clinically presents most often as a chronic and ultimately fatal viral disease of Psittaciformes. While acute forms of the disease can occur in nestling and fledgling birds, the incubation period can be very long, with the slow development of feather dystrophy as molting progresses. All parrots, lorikeets, and cockatoos are considered susceptible to infection,[1,2] and there is evidence of it occurring naturally in wild birds for more than 120 years in Australia, where it is recognized as the main disease threat to many critically endangered birds such as the orange-bellied parrot *(Neophema chrysogaster)*. Increasing evidence suggests that the dispersion of wild-caught Australian parrot species such as the budgerigar *(Melopsittacus undulatus)* since the early 1840s has most likely resulted in the global spread of PBFD because it now affects a wide range of psittacine species in both wild and captive populations worldwide,[1,3-7]

Etiologic Agent

The virus that causes PBFD is beak and feather disease virus (BFDV) and despite many attempts, no method for cultivating BFDV in vitro has been successful, which impeded early research into the disease. The biologic characteristics, pathophysiology, and mode of replication have all been determined by studying the natural virus purified from the tissues of infected birds, by studying recombinant proteins, or by inferring from related circoviruses. The virus is a member of the family of Circoviridae[8] and is perhaps the simplest pathogen known to infect vertebrates. It is highly genetically diverse and prone to mutation[9–11] but relatively antigenically conserved based on serology.[12–14] Unlike other members of the *Circovirus* genus, BFDV is a hemagglutinating virus and has been shown to agglutinate erythrocytes from guinea pigs, geese, and many species of psittacine birds.[15–18] The disease is associated with ongoing massive viral excretion, a feature that can be readily detected with hemagglutination assay (HA) as an antigen detection diagnostic test.

Origins of Beak and Feather Disease Virus

The first recorded description of a feather loss syndrome that almost certainly was PBFD was in South Australia in 1907 in red-rumped grass parakeets *(Psephotus haematonotus)*. Affected birds were described as "quite healthy, except being destitute of feathers,"[19] and this was considered responsible for the decline of the species in the Adelaide Hills, since affected birds were likely to be more susceptible to predation. The use of terms such as "runners," or "hikers"[6] but more commonly "French molt" in historical records, particularly in reference to feather loss syndromes in budgerigars, probably included examples of PBFD as well as avian polyomavirus disease. Nevertheless, the disease has been recognized by aviculturists since the early 1970s.[20]

Until recently, it was thought that different BFDV genotypes or even distinct virus sub-types were responsible for, or at least associated with, disease in certain geographic areas or psittacine bird species. However, emerging consensus indicates that all psittacine birds are susceptible to a diversity of BFDV clades, with no clear association based on host–virus cospeciation. Within the order Psittaciformes as a whole, BFDV exhibits host-generalism with wide species susceptibility.[11]

Phylogenetic analysis of BFDV genomes strongly indicates that no one genotype can be considered more virulent than another; as such, it behaves like a viral quasispecies and host-generalist in the Psittaciformes, with shallow host-based divergence likely reflecting the dynamic ranges of interspecific transmission. Any effort to develop an attenuated strain for vaccination purposes is likely to be confounded by this feature. There is evidence that the Loriinae subfamily, which includes the lorikeets, lories, fig parrots, and budgerigars, may be the most robust or deeply adapted host of BFDV and are potentially super-distributors of this virus, at least throughout Australasia (Figure 2-7).

There is increasing viral genetic evidence that BFDV originated in the Australasian and not African or South American Psittaciformes.[1,21-23] While captive macaws, conures, and Amazon parrots are susceptible to BFDV infection,[9] the conspicuous paucity of unique BFDV genotypes from South American parrots suggests that the disease does not occur naturally in the wild in this region. Given the prominence of neotropical parrots in the North American and European aviculture, it seems likely that if it does occur in the

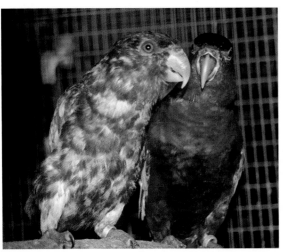

FIGURE 2-7 Abnormal and discolored plumage in a black-capped lory *(Lorius lory)* on the left with psittacine beak and feather disease. Affected contour feathers are abnormally yellow, while others are missing, including the primary flight feathers. While more than 200 different beak and feather disease virus (BFDV) genotypes have been detected, there are no distinct subtypes or strains, with only weak association with certain geographic areas or psittacine bird species. Emerging consensus indicates that all psittacine birds are susceptible to a diversity of BFDV clades. (Courtesy Dr. Brian Speer.)

wild in South America with an epidemiology similar to that in Australasia, then the disease would have been historically more frequently seen in shipments of wild-caught South American birds. This is because the less-than-ideal disease control in the pet bird trade during the height of exportation in the previous decades would have allowed ample exposure to any neotropical BFDV genotypes admixing from a variety of sources. Such genetic admixing has clearly been documented recently among captive psittacine flocks in Europe.[9] Recent evidence of BFDV infecting wild Cape Parrots in South Africa[7] is likely the result of a recent introduction, given the constrained degree of genetic diversity observed as well as the close relatedness of Cape Parrot isolates to BFDV genotypes from captive birds in Europe.

Features of differential disease expression—seen in Grey parrots at one end of a scale of susceptibility and in lorikeets and cockatiels at the other—are typical of the accentuated virulence seen when a virus switches from its preferred host to another.[24,25] There is evidence for this because BFDV jumps from one host species to another. In quasispecies theory, it is likely that a greater number of genetic variants occur as the most replicatively efficient variants compete within new hosts. This has been recently shown in PBFD-affected orange-bellied parrots[11] and cockatoos,[26] and an overall consequence of this might be the retention or enhancement of virulence across Psittaciformes as BFDV jumps flexibly from one host to another. In other words, the rich range in psittacine hosts probably counteracts any evolutionary trend toward viral attenuation.

Many avian circoviruses have been detected recently, some more pathogenic than others,[27-32] and many more are likely to be discovered serendipitously with the use of next-generation sequencing and metagenomic techniques. Circovirus DNA sequences present in a wide range of invertebrates, protozoans, plants, fungi, algae, and bacteria suggest a likely ancient coevolution of circoviruses with vertebrate hosts,[33,34] and this is likely to be true for the majority of birds. Indeed, the absence of a circovirus lineage in any extant psittacine species is somewhat puzzling, given the recent findings. Increasing evidence supports a post-Gondwanan origin of BFDV in the Australian species,[26] and there is fossil evidence that *Cacatua*[35] and the budgerigar have likely been present in Australia in their present forms for at least five million years.[36] Theoretically it is likely that BFDV has circulated with limited host-based divergence among the Australian Psittaciformes for at least this period. In contrast, there is no strong evidence of BFDV endemicity in native New Zealand parrot species prior to human colonization,[4] and the recent detection of PBFD in wild New Zealand birds is best explained by the introduction of this pathogen with the release of infected feral eastern rosellas *(Platycercus eximius)* from Australia. A similar scenario almost certainly occurred for the Norfolk Island green parrot.[37] The recent characterization of BFDV infection in captive New Caledonian lorikeets and parrots[21] is evidence of contemporary introductions of at least two BFDV lineages in Deplanche's rainbow lorikeets *(Trichoglossus haematodus deplanchii)* and the vulnerable New Caledonian parakeet *(Cyanoramphus saisseti)*. Given the relatedness of the Indonesian, Australian, and Polynesian BFDV genotypes, it seems most likely that continental Australia, or Sahul, has acted as a pathogen reservoir for island seeding in the South Pacific region. Within the Australian parrot species, there is a clinically well-recognized differential host susceptibility to PBFD. Lorikeets have never been reported with the same degree of advanced feather and beak dystrophy as is seen very commonly in sulfur-crested and other white cockatoos,[38] and there is anecdotal evidence that lorikeets frequently make complete clinical recoveries or at least regain relatively normal plumage. The majority of these recovered lorikeets may continue as BFDV carriers, excreting large viral titers in feces for months and possibly years. It is plausible that lorikeets disperse BFDV to the islands. This is supported by the results of a recent survey of captive birds in New Caledonia, which showed a strong infection bias to lorikeets,[21] but in the absence of more widespread sampling of wild birds, iatrogenic reasons, rather than natural expansion, will have to be held responsible in that case.

In the context of BFDV in the Australian landscape, a definitive understanding of disease modeling and population thresholds for a multihost disease such as PBFD may not be possible, given the large number of potential host species and conceivable parameters that could dynamically influence intraspecies and interspecies transmission rates alongside other factors such as abundance of important host reservoir species. Nevertheless, phylogenetic analysis of BFDV genomes strongly indicates that no one genotype can be considered more virulent than another, and as such, BFDV behaves like a viral quasispecies and host-generalist in Psittaciformes, with shallow host-based divergence likely reflecting dynamic ranges of interspecific transmission.

Transmission

The virus is excreted in feather dander and in feces. Consequently, high concentrations of the virus can be detected in liver tissue, bile, crop secretions, feces, and feathers.[18,39,40] Infection is most likely by oral and/or intracloacal ingestion of the virus, as demonstrated by experimental infection studies.[41] BFDV is suspected to be transmitted vertically[42,43] because BFDV DNA can be found in embryos from infected hens.[43] However, there is no experimental evidence that has conclusively confirmed vertical transmission rather than horizontal transmission to the embryo via cloacal secretions and nesting material. If vertical transmission occurs, it is unlikely to be a significant mechanism for circovirus maintenance in populations, since it is more likely to be a deep force for virus–host coevolution. Recent phylogenetic analyses provide little evidence to support strong host-based divergence. When considered in broader terms of disease ecology, BFDV behaves more as a resource-generalist with flexible host switching. This is much more likely facilitated by horizontal transmission and, at least in Australia, is most likely to occur in tree nest hollows, where there is strong competition between Psittaciformes and other birds for reproductive opportunities.[44-46] The ability of BFDV to persist in the environment,[47] along with the massively high titers excreted by PBFD-affected birds, supports this. As such the role of sequestration of BFDV genotypes within nest hollows, perhaps for many years, may be an important factor in extending the replication strategy of the virus along with re-entry of ancestral BFDV genotypes into host populations.

Clinical Signs

Juvenile or young adult psittacine birds are the most susceptible to PBFD, but birds of all ages can succumb to the disease. Birds kept in isolation for many decades can become infected when exposed to affected psittacine birds or contaminated areas. An acute form of the disease is well recognized in nestling or fledgling birds,[48] particularly in the Grey parrots (*Psittacus erithacus*),[49,50] which can die within a week of developing signs, and a more commonly encountered chronic form that can occur in all psittacine species. In acute disease, there is rapid development of depression associated with leukopenia, anemia, green diarrhea, biliverdinuria, and death due to hepatic necrosis. Acutely affected birds often become systemically ill and anorexic and/or regurgitate food. There may be pterylodynia with edematous and painful wing tips caused by inflammation, vasculitis, and subcutaneous edema. High viral titers can be detected in the liver and bile of affected birds, and some may die of liver failure without obvious feather lesions. Depending on the age of the nestling and thus the phase of feather development in individual pterylae, affected feathers may be shed all at once, or only the primary flight feathers may be affected, but this is usually seen in a bilaterally symmetric pattern. Fractures of the developing calamus and accompanying intrapulp hemorrhage are the predominant clinical findings. Affected feathers fracture at points of necrosis, usually before the feather has unsheathed.

The more commonly encountered manifestation of PBFD is a chronic disease with a slow subtle development and progression. As the molt progresses, dystrophic feathers replace normal ones, and the affected birds gradually lose plumage, often without other clinical signs of illness. The pattern of ongoing plumage damage is related to the stage of the molt that the bird is in when the disease first begins but is usually bilaterally symmetric and slowly progressive. Dystrophic

feathers are usually short and have one or more of the following characteristics: fault lines across the vanes, a thickened or retained feather sheath, blood within the calamus, an annular constriction of the calamus, or curling (Figure 2-8).

While some species such as the cockatiel, *Trichoglossus* lorikeets and New World psittacines appear to have an inherent resistance to BFDV infection or at least to the development of PBFD, if they become infected at all, others such as the gang gang cockatoo and black cockatoos (*Calyptorhynchus* spp.), which occupy specialist ecologic niches, seem more susceptible to succumbing, especially from the acute phase of infection (Figure 2-9).

In all Cacatuidae, the powder down feathers, or pulviplumes, are often the first feathers affected, and the ensuing lack of powder throughout the plumage can result in a glossy or dark pseudodiscoloration of the beak and claws and cause the plumage to become dull. PBFD-affected pulviplumes are fragile or develop an abnormally thickened outer sheath that fails to disintegrate. Powder down feathers may atrophy and create bare patches of affected skin. Claw abnormalities occur occasionally and generally develop well after feather and beak lesions become apparent. The beak can progressively

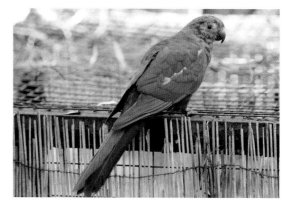

FIGURE 2-8 Wild Australian king parrot *(Alisterus scapularis)* with early clinical signs of psittacine beak and feather disease, with plumage deficits around the face and head.

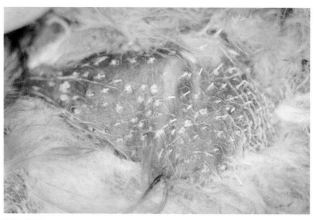

FIGURE 2-9 Powder down patch in a gang gang cockatoo *(Callocephalon fimbriatum)* with psittacine beak and feather disease (PBFD) demonstrated atrophic and dysplastic pulviplume feathers, which results in a loss of powder throughout the rest of the plumage.

elongate and/or develop fracture lines, and the affected rhamphotheca may slough off. In severe cases, necrosis of the oral epithelium and osteomyelitis can extend through to the esophagus and crop. On the extremities, PBFD-induced hyperkeratosis can cause the skin to appear excessively scaly, or it may be thickened and moist. Sunlight-exposed skin can become darkly pigmented. Chronic skin ulcers can occur at the elbows and wing tips. Chronically affected birds are predisposed to hypothermia, and secondary infections are common as a result of immunosuppression. These include cryptosporidiosis and bacterial, mycotic, and other viral infections. Most birds with chronic disease eventually have difficulty eating, lose weight, and die. In smaller grass parrots such as the *Psephotus* and *Neophema* species, apparently normal feathers that fall out or are easily plucked may be the only clinical sign. The first clinical sign in birds with green plumage may be the development of yellow feathers which may appear normal in other respects (Figure 2-10).

Clinical Pathology

The acute form of PBFD is associated with severe leukopenia in juvenile birds,[49,51,52] and chronically affected birds may have lower serum protein concentrations, characterized by low prealbumin and gammaglobulin concentrations.[53] The hematologic characteristics of juvenile long-billed corellas (*Cacatua tenuirostris*) were studied following experimental infection with BFDV and compared with vaccinated birds.[54] Significant differences in total and differential leukocyte concentrations, including heteropenia and lymphopenia, were demonstrated in BFDV-infected birds, but packed cell volume (PCV) and total serum protein (TSP) were not significantly affected.

Histopathology

Lesions within the skin and epidermis include multifocal epithelial cell necrosis, necrosis of distal pulp and hemorrhage into the distal shaft of feathers, and epidermal hyperplasia and hyperkeratosis.[20,41,55] There may also be infiltration of heterophils and lymphocytes into the pulp of some feathers. Basophilic intracytoplasmic inclusions can be found within macrophages in the feather pulp (see Figure 2-8), and some epithelial keratinocytes may contain intracytoplasmic or intranuclear inclusions.[20,56] Within the beak, degeneration and necrosis of

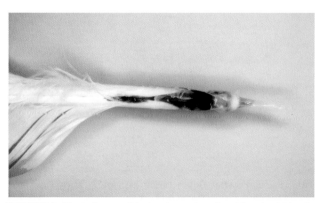

FIGURE 2-10 A dystrophic feather, showing blood within the calamus and annular constrictions of the calamus.

epithelial cells occur in the basal and intermediate cell layers. Chronic beak lesions are also associated with inflammation as a result of the presence of bacteria within the exudate and the keratinized layers of epithelium.[20]

The liver may be congested, with multifocal areas of necrosis of varying severity.[56] Characteristic basophilic inclusions may be present in Kupffer cells within the liver, and occasionally erythrophagocytosis may be seen in the liver and spleen. The thymus and bursa may show varying degrees of atrophy and necrosis. Focal aggregates of necrotic lymphocytes often contain macrophages with typical inclusions, and necrotic lymphocytes with intranuclear inclusions may also be visible.[20,56] Intracytoplasmic inclusion bodies within macrophages are variable in size and shape, and electron microscopic examination shows that they are composed of particles 17 to 20 nm in diameter arranged in a paracrystalline array.[20,41,55]

Immunohistochemistry and in situ hybridization[57] can be used to demonstrate BFDV antigens in a wide range of tissues,[58] but the best organs to assess are the bursa of Fabricius, feather follicles, spleen, esophagus, and crop. In some species, there appears to be differential expression in these tissues (Figure 2-11).

Diagnosis

The chronic form of PBFD can be diagnosed clinically with a high degree of certainty by careful physical clinical examination. Very few other diseases can mimic the bilaterally symmetric feather dysplasia seen in this disease, but endocrine conditions such as hypothyroidism should be considered in rare cases. Cases of feather plucking may be present, resulting in widespread iatrogenic plumage damage, so it is important to examine the feathers around the head and face area, where single birds cannot easily inflict self-trauma. In pairs or groups of birds, occasionally excessive allopreening might result in physical trauma to facial and head feathers that can mimic the lesions seen in PBFD. Surgical biopsy of skin and developing feather follicles has been used to detect histopathologic evidence of infection, but the sensitivity of detection is low unless chronic fulminate disease is present. In some species such as the grass parrots, *Neophema*, and *Psephotus* parrots, viral inclusions can be rare or difficult to confirm without immunohistochemistry (Figure 2-12).

In Australia, serology and antigen detection have proven to be valuable diagnostic tests for detecting and quantitating BFDV excretion and antibody responses, and when used in combination, different tests have proven extremely useful for understanding the impact of viral infection in individual birds and to identify potential false-positive and false-negative results.[13] While a number of antibody-detecting enzyme-linked immunosorbent assay (ELISA)–based tests[59,60] have been developed, they are not used extensively in diagnostic testing, primarily because the cross-reactivity between the immunoglobulin Y (IgY) of different psittacine birds is not known, and it is impossible to guarantee the validity of the assay when used with sera from other species. Hemagglutination inhibition (HI) avoids such issues and remains the gold standard for antibody detection.[14] HI assays tend to be technically simple and rapid and do not require anti-species-specific secondary antibodies or highly purified antigen. Antibody

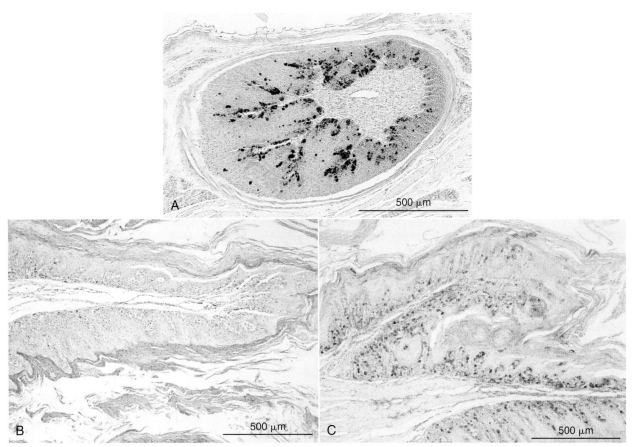

FIGURE 2-11 Typical strong positive immunohistochemistry reaction shown in the developing feather of a cockatoo with chronic psittacine beak and feather disease (PBFD) **(A)**. Beak and feather disease virus (BFDV) antigen can be detected in other organs such as the esophagus shown in a hematoxylin and eosin–stained section **(B)** from a gang gang cockatoo *(Callocephalon fimbriatum)*, which had areas of epithelial cell apoptosis and spongiosis. In the absence of characteristic botryoid amphomphilic intracytoplasmic inclusions, immunohistochemistry has shown a positive reaction to antigen **(C)**.

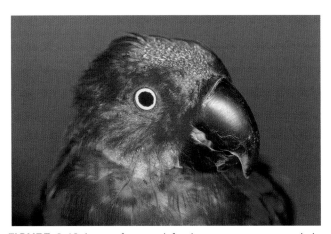

FIGURE 2-12 Loss of normal feather coverage around the head and face in a female eclectus parrot with abortive attempts at follicular regeneration, resulting in small atrophic and dysplastic feather stumps.

measurements using HI have reasonable precision if attention is paid to minimizing interassay variation by titrating standard virus and antibody activity against each other and against the erythrocytes from multiple birds prior to testing. Even so, HI assays are still prone to an appreciable amount of intertest variations, especially if performed infrequently or without standard reference antigen and sera.[61]

Along with HA and HI, polymerase chain reaction (PCR) testing has been used extensively for managing PBFD,[13] and in most countries, PCR testing has become the main method for detecting BFDV infection. As mentioned above, there is a wide variation in BFDV genetics, which has the potential to confound the PCR test design. Nevertheless, the BFDV *Rep* gene is relatively conserved,[1,62] and the PCR primer set P2-P4,[63] which targets this gene, has proven to be reliable for detecting BFDV DNA; even so, there are some rare genotypes that do not match perfectly with this primer set, and at least one study has revealed wide variations in diagnostic laboratory accuracy.[64] The PCR product from this diagnostic test covers a 700-nucleotide segment of the *Rep* gene, providing an ideal length for routine DNA sequencing,[65] which is useful for tracing the origin and establishment of infection in a flock.[66] This can be an important legal aspect of a diagnostic investigation. Within the diagnostic laboratory, it is also a useful step to monitor or identify potential sources of DNA contamination. Clinicians need to be aware that different laboratories might target slightly different parts of the BFDV genome or the capsid gene that has a higher degree of genetic diversity. Even for the same primer sequence set, they may use different PCR amplification conditions in their diagnostic assay, and the potential number of different variables that goes into designing a test protocol means that laboratory results from different laboratories should not be considered as equal.

In real-time PCR assays, primer dimers and other artefacts can result in false-positive interpretations. Other sources of false-positive PCR results include contamination of samples from the environment, especially if feathers are being collected, as well as amplicon contamination in the laboratory during DNA extraction. Copious shedding of BFDV occurs in the environment of PBFD-affected birds, and the risk of contamination of samples precludes the use of any material such as feathers exposed to the environment for meaningful PCR diagnosis in individuals that are not isolated for a prolonged period. Collection of bodily tissues such as blood is ideal for PCR testing. So it is important for clinicians to use and change gloves when handling and collecting samples from multiple birds. In the laboratory, a number of steps can be taken to investigate suspected false-positive reactions. First, the tests can be repeated using a second round of DNA extraction from the original submitted sample. Second, a separate PCR test that targets a different part of the viral genome, such as the capsid gene, can be used. Third, DNA sequencing can be done on the amplicons and compared with reference or positive controls. If the clinicians are suspicious of the results, they should contact the laboratory and ask for further validation of results.

Appropriate sample collection is important for determining the infection status of suspect birds. One study showed that in a flock of 56 peach-faced lovebirds (*Agapornis roseicollis*), of the 47 birds that were PCR positive on blood samples, only 10 were also positive on feather samples (Figure 2-13).[13]

While rarer than false-positive results, false-negative PCR results do occur. There are various reasons for this, but most importantly, the clinician needs to consider whether the sample collected was appropriate for the question being asked and if it has been appropriately stored. False-negative PCR results can occur due to a number of intralaboratory errors in technique, but more importantly, the degree of genetic variation that occurs in BFDV can lead to errors in primer annealing.

More recent studies in clinical research and diagnostics have used high-resolution DNA melt (HRM) curve analysis for routinely identifying differences in genetic sequences.[67] Newer-generation PCR machines can do this automatically as part of the diagnostic analysis. The melting profile of a PCR product is dependent on length, sequence divergence, guanine-cytosine (GC) content, and heterozygosity and is an accurate, robust, and cost-effective alternative to existing methods for genotypic differentiation of BFDV. Compared with sequencing, the technique is faster, and results can be obtained within 5 hours from receipt of blood or feather specimens.[68]

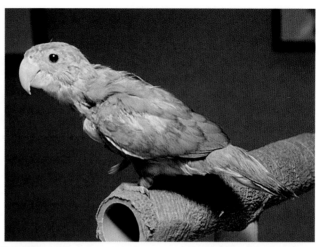

FIGURE 2-13 A peach-faced love bird (*Agapornis roseicollis*) with advanced clinical signs of plumage deficits due to PBFD. (Courtesy Dr Brian Speer.)

Management of Disease and Treatment

Individuals within many species may make full recoveries from clinical PBFD. For example, lorikeets (*Trichoglossus* sp.) and Eclectus parrots (*Eclectus* sp.) often develop protective HI titers alongside cessation of virus excretion. The immunologic mechanisms that control whether or not a bird succumbs to full-blown disease or recovers from subclinical infection is not well understood. Successful therapeutic regimes are likely to be developed but almost certainly will have a higher rate of success in subclinically infected birds rather than those with chronic disease. Current therapeutic options for PBFD are mainly supportive. Birds with chronic BFDV can live for many years, even after the development of significant beak lesions.

There have been few studies on possible therapeutic interventions for PBFD. Interferon alpha (IFN-α)–modulatory CpG sequences have been described in other circoviruses and likely also exist within BFDV. These oligodeoxyribonucleotides (ODNs) have been shown to have both inhibitory and stimulatory effects on the induction of IFN-α and an inhibitory effect on the production of tumor necrosis factor alpha (TNF-α) in natural interferon-producing cells,[69-71] independent of viral replication or the presence of capsid proteins. Cytokines show promise for the treatment of many viral diseases, and the use of chicken IFN-γ has been promoted anecdotally. Interferon of avian origin is not yet commercially available, and its efficacy for the treatment of chronic cases is yet to be investigated, especially in light of findings that IFN-γ may enhance circovirus replication in cell culture.[72]

In one case, treatment with b-(1,3/1,6)-D-glucan from oyster mushroom was claimed to have cleared BFDV DNA from four out of the six BFDV-infected horned parakeets (*Eunymphicus cornutus*), and four subclinically affected Major Mitchell cockatoos (*Lophochroa leadbeateri*) some 9 months after the treatment commenced.[73] However, the absence of BFDV DNA in blood should not lead to the conclusion that an effective clearance because an insufficient number of birds were treated, no control group was included, and no evidence that absence of BFDV DNA was not simply a result of the development of an appropriate antibody response was provided.

Prevention and Control

It is presumed based on its physicochemical characteristics that BFDV is resistant to extremes of temperature and various chemical disinfectants.[18] However, disinfection using peroxide compounds (Virkon S) has been recommended for use in captive breeding programs of endangered psittacine species.[74] Strict quarantine and diagnostic screening of new additions to the flock, using a combination of assays to detect potentially infected birds, is recommended. In countries where free-flying PBFD-infected birds may exist, prevention of access to the flock by wild birds is important, as is prevention of contamination of the flock by feces from wild birds. Stringent hygiene protocols should be in place, including regular cleaning with an appropriate disinfectant such as Virkon S in a 1% solution, which has been shown to inactivate nonenveloped viruses and bacterial spores.

Currently, there is no commercially available vaccine for BFDV. An experimental inactivated vaccine using inactivated virus or recombinant proteins has been shown to be effective.[75,76] As no cell culture system has been developed to grow the virus successfully in vitro, recombinant techniques show the most promise for the development of effective vaccines that may be produced on a large scale. Recombinant capsid proteins, expressed in bacterial and insect cell–based systems have been proposed for use in diagnostic tests and vaccines for BFDV.[77,78] It should be noted, however, that vaccination does not prevent viral replication,[79,80] so effective control of PBFD will always depend on a combination of diagnostic testing, hygiene measures, and the maintenance of high levels of flock immunity.

REFERENCES

1. Bassami MR, Ypelaar I, Berryman D, et al: Genetic diversity of beak and feather disease virus detected in psittacine species in Australia, *Virology* 2792:392–400, 2001.
2. Ritchie PA, Anderson IL, Lambert DM: Evidence for specificity of psittacine beak and feather disease viruses among avian hosts, *Virology* 3061:109–115, 2003.
3. Raidal SR, McElnea CL, Cross GM: Seroprevalence of psittacine beak and feather disease in wild psittacine birds in New South Wales, *Aust Vet J* 704:137–139, 1993.
4. Ha HJ, Anderson IL, Alley MR, Spet al:. The prevalence of beak and feather disease virus infection in wild populations of parrots and cockatoos in New Zealand, *N Z Vet J* 555:235–238, 2007.
5. Clout MN, Merton DV: Saving the Kakapo: the conservation of the world's most peculiar parrot, *Bird Conservat Int.* 803:281–296, 1998.
6. Layton F: Runners or hikers in budgerigars, *Central Queensland Herald (Rockhampton)* 7357:11, 1936.
7. Regnard GL, Boyes RS, Martin RO, et al: Beak and feather disease viruses circulating in Cape parrots *(Poicepahlus robustus)* in South Africa, *Arch Virol* 160(1):47–54, 2015.
8. Bassami MR, Berryman D, Wilcox GE, et al: Psittacine beak and feather disease virus nucleotide sequence analysis and its relationship to porcine circovirus, plant circoviruses, and chicken anaemia virus, *Virology* 2492:453–459, 1998.
9. Julian L, Piasecki T, Chrząstek K, et al: Extensive recombination detected amongst Beak and feather disease virus isolates from breeding facilities in Poland, *J Gen Virol* 941086–941095, 2013.
10. Duffy S, Holmes EC: Phylogenetic Evidence for rapid rates of molecular evolution in the single-stranded DNA begomovirus tomato yellow leaf curl virus, *J Virol* 822:957–965, 2008.
11. Sarker S, Patterson EI, Peters A, et al: Mutability dynamics of an emergent single stranded DNA virus in a naïve host, *PLoS One* 9(1):e85370, 2013.
12. Shearer PL, Bonne N, Clark P, et al: Beak and feather disease virus infection in cockatiels *(Nymphicus hollandicus)*, *Avian Pathol* 371:75–81, 2008.
13. Khalesi B, Bonne N, Stewart M, et al: A comparison of haemagglutination, haemagglutination inhibition and PCR for the detection of psittacine beak and feather disease virus infection and a comparison of isolates obtained from loriids, *J Gen Virol* 863039–863046, 2005.
14. Raidal SR, Sabine M, Cross GM: Laboratory diagnosis of psittacine beak and feather disease by hemagglutination and hemagglutination inhibition, *Aust Vet J* 704:133–137, 1993.
15. Kondiah K, Albertyn J, Bragg RR: Beak and feather disease virus haemagglutinating activity using erythrocytes from African grey parrots and brown-headed parrots, *Onderstepoort J Vet Res* 723:263–265, 2005.
16. Sanada N, Sanada Y: The sensitivities of various erythrocytes in a haemagglutination assay for the detection of psittacine beak and feather disease virus, *J Vet Med* S 476:441–443, 2000.
17. Sexton N, Penhale WJ, Plant SL, et al: Use of goose red blood cells for detection of infection with psittacine beak and feather disease virus by haemagglutination and haemagglutination inhibition, *Aust Vet J* 7110:345–347, 1994.
18. Raidal SR, Cross GM: The haemagglutination spectrum of psittacine beak and feather disease virus, *Avian Pathol* 23621–23630, 1994.
19. Ashby E: Parakeets moulting, *Emu* 193–194, 1907.
20. Pass DA, Perry RA: The pathology of psittacine beak and feather disease, *Aust Vet J* 613:69–74, 1984.
21. Julian L, Lorenzo A, Chenuet JP, et al: Evidence of multiple introductions of beak and feather disease virus into the Pacific islands of Nouvelle-Caledonie (New Caledonia), *J Gen Virol* 93 Pt 11:2466–2472, 2012.
22. Massaro M, Ortiz-Catedral L, Julian L, et al: Molecular characterisation of beak and feather disease virus (BFDV) in New Zealand and its implications for managing an infectious disease, *Arch Virol* 1579:1651–1663, 2012.
23. Varsani A, Regnard GL, Bragg R, et al: Global genetic diversity and geographical and host-species distribution of beak and feather disease virus isolates, *J Gen Virol* 92 Pt 4:752–767, 2010.
24. Hawley DM, Osnas EE, Dobson AP, et al: Parallel patterns of increased virulence in a recently emerged wildlife pathogen, *PLoS Biol* 115:e1001570, 2013.
25. Osnas EE, Dobson AP: Evolution of virulence in heterogeneous host communities under multiple trade-offs, *Evolution* 662:391–401, 2012.
26. Sarker S, Ghorashi SA, Forwood JK, et al: Phylogeny of beak and feather disease virus in cockatoos demonstrates host generalism and multiple-variant infections within Psittaciformes, *Virology* 460-461:72–82, 2014.
27. Phenix KV, Weston JH, Ypelaar I, et al: Nucleotide sequence analysis of a novel circovirus of canaries and its relationship to other members of the genus Circovirus of the family Circoviridae, *J Gen Virol* 822805–822809, 2001.
28. Halami MY, Nieper H, Muller H, et al: Detection of a novel circovirus in mute swans *(Cygnus olor)* by using nested broad-spectrum PCR, *Virus Res* 1321(2):208–212, 2008.
29. Todd D, Fringuelli E, Scott AN, et al: Sequence comparison of pigeon circoviruses, *Res Vet Sci* 842:311–319, 2008.
30. Smyth JA, Todd D, Scott A, et al: Identification of circovirus infection in three species of gull, *Vet Rec* 1597:212–214, 2006.
31. Stewart ME, Perry R, Raidal SR: Identification of a novel circovirus in Australian ravens *(Corvus coronoides)* with feather disease, *Avian Pathol* 35(2):86–92, 2006.

32. Johne R, Fernandez-de-Luco D, Hofle U, et al: Genome of a novel circovirus of starlings, amplified by multiply primed rolling-circle amplification, *J Gen Virol* 871189–1195, 2006.

33. Gibbs MJ, Weiller GF: Evidence that a plant virus switched hosts to infect a vertebrate and then recombined with a vertebrate-infecting virus, *Proc Natl Acad Sci U S A* 9614:8022–8027, 1999.

34. Delwart E, Li L: Rapidly expanding genetic diversity and host range of the Circoviridae viral family and other Rep encoding small circular ssDNA genomes, *Virus Res* 1641–1642:114–121, 2012.

35. Boles WE: A New cockatoo (Psittaciformes, Cacatuidae) from the Tertiary of Riversleigh, Northwestern Queensland, and an evaluation of rostral characters in the systematics of parrots, *Ibis* 1351:8–18, 1993.

36. Boles WE: A budgerigar *Melopsittacus undulatus* from the Pliocene of Riversleigh, north-western Queensland, *Emu* 9832–9835, 1998.

37. Stevenson P, Yorkston P, Greenwood D: Draft Interim Plan. Green Parrot Recovery Program 1995-96. In: Norfolk Island Conservancy ANCA, editor: *Commonwealth of Australia (1993-1998)*, Canberra, Australia, 1995, Australian Nature Conservation Agency.

38. Pass DA, Perry RA: The pathology of psittacine beak and feather disease, *Aust Vet J* 613:69–74, 1984.

39. Ritchie BW, Niagro FD, Latimer KS, et al: Haemagglutination by psittacine beak and feather disease virus and the use of haemagglutination inhibition for the detection of antibodies against the virus, *Am J Vet Res* 52:1810–1815, 1991.

40. Ritchie BW, Niagro FD, Latimer KS, et al: Routes and prevalence of shedding of psittacine beak and feather disease virus, *Am J Vet Res* 5211:1804–1809, 1991.

41. Wylie SL, Pass DA: Experimental reproduction of psittacine beak and feather disease/french moult, *Avian Pathol* 16269–16281, 1987.

42. Ritchie BW, Harrison G, Harrison L, editors: *Avian medicine: principles and application*, Lakeworth, FL, 1994, Wingers Publishing Inc.

43. Rahaus M, Desloges N, Probst S, et al: Detection of beak and feather disease virus DNA in embryonated eggs of psittacine birds, *Veterinarni Medicina* 531:53 58, 2008.

44. Heinsohn R, Murphy S, Legge S: Overlap and competition for nest holes among eclectus parrots, palm cockatoos and sulphur-crested cockatoos, *Aust J Zool* 511:81–94, 2003.

45. Legge S, Heinsohn R, Garnett S: Availability of nest hollows and breeding population size of eclectus parrots, *Eclectus roratus*, on Cape York Peninsula, Australia, *Aust Wildlife Res* 312:149–161, 2004.

46. Saunders DA, Smith GT, Rowley I: The availability and dimensions of tree hollows that provide nest sites for cockatoos (Psittaciformes) in Western Australia, *Aust Wildlife Res* 9541–9546, 1982.

47. Raidal SR, Cross GM: The hemagglutination spectrum of psittacine beak and feather disease virus, *Avian Pathol* 234:621–630, 1994.

48. Raidal SR, Cross GM: Acute necrotizing hepatitis caused by experimental infection with psittacine beak and feather disease virus, *J Avian Med Surg* 936–940, 1995.

49. Doneley RJT: Acute beak and feather disease in juvenile African Grey parrots—an uncommon presentation of a common disease, *Aust Vet J* 814:206–207, 2003.

50. Schoemaker NJ, Dorrestein GM, Latimer KS, et al: Severe leukopenia and liver necrosis in young African grey parrots *(Psittacus erithacus erithacus)* infected with psittacine circovirus, *Avian Dis* 442:470–478, 2000.

51. Schoemaker NJ, Dorrestein GM, Latimer KS, et al: Severe leukopaenia and liver necrosis in young African grey parrots *(Psittacus erithacus erithacus)* infected with psittacine circovirus, *Avian Dis* 44470–44478, 2000.

52. Stanford M: Interferon treatment of circovirus infection in grey parrots *(Psittacus e erithacus)*, *Vet Rec* 154435-154436, 2004.

53. Jacobson ER, Clubb S, Simpson C, et al: Feather and beak dystrophy and necrosis in cockatoos: clinicopathologic evaluations. *J Am Vet Med Assoc* 1899:999–1005, 1986.

54. Bonne N, Clark P, Shearer P, et al: Hematology of vaccinated and non-vaccinated long-billed corellas following infection with beak and feather disease virus (BFDV), *Comparat Clin Pathol* 18353–18359, 2009.

55. McOrist S, Black DG, Pass DA, et al: Beak and feather dystrophy in wild sulphur crested cockatoos *(Cacatua galerita)*, *J Wildlife Dis* 202:120–124, 1984.

56. Raidal SR, Cross GM: Acute necrotizing hepatitis caused by experimental infection with psittacine beak and feather disease virus, *J Avian Med Surg* 936–940, 1995.

57. Ramis A, Latimer KS, Niagro FD, et al: Diagnosis of psittacine beak and feather disease (PBFD) viral infection, avian polyomavirus infection, adenovirus infection and herpesvirus infection in psittacine tissues using DNA in situ hybridization, *Avian Pathol* 234:643–657, 1994.

58. Latimer KS, Rakich PM, Kircher IM, et al: Extracutaneous viral inclusions in psittacine beak and feather disease, *J Vet Diagn Invest* 23:204–207, 1990.

59. Ritchie BW, Niagro FD, Latimer KS, et al: Production and characterisation of monoclonal antibodies to psittacine beak and feather disease virus, *J Vet Diagn Invest* 413–418, 1992.

60. Shearer PL, Sharp M, Bonne N, et al: A blocking ELISA for the detection of antibodies to psittacine beak and feather disease virus (BFDV), *J Virol Methods* 1581–1582:136–140, 2009.

61. Cross G: Hemagglutination inhibition assays, *Semin Avian Exot Pet Med* 111:15–18, 2002.

62. Heath L, Martin DP, Warburton L, et al: Evidence of unique genotypes of beak and feather disease virus in southern Africa, *J Virol* 7817:9277–9284, 2004.

63. Ypelaar I, Bassami MR, Wilcox GE, et al: A universal polymerase chain reaction for the detection of psittacine beak and feather disease virus, *Vet Microbiol* 681–682:141–148, 1999.

64. Olsen G, Speer B: Laboratory reporting accuracy of polymerase chain reaction testing for psittacine beak and feather disease virus, *J Avian Med Surg* 233:194–198, 2009.

65. Sanger F, Nicklen S, Coulson AR: DNA sequencing with chain-terminating inhibitors, *Biotechnology* 24104–24108, 1992.

66. Kundu S, Faulkes CG, Greenwood AG, et al: Tracking viral evolution during a disease outbreak: the rapid and complete selective sweep of a circovirus in the endangered Echo parakeet, *J Virol* 869:5221–5229, 2012.

67. Sarker S, Ghorashi SA, Forwood JK, et al: Rapid genotyping of beak and feather disease virus using high-resolution DNA melt curve analysis, *J Virol Methods* 208:47–55, 2014.

68. Sarker S, Ghorashi SA, Forwood JK, et al: Rapid genotyping of beak and feather disease virus using high-resolution DNA melt curve analysis, *J Virol Methods* 208:47-55, 2014.

69. Hasslung F, Berg M, Allan GM, et al: Identification of a sequence from the genome of porcine circovirus type 2 with an inhibitory effect on IFN-alpha production by porcine PBMCs, *J Gen Virol* 842937–842945, 2003.

70. Stevenson LS, McCullough K, Vincent I, et al: Cytokine and C-reactive protein profiles induced by Porcine Circovirus Type 2 experimental infection in 3-week-old piglets, *Viral Immunol* 192:189–195, 2006.

71. Wikstrom FH, Meehan BM, Berg M, et al: Structure-dependent modulation of alpha interferon production by porcine circovirus 2 oligodeoxyribonucleotide and CpG DNAs in porcine peripheral blood mononuclear cells, *J Virol* 8110:4919–4927, 2007.

72. Meerts P, Misinzo G, McNeilly F, et al: Replication kinetics of different porcine circovirus 2 strains in PK-15 cells, foetal cardiomyocytes and macrophages, *Arch Virol* 150427–150441, 2005.

73. Tomasek O, Tukac V: Psittacine circovirus infection in parakeets of the genus *Eunymphicus* and treatment with B-(1,3/1,6)-D-Glucan, *Avian Dis* 514:989–991, 2007.

74. Cross GM: *Draft threat abatement plan for psittacine circoviral (beak and feather) disease affecting endangered psittacine species*, Canberra, Australia, 2004, Department of the Environment and Heritage, Commonwealth of Australia.

75. Raidal SR, Firth GA, Cross GM: Vaccination and challenge studies with psittacine beak and feather disease, *Aust Vet J* 70437–70441, 1993.

76. Raidal SR, Cross GM: Control by vaccination of psittacine beak and feather disease in a mixed flock of *Agapornis* sp., *Aust Vet Pract* 24178–24180, 1994.

77. Johne R, Raue R, Grund C, et al: Recombinant expression of a truncated capsid protein of beak and feather disease virus and its application in serological tests, *Avian Pathol* 333:328–336, 2004.

78. Heath L, Williamson A, Rybicki EP: The capsid protein of beak and feather disease virus binds to the viral DNA and is responsible for transporting the replication-associated protein into the nucleus, *J Virol* 8014:7219–7225, 2006.

79. Bonne N, Shearer P, Sharp M, et al: Assessment of recombinant beak and feather disease virus (BFDV) capsid protein as a vaccine for psittacine beak and feather disease (PBFD), *J Gen Virol* 90(apt 3): 640–647, 2009.

80. Shearer P, Bonne N, Clark P, et al: A blocking ELISA for the detection of antibodies to psittacine beak and feather disease virus (BFDV). *J Virol Methods* 158(1–2):136–140, 2009.

AN OVERVIEW OF AVIAN INFLUENZA IN DOMESTIC AND NONDOMESTIC AVIAN SPECIES

Darrel K. Styles

Influenza poses significant disease risk to both animal and public health, causing extensive morbidity and sometimes high mortality. Influenza may cause global pandemics such as the recent 2009 H1N1 pandemic, and avian influenza results in the loss of billions of dollars of poultry yearly, hence the older term for its disease "fowl plague." While biologics are useful in limiting the spread of influenza, the rapid rate of viral evolution and its ability to elude the immune response make it a challenging disease to control. This chapter is intended to provide a cursory overview of influenza virology and disease dynamics and discuss the disease risk and sequelae in both domestic and wild avian species.

Influenza viruses belong to the family Orthomyxoviridae and are enveloped, single-stranded negative-sense ribonucleic acid (RNA) viruses with segmented genomes consisting of eight gene segments coding for 11 known proteins. These viruses are broadly subdivided into types A, B, and C. Type A influenza viruses are further classified into subtypes based on the major antigenic proteins that festoon the viral capsid, namely, hemagglutinin (H or HA) and neuraminidase (N or NA). These two proteins provide the basis for the subtype nomenclature (e.g., H5N1, H3N2, and H7N9), because there are 16 recognized HA and 9 NA confirmations that occur in different combinations and comprise a range of avian influenza subtypes. Avian influenzas are widely distributed in waterfowl and shorebirds, which are considered the natural hosts for influenza viruses.[1,2] However, recent reports have described bat species as being hosts for two novel strains, H17N10 and H18N11, showing that influenza virus host diversity extends beyond avian species.[3,4] Type A influenza viruses are antigenically diverse and express a cosmopolitan host preference. These viruses may affect many avian species and a broad range of mammals, including, but not limited to, humans, swine, horses, dogs, ferrets, bats, and marine mammals. Clinically, influenza A viruses are responsible for outbreaks, epidemics, and pandemics.

Type B influenza viruses are also further classified into subtypes and express a more restricted host range, which includes humans, seals, and, experimentally, ferrets. Influenza B viruses typically cause outbreaks and epidemics but not pandemics. Type C influenza viruses are the least antigenically diverse and are largely confined to humans, although both canine and swine infections and experimental infections in ferrets have been reported. Therefore influenza C viruses cause outbreaks and highly localized epidemics but are not involved in pandemics.

BIOLOGY OF TYPE A INFLUENZA VIRUSES

Avian influenza viruses (AIVs) are Type A influenza viruses and are thought to be the progenitor of all influenza A viruses regardless of their host species. AIVs are found in waterfowl and shorebirds globally, and these species are the natural reservoirs for the virus. AIVs may adapt to mammalian species and become established in those populations; however, how this occurs has not been well elucidated, although there may be select evolutionary mechanisms by which this transition occurs.

Type A influenza viruses are highly subject to mutation and evolution, and primarily change by two mechanisms, antigenic drift and antigenic shift. Antigenic drift occurs because the virus' RNA polymerase has no proofreading function; therefore substitutions are introduced resulting in a somewhat predictable error rate between 1×10^{-3} and 8×10^{-3} substitutions per site per year.[8] Antigenic drift may contribute to the agent's ability to elude the host immune response, but generally it does not result in significant virulence changes in the virus. By contrast, antigenic shift can radically change the virus' pathogenic potential. Antigenic shift generally occurs by reassortment of heterologous influenza virus gene segments when the host is co-infected with two different influenza subtypes. The influenza genome is segmented and the gene segments of different influenza viruses can reassort to create unique viruses.[8] For example, if a host is co-infected with H5N1 and H3N2, then new reassortant viruses such as H5N2 and H3N1 can result. Antigenic shift can greatly increase virulence or host adaptation in a single viral generation. This shift may potentially advance zoonotic potential and certainly enhances the ability to elude the host immune response.

VIROLOGY, PATHOBIOLOGY, AND ECOLOGY OF AVIAN INFLUENZA VIRUSES

Type A influenza viruses attach to a host's respiratory or gastrointestinal (GI) epithelial cell's sialic acid receptor by means of their hemagglutinin protein. Mammalian adapted influenza viruses and AIVs demonstrate different receptor preferences for the confirmation of the terminal galactose on the polysaccharide chain of the sialic acid. AIVs prefer this terminal sugar to be in an α-2,3 orientation, whereas mammalian adapted influenza viruses prefer an α-2,6 orientation. This specificity helps to partially explain host preferences for these viruses. Avian species have a greater density of α-2,3 receptors on their epithelial surfaces, whereas mammals have a greater density of α-2,6. However, mammals do possess α-2,3 receptors of variable concentration, and in humans, these are typically found in the lower respiratory tract. This is one of the possible pathways for avian influenza viruses to infect mammalian hosts. Swine have demonstrated the potential for being readily infected with both avian and mammalian strains, and this has, in part, been attributed to receptor sialobiology.[8] Therefore, swine have been postulated to be the "mixing vessels" for avian and mammalian strains and capable of adapting avian strains to mammals. However, other findings suggest that the distribution of receptor type in swine is not dissimilar to humans; hence the mechanism(s) for avian strain adaptation to mammals is more complex than receptor biology alone. Quail have also been postulated to play a similar role in this type of adaptation scheme; however, whether this might occur has not been established.[9]

Once the influenza virus hemagglutinin protein has been bound to the sialic acid receptor with the carbohydrate moiety in the appropriate confirmation for that virus and species, an essential enzymatic cleavage of the hemagglutinin protein must occur in order for the virus to enter the host cell. This cleavage has important implications for AIV virulence, which will be discussed later.

AIVs are further classified by their pathogenic potential for poultry, namely, highly pathogenic avian influenza (HPAI) and low pathogenicity avian influenza (LPAI). Therefore, when designating an avian influenza virus, the HA/NA subtype designation is preceded by its pathogenic potential (e.g., HPAI H5N1, LPAI H7N9). HPAI infection typically causes severe illness and death in avian species, but the clinical signs of LPAI range from subclinical to mild, depending on the species infected and the strain of virus. Clinical signs described in susceptible chickens infected with HPAI include ocular and nasal discharges, coughing, snicking and dyspnea, swelling of the sinuses and/or head, apathy, reduced vocalization, marked reduction in feed and water intake, cyanosis of the unfeathered skin, wattles and comb, incoordination, nervous signs, diarrhea, and acute death. In laying birds, additional clinical features include a marked drop in egg production, usually accompanied by an increase in numbers of poor-quality eggs. None of these signs is considered to be pathognomonic for HPAI infection. LPAI viruses that normally cause only mild or no clinical disease in poultry can result in more severe disease if concurrent infections or adverse environmental factors are present. LPAI infections in poultry are often detected serologically with hemagglutination inhibition (HI) assays, agar gel immunodiffusion tests (AGIT), and enzyme-linked immunosorbent assays (ELISA). Virus isolation with LPAI viruses can be challenging, but often partial sequencing for characterization can be accomplished by molecular methods such as reverse transcriptase polymerase chain reaction (RT-PCR). By contrast, birds with HPAI may succumb to disease before seroconversion and molecular testing (e.g., RT-PCR) and sequencing and/or virus isolation is used to characterize the virus.[10,11]

Domestic poultry and other birds are usually infected by LPAI from spillover from infected wild migratory waterfowl. While such events typically result in a mild or asymptomatic infection, LPAIs of the H5 and H7 subtype are subject to mutation in land-based poultry (e.g., chickens, turkeys) and can evolve into highly pathogenic strains. All currently known HPAI viruses are restricted to subtypes H5 and H7 (although not all H5 and H7 are highly pathogenic; in fact, most are LPAI viruses). HPAI virus infections may cause high flock mortality up to 100%. Some subtypes of HPAI viruses have become adapted to wild migratory waterfowl and may crossover directly into poultry from that compartment.

Commercial poultry in the United States is subjected to rigorous surveillance for LPAI and HPAI; infection in commercial poultry is usually detected through this routine serologic or molecular surveillance for subclinical infections or by clinical illness and production losses. Commercial flocks showing clinical signs consistent with avian influenza are subjected to extensive diagnostics and may be depopulated if an H5 or H7 subtype is detected. LPAI infection of land-based poultry is largely confined to the respiratory tract, unless the infection is exacerbated, whereas in waterfowl it is largely subclinical and confined to the gastrointestinal tract.[5] This tissue tropism is a result of the necessary enzymes being present in the target cells to cleave the hemagglutinin protein after attachment, typically confined to the avian intestinal or respiratory tract. LPAI viruses have a single cleavage point within their HA protein that helps to convey this cell-type specificity where only the target cells (e.g., GI tract) possess the necessary enzymes to cleave the HA protein and allow ingress. By contrast, HPAI viruses have multiple basic amino acid cleavage points within their HA protein, which permits an array of cell types to actively cleave the HA protein. Therefore, HPAI viruses are systemic in nature and infect multiple organ systems.

DIAGNOSIS

Identification of the Agent

Samples of oropharyngeal and cloacal swabs, feces, or specimens from dead birds can be submitted for virus isolation. RT-PCR, targeting one or more segments of the virus genome (usually the matrix protein, HA, and NA) offers accurate and rapid results.[12,13] The matrix or M protein is a highly conserved protein across all subtypes of influenza, and a PCR-positive result suggests that there is an influenza A virus in the sample. Subtyping the virus may be accomplished by HI and neuraminidase inhibition tests against a battery of polyclonal or monospecific antisera to each of the 16 hemagglutinin (H1–16) and 9 neuraminidase (N1–9) subtypes of influenza A virus. However, sequencing is more frequently used in determining virus subtype. Pathogenicity is determined by inoculation of live susceptible chickens in a virus-secure biocontainment laboratory to determine the intravenous pathogenicity index (IVPI), which defines the threshold for HPAI designation when the mortality rate is 75% or greater, and/or by sequencing the H5 or H7 gene and determining whether the genes possess the multiple basic amino acid cleavage sites common to all HPAI viruses.[14–16]

Serology

Serological diagnostics have been validated for poultry species, but may not be fully applicable across the range of avian species that may be examined. Some pen-side antigen capture tests have demonstrated effectiveness for detection of avian influenza virus both in terms of sensitivity and specificity.[17] ELISA assays that have been validated for veterinary use are preferred for veterinary diagnostic laboratories. AGITs are used to detect antibodies to the conserved nucleocapsid and matrix antigens of influenza A viruses, and are therefore used as general screening tools for domestic poultry monitoring.[18,19] AGITs may be less reliable for detection of antibodies to influenza A in species of birds other than domestic poultry, so results from nondomestic species should be carefully interpreted.[20] HI tests can be used in diagnostic or screening serology; however, these tests also may lack sensitivity because of the subtype specificity of the hemagglutinin used. ELISA is used to detect antibodies to influenza type A–specific antigens in either species-dependent (indirect) or species-independent (competitive) test formats.

REPORTABLE (NOTIFIABLE) AVIAN INFLUENZA

Infection of poultry by H5 or H7 strains is considered to be a reportable disease to State and Federal animal health authorities. Older regulatory language refers to infection of poultry by H5 or H7 subtypes as "notifiable," but this language is considered obsolete by the World Organization for Animal Health (OIE), which provides regulatory guidance for the international trade of animal commodities. OIE defines avian influenza for its purposes in the Terrestrial Code Chapter 10.4, which is paraphrased as "infection of poultry caused by any influenza A virus of subtype H5 or H7; HPAI viruses demonstrate an IVPI of 1.2 (75% mortality) or greater or possesses multiple basic amino acid cleavage sites within their HA protein." LPAI viruses are considered to be all other H5 or H7 viruses in poultry that cannot be classifed as HPAI viruses by the aforementioned criteria. Infection of commercial poultry by non-H5 or non-H7 LPAI subtypes (e.g., H1, H3) is not immediately reportable, but these LPAI viruses may cause mild disease or production loss. Detection of any HPAI strain in commercial poultry is immediately reportable to regulatory authorities and has a swift and direct impact on the interstate and international movement of poultry commodities. All poultry infected with or exposed to HPAI, and some classes of poultry infected with LPAI H5 or LPAI H7, are quarantined and depopulated to control the spread of the disease or prevent evolution into a more dangerous strain.

ZOONOTIC POTENTIAL OF AVIAN INFLUENZA VIRUSES

While influenza infects a broad range of avian species, outbreaks in domestic poultry remain the primary concern due to the potential for the H5 and H7 subtypes to evolve into highly pathogenic strains. Zoonotic transmission is also a possibility with some subtypes of avian influenza, which—if they could achieve sustained lateral transmission in people—might result in a pandemic.[6] Both HPAI H5 and HPAI H7 subtypes have demonstrated the potential for zoonotic transmission. This is exemplified by the emergence of the virulent genotypes of the

Asian strains of HPAI H5N1 in 1996, which have caused an epizootic extending from a pan-Asian distribution to parts of Africa and resulted in scores of human cases and fatalities. However, LPAI viruses such as LPAI H7N9 and LPAI H9N2 have also exhibited zoonotic behavior. LPAI H7N9 emerged in China in 2013 and is sustaining ongoing infections, which are characterized by land-based poultry subclinically infected by LPAI H7N9 and are being transmitted to people, resulting in human illness and fatalities.[7] How avian influenza viruses adapt to mammals is not well understood, but the potential for emergence of zoonotic or pandemic strains exists within the avian population.[21] It has been speculated that virulence changes occur when the viruses attempt to adapt to novel hosts (e.g., land-based poultry, mammals).

AVIAN INFLUENZA IN BIRDS OTHER THAN WATERFOWL AND POULTRY

For purposes of this discussion, the nondomestic avian species that will be addressed are psittacines, passerines, Columbiformes, Accipitriformes, and ratites. Avian influenza has been reported in a number of different bird species.[22] However, these were likely coincidental infections resulting from spillover from either infected waterfowl (the natural hosts) or infected domestic poultry.[23] Epidemiological data suggest that LPAI and some HPAI viruses may spread from wild waterfowl along their migratory route to domestic birds such as chickens, turkeys, or even ostriches. However, HPAI had rarely been detected in any wild bird species until the appearance of the current pathogenic clades of Eurasian HPAI H5N1 that emerged in 1996 and then re-emerged with the more modern pathogenic clades in 2003.[24] Since 2003, HPAI H5N1 has been detected in a number of avian species other than wild waterfowl and domestic poultry, which is likely due to the magnitude of the epizootic across Asia and extending into Africa.

Occasionally, raptor and passerine species are incidentally infected by spillover from the infected domestic poultry compartment or infected wild waterfowl. This transmission can occur indirectly through the contaminated environment (passerines) or directly through consumption of infected poultry or waterfowl (raptors). Columbiforms appear to be highly resistant to avian influenza virus infection and are not considered to be a high-risk species.

Pet Bird Species

Because psittacines figure prominently in pet bird culture, they will be the focus of this discussion, but the findings are largely applicable to other conventional pet bird species. Parrots have been reported to have been infected with HPAI H5N1, HPAI H5N2, and LPAI H9N2, as well as other LPAI subtypes.[25-28] However, these infections have likely occurred because of housing the birds in close proximity to infected poultry, waterfowl, or other avian species that are shedding virus. Situations that are associated with pet bird species being infected with avian influenza include trapping of wild caught birds that may be exposed to infected poultry or other infected species in places like the live-bird markets that are common in the developing world.

Psittacines would not normally encounter high-risk influenza species in the wild, and experimental studies have shown that avian influenza virus infection and transmission is not efficient in parrots. However, avian influenza infection can cause serious disease or death in pet bird species and can mimic the clinical signs of other viral diseases (e.g., Newcastle, avian polyomavirus).[25] Neotropical parrots were infected when being co-housed in a quarantine station with infected bulbuls and vireos from Asia (which may have originated from live-bird market environments), resulting in the depopulation of the station. The infection of these passerines likely occurred in the exporting country through exposure to infected poultry or waterfowl prior to export and the virus was then transmitted to the psittacines.

Psittacines can be treated palliatively for avian influenza (including HPAI infections), and there is a case where an infected pet parrot was isolated and supported until it cleared the infection.[25] While some subtypes of avian influenza have been shown to be zoonotic, parrots have been experimentally infected with avian influenza, including HPAI H5N1 and the zoonotic LPAI N7N9; but it is questionable how efficient these birds could be as vectors of avian influenza to other birds or animals.[22]

CURRENT HPAI DYNAMICS IN THE WORLD

Eurasian HPAI H5N1 continues to cause disease in both domestic poultry and wild birds across Asia and parts of Africa. It also continues to cause infections in humans, but to date has not increased in virulence or transmission potential in regard to its zoonotic capacity. However in Asia, HPAI H5N1 over the past decade or so has generated a number of reassortants including H5N2, H5N3, H5N5, H5N6, and H5N8. Of these reassortants, Eurasian HPAI H5N6 and H5N8 have proven to be particularly robust. This clade of Eurasian H5 viruses appears to be uniquely adapted to select species of dabbling ducks (genus *Anas* spp.) where the birds manifest infection asymptomatically and serve as reservoirs of the viruses without consequence. Eurasian HPAI H5N8 (EA H5N8) has spread to much of Asia and even made incursions into Europe in late 2014. EA H5N8 reached North America sometime in late 2014 and was detected in the United States in December 2014. Presumably, EA H5N8 arrived in wild migratory waterfowl from Asia during the migration season in 2014 via the Pacific flyway along the Aleutian chain. Shortly after EA H5N8's arrival, it reassorted with an endemic LPAI N2 virus to create Eurasian/North American HPAI H5N2 (EA/NA H5N2). Both EA H5N8 and EA/NA H5N2 have been detected in wild birds and domestic poultry in the Pacific, Central, and Mississippi flyways of the United States. Only the Atlantic or Eastern flyway has no reported detections to date (May 2015). EA H5N8 has also generated another reassortant, EA/NA HPAI H5N1, but this virus has only been found in a single wild bird and has not been detected since. These viruses appear to be moving in subclinically infected dabbling duck (mallards and their relatives) species and precipitating outbreaks in both commercial and backyard poultry, which intensified during the spring migration period of 2015. Disease in the wild bird population is rare (the viruses have only been detected in a few species other than dabbling ducks) but the dynamics of these viruses are still being studied in the many different avian species that are being exposed. However, both captive and wild raptors feeding on infected waterfowl have died from the disease in the United States, thus generating extreme concern within the falconry community. These Eurasian H5 viruses will likely persist in the wild migratory waterfowl compartment and may spread throughout all U.S. flyways at an increased prevalence in the fall of 2015, exposing both domestic poultry and other avian species to infection. What the ultimate fate of these Eurasian H5 viruses will be in North America is uncertain. They could potentially attenuate over time or be subsumed into the larger endemic LPAI community. Nevertheless, all holders of birds should be implementing good biosecurity practices and should notify their state animal health officials if diseased or dead birds are observed.

VACCINATION

Vaccination for avian influenza is strictly controlled in the United States by state and federal authorities because of the impact that seropositive birds may have on interstate and international commerce. Vaccination for LPAI (e.g., H1, H3) does occur in the United States for some species such as turkeys. However, vaccination for any H5 or H7 subtype is highly restricted to a case-by-case basis.

Nondomestic birds, including parrots, were vaccinated in zoos in Europe during the HPAI H5N1 crisis in the mid-2000s.[29] However, the likelihood of any nondomestic pet bird housed outdoors in a secure enclosure (excluding waterfowl and galliforms) being infected by a wild migratory waterfowl is low. Therefore, vaccination may provide no more additional protection of outdoor caged birds than does adequate biosecurity. Moreover, the performance of many vaccines and the vaccination schedule in nonpoultry species is not well defined. Therefore, vaccination of nondomestic avian species is done only under extreme situations.

There are many platforms of avian influenza vaccine available, ranging from inactivated (killed) to modified-live vectored vaccines. However, only inactivated or nonreplicating vectored vaccines would likely be recommended for nondomestic species should they become eligible for vaccination.

SUMMARY

Avian influenza is a complex virus that will continue to be a challenge to poultry production and other avicultural operations for the foreseeable future. The high mutability of the virus complicates vaccination efforts, but biosecurity practices coupled with surveillance and depopulation of infected birds helps control any outbreaks. While avian influenza has been detected in pet bird species, it is usually the result from spillover from the infected waterfowl or poultry compartments and does not naturally circulate in pet bird species in the wild. The risk that avian influenza poses to pet birds is largely a function of the potential exposure to infected high-risk species and disruptions in commerce caused by the presence of the disease.

REFERENCES

1. Scholtissek C: Molecular evolution of influenza viruses, *Virus Genes* 11:209–215, 1995.
2. Zambon MC: Epidemiology and pathogenesis of influenza, *J Antimicrob Chemother* 44(Suppl B):3–9, 1999.
3. Tong S, Li Y, Rivailler P, et al: A distinct lineage of influenza A virus from bats, *Proc Natl Acad Sci USA* 109:4269–4274, 2012.
4. Tong S, Zhu X, Li Y, et al: New world bats harbor diverse influenza a viruses, *PLoS Pathog* 9:e1003657, 2013.
5. Capua I, Alexander DJ: Avian influenza infection in birds: a challenge and opportunity for the poultry veterinarian, *Poult Sci* 88:842–846, 2009.
6. Center for Disease Control and Prevention. Spread of avian influenza viruses among birds. Department of Health and Human Services 2008. Available from: http://www.cdc.gov/flu/avian/gen-info/spread.htm. 2008.
7. Chen Y, Liang W, Yang S, et al: Human infections with the emerging avian influenza A H7N9 virus from wet market poultry: clinical analysis and characterisation of viral genome, *Lancet* 381:1916–1925, 2013.
8. Taubenberger JK, Kash JC: Influenza virus evolution, host adaptation and pandemic formation, *Cell Host Microbe* 7: 440–451, 2010.
9. Thontiravong A, Kitikoon P, Wannaaratana S: Quail as a potential mixing vessel for the generation of new reassortant influenza A viruses, *Vet Microbiol* 160:305–313, 2012.
10. Hecker RA, McIsaac M, Chan M, et al: Experimental infection of emus *(Dromaiius novaehollandiae)* with avian influenza viruses of varying virulence: clinical signs, virus shedding and serology, *Avian Pathol* 28:13–16, 1999.
11. Kishidal N, Sakoda Y, Isoda N et al: Pathogenicity of H5 influenza viruses for ducks, *Arch Virol* 150:1383–1392.
12. Altmuller A, Kunerl M, Muller K, et al: Genetic relatedness of the nucleoprotein (NP) of recent swine, turkey and human influenza A virus (H1N1) isolates, *Virus Res* 22(1):79–87, 1992.
13. Spackman E, Senne DA, Myers TJ, et al: Development of a real-time reverse transcriptase PCR assay for type A influenza virus and the avian H5 and H7 hemagglutinin subtypes. *J Clin Microbiol* 40:3256–3260, 2002.
14. Munch M, Nielsen L, Handberg K, et al: Detection and subtyping (H5 and H7) of avian type A influenza virus by reverse transcription-PCR and PCR-ELISA, *Arch Virol* 146: 87–97, 2001.
15. Starick E: Type- and subtype-specific RT-PCR assays for avian influenza viruses, *J Vet Med* 47(4):295–301, 2001.
16. Suarez D: Molecular diagnostic techniques: can we identify influenza viruses, differentiate subtypes and determine pathogenicity potential of viruses by RT-PCR? In: *Proceedings of the Fourth International Symposium on Avian Influenza*, 1998, pp 318–325.
17. Woolcock PR, Cardona CJ: Commercial immunoassay kits for the detection of influenza virus type A: evaluation of their use with poultry, *Avian Dis* 49:477–481, 2005.
18. Lu HG: A longitudinal study of a novel dot-enzyme-linked immunosorbent assay for detection of avian influenza virus, *Avian Dis* 47:361–369, 2003.
19. Slemons RD, Bruth M: Rapid antigen detection as an aid in early diagnosis and control of avian influenza. In: Swayne DE, Slemons RD, editors: Proceedings of the Fourth International Symposium on Avian Influenza, Athens, Georgia, 1998, pp 313–317.
20. Swayne DE, Senne DA, Beard CW: Influenza. In: Swayne DE, Glisson JR, Jackwood MW, et al, editors: *Isolation and identification of avian pathogens*, ed 4, Kennett Square, PA, 1998, American Association of Avian Pathologists, pp 150–155.
21. Watanabe T, Zhong G, Russell C, et al: Circulating avian influenza viruses closely related to the 1918 virus have pandemic potential, *Cell Host Microbe* 15:692–705, 2014.
22. Stallknecht D, Shane S: Host range of avian influenza virus in free-living birds, *Vet Res Comm* 12:125–141, 1988.
23. Vandergrift K, Sokolow S, Kilpatrick A: Ecology of avian influenza viruses in a changing world, *Ann NY Acad Sci* 1195:113–128, 2010.
24. Li K, Guan Y, Wang J, et al: Genesis of a highly pathogenic and potentially pandemic H5N1 virus in eastern Asia, 430:209–213, 2004.
25. Hawkins M, Crossley B, Osofsky A, et al: Avian influenza A virus subtype H5N2 in a red-lored Amazon parrot, *J Am Vet Med Assoc* 228:236–241, 2006.
26. Pillai S, Suarez D, Pantin-Jackwood M, et al: Pathogenicity and transmission studies of H5N2 parrot avian influenza virus of Mexican lineage in different poultry species, *Vet Microbiol* 129:48–56, 2008.
27. Mase M, Imada T, Y Sanada, et al: Imported parakeets harbor H9N2 influenza A viruses that are genetically closely related to those transmitted to humans in Hong Kong, *J Virol* 75:3490–3494, 2001.
28. Jones J, Sonnberg S, K Zeynep, et al: Possible role of songbirds and parakeets in transmission of influenza A(H7N9) virus to humans. *EID* 20:380–385, 2014.
29. Lecu A, De Langhe C, Petit T, et al: Serologic response and safety to vaccination against avian influenza using inactivated H5N2 vaccine in zoo birds, *J Zoo Wild Med* 40:731–743, 2009.

ASPERGILLOSIS

An Martel

Aspergillosis is one of the most frequently occurring mycotic diseases in birds and is caused by infection by the genus *Aspergillus*. Although other *Aspergillus* species such as *A. flavus, A. niger, A. glaucus, A. nidulans, A. terreus, A. clavatus, A. oryzae, A. ustus,* and *A. versicolor* have been isolated from patients with aspergillosis, *A. fumigatus* is the predominant species of this airborne infection.[1] The pathogenesis of this respiratory disease is still poorly understood. Acute or chronic disease can occur, varying in spectrum from local involvement to systemic dissemination. Although epizootics as flock diseases with severe mortality from brooder-borne or litter-sourced infection can occur, in most cases, only an individual is infected.

ETIOLOGY

A. fumigatus is a ubiquitous saprophytic ascomycetous fungus, which is identified on the basis of its macromorphology and micromorphology. The macromorphology comprises the features that can be observed with the naked eye or the stereomicroscope. Colonies are dark blue-green in color (Figure 2-14) and consist of a dense felt of conidiophores, intermingled with aerial hyphae.[2] Hyphae are the main mode of vegetative growth and are collectively called a *mycelium*.[3] To examine the micromorphology, a smear is stained with lactophenol blue or new methylene blue staining (Figure 2-15). The conidial heads (conidiophores or fruiting bodies) are columnar, resembling a "holy water sprinkler."[4] Conidiophores are specialized hyphae with a swollen end, known as *vesicle* (15–30 μm in diameter), from which the green phialides (5 to 9 μm length) directly arise. A chain of green smooth-walled conidia (2 to 3 μm in diameter) emerges from each phialide.[3]

A. fumigatus is a rapidly growing fungus and is thermophilic, with growth occurring at temperatures as high as 55° C, and survival at temperatures up to 70° C.[3,5] It grows rapidly on

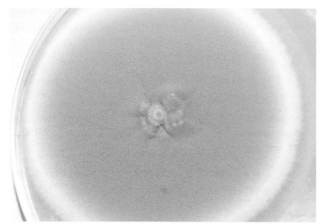

FIGURE 2-14 *Aspergillus fumigatus* culture grown on Sabouraud dextrose agar plate.

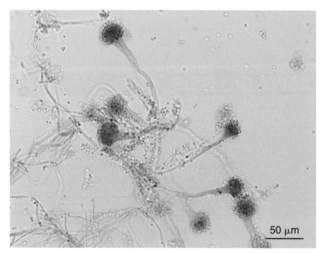

FIGURE 2-15 Lactophenol blue stain of a smear.

Sabouraud dextrose agar (see Figure 2-14), Czapek yeast agar or potato dextrose agar at 25° C to 37° C. Colonies develop a diameter of approximately 3 to 4 cm in 7 days. A young *A. fumigatus* colony is white but turns green to dark blue-green after a few days of growth due to sporulation. As the colony matures, conidial masses become gray-green, but the colony edge remains white (see Figure 2-14).

DISEASE PREDISPOSITION

The major risk factors for an *Aspergillus* infection are exposure to an overwhelming number of conidia and/or immunosuppression of the host. An overwhelming amount of spores can rapidly develop in a warm humid environment with poor ventilation and poor sanitation.[4,6,7] Besides, improperly stored feeds can be a source of fungal pathogens (*A. fumigatus*, *A. flavus*, *A. glaucus*, and *A. niger*).[8,9] In those feeds, not only the fungi but also immunosuppressive mycotoxins such as zearalenone, trichothecenes, aflatoxins, and/or fumonisins can be present.[10,11] Intensive production strategies, severe genetic manipulation, and inadequate management and husbandry practices of domestic birds may also weaken the immunologic

defense.[12,13] Other immunosuppressive factors that can predispose birds to aspergillosis include administration of tetracyclines, vaccination (e.g., against infectious bursal disease, infectious bronchitis, or Newcastle disease), overcrowding, shipping, quarantine or capture of wild birds, starvation, thermal discomfort, migration, inbreeding, *Psittacine circovirus* infection, lymphoproliferative disorders, toxicosis (e.g., heavy metals, being oil soaked), traumatic injuries, and reproductive activity.[1]

All bird species are considered particularly susceptible to aspergillosis, probably because of the anatomic and physiologic characteristics of the avian respiratory system compared with those of mammals and humans. These characteristics include the high average body temperature (38° to 45° C), which is favorable for the growth of thermophilic fungus; the absence of an epiglottis, which otherwise prevents particles from reaching the lower respiratory tract; the lack of a diaphragm, which disables a strong cough reflex; the limited distribution of ciliated epithelium through the respiratory tract; a greater respiratory surface area and a thinner air-blood capillary barrier; and the presence of an air sac system, which widely extends throughout most of the body.[7,12] The warm and oxygenated air sacs provide a favorable condition for the vegetative growth and even sporulation of *Aspergillus*.[7] In addition, the unidirectional air flow in the lungs and the bidirectional air flow in the air sacs hinder the elimination of inhaled particles.[14] The paucity of free respiratory macrophages in the avian respiratory system is also assumed to obstruct the respiratory immunity against respiratory pathogens, but this might be compensated by the phagocytic epithelial cells in the atria and infundibula, the pulmonary intravascular macrophages, and subepithelial macrophages, which can be efficiently translocated to the epithelial surface.[12,13,15-19]

A. fumigatus infections have been observed in a wide number of taxonomic orders, including Accipitriformes, Anseriformes, Charadriiformes, Ciconiiformes, Columbiformes, Falconiformes, Galliformes, Gruiformes, Gaviiformes, Passeriformes, Psittaciformes, Rheiformes, Sphenisciformes, Strigiformes, Struthioniformes, and Tinamiformes.[1] Although every bird species is intrinsically susceptible to the disease, some authors report some species to be more susceptible than others. Based on empirical data, several authors claim that birds of prey, especially gyrfalcon (*Falco rusticollis*) and hybrids, rough-legged hawk (*Buteo lagopus*), and red-tailed hawk (*Buteo jamaicensis*) are highly susceptible to aspergillosis.[7,21,22] In psittacines, the Grey parrot (*Psittacus erithacus*), the blue-fronted amazon (*Amazona aestiva*), and pionus parrots (*Pionus* spp.) seem highly susceptible.[4] Another group of birds considered extremely susceptible to infection are seabirds. Although there are a few sporadic cases reported for these birds in the wild, the incidence increases substantially in birds coming into captivity to be rehabilitated.[23,24] There have been a number of documented cases of aspergillosis in penguins, either during rehabilitation or in zoologic settings.[25-27] Most of these data are coming from observations of the prevalence of aspergillosis in avian clinics and zoos. Limited experimental studies concerning the true susceptibility of these presumptively highly susceptible species have been conducted. Because of the lack of scientific research in this area, it is not clear if these highly susceptible birds are intrinsically more susceptible to aspergillosis or if other factors such as stress renders them more vulnerable to develop the disease. Van Waeyenberghe[28] demonstrated that there was no difference in species susceptibility between 8-month-old Gyr-Saker hybrid falcons and pigeons to a single-dose exposure of 10^7 *A. fumigatus* conidia, supporting the latter hypothesis.

PATHOGENESIS OF ASPERGILLOSIS

Because of continuous inhalation of the ubiquitously present and small-sized *A. fumigatus* conidia, the respiratory system is primarily affected, although other body sites such as the eye or skin can be infected as well.[4,7,29-33] Some inhaled *A. fumigatus* conidia are not trapped in the nasal cavity and trachea and are therefore able to colonize the lungs and air sacs.[34] The tracheal bifurcation can also be infected due to conidia deposition in the narrow lumen. The consequences of colonization of *A. fumigatus* conidia ultimately depend on the interaction between the host immune system and the fungus.[35]

The *A. fumigatus* conidia that colonize the lung get embedded in the atria and in parts of the infundibula in the parabronchus and are first attacked by the phagocytic epithelial cells, subepithelial macrophages, and intravascular macrophages.[12,13,18,34] If the conidia overwhelm the immune defense, they break dormancy and start germinating by mitotic divisions.[4,36] Germination switches the fungal morphotype from unicellular conidia to multicellular hyphae, which extend and enable tissue invasion.[35] As the hyphae invade, tissues necrotize, and plaques are formed in the lung and respiratory tract and obstruct the trachea or bronchi or fill an air sac.[4] Occasionally, sporulation occurs in the aerated spaces of lungs and air sacs (Figure 2-16).[37,38]

Because hyphae are tissue invasive, extension of the infection can occur through the air sac wall to adjacent tissues and organ systems. In addition, hematogenous spread can occur.[39] In this circumstance, hyphae as well as host cells play a role in the hematogenous spread of infection. Conidia can become attached to erythrocytes or be ingested by respiratory macrophages and then carried by the bloodstream and the lymph stream to other organs.[40,41]

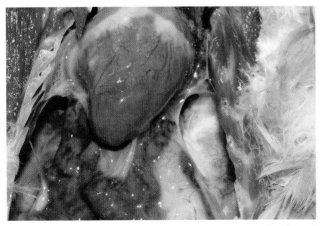
FIGURE 2-16 *Aspergillus fumigatus* granuloma in the air sacs of a Grey parrot.

Tissue reactions to *A. fumigatus* infections in birds can be granulomatous and/or infiltrative, depending on the immune status of the bird. The granulomatous form is characterized by a necrotic center containing hyphae and/or heterophils surrounded by abundant inflammatory cells, including giant cells, macrophages, and lymphocytes, and encapsulated by an outer layer of fibrous connective tissue. Neither exudative inflammation nor vascular lesions are seen in the neighboring tissues.[1] The infiltrative types of tissue reaction include exudative cellular inflammation with giant cells, macrophages, heterophils, and lymphocytes. In this type, the fungus frequently invades blood vessels and forms aggregates of radiating hyphae containing a large number of conidiophores and conidia without forming structured granuloma due to T-cell suppression.[1]

Host Immune Response to Aspergillosis

Both cellular and humoral immunity are involved in the bird's immune response to infection. Macrophages and heterophils play the primary role in phagocytizing the invading *A. fumigatus* conidia and hyphae, followed by antibody reactions for adaptive immunity.[42,43]

The respiratory macrophages form the early immune defense against *A. fumigatus* infection in birds.[42] Birds lack free respiratory macrophages in the respiratory system.[13,15,16] Instead, respiratory macrophages are present in the epithelia and the subepithelial interatrial septa of the atria and infundibula and can be reinforced by the pulmonary intravascular macrophages.[12,15,18,44] These macrophages can transmigrate from the epithelia and the interatrial areas or the vascular system into the air surface and play an important role in the removal of particles or pathogens from the air.[12,13,18-20] In vitro studies with *Aspergillus* conidia and avian macrophages demonstrate that they may prevent early establishment of infection unless the number of *A. fumigatus* conidia exceeds the macrophage killing capacity, leading to intracellular germination and lysis of the phagocytic cells, which may contribute to colonization of the respiratory tract.[45]

Immunosuppressive agents such as mycotoxins, frequently present in parrot feeds,[11] can alter the macrophage functions. It has been demonstrated that the mycotoxin T-2, on the one hand, impairs the antifungal activities of chicken macrophages against *A. fumigatus* conidial infection; on the other hand, it stimulates a proinflammatory response in infected macrophages, which might compensate for the observed macrophage functional impairment.[46] However, fungal growth in the presence of T-2 induces a stress response in *A. fumigatus*. The net outcome of decreased macrophage defense, increased proinflammatory response, and induction of fungal stress in birds exposed to T-2 is an overall exacerbation of aspergillosis.[47]

The avian immune response is regulated by cytokines, which can be produced by virtually every cell type, and chemokines are a group of cytokines that regulate leukocyte traffic. Recruitment of leukocytes (e.g., macrophages, heterophils, and dendritic cells) to the infection cite is primarily mediated by the interaction between the circulating leukocytes and the chemokines released from the infection cite.[48] Instead of the oxidative mechanisms used in neutrophils, heterophils use cationic proteins, hydrolases, and lysozymes to kill fungal hyphae, but more research is needed to elucidate the fungal killing mechanisms in avian heterophils.[7]

Also, the avian adaptive immune response against aspergillosis is poorly known.[49] A study of the humoral response of pigeons to *A. fumigatus* antigens showed an early rise of immunoglobulin M (IgM) and a later rise of IgG following injection of *A. fumigatus* culture filtrate.[21,50-53]

Aspergillus fumigatus Virulence Factors

Most airborne fungi rarely cause disease. This suggests that *A. fumigatus* produces specific virulence factors that are important for the fungus to colonize avian tissues. In humans, several factors, including phospholipase, protease, elastase, and gliotoxin, play a role in the pathogenesis of aspergillosis.[54-56] The relevance of these factors in avian aspergillosis is not well known because research concerning this subject in birds is minimal. One study conducted in turkeys revealed marked variability in pathogenicity between several *A. fumigatus* isolates.[57] Other studies in turkeys have considered that gliotoxin may be involved in the pathogenesis of aspergillosis.[58,59]

CLINICAL SIGNS AND LESIONS

Clinical manifestations of aspergillosis depend on the infection dose, the pathogen distribution, pre-existing disease, and the immune response of the bird. The disease may be either localized or diffuse but often causes a progressive illness leading to mortality if untreated. Although aspergillosis is predominantly a disease of the respiratory tract, any organ can be infected.[60] Avian aspergillosis is distinguished into two forms: acute and chronic.[1]

The *acute form* is thought to be caused by exposure to an overwhelming number of *Aspergillus* conidia.[61] Onset of clinical disease is rapid. The acute signs include dyspnea, anorexia, tail bobbing, open mouth breathing, and gasping. Potential general signs are acute depression, inappetence, vomiting, crop stasis, ascites, polydipsia, polyuria, and cyanosis. Death usually occurs within 7 days.[4,61,62] At necropsy, a white mucoid exudate and marked congestion of the lungs and air sacs can be noted. Although multiple foci of pneumonic nodules may be present, because of the rapid progress of the disease, large pulmonary granulomas are frequently absent. The *chronic form* is generally associated with immune suppression as a localized or disseminated disease.[62] The chronic signs include decreased appetite, lethargy, weight loss, change or loss of voice, cough, open beak breathing, cyanosis, polyuria, depression, and vomiting.[61,62] With the exception of *mycotic tracheitis*, little, if any, respiratory sign is seen at the beginning of the disease.[61,63] In case of tracheitis, a milky white tracheal discharge, loss of voice, and the occasional cough can be observed.[61,63] *Airsacculitis* with extension to the lungs, is the most frequently encountered form of the disease.[6] Aspergillomas may be found throughout the entire respiratory tract (see Figure 2-16; Figure 2-17).

Localized aspergillosis involving the upper respiratory tract often presents as chronic rhinitis and sinusitis (Figure 2-18), possibly accompanied by malformation of the nostrils, beak, and cere and a purulent nasal discharge.[33] Wheezing respiratory sounds may be caused by the formation of rhinoliths or oronasal granulomas obstructing the upper airways.

Mycotic keratitis can cause blepharospasm, photophobia, periorbital swelling, turbid discharge, swollen and adhered

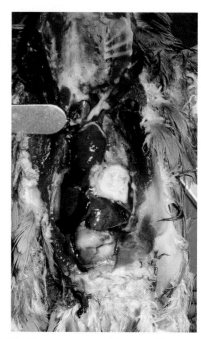

FIGURE 2-17 Air sac aspergilloma. (Courtesy Dr. Brian Speer.)

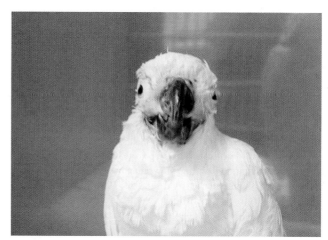

FIGURE 2-18 Chronic sinusitis in a citron crested cockatoo. (Courtesy Dr. Scott Ford.)

eyelids, cloudy cornea, and cheesy yellow exudates within the conjunctival sac.[30,31] Fungal infections of the eye are rare in birds, and most reported cases result from the extension of pre-existing upper respiratory infections, although ocular trauma and corticosteroid therapy are other predisposing factors.[30,31,64]

Encephalitic and meningoencephalitic lesions may occur with *disseminated aspergillosis*. Depression, unilateral wing drooping, paralysis, ataxia, weakness or general disinclination to move, unsteady gait, falling on the side or back, torticollis, and tremors are potential neurologic signs caused by *Aspergillus* infection.[65-67]

Epidermal cysts associated with *A. fumigatus* have been described in the comb of a silky bantam chicken.[32] Although necrotic granulomatous dermatitis from which *A. fumigatus* was isolated has been described in chickens, *cutaneous lesions* caused by *Aspergillus* occur rarely in avian species.[68]

DIAGNOSIS

Because the clinical signs of aspergillosis are nonspecific, the diagnosis of the disease is difficult.[39] Moreover, there is no single test that provides certainty. Most of the time, the diagnosis relies on an accumulation of evidence from history, clinical presentation, hematology and biochemistry, serologic tests, radiographic changes, endoscopy, and culture of the fungus.[53] Anamnesis can reveal a stressful event , some underlying environmental factors, and/or an immunosuppressive condition or treatment.[63] It may also reveal chronic debilitation, weight loss, voice change, and exercise intolerance.[4] Since clinical signs are nonspecific and depend on which aspergillosis form a bird develops and which organs are involved, aspergillosis should be included in the differential diagnosis of most respiratory tract diseases as well as systemic diseases.[39,53]

Unfortunately, aspergillosis is frequently diagnosed at postmortem examination, often based on identifying characteristic caseous nodules in the lungs or plaques in the air sacs, followed by cytologic and histologic examinations of the lesions and culturing of the fungus.

Hematology and Serum Chemistry

Hematology and serum chemistry in birds is considered rather indicative than diagnostic of any particular disease.[53] Leukocytosis of 20,000 to more than 100,000 white blood cells per microliter, heterophilia with a left shift (degenerative shift), monocytosis and lymphopenia, nonregenerative anemia, and increased serum total proteins are described in birds with aspergillosis.[b] An increase in β-globulins and an increase of β-globulins and/or γ-globulins can be noticed in acute and chronic infections, respectively. Multiple studies in birds stated a decreased concentration of albumin and a decreased A/G ratio as the most marked electrophoretic changes with aspergillosis.[70–72] In falcons with aspergillosis, lower prealbumin values were noted compared with healthy falcons.[73,74] However, immune-suppressed birds may have hypoproteinemia, and white cells may be in the normal range.[71,72,75]

Serum biochemical changes in specific organ parameters will vary, depending on the organ system affected, and are not specific to aspergillosis.

Antibody and Antigen Detection

Although humoral immunity is generally considered to have less importance than cellular immunity in fungal infections, it is possible to use the antibody response as a diagnostic aid.[57] However, in the acute stage, the antibody production trails behind antigen exposure by 10 to 14 days, and in case the bird is immunosuppressed, the low antibody production results in false-negative results.[21,51] In these cases, detection of circulating *Aspergillus* antigen in serum may be more helpful.[71] Also, high antibody titers against *Aspergillus* antigen have been demonstrated in healthy as well as in *A. fumigatus*-infected raptors.[74,76] Overall, negative serologic test results

do not rule out aspergillosis, and positive test results are only considered diagnostic by accumulation of evidence from other diagnostic aids.

Counter-immunoelectrophoresis is a technique that detects precipitating antibodies against *Aspergillus* spp. with the use of metabolic or somatic *A. fumigatus* antigens. The number and intensity of the precipitation vary in function of the precipitant antibody concentration.[77] Precipitating antibodies against *Aspergillus* spp. can also be measured by agar gel immunodiffusion.[57] Both tests, however, result in a poor sensitivity, possibly because of the requirement of a higher antibody concentration than commonly found in patients.[76]

An indirect enzyme-linked immunosorbent assay (ELISA) has been developed to detect antibodies against *Aspergillus* spp. (The Raptor Center at the University of Minnesota, Minneapolis, MN). Although false-negative results can occur, this assay appears to be a useful clinical tool, especially in the detection of subclinical cases of aspergillosis.[69,78] In a report of 23 falconiform birds with confirmed aspergillosis, 43% of the birds had moderate to marked antibody titers, whereas 22% had negative titers. In contrast, in the same study, the owls with confirmed aspergillosis had negative antibody titers.[78] In a study of captive penguins with confirmed aspergillosis, many birds had increased titers, and only 20% had negative antibody titers.[69] The indirect ELISA is limited by the inability of the conjugated antibodies to cross-react with all avian orders.[21,51]

A commercial direct ELISA Platelia *Aspergillus* kit (Bio-Rad, France), which was developed for humans, detects the fungal antigen galactomannan, a major cell wall constituent of *Aspergillus* species, in serum using rat monoclonal antibodies. Galactomannan levels have been 2.6-fold elevated in psittacines with aspergillosis.[79] False-positive results do occur[77,80] and may be explained by the cross-reaction with antigens of other organisms, feeding soybeans, and the use of beta-lactam antibiotics.[81–83] In addition, the sensitivity of this serologic test appears to be low to moderate.[71,77,84] Possible reasons for false-negative results are not well known. Cray[71] hypothesized that necrotic areas that are not nutrient or oxygen rich may decrease the amount of released galactomannan. Also, since galactomannan antigens are large, a degree of angioinvasion may be necessary for the antigen to reach the circulation. Finally, the report suggested that antibodies may bind to galactomannan reducing the test sensitivity.

Concentrations of (1→3)-ß-D-glucan in plasma samples have been shown to be significantly higher in aspergillosis-positive birds than in aspergillosis-negative birds, with the highest averaged values in infected sea birds, followed by companion birds, and raptors.[85]

In birds with aspergillosis confirmed by necropsy, the *Aspergillus* toxin fumigaclavine A (FuA) has been detected in air sac samples with the use of an enzyme immunoassay (EIA).[86,87] Little is known whether this EIA can be used in serum or plasma samples of birds. One study on experimentally infected falcons was not able to demonstrate FuA in blood samples.[74]

Radiology

Lateral radiography and ventrodorsal radiography are part of the routine clinical examination of a sick bird. Radiographic changes noticed in aspergillosis patients can be bronchopneumonia with a prominent parabronchial pattern; thickening of

---

[b]References 4,53,61,63,66,69.

the air sac walls, reducing the detail in the coelomic cavity; distinct nodular lesions; and/or air sac hyperinflation as a result of airway obstruction or loss of air sac compliance.[62] Although intraluminal granulomas of the syrinx, trachea, and main stem bronchi are fairly common, they can be seldom visualized radiographically.[6] Organ enlargement can be noticed in systemic disease. A disadvantage is that radiographic features indicating an *Aspergillus* spp. infection are only obvious in the late phase of the disease. In addition, the changes of pneumonia and consolidating airsacculitis are nonspecific, leading to a broad differential diagnosis that includes bacterial pneumonia, hypovitaminosis A, pulmonary hemorrhage or infarction, and neoplasia.[62]

Other imaging techniques such as computed tomography (CT) or magnetic resonance imaging (MRI) avoid the superposition of overlying structures and can be useful for demonstrating small lesions that are not visible on radiographs. However, the definitive diagnosis of aspergillosis still requires identification by biopsy, histopathology and/or cytology, or culture.[6]

Polymerase Chain Reaction

Polymerase chain reaction (PCR) assays have been developed for the diagnosis of human aspergillosis. Few reports of different PCR assays (including real-time PCR) tested on heparinized whole blood, tracheal washings, air sac fluids, respiratory tract granulomas, and (biopsy) tissue samples from birds support the value of this assay for the diagnosis of avian aspergillosis.[39,71]

Endoscopy

By using endoscopy, the respiratory tract, including choanal opening, glottis, trachea, syrinx, lung, and air sacs, and the coelomic cavity, can be evaluated. With this invasive technique, the lesions can be visualized and the extent as well as the progress of infection during treatment can be followed up (Figure 2-19).[21,53] Tracheal endoscopy is useful to visualize a lesion (e.g., a plaque or white discharge) occluding the trachea or syrinx (Figures 2-20 and 2-21). The use of bronchoscopy is limited by the size of the bird. Samples for culture,

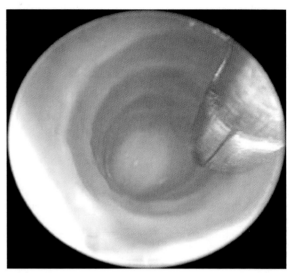

FIGURE 2-20 White discharge occluding the trachea as visualized by tracheal endoscopy. (Courtesy Dr. Brian Speer.)

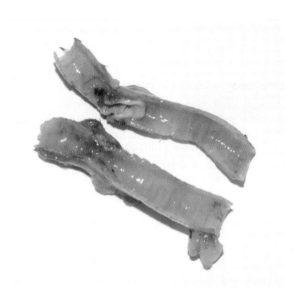

FIGURE 2-21 Aspergilloma of the syrinx in a mallard duck *(Anas platyrhynchos)*.

cytology, or histology should be taken directly with biopsy forceps or via air sac lavage.[4]

Cytology

Cytologic evaluation of clinical samples can aid the diagnosis of aspergillosis. Squash preparations are prepared and stained with lactophenol cotton blue of methylene blue stain. Conidiophores and hyphae can be identified.

Histopathology

Histologic characteristics can be indicative for aspergillosis (Figure 2-22), but because in-vivo hyphae of hyaline filamentous fungi are very similar and their in situ manifestations are not pathognomonic, this technique does not allow fungal species identification.[71,88] To identify *Aspergillus* spp. PCR or immunohistochemistry could be used using monoclonal or polyclonal antibodies.[67,88-91]

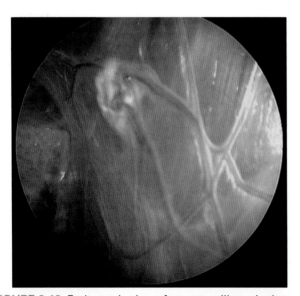

FIGURE 2-19 Endoscopic view of an aspergilloma in the cranial thoracic air sac of a hybrid falcon *(Falco rusticolis x F. cherrug)*.

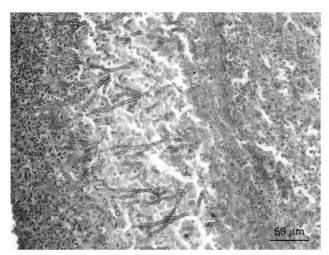

FIGURE 2-22 Hematoxylin and eosin staining from aspergilloma in a peacock.

Confirming the Diagnosis: Fungal Culture

Isolation of the fungus is considered the gold standard of an etiologic diagnosis of aspergillosis. However, it is important to mention that isolating the fungus alone is not confirming the infection because *Aspergillus* fungi are ubiquitous and can be a contaminant. An abundant culture from any organ is considered diagnostic. However, depending on the sample place (e.g., trachea swab), a negative culture does not rule out aspergillosis.[21]

TREATMENT

Treating avian aspergillosis is a challenge because of the limited knowledge regarding the pharmacokinetics of antifungal agents in different bird species; the presence of granulomatous inflammation, which makes it difficult for the drug to reach the fungus; the presence of concurrent disease and/or immunosuppression; and the late stage at which birds mostly are presented.[1] Prolonged antifungal therapy for periods up to 4 to 6 months or even greater is often necessary for treatment success.

Topical therapy after debulking the granulomatous lesions, in combination with an early, systemic antifungal therapy is recommended when the lesions can be easily removed. In most patients, however, granulomatous lesions are difficult to remove because of their location and/or extent. In these cases, only systemic antifungal therapy can be applied. Topical therapy can be administered through nebulization, nasal or air sac flushing, and endoscopic or surgical irrigation of abdominal cavities or lesions, while systemic therapy can be administered intravenously or orally.[4,6] A summary of the administration routes and doses of antifungal agents for birds is presented in Table 2-4.

Polyenes

Amphotericin B is a polyene macrolide that acts by binding to ergosterol, which is the principal sterol in the cell membrane of the fungus. This binding alters membrane permeability, causing leakage of sodium, potassium, and hydrogen ions and leads eventually to cell death.[92-94] In mammals, amphotericin B is nephrotoxic because of the binding to mammalian sterols (e.g., cholesterol) in the cell membrane. Pharmacokinetic studies with amphotericin B conducted in domestic turkeys and three raptor species reported that the half-life is much shorter than in mammals.[95] This finding may be responsible for the lack of nephrotoxicity in avian species in contrast to mammals.[80] Despite this fact, clinicians are still advised to monitor the renal function of their avian patients. Amphotericin B is fungicidal to a variety of organisms, including *Aspergillus* spp.[94] Native reduced susceptibility of *A. terreus* and *A. flavus* and acquired resistance in *A. fumigatus* to amphotericin B is documented.[96,97]

TABLE 2-4
Summary of the Administration Routes and Doses of Antifungal Agents Used for Treatment of Avian Aspergillosis

Antifungal Agent	Administration Route	Dose
Amphotericin B	Intravenous	1.5 mg/kg q8h 3–7 days (most species)[93,99]
	Intratracheal/nasal flush	1 mg/kg q8-12h, dilute to 1 mL with sterile water (psittacines, raptors)[114,115]
	Nebulized	7 mg/mL 15 min q12h (most species)[116]
Clotrimazole	Nasal flush	1% solution[93]
	Nebulized	1% solution, 30–60 min[116]
Enilconazole	Nebulized	0.1 mL/kg in 5 mL sterile water, 30 minutes q24h 5 days on/2 days off (raptors)[117]
Itraconazole	Oral	5–10 mg/kg q12-24h (toxicity is reported in Grey parrots: recommended dose for this species 2.5–5 mg/kg PO 24h)[114,118]
Ketoconazole	Oral	10–30 mg/kg q12h 21 days[99]
Terbinafine	Oral	15–30 mg/kg q12h[105]
	Nebulized	1 mg/mL solution (can be combined with itraconazole)[119]
Voriconazole	Oral	10 mg/kg q12h (chickens, pigeons, Grey parrots)[100,107,108]
		12–18 mg/kg q12h (Grey parrots)[120]
		12.5 mg/kg q12h (falcons)[121]

mg/kg, Milligrams per kilogram; mg/mL, milligrams per milliliter; min, minutes; q8h/q12h/q24h, every 8/12/24 hours; PO, orally; q8-12h, every 8 to 12 hours.

Amphotericin B has been used to treat both systemic and topical fungal infections in birds. It can be administered intratracheally, intravenously, in sinus flushes, and through nebulization. Topically, the drug can be very irritating to tissue, and to reduce the risk of iatrogenic sinusitis or tracheitis, the drug must be diluted in water (saline inactivates amphotericin B).

Azoles

Azoles inhibit the enzyme cytochrome P450-dependent 14-α-sterol demethylase, required for the conversion of lanosterol to ergosterol.[75,98] Exposed fungi become depleted of ergosterol and accumulate 14-α-methylated sterols. This causes disruption of membrane structure and function, thereby inhibiting fungal growth.[98] Vertebrates have slightly different cytochrome P450 enzymes compared with fungi. The relative toxicity of the drug depends on the specificity for binding the fungal enzyme instead of the vertebrate one.[93] The side effects of the azole family of drugs in general are anorexia, vomiting, and liver alterations.[99] With the exception of voriconazole, azoles are known to be fungistatic at the doses used in birds and need several days to reach steady-state concentrations.[61,80,93,100] Hence, months of therapy are often required to cure patients. Itraconazole (first-generation triazole) and voriconazole (second-generation triazole) are the azoles most thoroughly studied in birds. Pharmacokinetic studies with itraconazole were conducted in pigeons, amazon parrots, red-tailed hawks, and ducks.[7,94,101-104] These studies documented species-dependent variability, suggesting that different dosage regimens of itraconazole may be required for various species of birds. Grey parrots are reportedly more sensitive to itraconazole and may exhibit adverse drug effects (anorexia, depression, and death) at normal dosage levels. For voriconazole, a high interindividual variability, dose-dependent pharmacokinetics, and a possible induction of liver enzymes were found in raptors and Grey parrots.[100,105,106] In chickens, the bioavailability of orally administered voriconazole was found to be poor.[107] Compared with itraconazole, voriconazole shows good distribution to the tissues in which *A. fumigatus* is mostly located: the respiratory tract and the brain. Moreover, voriconazole may be a valuable alternative in Grey parrots that do not tolerate itraconazole.[105,108] Compared with amphotericin B, voriconazole has the advantage that it can be administered orally in addition to intravenously, which makes this drug suitable for long-term use in birds. However, since liver toxicity was observed in studies in racing pigeons, blood biochemistry should be closely monitored for potential side effects.[100] To maximize drug concentrations in the lungs, the upper respiratory system (nose and sinuses), and skin (in case of dermal aspergillosis) and to minimize adverse effects, topical treatment for localized aspergillosis is preferable to oral or intravenous treatment. However, it has been shown that nebulizing the intravenous formulation of voriconazole does not provide good plasma or lung concentrations in racing pigeons.[100] Nebulization of a nanosuspension of itraconazole is well tolerated by pigeons.[109] In poultry, enilconazole fumigation is frequently used to treat infected chicks and the litter. Acquired resistance of *A. fumigatus* strains to azoles is increasingly reported.[97,110]

Allylamines

Allylamines (terbinafine) act by inhibiting the ergosterol synthesis by interfering with squalene epioxidase, another key enzyme in the biosynthesis of ergosterol. In common with other antifungal agents that interfere with the biosynthesis of ergosterol, allylamines result in ergosterol depletion and accumulation of toxic sterols.[105] In pharmacokinetic studies in Grey parrots (15 and 30 milligrams per kilogram [mg/kg]) and raptors, no therapeutic concentrations were achieved in the plasma.[105] Despite these findings, some reports document successful treatment in birds using terbinafine or terbinafine combined with itraconazole, at a dosage of 15 milligrams per kilogram (mg/kg) orally every 12 hours.[105]

PREVENTION

In order to prevent aspergillosis, it is important to minimize the risk factors, which are an overload of spores and immunosuppression. Birds at high risk for aspergillosis can be treated prophylactically with antifungals during the risk period. In the presence of live animals, nebulization of facilities with commercial disinfectants is frequently used to lower the environmental load of *Aspergillus* spp. and the risk of infection.

A number of vaccination strategies have been attempted in birds, with the use of different preparations of vaccines, but the results have been inconsistent.[99,111,112] The use of the immunostimulant levamisole did not decrease aspergillosis associated lesions in turkeys.[102] In humans, clinical improvement of aspergillosis is documented after adding interferon-gamma and granulocyte-macrophage colony stimulating factor to the antifungal treatment.[113] Whether the favorable effect of these products could have value in future treatment protocols for avian aspergillosis is not known.

REFERENCES

1. Beernaert LA, Pasmans F, Van Waeyenberghe L, et al: *Aspergillus* infections in birds: a review, *Avian Pathol* 39:325–321, 2010.
2. de Hoog GS, Guarro J, Gené J, et al: Hyphomycetes genus: *Aspergillus*. In de Hoog GS, Guarro J, Gene J, Figueras MJ, editors: *Atlas of clinical fungi*, ed 2, Utrecht, The Netherlands, 2000, Centraal bureau voor Schimmelcultures and Universitat Rovira i Virgili, pp 442–518.
3. Klich MA: *Identification of common Aspergillus species*, Utrecht, 2002, Centraal bureau voor schimmelcultures.
4. Oglesbee BL: Mycotic diseases. In Altman RB, editor: *Avian medicine and surgery*, cd 1, Philadelphia, PA, 1997, W.B. Saunders Company, pp 323–361.
5. Latgé JP: *Aspergillus fumigatus* and aspergillosis, *Clin Microbiol Rev* 12:310–350, 1999.
6. Phalen DN: Respiratory medicine of cage and aviary birds, *Vet Clin N Am Exot Anim Pract* 3:423–452, 2000.
7. Tell LA: Aspergillosis in mammals and birds: impact on veterinary medicine, *Med Mycol* 43:S71–S73, 2005.
8. Khosravi AR, Shokri H, Ziglari T, et al: Outbreak of severe disseminated aspergillosis in a flock of ostrich (*Struthio camelus*), *Mycoses* 51:557–559, 2008.

9. Simpson VR, Euden PR: Aspergillosis in parrots, *Vet Rec* 128: 191–192, 1991.

10. EFSA: Scientific opinion on risks for animal and public health related to the presence of nivalenol in food and feed, *EFSA J* 11:3262, 2013.

11. Li S, Ediage EN, De Saeger S, et al: Occurrence and pathology of mycotoxins in commercial parrot feeds, *World Mycotoxin J* 6:449–453, 2013.

12. Maina JN: Some recent advances on the study and understanding of the functional design of the avian lung: morphological and morphometric perspectives, *Biol Rev* 77:97–152, 2002.

13. Nganpiep LN, Maina JN: Composite cellular defence stratagem in the avian respiratory system: functional morphology of the free (surface) macrophages and specialized pulmonary epithelia, *J Anat* 200:499–516, 2002.

14. Toth TE: Nonspecific cellular defense of the avian respiratory system: a review, *Dev Comp Immunol* 24: 121–139, 2000.

15. Ficken MD, Edwards JF, Lay JC: Induction, collection, and partial characterization of induced respiratory macrophages of the turkey, *Avian Dis* 30:766–771, 1986.

16. Maina JN, Cowley HM: Ultrastructural characterization of the pulmonary cellular defences in the lung of a bird, the rock dove, Columba livia. *P Ro Soc B-Biol Sci* 265:1567–1572, 1998.

17. Toth TE, Siegel PB: Cellular defense of the avian respiratory tract: paucity of free-residing macrophages in the normal chicken, *Avian Dis* 30:67–75, 1986.

18. Reese S, Dalamani G, Kaspers B: The avian lung-associated immune system: a review, *Vet Res* 37:311–324, 2006.

19. Kiama SG, Adekunle JS, Maina JN: Comparative in vitro study of interactions between particles and respiratory surface macrophages, erythrocytes, and epithelial cells of the chicken and the rat, *J Anat* 213:452–463, 2008.

20. Mutua PM, Gicheru MM, Makanya AN, et al: Comparative quantitative and qualitative attributes of the surface respiratory macrophages in the domestic duck and the rabbit, *Int J Morph* 29:353–362, 2011.

21. Redig PT: Diagnosis of avian aspergillosis, *Proc Annu Conf Assoc Avian Vet* 355–357, 1994.

22. Joseph V: Aspergillosis in raptors, *Semin Avian Exotic Pet* 9:52–58, 2000.

23. White FH, Forrester DJ, Nesbitt SA: *Salmonella* and *Aspergillus* infections in common loons overwintering in Florida, *J Am Vet Med A* 169:936–937, 1976.

24. Daoust PY, Conboy G, McBurney S, et al: Interactive mortality factors in common loons from Maritime Canada, *J Wildlife Dis* 34:524–531, 1998.

25. Carrasco L, Lima Jr JS, Halfen DC, et al: Systemic aspergillosis in an oiled Magallanic penguin *(Speniscus magellanicus)*, *J Vet Med* 48:551–554, 2001.

26. Khan ZU, Pal M, Paliwal DK, et al: Aspergillosis in imported penguins, *Sabouraudia* 15:43–45, 1977.

27. Flach EJ, Stevenson MF, Henderson GM: Aspergillosis in gentoo penguins *(Pygoscelis papua)* at Edinburgh Zoo, 1964 to 1988, *Vet Rec* 126:81–85, 1990.

28. Van Waeyenberghe L, Fischer D, Coenye T, et al: Susceptibility of adult pigeons and hybrid falcons to experimental aspergillosis, *Avian Pathol* 41:563–567, 2012.

29. Latgé JP: *Aspergillus fumigatus* and aspergillosis, *Clin Microbiol Rev* 12:310–350, 1999.

30. Beckman BJ, Howe CW, Trampel DW, et al: *Aspergillus fumigatus* keratitis with intraocular invasion in 15-day-old chicks, *Avian Dis* 38:660–665, 1994.

31. Hoppes S, Gurfield N, Flammer K, et al: Mycotic keratitis in a blue-fronted amazon parrot *(Amazona aestiva)*, *J Avian Med Surg* 14:185–189, 2000.

32. Suedmeyer WK, Bermudez AJ, Fales WH: Treatment of epidermal cysts associated with *Aspergillus fumigatus* and *Alternaria* species in a silky bantam chicken, *J Avian Med Surg* 16: 133–137, 2002.

33. Tsai SS, Park JH, Hirai K, et al: Aspergillosis and candidiasis in psittacine and passeriform birds with particular reference to nasal lesions, *Avian Pathol* 21:699–709, 1992.

34. Fedde MR: Relationship of structure and function of the avian respiratory system to disease susceptibility, *Poultry Sci* 77:1130–1138, 1998.

35. Ben-Ami R, Lewis RE, Kontoyiannis DP: Enemy of the (immunosuppressed) state: an update on the pathogenesis of *Aspergillus fumigatus* infection, *Br J Haematol* 150:406–417, 2010.

36. Momany M, Taylor I: Landmarks in the early duplication cycles of *Aspergillus fumigatus* and *Aspergillus nidulans*: polarity, germ tube emergence and septation, *Microbiology* 146:3279–3284, 2000.

37. Cacciuttolo E, Rossi G, Nardoni S et al: Anatomopathological aspects of avian aspergillosis, *Vet Res Commun* 33:521–527, 2009.

38. Nardoni S, Ceccherelli R, Rossi G, et al: Aspergillosis in *Larus cachinnans micaellis*: survey of eight cases, *Mycopathologia* 161:317–321, 2006.

39. Dahlhausen B, Abbott R, VanOverloop P: Rapid detection of pathogenic Aspergillus species in avian samples by Real-Time PCR assay: a preliminary report, *Proc 25th Annu Conf Assoc Avian Vet* 37–40, 2004.

40. Richard JL, Thurston JR: Rapid hematogenous dissemination of *Aspergillus fumigatus* and *Aspergillus flavus* spores in turkey poults following aerosol exposure, *Avian Dis* 27:1025–1033, 1983.

41. van Veen L, Dwars RM, Fabri THF: Mycotic spondylitis in broilers caused by *Aspergillus fumigatus* resulting in partial anterior and posterior paralysis, *Avian Pathol* 28:487–490, 1999.

42. Arné P, Thierry S, Wang D, et al: *Aspergillus fumigatus* in poultry, *Int J Microbiol*: 2011;2011:746356.

43. Richard JL, Cutlip RC, Thurston JR, et al: Response of turkey poults to aerosolized spores of *Aspergillus fumigatus* and aflatoxigenic and nonaflatoxigenic strains of *Aspergillus flavus*, *Avian Dis* 25:53–67, 1981.

44. Klika E, Scheuermann DW, De Groodt-Lasseel MH, et al: Pulmonary macrophages in birds (barn owl, *Tyto tyto alba*), domestic fowl *(Gallus gallus f. domestica)*, quail *(Coturnix coturnix)*, and pigeons *(Columbia livia)*, *Anat Rec* 246:7-97, 1996.

45. Van Waeyenberghe L, Pasmans F, D'Herde K, et al: Germination of *Aspergillus fumigatus* inside avian respiratory macrophages is associated with cytotoxicity, *Vet Res* 43:32–36, 2012.

46. Li S, Pasmans F, Croubels S, et al: T-2 toxin impairs antifungal activities of chicken macrophages against *Aspergillus fumigatus* conidia but promotes the pro-inflammatory responses, *Avian Pathol* 42: 457–463, 2013.

47. Li S, Dhaenens M, Garmyn A, et al: Exposure of *Aspergillus fumigatus* to T-2 toxin results in a stress response associated with exacerbation of aspergillosis in poultry, *World Mycotoxin J* in press.

48. Kaiser P, Stäheli P: Avian cytokines and chemokines. In Davison F, Kaspers B, Schat KA, editors: *Avian immunology*, London, U.K., 2008, Elsevier, pp 203–222.

49. Kaspers B, Kothlow S, Butter C: Avian antigen presenting cells. In Davison F, Kaspers B, Schat KA, editors: *Avian immunology*, London, U.K., 2008, Elsevier, pp 183–202.

50. Martinez-Quesada J, Nieto-Cadenazzi A, Torres-Rodriguez JM: Humoral immunoresponse of pigeons to *Aspergillus fumigatus* antigens, *Mycopathologia* 124:131–137, 1993.

51. Brown PA, Redig PT. Aspergillus ELISA: a tool for detection and management, *Proc Annu Conf Assoc Avian Vet* 295–300, 1994.

52. Davidow EB, Joslin J, Collins DM, et al: Serial *Aspergillus* antibody levels and serum protein electrophoresis as diagnostic and treatment monitoring technique in Humboldt penguins *(Spheniscus humboldti)*, *Proc Annu Conf Assoc Zoo Vet* 31–35, 1997.

53. Jones MP, Orosz SE: The diagnosis of aspergillosis in birds, *Semin Avian Exotic Pet* 9:52–58, 2000.

54. Gardiner DM, Waring P, Howlett BJ: The epipolythiodioxopiperazine (ETP) class of fungal toxins: distribution, mode of action, functions and biosynthesis, *Microbiology* 151:1021–1032, 2005.

55. Sugui JA, Pardo J, Chang YC, et al: Gliotoxin is a virulence factor of *Aspergillus fumigatus*: gliP deletion attenuates virulence in mice immunosuppressed with hydrocortisone, *Eukaryot Cell* 6:1562–1569, 2007.

56. Rementeria A, López-Molina N, Ludwig A, et al: Genes and molecules involved in *Aspergillus fumigatus* virulence, *Revista Iberoamericana de Micología* 22:1–23, 2005.

57. Peden WM, Rhoades KR: Pathogenicity differences of multiple isolates of *Aspergillus fumigatus* in turkeys, *Avian Dis* 36:537–542, 1992.

58. Richard JL, Peden WM, Williams PP: Gliotoxin inhibits transformation and its cytotoxic to turkey peripheral blood lymphocytes, *Mycopathologia* 126:109–114, 1994.

59. Richard JL, Dvorak TJ, Ross PF: Natural occurrence of gliotoxin in turkeys infected with *Aspergillus fumigatus*, Fresenius, *Mycopathologia* 134:167–170, 1996.

60. Dahlhausen RD. Implications of mycoses in clinical disorders. In Harrison GJ, Lightfood TL, editors: *Clinical avian medicine*, Palm Beach, FL, 2006, Spix Publishing, pp 691–704.

61. Vanderheyden N: Aspergillosis in psittacine chicks, *Proc Annu Conf Assoc Avian Vet* 207–212, 1993.

62. McMillan MC, Petrak ML: Retrospective study of aspergillosis in pet birds, *J Assoc Avian Vet* 3:211–215, 1989.

63. Jenkins J: Aspergillosis, *Proc Annu Conf Assoc Avian Vet* 328–330, 1991.

64. Kern TJ: Exotic animal ophthalmology. In Gelatt KN, editor: *Veterinary ophthalmology*, ed 3, Philadelphia, PA, 1999, Lippincot, Williams and Wilkins, pp 1273–1305.

65. Forbes NA: Aspergillosis in raptors, *Vet Rec* 128:263, 1991.

66. Forbes NA: Diagnosis of avian aspergillosis and treatment with itraconazole, *Vet Rec* 130:519–520, 1992.

67. Jensen HE, Christensen JP, Bisgaard M, et al: Immunohistochemistry for the diagnosis of aspergillosis in Turkey poults, *Avian Pathol* 26:5–18, 1997.

68. Ghazikanian GY: An outbreak of systemic aspergillosis caused by *Aspergillus flavus* in turkey poults, *J Am Vet Med Assoc* 194:1798, 1989.

69. Reidarson TH, McBain J: Serum protein electrophoresis and *Aspergillus* antibody titers as an aid to diagnosis of aspergillosis in penguins, *Proc Annu Conf Assoc Avian Vet* 61–64, 1995.

70. Cray C, Tatum LM: Applications of protein electrophoresis in avian diagnostics, *J Avian Med Surg* 12:4–10, 1998.

71. Cray C, Watson T, Rodriguez M, et al: Application of galactomannan analysis and protein electrophoresis in the diagnosis of aspergillosis in avian species, *J Zoo Wildlife Med* 40:64–70, 2009.

72. Ivey ES: Serologic and plasma protein electrophoretic findings in seven psittacine birds with aspergillosis, *J Avian Med Surg* 14:103–106, 2000.

73. Kummrow M, Silvanose C, Di Somma A, et al: Serum protein electrophoresis by using high-resolution agarose gel in clinically healthy and *Aspergillus* species-infected falcons, *J Avian Med Surg* 26:213–220, 2012.

74. Fischer D, Van Waeyenberghe L, Cray C, et al: Comparison of diagnostic tools for the detection of aspergillosis in blood samples of experimentally infected falcons, *Avian Dis* 58(4):587–598, 2014.

75. Flammer K, Orosz S: Avian mycoses: managing these difficult diseases, *Proc Annu Conf Assoc Avian Vet* 153–163, 2008.

76. Cray C, Watson T, Arheart KL: Serosurvey and diagnostic application of antibody titers to *Aspergillus* in avian species, *Avian Dis* 53:491–494, 2009.

77. Le Loch G, Deville M, Risis E, et al: Evaluation of the serological test *Platelia Aspergillus* for the diagnosis of aspergillosis, *Proc Eur Assoc Avian Vet Conf* 260–266, 2005.

78. Redig PT, Orosz S, Cray C: The ELISA as a management guide for aspergillosis in raptors, *Proc Annu Conf Assoc Avian Vet* 99–104, 1997.

79. Cray C, Reavill D, Romagnano A, et al: Galactomannan assay and plasma protein electrophoresis findings in psittacine birds with aspergillosis. *J Avian Med Surg* 23:125–135, 2009.

80. Orosz S, Martel A: Avian mycoses, *Proc Eur Assoc Avian Vet Conf* 249–259, 2009.

81. Stynen D, Sarfati J, Goris A, et al: Rat monoclonal antibodies against *Aspergillus* galactomannan, *Infect Immunity* 60:2237–2245, 1992.

82. Murashige N, Kami M, Kishi Y, et al: False-positive results of *Aspergillus* enzyme-linked immunosorbent assays for a patient with gastrointestinal graft-versus-host disease taking a nutrient containing soybean protein, *Clin Infect Dis* 40:333–334, 2005.

83. Viscoli C, Machetti M, Cappellano P, et al: False-positive galactomannan platelia *Aspergillus* test results for patients receiving piperacillin-tazobactam, *Clin Infect Dis* 38:913–916, 2005.

84. Arca-Ruibal B, Wernery U, Zachariah R, et al: Assessment of a commercial sandwich ELISA in the diagnosis of aspergillosis in falcons, *Vet Rec* 158:442–444, 2006.

85. Burco JD, Ziccardi MH, Clemons KV, et al: Evaluation of Plasma $(1\rightarrow3)$ β-D-glucan concentrations in birds naturally and experimentally infected with *Aspergillus fumigatus*, *Avian Dis* 56:183–191, 2011.

86. Latif H: *Development and application of an enzyme immunoassay for the detection of mycotoxin fumigaclavine A*, Giessen, Germany, 2010, Veterinary Faculty, Justus Liebig University.

87. Latif H, Curtui V, Ackermann Y, et al: Production and characterization of antibodies against fumigaclavine A, *Mycotox Res* 25:159–164, 2009.

88. Kaufman L, Standard PG, Jalbert M, et al: Immunohistologic identification of *Aspergillus* spp. and other hyaline fungi by using polyclonal fluorescent antibodies, *J Clin Microbiol* 35:2206–2209, 1997.

89. Carrasco L, Bautista MJ, de las Mulas JM, et al: Application of enzyme-immunohistochemistry for the diagnosis of aspergillosis, candidiasis and zygomycosis in three lovebirds, *Avian Dis* 37:923–927, 1993.

90. Beytut E, azcan K, Erginsoy S: Immunohistochemical detection of fungal elements in the tissues of goslings with pulmonary and systemic aspergillosis, *Acta Vet Hung* 52:71–84, 2004.

91. Beytut E: Immunohistochemical diagnosis of aspergillosis in adult turkeys, *Turk J Vet Anim Sci* 31:99–104, 2007.

92. Lyman CA, Walsh TJ: Systemically administered antifungal agents. A review of their clinical pharmacology and therapeutic applications, *Drugs* 44:9–35, 1992.

93. Flammer K: An overview of antifungal therapy in birds, *Proc Annu Conf Assoc Avian Vet* 1–4, 1993.

94. Orosz SE, Frazier DL: Antifungal agents: a review of their pharmacology and therapeutic indications, *J Avian Med Surg* 9:8–18, 1995.

95. Redig PT, Duke GE: Comparative pharmacokinetics of antifungal drugs in domestic turkeys, red-tailed hawks, broad-winged hawks, and great-horned owls, *Avian Dis* 29:649–661, 1985.

96. Aruajo R, Pina-Vaz C, Rodriguez AG: Susceptibility of environmental versus clinical strains of pathogenic *Aspergillus*, *Int J Antimicrob Agents* 108–111, 2007.

97. Ziolkowska G, Tokarzewski S, Nowakiewicz A: Drug resistance of *Aspergillus fumigatus* strains isolated from flocks of domestic geese in Poland, *Poultry Sci* 93:1106–1112, 2014.

98. Van den Bossche H, Willemsens G, Cools W, et al: Hypothesis on the molecular basis of the antifungal activity of N-substituted imidazoles and triazoles, *Biochem Soc T* 11:665–667, 1983.

99. Bauck L, Hillyer A, Hoefer H: Rhinitis: case reports, *Proc Annu Conf Assoc Avian Vet* 134–139, 1992.

100. Beernaert LA, Baert K, Marin P, et al: Designing voriconazole treatment for racing pigeons: balancing between hepatic enzyme auto induction and toxicity, *Med Mycol* 47:276–285, 2009.

101. Orosz SE, Schroeder E, Frazier DL: Itraconazole: a new antifungal drug for birds, *Proc Annu Conf Assoc Avian Vet* 13–16, 1994.

102. Perelman B: Evaluation of azole anti-mycotic agents using an experimental model of aspergillosis in turkey poults, *Proc Eur Conf Avian Med Surg* 120–126, 1993.

103. Lumeij JT, Gorgevska D, Woestenborghs R: Plasma and tissue concentrations of itraconazole in racing pigeons (*Columba livia domestica*), *J Avian Med Surg* 9:32–35, 1995.
104. Jones MP, Orosz SE, Cox SK, et al: Pharmacokinetic disposition of itraconazole in red-tailed hawks (*Buteo jamaicensis*). *J Avian Med Surg* 14:15–22, 2000.
105. Flammer K: Antifungal drug update, *Proc Conf Ass Avian Vet* 3–6, 2006.
106. Schmidt V, Demiraj F, Bailey T, et al: Plasma concentrations of voriconazole in falcons, *Proc Annu Conf Assoc Avian Vet* 323–326, 2006.
107. Burhenne J, Haefeli WE, Hess M, et al: Pharmacokinetics, tissue concentrations, and safety of the antifungal agent voriconazole in chickens, *J Avian Med Surg* 22:199–207, 2008.
108. Scope A, Burhenne J, Haefeli WE, et al: Pharmacokinetics and pharmacodynamics of the new antifungal agent voriconazole in birds, *Proc Eur Assoc Avian Vet Conf* 217–221, 2005.
109. Krautwald-Junghanns ME, Schmidt V, Vorbrüggen S, et al: Inhalative nanosuspensions – the future of avian antimycotic therapy? *Proc Int Conf Avian Herp Exot Mammal Med* 232, 2013.
110. Beernaert LA, Pasmans F, Van Waeyenberghe L, et al: Avian *Aspergillus fumigatus* strains resistant to both itraconazole and voriconazole, *Antimicrob Agents Ch* 53:2199–2201, 2009.
111. Richard JL, Peden WM, Sacks JM: Effects of adjuvant-augmented germling vaccines in turkey poults challenged with *Aspergillus fumigatus*, *Avian Dis* 35:93–99, 1991.
112. Meredith A: Prophylactic administration of itraconazole for the control of aspergillosis in Gentoo penguins (*Pygoscelis papua*), *Proc Eur Conf Assoc Avian Vet* 227–232, 1997.
113. Bandera A, Trabattoni D, Ferrario G, et al: Interferon-gamma and granulocyte-macrophage colony stimulating factor therapy in three patients with pulmonary aspergillosis, *Infection* 36:368–373, 2008.
114. Redig P: Medical management of birds of prey. In Samour J, editor: *Avian medicine*, London, U.K., 2000, Harcourt Publishers, pp 275–291.
115. Ritchie BW, Harrison GJ. Formulary. In Ritchie BW, Harrison GJ, Harrison LR, editors: *Avian medicine: principles and application*, Lake Worth, FL, 1997, Wingers Publishers, pp 227–253.
116. Tully TN Jr.: Birds. In Mitchell MA, Tully TN Jr., editors: *Manual of exotic pet practice*, St. Louis, MO, 2009, Saunders, pp 250–298.
117. Heatley JJ, Gill H, Crandall L, et al: Enilconazole for treatment of raptor aspergillosis, *Proc Annu Conf Assoc Avian Vet* 287–288, 2007.
118. Orosz SE, Jones MP, Cox SK, et al: Pharmacokinetics properties of itraconazole in blue-fronted Amazon parrots (*Amazona aestiva aestiva*), *J Avian Med Surg* 10:168–173, 1996.
119. Rabadaugh SC, Lindstrom JG, Dahlhausen B: The use of terbinafine hydrochloride in the treatment of avian fungal disease, *AAV Clin Forum* 2007;2007:5-7.
120. Flammer K, Nettifee-Osborne JA, Webb DJ, et al: Pharmacokinetics of voriconazole after oral administration of single and multiple doses in African grey parrots (*Psittacus erithacus timneh*), *Am J Vet Res* 69:114–121, 2008.
121. Schmidt V, Demiraj F, Di Somma A, et al: Plasma concentrations of voriconazole in falcons, *Vet Rec* 161:265–268, 2007.

COCCIDIAL DISEASES OF BIRDS

James F. X. Wellehan Jr.

BIOLOGY OF COCCIDIA

Coccidia are one of the groups of single-celled parasitic eukaryotes in the phylum Apicomplexa. The Apicomplexa may be distinguished by the presence of an apicoplast, an organelle derived from an endosymbiont much like a mitochondrion or chloroplast. This organelle is essential for the organism's survival and serves as a useful drug target. Related noncoccidial Apicomplexa include the hemosporidians (e.g., *Plasmodium*, *Leucocytozoon*) and the piroplasms (e.g., *Babesia*, *Theileria*). Within the Apicomplexa, the taxa known as coccidia include the families Cryptosporidiidae, Eimeriidae, and Sarcocystidae. Initial morphologic identification has resulted in a number of errors in coccidian taxonomy that have been revealed with deoxyribonucleic acid (DNA) sequence-based phylogeny. Evidence has emerged that the Cryptosporidiidae are more closely related to other apicomplexan taxa than to the Eimeriidae and Sarcocystidae,[1] and this is reflected in their biology and medical treatment. However, for the purposes of this discussion, these three families and their members affecting the Dinosauria will be discussed.

An important consideration when dealing with coccidia is the life cycle of the organism. Some taxa have direct life cycles, involving only one definitive host, whereas others have indirect life cycles, utilizing an intermediate host for asexual reproduction and a definitive host for sexual reproduction. Although some pathology such as causing diarrhea may help with transmission, killing the definitive host is typically disadvantageous for a parasite; it loses its breeding habitat. Coccidian evolution therefore involves significant selective pressure against killing definitive hosts. However, when the parasite is in the intermediate host, the life cycle is most typically completed by the definitive host eating the intermediate host. A bird with encephalitis caused by *Toxoplasma gondii* is more likely to be eaten by a cat. Causing significant disease in the intermediate host may therefore be advantageous, and the most significant pathology is seen in intermediate hosts. Management of coccidial disease in an avian collection requires knowledge of the life cycle; management of coccidia with indirect life cycles is centered on separating intermediate and definitive hosts, whereas management of coccidia with direct life cycles centers on hygiene. It is therefore crucial to properly identify coccidian species for effective management.

CRYPTOSPORIDIIDAE OF BIRDS

The family Cryptosporidiidae contains one genus, *Cryptosporidium*. Cryptosporidiidae are more closely related to other apicomplexan taxa than to the Eimeriidae and Sarcocystidae,[1] and this is reflected in their biology and response to pharmacologic therapy. Cryptosporidia develop on the apical surface of the epithelium in the gastrointestinal, respiratory, and urinary tracts. All cryptosporidia have direct life cycles. Management centers on exclusion of *Cryptosporidium* spp. from collections through quarantine surveillance and by disinfection of contaminated areas. *Cryptosporidium* spores are exceptionally stable in the environment; they are not very susceptible to ultraviolet disinfection, and even 6% bleach with a 2-hour contact time was shown to only result in 92.7% reduction. Chloro-m-cresol was more effective.[2] Cleaning should involve as much mechanical removal of feces as possible.

There are many species of *Cryptosporidium* with significantly different clinical implications. The vast majority of *Cryptosporidium* spp. seen in birds are still unnamed. Morphologic species identification is not reliable, and sequence-based techniques are needed to differentiate species.[3] The known species of *Cryptosporidium* form two clades, one with gastric tropism and one with primarily intestinal tropism (and sometimes respiratory or urinary tropism), indicating that the site of infection has had greater long-term fidelity than host species.[4] This is useful for the prediction of the site of infection of unknown species lacking histologic data; *Cryptosporidium* avian "genotype IV" has only been identified through fecal surveillance but would be expected to be gastrotropic.[5] Knowledge of the site of infection of a given *Cryptosporidium* spp. is also important for diagnostic sampling. Gastric lavage was found to be a better sample for detection of *C. serpentis*, a gastrotropic species found in snakes compared with cloacal swabs; this would not be expected for a species tropic for the cloaca.[4] Gastrotropic *Cryptosporidium* spp. tend to be associated with decreased appetite, weight loss, and chronic vomiting.[5] Enterotropic *Cryptosporidium* spp. tend to be primarily associated with weight loss and diarrhea. *Cryptosporidium* spp. tropic for the urinary tract have been associated with gout and renal failure.[5] *Cryptosporidium* spp. tropic for the respiratory tract have been associated with respiratory distress, otitis, and ocular disease.[6]

Cryptosporidium spp. vary significantly in their host specificity; some are highly tropic for one host taxon, whereas others have a broad host range. Within species infecting bird hosts, *C. meleagridis*, an enterotropic species first described in turkeys, has the broadest known host range.[5] Initially discovered in turkeys, it affects a wide range of avian species, including parrots, chickens, partridges, and columbiform birds, and has also been reported in dogs, cattle, pigs, rabbits, and rodents, and is zoonotic.[5–8] In companion psittacines, most infections are caused by species that have yet to be named. Specifics of select species may be seen in Table 2-5.

EIMERIIDAE OF BIRDS

The family Eimeriidae contains several different genera, not all of which have proven to be valid when further examined with sequence data. The clinically relevant genera in avian hosts include *Caryospora*, *Eimeria*, and *Isospora*. Eimeriidae typically have direct life cycles but may facultatively have indirect life cycles as well. There are diverse species with significantly different clinical implications. Specifics of select taxa may be seen in Table 2-6.

Caryospora are an Eimeriid genus with both direct and indirect life cycles, containing more than 25 species. Oocysts have a single sporocyst with eight sporozoites. Carnivorous birds and other carnivorous reptiles serve as definitive hosts, in which *Caryospora* spp. replicate in the intestines. Known intermediate hosts are typically prey mammals, in which extraintestinal tissue cysts may be in the skin. However, birds may also be directly infected with oocysts shed by another bird.[9] Clinical signs in carnivorous birds center around enteritis, with weight

TABLE 2-5
Select Cryptosporidiidae Infecting Birds

Species	Site	Known Affected Species
C. galli	Gastric	Diverse avian species
C. "avian genotype III"	Gastric	Psittacines, passerines, gulls
C. meleagridis	Intestinal	Diverse vertebrates, zoonotic
C. baileyi	Respiratory, ocular	Diverse avian species
C. "avian genotype V"	Urinary tract, cloaca	Psittacines, green iguana

loss and diarrhea being the most commonly seen signs. Management is focused on the exclusion of *Caryospora* spp. from collections through quarantine surveillance, disinfection of contaminated areas, and breaking the life cycle by obtaining food animals that are free of *Caryospora*. Mammals beyond those normally preyed upon by birds may be intermediate or aberrant hosts; dogs and pigs are susceptible to *Caryospora* dermatitis, and the concern of possible zoonotic infection exists.[10]

Eimeria is a diverse eimeriid genus with direct life cycles, containing more than 200 species infecting birds. Oocysts have four sporocysts, each of which contains two sporozoites. Most species replicate in intestinal epithelium, but some species replicate in renal tubular epithelium, and disseminated visceral infections are a significant problem in cranes. Management focuses on the exclusion of *Eimeria* spp. from collections through quarantine surveillance and disinfection of contaminated areas.

Eimeria spp. tend to be very host specific, and host jumping between distantly related avian taxa is rare. However, there are potential concerns for transmission between more closely related taxa; *E. dunsingi*, first identified in budgerigars with intestinal coccidiosis, has been found to be capable of infecting the enterocytes of musk lorikeets.[5,10] In the case of enterotropic species, disease tends to be most significant in young or otherwise compromised birds; co-infections with agents such as adenoviruses may play significant roles in disease manifestation. Infections in otherwise healthy adult animals are often subclinical. Nephrotropic *Eimeria* infection may result in signs such as weakness, depression, and wasting and has been associated with mortality events, but many infections may be subclinical.[11]

The most significant eimerian pathology is seen with disseminated visceral coccidiosis in cranes, with *E. reichenowi* and *E. gruis* being the most common etiologies. These agents appear to infect all crane species. Cranes may display weakness, lethargy, diarrhea, and oral granulomas. Again, subclinical infections are also common. Necropsy may reveal additional disseminated granulomas, most commonly in the liver. Infection is disseminated via the peripheral blood monocytes and can be seen on a blood smear, bearing significant resemblance to extraintestinal *Isospora* infection in passerines. Oocysts are then produced in both the lungs and the intestine.

Isospora is a diverse eimeriid genus with direct life cycles. Oocysts have two sporocysts, each of which contains four sporozoites. However, molecular sequence data have shown

TABLE 2-6

Select Eimeriidae Infecting Birds

Species	Site in Avian Host	Known Affected Species	Life Cycle	Intermediate Host	Notes
Caryospora sp.	Intestinal	Carnivorous birds	Indirect or Direct	Typically small mammals	Potentially zoonotic
Eimeria dunsingi	Intestinal	Budgerigar, Musk lorikeet, Musschenbroek's lorikeet	Direct	None	No sequence data
E. psittacina	Unknown, likely intestinal	Budgerigar	Direct	None	No sequence data
E. haematodi	Unknown, likely intestinal	Rainbow lorikeet	Direct	None	No sequence data
E. aestivae	Unknown, likely intestinal	Blue-fronted Amazon	Direct	None	No sequence data, morphologically similar to *E. aratinga*
E. amazonae	Unknown, likely intestinal	Yellow-crowned amazon	Direct	None	No sequence data, morphologically similar coccidian seen in blue-fronted Amazon
E. ochrocephalae	Unknown, likely intestinal	Yellow-crowned amazon	Direct	None	No sequence data
E. aratinga	Unknown, likely intestinal	Orange-fronted conure	Direct	None	No sequence data, morphologically similar to *E. aestivae*
E. ararae	Unknown, likely intestinal	Blue-and-gold macaw	Direct	None	No sequence data
E. auritusi	Renal	Double-crested cormorant	Direct	None	
E. truncata	Renal	Canada goose, Lesser snow goose, gray-lag goose	Direct	None	No sequence data
E. reichenowi	Disseminated	Cranes	Direct	None	
E. gruis	Disseminated	Cranes	Direct	None	
Isospora greineri	Disseminated	Superb starlings	Direct	None	
I. superbusi	Disseminated	Superb starlings	Direct	None	

conclusively that what was formerly considered *Isospora*, based on sporulation patterns, consisted of two evolutionarily distinct groups. The presence or absence of Stieda bodies, the use of paratenic hosts, and reptilian or mammalian host specificity are more phylogenetically informative than the number of sporocysts or sporozoites for these genera.[12] All former *Isospora* spp. of mammals are members of the Sarcocystinae, not the Eimeriidae, and were moved into the new genus *Cystoisospora*. All true *Isospora* spp. utilize reptilian hosts, including the Dinosauria (birds). The diversity of *Isospora* has not been well defined; although there are over 140 species in birds referred to in the literature, much of this is based on the likely incorrect assumption of host specificity; experimental data have shown that *Isospora* infection in evening grosbeaks could be transmitted to other passerine species but not to ducks.[13] There are only 10 named true *Isospora* spp. for which sequence data are currently available; the majority of publically available sequence data is not associated with named organisms. Most species replicate in intestinal epithelium, but some species have extraintestinal stages that may be associated with significant pathology. Species with extraintestinal stages are found in passerine birds and were formerly known as *Atoxoplasma* but have now been shown not

to be distinct from *Isospora*.[12] Similar to *E. reichenowi* and *E. gruis* in cranes, after initial infection in the small intestine, the peripheral blood mononuclear leukocytes are infected, and the infection is disseminated to other tissues, especially the liver and the lungs. Transmission is primarily by the fecal–oral route, but it has been hypothesized that hematophagous arthropods may also serve as vectors. Systemic isosporosis has been recognized as important in passerines, having caused significant mortality in captive populations of the endangered Bali mynah.

SARCOCYSTIDAE OF BIRDS

The family Sarcocystidae contains several different genera, not all of which have proven to be valid when further examined. The clinically relevant genera in avian hosts include *Sarcocystis*, *Toxoplasma*, and *Neospora*. Sarcocystidae typically have indirect life cycles, although some species may be facultatively direct in their definitive hosts. There are diverse species with significantly different clinical implications. Specifics of select taxa may be seen in Table 2-7.

Sarcocystis are a sarcocystid genus with obligate indirect life cycles, containing more than 120 known species. Some species

TABLE 2-7

Select Sarcocystidae Infecting Birds

Species	Site in Avian Host	Known Affected Avian Species	Definitive Host	Intermediate Host	Notes
Sarcocystis falcatula	Disseminated	Diverse avian hosts	Virginia opossum	Diverse birds	
Sarcocystis calchasi	Intestinal in hawks, disseminated in other species	Pigeons, parrots	Hawks	Diverse birds	Likely further avian hosts susceptible
Toxoplasma gondii	Disseminated	Diverse avian hosts	Cats	Diverse animals	Zoonotic
Neospora caninum	Disseminated	Passerines, parrots, pigeons	Dogs	Diverse animals	Galliform birds not susceptible

utilizing raptors as definitive hosts were formerly known as *Frenkelia* but have now been shown not to be distinct from *Sarcocystis*.[14,15] Oocysts have two sporocysts with four sporozoites, similar to *Isospora* in the Eimeriidae. Carnivorous or omnivorous vertebrates serve as definitive hosts, in which *Sarcocystis* spp. replicate in the intestines. Clinical disease in definitive hosts includes enteritis, with weight loss and diarrhea being the most common signs. Definitive host ranges tend to be more limited than intermediate host ranges. Intermediate hosts are prey animals, in which initial stages replicate in blood vessels, followed by the development of sarcocysts in tissues, commonly muscle. Sarcocysts are often grossly visible and may appear as white streaks in muscle. The most significant disease is seen in intermediate hosts, in which signs may include depression and sudden death. The most clinically significant species of *Sarcocystis* seen in birds are *S. falcatula*, which uses Virginia opossums as definitive hosts, and *S. calchasi*, which uses hawks in the genus *Accipiter* and possibly *Buteo* as definitive hosts.[16] Management focuses on excluding *Sarcocystis* spp. from collections through separation of definitive hosts and their feces from intermediate hosts. It is not uncommon for Virginia opossums or hawks to perch on top of outdoor avian enclosures, and thus their feces fall inside.

Toxoplasma is a sarcocystid genus with a facultatively indirect life cycle, containing one species, *T. gondii*. Cats are the definitive hosts. *T. gondii* has very little specificity for intermediate hosts and is a zoonotic disease. All avian species should be considered susceptible intermediate hosts; those that ingest other intermediate hosts or cat feces are at greater risk, and pigeons and canaries are most likely to present with clinical disease.[16a] Clinically, toxoplasmosis may mimic systemic isosporosis in passerines. Management focuses on excluding *T. gondii* from collections through exclusion of cats and cat feces and, in the case of carnivorous and omnivorous birds, exclusion of potential other intermediate hosts that may be ingested.

Neospora is a sarcocystid genus with a facultatively indirect life cycle, containing two species, *N. caninum* and *N. hughesii*. Dogs are the definitive hosts. Although ruminants are the best-studied intermediate hosts, diverse species may be infected. It is not known to be zoonotic. One of four experimentally infected pigeons died with these organisms found in the lungs, heart, central nervous system, liver, spleen, and kidney.[17] *Neospora* has also been identified in wild parrots and passerines; however, quail are resistant to infection.[18]. Management centers around

excluding *Neospora* from collections through the exclusion of dogs and dog feces and, in the case of carnivorous and omnivorous birds, exclusion of other potential intermediate hosts that may be ingested.

DIAGNOSIS OF COCCIDIAL DISEASES

When dealing with coccidian species that utilize birds as definitive hosts, fecal flotation is often the best screening test, especially for strictly enteric species. There are circadian differences in the shedding of at least some coccidia; *I. lesouefi* in regent honeyeaters was identified in 21% of fecal samples shed in the morning and 91% of samples shed in the afternoon.[19] This timing has been observed in other *Isospora* spp., and afternoon fecal samples should be chosen. *Cryptosporidium* spp. have relatively few distinguishing features, but do stain acid-fast positive unless they have been formalin fixed, so an acid-fast stain may improve detection. When dealing with gastrotropic *Cryptosporidium* spp., a gastric wash is preferable to a fecal sample; this is reversed for intestinal species. For species that are found in peripheral blood, such as *Toxoplasma*, *Isospora* spp. in passerines, or *Eimeria* spp. in cranes, examination of blood smears is helpful for detection. Organisms may be seen in mononuclear leukocytes. After identification in blood, gastric wash, or feces, species identification is indicated to determine the life cycle for disease management.

Diagnosis of coccidiosis in indirect hosts is significantly more challenging. The first sign seen in indirect hosts is often death, and a necropsy may be the first feasible diagnostic test. With *Sarcocystis* spp., light-colored sarcocysts may or may not be visible in the muscle on gross examination, but typically nothing specific is seen without histopathology. It is important to collect a set of tissues in formalin for histopathology as well as a set of tissues frozen without formalin for additional diagnostics, as indicated by histopathology. Once a coccidian agent has been identified histopathologically, species identification is indicated to determine the life cycle for disease management.

Historically, morphologic identification was used for coccidian identification, but this resulted in numerous errors. Organisms now known to be in two different families had been classed as *Isospora*, and *Cryptosporidium* spp. cannot be reliably differentiated morphologically.[3] With carnivorous birds, it is not uncommon to see pass-through in the feces of coccidia from prey that are clinically irrelevant.

Immunodiagnostics are also possible in some cases. However, especially in avian species whose coccidial diversity has not been well studied, there is concern of nonspecific cross-reactivity of antibodies against as-yet unstudied, but antigenically related, species. Although antibody cross-reactivity does correlate with genetic distance, small genetic distances may be highly clinically significant.

DNA-based methods are the diagnostic modality of choice. The methods most commonly used are based on polymerase chain reaction (PCR). Primers may be designed to be very specific for a given species or even strain or may be designed for regions conserved across a wider taxonomic group. Pan-coccidial primers have been used to discover diverse novel taxa.[20,21] Validation of primers is critical, and laboratories should provide a peer-reviewed publication on the validation of a given primer set for diagnostic use to clinicians for evaluation. Once a PCR product has been amplified, it is then essential to validate that product. Older methods included gel electrophoresis, restriction digestion, and SYBR-green real-time PCR. None of these methods sufficiently identifies the sequence of the product, and they should not be considered acceptable. Acceptable methods of product identification for diagnostic use include DNA sequencing and probe hybridization quantitative PCR (qPCR, or TaqMan real-time PCR).

DNA sequencing provides not only the possibility of identifying known organisms but also the characterization of novel organisms by comparison to reference sequences and subsequent phylogenetic analysis. Although capable of identifying novel organisms, it is slower and more labor intensive than probe hybridization qPCR.

Probe hybridization qPCR involves a probe with a dye that matches the expected sequence between the two primers. With proper temperature and salt conditions, the probe will not bind unless it matches perfectly. This allows the product to be validated while the PCR is running. The more of the target DNA in the sample, the fewer rounds of PCR are required to release a threshold amount of dye. This can be measured against a standard curve of known amounts of target DNA, enabling measurement of the amount of target DNA in a sample. Knowing the amount of target pathogen in a lesion may be important for assessing clinical significance. When well designed and properly validated to ensure the assay specifically identifies only the target DNA, probe hybridization qPCR can be a sensitive, specific, rapid, quantitative, and relatively inexpensive test. Proper validation is critical, and laboratories should provide a peer-reviewed publication on the validation of a given probe hybridization qPCR assay for diagnostic use to clinicians for evaluation.

TREATMENT OF COCCIDIAL DISEASES

Central to any coccidial treatment and control plan is an understanding of the life cycle of the species and appropriate management changes. Without appropriate management changes, pharmacologic therapy will fail. For species with indirect life cycles, removing access to other hosts in the life cycle is critical. Coccidial species utilizing the avian species of concern as a definitive host require strict hygiene to prevent reinfection; moving birds to a simpler,

more easily cleaned enclosure may be necessary. *Cryptosporidium* spp. are especially stable in the environment and resistant to many disinfectants.[22] Peroxide-based disinfectants are the most effective without resorting to toxic agents such as gluteraldehyde. Disinfection should focus on mechanical removal of all feces. Drying will reduce coccidial persistence, and ultraviolet irradiation is also helpful for disinfection.[23]

As eukaryotic parasites, coccidia have diverged more recently from animals compared with bacteria. Antimicrobial drugs target biochemical differences between a pathogen and a host, and there are fewer differences between a coccidian and an animal than between a bacterium and an animal. There are therefore fewer options for classes of anticoccidial drugs than for antibacterial drugs, and available drugs are often more toxic. Pharmacologic therapy of coccidia needs to be done with discretion; overuse of anticoccidial drugs in poultry has resulted in extensive resistance,[24] and indiscriminate use will rapidly lead to resistant coccidia in a collection. Empirically, a good choice for pharmacologic therapy of Eimeriidae or Sarcocystidae is toltrazuril or toltrazuril sulfone (ponazuril). Toltrazuril is a triazine anticoccidial drug.[25] It is thought to act on the apicoplast, an apicomplexan-specific organelle, and affected organisms develop vacuoles and degenerate. It appears to be a relatively safe drug, and significant adverse effects have not been observed in pharmacokinetic studies in mammals.[26] Pharmacokinetic studies in chickens have shown the half-life of toltrazuril sulfone, the active and longest-lasting metabolite, to be approximately 15 hours,[27] and doses of 5 to 20 mg/kg daily have been suggested.

Pharmacologic therapy of *Cryptosporidium* is more problematic; there is no available drug with very good efficacy and safety data. Monensin, salinomycin, alborixin, lasalocid, trifluralin, and nicarbazin have some activity in vitro.[28] Toltrazuril, spiramycin, and halofuginone have been used in stone curlews with *C. parvum*,[29] and azithromycin has been used in scops owls with *C. baileyi*,[30] but there were no control animals to evaluate efficacy or safety.

REFERENCES

1. Barta JR, Ogedengbe JD, Martin DS, et al: Phylogenetic position of the adeleorinid coccidia (Myzozoa, Apicomplexa, Coccidia, Eucoccidiorida, Adeleorina) inferred using 18S rDNA sequences, *J Eukaryot Microbiol* 59:171–180, 2012.
2. Shahiduzzaman M, Dyachenko V, Keidel J, et al: Combination of cell culture and quantitative PCR (cc-qPCR) to assess disinfectants efficacy on *Cryptosporidium* oocysts under standardized conditions, *Vet Parasitol* 167:43–49, 2010.
3. Fall A, Thompson RA, Hobbs RP, et al: Morphology is not a reliable tool for delineating species within *Cryptosporidium*, *J Parasitol* 89:399–402, 2009.
4. Griffin C, Reavill DR, Stacy BA, et al: Cryptosporidiosis caused by two distinct species in Russian tortoises and a pancake tortoise, *Vet Parasitol* 170:14–19, 2010.
5. Ravich ML, Reavill DR, Hess L, et al: Gastrointestinal Cryptosporidiosis in Captive Psittacine Birds in the United States, *J Avian Med Surg* 28:297–303, 2014.
6. Curtiss JB, Leone AM, Wellehan JFX, et al: Renal and cloacal cryptosporidiosis (*Cryptosporidium* avian genotype V) in a Major Mitchell's cockatoo (*Lophochroa leadbeateri*), *J Zoo Wildlife Med* 2015.

7. Gharagozlou MJ, Nouri M, Pourhajati V: Cryptosporidial infection of lower respiratory tract in a budgerigar (Melopsittacus undulatus), Arch Razi Institute 69: 95–97, 2013.

8. Pedraza-Diaz S, Amar CF, McLauchlin GL, et al: Cryptosporidium meleagridis from humans: molecular analysis and description of affected patients, J Infect 42:243–250, 2001.

9. Volf J, Modrý D, Koudela B: Experimental transmission of Caryospora kutzeri (Apicomplexa: Eimeriidae) by rodent hosts, Folia Parasitol (Praha) 48:11–14, 2001.

10. Euzeby J: Une parasitose zoonosique potentielle: la dermatite coccidienne à Caryospora, Bull Acad Natle Méd 175:1367–1375, 1991.

11. Gartrell BD, O'Donoghue P, Raidal SR: Eimeria dunsingi in free living musk lorikeets (Glossopsitta concinna), Aust Vet J 78:717–718, 2000.

12. Yabsley MJ, Gibbs SEJ: Description and phylogeny of a new species of Eimeria from double crested cormorants (Phalacrocorax auritus) near Fort Gaines, Georgia, J Parasitol 92:385–388, 2006.

13. Barta JR, Schrenzel MD, Carreno R, et al: The genus Atoxoplasma (Garnham 1950) as a junior objective synonym of the genus Isospora (Schneider 1881) species infecting birds and resurrection of Cystoisospora (Frenkel 1977) as the correct genus for Isospora species infecting mammals, J Parasitol 91:726–727, 2005.

14. Khan RA, Desser SS: Avian Lankesterella infections in Algonquin Park, Ontario, Can J Zool 49:1105–1110, 1971.

15. Modrý D, Votýpka J, Svobodová M: Note on the Taxonomy of Frenkelia microti (Findlay & Middleton, 1934) (Apicomplexa: Sarcocystidae), Syst Parasitol 58:185–187, 2004.

16. Rimoldi G, Speer B, Wellehan JFX, et al: An outbreak of Sarcocystis calchasi encephalitis in multiple psittacine species within an enclosed zoological aviary, J Vet Diagn Investig 25:775–781, 2013.

16a. Dubey JP: A review of toxoplasmosis in wild birds, Vet Parasitol 106:121–153, 2002.

17. Mineo TW, Carrasco AO, Marciano JA, et al: Pigeons (Columba livia) are a suitable experimental model for Neospora caninum infection in birds, Vet Parasitol 159:149–153, 2009.

18. de Oliveira UV, de Magalhães VC, Almeida CP, et al: Quails are resistant to infection with Neospora caninum tachyzoites, Vet Parasitol 198:209–213, 2013.

19. Morin-Adeline V, Vogelnest L, Dhand NK, et al: Afternoon shedding of a new species of Isospora (Apicomplexa) in the endangered Regent Honeyeater (Xanthomyza Phrygia), Parasitology 138:713–724, 2011.

20. Innis, CJ, Garner MM, Johnson AJ, et al: Antemortem diagnosis and characterization of nasal intranuclear coccidiosis in tortoises, J Vet Diagn Investig 19:660–667, 2007.

21. Wünschmann A, Wellehan JFX, Armien AG, et al: Renal infection by a new coccidian genus in big brown bats (Eptesicus fuscus), J Parasitol 96:178–183, 2010.

22. Barbee SL, Weber DJ, Sobsey MD, etb al.: Inactivation of Cryptosporidium parvum oocyst infectivity by disinfection and sterilization processes, Gastrointest Endosc 49:605–611, 1999.

23. Connelly SJ, Wolyniak EA, Williamson CE, et al: Artificial UV-B and solar radiation reduce in vitro infectivity of the human pathogen Cryptosporidium parvum, Environ Sci Technol 41:7101–7106, 2007.

24. Stephan B, Rommel M, Daugschies A, et al: Studies of resistance to anticoccidials in Eimeria field isolates and pure Eimeria strains, Vet Parasitol 69:19–29, 1997.

25. Mitchell SM, Zajac AM, Davis WL, et al: The effects of ponazuril on development of apicomplexans in vitro, Eukaryot Microbiol 52: 231–235, 2005.

26. Dirikolu L, Karpiesiuk W, Lehner AF, et al: Toltrazuril sulfone sodium salt: synthesis, analytical detection, and pharmacokinetics in the horse, J Vet Pharmacol Ther 35:265–274, 2011.

27. Kim M-S, Park B-K, Hwang Y-H, et al: Pharmacokinetics and metabolism of toltrazuil and its major metabolites after oral administration in broilers, J Poultry Sci 50:257–261, 2013.

28. Armson A, Meloni BP, Reynoldson JA, et al: Assessment of drugs against Cryptosporidium parvum using a simple in vitro screening method, FEMS Microbiol Lett 178:227–233, 1999.

29. Zylan K, Bailey T, Smith HV, et al: An outbreak of cryptosporidiosis in a collection of stone curlews (Burhinus oedicnemus) in Dubai, Avian Pathol 37:521–526, 2008.

30. Molina- López RA, Ramis A, Martin-Vazquez S, et al: Cryptosporidium baileyi infection associated with an outbreak of ocular and respiratory disease in otus owls (Otus scops) in a rehabilitation centre, Avian Pathol 39:171–176, 2010.

MACRORHABDOSIS

David Phalen *

HISTORY AND DESCRIPTION OF *MACRORHABDUS ORNITHOGASTER*

Macrorhabdus ornithogaster is an anamorphic ascomycetes yeast that has only been found to grow at the junction of the proventriculus and ventriculus in birds.[1] It was first recognized in the early 1980s in the United States in budgerigars and was thought to be a yeast.[2] Concurrent investigations in the Netherlands described it in canaries and incorrectly concluded it was a bacterium and gave it the name *Megabacterium*, which continues to be used improperly to the present.[3] A subsequent study claimed to be able to isolate the organism from budgerigar stomachs by using traditional bacterial isolation methods; however, the authors of that study did not characterize their isolate sufficiently, and subsequently it was shown that the isolate that was described in this study was a bacterium and not *M. ornithogaster*.[4]

The true nature of *M. ornithogaster* was only conclusively demonstrated recently. Studies in Australia demonstrated that it was not sensitive to antibiotics but was sensitive to amphotericin, suggesting that it was, in fact, a fungus.[5] It was shown to stain for chitin, a protein that is only produced by eukaryote organisms, thus proving that it was not a bacterium. Investigators were then able to purify the organism and sequence portions of the deoxyribonucleic acid (DNA) that code for ribosomal ribonucleic acid (RNA). Comparing this sequence to other known yeast it was then shown that *M. ornithogaster* was not only a novel species of yeast but, in fact, was the only known representative of an entirely new genus of yeasts.[1]

It can infect many species of birds.[4] There is convincing evidence *M. ornithogaster* can cause disease in its host, but it is also clear that many birds live with this organism without obvious signs. The only effective treatments for *M. ornithogaster* are a few antifungal drugs and these drugs do not always lend themselves to large-scale flock treatment. Because *M. ornithogaster* was thought to be a bacterium (*Megabacterium*) for more than 20 years, many assumptions about this organism's biology have subsequently proven to be untrue. Continued referencing

---

*This chapter is a modified version of Phalen DN: Update: diagnosis and management of *Macrorhabdus ornithogaster* (formally Megabacteria). Vet Clin North Am Exot Anim 17(2):203–210, 2013.

of some of these flawed studies and anecdotal reports often creates confusion for veterinarians and bird owners alike.[4]

HOST RANGE

The reported host range of *M. ornithogaster* includes a wide range of psittacine birds, passerine birds, poultry, and other species. It has a worldwide distribution and is found in both wild and captive birds.[4,6]

The species of psittacine birds most commonly infected with *M. ornithogaster* are the budgerigar (*Melopsittacus undulates*), lovebirds (*Agapornis* sp.), and to a lesser extent cockatiels (*Nymphicus hollandicus*). Infection has also been reported to be common in parrotlets (*Forpus* sp.). In wild Australian birds, the organism is commonly found in recently fledged Galahs (*Eolophus roseicapilla*) and Corellas (*Cacatua* sp.) with chronic diarrheal disease and weight loss. These birds have other intestinal parasites and at least some have concurrent infections with the psittacine beak and feather disease virus. The full host range of *M. ornithogaster* in psittacine birds is unknown, and infection should be considered in any species of psittacine birds presenting with gastrointestinal signs.[4]

Passerine species infected with *M. ornithogaster* include pet canaries (*Serinus canaria*), zebra finches (*Taeniopygia guttata*), and Gouldian finches (*Erythrura gouldiae*). It has also been found in a range of wild European finches and the sisken (*Carduelis spinus*), and in feral European goldfinches (*Carduelis carduelis*), and wild-caught feral European goldfinches and green finches (*Carduelis chloris*) captured for the pet trade in Australia.[4]

M. ornithogaster infections have now been reported in chickens (*Gallus gallus*) on four continents—Europe, North and South Americas, and Australia. Other gallinaceous birds reported to be infected with *M. ornithogaster* include the gray partridge (*Perdix perdix*), the Japanese quail (*Coturnix japonica*), domestic turkey (*Meleagris gallopavo*), chukar partridge (*Alectoris chukar*), and guinea fowl (genus and species not reported). Infection has also been reported in ducks, geese, and ibis, although no supporting evidence on how the diagnosis was made in ibis was provided. Recently, *M. ornithogaster* has been reported in captive raised greater rheas (*Rhea americana*). Morphologically, these organisms are consistent with those that have been reported in other species. However, they still remain to be characterized by molecular techniques.[4,6]

There are two reports of an organism resembling *M. ornithogaster* infecting the upper respiratory tract of a dog and a cat. These organisms were never described, and given that *M. ornithogaster* is microaerophilic, its growth on a respiratory epithelium does not seem plausible. Recent infection attempts in mice provide additional evidence that *M. ornithogaster* cannot grow in mammals.[7]

Isolation attempts from stomach contents of greater rheas by using growth conditions that are inconsistent with the metabolic requirements of *M. ornithogaster* have resulted in the isolation of a small motile organism, which the investigators suggest is *M. ornithogaster*. This uncharacterized organism has been shown to be able to colonize the stomach of mice. Given that this organism grows in conditions that are incompatible for *M. ornithogaster* growth, that it has morphologic characteristics that have never been seen in *M. ornithogaster* either in vivo or in vitro, and that it has never been

characterized genetically, it is the author's opinion that the conclusion that this organism is *M. ornithogaster* is premature and is likely to be incorrect.[6]

CLINICAL MANIFESTATIONS

The signs of *M. ornithogaster* in birds include vomiting, regurgitation, diarrhea, and chronic weight (Figure 2-23). Disease has been seen in young and adult birds. Disease in budgerigars occurs most commonly in middle-aged birds. An acute hemorrhagic disease has been reported in parrotlets. Weight loss, anorexia, melena, and anemia are commonly seen in cockatiels and occasionally in other species that have gastric ulceration secondary to *M. ornithogaster* infection. Canaries and other finches with *M. ornithogaster* infections are often found dead with no premonitory signs but are generally emaciated, which suggests that they had been ill for at least a few days prior to death.[4]

DIAGNOSIS IN THE LIVE BIRD

Detection of *M. ornithogaster* infection in the live bird is most commonly done by microscopic examination of feces. Feces made into a slurry with water or saline can be scanned for *M. ornithogaster* using 40× magnification. Alternatively, fecal smears can be stained with a quick stain or Gram stain. A rapid way of concentrating *M. ornithogaster* and separating it from other solid matter in feces is to homogenize a dropping with approximately 20 times its volume of physiologic saline in a small tube, let it sit for 10 seconds, and then examine a small drop of the suspension collected from the meniscus. As *M. ornithogaster* takes longer to settle than most other material in feces, it is more easily seen in wet preparations after this treatment.[4] A polymerase chain reaction (PCR) assay to detect *M. ornithogaster* in feces is also available in North America (Veterinary Molecular Diagnostics, Milford, OH).

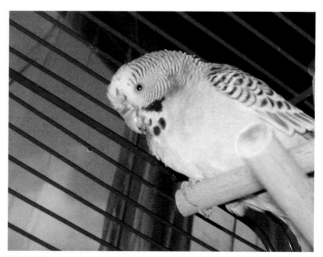

FIGURE 2-23 Budgerigar with *Macrorhabdus* infection and a history of vomiting. The pink stain on the feathers is from an antibiotic that had been vomited after the owner had attempted home treatment.

M. ornithogaster is a long, slender, straight stiff rod with rounded ends when it is found in feces (Figures 2-24 and 2-25). In some circumstances, the long rod may bend slightly in a gentle curve. Y-shaped organisms can be seen (see Figure 2-25), but extremely rarely. Viewed directly in a wet mount, small, oblong, refractile structures found at regular intervals are readily seen. These structures are the nuclei. The nuclei stain with Giemsa stains. *M. ornithogaster* ranges in length from 20 to 80 µm and is consistently 2 to 3 µm in width. The organisms often stain poorly with quick stains and the Gram stain instead of staining uniformly with only pickup small droplets of the stain. When they do stain well, they are gram positive and stain dark blue with quick stains (Figure 2-26). Unlike bacteria and other yeasts, the contents of the cell stain, but not the cell wall.

It is the author's impression that they do not stick well to glass slides unless the slide has been heat fixed. It is also the author's impression that heat fixing makes them more likely to stain uniformly.

Birds infected with *M. ornithogaster* may shed the organism in low numbers, in large numbers, or not at all. It has been the author's experience that the majority of birds that exhibit disease as the result of *M. ornithogaster* infection will be shedding large numbers of organisms. However, this may not always be the case, and the absence of *M. ornithogaster* in feces does not completely rule out infection.[4]

There can be other things in feces that resemble *M. ornithogaster* (Figure 2-27). An unknown structure commonly seen by the author in the droppings of many birds is approximately the size of *Macrorhabdus* but has a straight not rounded

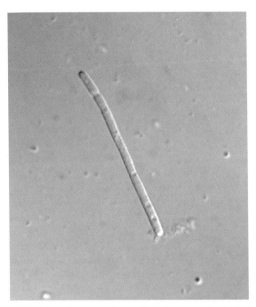

FIGURE 2-24 Unstained *Macrorhabdus ornithogaster*. Original magnification 100×.(With permission from Phalen DN: Update: diagnosis and management of *Macrorhabdus ornithogaster* (formally Megabacteria), *Vet Clin North Am Exot Anim* 17:(2):203–210, 2013.)

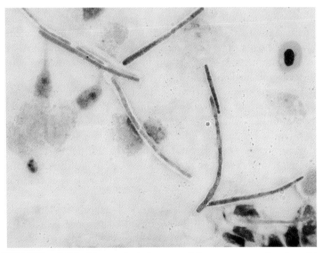

FIGURE 2-26 *Macrorhabdus ornithogaster* stained with Gram stain. Original magnification 100×. (With permission from Phalen DN: Update: diagnosis and management of *Macrorhabdus ornithogaster* (formally Megabacteria), *Vet Clin North Am Exot Anim* 17:(2):203–210, 2013.)

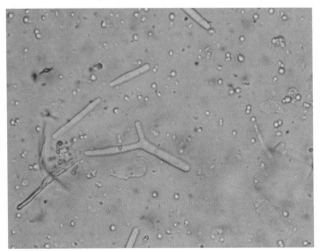

FIGURE 2-25 Unstained wet mount of *Macrorhabdus ornithogaster* showing typical rod-shaped organisms and an unusual Y-shaped organism. Original magnification 100×.

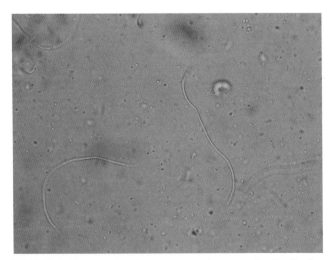

FIGURE 2-27 Unstained wetmount photograph of a finding that may be misinterpreted as *M. ornithogaster*. Other things can be found in the feces that may resemble *M. ornithogaster*, including unknown organisms or structures and filamentous bacteria.

terminal end that appears to be the result of the structure breaking off of something larger. *M. ornithogaster* always has rounded ends. Filamentous gram-positive bacteria can also approach the size of *M. ornithogaster*. These bacteria, however, are often segmented, are thinner than *M. ornithogaster*, generally curve back and forth, and thus are readily distinguished from *M. ornithogaster*.

POSTMORTEM DIAGNOSIS

M. ornithogaster infection is readily made at postmortem examination. A saline preparation of a scraping of junction (isthmus) of the proventriculus and the ventriculus will demonstrate the organisms and they will generally be abundant. *M. ornithogaster* is also readily demonstrated in hematoxylin and eosin–stained sections of the isthmus. It is eosinophilic and is found forming the characteristic log-jam pattern on the surface of and between the mucosal glands. Because it is a fungus, it stains with silver stains and the periodic acid–Schiff stain.[1]

Showing that *M. ornithogaster* infection has contributed to a bird's death, however, requires more proof than just finding the organism. Budgerigars and passerines with disease caused by *M. ornithogaster* will grossly have a thickened mucosa of the proventriculus, and there will be increased mucus in the lumen. Some birds may have one or more bleeding ulcers of the proventriculus. In birds with clinical signs caused by *M. ornithogaster* infection, growth extends beyond the isthmus into the proventriculus and the koilin of the ventriculus and may disrupt the structure of the koilin. Lymphoplasmacytic inflammation is common in birds with heavy *M. ornithogaster* growth but is less likely in birds with minimal superficial colonization by the organism.[4]

GROWTH IN VITRO

M. ornithogaster is readily grown in vitro given the correct substrate and conditions. It must be provided with a microaerophilic environment and grown in a medium with a pH between 3 and 4. Traditional cell culture media containing up to 20% fetal bovine serum and 1% to 5% glucose or sucrose has been shown to support its growth. Its optimal growth temperature is 42° C. Addition of antibiotics to the growth media is recommended to prevent the overgrowth of bacteria. It can be cultured from the isthmus scrapings or from feces.[8]

TREATMENT

A few treatment trials have been performed in birds with *M. ornithogaster* infection.[4] In many of these trials, the measure of successful treatment was the cessation of *M. ornithogaster* shedding in feces, as opposed to the less common trial in which treated birds were killed and the stomach examined directly.[4,5,9] Although it is likely that the cessation of shedding may be the result of a cure, it is also possible that some of these treated birds may have remained infected at low levels.

Amphotericin B is used widely to treat *M. ornithogaster* and appears to be effective and safe when administered orally by gavage and, in some circumstances, in water. Various dosages have been recommended. The author has used 100 milligrams per kilogram (mg/kg), twice a day for 14 days, with direct oral administration but has been gradually reducing the amount and is now using 25 mg/kg, twice a day for 14 days, with apparent success. Success of treatment has been judged by the rapid cessation of *M. ornithogaster* shedding and resolution of signs. Amphotericin B can be purchased as a powder (Gallipot, St. Paul, MN) and compounded into a formula that can be given orally. The 2.5% water-soluble powder from Vetafam (3 Bye Street Wagga Wagga, NSW, Australia) that has been used extensively in the past is no longer available at the time of this writing. There is one report of resistance of *M. ornithogaster* to amphotericin B. It is not known how widespread the resistance may be.[4]

The ability of nystatin to kill *M. ornithogaster* may vary from strain to strain. In vitro trials by Bradely et al showed that *M. ornithogaster* is sensitive to nystatin at concentrations of 0.1 units per milliliter (units/mL).[10] In one clinical trial, the authors also saw a cessation of *M. ornithogaster* shedding after treatment with nystatin. In a recent study, a flock of budgerigars was treated with nystatin at 3,500,000 international units per liter (IU/L) of drinking water for 2 days, followed by 2,000,000 IU/L for 28 days.[9] Some birds in this study were euthanized at the end of treatment and were found to be free of infection. Resistance of some strains of *M. ornithogaster* to nystatin has been reported following clinical trials performed by others.[5]

Research by Bradley et al[10] has shown that *M. ornithogaster* cultured in vitro is highly sensitive to sodium and potassium benzoate and sodium sorbate. Treatment attempts with sodium benzoate in drinking water in live birds have been studied by the author and others.[4] The author's experiences have not been uniformly successful, and in many cases, shedding and clinical signs have not resolved.[4] The reason for the failure of treatment in these instances is not known, but inadequate consumption of the treated water may be to blame. In another trial in which a flock of breeding budgerigars were treated, *M. ornithogaster* shedding stopped, but some of the treated birds died. The cause of the deaths was not determined but could have been the result of sodium toxicity. Water consumption in the treated budgerigars was very high because they were feeding young and because it was the middle of the summer and day time temperatures were very high.[4] The use of potassium benzoate has not been studied, but it may be safer than sodium benzoate because it is more difficult for potassium toxicity to result from ingested potassium than it is for sodium toxicity to result from ingested sodium. The use of any of these chemicals requires additional research before they can be recommended for routine use. There are many potential sources of sodium and potassium benzoate. The product used by the author is purchased as a 99% pure product (Sigma-Aldrich, St. Louis, MO).

Fluconazole has been used to effectively treat *M. ornithogaster* in experimentally infected chickens at dosage of 100 mg/kg. In trials in budgerigars, this dosage rate was found to be toxic and a lower dosage was not effective. Gentian violet was found to prevent *M. ornithogaster* growth in vitro. Gentian violet at moderate concentrations, however, was found to be toxic to budgerigars (Phalen, unpublished information, 2005).

CONCLUSION

M. ornithogaster is found in many species of birds around the world. It can be a significant cause of both morbidity and mortality. Detecting the infection in the live bird requires the direct observation of the organism in feces or its detection by PCR; however, these assays are not so sensitive that a negative result rules out infection. Diagnosis is readily made at postmortem examination of scrapings of the isthmus and histopathology of the proventriculus and ventriculus. The only consistently proven treatment for infected birds is direct oral administration of amphotericin B, although nystatin and sodium benzoate may also be effective under some circumstances.

REFERENCES

1. Tomaszewski EK, Logan KE, Kurtzman CP, et al: Phylogenetic analysis indicates the "megabacterium" of birds is a novel anamorphic ascomycetous yeast, *Macrorhabdus ornithogaster*, gen. nov., sp. nov, *Int J Sys Evol Micro* 3:1201–1205, 2003.
2. Hargreaves RC: A fungus commonly found in the proventriculus of small pet birds. In *30th Western Poultry Disease Conference and 15th Poultry Health Symposium*, Davis, CA, 1981, University of California at Davis,. pp 75–76.
3. van Herck H, Duijser T, Zwart P, et al: A bacterial proventriculitis of canaries, *Avian Pathol* 13:561–572, 1984.
4. Phalen DN: Update: diagnosis and management of *Macrorhabdus ornithogaster* (formally *Megabacteria*), *Vet Clin North Am Exot Anim* 17:(2):203–210, 2013.
5. Filippich LJ, Perry RA: Drug trials against Megabacteria in budgerigars (*Melopsittacus undulatus*), *Aust Vet Practit* 23:184–189,1993.
6. Martins NRS, Horta AC, Siqueira, AM, et al: *Macrorhabdus ornithogaster* in ostrich, rhea, canary, zebra finch, free range chicken, turkey, guinea-fowl, columbina pigeon, toucan, chuckar partridge and experimental infection in chicken, Japanese quail and mice, *Arq Bras De Med Vet Zootech* 58:291–298, 2006.
7. Hanafusa Y, Costa E, Phalen DN: Infection trials in mice suggest that *Macrorhabdus ornithogaster* is not capable of growth in mammals, 51:669–672, 2013.
8. Hanafusa Y, Bradley A, Tomaszewski EK, et al: Growth and metabolic characterization of *Macrorhabdus ornithogaster*, *J Vet Med Diag* 19:256–265, 2007.
9. Kheirandish R, Salehi M: Megabacteriosis in budgerigars: diagnosis and treatment, *Comp Clin Pathol* 20:501-505, 2011.
10. Bradley A, Yasuka H, Phalen DN: *Macrorhabdus ornithogaster*: inhibitory drugs, oxygen toxicity and culturing from feces. USDA sponsored summer research program. Athens, GA, July 2005.

CHLAMYDIOSIS (PSITTACOSIS)

Lorenzo Crosta, Alessandro Melillo, Petra Schnitzer
Chlamydiosis is an infectious disease of birds and mammals, including human beings. The disease is so well known in psittacine birds that it has been named after them (psittacosis).

There are several ways to diagnose psittacosis, but many diagnostic approaches that are commonly used only provide degrees of inductive strength to the argument for the diagnosis rather than confirmatory diagnosis. In fact, a generalized disease with clinical signs related to the respiratory, digestive, and nervous systems; leukocytosis with heterophilia; and elevated liver leakage enzymes is rather common in several diseases of psittacines and not specific to chlamydiosis.

DEFINITION

Avian chlamydiosis is an infectious disease; it is contagious, most often systemic, and sometimes deadly. The causative organism is the intracellular, gram-negative bacterium *Chlamydia psittaci* (until recently controversially named *Chlamydophila psittaci*). Depending on the particular strain involved and the host species, chlamydiosis can present with different clinical features that may range from lethargy and anorexia, to ocular and nasal discharge, diarrhea, and green to yellow-green feces.[1]

HISTORICAL DATA

The disease which was already named psittacosis in the 1940s was differentiated into "ornithosis," used to describe the disease when nonpsittacine birds were infected and "psittacosis" when psittacines were affected or when another nonavian species was infected by a parrot.[2] This subdefinition was made on the presumption that the human form of the disease acquired from infected chickens or pigeons is less serious than the clinical form deriving from infected psittacines. Currently, we know this is not true, and often the human infections originating from turkey strains of *C. psittaci* may be even more serious.[3]

ETIOLOGY

The systematic of the order *Chlamydiales* was revised in the late 1990s, and the old name *Chlamydia psittaci* was reclassified as *Chlamydophila psittaci*.[4] However, this reclassification has always been debated, and in 2009, a subcommittee of the International Committee on Systematics of Prokaryotes re-examined the taxonomy and nomenclature issues, and a decision was made to again merge species in the genus *Chlamydophila* into *Chlamydia*.[5]

To date, the family *Chlamydiaceae* comprises nine species in the genus *Chlamydia*: (1) *C. trachomatis*, a causative agent of sexually transmitted and ocular diseases in humans; (2) *C. pneumoniae*, which causes atypical pneumonia in humans and is associated with diseases in reptiles, amphibians, and marsupials; (3) *C. suis*, found only in pigs; (4) *C. muridarum*, found in mice; (5) *C. felis*, the causative agent of keratoconjunctivitis in cats; (6) *C. caviae*, whose natural host is the guinea pig; (7) *C. pecorum*, the etiologic agent of a range of clinical disease manifestations in cattle, small ruminants, and marsupials; (8) *C. psittaci*, comprising the avian subtype and etiologic agent of psittacosis in birds and humans; and (9) *C. abortus*, the causative agent of ovine enzootic abortion.[6]

To summarize, *C. psittaci* is a gram negative bacterium, is an intracellular obligate parasite, has specific energy needs, and cannot move. It differs from more conventional bacteria for several reasons. However, as deeper studies are carried on and new techniques come into the hands of dedicated researchers, it is becoming clear that some facts, which were considered unequivocal in the past such as the inability of *C. psittaci* to form compounds rich in energy, for example, adenosine triphosphate (ATP), are no longer valid.

C. PSITTACI REPLICATION CYCLE

The replication cycle starts with the attachment to, and penetration of, a target cell (mainly columnar epithelial cells of mucous membranes and mononuclear macrophages),[7] by the infecting and cytotoxic elementary bodies (EBs); they contain deoxyribonucleic acid (DNA) and measure about 300 nanometers (nm) (0.3 micrometer [μm]). The EBs represent the form that chlamydiae, as a group, use to survive outside the host cell. Since they cannot move by themselves, they attach to the microvilli of the epithelial cells and enter by endocytosis (Figure 2-28). The receptor site on the membrane is very specific and is identified in the major outer membrane protein (MOMP) of the EBs; in fact, the MOMP is found only on the EB. Once endocytosis has occurred, the EB is enveloped by a membrane produced by the host cell to form a vesicle. Through a mechanism not yet known, *Chlamydia* inhibits the fusion between this new vesicle (or vacuole) and lysosomes, thereby preventing the formation of a phagolysosome and then the digestion of the agent, particularly in macrophages.

At this point, protected by the vesicle (Figure 2-29), the EB of *C. psittaci* starts a reorganization process, during which the EB, which was metabolically inert, goes through some intermediate forms, to be transformed in the larger (0.5–1.5 μm) and metabolically active reticulated body (RB) (Figure 2-30).

It must be remembered that growth and propagation of RB requires a high-energy source, and for this purpose, the

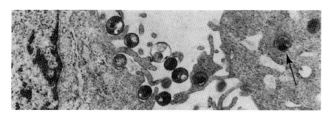

FIGURE 2-28 Chlamydial elementary bodies are shown attaching to the microvilli of epithelial cells on this electron microscopic image. (From Harrison GJ, Ritchie BW, Harrison LR: *Avian Medicine: Principles and Application,* Lake Worth, FL, 1994, Wingers Publishing.)

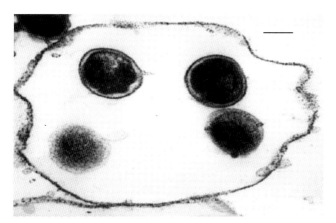

FIGURE 2-29 Elementary body of *C. psittaci* beginning reorganization. (Source: http://chlamydiae.com/twiki/bin/view/Cell_Biology/GrowthCycle. Electronic micrograph by Michael Ward. From Ward ME: The chlamydial developmental cycle. In Baron AL: *Microbiology of Chlamydia,* 1988, CRC Press.)

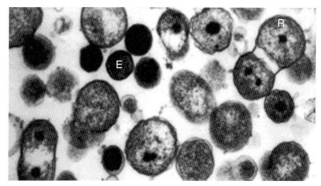

FIGURE 2-30 Elementary bodies (E) being transformed into the larger, metabolically active reticulated bodies (R). (Source: http://chlamydiae.com/twiki/bin/view/Cell_Biology/GrowthCycle. Electronic micrograph by Michael Ward.)

RB sprouts special projections. These are able to cross the membrane of the intracytoplasmic vacuole (the protection of the EB), allowing the uptake of substances from the host cell: most important, the mitochondrial ATP is transferred with the help of an ATP–ADP (adenosine diphosphate) translocase produced by *C. psittaci*.[7] However, it has recently been discovered that *C. psittaci* has more metabolic capabilities than previously believed. Principally among these was the discovery that *Chlamydia* has a nearly complete peptidoglycan synthesis pathway. This discovery confirmed previous work showing that chlamydial development is highly sensitive to beta-lactam antibiotic treatment.[6] Furthermore, other analyses have also revealed that *Chlamydia* can also produce its own ATP, which contradicts previous thoughts that *Chlamydia* was entirely dependent on the host cell's energy reserves. The RB also contains a genus-specific antigen (lipopolysaccharide), which is also located on the surface of the host cell and, probably by increasing the viscosity of the cell wall, appears to protect the infected cell from the cytotoxic effects of T lymphocytes. The growth by binary fission of the RB leads to the formation of microcolonies of 100 to 500 *C. psittaci* cells, called also *inclusions* or *Levinthal-Cole-Lillie bodies* (LCL bodies). The duration of the propagation cycle depends on the *C. psittaci* strain and the type of host cell, but it generally takes from 20 to 40 hours.

During the last stages of the replication process, proteases produced by *C. psittaci* lyse the host cell (these enzymes are sensitive to antibiotics). Simultaneously, the enzyme system of the host is activated, with endotoxicosis of the host cell. This contributes to the release of a new generation of EBs. However, before cell lysis and exocytosis happen, the RB "matures" in its condensed form by concentrating the DNA and stabilizing the cell membrane, until the new EBs are completed and ready to leave the host cell. The whole cycle takes up to 48 hours (Figure 2-31). The enzyme systems mentioned previously destroy the host cell, but the EBs may be shed continuously. With this system, the host cell is permanently infected, maintaining its functions and replicating capabilities. Besides being very interesting, this mechanism is also strategically advanced because the EBs can infect various types of macrophages, after the initial entry through the epithelial cells. Furthermore, since *C. psittaci* can survive in the host cells during mitosis, it is able to infect the next generation of macrophages.

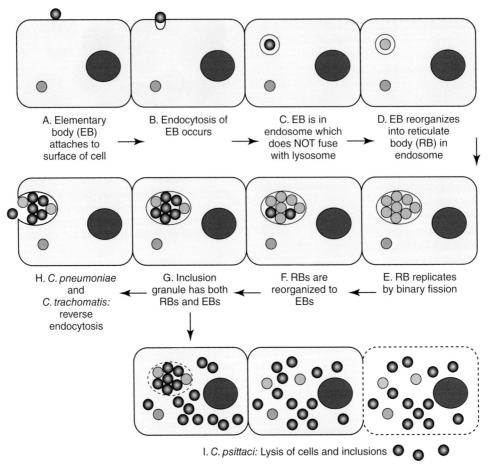

A. Elementary body (EB) attaches to surface of cell

B. Endocytosis of EB occurs

C. EB is in endosome which does NOT fuse with lysosome

D. EB reorganizes into reticulate body (RB) in endosome

H. *C. pneumoniae* and *C. trachomatis:* reverse endocytosis

G. Inclusion granule has both RBs and EBs

F. RBs are reorganized to EBs

E. RB replicates by binary fission

I. *C. psittaci:* Lysis of cells and inclusions

FIGURE 2-31 Replication life cycle of *Chlamydia psittaci*. (From Microbiology and Immunology on-line. University of South Carolina – School of Medicine.)

Under stress conditions, triggered by a range of factors, including the presence of antibiotics, the effects of cytokines such as γ-interferon, and the depletion of glucose and essential amino acids, chlamydial RBs may enter an alternative developmental stage, which involves the formation of large, pleomorphic cellular forms known as the aberrant bodies (ABs). The ABs will persist inside host cells, which led to the term "persistence," until the developmental trigger is removed or the nutrients are replaced. Importantly, in terms of treatment, in vitro studies have indicated that persistent chlamydial infections are refractile to standard antibiotic treatment.[6] This would explain why the idea that treatment of psittacosis with enough time to have some subsequent generations of macrophages replaced is no longer valid. The inhibition of the defense mechanisms of the infected animal, such as phagolysosomes and cytotoxic T lymphocytes, allow for the survival of *C. psittaci* inside the host cell. Even if specific lipoglycoproteins are stimulating the production of antibodies, this does not correlate with an immunologic protection. The hepatotoxic and nephrotoxic toxin, which disappears after *C. psittaci* enters into the host cell and which is linked to the presence of the MOMP, is able to stimulate the production of small quantities of antitoxin antibodies. Unfortunately, these toxins are not useful for the production of vaccines, as the antibodies are not protective and only indicate a previous exposure to *C. psittaci*. Thus, they can eventually be used for diagnostic purposes.

We may make the following conclusions from *Chlamydia psittaci* biology and replication strategy:

1. *C. psittaci* is able to inhibit the defense mechanisms of the host. This enables the infectious agent to survive inside the host cells during its propagation and may cause chronic, long-lasting (sometimes lifelong) infections. Some of those chronic infections cannot be treated adequately inside the host cell.
2. Inhibition of the phagolysosomes in the macrophages compromises the immune response. In birds that overcome the clinical disease, antibodies can be detected, but they are not able to protect the host from the infection.
3. The high variability of the different *C. psittaci* strains is determined by the MOMP, which defines receptor ability and toxic properties of a given strain and thus virulence of the strain and susceptibility of the host.
4. The persistence of *C. psittaci* in the macrophages of a given avian species is naturally selecting strains with low virulence for that species, which may still be much more virulent for other species.
5. Although the detection and discrimination between multiple repeat infections and a single chronic infection remain difficult, persistent infections have been associated with a range of chronic infections.

PATHOGENICITY

The pathogenicity of *C. psittaci* cannot be fully explained by the simple, direct damage to the host cell. In fact, the most important virulence factor is a toxin, intimately bonded to the outer membrane of the elementary bodies. This toxin is present in different amounts in the different *C. psittaci* strains. During the growth and replication of *C. psittaci* in a specific avian host, the bacterium can be modified, either in its structure or in its metabolism, and this will alter its antigenic profile and pathogenicity. The modification rate depends on the number of subsequent replication in a given species, and the surface of the new EBs contains "new" heterologous antibodies, which are supposed to be host-specific.[8] *Chlamydia* interspecific jumps, or spillovers—as may happen in quarantine stations, breeding facilities, or pet shops—can modify its physical–chemical characteristics, toxic components, and, virulence, also the host range.[9] However, these newly acquired characteristics are not necessarily permanent.

The clinical outcome of an infection depends largely on the relationship between the EBs and macrophages. A lytic and lethal reaction takes hold in phagocytic cells infected with a large number of virulent chlamydial particles. Low concentrations of virulent strains are rapidly inactivated by polymorphonuclear and mononuclear phagocytes. If the macrophage is damaged, the chances of chlamydial survival are reduced. Low concentrations of a nonvirulent strain will not stimulate an adequate lytic reaction, producing macrophages that are transformed into epithelioid cells, which remain infected chronically. The average lifespan of these epithelioid cells should be the index to determine the duration of treatment, but little or nothing is known about the lifespan of these cells in birds.[10] Further, during mitosis in the bone marrow, it is very likely that the infected macrophages transfer the chlamydial inclusion bodies in the next generation of macrophages.[11] The partial removal and phagocytosis in new macrophages promotes the selection of strains with low virulence for the species in question. However, these chronic infections facilitate the diffusion of a large number of chlamydiae that can potentially be very virulent for other avian species.[10]

RESISTENCE OF *C. PSITTACI*

The infectious elementary bodies, which can be stained with the Giemsa, Macchiavello, Gimenez, Stamp, or Castaneda stain, can survive out of the host (protected by organic material), and inside the host cells, for several weeks.[7] The tissue destruction induced by bacteria and the presence of feces inactivate the microorganism rapidly. On the other hand, the "free" EBs are relatively unstable in the environment and will be inactivated in a few days. *C. psittaci* is particularly sensitive to heat and is inactivated by relatively low concentrations of formaldehyde (1%), if the room temperature is above 20° C. Quaternary ammonium salts and lipid solvents are not a good choice for the elimination of *C. psittaci*. Its infectivity may, however, be eliminated in just a few minutes by using benzalkonium chloride.[12] Also, hydrogen peroxide has shown some efficacy against *C. psittaci*.

TRANSMISSION

C. psittaci can be detected in feces 10 days before the onset of clinical signs. A large number of chlamydial elementary bodies can be found, continuously or intermittently, in feces (up to 10^5 infectious units per gram of feces), urine, tears, nasal discharge, oropharyngeal mucus, and crop-milk (limited to Columbiformes) of infected birds. Unfortunately, not enough information is available about the period during which the clinically symptomatic birds or asymptomatic carriers can transmit the infection. In this way, a high concentration of bacterial particles can be aerosolized, and the wing flapping of a large number of birds in an enclosed collection can further facilitate this overhead suspension. Therefore, the infection can occur either by inhalation or by ingestion of these infectious particles. The following must always be kept in mind:

◆ Infection takes place very quickly.
◆ *C. psittaci* will replicate in the lungs, air sacs, and pericardium of infected birds, as soon as 24 hours after infection.
◆ Within 48 hours, *C. psittaci* is present in the bloodstream.
◆ After 72 hours, the infected birds are able to shed *C. psittaci* in the environment.

These facts by themselves can explain how the disease can spread rapidly within a closed group of animals.

It appears that when the infection takes place via the respiratory route, it spreads through the lungs and air sacs to other organs, resulting in a symptomatic disease. However, oral–intestinal infections are less likely to cause symptomatic chlamydiosis and more often lead to chronic, nonsymptomatic forms of the disease.

Vertical transmission, through the egg, has been demonstrated in the domestic duck,[13] in the black-headed gull (*Chroicocephalus (Larus) ridibundus*),[13] and in the budgerigar,[15] and it is suspected to occur in the turkey. Cockatiels (*N. hollandicus*), are frequent carriers of *C. psittaci* and can shed the agent through their feces for more than 1 year after an active infection. Ducks can shed *C. psittaci* in feces for 100 days and can harbor the bacterium for up to 170 days.[7] In any case, carriers may start eliminating the organism after a stressful event; the hypothesis that in a group of birds, the organism may be eliminated within 4 to 5 months has never been confirmed. Finally, it should be noted that while transmission through invertebrate vectors (mites and bloodsucking insects) is possible, direct transmission of *C. psittaci* from dogs, cats, horses, pigs, and humans to members of the same species does not seem to occur.[7]

CLINICAL FEATURES

Psittacosis is a highly heterogeneous disease. The clinical course has been described in detail in chickens and pet birds; however, well-documented cases in wild birds are less common, and usually it is assumed that the latter have simple respiratory signs.[16] Generally, acute, subacute, and chronic forms are described.[1] However, in these forms, overt clinical signs are often evident and include various combinations of respiratory signs, dyspnea, oculonasal discharge, anorexia, regurgitation, vomiting, and greenish diarrhea. On some occasions, psittacosis manifests in a more subtle way. In these situations, clinical signs may range from a simple conjunctivitis to neurologic symptoms such as tremors or torticollis;

sometimes nonspecific signs such as loss of productivity of the flock are present, or sudden deaths occur, with no prodromal signs.

To help overcome the difficulties that may be encountered in the diagnosis, given also the legal implications of the disease, the National Association of State Health Veterinarians (NASPHV), the Centers for Disease Control and Prevention (CDC), and the Council of State and Territorial Epidemiologists (CSTE) have established national case definitions for epidemiologic surveillance of psittacosis in the United States. The most up-to-date case definitions were published in 2010.

AVIAN CHLAMYDIOSIS

The usual incubation period of *C. psittaci* ranges from 3 days to several weeks. However, active disease can appear with no identifiable exposure or risk factor. Clinical signs of chlamydiosis in birds are often nonspecific and include lethargy, anorexia, and ruffled feathers. Other signs include serous or mucopurulent ocular or nasal discharge, conjunctivitis, diarrhea, and excretion of green to yellow-green urates. Severely affected birds may become anorectic and produce sparse, dark green droppings, followed by emaciation, dehydration, and death. Whether the bird has acute or chronic signs of illness or dies depends on the species of bird, virulence of the strain, infectious dose, stress factors, age, and extent of treatment or prophylaxis.

Case Definitions in Birds

Clinical signs may be subtle or not always evident in infected birds.

A confirmed case of avian chlamydial infection is defined on the basis of one of the following:
- Isolation of *C. psittaci* from a clinical specimen
- Identification of chlamydial antigen in the bird's tissues by use of immunofluorescence (fluorescent antibody)
- A fourfold or greater change in serologic titer in two specimens from the bird obtained at least 2 weeks apart and assayed simultaneously at the same laboratory
- Identification of Chlamydiaceae within macrophages in smears or tissues (e.g., liver, conjunctival, spleen, respiratory secretions) stained with Gimenez or Macchiavello stain

A probable case of avian chlamydial infection is defined as compatible illness and one of the following:
- A single high serologic titer in a specimen obtained after onset of clinical signs
- Chlamydiaceae antigen (identified by use of enzyme-linked immunosorbent assay [ELISA], PCR or fluorescent antibody) in feces, a cloacal swab specimen, or respiratory tract or ocular exudates

A suspected case of avian chlamydial infection is defined as one of the following:
- A compatible illness that is not laboratory confirmed but is epidemiologically linked to a confirmed case in a human or bird
- A bird with no clinical signs and a single high serologic titer or detection of chlamydial antigen
- Compatible illness with positive results from a nonstandardized test or a new investigational test
- Compatible illness that is responsive to appropriate therapy

PSITTACOSIS IN HUMANS

As mentioned earlier, psittacosis is a zoonosis, and the level of attention to this disease may vary in different countries or states. In humans, the first symptoms of disease tend to appear after an incubation period of 5 to 14 days, but on occasion, periods of more prolonged incubation have been observed (up to a month).

The first systemic manifestations can be nonspecific: fever, chills, headache, muscle aches, dry cough, and symptoms related to the upper respiratory tract. Usually, involvement of the lungs is detected radiographically, with evidence of pulmonary consolidation. However, the disease can affect organs that do not belong to the respiratory system, such as the liver, myocardium, skin, and brain. Coughing, when present, is usually a late symptom, generally with little mucopurulent expectorate. Sometimes, slowed heartbeat, chest pain, and splenomegaly can be observed, and myocarditis, encephalitis, and thrombophlebitis may occur as complications, or recurrences.

Psittacosis can be suspected in people who, in addition to presenting symptoms compatible with the disease, have had contact with birds. The diagnosis is confirmed with the isolation of the infectious agent from sputum, blood, or tissues. The analysis must be carried out in laboratories with appropriate protective measures. The etiologic diagnosis may be difficult in patients who have been treated with broad-spectrum antibiotics. People in direct contact with wild, domestic, or captive birds, such as owners and breeders of exotic birds, workers in poultry farms or poultry meat processing plants, avian veterinarians and veterinary support staff, and so on are considered to be at risk. Case definitions have been published for humans, as well:

A (human) patient is considered to have a confirmed case of psittacosis if clinical illness is compatible with psittacosis and the case is confirmed by a laboratory with the use of one of two methods:
- Isolation of *C. psittaci* from respiratory specimens (e.g., sputum, pleural fluid, or tissue) or blood
- Fourfold or greater increase in antibody (immunoglobulin G [IgG]) against *C. psittaci* by use of complement fixation (CF) or microimmunofluorescence (MIF) between paired acute-phase and convalescent-phase serum specimens obtained at least 2 to 4 weeks apart.

A (human) patient is considered to have a probable case of psittacosis if the clinical illness is compatible with psittacosis and one of the two following laboratory results is present:
- Supportive serology (e.g., *C. psittaci* antibody titer [immunoglobulin M {IgM}] of ≥32 in at least one serum specimen obtained after onset of symptoms)
- Detection of *C. psittaci* DNA in a respiratory specimen (e.g., sputum, pleural fluid, or tissue) via amplification of a specific target by polymerase chain reaction (PCR) assay.

DIAGNOSIS

The diagnosis of psittacosis in the living animal cannot be made only on the basis of clinical suspicion but must be confirmed by a series of laboratory tests. This is very important given the zoonotic nature of the disease, which carries legal implications, especially in the case of human infection.

Clinical Diagnosis

Following clinical suspicion (clinical signs), the veterinary practitioner may use supportive diagnostic tools such as hematology, blood chemistry, radiology, and endoscopy. Further, the discovery of circulating antibodies, antigen, or both plays an important role in the diagnostic process. Even the response to specific therapy (ex juvantibus diagnosis) proves to be a fundamental diagnostic factor for the clinician.

From the perspective of hematology and blood chemistry, birds with psittacosis often show anemia (hematocrit <30%), marked leukocytosis (white blood cells [WBCs] >30,000) and heterophilia (>70% to 80%). Often there is an increase in the levels of aspartate aminotransferase (AST), lactate dehydrogenase (LDH), creatine phosphokinase (CPK), and bile acids. Radiographically (Figure 2-32) and endoscopically, there are often signs of pneumonia (Figure 2-33), airsacculitis (Figure 2-34), and splenomegaly, the last being often marked in macaws.

Isolation of *C. psitacci*

Theoretically, the preferred method for diagnosis is through isolation and identification of the living organism. However, because of the time needed, the need of flawless sampling methods, and the possible risks to laboratory personnel, often other techniques are preferred. These include the immunohistochemical staining of cytologic and histologic samples, as well as enzyme-linked immunosorbent assay (ELISA) and PCR, with their many variants.

However, the *OIE Manual of Diagnostic Tests and Vaccines Standards* outlines the various steps and methods to follow and apply for the correct diagnosis of psittacosis. Samples should be collected aseptically, avoiding contamination by other bacteria. In live birds, the best sites for the collection of samples are the throat and the choana, but fecal, cloacal, and conjunctival swabs can also be used, alone or in combination, as well as the peritoneal or air sac exudate.[17] Furthermore, to optimize the chances of isolating and cultivating *C. psittaci* from a living patient, choanal and cloacal samples should be collected for 3 to 5 consecutive days. The samples should be pooled and sent to the laboratory.[18,19]

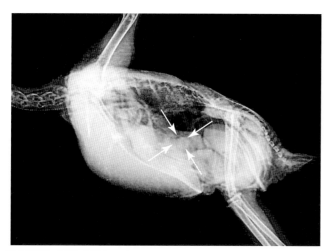

FIGURE 2-32 Mild splenomegaly in a red-tailed Amazon *(Amazona brasiliensis) (white arrows)* with chlamydiosis.

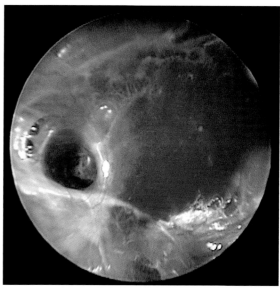

FIGURE 2-33 Pneumonia with congestion in a lovebird (*Agapornis* sp.).

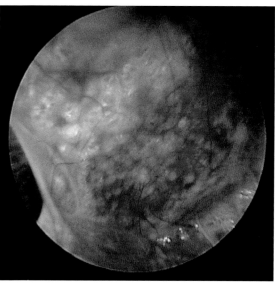

FIGURE 2-34 Airsacculitis with hemorrhage, in a blue-and-gold macaw *(Ara aurana)* with chlamydiosis.

There are specific transport media for Chlamydiae, for example, the GSP transport medium for Rickettsiae or the UTM (Coban). These media work well and carry added vancomycin, streptomycin, nystatin, and gentamicin to reduce contamination by other microorganisms. Moreover, these media can be used as diluents in the laboratory and to freeze chlamydia.[20]

Isolation of Chlamydiae in Eukaryotic Cell Cultures

Cell cultures are one of the best methods for the isolation of *C. psittaci*,[21] and there are different cell lines suitable for the purpose, such as BGM, McCoy, He-La, Vero, and others.[22] Normally, the cell lines contain antibiotics that do not inhibit the growth of *C. psittaci*. However, isolation is laborious and costly and has largely been replaced by other techniques such as PCR.

In the selection of equipment and materials for cell cultures, it is important to remember the following:

1. Chlamydiae can be identified by using direct immunofluorescence or other appropriate staining techniques.
2. The inoculum is usually centrifuged to increase its infectivity.
3. The sample may have to undergo a blind passage at 5 to 6 days to increase sensitivity of isolation.
4. The sample should be tested two or three times during each step.
5. *C. psittaci* may be infectious to humans.

Chlamydiae can be isolated on cells that replicate normally. Cells that are not able to replicate are preferred for isolation, since they can provide a greater amount of nutrients for the growth of organisms. Moreover, these cells can be monitored and observed for longer periods.

Cell cultures should be checked for the presence of Chlamydiae at regular intervals. This is generally done at day 2 or 3, as well as on day 5 or 6. Cultures that are negative on day 6 are harvested and replanted.

Several staining methods may be used to stain *C. psittaci* inclusions, but the preferred one is direct immunofluorescence, in which inclusions appear fluorescent green.[22-24] *C. psittaci* inclusions may also be demonstrated by using indirect immunofluorescence and immunoperoxidase.[22,24,25] Direct staining can be done with the Gimenez, Giemsa, Ziehl-Neelsen, or Macchiavello stain. With the exception of immunofluorescence, all the other techniques have the advantage of being suitable for a normal optical microscope.

Isolation on Embryonated Eggs

Chicken embryos can still be used for the isolation of *Chlamydia*. The standard procedure is to inject up to 0.5 milliliters (mL) of inoculum in the yolk sac of embryos of 6 or 7 days. The eggs are then incubated at 39° C rather than 37° C. In fact, the multiplication of Chlamydiae increases at high temperatures. The replication of the organism causes the death of the embryo in 3 to 10 days. If it does not happen, two other blind steps are done, at the end of which, if the embryo is still alive, the sample is declared negative. Infection with *Chlamydia* is determined by typical vascular congestion of the yolk membrane. These are collected and homogenized with a 20% suspension of SPG buffer, and then they are frozen or inoculated on eggs or cell cultures.[26] The organism can be identified by preparing an antigen from an infected yolk sac and then testing a smear with an appropriate staining method or with a serological test.

Histochemical Stains

Giemsa, Gimenez, Ziehl-Neelsen, and Macchiavello stains are normally used to stain the Chlamydiae on liver or spleen direct smears. Alternatively, a modified Gimenez (or Pierce-van der Kamp) stain can be used.

Immunohistochemical Staining

These techniques can be used for the identification of *C. psittaci* in cytologic or histologic preparations. The technique is more sensitive than standard histochemical staining, but some experience is required, since some cross-reactions with certain bacteria and fungi are to be expected. For these reasons, specific morphologic aspects have to be evaluated as well. Most of the common immunohistochemical staining can be adapted to obtain satisfactory results; however, the selection of the primary antibody is very important. Both monoclonal and polyclonal antibodies can be used. When having to work with Chlamydiae that have been inactivated by formalin, since formalin damages the antigen, it is better to use polyclonal antibodies. The *Chlamydia* strain that is used does not really matter, since the antibodies will react with antigens that are common to the whole group.

Enzyme-Linked Immunosorbent Assay

The ELISA technique has been widely advertised in the form of simple kits for the diagnosis of human chlamydiosis. These kits seek a lipopolysaccharide antigen (LPS), which is common to all the *Chlamydiae* and therefore will be able to identify all species of the group. Many commercial tests of this type were tested in birds, but no test has been officially approved.[27] One of the problems with these tests is that the chlamydial LPS has epitopes in common with other gram-negative bacteria and the frequent cross-reactions give many false-positive results. This problem seems to be overcome, or at least reduced, with the newest kits that use selected monoclonal antibodies (MAbs). However, these kits do not have high sensitivity, and they still need hundreds of antigen units to give a positive reaction. For this reason, many clinicians believe that the diagnosis of psittacosis in birds with antigen ELISA should be considered valid only if the reaction is very positive in symptomatic birds. Part of the reason is that a high number of false positives can be obtained; therefore, a positive ELISA antigen result in an individual nonsymptomatic bird should be considered not significant.

Polymerase Chain Reaction

The PCR technique is based on the identification of DNA (or RNA) sequences that are specific to a given organism[28,29] and has long been used for the diagnosis of *C. trachomatis* in humans, in whom it is considered highly sensitive and specific. Unfortunately, the test is not directly applicable to other Chlamydiae because it searches a plasmid that is present only on *C. trachomatis* and, therefore, cannot be used for the diagnosis of psittacosis in birds. A further problem lies in the variety of different samples used for the extraction of DNA in the veterinary field, such as oral, conjunctival, and cloacal swabs, as well as tissue samples.[30]

In recent times, PCR has replaced traditional methods as the preferred method for detecting chlamydial infections in humans and animals.[31,32] This method is reliable, rapid, and highly sensitive and can be used on nonviable specimens. Additional advantages include opportunities for subsequent speciation and fine-detailed molecular typing of isolates.

PCR assays targeting a variety of chlamydial genes are available, and a range of specificities and sensitivities has been reported. The most common amplification targets are genes encoding chlamydial 16S rRNA, 23S rRNA, and ompA (encoding MOMP). PCRs that target the 16S rRNA-23S rRNA region are generally able to amplify all members of the order Chlamydiales but make subsequent speciation difficult because of the conservation between species.[4] ompA has also been widely used but is highly variable; this makes selection of conserved PCR primers difficult, but the variability can be used for fine-detailed epidemiologic analysis of chlamydial outbreaks in animal populations.[6]

Serology Tests

Serologic tests are a great aid in the diagnosis of psittacosis, but they have a greater significance when used in association with other analyses and observations. Serologic assays are particularly valuable in cases with symptomatic populations and individual animals and to monitor response to treatment.[19,33]

Complement fixation test

Serology, particularly in the form of the complement fixation test (CFT), is still a convenient and commonly used technique for detecting present and past chlamydial infections in humans, cats, birds, cattle, and small ruminants. Although the sensitivity is significantly less than 100%, the ease of collection of blood samples and the availability of technology to perform these tests make these ideal for screening large numbers of samples (particularly suited to screen livestock).[6] The standard serologic test for chlamydial antibodies is the CFT. The modified direct CFT can be used with most sera. The antigen is a group-reactive lipopolysaccharide antigen present in all strains. The occurrence of high complement fixation titers in the majority of individuals in a flock with clinical signs is presumptive evidence of active infection. The demonstration of a fourfold increase in titer in an individual bird is considered to be diagnostic of a current infection.[20]

Other tests

Other serologic tests such as ELISA, latex agglutination, EB agglutination, microimmunofluorescence, and agar gel immunodiffusion tests can be used. These tests are of value in specific cases and may replace the CFT; however, comparisons of reliability and reproducibility are not yet available.[20]

Some trials of ELISA for the detection of antibodies against both *C. trachomatis* and *C. psittaci* indicate that in many cases these can replace the CFT.[34–37] However, the tests must be standardized and are not available for all avian species. However, some modified ELISA kit tests for research of anti–*C. psittaci* in parrots are already available commercially.[38,39]

Other possible diagnostic tests are agar gel immunodiffusion (AGID),[40] latex agglutination (LA), EB agglutination (EBA),[41,42] and micro-immunofluorescence (MIF) tests. AGID is less sensitive than complement fixation, although it is more easy and quicker to perform.[43] There is a correlation of 72.5% between latex agglutination and direct complement fixation. LA has a sensitivity of 39.1% and a specificity of 98.8%, compared with direct complement fixation.[43] This test searches both IgM and IgG (IgY), but it is more suitable for the detection of IgM. Therefore, it is recommended to be used for active or recent infections. The EBA can only identify IgM and is therefore indicated only for active infections. The MIF is easy and quick to perform, but unfortunately species-specific fluorescent sera are not always available.

THERAPY

The "traditional" treatment for avian chlamydiosis is based on the administration of tetracyclines for 45 days. The duration of treatment depends on the fact that the antibiotic cannot penetrate the macrophages and therefore cannot reach *C. psittaci* and neutralize it. During the 45-day treatment, at least two complete replicative cycles of avian macrophages take place, and during the division phase, the microorganism should be released from the cells and, if the plasma concentration of antibiotic is sufficiently high to inhibit *C. psittaci*, the organism should be eliminated.

Doxycycline is the accepted first-choice drug for treatment. This is probably because whatever the route of administration, doxycycline shows good bioavailability; furthermore, its absorption is not influenced by the intake of dietary calcium compared with other tetracyclines.[19] There are some established protocols, the most used being intramuscular injections of high doses of doxycycline (75 to 100 mg/kg) on days 0, 7, 7, 7, 7, 6, 5, and 5. The shortening of the interval between injections depends on the development of enzymatic mechanisms that facilitate the metabolism of the drug, which thus would not be able to maintain a therapeutically effective concentration in the last stages.

Also, the formulation of the finished drug, including the doxycycline salt and the vehicle used, affects its absorption. Thus, after various studies and clinical trials, the most used preparation is a product for human use (Vibravenös, Pfizer). Although it is a preparation for intravenous use, it has been demonstrated that it can be used intramuscularly in birds. Among other things, particularly in the case of untamed birds, it may be easier to bring the patient to the veterinarian (or administer the injection) every 5 to 7 days than to catch the bird(s) on a daily basis for a month and a half. The dose of doxycycline that is injected varies somewhat, and readers are encouraged to seek species-specific recommendations in the formulary of this text or others. Alternatively, doxycycline and other tetracyclines can be given orally via drinking water or medicated food or through direct administration.

Administration via drinking water is carried out at a concentration of 400 mg doxycycline hyclate per liter of water for cockatiels (*Nymphicus hollandicus*); for other species, the doxycycline concentration can be increased up to 600 mg/L.[19,20] Unfortunately, no data on the possible toxicity of this treatment regimen are available; however, the reported symptoms are depression, anorexia, biliverdinuria, and alteration of liver enzymes.[19]

Therapy with medicated food can give good results, especially because it is easier to control the intake of food compared with water. For this purpose, in the past, corn was soaked in a solution of chlortetracycline, but currently extruded and pelleted diets, with 1% chlortetracycline, are available. The drawback to this method is that the birds should already be accustomed to eating pelleted or extruded diets before the onset of treatment. For this reason, medicated food is often used for the prophylaxis of groups that are first adapted to the diet and for individual patients that already eat extruded or pelleted diets.[19] Direct, oral treatment is practical and easy to do, but it can cause minor gastrointestinal symptoms. The recommended dosage in parrots varies among studied species, with a generic recommendation from 25 to 50 mg/kg, every day.[19] Species-specific dosage recommendations are as follows: 25 to 35 mg/kg every 24 hours for cockatiels; 25 to 50 mg/kg for Senegal parrots and blue-fronted and orange-winged Amazon parrots; and 25 mg/kg every 24 hours for Grey parrots, Goffin's cockatoos, blue and gold macaws, and green-winged macaws. Precise dosages cannot be extrapolated for other species; however, 25 to 30 mg/kg every 24 hours is the recommended starting dosage for cockatoos and macaws. If the bird regurgitates or refuses orally administered doxycycline, another treatment method should be used.

In the past, it was hypothesized that a 3-week treatment can be as effective as a 45-day course of antibiotics. In addition, it was supposed that most treatment failures were not due to the drug or to the duration of therapy but to the microorganism.[44] Recent publications have demonstrated the possibility of shortening the treatment time to less than half (21 days), compared with the classic duration of 45 days, by administering oral doxycycline at lower doses (35 mg/kg) and with shorter intervals (24 hours).

Alternatively, fluoroquinolones (enrofloxacin) or macrolides (azithromycin) have been proposed for the treatment of avian chlamydiosis. Although results of early experimental studies suggested enrofloxacin as a potential alternative treatment, anecdotal use of enrofloxacin in clinical practice showed that many birds fail to eliminate infection.[45]

Macrolide antibiotics such as azithromycin and clarithromycin have been used for years to treat humans with *C. trachomatis* or *C. pneumoniae* infections.[45] The main advantage of the newest macrolides is their ability to enter the macrophages in an active form. For this reason, it has been theorized that azithromycin is a better drug for the treatment of long-term, chronic, or "persistent" infections, while the classic intramuscular doxycycline is a better choice for the acute clinical forms, with the classic psittacosis symptoms.

THE AVIAN CHLAMYDIOSIS CONNECTION: AN INFORMAL WORLD TOUR AS IT IS SEEN BY SURVEYED AVIAN VETERINARIANS

One of the most sensitive points about chlamydiosis is its zoonotic nature. The capability of this organism to infect humans has a great impact on the perception of the general public about the disease. Furthermore, depending on the geographic location in the world, several clinical aspects of psittacosis may vary. For example, these may include the prevalence of the agent in a given wild population of birds or the incidence of disease; the variety of captively maintained or domestic species that are presented for diagnosis and treatment; the treatments used by veterinarians; and the legal implications in a given country or region. All of these factors and more will influence many aspects of disease recognition, diagnosis, and treatment options put into play.

To get an idea about how often the disease is seen in practice, how it is managed, and how often it is reported, a small, informal Internet survey of several veterinarians around the world was conducted. The outcome is interesting, and the author (LC) is grateful to those participating colleagues who took the time to answer the questions. The questions included the following: (1) Do you see chlamydiosis cases? (2) If yes, which species are most commonly seen with the disease? (3) What are the predominant clinical signs that you see? (4) How is diagnosis made most often? (5) What is your most common therapeutic plan? (6) Have you seen or heard of cases in humans? (7) Is avian chlamydiosis (psittacosis) a notifiable (reportable) disease where you practice? The survey results are presented in Table 2-8.

The most common species recognized with the disease seemed to be the cockatiel *(Nymphicus hollandicus)*, followed by the budgerigar *(Melopsittacus undulatus)*. Larger parrots or other species were mentioned less often, and the frequency of these other species presenting with this disease may be dependent, at least in part, on the geographic location or the nature of practice exposure. The most commonly described clinical presentation included the "classic" upper respiratory form, with conjunctivitis and oculonasal discharge; this may or may not be combined with the other set of clinical signs—those associated with hepatic disease. In addition to clinical signs compatible with the disease, leading to a heightened index of suspicion, other diagnostics that play an important role in diagnosis included supportive clinical pathology and diagnostic imaging. PCR, performed on conjunctival, oral, and cloacal swabs, appears to be a commonly employed diagnostic tool. Serologically, Immunocomb, a commercially available modified ELISA antibody test, appears to be a fairly common test utilized in diagnosis (but this brand is not available everywhere in the world). A 45-day course of parenteral doxycycline seems to be widely used as the "standard treatment" for psittacosis, although orally administered azithromycin in some regions appears to be a common option. Differences of opinion and treatment options seem to exist with regard to the treatment method for small or larger psittacines and also for tame pet birds and breeding or avicultural specimens. Most of the surveyed practitioners reported having seen cases of human chlamydiosis. However, these appear to be infrequent, overall. Interestingly, two of the interviewed colleagues had suffered from psittacosis themselves. Other colleagues noted that their diagnoses in humans had been confirmed following their recommendations to see their physicians. There was concern expressed about lack of familiarity in some physicians with the disease, its diagnosis in humans, and treatment. The medicolegal aspects of notifiability, that is, the level and manner of notifiable diagnosis, with regard to chlamydiosis seem to vary . Each country seems to treat the problem differently, and even where there is a federation of different states (e.g., Australia, United States), those different states may apply different laws and regulations. In some countries, even if avian chlamydiosis is a notifiable disease, case definitions and the circumstances under which the disease should be reported vary. It appears advisable for avian veterinarians to obtain the relevant recommendations from the appropriate authorities in their area in order to most optimally pursue diagnosis (suspect, probable, or confirmed) and properly address human health concerns, where applicable. An example of case definitions (human and birds), with diagnosis and treatment options, can be found and downloaded in PDF format from the Centers for Disease Control (CDC) website: http://www.nasphv.org/Documents/Psittacosis.pdf.

REFERENCES

1. Andersen AA, Franson JC: Avian chlamydiosis. In Thomas NJ, Hunter DB, Atkinson CT, editors: *Infectious diseases of wild birds*, Ames, IA, 2007, Blackwell Publishing, pp 303–316.
2. Meyer KF: Phagocytosis and immunity in psittacosis, *Schweizerische Medizinische Wochenschrift* 71:436-438, 1941.

3. Office International des Epizooties: Avian chlamydiosis. In World Organisation for Animal Health: *Manual of standards, Diagnostic Tests and Vaccines*, Paris, France, 2000, World Organisation for Animal Health.

4. Everett et al: Emended description of the order Chlamydiales, proposal of Parachlamydiaceae fam. nov. and Simkaniaceae fam. nov., each containing one monotypic genus, revised taxonomy of the family Chlamydiaceae, including a new genus and five new species, and standards for the identification of organisms, *Int J Systemat Evolution Microbiol* 49:415–440, 1999.

5. Stephens RS, Myers G, Eppinger M, et al: Divergence without difference: phylogenetic and taxonomy of *Chlamydia* resolved, *FEMS Immunol Med Microbiol* 55:115–119, 2009.

6. Polkinghorne A: Chlamydiosis: the ignored zoonotic—chlamydia, the organism, *AAAV Austr Comm Proc* 2010.

7. Gerlach H: Chlamydia. In Ritchie BW, Harrison GJ and Harrison LR, editors: *Avian medicine and surgery: principles and application*, Lake Worth, FL, 1994, Wingers Publishing Inc., pp 984–996.

8. Allen I, et al: Host modification of chlamydiae: presence of an egg antigen on the surface of chlamydiae grown in the chick embryo, *J Gen Microbiol* 112:61–66, 1979.

9. Gylstorff I: Chlamydiales. In Gylstroff I, Grimm F, editors: *Vogelkrankheiten*. Stuttgart, Germany, 1987, Verlag Eugen Ulmer, pp 317–322.

10. Gerlach H: Chlamydia. In Harrison GJ, Harrison LR, editors: *Clinical avian medicine and surgery*, Philadelphia, London, Toronto, 1986, WB Saunders Co., pp 457–463.

11. Wyrick PB, et al: Biology of chlamydiae, *J Am Vet Med Assoc* 195:1507–1512, 1989.

12. Grimes JE, et al: Chlamydiosis (ornithosis). In Calnek BW, et al, editors: Diseases of poultry, 9th ed. Prescott, AZ, 1991, Wolfe Publishing, pp 311–325.

13. Illner F: Zur Frage der bertragung des Ornithosevirus durch das Ei, *Mb Vet Med* 17:116–117, 1962.

14. Reference deleted in pages.

15. Olsen GH, et al: A review of some causes of death of avian embryos, *Proc Assoc Avian Vet* , 106–111, 1990.

16. Burkhart RL, Page LA: Chlamydiosis (ornithosis, psittacosis). In Davis JW, Anderson RC, Karstad L, Trainer DO, editors: *Infectious and parasitic diseases of wild birds*, Ames, IA, 1971, Iowa State University Press, pp 118–140.

17. Andersen AA: Comparison of pharyngeal, fecal, and cloacal samples for the isolation of *Chlamydia psittaci* from experimentally infected cockatiels and turkeys, *J Vet Diagn Invest* 8:448–450, 1996.

18. CDC (Centers for Disease Control and Prevention): Compendium of measures to control *Chlamydia psittaci* infection among humans (psittacosis) and pet birds (avian chlamydiosis), 2010. Available from: http://www.nasphv.org/Documents/Psittacosis.pdf. 2010. Accessed Feb. 17 2015.

19. Tully TN: Update on *Chlamydophila psittaci, Semin Avian Exot Pet Med* 10(1):20–24, 2001.

20. Office International des Epizooties: *Manual of diagnostic tests and vaccines for terrestrial animals*, Paris, France, 2014, Office International des Epizooties.

21. Vanrompay D, Ducatelle R, Haesebrouck F: Diagnosis of avian chlamydiosis: specificity of the modified Gimenez staining on smears and comparison of the sensitivity of isolation in eggs and three different cell cultures, *J Vet Med B* 39:105–112, 1992.

22. Andersen AA: Chlamydiosis. In *A laboratory manual for the isolation and identification of avian pathogens*, 4th ed. Dubuque, IA, 1998, Kendall/Hunt Publishing.

23. Bevan BJ, Bracewell CD: Chlamydiosis in birds in Great Britain. 2. Isolations of *Chlamydia psittaci* from birds sampled between 1976 and 1984, *J Hyg Camb* 96:453–458, 1986.

24. Moore FM, Petrak ML: *Chlamydia* immunoreactivity in birds with psittacosis: localization of chlamydiae by the peroxidase antiperoxidase method, *Avian Dis* 29:1036–1042, 1985.

25. Andersen AA, Van Dusen RA: Production and partial characterization of monoclonal antibodies to four *Chlamydia psittaci* isolates, *Infect Immun* 56:2075–2079, 1988.

26. Andersen AA, Grimes JE, Wyrick PB: Chlamydiosis (psittacosis, ornithosis). In *Diseases of poultry*, 10th ed. Ames, IA, 1997, Iowa State University Press, pp 333–349.

27. Vanrompay D, Van Nerom A, Ducatelle R et al: Evaluation of five immunoassays for detection of *Chlamydia psittaci* in cloacal and conjunctival specimens from turkeys, *J Clin Microbiol* 32:1470–1474, 1994.

28. Tully TN: Update on *Chlamydophila psittaci*. A short comment. In Harrison GJ, Lightfoot T, et al, editors: *Clinical avian medicine*, Palm Beach, FL, 2006, Spix Publishing, Inc., pp 679–680.

29. Messmer T, Tully TN, Ritchie BW, et al: A tale of discrimination: differentiation of Chlamydiaceae by polymerase chain reaction. *Semin Avian Exotic Pet Med* 9:36–42, 2000.

30. Takashima I, Imai Y, Kariwa H, et al: Polymerase chain-reaction for the detection of *Chlamydia psittaci* in the feces of budgerigars, *Microbiol Immunol* 40:21–26, 1996.

31. Hewinson RG, Griffiths PC, Bevan BJ, et al: Detection of *Chlamydia psittaci* DNA in avian clinical samples by polymerase chain reaction, *Vet Microbiol* 54:155–166, 1997.

32. Isaza R, Murray MJ, Vanrompay D, et al: Round table discussion: use of PCR testing in diagnosing chlamydiosis, *J Avian Med Surg* 14:122–127, 2000.

33. Vanrompay D: Avian chlamydial diagnostics. In Fudge AM, editor: Laboratory medicine: avian and exotic pets, Philadelphia, PA, 2000, Saunders, pp 99–110.

34. Evans RT, Chalmers WSK, Woolcock PR, et al: An enzyme-linked immunosorbent assay (ELISA) for detection of chlamydial antibody in duck sera, *Avian Pathol* 12:117-124. 1983.

35. Lang GH: La chlamydiose du dindon: Diagnostic serologique par la methode ELISA, *Rec Med Vet* 160:763–771, 1984.

36. Pepin M, Bailly L, Souriau A, et al: An enzyme-linked immunosorbent assay (ELISA) for the detection of chlamydial antibodies in caprine sera, *Ann Rech Vet* 16:393-398. 1985.

37. Ruppaner R, Behymer DE, Delong WJ III, et al: Enzyme immunoassay of chlamydia in birds, *Avian Dis* 28:608–615, 1984.

38. Bendheim U, Wodowski I, Ordonez M et al: Entwicklung eines ELISA kit fur die antikorperbestimmung bei psittaziden. (The development of an ELISA-kit for antibody determination in birds including poultry and psittacines.) In *Proceedings of Deutsch Veterinarmedizinische Gesellschaft*, Munchen, Germany, 1994.

39. Lublin A, Leiderman E, Mechani S, et al: Influence of ambient temperature on shedding of *Chlamydia psittaci* in pigeons. In *Proceedings of the 4th Conference of the European Committee of the Association of Avian Veterinarians*, London, England, 1997.

40. Page LA: Application of an agar gel precipitin test to the serodiagnosis of avian chlamydiosis, *Proc Am Assoc Vet Lab Diagnosticians* 17:51–61, 1974.

41. Grimes JE, Tully TN Jr., Arizmendi F, et al: Elementary body agglutination for rapidly demonstrating chlamydial agglutinins in avian serum with emphasis on testing cockatiels, *Avian Dis* 38:822–831, 1994.

42. Grimes JE, Arizmendi F: Usefulness and limitations of three serologic methods for diagnosing or excluding chlamydiosis in birds, *J Am Vet Med Assoc* 209:747–750, 1996.

43. Grimes JE, Phalen DN, Arizmendi F: *Chlamydia* latex agglutination antigen and protocol improvement and psittacine bird anti-chlamydial immunoglobulin reactivity, *Avian Dis* 37:817–824, 1993.

44. Gerlach H: personal communication, Tenerife, Spain, 2000.

45. Sanchez-Migallon Guzman D, et al: Evaluating 21-day doxycycline and azithromycin treatments for experimental *Chlamydophila psittaci* infection in cockatiels (*Nymphicus hollandicus*), *J Avian Med Surg* 24(1):35–45, 2010.

TABLE 2-8

Summary of Findings from Informal Survey of Avian Chlamydiosis As It Is Seen by Avian Veterinarians in the World

1	Do you see Chlamydiosis cases?	Yes	Occasionally	Not as much as in years past	Yes	Yes, but not commonly	Yes	Yes
2	If yes, which species are most commonly seen with the disease?	Cockatiels	Small psittacines	Cockatiels, budgerigars	Red-Tailed hawks	Pigeons, budgerigars	Sun conures, cockatoos	Cockatiels, budgerigars, Grey parrots
		Occasionally large and wild parrots	Rarely larger parrots, particularly macaws	Less common large parrots		Parrot nurseries	Feral pigeons and wild sparrows	Amazons, macaws
3	What are the predominant clinical signs that you see?	Conjunctivitis, sinusitis	Generalized (systemic) disease, conjunctivitis	Oculonasal discharge, depression	Poor body condition, lethargy	Upper respiratory signs	Chronic weight loss, oculonasal discharge	Nonspecific signs of illness, hepatopathy
		Systemic disease, airsacculitis, hepatitis		Hepatopathy	Poor feather condition, oculonasal and respiratory signs	Hepatitis, sudden death	Chronic respiratory disease, hepatopathy	Respiratory signs, feather damaging behaviors
4	How is diagnosis made most often?	Clinical signs, serology (Immunocomb)	Clinical signs, serology and polymerase chain reaction (PCR); splenic biopsy	Clinical signs, serology (Immunocomb)	Clinical signs, PCR, necropsy	Clinical signs, PCR, necropsy	Clinical signs, PCR	Clinical signs, complete blood count (CBC), blood chemistries, serology (Immunocomb), PCR
5	What is your most common therapeutic plan?	Parenteral doxycycline (intramuscular [IM])	Large birds: Parenteral doxycycline (IM); small birds: enrofloxacin	Doxycycline IM or orally (PO)	Euthanasia	Doxycycline	Doxycycline, azythromicin	Parenteral doxycycline (IM) 45 days; azythromicin 3 weeks
6	Have you seen or heard of cases in humans?	Yes: co-workers	Yes: myself	Yes: but few	Yes: but many years ago	Yes: several	Yes: veterinarians	Yes: but unconfirmed ones
7	Is Avian chlamydiosis (psittacosis) a notifiable (reportable) disease where you practice?	Yes	No: there are no formal rules	No	Yes	No	Yes: there is a specific government manual	Yes

The authors would like to thank the following for their assistance: Dr. Roberto Aguilar (New Zealand); Dr. Marco Bedin (Italy); Dr. John Chitty (UK); Dr. Erica Couto (Brazil); Dr. Tânia de Freitas Raso (Brazil); Dr. Luis Flores Giron (Spain); Dr. Brett Gartrell (New Zealand); Dr. Alessandro Melillo (Italy); Dr. Deborah Monks (Australia); Dr. Andres Montesinos (Spain); Dr. Javier Origlia (Argentina); Dr. Adrian Petta (Argentina); Dr. David Phalen (Australia); Dr. Miguel Saggese (USA); Dr. Jaime Samour (Abu Dhabi, United Arab Emirates); Dr. David Sanchez-Migallon Guzman (USA); Dr. Brian Speer (USA); Dr. Kaset Sutasha (Thailand); and Dr. Kevin Turner (New Zealand).

Yes	Yes	Yes	Yes	Yes	Yes	Yes, approximately twice each year	Yes, but less often than in in the past	Yes
Quaker parakeets, blue fronted Amazons, Patagonian conures	Gray parrots, cockatiels	Cockatiels	Quaker parakeets, budgerigars	Blue-fronted Amazons, Quaker parakeets	Cockatiels, budgerigars	Macaws and Amazons	Amazons, conures, macaws	Eclectus parrots, budgerigars, sulfur-crested cockatoos
	Less common lovebirds		Amazona aestiva, *Cyanolyseus patagonicus*	Chickens, pigeons	Larger parrots	Less Greys and cockatiels	Less frequent lovebirds	Cockatiels, chickens
Upper respiratory signs	Conjunctivitis	Nonspecific signs of illness	Conjunctivitis, sinusitis	Conjunctivitis, nasal discharge, diarrhea	Conjunctivitis, rhinitis, acute or chronic hepatopathies	Conjunctivitis, nasal discharge	Weight loss, chronic hepatopathies, poor plumage quality, biliverdinuria	Lethargy, anorexia, conjunctivitis, respiratory signs, generalized ill thrift
Conjunctivitis, oculonasal discharge	Hepatopathies less often	Conjunctivitis, weight loss, diarrhea	General depression		Generalized ill-thrift, weight loss	Chronic weight loss, poor feathering		
Clinical signs, direct stain from swabs, serology (enzyme-linked immunosorbent assay [ELISA]), immunofluorescence	Clinical signs, PCR	Clinical signs, PCR	Clinical signs, direct stain from swabs, PCR	Clinical signs, PCR	Clinical signs, history, clinical pathology findings, diagnostic imaging, response to treatment, high antibody titer, PCR, immunofluorescence assay (IFA) or special stains of tissue samples	Clinical signs, clinical pathology findings, serology (Immunocomb), PCR	Clinical signs, CBC, protein electrophoresis, serology (Immunocomb), PCR	Clinical signs, CBC, blood chemistry, diagnostic imaging, serology (Immunocomb), ELISA antigen capture or PCR from choanal/cloacal swab, necropsy
Doxycycline	Doxycycline, enrofloxacin	Doxycycline, enrofloxacin, azythromicin	Doxycycline, enrofloxacin, azithromycin	Doxycycline, azithromycin	Parenteral doxycycline (IM) predominantly	Parenteral doxycycline (IM), 45 days	Pet birds: azithromycin PO; wild or aviary birds: doxycycline in water	Parenteral doxycycline (IM) for 6 Weeks; oral doxycycline as an alternative
Yes: several	Yes: few	Yes	Yes: particularly bird breeders	Yes: several	Yes: some	No	Yes: but not recently	Yes
No	Yes	Yes		Reportable	Reportable	Reportable	Reportable	Not notifiable

MYCOBACTERIOSIS

Angela Lennox

ETIOLOGY AND PREVALENCE

Mycobacterial infections have been described in companion, zoo, and free-ranging birds for many years. Strict eradication programs have nearly eliminated mycobacteriosis in commercial poultry flocks.[1] Mycobacterial infections consist of tuberculous and atypical nontuberculous species. Most infections in birds are atypical nontuberculous and involve species such as *Mycobacterium genavense*, and *M. avium*. A recent 2013 report described *M. genavense* as the most commonly identified species in psittacines.[2] Other atypical organisms include *M. marinum* and others.[3] Tuberculous mycobacteriosis, which is a major health concern in humans, is rarely reported in bird species.

Many different avian species have been affected with mycobacteriosis and include psittacines, passerines, waterfowl, and wild and zoo species. An earlier survey of pet psittacines birds suggested an overall infection prevalence of 0.5% to 14%, with the following species most commonly affected: brotogerid parakeets (*Brotogeris* spp.), Amazon parrots (*Amazona* spp.), budgerigars (*Melopsittacus undulates*), and Pionus parrots (*Pionus* spp.).[4] Similarly, a more recent updated review of 123 cases in psittacines indicated the most commonly affected psittacines were Amazon parrots (*Amazona* sp.), and gray-cheeked parakeets (*Brotogeris pyrrophterus*).[2] As these organisms are slow growing and disease is chronic, this tends to be a disease of older birds. There is no reported gender predilection.

EXPOSURE

Atypical mycobacterial organisms are commonly found in the environment, especially in water and soil. Organisms can survive in the environment for long periods. It is assumed that birds acquire atypical mycobacteriosis via ingestion of organisms in food or water or through contact with infected soil.[1,2] Although there are no confirmed cases of bird-to-bird transmission, outbreaks have occurred in free-ranging nonpsittacine birds, including an epizootic in free-ranging flamingos that resulted in 18,500 deaths within a short period. This outbreak was associated with malnutrition and other conditions resulting in immunodeficiency, in combination with dense populations and overwhelming exposure to organisms shed in feces.[5] In humans and some other species, immunocompromise or exposure to large numbers of organisms are a prerequisite for infection with atypical mycobacteriosis.[6] It is uncertain if immunocompromise is required for disease in individual captive birds.

Sporadic cases of tuberculous mycobacteriosis (*M. tuberculosis*) have been reported in birds, including a macaw, an Amazon parrot, and a canary.[7,8] In the case of the blue-and-gold macaw, the source was assumed to be an infected owner.[8] There are no current confirmed cases of transmission of any mycobacterial organism from birds to humans.

Routes of Infection and Pathogenesis

Many body systems can be infected, including the gastrointestinal (GI) tract, liver, respiratory tract, bone, dermis, and others, and this is likely related to the route of infection. A recent review of avian submissions indicated the liver was most commonly affected, followed by the spleen and then the GI tract.[2] Fatal *M. genavense* infection in the central nervous system (CNS) of a spectacled Amazon parrot (*Amazona albifrons*) has been described.[9]

After ingestion of organisms, the organisms infect the small intestine and the liver. Hematogenous spread leads to infection of the bone marrow, lungs, air sacs, spleen, gonads, and, rarely, kidney and pancreas.[2]

Inhalation of organisms may lead to pulmonary infections. Organisms may also enter wounds. The author noted a case of atypical mycobacteriosis associated with a wing web tattoo site used to indicate gender after surgical sexing.

Atypical nontuberculous infections tend to cause diffuse enlargement of the affected organ(s) secondary to macrophage accumulation within the organ parenchyma. The liver may appear enlarged and tan-colored, without visible granulomas, and the intestinal loops may be thickened. In contrast, *M. tuberculosis* infections tend to produce visible nodules containing epithelioid cells, giant cells, and heterophils. The cytoplasm of affected cells is filled with acid-fast organisms.[4]

CLINICAL PRESENTATION

Symptoms of mycobacteriosis are generally nonspecific and vary widely, depending on the length and severity of infection and the organ system affected. Birds can present with weight loss, poor feathering, polyuria, diarrhea, and abdominal distention. Birds with respiratory infections may present with abnormal respirations (rate or effort) and audible respiratory sounds. Some birds die acutely without recognized signs of illness. Less common physical examination findings can include lameness, cutaneous masses, and ocular lesions (Figures 2-35 through 2-37). Weight loss appears to be the most consistent finding in birds with mycobacteriosis. In many cases, birds fail to respond or only temporarily respond to routine antibiotic therapeutic choices.[4,10,11]

Because of the wide range of body systems affected and the chronic nature of the disease, the differential diagnosis list can be extensive and include numerous other infectious, neoplastic, or metabolic diseases. In cases of dermal or conjunctival masses, differential diagnoses include inflammation, infection, cysts, and neoplasia.

Supportive Laboratory Data and Diagnostic Findings

General diagnostic testing results are often nonspecific. Hemogram abnormalities vary; however, typical "textbook" disseminated mycobacteriosis in psittacine birds tends to produce moderate to marked increases in white blood cell numbers characterized by heterophilia and monocytosis. Reactive lymphocytosis can be present. Birds with impaired immunologic function or only localized disease may not exhibit leukocyte abnormalities. Packed cell volume (PCV) is often decreased as a result of chronic infection or inflammation; however, in some cases of primary respiratory mycobacteriosis, PCV can be greatly increased. These hematologic abnormalities can be present in many inflammatory and chronic disease conditions other than mycobacteriosis.[12,13]

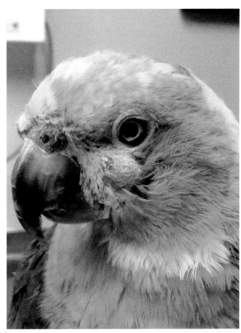

FIGURE 2-35 Left-sided view of a yellow-naped Amazon parrot *(Amazona auropalliata)* with facial and oral lesions confirmed as *Mycobacterium genavense*. (Courtesy Dr. Brian Speer.)

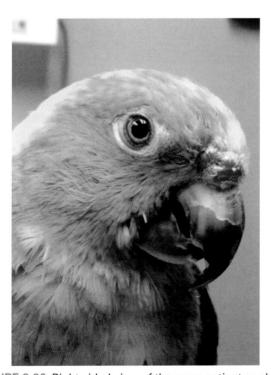

FIGURE 2-36 Right-sided view of the same patient as shown in Figure 2-35, yellow-naped Amazon parrot *(Amazona auropalliata)* with facial and oral lesions confirmed as *Mycobacterium genavense*. Note the asymmetry of the appearance of the lesions. (Courtesy Dr. Brian Speer.)

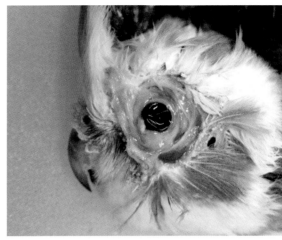

FIGURE 2-37 Necropsy images of a cockatiel *(Nymphicus hollandicus)* with *Mycobacterium genavense*–related conjunctivitis. (Courtesy Dr. Geoff Olsen.)

Hepatic mycobacteriosis can produce increases in concentrations of enzymes such as alanine aminotransferase (ALT), aspartate aminotransferase, (AST), and lactate dehydrogenase (LDH). However, these enzymes are also present in varying amounts in a variety of other tissues such as muscle, kidney, and heart. Therefore, increases may not truly reflect hepatocellular damage. Conversely, enzyme concentrations can be normal in the face of severe hepatic disease. If liver function has been compromised, hepatic mycobacteriosis may produce increased concentrations of serum bile acids. Plasma protein electrophoresis results are variable.[14–16]

Radiographic findings are also variable and can include evidence of enlarged liver and spleen, thickened intestinal loops, and pulmonary lesions. Infections of bone have produced lesions described as increased opacity of endosteal bone.[4,10]

In birds with GI infections, nonstaining bacterial rods may appear in fresh fecal cytologic samples. These samples can be submitted for acid-fast staining. It should be noted that since organisms can be present in food and water, presence of mycobacterial organisms in feces may not be proof of actual infection and disease, and the amount of fecal shedding can vary, resulting in impaired sensitivity and specificity of the fecal acid-fast test as a screening tool. Acid-fast positive organisms may be identified in other tissue samples as well, including cytologic preparations of liver or cutaneous masses.

CONFIRMATION OF DIAGNOSIS

Diagnosis of cutaneous forms of mycobacteriosis is often straightforward and is achieved by biopsy, cytology, histopathology, or all of these, with additional testing for organism identification. Diagnosis of internal forms of the disease (liver, kidney, spleen, or pulmonary) is significantly more difficult and, in the author's experience, is achieved after extensive workup, including biopsy of abnormal organs, followed by additional testing for organism identification (Figure 2-38). Many infections are identified at postmortem examination.[1]

Histopathology can reveal lesions consistent with mycobacteriosis but cannot confirm nor identify the species in question. Confirmatory diagnostic methods include polymerase

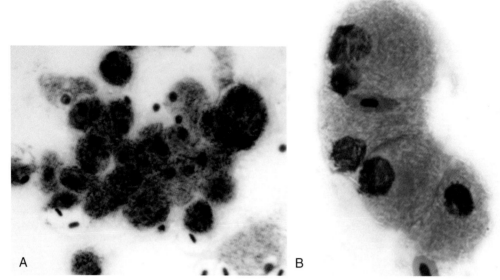

FIGURE 2-38 Specimens from a red-lored Amazon *(Amazona autumnalis).* **A,** Cytologic preparations of an intestinal aspirate demonstrating macrophages with acid-fast positive bacteria in the cytoplasm. Stain: Acid-fast blue. Objective 40×. **B,** Cytologic preparations of intestinal aspirate demonstrating macrophages with nonstaining rod-shaped bacteria in the cytoplasm. Stain May-Grunwald Giemsa. Oil Objective 100×. (Courtesy Dr. Drury Reavill.)

chain reaction (PCR) and culture and sensitivity of feces and target tissues. It should be noted that intradermal tuberculosis testing, as used in humans, correlates poorly with the presence of disease in psittacines.[1] PCR testing of specimens is the most useful diagnostic test both for confirmation of infection and for speciation of the organism in question, which, again, is a critical consideration when considering treatment. Samples include feces and fresh tissue specimens. PCR can detect very low numbers of organisms and provide rapid results. Many diagnostic laboratories now offer PCR for mycobacterial organisms in exotic species (Table 2-9). Some laboratories may have the ability to perform PCR on paraffin block tissues prepared from histopathology submissions, but many cannot. Therefore, practitioners should develop the habit of collecting, saving, and freezing additional biopsy tissue samples.

Culture of avian tissue and fecal samples for mycobacterial organisms is difficult. *M. avium* may require 1 to 6 months to grow, and *M. genavense* does not grow on conventional mycobacterial media.[1] Some human diagnostic laboratories are willing to provide culture and sensitivity of animal samples, which may guide treatment decisions (see Table 2-9). A study of Japanese quail experimentally inoculated with *M. avium* demonstrated that culture and PCR of target tissue samples were much more sensitive than either method used to detect organisms in fecal samples, respectively.[17]

TABLE 2-9
Specific Diagnostic Testing for Mycobacteriosis

Mycobacterium sp.: PCR	Research Associates Laboratory www.vetdna.com
Mycobacterium sp.: PCR	Veterinary Molecular Diagnostics www.vmdl.com
Mycobacterium sp.: PCR	Washington State University Animal Disease Diagnostic Laboratory www.waddl.vetmed.wsu.edu
Mycobacterium sp.: PCR *Mycobacterium* sp.: Culture and sensitivity	National Jewish Medical and Research Center, Denver, CO www.testmenu.com/NationalJewish Contact laboratory for submission instructions and availability

PCR, Polymerase chain reaction.

ZOONOTIC CONSIDERATIONS

Human infection with *M. tuberculosis* is of serious concern, and there are concerns worldwide about organisms resistant to some of the drugs used for treatment of this disease in humans. For these reasons, most experts recommend euthanasia of birds that are confirmed as being actively infected with *M. tuberculosis.* Despite this caution, a single case of successful treatment of a pet bird with *M. tuberculosis* has been described.[18] Atypical mycobacteriosis, however, is extremely rare in humans with normal, competent immune systems. In these cases, infection is often traced to overwhelming exposure, such as inhalation of organisms in water vapor from an improperly sanitized hot tub or spa. One recent report described 36 cases of "hot tub lung" and a single case of hypersensitivity pneumonitis reaction to *M. avium* in household water, likely acquired during routine showering.[6,19] Treatment in these cases was successful.

In contrast, atypical mycobacteriosis is common in immunocompromised human patients. Prior to the acquired immune deficiency syndrome (AIDS) epidemic (pre-1981), infections with *M. avium* complex were actually rare, with an estimated 3000 cases occurring worldwide per year. Most cases involved patients having undergone organ transplantation or suffering from hairy cell leukemia. Current recommendations for patients with AIDS include preventive treatment for atypical mycobacteriosis. Without preventive treatment, approximately 40% of patients with AIDS will eventually develop *M. avium* complex infections. In the early 1990s, *M. genavense* was also recognized as a cause of mycobacteriosis in patients with AIDS, although with much less frequency than *M. avium* complex.[20]

In humans, the source of atypical mycobacterial infection is most likely environmental, as organisms are common in food, water, and soil.[21] Humans with disseminated disease caused by *M. avium* complex and *M. genavense* typically have heavy infection of the GI tract, suggesting ingestion of the organisms as the primary route of exposure. Results of one study demonstrated DNA of *M. genavense* present in 25% of intestinal biopsy samples collected from patients without human immunodeficiency virus (HIV) infection.[22]

For these reasons, mycobacteriosis in pet birds caused by *M. avium* complex or *M. genavense* are unlikely to be a health risk to humans with normal immune systems. However, persons with HIV infection or other diseases impacting the immune system are likely at increased risk, especially when CD4 T-lymphocyte counts drop below normal.[21,23,24]

It is interesting to note that U.S. Government-sponsored publications, including the *Guidelines for the Prevention of Opportunistic Infections in Persons Infected with Human Immunodeficiency Virus*, published by the U.S. Public Health Service/Infectious Diseases Society of America (USPHS/IDSA) and similar publications from the CDC do not recommend avoidance of birds for prevention of mycobacteriosis to normal or immunocompromised persons.[25]

TREATMENT OF MYCOBACTERIOSIS

Both treatment successes and failures have been reported.[3,26,27] Prior to considering treatment, the organisms should be positively identified in order to rule out cases of *M. tuberculosis* and to help guide treatment decisions for birds with atypical mycobacteriosis. Birds with confirmed atypical mycobacteriosis should be treated on a case-by-case basis, keeping in mind overall condition and likelihood of treatment success, with input from the owner's physician. It should be kept in mind that treatment requires daily administration of a combination of medications for a year or longer, which may be difficult for many owners. Treatment with a single agent and incomplete or sporadic treatment of mycobacterial infections are both linked to development of resistant organisms and should be discouraged.[1]

Reviews of outcomes of large numbers of birds treated for mycobacteriosis with specific drug combinations at specific dosages are unavailable. Therefore, treatment is based on drug combinations used in humans and other animals for similar species. Without the benefit of culture and sensitivity (which is available but difficult and expensive), the practitioner is advised to research medications currently used for similar organisms in human patients. Drugs reported used for mycobacteriosis in birds include enrofloxacin, rifampin, ethambutol, clarithromycin, and others. Drug dosages are entirely extrapolated from other species (Table 2-10).

Publications in human medicine report that clarithromycin and ethambutol (with or without rifampicin) are commonly used to treat pulmonary *M. avium* complex in humans.[28] No known toxicities have been reported with the use of these drugs in psittacine birds.

The author has found improved owner compliance when selected antimycobacterial drugs are prepared by a compounding pharmacy in the smallest volume dose possible and mixed with powdered sugar. Food is removed the night before and the dose offered to the bird sprinkled on a small amount of a favorite moist table food. No other food is offered until the entire dose is consumed. Many birds require several weeks of "practice" before learning to eat the entire dose. However, birds accustomed to a single food item (e.g., seeds only) may be difficult to reliably medicate. One budgerigar refused to eat the powdered sugar. For this patient, medications were compounded in liquid form, and the bird was toweled and medicated daily. The owner admitted compliance was irregular with this method. Operant conditioning, where these patients undergoing long-term treatment can be trained to participate in their medication process can greatly facilitate treatment.

FOLLOW-UP

The diagnosis of disease can be challenging and so is judging response to therapy, especially when diagnosis was based on biopsy of an organ such as the liver. Clinical abnormalities may appear to resolve, and supportive clinical evidence such as changes in the hemogram may show marked improvement. Birds with GI forms of the disease may be screened for the presence of acid-fast bacteria; however, it should be kept in mind that shedding of mycobacterial organisms is sporadic.

In human medicine, patients are generally treated for a year or more, and in the case of humans with pulmonary disease, patients are released from treatment after being determined to be "culture negative" for 1 year. In the author's experience,

---

TABLE 2-10

Published Dosages of Antimycobacterial Drugs Used in the Treatment of Mycobacteriosis in Humans and Birds

Drug	Dosage (q24h)	
	Human Pediatric	Psittacine Bird
Clarithromycin	7.5–15 mg/kg	60 mg/kg
Clofazamine	1–2 mg/kg	6 mg/kg
Ciprofloxacin	10–15 mg/kg	80 mg/kg
Ethambutol	10–15 mg/kg	15–30 mg/kg
Isoniazid	10–20 mg/kg	30 mg/kg
Rifabutin		15–45 mg/kg
Rifampin	10 mg/kg	10–45 mg/kg
Streptomycin	20–40 mg/kg	20–40 mg/kg

Mg/kg, Milligrams per kilogram; q24h, every 24 hours.

treatment is continued for 1 year, and discontinued when the result of a follow-up biopsy of the target organ is negative; however, it should be kept in mind that a single biopsy can miss lesions. All patients finishing treatment for mycobacteriosis should be monitored carefully for any evidence of return of clinical signs.

CONCLUSION

Mycobacteriosis is an uncommon but well-recognized disease in companion psittacine birds. Molecular diagnostic techniques have improved the ability to confirm this disease in pet birds. Studies on efficacious therapeutic protocols in humans, and case reports of successful treatment in psittacine birds provide the avian practitioner with realistic treatment options. Although current research indicates that mycobacteriosis in psittacine birds is unlikely to represent a significant zoonotic risk, the potential risk cannot be ignored, particularly in the case of pet owners who may be immunocompromised.

REFERENCES

1. Tell LA, Woods L, Cromie RL: Mycobacteriosis in birds, *Rev Sci Tech Off Int Epiz* 20(1):180–203, 2001.
2. Palmieri C, Roy, P, Dhillion AS, et al: Avian mycobacteriosis in psittacines: a retrospective study of 123 cases, *J Comp Path* 148(203):126–138, 2013.
3. Hannon DE, Bemis DE, Garner MM: *Mycobacterium marinum* infection in a blue-fronted amazon parrot (*Amazona aestiva*), *J Avian Med Surg* 26(4):239–247, 2012.
4. Van Der Heyden N: Clinical manifestations of mycobacteriosis in pet birds, *Semin Avian Exotic Pet Med* 6:18–24, 1997.
5. Kock ND, Kock RA, Wambua J, et al: *Mycobacterium avium* related epizootic in free-ranging lesser flamingos in Kenya, *J Wild Dis* 35(2):297–300, 1999.
6. Mangione EJ, Huitt G, Lenaway D, et al: Nontuberculous mycobacterial disease following hot tub exposure, *Emerg Infect Dis* 7(6):1039–1042, 2001. Available from: www.cdc.gov/ncidod/eid/vol7no6.2001. Accessed Feb. 21, 2014.
7. Hoop RK: *Mycobacterium tuberculosis* infection in a canary (*Serinus canaria L.*) and a blue-fronted Amazon parrot (*Amazona amazona aestiva*), *Avian Dis* 46(2):502–504, 2002.
8. Washko RM, Hoefer H, Kiehn TE, et al: *Mycobacterium tuberculosis* infection in a green-winged macaw (*Ara chloroptera*): report with public health implications, *J Clin Microbiol* 36(4):1101–1102, 1998.
9. Gomez G, Saggase MD, Weeks BR, et al: Granulomatous encephalomyelitis and intestinal ganglionitis in a spectacled amazon parrot (*Amazona albifrons*) infected with *Mycobacterium genavense*, *J Comp Path* 144(2-3):219–222, 2011.
10. Van Der Heyden N: Mycobacteriosis. In Rosskopf W, Woerpel R, editors: *Diseases of cage and aviary birds*, Baltimore, MD, 1996, Williams and Wilkins, pp 568–571.
11. Phalen DN: Avian mycobateriosis. In Bonagura FD, editor: *Kirk's current veterinary therapy*, Vol. XIII. Philadelphia, PA, 2000, WB Saunders, pp 1116–1118.
12. Cooper JE: Avian microbiology. In Fudge AM, editor: *Laboratory medicine avian and exotic pets*, Philadelphia, PA, 2000, WB Saunders, pp 90–98.
13. Fudge AM: Avian complete blood count. In Fudge AM, editor: *Laboratory medicine avian and exotic pets*, Philadelphia, PA, 2000, WB Saunders, pp 90–98.
14. Janesch S: Diagnosis of avian hepatic disease, *Sem Av Ex Pet Med* 9(3):126–135, 2000.
15. Fudge AM: Avian liver and gastrointestinal testing. In Fudge AM, editor: *Laboratory medicine avian and exotic pets*, Philadelphia, PA, 2000, WB Saunders, pp 9–18.
16. Rosenthal K: Avian protein disorders. In Fudge AM, editor: Laboratory medicine avian and exotic pets, Philadelphia, PA, 2000, WB Saunders, pp 171–173.
17. Tell LA, Foley J, Needham ML, et al: Diagnosis of avian mycobacteriosis: comparison of culture, acid-fast stains, and polymerase chain reaction for the identification of Mycobacterium avium in experimentally inoculated Japanese quail (*Coturnix Coturnix japonica*), *Avian Dis* 47(2):444–452, 2003.
18. Schoemaker N, Wagenaar J: Diagnosis and treatment of a *Mycobacterium tuberculosis* infection in a red-lored Amazon (*Amazona autumnalis*), *Proc Eur Assoc Avian Vet* 24–26, 1999.
19. Marras TK, Wallace RJ, Koth LL, et al: Hypersensitivity pneumonitis reaction to *Mycobacterium avium* in household water, *Chest* 127(2):664–671, 2005.
20. Tortoli E, Brunello F, Cagni AE, et al: *Mycobacterium genavense* in AIDS patients, a report of 24 cases in Italy and review of the literature, *Eur J Epidemiol* 14(3):219–224, 1998.
21. Chaisson RE, Bishai WR: MAC and TB infection: management in HIV disease. *HIV clinical management*, Vol. 5, Medscape Inc., Available from: www.medscape.com/medscape/HIV/ClinicalMgmt/CM.v05/public/index-CM.v05.html. 1999. Accessed Oct. 21, 2014.
22. Kuijper EJ, de Witte M, Verhagen DW, et al: *Mycobacterium genavense* infection in two HIV-seropositive patients in Amsterdam, *Tijdschrift-voor-Geneeskunde* 142:970–972, 1998.
23. Haefner M, Funke-Kissling P, Pfyffer G: Clarithromycin, rifabutin and clofazimine for treatment of disseminated *Mycobacterium avium* complex disease in AIDS patients, *Clin Drug Invest* 17(3):171–178, 1999.
24. USPHS/IDS Guidelines for the prevention of opportunistic infections in persons infected with human immunodeficiency virus, *MMWR*48(No. RR-10). Available from: www.medscape.com/other/guidelines. 2002. Accessed Oct. 21, 2014.
25. Lennox AM: Antemortem diagnosis and treatment of mycobacteriosis in a budgerigar, *Proc Annu Conf Assoc Avian Vet* 425–426, 1999.
26. Van Der Heyden N: New Strategies in the treatment of avian mycobacteriosis, *Semin Av Ex Pet Med* 6(1):25–33, 1997.
27. Miwa S, Shirai M, Toyoshima M, et al: Efficacy of clarithromycin and ethambutol for mycobacterium avium complex pulmonary disease: a preliminary study, *Ann Am Thoracic Soc* 11(1):23–39, 2014.
28. Gordin FM, Sullam PM, Shafran SD, et al: A randomized, placebo-controlled study of rifabutin added to a regimen of clarithromycin and ethambutol for treatment of disseminated infection with *Mycobacterium avium complex. Clin Infect Dis* 28(5):1080–1085, 1999.

USUTU VIRUS

Johannes Thomas Lumeij

Usutu virus (USUV) is a mosquito-borne Flavivirus of African origin and belongs to the Japanese virus encephalitis group. Since it was identified as a cause of significant mortality in European blackbirds (*Turdus merula*) in Vienna in 2001, and because of the similarity to other members of the Japanese encephalitis antigenic complex, such as West Nile virus (WNV), it has received increased attention as an emerging epornitic with a zoonotic potential. The emergence and spread of USUV from Central Europe is well documented. So far, the risk for wild avian populations seems mainly limited to USUV-naïve European blackbirds, while of the captive populations, some species of USUV-naïve Strigiformes seem to be predisposed. The risk to humans seems limited to immunocompromised individuals. In healthy individuals, USUV may lead to a benign skin rash or seroconversion. The potential to spread to other than the African or Eurasian continents is unknown, but considering the similarity to WNV, this seems plausible.

THE VIRUS

Taxonomy and Description

The species USUV belongs to the family Flaviviridae and the genus *Flavivirus*. Other genera within the family Flaviviridae include *Hepacivirus* (hepatitis C virus) and *Pestivirus* (bovine viral diarrhea virus, border disease virus, and classic swine fever virus). The genus name *Flavivirus* is derived from the Latin word *flavus* (yellow) and refers to the jaundice seen in humans infected with one of the representatives of this group: the Yellow fever virus (YFV). Flaviviruses are single-stranded, enveloped ribonucleic acid (RNA) viruses of 40 to 65 nanometers (nm), with an icosahedral nucleocapsid. The positive-sense, single-stranded RNA of USUV contains approximately 11,000 bases. The entire *Flavivirus* genome is translated into a single polyprotein of 3400 amino acids. The USUV polyprotein contains three structural proteins, the capsid protein (C), the precursor membrane protein/membrane protein (prM/M) and the envelope protein (E), and seven nonstructural (NS) proteins with a regulatory function. The entire polyprotein is later cleaved into its components. In contrast to the alphaviruses, this process starts with the structural proteins in flaviviruses.[1,2] More than 70 different species of *Flavivirus* have been reported, some vectorborne and others without known vectors. Classification is primarily based on the type (or absence) of vector, and further classification is based on antigenic cross-reactivity.[3] Phylogenetic relationships have proven to match this antigenic based classification.[4,5] Those flaviviruses that are transmitted by bite from tick or mosquito had historically been classified together with alphaviruses and some other virus families as arboviruses (arthropod-borne). Well-known serocomplexes are the tickborne encephalitis group, including tickborne encephalitis virus (TBEV or FSMEV from German: Frühsommer Meningoenzephalitis Virus) and louping ill virus (LIV), the Yellow fever virus (YFV) group, the Dengue virus (DENV) group, and the Japanese encephalitis virus (JEV) serocomplex. Human infections with arboviruses are mostly incidental; humans are dead-end hosts because the virus replication is insufficient to reinfect the arthropods and continue the infectious cycle. Examples of exceptions are DENV and YFV. These viruses are so well adapted to the human host that an urban human–mosquito cycle without an animal host is possible, in contrast to the sylvatic cycle, in which monkeys are the reservoir host. The JEV serocomplex of flaviviruses has 11 representatives, of which JEV, Murray valley encephalitis virus (MVEV), St. Louis encephalitis virus (SLEV), and WNV are currently of most concern to humans. All members of this group have a bird–mosquito transmission cycle, and mammals are dead-end hosts. An exception to this is JEV, for which domestic pigs also serve as amplifying hosts. The subject of this section, USUV, is also a member of the JEV serocomplex but has hitherto only caused disease in a limited number of humans, whereas large-scale bird mortality seems associated with infections of virus-naïve avian populations. Alphaviruses are slightly larger (40 to 75 nm) than flaviviruses and differ in the organization of their genomes and protein synthesis. Examples of alphaviruses include Sindbis virus and Western-, Eastern-, and Venezuelan equine encephalitis viruses (SV, WEEV, EEEV, and VEEV).

Physical and Chemical Properties

Flaviviruses are inactivated by drying, organic solvents, low pH, and proteases. Procedures such as those applied to the production of plasma products that inactivate other flaviviruses (e.g., the use of solvents and detergents) are likely to be effective against USUV as well.[2] There are no specific studies on the stability of USUV.

Biologic Properties

Susceptible species

Apart from a wide range of avian species that can be affected by USUV, clinical infections have also been reported in humans. In some bird populations that have not been exposed to USUV infections previously, infections can lead to significant mortality. In humans, there have only been a limited number of documented cases of infections leading to clinical signs. The common (European) blackbird *(Turdus merula)* is the most widely reported affected species in areas where USUV has been recently introduced. Captive great gray owls *(Strix nebulosa)* were also commonly affected.[6,7] In Switzerland, the house sparrow *(Passer domesticus)* was commonly affected.[8] So far, clinical disease in birds seems mainly limited to representatives of the orders Passeriformes and (captive) Strigiformes. Apart from clinical infections in the aforementioned avian species, a number of avian species have shown seroconversion without clinical signs, notably rock pigeons *(Columba livia)*, mallards *(Anas platyrhynchos)*, and magpies *(Pica pica)*.[9]

The prevalence of USUV infection in specific avian species can be dependent not only on the virulence of the virus strain and host susceptibility but also on the innate preference by the mosquito vector for certain host species. Preference trials with adult female *Culex pipiens*, relating to the epidemiology of WNV in the United States, have shown that host-seeking *Cx. pipiens* were three times more likely to enter the American robin *(Turdus migratorius)*–baited traps compared with traps baited with the sympatric European starling *(Sturnus vulgaris)*.[10]

The mosquito–avian transmission cycle is dependent on the presence of an ornithophilic mosquito vector, in which virus replication and dissemination occurs to such a degree that virus transmission through infected saliva is possible. USUV has been isolated from a large variety of African mosquito species, including *Cx. perfuscus*, *Cx. quinquefasciatus*, *Aedes (Aedimorphus) minutus*, *Mansonia africana*, and *Coquillettidia aurites*,[11] but their vector role is unknown. Results from studies on *Cx. neavei* from Senegal strongly suggest this species acts as a vector for USUV.[12] The low abundance of *Cx. neavei* in inhabited areas in combination with the low anthropophily has been mentioned as a possible explanation for the rarity of reported USUV infections in humans in Africa. In Europe, USUV isolations have been reported mainly from

Cx. pipiens but also from *A. albopictus*.[13,14] For human infections to occur, the feeding pattern of the mosquitoes must be more opportunistic to enable the mosquitoes to act as bridge vectors between the avian populations, in which the infection is enzootic, and the human dead-end host. In Europe, *Cx. pipiens* is considered the most important vector. The *Cx. pipiens* taxonomic complex contains two distinct biotypes: (1) *pipiens* and (2) *molestus*. Although they are morphologically indistinguishable, they differ in physiology and behavior. *Cx. pipiens* requires a blood meal for each batch of eggs (anautogenous), is seasonally active and mainly ornithophilic, whereas *Cx. molestus* is autogenous, active throughout the year and mammophilic, especially anthrophilic.[15] In the northeastern United States, a large proportion of *Cx. pipiens* complex has been found to be a hybrid between both biotypes. These hybrids have lost their host specificity and have become opportunistic feeders, feeding both on birds and on humans. In Europe, the biotype *pipiens* is considered the most widespread, whereas the biotype *molestus* is only known from underground breeding sites. Hybridization between the biotypes has so far been reported only in a restricted number of places. It has been claimed that these opportunistic *Cx. pipiens* hybrids may have served as an important bridge between the avian and human populations and may have had a major contribution to the emergence and spread of WNV in the United States.[16] Likewise, *Cx. pipiens* hybrids might play a role in the transmission of USUV in Europe from birds to humans.

Cell cultures

Flaviviruses can be grown in both vertebrate and mosquito cell lines, but the susceptibility of cell cultures from different species varies.[17] Even cell lines from the same organ of a particular species may show differences in susceptibility. Often, multiplication of flaviviruses in cell lines does not result in alteration of the macromolecular structure, resulting in a persistent infection without a cytopathogenic effect (CPE). From a study conducted on vertebrate cell lines, it was concluded that the most appropriate cell lines for isolation and plaque reduction test for USUV are from the green monkey (Vero), the porcine kidney (PK15), and the goose embryo fibroblast (GEF). Although one would expect that avian cell lines are more susceptible to USUV than mammalian cell lines, it was found that chicken embryo fibroblast monolayers and chicken embryos seem resistant to USUV infection.[17] USUV from pooled trapped mosquitoes was successfully propagated with accompanying CPE in an *A. albopictus* C6/36 mosquito cell line.[18] Three human cell lines (human long adenocarcinoma epithelial A549, human epidermoid larynx carcinoma Hep-2, and human epidermoid oral carcinoma KB) were susceptible to USUV infection and developed a clear-cut CPE, comparable with that produced in Vero cells.[19]

Antigenic properties

The lipid bilayered viral envelope of Flaviviridae is composed of two proteins, of which protein E is the primary target of the immune response of the host. Protein E is the aspecific viral hemagglutinin responsible for seroconversion of infected individuals. The strong cross-reactivity of hemagglutinating antibodies to the various species within the *Flavivirus* family is a characteristic on which the various flaviviruses have been classified and it should come to no surprise therefore that it is impossible to make a species-specific diagnosis. A clinical diagnosis of acute *Flavivirus* infection, however, can be helpful to a clinician. Apart from the envelope glycoprotein, flaviviruses have other antigenic components and antibodies against the prM and NS1 proteins have also been reported.[20-23] Maternal antibodies from adult birds are transferred to their offspring through the egg yolk, where the antibody is absorbed and enters the circulatory system. USUV maternal antibodies were detectable up to 2 months in Ural owls (*Strix uralensis*).[24] Cross-reacting antibodies play an important role for both serologic diagnosis and the protection of individuals or populations, but our limited understanding of the inconsistent relationships within and between the various serocomplexes complicates serologic diagnosis and the prediction of protection.[25]

OCCURRENCE

History

USUV was first isolated in 1959 in South Africa by B.R. McIntosh from *Cx. neavei* (originally classified as *Cx. univittatus*, but renamed in 1971[26]) during a study on the prevalence of viruses in mosquito species. It was named after the Usutu river in Swaziland.[27] This South African reference strain is identified as SAAr 1776. Additional isolates were found in the following years in a variety of mosquitoes from a variety of African countries. Mosquito species involved include *Cx. perfusus*, *Mansonia africanus*, *M. autites*, and *A. minutus*. Apart from a report of USUV from a human patient in 1981 in the Central African Republic, followed by a second case in 2004 from Burkina Faso, USUV has been largely ignored by the scientific community, until it emerged in 2001 in central Europe as a cause of avian mortality, especially of Eurasian blackbirds, *Turdus merula*, and great gray owls, *Strix nebulosa*.[28] Later studies have shown the presence of USUV in a variety of other avian species in neighboring countries. Retrospective analysis of archived tissue samples from bird deaths in the Tuscany region of Italy in 1996[29] identified USUV. Partial sequencing confirmed identity with the 2001 Vienna strain and provided evidence for at least a 5-year earlier introduction of USUV into Europe than previously assumed.[7] Currently, USUV is considered enzootic in central Europe, with a mosquito–bird transmission cycle and the potential to spread to other geographic areas. The zoonotic potential in healthy human subjects seems to be limited to a transient skin rash, with possibly a more severe clinical course in immunocompromised patients. The first human cases outside Africa were seen in immunocompromised patients in Italy. These patients showed meningoencephalitis.[30,31] Seroepidemiologic studies in humans indicate that USUV can be endemic in certain areas with no signs of disease in infected people.

Geographic Range

USUV has been reported in a number of African countries, including Burkina Faso, Cote d'Ivoire, Uganda, Nigeria, Senegal, Morocco, and the Central African Republic. After its first documented European appearance in Italy in 1996,[7]

USUV-associated clinical disease in birds has been reported from Austria,[6] Hungary,[32] Switzerland,[8] Czech Republic,[33] Spain,[34-36] Germany,[37,38] and Belgium.[39] Neutralizing antibodies to USUV have also been found in birds from the United Kingdom,[40,41] Poland,[42] and Greece (Figure 2-39).[43] Considering the erratic results seen with *Flavivirus* serology, final conclusions about the presence or absence of USUV in these latter countries can be drawn after more specific confirmatory tests. There is also insufficient information to evaluate the USUV seropositive samples in the period from 2001 to 2005 from Germany. Seroconversion in horses[44] and neuroinvasive disease in humans have been reported from Croatia.[45] Phylogenetic analysis of the currently known complete USUV genome sequences from Africa, central Europe, and Spain has revealed that at least three distinct genetic clusters circulate in Europe.[46] USUV strains isolated from Africa showed an even greater genetic diversity.[47] The two distinct clusters circulating in Spain, which seem to differ in their virulence for avian hosts, are most likely independently introduced by migratory birds from Africa, whereas the central European cluster seems to be an independent introduction.[46] Seroconversion without clinical disease in birds from the British Isles, Poland, and Greece might indicate that the geographic distribution of USUV in Europe is wider than currently realized. However, the limitations of only serologic diagnosis should be kept in mind. A more definitive proof from these countries, in the form of virus isolation and identification, would be more convincing.

CLINICAL FINDINGS

In contrast to a number of avian species that seem highly susceptible to USUV infections and may show clinical signs, a wide range of avian species seems to show only seroconversion after infection with USUV without showing any clinical signs. Clinical signs may vary from nonspecific (immobility, ruffled plumage, half-closed eyes, and anorexia) to neurologic signs such as depression, ataxia, jerky movements, torticollis, and nystagmus, followed by mortality. A poor nutritional status has been reported in wild birds, whereas the nutritional status of captive birds was more variable.[8] This might be related to the more protected captive environment, where food is freely available to the affected individuals.

In humans, infections often go unnoticed, as can be concluded from finding neutralizing antibodies against USUV in clinically healthy blood donors from an endemic region in Italy[48,49] and from a blood donor in southwestern Germany.[50] In Austria, 52 out of 203 individuals from an endemic area who had developed a skin rash of unknown cause were seropositive against USUV, as concluded after finding neutralizing antibodies. In one of these patients, the USUV genome was detected by using PCR.[51] A more serious neuroinvasive form of USUV infection has been seen in two immunocompromised humans.

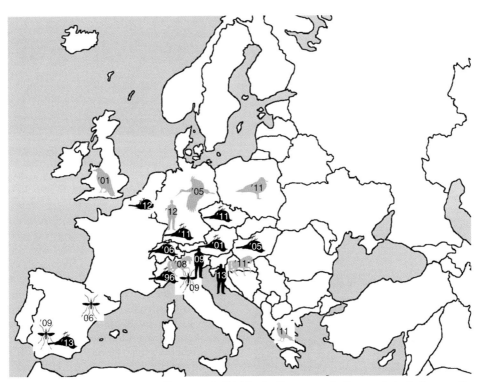

FIGURE 2-39 Usutu virus in Europe. Solid black silhouettes indicate clinical disease (in immunocompromised humans), USUV confirmed mortality (birds), or virus isolation (mosquitoes). The two USUV strains circulating in Spain are different from the Central European strain, which seems to have spread from Italy since 1996. Gray silhouettes indicate seroconversion only (birds, horses, or humans) and possible USUV circulation. Flavivirus serologic results should be interpreted with caution. The numbers indicate the year in which first occurrence was demonstrated.

PATHOLOGIC FINDINGS

Birds that have died from USUV infection may be in good body condition without obvious gross pathologic lesions, indicating peracute mortality. Splenomegaly, hepatomegaly, and pulmonary hyperemia may be seen in affected animals. Histopathologic examination of the cortex and brainstem may reveal multifocal neuronal degeneration and perineuronal clustering of glial cells. Cerebellar lesions may include degeneration of Purkinje cells, formation of glial shrubberies, lymphoplasmacytic perivascular cuffs, and mild degeneration and necrosis at the molecular–granular layer interface (Figure 2-40). A miliary pattern of liver necrosis and a scattered cellular necrosis may be seen in the myocardium (Figures 2-41 and 2-42).[52] Paraffin-embedded tissue can be processed for immunohistochemical staining by using rabbit USUV-specific antibody (Figure 2-43). However, with immunohistochemistry (IHC), there is still the potential for cross-reactivity with other flaviviruses. In situ hybridization (ISH) is based on the complementary pairing of labeled deoxyribonucleic acid (DNA) or RNA probes with USUV-specific nucleic acid sequences in tissue sections (Figure 2-44).

DIAGNOSTIC ASPECTS

Flavivirus infections cause a short-lived viremia of maximum 2 days. A serologic response follows after the viremic stage. Circulating immunoglobulin M (IgM) is produced within 6 days, followed by IgG. Identification of specific immunoglobulin M and seroconversion to IgG or a fourfold rise in titer between acute and convalescent sera taken 10 days apart indicate an acute infection.[1,2] The possibility of false-positive results should be borne in mind, as was demonstrated with IgM antibodies against WNV.[53,54] Individuals that have shown acute mortality are poor candidates for serologic diagnosis because they did not have enough time to seroconvert. Less vulnerable species are likely to show no clinical signs of disease and to still seroconvert, thereby providing an opportunity for serologic screening of populations.

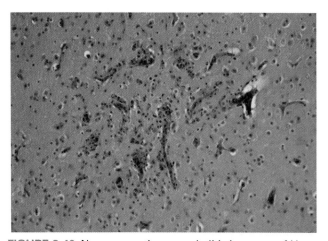

FIGURE 2-40 Nonsuppurative encephalitis in a case of Usutu virus infection, blackbird *(Turdus merula)*. Hematoxylin and eosin stain. Original magnification 203. (Courtesy Herbert Weissenböck, DVM, University of Veterinary Medicine, Vienna.)

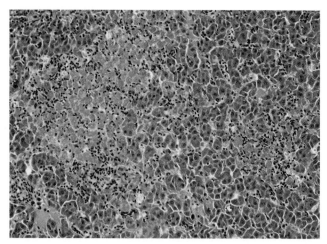

FIGURE 2-41 Irregularly demarcated liver necrosis in a case of Usutu virus infection, blackbird *(Turdus merula)*. Hematoxylin and eosin stain. Original magnification 20×. (Courtesy Herbert Weissenböck, DVM, University of Veterinary Medicine, Vienna.)

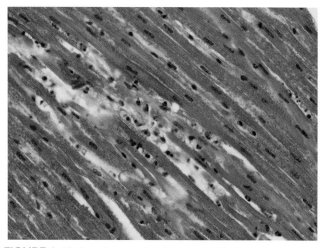

FIGURE 2-42 Focal necrosis of myocardial fibers in a case of Usutu virus infection, blackbird *(Turdus merula)*. Hematoxylin and eosin stain. Original magnification 40×. (Courtesy Herbert Weissenböck, DVM, University of Veterinary Medicine, Vienna.)

For initial serologic screening of populations for USUV, the hemagglutination inhibition test (HIT) can be used.[55,56] This test is not considered specific. Cross-reactions with other flaviviruses such as TBEV and WNV do occur, and distinction between USUV infections and other flavivirus infections are difficult. For confirmation of suspected cases, the more specific plaque reduction neutralization test (PRNT) can be used.[57] However, although the PRNT is considered the gold standard within the Flaviviridae family, cross-reactivity also occurs with the PRNT. All sera from a human cohort vaccinated with JEV and TBEV caused neutralization of LIV, and some sera also neutralized WNV, which was enhanced by YFV vaccination.[58] The specificity of the PRNT using WNV and USUV test sera has been investigated recently by using the USUV strain Blackbird Vienna 2001 and WNV topotype strain Eg-101. Cross-reactivity only occurred in sera with high titers to one of the viruses, to a titer of at least four dilutions steps less than the homolog

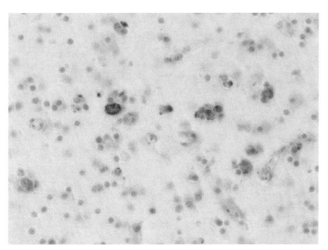

FIGURE 2-43 Usutu virus antigen demonstrated by immuno-histochemistry in the cytoplasm of neurons and glial cells in the brain of a blackbird *(Turdus merula)*. Original magnification 40×. (Courtesy Herbert Weissenböck, DVM, University of Veterinary Medicine, Vienna.)

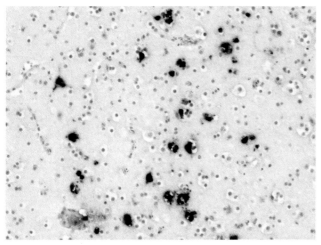

FIGURE 2-44 Usutu virus nucleic acid demonstrated by in situ hybridization within neurons and glial cells in the brain of a blackbird *(Turdus merula)*. Original magnification 20×. (Courtesy Herbert Weissenböck, DVM, University of Veterinary Medicine, Vienna.)

virus. Considering the broad antigenic cross-reactivity between different flaviviruses and therefore the erratic and unpredictable results from *Flavivirus* serology, other strains might yield different findings. Diagnostic experience with WNV has shown that a PRNT must be evaluated by testing neutralizing antibodies against a panel of related viruses. Based on experiences with WNV and considering the diversity and constant evolution of circulating strains, the choice of reference strains should include recent isolates that are known to circulate in the region, and the use of old strains should be avoided. Technical variations between different laboratories might also contribute to variations observed.[59]

The most reliable method to establish a causative diagnosis is reverse transcriptase (RT)-PCR. USUV-specific amplicons can be amplified by RT-PCR on unfixed or formalin-fixed paraffin-embedded brain tissue, and RT-PCR amplification

products can be sequenced and compared with already known USUV sequences available in Genbank.[7,60]

DIFFERENTIAL DIAGNOSIS

The most important differential diagnosis, both clinically and serologically, is an infection with another virus of the Japanese encephalitis complex. Apart from cross-reactions with other flaviviruses, nonspecific reactions may also occur.[53,54] Because flaviviruses might share the same vector, simultaneous infections with various viruses might occur, as has been shown for USUV and WNV. For this reason, it is important to rule out exposure to other flaviviruses through natural contact (travel history to *Flavivirus* endemic areas in humans; migratory patterns in birds) or vaccination status (YFV, TBEV, JEV) and to always use specific confirmatory tests.

EPIZOOTIOLOGY

Like WNV, USUV spreads in cycles between ornithophilic mosquito vectors and an avian reservoir host. Once the appropriate vector becomes infected, other susceptible hosts such as humans can be infected. They act as dead-end hosts, since viral replication is insufficient to cause reinfection of another vector. Humans, however, may transmit arboviruses through blood transfusions. Documentation of two cases of blood transfusion–induced WNV infection in humans has led to screening of blood donors for WNV and rejecting donors who have fever and headache during the week of blood donation. For USUV, blood transfusion–induced infection in humans has not been proven. Despite high arboviral titers in reservoir hosts, infections may remain subclinical.[61] For *Flavivirus* enzootics to occur, there must be a sufficient number of specific vectors and susceptible reservoir hosts.[62] Seasonal differences in prevalence are associated with climatic conditions that influence overwintering of vectors and migration patterns of reservoir hosts. Migration of birds may be a factor in reintroduction of new viruses in a specific region or spreading to new regions. Longitudinal studies with USUV in Austria in the period 2003–2006 have shown a year-to-year decrease in USUV-associated wild bird mortality since the initial outbreak in 2001, which was associated with an increasing proportion of seropositive wild birds. It has been hypothesized that the apparent disappearance of USUV-associated avian mortality in Austria can be explained by the rapid establishment of resident flock immunity. Other possible factors are climatic factors and decreased virulence. It has been shown, for example, that in American crows, the virulence of WNV is strain dependent.[63] The high percentage of seropositive birds (>50%) to a circulating arbovirus with an avian–mosquito transmission cycle, as observed by Meister et al,[24] has not been seen in other enzootic transmission cycles of flaviviruses so far and awaits further explanation.

Most of the European USUV epornitics have occurred in urban areas. It has been speculated that the presence of supervised avian collections or bird sanctuaries in urban areas would enhance the detection of new cases, whereas the abundance of predators in the wild would explain the absence of detection of outbreaks in rural areas. However, when the spatial distribution of blackbird mortality in Austria was plotted against the average number of hot days per year, a correlation between local environmental temperature and blackbird mortality became clear.[64] The emergence of USUV infections was mainly related to those regions around Vienna, where the number of hot days exceeds 10 days per year. This region of the district Lower Austria has the densest human population. Apart from the heat island effect of urban areas, it has been shown that urbanization favors the propagation of *Cx. pipiens* by the proliferation of artificial container habitats.[65] Through mathematic modelling, Rubel et al explained the multiseasonal dynamics of USUV infections in Austria.[66] In this model, the seasonal dynamics of mosquitoes and birds and the density-dependent avian–mosquito infection cycle was considered. USUV dynamics were mainly determined by the interaction between bird immunity and environmental temperature. Higher temperatures increase the reproduction and biting rate and decrease the extrinsic incubation period of mosquitoes. On the basis of this mathematic USUV avian–mosquito model, historical temperature recordings, as well as temperature predictions from global climate models from the Intergovernmental Panel on Climate Change (IPCC), both historical and future scenarios for R_0 were calculated. When R_0 is less than 1, the infection will die out in the long run, but if R_0 is greater than 1, the infection will be able to spread in a population. From 1900 until 2100, R_0 increased for the worst-case IPCC scenario with 0.61 per 100 years and for the best-case scenario with 0.51 per 100 years. For both scenarios R_0 would be consistently larger than one from 2040 onward, whereas it never reached values greater than 1 before 2000. This means that on the basis of this model, it is unlikely that undetected outbreaks would have occurred before 2000, whereas from 2040 onward, the disease will be endemic in the area. For the future, it can be predicted that the disease will become endemic in Austria from 2040 onward, and new outbreaks will occur in immunologically naive avian populations in other European countries, mainly in Passeriformes (blackbirds and house sparrows) and Strigiformes. Outbreaks can be expected during the peak of the *Cx. pipiens* reproductive season between mid-July and mid-September. Urban areas are predisposed because they cause the heat island effect and offer a wide variety of breeding sites for *Cx. pipiens* in the form of stagnant water pools, varying from birds baths to disposed car tires. Urban areas are probably more likely to show benign human infections because these areas are more likely to harbor the aforementioned opportunistic feeding *Cx. pipiens* hybrids. USUV epornitics that do occur in rural areas might go unnoticed because bird carcasses disappear relatively quickly as a result of the abundance of avian or mammalian scavengers.[67]

PROPHYLAXIS

Surveillance

To monitor USUV circulation in a specific region, several approaches have been used, including the use of sentinel animals (horses and chickens), virologic examination of dead wild birds, serologic examination of backyard poultry flocks and mosquito collection, and identification and testing for USUV in pooled mosquito samples. Serologic examination of sentinel animals should be done twice a year, that is, before and after the mosquito season. Considering the host specificity of USUV within the order Passeriformes, a targeted surveillance with special attention for dead blackbirds and house sparrows might prove to be more cost effective than a random search for USUV among all avian species. Although rock pigeons (*Columba livia*) and mallards (*Anas platyrhynchos*) have not been reported to be clinically affected, they have proven to be useful species for serologic examination.[9] It is important to be aware of the close antigenic relationship between various flaviviruses and take appropriate precautions to enable differentiation between the *Flavivirus* species. With regard to the low susceptibility of chicken embryos to USUV infections, and the limited pathogenicity of USUV for chickens,[68] it is questionable whether backyard chickens are the most appropriate species to act as sentinel animals. Considering the findings of Savini et al, feral pigeons (*Columba livia*) might be a better choice.

Vaccination

There is currently no specific USUV vaccine available, and the need is questionable. Although there are human vaccines available for a number of flaviviruses, including JEV, TBEV, and YFV, and an equine vaccine for WNV and sera raised against one of these agents may cross-react in serologic tests with other flaviviruses, cross-protection against USUV has not yet been reported. The cross-reactive properties of flaviviruses are potentially useful for the development of a broad-spectrum vaccine for emerging flaviviruses. However, a worsening of disease symptoms through a possible antibody-dependent enhancement effect should be carefully evaluated.

Mosquito Prevention

Since outbreaks are related to the avian–mosquito transmission cycle, captive susceptible avian collections can be protected against USUV (and other arbovirus) infections by mosquito control. Prevention of stagnant pools of water (in flower pots, gutters, buckets, pool covers, water dishes, discarded tires, birdbaths) has been advocated as a valuable method to reduce the number of breeding sites for the mosquito vector of WNV. *Cx. pipiens* is a lazy flier, and the lack of breeding sites in the vicinity may reduce the number of mosquitoes considerably. Cyclopoid crustaceans[69] or aquatic vertebrates such as fish[70] or terrapines[71] may be used to reduce larvae in pools or holding tanks that cannot be drained. Indoor housing during the mosquito season of immunologically naive Passeriformes and Strigiformes, including young birds and new additions, has been suggested as a method to protect valuable avian collections.[8] Mosquito screens on windows and doors can help keep mosquitoes outside. Air conditioning during the critical months may be an effective alternative to natural ventilation for climate control. Ectoparasites might also contribute to the spread of the disease. Although it is unknown whether the virus can replicate outside the specific *Culex* mosquito vector, it seems a wise precaution to treat susceptible avian collections on a regular basis against ectoparasites.

In addition to the above, humans can protect themselves from *Cx. pipiens* bites by dressing in loose-fitting, long-sleeved clothes, staying indoors at dusk and dawn, and using a 50% solution of N,N-Diethyl-meta-toluamide (DEET) on the bare skin. DEET is considered the most effective repellent against *Cx. pipiens* outdoors during these feeding periods.

Although dying black birds are inherent to nature and in general giving a symbolic meaning to finding deceased black birds can be categorized under superstition, the USUV-induced blackbird mortality can be considered a bad omen to what the future will bring with regard to climate change–related vectorborne diseases. Since USUV epornitics outside its former tropical range are linked to climate change and global warming, the most important consideration in combatting this and other emerging arbovirus epidemics is a global reduction of greenhouse gases. In an attempt to reduce the heat island effect of urban areas, a long-term heat island reduction strategy of planting shade trees and increasing urban albedo by using light-colored, highly reflective roof and paving materials should be included in the plans of city planners, environmental managers, and other decision makers.[72,73]

ACKNOWLEDGMENTS

Norbert Nowotny, PhD, Professor of Virology, Institute of Virology, University of Veterinary Medicine at Vienna, is gratefully acknowledged for critical reading of the manuscript.

Herbert Weissenböck, DVM, Dipl. ECPHM, Associate Professor Pathology and Forensic Veterinary Medicine, Department of Pathobiology, University of Veterinary Medicine, Vienna, is gratefully acknowledged for supplying Figures 2-40 through 2-44.

REFERENCES

1. Murray PR, Rosenthal KS, Pfaller MA: *Medical microbiology*. 7th ed., Philadelphia, PA, 2013, Saunders, Elsevier.
2. Blut A: Usutu virus, *Transfus Med Hemother* 41:73–82, 2014.
3. Porterfield JS: Antigenic characteristics and classification of Togaviridae. In Schlesinger RW, editor: *The togaviruses*, New York, 1980, Academic Press, pp 13–46.
4. Gaunt MW, Sall AA, de Lamballerie X, et al: Phylogenetic relationships of flaviviruses correlate with their epidemiology, disease association and biogeography, *J Gen Virol* 82:1867–1876, 2001.
5. Kuno G, Chang G-JJ, Tsuchiya KR et al: Phylogeny of the genus *Flavivirus*, *J Virol* 72:73–83, 1998.
6. Weissenböck H, Kolodziejek J, Url A, et al: Emergence of Usutu virus, an African mosquito-borne *Flavivirus* of the Japanese encephalitis virus group, central Europe, *Emerg Infect Dis* 8:652–656, 2002.
7. Weissenböck H, Bakonyi T, Rossi G, et al: Usutu virus, Italy, 1996, *Emerg Infect Dis* 19:274–277, 2013.
8. Steinmetz HW, Bakonyi T, Weissenböck H, et al: Emergence and establishment of Usutu virus infection in wild and captive avian species in and around Zurich, Switzerland - Genomic and pathologic comparison to other central European outbreaks, *Vet Microbiol* 148:207–212, 2011.
9. Savini G, Monaco F, Terregino C, et al: Usutu virus in Italy: an emergence or a silent infection? *Vet Microbiol* 151:264–274, 2011.
10. Simpson JE, Folsom-O'Keele CM, Childs JE, et al: Avian host-selection by *Culex pipiens* in experimental trials, *PLos One* 4:e7861, 2009.
11. Nicolay B, Diallo M, Boye CS, et al: Usutu virus in Africa, *Vector Borne Zoonotic Dis* 11:1417–1423, 2011.
12. Nicolay B, Diallo M, Faye O, et al: Vector competence of *Culex neavei* for Usutu virus, *Am J Trop Med Hyg* 86:993–996, 2012.
13. Calzolari M, Bonilauri P, Bellini R, et al: Evidence of simultaneous circulation of West Nile and Usutu viruses in mosquitoes sampled in Emilia-Romagna region (Italy) in 2009, *PLoS One* 5:e14324, 2010.
14. Calzolari M, Gaibani P, Bellini R, et al: Mosquito, bird and human surveillance of West Nile and Usutu viruses in Emilia-Romagna Region (Italy) in 2010, *PLoS One* 7:e38058, 2012.
15. Harbach RE, Harrison BA, Gad AM: *Culex (Culex) molestus* Forskal *(Diptera: Culicidae)*: Neotype designation, description, variation, and taxonomic status, *Proc Entomol Soc Wash* 86:521–542, 1984.
16. Reusken CBEM, de Vries A, Buijs J, et al: First evidence for presence of *Culex pipiens* biotype molestus in the Netherlands, and of hybrid biotype pipiens and molestus in Northern Europe, *J Vector Ecol* 35:210–212, 2010.
17. Bakonyi T, Lussy H, Weissenböck H, et al: In vitro host-cell susceptibility to Usutu virus. *Emerg Infect Dis* 11:298–301, 2005.
18. Jöst H, Bialonski A, Maus D, et al: Isolation of Usutu virus in Germany, *Am J Trop Med Hyg* 85:551–553, 2011.
19. Scagnolari C, Caputo B, Trombetti S, et al: Usutu virus growth in human cell lines: induction of and sensitivity to type I and III interferons, *J Gen Virol* 94:789–795, 2013.
20. Pincus S, Mason PW, Konishi E, et al: Recombinant vaccinia virus producing the prM and E proteins of yellow fever virus protects mice from lethal yellow fever encephalitis, *Virology* 187:290–297, 1982.
21. Chung KM, Thompson BS, Fremont DH, et al: Antibody recognition of cell surface-associated NS1 triggers Fc-gamma receptor-mediated phagocytosis and clearance of West Nile virus-infected cells, *J Virol* 81:9551–9555, 2007.
22. Colombage G, Hall R, Pavy M, et al: DNA-based and alphavirus-vectored immunisation with prM and E proteins elicits long-lived and protective immunity against the flavivirus Murrey Valley encephalitis virus, *Virology* 250:151–163, 1998.
23. Shu PY, Chen LK, Chang SF, et al: Dengue NS1-specific antibody responses: isotype distribution and serotyping in patients with Dengue fever and Dengue hemorrhagic fever, *J Med Virol* 62:224–232, 2000.
24. Meister T, Lussy H, Bakonye T, et al: Serologic evidence of continuing high Usutu virus (Flaviviridae) activity and establishment of herd immunity in wild birds in Austria, *Vet Microbiol* 127:237–248, 2008.
25. Calisher CH, Karabatsos N, Dalrymple JM, et al: Antigenic relationships between Flaviviruses as determined by cross-neutralization test with polyclonal antisera, *J Gen Virol* 70:37–43, 1989.
26. Jupp PG: The taxonomic status of *Culex (Culex) univittatus* Theobald *(Diptera: Culicidae)* in South Africa, *J Entomol Soc Southern Afr* 34:339–357, 1971.
27. Arbovirus catalogue. Centers for Disease Control and Prevention. Usutu virus (USUV). Available from: https://wwwn.cdc.gov/arbocat/VirusDetails.aspx?ID=503&SID=4. Accessed 07/23/2014.
28. Weissenböck H, Kolodziejek J, Fragner K, et al: Usutu virus activity in Austria, 2001–2002. *Microbes Infect* 5:1132–1136, 2003.
29. Mani P, Rossi G, Perrucci S, et al: Mortality of *Turdus merula* in Tuscany, *Selezione veterinaria* 39:749–753, 1998. Italian.
30. Cavrini F, Gaibani P, Longo G, et al: Usutu virus infection on a patient who underwent orthotopic liver transplantation, Italy, August–September 2009, *Euro Surveill* 14(pii):19448, 2009.
31. Pecorari M, Longo G, Gennari W, et al: First human case of Usutu virus neuroinvasive infection, Italy, August-September 2009, *Euro Surveill* 14(pii):19446, 2009.
32. Bakonyi T, Erdélyi K, Ursu K, et al: Emergence of Usutu virus in Hungary, *J Clin Microbiol* 45:3870–3874, 2007.
33. Hubálek Z, Rudolf I, Čapek M, et al: Usutu virus in blackbirds (*Turdus merula*), Czech Republic, 2011–2012, *Transbound Emerg Dis* 61:273–276, 2014.
34. Busquets N, Alba A, Allepuz A, et al: Usutu virus sequences in *Culex pipiens (Diptera: Culicidae)*, Spain, *Emerg Infect Dis* 14:861–863, 2008.
35. Höfle U, Gamino V, Fernández de Mera IG, et al: Usutu virus in migratory song thrushes, Spain. *Emerg Infect Dis* 19, 2013.
36. Vázquez A, Ruiz S, Herrero L, et al: West Nile and Usutu viruses in mosquitoes in Spain, 2008–2009. *Am J Trop Med Hyg* 85:178–181, 2011.
37. Becker N1, Jöst H, Ziegler U, et al: Epizootic emergence of Usutu virus in wild and captive birds in Germany, *PLoS One* 7:e32604, 2012.

38. Linke S, Niedrig M, Kaiser A, et al: Serologic evidence of West Nile virus infection in wild birds captured in Germany, *Am J Trop Med Hyg* 77:358–364, 2007.

39. Garigliany M-M, Marlier D, Tenner-Racz K, et al: Detection of Usutu virus in a bullfinch *(Pyrrhula pyrrhula)* and a great spotted woodpecker *(Dendrocopus major)*, *Vet J* 199:191–193, 2014.

40. Buckley A, Dawson A, Moss SR, et al: Serologic evidence of West Nile virus, Usutu virus and Sindbiss virus infection of birds in the UK, *J Gen Virol* 84:2807–2817, 2003.

41. Buckley A, Dawson A, Gould EA: Detection of seroconversion to West Nile virus, Usutu virus and Sindbis virus in UK sentinel chickens, *Virol J* 3:71, 2006.

42. Hubálek Z, Wegner E, Halouzka J, et al: Serologic survey of potential vertebrate hosts for West Nile Virus in Poland, *Viral Immunol* 21:247–253, 2008.

43. Chaintoutis SC, Dovas CI, Papanastassopoulou M, et al: Evaluation of a West Nile virus surveillance and early warning system in Greece, based on domestic pigeons, *Comp Immunol Microbiol Infect Dis* 37:131–141, 2014.

44. Barbic L, Vilibic-Cavlek T, Listes E, et al. : Demonstration of Usutu virus antibodies in horses, Croatia, *Vector Borne Zoonotic Dis* 13:772–774, 2013.

45. Vilibic-Cavlek T, Kaic B, Barbic L, et al: First evidence of simultaneous occurrence of West Nile virus and Usutu virus neuroinvasive disease in humans in Croatia during the 2013 outbreak. *Infection* 42:689–695, 2014.

46. Bakonyi TM, Busquets N, Nowotny N: Comparison of complete genome sequences of Usutu virus strains detected in Spain, Central Europe, and Africa, *Vector Borne Zoonotic Dis* 14:324–329, 2014.

47. Nikolay B, Dupressoir A, Firth C, et al: Comparative full length genome sequence analysis of Usutu virus isolates from Africa, *Virol J* 10:217, 2013.

48. Gaibani P, Pierro A, Alicino R, et al: Detection of Usutu-virus-specific IgG in blood donors from northern Italy, *Vector Borne Zoonotic Dis* 12:431–433, 2012.

49. Pierro A, Gaibani P, Spadafora C, et al: Detection of specific antibodies against West Nile and Usutu viruses in healthy blood donors in northern Italy, 2010/2011, *Clin Microbiol Infect* 19:E451–E453, 2013.

50. Allering L, Jöst H, Emmerich P, et al: Detection of Usutu virus infection in a healthy blood donor from south-west Germany, 2012, *Euro Surveill* 17(pii): 20341, 2012.

51. Weissenböck H, Chvala S, Bakonyi T, et al: Emergence of Usutu virus in central Europe: diagnosis, surveillance and epizootiology. In Takken W, Knols B, editors: *Emerging pests and vector-borne diseases in Europe*, Wageningen, The Netherlands, 2007, Wageningen Academic Publishers, pp 153–168.

52. Chvala S, Kolodziejek J, Nowotny N et al: Pathology and viral distribution in fatal Usutu virus infections of birds from the 2001 and 2002 outbreaks in Austria, *J Comp Pathol* 131:176–185, 2004.

53. Centers for Disease Control and Prevention. False-positive results with a commercially available West Nile virus immunoglobulin M assay — United States, 2008, *Morb Mortal Wkly Rep* 58:458–460, 2009.

54. Janusz KB, Lehman JA, Panella AJ, et al: Laboratory testing practices for West Nile virus in the United States, *Vector Borne Zoonotic Dis* 11:597–599, 2011.

55. Clarke DH, Casals J: Techniques for hemagglutination and hemagglutination-inhibition with arthropod-borne viruses, *Am J Trop Med Hyg* 7:561–573, 1958.

56. Chvala S, Bakonyi T, Bukovsky C, et al: Monitoring of Usutu virus activity and spread by using dead bird surveillance in Austria, 2003–2005, *Vet Microbiol* 122:237–245, 2007.

57. De Madrid AT, Porterfield JS: The flaviviruses (group B arboviruses): a cross-neutralization study, *J Gen Virol* 23:91–96, 1974.

58. Mansfield KL, Horton DL, Johnson N, et al: Flavivirus-induced antibody cross-reactivity, *J Gen Virol* 92:2812–2829, 2011.

59. Sambri V, Capobianchi MR, Cavrini F, et al: Diagnosis of West Nile virus human infections: overview and proposal of diagnostic protocols considering the results of external quality assessment studies. *Viruses* 5:2329–2348, 2013.

60. Johnson N, Wakeley PR, Mansfield KL, et al: Assessment of a novel real-time pan-Flavivirus RT-polymerase chain reaction, *Vector Borne Zoonotic Dis* 10:665–671, 2010.

61. Weaver SC, Barrett AD: Transmission cycles, host range, evolution and emergence of arboviral disease, *Nat Rev Microbiol* 2:789–801, 2004.

62. Day JF: Predicting St. Louis encephalitis virus epidemics: lessons from recent, and not so recent, outbreaks, *Annu Rev Entomol* 46:111–138, 2001.

63. Brault AC, Langevin SA, Bowen RA, et al: Differential virulence of West Nile strains for American crows, *Emerg Infect Dis* 10:2161–2168, 2004.

64. Brugger K, Rubel F: Simulation of climate-change scenarios to explain Usutu-virus dynamics in Austria, *Prev Vet Med* 88:24–31, 2009.

65. Townroe S, Callaghan A: British container breeding mosquitoes: the impact of urbanisation and climate change on community composition and phenology. *PLoS One* 9:e95325, 2014.

66. Rubel F, Brugger K, Hantel M, et al: Explaining Usutu virus dynamics in Austria: model development and calibration, *Prev Vet Med* 85:166–186, 2008.

67. Wobeser G, Wobeser AG: Carcass disappearance and estimation of mortality in a simulated die-off of small birds, *J Wildl Dis* 28:548–564, 1992.

68. Chvala S, Bakonyi T, Hacki R, et al: Limited pathogenicity of Usutu virus for the domestic chicken *(Gallus domesticus)*, *Avian Pathol* 34:392–395, 2005.

69. Soumare MK, Cilek JE: The effectiveness of *Mesocyclops longisetus* (Copepoda) for the control of container-inhabiting mosquitoes in residential environments, *J Am Mosq Control Assoc* 27:376–383, 2011.

70. Saleeza SN, Norma-Rashid Y, Sofian-Azirun M: Guppies as predators of common mosquito larvae in Malaysia, *Southeast Asian J Trop Med Public Health* 45:299–308, 2014.

71. Marten GG: Turtles. *J Am Mosq Control Assoc* 23(2 Suppl):221–224, 2007.

72. Xu HQ, Chen BQ: Remote sensing of the urban heat island and its changes in Xiamen City of SE China, *J Environ Sci (China)* 16:276–281, 2004.

73. Lei Zhao L, Lee X, Smith RG et al: Strong contributions of local background climate to urban heat islands, *Nature* 511:216–219, 2014.

CHAPTER 3

Neoplastic Diseases in Avian Species

Ashley Zehnder • Jennifer Graham • Drury R. Reavill • Alicia McLaughlin

The field of avian medicine has made great advances in recent years, particularly in the understanding and treatment of infectious diseases, anesthesia, analgesia, and nutrition for many species. However, as our patients are living longer and not dying from the infectious diseases that were so prevalent in the past, they are presenting more often with neoplastic disease. This is a close parallel to what is observed in humans and in other companion animals.

Unfortunately, avian patients present some unique challenges to the practitioner. They often present with advanced disease due to their excellent ability to hide signs of illness. They may be very small, making certain therapeutic options impractical. Case numbers are limited in the literature, and epidemiologic studies on avian cancer are lacking. This negatively impacts the veterinarian's ability to provide owners with accurate prognostic information and expected therapeutic outcomes.

There is improved research into the underlying genetic cause for many cancers in humans, and some of that research is also being evaluated in companion animals, primarily dogs and cats. Tools and criteria for monitoring therapeutic outcomes and side effects continue to improve. Clinical survey tools that can be used to gather data from patients across different institutions have been developed, allowing us to begin to apply more evidence-based research to the treatment of avian cancers. With these tools in hand, we are poised to take avian cancer care from therapies based on single case reports or anecdotal reports to something that better approaches the standards of care we observe in humans and other companion animals.

The goal of this chapter is not to provide an encyclopedic repetition of previously reported tumors in birds. We provide references to excellent reviews on the topic.[1-3] Rather, we wish to review the current standard of care for avian patients, identify areas of improvement, provide suggestions based on cancer care and research for other species, and hopefully set a new standard for effective diagnosis, monitoring, and therapeutics for avian cancer patients. Unfortunately, there is very little primary research in avian patients on this topic. Where applicable, we have pulled data from human and companion animal literature to fill in the gaps.

EMERGING TRENDS IN PATHOLOGY

As with veterinary clinical practice, pathology is an art, encompassing multiple variables, including the quality of the samples submitted, as well as the skill and experience of the pathologist. With tumor diagnostics, especially in the living patient, the pathologist has the additional charge of determining prognosis, contributing to possible therapeutic options, and possibly highlighting additional clinical support. Unfortunately, the pathologist often labors with unsuitable samples and inadequate, or worse, misleading histories. This degrades the quality of the results, especially in the field of avian medicine, where each case may provide valuable information about tumor behavior. For tumor diagnosis, there is a need for the clinician (primary clinician and oncologist) and pathologists to have a cooperative working relationship. Every submission adds to the collective knowledge about tumor behavior that can be applied to the individual case. The process of providing the best options for the patient starts with the attending clinician. The collected biopsy sample needs to be handled appropriately and the pertinent history conveyed to the pathologist.

Sample Collection

The method of collecting and handling the biopsy sample can introduce artifacts (Figure 3-1) that may complicate and/or obscure important lesions. Biopsies can be taken by means of surgical excision or incision, electrosurgery, punches, biopsy forceps, and needles. Electrosurgery can produce margin fragmentation and cautery artifact, which can affect the ability to accurately assess surgical margins for tumor removal. Dull cutting edges with punches and biopsy forceps can result in tissue crushing, splitting, and fragmentation of friable samples, and pseudocysts.[4] In particular, small biopsy samples need to be handled carefully. Extensive crush artifact (tissue forceps) (see Figure 3-1, *A*) and/or distortion of the tissues (excessive pulling) can make reading and interpretation impossible.

For many tumor samples, removing and submitting the entire mass and indicating the borders will help direct follow-up and possible additional therapies. The tissue specimen should be placed directly in 10% neutral buffered formalin unless inking or suturing of the cut margins is needed. There is approximately a 30-minute window of time to handle the fresh sample before autolysis or other artifacts develop. For borders, inking and suture placement are best done before fixation; however, both may also be done after fixation. Use of these markers can help orient the samples for specific evaluation of margins and to define areas of greatest concern. Inking should be performed with surgical ink or waterproof drawing ink (e.g., Higgins Waterproof Black India Ink). The tissues should be dry (gently blotted) before application, and the ink

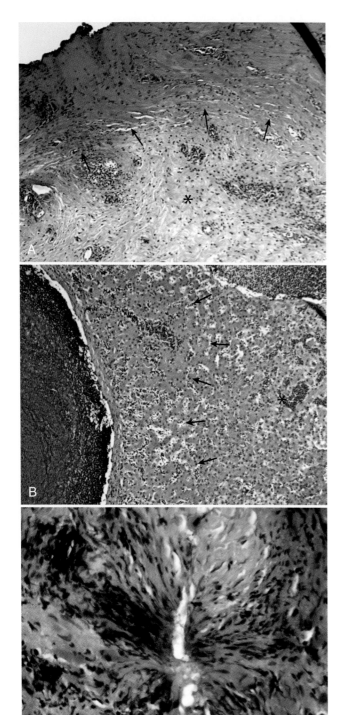

FIGURE 3-1 Common histologic artifacts in submitted samples. **A,** Heat artifact from use of cautery from a skin biopsy (10×). The arrows indicate the border between affected and unaffected tissue (*). Heat results in coagulation of the tissues, obscuring cellular details. **B,** Lesions from euthanasia solution in a liver section (10×). The arrows indicate the border between affected and unaffected tissue (*). The affected hepatocytes are swollen and eosinophilic. The blood vessel to the left is dilated and filled with necrotic cells. **C,** Tissue architecture changes due to crushing artifact (40×). This biopsy is collected from a squamous cell carcinoma; however, all the cells have been crushed rendering the sample nondiagnostic.

needs to dry (approximately 5 minutes) before placing the specimen in formalin. A cotton swab or wooden applicator works best for application of the ink. Black, yellow, and green are preferred colors for best visibility on hematoxylin and eosin (H&E) slides. Sutures can also be used to mark surgical margins or identify specific tissues (masses adjacent to the primary tumor, lateral, cranial, caudal sections) if more than one is submitted. The suture should be described by color, as suture types may not be familiar to laboratory personal.

Oversized specimens should be prefixed in formalin before shipping. Oversized samples are defined as those that do not fit into standard formalin jars and that are not expected to fix at a 1:15 to 1:20 tissue to formalin ratio. To enhance fixation of samples larger than 1 inch (2.5 cm) thick, the sections should be bread-loafed (partial parallel incisions 1 cm apart) after inking margins to enhance fixation. Small specimens (<0.5 mm) should be placed in screen tissue cassettes and the cassette dropped into the formalin jar to prevent damage during shipping. Gauze sponges, cardboard, or stapling the sample to wood depressors should be avoided, as these can result in damaged sections when laboratory personnel attempt to process the tissue. Thin flat tissue sections should be placed on a sponge (foam pad) within a tissue cassette. Larger sections can be sutured flat to a section of cardboard or wood depressor; however, needles should be avoided, as these pose a hazard to laboratory personnel.

Specific Sample Types

Bone tumors require special handling and interactions with the pathologist. Radiographic images add greatly to the diagnosis and may be the primary method to differentiate infection from neoplasia in avian species. As with domestic mammalian species, the site of collection of a bone tumor will affect the diagnosis. Peripheral sampling of a bone tumor results in a 54% chance of neoplastic tissues being present in the sample. Clinicians should note, however, that biopsies through lytic lesions run the risk of fracturing the bone, requiring additional surgery for repair. As with mammals, multiple biopsies enhance the probability of obtaining a diagnostic sample; however, this may not be an option in most avian patients.[5] Bone requires decalcification in order to be processed for histology. If the sections are small and the laboratory is not notified that the sample was from bone, these specimens can come out of the paraffin block during routine cutting and be lost.

Biopsies can become fragmented and less diagnostic when the tissues are of different consistencies. Hepatic lipidosis and bands of fibrosis within tumor masses can result in a fragmented sample. In these cases, a wedge biopsy of the liver mass is more likely to provide a diagnosis.[6] This is also true of tumors with extensive areas of hemorrhage and/or necrosis. Submission of the entire tumor mass is recommended, so additional sections can be processed if only necrotic areas are identified on the first evaluation. The entire mass is also recommended for margin checks.

Key Pathology History

Pathologists usually ask themselves if the proposed diagnosis is consistent with the clinical findings. If there are several possible differential diagnoses based on the morphology, the clinical information may help develop a list of the more probable diagnoses. Without any clinical history, there is no internal control or even a reason to contact the clinician for more information if the diagnosis seems uncomplicated. Providing a relevant, succinct history can be challenging but is crucial to aid the pathologist in a diagnosis. If the clinician produces the entire 50+ page history on the animal, it is inevitable that important details become obscured, especially in a busy commercial pathology service. The clinician should strive to provide succinct histories while including relevant details as described below (Box 3-1). It is important to identify the species and signalment of the bird. Some unusual tumors are more common in certain species, and other tumors are definitively linked to infectious disease agents. This makes species and signalment valuable information the clinician may need in order to direct any therapies or recommendations in a large collection or birds. Approximate age (hatchling, fledgling, young adult, aged) and sex should also be noted, as there are some tumor trends that are associated with these parameters.

The precise location of the mass is important. It makes a difference if the tumor is within the body cavity or on the skin. Also, the behavior of some tumors may vary, depending on where they arise. This is well described for some tumors in dogs and cats. For avian tumors, this information is not yet available, but associations may be found after collection and correlation of tumor location and outcome are done with retrospective studies. The rate of growth of the mass is also important information to provide and may help with selection of additional therapies.

The clinical history should describe any potentially lesion-associated clinical signs, previous biopsies, serum biochemistry results, complete blood count (CBC) results, imaging studies, and information regarding previous therapies. Frequently, tumors from the oral cavity or cloaca are associated with extensive inflammation and ulceration that can obscure the tumor itself. Therefore, it is important to perform a repeat biopsy of the masses that may have been previously diagnosed as inflammatory lesions and to note the sample as a repeat biopsy specimen. This holds true for any lesion that recurs after apparently effective antimicrobial therapy. Complete removal is a viable option for many lesions if they cannot be controlled with other therapies.[7]

BOX 3-1 KEY PATHOLOGY HISTORY POINTS

1. Patient signalment
   a. Species
   b. Age
   c. Sex
2. Lesion location
3. Rate of tumor growth, duration of time since lesion was first observed
4. Clinical history
   a. Associated clinical signs
   b. Previous biopsy results
   c. Previous therapies
   d. Clinical pathology abnormalities
   e. Imaging results

The axiom "If it is important enough to remove, it is important enough to determine what it is and submit the sample" should be followed. It is the rare client who will not, at some point, wonder what the mass might have been, especially if it recurs or the bird dies unexpectedly. In addition, although formalin-fixed tissues can be preserved indefinitely for a routine H&E as well as most other commonly used histochemical staining procedures, long-term storage in formalin will adversely affect additional tests such as immune diagnostics, polymerase chain reaction (PCR), and electron microscopy. In short, holding the samples can limit future diagnostic options.

The report contents

A full histologic description of tumors can be helpful for determining metastatic and invasive potential. Metastatic lesions in birds are rare but do occur occasionally (Table 3-1). The microscopic histology report generally includes such features as invasive or discrete growth, mitotic index, cell and nuclear shapes and sizes, nucleoli numbers and sizes, and supporting tissue reactions. Not only is this important for the individual's therapeutic options but it can also contribute valuable information in retrospective studies. A review of similar cases with detailed histologic descriptions may elucidate features that predict malignancy. For example, in malignant melanoma, which is uncommon in birds, the parameters of mitotic index, cellular atypia, and pigmentation are not correlated with malignancy. However, one study identified anisokaryosis and prominent nucleoli as possible predictors of malignant behavior.[8] More of these types of studies need to be performed on avian patients, as even among mammalian species these predictors do not apply across all species.

If the definitive diagnosis cannot unequivocally be determined on routine H&E evaluation, a presumptive diagnosis or differential diagnoses should be provided and possible additional diagnostic tests may be recommended. These additional tests can include differential stains, immunohistochemistry (IHC), PCR, or electron microscopy. In cases of a nondiagnostic sample, possible reasons why the sample failed to give a diagnosis should be provided in the comments.

Additional Tests

Special stains

There are a number of stains that can be applied to identify not only infectious disease agents such as fungi or acid-fast bacteria but also some tumors. For example, granular cell tumors, which are uncommon in birds, generally require additional stains for definitive diagnosis. The tumor cells are periodic acid–Schiff (PAS) positive and acid-fast negative. Additional testing such as electron microscopy and IHC also aid in the diagnosis. They are variably vimentin and desmin immunoreactive but negative for S100. Melanomas are another type of tumor that, if poorly differentiated or amelanotic, can be diagnosed with additional stains such as the Fontana-Masson stain for melanin. The cells have negative S100 immunoreactivity; however, unlike most mammalian melanomas, the avian tumors are also immunoreactive negative for Melan A. See Box 3-2 for an explanation of the special stains mentioned in this chapter.

IHC facilitates distinction between tumors with overlapping histologic features and enables finer reclassification of

TABLE 3-1

Reported Metastatic Tumors in Birds

Tumor Type	Species	Primary Tumor Site	Site of Metastasis	Reference
Adrenal carcinoma	Budgerigar *(Melopsittacus undulatus)*	Adrenal gland	Air sac, testicular capsule, kidney	104
Air sac carcinoma	Unspecified avian species	Air sac	Not provided	1
Biliary carcinoma/ adenocarcinomas	Budgerigar *(Melopsittacus undulatus)*	Liver	Not provided	3
Bile duct carcinomas	Unspecified avian species	Liver	Not provided	1
Cholangiocarcinoma	Adelie penguin *(Pygoscelis adeliae)*	Liver	Lung, pancreas, mesentery, and cloaca	105
Cholangiocarcinoma	Red-tailed hawk *(Buteo jamaicensis)*	Liver	Adrenal gland, lung, and left femur	106
Bronchial carcinoma	Grey parrot *(Psittacus erithacus)*	Lung	Humerus	107
Bronchial carcinoma	Red-shouldered hawk *(Buteo lineatus)*	Lung	Caudal air sac, Kidney, peritoneal surfaces	108
Chromophobic pituitary carcinomas	Budgerigar *(Melopsittacus undulatus)*	Pituitary	Liver, mid-brain, air sac	109
Fibrosarcoma	Budgerigar, rose-ringed parakeet, Amazon parrot	Skin	Not provided	3
Fibrosarcoma	Budgerigar *(Melopsittacus undulatus)*	Spleen	Not provided	3
Fibrosarcoma	Budgerigar *(Melopsittacus undulatus)*	Cloaca	Not provided	3
Fibrosarcoma	Budgerigar *(Melopsittacus undulatus)*	Intestine	Not provided	3
Fibrosarcoma	Grey parrot *(Psittacus erithacus)*	Unknown Not determined	Beak, syrinx, tibio-metatarsus	110
Fibrosarcoma	Cockatiel *(Nymphicus hollandicus)*	Lung	Liver	111
Hepatocellular carcinoma	Unspecified avian species	Liver	Not provided	1
Leiomyosarcoma	Budgerigar *(Melopsittacus undulatus)*	Unknown Not determined	Bone marrow, spleen, and liver	112
Hemangiosarcoma	Java sparrow	Metatarsal pad	Kidney, liver	113
Hemangiosarcoma	Unspecified avian species	Not provided	Not provided	1
Hemangiosarcoma	White turtle dove	Skin	Not provided	3
Hemangiosarcoma	Java sparrow *(Lonchura oryzivora)*	Foot—metatarsal pad	Kidney, liver	113
Hepatocellular carcinoma	Mynah	Liver	Not provided	3
Malignant melanoma	Macaroni penguin *(Eudyptes chrysolophus)*	Beak	Adrenal gland	114
Malignant melanoma	Red-tailed hawk *(Buteo jamaicensis)*	Adrenal gland	Lungs, liver, pancreas, skeletal muscle	114
Malignant melanoma	Mandarin duck *(Aix galericulata)*	Beak	Tissues in the neck	115
Malignant melanoma	Zebra finch *(Poephila castanotis)*	Coelom	Lung	116
Malignant melanoma	Pigeon *(Columba livia)*	Mucous membrane lower beak	Liver, kidney, spleen, and femur bone marrow	8
Malignant melanoma	Thick-billed parrot *(Rhynchopsitta pachyrhyncha)*	Beak	Lung liver spleen	7
Malignant melanoma	Merlin *(Falco columbarius)*	Adrenal gland	Liver, spleen, lung	117
Nephroblastoma	Budgerigar *(Melopsittacus undulatus)*	Kidney	Not provided	3
Osteosarcoma	Ring-necked dove *(Streptopelia risoria)*	Tibiotarsus	Lung	118
Ovarian/Oviduct adenocarcinoma	Unspecified avian species	Gonad	Not provided	1
Oviduct adenocarcinoma	Great tit *(Parus major L.)*	Oviduct	Intestine, pancreas, liver, kidney	119
Ovarian adenocarcinoma	Budgerigar *(Melopsittacus undulatus)*	Ovary	Not provided	3
Pancreatic adenocarcinoma	Cockatiel *(Nymphicus hollandicus)*	Pancreas	Surrounding tissues	120
Pancreatic adenocarcinoma	Unspecified avian species	Pancreas	Not provided	1
Pancreatic adenocarcinoma	Mynah	Pancreas	Not provided	3
Pancreatic carcinoma	Cockatiel *(Nymphicus hollandicus)*	Pancreas	Not provided	3
Pheochromocytoma	Budgerigar *(Melopsittacus undulatus)*	Adrenal gland	Liver, lung	121
Pituitary gland: Chromophobe adenocarcinoma	Budgerigar *(Melopsittacus undulatus)*	Pituitary gland	Not provided	3
Pituitary gland: Somatotroph carcinoma	Budgerigar *(Melopsittacus undulatus)*	Pituitary gland	Liver, midbrain, air sac	109

TABLE 3-1

Reported Metastatic Tumors in Birds—cont'd

Tumor Type	Species	Primary Tumor Site	Site of Metastasis	Reference
Proventricular adenocarcinoma	Unspecified avian species	Proventriculus	Not provided	1
Proventricular adenocarcinoma	Grey-cheeked parakeets (*Brotogeris pyrrhopterus*)	Proventriculus	Not provided	3
Proventricular adenocarcinoma	Budgerigar (*Melopsittacus undulatus*)	Proventriculus	Liver	122
Proventricular adenocarcinoma	Amazon parrot (*Amazona* species)	Proventriculus	Not provided	3
Pulmonary adenocarcinoma	Blue and gold macaw (*Ara ararauna*)	Lung	Vertebrae	123
Pulmonary carcinoma	Moluccan cockatoo (*Cacatua moluccensis*)	Lung	Vertebral column, humerus	124
Rhabdomyosarcoma	Yellow-headed caracara (*Milvago chimachima*)	Muscle region of proximal left humerus	Heart, lungs, and proventriculus	125
Rhabdomyosarcoma	Budgerigar (*Melopsittacus undulatus*)	Muscle	Not provided	3
Renal adenocarcinoma	Unspecified avian species	Kidney	Not provided	1
Renal adenocarcinoma	Budgerigar, Parakeet, Chestnut-eared finch	Kidney	Not provided	3
Renal carcinoma	Grey parrot (*Psittacus erithacus erithacus*)	Kidney	Lung, liver, heart, Sub cutis	126
Seminoma	Amazon green parrot (*Amazona* species)	Testicle	Not provided	3
Seminoma	Cockatiel (*Nymphicus hollandicus*)	Testicle	Liver	127
Seminoma	Guinea fowl (*Numida meleagris*)	Testicle	Liver, lungs, kidney, heart	128
Seminoma	Duck (*Anas platyrhynchos*)	Testicle	Liver, lung, pancreas, peritoneal	129
Seminoma	Pigeon (*Columba livia*)	Testicle	Liver, kidney	130
Sertoli cell tumor	Unspecified avian species	Gonad	Not provided	1
Squamous cell carcinoma	Montagu's harrier (*Circus pygargus*)	Oral cavity (hard palate)	Right tibia and radius, and lung	131
Squamous cell carcinoma	Salmon-crested cockatoo (*Cacatua moluccensis*)	Unknown	Bone, lungs, liver, and spleen	132
Squamous cell carcinoma (cutaneous)	Grey parrot (*Psittacus erithacus*)	Skin	Skin multiple sites (patagial and axilla)	133
Ventricular carcinoma	Unspecified avian species	Ventriculus	Not provided	1
Ventricular carcinoma	Sulfur-crested cockatoo (*Cacatua galerita*)	Ventriculus	Lungs	134

BOX 3-2 PATHOLOGY DEFINITIONS

1. **Periodic acid-Schiff (PAS)**: a staining method to detect polysaccharides such as glycogen, and mucosubstances such as glycoproteins, glycolipids, and mucins in tissues.
2. **S-100**: part of a protein family of low molecular weight that are used as markers for certain tumors and epidermal differentiation.
3. **Vimentin**: a type III intermediate filament protein that is expressed in mesenchymal cells and used as a sarcoma tumor marker.
4. **Desmin**: a type III intermediate filament found near the Z-line in sarcomeres and used to identify muscle.
5. **Fontana-Masson's stain**: a silver stain that stains argentaffin granules and melanin.
6. **Melan-A**: a melanoma-specific marker.
7. **GFAP**: a stain for glial fibrillary acidic protein, a protein found in glial cells and used to determine if a tumor is of glial origin.
8. **NSE**: neuron-specific enolase that is found in both normal and neoplastic cells of neuronal and neuroendocrine origin.
9. **von Willebrand Factor (Factor VIII-related antigen)**: antibody that specifically reacts with endothelial cells of normal and neoplastic blood and lymphatic vessels.
10. **PCNA**: proliferating cell nuclear antigen, a DNA clamp that acts as a processivity factor for DNA polymerase and is essential for replication. It is important for both DNA synthesis and repair and is used as a marker for cell proliferation.
11. **Ki-67**: a nuclear protein that is associated with and may be necessary for cellular proliferation. It is associated with ribosomal RNA transcription and is used as a marker for cell proliferation.

some cancers based on expression of specific proteins and carbohydrates. However, applying IHC stains for further characterization of avian tumors is complicated, as the previous melanoma example above illustrates. In additional examples, glial fibrillary acidic protein (GFAP) and neuron-specific enolase (NSE) did not stain internal controls (nervous tissues that are known to react to the stains), indicating that these two antibodies are unreactive in exotic avian species compared with mammals.[9] There are conflicting reports on whether antihuman von Willebrand factor antibodies (Factor VIII–related protein) have reactivity with avian tissue. The interpretation relies on internal positive controls (normal endothelial cells) to determine if there is a reaction.[10] IHC can also identify cell cycle markers that can be used to provide diagnostic and prognostic information. Examples include proliferating cell nuclear antigen (PCNA) and Ki-67.[11] Unfortunately, the clinical interpretation of these tests requires studies comparing normal versus neoplastic tissues in each species of interest. This may not be feasible with many pet birds.[12]

Lymphoma is one tumor type where increasing the use of IHC may someday provide more definitive diagnoses and prognoses. Currently, there are no known associations between tumor behavior and lymphoma classifications in birds, and validation of some of these markers for avian species remains to be done. The CD3 antigen (T lymphocyte marker) appears to react across most, if not all, avian species. B-cell and histiocytic cell markers vary; however, cases submitted to laboratories that maintain tissue blocks (formalin-fixed, paraffin-embedded [FFPE] tissue) collected from a variety of avian species may also have samples that can be used as controls to match the clinical case of concern. Most large commercial laboratories do not store FFPE blocks for more than a few years, and identifying blocks for control samples may not be possible at these facilities.

The electron microscope, which first revealed the existence of subcellular organelles, can incorporate ultrastructural features of differentiation into the diagnostic workup of difficult to diagnose neoplasms. For tumor types that are generally poorly differentiated or unusual, the finding of specific ultrastructural features may at least help determine tissue of origin.

Polymerase chain reaction

Molecular genetic analysis of tissue specimens is the latest innovation to contribute to the understanding of tumor etiologies. Tumor development due to a disease agent is well described in the literature.[13] Probably the best known avian viral examples are of avian sarcoma induced by Rous sarcoma virus (RSV) and Marek disease, a lymphoma induced by a herpesvirus in poultry.

In pet birds, some tumors such as mucosal papillomas have been associated with viral infections. The etiology of this lesion in New World parrots is felt to be psittacid herpesvirus (PsHV), identical or closely related to those that cause Pacheco disease. Mucosal papillomas have developed in some parrots that survived acute PsHV infection (Pacheco disease).[14] No herpesvirus or papillomavirus has been identified in the cloacal papillomas of cockatoos or cockatiels, suggesting that not all papilloma tumors arise from disease agents, or at least not the same agents.[15]

To obtain samples most likely to yield positive results, samples should be taken from the lesion itself. Given the possible infectious etiology of some tumors, preserving samples for further diagnostics can be important, both clinically and for research. Keeping current with the latest literature in avian medicine can help the practitioner identify researchers looking for specific materials and also identify the appropriate samples and/or handling restrictions. These samples are in addition to the FFPE tissue for diagnostic pathology, as this sample type is not ideal for molecular analyses. Representative fresh tissue samples can be collected and stored frozen, ideally in a $-80°$ C freezer or liquid nitrogen for years, although this type of storage is unlikely to be available to anyone outside of large research facilities or a university setting.[16] A non–frost-free standard freezer can be used to hold these samples in practice. Prefixation time (the time between tissue dissection and freezing or fixation) is a major factor that influences the integrity of banked samples. For most viral agents, tissues left in formalin more than 2 to 3 days will result in nondiagnostic negative findings, while FFPE and fresh frozen tissue may have viable material for years.[16]

Additional testing of tumor gene alterations or mutations has been described in the mammalian literature but not yet in pet birds. These genetic changes can affect the regulation of the cell cycle, apoptosis, or cell–cell and cell–matrix interactions (potential for metastasis). The methods used to detect these alterations vary considerably, depending on the type of mutation being sought. In general, alterations in gene number are best assessed by cytogenetic techniques (e.g., karyotype or fluorescence in situ hybridization [FISH]), alterations in deoxyribonucleic acid (DNA) sequence by molecular diagnostic techniques (e.g., PCR, sequence analysis), and structural rearrangements such as translocations may be detected by either method, depending on the rearrangement. Additionally, genome-wide association studies (GWASs) and next-generation sequencing are making it easier to link genetic alterations to diseases.

However, it is unlikely this work will be applied to our pet bird patients in the near future, as it generally requires significant funding to identify the genetic changes in a specific animal and tumor. As the costs of whole genome sequencing decrease and additional bird species are sequenced for the purposes of determining evolutionary genetic conservation, the ability to determine the presence or absence of cancer-associated mutations in avian clinical patients will improve. There are currently 14 avian genomes that can be viewed on the UCSC Genome browser, including three psittacine species (budgerigar [*Melopsittacus undulatus*], Puerto Rican parrot [*Amazona vittata*], and scarlet macaw [*Ara macao*]). A recent study examining the conservation of amino acid residues that are known to be oncogenic in human found that 21 of 29 oncogenic hotspots (72.4%) were fully conserved in all species examined, including the three available psittacine genomes.[17] This suggests that it may be valuable to see if the same activating mutations found in many human cancers are present in avian tumors as well. This would help guide the use of targeted cancer therapies in avian species.

With the explosion in our understanding of the factors that influence tumor formation, growth, and behavior, new testing modalities are arising. Understanding more about the specific tumor biology in the individual will hopefully lead to tailoring of therapies and improved prognosis.

CANCER DIAGNOSTICS

Staging

Signalment, history, and thorough physical examination are important parts of the initial clinical evaluation of avian patients with tumors. Since many tumors have a tendency to affect birds of a particular age, gender, or species, collection of this information is vital. Diet history can help identify potential risk factors for neoplasia related to malnutrition; for example, in epidemiologic studies, the intake of carotenoid-rich fruits and vegetables has been correlated with protection from some forms of cancer,[18] and it is suspected that chronic hypovitaminosis A may be a risk factor for development of squamous cell carcinoma in pet birds. Sex identification and reproductive history are important, since chronic egg laying is a risk factor for development of ovarian or reproductive cancers.[12] Previous infection with *Macrorhabdus ornithogaster* may increase the risk of proventricular adenocarcinoma in budgerigars, so a history of chronic macrorhabdiosis should not be overlooked.[19] Additionally, any chronic nonhealing wound, areas subject to repeated trauma, or any region prone to chronic inflammatory conditions may be at risk for development of neoplasia. Cardiovascular disease, particularly atherosclerosis, is common in aged female parrots, particularly the *Psittacus*, *Amazona*, and *Nymphicus* species, and could alter prognosis or a patient's ability to tolerate treatment.[20] It is important to rule out underlying (and potentially zoonotic) disease such as chlamydiosis or mycobacteriosis prior to the use of immunosuppressive agents.

For any avian species with a suspected tumor, histologic or cytologic diagnosis of the tumor is recommended to determine (if possible) the tissue of origin and grade of tumor. Cytology may help differentiate neoplastic from non-neoplastic lesions and may indicate tumor type. This is particularly true for tumors that are likely to exfoliate, such as lymphomas (Figure 3-2). However, accurate histogenesis and tumor grading require histology.[21] Special staining procedures, including IHC, may be needed to further determine various cellular antigens and cell of origin (as discussed above). Mitotic index may help determine tumor grade, but there is no clear evidence from the avian literature that mitotic index is prognostic. No one has yet established grading systems for avian tumors due to lack of data linking tumor grade with patient outcomes.

The tumor–node–metastasis (TNM) approach, developed by the World Health Organization (WHO), is used in mammalian species to stage solid tumors and has been adapted for evaluation of disseminated tumors such as lymphoma.[21] The "TNM" approach evaluates the primary tumor (T), presence or absence of metastatic disease in local, regional, and distant lymph nodes (N), and the presence or absence of metastatic disease within the rest of the body (M). Although birds lack lymph nodes, this general concept can be adapted using a "TM" approach to evaluate avian tumors to best determine extent of disease and determine treatment options. See Figure 3-3 for a "TM" algorithm approach for avian cancer patients. Because there is no clinical evidence to support the use of more precise

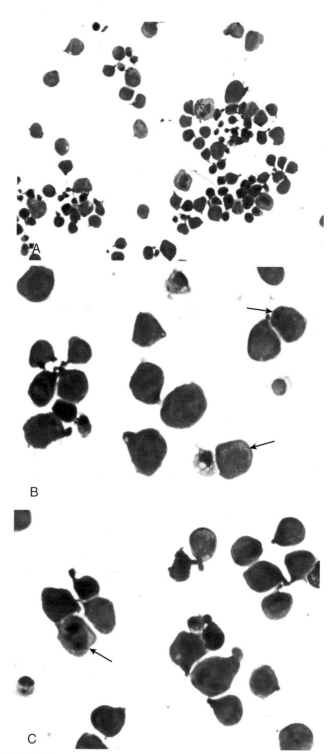

FIGURE 3-2 Cytologic diagnosis of lymphoma from coelomic fluid in a budgerigar presenting with hepatic failure and coelomic distension. Neoplastic effusion demonstrates atypical round cells with rare mitotic figures (**A**—500×), many cells with prominent nucleoli (**B**—1000×), and rare binucleation (**C**—1000×). (Image courtesy Angell Animal Medicine Center, Department of Pathology.)

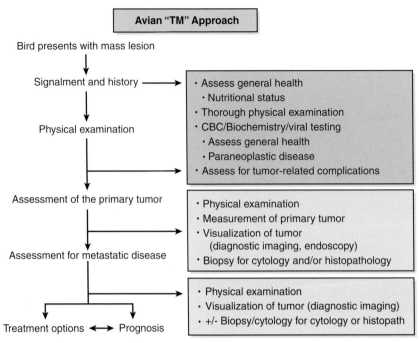

FIGURE 3-3 Diagrammatic approach to "TM" tumor staging in avian patients.

tumor scales such as those developed for specific tumors in humans and, to some degree, in companion animals, the authors recommend a more general staging technique that takes into account the overall health of the animal, in addition to details about the primary tumor and metastatic lesions. As we collect additional evidence on tumor descriptions along with outcome data, we can begin to make better predictions on prognosis based on tumors at their initial presentation and develop better staging systems.

Evaluation of the primary tumor (T)
The tumor is evaluated both in terms of size and invasiveness. The tumor is sampled by way of aspirates for cytologic diagnosis or biopsy for histologic diagnosis. In some situations,

complete surgical excision of the mass may be the best option for diagnosis and treatment if the disease is localized. The extent of the tumor can be evaluated by clinical examination of the patient, but the disease may extend beyond visible margins. Diagnostic imaging techniques, including plain and contrast radiography, ultrasonography, computed tomography (CT), magnetic resonance imaging (MRI), and endoscopy, can help assess the extent of the tumor, depending on the tumor site. Objective tumor descriptions, including specific locations and measurements in three planes whenever possible, should be recorded to monitor patient response. A general psittacine body map has been created for use in avian patients and can be printed out and added to the medical records for increased ease of tumor measurements (Figure 3-4).

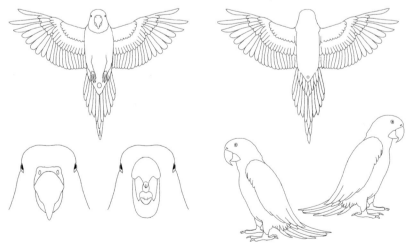

FIGURE 3-4 General psittacine body map for tumor mapping.

Evaluation for metastatic disease (M)

While the lung is generally the most common site for distant metastatic disease, other sites can include the skin, liver, kidneys, bone, brain or nervous tissue, and spleen. Physical examination may suggest metastases (e.g., cutaneous masses), but diagnostic imaging techniques, as described above, are generally required to evaluate for metastases. Multiple radiographic views can help evaluate for metastatic disease, but CT is more sensitive for evaluation of metastatic disease compared with radiography in other species. Radiography may reveal changes in the size or shape of the liver, spleen, and kidneys, but ultrasound-guided aspirates or endoscopic biopsies may be required to determine the extent of disease spread into these organs. It is important to remember that imaging alone does not necessarily prove that an identified lesion is a metastasis. There could be a nonmalignant cause, or there could be a secondary primary tumor. Either an aspirate or a biopsy is needed to definitively diagnose metastasis. Bone marrow aspiration is recommended for staging and diagnosing disseminated diseases such as lymphoma or leukemia. More advanced imaging modalities, including MRI, positron emission tomography (PET), and technetium-99 bone scans have been used to evaluate for metastatic disease in a variety of species.[22–25]

Clinical Pathology

Complete blood count

A CBC should be performed as part of a minimum database collection on any patient being evaluated for cancer diagnosis or treatment. Anemia or leukopenia could indicate bone marrow involvement or splenic disease. Chemotherapy agents are generally most toxic to rapidly dividing cells, so toxicity to the bone marrow and the gastrointestinal (GI) tract is a concern. CBC should be monitored, and treatment should be delayed if the heterophil count is too low. In mammals such as dogs and cats, a neutrophil count less than 2000 cells per microliter (cells/μL) indicates that treatment should be delayed, but to some degree this is agent dependent.[26]

Biochemistry

Similar to CBC, biochemistry profile is recommended as part of a minimum database collection. Renal or hepatic enzyme elevation may indicate organ involvement or dysfunction and may preclude the use of certain chemotherapeutic drugs. Nevertheless, it is important to remember that these tests rarely provide definitive information as to the type of cancer or the presence of metastasis.

Imaging modalities

Radiography of the thorax is valuable in determining the clinical stage of disease in mammals. To assess the lungs properly in mammals, three views should be obtained—both left and right lateral views, as well as a ventrodorsal (VD) view. These recommendations should be followed for avian patients as well. It is important to remember that pulmonary nodules less than 1 cm may not be detected on plain radiographs in mammals. Radiography enables limited soft tissue discrimination but may be valuable in screening for organomegaly or lytic bone lesions consistent with metastasis. Conventional radiography, preferably with high-detail film, may provide adequate diagnostic imaging for nasal and oral tumors, although the extent of disease may not be fully elucidated. Administration of contrast agents such as barium or iohexol or fluoroscopy may be helpful to delineate masses or organomegaly (Figure 3-5).

Ultrasonography allows for evaluation of the architecture of abdominal viscera and has largely replaced radiography in the staging of mammalian cancer patients. In addition, it carries no radiation risk to the patient or hospital personnel. If aspiration or biopsy of a mass within a body cavity is indicated, particularly if effusion is present, ultrasonography provides an accurate guide and a relatively safe and noninvasive means of obtaining a tissue or fluid sample. Ultrasonography is the imaging modality of choice for tumors of the heart because of the motion of this organ. In addition, ultrasonography may reveal the presence of a retrobulbar mass. It is important to note that ultrasonographic measurements of lesions are not considered very reliable for monitoring patient response. Again, it is important to note that ultrasonography does not provide a definitive diagnosis of metastasis, and sampling of a lesion is needed to be sure of the diagnosis.

CT has become more widely available for veterinary use, particularly at teaching institutions and large specialty practices. In some areas of the United States, imaging centers offer these services to local practitioners. The major advantage of CT and MRI over conventional radiography is their ability to provide a three-dimensional image and to discriminate between tissues that have only minor differences in radiodensity or intensity that would silhouette together on plain radiographs. They also have advantages over ultrasonography in the ability to image lesions that are shielded by bone or gas. Although MRI is very good at delineating soft tissue, it can be difficult to judge if there is bone involvement or extension of a tumor. CT is a better modality for this. For this reason, CT can be helpful to evaluate tumors within the nasal and oral cavities. CT is particularly useful when the veterinarian is trying to determine tumor margins prior to surgery or radiation therapy (RT) and to delineate important surrounding structures (see Figure 3-5). Contrast agents can be used to better delineate many tumors with both CT and MRI. According to literature sources, a dose of 2 milliliters per kilogram (mL/kg) of iodinated contrast should provide visualization of the kidneys and ureters within 10 to 20 seconds after administration, and the cloaca may be outlined in 2 to 5 minutes.[27] Complications of iodinated contrast media are generally related to increased osmolality, and caution should be used in patients with renal compromise, as there may be poor excretion of the contrast agent. CT imaging of the lungs can often be accomplished with controlled ventilation in mammals, thus ensuring increased sensitivity in detecting small pulmonary nodules, as well as enhanced discrimination of lesion location. This is done to limit motion artifact that can occur with breathing. Imaging is often essential in determining both resectability of a primary tumor and identification of suspected metastatic lesions. This information is crucial for devising an appropriate and rational treatment plan for the veterinary cancer patient.

MRI is often the modality of choice for imaging tumors of the brain and spine. Lesions of the brainstem may require MRI for diagnostic quality. In addition to CT, MRI is also useful when the veterinarian is trying to determine tumor margins prior to surgery or RT as MRI is often considered

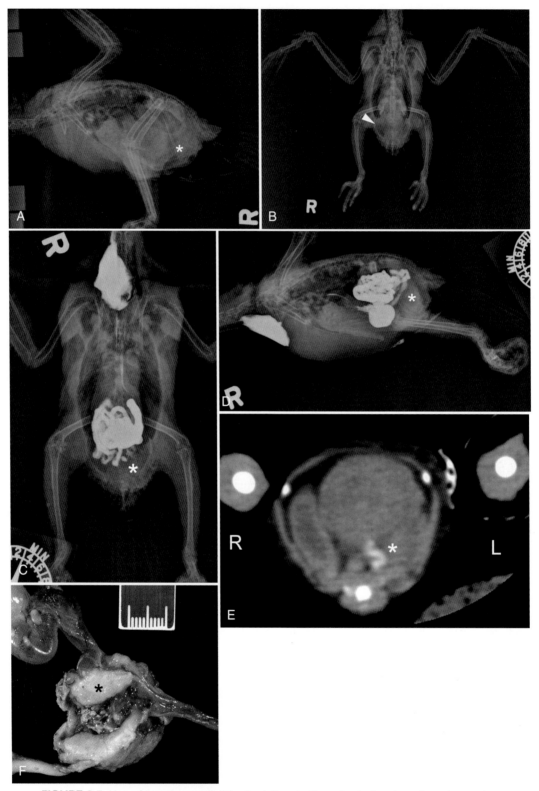

FIGURE 3-5 Use of imaging modalities to delineate the extent of a cloacal carcinoma in a 27-year-old female Green-cheeked Amazon parrot *(Amazona viridigenalis)* presenting for frank blood in the stool and a cloacal mass. On the lateral projection without contrast, there is loss of coelomic detail and increased soft tissue density near the cloaca **(A)**(*). On the VD projection without contrast, the mass is not clearly visible, but the abdominal air sac is reduced bilaterally **(B)** *(white arrowhead)*. Three hours after barium administration, a soft tissue mass (*) is seen displacing the intestines craniodorsally on the ventrodorsal **(C)** and lateral **(D)** projections. Computed tomography with nonionic contrast (120 mg iodine/kg) **(E)** was used to delineate the soft tissue extent of the mass and also allowed visualization of a dilated left ureter (*), suggesting partial obstruction by the mass. Gross necropsy image **(F)** of the cloacal mass (*). Note the dilated ureter proximal to the mass.

more sensitive for detecting tumor margins in soft tissues. However, due to cost and concerns over longer anesthesia, clinicians may choose CT with contrast over MRI to delineate tumors in areas of soft tissue. Due to the relatively slow speed of image acquisition, MRI has limited utility in imaging of the thoracic cavity in mammals due to movements of the heart and lungs.

Radioactive tracers can be used to identify active neoplastic lesions and metastases and are often paired with CT to aid localization. Radioisotopes may release two different types of radiation when they decay: gamma from single photon emitters and annihilation radiation from positron emitters.[28] Technetium-99m, a single photon emitter, is used in nuclear scintigraphy. It is primarily useful for determining the presence and extent of bony lesions and for examining blood flow to a lesion. One author's (JG's) institution has used Tech99 scanning paired with CT to detect active neoplastic lesions in a goose with osteosarcoma (Figure 3-6).

PET is used to evaluate the biochemical function or metabolic activity of a tumor by radiolabeling biologic substrates (i.e., glucose in fluorodeoxyglucose [FDG]-PET). This helps the clinician stage the tumor, plan surgery, evaluate response to therapy, and detect relapse of various neoplastic conditions.[23] PET was used to evaluate two cases of avian neoplasia, and normal PET image acquisition in Hispaniolan Amazon parrots has been described.[23] The authors recommend that dynamic scans be performed, starting immediately after radiopharmaceutical injection so that increased radioactivity

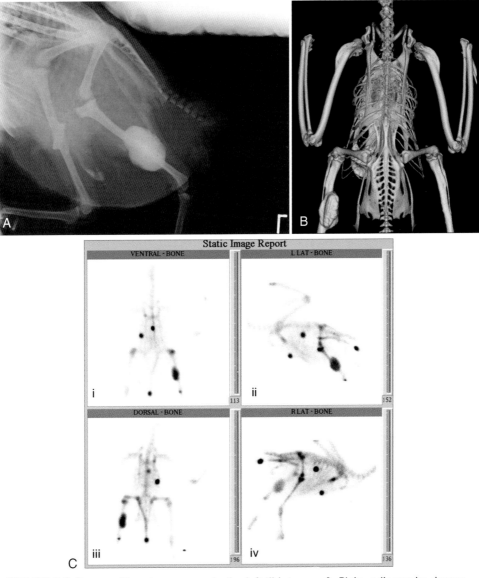

FIGURE 3-6 Goose with osteosarcoma in the left tibiotarsus. **A,** Plain radiographs demonstrating a large bony lesion in the mid-tibiotarsus. **B,** Three-dimensional reconstruction of the lesion using computed tomography. **C,** Technitium-99 scan using 0.167 GBq of 99m Tc-HDP injected intravenously. Subsequent static images of the body and proximal limbs were obtained during the bone phase of radiopharmaceutical distribution. Markedly increased radiopharmaceutical uptake is noted in the left tibiotarsus, left proximal tarsometatarsus, left stifle. There is also increased uptake in one of the right ribs, right coracoid, and keel.

due to metabolism or hypermetabolic lesions such as cancer can be differentiated from increased radioactivity due to reflux of fluid from the cloaca when evaluating the intestinal tract.

Cancer Therapeutics

Once clinicians have properly evaluated the primary lesions and the presence of metastatic disease, the next step is to design a treatment plan. The major considerations are the resectability of the primary tumor, the presence of multiple or distant lesions, technical or logistical concerns, and patient comorbidities. The authors have outlined the major decision points for creating a treatment plan in Figure 3-7. Avian practitioners are limited by some additional concerns, as basic issues such as obtaining repeated, dedicated venous access may not be possible. Avian patients can be very small, and they generally will require repeated anesthetic episodes for treatments such as chemotherapy, which poses more risk to birds than to dogs and cats, which do not require multiple anesthetic episodes. Additionally, avian patients may hide underlying illnesses and may be more susceptible to the immunosuppressive effects of corticosteroids, a common component of treatments for dogs and cats with certain lymphoid tumors. Clinicians need to work closely with owners to make sure they understand that nearly all the treatment recommendations made for avian patients are extrapolated from treatments designed for humans, dogs, or cats and that there is only rare primary research examining the effectiveness of cancer therapy in birds. It also is a great opportunity for pet bird owners to improve the care for all birds undergoing treatment for cancer by making sure they follow up with their veterinarians regularly and let the veterinarians know if their animal dies at home. Necropsies at the time of death may provide additional information to expand the knowledge about the behaviors of avian neoplasia. This chapter will focus on the most commonly utilized therapies—surgical resection, chemotherapy, radiation, cryotherapy, and a few other adjunctive therapies.

Surgical Resection

A recent survey of 85 cases of squamous cell carcinoma in birds reported an odds ratio of 7.48 (1.97 to 28.36) for complete or partial response in patients that had complete surgical excision. This means that the odds of a patient having a complete or partial response outcome for its tumor is 7.48 higher if that patient received complete surgical excision. No other treatment category had a significant odds ratio for these response categories.[29] This coincides with observations made in published case reports of cancer treatment in avian medicine. An informal survey of 39 single case reports in the avian tumor literature listing therapy and outcome revealed that 7 of 9 (78%) cases that listed only surgical resection as a therapy also reported complete response or a greater than 6-month survival. However, only 16 of 30 (54%) cases that used adjunctive therapies (with or without surgery) reported complete responses or long-term (>6-month) survival. The differences here are not statistically significant when evaluated with Chi-square analysis (p value 0.06), but it is reasonable to suggest cases that are treated by surgical resection alone are underreported in the literature, as clinicians tend to publish cases utilizing novel treatment strategies. Obviously, each case has its own set of circumstances, so the cases should not be directly compared, but most clinicians would agree (and the data above suggest) that complete surgical excision of a tumor yields the best hope for a cure. Basic oncologic principles should be adhered to, including using a separate surgical pack for tumor

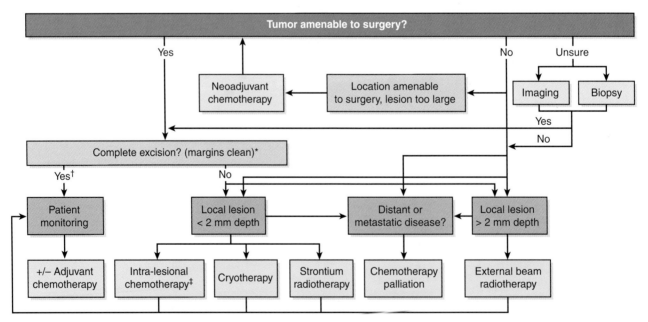

* Recommended histology be performed on all excised tumors.
† If tumor was high grade or there are metastases, adjunctive chemotherapy is indicated.
‡ May be appropriate for lesions > 2 mm in depth depending on location and proximity to nearby vital structures.

FIGURE 3-7 Decision tree for avian patients with neoplastic disease.

excision and surgical site closure and taking care not to seed the surrounding tissue with tumor cells. It is not clear yet what constitutes adequate margins for surgical resections in avian patients, but cut margins should be marked, either with appropriate ink, sutures, or staples and submitted for histologic examination (see recommendations above). The presence of tumor cells on the surgical margins is an indication for follow-up local therapies (if there is no evidence of distant disease) such as additional surgery or RT.

Chemotherapy

Consultation with an oncologist is strongly recommended prior to initiating chemotherapy. Oncologists used to working with dogs and cats may not understand the adaptations necessary for treating avian patients, but they are much more familiar with treatment protocols. Avian practitioners can work together with oncologists to craft the most appropriate treatment plan for each patient. Chemotherapy is indicated for the control of lesions that are unresectable or were resected with incomplete margins or for patients with distant, disseminated disease. Because chemotherapy is more likely to be beneficial when metastatic disease is at a microscopic level, it may best be used as adjuvant therapy following surgical resection of high-grade tumors before gross metastasis is detected. Chemotherapy can also be given in a neoadjuvant setting. Neoadjuvant treatments are used to reduce tumors that are too large to be surgically resected in order to make them amenable for later resection. Veterinarians administering chemotherapy need to be familiar with the chemotherapeutic agents used and of safety issues for themselves, owners, staff, and possible complications for their patients.[22] All drugs should be mixed under a fume hood by properly trained personnel. Women who are pregnant or attempting to become pregnant should avoid handling chemotherapeutics. Luer-Lok syringes should be used to avoid drug leakage, and closed chemotherapy systems that limit the risk of exposure are now available. All personnel handling drugs or patients receiving drugs should wear protective clothing, including gloves, eye protection, closed-toe shoes, and long sleeves. Pills should not be cut or split. All waste should be disposed of in appropriate containers. Clients should be told to wear gloves when administering any chemotherapeutic medication or cleaning waste from patients receiving chemotherapy.

Dosing

Chemotherapy dosing should be based on the maximum dose that has a small chance of severe toxicity.[26] Drug dosages are calculated by using body weight or body surface area (BSA). Although there is limited information available regarding the determination of BSA in exotic species, there are reports of using the formula for the area of a cylinder to estimate the BSA of birds. A formula that has been proposed for birds is: $M^2 = \text{Body weight (g)}^{2/3} \times K \times 10^{-4}$, where $K = 10.0$.[30] However, BSA-based dosing has not been validated in birds and may not have advantages over milligrams per kilogram (mg/kg) dosing. One recent study examined single-dose carboplatin pharmacokinetics across four species: domestic chickens (*Gallus gallus*), racing pigeons (*Columbia livia*), call ducks (*Anas platyrhynchos*) and English budgerigars (*Melopsittacus undulates*). In this study, the authors noted a good correlation ($R^2 > 0.97$) between elimination half-life ($T_{1/2el}$) and body weight (Antonissen et al, manuscript in preparation). When extrapolating from canine and feline chemotherapeutic drug dosing, it should be kept in mind that these doses may not be appropriate, and avian patients should be monitored closely for adverse side effects.

Monitoring

Chemotherapy agents are generally most toxic to rapidly dividing cells, so toxicity to bone marrow and the GI tract is a concern. CBC should be monitored weekly to biweekly, and treatment should be delayed if the heterophil count is too low. In mammals such as dogs and cats, a neutrophil count less than 2000 cells/μL indicates the need for delaying treatment.[26] A general rule is that treatment should be delayed for avian patients with a heterophil count less than 2000 cells/μL if a drug that is generally considered myelosuppressive is scheduled. If the drug is not considered myelosuppressive in other species, it may be possible to administer therapy as long as the heterophil count is 1500 cells/μL. A conservative rule is to administer antibiotics to any avian patient with a heterophil count below 2000 cells/μL. The Veterinary Cooperative Oncology Group has established common terminology criteria for adverse events following chemotherapy or biologic antineoplastic therapy in dogs and cats.[31] These documents define an adverse event as "any unfavorable and unintended sign, clinical sign, or disease temporally associated with the use of a medical treatment that may or may not be considered related to the medical treatment." This document can be used as a guideline for uniform terminology usage in recording adverse events in avian species following chemotherapy administration. A version of this document that has been modified for avian patients is provided (Table 3-2). It is important for clinicians to understand that they do not necessarily need to work out if the adverse event is a direct consequence of a treatment, but they should be recorded nonetheless. Adverse events are categorized by different body systems, with a separate category for clinical pathology. There is a grading scale that quantifies the severity of the observed effects. Generally, grade 1 is mild and may be subclinical, grade 2 is moderate, grade 3 is severe, grade 4 is life threatening, and grade 5 is death.

Commonly used chemotherapeutic agents

Table 3-3 lists avian case reports describing the use of the chemotherapeutic agents below and other adjuvant therapies.

Alkylating agents

Indications. Alkylating agents are used for the treatment of lymphoma and lymphoblastic leukemia, mast cell tumors, and occasionally combined with doxorubicin to treat mammary carcinoma and soft tissue sarcomas.

Mechanism of action of drugs. Alkylating agents act by cross-linking strands of DNA, particularly at the N-7 position of guanine. They are nonspecific for cell cycle phase and are thus active during most parts of the cell cycle. Alkylating agents in the classic family include nitrogen mustard, cyclophosphamide, chlorambucil, melphalan, busulfan, and ifosfamide. Other drugs classified as alkylating agents include the nitrosoureas (CCNU and BCNU), the tetrazines (DTIC, or dacarbazine), the aziridines (thiotepa and mitomycin C), and nonclassic alkylating agents such as procarbazine and hexamethylmelamine.

TABLE 3-2

Side Effect Monitoring Criteria for Avian Patients Receiving Chemotherapy or Radiation Treatments

Adverse Event	Grade 1	2	3	4	5
ALLERGIC/IMMUNOLOGIC EVENT					
Allergic reaction/ hypersensitivity	Transient erythema/ urticaria	Rash; urticaria; dyspnea	Hypotension; edema	Anaphylaxis	Death
Autoimmune reaction	Asymptomatic (se-rologic evidence), no intervention	Affecting nonessen-tial organ or func-tion (e.g., thyroid)	Affecting function of a major organ—reversible (e.g., anemia)	Reaction with life-threatening con-sequences	Death
Vasculitis (does not include perivascu-lar administration)	Mild—needs no intervention	Symptomatic, non-steroidal antiin-flammatory drugs (NSAIDs) indicated	Steroids may be considered	Ischemia, amputa-tion or surgical debridement indicated	Death
Other (specify)	Mild	Moderate	Severe	Life-threatening; disabling	Death
BLOOD/BONE MARROW					
Bone marrow cellu-larity	Mildly hypocellular; <25% reduction of cellularity from expected	Moderately hypocel-lular; 25%–50% re-duction of cellular-ity from expected	Severely hypocellular; >50% reduction of cellularity from expected	—	—
Packed cell volume (PCV)	PCV ≤15% below lower limit of normal (LLN)	PCV = 15%–30% be-low LLN	PCV = 30%–45% below LLN	PCV = >45% below LLN	
Heteropenia	Heterophils ≤25% below LLN	Heterophils 25–50% below LLN	Heterophils 50%–75% below LLN	Heterophils >75% below LLN	
Thrombocytopenia*	Mild	Moderate	Severe	Life-threatening	
Other (specify)	Mild	Moderate	Severe	Life-threatening; disabling	Death
CARDIAC					
Cardiopulmonary Arrest	—	—	—	Life-threatening	Death
Hypertension	Asymptomatic, transient (<24 hours), interven-tion not indicated	Recurrent or persis-tent (>24 hours) or symptomatic in-crease; monother-apy may be indi-cated	Requiring more than one drug or more intensive therapy	Life-threatening consequences (e.g., hypertensive crisis)	Death
Hypotension	Asymptomatic, intervention not indicated	Brief (<24 hours) fluid replacement or other therapy; no physiologic con-sequences	Sustained (>24 hours) therapy, resolves without persisting physiologic conse-quences	Shock (e.g., impair-ment of vital or-gan function)	Death
Myocarditis	—	—	Congestive heart fail-ure (CHF) respon-sive to intervention	Severe or refractory CHF	Death
Pericardial effusion (non-malignant)	Asymptomatic effusion	—	Physiologic conse-quences	Life-threatening; emergency inter-vention indicated	Death
Arrhythmia: indicate which type of ar-rhythmia along with the severity grade: Conduction abnormality/ atrioventricular (AV) heart block Supraventricular and nodal ar-rhythmia	Asymptomatic, intervention not indicated	Non-urgent medical intervention indi-cated	Incompletely con-trolled medically	Life-threatening (e.g., arrhythmia associated with CHF, hypotension, syncope, shock)	Death

TABLE 3-2

Side Effect Monitoring Criteria for Avian Patients Receiving Chemotherapy or Radiation Treatments—cont'd

Adverse Event	Grade				
	1	2	3	4	5
Ventricular arrhythmia					
Other (please specify)	Mild	Moderate	Severe	Life-threatening; disabling	Death
COAGULATION/HEMORRHAGE					
Coagulation deficit[†]	Mild	Moderate	Severe	Life-threatening	Death
Hematoma	Minimal signs, no intervention	Aspiration indicated	Transfusion indicated	Life-threatening	Death
Surgical hemorrhage	—	—	Requires transfusion	Life-threatening	Death
Spontaneous hemorrhage	Minimal signs, no intervention	Symptomatic, medical or minor surgical intervention indicated	Transfusion or operative intervention indicated	Life-threatening	Death
Petechiae/ ecchymoses	Few	Moderate	Generalized	—	—
DERMATOLOGIC					
Injection site reaction/extravasation changes	Pain; itching; erythema	Pain or swelling with inflammation or phlebitis	Ulceration or necrosis not requiring operative intervention	Ulceration or necrosis that requires operative intervention	—
Pruritus	Mild or localized	Intense or widespread	Intense, widespread and interfering with activities of daily living (ADLs)	—	—
Feather-damaging behavior (not previously present)	Mild or localized	Moderate, involving two or more areas	Complete removal of contour and down feathers	Self-mutilation	—
Rash	Mild, no intervention	Increasing erythema or ulceration, treatment indicated	Severe, requiring more complex intervention	—	—
Other (please specify)	Mild	Moderate	Severe	Life-threatening; disabling	Death
GASTROINTESTINAL					
Anorexia	Mild - treated with diet change or coaxing	Reduced intake with <5% weight loss	Longer than 2–5 days duration, weight loss >20%–30%, supportive feeding required	>5 days, life-threatening	Death
Colitis	Asymptomatic, hemoccult positive	Straining to defecate, frank blood or mucous in stool	Obvious discomfort, pain, change in defecation, signs of coelomitis	Bowel perforation or other life-threatening consequences	Death
Constipation	Mild, occasional symptoms	Persistent symptoms, needs medication	Increasing symptoms, manual evacuation of cloaca indicated	Life-threatening obstruction	Death
Diarrhea	Mildly increased fecal water content	Moderately increased stool frequency/ volume, fluid therapy indicated	Hospitalization and intravenous (IV) fluids indicated	Life-threatening, hypovolemic shock	Death
Dysphagia	Mild discomfort, does not affect eating	Altered dietary habits required, may require temporary subcutaneous (SC) fluids	Eating severely hampered, requires IV fluids and nutritional supplementation	Life-threatening (e.g., obstruction)	Death
Enteritis	Asymptomatic, radiographic evidence only	Clinical discomfort, blood or mucous in stool	Change in defecation frequency or ileus, evidence of coelomitis	Life-threatening (e.g., perforation, bleeding, ischemia, necrosis)	Death

Continued

TABLE 3-2

Side Effect Monitoring Criteria for Avian Patients Receiving Chemotherapy or Radiation Treatments—cont'd

Adverse Event	Grade				
	1	**2**	**3**	**4**	**5**
Mucositis/stomatitis	Mucosal erythema	Small ulcerations	Larger ulcerations with hemorrhage	Tissue necrosis with life-threatening hemorrhage	Death
Vomiting/ regurgitation	<3 episodes over 24 hours	<3 episodes over 1–5 days; 3–5 episodes in 24 hours; SC fluids indicated	>5 episodes in 24 hours, SC or IV fluids indicated	Life-threatening (e.g., hemody-namic shock)	Death
GENERAL/CONSTITUTIONAL					
Lethargy/fatigue	Mild	Moderate - interferes with ADL	Severely restricts ADL	Disabled, requires assist feeding	Death
Fever (in the absence of grade 3 or 4 het-eropenia)	1–2°C above normal	2–3°C	3–4°C	>4°C	Death
Weight loss	5%–15% below baseline	15%–25% below baseline	25%–35% below base-line	>35% decrease from baseline	Death
Dehydration	Increased oral in-take indicated	5%–10% SC fluids indicated	10%–12% IV fluids indicated	Hypovolemic shock	Death
HEPATOBILIARY/PANCREATIC					
Liver dysfunction	Asymptomatic, ab-normal biochemi-cal profile or bile acids	Symptomatic, single agent medical therapy indicated	More supportive care (SC or IV fluid), more complex medi-cal therapy	Severe signs; en-cephalopathy; coma	Death
Pancreatic insuffi-ciency	Asymptomatic, no intervention required	Mild, requires dietary supplementation	Moderate, weight loss and maldigestion evident	Life-threatening, re-quires intensive supportive care	Death
Pancreatitis	Asymptomatic, in-flammation or enzyme altera-tions on blood-work	Asymptomatic, single agent medical ther-apy indicated	More supportive care (SC or IV fluid), more complex medi-cal therapy	Life-threatening (e.g., circulatory failure, sepsis)	Death
Other (please specify)	Mild	Moderate	Severe	Life-threatening; disabling	Death
METABOLIC/LABORATORY					
Albumin (g/dL)	<Lower limit of normal (LLN)–1.0	0.9–0.5	<0.5	—	—
Aspartate amino-transferase (AST) (IU/L)	>Upper limit of normal (ULN)–1.5× ULN	>1.5 ULN–2.0× ULN	>2.0–10× ULN	>10× ULN	—
Bile Acids (μmol/L)	>ULN–1.5× ULN	>1.5 ULN–2.0× ULN	>2.0–10× ULN	>10× ULN	—
Calcium (total) (mg/dL)	<LLN–8.0	7.9–7.0	6.9–6.0	< 6.0	—
Calcium (ionized) (nmol/L)	<LLN–1.1	<1.1–1.0 nmol/L	<1.0–0.9 nmol/L	<0.9 nmol/L	—
CPK	>ULN–2.5× ULN	>2.5–5× ULN	>5–10× ULN	>10× ULN	—
Glucose (high) (mg/dL)	>ULN–300	301–500	501–800	>800	—
Hemoglobinuria	Present	—	—	—	—
Potassium (high)	>ULN–5.5 mmol/L	5.6–6.0 mmol/L	6.0–7.0 mmol/L	>7.0 mmol/L	—
Potassium (low)	<LLN–3.0 mmol/L	<3.0–2.5	<2.5	—	—
Uric acid	>ULN–10	11–20	21–30	>30	—
MUSCULOSKELETAL/SOFT TISSUE					
Muscle loss or weak-ness	Only evident on examination	Mild clinical signs, interferes with function	Moderate signs, inter-feres with ADL	Disabling; life-threatening	Death
Myositis	Mild pain, no func-tional deficit	Mild pain, interferes with function	Moderate pain, inter-feres with ADL	Disabling	—

TABLE 3-2

Side Effect Monitoring Criteria for Avian Patients Receiving Chemotherapy or Radiation Treatments—cont'd

Adverse Event	Grade				
	1	**2**	**3**	**4**	**5**
Soft tissue necrosis	—	Local wound care, medical intervention	Operative debridement or more invasive wound management	Life-threatening; requires graft or reconstruction	Death
Other (please specify)	Mild	Moderate	Severe	Life-threatening; disabling	Death
NEUROLOGIC					
Apnea	—	—-	Present	Intubation required	Death
Ataxia	—	Symptomatic, not interfering with ADL	Symptomatic, interfering with ADL	Disabling	Death
Encephalopathy	—	Mild signs not interfering with ADL	Signs interfering with ADL; hospitalization indicated	Life-threatening; disabling	Death
Neuropathy—cranial nerve (please specify)	Asymptomatic, only noted on examination	Symptomatic, not interfering with ADL	Symptomatic, interfering with ADL	Life-threatening; disabling	Death
Neuropathy—motor	Asymptomatic, only noted on examination	Symptomatic weakness, not interfering with ADL	Weakness, interfering with ADL	Life-threatening; disabling (e.g., paralysis)	Death
Neuropathy—sensory	Asymptomatic; loss of deep tendon reflexes or paresthesia but not interfering with function	Sensory alteration or paresthesia, interfering with function but not ADL	Sensory alteration or paresthesia interfering with ADL	Disabling	Death
Seizure	—	One generalized seizure; controlled by anticonvulsants or infrequent focal motor seizures not interfering with ADL	Seizures in which consciousness is altered; poorly controlled seizure disorder despite medical intervention	Seizures of any kind which are prolonged, repetitive, or difficult to control (e.g., status epilepticus, intractable epilepsy)	Death
Depressed level of consciousness	—	Somnolence or sedation not interfering with ADL	Obtundation or stupor; difficult to arouse	Coma	Death
Tremor	Mild and brief or intermittent but not interfering with function	Moderate tremor interfering with function, but not interfering with ADL	Severe tremor interfering with ADL	Disabling	—
OCULAR/VISUAL					
Keratitis	Abnormal ophthalmologic changes only; intervention not indicated	Symptomatic and interfering with function, but not ADL	Symptomatic and interfering with ADL; operative intervention indicated	Perforation or blindness	—
Retinal detachment	Exudative; no central vision loss; intervention not indicated	Exudative and some visual acuity loss but intervention not indicated	More severe exudative detachment; operative intervention indicated	Blindness	—
Uveitis	—	Anterior uveitis; medical intervention indicated	Posterior or pan-uveitis; operative intervention indicated	Blindness	—
Other (please specify)	Mild	Moderate	Severe	Disabling	—

Continued

TABLE 3-2

Side Effect Monitoring Criteria for Avian Patients Receiving Chemotherapy or Radiation Treatments—cont'd

Adverse Event	Grade				
	1	2	3	4	5
PULMONARY					
Acute respiratory distress syndrome (ARDS)	—	—	Intubation not indicated	Intubation indicated	Death
Aspiration	Asymptomatic; radiographic findings	Symptomatic; medical intervention indicated	Clinical or radiographic signs of pneumonia or pneumonitis	Life-threatening	Death
Dyspnea	Dyspnea on exertion, but demonstrates normal activity without tiring	Dyspnea on exertion	Dyspnea with ADL	Dyspnea at rest; intubation/air sac cannula indicated	Death
Edema, larynx	Asymptomatic edema by exam only	Symptomatic edema, no respiratory distress	Stridor; respiratory distress; interfering with ADL	Life-threatening; air sac cannula or intubation indicated	Death
Hypoxia	—	<Oxygen (O$_2$) saturation with exercise	<O$_2$ saturation at rest; continuous O$_2$ supplementation required	Life-threatening; intubation or ventilation required	Death
Other (please specify)	Mild	Moderate	Severe	Life-threatening	Death
RENAL/GENITOURINARY					
Urinary obstruction	Asymptomatic; radiographic or endoscopic finding	Symptomatic without hydronephrosis or renal dysfunction	Symptomatic, altered organ function; hydronephrosis; operative intervention indicated	Life-threatening; organ failure	Death
Renal dysfunction	Asymptomatic; elevations in uric acid	Mild dehydration, increased urine volume, temporary SQ fluid indicated	Chronic, requires ongoing fluid therapy and medical management	Progressive, nonresponsive to therapy	Death
Other (please specify)	Mild	Moderate	Severe	Life-threatening	Death
SECONDARY MALIGNANCY					
Secondary malignancy – possibly related to cancer treatment (Specify, ——)	—	—	Non–life-threatening benign tumor or malignancy	Malignant solid tumor, leukemia, or lymphoma	Death

*Due to the difficulty of obtaining accurate thrombocyte counts in many avian species, this is listed as a subjective rather than a quantitative measure.
†Due to a lack of defined parameters for clotting times for many species, this is a subjective measure based on clinical observation of coagulation deficits.

Dosing
Chlorambucil: 1 mg/bird PO 2×/wk[32]; 2 mg/kg PO 2×/wk[33]
Cyclophosphamide: 200 mg/m^2 IO q7d[34,35]
Side effects. Side effects seen with alkylating agents include myelosuppression, GI toxicity, and sterile hemorrhagic cystitis in mammals. Cyclophosphamide will lead to heteropenia and generalized bone marrow suppression in birds in experimental models.[36,37] Reversible changes in the liver and feather lesions were found in chickens that were given cyclophosphamide.[38] CCNU has been associated with thrombocytopenia and hepatic failure in mammals.
Monitoring. Evaluate for myelosuppression, hepatotoxicity, and renal toxicity.

Antitumor antibiotics
Indications. Antitumor antibiotics can be used for a wide variety of tumors, including osteosarcoma, mesenchymal and epithelial tumors, leukemias, and lymphomas.
Mechanism of action. Antitumor antibiotics or topoisomerase inhibitors include doxorubicin, daunorubicin, epirubicin, idarubicin, mitoxantrone, and bleomycin. Antitumor antibiotics are potent drugs, with doxorubicin being used most commonly in veterinary medicine. These drugs are generally administered intravenously (IV), although bleomycin has been administered intratumorally in a dog as well as subcutaneously in a ferret. Mechanisms of action include intercalation of DNA and interference with topoisomerase enzyme function.

TABLE 3-3

Reported Use of Chemotherapy and Other Adjunctive Therapies in Avian Cancer Patients

Tumor	Origin	Therapy	Outcome	Species [(Reference)]
Adenocarcinoma	Ovary	Conservatively managed by periodic coelomocentesis, supportive care, and gonadotropin-releasing hormone (GnRH) agonist administration; dose range = 1500–3000 μg/kg intramuscularly (IM) Lupron q2-3 weeks, 4.6 mg deslorelin at 4- to 6-month intervals (only one bird responded to implant).	Lifespan 9 months for one cockatiel, 25 months for another cockatiel.	Cockatiels *(Nymphicus hollandicus)*[135]
Adenocarcinoma	Pancreatic duct	Carboplatin 5 mg/kg intraosseously (IO) once q4 weeks, for a total of 3 doses.	Patient was asymptomatic for 1 year following treatment; mass eventually recurred, and patient was euthanized.	Green-winged macaw *(Ara chloroptera)*[136]
Adenocarcinoma	Exocrine pancreatic	Surgical removal, celecoxib 10 mg/kg orally (PO) q24hr.	Died 4.5 months postoperatively; metastatic lesions confirmed on necropsy.	Cockatiel *(Nymphicus hollandicus)*[120]
Adenocarcinoma	Renal	Carboplatin 5 mg/kg intravenously (IV) q30 days for 4 treatments.	Improved clinically after the first 3 carboplatin treatments; died 2 weeks after the 4th carboplatin treatment.	Budgerigar *(Melopsittacus undulatus)*[48]
Carcinoma	Bronchial, with osseous metastasis	Methylprednisolone 2 mg IM once (palliative).	Initial improvement in appetite after treatment; died 25 days later with evidence of metastatic disease.	Grey parrot *(Psittacus erithacus)*[107]
Carcinoma	Uropygial gland	Surgical removal, strontium probe (Sr-90) radiotherapy, 100 Gray (Gy) fractions administered twice, 1 week apart.	No recurrence 6 months after the final radiation treatment.	Grey parrot *(Psittacus erithacus)*[137]
Carcinoma	Bile duct	Carboplatin, two IV doses (1st dose 100 mg/m^2, 2nd dose 125 mg/m^2), administered 3 weeks apart.	No reported recurrence at 30 days after first treatment.	Yellow-naped amazon *(Amazona ochrocephala)*[49]
Fibrosarcoma	Facial	Surgical debulking, orthovoltage radiotherapy (4 Gy/fraction, administered three times per week, total of eleven treatments), and intralesional cisplatin (0.2 mL cisplatin injected into the tumor before the eighth and eleventh radiation treatments).	Remission ~29 months, with subsequent slow regrowth.	Blue and gold macaw *(Ara ararauna)*[138]
Fibrosarcoma, myxoid	Wing	Radiotherapy with telecobalt-60 unit (4 Gy/fraction, administered on an alternate-day schedule over 22 days for a total of ten treatments) and intratumoral cisplatin (total of 3 chemotherapy treatments given once weekly at a dose of 0.3 mg of cisplatin per cm^3 of tissue).	Complete tumor remission lasted 15 months until the macaw died of an unrelated cause.	Blue and gold macaw *(Ara ararauna)*[139]
Hemangiosarcoma	Beak	Local radiation therapy, unknown type.	Tumor-free for 6 months.	Swan[140]
Hemangiosarcoma	Wing	Cesium radiation (137 Cesium unit, 400-cGy fractions, three times per week, total of 10 treatments).	Died 8 weeks after completion of radiation course due to disseminated hemangiosarcoma.	Budgerigar *(Melopsittacus undulatus)*[141]

Continued

Tumor	Origin	Therapy	Outcome	Species (Reference)
Leukemia	Lymphocytic T-cell, chronic	Prednisone (1 mg/kg PO once a day), chlorambucil (1 mg/kg PO twice weekly, discontinued at 6 weeks due to thrombocytopenia), and cyclophosphamide (5 mg/kg PO four days per week).	Treatment was well tolerated, and the patient appeared to have a good quality of life throughout duration of therapy. Treatment was inadvertently discontinued for 5 weeks due to a natural disaster. Patient died 2 weeks after treatment was restarted. Metastatic disease was evident on necropsy.	Green-winged macaw (*Ara chloroptera*)[142]
Leukemia/ lymphoma	Lymphocytic	Vincristine sulfate (four weekly injections, unknown route; 0.5 mg/m² on week 1; 0.75 mg/m² on weeks 2–4), prednisone (0.45 mg/kg PO twice a day), and chlorambucil (1 mg PO twice weekly).	Euthanized approximately one month after the initial diagnosis due to declining condition. Concurrent pneumonia and cardiac failure complicated this case.	Peking duck (*Anas platyrhynchos domesticus*)[32]
Lipoblastomatosis or atypical papilliform xanthoma	Cutaneous, multifocal (feet/face in unfeathered skin)	Surgical removal and intralesional carboplatin (an unknown volume of a 10 mg/mL carboplatin suspension was injected into each lesion in two planes once weekly for two treatments).	No resolution. Lost to follow-up.	Graylag goose (*Anser anser*)[143]
Lipoma	Cutaneous	Supplementation of diets with L-carnitine at 1000 mg/kg.	Tumors decreased in size.	32 budgerigars (*Melopsittacus undulatus*)[97]
Lymphoma/ leukosis	Cutaneous B-cell	Vincristine (1 mg/kg IV every 1–3 weeks, total of 8 injections) and chlorambucil (2 mg/kg PO twice weekly for 17 weeks).	Complete remission at last reported evaluation, 8 years after discontinuation of therapy.	Umbrella cockatoo, (*Cacatua alba*)[33]
Lymphoma/ leukosis	Cutaneous	Multiple drug chemotherapy: prednisone (25 mg/m² PO once a day), vincristine (0.75 mg/m² IO once weekly), cyclophosphamide (200 mg/m2 IO once weekly), doxorubicin (30 mg/m² IO q 3 weeks), L-asparaginase (400 IU/kg IM once weekly), and alpha interferon (15,000 U/m² SQ every other day for 3 treatments). Diphenhydramine (2 mg/kg IO) and dexamethasone (1 mg/kg IM) were administered prior to all L-asparaginase and doxorubicin treatments to minimize risk of anaphylactic reactions.	The solid tumors slowly regressed; however, the bird remained leukemic.	Moluccan cockatoo (*Cacatua moluccensis*)[34]
Lymphoma	Conjunctiva, cutaneous T-cell	Dexamethasone SP 2 mg/kg IM once; prednisolone 1 mg/kg PO once a day.	Four months after starting treatment, owner reported that the bird was doing well. Lost to follow-up.	Red lored amazon (*Amazona autumnalis*)[144]
Lymphoma	Periocular	400 rads/fraction of orthovoltage teletherapy radiation, administered 3 days per week for a total of 10 treatments.	Survived 2 months following treatment, then was euthanized due to tumor recurrence and declining condition.	Grey parrot (*Psittacus erithacus*)[145]
Malignant melanoma	Mandibular beak	Megavoltage linear accelerator radiation (2.5 Gy/fraction, administered 5 days per week for 4 weeks, total of 20 treatments); piroxicam (0.3 mg/kg PO once a day) and cimetidine (5 mg/kg PO twice a day).	Died 11.5 weeks after initiation of radiation therapy and supportive care. Confirmed metastatic disease on necropsy.	Thick-billed parrot (*Rhynchopsitta pachyrhyncha*)[7]

TABLE 3-3

Reported Use of Chemotherapy and Other Adjunctive Therapies in Avian Cancer Patients—cont'd

Tumor	Origin	Therapy	Outcome	Species [Reference]
Osteosarcoma	Face/zygomatic arch	Debulking and doxorubicin (60 mg/m² IV once monthly). Patient was premedicated with 1 mg/kg diphenhydramine prior to each chemotherapy treatment to reduce the risk of anaphylaxis.	Remission ~20 months.	Blue-fronted amazon (*Amazona aestiva aestiva*)[40]
Osteosarcoma	Intraocular	Surgical removal, radiotherapy with Stabilipan orthovoltage unit (4Gy/fraction, administered three days per week for 6 weeks, total of 17 treatments)	Died two months after last radiation session; no necropsy performed.	Umbrella cockatoo (*Cacatua alba*)[146]
Pseudolymphoma	Cutaneous	Chlorambucil 20 mg/m² PO q14d, total of three treatments; repeated course three months later.	Neoplastic lesions recurred three months after the end of the first course of chemotherapy. Patient underwent a second round of chemotherapy, and afterwards remained in remission (last reported evaluation 2.5 years after discontinuation of therapy).	Blue and gold macaw (*Ara ararauna*)[147]
Sertoli cell tumor	Testicular	Carboplatin 15 mg/kg diluted in 25 mL of 5% dextrose, administered IV q5 weeks for 4 doses.	Improved starting 3 weeks after onset of chemotherapy, and maintained a good quality of life until 12 months after treatment, when the tumor recurred. No further treatment was attempted, and the patient gradually deteriorated and died 1 month later.	Mallard duck (*Anas platyrhynchos*)[148]
Squamous cell carcinoma	Casque	IV photodynamic therapy (Single dose of 0.3 mg/kg IV hexyl ether pyropheophorbide-a, followed by exposure of the neoplastic tissue to 665-nm light via a diode laser (tissue dose 100 joules/cm²) the next day). Treatment was repeated 8 weeks later.	Initial improvement, but the tumor was very locally invasive and never fully eliminated. The patient was euthanized 2 weeks after the second photodynamic therapy session due to declining condition and tumor recurrence.	Great hornbill (*Buceros bicornis*)[149]
Squamous cell carcinoma	Choana	Radiation (details not provided), two equal doses of 4 Gy administered using parallel opposed beams during each treatment, (8 Gy/treatment) for a total of 3 treatments.	The choanal mass was no longer visible by the 3rd radiation treatment. Two months later, the mass recurred, and the patient was euthanized. Metastatic disease was identified on necropsy.	Amazon (*Amazona species*)[150]
Squamous cell carcinoma	Choana	Intralesional cisplatin q7d for a total of 3 treatments (total dosage 0.2 mg/kg for the first treatment, and 0.9 mg/kg for the second and third treatments; doses administered both intralesionally and topically for all treatments).	No recurrence after second cryotherapy treatment (last reported evaluation was 13 months after discontinuation of therapy).	African penguin (*Spheniscus demersus*)[60]
Squamous cell carcinoma	Choana	Carboplatin (17.2mg/kg) for 4 doses 3–10 weeks apart.	Tumor slowly progressed, patient died at home 9 months after starting therapy.	Yellow-naped amazon (*Amazona auropalliata*)[151]

Continued

TABLE 3-3

Reported Use of Chemotherapy and Other Adjunctive Therapies in Avian Cancer Patients—cont'd

Tumor	Origin	Therapy	Outcome	Species [(Reference)]
Squamous cell carcinoma	Cutaneous	Repeated surgical removal, 9 sessions of localized topical liquid nitrogen cryotherapy.	Mass recurred multiple times over a 13-month period. Patient maintained good quality of life before dying of unrelated causes.	Cockatiel (Nymphicus hollandicus)[61]
Squamous cell carcinoma	Cutaneous (patagium and axillary skin)	Complete surgical removal of the patagial tumor.	Patient was euthanized one month post diagnosis due to declining condition.	Grey parrot (Psittacus erithacus erithacus)[133]
		Cisplatin 17.5 mg/m² administered intralesionally into the axillary tumor q7d for a total of 4 treatments.	The axillary tumor was found to be very locally invasive, but metastatic disease was not identified.	
Squamous cell carcinoma	Cutaneous (multicentric)	Cryotherapy tried previously (7 treatments), Carboplatin at 27mg/kg for 4 doses every 4 weeks.	Tumor progressed despite therapy, patient euthanized 3 months after start of therapy	Cockatiel (Nymphicus hollandicus)[151]
Squamous cell carcinoma	Cutaneous (multicentric)	Aldara first attempted for in-situ lesion, then Carboplatin at 24mg/kg for 9 doses every 3–4 weeks.	Survived approximately 1 year before dying at home	Spectacled amazon (Amazona albifrons)[151]
Squamous cell carcinoma	Mandibular beak	Surgical debulking, Cobalt-60 radiation (400 cGy/fraction, administered three times per week for a total of 12 treatments; a boost dose of 800 cGy was administered at week 20), and intralesional carboplatin (single dose of 30 mg/m² administered at week 29).	The neoplastic lesion was very locally invasive, and a severe multi-drug resistant bacterial infection developed at the site. The patient developed anemia and renal insufficiency as treatment progressed, possibly as a side effect of medications. Patient died 30 weeks after initiation of therapy. No metastatic lesions were identified.	Buffon's macaw (Ara ambigua)[152]
Squamous cell carcinoma	Neck	Cobalt-60 teletherapy radiation (dose not reported), intralesional cisplatin.	Intralesional carboplatin treatment resulted in complete regression after the tumor failed to respond to cobalt-60 teletherapy radiation.	Amazon parrot (Amazona ochrocephala)[50]
Squamous cell carcinoma	Patagium	Five photodynamic therapy treatments (Single dose of 0.3 mg/kg IV hexyl ether pyropheophobide-a, followed by exposure of the neoplastic tissue to 665 nm of diode laser light (100 joules/cm²) the next day; interval between treatments not reported.	Complete remission was not achieved, and the bird euthanized (date of euthanasia relative to diagnosis not reported).	Rose-ringed parakeet (Psittacula krameri)[153]
Squamous cell carcinoma	Toe (digit III)	Electrosurgery debulking and cobalt radiation therapy (opposing fields, 5 Gy/port, 10-Gy fractions, administered on day 0, 7, 21, 51, and 58), followed by amputation of the affected digit III.	No recurrence at the initial site following amputation. However, digit III on the opposite foot developed squamous cell carcinoma 3 years later and also had to be amputated. There was no recurrence of tumors at time of last reported evaluation, 1 month after the second amputation surgery.	American flamingo (Phoenicopterus ruber)[154]

TABLE 3-3

Reported Use of Chemotherapy and Other Adjunctive Therapies in Avian Cancer Patients—cont'd

Tumor	Origin	Therapy	Outcome	Species [(Reference)]
Squamous cell carcinoma	Uropygial gland	Surgical removal and intralesional carboplatin; dose not reported.	One bird had complete surgical removal of the uropygial gland, but died four months later of unknown causes. The other bird had incomplete gland removal, and the tumor regrew during therapy.	Cockatiel and budgerigar *(Nymphicus hollandicus, Melopsittacus undulatus)*[140]

Dosing. Doxorubicin: 2 mg/kg IV[39]; 30 mg/m^2 IO q2d[34]; 60 mg/m^2 IV q30d[40]

Side effects. Toxicities in mammals may include myelosuppression; GI signs; cardiac (doxorubicin), pulmonary (bleomycin), renal (doxorubicin in cats), and perivascular sloughing if extravasated; anaphylaxis; and alopecia. Cardiomyopathy has been induced experimentally using doxorubicin in birds.[41]

Monitoring. Evaluate for myelosuppression, anaphylaxis, cardiotoxicity, and renal toxicity.

Vinca alkaloids

Indications. Vinca alkaloids are indicated to treat lymphoma and other lymphoid tumors, mast cell tumors, and some sarcomas.

Mechanism of action. Plant alkaloids (vinca alkaloids, taxanes) are mitotic spindle poisons active in the G2 and M phases of cell division or are topoisomerase interactive agents (etoposide and teniposide). Vincristine and vinblastine are most commonly used, with new drugs such as teniposide and vinorelbine being used in human medicine. The use of the newer agents in the taxane class (paclitaxel and docetaxel) is being explored in veterinary medicine as these agents are highly effective in human medicine.[42,43] Previous formulations of paclitaxel used Cremophor EL as a solvent, which caused severe hypersensitivity reactions in dogs. A new formulation of paclitaxel made with water-soluble retinoid derivatives has received conditional approval from the U.S. Food and Drug Administration (FDA) in early 2014 for dogs with mammary carcinoma and squamous cell carcinoma.[44,45]

Dosing. Vincristine: 0.1 mg/kg IV q7-14 d[33]; 0.5 mg/m^2 IV, then 0.75 mg/m^2 q7d × 3 treatments in ducks[32]; 0.75 mg/m^2 IO q7d × 3 treatments in cockatoos.[34]

Side effects. The solvents in some taxanes are extremely anaphylactogenic and can cause myelosuppression and GI toxicity. Vincristine toxicities are generally mild, but perivascular reaction can occur. Myelosuppression can occur with vinblastine.

Monitoring. Monitor for myelosuppression and anaphylaxis.

Platinum products.

Indications. Platinum products can be used to treat osteosarcoma, carcinoma, other sarcomas, and mesothelioma.

Mechanism of action. Platinum agents are commonly used in veterinary medicine. They act by cross-linking DNA, generally at the guanine base. Cisplatin and carboplatin both appear to be effective and tolerable agents when used

intravenously or intratumorally for treatment of canine tumors. Cisplatin and carboplatin pharmacokinetics have been described in sulfur-crested cockatoos *(Cacatua galerita)*.[46,47] GI side effects, including transient regurgitation, were seen in these studies for up to 48 to 72 hours following drug administration. A more recent study has examined single-dose carboplatin pharmacokinetics across four species: domestic chickens *(Gallus gallus)*, racing pigeons *(Columbia livia)*, call ducks *(Anas platyrhynchos)*, and English budgerigars *(Melopsittacus undulates)*. The authors found that carboplatin elimination half-life ranged from 0.41 hours in English budgerigars to 1.16 hours in chickens. (Antonissen G et al, manuscript in preparation).

Dosing

Carboplatin: 5 mg/kg IV, IO over 3 min[47,48] 5 mg/kg, intralesionally, mixed with sesame oil at a concentration of 10 mg/mL[22]; 125 mg/m^2, IV (slow bolus) q14-21 d[49]

Cisplatin: 1mg/kg IV over 1 hr[46]

Side effects. Cisplatin is highly nephrotoxic and myelosuppressive in mammals and requires diuresis with administration. Carboplatin is not nephrotoxic but is renally cleared, so caution should be used in patients with renal insufficiency, and renal function should be closely monitored.

Monitoring. Monitor for myelosuppression and renal toxicity.

Antimetabolites

Indications. Antimetabolites are indicated to treat lymphoma and immune-mediated disease.

Mechanism of action. Antimetabolites act during the S phase of the cell cycle, usually by mimicking normal purines and pyrimidine. Drugs in the category include methotrexate and 5-fluorouracil (folic acid antagonists); azathioprine, mercaptopurine, and 6-thioguanine (purine antagonists); and cytosine arabinoside and gemcitabine (pyrimidine antagonists). The newest agent in this class to be used in veterinary medicine is the fluorinated cytidine analog gemcitabine. L-asparaginase, another antimetabolite, is an enzyme that inhibits lymphoma cells with a requirement for the preformed amino acid asparagine. Since normal cells are capable of making asparagine from other amino acids, and lymphoma cells generally cannot, L-asparaginase kills cancer cells without affecting normal cells. This drug is often listed in its own category, as it is specific for the G$_1$ phase of the cell cycle. Repeated dosing may result in delayed anaphylaxis as well as resistance to therapy.

Dosing. Asparaginase: 400 U/kg IM q7d[34]; 1650 U/kg SC once[35]

Side effects. Toxicities seen include myelosuppression and GI toxicity (especially methotrexate). Anaphylaxis and pancreatitis have been associated with the use of L-asparaginase.

Monitoring. Monitor for anaphylaxis and myelosuppression.

Intralesional chemotherapy

Intratumoral administration of chemotherapeutic agents is the simplest and most direct approach for treatment of accessible solid tumors. Slow-release formulations that allow prolonged local exposure of the tissue to high drug concentrations can optimize the pharmacokinetics of the drug at the site of the tumor. Intratumoral chemotherapy can be used alone or in combination with other treatment modalities, including surgery and radiotherapy. Collagen matrix has been used in companion animals and humans as a drug carrier. A water-in-sesame oil emulsion is a cost-effective drug carrier for use with cisplatin, carboplatin, and other antineoplastic drugs.[22,50] Strict safety rules should be observed concerning drug preparation, administration, and handling by caretakers.

Radiation/Strontium

Indications and staging considerations

Consultation with a radiation oncologist is recommended to coordinate a plan for RT. RT is effective for local control of certain types of cancer. Strontium-90 and external beam radiation can be used in birds.[22] External beam radiation can be used as a sole method of treatment or in combination with other tumor treatment modalities, such as surgery and chemotherapy. The radiation field is localized to the tumor, along with a margin of normal tissue to account for microscopic extension of disease. There are two main types of radiation therapy protocols: definitive and palliative. A definitive course of radiation therapy generally involves more

fractions and more acute normal tissue radiation side effects in mammals. A definitive course of radiation is generally chosen in mammals when the patient is anticipated to live for 1 year (or longer) after treatment. Palliative radiation therapy is chosen for patients with a decrease in quality of life (QOL) due to the tumor and not anticipated to have a good response to a full course of therapy (estimated to survive 2 to 6 months after treatment). Strontium-90 (Sr-90) has a 2- to 3-millimeter (mm) penetration depth. The active area of the probe that is placed on the surface of the tumor is approximately 8 mm. While overlapping circles of dose can be applied to treat a larger area, the total area that can be treated is limited and the larger the area the longer the treatment takes. Therefore, this modality of treatment is useful only for very small or superficial lesions such as some uropygial gland tumors or treating a surgical site post-tumor removal (Figure 3-8). Sr-90 radiation has been used to treat localized neoplasms of the orbit in humans, squamous cell carcinoma of the nasal planum in cats, small cutaneous mast cell tumors in cats,[51] and corneal pannus in dogs. Sr-90 radiation has also been used to treat conjunctival squamous cell carcinoma in a cockatoo and uropygial neoplasia in birds.[52]

Side effects

There are multiple reports of radiation treatment used in a variety of avian tumors with variable response to therapy. Typical acute side effects seen with radiation therapy in mammalian species include mucositis, dry or moist desquamation, and keratitis. Late radiation effects in mammals can include necrosis, fibrosis, nonhealing ulceration, central nervous system (CNS) damage, and blindness and is dependent on normal tissues being irradiated.[53] One other concern is that since radiation is a carcinogen, it is possible to develop a new tumor in the radiation field. This has been reported in humans and dogs. The potential for this to be an issue in avian medicine is not known, but if the risk is similar to that of other patients

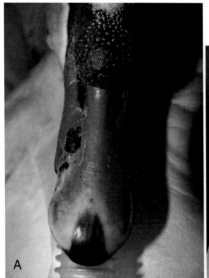
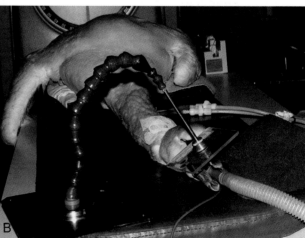

FIGURE 3-8 Strontium-90 therapy of a mute swan *(Cygnus olor)* with a beak hemangioma. **A,** The lesion is visible on the right rhamphotheca. **B,** Strontium-90 therapy was performed using 100 Gy/site over seven overlapping treatment areas to cover the entire lesion for 3.5 minutes each.

probably is in the range of 1% to 2%. Anecdotally, minimal observations of tissue radiation side effects are noted in avian patients. Interestingly, quail and chickens are among the least radiosensitive species with regard to whole body irradiation effects on bone marrow compared with other animals such as sheep, cattle, and swine.[54-56] A study examining tolerance doses of cutaneous and mucosal tissues in ring-necked parakeets *(Psittacula krameri)* for external beam megavoltage radiation revealed minimal radiation-induced epidermal histologic changes in the high-dose group receiving 72 Grays (Gy) in 4-Gy fractions.[57] Additionally, another study revealed that radiation delivered to the sinuses of macaws did not reach intended dose.[58] This implies that higher doses of radiation may be needed to produce equivalent response in avian patients compared with mammals, although the radiosensitivity of avian tumors is unknown. Long-term studies using Sr-90 in humans to treat pterygia and conjunctival lymphoma have shown minimal complications. Similarly, minimal complications have been reported with the use of SR-90 in canine, feline, and avian patients.[52]

Other/Adjunctive Therapies

Hormonal therapy

Hormones are used in the palliation of certain human and animal tumors. The most used hormones in veterinary medicine are corticosteroids, which are helpful in mast cell tumors, lymphomas, and lymphoid leukemias. The mechanism of action by which steroids kill cancer cells is thought to be through altered cellular transport of nutrients, induction of apoptosis (programmed cell death), and induction of cellular differentiation. The effects are generally short lived, and there is concern of inducing multidrug resistance to chemotherapeutics in lymphoid cancers. Birds are particularly susceptible to immunosuppression and secondary infection from the use of steroids. Prophylactic antibiotics and antifungals may be necessary when steroids or chemotherapeutics are administered to avian patients. Tamoxifen administration has not been evaluated for efficacy in cases of ovarian carcinoma, but antiestrogenic activity was suggested in one drug trial in budgerigars.[59] Gonadotropin-releasing hormone (GnRH) agonists (i.e., leuprolide acetate) have been effective empirically for reproductive disease in birds; however, confirmation of neoplasia (as opposed to cystic ovaries) has not occurred in anecdotal reports.

Cryotherapy

Cryotherapy for tumor treatment is reported infrequently in the avian literature.[60] It is a local therapy utilizing extreme cold produced by liquid nitrogen or argon gas and may have some utility in treating small, local lesions or residual disease postsurgical resection (Figure 3-9). Repeated treatments may be needed to achieve tumor control,[61] and patients should be monitored closely for recurrence. Treatment areas should be monitored for any related skin effects, but such side effects are rarely reported. Care should be taken if cryotherapy is used over areas of bone, as it can cause necrosis.

Phototherapy, hyperthermia, immunotherapy, nonsteroidal therapy, antiangiogenic agents, metronomic chemotherapy, and complementary and alternative therapy are other considerations for treatment of avian neoplasia.[22] Occasional reports of these treatments are described with avian patients,

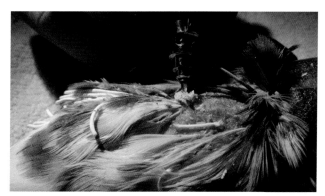

FIGURE 3-9 Cryotherapy for treatment of a squamous cell carcinoma in a cockatiel.

but application of mammalian concepts of these therapies is a reasonable option for avian tumors. Nonsteroidal antiinflammatory drugs (NSAIDs) inhibit cyclo-oxygenase which inhibits the formation of direct carcinogens, have antiangiogenic effects, and may prevent metastasis via inhibition of platelet aggregation. Certain antibiotics such as tetracycline derivatives (e.g., minocycline) may have antiangiogenic effects and may potentiate the efficacy of standard anticancer therapies,[62] although most studies to date have not shown benefit. Herbs described for use with human and mammalian patients with cancer include Asian mushrooms, curcumin, boswellia, bloodroot, and Yunnan baiyao.[63] Although the effects of these herbs on birds are largely unknown, toxicity has been described with the use of some herbs such as bloodroot in mammals. Below is a discussion on NSAIDs and milk thistle.

Nonsteroidal antiinflammatory drugs

Epidemiologic studies in humans have demonstrated a protective effect of chronic aspirin intake in the incidence of colorectal cancer.[64] Anti-inflammatory drugs to slow or stop tumor growth have shown promise in several animal model systems and clinical cancer cases. The majority of NSAIDs inhibit the isoforms of cyclo-oxygenase (COX-1 and COX-2) or are selective for one isoform. The NSAID piroxicam has activity against a variety of tumors in humans and dogs. Piroxicam is used in the treatment of transitional cell carcinomas (TCCs) of the urinary bladder and urethra in dogs and has also shown benefit in the treatment of some squamous cell carcinomas and mammary adenocarcinomas. Canine patients receiving piroxicam or meloxicam appear to have an improved QOL, with increased activity and alertness reported by owners.[64] Oral piroxicam has uncommonly been associated with GI ulceration and renal papillary necrosis in dogs. Meloxicam or other selective COX-2 inhibitors may be safer alternatives to piroxicam in the treatment of cancer, since they may reduce possible GI side effects due to increased COX-2 selectivity, but their effectiveness as an anticancer therapy is less well studied.

Milk thistle

In addition to providing liver support, milk thistle can be a helpful adjunct to consider for avian patients with cancer due to its role as an adjunct for cancer chemoprevention and treatment and to reduce side effects of treatment. Silymarin has led to a decrease in tumor incidence in rat models for colon, tongue, and bladder cancers.[63] It also inhibits the growth of human prostate cancer and lung cancer xenografts in mice. Derivatives from milk thistle protect the kidneys from cisplatin nephrotoxicity and radiation injury.[63] These derivatives may also protect the liver from CCNU (lomustine) toxicity and the heart from doxorubicin-induced lipid peroxidation. Milk thistle, when combined with omega-3 fatty acids, has reduced radionecrosis sites in cancer patients and has led to prolonged survival. Milk thistle potentiated antitumor effects of drugs such as cisplatin in both in vivo and in vitro studies.[63] Because milk thistle may inhibit certain isoforms of CYP450, consideration should be made when combining milk thistle with agents that rely on CYP450 metabolism. Dosing recommendation for birds is 50 to 75 mg/kg orally every 12 hours.[65]

Molecular Targeted Therapies

Historically, the mainstay therapies in cancer treatment have been drugs or other therapies that target cancer cells in a highly generalized manner, by killing rapidly dividing cells or killing all the cells in a particular area of the body affected by cancer. Although this strategy has certainly helped cure many patients, it fails to spare many of the body's normal cells and will often lead to treatment-limiting side effects. The ultimate goal of any cancer therapy is to kill cancerous cells while leaving normal, healthy cells intact. New generations of targeted therapies are often logically designed to target specific mutations or specific pathways that make a cell cancerous (Figure 3-10). The caveat to this new wave of innovation is that it becomes much more important to know what particular mutations are present in a cancer cell or what cellular pathways it is dependent on for survival. This may make it more difficult to translate new therapies emerging in human (as well as canine and feline) medicine without knowing how

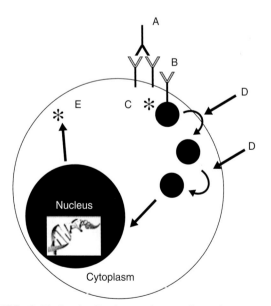

FIGURE 3-10 **A,** Antibody against cell surface receptor. **B,** Cell surface receptor. **C,** Small molecular inhibitor of cell surface receptor. **D,** Inhibitor of downstream pathway components. **E,** Inhibitor of gene fusion product.

cancer in avian species is alike and different. Below is a summary of the types of therapies that are being developed for use in humans and in companion animals so that clinicians know what types of therapies may be available for treating avian patients once more of the underlying tumor biology is understood.

There are two tyrosine kinase inhibitors approved for use in veterinary patients. The first is toceranib phosphate (Palladia), an inhibitor of the split-kinase family, which includes several growth factors implicated in cancer development: vascular endothelial growth factor receptor (VEGFR), platelet-derived growth factor receptor (PDGFR), c-kit, Flt-3, and others.[66] It was originally developed for use in the treatment of mast cell tumors with an activating c-kit mutation, but its role in antiangiogenic therapy is also being studied due to its inhibition of additional kinase family members.

The second is masitinib (Masivet), targeting primarily the mutated forms of the c-kit receptor (c-KitR), PDGFR, lymphocyte specific kinase (LCK), Lck/Yes-related protein (Lyn), fibroblast growth factor 3 (FGFR3), and focal adhesion kinase (FAK).[66] It is approved in veterinary medicine for the treatment of nonresectable canine mast cell tumors. It is also being researched in human oncology for the treatment of multiple cancer types (including GI stromal tumors, pancreatic tumors, and melanoma). It represents one of the only drugs approved for veterinary cancer patients but is not being used in clinical trials for human patients. A related tyrosine kinase inhibitor, imatinib (Gleevec) is approved for use in humans and is frequently used for treating certain leukemias and solid tumors. It is also used in dogs for mast cell tumors and sarcomas.[66] With all targeted therapies, it is important to know that the target is actually present in order to have hope of success. These drugs also can have significant toxicities and the effects on avian species are not yet studied to know if they will be safe and effective in these species.

General Recommendations for Clinicians Translating Therapies from Human, Canine, and Feline Medicine

Factors to consider when translating therapies in human, canine, and feline medicine to avian patients are as follows:
1. Patient size (vascular access)
2. Metabolism
3. Vascular support; renal or hepatic excretion
4. Risks of corticosteroids and immunosuppressive agents

Much of what is considered in avian oncology therapy is based on recommendations for humans and small animals such as dogs and cats. There are some important differences between avian and mammalian patients that must be kept in mind. Most notably, many avian patients presenting with tumors are small, and vascular access is challenging. Vascular access ports have been reported in avian patients and can be considered in situations where repeated vascular access is necessary. Birds have a renal portal system, and injection of chemotherapeutic drugs into leg vasculature should be generally avoided. Birds have a high metabolic rate compared with most mammals, but pharmacokinetic data on some chemotherapeutics in a limited number of avian species have been obtained, and the results do show that extrapolation of dosing regimens from mammals to avian species is at least a good starting point. As more information about response to therapy and adverse outcomes becomes available, our knowledge base will continue to expand. Any immunosuppressive therapy should be used with caution in avian species. Because of the relatively high number of zoonotic diseases reported in exotic species, this issue must be taken into consideration when using immunosuppressive therapy in birds or if owners are immunocompromised. Steroid therapy is not without risk of immunosuppression and secondary infection in avian patients. Prophylactic antibiotic and antifungal therapy may be prudent whenever immunosuppressive drugs are used in avian species.

Patient Monitoring and Side Effects

Introducing a standard of care

In avian medicine, there is a lack of standardization for clinicians to follow in terms of quantifying patient response and outcomes as well as accurately categorizing side effects. This lack of consistency and quantitative patient information greatly hinders the ability to combine cases from different institutions and also assemble larger case series to analyze population-level data for different types of cancers. There are great models for this type of patient monitoring in human, canine, and feline medicine. It is also crucial for clinicians to convey to owners the importance of regular checkups, even when patients are apparently doing well, and also in letting veterinarians know when patients die at home. Owners should be encouraged to allow necropsy, whenever feasible, as it may otherwise be hard to know if our therapies are truly effective or if there are subclinical side effects from therapy that we may not otherwise diagnose.

Assessing response to therapy

Since 2000, human oncologists have used a set of criteria (Response Evaluation Criteria in Solid Tumors [RECIST]) to objectively monitor primary tumors (target lesions) and lymph nodes and provide a standardized way to compare outcomes across multiple clinical trials and patient populations. These criteria received a major update in 2009 and are used in the majority of clinical trials.[67] The Veterinary Cooperative Oncology Group (VCOG) published an adapted version of these criteria for canine solid tumors in 2013.[68] Even in canine and feline oncology, these standards are not well established. However, there are a few basic guidelines that clinicians can adopt into their practice to make their patient assessments more quantitative and allow accurate patient assessments over time.

Basic RECIST guidelines address the following points: baseline tumor measurements, methods of tumor assessments, evaluation of tumor response, definitions of progression-free survival. Accurate, baseline tumor assessments are the key to objectively evaluating a patient's later response to therapy. It is recommended that measurements be taken as close as possible to the initiation of therapy. Lesions that are larger than 10 mm should be monitored either with caliper measurements (for cutaneous lesions) or imaging modalities for internal lesions (where feasible). Ultrasonography is not recommended for repeat tumor assessments if other options are available. Due to the imprecise nature of radiography and ultrasonography, only lesions measuring greater than 20 mm should be routinely monitored using these modalities. PET can be used to monitor response, but not for accurate lesion measurements. Consistency is also important when tracking

lesions. If caliper measurements are used, it is advisable that the same person perform those measurements at subsequent visits. CT is preferred over radiography; however, this is not always feasible due to concerns over cost and longer anesthesia times. If ultrasonography is used to monitor lesions, it is important to use the same radiologist for the scanning and use previous images to guide acquisition of new images so that they are obtained in the same plane. In the evaluation of patient response, clinicians should attempt to quantitate a patient's overall tumor burden in all measurable lesions. The longest diameters of target lesions (those that are measured repeatedly over time) are summed to obtain the "baseline sum diameters." This is the reference for assessing patient response.

There are four different potential patient outcomes to any cancer treatment: complete response, partial response, progressive disease, and stable disease. "Complete response" describes the complete disappearance of all target (measured) lesions. "Partial response" describes at least a 30% reduction in the sum of diameters of target lesions (using the baseline sum as a reference). "Progressive disease" describes the appearance of new lesions or a 20% or greater increase in the sum of diameters of target lesions. "Stable disease" describes less than 30% decrease or less than 20% increase in tumor burden. There are additional details regarding nontarget or nonmeasurable lesions, and the authors suggest reading the VCOG consensus document, mentioned earlier, for more information. Included in this chapter is a simple form that clinicians can include in a patient medical record to track tumor measurements over time (Figure 3-11).

SUPPORT OF AVIAN CANCER PATIENTS

Neoplasia and associated paraneoplastic syndromes can have devastating effects on the body. Both the avian clinician and the patient's owner should closely monitor QOL during treatment and/or palliative care. QOL is difficult to define and assess in patients that cannot verbally communicate their psychological well-being. The "five freedoms" (freedom from hunger and thirst, freedom from physical and thermal discomfort, freedom from pain and injury, freedom from fear and distress, and freedom to express normal behavior) have often been used to help define QOL in animals.[69]

Accurate evaluation of QOL requires a trained eye and careful history collection. This is even more important when assessing avian patients, since the default response to discomfort and illness in a prey species is to hide their symptoms. Adopting an objective method of measuring QOL can help keep perspectives clear while treating long-term illnesses and aid in decision making. A number of QOL questionnaires have been developed for use in dogs and cats.[70–72] A questionnaire that has been modified for use in birds is presented in Table 3-4.

We recommend that owners fill out this questionnaire (or one like it) during each follow-up visit with their veterinarians after their pets have been diagnosed with neoplasia. We also recommend that owners keep a daily QOL diary. In this diary, the owner records a pet's QOL each day on a scale of 1 to 10, with notes to clarify which behavioral cues were used to determine this score. Having this diary evaluated by the

Appendix: Tumor measurement

Animal ID: _____ Name: _____ Date: _____
         (Case #)   (DDMMYY)

Tumor Measurement

Visit: Week 1 ☐, Week 2 ☐, Week 3 ☐, Week 4 ☐, Week 5 ☐, Week ____ ☐ Unscheduled (DAY ____) ☐

Response Assessment Record: Tumor measurements using the longest diameter.

Tumor Location	Pre-enrollment size	Day of Visit Size	% Difference of Sums*
SUM:			

* % Difference of Sums = (Current sum − Baseline sum)/(Baseline sum) × 100.

Overall Response Based on Tumor Measurements	Date Assessed (DDMMYY)	Initials/Date (DDMMYY)
CR ☐ (completely gone) PR ☐ (≥30% decrease) PD ☐ (≥20% increase) SD ☐ (% diff. between -30% to +20%)		

☐ Not Done

Comments:

Examined by: _____ Date: _____
(Examining Veterinarian)   (DDMMYY)

Recorded by: _____ Date: _____
(if different than examined by)   (DDMMYY)

Confidential

FIGURE 3-11 Form for tumor outcome monitoring for patients.

TABLE 3-4

Quality of Life (QOL) Assessment Tool for Avian Cancer Patients

Avian QOL Questionnaire	Score Each Question 0-2. Higher Scores Indicate that QOL is being Affected more Significantly.	Score
1. Has your bird changed its normal routine since it was last evaluated?	(0) No (1) Yes, somewhat (2) Yes, significantly	
2. How much interaction is your bird having with your family/flock members?	(0) No change, normal interaction (1) Reduced interaction (1) Increased interaction (2) No interaction	
3. How much does your bird play with toys or engage in foraging behaviors?	(0) No change (1) Less frequently (1) Increased amount (2) Not at all	
4. How often do you think your bird feels pain?	(0) Never (1) Rarely (2) Frequently	
5. Does your bird seem more irritable than normal?	(0) No (1) Yes, somewhat (2) Yes, significantly	
6. Does your bird ever seem anxious or fearful?	(0) Never (1) Sometimes (2) Often	
7. Has your bird's body posture or mobility changed?	(0) No (1) Yes, somewhat (2) Yes, significantly	
8. Have your bird's vocalization habits changed?	(0) No (1) Yes, somewhat (2) Yes, significantly	
9. Does your bird still groom/preen itself normally?	(0) Yes (1) Somewhat (2) No	
10. Does your bird pluck or chew at feathers?	(0) Normal amounts (if a chronic feather plucker) (1) Increased amounts (1) Decreased amounts	
11. Does your bird still perch normally?	(0) No (1) Yes, somewhat (2) Yes	
12. Has your bird's appetite changed?	(0) No (1) Yes, somewhat (2) Yes	
13. Have your bird's urination/defecation habits changed?	(0) No (1) Yes, somewhat (2) Yes	
14. Does your bird ever vomit or have diarrhea?	(0) No (1) Rarely (2) Frequently	
15. Does your bird get tired easily?	(0) No (1) Yes, somewhat (2) Yes	
16. How is your bird sleeping?	(0) Normally (1) Somewhat normally (2) Badly	
Name five areas of life or life activities that have the biggest influence on your bird's life, and rank them in order of importance. Please indicate which of those activities your bird is still participating in. (0 = no, 1 = yes)	1 2 3 4 5	
On a scale of 1–10, how much do you think the disease is impacting your bird's quality of life?		
Total Score		

supervising veterinarian on a regular basis could help identify trends that would have otherwise gone unnoticed.

Pain Management

Cancer causes pain by invading tissues, inducing inflammation, and altering normal flow of neurologic signals and vasculature.[73] In addition, both surgical and medical treatments of cancer can induce pain. Pain management in cancer patients is a crucial part of maintaining adequate QOL. Multimodal analgesia is preferred, as noxious stimuli from the disease are usually impacting multiple body systems and may be caused by a variety of different processes; this also may allow for lower dosages of pain medications to be used.[74] Birds have been described as possessing primarily κ-receptors,[75] and they do not respond consistently to μ-opioid analgesics.[76–79] Otherwise, management of pain in birds is similar to that in other animals.

Pain management modalities that are commonly utilized in the treatment of avian cancer patients include opioids, NSAIDs, and anticonvulsant neuroleptics (e.g., gabapentin). Surgical analgesia such as amputation of a painful limb may also be instituted. The use of nerve blocks and low-dose N-methyl-D-aspartate (NMDA) receptor antagonists to help prevent windup pain in birds has been described.[80] Constant rate infusion of pain medications is currently not possible unless the patient is hospitalized but has been used for surgical and postsurgical analgesia.[74]

Other medications that may be considered in specific cases include tricyclic antidepressants, muscle relaxants or tranquilizers, and bisphosphonates.[81] Tricyclic antidepressants and muscle relaxants or tranquilizers may be helpful in alleviating dysphoria in cancer patients and, in some cases, may aid in treatment of chronic or neuropathic pain.[82] It is important to note that these medications have only been evaluated for safety in a select number of species (if at all), and efficacy studies are lacking. Further research is necessary to confirm whether these treatments should be recommended.

Bisphosphonates such as pamidronate have been used in cases of bone malignancy, in both humans and veterinary species, due to their inhibiting effects on osteoclast resorption, reducing bone loss and the risk of pathologic fractures from osteolytic lesions.[83] This class of drug may also have antineoplastic effects directly on the tumor cells themselves. Suggested dosage for pamidronate in dogs is 1 to 2 mg/kg intravenously, administered every 28 days.[84] An oral bisphosphonate alternative is alendronate, which has been dosed in dogs at 0.25 to 1.0 mg/kg per day for up to 3 years with no negative side effects.[85] Reported side effects in other species, although rare, include esophagitis, gastritis, changes in bone metabolism, and allergic reactions.

A single study evaluated short-term use of alendronate in laying hens at doses ranging from 0.01 mg/kg twice weekly to 1 mg/kg every other day, with different treatment groups starting therapy mid-lay and before the onset of lay.[86] Some hens on the highest doses of alendronate stopped laying eggs, produced eggs with reduced shell quality, and/or had decreased serum calcium concentrations. No other clinical side effects were noted. Pullets receiving alendronate during onset of follicular activity had a higher trabecular bone volume, compared with the control group, when necropsied after their first egg was laid. This study indicated that alendronate can affect bone volume, plasma calcium levels, and egg laying in chickens. At this time, no studies have been performed to evaluate the use of alendronate or other bisphosphonates in birds with bone neoplasia. Further studies are necessary to establish safe and efficacious doses for chickens and other species.

Nonpharmaceutical options that have been suggested as complementary alternative therapies for pain management in veterinary patients include housing adaptations to accommodate disabilities, thermal treatments (both cold and heat), massage, physical therapy, therapeutic exercise, acupuncture, and cold laser therapy.[87–89] These may have applications for use in certain patients; however, there are no peer-reviewed studies currently available to critically evaluate the safety or efficacy of these treatments in birds.

A number of factors have been noted to lower the pain threshold in humans, including insomnia, fatigue, boredom, anxiety, frustration, isolation, and fear of worsening pain.[90] Clinicians may be able to raise the pain threshold in their patients by eliminating or reducing these factors. Providing avian patients with an enriched home environment, adequate social structure, consistent administration of analgesics to prevent windup pain, and antipsychotic medications, as necessary, to alleviate anxiety and other behavioral disorders, should be part of the pain management protocol.

Refer to Chapter 20 of this text for more information on current analgesic therapy in avian patients.

Nutritional Support

Appropriate nutritional support is vital for cancer patients. Cancer cachexia (CC) is a well-known phenomenon that has been described in both humans and veterinary species.[91] It is considered the most common paraneoplastic syndrome in veterinary medicine.[92] CC causes significant changes in nutrient metabolism, leading to weight loss, muscle atrophy, loss of appetite, fatigue, immunosuppression, and decreased energy. Biochemical alterations induced by this syndrome include hyperlactemia, insulin resistance, hyperlipidemia, and depletion of protein stores.[93] CC is typically progressive and can significantly impact both longevity and QOL if it is not appropriately managed.[94] Although no studies have been published on whether or not cancer cachexia occurs in birds, it is probable that birds experience a similar syndrome, since progression of neoplasia in birds usually closely mirrors progression in other species.

A few general rules can be applied across species when selecting a diet for an avian patient with neoplasia. Recommendations for management of CC include feeding a highly digestible diet that is limited in simple carbohydrates, contains moderate amounts of highly bioavailable amino acids, and contains increased amounts of fat. Supplementing the diet with omega-3 polyunsaturated fatty acids (PUFAs), eicosapentaenoic acid (EPA), and docosahexaenoic acid (DHA) may be protective against some of the common metabolic abnormalities associated with CC and may improve response to treatment.[95] Omega-3 PUFAs can be generally recommended as a healthy supplement for avian patients, as these substances are also beneficial for cardiovascular, skeletal, and neurologic health.[96] Adequate amounts of insoluble fiber intake can improve GI health and promote normal GI flora, which may benefit patients undergoing cancer therapy.[92]

There is limited published information on the association between different dietary factors and cancer in avian species. A study in budgerigars with lipomas found that dietary supplementation with 1000 mg/kg L-carnitine caused a reduction in tumor size over a 102-day period.[97] This may have occurred due to alterations in metabolism associated with L-carnitine supplementation, as these tumors are commonly associated with obesity. Although L-carnitine supplementation should be considered in birds with lipomas, it is currently unknown if this amino acid derivative has any effect on other forms of avian neoplasia.

The impact of vitamins, minerals, and micronutrients on cancer risk and treatment has been extensively discussed in the human literature.[98] Carotenoids, selenium, folic acid, and vitamins A, C, E, and D have all been linked in certain studies to a reduction in cancer risk; however, many studies have produced conflicting information, and there is currently limited consensus on their correlation to cancer development.[99] As also mentioned later in this chapter, chronic vitamin A deficiency in birds may predispose them to developing squamous cell carcinomas. Growth of a number of cancers in humans has been correlated with increased serum iron content;[100] however, there is currently no information on whether or not this is applicable to avian species.

Feeding a diet that is high in a variety of fresh vegetables and fruits, contains a moderate amount of nut protein and whole grain cereals, and contains small amounts of omega-3-rich fish oils would provide most of the nutrients recommended for maintaining appropriate health in cancer patients.[101] Dietary decisions should always be made in light of species-specific requirements. It is important for owners not to make drastic diet changes that may affect overall intake. Any significant changes in diet should be made slowly, and patient weight should be monitored to ensure that the bird is getting enough nutrition. Clinicians must be sure to ask clients if they are providing supplements at home, as owners may leave this out of a routine diet history.

Regardless of which dietary supplements are elected for use in the cancer patient (if any), the patient must eat to benefit from nutritional support. Anorexia is a common side effect of pain and paraneoplastic syndromes. The use of appetite stimulants such as vitamin B (1 to 3 mg/kg, PO/IM, q24h or q7d) or benzodiazepines (diazepam 0.25 to 1.0 mg/kg IM/IV q24h ×2 to 3 days) may be helpful.[65,102,103] Warming the food prior to offering it to the patient and decreasing stress in the surrounding environment may improve food acceptance. Appropriate medical management of pain and nausea is an extremely important factor. Metoclopramide at 0.5 mg/kg orally, intramuscularly, or intravenously, every 8 to 12 hours, may be used to help decrease nausea, improve appetite, and improve normal GI motility.[65] Efficacy and safety of other antinausea medications have not been critically evaluated in birds as of yet.

If necessary, supplemental gavage feeding or placement of an esophagostomy or ingluviotomy tube could be performed for long-term nutritional management. A variety of critical-care liquid diets for birds are commercially available and can be used for nutritional supplementation via these methods. Volume and frequency of administration recommendations vary, depending on brand, the size of the patient, and the degree of nutritional support required. Gavage feeding is advantageous in many cases, as it does not require general anesthesia to be administered, requires no long-term maintenance, and is well tolerated by most avian patients. It is an excellent method of nutritional support for patients undergoing short bouts of anorexia. However, it is not a recommended feeding method for pet owners to utilize, due to the risks of aspiration, esophageal injury, and/or crop burns from improper administration techniques.

Esophagostomy or ingluviotomy tube placement is a straightforward, quick surgical procedure that may allow a chronically anorectic patient to receive appropriate nutrition for weeks to months without long-term hospitalization. Risks of tube placement include infection and removal of the tube by the patient if the tube is not secured well. Tube placement is not a good option if nausea and vomiting are not well controlled. The tube should always be flushed with water after administration of the liquid diet to reduce the risk of clogging.[103] Body condition scores should be closely monitored over time and the diet adjusted accordingly.

Client Support

Managing client communication is a critical part of the clinician's job description. Pet owners have an integral role to play in medical decision making, and if they are not adequately informed of the reasons behind clinical recommendations, this may negatively impact patient care. Veterinarians should actively seek to improve their communication skills with clients. Professional grief counseling should be offered to clients whose pets are suffering from terminal illnesses. Support groups for owners of pets with cancer are available online (www.veterinarywisdomforpetparents.com) and may also be found locally.

FUTURE DIRECTIONS AND ONGOING EFFORTS

Research into the diagnosis and treatment of avian cancer is still in its infancy. The current state of the literature is primarily single case reports, case series, and small clinical trials. Clinicians and researchers alike are hindered by several issues. We are dealing with small sample numbers distributed among many different institutions, most of which have very different record-keeping protocols and standard therapies. As avian clinicians, we may regularly see 15 to 20 different species. These different species often come from different continents, have different metabolisms, and demonstrate different responses to drugs used for cancer therapy. To address this, the authors are working on two main efforts. The first is a way to link avian clinicians, researchers, oncologists, and other professionals who want to work together on cancer projects. This effort is known as the Exotic Species Cancer Research Alliance (ESCRA), and the goal is to promote research into the underlying causes of cancer in all exotic and nondomestic species, not just birds. (Additional information may be found at www.escra.org.) The second effort is a collaboration with the Veterinary Information Network (VIN) to form an ongoing online repository, where clinicians can deposit information on their patients with cancer, including diagnosis, treatment, and outcomes. This database will be made available to clinicians and researchers who wish to find out more about a particular cancer or about cancers in a particular species.

It will take many years for avian and exotic cancer medicine to be supported by the kinds of research that support human and domestic companion animal oncology. However, it is imperative that clinicians realize the value of the patients they are treating and carefully document those cases, particularly the outcomes and side effects of therapy. Without proper case follow-up, it would be impossible to know what therapies are working and which may be causing more harm than good. The authors hope that this chapter has provided clinicians with additional tools to more quantitatively monitor their cancer patients and has laid a foundation for outcomes and side effects monitoring that can be revised and updated over time as we gain additional information.

ACKNOWLEDGMENTS

The authors would like to thank Michael S. Kent, MAS, DVM, DACVIM, DACVR, for manuscript review and editing; Laura Anne Swift, MPH, for statistical consultation on published case series; and the Veterinary Information Network for access to references.

REFERENCES

1. Garner M: Overview of tumors: section II. In Harrison GJ LT, editor: *Clinical avian medicine*, Palm Beach, FL, 2006, Spix Publishing, pp. 566–571.
2. Reavill D: Tumors of pet birds, *Vet Clin North Am Exot Anim Pract* 7:537–560, 2004.
3. Leach M: A survey of neoplasia in pet birds, *Sem Av Exotic Med* 1:52–64, 1992.
4. Kakarala K, Faquin WC, Deschler DG: A comparison of histopathologic margin assessment after steel scalpel, monopolar electrosurgery, and ultrasonic scalpel glossectomy in a rat model, *Laryngoscope* 120(Suppl 4):S155, 2010.
5. Wykes PM, Powers BE, Park RD: Closed biopsy for diagnosis of longbone tumors: Accuracy and results, *J Am Anim Hosp Assoc* 21:489–494, 1985.
6. Cole TL, Center SA, Flood SN, et al: Diagnostic comparison of needle and wedge biopsy specimens of the liver in dogs and cats, *J Am Vet Med Assoc* 220:1483–1490, 2002.
7. Guthrie AL, Gonzalez-Angulo C, Wigle WL, et al: Radiation therapy of a malignant melanoma in a thick-billed parrot (Rhynchopsitta pachyrhyncha), *J Avian Med Surg* 24:299–307, 2010.
8. Kajigaya H, Konagaya K, Ejima H, et al: Metastatic melanoma appearing to originate from the beak of a racing pigeon (Columba livia), *Avian Dis* 54:958–960, 2010.
9. Watson VE MJ, Cazzini P, Schnellbacher R, et al: Retrobulbar adenocarcinoma in an Amazon parrot, *J Vet Diagn Invest* 25:273–276, 2013.
10. Hanley C, Wilson, GH, Latimer, KS, et al: Interclavicular hemangiosarcoma in a double yellow-headed amazon parrot, *J Avian Med Surg* 19:130–137, 2005.
11. Ortego LS, Hawkins WE, Walker WW, et al: Detection of proliferating cell nuclear antigen in tissues of three small fish species, *Biotech Histochem* 69:317–323, 1994.
12. Johnson P, Giles JR: The hen as a model of ovarian cancer, *Nat Rev Cancer* 13:432–436, 2013.
13. Javier R, Butel JS: The History of tumor virology, *Cancer Res* 68:7693–7706, 2008.
14. Styles DK, Tomaszewski EK, Jaeger LA, et al: Psittacid herpesviruses associated with mucosal papillomas in neotropical parrots, *Virology* 325:24–35, 2004.
15. Gartrell BD, Morgan KJ, Howe L, et al: Cloacal papillomatosis in the absence of herpesvirus and papillomavirus in a sulphur-crested cockatoo (Cacatua galerita), *N Z Vet J* 57:241–243, 2009.
16. Sandusky G, Dumaual C, Cheng L: Review paper: human tissues for discovery biomarker pharmaceutical research: the experience of the Indiana University Simon Cancer.
17. Sundaram A, Zehnder A: Conservation of known oncogenes in nondomestic species, New Orleans, LA, 2014, Association of Avian Veterinarians.
18. Bendich A, Olson JA: Biological actions of carotenoids, *FASEB J* 3:1927–1932, 1989.
19. Garner MPL, Mitchell M: *Does Macrorhabdus ornithogaster predispose budgerigars to proventricular adenocarcinoma? Proc Annu Conf Assoc Avian Vet, 35th Annual*, New Orleans, 2014, p 311.
20. Beaufrere H, Ammersbach M, Reavill DR, et al: Prevalence of and risk factors associated with atherosclerosis in psittacine birds, *J Am Vet Med Assoc* 242:1696–1704, 2013.
21. Blackwood L: Approach to the cancer case: staging—how and why, Sao Paulo, Brazil, 2008, World Small Animal Veterinary Association World Congress.
22. Graham JE, Kent MS, Theon A: Current therapies in exotic animal oncology, *Vet Clin North Am Exot Anim Pract* 7:757–781, vii, 2004.
23. Souza MJ, Wall JS, Stuckey A, et al: Static and dynamic (18) FDG-PET in normal hispaniolan Amazon parrots (Amazona ventralis), *Vet Radiol Ultrasound* 52:340–344, 2011.
24. Stauber E, Holmes S, DeGhetto DL, Finch N: Magnetic resonance imaging is superior to radiography in evaluating spinal cord trauma in three bald eagles (Haliaeetus leucocephalus), *J Avian Med Surg* 21:196–200, 2007.
25. Krautwald-Junghanns M-E, Kostka VM, Dörsch B; Comparative studies on the diagnostic value of conventional radiography and computed tomography in evaluating the heads of psittacine and raptorial birds, *J Avian Med Surg* 12:149–157, 1998.
26. Kent M: The use of chemotherapy in exotic animals, *Vet Clin North Am Exot Anim Pract* 7:807–820, 2004.
27. Lumeij J: *Pathophysiology, Diagnosis and treatment of renal disorders in birds of prey. Raptor biomedicine III*, Lake Worth, FL, 2000, Zoological Education Network, Inc.
28. Coleman RE: Single photon emission computed tomography and positron emission tomography in cancer imaging, *Cancer* 67:1261–1270, 1991.
29. Zehnder A, Swift L, Sundaram A, et al: *Multi-institutional survey of squamous cell carcinoma in birds, Proc Assoc Avian Vet*, New Orleans, 2014, p 3.
30. Schmidt-Nielsen K: *Scaling, why is animal size so important?* New York, NY, 1984, Cambridge University Press.
31. Veterinary Cooperative Oncology Group: Common terminology criteria for adverse events (VCOG-CTCAE) following chemotherapy or biological antineoplastic therapy in dogs and cats v1.1, *Vet Comp Oncol*, 2011. doi: 10.1111/j.1476-5829.2011.00283.x.
32. Newell S: Diagnosis and treatment of lymphocytic leukemia and malignant lymphoma in a Pekin duck (Anas platyrhyncos domesticus), *J Assoc Avian Vet* 5:85–86, 1991.
33. Rivera S, McClearen JR, Reavill DR: Treatment of nonepitheliotropic cutaneous B-cell lymphoma in an umbrella cockatoo (Cacatua alba), *J Avian Med Surg* 23:294–302, 2009.
34. France M, Gilson S: *Chemotherapy treatment of lymphosarcoma in a Moluccan cockatoo, Proc Assoc Avian Vet*, 1993, pp 15–19.
35. Sacre BJ, Oppenheim YC, Steinberg H, et al: Presumptive histiocytic sarcoma in a great horned owl, *J Zoo Wild Med* 23:113–121.
36. Fulton RM, Reed WM, Thacker HL, et al: Cyclophosphamide (Cytoxan)-induced hematologic alterations in specific-pathogen-free chickens, *Avian Dis* 40:1–12, 1996.
37. Ficken MD, Barnes HJ: Effect of cyclophosphamide on selected hematologic parameters of the turkey, *Avian Dis* 32:812–817, 1988.
38. Ratnamohan N: Feather lesions in cyclophosphamide-treated chickens, *Avian Dis* 25:534–537, 1981.

39. Gilbert CM, Filippich LJ, Charles BG: Doxorubicin pharmacokinetics following a single-dose infusion to sulphur-crested cockatoos (Cacatua galerita), *Aust Vet J* 82:769–772, 2004.

40. Doolen M: *Adriamycin chemotherapy in a blue-fronted Amazon with osteosarcoma, Proc Annu Conf Assoc Avian Vet*, Boca Raton, 1994, pp 89–91.

41. Czarnecki CM: Doxorubicin (adriamycin)-induced cardiotoxicity in turkey poults: an animal model, *Comp Biochem Physiol C* 83:53–60, 1986.

42. Vaclavikova R, Soucek P, Svobodova L, et al: Different in vitro metabolism of paclitaxel and docetaxel in humans, rats, pigs, and minipigs, *Drug Metab Dispos* 32:666–674, 2004.

43. McEntree M: *Docetaxel and cyclosporine combination therapy for canine tumors*, 24th Annual Forum of the American College of Veterinary Internal Medicine Conference, 2006. Proceedings online.

44. von Euler H, Rivera P, Nyman H, et al: A dose-finding study with a novel water-soluble formulation of paclitaxel for the treatment of malignant high-grade solid tumours in dogs, *Vet Comp Oncol* 11:243–255, 2013.

45. Medicine FaDACfV: *FDA Provides important information to veterinarians about PACCAL VET-CA1 for treating cancer in dogs*, Silver Spring, MD, 2014, FDA.

46. Filippich LJ, Bucher AM, Charles BG: Platinum pharmacokinetics in sulphur-crested cockatoos (Cacatua galerita) following single-dose cisplatin infusion, *Aust Vet J* 78:406–411, 2000.

47. Filippich LJ, Charles BG, Sutton RH, et al: Carboplatin pharmacokinetics following a single-dose infusion in sulphur-crested cockatoos (Cacatua galerita), *Aust Vet J* 82:366–369, 2004.

48. Macwhirter P, Pyke D, Wayne J: Use of carboplatin in the treatment of renal adenocarcinoma in a budgerigar, *Exotic DVM* 4:11–12, 2002.

49. Zantop D: Treatment of bile duct carcinoma in birds with carboplatin, *Exotic DVM* 2:76–78, 2000.

50. Wilson G, Graham J, Roberts R, et al: *Integumentary neoplasms in psittacine birds: treatment strategies, Proc Assoc Avian Vet 21st Annual Conference*, Portland, OR, 2000, pp 211–214.

51. Turrel JM, Farrelly J, Page RL, et al: Evaluation of strontium 90 irradiation in treatment of cutaneous mast cell tumors in cats: 35 cases (1992–2002), *J Am Vet Med Assoc* 228:898–901, 2006.

52. Nemetz L, Broome M: *Strontium-90 therapy for uropygial neoplasia, Proc Annu Conf Assoc Avian Vet 25th Annual Conference*, New Orleans, 2004, pp 15–19.

53. Moore AS: Radiation therapy for the treatment of tumours in small companion animals, *Vet J* 164:176–187, 2002.

54. von Zallinger C, Tempel K: The physiologic response of domestic animals to ionizing radiation: a review, *Vet Radiol Ultrasound* 39:495–503, 1998.

55. Eisele GR: Bacterial and biochemical studies on gamma-irradiated swine, *Am J Vet Res* 35:1305–1308, 1974.

56. Broerse JJ, Macvittie T, editors: *Response of different species to total-body irradiation*, Boston, MA, 1984, Nijhoff.

57. Barron HW, Roberts RE, Latimer KS, et al: Tolerance doses of cutaneous and mucosal tissues in ring-necked parakeets (Psittacula krameri) for external beam megavoltage radiation, *J Avian Med Surg* 23:6–9, 2009.

58. Cutler D NJ, Shiomitsu K: *Measurement of therapeutic radiation delivery in military macaws*, Jacksonville, FL, 2013, Association of Avian Veterinarians Conference.

59. Lupu C: Evaluation of side effects of tamoxifen in budgerigars (Melopsittacus undulatus), *J Avian Med Surg* 14:237–242, 2000.

60. Ferrell ST, Marlar AB, Garner M, et al: Intralesional cisplatin chemotherapy and topical cryotherapy for the control of choanal squamous cell carcinoma in an African penguin (Spheniscus demersus), *J Zoo Wildl Med* 37:539–541, 2006.

61. McLaughlin A, Reavill D, Maas AK: Management of recurrent cutaneous squamous cell carcinoma in a cockatiel (Nymphicus hollandicus), *Proc Assoc Avian Vet 35th Annual Conference*, 2014, New Orleans, pp 341–346.

62. Teicher BA, Sotomayor EA, Huang ZD: Antiangiogenic agents potentiate cytotoxic cancer therapies against primary and metastatic disease, *Cancer Res* 52:6702–6704, 1992.

63. Robinson N: Complementary and alternative medicine for cancer. In Withrow S, Vail D, Page R, editors: *Withrow and MacEwan's small animal oncology*, St. Louis, MO, 2013, Saunders, pp 281–291.

64. Argyle D, Ljung BM, Turek M, et al: Cancer treatment modalities, *Decision Making Sm Anim Oncol* 69–128, 2008.

65. Hawkins MG, Ljung BH, Speer BL, et al: Nutritional/mineral support used in birds. In Carpenter JW, editor: *Exotic Animal Formulary*, ed 4, St. Louis, MO, 2013, Elsevier, p 306.

66. London CA: Tyrosine kinase inhibitors in veterinary medicine, *Top Companion Anim Med* 24:106–112, 2009.

67. Eisenhauer EA, Therasse P, Bogaerts J, et al: New response evaluation criteria in solid tumours: Revised RECIST guideline (version 1.1), *Eur J Cancer* 45:228–247, 2009.

68. Nguyen SM, Thamm DH, Vail DM, et al: Response evaluation criteria for solid tumours in dogs (v1.0): a Veterinary Cooperative Oncology Group (VCOG) consensus document, *Vet Comp Oncol* 2013 Mar 28. doi: 10.1111/vco.12032. [Epub ahead of print].

69. Wojciechowska JI, Hewson CJ: Quality-of-life assessment in pet dogs, *J Am Vet Med Assoc* 226:722–728, 2005.

70. Iliopoulou MA, Kitchell BE, Yuzbasiyan-Gurkan V: Development of a survey instrument to assess health-related quality of life in small animal cancer patients treated with chemotherapy, *J Am Vet Med Assoc* 242:1679–1687, 2013.

71. Freeman LM, Rush JE, Oyama MA, et al: Development and evaluation of a questionnaire for assessment of health-related quality of life in cats with cardiac disease, *J Am Vet Med Assoc* 240:1188–1193, 2012.

72. Budke CM, Levine JM, Kerwin SC, et al: Evaluation of a questionnaire for obtaining owner-perceived, weighted quality-of-life assessments for dogs with spinal cord injuries, *J Am Vet Med Assoc* 233:925–930, 2008.

73. Wilson J, Stack C, Hester J: Recent advances in cancer pain management, *F1000Prime Rep* 6:10, 2014.

74. Lichtenberger M, Ko J: Anesthesia and analgesia for small mammals and birds, *Vet Clin North Am Exot Anim Pract* 10:293–315, 2007.

75. Machin K: Avian analgesia, *Sem Av Exotic Med* 14:236–242, 2005.

76. Paul-Murphy JR, Brunson DB, Miletic V: Analgesic effects of butorphanol and buprenorphine in conscious African grey parrots (Psittacus erithacus erithacus and Psittacus erithacus timneh), *Am J Vet Res* 60:1218–1221, 1999.

77. Hoppes S, Flammer K, Hoersch K, et al: Disposition and analgesic effects of fentanyl in white cockatoos, *J Avian Med Surg* 17:124–130, 2003.

78. Guzman DS, Drazenovich TL, Olsen GH, et al: Evaluation of thermal antinociceptive effects after intramuscular administration of hydromorphone hydrochloride to American kestrels (Falco sparverius), *Am J Vet Res* 74:817–822, 2013.

79. Ceulemans SM, Guzman DS, Olsen GH, et al: Evaluation of thermal antinociceptive effects after intramuscular administration of buprenorphine hydrochloride to American kestrels (Falco sparverius), *Am J Vet Res* 75:705–710, 2014.

80. Shaver SL, Robinson NG, Wright BD, et al: A multimodal approach to management of suspected neuropathic pain in a prairie falcon (Falco mexicanus), *J Avian Med Surg* 23:209–213, 2009.

81. Gaynor JS: Control of cancer pain in veterinary patients, *Vet Clin North Am Small Anim Pract* 38:1429–1448, viii, 2008.

82. Merskey H: Pharmacologic approaches other than opioids in chronic non-cancer pain management, *Acta Anaesthesiol Scand* 41:187–190, 1997.

83. Veri A, D'Andrea MR, Bonginelli P, et al: Clinical usefulness of bisphosphonates in oncology: treatment of bone metastases, antitumoral activity and effect on bone resorption markers, *Int J Biol Markers* 22:24–33, 2007.

84. Fan TM, de Lorimier LP, O'Dell-Anderson K, et al: Single-agent pamidronate for palliative therapy of canine appendicular osteosarcoma bone pain, *J Vet Intern Med* 21:431–439, 2007.

85. Peter CP, Guy J, Shea M, et al: Long-term safety of the aminobisphosphonate alendronate in adult dogs. I. General safety and biomechanical properties of bone, *J Pharmacol Exp Ther* 276:271–276, 1996.

86. Thorp BH, Wilson S, Rennie S, et al: The effect of a bisphosphonate on bone volume and eggshell structure in the hen, *Avian Pathol* 22:671–682, 1993.

87. Corti L: Nonpharmaceutical approaches to pain management, *Top Companion Anim Med* 29:24–28, 2014.

88. MacFarlane PD, Tute AS, Alderson B: Therapeutic options for the treatment of chronic pain in dogs, *J Small Anim Pract* 55:127–134, 2014.

89. Members of the AAPMGTF, Hellyer P, Rodan I, et al: AAHA/AAFP pain management guidelines for dogs and cats, *J Feline Med Surg* 9:466–480, 2007.

90. Looney A: Oncology pain in veterinary patients, *Top Companion Anim Med* 25:32–44, 2010.

91. Nitenberg G, Raynard B: Nutritional support of the cancer patient: issues and dilemmas, *Crit Rev Oncol Hematol* 34:137–168, 2000.

92. Ogilvie GK: Interventional nutrition for the cancer patient, *Clin Tech Small Anim Pract* 13:224–231, 1998.

93. Kerl ME, Johnson PA: Nutritional plan: matching diet to disease, *Clin Tech Small Anim Pract* 19:9–21, 2004.

94. Ogilvie GK, Fettman M, Mallinckrodt CH, et al: Effect of fish oil, arginine, and doxorubicin chemotherapy on remission and survival time for dogs with lymphoma: a double-blind, randomized placebo-controlled study, *Cancer* 88:1916–1928, 2000.

95. Barber MD, Ross JA, Voss AC, et al: The effect of an oral nutritional supplement enriched with fish oil on weight-loss in patients with pancreatic cancer, *Br J Cancer* 81:80–86, 1999.

96. Petzinger C, Heatley JJ, Cornejo J, et al: Dietary modification of omega-3 fatty acids for birds with atherosclerosis, *J Am Vet Med Assoc* 236:523–528, 2010.

97. DeVoe R, Trogdon M, Flammer K: Preliminary assessment of the effect of diet and L-carnitine supplementation on lipoma size and body weight in Budgerigars, *J Avian Med Surg* 18:12–18, 2004.

98. Gonzalez CA, Riboli E: Diet and cancer prevention: contributions from the European Prospective Investigation into Cancer and Nutrition (EPIC) study, *Eur J Cancer* 46:2555–2562, 2010.

99. Greenwald P, Anderson D, Nelson SA, et al: Clinical trials of vitamin and mineral supplements for cancer prevention, *Am J Clin Nutr* 85:314S–317S, 2007.

100. Stevens RG, Graubard BI, Micozzi MS, et al: Moderate elevation of body iron level and increased risk of cancer occurrence and death, *Int J Cancer* 56:364–369, 1994.

101. Willett W: Diet and cancer, *The Oncologist* 5:393–404, 2000.

102. Gaskins LA, Massey JG, Ziccardi MH: Effect of oral diazepam on feeding behavior and activity of Hawaii amakihi (Hemignathus virens), *Appl Anim Behav Sci* 112:384–394, 2008.

103. Suarez D: Appetite stimulation in raptors. In Redig, P, Hunter B, editors: *Raptor Biomedicine*, Minneapolis, MN, 1993, University of Minnesota Press, pp 225–228.

104. Latimer K, Greenacre CB: Adrenal carcinoma in a budgerigar, *J Avian Med Surg* 9:141–143, 1995.

105. Renner MS, Zaias J, Bossart GD: Cholangiocarcinoma with metastasis in a captive Adelie penguin (Pygoscelis adeliae), *J Zoo Wildl Med* 32:384–386, 2001.

106. Hartup B, Steinberg H, Forrest L: Cholangiocarcinoma in a red-tailed hawk (Buteo Jamaicensis), *J Zoo Wild Med* 27:539–545, 1996.

107. André J, Delverdier M: Primary Bronchial carcinoma with osseous metastasis in an African grey parrot (Psittacus erithacus), *J Avian Med Surg* 13:180–186, 1999.

108. Greenlee JJ, Nieves MA, Myers RK: Bronchial carcinoma in a red-shouldered hawk (Buteo lineatus), *J Zoo Wildl Med* 42:153–155, 2011.

109. Langohr IM, Garner MM, Kiupel M: Somatotroph pituitary tumors in budgerigars (Melopsittacus undulatus), *Vet Pathol* 49:503–507, 2012.

110. Riddell C, Cribb PH: Fibrosarcoma in an African grey parrot (Psittacus erithacus). *Avian Dis* 27:549–555, 1983.

111. Burgmann P: Pulmonary fibrosarcoma with hepatic metastases in a cockatiel (Nymphicus Hollandicus), *J Assoc Avian Vet* 8:81–84, 1994.

112. Sasipreeyajan J, Newman JA, Brown PA: Leiomyosarcoma in a budgerigar (Melopsittacus undulatus), *Avian Dis* 32:163–165, 1988.

113. Nakano Y, Une Y: Hemangiosarcoma with widespread metastasis that originated on the metatarsal pad of a Java sparrow, *J Vet Med Sci* 74:621–623, 2012.

114. Kufuor-Mensah E, Watson GL: Malignant melanomas in a penguin (Eudyptes chrysolophus) and a red-tailed hawk (Buteo jamaicensis), *Vet Pathol* 29:354–356, 1992.

115. Reid HA, Herron AJ, Hines ME 2nd, et al: Metastatic malignant melanoma in a mandarin duck (Aix galericulata), *Avian Dis* 37:1158–1162, 1993.

116. Irizarry-Rovira AR, Lennox AM, Ramos-Vara JA: Malignant melanoma in a zebra finch (Taeniopygia guttata): cytologic, histologic, and ultrastructural characteristics, *Vet Clin Pathol* 36:297–302, 2007.

117. Barlow A, Girling TR: Malignant melanoma in a merlin (Falco columbarius), *Vet Rec* 154:696–697, 2004.

118. Lamb S, Reavill D, Wojcieszyn J, et al: Osteosarcoma of the tibiotarsus with possible pulmonary metastasis in a ring-necked dove (Streptopelia risoria), *J Avian Med Surg* 28:50–56, 2014.

119. Ojanen M, Orell M, Rasanen O: Metastaseous adenocarcinoma in the oviduct of a great tit (Parus major L.) preventing laying, *Acta Zool Pathol Antverp* 62:143–148, 1975.

120. Chen S, Bartick T: Resection and use of a cyclooxygenase-2 inhibitor for treatment of pancreatic adenocarcinoma in a cockatiel, *J Am Vet Med Assoc* 228:69–73, 2006.

121. Hahn KA, Jones MP, Petersen MG, et al: Metastatic pheochromocytoma in a parakeet, *Avian Dis* 41:751–754, 1997.

122. Snyder JM, Treuting PM: Pathology in practice. Adenocarcinoma of the proventriculus with liver metastasis and marked, diffuse chronic-active proventriculitis and ventriculitis with moderate M. ornithogaster infection in a budgerigar, *J Am Vet Med Assoc* 244:667–669, 2014.

123. Fredholm DV, Carpenter JW, Schumacher LL, et al: Pulmonary adenocarcinoma with osseous metastasis and secondary paresis in a blue and gold macaw (Ara ararauna), *J Zoo Wildl Med* 43:909–913, 2012.

124. Jones M, Orosz SE, Richman LK, et al. Pulmonary carcinoma with metastases in a moluccan cockatoo (Cacatua moluccensis), *J Avian Med Surg* 15:107–113, 2001.

125. Maluenda AC, Casagrande RA, Kanamura CT, et al: Rhabdomyosarcoma in a yellow-headed caracara (Milvago chimachima), *Avian Dis* 54:951–954, 2010.

126. Latimer K, Ritchie BW, Campagnoli RP, et al: Metastatic renal carcinoma in an African grey parrot (Psittacus erithacus erithacus), *J Vet Diagn Invest* 8:261–264, 1996.

127. Saied A, Beaufrere H, Tully TN Jr, et al: Bilateral seminoma with hepatic metastasis in a cockatiel (Nymphicus hollandicus), *J Avian Med Surg* 25:126–131, 2011.

128. Golbar H, Izawa T, Kuwamura M, et al: Malignant seminoma with multiple visceral metastases in a guinea fowl (Numida meleagris) kept in a zoo, *Avian Dis* 53:143–145, 2009.

129. Mutinelli F, Vascellari M, Bozzato E: Unilateral seminoma with multiple visceral metastases in a duck (Anas platyrhynchos), *Avian Pathol* 35:327–329, 2006.

130. Shimonohara N, Holland CH, Lin TL, et al: Naturally occurring neoplasms in pigeons in a research colony: a retrospective study, *Avian Dis* 57:133–139, 2013.

131. Ramis A, Gibert X, Majo N, et al: Metastatic oral squamous cell carcinoma in a Montagu's harrier *(Circus pigargus)*, *J Vet Diagn Invest* 11:191–194, 1999.

132. Pye G, Carpenter JW, Goggin JM, et al. Metastatic Squamous cell carcinoma in a salmon-crested cockatoo (Cacatua moluccensis), *J Avian Med Surg* 13:192–200, 1999.

133. Klaphake E, Beazley-Keane SL, Jones M, et al: Multisite integumentary squamous cell carcinoma in an African grey parrot *(Psittacus erithacus erithacus)*, Vet Rec 158:593–596, 2006.
134. Campbell T, Oliver T: Carcinoma of the ventriculus with metastasis to the lungs in a sulphur-crested cockatoo (Cacatua galerita), *J Avian Med Surg* 13:265–268, 1999.
135. Keller KA, Beaufrere H, Brandao J, et al: Long-term management of ovarian neoplasia in two cockatiels (Nymphicus hollandicus), *J Avian Med Surg* 27:44–52, 2013.
136. Speer B, Eckermann-Ross C: *Diagnosis and clinical management of pancreatic ductadenocarcinoma in a green-winged macaw*, 6th Proc Eur Conf Avian Med Surg and 4th Scientific ECAMS conference, 2001, pp 20–21.
137. Pignon C, Azuma C, Mayer J: *Radiation Therapy of uropygial gland carcinoma in psittacine species*, 32nd Annual Proc Assoc Avian Vet, Seattle, WA, 2011, p 263.
138. Ramsay E, Bos JH, McFadden C: Use of intratumoral cisplatin and orthovoltage radiotherapy intreatment of a fibrosarcoma in a macaw, *J Assoc Avian Vet* 42:408–412, 1998.
139. Lamberski N, Theon AP: Concurrent irradiation and intratumoral chemotherapy with cisplatin for treatment of a fibrosarcoma in a blue and gold macaw *(Ara ararauna)*, *J Avian Med Surg* 16:234–238, 2002.
140. Reavill D: *Pet bird oncology, 22nd Annual Proc Assoc Avian Vet*, Orlando, FL, 2001, Avian Specialty Advanced Program, pp 29–43.
141. Freeman K, Hahn KA, Adams WH, et al: Radiation therapy for hemangiosarcoma in a budgerigar, *J Avian Med Surg* 13:40–44, 1999.
142. Hammond EE, Guzman DS, Garner MM, et al: Long-term treatment of chronic lymphocytic leukemia in a green-winged macaw (Ara chloroptera), *J Avian Med Surg* 24:330–338, 2010.
143. Jaensch S, Butler R, O'Hara A, et al: Atypical multiple, papilliform, xanthomatous, cutaneous neoplasia in a goose (Anser anser), *Aust Vet J* 80:277–280, 2002.
144. Jones A, Kirchgessner M, Mitchell MA, et al: Diagnostic challenge, *J Exotic Pet Med* 16:122–125, 2007.
145. Paul-Murphy J, Lowenstine L, Turrel JM, et al: Malignant lymphoreticular neoplasm in an African gray parrot, *J Am Vet Med Assoc* 187:1216–1217, 1985.
146. Fordham M, Rosenthal K, Durham A, et al: Intraocular osteosarcoma in an umbrella cockatoo (Cacatua alba), *Vet Ophthalmol* 13(Suppl):103–108, 2010.
147. Kollias G, Homer B, Thompson JP: Cutaneous pseudolymphoma in a juvenile blue and gold macaw (Ara ararauna), *J Zoo Wild Med* 23:235–240, 1992.
148. Childs-Sanford SE, Rassnick KM, Alcaraz A: Carboplatin for treatment of a Sertoli cell tumor in a mallard (Anas platyrhynchos), *Vet Comp Oncol* 4:51–56, 2006.
149. Suedmeyer W, McCaw D, Turnquist S: Attempted photodynamic therapy of squamous cell carcinoma in the casque of a great hornbill, *J Avian Med Surg* 15:44–49, 2001.
150. Quesenberry K: Treatment of neoplasia. In Altman R, Clubb SL, Dorrestein GM, Quesenberry K, editors: *Avian medicine and surgery*, Philadelphia, PA, 1997, W.B. Saunders, pp 600–603.
151. Zehnder A, Hawkins M, Koski M, et al: *Therapeutic considerations for squamous cell carcinoma: an avian case series, 31st Annual Proc Assoc Avian Vet*, San Diego, 2010, p 711.
152. Manucy T, Bennett RA, Greenacre CB, et al: Squamous cell carcinoma of the mandibular beak in a buffon's macaw (Ara ambigua), *J Avian Med Surg* 12:158–166, 1998.
153. Suedmeyer WK, Henry C, McCaw D, et al: Attempted photodynamic therapy against patagial squamous cell carcinoma in an African rose-ringed parakeet (Psittacula krameri), *J Zoo Wildl Med* 38:597–600, 2007.
154. Abu J, Wunschmann A, Redig PT, et al: Management of a cutaneous squamous cell carcinoma in an American flamingo (Phoenicopterus ruber), *J Avian Med Surg* 23:44–48, 2009.

CHAPTER 4

Advancements in Nutrition and Nutritional Therapy

Elizabeth Koutsos • Stacey Gelis • Michael Scott Echols

FOUNDATIONS IN AVIAN NUTRITION

Elizabeth Koutsos

In 2011, over 8 million birds were kept as companion animals in over 3.5 million homes in the United States,[1] in addition to those kept in private breeding collections and zoos. Providing proper nutrition continues to be a challenge in the successful management of these animals. This review will focus on the nutrient requirements and general feeding principles for birds and recent advances that may enhance the management and well-being of these animals, with an emphasis on companion psittacine species.

FUNDAMENTALS OF NUTRITION

Animals require nutrients in their environment, provisioned through food or water, to provide the biochemical building blocks for life. In general, water, energy (derived from nutrients), amino acids and protein, fatty acids and lipids, and vitamins and minerals are required. For further details, an excellent overview of avian nutrition is available from Klasing.[1a] Unfortunately, the precise amount of a required nutrient for a given species is generally not known, except for some domesticated species used for food and fiber production (e.g., commercial poultry and other domesticated agricultural species). The paucity of information is because of the difficulty in measuring nutrient requirements of a species, which requires large numbers of animals, long-term and costly experiments, and invasive endpoints. These factors make it unlikely that nutrient requirements of many exotic species will ever be empirically determined. However, extrapolations and assumptions may be made to generate a "recommended" level of nutrient intake for less well-studied species. These extrapolations take into account the wild-type diet of the species, its gastrointestinal anatomy and physiology, and gustatory capacity, along with any data generated in that species or related species on nutrient requirements and known pathologies with nutritional basis. Nutrient recommendations, derived from these processes, serve as a benchmark and allow researchers and animal caretakers to focus on areas in which these assumptions do not seem appropriate.

Water

Water is essential, and requirements are generally higher in younger birds, larger birds, and in warmer environmental conditions. Hydration is extremely important in the success of young chicks. Moisture requirements are highest in the newly hatched altricial chick (greater than 80% moisture in the diet) and reduce over time, based on work on hand-reared cockatiels.[2] Similarly, in wild scarlet macaw chicks, moisture content of crop contents decreased significantly with increasing age.[3] A well-hydrated chick is evident by plumpness of skin, as opposed to a dehydrated chick in which the skin is generally tight and dry in appearance. Temperatures above a bird's thermoneutral zone will increase water requirements to account for evaporative losses of panting. For example, under thermoneutral conditions, adult parrots require ~2.4% of their body weight per day as water,[4] but this requirement may increase by as much as 12-fold in hot environments.[5] An important note about water: many birds will "play" with their water, resulting in highly variable levels of intake,[6] making the use of water as a vehicle for delivery of nutrients ill-advised. The delivery of medication via water should be limited to those medications for which pharmacokinetic data are available to support this method of administration.[7,8]

Energy

Energy is not an essential nutrient per se, but it is created from nutrients to drive biochemical processes. Birds generally have a higher level of energy expenditure than mammals,[9] and they require energy to maintain a certain basal metabolism rate (BMR) and thermoregulation, as well as energy for other activities such as movement (walking, running, flight, and swimming), perching, preening, eating, bathing and singing/calling, growth, reproduction, and molting.[10] There are several equations used to calculate BMR in passerines and non-passerines (Table 4-1) that all reflect the higher energy requirements of smaller birds compared with larger birds because of high mass-specific metabolic rates.[10] The energetic cost of thermoregulation is difficult to measure and may be offset by compensatory mechanisms like heat produced from shivering or energy conservation through torpor. However, cold environments may increase energy requirements up to four to eight times BMR, while hot environments may increase energy requirements one to two times BMR.[1,11] The energetic costs of other activities such as flight, foraging, and preening contribute to increased overall energy requirements[10] (Table 4-2). Finally, energy requirements for growth, reproduction, and molting increase energy demands. Growth requires approximately 13 kcal/g tissue on a dry matter basis,[1] although the energetic costs of adipose tissue deposition are substantially higher than that of lean tissue because of the varied water content of these tissues. Over the entire growth

TABLE 4-1

Basal Metabolic Rates of Passerines, Non-Passerines, and Psittacines[10]

	BMR (kcal/day)	Example of BMR of 100 g Bird (kcal/day)	Reference
Passerine	$0.744 \times$ (BW in grams)$^{0.713}$	19.84	11
	$114.7 \times$ (BW in kilograms)$^{0.73}$	21.36	75
Non-passerine	$0.510 \times$ (BW in grams)$^{0.724}$	14.30	11
	$73.6 \times$ (BW in kilograms)$^{0.73}$	13.70	75
Psittacine	$0.697 \times$ (BW in grams)$^{0.705}$	17.91	11

TABLE 4-2

Energetic Costs of Activity By Birds

Activity	Cost ($\times$ BMR)
Flight	
• Aerial species (e.g., swifts)	2.7-5.7
• Other birds, sustained flight	~11
• Gliding	2
Perching	
• Resting	1
• Alert	1.9-2.1
Preening	1.6-2.3
Eating	1.7-2.2
Singing/calling	2.9
Grooming/bathing	2.9

TABLE 4-3

Estimated ME Requirements for Adult Psittacines in Various Environments and Activity Levels[63]

Management Scenario	ME Requirement (kcal/day)
Indoor cage	$154.6 \times$ (BW in kilograms)$^{0.73}$
Indoor aviary	$176.6 \times$ (BW in kilograms)$^{0.73}$
Outdoor aviary in warm/ hot environment	$203.9 \times$ (BW in kilograms)$^{0.73}$
Outdoor aviary in cold environment	$226.1 \times$ (BW in kilograms)$^{0.73}$
Free ranging	$229.2 \times$ (BW in kilograms)$^{0.73}$

period, the energy required for growth is generally not more than 25% of the total energy requirement, but the energy needed for a particular stage of growth can be dramatically higher. For example, the energy (in metabolizable energy [ME]) requirement for growth of altricial chicks in the very early life stages can be more than double the energy needed for BMR because of the very fast growth rate and inability to thermoregulate.[1] Reproduction, like growth, will increase energy requirements, and most dramatically for hens laying a large number of eggs with a short interval between clutches. Energetic costs of reproduction can range from 39% of BMR in raptors to more than 180% in some waterfowl species.[12] Finally, the energy requirements for molt can be significant because of the high amount of cysteine in feathers compared with its concentration in other tissues and food, and thus inefficient use of protein substrate to generate the amount of cysteine needed for feather deposition. The energy required for molt (kcal ME/g feather mass/day) is estimated at 64.5 times BMR. Examples of variations in energy requirements from environment and activity in psittacines are found in Table 4-3.

Energy can be supplied by lipid, protein, or carbohydrate, and a bird's wild-type feeding strategy (e.g., carnivore, omnivore, herbivore) can be used to predict the primary energy source for which that bird is metabolically adapted. The amount of food required to meet energy demands varies depending on the energy content of the food and the bird's ability to utilize the source of energy. For example, a carnivorous bird may be poorly adapted to utilize the energy available from starch-based diet items because of low endogenous amylase activity. Even within a category of foodstuffs (e.g., seeds) efficiency of energy utilization will vary,[13,14]

making it important to use measurements like ME rather than gross energy to predict energy content of the diet. Finally, it is generally assumed that animals will eat to meet their energy requirements, but clearly birds in captivity can be predisposed to overeat energy and become overweight and obese (see Obesity).

Amino Acids and Protein

Amino acids, the building blocks of proteins, can be synthesized ("nonessential") or may be required in the diet ("essential" or "conditionally essential"). Birds require 12 essential amino acids plus a source of nitrogen for synthesis of nonessential amino acids. Requirements vary by life stage; reproduction will increase protein requirements, and some birds appear to time their reproductive output with increased protein availability.[15,16] Growth will also significantly increase protein requirements, particularly for altricial chicks in the early life stages.[2]

There are also differences in protein needs because of dietary feeding strategy. Frugivorous birds have lower rates of nitrogen losses compared with granivorous birds[17] and thus have lower protein requirements. For example, rainbow lorikeets require less than 3% crude protein from a high-quality protein source,[18] while cockatiels at maintenance require 11% crude protein when protein is sourced from high-quality ingredients.[6] Larger psittacines likely have higher protein requirements than smaller birds, but may not reach the level of protein requirement determined for intensively produced agricultural species.[1,19] In all species, protein restrictions during growth are visible because of the essentiality of protein for feather and muscle production and resulting lower growth rates and feather production in cases of deficiency or imbalance. In adult birds at maintenance, protein restriction may be less apparent. Excess dietary protein is less likely to be a concern, although it has been discussed regarding gout in granivorous birds. However, in cockatiels, high dietary protein (up to 70%) was not associated with any clinical pathology, because birds were able to upregulate enzymes associated with amino acid catabolism and uric acid synthesis. Further, high levels of blood uric acid were not associated with kidney pathology,[6] demonstrating the ability of granivorous birds to metabolically adapt to various dietary protein levels. More important than the amount of dietary protein is likely the transition time for a bird to metabolically adapt to varying protein levels. Carnivorous birds, on the other hand, have higher rates of protein degradation and thus higher protein requirements to meet their needs for gluconeogenesis from amino acid sources.[20] These birds are unable to effectively downregulate amino acid catabolism and thus cannot adapt to low dietary protein levels.

Essential Fatty Acids and Lipids

Essential fatty acids and lipids are required for energy production, cell membrane synthesis, intracellular signaling molecules, and hormone production. Little data exist concerning the fatty acid requirements of psittacines, and poultry guidelines of 1% linoleic acid and 4% to 5% total dietary lipid are generally used as a reference.[20a] However, more recent research suggests a significant role of omega-3 fatty acids in psittacine health and well-being (see Atherosclerosis), and it is likely that birds that evolved to eat marine-based organisms (plant or animal origin) have an obligatory requirement for omega-3 fatty acids.

Vitamins

A number of water-soluble and fat-soluble vitamins are essential for birds, although fat-soluble vitamins are often of greater concern because of their potential for toxicity and lower range of safety between deficiency and toxicity. For example, vitamin A deficiency is commonly reported in birds fed seed-based diets,[21] and supplementation may be offered in powder form (e.g., coating the seeds) or in the water. However, vitamin A toxicity also is a real concern; toxicity occurs quite rapidly in adult cockatiels fed a 100,000 IU of vitamin A per kilogram diet, and is characterized by dramatically altered vocalization patterns and deterioration of feather quality and muscle mass. Vitamin A toxicity can also occur at modest levels of intake. Cockatiels fed 10,000 IU vitamin A/kg had impaired antibody responses, modified vocalizations, and hyperexcitability.[22] This level of vitamin A is not uncommon in formulated pellets and is certainly achieved with routine vitamin supplementation of water or seeds. In contrast, cockatiels not fed vitamin A maintained reasonable liver vitamin A levels for 2 years, demonstrating the degree to which vitamin A is conserved. However, these birds did have impaired antibody responses prior to any other clinical signs of vitamin A deficiency.[22] Nectarivorous birds have also been reported to be susceptible to vitamin A toxicity, resulting in reduced fertility, increased embryonic deaths and high hatchling mortality, and compromised feather condition (lorikeets[23]). β-Carotene can serve as a precursor to vitamin A, and can serve as a safer alternative to potential toxic vitamin A in psittacines.[24] Insectivorous birds are at risk for vitamin A deficiency from the negligible levels

of vitamin A in commercially available insects such as crickets and mealworms,[25] and it is likely that β-carotene and other provitamin A carotenoids also may serve as the preferential vitamin A source for these species.

Vitamin D is of concern in birds, because of its critical role in calcium metabolism, bone mineralization, and reproduction. Vitamin D can be found in plants (ergocalciferol and vitamin D_2) or in animal sources (cholecalciferol and vitamin D_3). Adult cockatiels were unable to utilize vitamin D_2 to maintain blood vitamin D levels (E.A. Koutsos, unpublished observations), suggesting that vitamin D_3 is the bioactive dietary source, similar to that seen in poultry.[26] Birds may be able to synthesize adequate vitamin D from UV exposure (e.g., Grey parrots[27]), but this is highly dependent on the time of exposure, the amount of exposed skin, and the skin's pigmentation level. Little research has been conducted with nonpoultry species to clearly identify the potential for endogenous production of vitamin D_3.[1]

Minerals

Essential minerals include macrominerals (calcium and phosphorus), electrolytes (sodium, potassium, magnesium, and chloride), and micro and trace minerals (iron, zinc, copper, manganese, cobalt, and selenium). Calcium is generally the primary concern for birds because of high requirements of egg-shell formation and bone development, and because of the variable levels of calcium in typical diet items. Disorders of calcium metabolism are common in psittacines fed seed-based diets and kept indoors,[27] because seeds generally contain very low levels of calcium.[28] Plant-based sources of calcium (such as spinach) may contain oxalic acid, which binds calcium and reduces bioavailability.[29] Calcium is also a concern for insectivorous birds because commercially available insects such as crickets and mealworms are very deficient in calcium and have an inverse calcium to phosphorus (Ca:P) ratio.[25] This balance can be corrected by feeding the insects a supplement high in calcium prior to being offered as a diet item ("gut loading").[30] Calcium deficiency may lead to egg binding in females and impaired bone development in juveniles.[28]

Zinc is also of concern in captive managed avian species, generally because of the risk of zinc toxicosis as a result of ingestion of galvanized cage wire or other zinc-containing foreign bodies.[31] Signs of toxicity include depression, lethargy, anorexia, and weight loss. Plasma zinc can be used as a diagnostic tool, but diurnal fluctuations in its concentration require multiple sampling points for a secure diagnosis[32] and there is considerable variation across species,[33] making diagnosis of zinc toxicity difficult.[34]

Finally, iron is a concern for avian species that are susceptible to iron storage disease (ISD). Granivorous psittacines are not generally susceptible to ISD, but frugivorous avian species such as toucans, birds of paradise, quetzals, tanagers, hornbills, and manakans are well known for their susceptibility, as are some frugivore/insectivore species including mynahs and starlings. It is thought that these species evolved to eat foods that are low in iron and thus have very efficient iron absorption with little ability to downregulate iron uptake when dietary supply is abundant. Excess dietary iron is then stored in the liver, primarily in hepatocytes, in the form of hemosiderin.[35] Clinical signs of ISD include weight loss; abdominal distension; ascites;

and enlargement of liver, heart, and spleen. Typically hematology and serum biochemistry provide little diagnostic value. Diets containing low levels of bioavailable iron can delay or prevent ISD in susceptible species. Levels between 25 and 50 mg iron/kg dry matter are often recommended, although it is likely that these levels are inadequate for laying females and growing chicks. Adding compounds that decrease iron bioavailability such as tannins has been tried with some success, but these compounds may also reduce bioavailability of other minerals and should be used with caution. Organic acids such as citric acid and vitamin C (ascorbic acid) enhance absorption of iron; provision of foods high in these compounds at the same time as iron-containing diet items should be avoided.[35]

Other Dietary Components

In addition to the nutrients defined as *essential*, some nutrients or compounds may be beneficial. For example, carotenoids affect pigmentation of many avian species and can be required for normal mate selection. Additionally, carotenoids have been demonstrated to have immunomodulatory effects in birds including increased antibody responses, increased wing web swelling in response to phytohemagglutinin (and modified timing of this response) (see Chapter 11), and reductions in indices of systemic inflammation.[36,37] Further, lutein, a common dietary carotenoid, interacts with dietary fat sources to affect gene expression for inflammatory mediators.[38] Many carotenoids would be found in wild-type diets as components of plant and animal food items; thus, carotenoid supplementation of the diet is likely beneficial to most birds for some or all of the reasons noted earlier.

CURRENT ISSUES IN AVIAN NUTRITION

Obesity

Obesity is a major concern in captive avian species[39] (Figure 4-1). As discussed earlier, the energetic requirements of captive birds are greatly reduced compared with their wild counterparts. The two most common activities by free-living birds are feeding/foraging and actively perching (as opposed to sleeping on a perch), and although the proportion of each of these in a day varies with seasons and by species, the combination of these activities can take up as much as 56% to 90% of daytime activity.[11] Thus birds are adapted for long periods of feeding and foraging, and when this significant proportion of the day is dedicated to feeding in the captive environment, energy intake will be greater than energy requirements, resulting in obesity. Specific nutritional causes of obesity have also been examined in addition to overconsumption of energy. For example, sulfur amino acid deficiency (methionine or cysteine) has also been associated with fatty liver and obesity,[40,41] and is commonly seen in south American psittacine species that are fed high-fat seed- and nut-based diets that are deficient in methionine.[41]

Methods to prevent or reduce obesity generally include caloric restriction, but care must be taken to provision other activities to compensate for the reduced time eating or foraging, or stereotypic behaviors will likely result (see Food-Based Enrichment). Other interventions include ensuring the diet is nutritionally balanced to begin with to prevent incidence of

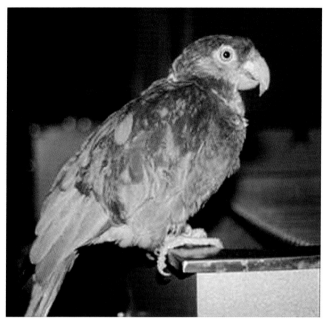

FIGURE 4-1 Delayed molt associated with obesity in a Green-cheeked amazon *(Amazona viridigenalis)*. Note the old, worn and blackened contour feathers. (Photo courtesy B. Speer.)

nutrient deficiencies or imbalances resulting in obesity independent of excess caloric intake. l-Carnitine has also been used as a therapeutic treatment for obesity. Lipomas, associated anecdotally with obesity, were reduced in size in budgerigars fed commercial pellets supplemented with l-carnitine (1000 mg/kg pellet) compared with birds fed unsupplemented pellets or seeds.[42]

Nutrition and Feather-Damaging Behaviors

Self-inflicted feather damage is a major issue in companion bird species[43,44] (Figure 4-2) (see Chapter 5). Often, "boredom" is cited as a cause for feather-damaging behaviors, and although the underlying basis is multifactorial, there are several nutritional components that may impact feather-damaging behaviors. First, as mentioned in relation to obesity, foraging behaviors are natural for birds in their wild environment and generally limited in captivity. Feather picking in some birds may result from lack of foraging opportunities; stereotypic feather picking developed in parrots when they were housed in unenriched environments, while birds housed with enrichment in the form of foraging opportunities and physical cage complexity had significant improvement in feather condition.[45] Nutrition and food-based enrichment is discussed later.

Frank nutrient deficiency or toxicity may also be implicated in some feather-damaging behaviors. For example, vitamin A deficiency results in dermatological symptoms, including rough scaly skin and poor feather quality,[46] which may lead to excess grooming behaviors and feather-damaging behaviors. Deficiencies of other nutrients including niacin, riboflavin, zinc, pantothenic acid, biotin, salt, sulfur-containing amino acids, arginine, and folic acid can cause dry flaky skin that may induce feather-damaging behaviors.[41,46]

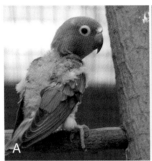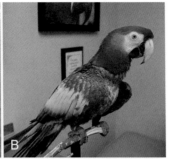

FIGURE 4-2 Examples of feather damaging behavior in (A) lovebird (*Agapornis* sp.) and (B) scarlet macaw (*Ara macao*). (Photos courtesy B. Speer.)

Atherosclerosis

Atherosclerosis is commonly found in birds, particularly in Galliformes, Columbiformes, Anseriformes, and Psittaciformes.[47] The reported prevalence of atherosclerosis in psittacines is highly variable, and ranges from 2% to 92%, depending on the species and method of diagnosis.[48] Susceptibility is increased with a number of factors including age (greater than 20 years of age or older),[49] body size (larger more than smaller),[47] sex (female more than male),[48] and species (higher incidence in Grey parrots, Amazon parrots, and cockatiels). Additionally, birds with reproductive or hepatic disease have increased likelihood of advanced atherosclerosis.[48] Nutrition-based risk factors for atherosclerosis include diets low in polyunsaturated fatty acids (PUFA) and high in saturated fatty acids, high-fat diets enriched in linoleic acid,[47] and diets rich in cholesterol (see Chapter 6).[50]

Dietary fiber, which effectively modulates cholesterol absorption and excretion in mammals, has been investigated in birds with little impact. Psyllium did not affect plasma cholesterol concentration of Grey parrots.[51] Dietary pectin in chickens increases rate of passage and thus may reduce caloric intake and reduce atherosclerosis risk similar to the effects of food restriction.[50]

In contrast, the association between fatty acid nutrition and atherosclerosis appears to be clinically significant. Diets rich in saturated fatty acids increased plasma cholesterol in Grey parrots, while diets with similar fat levels but composed of more PUFAs did not increase plasma cholesterol.[47] More recently, effects of omega-3 fatty acid nutrition have been examined in psittacines. Tissue levels of α-linolenic acid (ALA; omega-3 fatty acid) were correlated with reduced severity of atherosclerosis.[51] Dietary ALA is reflected in the blood of parrots, demonstrating successful absorption of this fatty acid. Further, higher blood levels of ALA were associated with higher blood levels of the longer chain omega-3 PUFA, eicosapentaenoic acid (EPA), and docosahexaenoic acid (DHA), demonstrating some capacity for elongation and desaturation of ALA.[52] However, the supplementation of ALA did not impact blood cholesterol or triglycerides in cockatiels or monk parrots, while fish oil (a source of EPA and DHA) did result in lowered blood triglycerides and cholesterol (see Chapter 6).[52] These lowered blood lipid parameters may result in reduced atherosclerosis risk and therefore omega-3 fatty acids, and particularly long chain EPA and DHA sources may present a good dietary intervention strategy for psittacines.

Most psittacine diets are highly enriched in omega-6 fatty acids and limited in omega-3 fatty acids of any kind. Domesticated foodstuffs used to make complete pellets, such as corn and soybean meal, are composed predominantly of omega-6 fatty acid (primarily linoleic acid). Flaxseed is a source of ALA, but is less commonly used in feed manufacturing because of susceptibility to oxidative rancidity. Many seeds and nuts commonly fed to psittacines have not been tested for fatty acid profiles, but for those that have been tested ALA content is relatively low.[53] Some fruits and vegetables have modest amounts of ALA (Table 4-4). Sources of the longer chain omega-3 fatty acids, EPA, docosapentaenoic acid, and DHA, are limited to fish and other marine products and algal-based sources.[54] However, palatability of fish oil is a major issue when considering supplementation.

SELECTING APPROPRIATE DIETS FOR BIRDS

Current Methods for Diet Selection

Feeding trends and recommendations from the late 1970s through the late 1990s document the transition from seed-based diets to seeds with supplements (which unfortunately are generally ineffective at correcting the deficiencies inherent in seed-based diets) to table food-based diets (which also are generally ineffective at providing balanced nutrition) culminating in production of manufactured bird diets.[55] Some examples of nutrient composition of seeds, typical supplemental food items, and pellets are listed in Table 4-4.

The selection of diets for companion birds by their owners/managers is generally made based on food item availability, cost, and preference of the bird and the owner. Many owners are reluctant to feed commercially prepared pellets because of their uniform appearance and lack of variety and similarity to perceived wild-type diets.[56] However, we know that data on wild-type diets of psittacines are often limited because of the difficulty of accurately monitoring food intake in flighted animals that often inhabit territories that are difficult to study.[57] Further, commercially available seeds do not provide similar nutrient profiles to wild seeds, are deficient in lysine and methionine, and contain very high levels of omega-6 fatty acids relative to wild seeds.[57] Additionally, seeds are often husked by psittacines before swallowing, resulting in a lower level of fiber, calcium, and manganese and a greater level of protein, fat, and phosphorus than determined from whole-seed analysis.[58]

The common method of presenting food for companions birds is to offer large quantities of a variety of food items and allow the bird to select its intake patterns. Unfortunately, for the most part, animals do not exhibit nutritional wisdom when selecting dietary ingredients, making this feeding program unlikely to achieve appropriate nutrition, which has been repeatedly demonstrated in birds. When offered seeds or table food, psittacines have been reported to have deficient intakes of vitamin A, vitamin D_3, calcium, protein (table food), and energy (table food) and excessive intake of fat (seeds).[59] Kakapo hens select a diet that is deficient in essential fatty acids, even when diet options containing sufficient nutrient

TABLE 4-4

Example Nutrient Content of Common Food Items Fed to Companion Psittacines, Including a Complete Diet Consisting of Pellets, Fruits, Vegetables, Nuts, and Seeds

Nutrient[a]	Green Peas, Raw	Broccoli, Raw	Sweet Potato, Cooked, no Skin	Apple, w/skin	Blueberries	Peanuts, Raw	Sunflower Seeds, no Hulls	Commercial Pellet[b]	Complete Blend[c]	Nutrient Rec.[d]
Moisture (%)	79	89	76	86	84	7	5	10	23	—
Gross energy (kcal/kg)	3832	3178	3716	3601	3610	6064	6130	—	—	—
Calculated ME (kcal/kg)[e]	3451	3388	3336	3510	3554	6046	5710	2970	3084	2900
Crude protein (%)	25.6	26.4	8.3	1.8	4.7	27.6	21.8	17.8	16.6	15.8
Methionine (%)	0.39	0.36	0.10	0.01	0.08	0.33	0.52	0.56	0.47	0.56
Methionine + cysteine (%)	0.70	0.62	0.19	0.01	0.13	0.67	0.99	0.90	0.76	1.00
Lysine (%)	1.50	1.26	0.24	0.08	0.08	0.97	0.98	0.89	0.81	1.00
Crude fat (%)	1.9	3.5	0.6	1.2	2.1	52.7	54.0	7.4	8.1	—
Linoleic acid (%)	0.72	0.20	0.25	0.30	0.56	15.67	24.19	3.11	3.20	1.11
Omega-3 fatty acids (%)	0.17	0.00	0.00	0.06	0.37	0.02	0.08	0.67	0.52	—
Ash (%)	4	8	6	1	2	2	3	5	5	—
Total carbohydrate (%)	68	62	86	96	92	17	10	66	65	—
Crude fiber (%)	24	24	14	17	15	9	9	3	6	—
Sugars (%)	27	16	27	72	63	4	3	2	9	—
Ca (mg/kg)	1183	4393	1569	416	380	984	819	1000	1076	16
P (mg/kg)	5109	6168	2230	762	760	4021	6928	854	1388	—
Nonphytate P (mg/kg)[f]	2758	4934	1699	—	—	1729	—	500	940	500
Fe (mg/kg)	70	68	28	8	18	49	55	269	210	89
Cu (mg/kg)	8	5	7	2	4	12	19	14	12	9
Mn (mg/kg)	19	20	21	2	21	21	20	102	80	67
Zn (mg/kg)	59	38	13	3	10	35	52	113	91	44
Se (mg/kg)	0.09	0.23	0.01	0.00	0.00	0.01	0.56	0.57	0.45	0.17
Mg (mg/kg)	1561	1963	1115	346	380	1797	3411	2186	1931	667
Na (mg/kg)	237	3084	1486	69	63	193	94	1333	1186	1667
K (mg/kg)	11542	29533	19612	7410	4877	7540	6770	7144	8277	3333
Vitamin C (mg/kg)	1892	8336	809	319	614	0	15	328	695	—
Thiamin (mg/kg)	13	7	4	1	2	7	16	13	11	2
Riboflavin (mg/kg)	6	11	4	2	3	1	4	13	11	4
Niacin (mg/kg)	99	60	61	6	26	129	87	78	71	39
Pantothenic acid (mg/kg)	5	54	36	4	8	19	12	26	24	11
Pyridoxine (mg/kg)	8	16	12	3	3	4	14	11	10	4
Folate (mg/kg)	3	6	0	0	0	0	2	4	4	1
Choline (mg/kg)	1343	1748	541	235	380	561	578	1556	1339	1444
Vitamin B$_{12}$ (µg/kg)	0	0	0	0	0	0	0	37	28	11
Vitamin A (IU/kg)	0	0	0	0	0	0	0	9436	7077	1667
β-Carotene (mg/kg)	21	34	475	2	0	0	0	11	25	—
Vitamin D (IU/kg)	0	0	0	0	0	0	0	2000	1500	222
Vitamin E (mg/kg)	6	73	29	12	36	89	349	194	160	11
Vitamin K (mg/kg)	1	9	0	0	0	0	0	3	3	1

[a]Nutrients expressed on a dry matter basis, except for moisture, and data from USDA[76] unless otherwise noted.

[b]Sample commercial pellet is Mazuri Parrot Maintenance Pellet 56A8: http://www.mazuri.com/product_pdfs/56A8.pdf.

[c]Complete blend consists of 75% pellet, 3% peas, 4% broccoli, 3% sweet potatoes, 5% apple, 3% blueberries, 2% peanuts, and 5% sunflower seeds.

[d]Nutrient recommendations from NRC Poultry[20b] and converted to dry matter basim for growing broiler chickens.

[e]ME (kcal/100 g) calculated as (3.5 × % carbohydrate) + (3.5 × % protein) + (8.5 × % lipid).

[f]Nonphytate P levels.[77-80] When nonphytate P levels were not available, total P was used to calculate P contribution to the complete blend.

levels are presented.[60] Grey parrots, when offered food items that could result in balanced nutrition, self-selected a diet deficient in numerous vitamins, minerals, and amino acids.[58] Amazon parrots offered a mix of seed, produce, and formulated pellets chose diets that were in gross excess of lipids and deficient in calcium.[61] Sodium and iron intake on these diets were below poultry recommendations but may not be deficient for psittacines.[61] Self-selection in conures resulted in diets high in fat and imbalanced in calcium and phosphorus.[62] The examples are numerous and the end result is always similar—self-selection by birds generally results in nutrient imbalances.

In an effort to balance the often preferred food items (seeds), vitamins and minerals are added to the water or to the seeds themselves. Both of these practices are ill-advised because of the natural behaviors of psittacines. As described earlier, water consumption varies significantly by individual and in response to environmental temperature, resulting in significant risk of toxicosis or deficiency when vitamins and minerals are supplemented in the water.[63] Second, as previously mentioned, husking of seeds makes vitamin and mineral coatings inadvisable because most will not be ingested.[58]

Another major issue with feeding balanced nutrition is the neophobia common in most companion bird species and difficulty transitioning them from preferred/known food items to balanced sources of nutrition. To address this concern, it is important that a large variety of foods are provided during the weaning period to ensure that birds are exposed to and willing to consume a wide variety of food items,[57] as early exposure can reduce neophobia.[64]

Current Diet Recommendations for Psittacines

Current dietary recommendations are to provide psittacines with a diet containing a mixture of commercially prepared pellets and fruits and vegetables at specific dietary proportions (i.e., not *ad libitum* for all diet components). Recommendations include 80% pellets:20% fruits and vegetables (dry weight),[65] 75% pellets:25% produce (dry weight),[61] and 60% produce (fresh weight):40% pellets.[58] All of these recommendations are based on the combination of a complete and balanced pelleted ration with fresh food supplementation with low levels of seed supplementation. This feeding strategy has resulted in higher fledging success[58] and reduced energy consumption compared with a seed-based diet.[66] Provisioning of multiple food items in addition to pellets is more likely to replicate wild-type feeding strategy in which most psittacines consume a wide variety of food items that may vary seasonally.[6,58,66] Finally, provisioning multiple food items (at specific dietary ratios) offers the benefits of each component (e.g., moisture from fruits, fiber from vegetables, balanced vitamin and mineral nutrition from pellets, and physical manipulation from seeds and nuts) that may not be achieved in the absence of that diet item. In the absence of pellets some other balanced diet items would be needed and may be in the form of a prepared "cake" or foodstuff balanced for another species (e.g., poultry).

Food-Based Enrichment

Recent research has examined the effect of diet particle size on parrot behaviors. In the wild, psittacines spend considerable amounts of time foraging. For example, crimson rosellas spent 67% of their time feeding and foraging[67] and Puerto Rican amazons forage for 4 to 6 hours per day.[45] In contrast, captive orange-winged amazons spent approximately 30 min of the day foraging for food,[68] because foraging opportunities are greatly reduced due to cage/aviary size and the resultant reduction in energy requirements and thus food intake, as described previously. It is thought that many stereotypic behaviors, including feather-damaging behaviors, are at least in part a result of austere captive environments[69] (see Chapter 5) and many enrichment devices for birds are thought to serve as substrates for foraging time that the bird would spend in the wild (see Chapter 5).[70] Offering seeds does not alleviate this concern; there was no difference in time spent foraging and feeding in parrots offered pellets or seeds.[71] However, feeding oversized pellets resulted in significantly increased time spent foraging and feeding—approximately five times longer than "traditional" sized pellets (178 minutes per day or 26% of the birds' daytime activity versus 36 minutes per day or 6% of the birds' daytime activity).[68] Even when traditional sized pellets were freely available, orange-winged amazons were highly motivated to work for larger sized pellets, as quantified by willingness to lift significant weight (up to 1.5 times their body weight) to access larger sized pellets.[72] Thus, modifying the size of the pellet offered can significantly impact the activity budget of captive birds thus reducing risk of stereotypic behaviors such as feather picking.[73,74]

Additional methods of providing food-based enrichment or foraging opportunities include scattering foraging food items on cage bottoms or exhibit floors; use of branches, leaves, or clean shavings to hide foraging food items; and providing whole nuts (which require time and energy investment to crack and dehull).[21] Nonfood-based enrichment is also beneficial for promoting natural behaviors and increasing energy expenditure. Toys, mirrors, baths, special perches, flights, bells, nests, routine training, feeder puzzles, and other options provide time expenditures to compensate for the loss of time spent foraging (see Chapter 5).[21]

SUMMARY

The science of nutrition has grown exponentially in the last 100 years, such that we have a good comprehension of the wide array of essential nutrients and the clinical signs of frank deficiency or toxicosis. However, information on the precise nutrient requirements of exotic avian species is unlikely to ever be complete, thus extrapolations and assumptions will continue to play a role in avian nutrition. It is clear that birds will not self-select nutritionally balanced diets, so the responsibility for providing proper nutrition falls on caretakers and their advisors. Offering large quantities of a variety of food items is not a recommended practice, nor is supplementation of seeds (via powder or water supplementation) to try to balance this type of diet. Current recommendations for psittacines require the majority of the diet to be based on a nutritionally complete pellet with supplemental vegetables and fruit and a small proportion of species-appropriate seeds or nuts. Recent research examining particle size of pellets may advance our ability to provide food-based enrichment and thus alleviate stereotypic behaviors that occur in captive birds.

REFERENCES

1. AVMA U: *Pet Ownership & Demographics Sourcebook*, Schaumberg, IL, 2012, American Veterinary Medical Association.

1a. Klasing KC: *Comparative avian nutrition*, New York, 1998, CAB International.

2. Roudybush TE, Grau CR: Food and water interrelations and the protein requirement for growth of an altricial bird, the Cockatiel (Nymphicus hollandicus), *J Nutr* 116:552–559, 1986.

3. Brightsmith DJ, McDonald D, et al: Nutritional content of the diets of free-living scarlet macaw chicks in southeastern Peru, *J Avian Med Surg* 24(1):9–23, 2010.

4. MacMillen R, Baudinette R: Water economy of granivorous birds: Australian parrots, *Funct Ecol* 704–712, 1993.

5. Weathers WW, Caccamise, DF: Temperature regulation and water requirements of the monk parakeet, Myiopsitta monachus, *Oecologia* 18(4):329–342, 1975.

6. Koutsos EA, Smith J, et al: Adult cockatiels (Nymphicus hollandicus) metabolically adapt to high protein diets, *J Nutr* 131(7):2014–2020, 2001.

7. Powers LV, Flammer K, et al: Preliminary investigation of doxycycline plasma concentrations in cockatiels (Nymphicus hollandicus) after administration by injection or in water or feed, *J Avian Med Surg* 23–30, 2000.

8. Flammer K, Whitt-Smith D, et al: Plasma concentrations of doxycycline in selected psittacine birds when administered in water for potential treatment of Chlamydophila psittaci infection, *J Avian Med Surg* 15(4):276–282, 2001.

9. Rezende EL, Swanson DL, et al: Passerines versus nonpasserines: so far, no statistical differences in the scaling of avian energetics, *J Exp Biol* 205(1):101–107, 2002.

10. Goldstein DL: Estimates of daily energy expenditure in birds: the time-energy budget as an integrator of laboratory and field studies, *Am Zool* 28(3):829–844, 1988.

11. McNab BK: Ecological factors affect the level and scaling of avian BMR, *Comp Biochem Physiol A Mol Integr Physiol* 152(1):22–45, 2009.

12. Ricklefs R: Energetics of reproduction in birds, *Avian Energet* 15:152–192, 1974.

13. Earle KE, Clarke NR: The nutrition of the budgerigar (*Melopsittacus undulatus.*, *J Nutr* 121(Suppl 11):S186–S192, 1991.

14. Underwood M, Polin D, et al: Short term energy and protein utilization by budgerigars (Melopsittacus undulatus) fed isocaloric diets of varying protein concentrations, *Proceedings of the Association of Avian Veterinarians* 1991, pp 27–237.

15. Sailaja R, Kotak VC, et al: Environmental, dietary, and hormonal factors in the regulation of seasonal breeding in free-living female Indian rose-ringed parakeets (Psittacula krameri), *Horm Behav* 22(4):518–527, 1988.

16. Williams TD: Variation in reproductive effort in female zebra finches (*Taeniopygia guttata*) in relation to nutrient-specific dietary supplements during egg laying, *Physiol Zool* 1255–1275, 1996.

17. Pryor GS: Protein requirements of three species of parrots with distinct dietary specializations, *Zoo Biol* 22:163–177, 2003.

18. Frankel TL, Avram DS: Protein requirements of rainbow lorikeets, Trichoglossus haematodus, *Aust J Zool* 49:435–443, 2001.

19. Carciofi AC, Sanfilippo LF, et al: Protein requirements for blue-fronted amazon (Amazona aestiva) growth, *J Anim Physiol Anim Nutr (Berl)* 92(3):363–368, 2008.

20. Migliorini R, Linder C, et al: Gluconeogenesis in a carnivorous bird (black vulture), *Am J Physiol* 225(6):1389–1392, 1973.

20a. NRC, editor: *Nutrient requirements of poultry*, Washington, DC, 1994, National Academy Press.

21. Bauck L: Nutritional problems in pet birds, *Semin Avian Exot Pet Med* 4(1)3–8, 1995.

22. Koutsos EA, Tell LA, et al: Adult cockatiels (Nymphicus hollandicus) at maintenance are more sensitive to diets containing excess vitamin A than to vitamin A-deficient diets, *J Nutr* 133(6):1898–1902, 2003.

23. McDonald D: Nutritional status of wild psittacines: optimizing the balance of fat-soluble vitamins, *Advances in companion bird nutrition, Avian Nutrition Seminar*, Oberschleibheim, Germany, 2004.

24. Koutsos EA, Klasing KC: Vitamin A nutrition of growing cockatiel chicks (Nymphicus hollandicus), *J Anim Physiol Anim Nutr* 89(11–12): 379, 2005.

25. Finke MD: Complete nutrient content of four species of feeder insects, *Zoo Biol* 32(1):27–36, 2013.

26. Hoy DA, Ramberg Jr CF, et al: Evidence that discrimination against ergocalciferol by the chick is the result of enhanced metabolic clearance rates for its mono-and dihydroxylated metabolites, *J Nutr* 118(5):633–638, 1988.

27. Stanford M: Calcium metabolism in psittacine birds: the effects of husbandry, *Advances in companion bird nutrition, Avian Nutrition Seminar*, Oberschleibheim, Germany, 2004.

28. Stanford M: Calcium metabolism. In Harrison GJ, Lightfoot T, editors: *Clinical avian medicine*, Palm Beach, FL, 2006, Spix Publishing.

29. Weaver CM, Martin BR, et al: Oxalic acid decreases calcium absorption in rats, *J Nutr* 117(11):1903–1906, 1987.

30. Finke M: Gut loading to enhance the nutrient content of insects as food for reptiles: a mathematical approach, *Zoo Biol* 22:147–162, 2003.

31. Romagnano AC, Grindem B, et al: Treatment of a hyacinth macaw with zinc toxicity, *J Avian Med Surg* 85–189, 1995.

32. Rosenthal KL, Johnston MS, et al: Psittacine plasma concentrations of elements: daily fluctuations and clinical implications, *J Vet Diagn Invest* 17(3):239–244, 2005.

33. Puschner B, Judy LS, et al: Normal and toxic zinc concentrations in serum/plasma and liver of psittacines with respect to genus differences, *J Vet Diagn Invest* 11(6):522–527, 1999.

34. Fudge AM, Speer B: Selected controversial topics in avian diagnostic testing, *Semin Avian Exot Pet Med* 10(2):96–100, 2001.

35. Klasing KC, Dierenfeld ES, et al: Avian iron storage disease: variations on a common theme. *J Zoo Wildl Med* 43(Suppl 3):S27–S34, 2012.

36. Koutsos EA, Lopez JGC, et al: Carotenoids from in ovo or dietary sources blunt systemic indices of the inflammatory response in growing chicks (Gallus gallus domesticus), *J Nutr* 136:1027–1031, 2006.

37. Koutsos EA, Lopez JCG, et al: Maternal and dietary carotenoids interactively affect cutaneous basophil responses in growing chickens (Gallus gallus domesticus), *Comp Biochm Physiol B* 147:87–92, 2007.

38. Selvaraj R, Klasing KC: Lutein and eicosapentaenoic acid interact to modify iNOS mRNA levels through the PPARgamma/RXR pathway in chickens and HD11 cell lines, *J Nutr* 136:1–7, 2006.

39. La Bonde J: Obesity in pet birds—the medical problems and management of the avian patient, *Proceedings of the Annual Conference of the Association of Avian Veterinarians*, 1992.

40. Butler E: Fatty liver diseases in the domestic fowl—a review, *Avian Pathol* 5(1):1–14, 1976.

41. Harrison GJ, McDonald D: Nutritional considerations section II. In Harrison GJ, Lightfoot TL, editors: *Clinical avian medicine*, Palm Beach, FL, 2006, Spix Publishing, pp 108–140.

42. De Voe RS, Trogdon M, et al: Preliminary assessment of the effect of diet and l-carnitine supplementation on lipoma size and body-weight in budgerigars (Melopsittacus undulatus), *J Avian Med Surg* 18(1):12–18, 2004.

43. Seibert LM: Feather-picking disorder in pet birds, *Manu Parrot Behav* 255–265, 2006.

44. van Zeeland YRA, Spruit BM et al: Feather damaging behaviour in parrots: a review with consideration of comparative aspects, *Appl Anim Behav Sci* 121(2):75–95, 2009.

45. Meehan C, Millam J, et al: Foraging opportunity and increased physical complexity both prevent and reduce psychogenic feather picking by young Amazon parrots, *Appl Anim Behav Sci* 80(1):71–85, 2003.

46. Burgmann PM: Common psittacine dermatologic diseases, *Semin Avian Exot Pet Med* 4(4):169–183, 1995.

47. Bavelaar F, Beynen A: Atherosclerosis in parrots. A review, *Vet Q* 26(2):50–60, 2004.

48. Beaufrere H, Ammersbach M, et al: Prevalence and risk factors in psittacine atherosclerosis: a multicenter case-control study, *J Am Vet Med Assoc* 242(12):1696–1704, 2013.

49. Pilny AA, Quesenberry KE, et al: Evaluation of Chlamydophila psittaci infection and other risk factors for atherosclerosis in pet psittacine birds, *J Am Vet Med Assoc* 240(12):1474–1480, 2012.

50. Petzinger C, Bauer JE: Dietary considerations for atherosclerosis in common companion avian species, *J Exot Pet Med* 22(4):358–365, 2013.

51. Bavelaar F, Beynen A: Severity of atherosclerosis in parrots in relation to the intake of α-linolenic acid, *Avian Dis* 47(3):566–577.

52. Heinze C, Hawkins M, et al: Effect of dietary omega-3 fatty acids on red blood cell lipid composition and plasma metabolites in the cockatiel, Nymphicus hollandicus, *J Anim Sci* 90(9):3068–3079, 2012.

53. Kris-Etherton P, Taylor DS, et al: Polyunsaturated fatty acids in the food chain in the United States, *Am J Clin Nutr* 71(1):179S–188S, 2000.

54. Nettleton J: Omega-3 fatty acids: comparison of plant and seafood sources in human nutrition, *J Am Diet Assoc* 91(3):331–337, 1991.

55. Harrison G: Twenty years of progress in pet bird nutrition, *J Am Vet Med Assoc* 212(8):1226–1230, 1998.

56. Bauck L: Psittacine diets and behavioral enrichment, *Semin Avian Exot Pet Med* 7(3):135–140, 1998.

57. Peron F, Grosset C: The diet of adult psittacids: veterinarian and ethological approaches, *J Anim Physiol Anim Nutr (Berl)* 98(3):403–416, 2014.

58. Ullrey DE, Allen ME, et al: Formulated diets versus seed mixtures for psittacines, *J Nutr* 121(Suppl 11):S193–S205, 1991.

59. Hess L, Mauldin G, et al: Estimated nutrient content of diets commonly fed to pet birds, *Vet Rec* 150(13):399–404, 2002.

60. Body DR, Powlesland RG: Lipid composition of a clutch of kakapo (Strigops habroptilus) (Aves:Cacatuidae) eggs, *NZ J Zool* 17:341–346, 1990.

61. Brightsmith DJ: Nutritional levels of diets fed to captive Amazon parrots: does mixing seed, produce, and pellets provide a healthy diet? *J Avian Med Surg* 26(3):149–160, 2012.

62. Carciofi AC, Duarte JMB, et al: Food selection and digestibility in yellow-headed conure (Aratinga jandaya) and golden-caped conure (Aratinga auricapilla) in captivity, *J Nutr* 136(7):2014S–2016S, 2006.

63. Koutsos EA, Matson KD, et al: Nutrition of birds in the order psittaciformes: a review, *J Avian Med Surg* 15:237–275, 2001.

64. Fox RA, Millam JR: Novelty and individual differences influence neophobia in orange-winged Amazon parrots (Amazona amazonica), *Appl Anim Behav Sci* 104(1):107–115, 2007.

65. Reid RB, Perlberg W: Emerging trends in pet bird diets, *J Am Vet Med Assoc* 212:1236–1237, 1998.

66. Kalmar I: *Features of psittacine birds in captivity: focus on diet selection and digestive characteristics*, PhD thesis, 2011, Ghent University.

67. Magrath RD, Lill A: Age related differences in behavior and ecology of crimson rosellas during the non-breeding season, *Aust Wildl Res* 12:299–306, 1985.

68. Rozek JC, Danner LM, et al: Over-sized pellets naturalize foraging time of captive Orange-winged Amazon parrots (Amazona amazonica), *Appl Anim Behav Sci* 125(1):80–87, 2010.

69. Garner JP, Meehan CL, et al: Stereotypies in caged parrots, schizophrenia and autism: evidence for a common mechanism, *Behav Brain Res* 145(1):125–134, 2003.

70. Kim LC, Garner JP, et al: Preferences of Orange-winged Amazon parrots (Amazona amazonica) for cage enrichment devices, *Appl Anim Behav Sci* 120(3):216–223, 2009.

71. Wolf P, Graubohm S, et al: Experimental data on feeding extruded diets in parrots, *Proceedings of the Joint Nutrition Symposium* Antwerp, Belgium, 2002.

72. Rozek JC, Millam JR: Preference and motivation for different diet forms and their effect on motivation for a foraging enrichment in captive orange-winged Amazon parrots (Amazona amazonica), *Appl Anim Behav Sci* 129(2):153–161, 2011.

73. Miller KA, Mench JA: The differential effects of four types of environmental enrichment on the activity budgets, fearfulness, and social proximity preference of Japanese quail, *Appl Anim Behav Sci* 95(3):169–187, 2005.

74. Lumeij JT, Hommers CJ: Foraging "enrichment" as treatment for pterotillomania, *Appl Anim Behav Sci* 111(1):85–94, 2008.

75. Aschoff J, Pohl H: Rhythmic variations in energy metabolism, *Federation Proceedings* 1969, pp 1541–1552.

76. USDA: U.S. Department of Agriculture, Agricultural research service. USDA National Nutrient Database for Standard Reference, Release 19, *Nutrient Data Laboratory Home Page*, 2006. http://www.ars.usda.gov/nutrientdata.

77. Hickling D: *Canadian feed peas industry guide*, Winnipeg, Manitoba, 2003, Pulse Canada.

78. Deshpande S: *Handbook of food toxicology*, Boca Raton, FL, 2012, CRC Press.

79. Harland B, Oberleas D: Phytate in foods, *World Rev Nutr Diet* 52:235–259, 1987.

80. Ravindran V, Ravindran G, et al: Total and phytate phosphorus contents of various foods and feedstuffs of plant origin, *Food Chem* 50(2):133–136, 1994.

ADVANCEMENTS IN NUTRITION OF LORIDAE

Stacey Gelis

With approximately 53 species, the subfamily Loriinae, which contains 11 genera, is spread across Australasia and the Pacific.[1] These birds inhabit a variety of habitats within this area, ranging from arid to tropical and from coastal lowland to cool highlands. They vary in size from 13 to 31 cm and weigh between 16 to greater than 250 g.[2,3]

Wild lorikeets obtain their carbohydrates predominately from the simple sugars in nectar and their protein from pollen found in flowering plants such as eucalypts (Figure 4-3). Lesser roles are filled by lerp, manna, honeydew, fruits, and seeds as carbohydrate sources and by insects as protein sources.[4-6] Lorikeets tend to be opportunistic feeders in the wild and may travel significant distances to locate suitable food sources. We know, for example, that rainbow lorikeets (*Trichoglossus haematodus moluccanus*; Figure 4-4) in Australia may feed on 43 species of food plants.[7] The planting of nonindigenous native flowering plants in suburban gardens and parks has allowed them to extend their range further south on a permanent basis.[8] In the same study, Musk lorikeets (*Glossopsitta concinna*) exploited 24 plant species. A study of Stephen's lory (*Vini stepheni*) on the isolated Henderson (Pitcairn) Island revealed that 15 species of plants were utilized as food sources.[9] However, there is a dearth of information about the feeding ecology of most species. Therefore, extrapolation from the limited data available on lorikeet nutrition from the few species studied, both in the wild and in captivity, and applying it to all species of Loriinae is fraught with potential dangers.

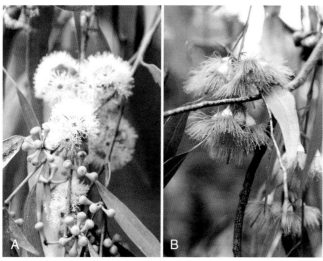

FIGURE 4-3 *Eucalyptus crebra* **(A)** and *leucoxylon* **(B)** are two species of flowering eucalypts that provide nectar and pollen to foraging lorikeets in southeastern Australia.

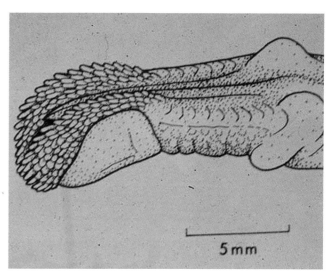

FIGURE 4-5 The lorikeet tongue possesses papillae at its tip, which can be everted to aid the harvesting of nectar and pollen.

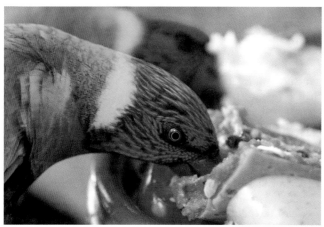

FIGURE 4-4 The Australian rainbow lorikeet *(Trichoglossus haematodus moluccanus)* is one of the most popular and successfully bred lorikeet species in captivity worldwide.

ANATOMICAL ADAPTATIONS TO NECTARIVORY

Lories and lorikeets have thinner and structurally weaker beaks than similarly sized granivorous parrots.[10] Because they are primarily nectar and pollen feeders, they do not require the beak strength to crack seeds or nuts like other parrots. However, their beaks have sufficient strength to inflict injuries on their handlers (personal observation).

The tongue is modified to aid in the harvesting of nectar and pollen (Figure 4-5). It is muscular and extensible and has a specialized brush tip that contains a cluster of threadlike papillae. The papillae increase the surface area of the tongue and may also create a capillary effect, increasing the speed of nectar extraction.[10,11]

The distal esophagus of lorikeets contains less mucin-secreting glands than seed-eating psittacine species because they have less need to lubricate food items, given

their nectarivorous diet.[12] The proventriculus has compound glands arranged in longitudinal rows with gland-free space to allow for the distension of the glandular stomach. This may be an adaptation to pollen digestion. The intermediate zone (zona intermedia) lies between the proventriculus and ventriculus. This zone has mucous glands replacing the compound glands of the proventriculus and also lacks the koilin layer of the ventriculus.[12] The intermediate zone is longer in the Loriinae than in seed-eating parrots.[11] The proposed adaptive advantage of this trait is that it aids storage of pollen, giving more time for chemical digestion and extraction of the contained amino acids.[12,13] The ventriculus is characterized by a comparative reduction in the mass of the gizzard muscle (Figure 4-6). This is most noticeable in *Glossopsitta* species, where the gizzard is barely recognizable. In contrast, rainbow lorikeets have a relatively muscular gizzard, reflecting their more generalized diet, which may contain seeds and hard-bodied insects.[14,15] The gizzard of the nectarivorous swift parrot *(Lathamus discolor)* is also more muscular than that of similar sized lorikeets, suggesting it is better able to utilize harder food sources and its similarity to lorikeets is more a result of convergent evolution. Gizzard musculature can hypertrophy or atrophy over time to adapt to seasonally available food sources. The koilin layer of the gizzard is thin and lacks striae, which are thought to aid the mechanical disruption of the insect exoskeleton in insect-eating species. Figure 4-6 illustrates the ventriculus and proventriculus of a wild rainbow lorikeet.

The proventricular and pyloric openings of the lorikeet gizzard both lie in the median plane. This allows rapid passage of ingesta, increasing absorption of nectar, and quicker passage of pollen to the intestine where most pollen digestion occurs. This is not the case with other parrots.[14]

The intestinal tract is reported to be shorter than in similar sized granivores or herbivores, and this is thought to be an adaptation resulting from the highly digestible diet.[13,14] However, this is refuted by the work of Schweizer et al[12] who

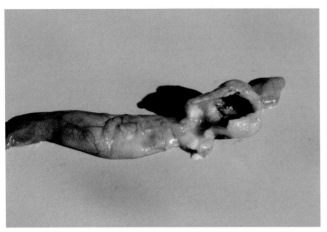

FIGURE 4-6 The glandular proventriculus (left) and relatively thin-walled ventriculus and thin koilin layer of a wild musk lorikeet.

found no difference in intestinal length between nectarivorous and seed-eating parrots. The cecae are relatively undeveloped, most probably because of the low fiber content of their diet.

The high moisture content of much of their food means that lories and lorikeets must consume a large volume of food to meet their energy requirements. This results in rapid transit times of food through the gastrointestinal tract and in the production of large volumes of feces. Because of the high moisture content of their food, the droppings also contain a great deal of moisture. These birds have evolved a very forceful way of expelling their droppings, which is thought to prevent soiling of feathers around the cloaca. Honeyeaters have adapted to the large fluid loads resulting from ingesting nectar diets by producing large volumes of dilute urine.[16] When ingesting concentrated diets, honeyeaters have a massive capacity for tubular reabsorption of water (greater than 90%) with little effect on glomerular filtration rate. Kidney architecture also differs between honeyeaters and other passerines enabling them to resorb a large proportion of solutes and water from the glomerular filtrate.[17]

There are also differences in the anatomy of wet-zone and arid-zone honeyeaters. The renal medulla of arid-zone honeyeaters has a higher percentage and absolute surface area of capillaries than those of wet-zone honeyeaters, allowing for more efficient water conservation.[18] Whether these renal modifications also occur in lories and lorikeets is unknown at this stage.

Lories and lorikeets typically possess a tight, glossy plumage thought to minimize feather soiling by nectar.

THE ROLE OF SUGARS AND STARCHES IN CARBOHYDRATE METABOLISM IN LORIKEETS

Nectar from flowering plants is a sugar-rich food that provides the major energy source for lorikeets and other nectarivorous species. However, it provides very low levels of amino acids, vitamins, and trace minerals.[4] Sugars make up nearly 100% of the dry weight of nectar.[19] The three main sugars include sucrose and its constituents, namely fructose

and glucose in equal amounts. These sugars can all be digested efficiently by lorikeets.[4] Xylose is found in nectar of Proteaceae and appears to be inefficiently digested by most nectarivores.[20,21] Sugar concentrations in nectar of Australian food plants that are bird pollinated vary between 15 and 35% wt/wt (weight/weight) sugar.[22,23] Nicolson and Fleming[24] suggested the approximate average nectar concentration of bird-pollinated plants was 23% wt/wt sugar or 0.75 mol/L for honeyeaters. This differs from plants relying on insect pollinators, which have higher sugar concentrations (30% to 74% sugar in nectar for honeybees).

The gross energy value of nectar has been reported to be 16.7 kJ/g.[19] Nectar flows vary between species but each flower of *Eucalyptus* and *Callistemon* can produce up to 5 ml of nectar during its lifespan.[4,25] Flowers of these species usually last 10 to 30 days. In one study, red lories (*Eos bornea*) (Figure 4-7) showed a preference for sucrose over glucose or fructose when fed nectars of low sugar concentrations (0.25 mol/L), but had no preference between the three sugars at higher concentrations (0.73 mol/L).[26] This was found to be similar to other non-psittacine nectarivores such as sunbirds, sugarbirds, honeyeaters, and hummingbirds.[27-29] These findings were explained in terms of energy profitability—a 0.25 mol/L sucrose solution yields more than double the energy of a 0.25 mol/L solution of glucose. However, this is in direct contrast to another study[30] in which rainbow lorikeets preferred a 1:1 glucose:fructose solution over an energetically equivalent sucrose solution when dilute nectars (less than 0.75 mol/L) were fed, but changed preference to sucrose when concentrated nectars (1 and 2 mol/L) were fed. At diets around the average concentration of natural nectars (23% sugar or 0.75 mol/L), rainbow lorikeets showed a significant hexose preference. The possible explanations for these findings are as follows:

1. At low sugar concentrations, with rapid gut transit times, hexose is much easier to absorb than sucrose, perhaps because of reduced sucrose hydrolysis efficiency.[30] The fact that rainbows preferred hexose at mid concentrations whereas New Holland honeyeaters and red wattlebirds

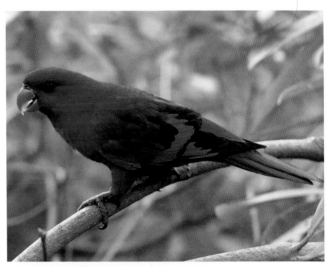

FIGURE 4-7 The red lory (*Eos bornea*) from Indonesia is another popularly kept species.

showed no preference was potentially attributed to decreased sucrase activity in rainbow lorikeets. However, sucrase levels have been found by some workers to be quite high in this species.[31]

2. At high sugar concentrations, sucrose may be preferred to hexose because hexose solutions have twice the osmolality of equicaloric sucrose solutions, which may make excretion of built up wastes more difficult and potentially result in dehydration, or require increased water intake.[32,33]

These preferences may also merely reflect the situation in nature and what birds are used to, i.e., natural nectars tend to contain more hexose when dilute and more sucrose when concentrated.[34] There may also be differences in taste perception by the birds between different sugar sources in nectars at different concentrations.

The apparent contradiction between the red lory study[26,27] and the rainbow lorikeet study[30] is, according to Fleming, because of experimental design. Hexose nectars made up on a percentage wt/wt basis actually only contain 95% of the energy content of sucrose solutions.[34] However, sugar solutions made up and matched on a molarity basis (expressed as mol/L), as was the case with Downs' work, resulted in the hexose nectars having only half the energy value of the sucrose nectar. Therefore, any sucrose preference observed was most likely an energy preference, particularly with dilute nectars. Brown et al[35] summarized these issues in stating that when comparing "equivalent" sugar solutions, the equivalence needs to be expressed either in terms of number of molecules in solution (equimolar), weight of each sugar in solution, or amount of energy in each solution (equicaloric). Changes in sugar preferences are usually only significant when birds are fed equicaloric low-sugar concentration nectars, where hexoses are preferred over sucrose.[34,35] Some of the earlier work on sugar preferences in lorikeets[26] would ideally need to be repeated comparing equicaloric sugar solutions.

The role of raffinose has been discussed as a fiber source rather than an energy source because it is assumed, but not proven, that lorikeets are unable to digest raffinose sugars efficiently. It is proposed that raffinose sugars potentially promote the colonization of bifidobacteria and lactobacillus in the lorikeet intestinal tract. This may have the benefit of inhibiting clostridial and other pathogenic infections.[5] However, the amount of raffinose sugars in most nectars is negligible (less than 1%). They are more likely to be encountered in wild plant and insect exudates and make up 5% to 10% of lerp and 37% to 48% of manna,[36] which are also eaten to various degrees by lorikeets. The role of raffinose sugars as prebiotics needs further investigation.

Lerp, the waxy protective scale secreted by psyllid insects, is composed of polymers of glucose (90%) and water (10%). Manna, the sugary exudate from damaged eucalypt leaves or woods, is composed of about 60% sugars, 16% water, and 20% pectin and uronic acids. Manna, lerp, and honeydew (the sugary excretion of nymphal insects) are all primarily carbohydrate sources and are supplementary food items upon which lorikeets occasionally forage.[37] They form a more significant proportion of the diet of the other Australian nectarivorous psittacine, the swift parrot, *L. discolor*.

Sugars in general have a very high degree of digestibility in lorikeets and are almost completely digested.[26,38] The digestibility of starch in artificial nectars appears to be similar to that recorded for granivorous psittacines fed seeds.[38] This is not surprising, given that most starch sources in artificial nectars are cereal based. Captive lorikeets maintained solely on artificial nectar with low protein showed weight loss and reduced activity compared with those fed artificial nectar supplemented with protein, which maintained weight.[39] The protein content of this supplement was 15.4% protein, most of which was derived from skim milk (Complan.com).[40]

PROTEIN REQUIREMENTS AND THE ROLE OF POLLEN AND INSECTS AS PROTEIN SOURCES

Many studies report lorikeets feeding on flowers, but few distinguish between nectar and pollen intake. This is because many of these studies are observation based, rather than relying on analysis of crop contents. There was some debate as to whether lorikeets could satisfy their energy requirements from nectar alone,[11] but this was refuted by the observations of Hopper and Burbidge[41] who saw purple-crowned lorikeets harvesting the flowers of *Eucalyptus buprestium* at the rate of one flower every 1 to 3 seconds, which is ample time to meet both their energy and nitrogen requirements.

Active pollen harvesting has been recorded in rainbow and purple-crowned lorikeets and in swift parrots.[4,11,14,41] The tip of a lorikeet's muscular tongue can compress the anthers of the flowers against its hard palate. In this way large amounts of pollen can be extracted from the flowers in a short period of time.

Pollen is considered the main protein source in lorikeet diets. Insect consumption is variable between species, but appears to be more important in honeyeaters than it is in lories and lorikeets.[8,11,37,42,43] Stomach contents of lorikeets contain few insects when the birds are harvesting nectar and pollen,[11,43] and lorikeets do not catch insects when suitable flowers are available.[44] The poorly developed lorikeet gizzard makes it unlikely that they could break down the hard chitinous exoskeleton of many insects. A notable exception is the Stephen's lory (*V. stepheni*), which ingests a considerable amount of lepidopteran larvae (soft bodied) found on the sporangia of *Phymatosorus* ferns.[9] Accidental ingestion of insects while feeding on flowers is also likely. Grubs of unidentified species have been identified in the gizzard of several musk lorikeets (*G. concinna*), dusky lories, and in a red-collared lorikeet (*Trichoglossus haematodus rubritorquis*) (Figure 4-8).[6,45] Soft-bodied *Homoptera* insects, psyllids, *Thysanoptera*, and *Diptera* adults and larvae have been found in the crops of the Papuan lory (*Charmosyna papou*).[2,46] Caterpillars were found in the crop of yellow-bibbed lories (*Lorius chlorocercus*) (Figure 4-9), and musk lorikeets.[2] Other unidentified small insects have been found in the crops of red lories (*E. bornea*), Ponape lories (*Trichoglossus rubiginosus*), and black-capped lories (*Lorius lory*; Figure 4-10). Invertebrates, lerp, and insect galls made up 9% of the feeding records of rainbow lorikeets and 4.8% of feeding records for musk lorikeets in one study.[8]

Pollens contain between 16 and 30% protein on a dry matter basis and contain a diverse amino acid profile.[47–49] *Banksia* pollen contains 33% protein, *Eucalyptus* pollen contains 25% (22% to 30%) protein, and Acacia pollen contains 24% protein.[50] *Hibiscus* pollen contains 19.1% protein.[38] All these

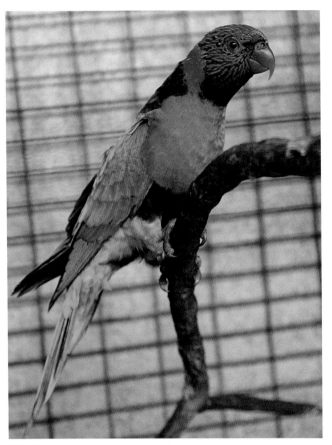

FIGURE 4-8 The red-collared lorikeet *(Trichoglossus rubritorquis)*, like many lorikeets, ingests insects while harvesting pollen and nectar from flowers.

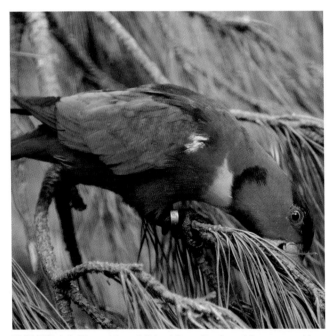

FIGURE 4-9 The yellow-bibbed lory *(Lorius chlorocercus)* has been found to consume caterpillars and other insects during foraging.

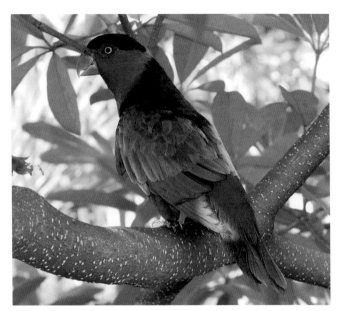

FIGURE 4-10 The black-capped lory *(Lorius lory)* is a relatively omnivorous species.

species are commonly utilized as food sources by lorikeets. In contrast, pollen from the Black She-oak *(Casuarina littoralis)* contains only 12.5% crude protein.[51] Crude protein in processed pollens are reported to vary between 7 and 40% despite the fact that pollens processed by bees have increased carbohydrate and water content, which should decrease the crude protein content.

Eucalyptus and *Banksia ericifolia* pollen contain adequate levels of all amino acids except methionine[51-54] and possibly isoleucine and valine.[51] Their amino acid composition is similar to vitellogenin of egg yolk, considered to be a high-quality, highly digestible protein.[4] Interestingly, methionine is also the one amino acid that rainbow lorikeets rejected when given diets offering a choice of four separate amino acids.[55]

Pollen digestibility figures vary widely and appear to be contradictory. Early reports suggested that *Eucalyptus calophylla* pollen digestibility was very low in lorikeets, with only 4.5% digested by adult green-naped lorikeets *(Trichoglossus haematodus haematodus)* (Figure 4-11) and 6.6% by adult Australian rainbow lorikeets *(T. haematodus moluccanus)*, but increased up to 26% in nestlings. The digestibility of *Prunus* pollen by adults of either species was less than 4%.[56] Delia and Frankel[57] showed that mixed *Eucalyptus* pollen had a digestibility of 17.4% in rainbow lorikeets, again a fairly low figure. The low digestibility was thought to be because of the difficulty in penetrating the outer exine shell of the pollen granules. It is thought that pollen digestion relies on direct enzymatic action through the pores of the outer exine shell and also changed osmotic pressures, which cause the pores of the pollen grain to open.[56,58,59] Pollen digestibility appears to be maximized in the presence of nectar.[60] This may result from the hypertonicity of the nectar having an osmotic effect, which causes leaching of free amino acids from the pollen granules through the pores into the bird's intestinal tract.

These data are at variance to the observations of Wooller et al[61] who observed that up to 48% of the naturally ingested *Hakea* pollen granules in the large intestine of wild

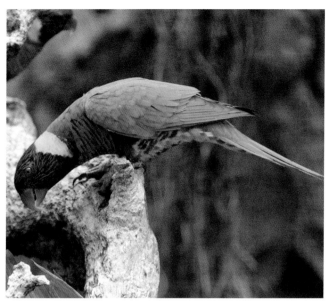

FIGURE 4-11 The green-naped lorikeet *(Trichoglossus hae-matodus haematodus)* was found to have limited ability to digest bee-processed *Eucalyptus calophylla* pollen.

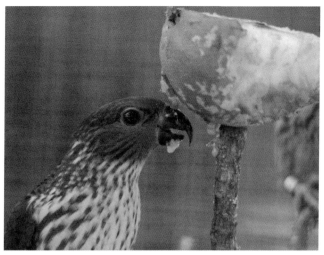

FIGURE 4-12 The Goldie's lorikeet *(Psitteuteles goldiei)* was found to digest over 50% of ingested *Hibiscus* pollen.

purple-crowned lorikeets *(Glossopsitta porphyrocephala)* were empty. Similarly, Gartrell and Jones[62] found that musk lorikeets and the co-evolved nectarivorous swift parrot *(L. discolor)* were similarly efficient at digesting pollen of two *Eucalyptus* species *(E. globulus* and *E. ovata).* Both of these studies utilized pollen that was taken directly from the flower, both fresh and frozen, and not bee-modified pollen, which is often utilized in captive feeding studies. Pollen harvested by bees has carbohydrates and water added, resulting in a conglomerated pollen that is a much larger molecule. Human and Nicolson[63] found that aloe pollen *(Aloe greatheadii* var. *davyana)* collected and stored by bees resulted in an increased water (13% to 21% wet weight) and carbohydrate (35% to 61% dry weight) content and a decreased protein (from 51% to 28% dry weight) and lipid (from 10% to 8%) content when compared with fresh pollen taken from the flower. Using bee-modified pollen may account for the differences noted by Brice et al[56] and Delia and Frankel.[57] Alternatively, there may be differences in the physiology and digestive capabilities of rainbow lorikeets compared with the purple-crowned and musk lorikeets, but given their close evolutionary relationship and the efficient digestion of pollen by the more distantly related swift parrot, this seems less likely. Wolf et al[38] found a high protein digestibility when using *Hibiscus* pollen of 51.6% in Goldie's *(Trichoglossus goldiei)* (Figure 4-12) and 56.3% in Rainbow lorikeets *(T. haematodus haematodus).* This study does not clarify whether the pollen used was bee pollen or natural pollen.

Pollen digestibility may also depend on pollen viability. Arnould[64] found that unviable *Banksia* pollen was digested more readily (43% to 61%) than live pollen (18% to 22%) by eastern pygmy possums *(Cercartetus nanus).* Not only was pollen found to be variably digested, but protein digestion overall was found to be low in lorikeets. Frankel and Avram[65] found that protein digestibility in rainbow lorikeets was only 13.3%, but they used egg-white protein as their protein source. Egg whites are lower in proline and histidine than several *Eucalyptus* species, which may account for its decreased digestibility.[65]

Further research by Delia and Frankel[57] found that digestibility of egg white to be only 4.3% and did not significantly increase when casein was added (5.6%), and that the digestibility of a commercial nectar product with a whey/casein protein base (Wombaroo Lorikeet and Honeyeater Food) was higher (7.3%) but not significantly so. In contrast the protein metabolizability of mixed *Eucalyptus* pollen in the same study was 17.4%. These figures suggest that the protein metabolizability of artificial protein sources by rainbow lorikeets is relatively low.

Lower protein digestibility may be from the lower pepsin activity found in lorikeets when compared with 3-week-old layer chickens.[66] Pepsin is the proventricular enzyme that begins protein digestion in the body. Optimum pH for pepsin activity in the rainbow lorikeet is similar to that in the chicken (pH 2.5 to 3.2). However, in the same study, the general proteolytic activity of the pancreatic proteases (trypsin, chymotrypsin, and carboxypeptidase A) was not different between the two species. However, no studies were performed on the activity of the small intestinal proteases such as glycyl-l-leucine dipeptidase and leucine aminopeptidase N in the rainbow lorikeet. The difference in pepsin activity in this study may possibly be attributable to the different physiological states of the two species, since the lorikeets were adults and the chickens were juveniles experiencing rapid growth, where demand for protein would be expected to be higher.

Low protein metabolizability may not only be from low proventricular pepsin activity. It may also be compounded by a rapid gastrointestinal transit time of food. The presence of free amino acids rather than protein in nectar may mean that high pepsin activities are not required in lorikeets. However, as stated earlier, nectar contains less than 1% protein and is inadequate as a sole dietary protein source for lories. The higher digestibility of pollen by nestlings suggests that pollen may be a useful addition for birds rearing young.

Dietary protein requirements of lorikeets are reported to be lower than those of similar-sized granivorous parrots.[65,67] This may reflect the large volume of food eaten and the rapid passage time in the gut. Therefore, although the concentration in the food may be low, the total amount absorbed over the course of the day may meet requirements.

It has been calculated by Frankel and Avram[65] that rainbow lorikeets require as little as 2.8% protein if the protein is high quality and readily digestible, or 8.6% protein for less digestible pollen (4.5% digestibility), to fulfill maintenance requirements. This equates to a daily pollen consumption of 5 to 6 g dry matter per day for a 150 g bird. Similarly, Pryor[58] established that red lories require at least 1% crude protein dry matter in their diet to maintain body mass.

The protein requirements of lories and lorikeets, however, may also be species dependent. For example, Cornejo and Clubb[68] found that captive *Chalcopsitta* spp. (Figure 4-13) and *Lorius* spp. (Figure 4-14) both chose diets higher in protein and with better amino acid profiles than did *Trichoglossus* spp. or *Eos* spp. However, the total protein concentration ingested was just under the estimated minimum value and the digestibility of this protein was not determined. It is uncertain if these results reflect a true higher protein requirement by these species, or merely reflect a taste preference or a learned preference for the high-protein dietary items within the foods offered. If using pollen as a feeding supplement, the source of the pollen and its amino acid profile both need to be considered.

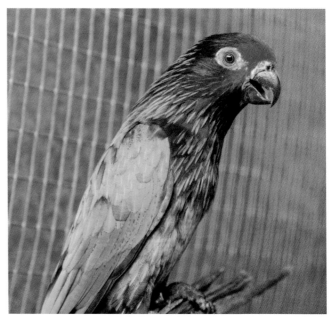

FIGURE 4-13 *Chalcopsitta* species such as the yellow-streaked lory *(C. scintillata)* exhibited a preference for higher protein diets in one captive trial.

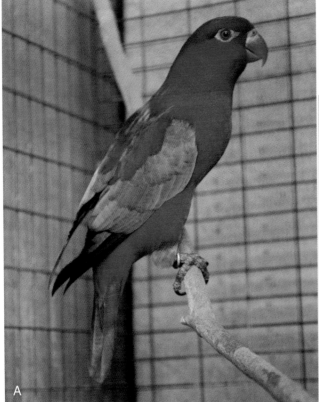

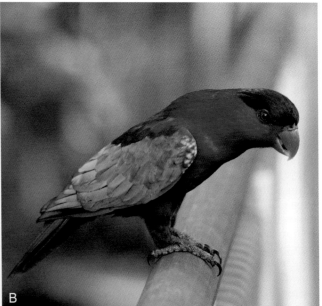

FIGURE 4-14 Two *Lorius* species that also chose higher protein diets in one captive study. **A,** The chattering lory *(Lorius garrulus),* a commonly kept lory species. **B,** The purple-naped lory *(Lorius domicella)* is a much prized but uncommonly kept species in captivity.

DIETARY FATS AND OTHER NUTRIENTS OBTAINED FROM POLLEN

The role of fats in lorikeet diets has not been well investigated. Fats make up between 1% and 20% dry matter of pollen, with triglycerides and phospholipids predominating.[4,69] These figures do not include the indigestible long-chain lipids found in the cell wall. Dietary fat is most likely sourced from pollen, native fruits, and insects.[5] The minimum crude fat recommended is 4%,[70] which is similar to the amount consumed in food in at least one study[68] and also the amount on several commercial lorikeet food products. The actual fatty acid requirements of lories and lorikeets have yet to be determined.

Pollens contain 4% to 10% carbohydrates, which consist of starch, fructose, glucose, and sucrose but are considered to be an insignificant source of energy for nectarivores compared with nectar. Pollens also contain vitamin C, vitamin E, B vitamins, and carotenoids (vitamin A precursors), which give pollen its yellow color. The exact amounts of these nutrients vary.[4] Minerals make up 2.5% to 6.5% dry matter of pollen. These largely consist of nitrogen, phosphorus, calcium, sulfur, sodium, and magnesium and trace amounts of iron and boron.[4,71]

THE ROLE OF FRUITS IN THE DIET OF WILD LORIES AND LORIKEETS

Native fruits make up a small percentage of the dietary items found in the crops of wild lories and lorikeets[2] and likely represent a seasonal food source. Lorikeets have been observed feeding on native figs (*Moraceae*), *Schefflera*, *Podocarpus* spp., and mistletoe berries,[2,4,5] although in many cases the species of fruit are not identified. Lorikeets will also raid domestic fruit crops and quickly adapt to this food source.[2,3]

There are substantial differences between native and domestic fruits. Some native Australian fruits have marginally higher protein but can have significantly higher fat values than domesticated fruits. However, there is the potential for decreased availability of this protein in fruits containing high tannin levels.[5] Domesticated fruits are higher in simple sugars and water and have poor protein levels. The fiber content of some wild fruits is similar to that of some vegetables.[5]

Fruits tend to contain low levels of calcium, but native figs contain calcium levels that fall within the recommended range for psittacines[72] and have a high calcium:phosphorus (Ca:P) ratio.[5] Domestic figs, on the other hand, remain calcium deficient but still maintain a positive Ca:P ratio. Fruits in general provide good levels of provitamin A and vitamin C and have low levels of iron. Native fruits have lower vitamin C levels than domestic fruits.

THE ROLE OF SEEDS IN THE DIET OF WILD LORIKEETS

Although lories and lorikeets are considered to be primarily pollen and nectar feeders, seeds are also opportunistically consumed by many species. Small seeds of unidentified plant species have been found in the crop of many lorikeet species including yellow-bibbed lories (*Lorius chlorocercus*)

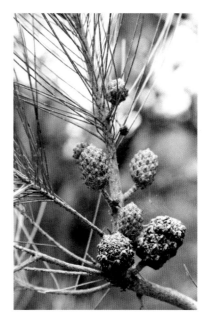

FIGURE 4-15 The small seeds produced by the cones of *Casuarina* and *Allocasuarina* plants are opportunistically eaten by several lorikeet species.

and Stella's lorikeets (*C. papou*).[2,46] Most seeds are described as small.

The small seeds of *Casuarina* trees are favored at particular times of the year by several lorikeet species (Figure 4-15). Rainbow lorikeets are frequently seen to feed on these seeds at certain times of the year when other favored food plants are not flowering.[3,45] *Casuarina* feeding has also been observed in green-naped lorikeets and in Kuhl's or Rimitara lories (*Vini kuhlii*).[3] The nutritional composition of various natural lorikeet food sources are summarized in Table 4-5.

ENERGY REQUIREMENTS OF LORIKEETS

Smaller lorikeet species seem to have a relatively higher energy requirement than do larger species. Mitchell's lorikeets have a relatively higher energy intake (883 kJ ME/kg, 0.75 body weight [BW]/day) than green-naped lorikeets (784 kJ ME/kg, 0.75 BW/day). The figures given are for medium dilution nectars but the results are the same for all dilutions.[73] Goldie's lorikeets have a relatively higher energy requirement (0.86 MJ ME/kg, 0.75 BW/day) than do green-naped lorikeets (0.65 MJ ME/kg, 0.75 BW/day).[38]

In green-naped lorikeets fed apple and nectar, energy intake was similar regardless of the degree of dilution of nectar. Feeding solely dilute nectar to this species resulted in a considerable decrease in energy intake. Increasing dilutions of nectar resulted in increased consumption of both nectar and apples. In Mitchell's lorikeets, in contrast, adding apple to dilute nectar resulted in a substantial increase in energy intake. Feeding solely dilute nectar resulted in only a slight decrease in energy intake.[73] In both subspecies, increasing dilution of nectar and feeding apples significantly decreased protein and thiamine intake and decreased the Ca:P ratio.[73]

TABLE 4-5

Nutritional Composition of Food Items Commonly Ingested by Wild Lorikeets (expressed as % DM)[4,5]

Food Source	% Protein	% Carbohydrate	% Fat	% Ash (Minerals)
Pollen	16-30	4-10	1-20	2.5-6.5
Nectar	<2	<99	0	Neg*
Manna	<0.2	60	0	Neg*
Honeydew	2.6	33	0	11.4
Lerp	0	90	0	Neg*
Fruit (domestic)	1-14	73-79	1-5	2-7
Native Australian Figs (*Ficus* spp.)	4-15	48	3-6	6

DM, Dry matter.
*Denotes negligible amounts.

WATER INTAKE IN RELATION TO DIET

Lorikeets drink only small amounts of water when fed high-moisture content foods. Conversely, water intake is maximized when pollen is the main dietary source.[38] However, this study does not measure total water intake in relation to the bird's bodyweight or to its calculated daily requirement. This information would be useful to determine whether high dry matter diets place any physiological stress on lorikeets, particularly when fed long term. Nectars are hypertonic relative to plasma,[74] so nectivores must consume fresh water either in food or separately on a regular basis to prevent dehydration.[4]

Kalmar et al[73] found that drinking water consumption in Mitchell's and green-naped lorikeets remained relatively constant and independent of nectar dilution or the provision of apple to the diet. Therefore, the total water intake for both species was increased when birds were fed dilute diets. Kalmar et al[73] also noted that the smaller subspecies (Mitchell's lorikeet) had a significantly higher intake of drinking water than did the green-naped lorikeet. There was no such correlation when total water intakes of the smaller Goldie's lorikeet were compared with the larger rainbow lorikeet in the study by Wolf et al.[38]

The nature of the droppings produced also changed depending on the moisture content of the diet fed.[38] Birds fed nectar produced droppings that were "beige, soft, and poorly shaped" and had a dry matter content of only 8%; those fed apples had watery droppings (2% dry matter), while those fed pollen produced well-formed droppings (30% dry matter) with a clear demarcation between urine, urates, and feces. These droppings were comparable to those produced by seed-fed granivores.[75] However, there are no studies that analyze what constitutes a "normal" dropping for wild lorikeets. If, as expected, this is dependent upon the local dietary sources, then a study showing the frequency with which droppings of varying consistencies are produced would provide valuable information in this area. Comparisons between renal and large intestinal anatomy and physiology between lorikeets and psittacine granivores would also further our knowledge in this field.

OTHER CONSIDERATIONS

Lorikeets eat approximately 10% to 15% of their body weight as a dry weight under captive maintenance conditions. The lower figures were seen with birds on apple diets while the higher figures correspond to feeding pollen.[11,38,39] These figures are slightly higher than those for similarly sized granivores (dry matter intake 7% to 12%).

Most seed-eating parrots have digestibility of organic matter of 75% to 90% on conventional diets.[38] The figures for lorikeets are approximately similar and diet dependent.[38] For example, digestibility of pollen was 55% for rainbow and Goldie's lorikeets, 82% for nectar, and greater than 90% for apples.

FEEDING PREFERENCES OF CAPTIVE LORIKEETS

Historically, the species of lorikeets that have adapted best to captivity have been the ones more adaptable in terms of diet and are less specialized in their needs. Hence the *Trichoglossus* spp., which have in the past even been maintained on an almost exclusively seed diet, have had a longer avicultural history than the more specialized nectar feeders such as *Glossopsitta* and *Charmosyna* spp.[3,76] In the Solomon Islands, yellow-bibbed lories (*Lo. chlorocercus*) were more popular as pet birds and survived well on a basic diet of sweet potatoes. In contrast, cardinal lories (*Chalcopsitta cardinals*), another island endemic, would rarely survive more than 12 months on this diet.[3]

Data gathered from feeding preferences shown by captive birds can also provide useful information. However, such data can be skewed because of the preferences formed by exposure to limited food types and by food-preference bias by parental birds and cage mates. Nearly all lorikeet species accept a nectar supplement in captivity.[3,30,38,65,68] Fruit is preferred to vegetables. In a study of 15 species of lories and lorikeets belonging to four genera (*Trichoglossus, Eos, Lorius,* and *Chalcopsitta*), apples and oranges were the favored fruits, with *Trichoglossus* species also favoring pears.[68] In the same study, *Chalcopsitta* spp., and to a lesser extent Lorius spp., had higher protein and essential amino acid values in the food they consumed than did *Eos* and *Trichoglossus* spp. Whether this reflects an increased requirement in these species or is because of other factors related to the diet offered is unclear.

Green foods in the form of chickweed, dandelion, and half-ripe seed heads have been eaten by many species of lories and lorikeets.[77] Green food is actively sought by breeding

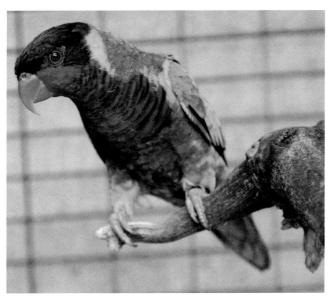

FIGURE 4-16 The ornate lorikeet *(Trichoglossus ornatus)* has been recorded eating green food in captivity, particularly while feeding young.

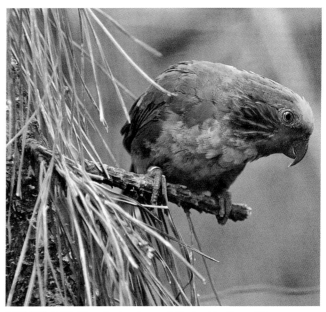

FIGURE 4-17 The diminutive red-flanked lorikeet *(Charmosyna placentis)*, although considered a specialized nectar feeder, has been observed eating small seeds in captivity.

birds and fed to youngsters. Whiskered lorikeets *(Oreopsittacus arfaki)*, in particular, seem to seek and eat large quantities of green foods when offered.[3,78] Other lorikeet species that have been recorded to eat green food, particularly when rearing young, include members of the *Eos, Trichoglossus* (Figure 4-16), *Neopsittacus*, and *Charmosyna* genera[3] and Mount Apo lorikeets *(Trichoglossus johnstoniae)*[79] and Stella's lorikeets *(C. papou)*.[46]

Seeds are also ingested periodically by various lorikeet species but are an important dietary item for Musschenbroek's lorikeet *(Neopsittacus musschenbroekii)*, emerald lorikeet *(Neopsittacus pullicauda)*, and the iris lorikeet *(Trichoglossus iris)*.[3,80,81] Other species that have been observed to eat seed in captivity include the red-flanked lorikeet *(Charmosyna plecentis)* (Figure 4-17), Stella's lorikeet (Figure 4-18), and most *Trichoglossus* spp., including Goldie's lorikeet *(T. goldiei)*, rainbow lorikeet *(T. haematodus* spp.), scaly-breasted lorikeet *(T. chlorolepidotus)*, and the Mount Apo lorikeet *(T. johnstoniae)*. Low[3] commented that the only species that reject *Casuarina* cones and seeds are the members of the *Chalcopsitta* genus.

Soft-bodied insects are also actively sought by many species. Blue-crowned lorikeets *(Vini australis)* and blue-streaked lories *(Eos reticulata)* actively seek out and eat mealworms.[82,83] Other species such as red-flanked lorikeets, Goldie's lorikeets, and emerald lorikeets have all been observed eating mealworms[81] and Musschenbroek's lorikeets seek wax moth larvae when young are in the nest.[80] No doubt many species will ingest insects when given the opportunity, especially when rearing young.

Several breeders have commented that certain species of lorikeets fare better when kept on low-protein diets in captivity. These species include members of the genera *Charmosyna* and *Chalcopsitta* and the whiskered lorikeet.[3,84] There is little scientific proof for these statements, which are based solely on observation and experiences in captivity by these breeders.

In general, from experiences with captive birds, the *Trichoglossus* spp., the dusky lory *(Pseudeos fuscata)* (Figure 4-19), and

the yellow-bibbed lory are considered more omnivorous in their dietary preferences than many other species of lories and lorikeets.[3] These feeding preferences are summarized in Table 4-6.

POTENTIAL PROBLEMS WITH CAPTIVE DIETS

Lack of Scientific Formulation

Many lories and lorikeets in captivity are fed home-made diets utilizing cereal-based ingredients and sugars. These have been developed over time and are based on aviculturists' experience rather than any scientific basis. The range of ingredients used and the individual adjustments made may vary from breeder to breeder. The end result is highly variable, and the nutritional composition of the diet fed, including total energy and amino acid composition, is largely unknown. Some of these diets have even been produced and sold commercially as dry powder or nectar diets, again with no scientific basis. Despite these limitations, many of these home-made diets are reported to be successfully used across a broad range of species.[84,85]

If these nectars are too dilute they will pass through the gut more quickly with less time for digestion and absorption of the nutrients within them. Therefore, diluting nectars as a means of effecting weight loss is likely to lead to nutritional deficiencies. Dilute nectars are also prone to spoilage because they have free water available, which allows bacteria to multiply. Nectars in the wild have a sugar concentration of 20% to 25% wt/vol, and those in captivity should mirror this. Producing nectars of the correct osmolality produces a bacteriostatic effect by depriving bacteria of available water. This acts as a natural preservative for the nectar. At the other extreme, nectars that are too hyperosmolar, such as those that contain mostly fructose or glucose, may cause osmotic water loss from the body and cause dehydration in birds. The ideal osmolality is 20% to 25% wt/vol as commonly occurs in natural nectars.

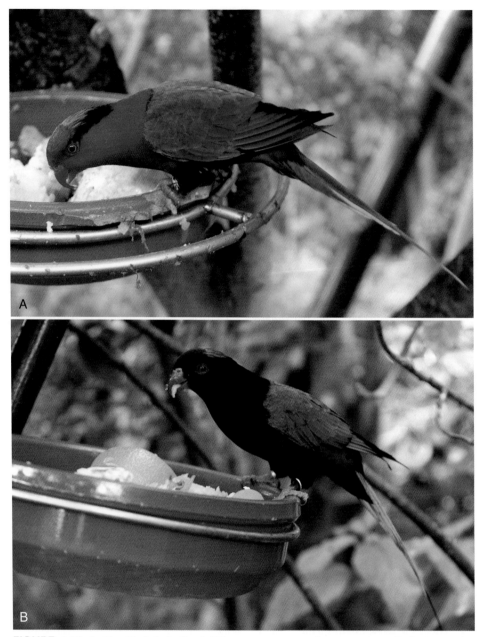

FIGURE 4-18 **A,** The Stella's lorikeet *(Charmosyna papou)* occurs naturally in two color morphs within its range. **A,** The red morph is more common at lower altitudes. **B,** Melanistic morph, which is found more commonly at higher altitudes within its range. Mixed red and melanistic pairs can be found at mid altitudes.

Some breeders supplement protein by using high-protein cereals with the mistaken belief that this may help counteract problems with feather plucking. Nectars are by nature low in protein; thus birds consume large volumes of them over the course of a day. There is no evidence that increasing the protein content of nectars will increase protein absorption in adults, but this may be beneficial for nestlings since they have a greater capacity for protein digestion, as mentioned previously.

Pollens are often touted as the ideal way of providing protein to lorikeet diets. As stated earlier, the suitability of these as dietary additions may depend on the species of plant from

which the pollen is derived and whether the pollen is natural or bee pollen. Questions also remain regarding the digestibility of each pollen species, which may be dependent upon how the pollen is fed. Some pollens are also very bitter, thereby totally unpalatable to lorikeets.

Many, but not all, commercial nectars are at least formulated by nutritionists. The end product is of known nutritional composition, assuming that quality control is high, which is not always the case. Known nutritional requirements for lorikeets are limited and much of this information is extrapolated from other psittacines or even poultry. How these figures apply to the large range of lory and lorikeet species

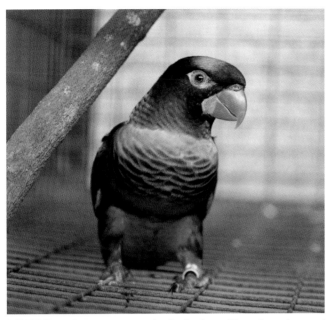

FIGURE 4-19 The monotypic dusky lory *(Pseudeos fuscata)* appears to be one of the more omnivorous lorikeet species.

kept in captivity is unknown. In addition, the nutritional requirements of nestlings are different compared with adults, but there are few manufacturers who produce separate diets to account for these differences (e.g., The Dutch company AVES Product produces Loristart for rearing young lories and Lorinectar for adults).

However, there is great variability between the differing commercial products. Those with low-energy value or low digestibility will result in the production of a greater volume

of droppings, which will necessitate more frequent cleaning if adequate hygiene is to be maintained.

Most people supplement lory diets with fresh fruit, with apple as the most popular kind.[68,76,85] The addition of fruit acts to dilute the total nutritional intake of the bird, since most domestic fruits are high in sugar—but not as high as most nectars—and low in protein, essential fatty acids, minerals, and some vitamins, as stated earlier.

Dry Powdered Diets versus "Nectar" Diets

There has been a trend in some countries to create dry diets for these birds. These diets were initially developed to minimize the risk of food spoilage and consequent outbreaks of bacterial and fungal infections, which periodically occurred in collections fed nectar-based diets.[76] They also resulted in firming up the droppings produced by the birds, which was seen as an advantage by the pet industry in making these birds more popular as pet birds.[86] In the author's opinion, droppings from birds fed on predominately dry diets tend to stick more to the aviary structure and can be much harder to clean, especially once dried.

Unlike nectars, dry diets do not suffer from the settling of ingredients, particularly during hot weather, which may result in the birds only ingesting the dilute liquid portion of the nectar while the more solid ingredients are left in the bottom of the food dish. Another advantage of dry foods is that they are less attractive to bees and wasps, but ants are still attracted to the high sugar content of these foods. These dry foods have been successfully used for the keeping and breeding of Australian lorikeets,[76,85] but have been less successful with many of the other lorikeet species. Issues with maintaining adequate hydration in birds fed dry-based diets, even in the presence of *ad libitum* drinking water, may

TABLE 4-6
Some Observed Dietary Preferences Excluding Pollen and Nectar

Insects	Greenfeed	Seeds	Protein levels	Most Omnivorous Species
Wild	Species eating Green-	*Neopsittacus* spp.*	Choose high pro-	*Trichoglossus* spp.
Stephen's lory	feed include:	Iris lorikeet*	tein diets:	Dusky lory
Musk lorikeet	Whiskered lorikeet	*Trichoglossus* spp.	*Chalcopsitta* spp.	Yellow-bibbed lory
Rainbow lorikeet	*Eos* spp.	including:	*Lorius* spp.	
Red-collared lorikeet	*Trichoglossus* spp. in-	Rainbow lorikeet		
Papuan lory	cluding Mount Apo	Scaly-breasted		
Yellow-bibbed lory	lorikeet	lorikeet		
Black-capped lory	*Neopsittacus* spp.	Mount Apo lorikeet		
Red lory	*Charmosyna* spp. in-	Goldie's lorikeet		
Ponape lory	cluding Stella's lori-	*Charmosyna* spp.		
Dusky lory	keet	including:		
		Stella's lorikeet		
		Red-flanked lorikeet		
Captive			Require lower pro-	
Blue-crowned lorikeet			tein diets:	
Blue-streaked lories			*Charmosyna* spp.	
Red-flanked lorikeet			including	
Goldie's lorikeet			Stella's lorikeet	
Emerald lorikeet			and red-flanked	
Musschenbroek's lorikeet			lorikeet	

Please note that these are observations only and in some cases not scientifically verified.

be placing physiological stresses on species that are less adapted to arid habitats.

Increased intake of dry foods may result in slower gut transit times of food, since nutrient digestion is maximized when foods are dissolved in water.[86] If dry foods take longer to digest, intake of many essential nutrients, not just energy, may be impaired resulting in nutritional deficiencies and potentially weight loss. There is a lack of published information on feeding dry diets to lorikeets in terms of digestibility.

Specific Health Problems Resulting from Lorikeet Diets

There are several health-related issues resulting directly or indirectly from the diet fed to lorikeets. The high sugar content of the diet can lead to yeast/fungal and bacterial infections. This is evident in many postmortem findings by the author, even if only as a terminal event. Similarly, the sticky and moist nature of the droppings and the high sugar content of the nectar, dry food, and fruits fed can provide an ideal environment for bacteria and yeast to proliferate on aviary structures if suitable hygiene practices are not maintained. The high energy content of most diets combined with a lack of activity in a captive situation can lead to obesity-related disorders, including but not limited to fatty liver disease and infertility. High iron content found in many human cereals and other foods used in lorikeet diets can lead to iron accumulation in various organs, but particularly in the liver, and iron storage disease. The exact nature of this problem in susceptible species requires further investigation, in particular the presence and activity of enzymes involved in iron homeostasis such as hepcidin, ferroportin, and hephaestin. High dietary vitamin A levels may also aid iron absorption and contribute to this problem.[5]

There is some evidence that captive diets may contain excessive amounts of preformed vitamin A leading to hypervitaminosis A.[87-89] A study of wild rainbow lorikeets showed them to have hepatic vitamin A concentrations between 29 and 56 mg/kg, which was much lower than captive rainbow, purple-crowned, and musk lorikeets whose hepatic vitamin A levels varied between 97 and 4093 mg/kg when fed commercial nectar mixes containing up to 9990 IU vitamin A/kg.[88,90] It was also demonstrated that wild birds transferred to formulated diets had rapid increases in hepatic vitamin A levels of 90 mg/kg after 1 month rising to 588 mg/kg after 6 months. Clinical signs of hypervitaminosis A noted in lorikeets include problems with breeding and embryonic mortality; feather, skin, and beak condition and pigmentation; liver disease; and death. Increased susceptibility to infections and vitamin E deficiency were also implicated.[88,89]

Although dietary vitamin A requirements for poultry and pet birds have been set at 2500 to 5000 IU/kg of food,[70] cockatiels have been found to have lower requirements of 2000 IU/kg.[90] No exact studies have been performed on lorikeets. However, it is suspected that their requirements may be even lower than this, with levels as low as 1000 IU/kg suggested as possibly toxic.[87] Lower dietary vitamin A levels supplemented with dietary vitamin A precursors may be a more suitable form of supplementation. This may also allow for adequate absorption of other fat-soluble vitamins such as vitamin E, which otherwise would suffer from competitive inhibition by high dietary vitamin A levels. It has

been suggested that nectarivorous birds rely on provitamin A carotenoids for their vitamin A requirements and would ingest very limited amounts of preformed vitamin A. McDonald and Oldfield[87] have even suggested that in the absence of data identifying whether lorikeets have a requirement for preformed vitamin A, (retinol) their diets should only be supplemented with 0.15% spirulina (1440 mg/kg β-carotene), which is sufficient to support the vitamin A requirements of cockatiels.[91]

CONCLUSION

Although nectar and pollen make up the bulk of lorikeet diets, supplemented with fruits, seeds, insects, lerp, manna, and honeydew, the exact nutritional requirements for each species is largely unknown. Therefore, the marketing of commercial lorikeet diets as "complete" foods is misleading. The use of home-made diets results at best in the feeding of foods of unknown nutritional composition, and at worst in malnutrition and associated diseases. Despite this, some of these appear to be successfully used with many species.

Even if the exact diet for each species in the wild could be accurately determined, its applicability to captive birds may be limited by the greatly reduced energy demands of birds kept in captivity.

Human-based foods need to be carefully considered before being used in captive lorikeet diets. Issues such as protein digestibility, levels of preformed vitamin A, iron, and total energy content and fluid content all need to be addressed and explored further.

REFERENCES

1. Collar NJ: Family Psittacidae. In Del Hoyo J, Elliott A, Sargatal J, editors: *Handbook of birds of the world*, Barcelona, Spain, 1997, Lynx Edicions, Vol 4, pp 280-470.
2. Forshaw JM: *Parrots of the world*, ed 3, Willoughby, 1998, Lansdowne Editions & Weldon Publishing.
3. Low R: *Hancock house encyclopedia of the lories*, Surrey, British Columbia, Canada, 1998, Hancock House Publishers.
4. Gartrell BD: The nutritional, morphologic and physiologic bases of nectarivory in Australian birds, *J Avian Med Surg* 14(2):85–94, 2000.
5. McDonald D: Feeding ecology and nutrition of Australian lorikeets, *Semin Avian Exotic Pet Med* 12 (4):195–204, 2003.
6. Pratt TK, Beehler BM: *Birds of New Guinea*, ed 2, Princeton, NJ, 2015, Princeton University Press.
7. Cannon CE: The diet of lorikeets *Trichoglossus* spp. in the Queensland-New South Wales border region, *Emu* 84:16–22, 1984.
8. Smith J, Lill A: Importance of eucalypts in exploitation of urban parks by rainbow and musk lorikeets, *Emu* 108(2):187–195, 2008.
9. Trevelyan R: The feeding ecology of Stephen's lorry and nectar availability in its food plants. In Benton TG, Spencer T, editors: *The Pitcairn Islands: biogeography, ecology and prehistory, Biol J Linnean Soc* 56:185–197, 1995.
10. Holyoak DT: Comments on taxonomy and relationships in the parrot subfamilies Nestorinae, Loriinae and Platycercinae, *Emu* 73: 157–176, 1973.
11. Churchill DM, Christensen P: Observations on pollen harvesting by brush-tongued lorikeets, *Aust J Zool* 18:427–437, 1970.
12. Schweizer M, Guntert M, Seehausen O, et al: Parallel adaptations to nectarivory in parrots, key innovations and the diversification of the

Loriinae, *Ecol Evol* 4(14):2867–2883, 2014, doi:10.1002/ece3.1131. Accessed July 20, 2014.

13. Guntert M: Morphologische untersuchungen zur adaptiven radiation des verdauungstraktes bei papageien (Psittaci), *Zool Jahrb Abt Anat Ontog Tiere* 106:471–526, 1981.

14. Richardson KC, Wooller RD: Adaptations of the alimentary tracts of some Australian lorikeets to a diet of pollen and nectar, *Aust J Zool* 38:581–586, 1990.

15. Gartrell BD, Jones SM, Brereton RN et al: Morphological adaptations to nectarivory in the swift parrot, *Lathamus discolor*, *Emu* 100:274–279, 2000.

16. Goldstein DL, Bradshaw SD: Renal function in red wattlebirds in response to varying fluid intake, *J Comp Physiol* 168:265–272, 1998.

17. Casotti G, Richardson KC, Bradley JS: Ecomorphological constraints imposed by the kidney component measurements in honeyeater birds inhabiting different environments, *J Biol* 231:611–625, 1993.

18. Casotti G, Richardson KC: A qualitative analysis of the kidney structure of meliphagid honeyeaters from wet and arid environments, *J Anat* 182:239–247, 1993.

19. Luttge U: Chemical composition of nectars. In Luttge U, Pitman MG, editors: *Transport in plants II. Tissues and organs. Part B*, Berlin, 1976, Springer-Verlag, pp 249–251.

20. Jackson S, Nicolson SW, Lotz CN: Sugar preferences and "side bias" in cape sugarbirds and lesser double-collared sunbirds, *Auk* 115:156–165, 1998.

21. Nicolson SW, Vanwyk BE: Nectar sugars in Proteaceae-patterns and processes, *Aust J Botany* 46:489–504, 1998.

22. Pyke GH: The foraging behaviour of Australian honeyeaters: a review and some comparisons with hummingbirds, *Aust J Ecol* 5:343–369, 1980.

23. Paton DC: The diet of the New Holland honeyeater, *Phyliodonyris novaehollandiae*, *Aust J Ecol* 7:279–298, 1982.

24. Nicolson SW, Fleming PA: Nectar as food for birds: the physiological consequences of drinking dilute sugar solutions, *Plant Syst Evol* 238:139–153, 2003b.

25. Christidis L, Boles WE: *The taxonomy and species of birds of Australia and its territories*, RAOU monograph no.2, Melbourne, Australia, 1994, Royal Australasian Ornithologists Union.

26. Downs CT: Sugar preference and apparent sugar assimilation in the red lory, *Aust J Zool* 45:613–619, 1997.

27. Downs CT, Perrin MR: Sugar preferences of some southern African nectarivorous birds, *Ibis* 138:455–459, 1996.

28. Martinez del Rio C: Sugar preferences in hummingbirds: the influence of subtle chemical differences on food choice, *Condor* 92:1022–1030, 1990.

29. Mitchell RJ, Paton DC: Effects of nectar volume and concentration on sugar intake rates of Australian honeyeaters (Meliphagidae), *Oecologia* 83:238–246, 1990.

30. Fleming PA, Xie S, Napier K, et al: Nectar concentration affects sugar preferences in two Australian honeyeaters and a lorikeet, *Funct Ecol* 22(4):599–605, 2008.

31. Rich G: Wombaroo food products, Glen Osmond, South Australia, 5064, 2011.

32. Fleming PA, Nicolson SW: Osmoregulation in an avian nectarivore, the white-bellied sunbird *Nectarinia talatala*: response to extremes of diet concentration, *J Exp Biol* 206:1845–1854, 2003.

33. Fleming PA, Gray DA, Nicholson SW: Osmoregulatory response to acute diet change in an avian nectarivore: rapid dehydration following water shortage, *Comp Biochem Physiol A Mol Integr Physiol* 138:321–326, 2004.

34. Lotz CN, Schondube JE: Sugar preferences in nectar- and fruit-eating birds: behavioural patterns and physiological causes, *Biotropica* 38:3–15, 2006.

35. Brown M, Downs CT, Johnson SD: Sugar preferences of nectar feeding birds–a comparison of experimental techniques, *J Avian Biol* 39:479–483, 2008.

36. Basden R: The occurrence and composition of manna in *Eucalyptus* and *Angophora*, *Proc Linn Soc NSW*, 90(2):152–156, 1965.

37. Brooker MG, Braithwaite RW, Estbergs JA: Foraging ecology of some insectivorous and nectarivorous species of birds in forests and woodlands of the wet-tropics of Australia, *Emu* 90:215–230, 1990.

38. Wolf P, Hablich A-C, Burkle M, et al: Basic data on food intake, nutrient digestibility and energy requirements of lorikeets, *J Anim Phys Anim Nutr* 91:282–288, 2007.

39. Cannon CE: Observations on the food and energy requirements of rainbow lorikeets, *Trichoglossus haematodus* (Aves:Psittacidae), *Aust Wildl Res* 6:337–346, 1979.

40. Complan website <www.complan.com>. Accessed Dec 2, 2011.

41. Hopper SD, Burbidge AA: Feeding behaviour of a purple-crowned lorikeet on flowers of *Eucalyptus prestium*, *Emu* 79:40–42, 1979.

42. Ford HA, Noske S, Bridges L: Foraging of birds in eucalypt woodland in north-eastern New South Wales, *Emu* 86:168–179, 1986.

43. Paton DC: The significance of pollen in the diet of the new Holland honeyeater, *Phylidonyris novaehollandiae* (Aves:Meliphagidae), *Aust J Zool* 29:217–224, 1981.

44. Cleland JB: Examination of contents of stomachs and crops of Australian birds, *Emu* 11:79–95, 1911.

45. Cleland JB: Lorikeets and the flowering of eucalypts, *S Aust Ornithol* 25:106–107, 1927.

46. Bosch J: The Papuan lory, *Charmosyna papou* (Scopoli) with particular details of the Mount Goliath or Stella lory, *Charmosyna papou goliathina* (Rothschild and Hartert), *Lori J Int* 3:49–72, 1994.

47. Turner V: *Banksia* pollen as a protein source in the diet of two Australian marsupials: *Cercartetus nanus* and *Tarsipes rostratus*, *Oikos* 43:53–61, 1984a.

48. Turner V: Eucalyptus pollen in the diet of the feathertail glider, *Acrobates pygmaeus*, *Aust Wild Res* 11:77–81, 1984b.

49. Stace P: Pollen quality-heath leaved *Banksia*, red cobbed *Banksia*, *Banksia ericifolia*, *Australas Beekeeper* 89:97–98, 1987.

50. Somerville DC: *Nutritional value of bee collected pollens*, Victoria, Australia, RIRDC, 2001.

51. Somerville DC and Nicol HI: Crude protein and amino acid composition of honey bee-collected pollen pellets from south-east Australia and a note on laboratory disparity, *Aust J Exp Agr* 46:141–149; 2006.

52. Bell RA, Thornber EJ, Seet JLL, et al: Composition and protein quality of honeybee-collected pollen of *Eucalyptus marginata* and *Eucalyptus calophylla*, *J Nutr* 113:2479–2484, 1983.

53. Van Tets IG: Can flower-feeding marsupials meet their nitrogen requirements on pollen in the field? *Aust Mamm* 20:383–390, 1998.

54. Van Tets IG, Hulbert AJ: A comparison of the nitrogen requirements of the eastern pygmy possum, *Cercartetus nanus*, on a pollen and on a mealworm diet, *Physiol Biochem Zool* 72(2):127–137, 1999.

55. Frankel TL: Faculty of Science, Technology and Engineering, School of Life Sciences, Department of Agricultural Sciences, La Trobe University, Bundoora, Melbourne. Accessed March 5, 2012.

56. Brice AT, Dahl KH, Grau CR: Pollen digestibility by hummingbirds and psittacines, *Condor* 91:681–688, 1989.

57. Delia D, Frankel TF: Protein digestion in rainbow lorikeets, *Trichoglossus haematodus*, *Asia Pac J Clin Nutr* 14(Suppl):S117, 2005.

58. Pryor GS: Protein requirements of three species of parrots with distinct dietary specializations, *Zoo Biol* 22:163–177, 2003.

59. Fleming PA, Moore TL: Do experimental methods affect estimates of pollen digestion by birds?, *Aust J Zool* 59 (6):407–415, 2012.

60. Roulston TH, Cane JH: Pollen nutritional content and digestibility for animals, *Plant Syst Evol* 222(1–4):187–209, 2000.

61. Wooller RD, Richardson KC, Pagendham CM: The digestion of pollen by some Australian birds, *Aust J Zool* 36:357–362, 1998.

62. Gartrell BD, Jones SM: Eucalyptus pollen grain emptying by two Australian nectarivorous psittacines, *J Avian Biol* 32:224–230, 2001.

63. Human H, Nicolson SW: Nutritional content of fresh bee-collected and stored pollen of *Aloe greatheadii* var. *davyana* (Asphodelaceae), *Phytochemistry* 67:1486–1492, 2006.

64. Arnould J: *Aspects of the diet of the eastern pygmy-possum Cercartetus nanus* (Desmarest., B.Sc. Hons Thesis, Monash University, Melbourne, Australia, 1986.

65. Frankel TL, Avram D: Protein requirements of rainbow lorikeets, *Trichoglossus haematodus*, *Aust J Zool* 49:435–443, 2001.

66. Delia D, Frankel TL: The activity of proteolytic enzymes in the rainbow lorikeet (*Trichoglossus haematodus*), *Proc Comp Nutr Soc* 27–31, 2006.

67. Grau CR, Roudybush TE: Protein requirement of growing cockatiels, *Proceedings of the 34th western poultry disease conference, March 3–6*, 107–108, 1985.

68. Cornejo J, Clubb S: Analysis of the maintenance diet offered to lories and lorikeets (Psittaciformes:Loriinae) at Loro Parque Fundacion, Tenerife, *Int Zoo Yearb*, 39:85–98, 2005.

69. Somerville DC: Lipid content of honey bee-collected pollen from south-east Australia, *Aust J Exp Agr* 45:1659–1661, 2005.

70. Brue RN: Nutrition. In Ritchie BW, Harrison GJ, Harrison LR, editors: *Avian medicine: principles and application*, Lake Worth, FL, 1994, Wingers Publishing, pp 63–95.

71. Somerville DC, Nicol HI: Mineral content of honey bee-collected pollen from southern New South Wales, *Aust J Exp Agr* 42:1131–1136, 2002.

72. Rosset KK, Hassler DN, Phalen DN: Determination of safe and adequate dietary calcium and vitamin D3 concentrations in a companion parrot. In *Proc AAV*, 239–242, 2000.

73. Kalmar ID, van Loon M, Burkle M, et al: Effect of dilution degree of commercial nectar and provision of fruit on food, energy and nutrient intake in two rainbow lorikeet subspecies, *Zoo Biol* 28:98–106, 2009.

74. Skadhauge E: *Osmoregulation in birds*, New York, 1981, Springer-Verlag.

75. Graubohm S: Comparative investigations on the chemical composition, palatability and digestibility of formulated, extruded diets for amazons, grey parrots and cockatoos, dissertation, Tierarztl. Hochsch., Hannover, 1998.

76. Sindel S, Gill J: *Australian lorikeets*. Experiences in the field and aviary, Austral, New South Wales, Australia, 1987, Singil Press.

77. Bosch J: The fairy lorikeet *Charmosyna pulchella* (G.R. Gray), *Lori J Int* 4:49–72, 1995.

78. Jensen KS: Experiences with the whiskered lorikeet, *Oreopsittacus arfaki major*, *Lori J Int* 9:81–84, 2000.

79. Hubers J: The only lory species in the Philippines, the Mount Apo lorikeet, *Trichoglossus johnstoniae*, *Lori J Int* 11:46–48, 2002.

80. Low R: The Musschenbroek's lorikeet, *Neopsittacus musschenbroekii*, *Lori J Int* 9:73–96, 2000.

81. Wierda J: What do we have for dinner today?, *Lori J Int* 9:31–39, 2000.

82. Jensen KS: Blue crowned lorikeet, *Vini australis*, *Lori J Int* 11:38–41, 2002.

83. Kreis P: Breeding and keeping of blue-streaked lories, *Eos reticulata*, *Lori J Int* 11:42–44, 2002.

84. Hubers J: (2006). Psittacidae lories. In Holland G, editor: *Encyclopaedia of aviculture*, Surrey, British Columbia, Canada, 2006, Hancock House Publishers, pp 292–296.

85. Sindel S, Gill J: *Australian lorikeets*. Experiences in the field and aviary (rev ed), Austral, New South Wales, Australia, 2007, Singil Press.

86. Holsheimer JP: Nutrition of lories and lorikeets, *Lori J Int* 3:9–12, 1992.

87. McDonald DL, Oldfield T: Dietary vitamin A requirements of lorikeets: how much is too much?, *Proc AAV Aust Comm Kakadu*, 83–86, 2004.

88. Park F: Vitamin A toxicosis in a lorikeet flock, *Vet Clin Exot Anim* 9:495–502, 2006.

89. McDonald DL, Oldfield T: Suspected hypervitaminosis A in lorikeets maintained on commercially formulated nectars: a case study, *Proc AAV Aust Comm*, Manly, New South Wales, Australia, 2003.

90. Koutsos EA, Tell LA, Woods LW, et al: Adult cockatiels at maintenance are more sensitive to diets containing excess vitamin A than to vitamin A deficient diets, *J Nutr* 43(4):26–30, 2003.

91. Koutsos EA, Klasing KC: Vitamin A nutrition of cockatiels, *Joint Nutrition Symposium*. Antwerp, Belgium, 2002.

NAVIGATING THE NUTRACEUTICAL INDUSTRY: A GUIDE TO HELP VETERINARIANS MAKE INFORMED CLINICAL DECISIONS

Michael Scott Echols

The blended word *nutraceutical* was coined by Dr. Stephen DeFelice in 1989 and comes from the words *nutrition* and *pharmaceutical*.[1] The name itself may conjure up many ideas of the composition and quality of products in this category. While the term nutraceutical is loosely applied to dietary supplements, herbal products, and other supplemental nutrients, it may also include specific diets and specially processed foods (including beverages, soups, and cereals) sometimes referred to as *functional foods*.[2] Functional foods have been described as "provides the body with required amounts of vitamins, fats, proteins, carbohydrates, etc., needed for healthy survival."[1] One author proposed that "when functional foods aid in the prevention of disease(s) and/or disorder(s) other than anemia, it is called a nutraceutical."[1] There is clear overlap in these definitions as a functional food could potentially provide necessary nutrients for survival of one animal and at the same time prevent or even treat a disease in another animal (nutraceutical). In the United States, the term nutraceutical has no legal meaning. The Food and Drug Administration (FDA) would categorize most products sold as nutraceuticals as one of four possibilities: drug, dietary supplement, food, or food additive. Health Canada also does not formally define a nutraceutical or functional food. However, the Bureau of Nutritional Sciences, the Food Directorate of Health Canada, has proposed the following definitions:

> A nutraceutical is a product isolated or purified from foods that is generally sold in medicinal forms not usually associated with food. A nutraceutical is demonstrated to have a physiological benefit or provide protection against chronic disease. A functional food is similar in appearance to, or may be a conventional food, is consumed as part of a usual diet, and is demonstrated to have physiological benefits and/or reduce the risk of chronic disease beyond basic nutritional functions.[3]

In Canada, there are no regulations that deal specifically with nutraceuticals or functional foods. In Canada, these nutrition products fall under either *foods* or *drugs* according to the provisions of the Food and Drugs Act and Regulations.[3]

More details on regulations pertaining to nutraceuticals will be defined later.

For the purposes of this portion of the chapter, nutraceutical(s) will be the term used to collectively describe nutritional supplements, herbals, vitamins, minerals, functional foods, probiotics, or other products that might be considered a supplemental nutritional product used in the maintenance of health and/or prevention or treatment of diseases. Because the vast majority of nutraceutical research is centered on human medicine with a secondary emphasis on laboratory and production animal and pet (dog) industries, there is little information on the use of these products in pet birds. There is even less information on animal-labeled nutraceutical quality with almost no attention paid to pet bird products. Because of these limitations, this article will focus on the nutraceutical industry as a whole and not specifically on bird-related products. As this chapter will elucidate, the nutraceutical industry often has vague legal boundaries, very much like its product definition. The purpose herein is to equip veterinary professionals with a better understanding of the convoluted nutraceutical industry and help guide informed product selection when nutraceuticals are being considered.

THE MONETARY VALUE OF THE NUTRACEUTICAL INDUSTRY

The nutraceutical industry has grown significantly in the past 20 years. According to the National Health and Nutrition Examination Survey (also known as NHANES) from 1999 to 2000, over 50% of American adults reported using nutraceuticals within the past 30 days.[4] Cohen similarly reported in 2009 that more than half of the adult population in the United States takes nutraceuticals.[5] Although the market region was not specified, one estimate said that the nutraceutical industry exceeded $20 billion in sales in 2005.[4] In 2012, nutraceutical sales in the United States reached $30 billion.[6] In 2014 Cohen reported that Americans spent $32 billion on over 85,000 different combinations of nutraceuticals.[7] Specific to the European Union, multivitamin and multimineral supplements represent half of the food supplement market, accounting for an estimated €5 billion in 2005 and greater than €6 billion in 2012 sales.[8] The value estimates and population percentage using nutraceuticals range significantly between markets and the year(s) reported. However, multimillion to multibillion dollar estimates and one half to three quarters of the market population using nutraceuticals are commonly described.[9]

THE ROLE OF NUTRITION IN DISEASE PREVENTION AND TREATMENT

The news is everywhere describing the role of nutraceuticals in disease prevention and sometimes even as treatments. There are truths and mistruths regarding these headlines. The facts are that many impressive studies have shown the value of nutraceuticals, especially in humans. Some of these studies have their origin in animals, which naturally leads to some conclusions favoring their use in pets. The problem is that well-designed studies that focus on the use of select nutraceuticals for use in animals under realistic (clinical and not laboratory or research) situations are far fewer in number, and these are even more rare pertinent to birds.

Selecting Nutraceutical Studies: Which Studies Have More Merit?

Well-designed nutraceutical studies are often long term, involve a large number of test participants, and use levels of nutrition products that exceed basic maintenance needs. With few exceptions, most nutrition-related diseases result from chronic nutritional deficiencies or excesses. Chronic degenerative diseases (e.g., atherosclerosis, stroke, cancer, arthritis) are the leading causes of illness and death in humans in all developed nations. Current health-based research is primarily focused on cause, prevention, and treatment of these chronic diseases. This research has included the role of nutrition.

Long-term dietary changes are often needed to detect statistically significant changes when evaluating the effects of nutraceutical supplementation in large populations with chronic diseases. The definition is debatable, but in terms of human nutraceutical studies, *long term* tends to be at least 6 months if not years to decades. These types of studies are often expensive and take a long time to collect the necessary data prior to publication. Most animal and pet supplement studies are short term, ranging from weeks to months.

With humans there are many variables affecting one's diet that can positively or negatively alter results with nutraceutical studies. These confounders include variation in diet, illness, activity level, exogenous chemical exposure (e.g., prescription and nonprescription medications, environmental contaminants/toxins), other lifestyle factors, and placebo effect. The more prevalent the studied nutraceutical may be in the diet (e.g., vitamin D) the larger the participant sample size needed. Less commonly encountered nutrients (e.g., glucosamine and uncommon herbals) may require fewer participants to draw significant conclusions, because these items may not naturally be in one's diet. The vast majority of animal nutraceutical studies involve small sample sizes.

Last, and not accounting for product quality (discussed later), is the actual dose of the nutraceutical being studied. The Dietary Reference Intake (DRI) is the most recent set of dietary recommendations made by the Food and Nutrition Board of the Institute of Medicine and provides several types of reference values,[10] one of which is the Recommended Daily Allowance (RDA). The RDA was established during World War II as a set of guidelines to meet nutrition requirements for 97.5% of the healthy individuals in each life stage and sex group (as determined in the United States). DRI values are set to prevent gross acute nutritional deficiency diseases (RDA), excessive dosages (Tolerable Upper Intake Levels or "UL"), and other basic nutrient guidelines. However, the RDA was not designed to determine nutrient values beneficial in preventing or treating chronic degenerative diseases.

Short- and long-term studies that dose nutraceuticals on known DRI numbers (especially RDA values) typically do not have much impact on chronic degenerative diseases. Large population, long-term studies that explore higher nutrient values that are within the UL often result in the most significant findings relating nutraceuticals to prevention or treatment of chronic degenerative disease. These findings may be inconclusive, positive, or negative, but carry more statistical significance than studies using any combination of small sample sizes, short duration, or DRI (especially RDA) values. While there are nutrition guidelines for commonly kept companion animals, there is very little information relating to birds beyond poultry species. There are few long-term studies on nutraceuticals in animals in general, but they rarely explore their effects on chronic degenerative diseases.

Nutraceutical Studies in Humans

Numerous impressive studies evaluating nutraceutical use in humans have been published over the past two decades. As discussed previously, strong statistical power in nutraceutical research is based on minimizing confounders and having large sample sizes, long-term use, and appropriate (often higher than most DRI values) product levels. These types of studies are rarely possible in animals because of shorter life-spans, high study costs, and other factors.

Omega-3 fatty acids

Research on omega-3 fatty acid supplementation has been shown to reduce risks of certain cardiovascular diseases (coronary artery disease, arrhythmias, and hypertension),[11,12] chronic renal disease,[13–17] and autoimmune diseases (rheumatoid arthritis)[18] and are important to the development of nervous and reproductive systems in humans.[19,20] The studies are seemingly endless, but point to the value of this one nutrient (omega-3 fatty acids) and its positive effects on significant diseases in humans.

Vitamin D

Vitamin D has been emerging in the literature as an extremely important nutrient. The fact that over 3000 binding sites for the vitamin D receptor have been found throughout the human genome (approximately 3% of the genome) supports the importance of this nutrient in gene regulation and ultimately disease expression.[21] Chowdhury et al[22] meta-analyzed 73 cohort studies (849,412 adult patients) and 22 randomized controlled trials (30,716 adult patients) reporting circulating vitamin D levels and/or vitamin D supplementation and causes of specific mortality outcomes. Their bottom line conclusions were as follows: (1) there is an inverse relationship between circulating 25-hydroxyvitamin D and risks of death from cardiovascular disease, cancer, and more and (2) vitamin D_3 supplementation significantly reduces overall mortality among older adults.[22]

Glucosamine

Two 3-year, randomized placebo-controlled studies using glucosamine sulfate showed that this nutrient alone improved symptoms (pain) and physical joint abnormalities over placebo in patients with osteoarthritis.[23,24] A combined total of 414 patients were given placebo or 1500 mg glucosamine sulfate daily. At the end of both studies, the glucosamine groups objectively showed no significant (radiographic) joint space narrowing whereas the placebo groups did.[23,24] Bruyere et al[25] more closely evaluated these two studies and specifically the results of 319 patients (of the 414 total) that were postmenopausal women. The authors concluded that results "demonstrated for the first time that a pharmacological intervention for osteoarthritis has a disease-modifying effect in this particular population, the most frequently affected by knee osteoarthritis."[25]

Folic acid and cyanocobalamin (vitamin B_{12})

A 2001 prospective study projected the health and economic impact of supplementing patients with known coronary heart disease (CHD) with folic acid and cyanocobalamin (vitamin B_{12}) above and beyond grain fortification.[26] The authors concluded that supplemental folic acid and B_{12} would reduce 310,000 CHD deaths over a 10-year period compared with current grain fortification levels. Additionally, the authors predicted that the supplement strategy would save $2 billion in medical costs.[26] These predictions and clinical statements by the authors could easily impress upon the public the value of the nutraceutical industry.[27,28] In a scientific review of studies on nutritional supplementation and disease from 1966 to 2002, the authors made the following conclusions[27]: "Inadequate intake of several vitamins has been linked to chronic diseases, including coronary heart disease, cancer and osteoporosis." and "Many physicians may be unaware of common food sources of vitamins or unsure which vitamins they should recommend for their patients." The authors then made the following clinical statements[28]: "Suboptimal folic acid levels, along with suboptimal levels of vitamins B_6 and B_{12}, are a risk factor for cardiovascular disease, neural tube defects, and colon and breast cancer; low levels of vitamin D contribute to osteopenia and fractures; and low levels of the antioxidant vitamins (vitamins A, E and C) may increase the risk for several chronic diseases." and "it appears prudent for all adults to take vitamin supplements." That support may be appropriate, overzealous, or inaccurate, depending on how it is presented.

Nutritional Supplement Studies in Animals

While there are not as many clinical studies on nutritional supplements in animals or such strong recommendations as noted earlier, animal and human literature are closely linked. This is partially fueled by the need for animal models for human diseases. Perhaps even more pressing is the desire to find disease prevention and treatment alternatives for the animals in our care. As discussed previously, the refereed literature does support some specific aspects of nutraceutical use. Similar or sometimes unrelated benefit claims are often carried over from human sources and applied to animal food and nutraceutical products. These claims may or may not have any correlation to published studies. As in human literature, there are numerous studies evaluating omega-3 fatty acids, glucosamine, vitamins, minerals, and other nutraceuticals in pets. However, good controlled studies on nutraceuticals that have clinical applications remain limited in most animals. Additionally, few toxicity or even optimal nutraceutical levels are reported.

Currently a disproportionately large number of nutraceutical animal studies evaluate omega series fatty acids. Much like in human literature, omega-3 fatty acids have been shown to favorably modify some renal diseases and have anti-arrhythmic effects as reported in (primarily) canine studies.[29–35] In terms of companion animals, the (primarily) canine literature includes studies demonstrating benefit of omega-3 fatty acids with atopic dermatitis and other "allergic" skin diseases, improving overall immune function, decreasing cancer cachexia, and prolonging disease-free intervals in dogs with neoplasia, decreasing joint inflammation, and improving eye and brain development.[35–47]

Most of the published nutraceutical work in avian species relates to nutritional needs of developing poultry and/or improving production standards (e.g., weight gain, egg laying). These studies tend to involve vitamins, minerals, probiotics, and enzymes, and are infrequently critically applied to companion or aviary birds. Newer studies evaluating omega-series fatty acids, involving pet and production birds, offer insights as to how some nutraceuticals can benefit captive avian species. Under various conditions, omega-3 fatty acid supplementation may positively alter body fatty acid composition, decrease serum triglycerides and cholesterol, increase bone mineral density and thickness, relate to and improve brain development and learning, decrease risk of select cancers and their development, decrease associated risk of atherosclerosis, and improve hepatic metabolism and egg laying.[48–58] While the purpose of this chapter is to better explain the nutraceutical industry and not specific products for use in animals, these referenced studies show increased interest in critically evaluating select products in birds. It is likely that with time, well designed nutraceutical studies in birds will increase in the refereed literature.

NUTRACEUTICAL INDUSTRY REGULATION

United States

While dietary supplements are "intended to supplement a normal diet" they are unlike drugs, which require FDA regulation.[59] This lack of FDA regulation has brought up serious concerns within the industry.

Nutraceuticals are legally defined as *foods* according to the Dietary Supplement Health and Education Act (DSHEA) of 1994.[60] The regulations governing dietary supplement manufacturing are for food-grade products and mimic the guidelines for the production of candies, pizza, and so forth. As a result, dietary supplements are not required to go through rigorous testing and guarantees like over the counter (OTC) drugs. These guarantees include proving potency (what is on the label is in the bottle), disintegration (the product will dissolve in a time considered normal for digestion), and uniformity (each pill, bottle, and lot are the same). Also, unlike OTC drugs, there is no requirement that supplement manufacturers demonstrate product efficacy or safety prior to market sale.[61]

According to the Federal Food, Drug, and Cosmetic Act, "foods are products used for food while drugs are products intended to diagnose, treat, cure or prevent disease."[60] Furthermore, foods are "assumed to be safe" and are "eaten primarily for taste, aroma, and nutritive value." Drugs are "intended for therapeutic benefits, and must be proven in clinical trials to provide those benefits."

DSHEA was established to be the first "regulatory structure that applies specifically to dietary supplements."[60] This act has proven to be a watershed for the dietary supplement industry in the United States and has significantly helped drive the continued expansion of the market. While it may seem that DSHEA has provided a regulatory structure for the supplement industry (and it has to some degree), this act has not necessarily guaranteed protection to the consuming public. DSHEA has grandfathered in all dietary supplement ingredients marketed in the United States before October 15, 1994, just as food additive amendments grandfathered in food additives already on the market before 1958. Before marketing a supplement containing a new dietary ingredient, the manufacturer must determine that the ingredient is "reasonably expected to be safe." However, no formal approval by the FDA is required prior to marketing the new dietary ingredient.[60]

DSHEA added new safety provisions specifying that a dietary supplement is adulterated if it presents a significant or unreasonable risk of illness or injury when used according to label directions. DSHEA provides that the FDA will bear the burden of proof in any court action claiming that a product is adulterated. This has always been the FDA's burden in a formal enforcement action.[60] The DSHEA assumes that nutraceuticals are safe until proven otherwise, creating a façade of safety for both legal and illegal dietary supplements.[7,62] In essence DSHEA helped spawn the massive growth of the dietary supplement industry by grandfathering in products and limiting regulation. The FDA is not required to regulate nutritional supplements and it becomes the FDA's burden to prove fault with the product in question. In this light, DSHEA presents serious obstacles to the FDA's ability to detect and eliminate contaminated supplements.[5]

New Rules from the United States Department of Agriculture

In June 2007, the United States Department of Agriculture (USDA) issued the final rule establishing regulations to require current good manufacturing practices (cGMPs) for dietary supplements. The cGMP's final rule requires that proper controls are in place for dietary supplements so that they are processed in a consistent manner and meet quality standards.[63] These cGMPs apply to all domestic and foreign companies that manufacture, package, label, or hold dietary supplements, including those involved with the activities of testing, quality control, packaging and labeling, and distributing them in the United States. This rule establishes cGMPs for industry-wide use that require that dietary supplements are manufactured consistently regarding identity, purity, strength, and composition. The requirements also include provisions related to the design and construction of physical plants that facilitate maintenance, cleaning, proper manufacturing operations, quality control procedures, testing final product or incoming and in-process materials, handling consumer complaints, and maintaining records.

While the rules have been set in place, an enforcement policy has not been established (other than for products containing unapproved regulated substances). Whether or not dietary supplement manufacturers will adhere to these new guidelines has been called into question. Per Harel et al, the "FDA has found violations of good manufacturing practices to be rampant in nearly half of the domestic dietary supplement firms it has inspected."[64] Additionally noted was that a "recent investigation by the Office of the Inspector General determined that the FDA does not possess accurate contact information for 20% of supplement manufacturers."[64] Cohen noted that while manufacturers in the United States are required to report supplement-associated adverse events to the FDA, "the great majority of the estimated 50,000 adverse events that occur annually remain unreported."[5] Clearly, the manufacturing deficits (and consequences described later in this chapter) are significant and pervasive.

Permissible Health Claims

Contrary to claims often published on labels, the FDA only allows a small number of health claims by manufacturers of nutraceutical products.[65] At least in the United States, any claims beyond those specifically spelled out by the FDA are nonpermissible. These claims primarily pertain to human health. This means that animal health claims listed on products marketed for pets are also, primarily, nonpermissible.

Canada

Under the Canadian Food and Drugs Act and Regulations, nutraceuticals would by default fall into either a food or drug category.[3] A food is defined as "any article manufactured, sold or represented for use as food or drink by man, chewing gum, and any ingredient that may be mixed with food for any purpose whatever."[3] A drug is defined as "any substance or mixture of substances manufactured, sold or represented for use in the diagnosis, treatment, mitigation or prevention of a disease, disorder, abnormal physical state, or the symptoms thereof, in man or animal, restoring, correcting or modifying organic functions in man or animal or, disinfection in premises in which food is manufactured, prepared or kept."[3] Based on the claims of many products, nutraceuticals may be defined as drugs in Canada. Canadian drugs authorized for sale must meet regulatory requirements for efficacy and carry a Drug Identification Number or General Public number on the label. Specifically, this number is located on the label of any drug product that has been approved for sale. It indicates that a product has undergone and passed a review of its formulation, labeling, and instructions for use. Because a nutraceutical product may have a role in modifying the course of a disease, manufacturers have two options: (1) market their product with no health claims or (2) follow stringent regulatory requirements for drugs. In relation to the rest of the developed world, Canadian regulations and policies are approximately equivalent to the European Union and the Australia and New Zealand Food Authority, but are more restrictive than in the United States and Japan.[3]

Other Countries

Most, if not all, developed countries mention or have specific provisions and/or laws that pertain to nutraceuticals. The Japanese Nutrition Improvement Law, Australia and New Zealand Food Authority, and the General Principles of Food Law in the European Union article outline specific guidelines relating (either directly or indirectly) to nutraceuticals in their respective country or region. The Codex Alimentarius Commission is the intergovernmental food standards setting organization with 162 member countries and also has some guidelines pertaining to nutraceuticals. For specific details about rules and regulations concerning nutraceuticals in markets not mentioned, the reader is encouraged to contact national governmental departments that handle foods or specifically nutraceuticals.

CURRENT RESEARCH ON THE QUALITY OF NUTRACEUTICALS

Numerous studies on product quality have unfortunately brought up serious concerns. Foster outlined a long history of nutraceutical adulteration that goes back nearly 2000 years, and the issue of questionable product quality is not new.[66] However, presently we now have readily available testing methodologies and published research that more clearly proves or disputes nutraceutical product quality claims. The laws governing nutraceuticals within countries or regions and pertinent to the type of product in question can vary dramatically. Regulations on nutraceuticals sold within North America are generally considered to be poor. Russell et al wrote that glucosamine supplements sold in Canada are "not subject to even rudimentary checks on purity."[67] In contrast glucosamine is regarded as a medication in Europe and is "thus subject to the usual quality controls."[67] These types of variables must be considered in product choice and use, as quality controls may vary significantly between markets. In addition to regulations pertinent to the product in the country of sale are the laws within the country of origin. Some products are manufactured with different standards for differing countries of sale, even by the same company. Although some studied products manufactured in China had higher levels of mercury and aluminum compared with samples originating from other countries,[5,9] these types of product quality issues appear to be prevalent throughout the industry.

Recalls

At least in the United States, the FDA may recall nutraceuticals based on manufacturer spot inspections, adverse event reports generated by consumers and physicians, tips of potentially adulterated products by retailers, and more.[64] Because nutraceuticals are not required to undergo stringent FDA review prior to reaching market, problems are often identified long after products have been sold to the public. While not regulated as drugs, nutraceuticals are categorized in FDA Enforcement Reports if found to contain unapproved regulated substances.[64] The FDA initiates class I drug recalls when the product contains a drug that has a reasonable possibility of causing serious adverse health consequences or death.[68] From January 1, 2004 through December 19, 2012, approximately half (237 of 465 [51%]) of all FDA class I drug recalls involved nutraceuticals adulterated with banned pharmaceuticals.[64] Of the recalled nutraceuticals, 175 (74%) were manufactured in the United States. Most of these recalls involve drug-contaminated sexual enhancement, body building, and weight loss nutraceuticals and do not necessarily pertain to animal products.[64] Recent research by Cohen et al showed that 18 of 27 (67%) previously FDA-recalled nutraceuticals still contained at least one pharmaceutical adulterant. The nutraceuticals were still available for sale and were selected for the study at least 6 months after the recall. Seventeen of the previously recalled products (63%) still contained the same drug adulterant originally identified by the FDA.[68]

Adulteration versus Contamination

Many of the studies that evaluate nutraceuticals for extra-label ingredients describe adulteration and/or contamination. These are two very different issues that affect nutraceuticals. Whitsitt et al distinguished the two terms:

> Adulteration—to make impure by adding foreign, extraneous, poisonous, insanitary, or inferior substances/ingredients to a food product; a food is adulterated if it fails to meet federal standards. Contamination—an element, substance, compound, or mixture which upon exposure is reasonably anticipated to cause serious medical conditions; a chemical, biological, radiological, degradant, or decomposition material, waste material, or physical element which makes food unfit for human consumption.[6]

In essence, adulteration involves the purposeful addition of an undeclared ingredient and contamination results from accidental inclusion of undeclared ingredients.

Vitamins and minerals

Vitamins and mineral nutraceuticals are those composed primarily of generally recognized micronutrients considered essential for life and may include trace and ultratrace nutrients. The nutrients may be represented as pure (such as vitamin B_{12} or cobalamin) or as a complex with another nutrient, nutrients, or non-nutrient carrier (such as calcium as calcium carbonate). Vitamins and minerals are generally listed by their common name (iodine), chemical name (potassium iodide), amount (e.g., μg, mg, g, IU) and relation to the daily value (DV; or average levels of nutrients for a person eating 2000 calories a day). Serving size and/or dosing recommendations are usually listed. Of course many of these DVs are not established for animals or listed on pet product labels. Specific forms of ingredients (i.e., d- or dl-α-tocopherol) may be named in the supplement facts or ingredient section of the label.[4] Common formulations include tablets, dry and gel capsules, free powder, and stick powder. In one review of vitamin E capsules from large chain pharmacies and specialty food retail stores in Toronto, 59% to 158% variation from label claim was noted, and only one product was within 10% of its stated dose.[69] Ninety percent of 27 products of calcium supplements sold in Pakistan exceeded California daily dose limits of lead.[70] Elevated lead, strontium, aluminum, cadmium, copper, and/or arsenic were found in tested calcium supplements, multiminerals, and multivitamins in a number of studies, many with lead levels exceeding California lead limits.[71-76] Failure for vitamin supplements to dissolve (meet dissolution standards) has been described with folic acid.[77,78]

Fatty acids

The omega series (primarily omegas 3, 6, and 9) fatty acids have been intensively studied and recognized for their primary and secondary roles in many biochemical reactions and health parameters. Depending on the specific form and the animal in question, the omega series fatty acids are often considered essential as the body must obtain either their precursor or final form from the diet. For example, docosahexaenoic acid (DHA) and eicosapentaenoic acid (EPA), also known as the "fish oils," are considered truly essential to domestic cats who cannot convert these fatty acids from the plant-based precursor α-linolenic acid (ALA). As a general rule the more herbivorous the animal the better its conversion from ALA to DHA and/or EPA. The converse is true of carnivorous animals who are generally poor converters.

Omega-6 series fatty acids (linoleic acid [LA] is the principle physiologic form and comes primarily from plant-based sources and plant-eating animal tissue) often have opposing functions to omega-3 series fats. Omega-9 series fatty acids (including oleic acid and erucic acid) commonly come from plant oils and animal fat. Omega-9 fatty acids are often not considered essential because many animals can construct these fats from unsaturated fat. Studies on omega-3 and omega-6 fatty acid supplementation are extensive in mammals. Additionally, there are numerous studies on both fatty acid types in birds, primarily in poultry species. The value and role(s) of omega-9 fatty acids in birds have yet to be clearly defined.

Omega series fatty acids are most often listed by their form (e.g., ALA, DHA, LA) and in milligram amounts. Serving size and/or dose recommendations are often included. These fatty acids may be packaged in gel capsules (preferred form for stability reasons), gel sticks, dry powder, pump and pour-on bottles, and more. DHA and EPA are highly unstable and currently best kept in gel capsules. All fatty acid supplements should be stored in dark cool locations and in tightly sealed bottles or capsules to slow oxidation.

With some exceptions, most studies on fatty acid quality pertain to contaminants. In particular, persistent organic pollutants (POPs) are of greatest concern as these toxic compounds bioaccumulate and biomagnify in animal tissues, particularly marine species.[19] While plants can also contain POPs, these organic compounds are typically deposited on the leafy portions of the plants and are not bioaccumulative and do not magnify as is common with predator species.[19] POP exposure is associated with a host of problems including endocrine disruptions; cancer; and neurobehavioral, reproductive, and developmental disturbances in humans and animals.[19,20] Contamination with polychlorinated biphenyls, organochlorinated pesticides, polybrominated diphenyl ethers, pristine, squalene, unresolved complex mixtures, aryl hydrocarbon receptor agonist (digoxin-like), polychlorinated dibenzo-p-dioxins/furans was noted in a number of studies of fish oils and omega-3 fatty acid supplements.[20,79-84] In 2004 ConsumerLab.com, an independent reviewer of nutraceuticals, reported that 6 of 20 omega-3 fatty acid products did not contain the label-stated amount of one or more essential fatty acids. The website stated "two of the products that failed made claims on their labels that their 'potency' had been 'tested' or 'verified'."[85] In a 2014 revised review of 30 omega-3 fatty acid supplements, ConsumerLab.com reported that five products failed to meet basic quality testing.[86]

Botanicals

Botanical, plant-based, or *herbal* nutraceuticals are those derived primarily from plants or less commonly fungi (while not truly plants). Botanicals are often listed by the common and scientific name of the ingredients and include which portion of the plant or fungi (e.g., leaf, stem, root) and in which form (e.g., whole, crushed, powdered, suspended, extracted). Some labels will include the active ingredient associated with the botanical product. The active ingredient(s) may or may not be known, because many botanicals are taken for a wide range of potential benefits. Serving size and/or dosing recommendations are also commonly listed. Sometimes the proven or known active ingredient is listed in addition to the genus and species of the plant/fungus. Total weight (usually milligrams or grams) is given for a specified dose. Common formulations include capsules, powder, gel capsules, liquid extracts, and free (whole or part form) product. Of the nutraceutical groups presented in this chapter, botanicals tend to have a higher rate of problems including inaccurate labeling, and contamination. Authors of papers studying botanicals (and other nutraceuticals) often comment on the poor quality of the products examined. Standardization of ingredients is inherently a serious and challenging problem. As Garrard et al pointed out, standardization of herbal ingredients may be "a practical impossibility."[87] Plants are composed of a number of chemical components, each of which has varying levels of biological activity. The portion of the plant used, growing and harvest conditions, and formulation (e.g., tea, extract, tablet) can all affect biologic activity. Garrard et al further stated "on a gram-per-gram basis, even products using the same plant parts may not be bioequivalent."[87]

For example, the authors of an Echinacea study came to the following conclusion: "Echinacea from retail stores often does not contain the labeled species. A claim of 'standardization' does not mean the preparation is accurately labeled, nor does it indicate less variability in concentration of constituents of the herb."[88] Bennet and Balick found that in a PubMed search of 100 titles or abstracts on medicinal plants, 20% contained taxonomic errors.[89] These errors may seem minor, but they actually make it impossible to search electronic databases for information on species. As stated by the authors, "An inexcusable error is to misspell binomials." Misspellings, lack of author citations, and other problems noted by the authors confound clinical studies and their interpretation, which dramatically decreases their scientific value. While some studies cite vouchers and botanical specimens deposited in herbaria, many recent investigations do not. Voucher specimens are essential to medicinal plant studies and are considered more important than correct identification, because erroneous scientific names can be modified to reflect new taxonomic circumscriptions.[89] Regardless of how well the study was designed or results reported, taxonomic errors can make it impossible to interpret the data of botanical studies because the substance studied may not truly be known.[90] Label claim versus actual ingredients varied widely in studies of saw palmetto products, ranging from 9.9% to 460.4%[91] and 2.6% to 241%.[69] Forty-three percent of mixed herbal products were consistent with a benchmark in ingredients and daily dose, 20% in ingredients only, and 37% were either not consistent or label information was insufficient.[87] Only 52% of the preparations of Echinacea contained the species listed, while 47% failed to contain the specific species noted on the label.[88] Ten percent of the products studied contained no Echinacea whatsoever. In a study of label claim versus actual ingredients of American skullcap (*Scutellaria teriflora* [SLDS]) and Chinese skullcap (*Scutellaria baicalensis)*, the authors concluded that "consumers cannot depend on manufacturers and distributors for the quality SLDS, and should not use SLDS until all the SLDS in the US market are properly regulated and tested."[92] Seventy-five percent of mixed botanical products exceeded the Chinese limit for inorganic arsenic in dietary supplements.

In addition to reported pharmaceutical adulterants causing serious health conditions, the effects of harmful botanical contaminants in nutraceuticals has to be considered.[5,7] Synthetic hypertensive drugs were found adulterating antihypertensive botanicals in 26% of the studied 35 products.[92] In one circumstance of digoxin toxicosis after consumption of contaminated botanical dietary supplements, the authors made the following comment: "the FDA bear the burden of proof that a marketed dietary supplement presents a serious or unreasonable risk under the conditions of use on the label or as commonly consumed" and "this requirement is in contrast to what is required of drugs, which must be shown to be safe and effective for a particular indication before they are approved for marketing."[93]

Miscellaneous nutraceuticals

This last category covers nutraceuticals that do not neatly fit into vitamins and minerals, fatty acids, or botanicals. Because of their popularity, joint health and probiotic products are discussed in this section. Homeopathic remedies are specifically excluded from this discussion because of the nature of their makeup, consisting of significantly diluted ingredients (in an alcohol or other base to create a "mother tincture") to the point that they may be nondetectable. As a result, homeopathics are difficult to test, especially since their ingredients may be largely undetectable. This is not to say that homeopathic products have no value, but they are excluded for these reasons.

Joint health product labels are similar to those of vitamins and minerals. Joint health products generally list the serving size and/or dosing recommendations, common name of the ingredients (shark cartilage), chemical name (chondroitin sulfate), amount (most often milligrams or grams), and relation to the DV, which is usually nothing because DVs have not been established for most of the *active* ingredients of joint health products. As described earlier, most of these DVs are not established for animals or pets, and they are not listed on pet product labels. Specific forms or sources of ingredients (vegetarian glucosamine [HCL]) may be named in the supplement facts or ingredient section of the label. Common formulations include tablets, dry and gel capsules, and free powder. In label claims versus ingredient studies of oral glucosamine products for horses, tested contents ranged from 0% to 221% of label claim. 61% were considered adequate based on tested amount and label claim, and 17% of the products had less than 30% of the label claim.[94] In another study of 14 glucosamine products, ingredients ranged from 25% to 115% label claim, 53% had less than 40% of label claim, and two of the three most expensive products had less than 10% of label claim.[95] Similar inconsistency was found in a Canadian study of 14 products, with 41% to 108% range from label claim, and all but two products had less than 67% of label claim.[67] In a study of 16 products of shark cartilage powder, 15 of 16 (94%) had cyanobacterial neurotoxin b-*N*-methylamino-l-alanine levels from 86 to 265 µg/g dry product, and all samples had *N*-(2-aminoethyl) glycine, 2,4-diaminobutyric acid, and mercury.[96] After reviewing chondroitin nutraceuticals, Volpi wrote:

> Due to the poor chondroitin sulfate quality of some nutraceuticals, we conclude that stricter regulations regarding their quality control should be introduced to guarantee the manufacture of high quality products for nutraceutical utilization and to protect customers from low-quality, ineffective and potentially dangerous products.[97]

Probiotic labels most often list the serving size and/or dosing recommendations, bacterial component(s) genus, and sometimes species (*Lactobacillus)*, strain (Bifidobacterium BB-12), and amount per serving (in terms of cells or colony-forming bacteria). Weese noted that strain identification is important as "beneficial effects can vary among strains of a given species."[98] Probiotics may be sold as pills, tablets, free, stick powders, and more. Drago et al noted many studies evaluating the quality of South African, Australian, American, Asian, and European probiotics show widespread lack of accuracy and identification of tested microorganisms and "many products were labeled with fictitious names or bacteria were misidentified or strain identity was often missing."[99] In one probiotic study, 33% of the products tested contained the bacteria listed, and only 56% contained sufficient bacterial for a probiotic effect. Thirty-three percent of the studied products contained no detectable bacteria. Somewhat similar findings have been also reported in other studies comparing label claims versus actual ingredients[99,100] or label scrutiny-only studies.[98]

As with botanicals and all of the other nutraceuticals, many authors make similar comments about the poor quality of the products they have specifically studied. ConsumerLab.com has specifically evaluated glucosamine and/or chondroitin-containing pet products. According to the report, the following statement was made: "Shockingly, no chondroitin sulfate could be detected in two pet supplements despite each displaying a 'guaranteed analysis' showing a significant amount of chondroitin sulfate."[101] Several years later (2007), ConsumerLab.com performed a similar study of joint products. This time, 73% of the chondroitin-containing products failed. Three of the six veterinary/pet joint health products failed because only 47.2, 2.1, and 0.7% of the label claim of chondroitin was actually in the product.[102]

THE EFFECT OF POOR NUTRACEUTICAL QUALITY ON RESEARCH

It is indisputable that proper nutrition is an essential component to health. With the well-documented problems pertaining to nutraceutical product quality, the validity of studies using these products needs to be questioned. There are several aspects to research studies that ensure obtaining reliable results, including but not limited to a proper research method that is reproducible, controls for variables, and limits bias. Specific to nutraceutical research and assuming proper methodology and other factors are controlled, the studied product must contain known and standardized ingredients. This single variable, given its due attention, can invalidate research studies that use nutraceuticals as part of their study design. Unless the nutraceutical composition is somehow validated and contaminants controlled, research using nonpharmaceutical grade nutraceuticals should be expected to have more potentially significant variable findings between comparable studies. Yetley commented that "label declarations of vitamin mineral content are often used as surrogates for actual levels."[103] Additionally the author noted that bioavailability and bioequivalence for nutraceuticals lack standard scientific and regulatory definitions, dissolution guidelines are voluntary, and drug–nutraceutical interactions are poorly researched. Because of these significant variables, Yetley concluded that it is "problematic" to directly compare results across (nutraceutical) studies.[103] The simple fact is that research using nonvalidated products is difficult to interpret. Oke et al made the comment "variable quality of supplements could hamper both objective and anecdotal assessment of the efficacy of commercial glucosamine products in clinical studies."[94] While the comment was directed to a specific type of nutraceutical (glucosamine), the statement is applicable to any such products used in research. Research evaluating nutraceutical research (meta-analyses) is becoming more common as a means to produce statistically stronger results than those accomplished via individual studies. Even with these analyses, heterogeneity in results between studies has been attributed to poor product quality and bias.[104,105]

HOW TO SELECT HIGH QUALITY NUTRACEUTICALS

Nutraceuticals are subject to cGMPs, which are very different from drug GMPs. DSHEA has placed nutraceuticals under the general umbrella of foods and not drugs. As a simplified comparison between foods and drugs, there is no guarantee how much icing will be on a cupcake, but a 500 mg amoxicillin tablet should contain 500 mg of amoxicillin (within an acceptable and published tolerance range).

According to the FDA's website[106]:

Under DSHEA, a firm is responsible for determining that the dietary supplements it manufactures or distributes are safe and that any representations or claims made about them are substantiated by adequate evidence to show that they are not false or misleading. This means that dietary supplements do not need approval from FDA before they are marketed.

Except in the case of a new dietary ingredient, where premarket review for safety data and other information is required by law, a firm does not have to provide FDA with the evidence it relies on to substantiate safety or effectiveness before or after it markets its products.

There is no authoritative list of dietary ingredients that were marketed before October 15, 1994. Therefore, manufacturers and distributors are responsible for determining if a dietary ingredient is 'new,' and if it is not, for documenting that the dietary supplements its sells, containing the dietary ingredient, were marketed before October 15, 1994.

With the minimal regulation, lack of enforcement, and reliance upon the nutraceutical manufacturer to inform the public about product safety and efficacy, there are some steps that consumers can take to try to assure safety and guaranteed content above and beyond the manufacturer's guarantee:

1. *Look for the "Meets USP Specifications for Potency, Uniformity and Disintegration, Where Applicable" label on the nutraceutical as a minimum.* These guidelines are voluntarily met by nutraceutical manufacturers. According to their website "The U.S. Pharmacopeial Convention (USP) is a scientific nonprofit organization that sets standards for the identity, strength, quality, and purity of medicines, food ingredients, and dietary supplements manufactured, distributed, and consumed worldwide. USP's drug standards are enforceable in the United States by the FDA, and these standards are used in more than 140 countries."[107] USP is the single most universally recognized standards organization and has even set standards, such as disintegration and dissolution, for most nutritional supplements.[103] While some nutritional supplements (particularly herbal/plant-based products) do not yet have complete USP standards, following USP guidelines implies that the manufacturer is making efforts to guarantee that what is on the label is in the product (potency); the product will dissolve in a time normal for digestion (disintegration); and that each pill, capsule, and so forth is the same throughout the bottle and product lot (uniformity).[108]

2. *Determine if the company manufacturing the supplements follows GMPs for drug standards, and not just food or nutraceutical standards.* This is voluntary on the part of supplement manufacturers. According to DSHEA, supplement manufacturers are

required to follow food GMPs. The newer FDA rules (as of 2007) set cGMP standards for nutraceuticals, which again are intended to ensure basic safety. However, the most current cGMPs do not guarantee the standards set by drug GMPs. The FDA nutraceutical guidelines are found under 21 CFR Part 111.[109] Specifically, they determine whether the supplement manufacturer follows the Code of Federal Regulations (21 CFR) Parts 210 and 211—the drug grade manufacturing codes.[110,111]

3. *Determine if the supplement manufacturer is currently regulated, reprimanded, or otherwise inspected by a governmental agency.* Depending on the country of sale, governmental regulation may be required, result from prior failed inspections, or be requested by the nutraceutical company. For example, nutraceutical manufacturers selling products in Australia are required by the Therapeutic Goods Administration (TGA) to follow GMPs similar to the FDA's drug GMPs. TGA regularly inspects and audits a nutraceutical manufacturer's facilities and company (if separate) if they sell products within Australian markets. Consumers can ask for current certificates of any applicable governmental inspections.

   If a facility has received a governmental warning or recall, you can often find out via the Internet. Consumer-Lab.com has compiled a list of recalls and FDA warning letters pertaining to dietary supplement manufacturers that can be found at www.consumerlabs.com/recalls.asp.[112] You can also go directly to the FDA's Inspections, Compliance, Enforcement, and Criminal Investigations web page.[113] The FDA openly displays warning letters written to companies and manufacturers in violation, many of which are directed at nutraceutical manufacturers and parent companies. Although rare, some nutraceutical companies may voluntarily apply for governmental inspection in markets that do not require such action. Even though the FDA does not generally regulate nutraceuticals, a company can become a U.S. FDA drug-approved establishment for the manufacture of pharmaceuticals if willing to meet all of the necessary requirements. These "FDA-approved" companies may not manufacture pharmaceuticals but must uphold the same standards as FDA-approved drugs for their nutraceuticals. Consumers can contact nutraceutical manufacturers to see if they claim to follow additional governmental standards and obtain proof of issuance.

4. *Look for companies that have third-party verification.* Most nutraceutical manufacturers have various quality control production standards. Many are set in the cGMP or other governmental mandated standards. These in-house standards are important. However, it is entirely at the manufacturer's discretion to determine what those standards are and if they are actually met. Whether good or bad, in-house quality control standards are at great risk of bias. Companies that submit their products and manufacturing plant to third-party evaluation and verification provide better evidence of product quality to the public. Several companies have created dietary supplement testing and verification programs to fill this need. Of the numerous verification programs currently available, the following are subjectively better recognized:

NSF Certification

The NSF was founded in 1944 and acts an "an independent, accredited organization, (we) develop standards, and test and certify products and systems." Several levels of NSF testing are available and it arguably has the most stringent requirements for a company to pass certification. Two to three levels of certification pertain to most nutraceuticals.

NSF Dietary Supplement Certification "ensures that dietary supplements do not contain unacceptable levels of contaminants."[114] This program is the least stringent but acts as a safeguard against unsafe product contamination for participating companies.

The NSF Certified for Sport "program certifies that what is on the label is in the bottle and that the product does not contain unsafe levels of contaminants" and "banned or prohibited substances such as narcotics, steroids, stimulants, hormones and other related substances along with diuretics and other masking agents."[115] The NSF Certified for Sport program has been adopted by numerous professional, Olympic, and collegiate athletic programs as a way to protect their athletes from poor product quality and banned substances that could harm one's body and career. Products Certified for Sport are regularly tested in batches and stored for later additional testing as needed. This program is currently the most comprehensive third-party testing for dietary supplements (whether for athletes or the general public). Participating companies can be found on the NSF Certified for Sport Products website.[116]

Companies can also submit to become an "NSF-Certified GMP Facility." Participating companies can be found by going to http://info.nsf.org/Certified/GMP/.[117] NSF-certified products may or may not bear the NSF mark. The mark is a paid requirement and does not imply any additional testing over other participating products not bearing the mark. NSF charges manufacturers for their services.

USP Verification Services

USP offers two levels of verification that may apply to most nutraceuticals. This is the same company that sets standards for pharmaceuticals and nutraceuticals outlined above. The USP Dietary Supplement Verification Program is a "voluntary program open to manufacturers of dietary supplement finished products from around the world."[118] The USP Verified Dietary Ingredients program "verifies active and inactive ingredients used in the manufacture of dietary supplements, including: amino acids, botanical extracts, nonbotanicals, fine chemicals, vitamins and minerals."[119]

With both USP Dietary Supplement Verification Program and USP Dietary Verified Ingredients, participating companies pay for the service and can show the appropriate mark on the product's container.

Both the NSF and USP programs do not specifically test pet nutraceuticals or necessarily all of a participating company's products. However, companies that do go through one or more of the above certifications are participating in verification above and beyond what is required. Additionally, products produced in the same facility at approximately the same time as those that pass the above testing can reasonably be assured to be of similar quality. Products produced in different facilities as those that pass this testing may have different production quality standards.

Other Nutraceutical Testing Organizations

Informed-Choice (informed-choice.org) "is a quality assurance program for sports nutrition products, suppliers to the sports nutrition industry, and supplement-manufacturing facilities. The program certifies that all nutritional supplements and/or ingredients that bear the Informed-Choice logo have been tested for banned substances by the world class sports anti-doping lab, LGC."[120] The website can be searched for participating companies. Fewer companies participate in Informed-Choice testing compared with the other programs mentioned, putting those companies in a more "elite" category. Pet supplements are not evaluated. However, Informed-Choice testing does offer insight into companies that might also produce nutraceuticals for animals.

ConsumerLab.com is a popular, paid subscription-based company that randomly tests a variety of parameters of commercially available nutraceuticals. Their mission is "to identify the best quality health and nutritional products through independent testing."[121] Nutraceuticals are randomly pulled "off the shelf" and tested for potency, contaminants, labeling infractions, and/or more features and conveniently grouped by product type. Specific products, manufacturers, and recalls can be searched through the website. While most of the products tested are for the human market, some pet nutraceuticals are examined and results reported. Because of the random testing, there are often inconsistent nutraceutical brands reported on sequential reports. Additionally, the same product may pass the ConsumerLab.com tests on one report and fail on another. This only highlights manufacturing inconsistencies that seem to be common with some nutraceuticals. However, the website serves as a good resource for consumers to scan many currently available products.

The National Animal Supplement Council (NASC) is a "non-profit industry group dedicated to protecting and enhancing the health of companion animals and horses throughout the United States."[122] Per their website "Purchasing products from NASC members is the best way consumers can support efforts to improve the quality of animal health supplements and ensure the continued availability of these products in the US market." While manufacturers must submit to a successful independent facility audit, specific product testing for potency, contaminants, and the like is not part of the program.

SUMMARY

There is, justifiably, tremendous interest in the role of nutraceuticals and disease prevention and even treatment. The interest has been generated by the wealth of studies supporting conscientious nutritional supplement use in humans and to a lesser degree in companion animals. This, along with an ever-increasing human animal bond, has driven consumers to look for preventative measures and alternative health-care solutions that frequently include nutraceuticals for family companion and other animals.

Consumers and researchers need to be educated in their choices of nutraceuticals. In reality, most nutraceuticals are not manufactured, researched, marketed, regulated, or enforced in the same manner as are drugs. Limited studies on potency, contaminants, adulterants, toxicities, and true benefits currently limit those nutraceuticals that would be considered safe and efficacious for companion animals. Those that can educate themselves and consumers and guide selection and use of reliable and guaranteed nutraceuticals stand to gain from this incredible market in terms of personal and patient health, research, and even financial gain. Future studies will likely greatly expand our knowledge of this field and interested readers are encouraged to stay current with the literature.

Disclosure from the Author

The author has been directly involved with various aspects of the nutraceutical industry including as a paid consultant, product distributor, and educator for numerous organizations (private and industry-specific companies, secondary education schools, nonprofits, and more) dealing with human and animal health. The author declares no known association with any regulatory body that may directly or indirectly affect the nutraceutical industry. Every effort was made to provide a balanced and thorough review of the industry with the intent to give veterinary professionals the tools necessary to make informed decisions about product selection and use.

REFERENCES

1. Kalra EK: Neutraceutical—definition and introduction, *AAPS Pharm Sci* 5:27–28, 2003.
2. *Wikipedia*: *Nutraceutical*. <http://en.wikipedia.org/wiki/Nutraceutical>. Accessed Nov 15, 2014.
3. *Health Canada*: *Policy paper–nutraceuticals/functional foods and health claims on foods*. <http://www.hc-sc.gc.ca/fn-an/label-etiquet/claims-reclam/nutra-funct_foods-nutra-fonct_aliment-eng.php>. Archived June 24, 2013. (Accessed Dec 13, 2014.)
4. Roseland JM, Holden JM, Andrews KW, et al: Dietary supplement ingredient database (DSID): preliminary USDA studies on the composition of adult multivitamin/mineral supplements, *J Food Compost Anal* 21:S69–S77, 2008.
5. Cohen PA: American roulette—contaminated dietary supplements, *New Engl J Med* 361:1523–1525, 2009.
6. Whitsitt V, Beehner C, Welch C: The role of good manufacturing practices for preventing dietary supplement adulteration, *Anal Bioanal Chem* 405:4353–4358, 2013.
7. Cohen PA: Hazards of hindsight—monitoring the safety of nutritional supplements, *New Engl J Med* 370:1277–1280, 2014.
8. Droz N, Marques-Vidal P: Multivitamins/multiminerals in Switzerland: not as good as it seems, *Nutr J* 13:24, 2014.
9. Genuis SJ, Schwalfenberg G, Siy AK, et al: Toxic element contamination of natural health products and pharmaceutical preparations, *PLoS One* 7:e49676, 2012.
10. Institute of Medicine Committee to Review Dietary Reference Intakes for Vitamin D and Calcium, *Dietary reference intakes for calcium and vitamin D*, Washington, DC, 2011, National Academies Press.
11. O'Keefe JH, Harris WS: From Inuit to implementation: omega-3 fatty acids come of age, *Mayo Clinic Proc* 75:607–614, 2000.
12. Albert CM, Campos H, Stampfer MJ, et al: Blood levels of long-chain n-3 fatty acids and the risk of sudden death, *NEJM* 346:1113–1118, 2002.
13. Leng GC, Lee AJ, Fowkes FGR, et al: Randomized controlled trial of gamma-linolenic acid and eicosapentaenoic acid in peripheral arterial disease, *Clin Nutr* 17:265–271, 1998.
14. Singh RB, Niaz MA, Sharma JP, et al: Randomized, double-blind, placebo-controlled trial of fish oil and mustard oil in patients with suspected acute myocardial infarction: the Indian experiment of infarct survival-4, *Cardiovasc Drugs Ther* 11:485–491, 1997.

15. Donadio JV, Larson TS, Bergstralh EJ, et al: A randomized trial of high-dose compared with low-dose omega-3 fatty acids in severe IgA nephropathy, *J Am Soc Nephrol* 12:791–799, 2001.

16. Cappelli P, Di Liberato L, Stuard S, et al: N-3 polyunsaturated fatty acid supplementation in chronic progressive renal disease, *J Nephrol* 10:157–162, 1997.

17. von Schacky C, Angerer P, Kthny W, et al: The effect of dietary Ω-3 fatty acids on coronary atherosclerosis a randomized, double-blind, placebo controlled trial, *Ann Intern Med* 130:554–562, 1999.

18. Volker D, Fitzgerald P, Major G, et al: Efficacy of fish oil concentrate in the treatment of rheumatoid arthritis, *J Rheumatol* 27:2434–2346, 2000.

19. Martí M, Ortiz X, Gasser M, et al: Persistent organic pollutants (PCDD/Fs, dioxin-like PCBs, marker PCBs, and PBDEs) in health supplements on the Spanish market, *Chemosphere* 78:1256–1262, 2010.

20. Rawn DFK, Breakell K, Verigin V, et al: Fish oil supplements on the Canadian market: polychlorinated dibenzo-*p*-dioxins, dibenzofurans, and polybrominated diphenyl ethers, *J Food Sci* 74:T31–T36, 2009.

21. Ramagopalan SV, Heger A, Berlanga AJ, et al: A ChIP-seq defined genome-wide map of vitamin D receptor binding: associations with disease and evolution, *Genome Res* 20:1352–1360, 2010.

22. Chowdhury R, Kunutsor S, Vitezova A, et al: Vitamin D and risk of cause specific death: systematic review and meta-analysis of observational cohort and randomised intervention studies, *BMJ* 348:g1903, 2014, doi:10.1136/bmj.g1903.

23. Pavelka K, Gatterova J, Olejarova M, et al: Glucosamine sulfate use and delay of progression of knee osteoarthritis: a 3-year, randomized, placebo-controlled, double blind study, *Arch Intern Med* 162:2113–2123, 2002.

24. Reginster JY, Deroisy R, Rovati LC, et al: Long-term effects of glucosamine sulphate on osteoarthritis progression: a randomized, placebo-controlled clinical trial, *Lancet* 357:251–256, 2001.

25. Bruyere O, Pavelka K, Rovati LC, et al: Glucosamine sulfate reduces osteoarthritis progression in postmenopausal women with knee osteoarthritis: evidence from two 3-year studies, *Menopause* 11:138–143, 2004.

26. Tice JA, Ross E, Coxson PG, et al: Cost-effectiveness of vitamin therapy to lower plasma homocysteine levels for the prevention of coronary heart disease, effect of grain fortification and beyond, *JAMA* 286:936–943, 2001.

27. Fletcher RH, Fairfield KM: Vitamins for chronic disease prevention in adults, scientific review, *JAMA* 287:3116–3126, 2002.

28. Fletcher RH, Fairfield KM: Vitamins for chronic disease prevention in adults, clinical applications, *JAMA* 287:3127–3129, 2002.

29. Brown SA, Brown CA, Crowell WA, et al: Beneficial effects of chronic administration of dietary Ω-3 polyunsaturated fatty acids in dogs with renal insufficiency, *J Clin Lab Med* 131:447–455, 1998.

30. Brown SA, Brown CA, Crowell WA, et al: Effects of dietary polyunsaturated fatty acids supplementation in early renal insufficiency in dogs, *J Lab Clin Med* 135:275–286, 2000.

31. Brown SA: Effects of dietary lipids on renal function in dogs and cats, *1998 Purina Nutrition Forum*, June 4–6, St Louis, MO, 1998.

32. Plantinga EA, Everts H, Kastelein AM, et al. Retrospective study of the survival of acts with acquired chronic renal insufficiency offered different commercial diets, *Vet Rec* 157:185–187, 2005.

33. Rosenberg I: Commentary, *NEJM* 346(15):1102–1103, 2002.

34. Billman GE: A comprehensive review and analysis of 25 years of data from an in vivo canine model of sudden cardiac death: implications for future anti-arrhythmic drug development, *Pharmacol Ther* 111:808–835, 2006.

35. Bauer JE: Responses of dogs to dietary omega-3 fatty acids, *JAVMA* 231:1657–1661, 2007.

36. Hall JA, Tooley KA, Gradin JL, et al: Effects of dietary n-6 and n-3 fatty acids and vitamin E on the immune response of healthy geriatric dogs, *AJVR* 64:762–772, 2003.

37. Gueck T, Seidel A, Baumann D, et al: Alterations of mast cell mediator production and release by gamma-linolenic and docosahexaenoic acid, *Vet Dermatol* 15:309–314, 2004.

38. Scott DW, Miller WH, et al: *Muller and Kirk's small animal dermatology*, ed 6, Philadelphia, PA, 2001, W.B. Saunders, pp 543–666.

39. Nesbitt GH, Freeman LM, Hannah SS: Effect of n-3 fatty acid ratio and dose on clinical manifestations, plasma fatty acids and inflammatory mediators in dogs with pruritus, *Vet Dermatol* 14:67–74, 2003.

40. Scott DW, Miller WH, Reinhart GA, et al: Effect of an omega-3/omega-6 fatty acid-containing commercial lamb and rice diet on pruritus in atopic dogs: results of a single-blinded study, *Can J Vet Res* 61:145–153, 1997.

41. Saevik BK, Bergvall K, Holm BR, et al: A randomized, controlled study to evaluate the steroid sparing effect of essential fatty acid supplementation in the treatment of canine atopic dermatitis, *Vet Dermatol* 15:137–145, 2004.

42. Mueller RS, Fieseler KV, Feltman MJ, et al: Effect of omega-3 fatty acids on canine atopic dermatitis, *J Small Anim Pract* 45:293–297, 2004.

43. Kearns RJ, Hayek MG, Turek JJ: Effect of age, breed and dietary omega-6 (n-6): omega-3 (n-3) fatty acid ratio on immune function, eicosanoid production, and lipid peroxidation in young and aged dogs, *Vet Immunol Immunopathol* 69:165–183, 1999.

44. Mueller RS, Rosychuk RA, Jones LD: A retrospective study regarding the treatment of lupoid onychodystrophy in 30 dogs and literature review, *JAAHA* 39:139–150, 2003.

45. Roudebush P, Davenport DJ, Novotny BJ: The use of neutraceuticals in cancer therapy, *Vet Clin Small Anim Pract* 34:249–269, 2004.

46. Ogilvie GK, Fettman MJ, Mallinckrodt CH, et al: Effect of fish oil, arginine and doxorubicin chemotherapy on remission and survival time for dogs with lymphoma, *Cancer* 88:1916–1928, 2000.

47. Waldron MK, Spencer AL, Bauer JE: Role of long-chain polyunsaturated n-3 fatty acids in the development of the nervous system of dogs and cats. In Heinemann KM, Bauer JE, editors: docosahexaenoic acid and neurological development in animals, *JAVMA* 228:700–705, 2006.

48. Schiavone BA, Romboli I, Chiarini R, et al: Influence of dietary lipid source and strain on fatty acid composition of Muscovy duck meat, *J Anim Physiol A Anim Nutr (Berl)* 88:88–93, 2004.

49. Liu W-M, Lai S-J, Lu L-Z, et al: Effects of dietary fatty acids on serum parameters, fatty acid compositions, and liver histology in Shaoxing laying ducks, *J Zhejiang Univ Sci B (Biomed Biotechnol)* 12:736–743, 2011.

50. Liu D, Veit HP, Wilson JH, et al: Long-term supplementation of various dietary lipids alters bone mineral content, mechanical properties and histologic characteristics of Japanese quail, *Poult Sci* 82:831–839, 2003.

51. Baird HT, Eggett DL, Fullmer S: Varying ratios of omega-6:omega-3 fatty acids on the pre- and postmortem bone mineral density, bone ash, and bone breaking strength of laying chickens, *Poult Sci* 87:323–328, 2008.

52. Speake BK, Wood NAR: Timing of incorporation of docosahexaenoic acid into brain and muscle phospholipids during precocial and altricial modes of avian development, *Comp Biochem Physiol B Biochem Mol Biol* 141:147–158, 2005.

53. Petzinger C, Heatley JJ, Cornejo J, et al: Dietary modification of omega-3 fatty acids for birds with atherosclerosis, *JAVMA* 236:523–528, 2010.

54. Fronte B, Paci G, Montanari G, et al: Learning ability of 1-d-old partridges (*Alectoris rufa*) from eggs laid by hens fed with different n-3 fatty acid concentrations, *Br Poult Sci* 49:776–780, 2008.

55. Ansenberger K, Richards C, Zhuge Y, et al: Decreased severity of ovarian cancer and increased survival in hens fed a flaxseed-enriched diet for 1 year, *Gynec Oncol* 117:341–347, 2010.

56. Newman RE, Bryden WL, Fleck E, et al: Dietary n-3 and n-6 fatty acids alter avian metabolism: metabolism and abdominal fat deposition, *Br J of Nutr* 88:11–18, 2002.

57. Liu WM, Jhang J, Lu LZ, et al: Effects of perilla extract on productive performance, serum values and hepatic expression of lipid-related genes in Shaoxing ducks, *Br Poult Sci* 52:381–387, 2011.

58. Petzinger C, Larner C, Heatley JJ, et al: Conversion of a-linolenic acid to long-chain omega-3 fatty acid derivatives and alterations of HDL density subfractions and plasma lipids with dietary polyunsaturated fatty acids in Monk parrots (*Myiopsitta monachus*), *J Anim Physiol Anim Nutr* 98:262–270, 2014.

59. Russell L, Hicks GS, Low AK, et al: Phytoestrogens: a viable option?, *Am J Med Sci* 324:185–188, 2002.

60. Dickinson A: *Before and after DSHEA*, Washington DC, 1999, Council for Responsible Nutrition.

61. Katz MH: How can we know if supplements are safe if we do not know what is in them?, *JAMA Intern Med* 173:928, 2013.

62. Cohen P: Contaminated dietary supplements. Letter to the editor, *New Engl J Med* 362:274, 2010.

63. *U.S. Food and Drug Administration*: Dietary supplement current good manufacturing practices (cGMPs) and interim final rule (IFR) facts. <http://www.fda.gov/Food/GuidanceRegulation/CGMP/ucm110858.htm>, 2007. (Accessed December 13, 2014.)

64. Harel Z, Harel S, Wald R, et al: The frequency and characteristics of dietary supplement recalls in the United States, *JAMA Intern Med* 173:926–928, 2013.

65. *Food and Drug Administration*: *Guidance for industry: a food labeling guide (11. Appendix C: Health Claims)*. <http://www.fda.gov/Food/GuidanceRegulation/GuidanceDocumentsRegulatoryInformation/LabelingNutrition/ucm064919.htm>, 2013. (Accessed Dec 13, 2014.)

66. Foster S: A brief history of adulteration of herbs, spices, and botanical drugs, *HerbalGram* 92:42–57, 2011.

67. Russell AS, Aghazadeh-Habashi A, Jamali F: Active ingredient consistency of commercially available glucosamine sulfate products. *J Rheumatol* 29:2407–2409, 2002.

68. Cohen PA, Maller G, DeSouza R, et al: Presence of banned drugs in dietary supplements following FDA recalls, *JAMA* 312:1691–1693, 2014.

69. Feifer A, Fleshner NE, Klotz L: Analytical accuracy and reliability of commonly used nutritional supplements in prostate disease, *J Urol* 168:150–154, 2002.

70. Rehman S, Adnan M, Khalid N, et al: Calcium supplements: an additional source of lead contamination, *Biol Trace Elem Res* 143:178–187, 2011.

71. Da Silva E, Jakubovic R, Pejović-Milić A, et al: Aluminium and strontium in calcium supplements and antacids: a concern to haemodialysis patients?, *Food Addit Contam Part A Chem Anal Control Expo Risk Assess* 27:1405–1414, 2010.

72. Mattos JCP, Hahn M, Augusti PR, et al: Lead content of dietary calcium supplements available in Brazil, *Food Addit Contam* 23:133–139, 2006.

73. Kim M, Kim C, Song I. Analysis of lead in 55 brands of dietary calcium supplements by graphite furnace atomic absorption spectrometry after microwave digestion, *Food Addit Contam* 20:149–153, 2003.

74. Scelfo GM, Flegal AR: Lead in calcium supplements, *Environ Health Perspect* 108(4):309–313, 2000.

75. Korfali SI, Hawi T, Mroueh M: Evaluation of heavy metals content in dietary supplements in Lebanon, *Chem Cent J* 7(1)10, 2013.

76. Genuis SJ, Schwalfenberg G, Siy AK, et al: Toxic element contamination of natural health products and pharmaceutical preparations, *PLoS One* 7 e49676, 2012.

77. Giebe K, Counts C: Comparison of Prenate Advance with other prescription prenatal vitamins: a folic acid dissolution study, *Adv Ther* 17:179–183, 2000.

78. Hoag SW, Ramachandruni H, Shangraw RF: Failure of prescription prenatal vitamin products to meet USP standards for folic acid dissolution, *J Am Pharm Assoc* NS37:397-400. 1997.

79. Rawn DFK, Breakell K, Verigin V, et al: Persistent organic pollutants in fish oil supplements on the Canadian market: polychlorinated

80. Kleiner AC, Cladis DP, Santerre CR: A comparison of actual versus stated label amounts of EPA and DHA in commercial omega-3 dietary supplements in the United States, *J Sci Food Agric* 95(6):1260–1267, 2014, doi:10.1002/jsfa.6816.

81. Jacobs MN, Covaci A, Gheorghe A, et al: Time trend investigation of PCBs, PBDEs, and organochlorine pesticides in selected n-3 polyunsaturated fatty acid rich dietary fish oil and vegetable oil supplements; nutritional relevance for human essential n-3 fatty acid requirements, *J Agric Food Chem* 52:1780–1788, 2004.

82. Reid A-J, Budge SM: Identification of unresolved complex mixtures (UCMs) of hydrocarbons in commercial fish oil supplements, *J Sci Food Agric* 95(2)423–428, 2015, doi:10.1002/jsfa.6741.

83. Bourdon JA, Bazinet TM, Arnason TT, et al: Polychlorinated biphenyls (PCBs) contamination and aryl hydrocarbon receptor (AhR) agonist activity of omega-3 polyunsaturated fatty acid supplements: implications for daily intake of dioxins and PCBs, *Food Chem Toxicol* 48:3093–3097, 2010.

84. Martí M, Ortiz X, Gasser M, et al: Persistent organic pollutants (PCDD/Fs, dioxin-like PCBs, marker PCBs, and PBDEs) in health supplements on the Spanish market, *Chemosphere* 78:1256–1262, 2010.

85. *Consumerlab.com*: *Fish oil and omega-3 fatty acid supplements review*. <www.consumerlabs.com/results/omega3.asp>. (Accessed August 1, 2004.)

86. *Consumerlab.com*: *Fish oil and omega-3 fatty acid supplements review*. <https://www.consumerlab.com/reviews/fish_oil_supplements_review/omega3/>. (Accessed November 30, 2014.)

87. Garrard J, Harms S, Eberly LE, et al: Variations in product choices of frequently purchased herbs, *Arch Intern Med* 163:2290–2295, 2003.

88. Gilroy CM, Steiner JF, Byers T, et al: Echinacea and truth in labeling, *Arch Intern Med* 163:699–704, 2003.

89. Bennett BC, Balick MJ: Phytomedicine 101: plant taxonomy for preclinical and clinical medicinal plant researchers, *J Soc Integr Oncol* 6:150–157, 2008.

90. Foster S: Exploring the peripatetic maze of black cohosh adulteration: a review of the nomenclature, distribution, chemistry, market status, analytical methods, and safety, *HerbalGram*, 98:32–51, 2013.

91. Sun J, Chen P: A flow-injection mass spectrometry fingerprinting method for authentication and quality assessment of *Scutellaria lateriflora*-based dietary supplements, *Anal Bioanal Chem* 401:1577–1584, 2011.

92. Lu YL, Zhou NL, Liao SY, et al: Detection of adulteration of antihypertension dietary supplements and traditional Chinese medicines with synthetic drugs using LC/MS, *Food Addit Contam Part A Chem Anal Control Expo Risk Assess* 27:893–902, 2010.

93. Slifman NR, Obermeyer WR, Musser SM, et al: Contamination of botanical dietary supplements by *Digitalis lanata*, *NEJM* 339:806–811, 1998.

94. Oke S, Aghazadeh-Habash A, Weese JS, et al: Evaluation of glucosamine levels in commercial equine oral supplements for joints, *Equine Vet J* 38:93–95, 2006.

95. Adebowale AO, Cox DS, Liang Z, et al: Chondroitin sulfate content in marketed products and the caco-2 permeability of chondroitin sulfate raw materials, *J Am Nutraceutical Assoc* 3:37–44, 2000.

96. Mondo K, Glover WB, Murch SJ, et al: Environmental neurotoxins b-N-methylamino-l-alanine (BMAA) and mercury in shark cartilage dietary supplements, *Food Chem Toxicol* 70:26–32, 2014.

97. Volpi N: Quality of different chondroitin sulfate preparations in relation to their therapeutic activity, *J Pharm Pharmacol* 61:1271–1280, 2009.

98. Weese JS: Evaluation of deficiencies in labeling of commercial probiotics, *Can Vet J* 44:982–983, 2003.

99. Drago L, Rodighiero V, Celeste T, et al: Microbiological evaluation of commercial probiotic products available in the USA in 2009, *J Chemother* 22:373–377, 2010.

100. Weese JS: Microbiologic evaluation of commercial probiotics, *JA-VMA* 220:794–797, 2002.

101. *Consumerlab.com*: *glucosamine, chondroitin and MSM supplements for joint health.* <http://consumerlabs.com/results/gluco.asp>. (Accessed August 22, 2004.)

102. *Consumerlab.com*: *glucosamine, chondroitin and MSM supplements for joint health.* <http://consumerlabs.com/results/gluco.asp>. (Accessed September 22, 2007.)

103. Yetley EA: Multivitamin and multimineral dietary supplements: definitions, characterization, bioavailability, and drug interactions, *Am J Clin Nutr* 85(Suppl):269S–276S, 2007.

104. Ericksen P, Bartels EM, Altman RD, et al: Risk of bias and brand explain the observed inconsistency in trials on glucosamine for symptomatic relief of osteoarthritis: a meta-analysis of placebo-controlled trials, *Arthritis Care Res* 66:1844–1855, 2014.

105. Little DR, Jeanson ML: DNA barcode authentication of saw palmetto herbal dietary supplements, *Sci Rep* 3:3518, 2013.

106. *U.S. Food and Drug Administration*: *Q and A on dietary supplements.* <http://www.fda.gov/Food/DietarySupplements/QADietarySupplements/ucm191930.htm>. (Accessed December 14, 2014.)

107. *U.S. Pharmacopeial Convention*: *about.* <http://www.usp.org/>. (Accessed December 14, 2014.)

108. *U.S. Food and Drug Administration*: *Code of Federal Regulations Title 21, Part 210—current good manufacturing practice in manufacturing, processing, packing, or holding drugs; general.* <http://www.accessdata.fda.gov/scripts/cdrh/cfdocs/cfcfr/CFRSearch.cfm?fr=210.1>. (Accessed December 14, 2014.)

109. *U.S. Food and Drug Administration*: *CFR–Code of Federal Regulations Title 21.* <http://www.accessdata.fda.gov/scripts/cdrh/cfdocs/cfCFR/CFRSearch.cfm?CFRPart=111>. (Accessed December 14, 2014.>

110. *U.S. Food and Drug Administration*: *CFR–Code of Federal Regulations Title 21, Part 210.* <http://www.accessdata.fda.gov/scripts/cdrh/cfdocs/cfcfr/CFRSearch.cfm?CFRPart=210>. (Accessed December 14, 2014.)

111. *U.S. Food and Drug Administration*: *CFR–Code of Federal Regulations Title 21, Part 211.* <http://www.accessdata.fda.gov/scripts/cdrh/cfdocs/cfcfr/CFRSearch.cfm?CFRPart=211>. (Accessed December 14, 2014.)

112. *Consumerlab.com*: *recalls and warnings.* <www.consumerlabs.com/recalls.asp>. (Accessed December 14, 2014.)

113. *U.S. Food and Drug Administration*: *Inspections, compliance, enforcement, and criminal investigations.* <http://www.fda.gov/ICECI/EnforcementActions/WarningLetters/default.htm>. (Accessed Nov 27, 2014.)

114. *NSF International*: *Dietary supplement certification: quality and safety provider.* <http://www.nsf.org/services/by-industry/dietary-supplements/dietary-supplement-certification/>. (Accessed December 14, 2014.)

115. *NSF International*: *Sports supplement screening–Certified for Sport.* <http://www.nsf.org/services/by-industry/dietary-supplements/sports-supplement-screening>. (Accessed December 14, 2014.)

116. *NSF International*: *Certified for sport products.* <http://www.nsfsport.com/listings/certified_products.asp>. (Accessed December 14, 2014.)

117. *NSF International*: *Search for NSF certified GMP facilities.* <http://info.nsf.org/Certified/GMP/>. (Accessed December 14, 2014.)

118. *U.S. Pharmacopeial Convention*: *For manufacturers.* <http://www.usp.org/usp-verification-services/usp-verified-dietary-supplements/manufacturers#processincludes>. (Accessed December 14, 2014.)

119. *U.S. Pharmacopeial Convention*: *USP verified dietary ingredients.* <http://www.usp.org/usp-verification-services/usp-verified-dietary-ingredients>. (Accessed December 14, 2014.)

120. *Informed-Choice*: *What is informed-choice?.* <http://www.informed-choice.org/>. (Accessed December 14, 2014.)

121. *Consumerlab.com*: *Home page.* <http://www.consumerlab.com/>. (Accessed December 14, 2014.)

122. *National Animal Supplement Council*: *About page.* <http://nasc.cc/index.php?option=com_content&task=view&id=40&Itemid=80>. (Accessed December 14, 2014.)

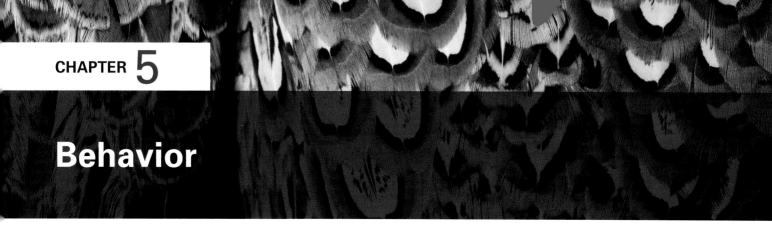

CHAPTER 5

Behavior

Yvonne R. A. van Zeeland • Susan G. Friedman • Laurie Bergman

Parrots are one of the most popular avian species kept as pets across the world. Currently, over 80 million pet birds are kept in the United States, Europe, and Australia combined.[1–3] In the United States, the great majority of these birds belong to the order Psittaciformes (~75% ≈15 million).[3] When provided proper living conditions and care, parrots can make good pets. They are skilled problem solvers, fast learners, and social, affectionate creatures who can form strong bonds with their caregivers. However, because of their intelligence and social nature, they require a complex environment that provides a lot of stimulation, both physical and mental. In addition, they need early and ongoing socialization, and basic training to learn the skills needed to mature into successful pets. These provisions may be easier said than done. Many caregivers purchase parrots unaware of their special needs. As a result, parrots often learn undesirable behaviors such as biting, excessive vocalization, and self-mutilation. This in turn leads many caregivers to have their parrots euthanized or relinquish them to a shelter or sanctuary.[4–7] Education and timely, skilled intervention can prevent these dire outcomes.

Veterinarians can play a vital role educating owners about parrot behavior, including how to prevent and ameliorate behavior problems effectively and humanely. However, to do so requires that veterinarians gain expertise in learning and behavior principles and procedures, and integrate this knowledge into their daily practice with avian patients and clients. The benefits for patients and clients will be profound, improving parrot health, quality of life, the human animal bond, and doctor-client-patient relationships.

One example of the benefits of integrating the behavioral and medical models within veterinary practice is the recent development of low-stress handling procedures. Although the traditional "capture and restraint" approach may get the job done more quickly, it can also result in unnecessarily high levels of patient stress, immediate and lasting fear reactions that pose a risk to the bird and the handler, misleading examination and diagnostic test results, and reduced owner compliance to a prescribed treatment. Further, veterinary staff can advocate and support caregivers learning how to teach their birds cooperative medical and husbandry procedures, such as toweling, wing trimming, nail clipping, stepping on and off a scale, and taking in oral medication, any of which can save time as well as increase positive outcomes.

Improved diagnosis, treatment, and prevention of infectious and nutritional diseases have led to a shift in presenting conditions in many veterinary practices, such as an increase in metabolic and neoplastic conditions. Similarly, behavioral complaints have shifted to the top of the list of client concerns. Veterinarians are often the first point of contact for clients reporting biting, screaming, feather damaging, mutilating, stereotypy, excessive egg-laying, and cloacal prolapse.[7,8] Unfortunately, by the time many clients consult with their veterinarians, behavior problems have been present for so long that it is difficult to accomplish rapid or simple resolutions. Thus, early assessment and intervention of behavior problems are integral in achieving successful outcomes, and veterinarians can and should be called upon to contribute to the goal of behavioral wellness for their patients.

This chapter provides an overview of companion bird behavior topics, which are discussed from various perspectives (i.e., medical, ethological, and behavioral). An emphasis throughout the chapter is on learning solutions and enrichment, from the field of applied behavior analysis. The topic of psychotropic drugs, although not recommended as a stand-alone treatment, is also presented. Common behavioral problems are described and current trends in assessment and intervention (behavioral model) and etiology, diagnosis, and treatment (medical model) are also explored. Companion bird behavior is by its very scope far bigger than this chapter allows. As such, the authors hope to provide a solid introduction of the key considerations, principles, and procedures available to veterinarians committed to including behavior therapy in their daily practice when dealing with an avian species.

WHAT IS BEHAVIOR?

Most behaviorists, ethologists, and veterinarians have an intuitive sense of what "behavior" is. A survey among members of three behavior-focused scientific societies with regard to their understanding of the term, however, showed that there is widespread disagreement as to what qualifies as behavior.[9] Based on the results of this survey and a meta-analysis of the scientific literature, a new definition was subsequently proposed. This definition stated that "behavior is the internally coordinated responses (actions or inactions) of whole living organisms (individuals or groups) to internal and/or external stimuli, excluding responses more easily understood as developmental changes."[9] This definition implies that behavior includes all responses of the organism (or organisms) to stimuli, regardless of whether these are internal or external, conscious or subconscious, overt (i.e., behavior that can be directly observed by others, such as preening, eating, and drinking) or covert (i.e., behavior that can only be directly observed by the individual itself, such as thinking and feeling), and voluntary or involuntary. Although the definition includes both overt and covert behaviors, the usefulness of covert behaviors is limited by our inability to directly measure and accurately interpret private events. In a scientific context, in which the goal is to explain phenomena by identifying observable, physical events that produce them, behavior is anything that an animal does that can be observed. Similarly, a scientific approach to behavior requires a description of what the animal does instead of what the animal is or has. The notion of being or having behavior (i.e., labeling a person or an animal) infers largely untestable theories about the mental processes behind the behavior. As a result, it may get in the way of identifying solutions to modify the behavior (Box 5-1).[10] Examples of constructs or labels that are commonly used when dealing with parrots are "territorial," "dominant," "hormonal," "asocial," or "spoiled." Veterinarians and behaviorists are advised to reconsider the use of such labels and describe instead observable behavior and conditions as objectively as possible, and they should encourage their clients to do the same. For example, the term "territorial" is often used to describe a bird that bites, or, even worse, the biting bird is referred to as "being territorial because it is hormonal." These constructed labels imply that behavior is a characteristic or personality trait of the animal, whereas the observable description, for example, biting, describes the action the animal performs, given a specific context (e.g., caregivers thrust their hands toward the birds' feet while the birds are in their cage). In the situation where biting is described, the intervention may subsequently focus on a change of the conditions to replace the biting. In the situation where the bird is referred to as being "territorial," however, the problem is inside the animal, independent of conditions without a solution being ready at hand.[11]

Although it is true that behavior is partly inherited (innate behaviors), learning—defined as behavior change due to experience—greatly accounts for the behavior animals display.[12] Both processes—inheritance and learning—work toward a similar goal, that is, the ability of the animal to adapt to pressure from the environment. Genetic processes occur at a species level, via natural selection over generations.[13] Learning processes, however, occur at the individual level, where behavior is selected by the outcomes of behaving.[14]

BOX 5-1 LIABILITIES WITH THE USE OF LABELS TO DESCRIBE BEHAVIOR[11]

1. Labels are based on circular reasoning that is not scientifically verifiable.
2. Labels become self-fulfilling prophecies.
3. Labels predispose us to using ineffective, forceful, or harmful strategies.
4. Labels create a false sense of having explained behavior, when all we have done is given it a name.
5. Labels end the search for actual causes we can do something about.
6. Labels provide excuses to get rid of the pet.

The behavior of animals in a captive setting directly impacts the quality of their lives, their interactions with their caregivers, their health, and the probability of veterinarians maintaining long-term doctor–client–patient relationships. It is known that training captive bird species to cooperate with medical procedures can lead to a decrease in risks associated with physical evaluations or medical procedures, reduce expenses associated with maintenance and preventative health procedures, and allow for a more complete patient evaluation. A behaviorally competent bird is a less fearful bird, and this leads to less stress and more valid laboratory results, fewer misdiagnoses, and errors of both overtreatment and undertreatment of the patient.

EXPLAINING BEHAVIOR USING TINBERGEN'S FOUR QUESTIONS

Many of the current ideas, concepts, and explanations regarding animal behavior have been derived from the work of Nikolaas Tinbergen, Karl von Frisch, and Konrad Lorenz. In 1973, these three biologists won the Nobel Prize in Physiology or Medicine for their groundbreaking studies on inherited behavior patterns, including causation, development, evolution, and functionality.[15] Tinbergen, in particular, laid the basis for a conceptual framework to study animal behavior, which included four complementary categories of explanations for behavior (Box 5-2)[16]:

1. *Ontogeny (Development):* explanations related to the formation or sequential changes of a trait or behavior of an organism in the various stages of its life, describing the translation of genotype to phenotype and the development of an organism across its life span, including the environmental factors that play a role in this process
2. *Mechanism (Causation):* explanations related to the anatomy, physiology, and regulation of a trait or behavior, describing both the stimuli that elicit a behavioral response as well as the response mechanisms at the molecular, physiologic, neuroethologic, cognitive, and social levels
3. *Phylogeny (Evolution):* explanations for the sequential changes in the behavior of a species across time, describing the history of a trait or typical behavior based on its genotype and phenotype, including how and why it evolved in this way (and not otherwise) throughout time, how this development compares with the development of similar behaviors in other related species, or both
4. *Adaptation (Function):* explanations for the evolutionary function of the traits or behavior of a species, including the ways in which variations in this trait or behavior have affected the species' chances of survival or reproduction

The first two categories together are summarized as the "proximate explanations" for a behavior, that is, how an organism functions. The latter two consist of "ultimate explanations," that is, how and why a species came to its current form. Since these explanations are all complementary, rather than exclusionary, to each other, all of the above-mentioned factors may be taken into consideration to explain why the individual is behaving in a certain way. For the individual parrot in the clinic, this therefore implies that the traits of the species, the individual's development and its response mechanisms, and the stimuli that elicit these mechanisms may all be addressed.

BOX 5-2 TINBERGEN'S FOUR QUESTIONS TO EXPLAIN BEHAVIOR

		Diachronic versus Synchronic Perspective	
		Dynamic View Explanation of Current Form in Terms of a Historical Sequence	**Static View Explanation of the Current Form of Species**
How vs. Why Questions	**Proximate view** How an individual organism's structures function	*Ontogeny (development)* Developmental explanations for changes in individuals, from DNA to their current form	*Mechanism (causation)* Mechanistic explanations for how an organism's structures work
	Ultimate (evolutionary) view Why a species evolved the structures (adaptations) it has	*Phylogeny (evolution)* The history of the evolution of sequential changes in a species over many generations	*Adaptation (function)* A species trait that solves a reproductive or survival problem in the current environment

Source: http://en.wikipedia.org/wiki/Tinbergen's_four_questions.

DOMESTICATED OR WILD? THE TRUE NATURE OF PARROTS

The first reports on parrots kept as pets probably date back as early as 2500 years ago when Alexander the Great presumably brought back Alexandrine parakeets *(Psittacula eupatria)* from his voyages to the Far East during the fourth century BC.[17–19] Trading in live birds, however, did not commence until the fifteenth or the sixteenth century, when European explorers brought back new parrot species from their voyages to Asia, America, and later also Australia.[17–19] By the end of the nineteenth century, the first steps toward domestication were taken when the first smaller parakeet species, most noticeably budgerigars *(Melopsittacus undulatus)* and cockatiels *(Nymphicus hollandicus)*, were successfully bred in captivity (Figure 5-1).[17,20] In most other psittacine species, it took until the 1970s and early 1980s for captive breeding programs to become successful.[21,22] Despite these breeding successes in captivity, however, domestication (the process whereby a population of living organisms adapts to a captive living environment through genetic changes occurring over

generations as well as environmentally induced developmental events that occur within the lifetime of an individual[23]) of parrots is still considered to be in its infancy; most parrots are only one or two generations removed from their wild counterparts and have not yet undergone the selection process that precedes true domestication.[24–26] Parrots therefore likely have retained most, if not all, of their wild instincts and needs. These instincts and needs shape, in part, their behavioral responses in captivity. In addition, they may predispose the parrots to experience stress or frustration when the parrots' captive living environments limit their ability to express their species-typical behaviors.[4,27] In addition, many of the wild behaviors displayed by captive parrots under captive circumstances that are considered undesirable by the owner are innate to the bird and therefore difficult to suppress. As a result, the bird will continue to perform the behaviors in the absence of reinforcers and may even be considered genetically contra-prepared to suppress these behaviors.[14,28] It is therefore important to consider the various biologic traits and characteristics of parrots in the wild, as well as the environmental conditions that elicit and shape these behaviors. Both may be of great help when trying to predict and manage parrot behaviors, adapt the parrots' captive living environment to meet their needs, and help owners and caregivers to set reasonable expectations for their parrot's behavior.

Characteristics, Behavior, and Activity Patterns of Parrots in the Wild

Of the various behaviors performed by parrots, many appear relatively conserved across the entire range of free-living members of the order of Psittaciformes, with little variability in the way they are performed. These behaviors therefore represent the so-called species-typical behaviors or "modal action patterns." These modal action patterns are part of the parrots' natural history and genetic endowment and allow parrots to adapt to their free-ranging living environment, serving important functions related to the survival and reproduction of the species.[29,30] Many of these behaviors are thought to be innate, thereby being relatively difficult to modify with environmental arrangement and also occurring in nondomesticated captive parrots. Learning is also innate to every animal. This implies that parrots can (and will) change behaviors based on consequences, which indicates that even relatively conserved behaviors can be flexible to some degree.

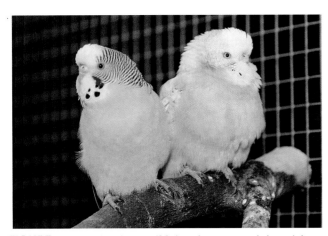

FIGURE 5-1 Budgerigars *(Melopsittacus undulatus)* have been bred in captivity with success since the nineteenth century. Similar to other small psittacine birds (e.g., cockatiels, lovebirds), budgerigars come in different colors, shapes, and sizes. Green *(left)* is the wild type. The blue budgerigar on the right is a color mutant. (Photo courtesy Nico Schoemaker.)

Thus, parrots can be flexible in their behaviors and learn to adapt to their captive living environment, as long as caregivers are knowledgeable about the processes underlying behavior change. Nevertheless, knowledge of the parrot's species-typical behaviors and the circumstances that elicit and shape them can also be important tools to help predict, interpret, and manage parrot behavior in captivity.

Cognition, communication, and sensory perception

Parrots are highly social and communicative species, with a communication system consisting of an extensive range of highly distinct vocalizations. These most likely belong to the most complex systems reported in the animal kingdom. Already in the nest, chicks start to learn these vocalizations from both parents and other flock members, including how to discriminate and identify individual calls to correctly interpret information conveyed by other birds.[31,32] Unrelated newly hatched budgerigars, for example, produce comparable vocalizations at first but mimic vocalizations of their parents within 3 weeks' time. This enables both parents and offspring to recognize and respond to calls produced by their relatives while ignoring others.[33,34]

Within and between species, several distinct regional dialects exist, with parrots from adjacent areas capable of producing and recognizing neighboring dialects.[35–38] Each repertoire includes a variety of different vocalizations that may serve different functions. Such functions may include distress and alarm calls, food begging calls, agonistic or threat displays, courtship duets, and calls to coordinate movement or signal food.[31,32,38,39] In addition, many flock-dwelling species produce a wide range of vocalizations that primarily serve as contact calls.[31,32,39-41] Contact calls are commonly heard during peaks of flock activity, that is, just before the flock sets out to forage, shortly after their return to the roosting area, or at both times—activities that often coincide with sunset and sunrise. These vocalizations form an important tool to help locate other flock members and promote cohesion within the flock.[42,43] Besides vocalizations, posturing is also used as a way of communication with conspecifics. Behavioral displays of territoriality and breeding, for example, may be noted in various parrot species (Figure 5-2). Examples of these include filoerection, voluntary pupillary constriction and dilation, fanning of tail feathers, spreading of the wings, and beak lunging.[41,44-48]

To understand and master the communication skills necessary to function in a highly complex social structure such as that present in parrot species, a certain level of intelligence and cognition is needed. Other factors include the increased chances for survival when capable of interpreting, learning, cooperating, and conveying information; and the ability of the parrot to adapt to changing circumstances during its life course (which is especially important in long-lived species). Studies on cognitive capacities of Grey parrots (Psittacus erithacus erithacus) have shown that these birds are capable of learning and conveying simple associations. Moreover, they are able to understand concepts of relative size, quantities (including a zero-like concept), absence versus presence, and same versus different, as well as learning spatial location or mirror-mediated object discrimination.[49] Much of this categorical discrimination, learning, and recollection is critical for birds to function as sentinels. For this

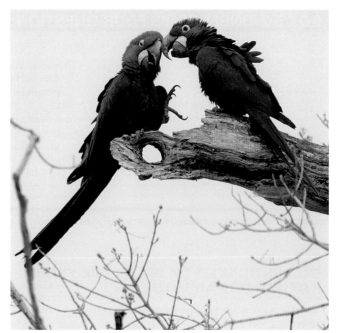

FIGURE 5-2 A hyacinth macaw (Anodorhynchus hyacinthinus) is pushing a conspecific from a branch in the Pantanal, Brazil. Note the territorial display of the "attacker" (on the right) as indicated by its fluffed feathers and its lunging with an open beak toward the "intruder" that is holding up its left foot open in the air at chest level as a means to defend itself. (Photo courtesy Nico Schoemaker.)

purpose, a bird needs to be able to screen and interpret information, whereby it can differentiate between "normal" situations and those that are potentially dangerous for the flock.[42,50,51]

Parrots rely heavily on their vision and hearing for detecting predators. In addition, these senses may help the birds to locate food, orient themselves in the environment, and allow communication with conspecifics. Tactile sensation is also well developed, with a variety of different sensory receptors, including those for touch, heat, and pain, distributed in the beak and skin. In contrast, smell and taste are less important for birds to obtain information about their surroundings.

The psittacine flock

Parrots in the wild typically live together in flocks, which allow for fast detection and avoidance of predators, whereby many birds keep a lookout for potential danger. At the slightest hint of danger, an alarm call is given, and the rest of the flock takes off, thus increasing the birds' chances of survival.[52] Besides predator avoidance, congregation in larger groups may be beneficial to parrots because it increases access to sexual partners, improves territorial defense against intruders, and increases foraging efficiency.[53,54] Flock size and composition may differ among the different parrot species and throughout the season, varying from small family groups of a few individuals to large flocks of hundreds or thousands of conspecifics or, occasionally, mixed groups of multiple species (Figure 5-3).[52,54-60] Much of the parrots' time is spent socially, when they engage in a variety of different behaviors aimed at

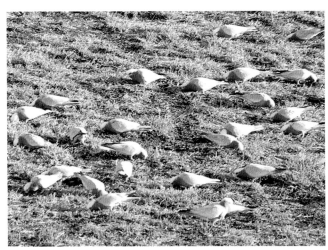

FIGURE 5-3 A flock of galah *(Eolophus roseicapilla)* is foraging together in a field in Australia. These and other cockatoo species are commonly found together in large flocks of several hundreds of individuals. (Photo courtesy Robert Doneley.)

predominantly directed toward the sexual partner, with which a strong, monogamous pair-bond is often formed.

Although parrots generally congregate in groups, various parrot species (e.g., Amazon parrots [*Amazona* spp.] and Macaws [*Ara* spp.]) may display territorial behavior during the breeding season in order to protect the nest site. This nest site is usually located in an excavated tree hole, cliff, or burrow (Figure 5-4, *A*). At the start of the breeding period, Amazon parrots and macaws typically form smaller groups consisting of a pair and their young and display more aggressive behavior toward conspecifics, whereby they chase and fight with each other. Other species (e.g., thick-billed parrots [*Rhynchopsitta* spp.], monk or Quaker parakeets [*Myiopsitta monachus*], and lovebirds [*Agapornis* spp.]) congregate in larger groups, building their nests in close proximity to each other (see Figure 5-4, *B*). In most parrot species, both the male and the female provide parental care to their altricial young, with social contact of nestlings restricted to interaction with the parents and siblings.[67-71] Once the chicks are weaned and fledged, the number and diversity of social interactions increase considerably as the young birds are placed in crèches. In these crèches, the chicks are introduced to other members of the flock and undergo an extensive socialization process.[69-72]

Foraging and feeding

In the wild, most parrots spend a considerable part of their daily activity budget on foraging. These activities start as soon as the sun rises, with many species regularly flying several miles per day to reach their feeding grounds and obtain their

communication (e.g., alarm calls to alert conspecifics about potential danger) or (direct) interaction with conspecifics. Examples of such social interactions include perching in close contact, allopreening, allofeeding, playing, courtship, and mating. All of these are important to maintain social bonds and may take up between 10% and 40% of the bird's time.[48,60-66] Of these behaviors, courtship and mating are

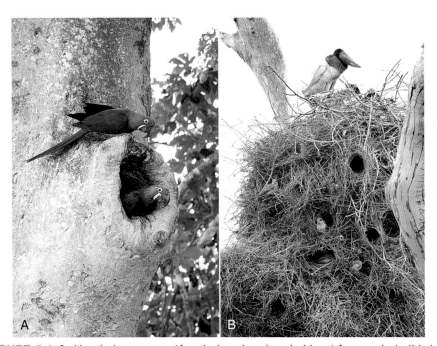

FIGURE 5-4 **A,** Hyacinth macaws *(Anodorhynchus hyacinthinus)* frequently build their nest in excavated tree holes. The feather quality may be affected by maneuvering in such a tight space, as can be seen by the macaw appearing from the hole. **B,** Monk parakeets *(Myiopsitta monachus)* commonly congregate during the breeding season, building their nests in close proximity to each other. These monk parakeets have built their nest under the nest of a Jabiru stork *(Jabiru mycteria)*. The combined nesting ensures protection for both species. The parakeets find protection in the large size of the stork, whereas the parakeets sound an alarm once a threat is visible, thereby also warning the Jabiru stork. (Photo courtesy Nico Schoemaker.)

daily food requirements.[42,47,52,58] Once the birds arrive at a feeding site, they typically engage in a wide variety of foraging behaviors (see Figures 5-3 and 5-5). Such foraging behaviors may include local search, identification, selection, procurement, manipulation, and consumption of food items such as fruits, seeds, nuts, insects, bark, nectar, and other plant materials.[42,57,73,74] Dependent on the species and season, the time invested on foraging and feeding behaviors may vary from 40% to 75% of the daytime, that is, 4 to 8 hours per day.[42,55,57,73,75] Similar to other activities, foraging and flying to and from these feeding grounds are activities that are performed with most of the group as a whole. As a result, large aggregates of parrots, composed of one or multiple species, can be found simultaneously at a feeding site. Other locations where such large groups have been sighted include areas with large water sources (e.g., waterfalls) that serve as drinking sites, and the *culpas* (clay-licks) in Mexico, Peru, and Brazil. Here, birds congregate along river banks to consume fine clay soil, which may both serve as a source of essential minerals (e.g., sodium) and protect the birds against (plant) toxins ingested via their diet (Figure 5-6).[54,76-78] Many of these feeding and drinking activities are often concentrated in the early

morning and late afternoon. A decrease in foraging activity is often seen during midday, when birds interrupt their activities and fly off to rest in the trees during the hottest parts of the day (Figure 5-7).[52,58,79]

Comfort behavior, rest, and activity

Parrots in the wild also spend time on locomotor behaviors, the so-called comfort behaviors, and sleep. The former includes behaviors such as climbing, walking, or flying. The zygodactyl feet of a parrot optimally adapt it to an arboreal life, allowing it to perch, climb, and walk across branches as well as grab and hold food in its foot in order to manipulate it with the beak (podomandibulation; Figure 5-8).[80] Parrots are less adapted to walking on a flat surface, which causes them to move slowly and clumsily on the ground. As a result, they generally prefer to fly rather than walk to escape from potential danger or to commute between feeding grounds and roosting areas.[18,58,62,73]

Comfort behaviors include activities that help maintain the feathers, the integument, and the musculoskeletal system of the bird and increase its physical comfort. Among the various comfort behaviors recognized in birds are (self) preening,

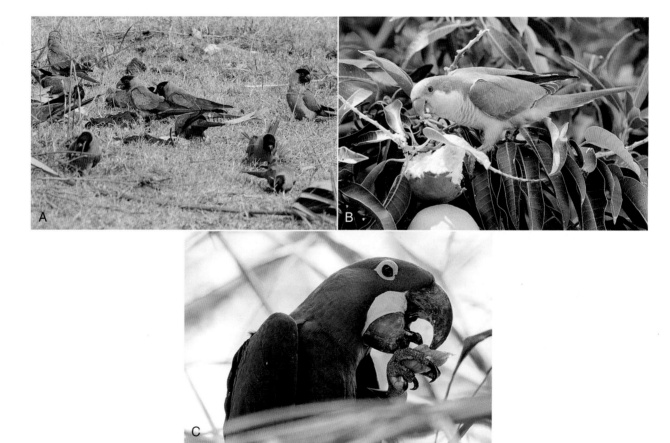

FIGURE 5-5 A, Nanday parakeets *(Aratinga nenday)* foraging for food in the fields of the Pantanal, Brazil. This type of activity may take up the greater part of the day for wild birds. **B,** Besides foraging on the ground, many psittacines will also forage in trees, as demonstrated by this Monk parakeet *(Myiopsitta monachus)*, which is eating a mango in the Pantanal, Brazil. **C,** Hyacinth macaws *(Anodorhynchus hyacinthinus)* commonly forage on their own, similar to this individual that was captured on camera while eating palm nut in the Brazilian Pantanal. (Photo courtesy Nico Schoemaker.)

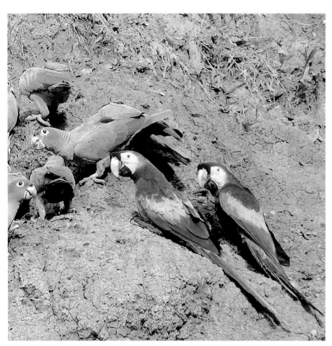

FIGURE 5-6 Mealy Amazon parrots *(Amazona farinosa farinosa)* and scarlet macaws *(Ara macao)* congregate at a clay-lick (also referred to as "culpa") along a river bank in Brazil. At these locations, birds of various species are often found together to consume fine clay soil. This soil consumption has been hypothesized to serve as a source of essential minerals (e.g., sodium) and protects the bird against ingested (plant) toxins. (Photo courtesy Scott Echols.)

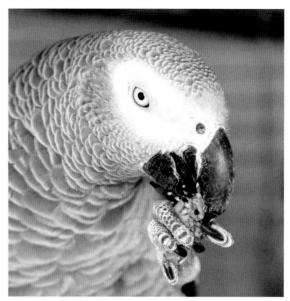

FIGURE 5-8 This Grey parrot *(Psittacus erithacus)* is holding food in its foot in order to manipulate it with the beak and consume the separate seeds. This activity is referred to as "podomandibulation" (see also Figure 5-5, *C*). (Photo courtesy Nico Schoemaker/Yvonne van Zeeland.)

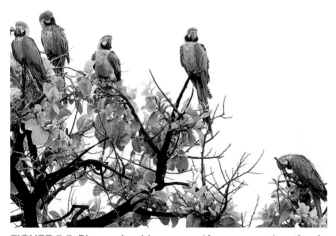

FIGURE 5-7 Blue-and-gold macaws *(Ara ararauna)* resting in the tree tops in the North Eastern part of the Pantanal, Brazil, after having foraged in the neighboring fields. (Photo courtesy Nico Schoemaker.)

bill-wiping, beak grinding and rasping, yawning, scratching, stretching, and bathing (Figure 5-9).[43,47,81,82] Bathing may take place in standing water (standing-water bathing) or in the rain (rain bathing), or the bird may rub its feathers against wet foliage (foliage bathing) (Figure 5-10).[83–86] Many of these comfort behaviors will be displayed during the sedentary

phases of the day, when the animal is not occupied with other essential activities such as foraging, drinking, or escaping a predator. Thus, these activities are often associated with either the beginning (e.g., grooming, beak grinding) or the end of a rest period (e.g., stretching), taking place in shorter bouts of a few seconds or longer bouts of several minutes.[43,81] Grooming or preening, in particular, may take up the greater portion of the waking hours when the parrot is not foraging. These preening behaviors are thought to serve an important function in optimizing plumage condition for flight, thermoregulation, waterproofing, camouflage, and communication. In addition, they play an important role in maintaining social relationships (e.g., through allopreening and during courtship displays). Preening behaviors may furthermore serve a function in comforting and soothing the bird by alleviating stress after a harrowing experience (de-arousal) or behavioral conflict (displacement behavior).[42,43,87,88]

Sleep and rest occupy a great portion of the day, as well.[58,62,73] As a social species, parrots usually sleep and rest simultaneously with the rest of the flock. In case of breeding pairs, the roosting site is usually located near or at the nest site, whereas nonbreeding birds generally roost on tree tops. As soon as dusk approaches, the birds will return from their feeding ground to these roosting areas, where they will sleep and rest until the next sunrise.[42,43,47,82] With most species of parrots coming from tropical or semitropical regions, where the day–night cycle approximates 12 hours of light and 12 hours of dark, respectively, parrots spend approximately half the time sleeping.[19] In addition, parrots will generally rest around noon, during the hottest parts of the day.[42,43,47,82] Typically, they will sleep while perched in an upright or somewhat lowered horizontal position with the body touching the perch and the head drooped because of decreased muscle tone (Figure 5-11, *A*). In case of prolonged sleep, which is

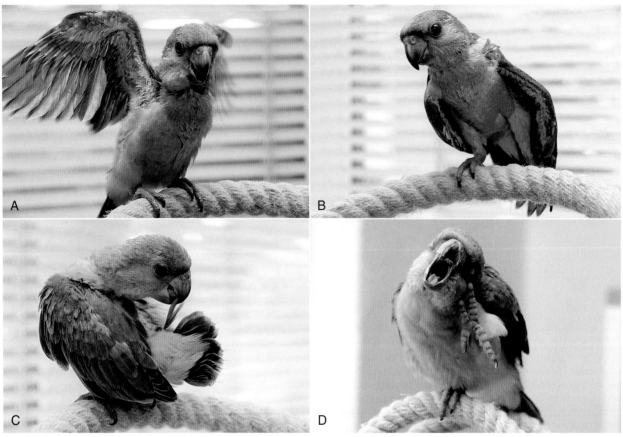

FIGURE 5-9 This young Senegal parrot *(Poicephalus senegalus)* demonstrates four different comfort behaviors (stretching the wings **[A]**, stretching a leg **[B]**, preening its feathers **[C]**, and yawning **[D]**). (Photo courtesy Ellen Uittenbogaard.)

considered important for brain restoration and memory formation, the birds may also turn the head 180 degrees, tucking it under the wing while staying perched on one or both feet (see Figure 5-11, *B*).[82,89,90] Similar to other bird species, parrots will engage in unihemispheric sleep, that is, a unique state during which one cerebral hemisphere sleeps while the other remains awake.[91] This physiologic phenomenon mitigates the fundamental conflict between sleep and staying awake and remaining vigilant to detect predators.

Characteristics and Consequences of the Parrot's Captive Living Environment

The typical companion parrot is likely to have many of the same instincts, behaviors, and needs as its conspecifics in the wild. Despite the similarities, many behaviors appear quite unique to a specific living environment. These adaptations to the specific living environment occur throughout the parrot's lifetime via the process of learning (see section Behavior: A Product of Previous Learning Experiences), thereby rendering the bird's behavior patterns flexible rather than rigid. This flexibility in behavior may be beneficial when adapting to the captive living environment. However, the parrots' captive living environment may contain features that they are evolutionarily counter-prepared to learn from. Conversely, domestically raised individuals may not have learned the right behaviors to prepare them for life in the wild.

One of the behavioral "needs" that seems to have been conserved in (captive) parrots is the need to forage. As has been shown in various studies, parrots display contra-freeloading (i.e., they choose to work for food even when the same food is freely available), suggesting they are motivated to forage.[80,92-94] This motivation, which is controlled by both physiologic and psychological parameters, can presumably only be fulfilled if an animal performs and experiences the consequences of both the appetitive and consummatory phases of feeding.[95-97] Unfortunately, many captive parrots have little to no opportunity to perform these behaviors: their food is often provided routinely in a food bowl at a predictable time and location in a readily available, easy-to-consume form, with no further need for the parrot to search or manipulate objects to obtain the food (Figure 5-12).[74] As a result, the time that captive parrots need to invest in foraging and food acquisition is significantly reduced, compared with wild conspecifics, and generally results in foraging times of less than an hour.[98,99]

In addition, many parrots are routinely denied flying and social contact with conspecifics, two other fundamental aspects of their natural behavior. Parrots kept as pets often spend the greater part of their lives confined to solitary housing in cages that do not accommodate flight and may even limit their ability to move around.[4,8,100] Even when allowed outside of their cage, parrots are restricted in their movement because owners often have their birds' flight feathers trimmed to prevent them from escaping or flying away (see Chapter 22).[101] The captive living environment may further prohibit the parrot from getting enough sleep. Ideally, pet parrots should be provided with a quiet, dark sleeping area (preferably a small sleeping cage that is separated from their daytime living area) and sufficient time for sleep. Specific data are, however, lacking on the quantity of sleep needed as well as the conditions under which sleep can best be provided. As a result, recommendations range from up to 12 hours in total darkness to allowing the bird downtime with the ability to take one or more short naps during the day. Periods of quiet time or quantifiable darkness, however, are often difficult to establish in a household situation where the parrot is generally kept in the main living area. The bird is often exposed not only to more hours of light per day compared with its wild counterparts but also to noises and visual stimulation from televisions, radios, and people talking and moving about the house.[82] Unless the bird is capable of adapting to these circumstances or the environment can be modified to enable the bird to obtain its required sleep, these disruptions can result in altered sleep cycles and have adverse effects on the bird's well-being.

Results of a study in Amazon parrots suggest that parrots need to be bathed, showered, sprayed, or misted at least on a weekly basis to allow expression of species-typical bathing behaviors that are elicited in response to rainfall (Figure 5-13).[86] The inability to engage in this or any of the other aforementioned natural behaviors may significantly decrease the bird's well-being. More importantly, these deficits may also predispose the bird to the development of physical and behavioral problems such as obesity (Figure 5-14) and abnormal repetitive behaviors (i.e., feather-damaging behavior [FDB] and oral and locomotor stereotypies).[8,25,100,102-107]

For birds that spend a great deal of their waking hours together with conspecifics and form strong, long-lasting

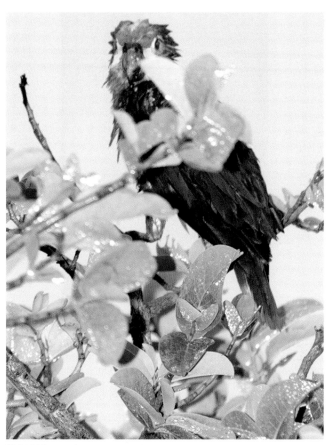

FIGURE 5-10 This blue-fronted Amazon parrot *(Amazona aestiva)* was found sitting on a tree after a heavy rain storm in Emas National Park, Brazil, being completely soaked in water. This demonstrates that parrots are used to a good soak of water. (Photo courtesy Nico Schoemaker.)

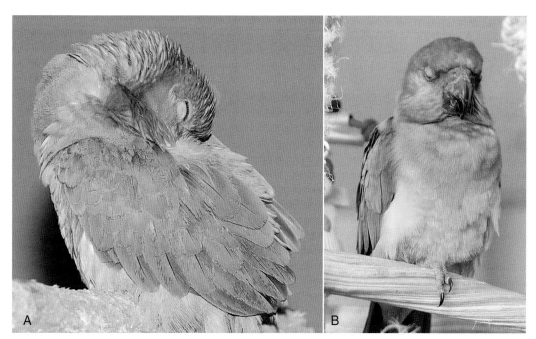

FIGURE 5-11 **A,** Senegal parrot *(Poicephalus senegalus)* showing the typical rest position with the head turned 180 degrees and tucked between the wings. **B,** Resting Senegal parrot *(Poicephalus senegalus)* with the eyes closed, a decreased muscle tone of the head and legs, and sitting on one leg. (Photo courtesy Ellen Uittenbogaard.)

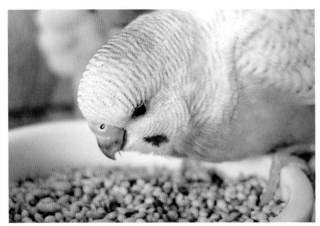

FIGURE 5-12 Many owners routinely provide readily available, easy-to-consume food in a food bowl. The budgerigar *(Melopsittacus undulatus)* in the image is provided enough seeds to eat for a couple of days. These circumstances limit the opportunities of psittacine birds to perform their species-typical foraging activities and reduce the time that is needed to consume the daily caloric intake to an absolute minimum. (Photo courtesy Ellen Uittenbogaard.)

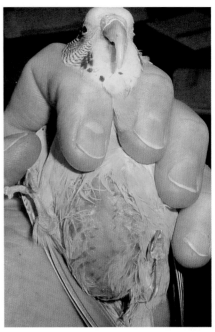

FIGURE 5-14 Severely obese budgerigar *(Melopsittacus undulatus)* with subcutaneous and even intracoelomic fat clearly visible through the thin skin. Also, note the abnormally long beak, which can be attributed to liver alterations such as hepatic lipidosis. (Photo courtesy Scott Echols.)

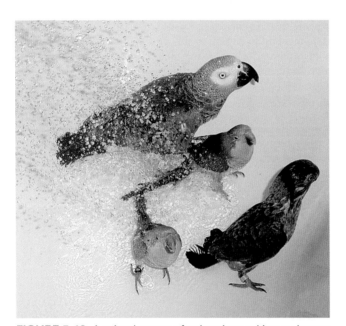

FIGURE 5-13 A mixed group of psittacines taking a shower in the bath tub. These birds clearly seem to enjoy their weekly bathing opportunity as they will actively go and sit under the water stream. Bathing, misting, or showering is considered an essential activity for parrots because it allows the bird to express natural bathing behaviors and promotes optimal skin and plumage condition. (Photo courtesy Ellen Uittenbogaard.)

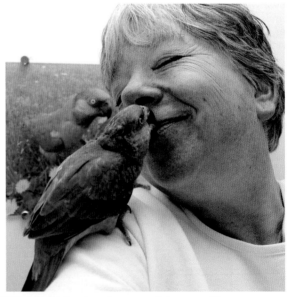

FIGURE 5-15 In the absence of conspecifics, parrots may also form strong bonds with humans, who may, partly, take over the role of a "life companion." Features that are indicative of such a bond include "kissing," preening the owner's hair (allopreening), and regurgitation of food to the owner. Although these activities are seemingly enjoyable, owners should take care to not encourage these activities too much because this may lead to inappropriate pair bond formation and behavior problems such as mate-related aggression or cloacal prolapse. (Photo courtesy Ellen Uittenbogaard.)

bonds with their mates, life without the company of conspecifics is likely to be stressful. In absence of conspecifics, parrots may also form strong bonds with humans and other animals, which may (in part) take over the role of a "life companion" (Figure 5-15). However, even when a surrogate human companion is available, parrots may still experience stress at times when he or she is (temporarily) gone (e.g., due to work, vacation, moving out, break up, death). In addition, the complexity of their communication, which human caregivers are often unfamiliar with, and the parrots' inability to interpret human signals predispose to miscommunication between parrots and their handlers. This, in turn, emphasizes the need for caregivers to invest time and energy in both teaching the parrots to interpret human signals and investing time to learn to interpret the parrot's signals. Learning to correctly interpret the birds' signals is challenging for many people because the birds' communication involves a complex system of different vocalizations and subtle changes in body posture. Such changes in body posture may include head, eye, and neck movements and wing, tail, leg, and foot gestures, all of which are used by the parrot to communicate its desires, intentions, and general comfort or discomfort with current events and conditions (Figure 5-16). Often, caregivers overlook or misinterpret the signals sent by the parrot, particularly those indicating any invasion of the parrot's personal space. Initial warnings to keep the person at a distance may include both subtle and more overt warnings such as raising of nape feathers, pupillary constriction and dilation, slight lifting of the wings, fanning of the tail feathers, holding a raised foot open at chest level, growling, and lunging with an open beak toward the "intruder."[48,108] Typically, the parrot will escalate to biting when the person does not recognize and respond to these warnings. Thus, it is important for the human handler to learn how to perceive, interpret, and respond to the parrot's signals. Variations in signals between bird species may, however, further complicate the ability of humans to fully understand the parrot's communication system. In addition, the species-typical nature of parrots' communication system suggests that birds of different species may not be able to fully communicate and understand each other without experience, potentially resulting in cross-species conflicts.[48,49]

A number of the innate behavior patterns displayed by wild parrots, including loud contact calls, wood chewing, tossing food, and biting to defend territories, are also displayed by companion birds under some captive conditions (Figure 5-17). Many of these behaviors are challenging to

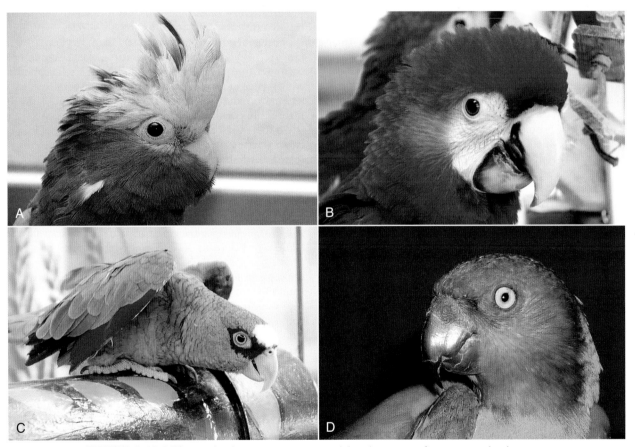

FIGURE 5-16 Different body postures are used by the parrot for communication purposes. These signals may have multiple meanings, varying from excitement to contentment. **A,** A raised crest and cranial placement of beard feathers in a galah *(Eolophus roseicapilla)* often indicate excitement and contentment, respectively. **B,** The raised feathers on the head of this young scarlet macaw *(Ara macao)* are an indication of alertness and excitement. **C,** This male white-fronted Amazon *(Amazona albifrons)* has a bent posture and quivering wings, which are often seen during courtship display or as an attempt to attract attention; if no quivering is seen, it can also be part of an aggressive display. **D,** Pinning of the eyes, as shown by this Senegal parrot *(Poicephalus senegalus)* can be a sign of aggression, excitement, nervousness, or pleasure. (Photo courtesy Ellen Uittenbogaard.)

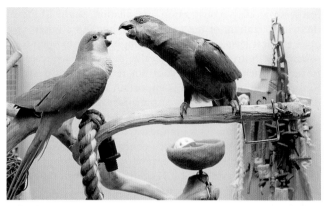

FIGURE 5-17 A Senegal parrot *(Poicephalus senegalus)* demonstrating territorial display, as indicated by the forward leaning motion and lunging toward the color mutant Monk parakeet *(Myiopsitta monachus)* with an open beak to prevent the latter from moving closer. (Photo courtesy Ellen Uittenbogaard.)

deal with for the owner, who unfortunately often responds incorrectly to the undesired behavior, thereby directly or indirectly reinforcing the behavior and further augmenting the problem.[109] For example, birds attempting to contact their caregiver may resort to persistent, loud, and excessive screaming or other attention-seeking behaviors. Owners often respond to these by verbally attempting to punish the bird, distracting it with its favorite food item or toy, covering the cage with a cloth (to contain the sound), or moving the bird (and its cage) to an isolated area. However, providing the bird with its favorite food item, toy, or attention often inadvertently positively reinforces the undesired behavior. Covering or moving the cage further enhances the bird's perceived sense of isolation. In the end, however, it is the future frequency of the behavior that provides evidence of effectiveness (or ineffectiveness). All of the aforementioned measures are likely to increase the bird's stress levels and the likelihood of the bird developing other abnormal behaviors and health problems. Whereas trained behaviors may easily be extinguished in the absence of reinforcers, innate behaviors may continue to persist despite the lack of reinforcement. As a result, these behaviors can be difficult to reduce. Thus, rather than attempting to reduce a behavior for which the bird has strong behavioral preparedness, the undesired behavior can best be prevented by changing the environment to better accommodate the bird's needs before the intensity of the behavior becomes problematic. For example, responding to the bird's natural contact call by whistling or talking to the bird when being in a different room may prevent screaming. In this situation, the bird no longer needs to start screaming as the normal contact call already results in the desired response (i.e., response back from the owner). Other examples include allowing the bird to climb out of the cage, rather than insisting that it step up, to prevent it from biting; offering smaller and more frequent meals to limit the amount of food wasted; and providing enrichment to the bird to prevent it from chewing the furniture or its feathers. Thus, accommodating the environment to the parrots' natural behavior should be considered an important tool to prevent and modify behavior that is considered undesirable by the caregiver and replace it with more appropriate, desirable behavior.[10]

The provision of toys and chewable items, however, does not guarantee success in preventing undesired behavior because its effect is highly dependent on the perceived value of the item to the bird. Many items only obtain their value once the parrot has discovered its benefits or if it has learned how to play with the object. If the item has no apparent value to the bird, it is often ignored. As a consequence, it does not serve its full potential as an outlet for exploratory, self-entertaining, and normal destructive behaviors such as chewing. Moreover, it remains questionable whether the physical stimulation, the toys and objects to chew and play with, and the social company of the caregiver in the captive environment can be sufficiently stimulating to satisfy the high intelligence and behavioral "needs" of most parrots.[4,24,49,100]

PSITTACINE BEHAVIORAL DEVELOPMENT—FROM NEONATE TO ADULT

The order of Psittaciformes consists of over 350 species, varying greatly in size and lifespan.[19,110] As a consequence, maturation rates also vary greatly among species, with smaller species generally maturing faster than larger parrot species.[19,111] Budgerigars and cockatiels, for example, fledge around 3 to 6 weeks, wean around 6 to 11 weeks, and enter adolescence at 4 to 7 months. In medium-sized species such as Amazon and Grey parrots, fledging, weaning, and sexual maturation occur at around 10 to 12 weeks, 12 to 16 weeks, and 3 to 4 years, respectively. Maturation takes the longest in larger species such as macaws, with fledging, weaning, and sexual maturation occurring at around 12 to 15 weeks, 16 to 20 weeks, and 4 to 5 years of age, respectively.[111] Because of this slow rate of maturation, owners of larger parrot species may not realize that their parrots' behaviors may change significantly over time. Thus, the owners may become confused and distraught once their parrots mature and start displaying adolescent behaviors such as courtship displays or territorial aggression. As a result, these owners, who are ignorant and unprepared for the behavioral changes accompanying avian adulthood, may complain that their parrot is "acting up," and they want it to return to its own sweet self again. In addition, many owners fail to realize that experiences during early childhood and adolescence have a significant influence on later behavior. It is thus vitally important to take into account the different developmental changes that parrots tend to go through and the factors that may influence its behavioral development.

Stages of Development in a Parrot's Life

The development of psittacine birds takes place according to a predictable path. In this development, various phases can be distinguished where the behavior and physical abilities of the bird develop parallel to each other and are greatly influenced by the arrangement of its environment (Table 5-1; Figure 5-18). For example, when the chick opens its eyes and begins to see, the provision of environmental enrichment further stimulates its visual acuity. Alternatively, the environment needs to be suitable for safe fledging once the chick's wings are fully feathered and it makes its first attempts to fly by flapping its wings and hovering over a perch. At this stage, the chick is also able to fully

TABLE 5-1

Developmental Phases During the Life of Psittacines*

Phase	Definition	(Physical) Characteristics	Behavioral Characteristics	Key Points for Adequate Care and Stimulation
Neonate	Period directly after hatching until opening of the eyes (altricial species)	Blind. Naked and poor thermoregulation. Unable to leave nest (≠ inactive). Fully dependent on parents for warmth and food.	Highly sensitive and responsive to various stimuli, including vocalizations, food, light, and touch Intense lighting may be detrimental to the developing eyes and also cause physiological distress, as indicated by display of behaviors such as flinching, hiding, and trembling. Gentle touch is readily accepted, with birds often immediately turning in the direction of the touch and moving around in circles until making contact with a sibling or parent to snuggle up against Open their beaks and gape upon gentle stroking of the rictus (the soft phalangeal [caudolateral] portions of the beak. Display pumping movements to ingest the food once it is regurgitated into the oral cavity. Produce begging sounds. Many behaviors are associated with a specific context: Snuggling (preceding sleeping) Pumping (preceding eating) Wiggling (preceding defecating). Ill, dehydrated, and/or hypothermic or hyperthermic chicks may show one or more of the following abnormalities: regurgitation, shivering, panting, crying, staying awake after feeding, and listlessness or hyperactivity.	When hand-raising (when parents are not able or willing to take care of the chick): Keep multiple chicks together. Provide daily physical contact with humans, including soft, gentle touches and handling. Cover chick with a towel that rests lightly on the neonate to mimic the parent's wing (helps quiet the chick after feeding). Provide darkened nest or container to mimic darkness of the nest inside the tree cavity. Optimal feeding schedule is sensitive to the chick's needs (usually once every 1 to 4 hours). Not adhering to these needs may pose unnecessary health risks (e.g., stunting, crop infections) and result in unnecessary stress in the chick.
Nestling or neophyte	Period starting at the time when the eyes open and pin feathers begin to develop until the time at which the chick makes its first attempt to fly	Eyes open. Nearsighted in initial phase. Developing (pin) feathers Lower susceptibility to temperature changes in the environment Development of long flight feathers triggers the chick to start flapping its wings. Still fed by parents or humans. Initiation of movement (jumping, hopping and parading around).	Imprinting (the process by which a young animal learns who its parents are and acquires several of its behavioral characteristics from them). Formation of a strong bond between the chick and its parents or a surrogate (e.g., human handler). Preference for dark corners initially, but with increased interest in their surroundings that coincides with the visual development. Looking at and moving toward objects, touching, and further exploring these objects. Start of socialization (period in which the chick is highly sensitive to stimuli and learns to visually recognize, accept, and interact with humans, animals, and objects) Exact time and length during which this developmental phase occurs in birds is currently unknown. May become quickly alarmed and display panic behaviors (trembling, trashing, backward flips) or fear cries when confronted by strange objects.	Provide a stimulating environment for the chick, including visual, tactile and auditory enrichment, as well as social interaction with humans and conspecifics. This allows the chick to get acquainted and accustomed to handling and a variable environment and decrease fearfulness at a later age. Examples of appropriate stimulation: Allow the bird to see outside. Allow the chick to listen to music. Talk to the chicks. Pick the chick up and carry it around in towels. Offer brightly colored objects or toys for exploration. Prevent overstimulation. Offer sufficient opportunity to prepare for flying, climbing, and landing. Provide preening toys to develop the chick's preening skills (especially when opportunities for allopreening [parents, siblings] are lacking). Initiation of training to promote behaviors that will benefit the bird and dissuade those that may be detrimental. Examples: Teach the chick to step up. Get the chick accustomed to handling.

Continued

TABLE 5-1

Developmental Phases During the Life of Psittacines—cont'd

Phase	Definition	(Physical) Characteristics	Behavioral Characteristics	Key Points for Adequate Care and Stimulation
Fledgling	Period in which the bird learns to fly	Development of the physical strength and dexterity to acquire and master the ability to fly. Chick is still food-dependent, although generally more keen on flying and less interested in food. Produces fewer begging sounds. Often weight loss observed, whereby the bird obtains a more streamlined, aerodynamic figure.	Chick makes first attempts to forage and feed independently. Time at which bird receives its first flying lessons from its parents and/or other flock members, including coordination of flight and landing. Exploration of toys, objects and food with the beak and tongue; biting, gnawing, and chewing on these items as well as on human hands. Development of play behaviors: Solicitation Play biting Play fighting Development of pair bonding behaviors: Allopreening Pseudocopulation Development of agonistic behaviors and fear to novel objects, noises or phenomena: Foot lifting Attack sliding Neck stretching Continued socialization. Acquire the social skills needed to interact and communicate with other flock members (including human handlers).	Continue to hand-feed the chick. Enable captive-born chicks to gain flying experience. Important for the bird's physical and emotional development and facilitates the weaning process. Gradual clips are recommended rather than the abrupt curtailment of flight if the owner wishes to have the bird's wings trimmed (see also Chapter 22). This allows the bird to develop sufficient strength, endurance, coordination, and confidence. Allow the bird to master flight in a dedicated area to reduce risks of injury. Provide additional (mental and physical) stimulation through opportunities to climb, forage, preen, bathe, shred, explore, and socially interact with humans or other birds. Prevents development of fear. Helps build confidence and independent play. Helps establish a long-term relationship between owner and bird. The more numerous and varied stimuli are to which a bird is exposed in this phase, the less likely it is to develop fears of objects, noises, or phenomena. Discourage the bird to bite or chew on human hands and fingers. Provide alternative chewing toys. Expose the bird to conspecifics. Stimulates development of normal behaviors. Increases potential for successful pair-bonding and breeding. Familiarize the parrots with human handling through regular touching, cuddling, and handling sessions (head, neck, and face are preferred). Touching toes, feet, legs, and wings may facilitate nail trimming and wing clipping. Learn behaviors that help the bird integrate in the "human flock." Examples: Stepping up Stepping down

Weanling	Period in which the bird (preferably gradually over a period of several weeks) learns to eat on its own	Bird learns to find and eat a variety of nutritious foods in sufficient quantities to survive.	Assist hand-reared birds by finger-feeding them warm, wet foods such as maize kernels and chunks of cooked pumpkin, carrots, yams, or mango, or offer pellets moistened with water or fruit juice. Do not ignore a bird that cries for food or allow it to go hungry. Instead, feed a moderate amount of hand-feeding formula and show how to forage and find its food. "Force-weaning" is discouraged because it can result in high-strung, hyper-responsive chicks that are prone to stress and become rigid in their eating habits. Force-weaning may lead to a multitude of behavioral problems, including phobias, chronic whining, and obsessive food-begging behaviors.
		Development of foraging and eating skills (exploring, manipulation of solid food items). Parents assist their young during the early phases of the weaning process. Feed large, more natural-sized food items. Present food to the chick in the beak or foot. Place food on the nest or perch to stimulate food-gathering behavior. Weaning may initially continue to beg and cry for food when parents start to ignore the begging behavior. Eventually chooses to start eating food unassisted.	
Juvenile or preadolescent	Period from the time when the bird is able to fly and eat on its own until puberty is reached	The bird is fully able to take care of itself (eating and drinking by itself). Time at which the bird can be safely separated from its parents and placed in a new home. Plumage may differ from that of the adult conspecifics; it may require one or several molts before the bird obtains its full adult feather coat.	Frequent baths and increased humidity may be beneficial to help alleviate discomfort because it helps soften the keratin sheaths of the pin feathers (thereby enabling them to open and be removed more easily). Perfect time for training and learning behaviors that are desirable when living together with humans. Exercise is important and may be encouraged by allowing them to fly or flap their wings, using movable perches and branches rather than stationary perches. Birds should be provided plenty of destructible toys and branches to encourage them to chew, shred, and pulverize these items as part of mental stimulation and beak exercise.
		Molt of feathers may be uncomfortable and make the bird irritable to touch (caution is advised when handling or stroking the bird!). The birds are curious and highly explorative. Easily learn and copy behaviors from others. As the birds mature, however, they may start refusing to cooperate.	
Adolescent (puberty)	Period during which hormonal changes occur which initiate the onset of sexual maturity and reproduction; onset of puberty not only varies per species but may also vary per individual	Hormonal changes that initiate the onset of sexual maturity	Provide materials and opportunities so that the bird can dissipate its energy in activities such as physical exercise, foraging, shredding, and play. Establish clear boundaries to help decrease unwanted behaviors. Unwanted behaviors often develop in this phase, particularly if owners are unprepared for the behavioral and temperamental changes that occur during this phase, thereby inadvertently rewarding these erratic behaviors.
		Increasing and fluctuating levels of sex hormones may result in the bird displaying sexual behaviors as well as signs of territoriality and/or aggression. Highly energetic birds. (Temporary) change in temperament is often observed.	

Continued

TABLE 5-1

Developmental Phases During the Life of Psittacines—cont'd

Phase	Definition	(Physical) Characteristics	Behavioral Characteristics	Key Points for Adequate Care and Stimulation
Adult	Period when hormonal fluctuations of puberty have subsided and the bird's behavior generally becomes calmer and more predictable		Calmer behavior. Less keen to try new things or travel. If socialized and trained properly early on in life, parrots can become docile and loving creatures that are well-adjusted to their life in a captive living environment. During the breeding season, birds may display a variety of reproductive behaviors including: Allopreening Allofeeding Mounting and copulatory movements Egg laying and incubation Territorial behavior to defend nesting area Birds sexually imprinted on humans, may reject other parrots as potential mates and choose a human partner instead. Display courtship and mating behaviors toward humans (e.g., regurgitation, masturbation). Display aggression toward other people. Similar behaviors may occur in parrots that are so-cialized with other parrots when a psittacine partner is lacking. Sexual frustration may lead to excessive vocalizations and feather-damaging behavior.	Refrain from touching the bird around the vent and lower back. Discourage courtship and mating behaviors displayed toward humans. Continue to provide enrichment and training for mental and physical stimulation.

*References 48,50,69,72,111,115-117,119-121,126,132-134,138,147,148,180,293,310.

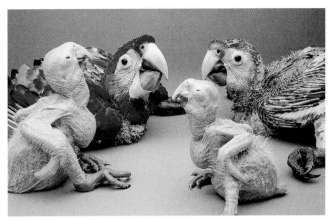

FIGURE 5-18 Scarlet macaw *(Ara macao)* chicks in different developmental stages. These birds are, from oldest to youngest, 48 days (1045 grams [g]), 37 days (965 g), 19 days (315 g), and 17 days (186 g). (Photo courtesy Joanne Abramson. Reprinted with permission from: Abramson J, Speer BL, Thomsen JB: *The large macaws: their care, breeding, and conservation*, Fort Bragg, CA, 1999, Raintree Publications.)

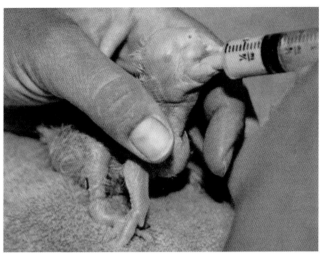

FIGURE 5-19 Hand-rearing has long been thought to be beneficial for strengthening the human–psittacine bond. Various studies have shown hand-rearing to be associated with display of abnormal behavior at older age as well. (Photo courtesy Joanne Abramson and Rick Droz. Reprinted with permission from: Abramson J, Speer BL, Thomsen JB: *The large macaws: their care, breeding, and conservation*, Fort Bragg, CA, 1999, Raintree Publications.)

interact with its environment and gains experiences that will have a significant impact on its responses later on in life.[112–115] Regardless of the stage—from neonate to adult—the parrot's living environment in captivity is largely controlled by humans. The level of control may, however, differ to some extent, dependent on the method of rearing (i.e., parent-raised or hand-reared). Under both circumstances, however, the role of human influence on the bird's living environment and, thus, its development underlines the importance of gaining insight into the various stages of development of the psittacine bird. This, in turn, will enable us to optimally rearrange the environment to its development and reinforce desirable companion characteristics and skills—two prerequisites for increasing the chances of the adult bird to thrive in captivity.

Factors Influencing the Behavioral Development of Parrots

Although the exact conditions under which chicks develop in the wild are largely unknown and likely vary between species, information about many critical developmental factors as well as information on behavioral development in other species can be derived from studies in captive-raised birds. The ontogenetic development of parrots in particular seems to be more comparable with that of the great apes than dogs and cats.[49] Two factors that are important to consider with respect to the development of a psittacine companion bird are (1) its socialization with humans and with other parrots; and (2) the degree of stimulation and enrichment provided in its rearing environment.

Socialization with parrots and humans

Being a social species, the visual, tactile, and auditory development of a parrot is greatly influenced by interaction with conspecifics such as parents and siblings.[72] In the case of captive rearing, humans also are part of the "flock," which requires parrots to become accustomed to physical contact and handling. For this purpose, hand-rearing (Figure 5-19) has long been the accepted method, as it is thought to help

strengthen the human–psittacine bond, thereby resulting in a bird that is more attached to humans and able to positively interact with people.[48] Hand-rearing and lack of interaction with conspecifics, however, can severely impact the emotional and social development of the captive psittacine bird and result in display of abnormal behaviors (see section Consequences of Hand-Rearing Psittacine Birds).

Stimulation and enrichment

Besides social contacts, the degree to which the bird is mentally and physically stimulated by its captive rearing environment will also influence the bird's development. The number and variety of the stimuli presented to the bird may significantly alter the risk of the bird developing phobias or anxiety disorders later on in life.[116,117] Such stimuli include not only a variety of (puzzle) toys and objects to shred and chew (Figure 5-20) but also visual, auditory, and tactile stimuli (e.g., trees, other animals, traffic noises, and radio or television sounds).[48,105,106,116] Although overstimulation should be avoided, especially in young birds, a moderate amount of novelty-related stress is considered important for the normal development of the chick. Such stress, resulting from exposure to novel objects and situations, enables the bird to cope with its ever-changing environment later on in life. Moreover, an overly safe, clean, and stable captive living environment in which such stressors are totally absent may predispose the birds to develop feather-damaging behavior or stereotypical behaviors.[48,106,118] Without the expenditure of physical or mental energy on foraging, initiating and maintaining contact with conspecifics, seeking shelter, and guarding against predators, birds may have more than enough time to spend on behaviors such as preening. This behavior may then be displayed in an exaggerated form and develop into an abnormal behavior such as feather-damaging behavior.[48,107]

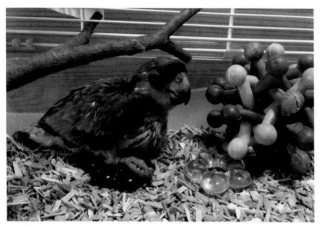

FIGURE 5-20 Novel objects being presented to a juvenile Senegal parrot *(Poicephalus senegalus)*. Provision of novel objects and enrichment at an early age stimulate the development of normal behavior and reduce stress from novelty later on in life. (Photo courtesy Ellen Uittenbogaard.)

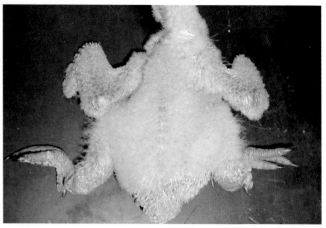

FIGURE 5-21 Malnutrition and excessive moving in the nest may lead to osteodystrophy and associated leg deformities as seen in this Grey parrot chick *(Psittacus erithacus)*. (Photo courtesy Michael Stanford.)

Consequences of Hand-Rearing Psittacine Birds

With the importation of wild parrots banned in many countries, hand-rearing chicks quickly became the predominant method of producing parrots for the pet trade. Traditionally, this method was promoted as the best available option to prepare the psittacine bird to its life as a pet, allowing it to be tamed and form a strong emotional and physical "bond" with its owner.[119,120] In addition, hand-rearing significantly decreased the cost and time investment for psittacine breeders, and prevented potential losses of chicks as a result of broken eggs, accidental injuries, and abuse or neglect by its parents. The brooding and rearing of chicks by the parents, however, have many advantages in terms of emotional and social development while also providing physical advantages. The limited movement of a group of chicks within the nest box, for example, provides them with the necessary support for the appendicular skeleton to develop properly. Chicks raised individually in incubators, in contrast, lack the support of the nest and siblings and frequently move around (allegedly in search of parental or sibling contact). This excessive moving around has been associated with a significantly higher incidence of bony deformations and osteodystrophy (Figure 5-21).[121]

To enable hand-rearing, chicks will often be hatched in an incubator or be removed from the nest and separated from their parents shortly after hatching (Figure 5-22). This disruption in parental care is suggested to be stressful and disrupt the normal behavioral and physiologic development of the bird.[120,122-124] For example, a study on growth rate differences between hand reared and parent-raised chicks showed slower growth rates in the hand-reared individuals.[125] Conversely, chicks hand reared by Abramson[126] showed growth rates and curves that exceeded that of their wild counterparts in many circumstances. Hand-rearing furthermore deprives chicks from the contact with conspecifics needed to establish normal social and sexual preferences.[127-129] If cross-fostered to other species or raised by humans, birds are more predisposed to imprint on or learn to identify with these foster

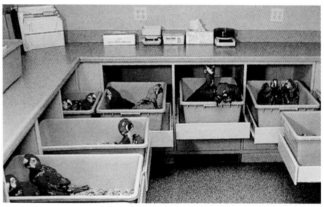

FIGURE 5-22 Some breeders incubate the eggs of their birds. Once these are hatched and the chicks are of an appropriate age, the birds are hand-reared in large nurseries. In this depicted nursery setting, the birds are group-housed with their conspecifics in large nest-bins, which, when pulled out as shown here, allows socialization with other adjacent youngsters. When the nest-bins are rolled in, the individual nest-bins are capable of providing a secure, darker nest-cavity location. (Photo courtesy Joanne Abramson and Rick Droz. Reprinted with permission from: Abramson J, Speer BL, Thomsen JB: *The large macaws: their care, breeding, and conservation*, Fort Bragg, CA, 1999, Raintree Publications.)

parents or caregivers, and may choose these as their preferred social and sexual partner after maturation.[129,130] As a rule of thumb, these concerns seem to manifest more often with cockatoo species (*Cacatua* spp.), as opposed to South American parrot species (macaws, Amazons, conures [*Aratinga* and *Pyrrhura* spp.]) but can be observed in individuals from any species. Imprinted or inappropriately reared birds may develop inappropriate reproductive behaviors as a result (e.g., impairment of normal copulatory behaviors and laying of eggs on the floor) and are less likely to successfully reproduce.[131] Effects may, however, differ between genders. For example, hand-rearing negatively impacted nest box inspections and egg fertility of the cock, whereas these parameters were unaffected in the hand-reared hens.[131] Thus, it appears hand-rearing may influence sexual imprinting in males more strongly than in females.[131] Social relationships may be disrupted as well, with hand-reared parrots displaying strong preference for social contact with humans and reduced interest in contact with conspecifics.[120,132,133] Parent-reared birds that have been tamed by occasional neonatal handling (i.e., five weekly 20-minute sessions), in contrast, exhibited approximately equal preference for human and conspecific companionship. This suggests that hand-rearing disrupts social preferences to a greater extent than taming.[120,134] Birds also differed in the extent and speed in which they learned human and species-typical vocalizations. Hand-reared birds were found to mimic human speech at an earlier age and to a greater extent than parent-reared birds. They remained unable, however, to produce the species-typical vocalizations until placed with normal vocalizing conspecifics for at least a week.[120] Most probably, these differences are the result of the level of social interaction, whereby the extensive exposure to human speech and human contact function as positive reinforcement. This, in turn, results in hand-reared chicks that quickly master the ability to talk.[49,120,135,136]

Parental separation and hand-rearing furthermore affect the development of other behaviors. Initially, hand-reared birds will display less neophobia (the avoidance of novel items by an animal[137]), as indicated by decreased latency times and overall decreased fear responses when presented with a novel object (Figure 5-23).[120,138] The effects, however, were only delayed, with no permanent alterations in the level of neophobia. At 1 year of age, both hand-reared and parent-raised birds (housed under similar conditions after weaning) were found to behave similarly when presented with a new object. These observations suggest that the differences may be a result of either delayed maturation or a more generalized habituation to novelty.[120,139] The lack of persistence of neophobia furthermore suggests neophobia to be plastic, with the birds remaining sensitive to environmental change well after weaning.[138] Such variability in behavior may be ecologically relevant for parrot species or individuals because it allows the birds to fine-tune their behavior to their environmental conditions. This may subsequently help decrease risks, for example, predation or ingestion of toxins, and increase the chances of finding unexploited foraging sites, nest sites, or mates. As a result, parrots that inhabit highly variable environments tend to be less neophobic than those that inhabit relatively constant, predictable environments.[140] Similar effects have also been observed in captivity, with frequent rotation and exposure to diverse environments significantly reducing neophobia in juvenile parrots.[117] These results emphasize the importance of regular rotation of enrichments over simple provision of enrichments. In fearful individuals, however, neophobia increased upon exposure to high levels of novelty,[117] which indicates that individual differences should always be taken into consideration when providing enrichment to a bird.

Aside from differences in development, birds are also more prone to develop abnormal behaviors as a consequence of hand-rearing. These include, but are not limited to, inappropriate sexual behaviors toward humans (e.g., regurgitation,

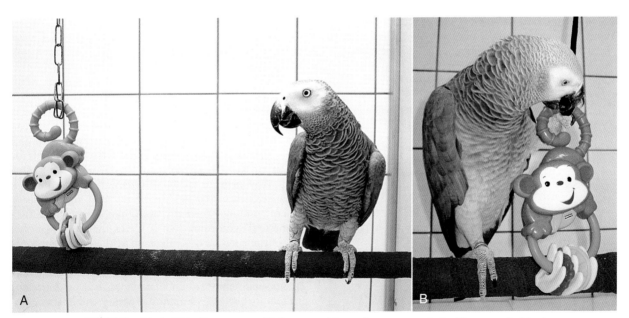

FIGURE 5-23 **A,** This Grey parrot *(Psittacus erithacus)* was presented with a novel object (a child's teething toy in the shape of a monkey). Although the bird did not panic, it was reluctant to approach this new toy. The reluctance to approach a novel object is referred to as "neophobia." **B,** This grey parrot *(Psittacus erithacus)* was presented with the same novel object as the parrot in Figure 5-23, A. Despite the fact that this bird had also never been in contact with the toy, it immediately approached this new toy and started to explore it with its beak and feet. (**A,** Photo courtesy Nico Schoemaker/Yvonne van Zeeland. **B,** Photo courtesy Kirsten van Bokhorst.)

courtship behavior), (territorial) aggression, (sudden onset of) phobic behaviors, excessive vocalizations, continued begging and whining for food (including delayed weaning), feather damaging behavior, and other stereotypies.[48,120,141-144] Many of these abnormal behaviors may develop as a result of so-called frustration (e.g., inability to sexually bond with humans) or to seek attention from the caregiver. As such, they appear similar to the "orphanage syndrome" or "relative attachment disorder" described in human children who have been deprived of affection and stability in their early childhood.[143-147]

Fortunately, increasing numbers of breeders are nowadays allowing parents to incubate, hatch, and raise their chicks themselves until fledging. Human interaction with these chicks may then either begin in the nest box ("co-parenting") or after the chicks have successfully fledged. Using these methods, the juvenile birds are accustomed to human handling via brief daily interactions while still also able to benefit from the interactions with their parents and siblings.[120,134,138] Particularly, the co-parenting technique appears successful at producing offspring that are less responsive to stress and well-socialized to both humans and parrots. In addition, this method increases the chances of the chicks displaying normal reproductive behaviors once they mature (because they had more intense contact with the parents and siblings than with humans[134,148]). Moreover, this often lowers the cost, time, and effort involved in successfully raising the chicks compared with conventional hand-rearing techniques.[120] Human contact with the neonate may, however, also increase the risk of abandonment, abuse, or infanticide.[48,120] As a result, the co-parenting technique may not be applicable to all species and individuals, especially those that appear prone to poor parenting.

If hand-rearing a psittacine chick is necessary, every attempt should be made to meet the physiologic, behavioral, and emotional needs of the bird throughout the various phases of its development (see section Stages of Development in a Parrot's Life). In addition, the risks of abnormal development may be lessened by raising neonates together rather than in individual enclosures.[111] Such crèches preferably consist of birds of a similar age and species (Figure 5-24). Mixed-species and mixed-age settings, however, may also yield good results, whereby the

young birds seek touching, sleep readily, play with, and are curious about others. Thus, the method poses as a suitable alternative that is widely accepted and used by breeders nowadays.[111]

BEHAVIOR: A PRODUCT OF PREVIOUS LEARNING EXPERIENCES

Besides evaluation from an ontogenetic, evolutionary, or physiologic level of analysis, behavior may also be understood in terms of learning processes, that is, behavior change as a result of experience. *Experience* is defined as contact with the environment, which can be classified into two broad categories of influence—antecedent and consequent events. Foremost among the different learning principles is the law of effect, whereby behavior is selected (or deselected) by the consequences or outcomes of behaving. Behaviors resulting in satisfying outcomes are more likely to be repeated, in contrast to those resulting in unsatisfying outcomes, which are less likely to occur. Thus, voluntary behavior is a function of its consequences.[149,150] This same concept also lies at the basis of behavior modification techniques known as "operant learning." Two key components of operant learning are reinforcement and punishment, which, respectively, result in an increase or decrease of the frequency in which behaviors are displayed.[151,152] The learning process may vary greatly among individuals, depending on previous experiences and the perceived value of the outcome, as well as the expertise with which these procedures are implemented. This emphasizes the importance of evaluating behavior separately for each individual in its specific context, rather than evaluating it solely on a species level. A similar individual assessment also lies at the heart of the field of applied behavior analysis (ABA), which focuses on the observable relation between an individual's behavior and the environment (antecedents and consequences) to predict and modify future behavior (see also section Applied Behavior Analysis).[10,11] Such analyses may greatly aid in our understanding and ability to intervene and ultimately change the behavior of an animal. Many pet owners, including those that own a parrot, however, are unaware of the fundamental principles of learning and behavior. As a result, they are often unable to provide a clear and objective description or recognize a pattern in their animals' behaviors. Only rarely do they realize that their birds' behaviors are a direct result of their own actions or the environment they provide to their birds.[10,11] In addition, owners unaware of the principles underlying learning may dislike the idea of "training" their parrots. Often, they believe this to be "unnatural" and think that it forces their birds to obey the will of their masters.[10,11] Because of these misconceptions, it is of utmost importance for veterinarians and behaviorists to understand the principles of ABA, explain these to their clients, and help them understand, analyze, and modify their parrots' behaviors, thereby increasing the chances for successful implementation of a proposed behavior modification strategy (see sections Applied Behavior Analysis; and Behavior Modification Therapy). Alternatively, veterinarians need to be aware of their limitations with regard to their knowledge about the learning and behavior change techniques. Rather than resorting to the use of psychoactive drugs or other intrusive methods as a first-choice intervention, they are advised to refer these clients and their patients to a

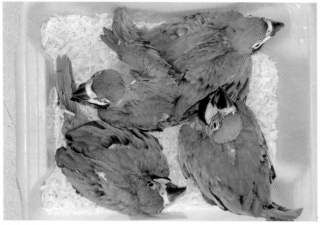

FIGURE 5-24 When neonates are raised together, as in the case of these blue-and-gold macaws (*Ara ararauna*), the risks of abnormal behavioral development are decreased. (Photo courtesy Lorenzo Crosta.)

behavior consultant or avian veterinarian who is familiar with treating avian behavior problems.

DIAGNOSIS OF BEHAVIOR PROBLEMS

Diagnosing and treating behavior problems can be one of the most challenging aspects of the veterinary profession. To be able to successfully diagnose a behavioral problem, veterinarians should be able to correctly analyze the animal's behavior and differentiate whether the behavior is normal, the result of learning, or a side effect of a medical problem. For this purpose, a sound understanding of the behavior and development of the species and the basic principles of learning theory are necessary (see sections Characteristics, Behavior and Activity Patterns of Parrots in the Wild; Psittacine Behavioral Development; Behavior: A Product of Previous Learning Experiences). Successful diagnosis of a behavioral problem furthermore requires the identification of all behavioral and medical signs and the circumstances under which the abnormal or undesirable behavior is displayed. The list of potential contributing factors for any behavioral problem is long, including a variety of infectious, toxic, nutritional, neoplastic, immune-mediated, metabolic, endocrine, behavioral, traumatic, and management-related conditions. As such, a complete diagnostic workup, consisting of an extensive and detailed history, full physical examination, and behavioral assessment, may be required.

Upon evaluating the information obtained from this medical and behavioral assessment, hypotheses regarding the underlying motivations and factors contributing to the onset and maintenance of the abnormal or undesirable behavior can be subsequently generated and tested. With no two individuals being exactly alike, each case should be considered as a "study of one," which warrants the formulation of a unique working hypothesis that is specifically tailored to the individual and its living environment.

Diagnostic Workup of a Behavioral Problem

When confronted with a parrot with abnormal or undesirable behavior, exclusion of medical conditions that might contribute to the observed behavioral signs is often the first step to be taken. In principle, any localized or systemic medical condition that affects brain function or results in pain, pruritus, irritation, or other type of discomfort to the parrot may initiate a change in behavior, resulting in, for example, aggression (biting), anxiety (screaming or sudden flailing around in the cage), or FDB. Concurrently, the initial aspects of behavioral assessment should be initiated as a portion of the foundational medical workup. If and when the physical assessment and diagnostic tests fail to identify an underlying medical condition that has a key contributing role in the problem behavior, implementing a more in-depth behavior analysis will be important. During that process, diligent efforts to identify the potential occasion-setting antecedents and reinforcing consequences that may have contributed to the onset and maintenance of the problem behavior can provide the working tools with which a behavior-change plan can be initially strategized.

The workup of a behavioral problem roughly involves the same systematic and critical thinking processes as those of a medical problem. The differences relate to what is being investigated and not to the framework of critical thought required. With medical problems, the investigation focuses primarily on internal pathologic processes that affect the animal's health, whereas the main focus during workup of behavior problems is placed on the animal's environment and how this affects the animal's behavior (i.e., external influences). In both, however, a similar sequence is followed, in which data are gathered (from the signalment, history, physical examination, or behavioral and environmental assessment), followed by compilation of a list of differential diagnoses or hypotheses as to why the behavior is occurring and the designing of a plan to test the aforementioned hypotheses (i.e., diagnose the problem or exclude [medical] causes) and treat the problem. Both require a critical assessment of the outcome (follow-up) and often a refinement of the treatment plan as further observational data become available.

Signalment

Similar to any other field of veterinary medicine, species, gender, and age may provide important clues regarding the potential origin of the abnormal or undesired behavior. For example, it is commonly believed that territorially associated aggression is more likely to occur in Amazon parrots and small macaw species,[153] whereas Grey parrots appear more prone to anxiety disorders or feather-damaging behavior (Figure 5-25).[154] In addition, certain behavioral problems may also be linked to a specific gender (e.g., territorial aggression is more likely to occur in male Amazon parrots, whereas problems related to egg laying obviously only occur in female birds).[153] Behaviors such as regurgitation or begging behavior may be considered normal when the parrot is relatively young but abnormal if the parrot still displays these as it grows older.[111,120] Similarly, certain behaviors may be linked to adolescence, puberty, and sexual maturation. The signalment may thus point toward specific problems or underlying causes, although these should always be interpreted with utmost care to prevent generalization and automatic labeling of a problem solely based on the bird's signalment, thereby limiting objective evaluation of the behavior.

History

Obtaining a thorough and comprehensive history is vital when presented with a parrot with a behavior problem as it may provide important clues regarding the potential underlying medical, behavioral, and environmental factors involved. To facilitate the history-taking process, standardized forms or questionnaires may be used (Box 5-3), especially with respect to data regarding housing, nutrition, social and environmental enrichment, daily routine, and the bird's background. By having the owner fill out these forms prior to the visit, data may be collected in a more organized, consistent, and timely manner while decreasing the odds of missing an important question.[155] A standardized form, however, can never replace the interactive questioning and discussion with the owner(s) as the spontaneous answers and responses as well as the nonverbal communication (e.g., body language, tone of voice) during such conversations may provide much additional information that cannot be obtained from a form.[155]

Taking a thorough history always starts with a detailed description of the abnormal or undesired behavior displayed

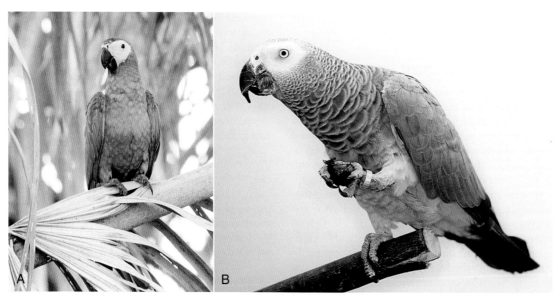

FIGURE 5-25 **A,** Territory-associated aggression is believed to occur more commonly in Amazon parrots and small macaw species, such as this red-bellied macaw *(Orthopsittaca manilata)*. **B,** Grey parrots *(Psittacus erithacus)* are considered predisposed to develop anxiety-related disorders or feather-damaging behavior. (Photo courtesy Nico Schoemaker.)

BOX 5-3 AVIAN BEHAVIORAL HISTORY FORM

Date of consultation:

Owner information:
Name:
Address:
Phone: (day)   (evening)
Email:
Who is the bird's primary caregiver?

Bird information:
Name of the bird:
Species:
Age: …. years/….. months   Unknown
Sex: Male/Female/Unknown
　If the sex is known, how was this determined?

Household information:
List all people in household and people who interact with bird on a regular basis:

Name	Age	Relationship (e.g., spouse, son, daughter, pet sitter, housecleaning service workers)

BOX 5-3 AVIAN BEHAVIORAL HISTORY FORM—cont'd

List other birds and/or pets in household (list these in the order in which they came into household; include the patient in this chronologic list as well):

Name	Species/Breed	Age Now	Age Acquired	Sex

Provide a brief description of the interaction between the birds (e.g., do they have vocal/visual/physical contact, share a cage)

Acquisition and rearing history:
Reason for acquisition:
    Acquired from (circle the answer that is applicable):
        Breeder/Pet Store/Previous Home (Re-homed bird)/Own bred/Shelter/Other (describe):
           If your bird is a re-homed bird, describe briefly below what is known about its previous home environment (e.g., married couple? children? length of time in home)
Your bird was (circle the answer that is applicable):
    Bred in captivity/Wild caught/Unknown
    Hand-raised/Parent-raised /Unknown rearing method
        If hand-raised, by whom? (e.g., breeder/you/unknown)
Raised with: siblings/similar-aged birds but different species/birds of other ages/unknown
At what age was your bird separated from its parents?
At what age was your bird re-homed to its new home?
Briefly describe the weaning process and stimuli (e.g., social contact and enrichment) the bird was confronted by during early life:

Husbandry:
Cage(s) and playpen:
◆ Size (approximate dimensions) and materials of which the cage is made
◆ When used (e.g., sleeping, daytime, outside)
◆ Location(s) (i.e., inside/outside, where in the house and where in the room)
◆ Cleaning (frequency, products, procedure of cleaning)
◆ Furniture in cage (include information on which types of enrichment are provided, which of these are used, frequency and way in which these are used, and how often these are changed, if applicable):
  ◆ Perches and other climbing materials/toys
  ◆ Bowls
  ◆ Chewing toys/materials
  ◆ Puzzle toys
  ◆ Foot toys
  ◆ Nest boxes
  ◆ Other

Nutrition:
◆ Diet: %'s fed (offered and % actually eaten)
  ◆ Main diet
  ◆ Treats and supplements (including which and how often provided)
  ◆ How fed (bowl, foraging enrichment)
  ◆ Water source (how provided and frequency of changing)

Sleep rhythm and lighting:
◆ Hours awake/asleep
◆ Hours light/dark
Cage covered: Yes/No
What type of lighting is available to your bird (e.g., daylight, UV-light, fluorescent light)

Feather care (bathing/misting/clipping):
◆ Do you provide your bird bathing/misting opportunities: Yes/No
  ◆ If yes:
    ◆ How often?
    ◆ Method?
    ◆ Bird's response to bathing/misting?
◆ Are wings routinely clipped? Yes/No
  ◆ If yes, how is the clipping performed?
◆ Does your bird come outside? Yes/No
  ◆ If yes, how often and where? (e.g., garden, park, friends/family)

Human/bird interaction:
◆ What tricks or commands does your bird know?
◆ Provide a brief description of the interaction between the bird and the people in the household (e.g., how often does the bird interact with the different people, characterize the interaction [cuddling/physical contact, playing/training, care and feeding])

Daily routine:
◆ Describe a typical day in your bird's life, starting with when and where bird wakes up in the morning. Be sure to include when, where, how, and who feeds bird, exercise/training/play (what type, how much, where), where bird is when people are not at home, where bird sleeps at night, and anything else you think is important (use additional pages as needed):

Behavior of your bird:
◆ Give a short description of your bird's behavior to the various people/animals/stimuli as mentioned below:
  ◆ How does your bird react to his/her daily caregiver?
  ◆ How does the bird react to familiar people (other than the daily caregiver)?
  ◆ How does the bird react to unfamiliar people?
  ◆ How does your parrot respond to other parrots?
  ◆ How does the bird react to new items or toys?
  ◆ How does the bird respond in a new environment (other than its familiar environment)?
◆ Does your bird allow petting?
  ◆ If yes, does it actively ask for it (e.g., by offering its head) or not?
◆ How does your parrot respond to handling (e.g., using a towel)?

Continued

BOX 5-3 AVIAN BEHAVIORAL HISTORY FORM—cont'd

Problem behaviors:
Indicate whether bird displays any of the following behaviors:

Behavior	No	Yes (indicate frequency in next columns)	Daily	Weekly	Monthly
Chronic egg laying					
Chewing/biting/tearing its own skin (self-mutilation)					
Damaging its own feathers (feather-damaging behavior)					
Destructive chewing of furniture or other materials in the environment					
Screaming					
Rubbing cloaca/vent on objects or people					
Regurgitating					
Repetitive behaviors such as somersaulting or weaving					
Hiding/trembling/trying to get away from people or other animals (fearful behavior)					
Lunging at/biting people or other animals					
Other (provide a description)					

Medical history:
Does your bird have any known medical conditions or physical problems?
  If yes, describe these briefly.
Does your bird take any medication?
  If yes, describe which, what dose, and how often?
Details regarding your bird's problem behavior:
◆ What is the behavior problem for which you are seeking advice?
◆ Did a specific event prompt you to address this problem now?
  ◆ If yes, describe this briefly.
◆ When did you first notice the problem, and what did the behavior "look like" at that time?
◆ When the problem first began, how frequently did it occur?
◆ How often does it occur now?

◆ Do you feel that there were any inciting factors?
  ◆ If yes, describe these briefly.
◆ How has the problem changed or developed over time?
◆ When does the problem behavior occur now?
◆ Do you feel that there are any specific situations that seem to "trigger" the behavior?
  ◆ If yes, describe these briefly.
Date of most recent incident of behavior:
Description of most recent incident of behavior:
How do you respond when your bird performs this problem behavior?
What, if anything, have you done to try to treat the problem (e.g., medical treatment, behavioral therapy, medications, supplements, herbs). Indicate if the attempted treatment made the problem better, worse, or if the behavior remained unchanged?

Treatment Attempted	Behavior Better	Behavior Worse	No Change in Behavior

by the parrot, including the age at onset; initial appearance and duration of existence of the problem; frequency, duration, severity, and timing of the bouts of problem behavior; progression and changes in pattern, frequency, intensity, and duration over time; and any previous corrective measures or treatments that have been tried to alter the behavior (including the parrot's responses to these). Besides the behavioral problems, the overall behavior of the animal should also be described, including its responses to family members and strangers, new situations, and other types of stimuli. The

veterinarian should always take into account the possibility that owners' descriptions may be tainted as they have their own interpretations of the behavior. If possible, it is therefore advised to have owners bring along video recordings of the parrot's behavior because these allow for objective evaluation of the behavior and can help provide further insight into the behavior and its origin and provide clues as to how the problem behavior might be managed or decreased.

Next, the parrot's living conditions, including its nutrition, physical and social environments, and daily routine are evaluated.

Photographs, a floor plan, and a video tour of the house may particularly be useful to form a complete and clear picture of the parrot's living environment. However, these can never be better than actually being in the parrot's living environment and observing it directly.[5] Factors of the living environment that may be evaluated include the size, construction, and cleanness of the cage, as well as the location and surroundings of the cage, including the presence (or lack) of any visual and auditory stimuli that may be perceived either as stimulating (e.g., people, toys) or threatening (e.g., loud noises, large objects, children, other animals). Particularly, the location of the cage has been shown to influence behavior. For example, cages placed in the center of a room or placed against a window or glass door compel the bird to continuously watch out for danger in every direction, never being able to let down its guard. Alternatively, placement near a doorway may startle a bird every time someone opens the door and enters the room.[118,155] Various toys and other types of enrichment may be provided to stimulate the bird's behavior (Table 5-2).

TABLE 5-2
Type of Enrichments that can be Provided to Parrots and Other Bird Species

Type of Enrichment*	Function
Sensory	Stimulates the parrot's visual, olfactory, auditory, tactile, and/or taste senses (e.g., radio, television)
Manipulatory	Can be manipulated by the feet and/or beak, thereby promoting investigatory behavior and exploratory play (e.g., foot toys [can be manipulated by the animal's feet] and chewing toys [can be manipulated or destroyed with the beak]
Environmental	Enhances the parrot's captive habitat with opportunities that change or add complexity to the environment (e.g., climbing toys [can be used for climbing, hanging, or swinging], branches, bushes, and plants
Puzzles	Stimulate the parrot's problem solving capabilities because they require the bird to analyze, solve, and complete a task to receive a reward (e.g., food)
Foraging/feeding	Encourage the animal to investigate, manipulate, and work for food, thereby mimicking the appetitive and consummative phases of feeding behavior, similar to a noncaptive environment (e.g., puzzle feeders, foraging trees, nuts)
Social	Provides the opportunity to interact with other animals (conspecifics or interspecifics) and/or humans
Training	Provides social interaction with humans and changes behavior using behavior modification techniques such as positive reinforcement and habituation

* Some items may serve multiple functions and can therefore be assigned to more than one group.

Preferably, at least one of each type should be available to the bird at all times. When evaluating the toys and enrichment provided to a bird, the type of toy, its size, materials, and suitability should be taken into account.[155,156] In addition, inquiries should be made into the frequency with which the toys are changed or replaced and, more importantly, whether and how (i.e., type of interaction, frequency, duration) the bird interacts with the toys and the enrichment it is provided with. Besides the bird's physical environment, its social environment and any interactions with people, animals, or other birds (including the type, frequency, and duration of those interactions) should also be evaluated. This may for example help identify whether the bird is bonded to a specific person or interacts with several people.[5] Last but not least, insight should be gained into the daily routine of the parrot (and its owner), including any day-to-day variations that may occur.[5]

Besides the current living environment, the background of the parrot is also important. Although it is not possible to go back in time and change these early experiences, it is important to realize that these may significantly affect the bird's confidence and sense of security as well as determine its overall flexibility and potential as a companion animal (see section Stages of Development in a Parrot's Life). Especially, the rearing technique (i.e., hand-rearing versus parent-rearing; solitary or together with siblings) and prior exposure to environmental enrichment may influence the way the chick interacts with, for example, conspecifics and humans. Moreover, it may also affect the occurrence of behavioral problems such as phobias, stereotypical behaviors, FDB, and aggression.[a] Information about the conditions under which the parrot was raised (including the age at which it was separated from its parents and siblings) thus needs to be obtained during the history taking. When dealing with a re-homed parrot, its living conditions in the previous home may also be of importance. These are, however, rarely known by the current owner, making it much more difficult to evaluate where the abnormal behavior originated from. Many owners often (wrongfully) assume that the bird must have been abused or neglected in its previous home. However, rather than taking the owner's word for it, veterinarians should draw their own conclusions about the prior situation of the bird.[155]

Obtaining honest and objective answers from the owner may prove difficult. In addition to (wrongful) assumptions about the bird's past, owners may often decide not to tell the truth but provide wishful answers instead. This may particularly be the case when asked leading questions or when they feel (in)directly accused of incorrect treatment of their parrot.[155] Thus, asking non-leading, open-ended questions and being sympathetic and nonjudgmental toward the owner provides the greatest chances of obtaining honest answers.

Physical examination and behavioral observations
A full physical examination, consisting of an observation of the patient followed by a hands-on examination, is performed to detect potential physical abnormalities that may suggest a potential underlying localized or generalized illness. For example, changes in the bird's mentation, plumage condition, and posture or stance may indicate presence of behavioral

[a]References 92,106,116,117,120,134,138,143,144,148.

problems or disease. Similarly, changes in the number or appearance of the droppings can suggest presence of an underlying kidney, liver, or intestinal problem. The hands-on examination, which should be performed in a manner that causes as little stress as possible, includes a closer inspection, palpation, and auscultation of the various structures. Abnormalities that are detected during this physical examination always warrant a closer examination (e.g., using magnifying glasses or surgical loupes) as well as concise documentation of the abnormalities in the patient's medical records.

In addition to a physical examination, the parrot's behavior may also be observed. This is often challenging as the new location and the presence of an observer may influence the bird's behavior. Because of this, observations are preferably performed in the parrot's own surroundings during a home visit, with as little disturbance of the normal behavior as possible; as an alternative, the observation may be performed with the bird at rest in a nonthreatening situation in the consultation room. Observations of behaviors are functionally prohibited by management practices such as transferring the bird directly from its carrier to physical restraint and/or conscious sedation or anesthesia. Although the presence of a behavior consultant or veterinarian in this home environment may also affect the parrot's behavior, it will generally do so to a lesser extent than when performing the observations in the unfamiliar surroundings of the veterinary clinic.[155,157] Video recordings of the animal's behavior may help to overcome the aforementioned limitations. This method allows recording of not only the interaction between the bird and owner without interference of a third party but also the bird's behavior when the owner leaves the room (e.g., in case of suspected separation anxiety). Thus, the technique offers a suitable and effective alternative to direct observations of the behavior.[155,157] Prior to making video recordings, owners should ensure that their birds are acclimatized to the camera to prevent fearful responses as a result of exposure to the camera. Similarly, owners should be discouraged to stage a situation that provokes an aggressive response just to get it on video. This may not only result in injuries to the owner but may also reinforce the bird to continue displaying aggressive behavior.

Direct observations of behaviors may best be performed at the beginning of a visit, shortly after or during the history taking. Preferably, the behaviors (including type, frequency, and duration) should be recorded within a defined period (e.g., 15 minutes) to enable monitoring of behavioral changes over time.[155,157] By observing the bird's behavior, additional information may be obtained about its personality, its responses to stimuli and commands, and its relationship and interaction with the owner. In addition, the owner's responses to the bird's behaviors may also be observed, which often provide important clues to the onset and maintenance of problem behaviors (see section Applied Behavior Analysis).[155]

Additional diagnostic testing

Depending on the findings from the history and concurrent behavioral assessment and physical examinations, a diagnostic workup may be performed. Conversely, not all problem behaviors require an in-depth diagnostic workup in all cases, and the key actionable diagnoses may already be apparent at the end of history taking and following observation and physical assessment of the patient. The types of additional testing performed should always be tailored to the individual bird, with selections based on the tentative diagnosis or differential diagnoses suspected in this patient. There rarely will be a standard diagnostic workup that fits all individuals, all species, and all problem behaviors. An overview of the various tests that may be considered or performed, in part, in select patients with behavioral abnormalities, including the types of diseases that may be diagnosed using these tests, is presented in Table 5-3.

Applied Behavior Analysis

ABA focuses on the environmental determinants of behavior, and behavior that occurs through the process of learning, that is, behavior change as a result of experience. ABA includes the comprehensive and scientific study of behavior in which hypotheses are generated regarding the environmental influences that account for a certain behavior (functional assessment), which may subsequently be tested and evaluated. This functional assessment is the first step to accurately assessing what is going on and why—two key factors in the development of a successful and effective behavioral intervention plan.[10,11]

The ABCs of behavior

Behavior never occurs randomly or independent of its environmental surroundings but always serves a function that is related to the (environmental) stimuli, events, and conditions that precede and follow it. Skinner described this three-term contingency, also known as the *ABCs of behavior*, as the smallest meaningful unit of behavior analysis (Box 5-4).[151,152] The three-way contingency indicates that no behavior can be understood without knowledge of the occasion that precedes a response (antecedents) and the consequences that immediately follow this response.[10,11]

Antecedents. Antecedents include the various stimuli, events, and conditions that immediately precede a behavior and influence the likelihood of a specific behavior occurring (rather than directly causing the behavior).[158,159] There are three classes of antecedents: setting events, motivating operations, and discriminative stimuli. Setting events are the context, conditions, and situational influences that affect behavior. For example, a small cage door or an unsteady hand may set the occasion for biting to escape the door or remove the hand. The relationship between setting events and problem behavior should be considered carefully as the environmental setting is often one of the easiest things to change. The goal is to remove the obstacles that make the "right" behavior harder to perform than the "wrong" behavior. Motivating operations (also known as "establishing operations") are antecedent events that temporarily alter the effectiveness of consequences. For example, a food treat that is only available for stepping on the hand will tend to be a stronger reinforcer than the same food when freely available throughout the day. Motivating operations is a broad category of antecedent influences that also includes past experience with reinforcers; personal space and physical obstacles; emotions such as fear, anxiety, and excitement; and the animals' learning history (e.g., ability and relationship with caregivers). Discriminative stimuli are the cues that signal the behavior–consequence contingency ahead. A stimulus becomes a cue for a particular behavior if the stimulus is repeatedly present when the

TABLE 5-3

Diagnostic Tests that may be Used to Aid in Identification of Physiological Correlates of Behavior Problems*

Diagnostic Test	Indications
Complete blood count and biochemistry	Hepatopathy, nephropathy, generalized infection or inflammatory process, diabetes mellitus, hypocalcemia
Toxicology	Suspected lead or zinc toxicosis. Collect heparinized whole blood (lead) or plasma/serum in non-rubber plastic or glass tubes
Thyroid-stimulating hormone test	Hypothyroidism
Fecal examination (cytology, including Gram staining, wet mount, and/or flotation)	Giardiasis (common in cockatiels), helminthic infection, coccidiosis (rare in parrots), candidiasis, *Macrorhabdus ornithogaster* infection (avian gastric yeast), bacterial overgrowth or dysbacteriosis
Radiology	Heavy metal intoxication, reproductive disorder (e.g., egg binding); hepatomegaly, splenomegaly, or renomegaly; proventricular dilatation disease; pneumonia; airsacculitis; neoplastic conditions; musculoskeletal disease (e.g., osteoarthritis, osteomyelitis, fractures, osteosarcoma)
Ultrasonography	Hepatomegaly, reproductive disorders (e.g., egg peritonitis, cystic ovary), neoplastic conditions, cardiac disease, ascites
Endoscopy	Airsacculitis, hepatopathy or nephropathy, splenomegaly, pancreatic disorders, reproductive disease
Skin scrapings	Ectoparasites, in particular mites (e.g., *Knemidokoptes*, *Metamichrolichus nudus*). Be careful not to tear the skin!
Impression smear, swab cytology, or tape strip	Bacterial or fungal dermatitis, dermatophytosis, *Malassezia*, *Candida*, ectoparasites (e.g., feather mites, lice), pox virus
Fine-needle aspiration	Skin neoplasia, xanthomatosis, feather follicle cyst, hematoma, bacterial dermatitis or abscess
Feather digest (using potassium hydroxide)	Ectoparasites (quill mites)
Feather pulp cytology	Bacterial or fungal folliculitis, psittacine beak and feather disease (PBFD) or polyomavirus infection, quill mites
Culture and sensitivity testing	Bacterial or fungal infection (e.g., dermatitis, folliculitis)
Skin and/or feather follicle biopsy (histopathology)	Various infectious, inflammatory and/or neoplastic skin diseases (e.g., PBFD, polyomavirus, bacterial and fungal folliculitis, quill mite infestation, xanthomatosis, squamous cell carcinoma, feather follicle cysts). A biopsy of an area that the bird is unable to reach may help to differentiate between psychogenic and inflammatory causes (i.e., no abnormalities versus presence of inflammation in the control biopsy) *Note:* Biopsy specimens may also be collected from other tissues and organs to detect abnormalities found with other diagnostic tests.
Intradermal skin testing	Hypersensitivity reactions, allergic skin disease. Thus far not found to be reliable because of the bird's diminished reaction to histamine
Tests for specific causative agents	Polymerase chain reaction (PCR) testing on whole blood, feather pulp, or tissue for PBFD PCR testing on fecal swab or tissue for presence of polyomavirus PCR on cloacal swab/feces and/or serologic testing for avian bornavirus (ABV) PCR on conjunctival/choanal/cloacal swab and/or serologic testing for *Chlamydia psittaci* Serology or galactomannan assay for *Aspergillus* (relative low sensitivity and specificity)

*When paired with behavior analysis, the two models of evaluation (medical and behavioral) can greatly enhance outcomes of intervention strategies.[157,191,266,281]

BOX 5-4 THE ABCs OF BEHAVIOR

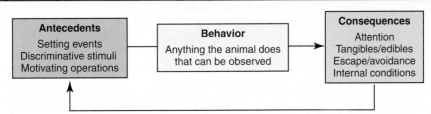

Three-Term Contingency of Antecedent–Behavior–Consequence

An *antecedent* is a stimulus, event, or condition that precedes a behavior and influences the likelihood that this behavior occurs.

A *behavior* is anything an individual does that can be unambiguously observed and operationally defined (i.e., overt behavior).

A *consequence* is the outcome that directly follows the behavior.

Looking at behavior from an ABC perspective lies at the basis of a comprehensive functional assessment of a behavior. It not only helps us understand why a behavior happens but also allows us to predict, influence, and change behavior (by changing the antecedents or consequences of the behavior).

behavior is reinforced. For example, a ringing doorbell can become a signal for loud vocalizations if the vocalizations result in social reinforcers when the bell rings. The strength of a stimulus to signal, or cue, for a particular behavior is related to the strength of the reinforcer that follows the behavior. To build strong cues, strong reinforcers should be delivered in the presence of the cues. If a behavior is reliably performed or suppressed in the presence of discriminative stimuli, it is considered to be under stimulus control.[160,161] However, even if strong stimulus control is present or antecedents are arranged in such a manner that a behavior is likely to occur, the animal ultimately always makes its own choice whether it will behave as expected or not based on past consequences and current conditons.[158]

Behavior. In ABA, behavior is defined as what an animal does in certain conditions. The main focus is on an evaluation of overt behaviors that may be unambiguously observed and operationally defined.[158] Thus, rather than focusing on what the animal is (i.e., labeling, see section What Is Behavior?), ABA is concerned with what the animal does that can be observed. By operationalizing the target behavior in as much detail as possible, it will often be easier to detect the environmental factors that influence this behavior, develop a behavior modification plan, and determine the effects of the intervention on the behavior. For example, the label "territorial" should be operationalized as "the bird lunges at my hand." For the purpose of detailed operationalization of behavior, behavior may be measured in terms of frequency, duration and magnitude, or latency (i.e., the length of time between the cue and the response).[162] Throughout the process of assessment and modification, the operational definition of the target may also be changed or amended, if needed, allowing for more precise evaluation and modification of the behavior.[163]

Consequences. Consequences are the outcomes produced by behavior (e.g., attention, tangible items, food or treats, escape or avoidance of an aversive stimulus, internal conditions). Consequences provide animals with essential feedback on the effectiveness of their behavior, thereby affecting the motivation and probability of the behavior occurring again in the future (as indicated by the law of effect; see section Behavior: A Product of Previous Learning Experiences).[158] Behaviors that produce valued outcomes tend to be repeated or increased, whereas those resulting in aversive consequences tend to be modified, decreased, or suppressed. Thus, an animal learns from the consequences of its actions; that is, it uses this information to alter its future behavior under similar antecedent circumstances, as needed. There are several ways to categorize consequences. Consequences may either increase or decrease the probability of behaviors they follow, thereby being referred to as either *reinforcers* (increasing the probability that a behavior occurs) or *punishers* (decreasing the probability that a behavior occurs). In addition to their effect on future behaviors, consequences may also be differentiated by operation, where the terms *positive* and *negative* have arithmetic meaning (not valence), that is, to add or subtract. When the behavior results in the addition of a stimulus (e.g., attention, tangible item, or sensory stimulation), it is called a *positive consequence*; when the behavior results in the removal of a stimulus, it is called a *negative consequence*. Finally, consequences can be categorized

as *primary* (unlearned or unconditional) or *secondary* (learned or conditional on being paired with a well-established reinforcer or punisher) through the process of classical conditioning (also known as "respondent conditioning" or "Pavlovian conditioning").[158,159,164]

Functional assessment

The ABCs of behavior form the basis of an analytic tool known as "functional assessment." The ABCs of behavior include (1) an operational definition of the behavior *(B);* and (2) hypothesized antecedents *(A)* and consequences *(C)* that are functionally related to the behavior. Identifying this three-term contingency helps us understand, predict, and modify behavior.[158] To conduct a proper functional assessment of a behavior, four steps need to be followed[10,11,158]:

1. Observe and operationally define the target behavior in unambiguous, objective (i.e., observable) terms. (What does the animal do that can be observed and measured?)
2. Identify the physical and environmental conditions in which the behavior is likely to occur. (What are general conditions/events that affect the target behavior [e.g., medical or physical problems, daily schedule, enclosure and surroundings, diet]. What are the immediate antecedents or predictors of this behavior [e.g., where, when, and with whom is the behavior most likely to occur], and under which circumstances does the behavior not occur?)
3. Identify the consequence (i.e., the immediate purpose) that the target behavior serves to the animal and thereby helps maintain the behavior. (What does the animal gain, escape, or avoid by behaving this way, and to what extent does the animal's natural environment support this behavior?)
4. Develop a summary statement that describes the relationship among the antecedents, behaviors, and consequences for each situation in which the behavior occurs.

Using this scaffolding, antecedents, behavior, and consequences, hypotheses can be generated regarding the circumstances under which the behavior is likely to occur and the function behavior has for the animal. In order to confirm these hypotheses, the environment may be rearranged systematically to create the different reinforcement contingencies that have been hypothesized. These contingencies can subsequently be presented independently to identify the effect of each condition on the behavior. When the behavior is dependent (contingent) on specific stimuli or events occurring in the animal's environment and the increases or decreases are dependent on the presence of this stimulus or event, a functional relationship exists between the behavior and the environment.

The hypothesis regarding the functional relationship between a target behavior and the environmental circumstances that set the occasion for and reinforce problem behavior will also help identify potential behavioral interventions (see section Treatment of Behavior Problems).[11,158]

Evaluation of the Findings

Once all the data have been collected, the obtained information should be carefully evaluated before a conclusion is drawn. In light of this evaluation, all relevant aspects, including those pertaining to the parrot's natural behaviors and development, should be taken into account. Based on this information, the veterinarian or behavior consultant should first assess whether there truly is a behavior problem or whether the behavior actually concerns normal behavior of a parrot, the latter requiring awareness to be created with the owner that the displayed behavior is part of the animal's natural history rather than a behavior problem per se. In addition, the evaluation may reveal management problems such as an inappropriate environment or inappropriate relationship between the parrot and its owner, which may warrant intervention to prevent future problems. If evaluation demonstrates a behavior problem to truly exist, evaluation of the obtained data may further help identify potential risk factors associated with the undesired behavior and allow for a customized intervention plan to be designed.

TREATMENT OF BEHAVIOR PROBLEMS

Behavior problems often develop because of the conditions that immediately precede the behavior, follow the behavior, or both. Often, antecedents are not set up for success, and consequences are inadvertently reinforcing to the bird's behavior, thereby maintaining or increasing the frequency with which this behavior is performed. Behavior is not repeated for any reason; behavior serves a function, which is to either gain something (i.e., positive reinforcement such as gaining attention or access to tangible items, sensory stimulation, or both) or to escape or avoid something (i.e., negative reinforcement such as removal of unwanted attention, aversive sensory stimulation, or a fear-eliciting tangible item).[163,165,166] To identify these reinforcing conditions, a functional assessment of the problem behavior (see section Applied Behavior Analysis) is necessary for identifying the potential reinforcers involved in the acquisition and maintaining of the problem behavior.[165–168]

Following the identification of the risk factors, antecedent cues and obstacles, and reinforcing outcomes, an intervention plan can be set up to replace or change the problem behavior. Prior to commencing this intervention, however, it should always be evaluated whether and which family members are willing to cooperate, and if so, to what extent they are prepared to make an effort to try and resolve the behavior problem by changing what they do or the conditions they provide to the bird.[155] Many behavior problems require the cooperation of all persons involved, with chances for a successful outcome decreasing significantly if one or multiple family members are unwilling or unable to adhere to an intervention plan. For example, if one of the family members is afraid of the parrot or frustrated to such an extent that he or she would prefer to relinquish or re-home the bird, that person is less likely to engage in positive interactions with the bird and participate in the behavior modification plan. Similarly, reinforcement of unacceptable behaviors by one person will likely counteract the measures undertaken to reduce the problem behavior, which would result in lack of improvement following the behavior modification plan. In addition, caregivers may not consider the behavior displayed by their parrot to be a problem, do not realize they are creating an untenable relationship with their parrot, or both until the behavior finally escalates. Many caregivers, for example, are flattered if their birds are highly dependent on them and consider them as their partners until the birds start displaying unacceptable behaviors such as excessive screaming,

aggression, and mutilation of feathers or skin. With such caregivers, awareness needs to be created first regarding the problematic nature of the behavior and their own role in its onset and maintenance. In addition, clients may need to be educated about the necessity and value of a behavioral intervention strategy, especially those averse to the idea of modifying their birds' behaviors as they consider this to be "training" and therefore "unnatural." Training may be, arguably, unnatural; however, learning is not only natural, it is also part of every animal's biologic imperative. Preferably, all family members are aware of the degree of their role in the process (not all interventions require the active participation of the entire family). With clear understanding of the roles in implementation of a behavior modification plan, there is an increased likelihood of the intervention leading to the desired change.[155]

To modify the parrot's behavior, various strategies may be considered, including teaching new, replacement behaviors, adaptations to the surroundings to create a more stimulating and suitable living environment, and, occasionally, use of psychoactive drugs. In case of suspected or confirmed medical problems, treatment should also be aimed at the underlying medical condition to increase the chances of resolving the behavioral issue. In various instances, however, eliminating the inciting medical event may not be sufficient, as the presence of reinforcing conditions may help maintain the problem behavior, eventually leading to habituation or ritualization of the behavior. When attempting to modify behavior, veterinarians are advised to start with the application of ABA principles and concurrent optimization of the parrot's diet and living conditions, where appropriate (antecedent arrangement). This approach is preferred, as the aforementioned methods are considered less intrusive than other methods such as the use of psychoactive drugs. In addition, if one is able to correctly identify and modify the environmental conditions that led to the development of the behavior in the first place, the use of ABA and environmental modifications are most likely to result in a successful outcome in the long term. Throughout the behavior modification therapy, close monitoring and regular rechecks of the bird are recommended, as new undesired behaviors as well as an augmentation of the initial problem behavior may be seen, subsequently warranting re-evaluation and adjustment of the intervention plan. Should the behavioral interventions fail or the bird appear less responsive to these, the use of psychoactive drugs may need to be considered as adjunctive therapy.

Tools and Techniques for Behavior Change

The building blocks of learning and therefore of behavior change are primarily based on operant learning, that is, voluntary learning, in which the animal learns that through its behavior, it is able to operate its environment and obtain a certain effect. Operant learning in principle consists of four basic elements upon which many different teaching techniques are based—positive reinforcement (known among lay people as "reward training") and negative reinforcement (also referred to as "escape training"), both of which result in an increase or maintenance of the target behavior; and positive and negative punishment, which result in a decrease or suppression of the behavior (Box 5-5). In addition to operant

---

BOX 5-5 CONSEQUENCES AND THEIR COMMON VERNACULAR: FUNCTION BY OPERATION AND COMMON TERMS

Animals behave to change their environment in some way. Consequences are the purpose served by behavior. As such, behaviors increase or decrease in the future, depending on the consequences the behavior has produced in the past. Consequences that function to increase future behavior are called *reinforcers*, and consequences that function to decrease future behavior are called *punishers*. The operation used to deliver consequences further refines our understanding of them. When the behavior results in the addition of a stimulus or event, the consequences that are contingently added to the environment are called *positive* (+), and when the behavior results in the removal of a stimulus or condition, the consequences that are contingently removed from the environment are called *negative* (−). These terms are used as in arithmetic, strictly mathematically (operations of addition and subtraction), with no emotional value or judgment implied. Thus, every consequence can be described along two different dimensions—function (increasing or decreasing) and operation (positive or negative). The terms in the cells in parentheses are the common lay equivalents of the scientific terminology.

		Function	
		Increase	**Decrease**
Operation	**Addition**	Positive reinforcement (rewards)	Positive punishment (discipline)
	Subtraction	Negative reinforcement (escape)	Negative punishment (fines)

---

learning, respondent learning and observational learning are other techniques commonly used to modify behavior.

Operant interventions to increase behavior: reinforcement

Reinforcement training should be the most commonly used technique to maintain or increase a behavior as a valued consequence is obtained following the behavior (positive reinforcement) or the behavior may be performed to avoid an aversive consequence (negative reinforcement). Although both positive and negative reinforcements increase or maintain behavior, they may exert different effects on the animal's engagement in the training. Whereas animals are often enthusiastic and excited to participate in training that results in positive reinforcement, thereby easily exceeding the minimum effort needed to obtain the reinforcer (increased discretionary effort), this minimum effort is seldom exceeded to avoid aversive stimuli with negative reinforcement training. Moreover, the use of aversive procedures may have detrimental side effects such as an increase in escape behaviors, generalized fear, apathy, and aggression.[169] Since these aversive effects are not seen with positive reinforcement, this technique should be considered the preferred strategy to use when designing a behavior-modification protocol (see also section

Behavior Modification Therapy), with several guidelines established to maximize its effect (Box 5-6).[170]

Factors affecting reinforcement. Several important factors may affect reinforcement learning, including the contingency and contiguity with which the reinforcer is presented. *Contingency* refers to the dependency with which the reinforcer is paired with the behavior, allowing the bird to link the two events (i.e., display of the behavior and presentation of the reinforcer). *Contiguity* refers to the temporal closeness of the behavior and the reinforcer, with learning occurring more quickly when the reinforcer is delivered immediately upon display of the behavior.[171,172]

Reinforcement learning is furthermore affected by the characteristics of the reinforcer, such as type, frequency, magnitude, and the relative availability of the reinforcer.[158] For example, small, frequent reinforcers tend to be more effective than large, occasional ones.[173,174] In addition, reinforcement learning may also be affected by the difficulty and specific characteristics of the task and by the animal's learning history.[158] Besides the general factors, individual differences may also account for the differences in learning among individuals.[158,163] A consequence that is reinforcing to one parrot may be neutral or aversive to another. As a result, arrangement of contingencies for behavior modification therapy

---

BOX 5-6 GUIDELINES FOR MAXIMIZING THE EFFECT OF REINFORCEMENT LEARNING[158,170]

- ◆ Define the target behavior operationally so that the description is observable and unambiguous.
- ◆ Arrange the antecedent environment to make the right behavior easy at first. Complexity can be faded in after the behavior is learned, as needed.
- ◆ Reinforce approximations, small steps, toward the complete target behavior.
- ◆ Reinforce behavior immediately as it occurs. Use a marker such as the word "good" to improve contiguity.
- ◆ Reinforce behavior contingently and consistently for fast learning and maintenance of target behaviors.
- ◆ For those few behaviors that need to persist in low reinforcement conditions, slowly thin the reinforcement schedule from continuous to intermittent.

- ◆ Deliver a quantity of reinforcers sufficient to maintain the behavior without causing rapid satiation.
- ◆ Select reinforcers appropriate to the individual. If the consequence does not strengthen the behavior it follows, it is not a reinforcer, de facto.
- ◆ Use a variety of reinforcers and reinforcing situations to maintain interest and motivation in an enriched environment.
- ◆ Provide opportunities to experience and learn new reinforcers by pairing neutral stimuli with well-established reinforcers.
- ◆ Identify, eliminate, reduce, or override competing contingencies by delivering stronger reinforcers.

should be tailored to the individual. Careful observation of the bird's favorite items, foods, activities, people, sounds, and locations may help determine its preferences and select an appropriate reinforcer.[158,163] Upon selection of the reinforcer, however, continued monitoring remains essential because the effects of the reinforcer can only be established by its effects on future behavior: if the behavior stops occurring, it could, by definition, not have been reinforced. Such a finding, therefore, indicates that the selected reinforcer is not truly acting as a reinforcer for this bird in this context.[158,163] Thus, reinforcers only include those consequences that actually do maintain or increase the frequency of a particular behavior that it follows and not those that we think should do so.

Primary and secondary reinforcers. Some consequences, especially those related to basic survival functions (e.g., food, water, and relief from heat or cold), are automatically reinforcing to all animals from the moment they are born and do not require prior pairing experience to function as behavior-increasing consequences. As a result, these consequences are referred to as "unconditional reinforcers" (or "unconditioned reinforcers") or "primary reinforcers." Once the animal starts interacting with its environment, the process of learning commences, with many initially neutral consequences becoming reinforcing by repeated pairing with existing reinforcers. These reinforcers are referred to as "conditional reinforcers" (or "conditioned reinforcers") or "secondary reinforcers" and may include consequences such as praise, petting, toys, and the sound of a whistle or clicker. Although both types of reinforcers have different advantages and disadvantages (Table 5-4), both are valuable in the context of training, with increasing numbers of available reinforcers providing us with greater opportunities to successfully influence and alter the bird's behavior.[14]

Schedules of reinforcement. Schedules of reinforcement are the rules that determine in which particular instance the behavior will be reinforced. In general, one of the following three schedules may be used when implementing a behavior-modification plan:

1. A continuous reinforcement (CRF) schedule, in which each and every occurrence of the target behavior is reinforced (i.e., a behavior-to-reinforcement ratio of 1:1). As a general rule, continuous reinforcement provides the clearest communication to the bird regarding the behavior that is being reinforced, thereby producing rapid learning. As a result, CRF is recommended for maintaining and increasing existing behaviors as well as teaching new behaviors.[158,170]

2. Extinction (EXT), in which no instance of the target behavior is reinforced (i.e., a behavior-to-reinforcement ratio of 1:0). By withholding the reinforcer that previously maintained a behavior, the rate of the behavior eventually will decrease to pre-reinforcement levels (which not necessarily implies total suppression). Although extinction can effectively help decrease undesired behavior, it is generally not considered easy to properly implement as a stand-alone technique (see section Extinction).

3. An intermittent schedule of reinforcement, in which only some instances of the target behavior are reinforced (i.e., a behavior-to-reinforcement ratio between 1:0 and 1:1). Generally, intermittent schedules can be arranged along two basic dimensions: (a) the frequency of responses following a target behavior (i.e., ratio schedules) or the amount of time that elapses between behavior and response (i.e., interval and duration schedules); and (b) the predictability of reinforcement, which may either be fixed (i.e., the ratio or interval is predetermined and does not change throughout the training) or variable (i.e., reinforcement fluctuates around a preset average, with the bird not knowing how many responses are needed, or how much time will elapse before the reinforcer will be presented upon displaying the target behavior). As a result, four basic types of intermittent schedules of reinforcement can be distinguished: fixed ratio (FR), variable ratio (VR), fixed interval (FI), and variable interval (VI) schedules (Box 5-7). Intermittent schedules generally result in higher persistence of behavior compared with continuous schedules under conditions of extinction or limited reinforcement. This also provides an explanation for the persistence of many of the problem behaviors seen in pet birds, as reinforcement often occurs on an unpredictable, intermittent basis.[158]

TABLE 5-4
Strengths and Limitations of Primary and Secondary Reinforcers

Primary or Unconditioned Reinforcers	Secondary or Conditioned Reinforcers
Generally quite powerful	Generally weaker
Do not rely on association with other reinforcers	Rely on pairing with other reinforcement, at least in the initial phase
Few in number	Large variety, with possibility to generate new reinforcers continuously throughout the bird's life by association with other reinforcers
Increased susceptibility to temporary loss of effectiveness due to satiation	Less susceptible to satiation, tend to hold their value longer
Generally applicable in a limited number of situations	Can generally be applied in a wider variety of situations
More difficult to control contiguity	Can be delivered with less disruption and better contiguity

BOX 5-7 DIAGRAM OF THE DIFFERENT KINDS OF INTERMITTENT REINFORCEMENT SCHEDULES

	Fixed	Variable
Ratio	Completion of a constant number of responses	Completion of a changing number of responses
Interval	Reinforces the first response after a constant amount of time	Reinforces the first response after a changing amount of time

Operant Interventions to Decrease Behavior: Punishment

In some situations, the frequency of a behavior may need to be decreased. Preferably, a combination of extinction (of the problem behavior to baseline levels) and reinforcement learning (of alternative or incompatible behavior), referred to as "differential reinforcement" (see section Differential Reinforcement), is used. Occasionally, punishment strategies may also be used to decrease or suppress the problem behavior. Both positive (i.e., the behavior is followed by presentation of an aversive stimulus) and negative (i.e., the behavior is followed by removal of something of value from the environment) punishment can be applied. Negative punishment (which includes procedures such as time-out from positive reinforcement) is generally preferred over positive punishment because taking away something of value is generally considered less aversive than administering something noxious or aversive. However, this may not be the case for every individual.

Similar to reinforcement, the effectiveness of particular punishers varies for each individual and is highly dependent on the contingency and contiguity between the target behavior and its consequence, the characteristics of the punisher, and the schedule with which the (primary or secondary) punisher is delivered.[158]

Punishment, however, does not teach an animal what it needs to do to be successful but only what it should not do. As a general rule, punishment should, therefore, be used in conjunction with positive reinforcement procedures, if at all, to strengthen desirable behaviors and maintain a reinforcing environment (this is called the "fair pairs rule").[158,175] In addition, mild punishment rarely results in long-lasting effects at any given level of behavioral suppression, thereby necessitating a trainer to resort to higher-intensity punishment, which generally exceeds the acceptable standards of ethical practice and induces aversive behaviors, including aggression, apathy, and fear.[169,176] If possible, negative reinforcement (which allows the animal to avoid an aversive stimulus by inducing escape behavior) is, therefore, preferred over positive punishment.

Time-out from positive reinforcement. Time-out from positive reinforcement includes the contingent, temporary removal of access to reinforcers. This procedure can be very effective but needs to be applied correctly (i.e., contingent, contiguous, and without inadvertent reinforcement of the behavior) in order to be effective. Time-out from access to reinforcement should be short, followed by an opportunity for the bird to perform the desired behavior with more

information at hand (Box 5-8).[158] As with all behavior change procedures, if the use of time-out from positive reinforcement does not result in a decrease of the problem behavior as a part of the behavior-change strategy, the delivery of the procedure(s) need to be re-evaluated.

Extinction. Extinction is the permanent removal of (specific) reinforcer(s) that maintains the problem behavior. Similar to time-out, the success of extinction as a strategy to decrease problem behavior is highly dependent on the fidelity with which the procedure is implemented. Several aspects, however, render the technique less useful when dealing with problem behaviors, including the following: (1) Prolonged time is needed for the procedure to take effect, especially if the behavior has been reinforced using intermittent reinforcement schedules (which is generally true for most problem behaviors); (2) many problem behaviors (e.g., extreme biting, screaming, or chewing on furniture) cannot simply be ignored (assuming that the caregiver's reaction is the maintaining reinforcer); (3) the frequency, intensity, and duration of the problem behavior may temporarily increase before a significant decrease in behavior occurs (called an "extinction burst"), with escalation of the behavior rarely being tolerated by caregivers, thereby resulting in reinforcement of the behavior at a new, often higher level of intensity; (4) various problem behaviors, especially those associated with frustration (e.g., aggression) are commonly elicited by extinction; (5) bootleg reinforcement (by uncontrolled reinforcers in the environment) may inadvertently strengthen the problem behavior; (6) spontaneous recovery of the problem behavior is common (although less likely to occur upon each successful re-application of extinction); and (7) resurgence of other, previously extinguished behaviors may occur.[158,170,177] On the whole, extinguishing a problem behavior is, therefore, most effective as a preventative strategy rather than a solution to a problem. In the situation where problem behaviors are well established, differential reinforcement of alternative behaviors is the better strategy (see section Differential Reinforcement).[158]

Classical conditioning (respondent learning)

Besides operant behavior, which is strengthened or weakened as a function of consequences, reflexive behavior is triggered by a stimulus. This behavior, referred to as "respondent behavior," comprises reflexive, involuntary behaviors that occur in response to a (natural) elicitor, for example, an eye blink occurs in response to a puff of air. Reflexive behavior is innate—that is, the response elicited by the stimulus is fully

---

BOX 5-8 GUIDELINES FOR EFFECTIVE IMPLEMENTATION OF TIME-OUT FROM POSITIVE REINFORCEMENT

Caution: Removing the bird to a time-out area itself is very likely to reinforce the problem behavior. Particularly in parrots, social reinforcers are very strong. As a result, the best implementation of time-out (TO) may be to not use it at all and instead work to redesigning the environment so that the right behavior is more reinforcing.

♦ Plan the TO location ahead of time to ensure the parrot can be placed there with clear contingency and immediacy upon performing the problem behavior. Turning away from the parrot may also be an effective way to create a TO.

♦ Increase the salience of the contingency between the behavior and the consequence by keeping the TO interval short (approximately 30 seconds to a few minutes).

♦ After the TO interval, the bird should always immediately be given the opportunity to practice the appropriate behavior, with the desired behavior being reinforced every time it is displayed.

♦ Allow the TO to do all the work in decreasing the problem behavior, without adding other consequences or emotional displays that may inadvertently reinforce the problem behavior (bootleg reinforcement).

functional right from the first exposure to the stimulus. As such, this type of behavior accounts for the reflexive aspects of emotions such as fear and joy. Rather than the bird learning how to be startled in response to an alarming stimulus, the alarming stimulus triggers a series of involuntary responses in the animal. Besides natural elicitors (e.g., a predator), animals may also learn to respond to a conditioned elicitor, as a result of pairing with other, well-established (natural) elicitors through a process known as "respondent learning." This type of learning, also referred to as "Pavlovian learning" or "classical or S-S (i.e., stimulus-stimulus) learning," accounts for the so-called irrational fear of things that do not actually pose a threat to the animal. For example, an unexpected spray of water used to shift an animal may result in an animal that is afraid of water, hoses, left-handed keepers, ponytails, and red caps. As another more complex example, an unexpected and fear-evoking capture-and-restraint experience for a pet bird may lead to an individual that is afraid of handlers, the carrier in which the bird is transported, veterinary personnel, laboratory jackets, and towels or other handling-associated and restraint-associated stimuli. When new elicitors are paired in this way with other learned elicitors, the process is called "higher-order conditioning."

Respondent learning comprises a process by which an innate response to an unconditioned, "biologically potent" stimulus (US) is elicited by a previously neutral stimulus (i.e., a stimulus that does not have any pleasant or aversive consequences). This is achieved by repeated pairings of the neutral stimulus with an existing stimulus–response set, which then becomes a conditioned stimulus (CS). In contrast to operant learning, respondent conditioning relies on the events occurring prior to the behavior (i.e., the antecedents), which automatically elicit the involuntary response. Thus, rather than being a function of its consequences, the behavior is a function of its antecedent stimuli. Moreover, respondent conditioning involves the learning of new triggers and not of new behaviors.

Although operant and respondent learning appear to be highly distinct processes, the reality is that they always occur simultaneously. Modal action patterns (e.g., courtship dances in birds), for example, are innate behavior patterns elicited by specific stimuli. However, these motor patterns can often be modified with ongoing experience, resulting in faster, more fluent and more effective action patterns and indicating that the behavior has both innate and learned properties. In contrast, learning of new behaviors by using operant learning may be complicated by the animal experiencing emotions, which are largely the result of respondent conditioning. Moreover, operant learning is often influenced by respondent conditioning. This inextricable intertwining of both learning processes is highly beneficial and important for successful implementation of many important teaching techniques, for example, clicker training (S-S learning, in which the animal learns that the clicker marks the right behavior and signals that a reinforcer will immediately follow). It is, however, also one of the more complex factors to account for in the treatment of problem behaviors such as phobias and fears.

Observational learning

Learning may also occur by providing another bird as a role model, that is, observational learning. In free-ranging parrots, other members of the flock generally serve as models for behavior. By observing the behavior of another bird and the consequences associated with the behavior, the parrot learns from the experiences of the other individual. The bird will subsequently repeat the behaviors that result in desired outcomes for the model and avoid others that result in less desired or negative outcomes (thereby also representing a form of operant behavior). This similar principle can also be applied in a captive setting, as demonstrated by the work of Irene Pepperberg with the Grey parrot Alex.[49] When applying this technique, one person serves as the trainer, while a second person (or bird) acts as the bird's model and demonstrates both correct and incorrect responses for which it is either reinforced or not. If the parrot subsequently displays the desired behavior, reinforcement of the behavior will be provided in a similar manner to that for the model.

Behavior Modification Therapy

To effectively modify the bird's behavior and solve a behavior problem, a veterinarian should have a basic understanding of the principles of learning and the know-how to conduct a functional assessment of the bird's behavior. Functional assessment of a behavior provides an important tool for developing and testing hypotheses about the environmental factors that control or reinforce the problem behavior, including its purpose or function for the animal. This is an essential first step toward the design and implementation of an effective behavior modification strategy. Behavior modification strategies are generally aimed at redesigning the antecedent and consequent environment so that the "right" behavior is easier and more reinforcing than the "wrong" behavior.[163]

Reducing the problem behavior is, however, not the only goal when designing a behavior modification strategy. A sound plan also consists of a redesign of the physical and social contexts of the living environment. This provides the bird with opportunities to replace the function served by the problem behavior with more acceptable, alternative behaviors. Moreover, it allows the bird to learn new skills that render the problem behavior less likely to occur. According to O'Neill et al (1997),[178] four conditions need to be met to increase the overall effectiveness and efficiency of a behavior modification strategy:

1. The behavior modification strategy should describe how the environment will be redesigned to promote and maintain appropriate behavior. Various aspects may be involved, including medications, diet, physical settings, schedules, exercise, training procedures, and the use of specified reinforcers and punishers. It is recommended to describe the proposed changes in as much detail as possible and include exactly what each family member is supposed to do and when.

2. A clear linkage should be present between the functional assessment and the intervention plan. The chances for success are highest when an animal is able to perform an alternative behavior that is functionally equivalent to the problem behavior. Thus, the strategy should focus on what the animal should do to achieve its goal rather than what it should not do.

3. The behavior modification strategy should be technically sound—that is, it should adhere to the scientific principles of learning to render the problem behavior irrelevant, ineffective, or inefficient. This can be accomplished by ensuring that the alternative behavior (a) provides the same or more reinforcement (thereby making the problem behavior irrelevant); (b) requires less effort or fewer responses (thereby making the problem behavior inefficient);

and (c) ensures that the problem behavior results in no or less reinforcement (thereby becoming ineffective).

4. The behavior modification strategy should fit the owner's routine, living conditions, values, resources, and skills. The best strategy should not only be effective in promoting the best outcome for the bird and its owners (both in the short term and the long term), but preferably also uses the most positive, least intrusive techniques to accomplish these goals.

As a general rule, teaching sessions should take place in uninterrupted sessions in a quiet training area. Dependent on the owner's opportunities and the bird's motivation and attention span, sessions may take place daily to several times per week, with each session lasting a few minutes or more. Additionally, given a choice between the different behavioral interventions available, selecting the most positive, least intrusive, and most effective strategy meets the highest standards of ethical practice (Box 5-9). As a result, antecedent changes and positive reinforcement procedures should always be tried before implementing negative punishment (removing positive reinforcers) or negative reinforcement (escape training). Positive punishment procedures, in which aversive stimuli are applied, should be used rarely, if ever. Finally, the latter three procedures should only be used as an adjunct to positive reinforcement strategies.[11,158,178a] These same types of ethical criteria should also be applied to any and all concurrent medical treatments being implemented.

Antecedent arrangement

Thoughtful arrangement of antecedent stimuli (see also section Environmental Adaptations As a Means of Antecedent Arrangement) is a very effective and practical method to solve behavior problems. Despite its practical applicability and efficacy, antecedent arrangement is a behavior-changing tool that is underused in practice. On the one hand, practitioners may easily overlook these obvious solutions to a behavior problem or downsize their specific implementation and follow-up with their recommendations. On the other hand, antecedent arrangement may be hindered by the owner's reluctance to implement these environmental changes (e.g., change the cage location, cage door size). Nevertheless, veterinarians are encouraged to use this behavioral tool in the initial approach of a behavior problem. Antecedent rearrangement may be accomplished through one of the following ways[163]:

1. *Altering or removing the antecedent stimulus that signals the opportunity for reinforcement.* Since behavior is maintained by reinforcement, removal of the stimulus that signals the opportunity to acquire reinforcement will make the behavior less likely to occur. In addition, antecedent stimuli may be changed to decrease the chances of the behavior occurring, new stimuli may be added to direct the bird's response, or both. These types of interventions are often very simple and generally require only small alterations to be made in the environment (e.g., if a bird bites when the owner wants to take it out of its cage and reaches for the bird with his or her hand, the biting may simply be avoided by not reaching for the bird in its cage with the hand but rather using a perch or allowing the bird to come out of the cage on its own).

2. *Changing the value of consequences through antecedent arrangement.* These antecedent arrangements, also called

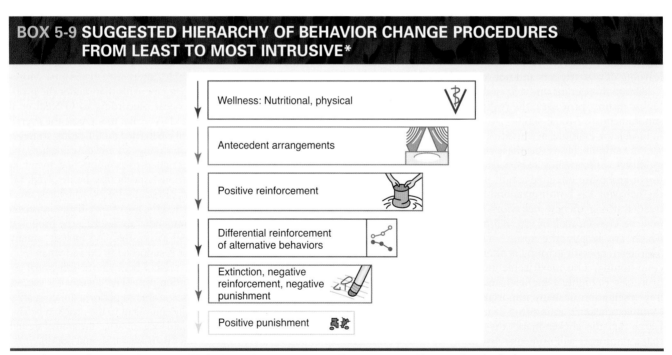

BOX 5-9 SUGGESTED HIERARCHY OF BEHAVIOR CHANGE PROCEDURES FROM LEAST TO MOST INTRUSIVE*

- Wellness: Nutritional, physical
- Antecedent arrangements
- Positive reinforcement
- Differential reinforcement of alternative behaviors
- Extinction, negative reinforcement, negative punishment
- Positive punishment

*Intrusiveness refers to the degree to which the learner has counter control. The goal is to use the procedure that is the least intrusive, effective alternative. Displayed here in this hierarchy, the premise that wellness and nutritional and physical health are evaluated and secured in a nonintrusive manner is a requisite. It is important for veterinarians and veterinary health care personnel to critically evaluate the degrees of intrusiveness of their contemplated medical or surgical procedures because considerable variation may be present. In the course of an experienced behavior practice, there may be situations in which a relatively more intrusive procedure is necessary for effective outcomes. In this case, a procedure that reduces the learner's control may be the least intrusive, effective alternative. The hierarchy is a cautionary tool to reduce both dogmatic rule-following and practice by familiarity or convenience. It offers an ethical checkpoint for veterinarians to carefully consider the process by which effective outcomes can be most humanely achieved on a case-by-case basis. Rationale such as "It worked with the last case!" is not enough. The evaluation and behavior change program of every animal should be a study of the individual (e.g., individual animal, setting, caregiver). Changing behavior is best understood as a study of one.

"motivating operations," increase or decrease the value of a reinforcer or the behavior that has led to the acquisition of this reinforcer in the past, thereby changing the motivation of the bird to perform a specific behavior (e.g., if a bird is working for special food treats, it is more likely to be motivated for work for those treats).[179]

Managing the consequences of a behavior

Managing the consequences of a behavior is the most common strategy employed when dealing with a behavior problem. To some, it may appear that the quickest and easiest way to reduce a problem behavior is to cease all reinforcement of that behavior.[163] After all, if the behavior is no longer reinforced (whereas it was in the past), the behavior will decrease and eventually return to baseline levels (i.e., before owners "supersized" the behavior with their unintended reinforcements). However, an extinction burst may be observed during which the frequency and intensity of the behavior increase to a maximum prior to its cessation. As a result, extinction is generally not implemented as a sole strategy but most often used in combination with other behavioral interventions such as differential reinforcement (see section Teaching Replacement Behaviors) so that another, more desired behavior is reinforced instead. Punishment is another alternative to decrease behavior. However, as discussed in the section titled Operant Interventions to Decrease Behavior, this strategy increases the chance of other, undesirable behavioral side effects such as aggression or fear.[163] It is therefore recommended that this risk be avoided and positive reinforcement of alternative, replacement behaviors or differential reinforcement strategies (the combination of positive reinforcement for the desired behavior and extinction for the undesired behavior) be chosen, whenever possible.

Teaching replacement behaviors: differential reinforcement

Problem behavior does not occur for no reason; rather, it serves a function to the parrot (e.g., to gain attention, items, activities, or sensory enrichment or to escape from aversive stimuli). By reinforcing a replacement behavior that serves a similar function as the problem behavior (but in a more appropriate way), problem behaviors can be successfully decreased without the behaviorally toxic side effects of punishment strategies. Once the new replacement behavior is mastered or an already fluent behavior is identified, the problem behavior can be extinguished by withholding the maintaining reinforcer. At the same time, the replacement behavior is reinforced consistently to at least the same extent or to an even greater extent than the problem behavior.

Differential reinforcement increases the rate of the replacement behavior rather than the problem behavior to obtain the reinforcer if the behaviors are functionally equivalent to the bird, or, preferably, the reinforcement obtained following the replacement behavior exceeds that of the problem behavior (i.e., the matching law). Thus, if the hypothesis about the function of the problem behavior was correct, the problem behavior will decrease. However, if the hypothesis was incorrect, the problem behavior will persist and sometimes even increase (rather than decrease) in frequency.[163,168]

Differential reinforcement strategies work best if the replacement behavior is a behavior that is already in the bird's behavioral repertoire. This will allow the owner and the bird to focus all their energy on replacement of the problem behavior with a desirable behavior, rather than having to spend energy on learning a new behavior first.[11,158,163] When birds have a narrow behavioral repertoire, it can sometimes be challenging to find a replacement behavior to use in a differential reinforcement program. As a result, antecedent arrangement and teaching of alternative behaviors first, prior to being able to properly implement a differential reinforcement procedure, may be necessary.

The many kinds of differential reinforcement. Differential reinforcement procedures combine extinction (during which one behavior is no longer reinforced) with positive reinforcement of another behavior. Because of the different schedules of reinforcement (i.e., no reinforcement versus high-rate positive reinforcement), the problem behavior will decrease and the desired behavior will increase in frequency. Various types of differential reinforcement exist, of which the three most commonly used schedules are[163]:

- Differential reinforcement of other behavior (DRO), during which the animal is reinforced for any behavior other than the problem behavior.
- Differential reinforcement of alternative behavior (DRA), during which the animal is reinforced for performing a particular alternative behavior that is either in the animal's repertoire or is specifically taught to the animal to serve as replacement behavior once mastered.
- Differential reinforcement of incompatible behavior (DRI), during which the animal is reinforced for engaging in a behavior that cannot be performed simultaneously with the problem behavior. As a result, this is one of the most powerful behavior reduction tools currently available to us.

Shaping, targeting, and cueing of behavior

Many behaviors occur only infrequently or not at all, thereby limiting the options to wait for the behavior to occur spontaneously. Shaping, also referred to as "differential reinforcement of successive approximations," is the technique to use when teaching new behaviors. Shaping is the procedure of reinforcing a graduated sequence of subtle changes toward the final behavior, starting with the closest response the bird already displays. In addition, shaping is used to change the dimensions of existing behaviors such as duration, rate, intensity, topography, and response time.[158] During the process of shaping, first the response that most closely resembles the target behavior and is already displayed by the bird is contingently reinforced. Once this behavior is performed without hesitation, reinforcement is withheld for that behavior, and the next closer approximation to the final behavior is reinforced. During this process, careful observation of the subtle, natural variations with which the behavior is displayed allows the observer to "catch" and reinforce the next closer approximation. This process of extinguishing one behavior (the mastered approximation) and reinforcing another behavior (the next closer approximation) is continued until the final target behavior is displayed and reinforced.[158] Should difficulties be experienced at any stage during the shaping process, the trainer should take a step back and repeat the previous successful step until this is performed without hesitation, or reinforce even smaller approximations toward the target behavior.

Once a target behavior is mastered, cues may also be added. To add a cue, the cue first needs to be introduced while the behavior is occurring. Next, the cue is gradually introduced earlier and earlier until it is signaled before the behavior. Finally, only cued instances of the behavior are reinforced, and all offered instances of the behavior are ignored (another example of differential reinforcement), thereby establishing the relationship between the cue and the behavior. Cues signal the availability of reinforcement contingent on the particular behavior cued. Therefore, to build strong cues, strong reinforcers have to be delivered. When a behavior is performed every time it is cued, it is said to be under stimulus control.

Targeting is the behavior of touching an object or mark with a designated body part (e.g., beak, wing, or foot), which can be easily taught to parrots using shaping (Figure 5-26). Targeting is considered an important basic skill for any parrot to master, as it allows caregivers a hands-off way to direct the bird's movements in a variety of situations, both inside and outside of the cage.

Systematic desensitization and counter-conditioning

Systematic desensitization, also known as "graduated exposure therapy," is used to reduce or extinguish an elicited (reflexive) emotional response (e.g., fear, aggression) to a conditioned stimulus (CS). It is one of the most commonly used techniques for the treatment of phobias and other anxiety disorders. Systemic desensitization involves a gradual and systematic exposure to a stimulus that subsequently results in an extinction of the conditioned emotional response to the stimulus. After identifying the fear-eliciting stimulus, the stimulus is presented to the animal in a low enough intensity, large enough distance, and for a short duration only so that no fear reaction is elicited. Subsequently, the intensity, proximity, or duration of the fear-eliciting stimulus may be increased in small, incremental steps. Eventually, this will result in the animal not reacting to the learned fear-eliciting stimulus and can be in close proximity without experiencing fear. Key to a successful implementation of this technique are the following: (1) The owner needs to be

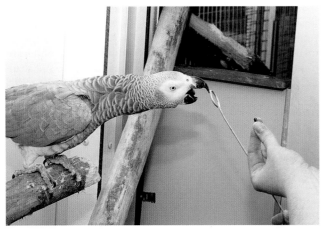

FIGURE 5-26 Targeting is the behavior of touching an object or mark with a designated body part (e.g., beak, wing, or foot), which can be easily taught to parrots. It is considered an important basic skill for any parrot and parrot steward to master, as it allows caregivers a hands-off way to direct the bird's movements in a variety of situations, both inside and outside of the cage. (Photo courtesy Nico Schoemaker/Yvonne van Zeeland.)

able to recognize what calm behavior looks like in the parrot by assessing the parrot's activities as well as its plumage, eyes, and the position of its head, torso, legs; (2) the fear-eliciting stimulus can be identified, reproduced, and controlled (not only in terms of distance, intensity, or duration but also in terms of its occurrence outside of the behavior modification sessions); (3) the stimulus is initially presented at a low enough duration and intensity or far enough distance to avoid eliciting a fear response; (4) the incremental steps are sufficiently small to prevent the triggering of a fearful response; and (5) advancement to the next step only occurs if the animal remains calm in the presence of the stimulus at that level. To boost its effectiveness, systematic desensitization may be combined with counter-conditioning. During this procedure, a positive (appetitive) stimulus is noncontingently paired with the aversive stimulus to change the value of the conditioned stimulus from CS− to CS+. As a result, rather than eliciting a fear response, the conditioned stimulus will elicit a positive emotional response.[154,180] Although counter-conditioning can also be applied as a single technique, it will only work if the "appetitive stimulus" triggers a response that is powerful enough to overcome the negative emotional response.

Response blocking or flooding

Response blocking, also commonly referred to as "flooding," is another technique to reduce a learned (conditioned) emotional response to a stimulus. Unlike systematic desensitization and counter-conditioning, however, the exposure to the fear-eliciting stimulus is not gradual; instead, it is presented at full strength, without any option for the animal to escape the stimulus. The exposure to the fear-eliciting stimulus subsequently needs to last until fear responses are no longer observed. Ending the session prior to complete extinction of the fear response in the presence of the trigger, however, may exacerbate the animal's fear during future exposures.[181,182]

Several aspects of this procedure indicate that it should not be used, especially given the less intrusive and effective alternative described above. Flooding completely eliminates the animal's ability to choose. Thus, it teaches the animal that its behavior has no effect on the environment. As a result, flooding often produces a condition termed "learned helplessness." This condition is characterized by the absence of an escape response even when the ability to escape or avoid the stimulus is restored. Learned helplessness can be hazardous under all conditions, including when the condition becomes generalized to situations other than the one in which it was induced. In addition, it has been demonstrated to produce a host of detrimental side effects such as immunosuppression and depression.[183,184]

Environmental Adaptations as a Means of Antecedent Arrangement

Environmental adaptations comprise an important part of any behavior modification plan. Thoughtful arrangement of the environment (i.e., antecedent arrangement; see also the appropriate section under Behavior Modification Therapy) may help provide the appropriate stimuli needed to perform natural behaviors and newly learned behaviors while reducing the occurrence of abnormal (repetitive) and problem behaviors and improving the parrots' well-being.[92,105,106,116,185] As a general rule, parrots are social animals that require daily attention and interaction with their caregivers, and the birds should be housed in an enclosure that is at least large enough to enable them to display their natural and learned behaviors. In addition, they should be provided with appropriate perches and toys to chew, manipulate, and play with, thereby stimulating their physical as well as behavioral and emotional well-being. The various aspects of the captive living environment that should be taken into account in the proposed environmental changes are discussed below.

Cages: Design, furnishing, and placement

Weaknesses in the structure, design, or delivery of these aspects of husbandry can result in impairment in a bird's ability to learn or lead to the onset of behavior problems, physical health issues, or both. Housing and enrichment of the environment can greatly affect the animal's behavior and well-being but are, nevertheless, components that are often ignored or weakly specified during routine wellness examinations. Furthermore, the ability for an owner to train the bird and enhance its emotional, behavioral, and physical welfare can also be mechanically blocked by many deficits in husbandry (see Chapter 22). Because of their status as prey species, it is important for parrots to have a place where they feel safe and secure. In captivity, the cage generally represents such a place. To provide the parrot with a proper sense of security, positioning of the cage in a location where it is open on all sides should be avoided. Instead, the cage should preferably be placed against the wall or in a corner of the room. This position guarantees that the bird at least has one direction where it does not need to be vigilant.[156,186] Placement near a window or a door may also cause stress because people may unexpectedly enter the visual field of the parrot. This may not only initiate a fear response but can also increase the risk for feather-damaging behavior.[118,186] Individual differences can, however, be present, depending on the personality of the bird. Some parrots, for example, may enjoy a window view that provides them with visual stimulation. Others may prefer the security of a solid wall. When a bird is placed partially against a window and partially against a solid wall, it is able to choose whether it prefers to be exposed to outside stimuli or not. The bird's personality should also be taken into account when deciding where to position the cage in the room. Extrovert parrots may prefer to be placed in the center of human activity and can start vocalizing excessively when positioned in a more isolated location. Anxious, fearful parrots may need a secure place away from high-traffic areas to avoid being startled and developing abnormal behaviors such as FDB.

Besides cage placement, the size, height, and shape of the cage are also important. Preferably, the cage should be as large as possible, providing the bird with ample space to flap its wings, climb, and move about comfortably, and, especially for macaws, should be tall enough to prevent damage to the tail from dragging.[156,186] Because parrots feel most secure in high places, the cage should be high enough to prevent the parrot from becoming frightened or insecure. Placing the cage too high, however, will hinder handling of the bird. To facilitate easy handling of the bird, cage doors should also open wide and preferably cover as much of the front as possible. The latter feature also eases the training of the parrot to step up and down in the cage, thereby decreasing the risk of problems with territorial aggression.[186]

Rectangular cages are generally preferred over round cages, since round cages do not provide a secure corner in

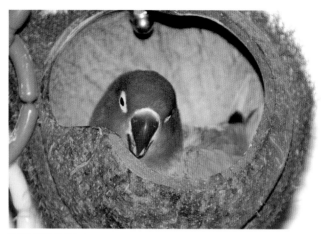

FIGURE 5-27 A coconut can provide a perfect hiding place for smaller psittacine species such as this Fischer's lovebird *(Agapornis fischeri)*. However, as the coconut may be perceived as an ideal nesting site, it may also stimulate territory-related aggression and sexual behaviors. (Photo courtesy Ellen Uittenbogaard.)

which the bird can retreat upon sensing danger. Hiding places may also be provided by wiring branches to the outside of the cage, placing a fabric cover over one corner, or placing wooden or cardboard boxes (or similar objects; Figure 5-27) in the enclosure (note: the latter may also inadvertently stimulate nesting behaviors!).[186] Cage bars should ideally be oriented horizontally, rather than vertically, to facilitate climbing and allow for easy arrangement of toys and other enrichment objects. However, care should be taken to not overcrowd the cage with perches or toys because these may also limit the ability of the bird to move around.

Several veterinarians and behaviorists recommend the use of two separate cages, one for the day and another for the night. This is suggested for reducing the onset of cage territoriality (biting to remove hands), and it promotes regular handling of the bird. In addition, the physical separation of the roosting and foraging areas provides the bird with a more "natural" environment.[186] In contrast to the day cage, which preferably is as large as possible with plentiful toys available, a night cage does not need to be big and can be sparsely furnished. It does, however, need to provide sufficient shelter for the bird and is preferably placed in a quiet, darkened room to enable the bird to obtain sufficient sleep. A carrier in which a perch is mounted fulfills these criteria and is commonly used for this purpose. The additional advantage is that the owner can teach the parrot to go into a carrier, thus training the bird to do so when it needs to be transported (e.g., to the veterinarian; Figure 5-28).

Perches

A newly purchased cage will generally be equipped with perches made of wood or plastic. Although these are generally easy to clean, the smooth surface and uniform diameter of such perches can be detrimental to the bird and increase the risk of pododermatitis.[186] However, the function of a perch extends beyond that of solely being a place to rest on, and those that are provided should be selected and provided with variety and goals of enrichment in mind. Natural branches (cleaned, not sprayed) from nontoxic trees (e.g., willow, maple,

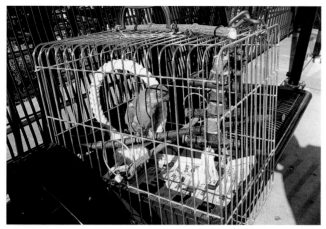

FIGURE 5-28 An example of a carrier in which a perch is mounted. This carrier may be used as a night cage and also as a carrier to transport the parrot in. The advantage of having a night cage that is also used as a carrier is that the parrot experiences less stress when it needs to be transported. (Photo courtesy Ellen Uittenbogaard.)

fig, grapevines) often are excellent perching materials because of their relative softness and variable diameter. This not only limits the risk of pododermatitis, but also provides the bird with a substrate for chewing. Similarly, sisal or 100% natural cotton ropes also make great perches. These items may also act as swings, thereby providing the bird with extra occupational activities.

Play stands or gyms

In addition to the cage, it is generally recommended to provide the parrot with at least one commercial or homemade "play stand," "gym," or freestanding perch away from the cage (Figure 5-29). Although allowing the parrot to roam around free in the house without supervision is ill-advised because of the potential dangers, supervised time outside of the cage is essential. This not only allows the parrot more freedom of choice and movement but also allows for an

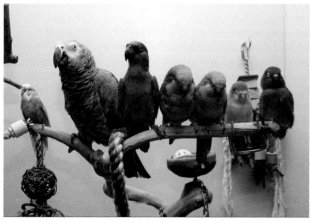

FIGURE 5-29 Supervised time outside of the cage is generally encouraged. A homemade "play stand," "gym," or freestanding perch away from the cage will not only allow the parrot more freedom and a change of scenery but will also provide the owner an excellent opportunity to handle and train the parrot. (Photo Courtesy Ellen Uittenbogaard.)

enriching change of scenery and provides an excellent opportunity for the owner to handle and train the parrot.

Toys and other environmental enrichment

Based on the parrot's natural behavior, foraging, chewing, and shredding appear to be important behaviors. Thus, suitable substrates and toys should be provided in the captive living situation to ensure the birds are able to perform these behaviors. Toys also provide a valuable means of encouraging psittacine development, promote learning, relieve stress, and keep the parrot occupied. Unfortunately, caregivers do not always understand the functionality of toys to the parrot. For example, owners may mention that they provided toys to their parrot but stopped giving these because "the bird chewed them up." Some owners may not understand that parrots may "ignore" a toy because it does not have innate value for the bird, thereby necessitating owners to shape interaction with the toy (see section Shaping, Targeting, and Cueing).

Although many different toys are nowadays available for purchase in pet stores, toys can also be made by owners themselves with little effort. This enables owners to keep the costs low while providing excellent opportunities to keep the parrot occupied. Examples of cheap, easy-to-make toys include (nontoxic) tree branches and twigs, paper cups, cardboard boxes, phone books, tongue depressors, and cotton-tipped applicators.[187,188] Parrot toys can be categorized into four types—chewing (destructible) toys, climbing toys, foot toys, and puzzle toys (Figure 5-30). However, an overlap in function may be present (e.g., a large nut may serve as both a foot toy and a chewing toy). A small number of toys, preferably one from each category, may be placed in the enclosure, although care should be taken to not compromise the parrot's ability to move around. In larger enclosures or aviaries, toys may be scattered throughout the enclosure to encourage the parrot to explore its territory. Ideally, toys are rotated on at least a weekly basis to keep the parrot engaged.[98,156,186] When placing new toys in the enclosure, gradual introduction of the toy may help avoid causing a fear response. In addition, systematic desensitization and counter-conditioning may be used if a fear response is displayed.

Generally, tree branches or destructible toys made of materials such as softwood, paper, or cardboard are preferred over indestructible toys made of materials such as acrylic, hardwood, or metal.[186,189,190] Not only will destructible toys help fulfill the parrot's motivation to chew and shred, but they may also reduce the risk of the bird starting to chew its own feathers or furniture (see Figure. 5-30, A). Similarly, toys with tassels may be useful to promote chewing and redirect social grooming in the absence of a cage mate.[186,190] Besides preferences with regard to hardness, type, and structure of materials, preferences may also exist for specific colors and sizes. For example, a preference for larger-sized items and yellow-colored ropes and wooden blocks was found in Amazon parrots.[80,189,190] Preferences may, however, differ between genders, ages, and species but even more so between individuals, depending on previous learning experiences. Thus, further research is needed to identify the preferred properties of a toy. For the individual bird, it is possible to evaluate its preferences. For this purpose, the bird may be placed in a confined area with a number of identical toys in different colors (e.g., wooden or plastic blocks or balls). By carefully observing the bird, it is possible to determine which colors the bird avoids, which it ignores, and which it

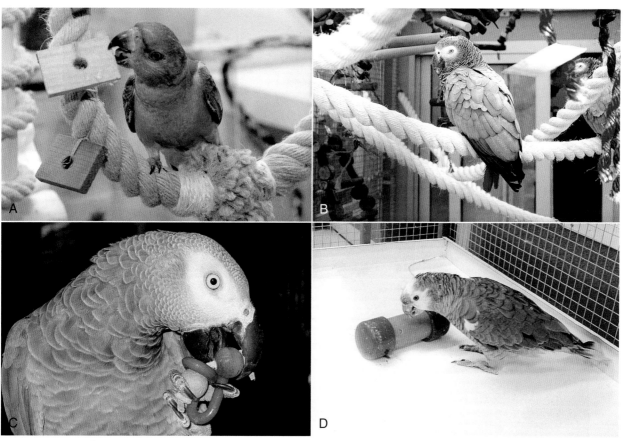

FIGURE 5-30 Four different categories of toys can be distinguished for parrots (i.e., chewing [destructible] toys, climbing toys, foot toys, and puzzle toys). **A,** The Senegal parrot in the top left image is demonstrating that wooden toys are nice to chew on and will be destroyed. **B,** The Grey parrot in the top right image has a lot of ropes in the aviary, which are ideal for climbing. **C,** The Grey parrot in the bottom left image has a toy in its foot and demonstrates that this toy not only makes a good foot toy but can also be used for chewing. **D,** The blue-fronted Amazon parrot in the bottom right image is using a custom-made pipe feeder from which pellets will drop onto the floor when the pipe is rolled over the floor, thus serving as a puzzle or foraging toy. (Photo courtesy Ellen Uittenbogaard/Nico Schoemaker/Yvonne van Zeeland.)

plays with. Repetition of the test is advised to confirm the found preferences. Subsequently, the colors of preference (i.e., the colors the parrot plays with) can be used to select items to be used in training sessions or as enrichment items in the bird's enclosure. It is important to realize that preferences for toys or certain characteristics are rarely fixed and may change over time depending on the reinforcement history.

Of the various types of enrichment that may be provided, items aimed at stimulation of foraging enrichment are in particular considered useful as these may help (1) increase activity; (2) provide cognitive stimulation and manipulative activities; (3) alleviate stress, frustration, and boredom; and (4) reduce and prevent aggression and abnormal repetitive behaviors, including stereotypies.[b] Compared with many of the other types of enrichment, which may lose their enriching effects quickly, foraging enrichment tends to remain stimulating to the animal for longer periods.[193] In addition, foraging

enrichment may help satisfy the parrot's behavioral "need" to manipulate items and forage (the latter being supported by the finding that parrots contra-freeload).[80,93,94,191]

Over the years, several enrichment strategies have been developed to stimulate foraging behavior and increase the foraging times of captive birds. These include (1) provision of smaller, more frequent meals in multiple locations (i.e., increase spatial or temporal variability of feeding); (2) scatter or hide food in the enclosure (i.e., increase search time); (3) provision of live prey to carnivorous or piscivorous species (i.e., increase capture time); (4) provision of foraging devices or puzzle feeders (i.e., increase extraction time and provide a mental challenge); (5) provision of vegetation, bones, ice blocks with food, whole food or carcasses, and so on (i.e., increase the time to process and ingest food); (6) increase of dietary fiber content (i.e., promote satiety); (7) feeding at irregular time intervals (i.e., decrease the predictability of feeding times); or a combination of two or more of the aforementioned options (Figure 5-31).[74,80,98,194-196] Recent studies have shown that foraging enrichments may effectively increase

---

[b]References 80,92,99,105,106,185,191,192.

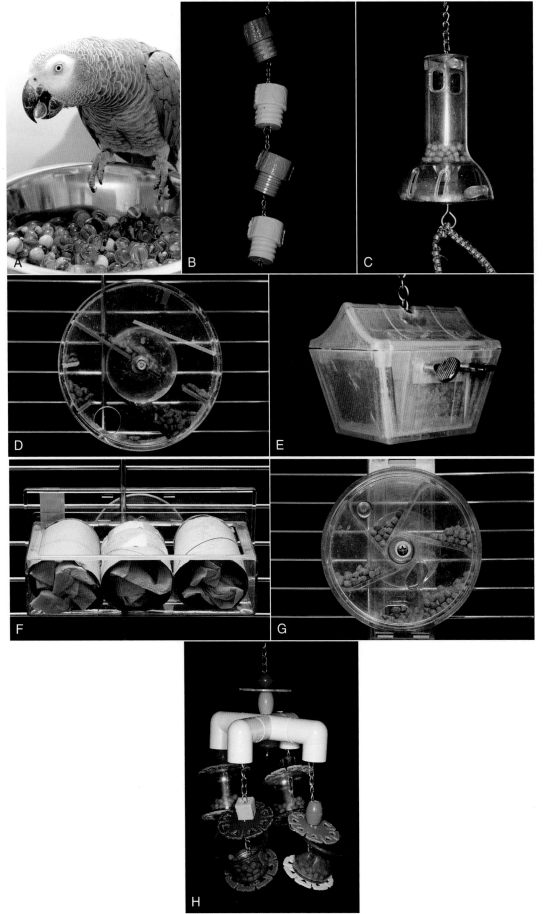

For legend see opposite page

FIGURE 5-31 **A,** Marbles can be great to hide food particles in between. The search between these marbles is very enriching, and as this Grey parrot *(Psittacus erithacus)* demonstrates, the marbles themselves can be stimulating to play with as well. Enrichments, or toys, can take many different forms. These images depict various types of commercial foraging toys that can be used to hide food and stimulate foraging activity. **B,** Turn 'n learn logs consisting of four opaque cups in which food can be hidden following which the bird needs to unscrew the cups to obtain the food (Nature's Instinct, Caitec Corporation, Baltimore, MD). In the beginning, the cups may be twisted loosely; once the bird gains more experience, cups may be tightened more. **C,** Foraging capsule, in which food can be placed, and the bird needs to pull down the platform and swing the toy around in order to obtain the food (Creative Foraging Systems, Caitec Corporation, Baltimore, MD). **D,** The Maze, which needs to be spun around by the bird in order to get the food out (Bell Plastic Bird Toys, Hayward, CA). **E,** Treasure chest, which requires parrots to unlock the chest in order to obtain the treats or food hidden inside (Nature's Instinct). **F,** Creative Foraging holder, in which cardboard compartmentalized boxes can be placed; these boxes can be shredded by the bird to obtain the food hidden inside (Creative Foraging Systems); toilet paper rolls make an excellent, cheap alternative to the commercially available boxes. **G,** Foraging maze, which has five compartments from which the bird needs to collect food via small holes at the front (Creative Foraging Systems). **H,** Four-way forager consisting of four clear plastic cups from which the bird has to retrieve the food hidden inside (Super Bird Creations, LLC, Grand Junction, CO). (**A,** Photo courtesy Nico Schoemaker/Yvonne van Zeeland. **B,** Reprinted from Van Zeeland YRA, Schoemaker NJ, Ravesteijn MM, et al: Efficacy of foraging enrichments to increase foraging time in grey parrots *(Psittacus erithacus erithacus), Appl Anim Behav Sci* 149:87–102, 2013.)

---

foraging times compared with baseline (i.e., a regular food bowl). Thus far, however, maximum foraging times of captive parrots provided with foraging enrichment have been found to not exceed 3 hours per day.[98,99,185,192] Thus, the ability to achieve foraging times comparable with that in the wild (i.e., 4 to 8 hours per day)[42] is currently limited. This inability to truly naturalize the foraging times of captive parrots may also partly explain why the provision of foraging enrichment often reduces, rather than eliminates, feather-damaging behaviors.[105,185]

Social enrichment

For flock birds such as parrots, companionship is vital and can be provided by humans, parrots, and other animals. Visual, vocal, and physical contact with humans or with other parrots are all considered important. Thus, lack of social contact may quickly result in the bird attempting to attract attention (e.g., by screaming excessively) or in stress and abnormal behaviors (e.g., feather-damaging behavior, fear).[197-199] Petting, cuddling, kissing, and allowing birds to climb onto the shoulder are generally considered activities that may encourage inappropriate

bond formation (see Figure 5-15). These should therefore be avoided, reduced, or only offered in specific, limited settings. In contrast, activities such as training, verbal games, dancing, and exercise are all considered activities that promote a healthy bond (Figure 5-32).[186] Particularly, training is considered an important tool to prevent behavioral problems and provide enrichment. Furthermore, it may help improve the human–avian bond, making the interaction more consistent, predictable, and stress-free (see section Behavior Modification Therapy).[186] Talking or whistling to the bird to maintain contact while out of sight may help discourage the bird from screaming. In addition, responding to the bird's soft calls reinforces low intensity contact calls, rather than loud, incessant screams (DRA). Likewise, radios or televisions or other types of background noises may provide the single pet parrot with vocal stimulation when the owner is away (Figure 5-33).[156]

The company of other birds may also be valued by parrots, especially by those that have been reared by their parents, with other birds, or both. Contact with conspecifics may vary from limited vocal contact, visual contact (e.g., when birds are placed in the same or an adjacent room or aviary), or both to

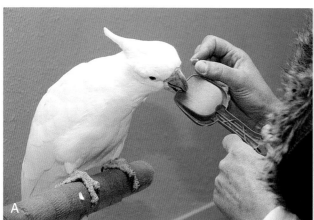
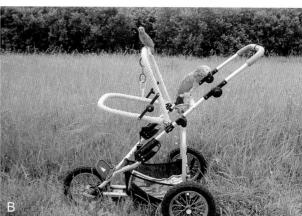

FIGURE 5-32 Providing a companion parrot with mental stimulation, in this case a form of target training **(A)** or taking them outdoors on a modified stroller **(B)**, promotes a healthy bond between the parrot and its owner. (Photo courtesy Ellen Uittenbogaard.)

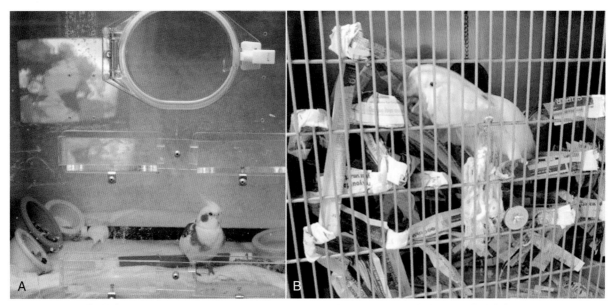

FIGURE 5-33 **A,** Cockatiel watching *Winnie the Pooh* in a hospital clinic. **B,** Moluccan cockatoo in a hospital cage setting with simple enrichments of newspaper and cardboard provided. (**A,** Photo courtesy Nico Schoemaker. **B,** Photo courtesy Melody Hennigh.)

more intense contact (e.g., when the cages are placed side by side, the birds are physically housed together or are allowed to interact with each other outside of their cages). Mutual preening, in particular, is considered important to promote social bonds and may be mimicked by humans by using the forefinger and thumb to make small "nibbling" actions on the head, neck, and breast (Figure 5-34). The lower back, inner thigh, and coelom should not be touched because this may not only function as a sexual stimulation but also increase the risk of hypersexual behaviors, inappropriate bond formation, or both (see section Reproduction-Related Behavior Problems; Figure 5-35).

Social contact with conspecifics has been shown to positively affect the welfare of parrots.[199] Moreover, the ability of birds to imitate one another (as used in observational or model-rival training) may be valuable when teaching a parrot new tricks or cues or to accept novel foods.[49,156] Parrots that have been imprinted on humans, however, may become aggressive or frightened when confronted with another bird. Thus, the parrot's previous experiences and rearing history need to be taken into account when weighing the risks and

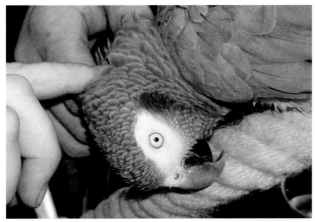

FIGURE 5-34 Mutual preening is important to promote social bonds, not only between birds but also between the bird and its owner. Preening should preferably focus on the head and neck area and not on other body parts as this may stimulate reproductive activity (see also Figure 5-35). (Photo courtesy Ellen Uittenbogaard.)

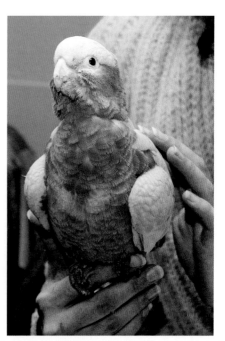

FIGURE 5-35 The owner of this adult male galah *(Eolophus roseicapilla)* is petting the back of this bird, not being aware that it actually can stimulate the bird sexually, thereby increasing the risk of reproduction-associated behavior problems in the bird. (Photo courtesy Ellen Uittenbogaard.)

benefits of the addition of a new bird to the household, and shaping may be required to introduce birds to one another.

Daily activity patterns

For parrots, it appears important to provide both an established framework of activity as well as some variation within this routine. Routine may help the parrot predict important events (i.e., regular times to eat, sleep, play, interact, and be alone). Variation in this routine (e.g., new toys, trips outside, and meeting new people), on the other hand, helps prevent stress in times that this routine is broken or changes to the environment are introduced. Preferably, a variation in routine is already started during the early life stages to allow the bird to get accustomed to change as early as possible.[156,186]

A basic routine consists of taking the bird out of its night cage in the morning, transferring it to its play gym or day cage, and practicing a similar routine at night. Preferably, the bird is placed back in its night cage at a regular time to allow it to get sufficient sleep (i.e., as many as 10 to 12 hours per day).[82] Moreover, it is recommended that the bird be placed in the night cage in a room away from human activity. Not moving the parrot to a designated sleeping area will otherwise result in a sleeping period that equals the time between the last person leaving the room at night and the first person entering the room in the morning. As a result, the parrot may be deprived of its much needed sleep, which may subsequently result in the increased possibility of behavior problems such as aggression, excessive screaming, and FDB.[200]

The feeding schedule is also important to consider in the daily activity pattern. Most commonly, parrots are fed ad libitum, allowing them to consume as much—often high-caloric—foods as they like, whenever they want to. This feeding schedule is, however, far from natural, with parrots in the wild spending a substantial part of their day foraging for food. These activities not only include the consummative (i.e., actual consumption of food) but also the procurement phase of feeding behavior (i.e., searching, exploring, and manipulating food). Feeding behavior can be stimulated by providing foraging enrichment to the parrot, for example, by providing food in meals (i.e., two times per day) rather than ad libitum (temporal distribution of food) or providing food in puzzle feeders (see section Toys and Other Environmental Enrichment).

Bathing

Many, but not all, of the captively maintained psittacines originate from tropical rainforest habitats. Hence, regular bathing (i.e., at least once a week, but preferably as a daily routine) is considered important for those species, from a psychological perspective. In addition, regular bathing is vital for the parrots' overall health, skin, and plumage, especially in homes with central heating with relative low humidity. Bathing can be provided in multiple ways, with each species and individual having its own preference.[86] Some birds enjoy conventional bathing in a bowl or bath, whereas others prefer being misted with a horticultural sprayer or showering together with the owner (see Figure 5-13). For birds that show escape or avoidance behaviors when an attempt is made to shower, mist, or bathe them, desensitization and counter-conditioning and shaping should be employed to teach the parrots to enjoy these daily water activities.

Wing trimming

Deflighting procedures, including the trimming of flight feathers to modify flight, is an intrusive maneuver that should be ethically balanced in the larger view of specific circumstances. The traditional approach of defaulting to the use of wing trimming procedures as a component of behavior modification is no longer a valid first option in most settings. Rather, the decision to deflight a bird should only be made after careful consideration of all relevant ethical, biologic, and environmental aspects (see Chapter 22), as well as available alternatives like adapting the environment to allow for safe indoor flight.

In some situations, safety of the bird and of the owner may warrant clipping of the bird's wing feathers; however, every environment is different and needs to be assessed on its own. Clipping may have several detrimental effects on the behavior of the bird, including, but not limited to, an increased risk of developing feather-damaging behaviors. Particularly, birds that have never been able to fly may lack self-confidence and display more escape and avoidance behaviors. Therefore, decisions to deflight a bird should not be made lightly or be considered an accepted protocol that can be applied out of its appropriate context.

Pharmacologic Intervention

Pharmacologic intervention using psychoactive or psychotropic drugs (i.e., drugs that cross the blood-brain barrier to induce alterations in mood, perception, consciousness, cognition, and behavior) is applied with increasing frequency within the veterinary field. Psychoactive drugs are considered particularly useful in patients that appear refractory to treatment with behavior modification therapy and environmental changes. They may also be useful in situations when the (aversive) stimulus cannot be controlled or avoided or when there is overwhelming fear, anxiety, or aggression.[201] The use of psychoactive drugs, however, is considered appropriate only when a (correct) behavioral diagnosis has been established and only when employing it as adjunctive therapy to appropriate behavior modification therapy, environmental adjustments, and adequate treatment of any concurrent medical illnesses.[202] Thus, prior to considering the use of psychoactive drugs, a complete behavioral and medical history taking, full physical examination, and baseline laboratory testing need to be performed in order to establish a definite or tentative diagnosis and provide a rationale for their use.[203] In addition, regular monitoring and follow-up of the patient (including history taking and physical examination) is advised to determine the efficacy of the treatment and evaluate the occurrence of potential adverse side effects from the drug.

Within the group of psychoactive drugs that have been used in parrots, the following classes may be distinguished: (1) anxiolytic drugs (e.g., diazepam),[202] (2) antipsychotic drugs (e.g., haloperidol, a dopamine antagonist),[204-206] (3) tricyclic antidepressants (e.g., amitriptyline, clomipramine, and doxepin),[202,207,208] (4) serotonin reuptake inhibitors (e.g., paroxetine and fluoxetine),[202,209,210] and (5) opioid antagonists (e.g., naltrexone),[202,211] (see Appendix 1, Table 10). In addition, the use of medroxyprogesterone acetate, or depot gonadotropin-releasing hormone (GnRH) agonists such as deslorelin or leuprolide acetate may be beneficial in patients with suspected sexual or hormone-related behavior problems (e.g., seasonal occurrence and presence of [hyper]sexual and nesting behaviors).[204,212-214] As with the psychotropic drugs, as discussed above, these treatments also are considered appropriate only when a behavioral diagnosis has been established and when used as adjunctive therapy to appropriate behavior modification, adequate treatment of any concurrent medical illnesses, or both.[202]

Unfortunately, for many of the psychoactive drugs, dose titration, pharmacokinetic, pharmacodynamic, and toxicity studies are lacking. Placebo-controlled clinical trials that have been performed to demonstrate the effectiveness of psychoactive drugs in psittacine birds are few in number. As a result, most of the current information on use of psychoactive drugs (including dosages, safety, and efficacy) in parrots is derived from anecdotal experience and expert opinion, single case reports, or uncontrolled clinical trials with small numbers of birds. Data on the use of psychoactive drugs are often extrapolated from studies on other animals or humans. Species differences may, however, be present, which could result in a lack of efficacy or onset of unexpected adverse events. Whenever using psychoactive drugs, veterinarians and owners should therefore be aware of the potential risks and outcomes that may reasonably be expected after treatment. For example, many psychoactive drugs will need at least 2 to 4 weeks to reach maximum efficacy. Gradual titration of the dose is recommended for the individual patient until clinical effects or side effects are noted.[201,202] Similarly, gradual tapering of the dose, rather than acute discontinuance, is recommended when attempting to wean the patient off a medication or to the lowest dose possible. This is generally accomplished by reducing the total daily dose by 25% every 3 weeks while keeping the dosing frequency the same.[201] In patients displaying severe side effects, however, immediate discontinuation of the drugs is warranted. Acute discontinuance may, however, increase the risk of adverse effects (i.e., withdrawal or discontinuation syndrome characterized by rebound anxiety and aggression or reoccurrence of the behavioral problem).[201,202] Similarly, coadministration of psychoactive drugs may result in undesired drug interactions. Thus, combined administration of psychoactive drugs warrants caution and awareness of the drug's targets and potential drug interactions that may occur. Furthermore, if a switch in medication is warranted, withdrawal of the initial drug is necessary before starting up the next, with at least two drug-free dosing intervals.[201,202]

The lack of registered drugs further complicates the use of psychoactive drugs in psittacine patients. As a result, treatment with psychoactive drugs is considered "off label," thus emphasizing the need to have the owner sign a consent form prior to dispensing the drug. Many of the psychoactive drugs also need compounding to enable their use in avian patients. This may pose additional challenges because the effects of compounding on storage and stability are largely unknown.[201,202] Other factors influencing the correct use of psychoactive drugs include the owner's ability or inability to administer the drugs and the acceptability of the drug (e.g., due to taste aversion, particularly in the case of bitter-tasting drugs).

Mechanism of action

Psychoactive drugs are thought to exert their effect through actions on the neurotransmitters in the central nervous system (CNS). Thus far, over 100 neurotransmitters have been identified. The most important ones include gamma amino butyric acid (GABA), acetylcholine (Ach) and the biogenic amines (monoamines), of which the last can be further subdivided into tryptophan-derived indoleamines (serotonin and melatonin) and tyrosine-derived catecholamines (dopamine, norepinephrine, and epinephrine) (Table 5-5). Following the depolarization of the presynaptic cell membrane, neurotransmitters are released into the synaptic cleft. These released neurotransmitters then bind to the receptors, which results in the transduction of the signal to the postsynaptic membrane. Signal transduction ceases again upon deactivation of the activity of the neurotransmitters. This may occur through enzymatic degradation, reuptake in the presynaptic cell via membrane channels, and activation of the autoreceptors (located on the presynaptic membrane) that block the continued release of the neurotransmitters.

Depending on the type of receptor involved, the release of the neurotransmitters may exert excitatory or inhibitory effects. With continued stimulation of the postsynaptic receptors by the neurotransmitters or psychoactive drugs (agonists), downregulation or hyposensitization of the receptors may occur. This downregulation is one of the proposed mechanisms of action of the so-called reuptake inhibitors, which prolong the effect of the neurotransmitters by blocking their reuptake. Alternatively, the receptors that are not stimulated by the neurotransmitters or are blocked by the drugs (antagonists) can become up-regulated or hypersensitive. Alterations in neurotransmitter concentrations and receptor activities result in physiologic and behavioral changes. The effects depend on the type of psychoactive drugs and neurotransmitters involved.

Drug selection

Selection of the appropriate drugs to use for a specific patient necessitates an accurate diagnosis of the behavioral problem of the patient as well as knowledge of drug efficacy and safety. Veterinarians therefore need to familiarize themselves with the indications and contraindications, mechanisms of action, and potential side effects of the various classes of psychoactive drugs. Selection of a psychoactive drug is primarily based on the type of behavioral problem that is present. However, other factors, including the species, age, sex and health status of the bird, cost, and ease of administration of the medication, may also be taken into account.[201,202] Generally, the preferred drug is the one that will likely be effective in treating the behavioral problem but has the least risk of causing side effects. In case this drug fails or results in unacceptable side effects, adjustment of the dose may be considered prior to switching to a different drug. Treatment failure warrants re-evaluation of the original diagnosis as well as the conditions of the drug use (e.g., has the drug been used sufficiently long for it to exert an effect?).

Drug classes

Over the years, a variety of different psychoactive drugs have become available on the veterinary and medical market. The effects (and thus the indications) of a psychoactive drug vary, depending on its chemical composition and the neurotransmitter(s) it targets. Based on their pharmacologic

TABLE 5-5

List of Neurotransmitters and their Respective Effects on Behavior

Neurotransmitter	Primary location	Metabolism	Function	Pathology
Acetylcholine	Wide distribution throughout the central nervous system (CNS) and the peripheral nervous system	Synthesized from acetate and choline; inactivated by acetylcholinesterase	Excitation via activation of muscarinic and nicotinic receptors Muscarinic stimulation: arteriole vasodilation, decreased heart rate and cardiac output, stimulation of the digestive system Nicotinic stimulation	Blockage of muscarinic receptors: atropine-like side effects (dry mouth, dry eye, pupil dilation, tachycardia, constipation, urinary retention) Depletion: cognitive decline, Alzheimer disease
Dopamine	Corpus striatum	Produced from L-dopa, stored in presynaptic vesicles. Inactivation by monoamine oxidase B (MAO B) and catechol-O-methyltransferase (COMT).	Coordination of motor activities (via extrapyramidal system)	Depletion: behavioral quieting, depression, extrapyramidal motor symptoms (muscle tremors, tics, motor restlessness ~ Parkinson disease) Excess: compulsive and stereotypical behaviors
Epinephrine	Widely distributed throughout the body and CNS	Secreted from the adrenal glands in response to norepinephrine	Sympathetic effects, dependent on type of receptor involved α-adrenergic activation: vasoconstriction, increased cardiac contractility, iris dilation, intestinal relaxation, pilomotor contraction, contraction of bladder and intestinal sphincters, inhibition of parasympathetic nervous system β-1 adrenergic activation: increased cardiac output β-2 adrenergic activation: vasodilation, bronchodilation, intestinal and uterine relaxation, dilation of coronary vessels	
Gamma amino butyric acid (GABA)	Wide distribution throughout the brain	Synthesized from glutamate	Inhibition, behavioral quieting	Depletion: seizure activity, Parkinson disease, fear and phobias
Norepinephrine	Widely distributed throughout the body and CNS	Formation by hydroxylation of dopamine. Breakdown by monoamine oxidase A (MAO A) and catechol-O-methyltransferase (COMT).		Depletion: depression Excess: mania
Serotonin	Mainly found in cells of the midline raphe	Synthesized from dietary tryptophan; inactivation by reuptake or breakdown by MAO	Modulation of sleep–wake cycle, mood, emotion, sexual behavior, and impulse control	Depletion: depression, anxiety, irritability, aggression, impulsiveness Excess: confidence, calmness, flexibility, resilience

effects, psychoactive drugs can be classified into the following classes:

1. Anxiolytics and sedatives, which act as CNS depressants and are primarily to reduce anxiety and anxiety-related symptoms and to calm the patient. In addition, many of these drugs also act as hypnotics that may help induce and maintain sleep. The class of anxiolytics and sedatives includes the following drugs: benzodiazepines (BZPs), barbiturates, buspirone, chloral hydrate, and zopiclone. Of these, the BZPs are the ones that are most commonly used, especially when long-term treatment is needed.

2. Antidepressants, which act directly or indirectly on various neurotransmitters, in particular serotonin and norepinephrine, and are prescribed in humans to treat depression. Among the antidepressants, the following categories may be identified: tricyclic antidepressants (TCAs), tetracyclic antidepressants (TeCAs), serotonin–norepinephrine reuptake inhibitors (SNRIs), selective serotonin reuptake inhibitors (SSRIs), reversible and irreversible (selective) monoamine oxidase inhibitors (MAOIs), and bupropion (a drug from the aminoketone family). Of these categories, TCAs and SSRIs are most commonly used in veterinary medicine.

3. Antipsychotics, which are primarily used in human medicine to treat psychosis (e.g., schizophrenia). Antipsychotics can be further subdivided into *typical antipsychotics*, including the phenothiazine, butyrophenone and thioxanthene derivatives, and diphenylbutylpiperidines, which specifically interact with the dopamine receptors and block their function; and *atypical antipsychotics*, including risperidone, loxapine, olanzapine, quetiapine, and clozapine, which not only function as dopamine antagonists but also interact with other receptors (including serotoninergic, histaminergic, adrenergic, and cholinergic receptors). This class of drugs is only rarely used by veterinary behaviorists.

4. Mood stabilizers, which are used to treat bipolar affective disorder and facilitate mood regulation in people experiencing alternating manic and depressive phases of the disease. The prototype of this class of medications is lithium. This class of drugs is even more rarely used in veterinary medicine than antipsychotics.

5. Psychoactive drugs used in the treatment of addictions. These include opioid antagonists, which help overcome endorphin-related or opioid-related addictions by blocking their euphoric effects.

Besides these psychoactive drugs, hormones, antihistaminergic drugs, and anticonvulsant drugs may also be used to alleviate behavior problems that are associated with increased levels of sex hormones, allergies, and neurologic dysfunction (e.g., epilepsy), respectively. The more commonly used drug classes in current avian medicine are discussed in more depth below.

Benzodiazepines. BZPs (e.g., diazepam, midazolam) are drugs that potentiate the effects of GABA by increasing the affinity of the GABA-A receptor for this inhibitory neurotransmitter. Because of their anxiolytic effects, BZPs are considered beneficial for short-term treatment of acute and intermittent behavior problems, particularly those involving fear, phobia, and anxiety, including fear-related aggression. In addition, BZPs have been used in the treatment of (acute episodes of) FDB and automutilation. Besides these behavioral indications, BZPs have sedative, appetite-stimulating, and anticonvulsant effects (with a rapid onset of action). As a result, BZPs are considered useful in the treatment of acute seizures or anorexia; to facilitate social interaction; and in situations where (temporary) sedation may be necessary, for example, to facilitate the acceptance of (Elizabethan) collars by the bird.[201,202,215] At low dosages, BZPs act as sedatives, whereas they act as anxiolytics at moderate dosages; and they act as hypnotics, facilitating sleep, at high dosages.

Although BZPs are generally considered safe, side effects have been reported. These may include sedation, ataxia,

muscle relaxation, hyperphagia, disinhibition of aggression, paradoxical excitation, and memory deficits. The last can cause BZPs to interfere with learning, thereby potentially affecting behavior modification therapy and training of the bird. In humans, long-term use has been reported to result in neutropenia, jaundice, anemia, and drug dependence. Because of the risk of drug dependence, gradual withdrawal of the drugs is recommended after chronic dosing.[216–218] In cats, BZPs have been associated with hepatic failure.[219,220]

As in humans, BZPs may be used concurrently with other psychoactive drugs, including TCAs and SSRIs. This combination is often used to alleviate panic attacks, since the BZPs help deal with the panic component of an anxiety (e.g., a panic attack displayed by an animal with separation anxiety at a time when the owner is preparing to leave). Coadministration of BZPs and SSRIs or TCAs may help to overcome the delayed efficacy of TCAs and SSRIs but could also be employed at times when the effectiveness of these drugs appears to be waning.[221,222] Dosages should, however, be adjusted accordingly in these instances because of increased risk of CNS depression resulting from concurrent administration of the various drugs.[201,202,223] Caution is furthermore warranted when using these drugs in obese patients and in those with renal or hepatic failure.[201,202]

Tricyclic antidepressants. TCAs potentiate the effects of biogenic amines to varying degrees. TCAs may either block the neurotransmitter reuptake (norepinephrine, serotonin) or act as competitive antagonists at the respective muscarinic acetylcholine, histaminergic H1, and α-1 or α-2 adrenergic receptors (acetylcholine, histamine, norepinephrine). Therapeutic effects are believed to result primarily from inhibition of norepinephrine and serotonin reuptake. However, blockage of α-adrenergic, antihistaminic, and anticholinergic activities is believed to account for the various side effects seen following administration of these drugs.[224] As TCAs exert their effect (in part) through downregulation of the receptors, their onset of action is delayed. Thus, clinical effects and improvement may not be noted until 2 to 4 weeks following start of treatment.[201,225]

Of the various TCAs available, clomipramine is the most commonly used and well-researched drug in the field of veterinary medicine. Clomipramine is most selective for serotonin reuptake inhibition. This makes clomipramine useful for treating compulsive disorders and potentially also for treating FDB.[201,207,208,226,227] A double-blind, placebo-controlled clinical trial in feather-plucking cockatoos supported these findings because a significant reduction in feather plucking behavior was observed at 3 and 6 weeks following start of treatment with clomipramine.[208] TCAs may also be indicated in the treatment of fear, phobia, anxiety, and aggression or to alleviate chronic neuropathic pain.[201,202] Amitriptyline and doxepin, which produce the strongest antihistaminergic effects, may be particularly useful to treat pruritus resulting from allergic conditions.[201,228] Both drugs have also been successfully used in the treatment of birds with an allergy-induced form of FDB.[225,229] However, no definite conclusions can be drawn at this time because of the lack of controlled studies on the efficacy of doxepin and amitriptyline in birds.

Because of their anticholinergic, antihistaminergic, and adrenergic effects, TCAs are generally considered to have narrow therapeutic safety, with no specific antidotes available for overdosing.[201] Side effects seen following TCA administration include tachycardia, mydriasis, decreased tear production, dry mouth, gastrointestinal (GI) upset, regurgitation, constipation, urine retention, change in appetite, change in glucose levels, sedation, lethargy, increased anxiety and aggression, ataxia, and seizures (resulting from lowering of the seizure threshold).[202,230-232] Side effects noted in a Grey parrot treated with clomipramine included increased wariness, anxiety, and increased appetite (at dosages of 4–9 mg/kg orally every 12 hours); and hallucinations (at dosages of 19 mg/kg orally).[233] A green-winged macaw (*Ara chloroptera*) and a Moluccan cockatoo (*Cacatua moluccensis*), however, already developed severe neurologic signs and died within a few days following the administration of 3 mg/kg clomipramine orally every 12 hours and 2 mg/kg imipramine orally every 12 hours, respectively.[202] These cases emphasize that caution should be exercised when administering these drugs to a bird because individual patients may respond differently to the treatment. Gradual dose titration and careful, continued monitoring for the presence of side effects are therefore recommended. Should the patient start displaying neurologic symptoms or unusual behavior, immediate discontinuation of the medication is warranted. Side effects noted following the administration of amitriptyline and doxepin include sedation, agitation (particularly in cockatoos), worsening of FDB, and increase in appetite.[225,229] In a blue-and-gold macaw (*Ara ararauna*) treated with 4 mg/kg clomipramine orally every 12 hours, extrapyramidal side effects, including disseminated dystonia (manifesting as pacing, head bobbing, and circling), intermittent ataxia, and coarse-muscle tremors, were noted.[234] This bird, however, had been treated with haloperidol just prior to the administration of clomipramine, which indicates that combined administration of psychoactive drugs should be done with caution. It is generally not advised to use TCAs in combination with MAOIs, antipsychotics, anticholinergics, antidepressants, barbiturates, and other CNS depressants, anticonvulsants, thyroid supplements, or antithyroid medications.[202] Similarly, the use of TCAs is contraindicated in patients with alterations in blood glucose levels (e.g., diabetes mellitus), adrenal or thyroid disorders, glaucoma, seizures, hepatic disease, or cardiac disease.[201,202]

Selective serotonin reuptake inhibitors. SSRIs exert their effect by producing a highly selective blockage of the serotonin reuptake at the presynaptic membrane, thereby increasing the availability of serotonin. In addition, SSRIs may increase the sensitivity of the postsynaptic receptors to serotonin. Indications for their use include compulsive and impulsive disorders (including FDB and automutilation), fear, phobias and anxiety-related disorders, and aggression.[201,202,235,236] Because of their mood-stabilizing effect, SSRIs are considered the preferred drugs for treating affective or anxiety-related disorders. Similar to TCAs, their onset of action is believed to be delayed. Thus, prolonged dosing for at least 2 to 6 weeks (in cats, clinical efficacy may already be seen within 1 to 2 weeks after initiation of treatment) is necessary to induce downregulation of the postsynaptic receptors and the associated clinical effects.[202] Because of their selectivity, which results in fewer side effects compared with TCAs and minimal to no effect on other neurotransmitter receptors, SSRIs are considered

safer.[237,238] Side effects reported in humans and animals are generally mild and may include lethargy, sedation, insomnia, loss of appetite, weight loss, nausea, diarrhea, mild ataxia, and potential lowering of seizure threshold.[236-239] Caution is warranted when using SSRIs in patients with seizures and alterations in blood glucose, although SSRIs generally appear to have limited effect on lowering the seizure threshold. SSRIs should not be administered in combination with MAOIs, TCAs, anticonvulsant drugs, and antipsychotic drugs because concurrent use of these drugs poses a risk for development of serotonin syndrome (a potentially fatal condition that is characterized by onset of one or more of the following symptoms: diarrhea; restlessness; extreme agitation, hyperreflexia, and autonomic instability with possible rapid fluctuations in vital signs; myoclonus, seizures, hyperthermia, uncontrollable shivering, and rigidity; and delirium, coma, status epilepticus, cardiovascular collapse, and death).[201,202,240]

Of the various SSRIs that are available (e.g., sertraline, citalopram, fluvoxamine, fluoxetine, paroxetine), paroxetine is one of the most potent and selective SSRIs. Paroxetine has little affinity for the adrenergic, dopaminergic, or histaminergic receptors. Furthermore, it has only a weak affinity for the cholinergic muscarinic receptors, thereby posing minimal risk of central and autonomous side effects.[241] Paroxetine has been found beneficial in treating phobias and FDB in birds. Several authors have recommended it as the drug of choice for treating these conditions.[201,202,242] However, reports concerning its efficacy are sparse and limited to case reports and anecdotal evidence, with no controlled clinical trials available to support these findings. Nevertheless, recently, a pharmacokinetic study was performed in Grey parrots that showed rapid distribution and elimination after intravenous administration of the drug.[210] Oral administration, in contrast, was relatively slow (Tmax: 5.9 ± 2.6 hours) and highly dependent on the formulation, with little to no uptake of paroxetine following administration of a commercial suspension. Oral administration of paroxetine hydrochloride dissolved in water, however, resulted in a low bioavailability of 31 ± 15%.[210] Following repeated administration, higher rates of absorption could be achieved, most likely as a result of saturation of the cytochrome P450–mediated first-pass metabolism. Based on the study in Grey parrots, a dose of 4 mg/kg paroxetine hydrochloride orally every 12 hours was found to result in plasma concentrations within the therapeutic range recommended for the treatment of depression in humans.[210] Large interindividual differences, however, were found upon evaluation of the plasma levels; these differences were hypothesized to be gender related.[210] Further clinical trials are needed to confirm these suspicions and to establish the effectiveness of the proposed dosing regimen in treating behavior problems in parrots.

An open (non–placebo-controlled) clinical trial was also performed with fluoxetine in feather-damaging birds, and the results showed an initial decline. However, relapses were seen in 12 of the 14 birds in the study.[209] Fluoxetine appeared beneficial in the treatment of toe chewing in a cockatiel,[243] suggesting that it has potential in the treatment of self-injurious behaviors. For this indication, one of the authors (YvZ) has also successfully used paroxetine in various bird species (particularly cockatoos). For the other SSRIs, no published information regarding their efficacy is available.

Dopamine antagonists. Dopamine receptor antagonists belong to the class of antipsychotics or neuroleptics. Their mode of action results in behavioral quieting or ataraxia (i.e., decreased emotional reactivity and relative indifference to stressful situations). In addition, they suppress spontaneous movements without affecting spinal and pain reflexes.[244] Antipsychotics have been used to treat schizophrenia, mania, violent behavior, and other psychotic disorders.[245] In veterinary medicine, "low-potency" antipsychotics (phenothiazine derivatives such as chlorpromazine) are commonly used as tranquilizers. "High-potency" antipsychotics (butyrophenone derivatives such as haloperidol) have been used to reduce compulsive behaviors in various animal species, including compulsive feather-damaging and self-injurious behavior.[204-206,244,246] Side effects may include hypotension, bradycardia, decreased seizure threshold, ataxia, sedation, extrapyramidal motor signs such as muscle tremors and ticks, and motor restlessness. Low-potency antipsychotics more frequently result in cardiotoxic side effects and sedation. High-potency antipsychotics, in contrast, are generally less sedative and hypotensive but do cause neurologic side effects (i.e., extrapyramidal signs).[244] These side effects have also been reported in birds.[201,205] Other side effects reported following the use of antipsychotics include depression, decreased appetite, regurgitation, ataxia, agitation, and excitability. Most of these side effects are primarily encountered in the first few days following initiation of treatment, with only few occurring in the long term (i.e., following treatment of several months up to years).[204-206] Anecdotally, haloperidol has been reported to result in sudden death in a hyacinth macaw (*Anodorhynchus hyacinthinus*) and a red-bellied macaw (*Orthopsittaca manilatus*).[205] Similarly, evidence suggests that Quaker parakeets and cockatoo species (e.g., umbrella [*Cacatua alba*] and Moluccan cockatoos) may be more sensitive to side effects. Caution and lowering of the dose may thus be warranted in these species.[205,247] Besides species differences in side effects, conflicting results have also been reported concerning the efficacy of antipsychotic drugs in the treatment of psittacine behavior problems. For example, favorable results were achieved following the use of haloperidol in automutilating cockatoos,[205,206,248] whereas no obvious improvement was seen in others.[204] Thus, further studies into dosing regimen and efficacy (including species differences therein) are needed to enable evidence-based decisions to be made on the use of antipsychotics in birds.

Phenothiazine derivatives (low-potency antipsychotics) may be combined with BZPs or SSRIs to provide an additive sedative effect. They should, however, not be used in conjunction with other antipsychotics because both have sedative and anticholinergic effects, thereby exacerbating each other's effects. Similarly, it is not advised to use high-potency antipsychotics with other psychoactive drugs such as TCAs, since their added effects may result in severe neurologic side effects.[234]

Opioid antagonists. Opioid or narcotic antagonists such as naloxone or naltrexone counteract the effects of endogenous opioids that are released during stress. Endogenous opioids activate the dopaminergic system, induce analgesia, and block pain, which are all factors believed to contribute in the onset of stereotypical and self-injurious behaviors.[249] By reversing the opioid-induced analgesia, opioid antagonists might have the potency to block the reinforcing effects of self-injurious behaviors. They have therefore been used to treat stereotypies and other compulsive or self-injurious behaviors in zoo and companion animals.[250-254] Opioid antagonists may, however, suppress these compulsive behaviors only for a short while, thereby only being beneficial in acute presentations when the behavior is not yet ritualized (i.e., shortly after their onset).[250-254] In parrots, opioid antagonists may be helpful to treat FDB and automutilation, especially when the behavior has not been present for more than 1 to 2 years.[211] A non–placebo-controlled clinical trial showed positive response in over 75% of birds (n = 41) treated with naltrexone for 1 to 6 months. However, a large number of these birds (n = 26) wore collars or restraint devices. The outcomes may thus have been biased, although in several individuals the collar was removed prior to the end of the trial.[211]

Opioid agonists (e.g., butorphanol) and antagonists provide analgesia. This analgesic effect may be advantageous in patients that are experiencing moderate to severe pain that may have been triggered by or resulted from self-injurious behaviors.[201] To establish whether pain is involved, a trial with an effective analgesic (opioid agonist/antagonist, nonsteroidal antiinflammatory drug [NSAID], or local anesthetic) may be warranted (see Chapter 20).

Possible side effects of opioid antagonists include increased anxiety and GI problems such as abdominal cramps, nausea, vomiting, and constipation. Opioid antagonists are contraindicated in patients with liver disease.[201]

Antihistaminergic drugs. Antihistaminergic drugs (e.g., diphenhydramine, hydroxyzine) block the physiologic effects of histamine by preventing it from binding to the postsynaptic H1 receptors. These receptors are responsible for the release of histamine mediators and recruitment of inflammatory cells that initiate an allergic response, including the onset of pruritus and increase in vascular permeability (see Chapter 11).[255] Antihistaminergic drugs may therefore be beneficial in the treatment of pruritus, as well as pruritus-associated self-trauma such as feather damaging or self-injurious behaviors.[201,256] One case report reported successful treatment of feather-damaging behavior in a red-lored Amazon parrot (*Amazona autumnalis*) following a combination treatment with hydroxyzine and eicosapentaenoic acid (DermCaps).[257] H1 receptor antagonists also have sedative, antinausea, anticholinergic, antiserotonergic, and local anesthetic (side) effects.[255] Caution is warranted when using antihistaminergic drugs concurrently with anticholinergic agents or CNS depressants or when using these drugs in patients with hepatic disease.[201,255]

Anticonvulsants: barbiturates and carbamazepine. Anticonvulsant drugs such as barbiturates (e.g., phenobarbital) are not commonly employed in behavioral medicine, unless an epileptic component that warrants long-term treatment is present (e.g., idiopathic epilepsy). Side effects are similar to those of BZPs, which have a wider therapeutic index. Barbiturate use is contraindicated in patients with hepatic disease (barbiturates are potent activators of the CYP-450 enzymes). Barbiturates should also not be used in patients receiving other CNS drugs (e.g., antipsychotics, antidepressants) because concurrent administration of these drugs may increase the risk of CNS and respiratory depression.[240] In addition, combined administration of paroxetine and phenobarbital, for example, may decrease plasma concentrations of paroxetine, thereby limiting its effects.[258]

Carbamazepine, an anticonvulsant drug that is structurally similar to the TCA imipramine, has mood-stabilizing properties. Because of these properties, carbamazepine may be useful in treating human patients with depression, mania, and explosive aggression. In birds, carbamazepine may likewise be useful to treat compulsive disorders (including FDB) and fear-related or frustration-related aggression. In birds with compulsive FDB or self-mutilation, carbamazepine may be used in combination with chlorpromazine or haloperidol, particularly during the initial first 2 weeks of treatment.[201] Side effects include mild sedation and other anticholinergic effects. Contraindications include renal, hepatic, cardiovascular, or hematologic disorders, including bone marrow suppression.

Hormone therapy. Drugs that alter sex steroidal hormone secretion may be beneficial in patients that display undesirable reproductive behaviors or behavior problems induced by hormonal changes and problems that have a cyclic or seasonal character. These include, but are not limited to, chronic egg laying, masturbation, seasonal aggression, and some FDBs.[202] Hormone therapy should be combined with behavioral and environmental interventions in order to prevent recurrence of problems in the future (see Chapters 12 and 14).

One of the more commonly used hormones in avian medicine is leuprolide acetate, a synthetic analog of GnRH. Similar to other GnRH agonists, leuprolide acetate inhibits gonadotropin secretion, thereby suppressing ovarian and testicular steroidogenesis and reducing hormone-related behaviors. As a result, leuprolide acetate has been used in the treatment of various reproduction-related disorders, including chronic egg laying, cystic ovarian and oviduct disease, egg yolk peritonitis, granulomas of the ovary and oviduct, cloacal prolapse, continued ovulation after salpingohysterectomy, FDB, aggression, and persistent sexually induced regurgitation. Anecdotal reports have suggested 73% overall improvement, with temporary resolution in 89% of chronic egg-laying psittacines.[259] As an alternative to injections with leuprolide acetate, implants containing the long-acting gonadotropin-releasing hormone agonist deslorelin may be used. These implants, which can be placed subcutaneously, have a longer-lasting effect (of up to several months; see Chapter 14). Over time, however, hormones may become less effective, thereby necessitating more frequent dosing and use of higher dosages.[201]

Medroxyprogesterone, a progestogen with antiandrogenic properties, is another drug that has previously been used to treat hormonal or reproduction-related disorders, including excessive egg laying, sexual behavior, and hormone-related FDB. Medroxyprogesterone may induce severe side effects, including lethargy, inappetence, weight gain, polyuria and polydipsia, diabetes mellitus, bone marrow suppression, adrenocortical suppression, tumor formation, hepatopathy, and death. Because of these serious side effects and the availability of other, safer alternatives, its use is generally now considered unnecessary. Human chorionic gonadotropin (hCG) also has been used in the past. It was found to only be moderately successful (i.e., 65% response rate) for treating aggression and FDB in female birds (and even less so in male birds). With the introduction of the more effective GnRH agonists, this drug has therefore also become obsolete.[260]

Monitoring and Follow-Up

Following the implementation of a behavior modification plan, it is vital to keep monitoring the patient and to evaluate the effects of the therapy. Preferably, the plan is implemented in a stepwise fashion. This enables each individual component of the plan to be evaluated separately for its effects. It also allows the veterinarian to gain insight into the extent to which a proposed intervention is responsible for an observed change in behavior. To evaluate the effect of the behavior modification plan, owners may be asked to keep a record of the bird's behavior. In this record, the frequency, severity, and timing of episodes of the problem behavior are tracked, including the factors that may influence the onset of this behavior. This not only helps document the effectiveness of the treatment but also facilitates a further defining of the problem in case the proposed treatment does not have the desired effects. Keeping a record may help keep the owner motivated to comply with the behavior modification plan, as it allows detection of gradual declines in frequency and severity of symptoms. Besides record keeping, regular (e.g., monthly to bimonthly) checkups in the clinic are advised to monitor the effects of the therapy on the bird's overall health and behavior. These checkups are especially important when drugs are included in the treatment plan. Checkups have also been found to be helpful in documenting changes in behavior, especially in birds displaying FDB or automutilation. During these checkups, photographs and feather scoring systems can be used to document dermatologic abnormalities (see section Feather Damaging Behavior–Prognosis and Monitoring). Comparison of photographs or feather scores of successive visits may subsequently help identify improvement in plumage condition or healing of skin lesions. Based on the aforementioned findings, adjustment of the behavior modification plan may then follow, if needed.

SPECIFIC BEHAVIOR PROBLEMS

Companion parrots with behavioral problems are frequently presented to the avian practitioner. Such problems may include biting, screaming, fear, FDB, and hypersexual behaviors (e.g., regurgitation, masturbation). According to a recent survey,[7] 71% of owners (n = 203) reported at least one problem behavior in their birds. Biting of humans was the most commonly reported problem (32%; n = 64), followed by screaming (17%; n = 35) and FDB (13%; n = 27). Approximately half the owners reporting behavioral issues in their birds considered these behaviors to be truly problematic. Help was sought by four fifths of these caregivers from either their veterinarian (52%; n = 33), behavior consultant (11%; n = 7), breeder (14%; n = 9), pet store (17%; n = 11), and friends and family (23%; n = 15). In contrast to the study among owners, FDB was reported as the predominant behavior problem encountered in the veterinary practice. Over 80% of participating veterinarians (69 of 84) even reported it as the most commonly seen behavior problem in practice, whereby at least one case per month was seen. The second-most and third-most common problems seen by veterinarians in practice included chronic egg laying (44%; 36 of 84) and aggression towards humans (30%; 24 of 79). Results from the surveys indicate that owners tend to seek veterinary advice in case of feather-damaging behavior and reproduction-related behaviors. The greater readiness of owners to seek veterinary help for these aforementioned problems may likely stem from the assumption that these behaviors must have an underlying medical cause. Screaming and biting are more likely to have a nonmedical, environmental component to them. As a result, it may be less obvious for owners to seek veterinary advice when trying to deal with these problems.[7] Nevertheless, it is considered important for veterinarians to question a parrot's owner routinely about problem behaviors, since this facilitates their early diagnosis and treatment. Of the various behavior problems that may be encountered, the following will be discussed in the sections below: self-injurious behaviors (including FDB and automutilation), reproduction-related behavior problems, anxiety-related disorders, aggression (biting), and excessive vocalizations (screaming).

Self-Injurious Behaviors: Feather-Damaging Behavior and Automutilation

Feather-damaging behavior (FDB), also referred to as feather-destructive behavior, feather plucking, feather picking, or pterotillomania,[157,185,261] is one of the most common and frustrating conditions to deal with in captive parrots. It has been estimated that approximately 10% to 15% of captive psittacine birds chew, bite, pluck, or pull their feathers (Figure 5-36), thereby inflicting localized or generalized damage to their plumage and preventing normal regrowth of feathers.[7,262,263] Damage always presents itself solely in the areas that can be accessed using their beak (i.e., neck, chest, flanks, inner thighs,

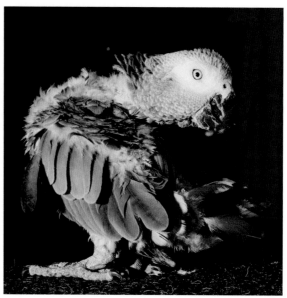

FIGURE 5-36 Grey parrot *(Psittacus erithacus)* in the process of removing a tail feather. Feather-damaging behavior is thought to occur in approximately 10% to 15% of captive parrots, with a higher incidence in Grey parrots and cockatoos. (Photo courtesy Nico Schoemaker/Yvonne van Zeeland.)

and wings).[215,261,264,265] When trauma to the skin and muscle is present, the condition is referred to as "automutilation."

Clinical signs in feather-damaging birds may vary from mild localized feather damage to completely bald areas and soft tissue damage (Figure 5-37). Chewed feathers generally have an irregular appearance, with barbs removed from the shaft, the ramus of the feather shaft split longitudinally, and

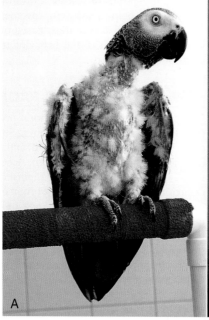
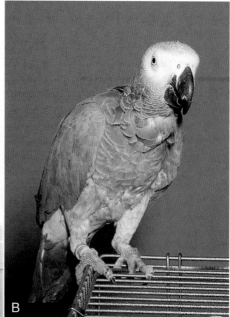

FIGURE 5-37 These two Grey parrots *(Psittacus erithacus)* demonstrate the typical appearance of a bird with self-inflicted feather-damaging behavior, as indicated by their normally feathered head. Severity of the feather damage may vary from case to case, resulting in more **(A)** or less **(B)** extensive loss of or damage to feathers. (Photo courtesy Nico Schoemaker/Yvonne van Zeeland.)

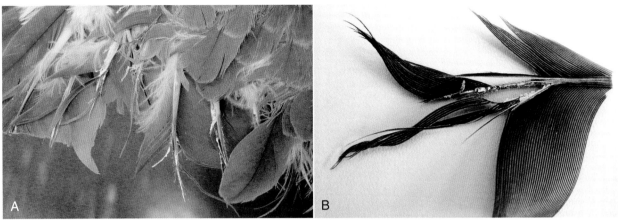

FIGURE 5-38 **A** and **B,** Chewed and frayed feathers often have an irregular appearance, as can be seen in these feathers. (Photo Courtesy Nico Schoemaker/Yvonne van Zeeland.)

V-shaped wedges being cut out of the top of the feathers (Figure 5-38). Plucking of feathers most commonly occurs on the chest, ventral wing surface, and inner thighs.[265,266] Feather chewing appears to primarily affect the larger primary and tail feathers.[265] Depending on the species, self-mutilation will often be localized to specific areas. Cockatoos, for example, often present with severe self-mutilation of feathers, skin, and muscles of the breast or patagium (Figure 5-39). Amazon parrots appear to primarily traumatize the feet and legs (a condition referred to as Amazon foot necrosis). In lovebirds, the patagium, neck, axillary region, and back are commonly affected (a condition known as chronic ulcerative dermatitis; Figure 5-40).[267] Quaker parakeets often self-mutilate the neck and chest area (Figure 5-41) and do it to such an extent that

the injuries become fatal (e.g., in case of damage to the crop and the jugular vein).[267]

In many cases, the consequences of this self-inflicted feather damage may be solely aesthetic. However, medical issues may also arise as a result of alterations to the birds' thermoregulatory abilities and metabolic demands, hemorrhage, and (secondary) infections.[215,264,265]

Species, age, and gender predilections

Although noted in all psittacine birds, Grey parrots and cockatoos are especially considered to be at risk. Odds of FDB in these species were, respectively, 8 and almost 13 times higher than in other species, with reported prevalence of around 40%.[198,263,268-270] Other species that are varyingly

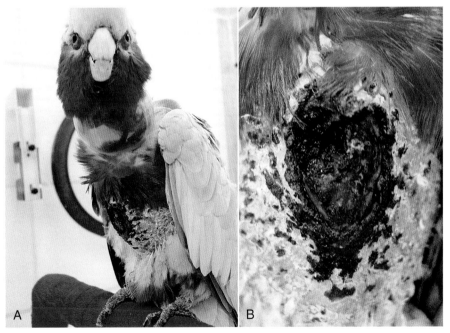

FIGURE 5-39 **A,** In cockatoos, besides feather damage, automutilation is also commonly encountered. Generally, the pectoral region is affected, as can be seen in this galah *(Eolophus roseicapilla)*. **B,** Close-up of the wound in the pectoral area of the galah from Figure 5-39, *A.* Besides the skin, the underlying tissues may also be damaged, which may be exacerbated by an infection. (Photo courtesy Nico Schoemaker/Yvonne van Zeeland.)

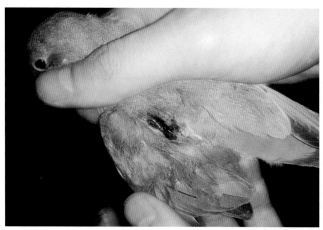

FIGURE 5-40 Chronic ulcerative dermatitis, or wing-web dermatitis, is a condition that is commonly encountered in lovebirds, as seen in this peach-faced lovebird *(Agapornis roseicollis)*. Many treatment options have been proposed, but none has been scientifically proven to be effective.

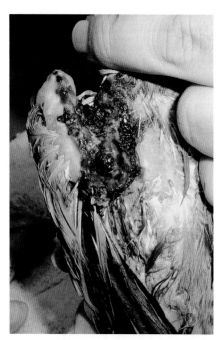

FIGURE 5-41 Quaker parrot with severe automutilation. Occasionally the self-inflicted trauma may be so severe that death results. Unfortunately, a singular cause of this type of self-injurious behavior remains to be elucidated. (Photo courtesy Scott Echols.)

reported as predisposed to FDB include macaws, Eclectus parrots *(Eclectus roratus)*, gray-cheeked parakeets *(Brotogeris* spp.), Quaker parakeets, and conures.[198,263,264,271] In contrast, FDB appears less common in Amazon parrots, cockatiels, and budgerigars.[198,263,268] Automutilation has often been reported to occur concurrently with FDB, with an overall higher incidence reported in cockatoo species (see Figure 5-39).[266] In addition, different mutilation syndromes have been described in lovebirds, Quaker parakeets, and Amazon parrots.[267,272]

Other predisposing factors for FDB include age and sex, with FDB suggested to occur more often in adolescent and adult female birds.[107,118,263,270] A recent pilot study in healthy and feather-damaging Grey parrots from a refuge suggested that FDB occurs predominantly in individuals demonstrating a proactive coping strategy (i.e., an active, fight-or-flight behavioral response).[273] This coping strategy is characterized by higher levels of aggression and territorial control, fast and superficial exploration of the environment, and an overall rigid and routine-like behavior. Preliminary findings of the study suggest a potential role for behavior tests to be performed in order to establish whether a parrot is at risk for developing FDB.[273] However, the number of birds included in this study was low (n = 22). In addition, no longitudinal data were obtained. Thus, further (prospective, longitudinal) studies with larger cohorts are needed to confirm whether a correlation (i.e., not necessarily a causal relationship) exists between coping style and FDB or the susceptibility to develop this behavior.

Although FDB is often self-inflicted, birds may sometimes also pluck the feathers of their cage mates or offspring if group-housed. In these situations, the head and face generally appear to be the primary target areas (Figure 5-42).[274,275]

Etiologic considerations

FDB is considered a multifactorial behavior, in which various medical, genetic, psychological, neurobiologic, and socioenvironmental factors may play a role (Table 5-6).[107,261,276] Similar factors may also play a role in automutilation, although for many of the species-specific self-mutilation syndromes, no clear linkage to any of the presumed etiologies has been identified.

Numerous medical conditions have been associated with self-injurious behaviors, but a reliable causal relationship has not been demonstrated. Any disease causing pain, discomfort, irritation, and pruritus may result in development of FDB or

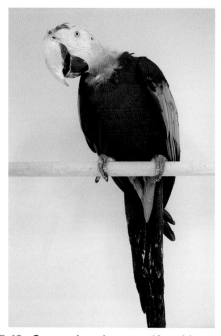

FIGURE 5-42 Green-winged macaw *(Ara chloropterus)* with feather loss on the head as a result of plucking by its partner. (Photo courtesy Nico Schoemaker.)

TABLE 5-6

Factors Suggested to be Involved in Onset and Maintenance of Feather-Damaging Behavior and Automutilation in Parrots

Medical	Socioenvironmental	Genetic / Psychological / Neurobiologic (Internal Factors)
• Ectoparasites (e.g., *Knemidokoptes* [in budgerigars], *Myialges*, red mites [*Dermanyssus*], feather or quill mites, lice) • Bacterial or fungal dermatitis and/or folliculitis (including *Staphylococcus*, *Mycobacterium*, *Aspergillus*, *Trichophyton*, *Microsporon*, *Candida*, *Malassezia*) • Viral disease (e.g., polyomavirus) (particularly in budgerigars, lovebirds with cutaneous ulcerative disease), psittacine beak and feather disease, papillomavirus, avipoxvirus • Feather dysplasia (e.g., polyfolliculitis in lovebirds) • Skin neoplasia (e.g., xanthoma, lipoma, squamous cell carcinoma) • Hypersensitivity, skin allergy (blue-and-gold macaws appear more prone); contact dermatitis (Amazon foot necrosis) • Airsacculitis, pneumonia • Chlamydiosis • Proventricular dilatation disease (PDD) • Gastrointestinal disorders such as colic, endoparasitism (particularly giardiasis in cockatiels) • Liver, pancreatic and/or renal disease • Hypocalcemia • Endocrine disease (e.g., hypothyroidism, diabetes mellitus) • Reproductive disease (e.g., egg binding, cystic ovaries) • Heavy metal toxicosis (e.g., lead, zinc) • Obesity and associated conditions such as lipemia and hepatic lipidosis (e.g., Quaker parakeets with self-mutilation) • Orthopedic disorders (e.g., osteosarcoma, fracture, osteomyelitis)	• Nutritional deficiencies (e.g., hypovitaminosis A) and/or dietary imbalances • Small cage or poor cage design with little space for the parrot to move around • Overcrowding • Social isolation • Lack of opportunities to perform species-specific behaviors in the captive living environment (e.g., foraging) • Sudden changes or unpredictable environment • Airborne and/or topical toxins, including cigarette smoke, scented candles, air fresheners, hand lotions and creams • Low humidity levels, lack of bathing opportunities • Abnormal photoperiod • Poor wing trim • Trauma (e.g., tail avulsion, split sternum, damage to blood feathers)	• Genetic • Temperamental traits (proactive response) • Hand-rearing and imprinting on humans • Poor socialization at earlier age • Boredom from insufficient mental or physical stimulation • (Sexual) frustration (e.g., because of inability to perform species-specific behaviors) • Stress from inability to perform species-specific behaviors and/or (repeated or chronic) exposure to aversive stimuli and/or sudden changes (redirected or displacement behavior; de-arousal) • Anxiety or phobias (e.g., separation anxiety, exposure to aversive stimuli) • Sleep deprivation as a result of irregular or abnormal photoperiods • Hormonal influences, reproduction-related behavior (often, but not always seasonal appearance) • Attention-seeking behavior; reinforced by actions of the owner (learned behavior) • Habituated, ritualized, and/or intrinsically reinforced behavior • Abnormal repetitive behavior resulting from neurotransmitter deficiencies and/or excesses (e.g., serotonin, dopamine, endorphins), similar to obsessive-compulsive or impulsive disorders

automutilation. This may include both primary feather and skin diseases as well as systemic diseases (see Table 5-6).[107,266] In case of systemic disease, feather damage may either be diffuse and generalized or localized directly over the region of discomfort. Renal disease, for example, appears to, at times, induce self-injurious behaviors in the region of the synsacrum.[277,278] Hepatic disease may either induce feather or skin damage that is limited to the ventral portion of the body or follows a more diffuse, generalized pattern.[279,280] Similarly, contact dermatitis (resulting from contact with substances such as nicotine, hand lotion, or other residues on the owner's hands or arms) may be suspected when lesions are restricted to the feet or legs (as in Amazon foot necrosis).[267] Lack of regrowth of feathers may indicate the presence of an endocrine disease (e.g., hypothyroidism) or a viral disease (e.g., psittacine beak and feather disease [PBFD]). A seasonal recurrence of FDB could suggest hormonal influence or the influence of other factors that are limited to a specific season (e.g., climate, humidity).

In addition to substantiated medical conditions, features of the environment are predictive (correlates) of FDB

(see Table 5-6). A small cage or poor cage design, for example, may result in damage to the feathers, particularly the primaries and tail feathers. As a result, the bird may remove the damaged feathers, which should actually be considered normal behavior. Other environmental risk factors that have been implicated in FDB include nutritional deficiencies and dietary imbalances, airborne and topical toxins, and low humidity levels.[107,281] Two recent nested case-control studies tried to identify the nonmedical risk factors associated with FDB in parrots.[269,270] Both, however, used survey results as the basis of their statistical analyses, thereby rendering it impossible to (1) ascertain that the included cases truly involved "primary" FDB (rather than FDB secondary to underlying medical conditions); (2) exclude potential confounding factors (as historical relationships between the onset of FDB and the presence of the identified risk factors were unknown); and (3) obtain further detailed and qualitative information about the parrots' living environment. In addition, group sizes were often too small to allow for statistical analysis of all hypothesized risk factors. It is therefore difficult to draw any real conclusions from these studies. These results, however, do emphasize the importance of conducting further longitudinal and experimental case-control studies to explore whether causal relationships truly exist between the risk factors identified in these studies and the onset of FDB.

Several hypotheses exist concerning the motivational and etiologic backgrounds of nonmedical FDB. Confinement and limited or no access to essential stimuli may, for example, result in the bird's inability to engage in species-typical behaviors, thereby inducing stress, boredom, and frustration. Particularly, the lack of social interaction (with either humans or other birds) or a sexual partner (especially in reproductively active birds), deprivation of locomotor activities, and foraging opportunities are thought to play a role.[105,198,199,270] Of these factors, only the lack of foraging opportunities has clearly been linked to FDB.[105,185] The onset of FDB in the absence of foraging opportunities may, in part, be a result of an altered time budget (i.e., foraging times decrease from approximately 5 to 8 hours in the wild to approximately 1 hour in captivity).[42,98] Alternatively, several studies have demonstrated that parrots are motivated to forage and will contra-freeload, which suggests that foraging may be a "behavioral need."[93,94,191]

Besides the lack of appropriate stimuli, the presence of aversive stimuli and sudden changes in the environment (lack of predictability) may result in anxiety and stress and subsequent self-injurious behaviors.[266,282] Birds may also experience stress from abnormal photoperiods (resulting in either sleep deprivation or prolonged sleep periods), overcrowding, and lack of routine.[261,269] As a result, FDB or automutilation may develop as a means with which the bird attempts to cope with these negative affective states, in which the self-injurious behavior serves as a tension-release mechanism. De-arousal may subsequently result from redirection of the motivation toward the feathers or skin (redirected behavior) or performance of comforting grooming behavior (displacement activity).[87,88] The hypothesis that chronic stress is involved is further supported by the finding that feather-damaging Grey parrots had higher resting fecal corticosterone levels compared with nondamaging individuals.[283]

In the aforementioned situations, FDB may be considered a maladaptive behavior, resulting from the attempts of the animal to cope with an inadequate environment (either because of lack of appropriate stimuli, the presence of aversive stimuli, or a combination of both). In this light, any abrupt change to the environment should be considered a potential stressor and a contributing factor to the onset or maintenance of self-injurious behavior. The results of one survey support this assumption, with up to two thirds of owners reporting a change in the household at the time of onset of FDB.[270] Of particular importance are changes in the family structure or social bonds (i.e., additions or deletions of family members, parrots, or other pets to the household). In addition, changes in the physical environment, housing, daily routine, and climate may play a role.[107,270,282] Owners should be aware that they may themselves also affect the onset and maintenance (or deterioration) of self-injurious behaviors by (unconsciously or unwillingly) reinforcing the behavior.

In case of prolonged deprivation of appropriate stimuli or continued presence of aversive stimuli, the behavior may eventually develop into abnormal repetitive behavior (ARB), which includes both stereotypical behaviors and impulse control disorders. In ARBs, changes in the neurochemistry and

neuroanatomy of the bird may lead to persistence of the behavior, even in the absence of the original stressors or environmental deficits.[284] However, the current living environment is not the only factor that is thought to play a role in this process. The early living environment (including the method used to raise the chick) may also greatly affect the behavioral development of the individual and the occurrence of abnormal behaviors such as FDB.[120,138,143,144,148] It has therefore been suggested that FDB may also represent malfunctional behavior, resulting from abnormal brain development and altered neurochemistry. Although the latter should not be considered a separate entity from maladaptive behavior per se, the ability to distinguish between the two may be important when considering the success of future therapeutic interventions. Maladaptive behaviors may benefit from changes to the environment that help optimize the bird's living conditions. However, malfunctional behaviors may not respond to these measures, and more likely the use of psychopharmaceutic drugs may be required to reduce these behaviors.

Diagnostic workup

As a general rule, it first needs to be established whether the feather damage is (1) inflicted by the bird itself (or its cage mate) or (2) a result of a medical-related or environment-related condition that causes loss or damage to the bird's plumage irrespective of its behavior. It may, however, not always be possible to reliably determine whether the damage is, indeed, self-inflicted. First, birds are often left unobserved throughout a specific portion of the day, which limits the owner's ability to properly observe the bird's behavior. Second, it is often difficult for the owner to distinguish FDB from normal preening behavior.[92]

If one is able to confirm that the feather damage or loss is self-inflicted, the next challenge is to identify whether the condition (1) primarily originates from a medical condition; (2) results from husbandry, management, or nutrition-related issues; (3) should be regarded as a primary behavioral problem (i.e., psychogenic FDB); or (4) is the result of a combination of two or more of the above. For this purpose, thorough history taking and a complete physical examination are deemed essential.

The history should include information regarding (1) the onset, duration, and progression of FDB or automutilation (including any socioenvironmental changes associated with it); (2) the time of day or year when the behavior is most intense; (3) the way the behavior is manifested (including eliciting and terminating stimuli and response of the owner to the behavior); and (4) the type of treatments initiated (including responses to these treatments). In addition, information should be obtained about (1) the housing conditions and living environment; (2) the type, duration, and frequency of social interactions with other birds and human caregivers; (3) nutrition, including provision of foraging enrichment; (4) early life experiences, including rearing method (parent-rearing versus hand-rearing), weaning age, socialization with humans and birds, adverse events experienced during sensitive periods of development, source from where the bird was obtained, and potential previous homes; and (5) general condition of the bird, including presence of other medical or behavioral problems that may potentially be associated with FDB or automutilation.

During the physical examination, a thorough dermatologic examination of the skin and feathers is warranted. This may help confirm the self-inflicted nature of the feather damage and loss evidenced by the absence of feather abnormalities on the head (see Figure 5-37).[261] Location (including symmetry or sidedness; Figure 5-43) and extent of the damage, the type of feathers involved, and the type of damage inflicted by the bird should all be noted. Documenting the physical changes may be valuable to determine whether and which medical conditions may potentially underlie the abnormal behavior. In addition, it may facilitate the monitoring of any changes that occur over time (see section Prognosis and Monitoring). Occasionally, owners may report that the bird constantly preens and chews its feathers without visible damage to the feathers present. This may indicate an inexperienced owner who is unfamiliar with the normal behavior of a parrot, including the time spent on daily grooming.[157] In other instances, owners will incorrectly designate the apterylae (spaces between the feather tracts [pterylae]) as signs of feather damage.[157]

In addition to the history taking and physical examination, diagnostic skin and feather samples may be collected (see Table 5-3). If an underlying systemic cause is suspected based on the history and clinical examination, the diagnostic workup may be further expanded with procedures such as hematologic and biochemical blood panels, urinalysis, diagnostic imaging, and endoscopy, with choices tailored to the differential diagnoses that apply to the individual bird (see section Diagnostic Workup of Behavior Problems; and Table 5-3).[157,285] Although intradermal skin testing for the diagnosis of allergic skin

disease has been described, it has thus far been found unreliable. This may be attributed in part to the birds' diminished intradermal reaction to histamine.[286,287] Definite diagnosis of allergic skin disease may therefore be difficult, although the collection of paired skin biopsies from affected and unaffected areas of the same patient may identify the presence of inflammation consistent with delayed-type hypersensitivity reaction.[288,289] If the above-mentioned tests, when indicated, fail to identify a medical problem, a primary psychological or behavioral origin of the disorder becomes likely. It then becomes important to identify the potential underlying settings or stimuli (antecedents) and reinforcing factors (consequences) that may have contributed to the onset and maintenance of the self-injurious behavior (see section Applied Behavior Analysis).[158] Given the multifactorial nature of the problem and the potential for learned consequential reinforcing value, a concurrent medical and behavioral investigation is often more balanced than a therapy focused on one or the other.

Therapeutic considerations

The therapeutic approach to FDB or automutilation in the individual bird will largely depend on the findings from the history taking, physical examination, initial behavioral assessment, and diagnostic tests. An initial therapeutic plan will often be aimed at correction of the diet and modification of the bird's housing and living conditions to address any environmental factors that may be involved (antecedent arrangement).

If any medical issues are identified or highly suspected to be strong contributors to the problem behavior, these should be appropriately addressed. For example, the use of topical and systemic antibiotics, antifungal medications, and antiparasitic drugs may be indicated to treat any underlying or secondary parasitic or infectious disease. In cases with a tentative diagnosis of hypersensitivity (e.g., based on histologic findings), treatment should preferably be aimed at dietary and environmental modifications that decrease or eliminate exposure to the suspected allergen(s). In addition, the use of antihistamines and corticosteroids may be considered, the latter with extreme caution because of their profound immunosuppressive effects.[257] All medical treatments always need to be assessed for their true need and are preferably implemented together with sound behavioral considerations (i.e., using the most ethical, least intrusive methods possible), as described below.

Promoting a more stimulating environment is an important part—if not the primary focus—of any treatment regimen implemented to reduce FDB.[107] Stimulation may be provided by means of social contact, perches, chewing toys, puzzle feeders, and other forms of environmental enrichment. In particular, foraging enrichment has been shown to effectively reduce FDB.[105,185,191] Providing such enrichment may be as simple as providing complex food items (e.g., corn on the cob, pineapples, or pomegranates), providing food in larger chunks or pellets, using multiple feeding stations, scattering food through the enclosure, and mixing of food with inedible items (see Figure 5-31, *A*).[98,99] Owners may also use paper bags, cardboard boxes, plastic bottles, and other materials to create their own foraging toys. Alternatively, they may buy one or more foraging devices and puzzle feeders to provide food in a more challenging manner (see Figure 5-31, *B*

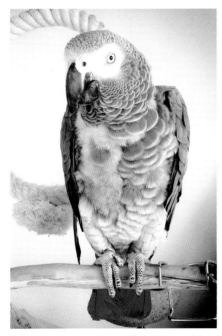

FIGURE 5-43 This Grey parrot *(Psittacus erithacus)* started damaging its feathers after a family member had died. This image clearly demonstrates a unilateral nature of the feather damage of the pectoral pterylae *(only on the right side)*. Distribution of the damaged feathers provides information on the difference between the direct etiologies of feather damaging behavior, which is important to address the condition in a manner tailored to the appropriate underlying cause. (Photo courtesy Ellen Uittenbogaard.)

to *H*). Frequently, owners may need to shape interaction with the toys through positive reinforcement (R+) in order to train the parrot to use the toys independently.

Behavior modification techniques should be employed to replace the behavior of the bird with other, more desirable behaviors (see section Behavior Modification Therapy).[10,198,290] In addition, training may be initiated to provide the bird with a mentally stimulating challenge or task. Both techniques provide excellent opportunities for the bird to gain more control over its environment and enable the bird to make its own choices. As a result, these techniques may be beneficial to reduce FDB, through (1) providing the bird with alternative activities (DRA/DRI); and (2) alleviating stress resulting from a lack of environmental control (which may have initiated FDB in the first place). In order for these techniques to work, however, the owner has to be willing and able to employ the techniques in a proper and consequent manner.

Other treatment options include the use of Elizabethan collars and neck braces (Figure 5-44); fabric "ponchos," "jackets," or "vests" (Figure 5-45); and local application of foul-tasting substances. These interventions, however, only provide a mechanical barrier and are therefore primarily aimed at preventing the symptoms rather than eliminating the underlying cause. Additionally, these methods are considered intrusive and offer only punishment strategies unless paired with counterconditioning measures. As a result, the authors only recommend these as a temporary measure to stop the birds from automutilating themselves and to temporarily stop the cycle of habitual FDB while alternative behaviors are identified, taught, and reinforced. The traditional justification for the use of these methods to "break the habit by response blocking," however, no longer holds validity in the current science of behavioral medicine and behavior change.

In case a collar or vest is deemed essential, it may be helpful to administer a tranquilizer such as midazolam (0.3–0.5 mg/kg, intramuscularly) to help facilitate placement and acceptance. In addition, the devices should ideally be applied in-house, with the patient hospitalized for the purpose

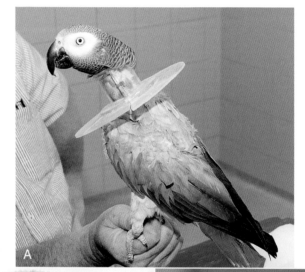

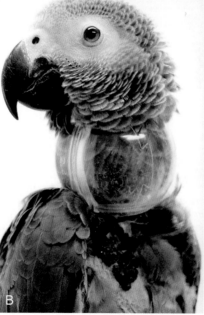

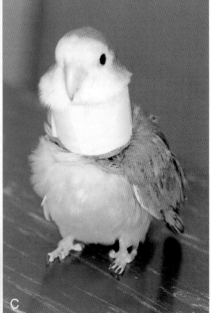

FIGURE 5-44 **A,** Many different types of Elizabethan collars are available for parrots and are preferably only used as a component of treatment if the parrot is automutilating. The collar this Grey parrot *(Psittacus erithacus)* is wearing has an extension that prevents the bird from reaching even the most distal areas of its body. A great disadvantage is that these collars commonly weigh around 20% of the body weight of the birds and prevent normal preening behavior and other important maintenance behaviors of the bird. **B,** In this Grey parrot *(Psittacus erithacus)* a ball-shaped collar is used to prevent the parrot from chewing on the esophageal tube, which was placed because of an extensive crop burn. The great advantage of this "ball" collar is that the curvature of the neck fits within the inner side of the ball. These collars are therefore often better tolerated compared with the one shown in Figure 5-45, *A.* The disadvantage is that the birds can still reach the feet and parts of the wings when wearing these types of collars. Neither of these mechanical blocking devices should be viewed as acceptable substitutes for appropriate pain management of these types of wounds and for promoting alternative chewing behaviors. **C,** Besides the commercially available Elizabethan collars, homemade collars are also frequently used. The collar that this lovebird is wearing was made out of insulation tubing that is used to protect warm-water pipes. These collars are not only very inexpensive, but they are easy to make, lightweight, effective, and well tolerated by the birds. (**A,** Photo courtesy Yvonne van Zeeland. **B** and **C,** Photos courtesy Nico Schoemaker/ Yvonne van Zeeland.)

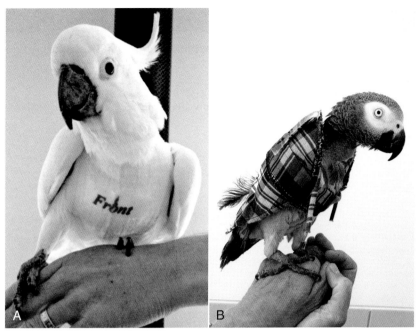

FIGURE 5-45 **A,** Alternatives to the use of Elizabethan collars are "ponchos" or "socks," which owners frequently fabricate themselves. Alternatively, socks can also be purchased online and customized to the size and color of the parrot, as is the case with this sulfur-crested cockatoo. These garments provide a safe, nonrestrictive and comfortable alternative to collars. Moreover, a "sock" helps protect against heat loss that may occur as a result of lack of insulating contour and down feathers. Birds generally tolerate "socks" surprisingly well, as this sulfur-crested cockatoo (*Cacatua sulphurea*) demonstrates. **B,** In case of automutilation of wings, socks will not suffice. However, a jacket, such as the one that was made by the owner of this Grey parrot, may be helpful to protect the wing area from further damage inflicted by the parrot's beak. (**A,** Courtesy Suzanne Freeman (www.thesockbuddy.com). **B,** Photo courtesy Nico Schoemaker/Yvonne van Zeeland.)

of observation and habituation to the device. The benefit of hospitalization is that it enables adjustments to the device or the environment to be made to facilitate its acceptance and comfort, if needed.

Pharmacologic intervention, in particular, is considered helpful in birds that appear refractory to treatment with behavior modification therapy and environmental changes, especially those with severe forms of self-mutilation (e.g., cockatoos). Options include (1) anxiolytic drugs such as diazepam[202]; (2) antipsychotic drugs such as haloperidol[204–206]; (3) TCAs such as clomipramine, amitriptyline, or doxepin (amitriptyline and doxepin tend not to have strong antianxiety or antiobsessional effects in humans, which renders them less preferred as a first-choice drug compared with clomipramine, unless antihistaminergic effects are warranted)[202,207,208]; (4) SSRIs such as paroxetine and fluoxetine[202,209,210]; and (5) opioid antagonists such as naltrexone[202,211] (see Appendix 1, Table 10). In cases of suspected sexual or hormonally related FDB (e.g., seasonal occurrence and presence of [hyper]sexual and nesting behaviors), treatment may be initiated with a targeted behavior-change strategy, or this may be aided with the use of depot GnRH-agonists such as deslorelin or leuprolide acetate. Pharmacologic intervention should never be a stand-alone option, however, but always needs to be followed by a more complete behavior-change strategy.[54]

Prognosis and monitoring

Because of the frequent inability to determine the antecedents and consequences that are associated with FDB and automutilation, the chronicity and ritualization of the behavior, and the overall lack of scientific evidence regarding the efficacy of the various therapeutic interventions, management of the condition often proves to be challenging. To evaluate whether therapeutic interventions elicit any effect, continued monitoring and adequate follow-up of the patient are essential. Although direct behavioral observations are possible,[92] these rarely appear reliable. Photographs, however, are easily taken by caregivers and provide an excellent tool to track the changes in plumage condition, which serves as an indirect measure of the severity of FDB. To assess plumage condition, feather scoring systems may be used. These provide a reliable and practical alternative to direct evaluation, enabling longitudinal monitoring of changes in the plumage condition (and thus the effects of specific interventions) (Box 5-10).[105,291] Plumage condition may either be assessed using photographs or during live visual inspection of the plumage in the clinic (e.g., during a checkup visit). When evaluating the parrot's plumage, intervals of at least 4 weeks (but preferably longer) should be allowed to ensure that sufficient time has elapsed for the feathers to regrow. A temporary setback, however, may occasionally be seen, during which the bird may seriously damage its plumage in a single plucking bout, and this could

BOX 5-10 FEATHER SCORING SYSTEM (VAN ZEELAND et al, 2013)[291]

(A) Score Determination Table for Coverts and Down Feathers; Used for Chest/Neck/Flank, Back, Legs, and Dorsal and Ventral Surface of Wings

COVERTS	No Down Removed	<50% of Down Removed	>50% of Down Removed	All Down Removed
		DOWN FEATHERS		
All Coverts Intact	100	85	70	60
Fraying or Breakage	95	80	65	55
<25% of Coverts Removed	90	75	60	50
25%–50% of Coverts Removed	80	65	50	40
50%–75% of Coverts Removed	70	55	40	30
75%–90% of Coverts Removed	60	45	30	20
>90% of Coverts Removed	50	35	20	10

The percentage of damage to the covert and down feathers is assessed for each body part separately.
Deduct 10 points from the score if skin damage is present.

Total body plumage score (0-100)[aa] = 0.25 × chest/flank + 0.17 × back + 0.10 × legs + 0.28 × dorsal wings + 0.20 × (ventral wings).

[aa]To determine the total body plumage score, the scores for each body part are corrected for their relative body surface percentage, similar to scoring systems used in human burn victims. These percentages (expressed as % of the total body surface area excluding the surface area of the head and unfeathered parts of the legs) were determined in six Grey parrots. Mean (± SD) values for the various body parts were 25 ± 1.2% (chest/neck/flank), 17 ± 1.5% (back), 10 ± 1.2% (legs), 28 ± 2.2% (dorsal wing surface, up to the level of the tertiaries) and 20 ± 1.9% (ventral wing surface, up to the level of the tertiaries).

(B) Score Determination for Flight Feathers; Used for Tail, Primary and Secondary Feathers (Wings)

Score	Description
0	Flight feather with signs of fraying and/or breakage over >50% of the original length
1	Flight feather with signs of fraying and/or breakage over <50% of the original length
2	Flight feather with little or no damage present

Damage to individual flight feathers is assessed.

Total flight feather score (0-100)[bb] = (primary + secondary feathers left wing) + (primary + secondary feathers right wing) + (tail feathers).

[bb]The maximum score is dependent on total number of flight feathers of the bird. In general, each wing has 10 primary feathers and 10 secondary feathers (remiges), whereas the tail has 10-12 flight feathers (rectrices). As each individual flight feather is awarded a score from 0-2, the score will range from 0-40 for each wing and from 0-20 (or 0-24 in the case of 12 tail feathers) for the tail, respectively.

have a significant impact on the plumage condition. In these situations, plumage scoring systems may not provide a reliable measurement. Thus, rather than using plumage scoring conditions as a single measure, veterinarians are advised to also inquire about any changes in the bird's behavior (e.g., engagement with the environment, social activities, change in time budget) to assess its quality of life.

Prognoses may vary considerably and depend on many factors, including the severity, duration, and ritualization of the behavior. On some occasions, repeated or vigorous plucking or biting may have resulted in permanent damage to the feather follicle, thereby preventing normal regrowth of feathers despite a decrease in FDB. The prognosis for many of the self-mutilation syndromes can unfortunately be poor, with treatment often being unrewarding and recurrence commonly reported. Because of the chronicity and severity of the problem, owners may end up electing euthanasia over continued treatment of the problem.

Reproduction-Related Behavior Problems

Many of the commonly observed behavior problems in pet parrots are believed to be related to reproduction and the associated hormonal changes resulting from the activation of the hypothalamic-pituitary gonadal (HPG) axis.[292,293] Such behaviors may include (1) (inappropriate) pair bond formation (i.e., affinity for a single person; see Figures 5-15 and 5-35); (2) territorial or mate-related aggression; (3) courtship regurgitation (to a bonded bird, humans, or items such as a mirror; Figure 5-46); (4) cavity seeking (i.e., seeking small, dark hideaways; Figure 5-47); (5) nest building (including shredding of paper or other bedding; Figure 5-48); and (6) copulatory behaviors (i.e., displaying a receptive posture,

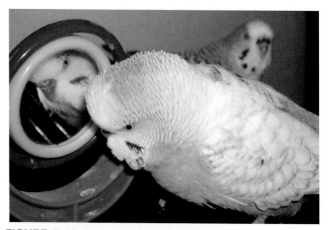

FIGURE 5-46 Mirrors are frequently provided to birds, as for this budgerigar *(Melopsittacus undulatus)*, to give them a surrogate companion. Unfortunately, this may stimulate courtship behavior, and regurgitation is frequently the first and foremost sign to be seen. (Photo courtesy Ellen Uittenbogaard.)

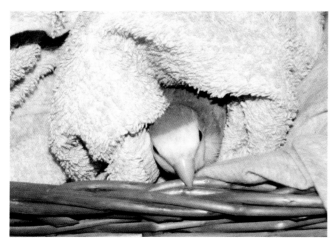

FIGURE 5-47 Many psittacines, such as this peach-faced lovebird *(Agapornis roseicollis)*, love to crawl into small, dark hideaways. Towels may provide an ideal space to hide in. Interpretive caution is required should the bird's behavior suggest that it perceives such types of enrichments as a nesting site. (Photo courtesy Ellen Uittenbogaard.)

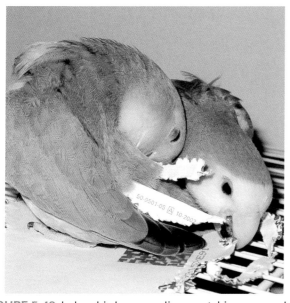

FIGURE 5-48 In lovebirds, a peculiar courtship or reproductive behavior is seen. During the breeding season, peach-faced lovebirds *(Agapornis roseicollis)* tuck long pieces of nest material across their back secured by the feathers of the lower back. This behavior is also displayed in the wild by several species of lovebirds, which use this technique to transport leaf litter, bark, and twigs for elaborate nest construction. (Photo courtesy Ellen Uittenbogaard.)

panting, and actual copulation such as by rubbing the cloaca against a toy).[293] Female birds, especially those of smaller-sized species (e.g., budgerigars, cockatiels, or lovebirds), may also lay large numbers of eggs over extended periods. Egg laying may continue up to a point where the bird's reserves become depleted and it collapses, or the bird develops egg binding or egg-related peritonitis.[294-296] The reproductive

drive can lead to behaviors that are considered problematic by the owner. Such behaviors may include incessant screaming, FDB, sudden aggression toward favored (or nonfavored) humans, and destructive attempts to excavate nests in furniture such as closets or drawers.[153,264,293] In addition, chronic reproductive stimulation has been considered a risk factor for developing cloacal prolapse, especially in (male) umbrella and Moluccan cockatoos (Figure 5-49).[297-299]

In the wild, activation of the HPG axis, resulting in the expression of most of the aforementioned reproductive behaviors, is regulated by a multiplicity of environmental cues such as photoperiod, temperature, rainfall, food availability, and the presence of nesting material or a mate.[292,300-302] Furthermore, reproductive activity may be enhanced by the behavioral interactions within the flock, specifically those that enhance pair bond formation (e.g., regurgitation, allofeeding, allopreening, nest building and inspection, courtship behavior, and copulation).[292] In contrast to birds in the wild, however, pet birds in captivity are not subjected to many of the limiting factors that are normally present in their natural environment. Moreover, they are often provided with several environmental and behavioral cues that may trigger the HPG axis and stimulate reproduction (see Chapter 12). These stimuli include (1) varied, nutrient-rich diets; (2) nesting materials (e.g., newspaper) and an appropriate nesting site; and (3) a perceived mate (the owner) that "feeds" and "preens" them, thereby encouraging the formation of a pair bond (see Figures 5-15 and 5-35).[293] The latter particularly applies to hand-reared birds that are imprinted on humans. The abundance of one or more of the aforementioned environmental

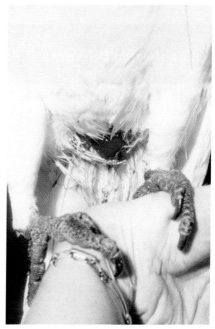

FIGURE 5-49 Sexual behavior, specifically rubbing the cloaca on surfaces and continued straining, may be predisposing factors for the development of a cloacal prolapse, which is commonly seen in cockatoos such as this umbrella cockatoo *(Cacatua alba)*. (Photo courtesy Nico Schoemaker/Yvonne van Zeeland.)

cues and pair bond activities stimulate reproductive activity, including any associated clinical and behavioral problems subsequently.

Diagnostic workup

The display of reproduction-related behaviors, first and foremost, warrants a bird to be sexually mature. The age at which this occurs is highly dependent on the species. Captive-bred parrots, however, may sometimes display sexual behaviors at earlier ages compared with their wild counterparts. For example, wild Eclectus hens generally will not lay eggs until they are about 6 years old but have been reported to start laying eggs at 3 years of age in captivity.[147] Besides age, certain reproduction-related behavior problems may also be linked to a specific gender or species (Table 5-7).

The history of a bird with reproduction-related behavior problems often reveals a concomitant display of normal reproductive behaviors. Often, there is a seasonal occurrence of the behavioral problem linked to the breeding season of the particular species. However, if the bird is exposed to unnatural photoperiods, the behavior may also occur year-round.[293] The history may reveal the presence of environmental stimuli that are known to trigger reproductive behavior. Such triggers can include (1) the provision of calorie-rich food items (e.g., sunflower or safflower seeds, millet seed, nuts, pasta, bread, corn, beans, peas) or fruit (e.g., apples, grapes, citrus, banana); (b) availability of nesting materials and a mate; and (3) exposure to prolonged photoperiods as a result of artificial lighting.[147,293] In addition, owners may—unconsciously—stimulate creation of a strong but inappropriate bond by stroking the bird (particularly on the back), feeding it by hand or mouth, and cuddling it. This may result in the bird favoring a specific person, and this appears more likely to occur in birds that have been hand-reared.

In cockatoos with cloacal prolapse, characteristic—albeit speculated—historical findings include hand-rearing; delayed weaning; bonding to a specific person; and display of behaviors such as continued begging for food, sexual arousal, and tendency to hold feces for a prolonged period (which may have been stimulated further by potty training by the owner).[147] These behaviors may stimulate prolonged and recurrent cloacal straining; subsequent cloacal stretching, dilatation, and prolapse (see Figure 5-49); and distension and flaccidity of the cloacal sphincter.

Whenever reproduction-related behaviors are suspected, a hormone panel may be requested to confirm or rule out increases in the levels of sex steroids. Additionally, a gender determination through polymerase chain reaction (PCR) methods, or endoscopy, during which the gonads can be visualized, may be performed.[157,292] A diagnostic workup may be warranted to exclude or diagnose underlying or secondary medical problems (see Table 5-3).

Therapeutic considerations

Treatment and prevention of reproduction-related disorders generally requires modifications to the bird's living environment as well as changes to the owner–bird relationship (see Chapter 12) (i.e., antecedent rearrangement; see section Behavior Modification Therapy). Environmental changes that may help deter the reproductive drive include the following[292,293,302,303]:

1. Adjustment of the photoperiod to a regular day–night rhythm appropriate for the species involved
2. Adjusting the diet by varying the foods offered, limiting the intake of calorie-rich food items, conversion to a formulated diet supplemented with vegetables, limiting food and caloric intake by providing food in meals, and encouraging foraging-related activities
3. Control shredding and nest building by removing materials that can serve as substrate for these activities (e.g., paper, cardboard) and replacing these behaviors with alternatives appropriate for the species and individual
4. Curtailing cavity seeking behaviors by removing the nest block; prohibiting the bird from wandering around; limiting access to areas that are favored for nesting activities, such as a closet, a drawer, or a blanket or the owner's clothes; and replacing cavity seeking behaviors with nonreproductively stimulating alternative activities
5. Curtailing courtship and other pair-bonding activities by removing the mate or object of affection (e.g., mirror) and replacing these behaviors with nonreproductively stimulating alternative activities
6. Provide opportunities for physical exercise (e.g., flight) and specifically working to reinforce and add to these behaviors

The vast majority of these standard environmental modifications can result in levels of deprivation that are too severe and that cascade into other problems. Although effective, in part at least, they are often stress evoking and less ethical unless balanced with a replacement strategy of alternative stimulation and behavior that results in a similar function for the parrot. Without this concurrent teaching and reinforcement of alternative behaviors, deprivational

---

TABLE 5-7

Reproduction-Related Behaviors or Behavior Problems of *Psittacine* Species

Behavior Problem	Species Predisposition
Cloacal prolapse	Cockatoos, in particular umbrella and Moluccan cockatoos[147]
Excessive egg laying	Parakeets and smaller parrot species, including budgerigars, lovebirds, and cockatiels[294-296]
Inappropriate pair-bond formation	All species, particularly hand-raised individuals[143,144,147]
Nest building, cavity seeking, including shredding/destruction of furniture	All species
Regurgitation of food toward people or objects	All species
Reproductive-related feather-damaging behavior and/or automutilation	Cockatoos, macaws, conures, Grey-cheeked parakeets[264]
Territorial- or mate-related aggression	Amazon parrots, cockatoos, (miniature) macaws, Grey parrots, conures, Quaker parakeets, lovebirds[153]

(i.e., withholding a functional behavior) or punishment (i.e., reducing a functional behavior without offering an alternative) strategies are considered neither ethical nor effective in the long term.

Besides modifications to the environment, owners should try to prevent their parrots from becoming excessively bonded to a specific person. This can be accomplished by ensuring that the parrot receives reinforcement for non–reproduction-associated behaviors from others beside the perceived mate. Although this can facilitate more normal flock behaviors, often these also can be taught when alternative human interaction is not readily available outside of a one-person relationship. Physical contact needs to be kept to a minimum, while reinforced appropriate social interactive and food acquisition behaviors are emphasized. Stroking of the back and tail, in particular, should be avoided because this may stimulate sexual behaviors, particularly when performed repetitively and often. Similarly, hand feeding the parrot warm foods and cuddling the parrot close to the body should be avoided. Instead, owners should replace these displays of affection with providing interaction through training and exercise, which may also be helpful to teach the parrot valuable new skills and cues.

Other therapeutic modalities that may be effective in treating hormonal or reproduction-related disorders include hormone therapy using GnRH agonists (e.g., leuprolide acetate, deslorelin). These medications may temporarily alleviate hormone-related behavior problems or medical problems such as egg laying (see Chapter 12).[212-214,304] In some cases, surgical intervention (e.g., salpingohysterectomy, orchiectomy, cloacoplasty, or cloacopexy) may be considered, particularly if medical issues arise (e.g., in birds with cloacal prolapse, egg binding or egg yolk peritonitis) (see Chapters 7, 12, and 21).[305,306] However, if the environment retains the triggers for reproductive stimulation, the problems are likely to recur despite medical or surgical management. Thus, environmental triggers must effectively be dealt with before long-term effects can be achieved.

Anxiety-Related Disorders: Fears and Phobias

Anxiety disorders are characterized by "feelings of anxiety and fear."[307] In human psychology, various forms of anxiety disorders have been identified, including generalized anxiety disorder, phobias, social anxiety disorder, and panic disorder.[307] As in humans, fears and phobias may be observed also in animals. Parrots, in particular, are often reported as species that have a tendency to be neophobic and experience fear when confronted by new and potentially threatening stimuli (e.g., new toys, strangers, other animals such as a cat or dog).[147,180] Research has shown, however, that novelty-related anxiety is largely a result of a stimulus-deprived rearing environment (in specific limited exposure to new objects), although differences may be observed among individuals and items (i.e., dependent, in part, on the object's properties).[117]

Fear, in general, manifests itself through a fight-flight-or-freeze response, with parrots instinctively responding to a perceived threat by flying away. If escape is impossible (e.g., because the bird's wings are trimmed or the bird is trapped in its cage), the bird may respond by biting in an attempt to defend itself (see section Aggression and Biting). If any of

these behaviors is effective in avoiding the threatening stimulus, the behavior is likely to occur again upon the next confrontation with the threatening stimulus (i.e., the law of effect). Moreover, fear may become generalized as a result of higher-order learning. As a result, the bird may begin to display anxiety-related behaviors when confronted by other nonthreatening situations, objects, or humans that were present at the time of the precipitating event. Furthermore, the birds may overreact to noise, movement, or even eye contact with humans. In these situations, where a nonthreatening stimulus is perceived as threatening by the bird, the definition of the term *phobia* (i.e., an unfounded or unreasonable dread or fear[307]) would likely apply.[147,154]

In the case of phobia, the irrational fear may relate to a specific person, animal, object, or situation (specific phobia) or apply to a broader range of people, animals, objects, or situations (generalized phobia or generalized anxiety disorder). Typically, a parrot with generalized phobia or fear is a young (juvenile or adolescent), high-strung bird that—through the process of higher-order learning and generalization of fear (see section Classical Conditioning)—will seemingly suddenly overreact to humans or objects as if they were deadly predators. The bird may respond by flailing around in the cage, screaming, and trying to escape upon being approached. During its frantic efforts to escape, the bird would often break its feathers and sustain considerable soft tissue injuries to the keel, wing tips, or tail.[180,308] Some species appear more prone to developing fears or phobias, including smaller-sized cockatoos (e.g., rose-breasted *[Eolophus roseicapillus]*, citron-crested *[Cacatua sulphurea citrinocristata]*, and triton *[C. s. triton]* cockatoos), *Poicephalus* parrots (e.g., Meyers *[P. meyeri]* and Senegal *[P. senegalus]* parrots), Grey parrots, and Eclectus parrots.[147,154] Besides these species tendencies, developmental problems are suspected to be the very basis of phobic behaviors. These may be the result of poor socialization (e.g., limited handling or solitary housing) or a suboptimal living environment (e.g., insufficient enrichment and stimulation or overexposure to light) at an early age.[c] Particular events—especially those including physical or psychological trauma such as poor wing trimming, aggressive capture and restraint techniques, abuse, or other forms of punishment—may further act as stressors and triggering or exacerbating the fear.[147,180]

Conditioning the fear response

It is not uncommon for a fearful parrot to learn about new stimuli for reflexive fear responses through the process of respondent learning, in which neutral stimuli may become aversive by (repeated) pairing with unpleasant stimuli.[154,182] For example, the approaching hand of the owner may become associated with restraint or the forced administration of foul-tasting medication. Often, however, a single trial is sufficient to condition a strong fight-flight-or-freeze response. This single-trial learning particularly occurs in cases of extremely frightening situations, some of which may include visits to the veterinary clinic.[154] Undoing this conditioning is, however, much more difficult, and it often takes repeated, systematic, favorable experiences to overcome the conditioned fear response

---

[c]References 17,113,114,117,138,148.

(i.e., respondent extinction). It is therefore important that veterinarians approach a bird—especially a fearful individual—cautiously and handle it with the utmost care. Impressively, many companion parrots with learned fear can become less fearful when only annual examinations and carefully balanced low-stress handling methods are employed. Careful observations and notes as to what behaviors were seen and what stimuli they were associated with can offer great value in handling future visits and in conducting discussions with owners. Moreover, owners may also exacerbate the animal's fear by overreacting and hysterically rushing over to the parrot to reassure it, thereby terrorizing a frightened bird even more. Thus, veterinarians should help their clients realize that they may actually worsen the situation by displaying signs of distress or even when trying to reassure the bird (e.g., by petting it or telling the bird "it's okay").

Besides respondent learning, fear responses may also become conditioned through avoidance learning or negative reinforcement (see section Tools and Techniques for Behavior Change). In this context, removal of the threatening stimulus (e.g., by moving the bird away from the fear-evoking stimulus or providing it shelter) acts as a reinforcer for the operant learned fear response.[182] The operant learned fear response, in this regard, is distinguished from the respondent fear reaction, which cannot be operantly conditioned.

Fear responses may be further enhanced through learning if the fear-evoking stimulus is of short duration or if escape from the stimulus is possible. In these situations, birds may perceive their fear response to be "successful" as the threat is eliminated (even if the removal is independent of their own actions). Moreover, birds may learn to display a fear response in situations where they are not frightened because this enables them to control the situation to achieve their goal (e.g., to keep people from approaching it).[154]

Diagnostic workup

Similar to other behavior problems, a functional assessment of the behavior may help determine the operant functions of the fear response. Careful observation is also needed to identify stimuli that elicit respondent fear reactions. Video recordings, in particular, may be very helpful because these allow the parrot's behavior and body language to be observed in the bird's own environment rather than in a strange environment and with a stranger present.

Therapeutic considerations

In general, there are three well-established procedures to reduce respondent fear, including (1) systematic desensitization; (2) counter-conditioning; and (3) response blocking (flooding). Flooding is often ill-advised because of the negative side effects associated with this type of therapy (see section Behavior Modification Therapy—Response Blocking or Flooding). The other two techniques are commonly used in conjunction with one another (see section Behavior Modification Therapy—Systematic Desensitization and Counter-Conditioning). Training with the use of operant techniques may further provide an essential adjunct to a desensitization and counter-conditioning protocol. Moreover, operant learning via training empowers the animal to make its own choices and control its living environment, thereby increasing the bird's behavioral success and reducing the fear.

In more extreme or refractory cases, anxiolytic drugs (e.g., BZPs, butyrophenones, TCAs, or a combination thereof) may be given in conjunction with behavior modification therapy. This may help speed up the process and reduce anxiety to a level at which the bird is capable of learning.[147,154] The owner and the attending veterinarian will, however, have to work to find a way to administer the drugs without resistance or further augmentation of stress. Any distress from handling, restraint, or forceful administration of the medication may otherwise evoke or increase the fear response. The use of a food vehicle to administer medications, which would eliminate the need for handling or restraint, may be a helpful consideration for many birds (Figure 5-50).

Rehabilitation of birds with xenophobia (fear of strangers), neophobia (fear of new things), or generalized anxiety disorder can be difficult and generally requires considerable time and patience from the owner, who needs to learn to relax and approach the bird calmly and patiently. Any misinterpretation or mishandling of the bird may worsen the situation and heighten the parrot's anxiety or reinforce the bird's frantic behavior.[309] Building a trustworthy relationship may be achieved by the process of systematic desensitization and counter-conditioning, during which the bird will learn to stop responding to a neutral stimulus (i.e., presence of the owner in proximity to the bird) through gradual exposure.[154] When habituating a bird to a

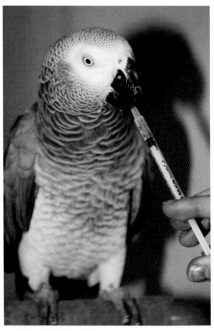

FIGURE 5-50 Medications are commonly prescribed as part of a treatment plan for sick parrots. Unfortunately, many owners are not experienced in administering medications to their birds, which often results in difficulties experienced by the owner when having to administer drugs to their birds. This may not only result in poor therapeutic compliance, but forceful administration of drugs is likely to be detrimental to the owner–bird relationship, resulting in, for example, stress, aggression, and fear in the bird. Operant learning techniques (shaping and positive reinforcement) can help teach the birds to voluntarily take in their medication, as demonstrated by this Grey parrot (*Psittacus erithacus*). (Photo courtesy Nico Schoemaker/Yvonne van Zeeland.)

stimulus, an owner should be seated or standing as close to the bird as possible without evoking a fear response. Additionally, he or she should be sure to not make any direct eye contact (because this may be perceived as threatening by the bird). The owner may, however, talk, sing, or read aloud quietly and occasionally look at the bird. Eye contact should always be brief, with the owner quickly turning away the eyes and head from the bird again to negatively reinforce the calm behavior.[141,154,308] Over time, the owner may gradually move closer to the cage and look at the bird for a longer time, thereby systematically desensitizing the bird to his or her presence close to the bird. In addition, the owner may provide treats to the parrot (if the bird is not too frightened to take these). As a result, the proximity of the owner will likely be associated with a more pleasant response (i.e., counter-conditioning). Other tools that may be helpful to rehabilitate a parrot with phobias include (1) dimming of the lights (many birds with phobias appear more comfortable in low-light conditions); (2) turning on soft music (which is often more soothing than total silence); and (3) empowering the bird by having it make its own choices on when and how to interact with others (which is equally critical to behavioral health as food and water are to physical health). Desensitization procedures should always be employed without force or pressure, allowing the bird to progress at its own speed.[154] In some cases, the use of anxiolytic drugs may prove helpful or even necessary, provided that stress-free administration is possible. These should, however, primarily be used following correct diagnosis and the absence of any ill-effects from behavior intervention techniques such as those described above. As a result, veterinarians are encouraged to consult or refer, prior to routinely prescribing these drugs, particularly as a first-choice level of intervention.

Preventive measures

As with any behavior problem, prevention of problems is the best strategy. Prevention of development of fears and phobias begins in the neophyte and continues throughout the socialization phase. Both breeder and owner play an essential role in the socialization process, as their actions help build a steady and trustworthy relationship with the bird and ensure the development of a confident and independent bird. The role of the veterinarian in facilitating and ensuring these key processes during new bird examinations is essential for developing and consolidating functional immunization from many behavior problems. Specific socialization processes that have value include the following:

- Nurturing the bird's self-confidence and individual potential during early development (see section Psittacine Behavioral Development)
- Allowing the bird to fledge normally and develop flight skills, followed by gradual clipping of the wings (if necessary) to enhance the bird's self-confidence[310]
- More balanced feeding and weaning schedules, which are based on the bird's development rather than the caregiver's convenience
- Establishing clear and consistent behavioral guidelines in the new home
- Teaching or facilitating the learning of normal self-maintenance behaviors, including feather care, foraging, and social interactions, preferably through contact with other birds

- Encouraging self-sufficiency in the bird through independent play
- Training through positive reinforcement rather than negative reinforcement or punishment strategies
- Empowering the bird by allowing it to make choices and control its environment[147]

Aggression and Biting

In animals, "aggression" often refers to behaviors that are displayed to protect a valuable resource or serve as a measure to protect the individual (self-defense) or group (e.g., to maintain integrity within the group or repel possible intruders).[157] In parrots, aggression often takes the form of biting or lunging at a person or another bird, with their strong jaws and hooked bill capable of inflicting serious pain and injuries (Figure 5-51). In general, parrots are not naturally frequent users of aggressive behavior to meet their goals. As observed in wild parrots, the beak is mainly used for eating, preening, and social interaction and not for attacking other flock members. Instead, parrots use complex body language, feather position, and vocalization to express themselves in conflict situations and fly away rather than engage in an actual combat.[147,311,312] Parrots should thus be considered animals that will use biting only as a last resort for removing aversive stimuli, protecting themselves, and guarding their resources. Because of their high intelligence and great learning capabilities, however, parrots may quickly learn that these displays of aggression are highly effective in accomplishing their goals (especially when their wings are trimmed and they have no option to escape by flying away). As a result, the frequency and intensity with which a parrot bites may quickly increase, thus becoming increasingly problematic for the owner. This

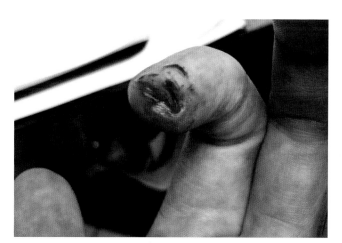

FIGURE 5-51 Any bird will try to defend itself when confronted by a threatening stimulus. Parrots will generally choose to escape or avoid danger, if possible, and only resort to biting if there is no means of escape. In the veterinary clinic, the risk of staff being bitten may be higher because the bird is in an unfamiliar area and is often confronted by aversive stimuli from which it cannot escape. As a result, it may more easily feel threatened and bite, compared with its normal behavior in the comfort of its own home surroundings. Low-stress handling techniques help with better handling and restraint experiences and can greatly reduce risk of harm to the staff, the owners, and the birds themselves. (Photo courtesy Brenna Fitzgerald.)

cycle of increased biting may continue to a point where the owner considers the problem to be severe enough to present the bird for evaluation to a veterinarian or a behavior consultant. Occasionally, biting may take on such a severe form that the owner will consider re-homing the bird or relinquishment to a shelter. Thus, timely and appropriate intervention is necessary to successfully deal with this problem and achieve a favorable outcome for both the owner and the bird.

Classification of aggression

Although aggression may have overlapping and interacting etiologies, categorization of the problem may be helpful when seeking to determine the settings and consequences that cause and reinforce the behavior and when developing a treatment plan. As in other animals, aggression in parrots can be subdivided into a number of categories based on etiology. According to Welle,[153] the following broad categories may be distinguished:

- *Fear-related aggression*, characterized by displays of aggression in combination with signs that indicate fear (e.g., withdrawal or passive and avoidance behaviors). With parrots being a prey species, fear is often an important motivator for biting that the parrot resorts to in order to defend itself. Usually, a bird with fear-related aggression only bites when it is being cornered or caught. Immediately following the bite, it will try to retreat rather than attack and chase the victim. Birds with fear-related aggression may produce fear-related vocalizations, including growling and screaming prior to, during, or following the biting. They may also be reluctant to leave the cage and may start to cower, pant, or thrash about when the cage is approached.[153] Fear-related aggression appears more common in wild-caught birds, particularly Grey parrots, but there are no age or sex predilections.[153] Other proposed predisposing factors include inadequate or poor socialization, lack of enrichment and stimulating environments at an early age, excessive wing trimming (resulting in frequent falls and diminished self-confidence) and abuse.[138,153,154]
- *Territorial aggression*, characterized by displays of aggression related to a specific location (e.g., the nest box, feeding station, cage, play gym, or other living area). Territorial aggression is common in breeding birds and serves a function to protect the nest. In captivity, it often only occurs in a defined area, with the aggression intensifying upon a person approaching the perceived territory. Territorial aggression appears particularly common in male individuals of certain parrot species, including Quaker parakeets, conures, miniature macaws, Grey parrots, and Amazon parrots.[153] In addition, one of the authors has frequently come across territorial aggression in female lovebirds. Territorial instincts may particularly be increased if the parrot is confined to a standard, small-sized living environment (cage). Occasionally, birds may also display territorial aggression when provided ample space to roam around freely because they have come to consider the space as their territory.
- *Mate-related aggression*, characterized by displays of aggressive behavior in the proximity of a favorite person or mate that is being approached by a third party (e.g., family member, other bird). Mate-related aggression commonly occurs in hand-raised individuals of parrot species such as Amazon parrots, macaws, cockatoos, and Quaker parakeets.[153] Male birds seem to be more commonly affected, with the aggressive behavior generally starting when the birds become sexually mature and worsening during the breeding season.[153] Aggression is often directed toward the rival. However, if this person or bird is out of reach, the aggression may also be directed toward the mate or the favorite person (i.e., redirected aggression). Unlike other types of aggression, birds with mate-related aggression will often chase or actively attack their victims, without an actual threat being present or easily recognized by the observers.[313] At other times, the bird may show affectionate displays, particularly toward the favorite person.
- *Redirected aggression*, which occurs when the object that the bird intends to bite is out of reach, thereby resulting in the bird biting someone or something that is close by. Rather than being a diagnosis on its own, redirected aggression serves as a mechanism to modify other types of aggression, most often mate-related aggression (as the bonded person is often close by). To treat the problem, the type of aggression underlying the redirected aggression needs to be identified and properly addressed.
- *Conditioned aggression*, which describes aggression that is conditioned through the desired consequences that the bird achieves by displaying this behavior (i.e., positive or negative reinforcement). For example, a bird can easily learn to lunge or bite a person in order to achieve the consequence that the person backs away from the bird, cage, or mate (negative reinforcement). In addition, the bird may bite out of frustration if the owner does not meet the parrot's expectations, with the owner inadvertently reinforcing the behavior if it then acts according to the parrot's expectations. Although this type of behavior may occur in any species and at any age, it has been suggested that it occurs more commonly in adult male birds of larger species such as Amazon parrots and macaws.[153] It appears more common in birds owned by people who have little experience with birds, most likely because these owners are more likely to be intimidated by the bird's size. Often, the bird tends to bite specific family members, especially those who are less confident and assertive around the bird. Biting also often occurs when these persons try to do something that the bird does not want them to do (e.g., get the bird off the shoulder, put it in the cage, stop petting).[153] Conditioned aggression is not uncommonly encountered in veterinary practice. In this context, the behavior often develops secondary to serial veterinary examinations, especially when forceful handling and restraints are the norm and fear-related aggressive behaviors have been effective for the bird in the past.

In addition to the aforementioned classes of aggression, aggression may occasionally also result from pain (resulting from trauma or medical conditions) and stress, which—together with fear-related aggression—can be classified as defensive forms of aggression.[314]

Diagnostic workup

Similar to most other behavior problems, the diagnosis of aggression in pet birds is based upon the behavioral history and direct observation of the bird's behavior, including an evaluation of the conditions that set the behavior in play and give it function, and the bird's responses under these conditions.

Aggressive behavior (e.g., biting and lunging) serves a function for the bird, or it would not persist in doing it. For example, biting effectively removes an imposing hand or offers an opportunity for the bird to escape being caged. As a result, a functional assessment of the behavior is important. In light of this, a detailed description of the aggression, the circumstances in which it occurs, and the owners' response to the behavior are considered critical.[153,313] To correctly identify potential antecedent stimuli and the consequences of the behavior, a comprehensive description of the bird's environment and social interactions may be useful. Seasonality of the problem may indicate aggression related to breeding activity and the presence of increased levels of sex hormones. These are motivating operations that increase the aversive quality of hands near cages. Similar to other reproduction-related behaviors, the diagnostic workup may subsequently include a hormone panel, gender determination, and endoscopy, during which the gonads can be visualized.[157,292] Alternatively, the history and physical examination may hint at the presence of an underlying medical condition that is causing pain, which may subsequently be diagnosed with the aid of several diagnostic tests (see Table 5-3). On rare occasions, aggression may warrant a neurologic examination because altered brain function may also result in behavioral changes, including aggression. In these patients, additional diagnostic testing, including computed tomography (CT) imaging, magnetic resonance imaging (MRI), or both, may be indicated (see Chapter 14).[157]

Besides a physical examination and history, direct behavioral observations can often help establish what type of aggression is present and under what circumstances it is manifested. These behavioral observations may also include an evaluation of the parrot's responses in different situations (e.g., approach of the cage, approach of a third party when the bird is with the owner). Preferably, behavioral observations are made in the home environment, since birds may behave differently in an unfamiliar setting such as the veterinary clinic. Many of these behaviors can be observed in the veterinary consultation room, if the environment is properly controlled. If these two options are not possible, video recordings of the bird's behavior at home may offer a suitable alternative to assess the behavior. Owners should, however, never attempt to stage a situation that provokes aggression because this may result in severe injuries to the owner and will likely reinforce the aggressive behavior.

Therapeutic considerations
Generally, parrots only resort to biting when other forms of communication do not result in the desired effect. Such signals may include the raising of a foot to fend off a hand, pushing a hand away with the beak, or backing away from the person or the hand. If a person ignores these signals, a bite may follow. Thus, biting can often be avoided by careful observation and interpretation of the parrot's body language, whereby people can learn to anticipate the various signals and avoid the bite with relative ease.[147] In addition, biting may often be prevented by (1) giving the parrot something on which to place its beak while stepping up onto the hand; (2) approaching the parrot with the hand from behind (and not approaching from the front); (3) wearing a protective glove; or (4) having the parrot step onto the perch, avoiding the hand

or arm altogether. By far, the most common explanation for biting is imposing hands that have in the past forced parrots to do something that is not reinforcing to them. Caregivers can be taught how to elicit the behaviors they need from their birds instead of relying on force and coercion.

Owners should always be made aware that parrots normally use their beaks as hands. If a person pulls away the hand when the parrot tries to reach for it, the bird may thus be inclined to grab the hand more quickly and forcefully, just to keep its balance or enable it to step up. Alternatively, biting behaviors may be reinforced by the owner's verbal response. In these aforementioned situations, biting may often be diminished quickly by simply holding the hand or arm steady in one position and reinforcing the parrot for good behavior (i.e., stepping up without biting).[154]

Treatment may vary, depending on the type of aggression involved. In case of fear-related aggression, gradual desensitization and counter-conditioning are the appropriate measures to reduce the fear response (see section Behavior Modification Therapy—Systematic Desensitization and Counter-Conditioning). Although these techniques may require a lot of time and patience from the owner to take effect, they may provide quick results when combined with a high-rate of positive reinforcement. In extreme cases, anxiolytic drugs (e.g., BZPs, butyrophenone) may be used to facilitate the behavior modification therapy. Punishment of fear-related aggression should be avoided at all times, as this may exacerbate the fear response.[153]

Behavior modification therapy for territorial aggression may consist of a combination of measures including (1) operant learning (e.g., teaching the step-up or other limited-contact behaviors such as target training); (2) the use of protected contact training, whereby the bird is conditioned while it remains inside its cage; (3) teaching an owner to safely but securely towel restrain a bird in case of emergency; (4) use of cages with wide opening doors and portable perches (to facilitate taking the bird out of the cage); and (5) measures aimed at making the bird less dependent on its cage.[153] Lowering cage dependency is commonly accomplished by providing the bird with a two-cage housing system consisting of a large, well-furnished cage or playpen for daytime activities and a smaller sleeping cage for the night. To transport the bird between the different enclosures, owners can let the bird step out of its cage to then have it step onto their arm or a perch for transportation to the other location.[153] Alternatively, owners may feed the parrot away from the cage or alter the configuration of surroundings to make the area outside the territory more attractive and decrease the territorial response.[153] Positive reinforcement of the parrot's voluntary departure of its territory will also be helpful. In some situations, using protected contact while working to desensitize and counter-condition the bird in its cage may be another viable option. Generally, these measures are sufficient to successfully reduce territorial aggression, without having to revert to the use of psychoactive drugs. Similarly, mate-related aggression rarely warrants use of psychoactive drugs as adjunctive therapy. However, hormones (e.g., leuprolide acetate, deslorelin) or surgery (e.g., orchiectomy) may sometimes be used to reduce the aggression associated with the sex hormones, thereby facilitating implementation of the remainder of the behavior-change plan.[214,293] Care should be taken to not pathologize normal behavior or endocrine cyclicity; however, behavior modification still should be considered the first and foremost method of choice for most circumstances. The main focus of this behavior modification should aim at having the bird establish a normal bond with the owner and proper socialization with other family members. The person with whom the bird has bonded should aim to develop a more platonic bond and avoid cuddling, petting, and shouldering (which may particularly be dangerous in case of a bite).[153] Alternatively, the other household members should engage in favorable social interactions with the bird (e.g., providing the bird with its favorite treats as a reinforcement for desired behaviors).[153] Safe, effective, and minimally intrusive use of towel restraint is also a prerequisite to appropriate handling of birds with mate-related aggression. If the owner is able to predict the aggression of the bird, it may be possible for the favored person to leave the room swiftly before the biting occurs, thereby removing the inciting cause for the aggression.[153] Although wing trimming may be considered a means to facilitate training and control the bird's actions, the use of these procedures should be limited and always ethically balanced in the larger view of the specific circumstances (see Chapter 22). Under no conditions should the owner hit, grab, or thump the parrot because this may escalate the aggression and result in the development of fear. Similarly, yelling or drama should be avoided because this may actually function to positively reinforce the behavior, thereby increasing rather than decreasing its occurrence. However, if the owner is consistent and confident in his or her interactions with the bird, the prognosis for successfully reducing aggressive behavior is generally considered fair. Long-term, established problems may have a more guarded prognosis with regard to the relationship between the owner and the bird. Occasionally, the bond may have been damaged to such an extent that re-homing the bird to a different owner is considered the single best option for both parties.[153]

In case of intraspecies aggression, individual housing and supervision of the birds when they are not confined often helps avoid the problem. Birds may learn to be more tolerant of one another if their cages are gradually placed closer together, in small enough increments as to keep the birds calm. Care should, however, be taken to prevent foot injuries (e.g., when one bird is loose and climbs onto the cage of the confined bird that subsequently bites in the foot of the other bird). Owners may also alleviate aggression by providing more space and extra resources, including additional perching space, multiple food and water bowls, and extra toys. In cockatoos, in which mate trauma is particularly common, wing trimming and the use of visual barriers or special nest boxes that have two entrance and baffled interiors may help prevent the male from attacking the female.[315] Alternatively, pairs may be separated temporarily (i.e., for several weeks up to several months or years, dependent on the severity of the attack) or permanently to break the cycle of aggression.[315] In some situations, training the birds (e.g., by having the birds fly around alone until tired, separating cages, making resources at each cage identical, teaching station behaviors and reinforcing these at high rates) has also been found successful to reduce aggression toward other parrots.[316]

Screaming or Excessive Vocalizations

The ability to imitate human words is one of the traits that render parrots, particularly Grey parrots, as popular and highly desired pets. However, when talking becomes screaming (i.e., high decibel, long-duration vocalizations), it is also one of the behaviors resulting in relinquishment of a parrot because the birds' loud and frequent vocalizations may quickly become problematic for the owners and their neighbors. Particularly the larger parrot species such as macaws and cockatoos can produce bursts of ear-piercing screams that last for several minutes. Although this can be extremely upsetting and annoying, people should remember that vocalizations are part of the normal behavior pattern of most parrots. In addition, these behaviors—although problematic for owners or their neighbors—are functional, that is, they serve a purpose for the animal.

The amount of "noise" produced varies greatly between species. Nevertheless, all parrots tend to vocalize loudly several times a day for periods of 5 to 15 minutes, especially at dawn and sunset.[42,43] In addition, many parrots learn to vocalize their "greeting" of the owner returning home from work or to "call" for the owner if he or she is out of sight. These vocalizations should be considered as contact calls, which are part of the normal behavior of a parrot and help them locate other flock members and promote flock cohesion.[31,39,40] Vocalizations may also serve as an alarm call produced in response to a threatening or aversive stimulus.[41] Thus, many vocalizations should be considered normal parrot behavior. However, screaming incessantly for hours on end is not normal and warrants investigation.

Occasionally, problems may arise from vocalizations that the bird has learned to imitate.[32] These may include words, phrases, and sounds (e.g., coughing, telephone sounds, microwave beeps, or a doorbell) that were accidentally or intentionally learned by the bird. These sounds may, for example, irritate or embarrass the owner (e.g., if the bird swears in front of others) or make the owner worry needlessly about the bird being sick (e.g., mimicked cough or sneeze) and turn to the veterinarian for help.[32] In these situations, the response of the family members often is the root cause of the bird repeating the words or sounds. For example, the words may have been uttered with a lot of emotion or at a high volume, thus being accentuated. Similarly, people's response to the bird's vocalization (e.g., laughter, yelling, or responding to the sound by walking to the door or looking for the telephone) can act as a reinforcer, thereby stimulating the bird to repeat the sound more often.[32]

Diagnostic workup

Similar to other behavior problems, a functional assessment of the behavior is necessary when dealing with parrots that vocalize excessively. This may help to establish what function the excessive vocalization serves for the bird—that is, what does the bird achieve by producing these sounds? For example, birds may vocalize when separated from the owner (when he or she has left the house or is out of sight). Initially, these sounds may consist of soft and calm contact calls, but soon they may progress to louder, more frequent calls, especially if no response is obtained. Alternatively, loud distress calls may be produced in combination with escape or avoidance behaviors if the bird is confronted by a threatening stimulus. In light of the functional assessment of the behavior, the circumstances under which the behavior occurs (e.g., time of day, week, or year; relationship to, for example, feeding time or activities in the house) should be noted. Particular attention should be paid to the stimuli immediately preceding the behavior, and the parrot's behavior and body language because these are an important part of a functional assessment that is needed to diagnose and treat behavior problems (see section Applied Behavior Analysis).[11,32,147] Moreover, it is important to evaluate how the owner responds to the screams (e.g., does the owner yell back, walk toward the cage, take the bird out of its cage, or give it a treat?) Such responses may unintentionally reward and thus reinforce the behavior, thereby often resulting in an escalation of the situation.

A thorough history will oftentimes reveal whether the vocalizations produced serve as contact calls (e.g., to get attention or in animals with separation anxiety) or as alarm calls (e.g., when confronted by large, new objects or new people in the house perceived as threatening). Occasionally, it may not be possible to clearly pinpoint the precipitating stimuli or the clear consequential value of the problem vocalizations. Often, further analysis of these situations will reveal a consequence that has positive reinforcing value to the bird—that is, the parrot has learned that it gets attention when it produces these sounds. Many times the attention received by the bird is intended to be negative and to stop the screaming (e.g., yelling or returning to the room where the bird is to "punish" it). However, if the problem continues or intensifies, the attempts clearly are not effective punishers and, in fact, may be functioning as a reinforcer of the behavior. An absence of alternatives, however, can be regarded equally important to the presence of reinforcers. Thus, in addition to identifying potential reinforcers for the problem behavior, it is also important to identify whether sufficient stimuli (alternatives) are known and available to the bird. These stimuli can function to provide the bird with distraction and enable it to perform alternative behaviors rather than scream for the caregiver's attention because of unavailability of other options.

Therapeutic considerations

The first step in treating excessive vocalization is proper education of the owners or caregivers of the birds, who should be aware that all parrots, even those bred in captivity, are essentially wild animals. As a result, many of their behaviors, particularly those that fall within the normal spectrum of the species, may be modified but cannot be fully eliminated. For example, owners should realize that birds normally vocalize in the morning and evening. Thus, chances to eradicate this behavior are limited but there is ample opportunity for owners to shape the behavior into a more acceptable form. For example, owners may provide the bird with opportunities to perform other activities such as providing the bird with a treat or new toy, or initiating a training session during which the bird is taught new sounds or words.[32] The toy or treat should, however, always be provided prior to the screaming episode to prevent the bird from learning that it earns this reward by screaming.[32]

As with many learned behaviors, learned vocalizations can be reduced through the process of extinction by ignoring them, provided that the attention received by the bird is the

maintaining reinforcer. Although ignoring unwanted vocalization is commonly considered, it is neither easy nor successful unless paired with other activities to replace the problem behavior. Extinction is often challenging and generally requires lots of patience, since extinction bursts may follow, with the slightest encouragement from the owner—even if unintentional—resulting in a relapse or worsening of the problem.[11,32] All family members should be aware that any response from them is also likely to reinforce the behavior. Consistency in their response is considered an essential part of a successful behavior modification plan, which may especially be difficult in a multiperson household. Because of the aforementioned reasons, it is often too difficult to reduce problem vocalizations with extinction alone. As a result, mild punishment strategies may sometimes be required. Such punishment strategies include the use of a "time-out" from social contact; that is, temporary withdrawal of attention from the parrot by turning away or leaving the room (see section Tools and Techniques for Behavior Change). Time-out from social contact, however, is only effective in the presence of alternative behaviors to screaming. Upon cessation of the screaming and the offering of an acceptable alternative vocal behavior (e.g., whistling a contact call), family members may re-enter the room or turn back and gently reward the bird with praise, a treat, or a toy. If the family members are not in the room when the bird starts screaming, they are encouraged to wait and do nothing until the parrot is quiet for a brief time or makes an acceptable type of vocalization. Only then may the family members re-enter the room and reward the bird to avoid reinforcing the loud screaming.[147]

If the screaming is suspected to function as a contact call, moving the cage to a location that promotes increased contact with the family members may help reduce the level and frequency of vocalizations. Alternatively, a hiding place or placement in a more sedentary location may be beneficial for parrots that produce distress calls. Having the owner maintain auditory contact (e.g., by whistling or talking) with the bird when he or she is elsewhere in the house and out of sight is another way to address and avoid "escalating" contact calls.

In birds with suspected separation anxiety (characterized by the observable onset of excessive vocalizations or destructive behaviors [including FDB] when being left alone), treatment should be aimed at reducing the bird's dependence on the owner. This may be accomplished by limiting and structuring the owner–bird interactions; providing the bird with alternatives to interaction with the owner (e.g., toys, puzzle feeders, nuts or whole fruits); and auditory or visual stimulation from a radio or television. In addition, the bird may be desensitized to the owner's departure and being left alone by a series of short departures that are brief enough to prevent the bird from becoming anxious or distressed. During such training sessions, the parrot should be provided with treats or toys that help promote alternative behaviors.[32] Similar distractions may be provided in cases where parrots scream when company arrives, preferably prior to the company entering the room and the parrot starting to vocalize.

Systematic desensitization and counter-conditioning are considered useful for treatment of distress calls. Prior to implementing these techniques, the stimulus that is provoking the excessive vocalization (e.g., a toy, cage furniture, person, or animal in the bird's immediate environment or visual field) needs to be identified and removed. Moreover, it is important to determine whether the excessive vocalization is, indeed, the result of a stressful situation. Determining the presence or absence of stress can be challenging, however, since not all birds necessarily vocalize excessively when stressed. In essence, not all excessive vocalizations need be distress calls, and not all necessarily have to indicate the presence or absence of stress. Operationalizing the behavior may, however, help clarify its purpose and its antecedent settings as well as the subsequent design of an intervention strategy.

To increase the chances of a successful outcome, owners should be careful to only reinforce "calm behavior" and not the anxious behaviors (e.g., by trying to reassure the bird when it shows signs of distress).[32,154] Similarly, it is essential to prevent the parrot from being pushed into a situation or interaction it is not comfortable with. Owners must also stay as relaxed and engaged as possible during the training sessions to teach the bird that the situation does not pose a threat. All of these measures may help the parrot become more relaxed and comfortable with the new situation.[32,154]

It is rare for screaming to become a stereotypical behavior (i.e., the screaming has become rigid and routine-like and is maintained by automatic reinforcement, whereby it will also be performed repetitively outside of an appropriate context). The distinction of a true stereotypical behavior is not a simple one, however, and as such, it may be prudent to consult or refer these patients to an (avian) behavior expert, if such problems are suspected. Should this appear to be the case, however, use of psychoactive drugs may be warranted.[32]

PREVENTION OF BEHAVIOR PROBLEMS AND THE VETERINARIAN'S ROLE

Once a behavior problem has arisen, intermittent and often unintentional reinforcement of the behavior may complicate the behavior modification process and hinder the successful extinction of the problem behavior. As a result, prevention is considered preferable over trying to cure an already existing behavior problem. Environmental enrichment, in particular, may provide a parrot with the necessary stimuli needed to perform its natural behaviors in captivity. This not only helps reduce problem behaviors but also improves the bird's well-being.[d] Upon providing enrichment to a bird, (individual) preferences for specific enrichment features (e.g., structure, hardness, color, size) may also be taken into account. So-called choice experiments may help unravel individual, species-related, gender-related, or age-related preferences for such features, thereby providing an empirical basis for the further development and refinement of enrichments. Generally, these experiments comprise preference studies, in which birds are offered a choice between two (sometimes more) options, thereby determining the bird's preference for alternative resources.[80,189,190,317] Unfortunately, choice experiments do not address the actual value and importance of a specific enrichment for the parrot.[318] The latter information can, however, be collected during so-called consumer demand studies. These types of studies allow objective measurement of an animal's motivation to gain access to a specific resource by

means of imposing a certain price to gain access to this resource.[97,319,320] By manipulating the costs to access the resource and observing how the animal changes its use of the resource as a result, the motivational strength for a specific resource can be quantitatively assessed and provides insight in its actual value.[319,321] A recent pilot study in Grey parrots showed the feasibility of a consumer demand setup to determine the parrot's motivation for specific resources.[322] Preliminary results suggest motivation to be highest for enrichments related to the natural behaviors that are most constrained in captivity (i.e., social enrichment, increased space, and foraging opportunity). For these enrichments, parrots paid prices (in energy and effort expenditure) similar to those paid for food,[322] thus indicating that these are highly valued or "desired," if not essential and "needed." However, the number of birds used in this study was small, which prevented drawing definitive conclusions at this stage. Nevertheless, results demonstrate that studies such as these may be particularly helpful to obtain valuable information on ways to optimize and expand the captive parrot's living environment.

The critical role of both the current living environment and the living environment in early life warrants special attention to be paid to proper housing, nutrition, and care to prevent behavior problems. Unfortunately, many owners will only consult a veterinarian after a (behavioral or medical) problem has arisen and already is well established. Veterinarians are therefore encouraged to liaise with breeders and pet stores to encourage owners to obtain a postpurchase examination during which basic husbandry advice may be provided.

Behavior classes provide an alternative support to (1) help owners gain better understanding of their birds' behavior; (2) improve the interaction and establishment of a healthy bond between the owner and the bird; (3) provide an opportunity for proper socialization; and (d) teach owners how to train their birds on good behavior by using the least intrusive, most effective learning techniques.[323] These training sessions will not only empower the parrots (by teaching them how they can operate their environment) but also empower owners (by teaching them how they can change the bird's behavior). This not only reduces the likelihood of a problem behavior occurring in the first place but also increases the likelihood of successful intervention when problem behaviors do arise, since the owner is more likely to intervene in an early stage and reverse the behavior. Behavior classes also help owners accustom their parrots to the clinic setting without having unpleasant procedures performed. Simultaneously, owners may be trained on various procedures such as towel restraint, weighing, administration of medications, or nail and wing trimming. As a result, birds may become easier to handle during clinical examinations because they are already accustomed to being handled and not stressed by just being in the clinic.[323] Particularly in the last decade, it has become increasingly apparent that many medical procedures can be performed with less force or coercion. The less the force used during a procedure, the less likely it is that the veterinary consult will be traumatic for the bird (and its owner). Highly effective, minimally intrusive techniques not only include the use of gentle, non–fear-eliciting methods of capture and restraint but also teach the owner how to teach behaviors to the bird, to facilitate such procedures as drug administration or having the bird enter a crate without restraining the bird.

[d]References 99,105,106,116,185,194,199.

Depending on the owner's motivation and insight in behavior modification procedures, even more complex cooperative behaviors for clinical purposes can be taught. For example, one of the authors (YvZ) has worked with an owner to teach her Grey parrot to allow regular filing of the beak. This not only decreased the level of stress experienced by the bird during the procedure but also significantly reduced the frequency of clinic visits for beak trimming (Figure 5-52).

Besides encouraging more cooperative behaviors and exerting less force and coercion, veterinarians and technicians are also urged to carefully monitor the bird during restraint. This monitoring includes the regular evaluation of physiologic and behavioral parameters that may indicate stress (e.g., respiration rate, eye pinning, struggling). If signs of stress are observed, the examination may be temporarily stopped to allow the parrot to recover. In mildly stressed parrots, this may include a short break during which the parrot can be spoken to in a soft voice. In more severely stressed parrots, the bird may need to be released from restraint altogether before resuming the procedure. Under these circumstances, the bird is preferably released into its carrier. Meanwhile, the owner is instructed to not force any attention on the animal immediately following the event to decrease the likelihood of the bird establishing a connection between the two events. Other measures that help minimize stress include (1) the establishment of a separate waiting room in which birds can be separated from predatory cats and barking dogs; (2) speaking in a soft, modulated tone; (3) moving slowly and cautiously toward the patient; (4) the use of conscious sedation in select cases; and (5) observing the bird from a distance during the initial phase of the consultation rather than confronting the bird immediately.

Through careful observation in the clinic (e.g., during the visit or hospitalization), the veterinary staff can gather valuable information about the bird's behavior and its bond with its owner. They may subsequently use this information to identify and address any behavioral issues that are present. By helping the owner prevent or resolve behavioral issues using the least intrusive and most effective techniques, the

veterinary staff can be valuable in preserving the long-term relationship between the owner and the bird. In addition, their efforts may help establish a long-term association between the owner and the clinic that may last for the parrot's lifetime. Veterinarians and their staff are therefore encouraged to carefully evaluate their own behaviors when it comes to their interactions with both clients and their birds, being aware that "learning happens to anyone, everywhere, and anytime" and that "no behavior is without consequences."

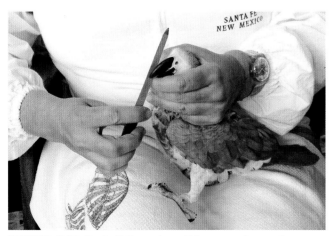

FIGURE 5-52 By building of confidence and trust between owner and animal, in this case a Grey parrot *(Psittacus erithacus)*, many tasks can be performed at home, without inflicting any stress to the animal. In the case of this bird, the owner regularly files the beak so that a beak trim by the veterinarian is no longer needed. (Photo courtesy of Ellen Uittenbogaard.)

REFERENCES

1. Australian Companion Animal Council (ACAC): *Australians and their pets: the facts*, 2009. http://www.acac.org.au/pdf/PetFactBook_June-6.pdf. Accessed January 6, 2014.
2. European Pet Food Industry Federation (FEDIAF): *Facts and figures*, 2012. http://www.fediaf.org/facts-figures/. Accessed January 6, 2014.
3. American Pet Products Association (APPA): *APPA national pet owners survey 2013-2014*, 2014. http://www.americanpetproducts.org/pubs_survey.asp. Accessed January 7, 2014.
4. Engebretson M: The welfare and suitability of parrots as companion animals: a review, *Anim Welfare* 15:263–276, 2006.
5. Meehan CL: *National parrot relinquishment research project 2003-2004*, 2007. http://www.thegabrielfoundation.org/documents/NPRRPReport.pdf. Accessed July 1, 2014.
6. Hoppes S, Gray P: Parrot rescue organizations and sanctuaries: a growing presence in 2010, *J Exotic Pet Med* 19:133–139, 2010.
7. Gaskins LA, Bergman L: Surveys of avian practitioners and pet owners regarding common behavior problems in psittacine birds, *J Avian Med Surg* 25:111–118, 2011.
8. van Hoek CS, ten Cate C: Abnormal behavior in caged birds kept as pets, *J Appl Anim Welf Sci* 1:51–64, 1998.
9. Levitis DA, Lidicker WZ Jr, Freund G: Behavioural biologists do not agree on what constitutes behaviour, *Anim Behav* 78:103–110, 2009.
10. Friedman SG, Edling TM, Cheney CD: Concepts in behavior—Section I, the natural science of behavior. In Harrison GJ, Lightfoot TL, editors: *Clinical avian medicine*, Vol 1, Palm Beach, FL, 2006, Spix Publishing, pp 46–59.
11. Friedman SG: A framework for solving behavior problems: functional assessment and intervention planning, *J Exotic Pet Med* 16:6–10, 2007.
12. Mazur JE: *Learning and behavior*, Upper Saddle River, NJ, 2002, Prentice Hall/Pearson Education.
13. Staddon JE: *Adaptive behaviour and learning*, Cambridge, U.K., 1983, Cambridge University Press Archive.
14. Chance P: *Learning and behavior*, Boston, MA, 2013, Cengage Learning.
15. Nobel Media AB: *The Nobel Prize in physiology or medicine*, 1973. http://www.nobelprize.org/nobel_prizes/medicine/laureates/. Accessed January 7, 2014.
16. Tinbergen N: On aims and methods of ethology, *Zeitschrift für Tierpsychologie* 20:410–433, 1963.
17. Silva T: *Psittaculture: breeding, rearing and management of parrots*, Surrey, U.K., 1991, Birdworld.
18. Collar NJ: Family psittacidae (parrots). In del Hoyo J, Elliott A, Sargatal J, editors: *Handbook of the birds of the world*, Vol 4, Barcelona, Spain, 1997, Lynx Edicions, pp 280–477.
19. Forshaw JM: *Parrots of the world*, Princeton, NJ, 2010, Princeton University Press.
20. Haupt T, Mancini JR: *Cockatiels*, Hauppauge, NY, 2008, Barron's Educational Series.
21. Schubot RM, Clubb KJ, Clubb SL, et al: *Psittacine aviculture: perspectives, techniques and research*, West Palm Beach, FL, 1992, Aviculture Breeding and Research Center.
22. Lindholm J: An historical review of parrots bred in zoos in the USA, *Avicultur Mag* 105:145–184, 1999.

23. Price EO: Behavioral aspects of animal domestication, *Q Rev Biol* 59:1–32, 1984.

24. Davis C: Appreciating avian intelligence: the importance of a proper domestic environment, *J Am Vet Med Assoc* 212:1220–1221, 1998.

25. Graham DL: Pet birds: historical and modern perspectives on the keeper and the kept, *J Am Vet Med Assoc* 212:1216–1219, 1998.

26. Price EO: Behavioral development in animals undergoing domestication, *Appl Anim Behav Sci* 65:245–271, 1999.

27. Kalmar ID, Janssens GP, Moons CP: Guidelines and ethical considerations for housing and management of psittacine birds used in research, *ILAR J* 51:409–423, 2010.

28. Breland K, Breland M: The misbehavior of organisms, *Am Psychol* 16:681–684, 1961.

29. Thorpe WH: The ibis: the learning abilities of birds, *Ibis* 93:1–52, 1951.

30. Moltz H: Contemporary instinct theory and the fixed action pattern, *Psychol Rev* 72:27–47, 1965.

31. Farabaugh SM, Dent ML, Dooling RJ: Hearing and vocalizations of wild-caught Australian budgerigars (Melopsittacus undulatus), *J Comp Psychol* 112:74–81, 1998.

32. Bergman L, Reinisch US: Parrot vocalization. In Luescher AU, editor: *Manual of parrot behavior*, Ames, IA, 2006, Blackwell Publishing, pp 219–223.

33. Brittan-Powell EF, Dooling RJ, Larsen ON, et al: Mechanisms of vocal production in budgerigars (Melopsittacus undulatus), *J Acoust Soc Am* 101:578–589, 1997.

34. Brittan-Powell EF, Dooling RJ, Farabaugh SM: Vocal development in budgerigars (Melopsittacus undulatus): contact calls, *J Comp Psychol* 111:226–241, 1997.

35. Wright TF: Regional dialects in the contact call of a parrot, *Series B Biol Sci* 263:867–872, 1996, In Proceedings of the Royal Society of London.

36. Wanker R, Fischer J: Intra-and interindividual variation in the contact calls of spectacled parrotlets (Forpus conspicillatus), *Behavior* 138:709–726, 2001.

37. Wright TF, Wilkinson GS: Population genetic structure and vocal dialects in an Amazon parrot, *Proc Biol Sci* 268:609–616, 2001.

38. May DL: *The vocal repertoire of grey parrots (Psittacus erithacus) living in the Congo basin* [PhD thesis], Tucson, AZ, 2004, University of Arizona.

39. Fernández-Juricic E, Martella MB, Alvarez EV: Vocalizations of the blue-fronted Amazon (Amazona aestiva) in the Chancaní reserve, Córdoba, Argentina, *Wilson Bull* 100:352–361, 1998.

40. Martella MB, Bucher EH: Vocalizations of the Monk parakeet, *Bird Behav* 8:101–110, 1990.

41. Pidgeon R: Call of the galah (Cacatua roseicapillus) and some comparisons with four other species of Australian parrots, *Emu* 81:158–168, 1981.

42. Snyder NF, Wiley JW, Kepler CB: *The parrots of Luquillo: natural history and conservation of the Puerto Rican parrot*, Camarillo, CA, 1987, Western Foundation of Vertebrate Zoology.

43. Rowley I: *Behavioural ecology of the Galah, Eolophus roseicapillus, in the wheatbelt of Western Australia*, Chipping Norton, Australia, 1990, Surrey Beatty & Sons.

44. Morris D: The feather postures of birds and the problem of the origin of social signals, *Behavior* 9:75–113, 1956.

45. Serpell J: Duets, greetings and triumph ceremonies: analogous displays in the parrot genus Trichoglossus, *Zeitschrift für Tierpsychologie* 55:268–283, 1981.

46. Serpell J: Visual displays and taxonomic affinities in the parrot genus Trichoglossus, *Biol J Linn Soc* 36:193–211, 1989.

47. Winninghaus J, Downs CT, Perrin M, et al: Abundance and activity patterns of the Cape parrot (Poicephalus robustus) in two Afromontane forests in South Africa, *Afr Zool* 36:71–77, 2001.

48. Lightfoot T, Nacewicz C: Psittacine behavior. In Bradley Bays T, Lightfoot T, Mayer J, editors: *Exotic pet behavior*, St. Louis, MO, 2006, Saunders, pp 51–101.

49. Pepperberg IM: *The Alex studies: cognitive and communicative abilities of grey parrots*, Cambridge, MA, 2009, Harvard University Press.

50. Levinson S: The social behavior of the White-fronted Amazon (Amazona albifrons). In Pasquier RF, editor: *Conservation of new world parrots*, Washington DC, 1980, Smithsonian Institution Press, pp 403–417.

51. Yamashita C: Field observations and comments on the Indigo macaw (Anodorhynchus leari), a highly endangered species from Northeastern Brazil, *Wilson Bull* 99:280–282, 1987.

52. Gilardi JD, Munn CA: Patterns of activity, flocking, and habitat use in parrots of the Peruvian Amazon, *Condor* 100:641–653, 1998.

53. Wilson EO: *Sociobiology*, Cambridge, MA, 1975, Belknap Press.

54. Enkerlin-Hoeflich EC, Snyder NF, Wiley JW, et al: Behavior of wild Amazona and Rhynchopsitta parrots, with comparative insights from other psittacines. In Luescher AU, editor: *Manual of parrot behavior*, Ames, IA, 2006, Blackwell Publishing, pp 13–25.

55. Westcott D, Cockburn A: Flock size and vigilance in parrots, *Aust J Zool* 36:335–349, 1988.

56. Chapman CA, Chapman L, Lefebvre L: Variability in parrot flock size: possible functions of communal roosts, *Condor* 91:842–847, 1989.

57. May DL: Grey parrots of the Congo basin forest, *PsittaScene* 13:8–10, 2001.

58. Symes C, Perrin M: Daily flight activity and flocking behaviour patterns of the Greyheaded parrot Poicephalus fuscicollis suahelicus Reichenow 1898 in Northern Province, South Africa, *Trop Zool* 16:47–62, 2003.

59. Masello JF, Pagnossin ML, Sommer C, et al: Population size, provisioning frequency, flock size and foraging range at the largest known colony of Psittaciformes: the burrowing parrots of the North-Eastern Patagonian coastal cliffs, *Emu* 106:69–79, 2006.

60. Seibert LM: Social behavior of psittacine birds. In Luescher AU, editor: *Manual of parrot behavior*, Ames, IA, 2006, Blackwell Publishing, pp 43–48.

61. Trillmich F: Spatial proximity and mate-specific behaviour in a flock of budgerigars (Melopsittacus undulatus; Aves, Psittacidae), *Zeitschrift für Tierpsychologie* 41:307–331, 1976.

62. Pitter E, Christiansen MB: Behavior of individuals and social interactions of the Red-fronted macaw Ara rubrogenys in the wild during the midday rest, *Ornitologia Neotropical* 8:133–143, 1997.

63. Arrowood PC: Duetting, pair bonding and agonistic display in parakeet pairs, *Behavior* 106:129–157, 1988.

64. Garnetzke-Stollmann K, Franck D: Socialisation tactics of the Spectacled parrotlet (Forpus conspicillatus), *Behavior* 119:1–29, 1991.

65. Harrison G: Perspective on parrot behavior. In Ritchie BW, Harrison GJ, Harrison LR, editors: *Avian medicine: principles and application*, Lake Worth, FL, 1994, Wingers Publishing, pp 96–108.

66. Seibert LM, Crowell-Davis SL: Gender effects on aggression, dominance rank, and affiliative behaviors in a flock of captive adult cockatiels (Nymphicus hollandicus), *Appl Anim Behav Sci* 71:155–170, 2001.

67. Heinsohn R, Murphy S, Legge S: Overlap and competition for nest holes among Eclectus parrots, palm cockatoos, and sulphur-crested cockatoos, *Aust J Zool* 51:81–94, 2003.

68. Brightsmith DJ: Competition, predation and nest niche shifts among tropical cavity nesters: phylogeny and natural history evolution of parrots (Psittaciformes) and trogons (Trogoniformes), *J Avian Biol* 36:64–73, 2005.

69. Spoon TR: Parrot reproductive behavior, or who associates, who mates, and who cares. In Luescher AU, editor: *Manual of parrot behavior*, Ames, IA, 2006, Blackwell Publishing, pp 63–77.

70. Taylor S, Perrin MR: Aspects of the breeding biology of the brown-headed parrot Poicephalus cryptoxanthus in South Africa, *Ostrich J Afr Ornithol* 77:225–228, 2006.

71. Parr M, Juniper T: *Parrots: a guide to parrots of the world*, London, U.K., 2010, Bloomsbury Publishing.

72. Wanker R, Bernate LC, Franck D: Socialization of spectacled parrotlets Forpus conspicillatus: the role of parents, crèches and sibling groups in nature, *J für Ornithologie* 137:447–461, 1996.

73. Margrath RD, Lill A: Age-related differences in behaviour and ecology of crimson rosellas, Platycercus elegans, during the non-breeding season, *Aust Wildl Res* 12:299–306, 1985.

74. Bauck L: Psittacine diets and behavioral enrichment, *Sem Avian Exotic Pet Med* 7:135–140, 1998.

75. Renton K: Lilac-crowned parrot diet and food resource availability: resource tracking by a parrot seed predator, *Condor* 103:62–69, 2001.

76. Gilardi JD, Duffey SS, Munn CA, et al: Biochemical functions of geophagy in parrots: detoxification of dietary toxins and cytoprotective effects, *J Chem Ecol* 25:897–922, 1999.

77. Brightsmith DJ, Taylor J, Phillips TD: The roles of soil characteristics and toxin adsorption in avian geophagy, *Biotropica* 40:766–774, 2008.

78. Lee AT, Kumar S, Brightsmith DJ, et al: Parrot claylick distribution in South America: do patterns of "where" help answer the question "why"? *Ecography* 33:503–513, 2010.

79. Emison W, Nicholls D: Notes on the feeding patterns of the long-billed corella, sulphur-crested cockatoo and galah in Southeastern Australia, *South Austral Ornithologist* 31:117–121, 1992.

80. Rozek JC, Millam JR: Preference and motivation for different diet forms and their effect on motivation for a foraging enrichment in captive orange-winged Amazon parrots (Amazona amazonica), *Appl Anim Behav Sci* 129:153–161, 2011.

81. Lefebvre L: The organization of grooming in budgerigars, *Behav Proc* 7:93–106, 1982.

82. Bergman L, Reinisch US: Comfort behavior and sleep. In Luescher AU, editor: *Manual of parrot behavior*, Ames, IA, 2006, Blackwell Publishing, pp 59–62.

83. Slessers M: Bathing behavior of land birds, *Auk* 87:91–99, 1970.

84. Dawson P: Foliage bathing of fig-parrots, *Sunbird J Queensland Ornithol Soc* 3:66, 1972.

85. Smith G: Systematics of parrots, *Ibis* 117:18–68, 1975.

86. Murphy SM, Braun JV, Millam JR: Bathing behavior of captive orange-winged amazon parrots (Amazona amazonica), *Appl Anim Behav Sci* 132:200–210, 2011.

87. Delius JD: Preening and associated comfort behavior in birds, *Ann N Y Acad Sci* 525:40–55, 1988.

88. Spruijt B, Van Hooff J, Gispen W: Ethology and neurobiology of grooming behavior, *Physiol Rev* 72:825–852, 1992.

89. Ayala-Guerrero F, Perez M, Calderon A: Sleep patterns in the bird Aratinga canicularis, *Physiol Behav* 43:585–589, 1988.

90. Ayala-Guerrero F: Sleep patterns in the parakeet Melopsittacus undulatus, *Physiol Behav* 46:787–791, 1989.

91. Rattenborg NC, Amlaner CJ, Lima SL: Behavioral, neurophysiological and evolutionary perspectives on unihemispheric sleep, *Neurosci Biobehav Rev* 24:817–842, 2000.

92. Van Hoek CS, King CE: Causation and influence of environmental enrichment on feather picking of the crimson-bellied conure (Pyrrhura perlata perlata), *Zoo Biol* 16:161–172, 1997.

93. Van Zeeland YRA, Schoemaker N, Lumeij J: Contrafreeloading in grey parrots, *Proc Ann Conf Assoc Avian Vet*, San Diego, 2010.

94. Joseph L: Contrafreeloading and its benefits to avian behavior, *Proc Ann Conf Assoc Avian Vet* 399–401, 2010.

95. Collier G, Rovee-Collier C: A comparative analysis of optimal foraging behavior: laboratory simulations. In Kamil AC, Sargent TD, editors: *Foraging behavior: ecological, ethological, and psychological approaches*, New York, 1981, Garland Press, pp 39–76.

96. Hughes B, Duncan I: The notion of ethological "need," models of motivation and animal welfare, *Anim Behav* 36:1696–1707, 1988.

97. Jensen P, Toates F: Who needs "behavioural needs"? Motivational aspects of the needs of animals, *Appl Anim Behav Sci* 37:161–181, 1993.

98. Van Zeeland YRA, Schoemaker NJ, Ravesteijn MM, et al: Efficacy of foraging enrichments to increase foraging time in grey parrots (Psittacus erithacus erithacus), *Appl Anim Behav Sci* 149:87–102, 2013.

99. Rozek JC, Danner LM, Stucky PA, et al: Over-sized pellets naturalize foraging time of captive orange-winged Amazon parrots (Amazona amazonica), *Appl Anim Behav Sci* 125:80–87, 2010.

100. Meehan C, Mench J: Captive parrot welfare. In Luescher AU, editor: *Manual of parrot behavior*, Ames, IA, 2006, Blackwell Publishing, pp 301–318.

101. Hesterman H, Gregory N, Boardman W: Deflighting procedures and their welfare implications in captive birds, *Anim Welfare* 10:405–419, 2001.

102. Keiper RR: Causal factors of stereotypies in caged birds, *Anim Behav* 17:114–119, 1969.

103. Lantermann W: *Verhaltensstörung bei Papageien. Entstehung, Diagnose, Therapie, Broschiert*, Germany, 1999, Enke.

104. Garner JP, Mason GJ, Smith R: Stereotypic route-tracing in experimentally caged songbirds correlates with general behavioural disinhibition, *Anim Behav* 66:711–727, 2003.

105. Meehan C, Millam J, Mench J: Foraging opportunity and increased physical complexity both prevent and reduce psychogenic feather picking by young Amazon parrots, *Appl Anim Behav Sci* 80:71–85, 2003.

106. Meehan C, Garner J, Mench J: Environmental enrichment and development of cage stereotypy in orange-winged Amazon parrots (Amazona amazonica), *Dev Psychobiol* 44:209–218, 2004.

107. Van Zeeland YR, Spruit BM, Rodenburg TB, et al: Feather damaging behaviour in parrots: a review with consideration of comparative aspects, *Appl Anim Behav Sci* 121:75–95, 2009.

108. Jordan T: *Understanding your bird's body language*, August 31, 1997, Winged Wisdom Pet Bird Magazine. http://www.birdsnways.com/wisdom/ww15eii.htm

109. Speer B: Normal and abnormal parrot behavior, *J Exotic Pet Med* 23:230–233, 2014.

110. Brouwer K, Jones M, King C, et al: Longevity records for Psittaciformes in captivity, *Int Zoo Yearbook* 37:299–316, 2000.

111. Lightfoot TL: Concepts in behavior—Section II: early Psittacine behaviour and development. In Harrison GJ, Lightfoot TL, editors: *Clinical avian medicine*, Vol 1, Palm Beach, FL, 2006, Spix Publishing, pp 60–72.

112. Nicol C, Pope S: A comparison of the behaviour of solitary and group-housed budgerigars, *Anim Welfare* 2:269–277, 1993.

113. Sheehan KL: *The effects of environmental enrichment and post-natal handling on the development, emotional reactivity and learning ability of juvenile Nanday conures (Nandayus nenday)* [MS thesis], West Lafayette, IN, 2001, Purdue University.

114. Luescher A, Sheehan K: Rearing environment and behavioral development of psittacine birds, *Cur Issues Res Vet Behav Med* 35–41, 2005.

115. Linden PG, Luescher AU: Behavioral development of psittacine companions: neonates, neophytes, and fledglings. In Luescher AU, editor: *Manual of parrot behavior*, Ames, IA, 2006, Blackwell Publishing, pp 93–111.

116. Meehan C, Mench J: Environmental enrichment affects the fear and exploratory responses to novelty of young Amazon parrots, *Appl Anim Behav Sci* 79:75–88, 2002.

117. Fox RA, Millam JR: Novelty and individual differences influence neophobia in orange-winged Amazon parrots (Amazona amazonica), *Appl Anim Behav Sci* 104:107–115, 2007.

118. Garner JP, Meehan CL, Famula TR, et al: Genetic, environmental, and neighbor effects on the severity of stereotypies and feather picking in orange-winged Amazon parrots (Amazona amazonica): an epidemiological study, *Appl Anim Behav Sci* 96:153–168. 2006.

119. Millam J: Neonatal handling, behaviour and reproduction in orange-winged Amazons and cockatiels, *Int Zoo Yearbook* 37:220–231, 2000.

120. Fox R: Hand-rearing: behavioral impacts and implications for captive parrot welfare. In Luescher AU, editor: *Manual of parrot behavior*, Ames, IA, 2006, Blackwell Publishing, pp 83–92.

121. Harcourt-Brown N: Development of the skeleton and feathers of dusky parrots (Pionus fuscus) in relation to their behaviour, *Vet Rec* 154:42–48, 2004.

122. Capitanio JP: Behavioral pathology, *Comp Primate Biol* 2:411–454, 1986.

123. Vázquez DM: Stress and the developing limbic–hypothalamic–pituitary–adrenal axis, *Psychoneuroendocrinology* 23:663–700, 1998.

124. Levine S: Primary social relationships influence the development of the hypothalamic–pituitary–adrenal axis in the rat, *Physiol Behav* 73:255–260, 2001.

125. Navarro A, Castanon I: Comparative study of the growth rates of hand-raised and parent-raised psittacids in Loro parque fundacion, *Cyanopsitta* 60:12–18, 2001.

126. Abramson J, Speer BL, Thomsen JB: *The large macaws: their care, breeding, and conservation*, Fort Bragg, NC, 1995, Raintree Publications.

127. Immelmann K: Sexual and other long-term aspects of imprinting in birds and other species, *Adv Study Behav* 4:147–174, 1972.

128. Immelmann K: Ecological significance of imprinting and early learning, *Annu Rev Ecol Syst* 6:15–37, 1975.

129. Rowley I, Chapman G: Cross-fostering, imprinting and learning in two sympatric species of cockatoo, *Behavior* 96:1–16, 1986.

130. Klinghammer E: Factors influencing choice of mate in altricial birds. In Stevenson HW, Hess EH, Rheingold HL, editors: *Early behavior: comparative and developmental approaches*, New York, 1967, Wiley, pp 5–42.

131. Myers S, Millam J, Roudybush T, et al: Reproductive success of hand-reared vs. parent-reared cockatiels (Nymphicus hollandicus), *Auk* 105:536–542, 1988.

132. Preiss H, Franck D: Verhaltensentwicklung isoliert handaufgezogener rosenköpfchen (Agapornis roseicollis [Vieillot]), *Zeitschrift fuÈr Tierpsychologie* 34:459–463, 1974.

133. Sistermann R: *Untersuchung zur sexuellen prägung handaufgezogener grosspapageien*, Aachen, Germany, 2000, Institut für Biologie II/Lehrstuhl für Zoologie-Tierphysiologie.

134. Aengus WL, Millam JR: Taming parent-reared orange-winged Amazon parrots by neonatal handling, *Zoo Biol* 18:177–187. 1999.

135. West MJ, King AP: Mozart's starling, *Am Sci* 78:106–114, 1990.

136. Pepperberg IM, Naughton JR, Banta PA: Allospecific vocal learning by grey parrots (Psittacus erithacus): a failure of videotaped instruction under certain conditions, *Behav Process* 42:139–158, 1998.

137. Meaney MJ: Maternal care, gene expression, and the transmission of individual differences in stress reactivity across generations, *Annu Rev Neurosci* 24:1161–1192, 2001.

138. Fox RA, Millam JR: The effect of early environment on neophobia in Orange-winged Amazon parrots (Amazona amazonica), *Appl Anim Behav Sci* 89:117–129, 2004.

139. Francis DD, Diorio J, Plotsky PM, et al: Environmental enrichment reverses the effects of maternal separation on stress reactivity, *J Neurosci* 22:7840–7843, 2002.

140. Mettke-Hofmann C, Winkler H, Leisler B: The significance of ecological factors for exploration and neophobia in parrots, *Ethology* 108:249–272, 2002.

141. Blanchard S: Working with phobic parrots, *Companion Parrot Quart* 54:43, 2001.

142. Clark P: A vicious cycle: helping the anxious parrot, *Companion Parrot Quart* 54:70–79, 2001.

143. Schmid R: *The influence of the breeding method on the behaviour of adult African grey parrots* [PhD thesis], Bern, Switzerland, 2004, Universität Bern.

144. Schmid R, Doherr MG, Steiger A: The influence of the breeding method on the behaviour of adult African grey parrots (Psittacus erithacus), *Appl Anim Behav Sci* 98:293–307, 2006.

145. American Psychiatric Association: *Diagnostic and statistical manual of mental disorders DSM-IV*, Washington DC, 1994, American psychiatric association.

146. Kaplan H, Sadock B, Grebb J: *Synopsis of psychiatry*, ed. 7, Philadelphia, PA, 1994, Williams & Wilkins.

147. Wilson L, Lightfoot T: Concepts in behavior—Section III: Pubescent and adult psittacine behavior. In Harrison GJ, Lightfoot TL, editors: *Clinical avian medicine*, Vol 1, Lake Worth, FL, 2006, Spix Publishing, pp 73–83.

148. Collette J, Millam J, Klasing K, et al: Neonatal handling of Amazon parrots alters the stress response and immune function, *Appl Anim Behav Sci* 66:335–349, 2000.

149. Thorndike EL: Animal intelligence: an experimental study of the associative processes in animals, *Psychol Monogr Gen Appl* 2:1–109, 1898.

150. Thorndike EL: *Animal intelligence: experimental studies*, London, U.K., 1911, Macmillan.

151. Skinner BF: *The behavior of organisms: an experimental analysis*, Oxford, U.K., 1938, Appleton-Century.

152. Skinner BF: Selection by consequences, *Science* 213:501–504, 1981.

153. Welle KR, Luescher AU: Aggressive behavior in pet birds. In Luescher AU, editor: *Manual of parrot behavior*, Ames, IA, 2006, Blackwell Publishing, pp 211–217.

154. Wilson L, Luescher AU: Parrots and fear. In Luescher AU, editor: *Manual of parrot behavior*, Ames, IA, 2006, Blackwell Publishing, pp 225–231.

155. Welle KR, Wilson L: Clinical evaluation of psittacine behavioral disorders. In Luescher AU, editor: *Manual of parrot behavior*, Ames, IA, 2006, Blackwell Publishing, pp 175–193.

156. Evans M: Environmental enrichment for pet parrots, *In Pract* 23:596–605, 2001.

157. Orosz SE: Diagnostic workup of suspected behavioral problems. In Luescher AU, editor: *Manual of parrot behavior*, Ames, IA, 2006, Blackwell Publishing, pp 195–210.

158. Friedman S, Martin S, Brinker B: Behavior analysis and parrot learning. In Luescher AU, editor: *Manual of parrot behavior*, Ames, IA, 2006, Blackwell Publishing, pp 147–163.

159. Kazdin AE: *Behavior modification in applied settings*, Long Grove, IA, 2012, Waveland Press.

160. Hearst E, Besley S, Farthing GW: Inhibition and the stimulus control of operant behavior, *J Exp Anal Behav* 14:373–409, 1970.

161. Yarczower M, Curto K: Stimulus control in pigeons after extended discriminative training, *J Comp Physiol Psychol* 80:484–489, 1972.

162. Martin P, Bateson PPG: *Measuring behaviour: an introductory guide*, Cambridge, U.K., 1993, Cambridge University Press.

163. Farhoody P: A framework for solving behavior problems, *Vet Clin N Am Exot Anim Pract* 15:399–411, 2012.

164. Pavlov IP: *Conditioned reÔçexes. An investigation of the physiological activity of the cerebral cortex*, London, U.K., 1927, Oxford University Press.

165. Carr EG: The motivation of self-injurious behavior: a review of some hypotheses, *Psychol Bull* 84:800–816, 1977.

166. Iwata BA, Pace GM, Dorsey MF, et al: The functions of self-injurious behavior: an experimental-epidemiological analysis, *J Appl Behav Anal* 27:215–240, 1994.

167. Day RM, Rea JA, Schussler NG, et al: A functionally based approach to the treatment of self-injurious behavior, *Behav Modif* 12:565–589, 1988.

168. Cooper JO, Heron TE, Heward WL: *Applied behavior analysis*. Upper Saddle River, NJ, 2007, Pearson, Merrill, Prentice Hall Publishers.

169. Azrin NH, Holz WC: Punishment. In Honig WK, editor: *Operant behavior: areas of research and application*, East Norwalk, CT, 1966, Appleton-Century-Crofts, pp 380–447.

170. Sulzer-Azaroff B, Mayer GR: *Behavior analysis for lasting change*, New York, 1991, Holt, Rinehart & Winston.

171. Lattal KA: Contingency and behavior analysis, *Behav Analyst* 18:209–224, 1995.

172. Elsner B, Hommel B: Contiguity and contingency in action-effect learning, *Psychol Res* 68:138–154, 2004.

173. Schneider JW: Reinforcer effectiveness as a function of reinforcer rate and magnitude: a comparison of concurrent performances, *J Exp Anal Behav* 20:461–471, 1973.

174. Todorov JC, Hanna ES, Neves Bittencourt de Sá MC: Frequency versus magnitude of reinforcement: new data with a different procedure, *J Exp Anal Behav* 41:157–167, 1984.

175. White OR, Haring NG: *Exceptional teaching*, Indianapolis, IN, 1980, Merrill Publishing Company.

176. Sidman M: *Coercion and its fallout*, Boston, MA, 1989, Authors Cooperative.

177. Alberto PA, Troutman AC: *Applied behavior analysis for teachers*, London, U.K., 2012, Pearson Higher Education.

178. O'Neill R, Horner R, Albin R, et al: *Functional assessment and program development for problem behavior*, Pacific Grove, CA, 1997, Cole Publishing Company.

178a. Friedman SG: What's wrong with this picture? Effectiveness is not enough, *Good Bird Magazine* 4(4):12–18, 2008.

179. Michael J: Distinguishing between discriminative and motivational functions of stimuli, *J Exp Anal Behav* 37:149–155, 1982.

180. Wilson L: Phobic psittacines: an increasing phenomenon, *Proc Annu Conf Assoc Avian Vet* 125–131, 1998.

181. Staub E: Duration of stimulus-exposure as determinant of the efficacy of flooding procedures in the elimination of fear, *Behav Res Ther* 6:131–132, 1968.

182. Friedman SG, Haug LI, Tynes VV: From parrots to pigs to pythons: universal principles and procedures of learning. In Tynes VV, editor: *Behavior of exotic pets*, Ames, IA, 2010, Wiley, pp 190–205.

183. Maier SF, Seligman ME: Learned helplessness: theory and evidence, *J Exp Psychol Gen* 105:3–46, 1976.

184. Laudenslager ML, Ryan SM, Drugan RC, et al: Coping and immunosuppression: inescapable but not escapable shock suppresses lymphocyte proliferation, *Science* 221:568–570, 1983.

185. Lumeij JT, Hommers CJ: Foraging "enrichment" as treatment for pterotillomania, *Appl Anim Behav Sci* 111:85–94, 2008.

186. Luescher U, Wilson L: Housing and management considerations for problem prevention. In Luescher AU, editor: *Manual of parrot behavior*, Ames, IA, 2006, Blackwell Publishing, pp 291–299.

187. Porter K: *The parrot enrichment activity book*, Vol 1.0, 2014. http://www.parrotenrichment.com. Accessed November 23, 2014.

188. Porter K: *The parrot enrichment activity book*, Vol 2.0, 2014. http://www.parrotenrichment.com. Accessed November 23, 2014.

189. Kim LC, Garner JP, Millam JR: Preferences of Orange-winged Amazon parrots (Amazona amazonica) for cage enrichment devices, *Appl Anim Behav Sci* 120:216–223, 2009.

190. Webb NV, Famula TR, Millam JR: The effect of rope color, size and fray on environmental enrichment device interaction in male and female orange-winged Amazon parrots (Amazona amazonica), *Appl Anim Behav Sci* 124:149–156, 2010.

191. Coulton L, Waran N, Young R: Effects of foraging enrichment on the behaviour of parrots, *Anim Welfare* 6:357–363, 1997.

192. Elson H, Marples N, Wehnelt S, et al: How captive parrots react to foraging enrichments, *Proc 3rd Annu Symp Zoo Res* 1–8, 2001.

193. Shyne A: Meta-analytic review of the effects of enrichment on stereotypic behavior in zoo mammals, *Zoo Biol* 25:317–337, 2006.

194. Newberry RC: Environmental enrichment: increasing the biological relevance of captive environments, *Appl Anim Behav Sci* 44: 229–243, 1995.

195. Echols MS: *Foraging and enrichment webinar*, 2015. http://lafeber.com/vet/foraging-and-enrichment-webinar/. Accessed March 09, 2015.

196. Young RJ: *Environmental enrichment for captive animals*, Oxford, U.K., 2008, Blackwell Publishing.

197. Chitty J: Feather plucking in psittacine birds 2. Social, environmental and behavioural considerations, *In Pract* 25:550–555, 2003.

198. Seibert LM: Feather-picking disorder in pet birds. In Luescher AU, editor: *Manual of parrot behavior*, Ames, IA, 2006, Blackwell Publishing, pp 255–265.

199. Meehan C, Garner J, Mench J: Isosexual pair housing improves the welfare of young Amazon parrots, *Appl Anim Behav Sci* 81:73–88, 2003.

200. Wilson L: Sleep: how much is enough for a parrot, *Pet Bird Rep* 43:60–62, 1999.

201. Martin KM: Psittacine behavioral pharmacotherapy. In Luescher AU, editor: *Manual of parrot behavior*, Ames, IA, 2006, Blackwell Publishing, pp 267–279.

202. Seibert LM: Pharmacotherapy for behavioral disorders in pet birds, *J Exot Pet Med* 16:30–37, 2007.

203. Crowell-Davis SL, Murray T: *Veterinary psychopharmacology*, Ames, IA, 2008, Blackwell Publishing.

204. Iglauer F, Rasim R: Treatment of psychogenic leather picking in psittacine birds with a dopamine antagonist, *J Small Anim Pract* 34:564–566, 1993.

205. Lennox A, VanDerHeyden N: Haloperidol for use in treatment of psittacine self-mutilation and feather plucking, *Proc Annu Conf Assoc Avian Vet* 119–120, 1993.

206. Lennox A, VanDerHeyden N: Long-term use of haloperidol in two parrots, *Proc Annu Conf Assoc Avian Vet* 133–137, 1999.

207. Ramsay EC, Grindlinger H: Use of clomipramine in the treatment of obsessive behavior in psittacine birds, *J Assoc Avian Vet* 8:9–15, 1994.

208. Seibert LM, Crowell-Davis SL, Wilson GH, et al: Placebo-controlled clomipramine trial for the treatment of feather picking disorder in cockatoos, *J Am Anim Hosp Assoc* 40:261–269, 2004.

209. Mertens P: Pharmacological treatment of feather picking in pet birds, *Proc First Int Meet Vet Behav Med* 209–211, 1997.

210. Van Zeeland YRA, Schoemaker NJ, Haritova A, et al: Pharmacokinetics of paroxetine, a selective serotonin reuptake inhibitor, in grey parrots (Psittacus erithacus erithacus): influence of pharmaceutical formulation and length of dosing, *J Vet Pharmacol Ther* 36:51–58, 2013.

211. Turner R: Trexan (naltrexone hydrochloride) use in feather picking in avian species, *Proc Assoc Avian Vet* 116–118, 1993.

212. Ottinger MA, Wu J, Pelican K: Neuroendocrine regulation of reproduction in birds and clinical applications of GnRH analogues in birds and mammals, *Sem Avian Exot Pet Med* 11:71–79, 2002.

213. Forbes NA: The use of GnRH implants in the treatment of sexual derived behavioural abnormalities in birds, *Proc Eur Assoc Avian Vet* 119–122, 2009.

214. Mans C, Pilny A: Use of GnRH-agonists for medical management of reproductive disorders in birds, *Vet Clin N Am Exot Anim Pract* 17:23–33, 2014.

215. Galvin C: The feather picking bird. In Kirk, RW, editor: *Current veterinary therapy VIII. Small animal practice*, Philadelphia, PA, 1983, WB Saunders, pp 646–652.

216. Edwards JG: Adverse effects of antianxiety drugs, *Drugs* 22: 495–514, 1981.

217. Oyesanmi O, Kunkel EJ, Monti DA, et al: Hematologic side effects of psychotropics, *Psychosomatics* 40:414–421, 1999.

218. Uzun S, Kozumplik O, Jakovljević M, et al: Side effects of treatment with benzodiazepines, *Psychiatria Danubina* 22:90–93, 2010.

219. Center SA, Elston TH, Rowland PH, et al: Fulminant hepatic failure associated with oral administration of diazepam in 11 cats, *J Am Vet Med Assoc* 209:618–625, 1996.

220. Moreau R, Overall K, Van Winkle T: Acute hepatic necrosis and liver failure associated with benzodiazepine therapy in six cats, 1986–1995, *J Vet Emerg Crit Care* 6:13–20, 1996.

221. Simon NM, Safren SA, Otto MW, et al: Longitudinal outcome with pharmacotherapy in a naturalistic study of panic disorder, *J Affect Disord* 69:201–208, 2002.

222. Pollack MH: The pharmacotherapy of panic disorder, *J Clin Psychiatry* 66:23–27, 2005.

223. Lasher T, Fleishaker J, Steenwyk R, et al: Pharmacokinetic pharmacodynamic evaluation of the combined administration of alprazolam and fluoxetine, *Psychopharmacology* 104:323–327, 1991.

224. Crowell-Davis SL: Tricyclic antidepressants. In: Crowell-Davis SL, Murray T, editors: *Veterinary psychopharmacology*, Ames, IA, 2006, Blackwell Publishing, pp 179–206.

225. Eugenio C: Amitriptyline HCl: clinical study for treatment of feather picking, *Proc Annu Meet Assoc Avian Vet* 133–135, 2003.

226. Hewson CJ, Luescher UA, Parent JM, et al: Efficacy of clomipramine in the treatment of canine compulsive disorder, *J Am Vet Med Assoc* 213:1760–1766, 1998.

227. Overall KL, Dunham AE: Clinical features and outcome in dogs and cats with obsessive-compulsive disorder: 126 cases (1989–2000), *J Am Vet Med Assoc* 221:1445–1452, 2002.

228. Gupta M, Gupta A: The use of antidepressant drugs in dermatology, *J Eur Acad Dermatol Venereol* 15:512–518, 2001.

229. Johnson C: Chronic feather picking: a different approach to treatment, *Proc Annu Meet Assoc Avian Vet* 125–142, 1987.

230. Jenike MA, Baer L, Greist JH: Clomipramine versus fluoxetine in obsessive-compulsive disorder: a retrospective comparison of side effects and efficacy, *J Clin Psychopharmacol* 10:122–124, 1990.

231. Vandel P, Bonin B, Leveque E, et al: Tricyclic antidepressant-induced extrapyramidal side effects, *Eur Neuropsychopharmacol* 7:207–212, 1997.

232. Pacher P, Kecskemeti V: Cardiovascular side effects of new antidepressants and antipsychotics: New drugs, old concerns? *Curr Pharm Des* 10:2463–2475, 2004.

233. Juarbe-Díaz SV: Animal behavior case of the month, *J Am Vet Med Assoc* 216:1562–1564, 2000.

234. Starkey SR, Morrisey JK, Hickam HD, et al: Extrapyramidal side effects in a Blue and gold macaw (Ara ararauna) treated with haloperidol and clomipramine, *J Avian Med Surg* 22:234–239, 2008.

235. Boyer W: Potential indications for the selective serotonin reuptake inhibitors, *Int Clin Psychopharmacol* 6:5–12, 1992.

236. Crowell-Davis S, Murray T: Selective serotonin reuptake inhibitors. In Crowell-Davis SL, Murray T, editors: *Veterinary psychopharmacology*, Ames, IA, 2006, Blackwell Publishing, pp 80–110.

237. Anderson IM: Selective serotonin reuptake inhibitors versus tricyclic antidepressants: a meta-analysis of efficacy and tolerability, *J Affect Disord* 58:19–36, 2000.

238. Brambilla P, Cipriani A, Hotopf M, et al: Side-effect profile of fluoxetine in comparison with other SSRIs, tricyclic and newer antidepressants: a meta-analysis of clinical trial data, *Pharmacopsychiatry* 38:69–77, 2005.

239. Marks DM, Park M, Ham B, et al: Paroxetine: safety and tolerability issues, *Exp Opin Drug Saf* 7:783–794, 2008.

240. Sadock BJ, Sadock VA: *Kaplan and Sadock's pocket handbook of clinical psychiatry*, Philadelphia, PA, 2010, Lippincott Williams & Wilkins.

241. Hyttel J: Pharmacological characterization of selective serotonin reuptake inhibitors (SSRIs), *Int Clin Psychopharmacol* 9:19–26, 1994.

242. Kearns K. Paroxetine therapy for feather picking and self-mutilation in the Waldrapp ibis (Geronticus eremita), *Proc Assoc Zoo Vet Am Assoc Wildl Vets* 254–255, 2004.

243. Seibert LM: Animal behavior case of the month, *J Am Vet Med Assoc* 224:1762–1764, 2004.

244. Seibert LM: Antipsychotics. In Crowell-Davis SL, Murray T, editors: *Veterinary psychopharmacology*, Ames, IA, 2006, Blackwell Publishing, pp 148–165.

245. Glick ID, Murray SR, Vasudevan P, et al: Treatment with atypical antipsychotics: new indications and new populations, *J Psychiatr Res* 35:187–191, 2001.

246. Luescher A: Compulsive behavior: recognition and treatment, *Proc Annu Conf Am Assoc Zoo Vets* 398–402, 1998.

247. Ritchie BW, Harrison GJ: Formulary. In Ritchie BW, Harrison GJ, Harrison LR, editors: *Avian medicine: principles and application*, Lake Worth, FL, 1994, Wingers Publishing, pp 227–253.

248. Welle K: A review of psychotropic drug therapy, *Proc Annu Conf Assoc Avian Vet* 121–123, 1998.

249. Landsberg GM, Hunthausen WL, Ackerman LJ: Behavior problems of the dog and cat, Vol 3, St. Louis, MO, 2012, Saunders.

250. Brown S, Crowell-Davis S, Malcolm T, et al: Naloxone-responsive compulsive tail chasing in a dog, *J Am Vet Med Assoc* 190:884–886, 1987.

251. Dodman NH, Shuster L, White SD, et al: Use of narcotic antagonists to modify stereotypic self-licking, self-chewing, and scratching behavior in dogs, *J Am Vet Med Assoc* 193(7):815–819, 1988.

252. White SD: Naltrexone for treatment of acral lick dermatitis in dogs, *J Am Vet Med Assoc* 196:1073–1076, 1990.

253. Kenny DE: Use of naltrexone for treatment of psychogenically induced dermatoses in five zoo animals, *J Am Vet Med Assoc* 205:1021–1023, 1994.

254. Dodman NH, Shuster D: *Psychopharmacology of animal behaviour disorders*, Malden, MA, 1998, Blackwell Science.

255. Scott D, Miller W: Antihistamines in the management of allergic pruritus in dogs and cats, *J Small Anim Pract* 40:359–364, 1999.

256. Gould W: Caring for pet birds' skin and feathers, *Vet Med* 90:53–63, 1995.

257. Krinsley M: Use of dermcaps liquid and hydroxyzine HCl for the treatment of feather picking, *J Assoc Avian Vet* 7:221, 1993.

258. Aranow A, Hudson JI, Pope Jr HG, et al: Elevated antidepressant plasma levels after addition of fluoxetine, *Am J Psychiatry* 146:911–913, 1989.

259. Zantop D: Using leuprolide acetate to manage common avian reproductive problems, *Exotic DVM* 2:70, 2000.

260. Lightfoot T: Feather "Plucking," In *Proceedings of the Atlantic Coast Veterinary Conference*, Atlantic City, NJ, 2001.

261. Harrison GJ: Disorders of the integument. In Harrison GJ, Harrison LR, Ritchie BW, editors: *Clinical avian medicine and surgery*, Philadelphia, PA, 1986, WB Saunders, pp 509–524.

262. Grindlinger HM: Compulsive feather picking in birds, *Arch Gen Psychiatry* 48:857, 1991.

263. Kinkaid HMY, Mills DS, Nichols SG, et al: Feather-damaging behaviour in companion parrots: an initial analysis of potential demographic risk factors, *Avian Biol Res* 6:289–296, 2013.

264. Rosskopf W, Woerpel R: Feather picking and therapy of skin and feather disorders. In Rosskopf W, Woerpel R, editors: *Diseases of cage and aviary birds*, ed 3, Baltimore, MD, 1996, Williams & Wilkins, pp 397–405.

265. Nett CS, Tully T: Anatomy, clinical presentation, and diagnostic approach to feather-picking pet birds, *Comp Cont Educ Pract Vet* 25:206–219, 2003.

266. Rosenthal K: Differential diagnosis of feather-picking in pet birds, *Proc Assoc Avian Vet* 108–112, 1993.

267. Schmidt RE, Lightfoot TL: Integument. In Harrison GJ, Lightfoot TL, editors: *Clinical avian medicine*, Palm Beach, FL, 2006, Spix Publishing, pp 395–409.

268. Briscoe J, Wilson L, Smith G: Non-medical risk factors for feather picking in pet parrots, *Proc Assoc Avian Vet* 131, 2001.

269. Gaskins LA, Hungerford L: Nonmedical factors associated with feather picking in pet psittacine birds, *J Avian Med Surg* 28:109–117, 2014.

270. Jayson SL, Williams DL, Wood JL: Prevalence and risk factors for feather plucking in African grey parrots (Psittacus erithacus erithacus and Psittacus erithacus timneh) and cockatoos (Cacatua spp.), *J Exot Pet Med* 23:250–257, 2014.

271. Jenkins JR: Feather picking and self-mutilation in psittacine birds, *Vet Clin N Am Exot Anim Pract* 4:651–667, 2001.

272. Rubinstein J, Lightfoot T: Feather loss and feather destructive behavior in pet birds, *J Exot Pet Med* 21:219–234, 2012.

273. Van Zeeland YRA, van der Aa MMJA, Vinke CM, et al: Behavioural testing to determine differences between coping styles in grey parrots (Psittacus erithacus erithacus) with and without feather damaging behaviour, *Appl Anim Behav Sci* 148:218–231, 2013.

274. Wedel A: Verhaltensstörungen. In Wedel A, editor: *Ziervogel—Erkrankungen, Haltung, Fütterung*, Vienna, Austria, 1999, Parey-Verlag, pp 283–286.

275. Bays TB, Lightfoot T, Mayer J: *Exotic pet behavior: birds, reptiles, and small mammals*, St. Louis, MO, 2006, Saunders.

276. Welle K: Clinical approach to feather picking, *Proc Annu Conf Assoc Avian Vets* 119–124, 1999.

277. Pollock C: Diagnosis and treatment of avian renal disease, *Vet Clin N Am Exot Anim Pract* 9:107–128, 2006.

278. Burgos-Rodríguez AG: Avian renal system: clinical implications, *Vet Clin N Am Exot Anim Pract* 13:393–411, 2010.

279. Davies RR: Avian liver disease: etiology and pathogenesis, *Sem Avian Exot Pet Med* 9:115–125, 2000.

280. Grunkemeyer VL: Advanced diagnostic approaches and current management of avian hepatic disorders, *Vet Clin N Am Exot Anim Pract* 13:413–427, 2010.

281. Koski MA: Dermatologic diseases in psittacine birds: an investigational approach, *Sem Avian Exot Pet Med* 11:105–124, 2002.

282. Westerhof I, Lumeij J: Feather picking in the African grey parrot, *Proc Eur Symp Bird Dis* 98–103, 1987.

283. Owen D, Lane J: High levels of corticosterone in feather-plucking parrots (Psittacus erithacus), *Vet Rec* 158:804–805, 2006.

284. Garner J: Perseveration and stereotypy: systems-level insights from clinical psychology. In Mason GJ, Rushen J, editors: *Stereotypic animal behaviour: fundamentals and applications to welfare*, ed 2, Oxfordshire, U.K., 2006, CAB International, pp 121–152.

285. Lamberski N: A diagnostic approach to feather picking, *Sem Avian Exot Pet Med* 4:161–168, 1995.

286. Colombini S, Foil CS, Hosgood G, et al: Intradermal skin testing in Hispaniolan parrots (Amazona ventralis), *Vet Dermatol* 11: 271–276, 2000.

287. Nett C, Hodgin E, Foil C, et al: A modified biopsy technique to improve histopathological evaluation of avian skin, *Vet Dermatol* 14:147–151, 2003.

288. Rosenthal KL, Morris DO, Mauldin EA, et al: Cytologic, histologic, and microbiologic characterization of the feather pulp and follicles of feather-picking psittacine birds: a preliminary study, *J Avian Med Surg* 18:137–143, 2004.

289. Garner MM, Clubb SL, Mitchell MA, et al: Feather-picking psittacines: histopathology and species trends, *Vet Pathol* 45:401–408, 2008.

290. Davis C: Basic considerations for avian behavior modification, *Sem Avian Exot Pet Med* 8:183–195, 1999.

291. Van Zeeland YRA, Bergers MJ, van der Valk L, et al: Evaluation of a novel feather scoring system for monitoring feather damaging behaviour in parrots, *Vet J* 196:247–252, 2013.

292. Pollock CG, Orosz SE: Avian reproductive anatomy, physiology and endocrinology, *Vet Clin N Am Exot Anim Pract* 5:441–474, 2002.

293. Van Sant F: Problem sexual behaviors of companion parrots. In Luescher AU, editor: *Manual of parrot behavior*, Ames, IA, 2006, Blackwell Publishing, pp 233–245.

294. Joyner K: Theriogenology. In Ritchie BW, Harrison GJ, Harrison LR, editors: *Avian medicine: principles and application*, Lake Worth, FL, 1994, Wingers, pp 748–804.

295. Romagnano A: Avian obstetrics, *Sem Avian Exot Pet Med* 5:180–188, 1996.

296. De Matos R, Morrisey JK: Emergency and critical care of small psittacines and passerines, *Sem Avian Exot Pet Med* 14:90–105, 2005.

297. Minsky L, Petrak ML: Diseases of the digestive system. In Petrak ML, editor: *Diseases of cage and aviary birds*, ed 2, Philadelphia, PA, 1982, Lea & Febiger, pp 432–443.

298. Avgeris S, Rigg D: Cloacopexy in a sulphur-crested cockatoo, *J Am Anim Hosp Assoc* 24:407–410, 1988.

299. Ritzman TK: *Cloacal disorders: Diagnosis and treatment (V454)*, 2015. http://www.vin.com/proceedings/proceedings.plx?CID=WSAVA2002. Accessed March 09, 2015.

300. Shields K, Yamamoto J, Millam J: Reproductive behavior and LH levels of cockatiels (Nymphicus hollandicus) associated with photostimulation, nest-box presentation, and degree of mate access, *Horm Behav* 23:68–82, 1989.

301. Hudelson K: A review of the mechanisms of avian reproduction and their clinical applications, *Sem Avian Exot Pet Med* 5:189–198, 1996.

302. Millam J: Reproductive physiology. In Altman RB, Clubb SL, Dorrestein GM, editors: *Avian medicine and surgery*, Philadelphia, PA, 1997, WB Saunders, pp 12–26.

303. Millam JR: Reproductive management of captive parrots, *Vet Clin North Am Exot Anim Pract* 2:93–110, 1999.

304. Millam J, Finney H: Leuprolide acetate can reversibly prevent egg laying in cockatiels (Nymphicus hollandicus), *Zoo Biol* 13:149–155, 1994.

305. Echols MS: Surgery of the avian reproductive tract, *Sem Avian Exot Pet Med* 11:177–195, 2002.

306. Rosen LB: Avian reproductive disorders, *J Exot Pet Med* 21: 124–131. 2012.

307. American Psychiatric Association: *The diagnostic and statistical manual of mental disorders: DSM 5*, Washington DC, 2013, American psychiatric association.

308. Blanchard S: Phobic behavior in companion parrots. In *Proceedings of the Annual Conference of the International Avicultural Society*, Orlando, FL,1998, International Avicultural Society.

309. Wilson L: Behavior problems in pet parrots. In Olsen GH, Orosz SE, editor: *Manual of avian medicine*, St. Louis, MO, 2000, Mosby, pp 124–147.

310. Speer BL. The clinical consequences of routine grooming procedures, *Proc Annu Conf Assoc Avian Vets* 22–24, 2001.

311. Bradbury J: Vocal communication of wild parrots, *J Acoust Soc Am* 115:2373, 2004.

312. Zgurski J: The behavior of wild amazon parrots, *Companion Parrot Quart* 71, 2007.

313. Welle K: *Psittacine behavior handbook*, Bedford Hills, NY, 1999, Association of Avian Veterinarians.

314. Dodman N: Pharmacologic treatment of aggression on veterinary patients. In Dodman NH. Shuster D, editors: *Psychopharmacology of animal behavior disorders*, Malden, MA, 1998, Blackwell Publishing, pp 41–63.

315. Romagnano A: Mate trauma. In Luescher AU, editor: *Manual of parrot behavior*, Ames, IA, 2006, Blackwell Publishing, pp 247–253.

316. Friedman S: The S-files: Kathy: Reba: Chasing Kiki, 2015. http://www.behaviorworks.org/htm/articles_success_files.html. Accessed March 15, 2015.

317. Péron F, Hoummady S, Mauny N, et al: Touch screen device and music as enrichments to captive housing conditions of African grey parrots, *J Vet Behav Clin Appl Res* 7:e13, 2012.

318. Kirkden RD, Pajor EA. Using preference, motivation and aversion tests to ask scientific questions about animals' feelings, *Appl Anim Behav Sci* 100(1):29–47, 2006.

319. Cooper JJ, Mason GJ: The use of operant technology to measure behavioral priorities in captive animals, *Behav Res Method Instr Comp* 33:427–434, 2001.

320. Jensen MB, Pedersen LJ: Using motivation tests to assess ethological needs and preferences, *Appl Anim Behav Sci* 113:340–356, 2008.

321. Cooper J: Consumer demand under commercial husbandry conditions: practical advice on measuring behavioural priorities in captive animals, *Anim Welfare* 13:47–56, 2004.

322. Van Zeeland YRA: *The feather damaging grey parrot: an analysis of its behaviour and needs* [PhD thesis], Utrecht, The Netherlands, 2013, Utrecht University.

323. Welle KR: Behavior classes in the veterinary hospital: preventing problems before they start. In Luescher AU, editor: *Manual of parrot behavior*, Ames, IA, 2006, Blackwell Publishing, pp 165–174.

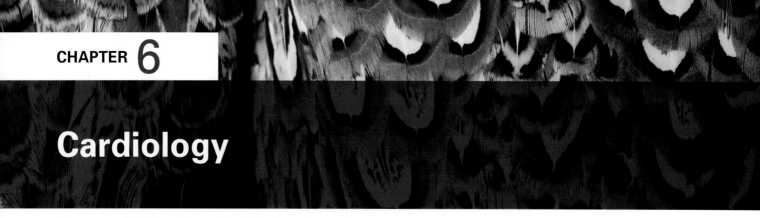

CHAPTER 6

Cardiology

Brenna Colleen Fitzgerald • Hugues Beaufrère

Cardiovascular disease has traditionally been thought to be a rare occurrence in companion birds, but a growing body of evidence collected over the last few decades indicates otherwise. Cardiovascular disease is frequently encountered in practice and poses a serious threat to the quality of life and longevity of many avian species. Successful intervention requires a foundational understanding of relevant anatomy and physiology, heightened awareness of risk factors and recognition of clinical disease states, accurate and timely diagnosis, and innovative treatment approaches. The latter should incorporate both available information specific to birds and components of therapy in human and small animal cardiovascular medicine.

Much of what is known of avian cardiovascular anatomy is based on the domestic fowl (*Gallus gallus domesticus*) and the pigeon (*Columba livia*). There have been relatively fewer investigations of psittacine anatomy specifically. Given that cardiovascular disease is commonly encountered in these species, which are regularly presented to the clinician, one objective of this chapter is to familiarize the reader with not only avian cardiovascular anatomy in general but also anatomic features of psittacine birds in particular, where known. This chapter will also present recognized disease states and their pathophysiology, clinical and pathologic features, and prevalence. Cardiovascular disease poses a particular diagnostic challenge, given the potential variability of its clinical manifestations (to include asymptomatic, slowly progressive disease) and the limited sensitivity of available investigative methods. In this chapter, we review current diagnostic options that can facilitate the detection of pathologic changes, with an emphasis on diagnostic imaging. Although the sparseness of pharmacologic data in avian species complicates effective medical management of cardiovascular disease, treatment approaches that have been reported, utilized by the authors, or show promise for future application are discussed.

ANATOMY AND PHYSIOLOGY

The high-performance cardiovascular system of birds has evolved to meet the high aerobic demands of flight and other intense activity by providing adequate oxygen transport with maximal efficiency. Although heart rate relative to body mass is lower in birds than in mammals, the avian heart is relatively larger and its stroke volume and cardiac output greater.[1,2] Heart rate can increase two to four times during flight.[2,3] The budgerigar (*Melopsittacus undulatus*) in flight has a cardiac output approximately seven times that of the dog during maximal exercise. Mean arterial pressure is higher in birds than in mammals, whereas total peripheral resistance is lower.[1,2] The anatomic and physiologic peculiarities of the avian cardiovascular system are summarized in Box 6-1.[2,4-6]

The Heart

The heart lies within the cranioventral coelom, its ventral surface in a concave indentation of the sternum, and its dorsal surface resting against the tracheal bifurcation (syrinx), the esophagus, and more caudally, the proventriculus (Figure 6-1).[4,6] The cardiac apex is enclosed within the lobes of the liver (Figure 6-2).[1,2] Adjacent respiratory structures include the paired, non-expansile lungs resting dorsal to the heart (see Figures 6-1 to 6-3), the cervical air sacs (singular in the fowl, paired in some psittacines[7]) and the unpaired clavicular air sac cranially, and the paired cranial thoracic air sacs laterally (see Figure 6-3). The clavicular air sac is large and complex, lying within the thoracic inlet and possessing numerous diverticula. Its intrathoracic diverticula surround the heart and the great vessels; suspend the esophagus, trachea, and syrinx; extend ventrally between the heart and the sternum; and pneumatize the sternum.[6,8,9] Extrathoracic diverticula extend from the thoracic inlet and among the structures of the thoracic girdle and shoulder, pneumatizing the constituent bones.[8] The position of these structures relative to the heart has great clinical relevance, given the potential for cardiovascular involvement in cases of primary respiratory disease.

The avian heart (Figures 6-4 to 6-6) is four-chambered, with left and right atria and left and right ventricles, each of which is composed of the endocardium, myocardium, and epicardium. The left ventricle perfuses the systemic circulation, and the right ventricle perfuses the pulmonary circulation. As resistance to blood flow is lower in the pulmonary circulation than in the systemic circulation, the right ventricle must produce less systolic pressure; it is smaller, and the myocardium is thinner than in the left ventricle. The wall of the left ventricle is two to three times thicker than that of the right ventricle and can generate four to five times the systolic pressure compared with the right ventricle.[1,2] The cone-shaped left ventricle extends to the cardiac apex, and its right wall forms the interventricular septum. The right ventricle is a crescent-shaped cavity that wraps around at least one half of the left ventricle.[1,2,10] Its free wall is continuous with the outer wall of the left ventricle, and it does not extend to the cardiac apex.[1,2,10]

These features have been demonstrated in morphologic studies of the psittacine heart where measurements of ventricular

BOX 6-1 CHARACTERISTICS OF THE AVIAN CARDIOVASCULAR SYSTEM DIFFERING FROM THOSE OF MAMMALS

Higher heart-to-body weight ratio

Higher stroke volume, arterial blood pressure, and cardiac output; lower total peripheral resistance

Tricuspid (poorly defined) left atrioventricular (AV) valve

Muscular unicuspid right AV valve

No chordae tendineae in the right AV valve

Muscular ring around the aortic valve

Ascending aorta on the right

Cartilage or ossification at base of aorta

Brachiocephalic arteries larger than aorta

Two cranial venae cavae

Most of myocardium vascularization derived from deep coronary arteries

No cerebral arterial circle of Willis

Renal portal system

Ring of Purkinje fibers around aorta and right AV valve

Depolarization of epicardium precedes endocardium

Negative cardiac mean electrical axis (except broilers, Pekin ducks)

Smaller cardiac muscle fibers

Absence of T-tubules in cardiac myocytes

Absence of M-bands connecting myosin filaments

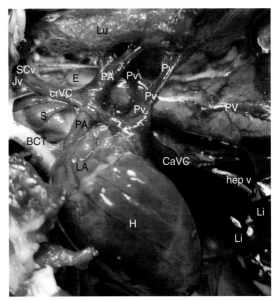

FIGURE 6-1 Heart in situ, left lateral view, blue-fronted Amazon parrot *(Amazona aestiva)*. The lungs (Lu), syrinx (S), esophagus (E), and proventriculus (PV) lie dorsal to the heart (H) and the two liver lobes (Li) caudally. Visible vascular structures are the left brachiocephalic trunk (BCT), pulmonary artery (PA), cranial vena cava (crVC), and pulmonary veins (Pv). The left cranial vena cava receives the left jugular vein (Jv) and subclavian vein (SCv). The left hepatic vein (hep v) is seen emptying into the caudal vena cava (CaVC), but the right hepatic vein is not readily visible in this image. LA, Left atrium.

lengths and myocardial thickness were collected for some species.[11,12] In one study (Table 6-1), the hearts were sectioned longitudinally, whereupon the lengths of both ventricles were recorded along with the thicknesses of the left and right ventricular free walls and interventricular septum at their midpoints (points *a*, *b*, and *c*; see Figure 6-6, *A*). To facilitate comparison, heart mass was considered relative to body mass and sternal length, and myocardial thickness was considered relative to sternal length and left ventricular length. In all birds, the myocardium was found to taper toward the cardiac apex, and the interventricular septum was widest at its midpoint. There were minimal differences in myocardial thicknesses between the two species, but both the left and the right ventricles were significantly shorter relative to sternal length in Australian king parrots *(Alisterus scapularis)* compared with those in budgerigars *(Melopsittacus undulatus)*.[11]

Another study (Table 6-2) examined the hearts of healthy, wild cockatoos belonging to three species: sulfur-crested cockatoos *(Cacatua galerita)*, rose-breasted cockatoos *(Eolophus roseicapilla)*, and long-billed corellas *(Cacatua tenuirostris)*. All birds were judged to be in excellent body condition, and the hearts free of either macroscopic or histologic lesions. Body mass and sternal length, as well as heart length, width, and height (in situ), were recorded for each bird. Later, the hearts were removed, weighed, and sectioned transversely (at the level indicated by the dashed line in Figure 6-5, *B*) and the thicknesses of the left and right ventricular free walls and interventricular septum measured. The relative thickness of the left ventricular wall was found to be greater in these birds than in the captive budgerigars and Australian king parrots of the previous study; this finding was considered indicative of superior cardiac fitness. Heart mass was found to correlate

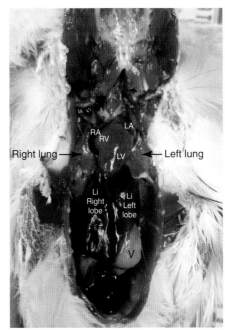

FIGURE 6-2 Heart in situ, ventral view, budgerigar *(Melopsittacus undulatus)*. Note the concave contour of the right side of the heart and the convex contour of the left side. The cardiac apex is enclosed within the left and right lobes of the liver (Li), and the left and right lungs are positioned dorsal to the heart. LA, Left atrium; LV, left ventricle; RA, right atrium; RV, right ventricle; V, ventriculus.

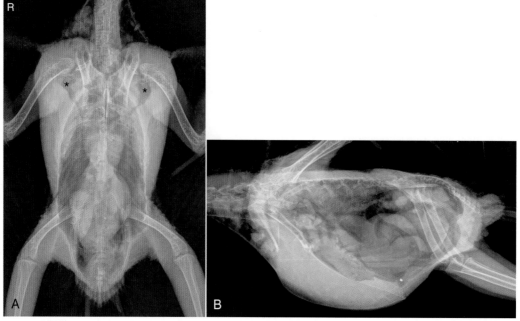

FIGURE 6-3 Digital superimposition of a latex cast of the lungs and air sacs over ventro-dorsal **(A)** and right lateral **(B)** radiographs of a medium-sized parrot, illustrating the position of these structures relative to the heart. The clavicular air sac *(blue)* occupies the cranioventral coelom, and its diverticula surround the heart and great vessels. Axillary diverticula are indicated by asterisks on the VD view. The lungs *(green)* are positioned dorsal to the heart, and the cranial thoracic air sacs *(red)* are positioned caudolaterally; caudal thoracic air sacs *(yellow)* and the abdominal air sacs *(magenta)* are also shown.

closely with body mass such that expected heart mass can be estimated by the following equation:

$$Heart\ mass\ (g) = 2.9 + 0.01 \times body\ mass\ (g)^{12}$$

The atria likely function principally as reservoirs for each ventricle rather than as active contributors to ventricular pressure.[2] They are separated from the ventricles externally by the fat-filled coronary groove and the main coronary arteries, and internally by fibrous rings (cardiac skeleton), which are well developed at the origin of the aorta, the pulmonary artery, and the right atrioventricular (AV) orifice.[6] A cardiac cartilage, sometimes mineralized, is present in the fibrous rings around the aorta[13] and the pulmonary arteries. The atrial muscle is composed of muscular bundles.[6] The right atrium is generally larger than the left and possesses a tubular recess (recessus sinister atrii dextri), which extends to the left dorsally to the aortic root.[4,5] Paired cranial venae cavae and the single caudal vena cava empty into the right atrium. In some species (e.g., chickens, crows, ostriches, kiwis), a sinus venosus is present, as in lower vertebrates, prior to the right atrium. It is not fully incorporated into its wall and presents a thin sinoatrial (SA) valve composed of two valvules. It receives blood from the caudal vena cava and the right cranial vena cava and is separated from the opening of the left cranial vena cava by the septum sinus venosi.[1,4] The left and right pulmonary veins open into the left atrium either separately (as in the domestic fowl) or combined into a common pulmonary vein outside the heart. In the fowl, the veins coalesce within the left atrium into a single vessel, whose opening protrudes into the left atrium and is guarded by the valve of the pulmonary vein.[1,14]

The left AV (mitral) valve is membranous and tricuspid (although the cusps are poorly defined) and is attached to papillary muscles via chordae tendineae (Figure 6-7). These are lacking in the right AV valve, which is unique to birds in that it consists of a spiral muscular flap composed of both atrial myocardium and ventricular myocardium (see Figures 6-4, *E*, and 6-6, *A* and *B*). This valve is also connected to the roof of the right ventricle by a muscle bundle and to the interventricular septum by a small and narrow membrane.[1,2,6] The closure mechanism of the right AV valve is poorly understood but is probably partially active, with contraction of the valve closing the AV orifice at the beginning of ventricular systole.[2] The pulmonary and aortic valves are composed of three semilunar cusps each, which are more rigid in the aortic valve (see Figures 6-6, *B* and 6-8).[1,2,10] The aortic valve is located at the root of the ascending aorta where, in contrast to mammals, a complete sphincterlike ring of myocardium is present; upon contraction, it may regulate left ventricular outflow and assist in closure of the rigid valvular cusps.[1,2]

Avian cardiomyocytes are smaller and more numerous than mammalian ones. Their large surface area relative to volume eliminates the need for transverse (T-)tubules, which, in the mammal, are invaginations of the sarcolemma essential in excitation–contraction coupling. A T-tubule system is therefore lacking in avian cardiomyocytes, where contacts between the sarcolemma and the sarcoplasmic reticulum occur instead at the cell surface. Also lacking are M-bands that connect myosin filaments in mammalian cardiac muscle.[1,2] The physiologic significance of these differences on the conduction velocity and the contractile properties of avian cardiomyocytes is poorly understood.[2]

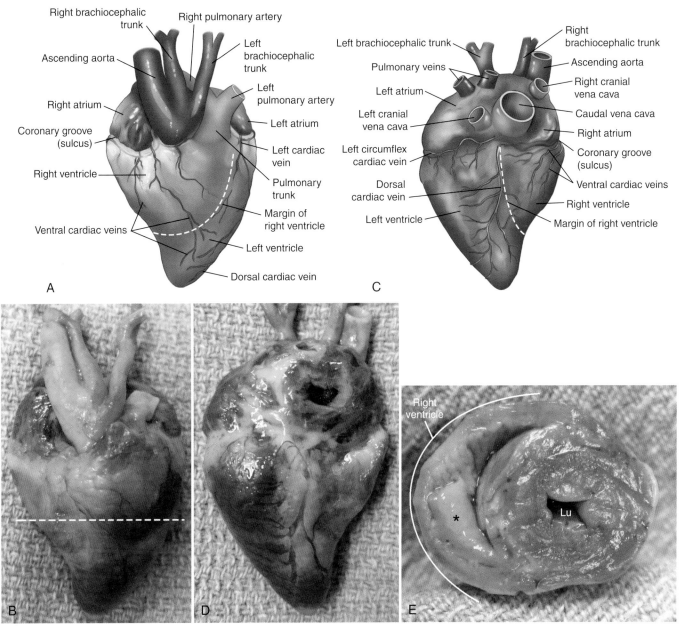

FIGURE 6-4 Heart of the domestic fowl *(Gallus gallus domesticus)*. **A** and **B,** Schematic representation and photograph of the ventral surface. **C** and **D,** The dorsal surface. Note: There is abundant coronary fat in this overconditioned hen. The opening of the left cranial vena cava is not visible in the dissection. **E,** Transverse section of the heart through the ventricles *(at the level of the dashed line in* **B***)* demonstrating the thick-walled left ventricle partially encircled by the thinner-walled right ventricle. The partially transected right atrioventricular valve *(asterisk)* is visible. Lu, Lumen.

Cardiac conduction system

The cardiac conduction system (Figure 6-9) of birds bears a close resemblance to that of mammals, consisting of the SA node, the AV node, and the bundle of His and its bundle branches. However, there are three bundle branches (left, right, and middle) and, unique to birds, an AV ring of Purkinje fibers surrounding the right AV opening and connecting to the muscular right AV valve. A figure-of-eight is formed as the middle bundle branch passes around the aorta and joins the AV ring. In the domestic fowl, the SA node lies between the openings of the right cranial and caudal venae cavae into the right atrium, and its pacemaker cells set the heart rate. The wave of excitation initiated in the SA node propagates through the atrial muscle and is transmitted to the ventricles via the AV node, which gives rise to the Purkinje fibers of the AV ring, the bundle of His, and the bundle branches. The location of the AV node is a subject of some debate but is most likely located at the right base of the interatrial septum. Left and right bundle branches emerge from the interventricular septum to supply the left and right

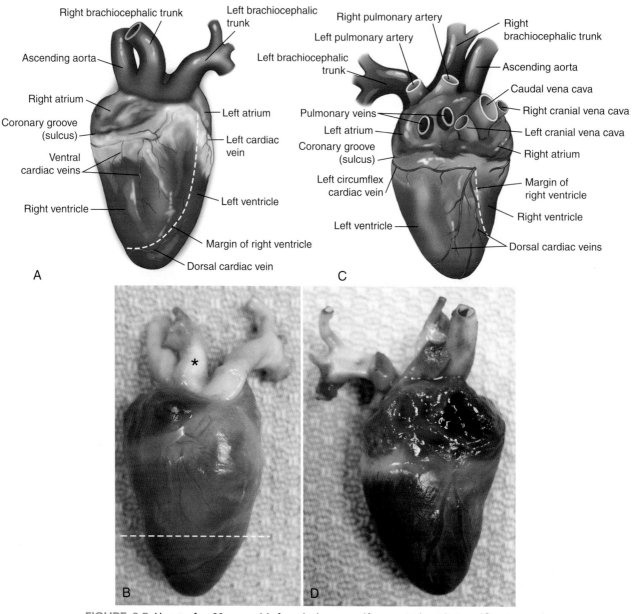

FIGURE 6-5 Heart of a 29-year-old, female lesser sulfur-crested cockatoo *(Cacatua sulphurea)*. **A** and **B**, Schematic representation and photograph of the ventral surface. **C** and **D**, The dorsal surface. Note: Yellow discoloration of the brachiocephalic trunks *(most notably the right, indicated by an asterisk)* reflects atherosclerotic lesions partially obstructing the lumen. The openings of the cranial venae cavae cannot be distinguished from that of the caudal vena cava in the dissection.

ventricles, following the tracts of the coronary arteries into the myocardium (periarterial Purkinje fibers).[1,2] Ventricular depolarization begins subepicardially and spreads through the myocardium to the endocardial surface, whereas the reverse is true in mammals; thus, the polarity of the major component of the electrocardiogram is negative in lead II.[2,15]

Pericardium

The heart is enclosed within a fibrous, relatively noncompliant pericardial sac (Figure 6-10), which normally contains a very small volume of serous fluid that serves to lubricate the movement of the heart within the pericardial sac. The outer fibrous layer of the pericardium is continuous with the adventitia of the great vessels, and attachments exist between the pericardium and the sternal plate, the hilus of the lungs, the adjacent air sacs, and the liver.[1,2,10,14,16] The last of these attachments is via the hepatopericardial ligament, which is continuous with the ventral mesentery caudally.[13,11] The heart is thereby well anchored within the cranioventral coelom (pericardial coelom) and its apex between the liver lobes and hepatic coelomic cavities.[1,2,10]

Vascular Anatomy

Coronary arteries and cardiac veins

The aorta is derived embryologically from the fourth aortic arch, and, unlike in mammals, the ascending aorta

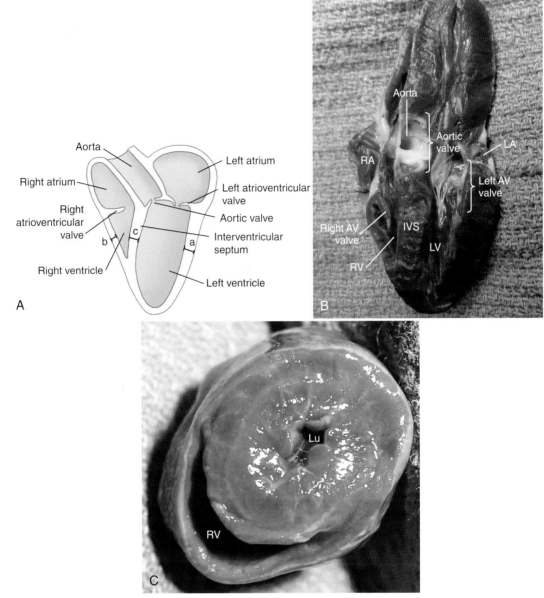

FIGURE 6-6 A, Schematic longitudinal section of the avian heart (a, b, c = points of measurement for myocardial thickness of the left ventricle, right ventricle, and interventricular septum, respectively, used to calculate ratios in Table 6-1, *B*). **B,** Longitudinal section of the heart of a hyacinth macaw *(Anodorhynchus hyacinthinus)* showing the left atrium (LA), left ventricle (LV), left atrioventricular (AV) valve, right atrium (RA), right ventricle (RV), muscular right AV valve, interventricular septum (IVS), aorta, and aortic valve. **C,** Heart of a military macaw *(Ara militaris)* sectioned transversely through the ventricles. The right ventricle (RV) is thin-walled and encircles approximately 50% of the left ventricle. Lu, Lumen. **(A,** Modified from: Pees M, Straub J, Krautwald-Junghanns M-E: Echocardiographic examinations of 60 African grey parrots and 30 other psittacine birds, *Vet Rec* 155(3):73–76, 2004; and Straub J, Valerius KP, Pees M, et al: Morphometry of the heart of budgerigars *(Melopsittacus undulatus)*, Alisterus parrots *(Alisterus s scapularis)* and common buzzards *(Buteo buteo)*, *Res Vet Sci* 72:147–151, 2002.)

curves to the right (Figure 6-11). It immediately gives rise to the left and right coronary arteries to supply the heart (see Figure 6-9). Each branches into a superficial and deep ramus near its origin; the superficial branches occupy the coronary groove, and the deep arteries provide most of the blood supply to the myocardium.[1,2,4,6] The right coronary artery is the largest in most species, and the coronary arteries anastomose frequently.[1] Blood is returned to the right atrium through several cardiac veins, most of which lie subepicardially and are externally visible (see Figures 6-4 and 6-5). These include the left cardiac vein, the right (or ventral) cardiac veins, the middle (or dorsal) cardiac

TABLE 6-1A

Mean ± Standard Deviation and Range (in parentheses) of Heart Mass, Heart Mass-to-Body Mass Ratio, and Ratios of the Left Ventricle (LV) Length to Sternal Length, Right Ventricle (RV) Length to Sternal Length, and LV Length to RV Length, for Healthy Individuals of Two Psittacine Species

	Budgerigar *(Melopsittacus undulatus)* (n = 14)	Australian King Parrot *(Alisterus scapularis)* (n = 5)
Heart mass (grams)	0.65 ± 0.1 (0.38–0.83)	1.62 ± 0.26 (1.24–1.94)
Heart mass to body mass (%)	1.5 ± 0.15 (1.2–1.8)	1.36 ± 0.18 (1.18–1.62)
LV length to sternal length (%)	38.3 ± 4.3 (29.7–45.6)	34.0 ± 3.9 (29.4–37.2)
RV length to sternal length (%)	29.9 ± 3.1 (25.3–34.5)	26.6 ± 3.1 (22.6–30.0)
LV length to RV length (%)	76.1 ± 5.2 (69.5–85.2)	78.2 ± 5.5 (69.9–84.9)

From Straub J, Valerius KP, Pees M, et al: Morphometry of the heart of budgerigars *(Melopsittacus undulatus)*, Alisterus parrots *(Alisterus s scapularis)* and common buzzards *(Buteo buteo)*, *Res Vet Sci* 2002;72:147–151.

TABLE 6-1B

Mean ± Standard Deviation of Midpoint Thickness of the Left Ventricle (LV) Free Wall, Right Ventricle (RV) Free Wall, and Interventricular Septum (IVS) Relative to Sternal Length and to LV Length for Healthy Individuals of Two Psittacine Species

	Budgerigar *(Melopsittacus undulatus)* (n = 14)	Australian King Parrot *(Alisterus scapularis)* (n = 5)
Thickness of LV free wall to sternal length (%)	8.7 ± 1.4	8.3 ± 1.6
Thickness of LV free wall to LV length (%)	23.9 ± 4.3	24.5 ± 5.3
Thickness of RV free wall to sternal length (%)	2.4 ± 0.6	2.2 ± 0.5
Thickness of RV free wall to LV length (%)	6.7 ± 1.7	6.5 ± 1.9
Thickness of IVS to sternal length (%)	7.3 ± 1.1	7.8 ± 1.4
Thickness of IVS to LV length (%)	18.8 ± 3.0	23.5 ± 6.7

From Straub J, Valerius KP, Pees M, et al: Morphometry of the heart of budgerigars *(Melopsittacus undulatus)*, Alisterus parrots *(Alisterus s scapularis)* and common buzzards *(Buteo buteo)*, *Res Vet Sci* 72:147–151, 2002.

TABLE 6-2

Mean ± Standard Deviation and Range (in parentheses) of Body Mass, Sternal Length, Heart Mass, Heart Width, Length, and Height in Situ, and Thickness of the Left Ventricle (LV) Free Wall, Right Ventricle (RV) Free Wall, and Interventricular Septum (IVS) for Healthy Individuals of Three Cockatoo Species

	Sulfur-Crested Cockatoo *(Cacatua galerita)* (n = 50)	Rose-Breasted Cockatoo *(Eolophus roseicapilla)* (n = 31)	Long-Billed Corella *(Cacatua tenuirostris)* (n = 3)
Body mass (g)	881.2 ±77.5 (648-1086)	368.9 ± 29.5 (307-437)	599.7 ± 63.3 (527-643)
Sternal length (mm)	73.4 ± 4.0 (63-82)	63.8 ± 2.2 (59-68)	66.7 ± 4.2 (62-70)
Heart mass (g)	8.7 ± 0.9 (5.8-11.0)	5.3 ± 0.5 (4.1-6.1)	8.6 ± 0.9 (7.6-9.3)
Heart width in situ (mm)	24.8 ± 1.9 (21.8-29.2)	20.0 ± 1.8 (17.7-27.3)	25.6 ± 2.0 (23.3-26.8)
Heart length in situ (mm)	31.0 ± 2.7 (23.9-39.4)	26.0 ± 2.2 (19.5-30.3)	32.9 ± 1.7 (31.8-34.8)
Heart height in situ (mm)	19.8 ± 2.2 (16.3-28.9)	16.0 ± 0.9 (14.1-18.0)	20.9 ± 1.3 (19.8-22.3)
Thickness of LV free wall (mm)	7.2 ± 0.7 (5.6-9.0)	6.6 ± 0.7 (5.3-8.3)	6.6 ± 0.5 (6.0-6.9)
Thickness of RV free wall (mm)	1.7 ± 0.3 (1.0-2.5)	1.5 ± 0.3 (0.9-1.9)	2.0 ± 0.17 (1.9-2.2)
Thickness of IVS (mm)	5.8 ± 0.8 (3.6-7.0)	6.4 ± 0.5 (4.3-6.0)	6.0 ± 0.1 (5.9-6.0)

Note: Heart width and height were measured at the level of the coronary sulcus and heart length from the coronary sulcus to the cardiac apex.
From Pees M, Zeh C, Filippich LJ, et al: Pathologisch-anatomische und morphometrische Untersuchungen am Herzen von wildlebenden Kakadus, *Tierärztliche Praxis Kleintiere* 6:300 306, 2014.

vein, and the left circumflex cardiac vein, the last two being largest.[1,4]

Ascending aorta—supply of the head, neck, and thoracic limbs

Following the coronary arteries, large, paired brachiocephalic trunks branch simultaneously from the ascending aorta (see Figure 6-11). These supply the large flight muscles through the subclavian arteries and are therefore larger than the aorta in many species of birds (including Psittaciformes)[13] (Figure 6-12, *A*); this is not so in the domestic fowl (see Figure 6-12, *B*). Each divides into common carotid and subclavian arteries. The common carotid arteries provide all of the blood supply to the head and neck, dividing into

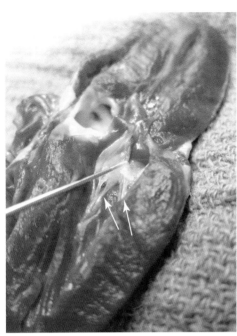

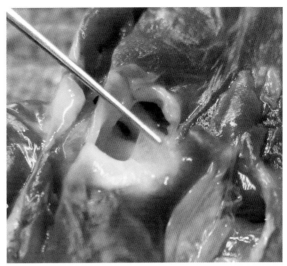

FIGURE 6-8 Longitudinal section of the heart of a hyacinth macaw *(Anodorhynchus hyacinthinus)* showing detail of the aortic valve with one of the three cusps elevated by the pointer.

FIGURE 6-7 Longitudinal section of the heart of a hyacinth macaw *(Anodorhynchus hyacinthinus)* showing the left atrioventricular valve (cusp elevated by a pointer) and chordae tendineae *(arrows)*.

internal carotid and vertebral arteries (see Figure 6-11), which ascend the neck and form numerous anastomoses. Among psittacine species, there is great variability in the arrangement of the internal carotid arteries. In some species (e.g., the cockatiel *[Nymphicus hollandicus]* and the budgerigar *[Melopsittacus undulatus]*), both the left and right internal

carotid arteries supply the head, whereas in others (e.g., the Grey parrot *[Psittacus erithacus]*, the Amazon parrots *[Amazona* spp.], the *Ara* macaws, and the *Aratinga* and *Pyrrhura* conures), this supply is provided only by the right internal carotid artery. Alternatively, the left internal carotid provides the great majority (in the lesser sulfur-crested cockatoo *[Cacatua sulphurea sulphurea]*) or entirety (in the greater sulfur-crested cockatoo *[Cacatua galerita galerita]* and the citron-crested cockatoo *[Cacatua sulphurea citrinocristata]*) of the blood supply to the head. Even in such unicarotid

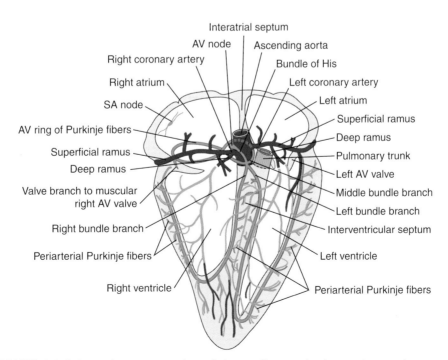

FIGURE 6-9 Schematic representation of the cardiac conduction system and coronary arteries. Cardiac conductive tissue is depicted in green and coronary arteries in red *(deep portions shaded)*.

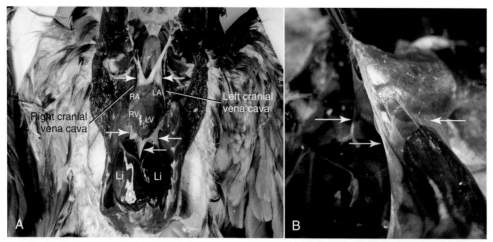

FIGURE 6-10 Pericardium and its attachments to adjacent structures *(arrows; the hepatopericardial ligament is indicated by the yellow arrow)*. **A,** Ventral view, Grey parrot *(Psittacus erithacus)*. **B,** Caudoventral view with fenestration made in the pericardium at the cardiac apex, scarlet macaw *(Ara macao)*. LA, Left atrium; LV, left ventricle; RA, right atrium; RV, right ventricle; Li, liver.

species, the internal carotid divides into left and right branches near the base of the skull, which go on to form an intercarotid anastomosis at the base of the brain. This anastomosis, present in virtually all species of birds, provides the collateral circulation afforded by the cerebral arterial circle of Willis in mammals. The left and right subclavian arteries supply the thoracic limbs and flight muscles, each giving off the pectoral trunk before continuing as the axillary artery. The axillary artery becomes the brachial artery, whose branches include the radial and ulnar arteries, which ultimately give rise to the metacarpal and digital arteries.[1,2,4]

Descending aorta—supply of the trunk, viscera, and pelvic limbs

In addition to paired intercostal and segmental synsacral arteries, the descending aorta gives off the following major branches (see Figures 6-11 and 6-13): the coeliac artery; the cranial mesenteric artery; the paired cranial renal, external iliac, and ischiatic arteries; the caudal mesenteric artery; and the internal iliac arteries. It terminates as the median caudal artery. In the male, testicular arteries arise from the cranial renal arteries, and in the female single or multiple ovarian arteries arise from either the left cranial renal artery or directly from the aorta. The middle and caudal renal arteries are branches of the ischiatic arteries. The pelvic limbs are supplied by the external iliac arteries (which continue into the thigh as the femoral arteries) and the larger ischiatic arteries, which continue as the popliteal and cranial tibial arteries before giving rise to the metatarsal and digital arteries (see Figure 6-11). Major branches of the descending aorta and tissues supplied by each are listed in Table 6-3.[1,2,4]

Pulmonary vasculature

The pulmonary trunk arises from the right ventricle and splits into right and left pulmonary arteries (Figure 6-14, *A*). These enter the lungs, along with the pulmonary veins and the primary bronchi, at the hilus (see Figure 6-14, *B*). The pulmonary arteries then divide into numerous interparabronchial arteries, which, in turn, give rise to the intraparabronchial

arterioles. These terminate in the extensive blood capillary network that interfaces with the air capillaries, where gas exchange occurs.[1,2,8,10]

Venous system

Cranial to the heart, the two cranial venae cavae receive blood from the jugular veins (draining the head and neck) and the subclavian veins (draining the thoracic limbs and pectoral region) (see Figures 6-1, 6-10, 6-12, and 6-14). In most species, the right jugular vein is larger than the left jugular vein and also receives blood from the left via an anastomosis at the base of the head.[1,2,4] Caudal to the heart, the caudal vena cava receives blood from the large left and right hepatic veins (see Figure 6-1) and the smaller middle hepatic veins. More caudally, the large common iliac veins drain the kidneys via the cranial and caudal renal veins. The common iliac veins are also joined by the external iliac veins draining the pelvic limbs (Figure 6-15).[1,4]

Renal portal system. An important peculiarity of the avian venous system is the renal portal system, which constitutes a ring formed by the cranial and caudal renal portal veins ventral to the kidneys (see Figure 6-15). The portal ring receives blood from the gut and the pelvic region (including the legs) through the external iliac veins, the ischiatic veins, the internal iliac veins, and the caudal mesenteric vein. This portal blood then passes through the renal parenchyma, mixing with postglomerular efferent arteriolar blood, before returning to the common iliac veins and the caudal vena cava via the renal veins. The proportion of venous blood that enters the kidney tissue depends on the action of the renal portal valve—a smooth muscle sphincter, with both sympathetic and parasympathetic innervation, that lies within each common iliac vein. Under sympathetic stimulation, the valves relax and open, diverting blood directly to the common iliac veins and the caudal vena cava, thereby bypassing the kidney tissue and increasing venous return directly to the heart. The venous flow may also be shunted into the internal vertebral venous sinus or to the hepatic portal system through the caudal mesenteric vein where flow can be bidirectional.[1,2,4,5]

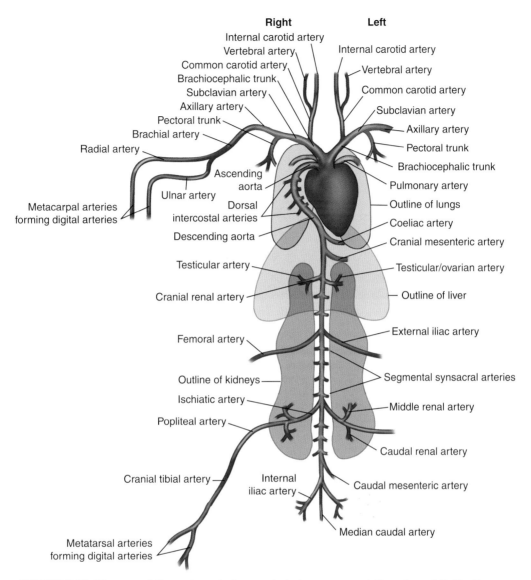

Right **Left**

Internal carotid artery
Vertebral artery
Common carotid artery
Brachiocephalic trunk
Subclavian artery
Axillary artery
Pectoral trunk
Brachial artery
Radial artery

Ascending aorta
Ulnar artery
Dorsal intercostal arteries
Descending aorta

Metacarpal arteries forming digital arteries

Testicular artery

Cranial renal artery

Femoral artery

Outline of kidneys

Ischiatic artery

Popliteal artery

Cranial tibial artery

Internal iliac artery

Metatarsal arteries forming digital arteries

Internal carotid artery
Vertebral artery
Common carotid artery
Subclavian artery
Axillary artery
Pectoral trunk
Brachiocephalic trunk
Pulmonary artery
Outline of lungs
Coeliac artery
Cranial mesenteric artery
Testicular/ovarian artery
Outline of liver
External iliac artery
Segmental synsacral arteries
Middle renal artery
Caudal renal artery
Caudal mesenteric artery
Median caudal artery

FIGURE 6-11 Diagram of the major arteries, ventral view, representative of most Psittaciformes (arrangement of internal carotid arteries reflects that of bicarotid species, for example, the cockatiel *[Nymphicus hollandicus]*). (Modified from King AS, McLelland J: Cardiovascular system. In King AS, McLelland J, editors: *Birds—their structure and function*, ed 2, London, UK, 1984, BaillièreTindall, pp 214–228; and Smith FM, West NH, Jones DR: The cardiovascular system. In Whittow GC, editor: *Sturkie's avian physiology*, ed 5, San Diego, CA, 2000, Academic Press, pp 141–231.)

Vascular microanatomy

Structurally the arteries can be classified into the elastic arteries, consisting of the aortic arch, the thoracic aorta up to the coeliac artery, the brachiocephalic trunks, and the extrapulmonary portions of the pulmonary arteries, with the muscular arteries comprising the remainder of the arterial system.[2,5] The elastic arteries act as a pressure reservoir redistributing the pulsatile input over time by expansion and recoil. These arteries expand smoothly over a range of pressure allowed by the compliance of elastin and the stiffness of collagen. The resilience of avian elastic arteries (ratio of the energy recovered to the energy needed to expand the vessel) is superior to that in mammals.[2] The walls of elastic arteries are composed of three layers: (1) the tunica intima, which is a single-cell layer of endothelial cells adjacent to the arterial lumen; (2) the tunica media, which is composed of concentric layers of collagen and elastic fibers composed of smooth muscle cells and elastin; and (3) the tunica adventitia, which is an outer layer of collagen fibers and connective tissue (Figure 6-16).[2,17] The intima is separated from the media by a poorly defined internal elastic lamina, which is itself separated from the adventitia by the external elastic lamina.[5,17] Muscular arteries have the same three tunicae, but the media is only composed of smooth muscle cells and elastin, and the adventitia is much thicker and has less compliance.[2]

Venous walls have the same organization as arterial walls, with a tunica intima, a tunica media, and a tunica adventitia.

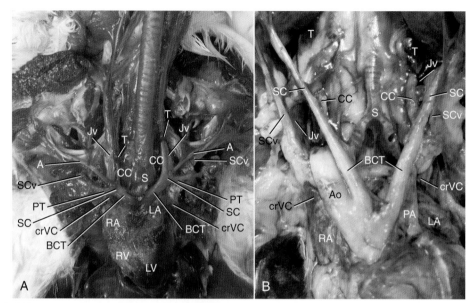

FIGURE 6-12 Major arteries and veins of the cervicothoracic region, ventral view, Moluccan cockatoo *(Cacatua moluccensis)* **(A)** in comparison with the domestic fowl *(Gallus gallus domesticus)* **(B)**. Note: In the cockatoo, discoloration of the venous structures and right heart is an artifact of euthanasia solution (pentobarbital sodium/phenytoin sodium) administered intravenously (right jugular vein). A, Axillary artery; Ao, ascending aorta; BCT, brachiocephalic trunk; CC, common carotid artery; crVC, cranial vena cava; Jv, jugular vein; LA, left atrium; LV, left ventricle; PA, pulmonary artery; PT, pectoral trunk (with a portion of pectoral musculature attached); RA, right atrium; RV, right ventricle; S, syrinx; SC, subclavian artery; SCv, subclavian vein; T, thyroid gland.

TABLE 6-3

Major Branches of the Descending Aorta and the Tissues Supplied

Coeliac artery	Liver, spleen, proventriculus, ventriculus, pancreas, portion of the intestine
Cranial mesenteric artery	Majority of the intestine, pancreas
Cranial renal arteries	Kidneys (cranial division), testes, ovary, oviduct (infundibulum, magnum)
External iliac arteries	Legs, oviduct (magnum)
Ischiatic arteries	Kidneys (middle and caudal divisions), legs, oviduct (magnum, uterus)
Caudal mesenteric artery	Rectum, cloaca
Internal iliac arteries	Pelvic walls, oviduct (uterus, vagina)
Median caudal artery	Tail

However, their walls are thinner, have less muscle tissue in the media, and have more connective tissue in the adventitia. Veins are capacitance vessels and contain about 60% to 80% of the total blood volume.[2]

Cardiovascular Control Systems

Systemic arterial blood pressure is a function of cardiac output and the resistance of the arterial system (Figure 6-17). Cardiac output is the product of heart rate and stroke volume; the former is set by the SA node, and the latter is determined by the inherent contractility of the cardiomyocytes, preload, and afterload. Preload is the end-diastolic volume of the ventricle that acts to stretch the myocardial fibers. Up to a point, increases in preload increase contractility by stretching the fibers to optimal precontraction length (Frank-Starling mechanism). Afterload is the resistance of the vasculature to ventricular ejection that increases ventricular wall stress, myocardial energy expenditure, and myocardial oxygen consumption. Afterload is determined by (1) impedance of the proximal aorta itself, (2) compliance (distensibility) of the elastic arteries, and (3) peripheral resistance to blood flow afforded primarily by small arteries and arterioles. The characteristic impedance of the proximal aorta increases with increased aortic stiffness and decreased radius, resulting in greater left ventricular afterload. Decreased compliance of elastic arteries, as well as increases in peripheral resistance (occurring with decreases in vessel radius), further contribute to afterload.[2,18]

Diastolic function has been minimally studied in birds but is presumed to be similar to that in mammals.[19] Diastolic performance (lusitropy) is a product of myocardial relaxation, which is an active process under autonomic control,[20] and ventricular compliance, which is a passive process dependent on the ability of the ventricular wall to distend. Compliance is subject to ventricular volume, geometry, and tissue characteristics. Ventricular filling is also determined by the AV pressure gradient, which is contingent on intravascular volume and peripheral vasodilation.[18]

Cardiac output and vascular resistance are regulated by a combination of neural, endocrine, and autoregulatory control

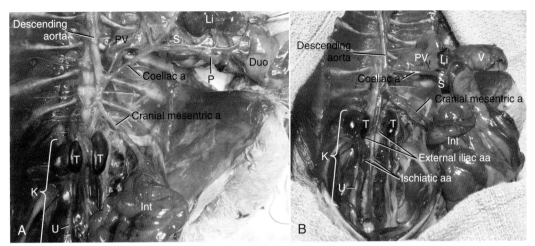

FIGURE 6-13 A and **B,** Descending aorta and branches, ventral view, Moluccan cockatoo *(Cacatua moluccensis)*. Note: The cranial renal arteries are not visible in these dissections. Duo, Duodenum; Int, intestine; K, kidney; Li, liver (partial); P, pancreas (splenic head); PV, proventriculus (partial); S, spleen; T, testis; U, ureter; V, ventriculus.

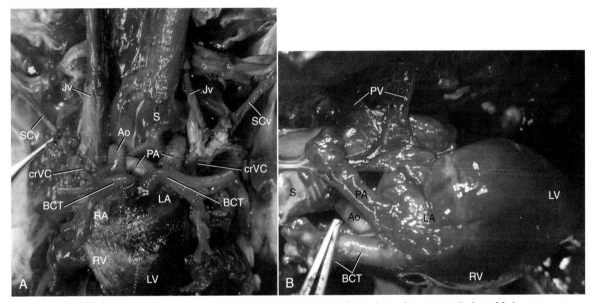

FIGURE 6-14 A, Major arteries and veins of the cervicothoracic region, ventral view, Moluccan cockatoo *(Cacatua moluccensis)*. The brachiocephalic trunks and their branches have been reflected ventrally to allow visibility of left and right pulmonary arteries and ascending aorta. **B,** Left pulmonary artery and veins, left lateral view, blue-fronted Amazon parrot *(Amazona aestiva)*. Note: In the cockatoo, discoloration of the venous structures, pulmonary arteries, and right heart is an artifact of euthanasia solution (pentobarbital sodium/phenytoin sodium) administered intravenously (right jugular vein). Ao, Ascending aorta; BCT, brachiocephalic trunk; crVC, cranial vena cava; Jv, jugular vein; LA, left atrium; LV, left ventricle; PA, pulmonary artery; PV, pulmonary vein; RA, right atrium; RV, right ventricle; S, syrinx; SCv, subclavian vein.

mechanisms, as well as humoral factors. The heart is innervated by both sympathetic and parasympathetic autonomic systems through the cardiac sympathetic nerve and the vagal nerve, respectively, and is also under the control of circulating catecholamines. Both epinephrine (EPI) and norepinephrine (NE) have positive inotropic, chronotropic, and lusitropic effects, acting primarily via β-adrenergic receptors. Unlike in mammals, NE is believed to be the more potent stimulant of the two. Parasympathetic activity, via acetylcholine (ACh) at cholinergic receptors, has reciprocal effects.[2,20]

In the periphery, vasoconstriction occurs by contraction of vascular smooth muscle, and it is muscle tone of the smallest arteries and arterioles that has the greatest influence on vascular resistance and alteration of blood flow.

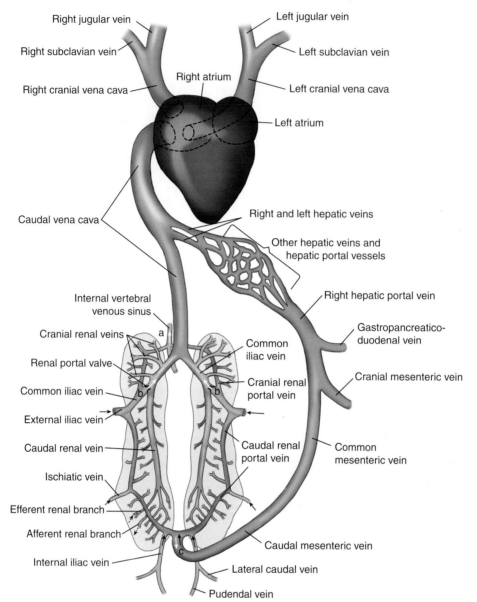

FIGURE 6-15 Diagram of the venous system including detail of the renal portal system (based on the domestic fowl [*Gallus gallus domesticus*]). Portal vessels and their afferent renal branches are shaded violet, whereas the renal veins and their efferent branches are shown in blue. Venous blood enters the portal ring through several veins *(black arrows)*; then it can (1) pass into the renal parenchyma via afferent branches, mix with postglomerular arterial blood, and enter the renal veins through their efferent branches; and/or (2) it can bypass the kidney tissue and return to the heart by various other routes *(white arrows)*: (a) the internal vertebral venous sinus, (b) the caudal vena cava via the common iliac veins and renal portal valves, or (c) caudal mesenteric vein toward the hepatic portal system. (Modified from King AS, McLelland J: Urinary system. In King AS, McLelland J, editors: *Birds—their structure and function*, ed 2, London, UK, 1984, BaillièreTindall, pp 175–186; and Sturkie PD: Heart and circulation: anatomy, hemodynamics, blood pressure, blood flow. In Sturkie PD, editor: *Avian physiology*, ed 4, New York, 1986, Springer-Verlag, pp 130–166.)

Vasoconstriction (and venoconstriction) are modulated by sympathetic tone and circulating catecholamines (EPI and NE acting via α-adrenergic receptors). Vasoconstriction is also mediated by activation of the renin–angiotensin–aldosterone system (RAAS); arginine vasotocin (AVT), which is the homolog of antidiuretic hormone in mammals;[2] and endothelin-1.[21] Vasodilation is mediated by increased parasympathetic tone. NE also has vasodilatory effects via β-adrenergic receptors, but these effects are usually secondary to α-adrenergic vasoconstriction. Nitric oxide (NO), released from vascular endothelial cells by parasympathetic activity and in response to shear stress,

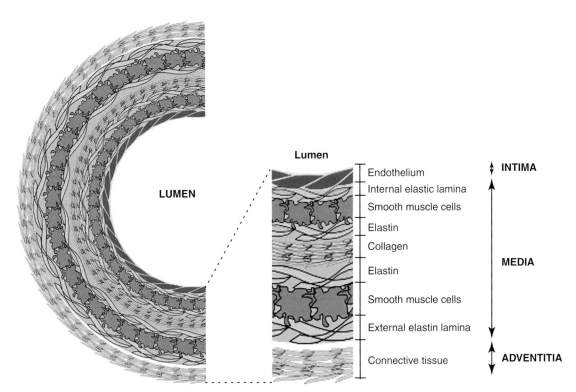

FIGURE 6-16 Schematic representation of the microanatomy of an avian elastic artery. The tunica media is composed of alternate layers of elastic laminae (smooth muscle cells between two sheets of elastin fibers) and collagen fibers.

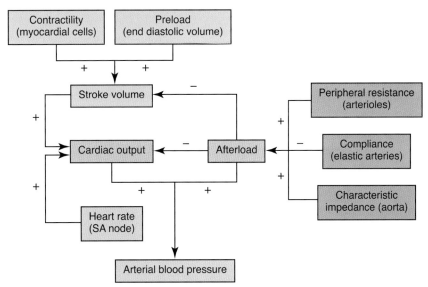

FIGURE 6-17 Factors determining arterial blood pressure. (Modified from de Morais HA, Schwartz DS: Pathophysiology of heart failure. In Ettinger SJ, Feldman EC, editors: *Textbook of veterinary internal medicine*, ed 6, St. Louis, MO, 2005, Saunders, pp 914–940.)

also effects vasodilation. Chemical factors, namely, increases in carbon dioxide and lactic acid levels and decreases in pH and oxygen levels, directly promote vasodilation to increase blood flow (functional hyperemia), oxygen delivery, and clearance of tissue metabolites when tissue metabolic rate increases or tissue ischemia occurs.[22]

CLINICAL DISEASE STATES

Atherosclerosis

Atherosclerosis is a chronic inflammatory and degenerative disease of the arterial wall, wherein the lumen narrows by progressive accumulation of inflammatory cells, fat, cholesterol, calcium, and cellular debris that forms fibrofatty atheromatous plaques within the intima. Potential complications include stenosis, ischemia, thrombosis, hemorrhage, and aneurysm.[23-25] Atherosclerosis is likely an underlying factor in the majority of noninfectious cardiovascular diseases diagnosed in pet birds and is undoubtedly the most common lesion of the cardiovascular system identified at postmortem examination in companion psittacine birds (Figure 6-18).

Pathophysiology

The etiology and development of atherosclerotic lesions can be broadly explained by the response-to-injury hypothesis, which postulates that damage to the endothelium lining the artery sets the stage for atherogenesis. Lesion formation involves endothelial dysfunction, damage, and oxidative stress, which promote increased endothelial permeability to lipoproteins and intimal adherence and migration of inflammatory cells (particularly monocytes). Subendothelial accumulation of lipoproteins, particularly oxidized low-density lipoproteins (LDL), further attracts monocytes, which, once within the subintimal space, differentiate into macrophages, internalize lipoproteins, and store cholesterol, thereby becoming foam cells. These cells eventually die by necrosis or apoptosis, resulting in further accumulation of extracellular lipid and necrotic debris. In this way, the process of intimal lipid accumulation, chemoattraction of macrophages, and formation of foam cells drives the progression of the atherosclerotic lesion and the eventual development of a necrotic core. Smooth muscle cells play a significant role in lesion development by proliferating and migrating into the intima and subintimal space and producing extracellular matrix components (including collagen and elastic fibers). This accounts for the formation of fibrous tissue, which, in advanced lesions, further enlarges the lesion and creates a fibrous cap overlying the lipid and necrotic core. Smooth muscle cells also accumulate cholesterol and become foam cells.[23-25]

Lesion characterization

In psittacines, lesions are characterized by accumulation of the components discussed above in the intima and luminal side of the vascular media (Figure 6-19). Lesions can be classified into seven types (I to VII); types I and II are considered early lesions (minimal changes characterized by increased numbers of foam cells, limited extracellular lipids

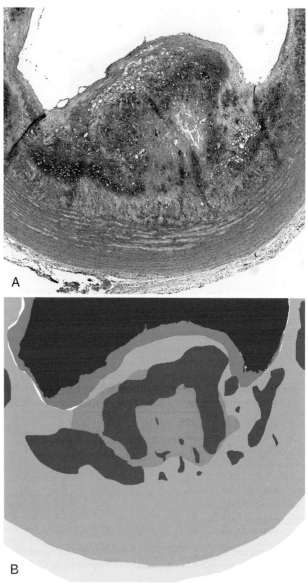

A

B

FIGURE 6-19 **A,** Calcific fibroatheroma (type V lesion) in the brachiocephalic trunk of an Amazon parrot (*Amazona* spp.). **B,** Schematic depiction of lesion composition. Red, arterial lumen; green, fibrous cap; gray, lipid; orange, lipidonecrotic core; blue, calcification; pink, normal tunica media; yellow, normal tunica adventitia. (From Beaufrere H: Avian atherosclerosis: parrots and beyond, *JEPM* 22(4):336–347, 2013.)

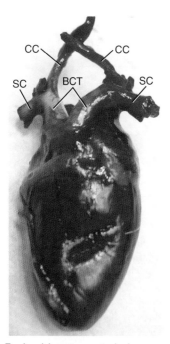

FIGURE 6-18 Excised heart, ventral view, peach-faced lovebird *(Agapornis roseicollis)* with advanced atherosclerosis of the brachiocephalic trunks (BCT), common carotid arteries (CC), and subclavian arteries (SC).

and calcium, and no disruption of arterial wall architecture), type III intermediate (with mild architectural disruption), and types IV to VII advanced (formation of a fibroatheromatous plaque by accumulation of lipid and cellular debris). Lesion type VI is distinguished from IV and V by the additional complication of fissure, hematoma, or thrombosis. Lesion type VII is a calcific lesion characterized by large calcium plaques and osseous metaplasia. Clinical signs are attributed to advanced lesions, whereas early and intermediate lesions are generally silent and subclinical. Unlike in humans, recognizable clinical disease is primarily the product of progressive, flow-limiting arterial stenosis, rather than that of thrombosis and hemorrhage of disrupted plaques, that results in thromboembolism and acute arterial obstruction. The difference is likely accounted for by the inability of the avian thrombocyte to form shear-resistant arterial thrombi and three-dimensional aggregates. Acute myocardial infarction is less likely in avian species than in humans because of the differences in avian coronary vasculature and the greater collateral circulation compared with that in humans.[23-25] In one study, advanced lesions were commonly characterized by severe arterial stenosis and occlusion, but atherothrombotic lesions, aortic dissection and rupture, and lesional hemorrhage were identified rarely (in 1.9% of lesions).[26]

Lesion location

Atherosclerotic lesions are most frequently recognized in the ascending aorta, brachiocephalic trunks, and pulmonary arteries (Figures 6-20 and 6-21). Although not as often appreciated, lesions also appear in peripheral vasculature, most notably the coronary arteries (Figure 6-22), carotid arteries, and descending aorta (Figures 6-23 and 6-24), as well as the subclavian arteries, coeliac artery (see Figure 6-24), and ischiatic arteries.[24,27,28] Coronary and aortic aneurysms have been known to arise secondary to atherosclerosis as a result of the decreased compliance of the affected vessels compared with normal elastic arteries.[24] A large coronary aneurysm developed secondary to coronary atherosclerosis in an umbrella cockatoo (*Cacatua alba*)[29] and an aortic aneurysm with severe atherosclerosis was reported in an Alexandrine parakeet (*Psittacula eupatria*).[30]

Prevalence and risk factors

Reported prevalence of atherosclerosis in psittacines varies widely (1.9% to 91.8%), with the highest recently reported among Amazons and Grey parrots (*Amazona* spp. and *Psittacus erithacus*, respectively).[24] The wide range of reported prevalence likely reflects the variations among studies in pathologic inclusion criteria, lesion severity, geographic areas, demographics, captive conditions, psittacine species, and the retrospective or prospective nature of the work. Most recently, prevalence and epidemiology of clinically relevant atherosclerotic lesions (types IV to VI) were investigated by review of over 7600 psittacine cases representing five genera. An overall prevalence of 6.8% was reported, but a significantly higher prevalence of advanced lesions was found among Grey parrots (having 275% the odds compared with other genera), Amazon parrots (having 183% the odds), and cockatiels (*Nymphicus hollandicus*) (having 146% the odds); cockatoos (*Cacatua* spp.) and macaws (*Ara* spp.) appeared less susceptible (Figure 6-25). There was a positive association between advanced atherosclerosis and increasing age, female sex, reproductive disease (predominately female), hepatic disease, and concurrent myocardial fibrosis.[26] These findings are subjectively consistent with the author's (BCF) experience in practice, where severe atherosclerosis is most often encountered in Grey and Amazon parrots over 20 years of age, followed by cockatiels, lovebirds (*Agapornis*

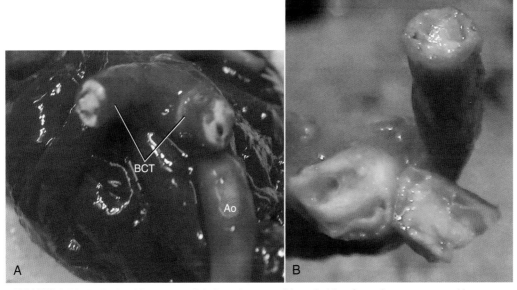

FIGURE 6-20 A, Excised heart, cranial view, 24-year-old, male blue-front Amazon parrot *(Amazona aestiva)* with advanced atherosclerosis of the ascending aorta (Ao) and brachiocephalic trunks (BCT). **B,** Detail of brachiocephalic trunks *(right sectioned longitudinally)* of the Amazon parrot demonstrating profound luminal stenosis.

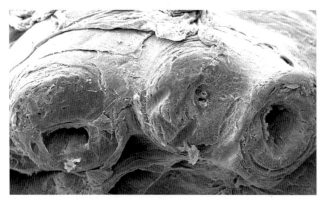

FIGURE 6-21 Scanning electron micrograph of advanced atherosclerosis and luminal stenosis of the ascending aorta and brachiocephalic trunks in a Quaker parrot *(Myiopsitta monachus).*

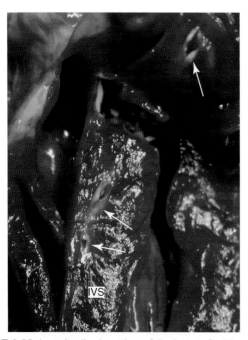

FIGURE 6-22 Longitudinal section of the heart of a 30-year-old, female military macaw *(Ara militaris)* showing atherosclerosis of an intramural coronary artery *(arrows)* in the interventricular septum (IVS).

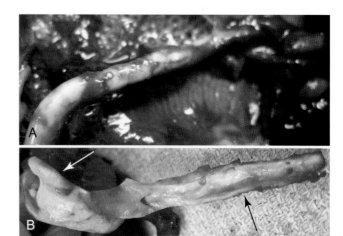

FIGURE 6-23 A, Advanced atherosclerosis of the descending aorta *(left lateral view)* in a 24-year-old, male blue-front Amazon parrot *(Amazona aestiva).* **B,** The ascending *(white arrow)* and descending *(black arrow)* aorta *(longitudinal section)* in a 28-year-old, male Grey parrot *(Psittacus erithacus).*

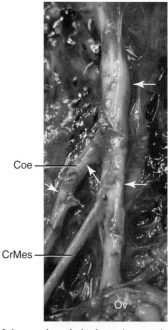

FIGURE 6-24 Atherosclerotic lesions *(arrows)* of the descending aorta and coeliac artery *(ventral view)* in a 30-year-old, female military macaw *(Ara militaris)*. Coe, Coeliac artery; CrMes, cranial mesenteric artery; Ov, ovary.

spp.), Eclectus parrots *(Eclectus roratus)*, cockatoos, and macaws.

In addition to age, female sex, and species, risk factors for development of atherosclerosis also include high-calorie and fat diets, dyslipidemia (e.g., hypercholesterolemia), and limited physical activity. The predisposition to the development of atherosclerosis in female psittacines likely relates to the profound effects of estrogen on lipid, protein, and calcium metabolism in reproductively active female birds. Estrogen promotes increased plasma total cholesterol, triglyceride, calcium, and protein levels, as well as the production of specific lipoproteins used to transport lipid from the liver (where lipogenesis predominately occurs in birds) to the developing yolk. These changes promote atherogenesis and may at least partially explain the association between reproductive tract disease and increased prevalence of advanced atherosclerotic lesions.[23,24] Species differences in plasma total cholesterol have been found to correlate with relative prevalence of severe atherosclerosis, with more susceptible genera having significantly higher total cholesterol levels. In a retrospective study, Grey parrots, Amazon parrots, and cockatiels had higher median plasma cholesterol levels relative to cockatoos, which, in turn, had significantly higher levels than macaws. Increasing high-density lipoprotein (HDL) levels, not LDL

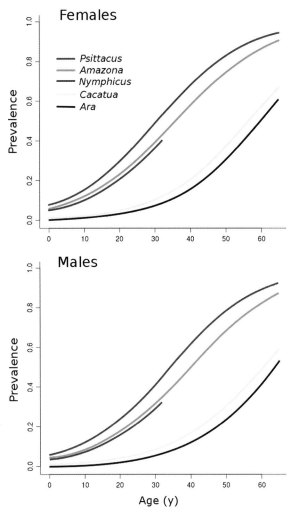

Females

- —— Psittacus
- —— Amazona
- —— Nymphicus
- —— Cacatua
- —— Ara

Males

Age (y)

FIGURE 6-25 Estimated prevalence of advanced atherosclerosis as a function of age, sex, and genus in 7683 psittacine birds representing five genera. (From Beaufrere H: Avian atherosclerosis: parrots and beyond, *JEPM* 22(4):336–347, 2013.)

demonstrate a significant difference in cholesterol and lipoprotein plasma concentrations between groups on pelletized or seed diets.[33] The intake in unsaturated fatty acids, especially omega-3 fatty acids, seems to protect against atherosclerosis in parrots.[34,35] The severity of atherosclerosis was found to negatively correlate with the muscle and adipose tissue content of α-linolenic acid in parrots.[34]

Diet-induced atherosclerosis has been demonstrated experimentally in budgerigars (*Melopsittacus undulatus*) and Quaker parrots. Budgerigars fed a 2% cholesterol diet developed advanced atherosclerotic lesions by 3 months, which further progressed by 6 months; hepatic lipidosis developed concurrently. In a recent study, Quaker parrots fed a 1% cholesterol diet developed severe dyslipidemia (plasma total cholesterol increased by a factor of 5 and LDLs by a factor of 15) and advanced atherosclerotic lesions in the aorta, brachiocephalic trunks, and coronary arteries within 4 months. The severity and cholesterol content of these lesions correlated significantly with plasma total cholesterol and LDL concentrations.[23] In the author's (BCF) experience, companion birds ultimately diagnosed with advanced atherosclerosis often have a long-term history of high-calorie and high-fat diets, regular provision of animal-based products (e.g., chicken bones, meat, and cheese), clinical obesity, and chronic reproductive activity (female birds).

The idea that dietary changes and relative lack of exercise associated with captivity contribute to prevalence of atherosclerotic disease in captive psittacines is supported by the findings of a recent study evaluating the hearts of 84 healthy, wild cockatoos. These birds had been euthanized in Australia as part of a control program and represented three species: 50 sulfur-crested cockatoos (*Cacatua galerita*), 31 rose-breasted cockatoos (*Eolophus roseicapilla*), and three long-billed corellas (*Cacatua tenuirostris*). All birds were in excellent body condition, and no lesions were found upon gross and histologic examinations of the myocardium and the great vessels (ascending aorta and brachiocephalic trunks).[12]

A possible association between *Chlamydia pneumoniae* infection and atherosclerosis has been investigated in multiple studies in humans but remains controversial.[36–38] The association between psittacine atherosclerosis and avian chlamydiosis is equally controversial and is probably not of great clinical significance.[24,26,39,40]

Atherosclerosis in other avian orders

Atherosclerosis has been described in almost all orders of birds.[41–45] Three large retrospective studies reported the prevalence of atherosclerosis in multiple avian orders (Table 6-4).[46–48] Most lesions were found not only in the major arteries but also in the carotid and coronary arteries. However, these prevalence data should be interpreted with caution because methods, inclusion criteria, and population demographics varied substantially among the reports, and there have since been changes in taxonomic classification. For instance, prevalence reported in Falconiformes actually included cases in the orders Falconiformes and Accipitriformes, cases belonging to Coraciiformes included cases from the orders of Coraciiformes and Bucerotiformes, and Struthioniformes may only have accounted for ostriches.

A report from the Oklahoma City Zoo documented a prevalence of 90% (65 of 72) of exotic birds with atherosclerosis with the most advanced lesions seen in Galliformes and

levels, correlated with greater atherosclerosis prevalence, suggesting that higher HDL levels may not be associated with reduced atherosclerosis risk, as it is in mammals. This may relate to the fact that most birds, including Psittaciformes, transport the majority of their cholesterol as HDL. Compared with other genera, Quaker parrots (*Myiopsitta monachus*) had the highest plasma cholesterol, triglyceride, and lipoprotein levels, although this could not be compared with the prevalence of atherosclerosis, as it has not been determined for this species as for the other genera. One possible explanation for these differences in plasma cholesterol and prevalence of atherosclerosis is that some species are poorly adapted to the dietary changes related to captivity and are less equipped to metabolize dietary lipids.[31]

The impact of diet on atherosclerosis and dyslipidemia has been investigated in a few studies. In a feed trial, Grey parrots fed a high-fat diet rich in saturated fatty acids had significantly higher plasma cholesterol than parrots on a low-fat diet or high-fat diet enriched in omega-6 unsaturated fatty acids (linoleic acid).[32] Another feed trial in Grey parrots did not

TABLE 6-4

Prevalence of Atherosclerosis in Different Avian Orders Kept in Zoologic Collections

Order	Garner[46]		Griner[48]		Finlayson[47]	
	N	%	N	%	N	%
Coraciiformes	199	6.5	110	8.0	19	31
Struthioniformes	136	5.0	78	1.3		
Falconiformes	282	4.2	129	10.8	30	53
Piciformes	205	3.4	138	12.3	23	22
Strigiformes	136	2.9	87	1.1		
Ciconiiformes	319	2.8	208	2.9	63	13
Psittaciformes	3678	2.6	1322	2.8	229	24
Galliformes	812	2.1	762	6.0	66	27
Gruiformes	258	1.9	229	1.7	27	19
Phoenicopteri- formes	275	1.8	56	3.6		
Columbiformes	305	1.6	186	12.4	28	9
Cuculiformes	64	1.5	64	0.0		
Anseriformes	1062	0.9	1047	3.1	131	19
Charadriiformes	249	0.8	256	1.6	40	12
Sphenisciformes	212	0.5	118	0.8	36	0
Passeriformes	1495	0.1	1300	2.4	168	7
Coliiformes	50	0.0	22	0.0		
Pelecaniformes	60	0.0	113	2.6		
Apodiformes	20	0.0	198	0.0		
Procellariiformes	6	0.0	43	0.0		
Gaviiformes	65	0.0	22	0.0		
Caprimulgiformes	15	0.0	1	100.0		
Unknown	46	2.0			59	19
Total	**9949**	**2.1**	**7689**	**3.0**	**919**	**21**

N, Total number of birds investigated; %, raw prevalence.

Ciconiiformes.[49] Atherosclerosis is also diagnosed with some frequency in wild birds. Out of 97 free-living birds examined in the United Kingdom and East Africa, 32 (33%) had evidence of atherosclerotic lesions, and 4 had evidence of advanced aortic lesions.[30] A report from Iraq found 10% of a sample of 100 wild pigeons with atherosclerotic lesions.[50]

Raptors. Atherosclerosis is the most common vascular disease reported in raptors, particularly older captive birds, but also free-ranging birds.[51] Postmortem examinations of 80 birds, predominately captive birds belonging to orders Falconiformes and Accipitriformes, revealed that 8% (10 of 80) had atherosclerotic lesions, as did 15.6% (7 of 45) of owls (Strigiformes), most of which were over 12 years old.[52] Another survey in captive birds of prey from the United Kingdom identified 7.6% (5 of 66) diurnal raptors with atherosclerosis, which was considered the cause of death in two Bonelli's eagles (*Aquila fasciata*).[53] A group of 50 black kites (*Milvus migrans*) at a large raptor collection in France (le parc du Puy du Fou) experienced severe loss from 2011 to 2012 as a result of atherosclerosis of the great vessels, which primarily manifested as acute deaths.[54] Myocardial infarction in association with advanced atherosclerosis was diagnosed in several birds, including a bald eagle (*Haliaeetus leucocephalus*), two white-backed vultures (*Gyps africanus*), and a Javan fishing owl (*Scotopelia* spp.).[30,47,48] Atherosclerosis precipitated ischemic cardiomyopathy in a red-tailed hawk (*Buteo jamaicensis*)[55] and ruptured aortic aneurysm in a crowned hawk-eagle (*Stephanoaetus coronatus*).[30,48]

A retrospective survey from Northern California found 1.5% (6 of 409) of free-living raptors diagnosed with atherosclerosis, a lower frequency than usually reported for these species in captivity.[56] In addition, atherosclerotic lesions were found in a population of wild Egyptian vultures (*Neophron percnopterus*).[57]

Galliformes. Chickens have been utilized as one avian model of atherosclerosis. They develop atherosclerotic lesions naturally in the aorta and coronary arteries, and cholesterol feeding accelerates the development of lesions.[58,59] Lesions are initially fibrous and can be induced in as little as 2 weeks.[60] Chickens are naturally hypercholesterolemic relative to most animal species and, like most birds, transport most of their cholesterol in HDL. Cholesterol feeding not only results in increased plasma total cholesterol but also shifts the lipoprotein profile to a predominance of very-low-density lipoprotein (VLDL) cholesterol.[61] In one study, addition of estradiol to the diet, particularly in combination with cholesterol, stimulated development of atherosclerotic lesions in both the aorta and the coronary arteries,[62] findings that contradicted those of previous studies suggesting estrogenic inhibition of atherogenesis in the coronary arteries.[63] Marek's disease virus (a herpesvirus) is known to promote lesion formation in the aorta, the coronary arteries, and the coeliac, gastric, and mesenteric arteries, most likely by altering lipid metabolism.[64]

Another model of atherosclerosis, Japanese quail (*Coturnix coturnix japonica*) develop diet-induced atherosclerosis, primarily in the intramyocardial coronary arteries, and myocardial infarction.[65-67] Susceptible and resistant strains are described. One strain is highly susceptible to diet-induced lesions, becoming hypercholesterolemic with a shift from HDL to VLDL and LDL as the main lipoproteins in the blood.[68,69] Increased levels of dietary cholesterol correlate with severity of lesions.[69]

Turkeys (*Meleagris gallopavo*) develop atherosclerosis naturally, and it can lead to aortic aneurysm,[70] although most cases of dissecting aortic aneurysms in turkeys are associated with copper deficiency.[71] An investigation of 157 wild male turkeys collected by hunters in the United States found atherosclerosis in 49.5% of arteries evaluated, with the greatest prevalence of lesions found in the aorta and ischiatic artery.[72]

Columbiformes. Pigeons have been used extensively as models in atherosclerosis research. The white Carneau (WC) pigeon is very susceptible to spontaneous development of atherosclerosis even on standard diets, whereas the show racer (SR) pigeon is relatively resistant. This difference in susceptibility lies at the level of the aortic wall, where an autosomal recessive genetic trait may be expressed by aortic smooth muscle cells.[73,74] On a standard grain diet (cholesterol-free), WC pigeons develop lesions in 3 to 4 years, mainly in the thoracic aorta at the bifurcation of the coeliac artery.[58,75,76] When atherosclerosis develops in the coronary arteries, lesions principally involve the intramyocardial coronary arteries and seem to develop independently from aortic lesions.[58] Complications associated with advanced lesions include hemorrhage, ulceration, mineralization, and thrombosis leading to myocardial ischemia.[58,73,77] As in most birds, the majority of cholesterol in pigeons is carried in HDL, but when pigeons are fed a cholesterol diet, total cholesterol and LDL increase by approximately 5 to 15 times.[61,78] Dietary cholesterol accelerates atherosclerotic lesion development in pigeons, in proportion to both the amount and duration of cholesterol feeding.[75]

Others. There are reports of atherosclerotic disease in a myriad of avian species. Myocardial infarction in association with advanced atherosclerosis was diagnosed in a concave-casqued hornbill *(Buceros bicornis)*, three pelicans *(Pelecanus* spp.), a tawny frogmouth *(Podargus strigoides)* that also had an arterial thrombus, and an Edward's pheasant *(Lophura edwardsi)*.[30,47,48] A review of 57 penguin pathology records over 5 years at SeaWorld identified 25 birds (44%) with atherosclerosis, and in four of the birds, it was considered the primary cause of death.[79] Ruptured aortic aneurysm caused by atherosclerosis has been reported in Antarctic penguins,[80] a flamingo *(Phoenicopterus* spp.) (Garner, written communication, May 2012), Sclater's crowned pigeon *(Goura sclaterii)*, Egyptian plover *(Pluvianus aegyptius)*, grey-winged trumpeter *(Psophia crepitans)*, and maned goose *(Chenonetta jubata)*.[30,48] Atherosclerosis with chondroid metaplasia was found in the ascending aorta of a pukeko *(Porphyrio melanotus)* with left-sided congestive heart failure,[81] and coronary atherosclerosis with focal mineralization was identified in a female greater hill mynah *(Gracula religiosa)* with right-sided congestive heart failure.[82] At the author's (BCF) practice, a large, nodular atherosclerotic lesion with chondroid dysplasia was found subtending the aortic valve in a yellow-billed magpie *(Pica nuttalli)* with myocardial degeneration and biventricular congestive heart failure.

Risk factors. Risk factors for atherosclerosis in nonpsittacine species are speculative, and its epidemiology has been less investigated. In raptors, the relative inactivity of captivity, increasing age, obesity, and rapid weight loss are presumed to contribute to atherosclerosis risk.[51] The common practice of feeding day-old chicks that have a large yolk sac rich in cholesterol may potentiate atherosclerosis in susceptible raptorial species (e.g., insectivorous raptors, falcons).[24] Likewise, development of atherosclerosis in chickens, quail, and pigeons is associated with increasing age and with elevated plasma total cholesterol and shifts in the lipoprotein profile induced by cholesterol feeding, but is at least partially contingent on predispositions of certain breeds or strains.[75] In chickens and turkeys, males are more prone to atherosclerosis than females, which may result, in part, from comparatively higher blood pressure in males.[71,83]

Non-atherosclerotic Aneurysm and Arterial Rupture

Other than atherosclerosis, causes of arterial aneurysm in birds include copper deficiency, hypertension, and fungal infection.[7,84-88] Also, spontaneous, idiopathic aneurysm formation is occasionally identified in companion birds,[10] as in one case of a 24-year-old, female blue-and-gold macaw *(Ara ararauna)* diagnosed at postmortem examination with a ruptured aneurysm of a midbrain artery.[28] Congenital cardiac aneurysms are also recognized, with left ventricular aneurysms seen in cockatiels *(Nymphicus hollandicus)* and in a blue-and-gold macaw,[10] and a right ventricular aneurysm reported in a pigeon.[89] A 14-year-old, female Moluccan cockatoo *(Cacatua moluccensis)* in apparently good health died suddenly and was presented to the author's (BCF) practice for necropsy. A ruptured right atrial aneurysm resulting in severe hemorrhage

into the coelom was identified. Nonatherosclerotic aneurysms with aortic dissection and rupture are mainly seen in ostriches *(Struthio camelus)* and turkeys.[a] The exact cause in these two species is not known, but systemic hypertension (common in meat-type turkeys, especially young males), genetic factors, connective tissue disorders, peas in the ration (toxin β-aminopropionitrile in peas will cause aortic rupture experimentally by interference with collagen formation), and dietary deficiencies notably in copper may contribute to the pathogenesis.[71,90-92] A copper-dependent enzyme is needed for connective cross-linking of collagen and elastin in the arterial wall.[10] A large saccular aneurysm of the ascending aorta associated with mycotic vasculitis *(Aspergillus* spp.) was identified in an adult common eider *(Somateria mollissima)*.[86] The author (BCF) has seen mycotic arteritis and severe erosion of the ascending aorta in a green-wing macaw *(Ara chloroptera)*, in which the great vessels were tightly encased by a fungal granuloma that formed within the clavicular air sac. It can be hypothesized that arterial rupture, potentially fatal, could occur subsequent to such fungal angioinvasion, although the authors are not aware of any case reports where this was specifically reported.

Heart Failure

Heart failure occurs when cardiac output becomes inadequate to maintain arterial blood pressure (manifested clinically by low-output signs of lethargy, depression, and weakness) and when the heart is unable to empty the venous reservoirs, manifested by vascular congestion and transudation of fluid within tissues and body cavities (congestive signs).[13,18,93-95] In the case of right-sided congestive heart failure, peripheral venous congestion, hepatic congestion, ascites, and pericardial effusion are often present (Figure 6-26, *A* through *F*).[b] Pulmonary edema and congestion of the pulmonary veins occur with left-sided congestive heart failure (Figure 6-27), and a combination of signs may be seen with biventricular failure.[13,93-96] Heart failure can further be characterized as systolic, diastolic, or a combination of the two. Systolic failure results from inadequate ventricular ejection and diastolic failure from inadequate ventricular filling. In either scenario, stroke volume and cardiac output decrease.[18]

Pathophysiology

Congestive heart failure is not a primary disease in itself, but an ultimate consequence of structural or functional abnormalities of the cardiovascular or pulmonary systems, compounded by the chronic effects of compensatory mechanisms (Box 6-2).[18] Not all cardiovascular disease necessarily leads to congestive heart failure, but it is a frequent clinical endpoint encountered in companion birds. The pathophysiology of congestive heart failure has been studied primarily in mammals but is likely similar across vertebrate taxons because of shared neuroendocrine regulatory pathways of circulation and hemodynamic constraints.[98]

In the mammalian model, heart failure can result from primary myocardial failure, ventricular pressure overload or volume overload, conduction disturbances, or diastolic

---

[a]References 70,71,84,85,87,88.
[b]References 7,13,41,82,93-97.

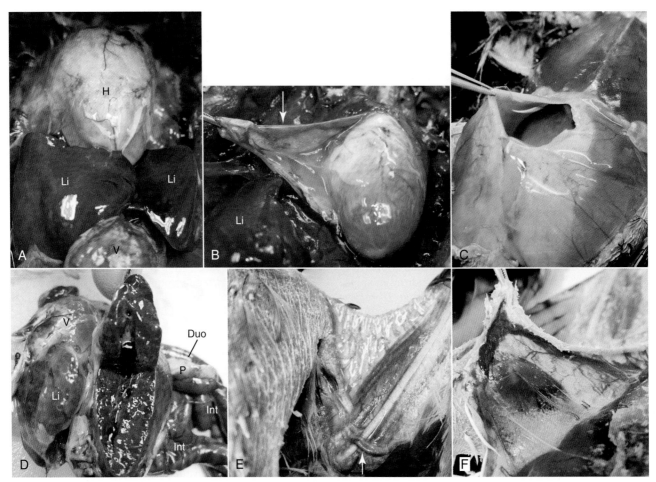

FIGURE 6-26 Right-sided congestive heart failure. **A** and **B**, Pericardial effusion, thickened pericardium *(arrow)*, and hepatic congestion in a 30-year-old, female military macaw *(Ara militaris)*, caudoventral view. **C**, Ascites in a 13-year-old, female yellow-billed magpie *(Pica nuttalli)*, caudoventral view. **D** to **F**, Hepatic venous congestion and peripheral venous congestion (in the face of severe tissue dehydration) in a 35-year-old, male Grey parrot *(Psittacus erithacus)*, sagittal section liver (right lobe), cutaneous ulnar vein (left wing; *arrow*), reflected skin (right inguinal area). Duo, Duodenum; H, heart; Int, intestine; Li, liver; P, pancreas; V, ventriculus.

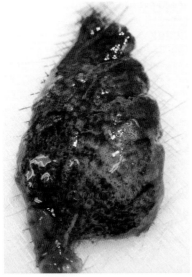

FIGURE 6-27 Left lung (dorsal aspect) of a 35-year-old, male Grey parrot *(Psittacus erithacus)* with pulmonary edema secondary to left-sided congestive heart failure.

dysfunction (Figure 6-28). Myocardial failure (Figure 6-29) can occur with either primary disease of the myocardium or secondary to chronic pressure or volume overload.[18] Pressure overload (Figure 6-30) results from outflow obstruction (e.g., from congenital or acquired valvular stenosis, narrowing of the aorta) or from systemic or pulmonary hypertension. The affected ventricles ultimately undergo concentric hypertrophy, in which the ventricular wall thickens, and a corresponding decrease occurs in chamber volume. Hypertrophy initially decreases wall stress and increases contractility, but eventual ischemia of the hypertrophied myocardium results in fibrosis and increased collagen content, impairing both systolic function and diastolic function. As myocardial failure progresses, the ventricle ultimately dilates. Volume overload (Figure 6-31) results from valvular insufficiency and abnormal communications between chambers. Increased end-diastolic volume not only has the positive effect of increasing stroke volume and cardiac output via the Frank-Starling mechanism but also has the negative consequence of increasing wall stress and pressure. The result is eccentric hypertrophy of the

BOX 6-2 DOCUMENTED CAUSES OF CONGESTIVE HEART FAILURE IN DOMESTIC, WILD, AND COMPANION BIRDS

Causes	References
Dilated cardiomyopathy	10,55,71,99,100
Hypertrophic cardiomyopathy	10,93,101
Ischemic cardiomyopathy	102
Cardiac infection	7,10,103,104
Nutritional causes	7,71
Toxic causes	105-108
Iron storage disease	109
Atherosclerosis	29,78,95,102,110
Systemic hypertension	71,108
Pulmonary hypertension	110-113
Pulmonary fibrosis or mycosis	13,93,97,114
Valvular insufficiency	41,71,81,82,113,115,116
Valvular stenosis	117
Septal defects	10,118-121
Arrhythmias	122
Pericardial effusion	123,124

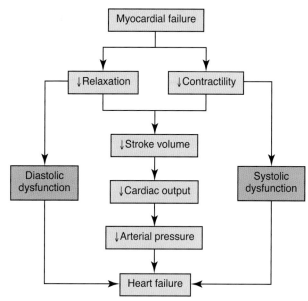

FIGURE 6-29 Steps by which myocardial failure progresses to heart failure. (Modified from de Morais HA, Schwartz DS. Pathophysiology of heart failure. In Ettinger SJ, Feldman EC, editors: *Textbook of veterinary internal medicine*, ed 6, St. Louis, MO, 2005, Saunders, pp 914–940.)

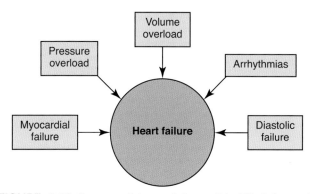

FIGURE 6-28 Causes of heart failure. (Modified from de Morais HA, Schwartz DS: Pathophysiology of heart failure. In Ettinger SJ, Feldman EC, editors: *Textbook of veterinary internal medicine*, ed 6, St. Louis, MO, 2005, Saunders, pp 914–940.)

affected ventricles, characterized by chamber enlargement and increased myocardial mass with little increase in wall thickness. This process is accompanied by decreased myocardial collagen, which not only improves diastolic function by increasing compliance but also leads to fiber slippage as the ventricle continues to dilate. Progression of disease sees further increases in wall stress and myocardial oxygen consumption, as well as pressure hypertrophy and fibrosis, eventually leading to myocardial failure and further chamber dilatation.[18]

Diastolic failure results from decreased ventricular compliance, abnormal myocardial relaxation, and cardiac tamponade or constrictive pericardial disease. Decreases in ventricular compliance occur with increased myocardial stiffness subsequent to myocardial infiltration, hypertrophy, fibrosis, and ischemia. The active process of relaxation is also impaired by myocardial hypertrophy and ischemia, as well as increases in afterload. Ventricular filling is diminished by obstruction of incoming veins, the atria, or the AV orifices

and is prematurely arrested by a constrictive pericardium or cardiac tamponade.[18]

Compared with mammals, birds are thought to have a greater propensity for developing pulmonary hypertension and right-sided congestive heart failure, rather than left-sided congestive heart failure, because of the morphology of the right AV valve, less deformable nucleated erythrocytes, and the rigid, nondistensible lungs, which limit the ability of the blood capillaries to expand and accommodate greater blood flow.[93,112]

Primary myocardial disease. The term *dilated cardiomyopathy* (DCM) refers to myocardial disease resulting in ventricular dilation, thinning of the myocardium, and systolic and diastolic dysfunction.[10] By definition, the condition cannot be fully explained by the effects of abnormal loading and so should not be confused with the chamber dilatation that develops as an endpoint of pressure or volume overload states.[125] Spontaneous DCM is a well-known disorder of 1- to 4-week-old turkey poults. The exact cause of the disease is unknown but is associated with rapid growth and production. Genetic factors, previous myocarditis, hypoxia during incubation, and other environmental and dietary factors have also been proposed to play a role in the etiology.[71,91,126] Characteristic gross findings include greatly dilated ventricles (right ventricle more so than left ventricle), and pericardial effusion, ascites, and pulmonary congestion and edema consistent with congestive heart failure. Histopathologic lesions include degeneration of myofibers with vacuolation, secondary endocardiosis, focal infiltration of lymphocytes, and secondary changes in the liver.[17,71] There are scant reports of DCM in other species of birds. There is one report of DCM in a whooper swan (*Cygnus cygnus*) with marked dilation of all cardiac chambers, diminished cardiac output, and arrhythmia,[100] and another of a captive red-tailed hawk (*Buteo jamaicensis*) with predominately right-sided DCM resulting in

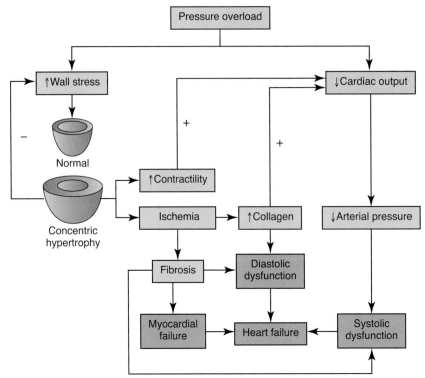

FIGURE 6-30 Steps by which pressure overload progresses to heart failure. (Modified from de Morais HA, Schwartz DS. Pathophysiology of heart failure. In Ettinger SJ, Feldman EC, editors: *Textbook of veterinary internal medicine*, ed 6, St. Louis, MO, 2005, Saunders, pp 914–940. The illustration of the hypertrophied ventricle was taken from the web: http://www.nature.com/nrcardio/journal/v8/n12/fig_tab/nrcardio.2011.154_F4.html. Source: Gjesdal O, Bluemke DA Lima JA: Cardiac remodeling at the population level—risk factors, screening, and outcomes, *Nat Rev Cardiol* 8:673-685, 2011.)

congestive heart failure. In both cases, the myocardium was histologically normal, and no specific cause could be identified.[55] DCM is scarcely reported in psittacines and is generally considered idiopathic.[10,93,94] Hypertrophic cardiomyopathy is usually the product of pressure and volume overload states[81,93,94,127] (cardiomyopathy of overload[18]), and will be discussed in the following sections.

Myocardial changes consistent with ischemic injury, including myocardial necrosis, inflammation, degeneration, and fibrosis, have been associated with atherosclerosis of the coronary arteries in psittacines.[27,128] Myocardial necrosis likely reflects recent injury, whereas degenerative and fibrotic changes reflect chronic, ongoing injury.[27] These changes have the potential to produce arrhythmias,[24,27] particularly considering the periarterial course of Purkinje fibers through the myocardium. Arrhythmias could result in sudden death, and systolic and diastolic myocardial dysfunction may ultimately culminate in congestive heart failure.[24] Acute myocardial infarction is thought to be rare, perhaps because of the different arrangement of the coronary arteries and the greater collateral circulation compared with that in humans. Ischemic cardiomyopathy and infarction have been reported in birds of prey and in pigeon and quail models of atherosclerosis.[48,65,77,102,129]

Myocardial disease may also be of infectious, metabolic, nutritional, neoplastic, or toxic[130] origin.[7,10] Myocarditis can be caused by a variety of infectious agents, including bacterial,

fungal, and viral pathogens, as well as protozoal and helminth parasites (Table 6-5). Bacterial infection may involve the epicardium, myocardium, or endocardium and occur by hematogenous spread or by extension from infected adjacent tissues. Fungal infection, most commonly by *Aspergillus* spp., can spread to the heart from the adjacent lungs and air sacs,[10,13] and disseminated infection by *Aspergillus* spp., *Candida* spp., and Zygomycetes can have cardiac involvement by angioinvasion and hematogenous spread.[10,131,132] Zygomycetes have a particular proclivity for vascular invasion. Thrombosing vasculitis was the predominant lesion in a blue-fronted Amazon parrot (*Amazona aestiva*) and a peach-faced lovebird (*Agapornis roseicollis*) with zygomycotic myocarditis.[131,132] Proventricular dilatation disease (PDD), for which avian bornavirus (ABV) has been recently identified as the etiologic agent,[133] is characterized histologically as lymphoplasmacytic infiltration of nerve ganglia throughout the body. Inflammatory infiltrates are frequently found in the epicardium and the myocardium,[7,13,93] particularly in proximity to Purkinje fibers, potentially precipitating arrhythmias and sudden death.[10,134,135] In one study, cardiac lesions were found in 79% of PDD cases.[135] Myocardial necrosis and fibrosis may also be associated with these lesions, and ventricular dilatation may be appreciated grossly.[10,134] In psittacines and finches, polyomavirus infection produces myocarditis with necrosis and hemorrhage, and intranuclear inclusion bodies

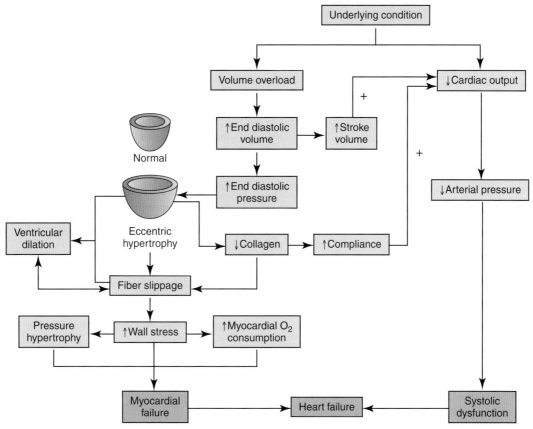

FIGURE 6-31 Steps by which volume overload progresses to heart failure. (Modified from de Morais HA, Schwartz DS. Pathophysiology of heart failure. In Ettinger SJ, Feldman EC, editors: *Textbook of veterinary internal medicine*, ed 6, St. Louis, MO, 2005, Saunders, pp 914–940. The illustration of the hypertrophied ventricle was taken from the web: http://www.nature.com/nrcardio/journal/v8/n12/fig_tab/nrcardio.2011.154_F4.html Source: Gjesdal O, Bluemke DA Lima JA: Cardiac remodeling at the population level—risk factors, screening, and outcomes, *Nature Reviews Cardiology* 8:673-685, 2011.)

can be seen within cardiomyocytes.[10] Myocarditis and necrosis caused by West Nile virus infection has been documented in several psittacine species and is a common feature of the disease in North American birds of prey.[136-138] Protozoal parasites, including *Sarcocystis* spp. and *Toxoplasma gondii*, have been reported to cause myocarditis and necrosis associated with protozoal cysts within cardiomyocytes.[7,10,139-141] *Sarcocystis falcatula*, for which the opossum is the definitive host, is known to cause severe disease in psittacines, which are considered accidental hosts. Cats are the definitive host for *T. gondii*, which causes myocardial disease in many species of birds, including psittacines. Birds housed outdoors are at potential risk by contact with feces of the definitive host and arthropod transport hosts (e.g., the cockroach).[10,141] Filarioid nematodes have been found in wild-caught cockatoos; in one case, adult worms belonging to the genus *Chandlerella* were found in the right atrium, renal veins, and hepatic veins of a Ducorps's cockatoo *(Cacatua ducorpsii)*, along with microfilariae within the capillaries of most major organs, including the myocardium. Focal hypertrophy of the endocardium and of the intima of myocardial vessels was noted, possibly the product of partial mechanical blockage by the organisms and turbulent blood flow.[10,142]

Visceral gout can affect the epicardium and the myocardium, where an inflammatory reaction variably accompanies urate deposition. Fatty infiltration into the myocardium associated with obesity may play a role in heart failure.[10,13] It has been the only pathologic finding in some cases of sudden death in obese pet birds.[10] Deficiencies of vitamin E and selenium are associated with myocardial degeneration, appearing grossly as white streaks, sometimes accompanied by pericardial effusion.[7,10] A fatal disease primarily characterized by myocardial degeneration has been reported in great billed parrots *(Tanygnathus megalorynchos)* along with skeletal muscle and neural lesions resembling those seen in poultry with vitamin E deficiency.[10] Cardiac and vascular mineralization can occur as a result of dietary calcium–phosphorous imbalance and vitamin D toxicity.[10,71]

Documented cardiotoxins in birds are summarized in Table 6-6. Furazolidone, a nitrofuran antibiotic, induces DCM in chicks, ducklings, and turkey poults when fed at a concentration of 300 parts per million (ppm) or greater.[7,71] Furazolidone-induced DCM in turkey poults is used as a model for human DCM. Systolic dysfunction results from altered ventricular geometry and shorter sarcomere lengths (thus limited utility of the Frank-Starling mechanism),

TABLE 6-5

Infectious Agents Reported to Cause Cardiovascular Lesions in Birds

- Pericarditis or epicarditis
  - *Listeria monocytogenes*
  - *Riemerella anatipestifer* (turkeys, ducks)
  - *Chlamydia psittaci*
  - *Mycoplasma gallisepticum*
  - *Salmonella* spp.
  - *Escherichia coli*
  - *Mycobacterium* spp.
  - *Erysipelothrix rhusiopathiae*
  - *Aspergillus* spp.
  - Reovirus
  - *Toxoplasma gondii*
  - *Trichomonas gallinae* (pigeons)
- Pericardial effusion
  - Fowl adenovirus C (serotype 4)
  - Reovirus
  - Polyomavirus
  - Highly pathogenic avian influenza virus (H5N1)
  - Parvovirus (geese, Muscovy ducks)
- Vasculitis
  - *Mycoplasma gallisepticum*
  - *Mycoplasma synoviae*
  - *Enterococcus* spp.
  - *Streptococcus* spp.
  - *Mycobacterium* spp.
  - *Aspergillus* spp.
  - Zygomycetes
  - Avian paramyxovirus I
  - Avian influenza virus
  - Eastern equine encephalitis virus
  - Marek's disease virus
- Intravascular or intracardiac parasites
  - *Trichomonas gallinae* (pigeons)
  - *Splendidofilaria* spp.
  - *Chandlerella* spp.
  - *Cardiofilaria* spp.
  - *Paronchocerca* spp.
  - *Sarconema* spp. (Anseriformes)
  - Schistosomes (Anseriformes)

- Myocarditis
  - *Escherichia coli*
  - *Salmonella* spp.
  - *Listeria monocytogenes*
  - *Pasteurella multocida*
  - *Mycobacterium* spp.
  - *Chlamydia psittaci*
  - *Aspergillus* spp.
  - *Candida* spp.
  - Zygomycetes
  - West Nile virus
  - Eastern equine encephalitis virus
  - Avian leucosis virus
  - Parvovirus (geese, Muscovy ducks)
  - Avian encephalomyelitis virus
  - Reovirus
  - Avian paramyxovirus I
  - Avian influenza virus
  - Polyomavirus
  - Proventricular dilation disease (Avian Bornavirus)
  - Psittacine poxvirus
  - *Sarcocystis* spp.
  - *Toxoplasma gondii*
  - *Atoxoplasma serini* (Passeriformes)
  - *Leucocytozoon* spp.
- Endocarditis
  - *Enterobacter cloacae*
  - *Enterococcus* spp.
  - *Streptococcus* spp.
  - *Staphylococcus* spp.
  - *Pasteurella multocida*
  - *Pseudomonas aeruginosa*
  - *Erysipelothrix rhusiopathiae*
  - *Lactobacillus jensenii*
  - *Escherichia coli*
  - Reovirus
  - *Toxoplasma gondii*
- Cardiac neoplasms
  - Marek's disease virus
  - Avian leucosis virus
  - Reticuloendotheliosis virus

whereas diastolic dysfunction is a product of greater collagen-based myocardial stiffness.[143] Myocardial degeneration and necrosis, fibrinoid necrosis of myocardial arterioles, and subsequent thrombosis and infarction are lesions frequently seen in waterfowl with lead toxicosis[144] and are also recognized in many other species of birds.[145]

Cardiac neoplasms include hemangioma and hemangiosarcoma, rhabdomyoma and rhabdomyosarcoma, fibrosarcoma, melanosarcoma, and lymphosarcoma. Whether histologically benign or malignant, cardiac tumors interfere with systolic and diastolic function. Other than in the heart, hemangiomas and hemangiosarcomas can appear anywhere but occur most often in the skin and subcutaneous tissue.[10] However, a hemangiosarcoma arising from the right internal carotid artery was reported in a double-yellow-headed Amazon parrot (*Amazona ochrocephala oratrix*).[158] In poultry, oncogenic viruses (see Table 6-5) can induce a variety of cardiac neoplasms, most notably lymphoma, which can be diffuse or nodular.[64]

The heart may be subject to traumatic injury in cases of sternal defect. Bifid sternum, a congenital defect in which the sternum is split longitudinally, has been reported in three Grey parrots (*Psittacus erithacus*) and an orange-winged Amazon parrot (*Amazona amazonica*).[159,160]

Pressure overload. Hypertrophic cardiomyopathy in psittacines most often develops secondary to chronic increase in afterload, which may be attributed to the arterial luminal stenosis and decreased compliance characteristic of atherosclerosis (see Figure 6-20, *A* and *B*) or to pulmonary hypertension related to atherosclerosis, chronic pulmonary disease, or left-sided congestive heart failure.[93-97,127] Compression of the great vessels can occur by accumulation of caseous debris in the clavicular air sac (as in the case of mycotic airsacculitis) (Figure 6-32) or by any mass encroaching on the heart base (Figures 6-33 and 6-34), which may also impair diastolic function. Atherosclerotic lesions of the ascending aorta and brachiocephalic trunks (Figure 6-35) have been correlated with myocardial

TABLE 6-6

Selected Cardiotoxins Recognized in Birds

Toxin	Effect	References
DIETARY AND PHYTOTOXINS		
Avocado (persin)	Pericardial effusion, myocarditis, myocardial degeneration and necrosis Congestive heart failure	105,146
Corn cockle (*Agrostemma githago*) (githagenin)	Pericardial effusion (hydropericardium)	106
Sweet pea (β-aminopropionitrile)	Aneurysm	92
Lily of the valley (glycosides)	Tachycardia, arrhythmias	147
Oleander (glycosides)	Tachycardia, arrhythmias	147,148
Kalanchoe (glycosides)	Tachycardia, arrhythmias	147
Cassia	Myocardial degeneration and necrosis	17
Crotalaria (pyrrolizidine, monocrotaline)	Ascites, pericardial effusion (hydropericardium)	106
Rapeseed (erucic acid, glucosinolate)	Ascites, pericardial effusion (hydropericardium), fatty changes of myocardium	106
Chocolate (theobromine, caffeine)	Tachycardia, hypertension, arrhythmias	147,149
Alcohol	Fatty changes	106
Moniliformin (*Fusarium* mycotoxin)	Myocardial degeneration and necrosis	108
Iron	Oxidative myocardial injury	82,150
Sodium	Congestive heart failure	90
Potassium	Arrhythmias, hypertrophy and degeneration of myofibers	17
Vitamin D$_3$	Cardiac and arterial mineralization, arrhythmias	17,106,151
ENVIRONMENTAL TOXINS		
Lead or zinc	Conduction abnormalities, pericardial effusion (hydropericardium)—geese, swans, myocardial necrosis, fibrinoid necrosis of blood vessels	106,144,152-154
Chlordane	Pericardial effusion (hydropericardium)	106
Organophosphates or carbamates	Bradycardia	153
Phenolic compounds or coal-tar derivatives	Vascular endothelial damage, pericardial effusion (hydropericardium), ascites	106
RODENTICIDES		
Alpha-naphthyl thiourea	Pericardial effusion (hydropericardium), myocardial degeneration	106
Sodium monofluoroacetate (compound 1080)	Pericardial effusion (hydropericardium)	106
Zinc phosphide	Pericardial effusion (hydropericardium), ascites	106
Cholecalciferol (vitamin D$_3$)	Myocardial mineralization, arrhythmias	151
IATROGENIC TOXINS		
Furazolidone (nitrofuran)	Dilated cardiomyopathy	106,107
Ionophores (monensin, salinomycin)	Myocardial degeneration and necrosis	17,106
Haloperidol	Bradycardia, hypotension	155
Lidocaine or bupivacaine	Arrhythmias, hypotension	156
Doxorubicin	Cardiomyopathy, arrhythmias	107,157

Note: Toxicities may vary by species, especially for plant toxins. Some toxin effects are poorly documented in birds.

hypertrophy and fibrosis and with pulmonary congestion and fibrosis; the incidence of fibrotic changes increases in proportion to atherosclerotic lesion severity.[96] Hypertrophic cardiomyopathy may have no accompanying histologic changes.[10]

Systemic arterial hypertension is common in young male turkeys and is considered one possible cause of left ventricular hypertrophy and congestive heart failure seen in 8-week-old to 14-week-old birds that die suddenly.[71] Young chicks and poults are susceptible to hypertension secondary to ingestion of excessive sodium in water or feed. This may result in severe ventricular hypertrophy (particularly of the right ventricle) and subsequent congestive heart failure.[108] Systemic hypertension has not been defined in psittacines[161] but is a probable disease entity in this group.[24] Ventricular

pressure overload can also stem from stenosis of the pulmonary or aortic valve, which, in psittacines, can result from chronic inflammation or metabolic disease.[13] Although valvular stenosis is considered uncommon in birds, congenital mitral and subvalvular aortic stenosis were identified as the cause of left-sided congestive heart failure in a mallard hybrid duck (*Anas* spp.). In that bird, mitral stenosis impaired ventricular filling and therefore diastolic function, while subvalvular aortic stenosis impaired systolic function.[117] Congenital aortic hypoplasia was diagnosed postmortem in a 6-month-old Moluccan cockatoo (*Cacatua moluccensis*) with biventricular congestive heart failure.[118] Left-sided congestive heart failure can also develop secondary to hepatic disease that increases afterload, particularly fibrotic

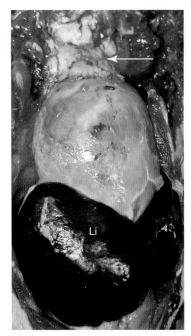

FIGURE 6-32 Right-sided congestive heart failure associated with a fungal granuloma *(arrow)* engulfing the great vessels *(ventral view)* in 31-year-old, female green wing macaw *(Ara chloroptera)* with severe pericardial effusion (20 mL volume) and marked hepatic congestion. Li, Liver.

conditions. Iron storage disease in mynah birds *(Gracula religiosa)* producing severe hepatic fibrosis has been associated with cardiomegaly, chamber dilatation, and thinning of the left ventricular myocardium.[109] An analogous scenario was seen by the author in a yellow-billed magpie *(Pica nuttalli)* with iron storage disease and associated hepatic fibrosis that developed biventricular congestive heart failure. However, a large atherosclerotic lesion at the level of the aortic valve likely contributed to left ventricular overload.

Cor pulmonale has been described in a Grey parrot subsequent to pulmonary arterial atherosclerosis and severe pulmonary hypertension.[110] Pulmonary hypertension secondary to chronic pulmonary interstitial fibrosis was identified in several species of Amazon parrots in the Netherlands, in many cases resulting in right ventricular hypertrophy and failure. In these birds, polycythemia developed as a consequence of chronic hypoxemia, creating further resistance to blood flow by increasing blood viscosity.[97] A similar scenario is seen with hypersensitivity pneumonitis of macaws, apparently most common in the blue-and-gold macaw *(Ara ararauna)* (see Chapter 11).[10,152-154] Cor pulmonale secondary to pulmonary mycosis has been documented in numerous cases[13,93,114] and has been seen on several occasions by the author (BCF) (Figure 6-36).

Pulmonary hypertension has been extensively investigated in the domestic fowl, as it plays a key role in ascites syndrome of growing broilers. The pathophysiology of avian heart failure has been most studied in the context of this disease, but not all findings may translate well to companion avian patients

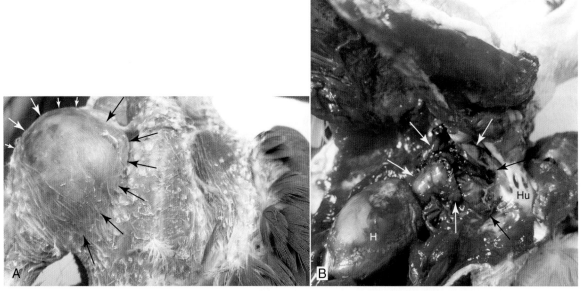

FIGURE 6-33 A, Hemorrhagic mass *(arrows)* involving the left shoulder of a 23-year-old, female blue-headed Pionus parrot *(Pionus menstruus) (dorsal view)*. **B,** The mass extending along the axillary diverticulum of the clavicular air sac to invade the cranial coelom and partially enclose the heart base *(left lateral view)*. Note: The hemorrhage extended into all air sacs, including the sternal diverticulum of the clavicular air sac, lungs, and upper airways. The position of the mass suggested an air sac origin, but histologically the mass could be identified only as a poorly differentiated unencapsulated infiltrative neoplasm. Discoloration of the right heart is an artifact of euthanasia solution (pentobarbital sodium/phenytoin sodium) administered intravenously (right jugular vein). H, Heart; Hu, humeral head.

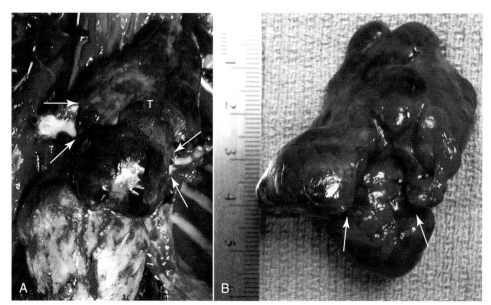

FIGURE 6-34 A, Large neuroendocrine tumor (probable parathyroid adenoma) enveloping the heart base and embedding the great vessels *(arrows)* and left common carotid artery of a 34-year-old, female green-wing macaw *(Ara chloroptera) (ventral view).* **B,** Caudoventral view of the excised tumor demonstrating grooves formerly occupied by the great vessels *(arrows).* H, Heart; T, tumor.

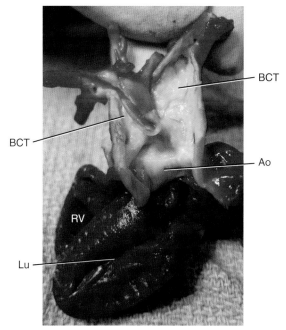

FIGURE 6-35 Concentric hypertrophy of the left ventricular myocardium *(longitudinal section)* in a 28-year-old, male Grey parrot *(Psittacus erithacus)* with left-sided congestive heart failure secondary to advanced atherosclerosis of the aorta and brachiocephalic trunks *(opened to demonstrate plaques).* Ao, Aorta; BCT, brachiocephalic trunk; Lu, lumen (left ventricle); RV, right ventricle.

because the pathogenesis involves a complex interaction of genetic factors, increased metabolic rate and rapid growth, and hypoxia.[111-113] Historically, it was hypothesized that broilers are susceptible to ascites syndrome, given the higher oxygen demands of rapid growth, coupled with small lungs relative to body size, insufficient pulmonary capillary capacity, and reduced respiratory efficiency that predispose to hypoxemia.[71,112,113] However, more recent evidence suggests that inadequate cardiac output related to a relatively small left ventricle and poor systolic function is the primary cause of pulmonary hypertension and hypoxemia, rather than inadequate pulmonary blood flow capacity. Chronic hypercapnia is also thought to contribute to pulmonary hypertension.[113] Environmental factors that exacerbate the condition are high altitude (where oxygen-hemoglobin binding affinity is reduced and hypoxia stimulates pulmonary vasoconstriction) and cold and hot temperatures, which increase oxygen demands. Polycythemia and increases in hemoglobin and hematocrit develop as a consequence of chronic hypoxemia, thereby increasing blood viscosity and rendering erythrocytes larger and less deformable. These changes increase resistance to blood flow in the lung and other tissues and therefore afterload. Right-sided dilatation and congestive heart failure follow right ventricular hypertrophy, including of the right muscular AV valve. Left atrial and ventricular dilatation, endocardiosis of the left AV valve, and pulmonary congestion and edema are also common pathologic findings.[71,112,113]

Volume overload. Congestive heart failure may also result from valvular insufficiency subsequent to valvular degeneration (endocardiosis) (Figure 6-37),[10,81,115,118,165] vegetative endocarditis,[13,29,94,103,155] congenital defect,[10,41,118,121] or ruptured chordae tendineae (Figure 6-38). Given the unique design of the muscular right AV valve, right-sided myocardial

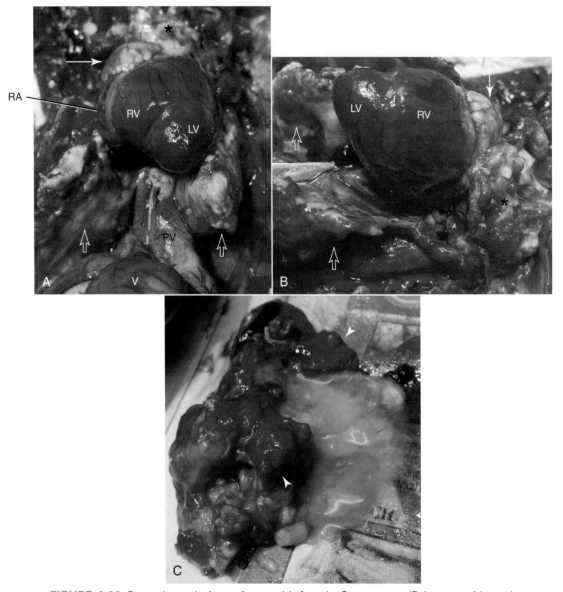

FIGURE 6-36 Cor pulmonale in an 8-year-old, female Grey parrot *(Psittacus erithacus)* with chronic, severe mycotic pneumonia and airsacculitis. **A** and **B,** Heart in situ *(caudoventral view* **[A]**; *right lateral view* **[B]).** Note the exudate-filled cardiac diverticulum of the clavicular air sac *(arrow),* the clavicular air sac exudates enveloping the great vessels *(asterisk),* and effacement of most lung tissue with fungal granulomas *(open arrows).* **C,** Excised lung, transected to expose exudate and mucoid debris within; note the narrow margin of grossly normal parenchyma *(arrowheads).* LV, Left ventricle; PV, proventriculus; RA, right atrium; RV, right ventricle; V, ventriculus.

hypertrophy can also produce valvular insufficiency as the valve itself thickens. Furthermore, as the right ventricle dilates, valvular insufficiency develops as a result of the fixed position of the valve extending from the ventricular wall.[7,13,90,93,166] These changes take place in ascites syndrome of broilers, which along with left AV valve insufficiency related to endocardiosis, further contribute to development of congestive heart failure.[71,113] Endocardiosis is a noninflammatory nodular thickening of the valves, which is generally considered idiopathic and most commonly affects the left AV valve.[10,17,71] Insufficiency of the left AV valve resulting from

endocardiosis has been reported in the Indian ringneck parakeet *(Psittacula krameri),* umbrella cockatoo *(Cacatua alba),* Indian hill mynah *(Gracula religiosa),* and pukeko *(Porphyrio melanotus).*[81,115,116,167]

Bacterial infection involving the heart, whether a consequence of bacteremia or local spread, can result in vegetative endocarditis.[7,10,103,104] Any condition producing turbulent blood flow within the heart may predispose to endocarditis.[7] The left AV valve is most consistently affected, but any valve can be involved, as can the chordae tendineae. Septic emboli can form and establish infection in any organ.[7,10] Numerous

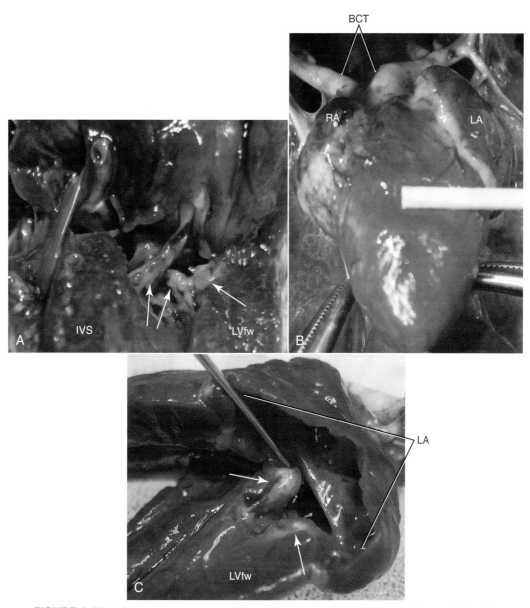

FIGURE 6-37 Valvular degeneration of the left AV valve *(arrows)* in a 64-year-old, male double yellow-headed Amazon parrot *(Amazona oratrix)* **(A)** and in a 17-year-old, male umbrella cockatoo *(Cacatua alba)* with marked left atrial dilatation, concurrent advanced atherosclerosis of the aorta and brachiocephalic trunks, and multifocal myocardial degeneration **(B** and **C)**. BCT, Brachiocephalic trunks; IVS, interventricular septum; LA, left atrium; LVfw, left ventricular free wall; RA, right atrium.

bacterial agents have been implicated in endocarditis (see Table 6-5). *Enterobacter cloacae* was isolated from peripheral and heart blood of a blue-and-gold macaw *(Ara ararauna)* with vegetative endocarditis of the left AV valve.[7,103]

Congenital anomalies producing volume overload in birds include atrial and ventricular septal defects, valvular deformities, and vascular malformations. An atrial septal defect was present in an inbred, 6-week-old Griffon vulture *(Gyps fulvus)* with biventricular congestive heart failure. The bird was the offspring of captive siblings.[121] Ventricular septal defects have been reported in the tundra swan *(Cygnus columbianus)*, Chinese goose *(Cygnopsis cygnoid)*, Houbara bustard *(Chlamydotis undulata)*, and ostrich *(Struthio camelus)*.[119,120,168] The ostrich

also had a defect in the left cranial vena cava.[168] Ventricular or atrial septal defects were diagnosed in eight of 111 Mississippi sandhill cranes *(Grus canadensis pulla)* in a mortality survey at the Patuxent Wildlife Research Center.[169] Ventricular septal defects and other cardiovascular malformations occur spontaneously in poultry but can also be induced experimentally in the chicken and turkey embryo by exposure to teratogenic agents and by improper incubation conditions and maternal nutritional deficiencies.[7,10,170,171] Among psittacines, cockatoos seem to be overrepresented, with ventricular septal defects documented most often in umbrella cockatoos *(Cacatua alba)* and also in the Moluccan cockatoo *(Cacatua moluccensis)*. Typically the defects are high, located just proximal to the

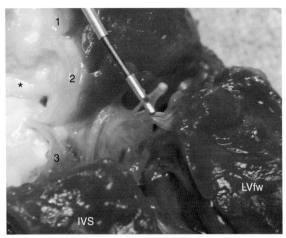

FIGURE 6-38 Insufficiency of the left atrioventricular valve resulting from torn chordae tendineae *(elevated by the pointer)* in a 30-year-old, female military macaw *(Ara militaris)* with concurrent advanced atherosclerosis *(asterisk)* and biventricular congestive heart failure. 1, 2, and 3, Aortic valve cusps; IVS, interventricular septum; LVfw, left ventricular free wall.

aortic and pulmonary valves, and result in biventricular congestive heart failure.[10,118] In one umbrella cockatoo, a ventricular septal defect was identified in combination with a persistent truncus arteriosus, wherein the aorta and pulmonary trunk arise as a single outflow vessel straddling both ventricles.[118] A congenital fissure of the right AV valve was reported in a blue-fronted Amazon parrot *(Amazona aestiva)* with right-sided congestive heart failure.[41]

Arrhythmias. Cardiac arrhythmias range from clinically insignificant events to life-threatening or terminal events.

Clinical signs may be absent or include weakness, syncope, or sudden death. Arrhythmias rarely constitute a primary disease process; they can develop secondary to cardiac chamber dilatation, myocarditis, or cardiomyopathy of any cause, as well as toxicoses, nutritional deficiencies, electrolyte imbalances, and various anesthetic agents.[7,19,172] They can be potentiated by catecholamine release, as occurs with handling stress and painful conditions.[7,173-175] Clinically significant cardiac arrhythmias likely represent the minority, but those producing hemodynamic instability and associated clinical signs warrant characterization and appropriate treatment.

Arrhythmias can be classified as excitability disturbances characterized by either increases or decreases in excitability (impulse formation) or as conduction disturbances characterized by impaired impulse transmission (blocks). Blocks are further characterized by anatomic location (SA node, AV node, bundle branches) and by degree: conduction is delayed in first-degree blocks, intermittent in second-degree blocks, and completely interrupted in third-degree blocks.[172] Escape beats and escape rhythms may be seen with severe bradyarrhythmias; they are of ectopic origin and perform an essential salvage function by preventing asystole at low heart rates. QRS morphology of ventricular escape beats may be abnormal (wide and bizarre), but these should not be confused with premature beats (additional beats added to already normal or rapid heart rate), because in the case of escape beats, antiarrhythmic therapy is contraindicated.[15,172]

Reported arrhythmias and their causes are summarized in Table 6-7. Of these, respiratory sinus arrhythmia, wandering pacemaker, and occasional sinus arrest and SA block can be considered physiologic in birds, related to increased vagal tone.[7,15,175,181] Supraventricular and ventricular premature complexes have been reported in apparently healthy, unanesthetized chickens and Amazon and Grey parrots.[175,181]

TABLE 6-7
Reported Cardiac Arrhythmias and Some Documented Causes in Birds[7,15,19,54,172–174,176–181]

Arrhythmias	Electrocardiographic Findings	Causes
EXCITABILITY DISTURBANCES		
Respiratory sinus arrhythmia	Heart rate increases with inspiration and decreases with expiration	Decreased vagal tone occurs with inspiration and increased tone with expiration: physiologic
Wandering pacemaker	Changing P wave morphology, +/−reduced PR interval	Shifting of the pacemaker site within the sinoatrial (SA) node or right atrium: physiologic
Sinus bradycardia	Low heart rate with normal sinus rhythm	Vagal stimulation,* anesthetic agents (halothane, methoxyflurane, isoflurane), acepromazine, xylazine, digoxin toxicity, acetylcholinesterase inhibitors (organophosphates, carbamates), polychlorinated biphenyl compounds, lead toxicosis, hypokalemia, hyperkalemia, thiamine (vitamin B_1) deficiency, vitamin E deficiency, hypothermia, compression of vagal nerve by neoplasms or other space-occupying masses
Sinus tachycardia	High heart rate with normal sinus rhythm; P wave may be superimposed on T wave (P on T phenomenon)	Sympathetic or catecholamine stimulation: exercise, pain, stress (physiologic); congestive heart failure, shock, hypotension, hypoxia, anemia, hypokalemia, avian influenza
Supraventricular premature complex (SPC)	Premature beat; change in P wave morphology, typically normal QRS complex morphology	Premature depolarization originating from an ectopic atrial focus: atrial dilatation or other structural abnormality, isoflurane, digoxin toxicity, avian influenza

TABLE 6-7

Reported Cardiac Arrhythmias and Some Documented Causes in Birds[7,15,19,54,172–174,176–181]—cont'd

Arrhythmias	Electrocardiographic Findings	Causes
Supraventricular tachycardia	Series of ≥3 SPCs more rapid than the sinus rate; intermittent or continuous	
Atrial fibrillation	Rapid, irregularly irregular rhythm; no normal P waves, typically normal QRS complexes	Atrial electrical disorganization with rapid, chaotic depolarizations: atrial dilatation, digoxin toxicity
Ventricular premature complex (VPC)	Premature beat; abnormal QRS complex morphology (wide and bizarre), normal P waves unrelated to abnormal QRS complexes, change in T wave morphology	Premature depolarization originating from an ectopic ventricular focus: myocardial infarction, hypoxia, anesthetic agents (halothane, isoflurane), digoxin toxicity, lead toxicosis, toxemia, hypokalemia, thiamine (vitamin B_1) deficiency, vitamin E deficiency, avian paramyxovirus 1, avian influenza
Ventricular tachycardia	Series of ≥3 VPCs more rapid than the sinus rate; intermittent or continuous	
Ventricular fibrillation	Irregular, bizarre waveforms; no recognizable P, QRS, or T waves	Ventricular electrical disorganization with chaotic depolarizations: severe, likely terminal cardiac disease, myocardial hypoxia, halothane, digoxin toxicity

CONDUCTION DISTURBANCES

Sinus arrest or SA block	Regular rhythm, absent ("dropped") P wave and following QRS, S-S interval twice normal, may see escape beat at very low heart rates; otherwise P waves and QRS complexes normal	SA node fails to depolarize (sinus arrest) or impulse fails to propagate beyond the SA node to depolarize the atria (SA block): increased vagal tone* (physiologic), atrial dilatation or other structural abnormality, isoflurane, digoxin toxicity, acetylcholinesterase inhibitors (organophosphates, carbamates), lead toxicosis, hypokalemia, hyperkalemia, thiamine (vitamin B_1) deficiency, vitamin E deficiency
First-degree atrioventricular (AV) block	Prolonged PR intervals	Delayed conduction through the AV node: increased vagal tone,* halothane, xylazine, digoxin toxicity; may be normal in some individuals
Second-degree AV block	Prolonged PR intervals, some P waves not followed by a QRS complex	AV conduction interrupted completely but intermittently: increased vagal tone,* isoflurane, dobutamine, digoxin toxicity, hypokalemia, thiamine (vitamin B_1) deficiency
Mobitz type 1	Progressively lengthening PR intervals prior to block (P wave without QRS complex), fixed ratio of P waves to QRS complexes	May be normal in racing pigeons, parrots, raptors
Mobitz type 2	Constant PR intervals, fixed ratio of P waves to QRS complexes	
Third-degree AV block	Normal P waves with no relation to ventricular escape rhythm (wide and bizarre QRS complexes at slow, fixed rate)	AV conduction interrupted completely and consistently: severe cardiac disease (cardiomyopathy, myocarditis), digoxin toxicity, hypokalemia
Bundle branch block	Increased duration and abnormal morphology of QRS complexes (wide and bizarre)	Delayed or interrupted conduction through one or more bundle branches, resulting in desynchronization of the ventricles: lead toxicosis

*Atropine responsiveness indicates a cause involving increased vagal tone.
Color-coding indicates relative clinical significance: gray, physiologic basis and/or clinically benign; orange, greater likelihood of pathologic basis and clinical disease; red, pathologic basis and high probability of severe clinical disease.

First-degree AV block and second-degree AV block (Mobitz type 1) may be found in healthy individuals of some species, the latter being recognized in chickens,[181] racing pigeons, Amazon and Grey parrots,[7,15,173] and one Muscovy duck (*Cairina moschata*).[174] They may occur with some frequency during anesthetic events and are unlikely to be clinically significant.[7,15,173-175] Second-degree AV block was seen in a clinically normal, 2-year-old Hispaniolan Amazon parrot (*Amazona ventralis*), in which no conclusive evidence of organic disease was found. Hypotensive episodes were documented during each block while the bird was anesthetized with isoflurane.[173]

Mobitz type 2 second-degree AV block may have greater clinical consequences and has the potential to progress to third-degree AV block.[15] A 30-year-old, female Moluccan cockatoo (*Cacatua moluccensis*) experiencing syncope was diagnosed with left ventricular dilatation and second-degree AV block (Mobitz type 2), which proved to be atropine responsive.[176] Third-degree AV block was identified in a 13-year-old Grey parrot, which died shortly after presentation and was diagnosed at postmortem examination with biventricular congestive heart failure and atherosclerosis of the great vessels.[7] Lead toxicosis in a galah *(Eolophus roseicollis)* was associated with marked bradycardia, sinus arrest, and left bundle branch block.[154] Syncopal episodes of several seconds, occurring a few times a month, occurred as a result of SA arrest in a 22-year-old Grey parrot. The underlying cause was not determined, although infectious myocarditis was suspected.[7] Atrial fibrillation developed subsequent to marked left atrial dilatation in a pukeko *(Porphyrio melanotus)* with left AV valve insufficiency and congestive heart failure.[81]

Compensatory mechanisms in heart failure. Congestive heart failure is the end result of chronic activation of compensatory mechanisms that are lifesaving in the short term by maintaining arterial blood pressure, but in the long term, are counterproductive and progressively deleterious (Figure 6-39). With compensation, cardiac output improves

at the expense of additional workload of the heart and vasculature; this state is termed "stable hyperfunction." With chronicity, this progresses to a state of "exhaustion and progressive cardiosclerosis" marked by ventricular myocardial dysfunction and damage, clinically apparent disease, and ultimately death.[18]

Decreases in cardiac output and arterial blood pressure are detected by chemoreceptors, baroreceptors, cardiac mechanoreceptors, and the renal juxtaglomerular apparatus. Low blood pressure activates numerous compensatory measures similar to those induced by blood loss and dehydration, initially preserving blood pressure. Principal players in this neuroendocrine activation are sympathetic tone, the RAAS, and AVT, which cause (1) increases in heart rate and contractility to increase cardiac output, (2) vasoconstriction to maintain arterial blood pressure, and (3) retention of water and sodium to increase circulatory volume, which, together with venoconstriction and opening of the renal portal valves, increases preload.[2,18] Longer-term results of increasing venous pressure are development of edema and effusions, whereas

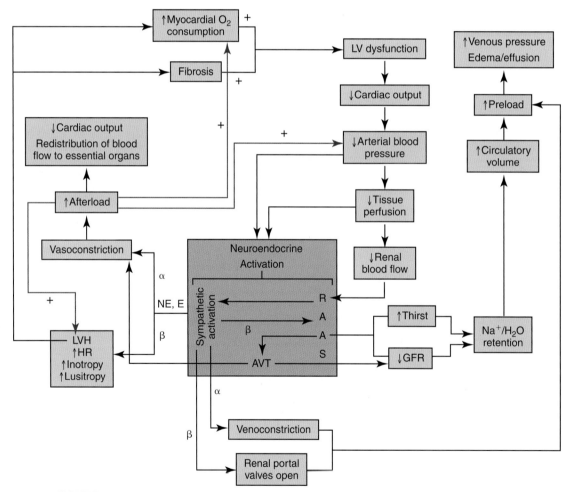

FIGURE 6-39 Compensatory mechanisms in congestive heart failure and their clinical consequences. α, Alpha-adrenergic receptor mediation; AVT, arginine vasotocin; β, beta-adrenergic receptor mediation; E, epinephrine; GFR, glomerular filtration rate; HR, heart rate; LV, left ventricle; LVH, left ventricular hypertrophy; NE, norepinephrine; RAAS, renin-angiotensin-aldosterone system. (Modified from de Morais HA, Schwartz DS: Pathophysiology of heart failure. In Ettinger SJ, Feldman EC, editors: *Textbook of veterinary internal medicine,* ed 6, St. Louis, MO, 2005, Saunders, pp 914–940.)

results of increasing afterload are decreased cardiac output (requiring redistribution of blood flow to essential organs), increased myocardial oxygen consumption, and ventricular hypertrophy, fibrosis, and progressive dysfunction.[18]

Immediately upon a decline in arterial blood pressure, parasympathetic tone decreases, and sympathetic tone and circulating catecholamines increase, thus exerting positive chronotropic, inotropic, and lusitropic effects[18] via β-adrenergic receptors; mediating vasoconstriction and venoconstriction via α-adrenergic receptors; and stimulating renin release from the renal juxtaglomerular apparatus by action at β-adrenergic receptors.[2] Renin is also released in response to decreased renal blood flow subsequent to systemic hypotension and hypovolemia and by decreased plasma sodium. Renin converts circulating angiotensinogen into angiotensin I, which, in turn, is converted into angiotensin II (AII) by angiotensin-converting enzyme (ACE). AII has myriad effects, including promotion of thirst, vasoconstriction and venoconstriction (by mediation of catecholamine release), the release of AVT,[182] and the production of the mineralocorticoid aldosterone, which causes sodium and water retention.[2,183] In mammals, AII and aldosterone are also known as mediators of inflammation, oxidative stress, and myocardial and vascular remodeling and fibrosis. AII contributes to the process of myocardial hypertrophy and has cytotoxic effects that incite cell necrosis. Promotion of fibroblast hypertrophy and increased collagen production by AII leads to fibrosis of the myocardium and vascular wall, and promotion of vascular smooth muscle cell growth by AII causes hyperplasia, hypertrophy, and apoptosis.[18] AVT, a product of the posterior pituitary homologous to mammalian antidiuretic hormone (ADH), is released in response to increases in plasma osmolality, hypotension, and AII. AVT induces vasoconstriction, decreases GFR by constriction of afferent glomerular arterioles, and promotes tubular water resorption.[2,182,184] A variety of vasodilatory agents, including the natriuretic peptides and nitric oxide, are released to counteract the effects of sympathetic activity and the RAAS, but their effects may be largely overridden in congestive heart failure.[18]

Prevalence
Overall, cardiac diseases have been recognized predominantly in poultry and companion psittacine birds, whereas they seem to be a relatively rare occurrence in other taxonomic groups. In large pathologic reviews of birds of prey, primary cardiovascular diseases were rarely reported outside of atherosclerosis.[48,185,186] Some disease entities reported more commonly in given taxonomic groups are listed in Table 6-8.

There are relatively few published studies examining the prevalence of cardiac disease in psittacines. These have had sample sizes ranging from 107 to 1322 birds and determined a prevalence between 5.2% and 36%.[13,48,93,187] Cardiac disease was recognized in 26 (9.7%) of 269 psittacine birds submitted for necropsy to Ohio State University, College of Veterinary Medicine, between 1991 and 1995. In 15 (58%) of these, congestive heart failure was ruled the cause of death, and in the remaining 11 (42%), cardiac lesions were considered incidental and secondary to systemic infectious diseases, including pulmonary aspergillosis, bacterial septicemia, avian polyomavirus (APV) infection, and PDD. In cases of right-sided congestive heart failure (10 birds), hepatic congestion, capsular fibrin, and ascites were consistently found. Pericardial

TABLE 6-8

Some Commonly Reported Cardiovascular Diseases and Lesions (Other Than Atherosclerosis) by Taxonomic Group[7,48,93]

Species	Common Cardiovascular Diseases
Psittacines	Congestive heart failure
Ducks, geese, swans	Vascular nematodes (schistosomes, filarioids)
Chickens, turkeys	Ascites syndrome, cardiomyopathies, infectious disease, aortic rupture
Ostriches	Aortic rupture
Birds of prey	Viral myocarditis (West Nile virus)

effusion was identified in three of these cases. Pulmonary congestion and edema were observed in cases of left-sided congestive heart failure (five birds), and birds with biventricular failure exhibited both hepatic and pulmonary lesions.[93]

In another study, 36% of 107 psittacine birds submitted for necropsy exhibited grossly visible abnormalities of the heart, great vessels, or both, whereas histologic changes in these tissues were found in 99% of birds; 15% had either myocardial hypertrophy or dilatation, and 60% had inflammatory infiltrates into the myocardium. Myocardial hemorrhage (19%), aortic chondroid metaplasia (21%), and myocardial fibrosis (10%) were also identified. Atherosclerosis of the great vessels was found in 13% of cases, and half of these also had calcification of the coronary arteries. Atherosclerotic disease and congestive heart failure accounted for the majority of noninfectious cardiovascular disease, and a similar spectrum of infectious disease states were identified as in the Ohio State study.[13]

In the author's (BCF) practice, cardiac disease most consistently is seen to take the form of congestive heart failure subsequent to advanced atherosclerotic disease, and as such, the represented age and species groups mirror those with higher prevalence of atherosclerosis. Cases of valvular insufficiency (including vegetative endocarditis), chronic pulmonary disease with probable hypertension, neoplasms or fungal granulomas encroaching on the heart base and great vessels, infectious myocarditis, cardiac arrhythmias, and congenital defects are encountered less frequently.

Pericardial Disease and Effusion
Pathophysiology
Pericardial effusion is characterized by an inappropriate accumulation of fluid within the pericardial sac. It can develop in birds as a result of inflammatory changes of the pericardium (pericarditis), trauma or aneurismal rupture, and cardiac or pericardial neoplasia or as a manifestation of metabolic derangements, toxic insult, or, commonly, right-sided congestive heart failure.[c] In some cases, an underlying cause cannot be identified, and the condition is ruled idiopathic. Depending on the etiology, the effusion may be a pure transudate, modified transudate, or an exudate.[d] Pure transudates accumulating within the pericardial sac (also termed *hydropericardium*) typically are the

---

[c]References 10,29,41,93,94,110,188,189.
[d]References 7,10,94,127,190,191.

result of increased vascular permeability or low vascular oncotic pressure, as occurs with vasculitis and hypoproteinemia, respectively.[7,10,127,190-192] Modified transudates accumulate with irritation or inflammation of the pericardium (pericarditis), hemorrhage into the pericardial sac (hemopericardium), or increased hydrostatic pressure, as occurs with central venous congestion subsequent to right-sided congestive heart failure.[110] Exudates may accumulate when infectious disease or neoplasia affects the heart, pericardium, or adjacent tissues, including the respiratory tract.[7,13,114,190,193]

Cardiac tamponade is defined as compression of the heart by a restrictive pericardium or accumulation of pericardial contents, resulting in impairment of ventricular filling (diastolic dysfunction), and subsequent decrease in stroke volume and cardiac output. Chamber filling requires positive intramural pressure (calculated as the difference of intracardiac pressure and intrapericardial pressure), but as intrapericardial pressure increases, intramural (filling) pressure progressively declines. Furthermore, given the Frank-Starling relationship between myocardial stretching and force of contraction, the systolic function of the underfilled cardiac chambers is diminished. The intramural pressure of the thinner-walled right ventricle is overcome more rapidly than that of the left. Therefore, cardiac tamponade results in right-sided congestive heart failure in advance of left-sided failure.[7,194] It follows that pericardial effusion that has developed secondary to right-sided congestive heart failure may precipitate decompensation.[7,94]

Cardiac tamponade may arise by constriction with a fibrotic pericardium subsequent to chronic, fibrinous pericarditis and adhesion to the epicardium.[7,113] When pericardial effusion is the cause of compression, the clinical severity of cardiac tamponade depends, in large part, on the rate at which the effusion develops. As the pericardium is relatively noncompliant, acute accumulations of even small fluid volumes can have profound hemodynamic effects.[7,194] Conversely, a more chronic onset of pericardial effusion allows time for expansion of the pericardial sac and compensatory physiologic mechanisms, including increased blood volume and heart rate via activation of the RAAS and sympathetic stimulation.[127,194]

Pericarditis and visceral gout. Infectious pericarditis and associated effusion can be a manifestation of systemic disease or occur as an extension of epicarditis, myocarditis, or inflammatory or infectious conditions affecting other adjacent tissues, including the air sacs, lungs, and liver. Bacterial, fungal, viral, and parasitic agents have been implicated (see Table 6-5),[7,10] with reported bacterial pathogens including *C. psittaci*, *Mycobacterium* spp., *Escherichia coli*,[e] *Listeria monocytogenes*,[7,192,197-199] *Salmonella* spp.,[7,192,197,200] *Riemerella anatipestifer*,[45] and *Erysipelothrix rhusiopathiae*.[201] In one study, gross evidence of pericarditis was found in 10% of *C. psittaci*–infected psittacine birds.[202] Fibrinous pericarditis is among the well-documented lesions of acute *C. psittaci* infection in psittacine species[190] and has also been documented in numerous other orders of birds, including Falconiformes,[203] Charadriiformes,[204] and Galliformes.[42,205] Pericarditis represents the most severe and persistent lesion

in domestic turkeys infected with virulent turkey strains of *C. psittaci*.[42] In cases of mycobacteriosis, in which *M. avium*, *M. tuberculosis*, and *M. genavense* have been the most commonly described isolates,[206,207] cardiovascular lesions typically involve the heart base or pericardium and manifest as nodular granulomas.[10,207] In an adult gang gang cockatoo (*Callocephalon fimbriatum*), mycobacterial infection resulted in granulomatous pericarditis and myocarditis with marked pericardial effusion and cardiac tamponade.[207]

Mycotic infection, most often with *Aspergillus* spp., can cause pericardial disease either by extension from the respiratory tract[7,13,94,192] or by hematogenous spread.[10,190] Pericardial effusion is a frequently reported gross finding in outbreaks of APV infection in budgerigars (*Melopsittacus undulatus*)[10,190,208,209] and is among the characteristic lesions of hemorrhagic nephritis enteritis of geese, which is caused by a polyomavirus phylogenetically distinct from psittacine polyomavirus.[210] Viral etiologies other than polyomavirus that are reported to cause pericardial disease and effusion in birds are psittacid herpesvirus (PsHV),[13] adenoviruses of the genus Aviadenovirus in fowl,[211-213] highly pathogenic avian influenza (H5N1),[214] parvovirus affecting geese and ducks,[215,216] and reoviruses in gallinaceous birds.[7,217] Parasitic infections of birds rarely produce pericardial lesions, but there are reports of *Toxoplasma gondii* infection causing fibrinous serositis in canaries (*Serinus canaria*)[190] and generalized *Trichomonas gallinae* resulting in granulomatous lesions in pigeons.[94,218] Filarioid nematodes have been identified in wild-caught cockatoos,[10,219] with one report of adult worms found in the pericardial sac of a red-vented cockatoo (*Cacatua haematuropygia*).[142]

Visceral gout frequently affects the pericardium (Figure 6-40), with urate deposition variably accompanied by a heterophilic inflammatory response. A turbid, flocculent pericardial effusion may also be present. Gout can grossly resemble

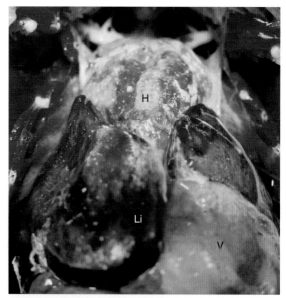

FIGURE 6-40 Visceral gout in a 16-year-old, female Grey parrot *(Psittacus erithacus)* with urate deposition visible on the pericardium and capsular surface of the liver *(caudoventral view)*. H, Heart; Li, liver; V, ventriculus.

---

[e]References 7, 44, 192, 193, 195, 196.

infectious pericarditis because both conditions cause pericardial thickening, but gout can be distinguished by its smooth, white plaques, in contrast to the yellowish, roughly-textured exudates of infectious pericarditis.[10,190,220]

Right-sided congestive heart failure. Pericardial effusion can result from systemic venous congestion in cases of right-sided congestive heart failure (see Figures 6-26, *A* and *B*, and 6-32).[f] Pericardial effusion was identified in an umbrella cockatoo (*Cacatua alba*) with right-sided congestive heart failure subsequent to severe atherosclerotic disease and aneurismal dilatation of the right coronary artery,[29] in a yellow-crowned Amazon parrot (*Amazona ochrocephala*) with right ventricular hypertrophy and polycythemia,[166] and in a blue-fronted Amazon parrot (*Amazona aestiva*) with insufficiency of the right AV valve resulting from a congenital defect.[41] Pericardial effusion was also present in a case of severe atherosclerosis, biventricular failure, and pulmonary and portal hypertension in a severe macaw (*Ara severa*).[95]

Others. Additional causes of pericardial effusion include hypoproteinemia,[7,10,94,127,165] toxin ingestion (see Table 6-6), neoplasia, and hemorrhage. Hemopericardium may occur with coagulopathy, trauma, atrial or aneurismal rupture, or neoplasia of the heart or pericardium.[g] There are no reports of primary pericardial tumors in companion birds,[10] but Lightfoot reported a case of hemangioma within the coelomic cavity of a juvenile Grey parrot, which involved numerous organs as well as the pericardium.[222] Hemopericardium and fibrinous epicarditis were identified in a case of ovarian hemangiosarcoma in an orange-winged Amazon parrot (*Amazona amazonica*), although the relationship between the two was undetermined.[221]

Prevalence

Pericardial disease in psittacine birds has been examined in a handful of studies and case reports. In one study, pericardial effusion, accompanied by moderate to marked hepatomegaly, was identified in 6% of 107 psittacine birds submitted for necropsy. Among these birds, pericardial effusion had occurred with infectious disease and visceral gout or was accompanied by right ventricular dilatation and ascites consistent with right-sided congestive heart failure. In 15% of birds with pericardial effusion, fibrinous pericarditis was identified in association with chlamydiosis, PsHV infection, respiratory tract mycosis, PDD, or bacterial septicemia.[13]

In a survey of 60 psittacines and birds of other taxonomic groups presented with varying degrees of illness over a 1-year period, five (8.3%) were diagnosed with pericardial effusion via echocardiography. These included one mallard duck (*Anas platyrhynchos*), three Grey parrots, and one blue-fronted Amazon parrot, all presenting with lethargy, weakness, and pectoral muscle wasting. In the Grey parrots, right ventricular dilatation, hepatic congestion, and ascites were also evident, consistent with right-sided congestive heart failure. Severe lower respiratory mycosis was diagnosed in all three birds. Low-grade pericardial effusion in the Amazon parrot, mentioned previously, had arisen secondary to right-sided congestive heart failure owing to incompetency of the right AV valve.[114]

In the author's (BCF) practice, 43 cases of pericardial disease, pericardial effusion, or a combination of both were reviewed. Infectious pericarditis was identified in 14 cases

(32%), including 3 cases of APV infection, 5 cases of aspergillosis with extension from the respiratory tract to the pericardium, 1 case of suspected chlamydiosis, 3 cases of bacterial pneumonia with extension to the pericardium, and 2 cases of bacterial sepsis. Visceral gout occurred in 12 cases (28%) and hypoproteinemia with transudation into the pericardial sac in 2 cases of hepatic failure. Pericardial effusion related to congestive heart failure (either right-sided or biventricular) occurred in 9 cases (20%). One cockatiel developed acute hemopericardium and died as a result of cardiac tamponade. Pericardial thickening was noted in a Grey parrot with multicentric lymphoma. In 5 birds (11%), pericardial effusion was ruled idiopathic.

DIAGNOSTIC METHODS

History, Clinical Signs, and Physical Examination Findings

Diagnosis of cardiovascular disease begins with careful history collection and thorough physical examination, to be performed in a manner in keeping with patient stability. Examination findings as well as relative predisposition to cardiovascular disease, given the species, breed (pertaining to poultry), age, gender, lifestyle, and diet, should be taken under consideration when formulating initial differential diagnoses and prioritizing diagnostic maneuvers. Clinical presentations of cardiovascular disease share many commonalities, particularly as more than one condition can exist concurrently, but there are distinguishing features of some disease states that warrant mention in the sections to follow. In companion birds, many cases are likely subclinical and go unrecognized for many years until well advanced. Clinical signs can have a subtle, insidious onset, with owners reporting progressively declining activity level, reduced appetite (to include refusal of favored items or "pickiness"), and waning interest in household activities, toys, and vocalizations that were historically of interest to the bird. Previously asymptomatic cardiovascular disease can manifest clinically following introduction of physiologic stressors such as concurrent disease or egg production that precipitate decompensation. In some cases, no premonitory signs are appreciated prior to sudden death.[24] Presenting complaints common to most forms of cardiovascular disease are lethargy, depression, weakness, reduced appetite, respiratory distress, and exercise intolerance.[h] Physical examination findings may include cachexia, tachypnea, dyspnea, harsh lung sounds, pallor or cyanosis, tachycardia, arrhythmia, systolic murmur, poor pulse quality or deficits, coelomic distension and ascites, peripheral edema, peripheral venous congestion, and altered mentation.

The physical examination should consist of two portions: a hands-off evaluation to be performed first to assess demeanor, posture and mobility, neurologic status, respiratory rate and character, and droppings, followed by a hands-on examination. The latter should be performed following a period of preoxygenation in patients with severe respiratory

[f]References 10,29,41,93,94,110,188,189.
[g]References 7,10,94,127,190,191,221.
[h]References 29,94,95,103,110,114,115,127,128,221,223-225.

compromise and may need to be completed in stages, with intervening initial supportive treatment, depending on the stability of the patient. In debilitated patients and companion birds that are familiar with and tolerant of handling, much of the physical examination can be performed with the bird standing, with minimal restraint necessary. Restrained birds should be held upright during physical examination to avoid additional respiratory or circulatory compromise that may occur with dorsal recumbency. Cardiac auscultation is a relatively insensitive tool, particularly with the rapid heart rates characteristic of birds, but subjective assessments of rate, rhythm, and sound quality can be made. Normal heart rates scale negatively with body weight and can increase up to four times the resting heart rate during flight, to which restraint may be comparable for some patients (Table 6-9). Cardiac auscultation is traditionally performed by placing a pediatric or neonatal stethoscope on the cranial keel, but by shifting to multiple locations along the keel, thoracic inlet, and dorsum, the clinician can identify the site of best audibility and increase the likelihood of detecting quiet, focal murmurs. A detectable murmur has been reported in many published cases of cardiac disease, but the absence of an audible murmur does not rule out cardiovascular pathology. Arterial pulses are best palpated at the medial aspect of the proximal antebrachium (superficial ulnar artery) and relative warmth of each extremity should also be subjectively assessed.

Atherosclerosis

Clinical signs of atherosclerotic disease are generally associated with diminished blood flow through stenotic arteries and vary depending on the vessels affected, severity of atherosclerotic lesions, and presence of concurrent disease, including cardiac disease and congestive heart failure.[24,27] Sudden death may occur as a result of a cerebral infarct, aneurysmal rupture, or a lethal cardiac arrhythmia secondary to myocardial ischemia. Patients are often presented for falling or collapsing, frequently accompanied by transient or persistent weakness and dysfunction of one or more limbs and with or without altered mentation, which the owners may describe as disorientation or confusion. Frequently, the owners report their birds exhibiting extension and rigidity of one leg

(and sometimes the ipsilateral wing), clenching of the toes, ataxia or difficulty perching, and tremors or convulsions. These signs are considered most consistent with stroke, but rarely is this confirmed diagnostically.[24,226] On the basis of the owners' descriptions, these events can be difficult to distinguish from seizure activity, and, indeed, seizures can occur subsequent to ischemic stroke.[226,227] Owners most often describe an acute onset, and in many instances, the bird seems to have recovered prior to the visit. Alternatively, there may be persistent neurologic abnormalities identified upon physical examination, including reduced mentation, blindness, anisocoria, seizures, vestibular signs, paresis of one or both pelvic limbs, and ataxia. Severe events may be accompanied by regurgitation and present with respiratory signs secondary to aspiration. In cases with concurrent congestive heart failure, dyspnea and exercise intolerance may be part of the history and appreciable upon physical examination, along with other congestive signs.

Intermittent claudication is a clinical manifestation of peripheral arterial disease wherein intermittent weakness and pain in the pelvic limbs is exercise-induced and resolves with rest. It has been suspected in a number of cases with compatible clinical signs,[96,227-229] including in a 25-year-old yellow-naped Amazon parrot (*Amazona auropalliata*) with severe atherosclerotic disease of the entire aorta and the external iliac arteries, extending to the ischiatic arteries.[230] The author (BCF) has seen numerous cases of recurrent or nonresolving dermatologic conditions (e.g., axillary or propatagial dermatitis, feather loss or abnormal growth, or self-inflicted feather damage or mutilation of the skin), wherein advanced atherosclerotic lesions were ultimately identified in vessels supplying the affected areas (Figure 6-41). The authors have therefore speculated that these conditions may develop secondary to tissue hypoperfusion or to associated pain or unusual sensations such as tingling and numbness. Further, it is possible that myocardial ischemia could produce angina pectoris as in human beings.[96]

Congestive heart failure

Birds with congestive heart failure present most consistently with respiratory embarrassment, as a result of intracoelomic air sac compression—caused by ascites and organomegaly—pulmonary edema, or a combination of the two. Some astute owners may note coelomic distention, which is among the congestive signs appreciable upon physical examination in cases of right-sided or biventricular failure. Hepatomegaly may also be apparent visually, with one or both lobes extending caudally beyond the sternal margin, or suggested upon palpation or transillumination of the coelom. Peripheral venous congestion is most easily appreciated by distention of the jugular and cutaneous ulnar veins. Edema, though a rarer finding, most often appears as swelling of the periorbital region or of the hocks and feet. In hospitalized patients receiving subcutaneous fluids, the first indication of circulatory compromise may be delayed absorption (>48 hours). Pericardial effusion inconsistently manifests as muffled heart sounds. In the case of cardiogenic pulmonary edema, increased respiratory noise is typically heard upon auscultation of the lung fields (cranial dorsum, parallel to the spine) in a calm bird, but characteristic "crackles and wheezes" are generally absent except in severe cases, and cough is exceptionally rare.

TABLE 6-9

Normal Heart Rates (Beats Per Minute) Expected for Most Species, at Rest and with Flight or Restraint, as a Function of Body Weight[5]

Weight (grams)	Heart Rate (Resting)	Heart Rate (Flight/ Restraint)	Factor Increase
25	380	909	2.4
50	329	815	2.5
100	284	731	2.6
200	245	655	2.7
300	226	615	2.7
400	213	588	2.8
500	203	568	2.8
1000	175	509	2.9
2000	152	457	3.0

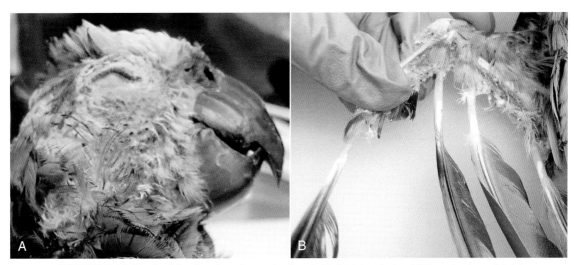

FIGURE 6-41 Marked feather loss from the head *(right lateral view)* **(A)** and wings *(right wing, ventral view)* **(B)**, with minimal replacement and dystrophic appearance of emerging pinfeathers, in a 24-year-old, male blue-front Amazon parrot *(Amazona aestiva)* with atherosclerotic lesions causing virtually complete obstruction of the brachiocephalic trunks (see Figure 6-20). Note: Feather loss progressed over a 6-month period, with no history of self-inflicted damage. Other clinical signs included periodic strokelike events, progressive weakness and ataxia, dull mentation, and seizures.

Pericardial effusion

Clinical manifestation of pericardial effusion depends on the underlying etiology and the rate of fluid accumulation. An acute onset of clinical signs would be expected with rapid development of pericardial effusion, as this would cause sudden, severe circulatory compromise as a result of cardiac tamponade. These birds may die suddenly or are presented in a profound state of debilitation and in respiratory distress. A more chronic onset would accompany slow accumulation of fluid over time because this would permit stretching and increased compliance of the pericardium. In this scenario, typical of right-sided congestive heart failure, birds may be asymptomatic for long periods. However, even in a well-compensated chronic case of pericardial effusion, clinical signs might become rapidly apparent when intrapericardial pressure ultimately overcomes cardiac filling pressure, producing an acute-on-chronic presentation.

A baseline diagnostic workup is appropriate in any patient presenting with clinical signs consistent with cardiovascular disease in order to begin to assess overall systemic health status. Key elements may include comprehensive serum biochemistry panel, complete blood count (CBC), and radiographic imaging (which may include imaging enhanced with contrast), ultrasonography, electrocardiography (ECG)[29,94] and blood pressure measurement[231] to further characterize the nature and extent of cardiovascular disease. Endoscopy[i] and advanced imaging, including computed tomography (CT) and magnetic resonance imaging (MRI),[233-235] also have application in the diagnosis and characterization of cardiovascular disease in some settings.

Clinical Pathology

Clinical pathology, overall, has a low sensitivity for specific cardiovascular disease. Abnormal findings are more often attributable to secondary effects on other organ systems, underlying primary disease processes, or concurrent, unrelated disease.

Biochemistries

In principle, disease affecting the myocardium may cause elevations in aspartate aminotransferase (AST), creatine kinase (CK), and lactate dehydrogenase (LDH).[7,94,236] The use of a cardiac muscle-specific CK isoenzyme (CK-MB) has been investigated in birds, and levels have been shown to significantly increase with furazolidone cardiotoxicosis in ducklings,[130] but this test is not readily available in clinical practice. Cardiac troponins T and I are cardiac regulatory proteins used as sensitive and specific markers of myocardial injury in humans.[55,237] They are detected by use of monoclonal antibodies,[237] but there are only 68% and 65% protein sequence homologies between chickens and humans for cardiac troponin T and I, respectively (BLAST Sequence Analysis Tool, Beaufrère, 2013). Therefore, sensitivity of this test for myocardial damage in birds may be suboptimal, and no reference ranges have been established.[55] Other biochemical abnormalities may be seen, depending on the systems secondarily or concurrently involved, particularly elevations in uric acid and bile acids, which reflect renal and hepatic functional impairments, respectively. These may occur as a consequence of renal hypoperfusion or hepatic congestion secondary to heart failure or as concurrent manifestations of an underlying disease process affecting multiple systems. Alternatively, hyperuricemia can be causally associated with cardiac disease (i.e., visceral gout), as can hypoproteinemia (which may result in pericardial effusion) and electrolyte disturbances (potassium, sodium, calcium, and magnesium), which can also produce cardiac arrhythmia.

Plasma lipids may offer some observational data pertinent to population-level risk factors for cardiovascular disease. An association between plasma lipid values, particularly plasma total cholesterol and HDL, and prevalence of atherosclerosis among certain psittacine genera has been shown, but the diagnostic value of a plasma lipid profile in assessing the relative atherosclerosis risk for an individual has not been established.[31] Hypercholesterolemia itself is neither necessary nor sufficient for a diagnosis of atherosclerosis, as birds with normal plasma cholesterol may have atherosclerotic disease,[28] whereas those with hypercholesterolemia may not.

Hematology

Hematologic changes, including elevated total white blood cell (WBC) count and shifts in the leukocyte differential are seen with many forms of inflammatory or infectious disease, as well as with stress, and can be seen in patients with cardiovascular disease.[238-240] Although no specific hematologic changes can be considered diagnostic, abnormalities reported in cases of cardiovascular disease in psittacine birds are leukocytosis, heterophilia, relative lymphopenia, and polycythemia.[29,166] Leukocytosis may be seen with bacterial myocarditis and valvular endocarditis, and with a number of concurrent or contributing systemic disease conditions, including, but not limited to, chlamydiosis, mycobacteriosis,[206] aspergillosis, or severe tissue necrosis secondary to trauma or neoplasia.[241] Polycythemia can result from chronic hypoxemia resulting from persistent ventilation/perfusion mismatch and increased oxygen demands.[97,162-164] If suspected, arterial blood gas analyses may help pinpoint an oxygenation problem.

Electrocardiography

ECG is an appropriate diagnostic step for characterization of arrhythmias and can provide information to suggest certain cardiac abnormalities, including chamber enlargement.[7,94,178] However, it must be used in conjunction with other diagnostic modalities, namely, imaging techniques, to diagnose specific cardiac disease. Severe pathology and mechanical dysfunction can exist in the absence of ECG changes.[7,15] ECG can also be valuable as part of anesthetic monitoring.[7,94] It is easier to perform an electrocardiographic examination on an anesthetized patient to avoid interference from movement and muscle tremors,[242] but patient stability, tolerance for handling, and the potential for anesthetic-related ECG alterations should be taken under consideration. ECG recording can, however, be accomplished in conscious birds,[7] particularly those that are accustomed to being handled or are weak and debilitated. Sedation represents another option; in recent years, protocols using benzodiazepines have been used with increasing regularity in companion birds,[243] but it is uncertain how these drugs may affect the ECG.

Instrumentation and technique

The electrocardiogram is obtained in the frontal plane by placing two cranial electrodes, one on each propatagium, and one (left) or two (right, ground) caudal electrodes on the inguinal skin web near the stifle.[7,175,178] Needle electrodes can be used or flat clips applied to the skin along with electrode gel.[94,175] The right thoracic limb (RA), left thoracic limb (LA), and left pelvic limb (LL) constitute the points of an equilateral triangle (Einthoven's triangle), wherein each side represents one of three bipolar leads (I, II, and III) (Figure 6-42). In lead I, LA is the positive pole and RA the negative pole; in lead II, LL is the positive pole and RA the negative pole; in lead III, LL is the positive pole and LA the negative pole. Additionally, three augmented unipolar leads (aVR, aVL, and aVF) are usually included in a standard examination. For each, one of the three limb electrodes is the positive pole (RA for aVR, LA for aVL, and LL for aVF) and an average of the

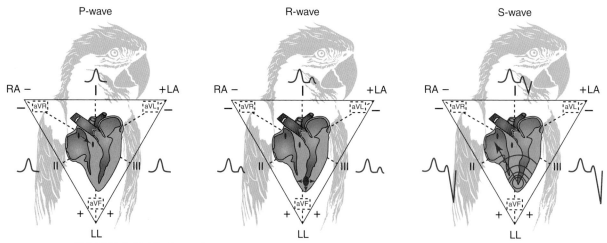

FIGURE 6-42 Einthoven's triangle, illustrating bipolar leads I, II, and III and augmented unipolar leads aVR, aVL, and aVF. Electrodes are placed on the right thoracic limb (RA), left thoracic limb (LA), and left pelvic limb (LL). Schematic representations of the electrical activity of the heart and the corresponding tracings in leads I–III are shown in red. Conduction proceeds from the sinoatrial node to the atrioventricular node, and atrial depolarization generates the P wave (positive deflection); ventricular depolarization begins, as represented by the R wave (positive deflection), and progresses to generate the S wave (negative deflection).

other two constitutes the negative pole. These six leads can also be represented with the Bailey's hexaxial system, where each lead axis is drawn passing through the central point in the triangle. This creates a circle with 30-degree segments and angle values assigned to the positive and negative pole of each lead; by convention, this begins with 0 degrees at the positive pole of lead I and proceeds clockwise (Figure 6-43).[7,15,175,178] An electrical impulse directed toward the positive pole of a given lead appears as a positive deflection on the electrocardiogram, whereas an impulse directed toward the negative pole appears as a negative deflection. An isoelectric lead is one to which the electrical impulse travels in a perpendicular direction, resulting in a recording of either no deflection or equal positive and negative deflections.[2,7,15]

Normal electrocardiogram deflections and mean electrical axis

The deflections on the normal avian electrocardiogram and their meanings are summarized in Table 6-10 and illustrated in Figure 6-42 and Figure 6-44. The first is the P wave, followed in some birds by a small depression in the beginning of the PR interval, known as the *Ta wave*. The QRS complex is more accurately described as an rS complex (or (Q)rS complex), given that the Q wave is typically absent, the R wave small, and the S wave the prominent deflection, which is negative in lead II for most birds. The ST segment is short or absent, and the S wave often merges into the T wave (ST-slurring). The ST segment, when present, is typically elevated above baseline.[7,15,175,242] Superimposition of the T wave on the following P wave (P-on-T phenomenon) is considered normal in some Amazon parrots (*Amazona* spp.) and Grey parrots (*Psittacus erithacus* and *P. timneh*).[7,15,175]

The ventricular mean electrical axis (MEA) is the direction of mean electrical activity during ventricular depolarization. Unlike in mammals, the ventricular MEA is negative in most birds, oriented along the body's long axis and near midline (close to −90 degrees), hence the negative polarity of the rS complex in lead II.[2,7,15,175,178] Broiler chickens[7,244] and Pekin ducks[245] are the exception, most often having a positive MEA.

Interpretation

Interpretation of the ECG should be methodical, following the same steps as those used in mammals: calculation of heart rate, evaluation of heart rhythm, measurement of complexes and intervals, and determination of the ventricular MEA.[7,15,175] Rapid heart rates of most patients necessitate the use of high paper speeds (preferably 100 to 200 millimeters per second [mm/s]) to best evaluate waveforms and obtain accurate measurements.[7,15,94,175] Electrocardiographic measurements are performed on lead II tracings and include duration (in seconds) and amplitude (in millivolts [mV]) of the P wave, duration of the PR interval, amplitude of the S wave, duration of the rS complex, amplitude of the T wave, and duration of the QT interval.[7,15,175] The MEA can be determined by using the isoelectric method and the Bailey's hexaxial system (see Figure 6-43). The first step is identification of the isoelectric lead, where either no deflections are seen or the sum of the (Q)rS deflections is zero. Second, the lead lying perpendicular to the isoelectric lead is found by referring to the hexaxial system diagram. The MEA lies along this perpendicular lead and is negative if the major deflection (rS complex) recorded in this lead is negative and positive if the major deflection is positive.[7,15] ECG reference intervals have been published for several species (Table 6-11). ECG alterations suggestive of pathology are summarized in Table 6-12, but their sensitivity and specificity should be considered low. Given that reference values do not exist for many species of birds, and there are likely age, sex, and breed differences, the practitioner should take care not to overinterpret small changes noted on the electrocardiogram.[2,7,15,178]

Blood Pressure

Arterial blood pressure is higher in birds than in most other vertebrates. Direct measurement is obtained by placing an

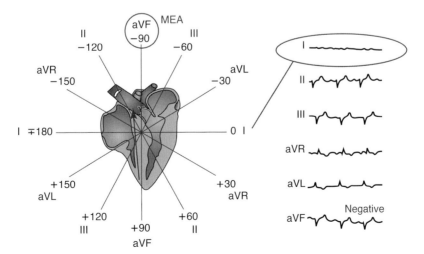

FIGURE 6-43 Determination of the ventricular mean electrical axis (MEA) (represented by the red vector) using the isoelectric method and the Bailey's hexaxial system. In this example, which is representative of most birds, lead I can be identified as the isoelectric lead, where net (Q)rS deflections are zero. The MEA lies along the lead perpendicular to lead I (aVF). Since the major deflection in lead aVF is negative, the MEA is −90 degrees.

Electrocardiogram (ECG) Segments and Their Significance During One Cardiac Cycle[2,7,15,178]

ECG Segment	Electrophysiologic meaning
P wave	Depolarization of the atria, conduction from sinoatrial (SA) to atrioventricular (AV) nodes
Ta wave	Repolarization of the atria (present in pigeons and some Galliformes and Psittaciformes)
PR interval	P wave, combined with the delay in conduction at the AV node
(Q)rS complex	Ventricular depolarization
ST segment	Period between the end of ventricular depolarization and beginning of ventricular repolarization
T wave	Repolarization of the ventricles
QT interval	rS complex and T wave: period of ventricular depolarization and repolarization

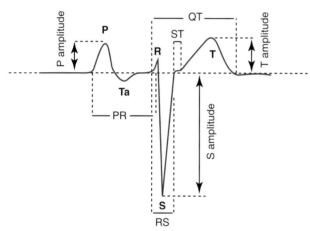

FIGURE 6-44 Schematic representation of a typical avian electrocardiographic complex in lead II (as it would appear with a paper speed of 200 millimeters per second [mm/s]) with depiction of measurement landmarks.

arterial catheter in the superficial ulnar artery (proximal medial antebrachium), deep radial artery (distal medial antebrachium), or external carotid artery. It is then connected to a pressure transducer and measured by an anesthetic monitor.[231,249-251] Direct arterial blood pressure values for selected species are displayed in Table 6-13.

Given that direct blood pressure measurement is challenging and often impractical in the clinical setting, indirect methods are most commonly used in veterinary practice to aid in the identification of hypertension and as part of anesthetic monitoring. Indirect blood pressure measurement can be obtained in birds using a Doppler ultrasonic flow detector placed on the wing or leg (over the superficial ulnar artery or cranial tibial artery, respectively), a cuff measured at 30% to 40% of the limb circumference, and a sphygmomanometer. However, it has been consistently demonstrated that values obtained with this method do not agree with

direct systolic blood pressure measurements and may therefore be of low clinical value as a diagnostic tool.[231,249,257] Limits of agreement were wide in a study in Hispaniolan Amazon parrots (*Amazona ventralis*) at −37 to 85 millimeters of mercury (mm Hg) and −14 to 42 mm Hg for wing and leg measurements, respectively.[231] In a study with subjects representing a variety of psittacine species, large variation was seen in repeated indirect blood pressure measurements, with the most variability attributable to the individual bird and to repeated cuff placement at the same site on the same individual.[257] Although these results indicated poor precision of indirect blood pressure measurements, they also suggested that monitoring of trends in the same bird during a single cuff placement such as during an anesthetic event, may be useful. In an experiment in red-tailed hawks (*Buteo jamaicensis*), indirect blood pressure measurements were found to be in disagreement with direct systolic blood pressure but in acceptable agreement with mean blood pressure (with limits of agreement of −9 to 13 mm Hg).[249] This suggests that the accuracy of indirect techniques may be higher in large birds. The oscillometric method of indirect blood pressure measurement has been found to be unreliable in all studied birds.[231,249]

In general, hypotension is defined as a systolic blood pressure lower than 90 mm Hg and a mean below 60 mm Hg. Values for hypertension have been poorly defined in birds but are expected to be higher than in mammals because of their greater blood pressure. Systolic values over 200 mm Hg have been proposed as hypertensive.[258]

Radiography

Radiographic imaging is generally an insensitive method to identify cardiovascular disease, but with practice, the clinician can expect to develop increased acuity, which would allow recognition of subtle changes and familiarity with species differences. Radiography allows for assessment of the size, contour, and radiodensity of the cardiac silhouette and the great vessels, including the aorta, brachiocephalic trunks, and pulmonary arteries and veins.[94,127,155,234] In large psittacines, by using high-resolution digital imaging, the common carotid and axillary arteries may be visualized on the ventrodorsal view, and some major branches of the descending aorta, namely, the coeliac and cranial mesenteric arteries, may be seen on the lateral view (Figure 6-45).

Use of sedation or anesthesia is often recommended in order to enable optimal patient positioning and diagnostic value.[233] The ultimate decision to use chemical restraint should be made on the basis of the need for optimal radiographic positioning balanced with the degree of patient debilitation, stress, and discomfort. Although general anesthesia facilitates patient positioning and reduces the risk of iatrogenic injury and motion artifact, it may be contraindicated in severely compromised patients.[234] In the author's (BCF) experience, sedation using a combination of butorphanol (1 to 2 mg/kg, intramuscularly [IM]) and midazolam (0.5 to 1.5 mg/kg, IM) provides an excellent alternative to general anesthesia with a wider margin of safety.

Cardiac silhouette and great vessels

Enlargement of the cardiac silhouette (Figure 6-46) can be seen with pericardial effusion, myocardial hypertrophy or inflammation, chamber dilatation, cardiac or pericardial

TABLE 6-11

Electrocardiographic (ECG) Reference Values for Selected Species, Taken in Lead II (Amplitude in mV, Duration in Seconds)[19,175,242,245-247]

Species	Racing Pigeon (*Columba livia*)	Amazon Parrots (*Amazona spp.*)	Grey Parrots (*Psittacus erithacus* and *P. timneh*)	Macaws (*Ara spp.*)	Cockatoos (*Cacatua spp.*)	Red-Tailed Hawk (*Buteo jamaicensis*)	Bald Eagle (*Haliaeetus leucocephalus*)	Pekin Duck (*Anas platyrhynchos domestica*)	Chicken (White Leghorn) (*Gallus gallus domesticus*)
N	60	37	45	41	31	11	20	50	72
Heart rate	160–300	340–600	340–600	255–555	259–575	80–220	50–160	200–360	180–340
P amplitude	0.4–0.6	0.25–0.60	0.25–0.55	0.03–0.47	0.13–0.53	−0.1–0.175	0.050–0.325		
P duration	0.015–0.020	0.008–0.017	0.012–0.018	0.009–0.021	0.009–0.025	0.020–0.035	0.030–0.060	0.015–0.035	0.035–0.043
PR interval	0.045–0.070	0.042–0.055	0.040–0.055	0.040–0.068	0.039–0.071	0.050–0.090	0.070–0.110	0.04–0.08	0.073–0.089
S amplitude	1.5–2.8	0.7–2.3	0.9–2.2	0.27–1.43	0.27–1.59	0.300–0.900	0.150–1.450	0.35–1.03	0.10–1.0
(Q)rS duration	0.013–0.016	0.010–0.015	0.010–0.016	0.002–0.030	0.014–0.026	0.020–0.030	0.020–0.040	0.028–0.044	0.02–0.028
T amplitude	0.3–0.8	0.3–0.8	0.18–0.6	0.12–0.80	0.17–0.97	0.000–0.300	0.050–0.200	0.04–0.40	0.03–0.28
QT interval	0.060–0.075	0.050–0.095	0.048–0.080	0.053–0.109	0.065–0.125	0.080–0.165	0.110–0.165	0.08–0.12	
MEA	−83 to −99	−90 to −107	−79 to −103	−76 to −87	−73 to −89	−50 to −110	−30 to −150	−160 to 95	−91 to −120

Note: To obtain a 95% reference interval, all published results in the form of mean ± SD were reported in the form of mean ± 2SD and in the form of mean ± SEM were reported as mean ± 2SEM√n; when only the range or a 95% reference interval was published, it was reported as is.

TABLE 6-12

Electrocardiographic (ECG) Alterations and Suggested Pathology[2,7,15,111,178,179,244,248]

Parameter	Alteration	Possible Pathologic Significance
P wave	Increased amplitude	Right atrial dilatation
	Increased duration	Left atrial dilatation
	Increased amplitude and duration	Biatrial dilatation
PR interval	Prolonged	Increased delay in conduction at the atrioventricular (AV) node (AV block)
(Q)rS complex	Prominent R wave in lead II	Right ventricular hypertrophy and/or dilatation
	Increased S wave amplitude in lead II	Left ventricular hypertrophy and/or dilatation
	Decreased S wave amplitude	Pericardial effusion
	Increased complex duration	Left ventricular hypertrophy and/or dilatation
T wave	Increased amplitude	Hyperkalemia
	Change in polarity in lead II	Myocardial hypoxia
QT interval	Increased duration	Isoflurane anesthesia
Ventricular mean electrical axis (MEA)	Axis deviation	Change in cardiac shape and/or position: right ventricular enlargement (usually right axis deviation); left ventricular enlargement (left or right axis deviation)

TABLE 6-13

Direct Arterial Blood Pressure [mean, (mean ± 2SD reference interval)] in Selected Species

Species	N	A/C	SAP (mm Hg)	MAP (mm Hg)	DAP (mm Hg)	Ref
Hispaniolan Amazon parrots *(Amazona ventralis)*	8	A (isoflurane)	133 (88–177)	117 (76–158)	102 (58–146)	180
Hispaniolan Amazon parrots *(Amazona ventralis)*	16	A (isoflurane)	163 (127–199)	155 (119–191)	148 (112–184)	231
Pigeons *(Columba livia)*	15	A (isoflurane)	93 (73–113)	82 (54–110)	72 (46–98)	253
Red-tailed hawks *(Buteo jamaicensis)*	8	C	220 (119–331)	187 (104–271)	160 (70–250)	254
Red-tailed hawks *(Buteo jamaicensis)*	6	A (sevoflurane)	178 (124–232)	159 (109–209)	143 (95–191)	249
Great horned owls *(Bubo virginianus)*	6	C	231.5 (157–306)	203 (146–260)	178 (128–228)	254
Bald eagles *(Haliaeetus leucocephalus)*	17	A (isoflurane)	195 (165–225)	171 (142–200)	148 (120–176)	250
Bald eagles *(Haliaeetus leucocephalus)*	17	A (sevoflurane)	144 (116–172)	139 (111–167)	134.5 (106–163)	250
Chickens *(Gallus gallus domesticus)*	40	A	141 (118–163)	136 (114–158)	131 (109–153)	255
Turkeys *(Meleagris gallopavo)*	20	C	302 (289–315)	253 (242–264)	204 (194–214)	251
Pekin ducks *(Anas platyrhynchos domestica)*	72	A	165 (138–192)	143 (111–174)	121 (85–157)	256

A, Anesthetized; C, conscious; DAP, diastolic arterial pressure; MAP, mean arterial pressure; SAP, systolic arterial pressure.
Note: Additional references available in *West's Zoo Animal and Wildlife Immobilization and Anesthesia,* 2nd Edition.[252]

masses, and aneurismal dilatation.[j] A rounded, globoid cardiac silhouette is suggestive of pericardial effusion, but accurate confirmation and differentiation between possible etiologies is impossible without echocardiography.[7,94,114,127,155] The size of the cardiac silhouette on the ventrodorsal view can be quantified by taking standardized measurements and calculating ratios relative to skeletal landmarks. Several techniques have been reported, but the most practical is measurement of the cardiac silhouette at its widest point on the ventrodorsal view, followed by comparison of this value with both the thoracic width at the same level and the length of the sternum (see Figure 6-46, *A* and *B*). In healthy, medium-sized psittacines of three species, the width of the cardiac silhouette on the ventrodorsal view was found to range between 51% and 61% of the thoracic width and

between 35% and 41% of the length of the sternum.[259] The ratio of cardiac width to thoracic width was found to be similar in Harris' hawks[260] but greater (up to 70%) in peregrine falcons *(Falco peregrinus),* in which the ratio decreased by 10% with positive pressure ventilation. In these birds, the ratio of cardiac width to a static variable—sternal width (measured at the same level)—was unaffected by respiratory movements and therefore proved more reliable as a predictor of cardiac width.[261] Sternal and thoracic widths can be used to calculate predictive reference intervals for the size of the cardiac silhouette in peregrine falcons *(Falco peregrinus),* red-tailed hawks *(Buteo jamaicensis),* screech owls *(Otus asio),* and Canada geese *(Branta canadensis)* using established regression equations.[261,262] However, these are of limited practicality, in part because measurement of sternal width becomes impossible if the sternal landmarks are obscured by an enlarged cardiac silhouette.

Increased radiodensity and tortuosity of the great vessels is suggestive, but not conclusive, of atherosclerosis.[29,94,95,128,228]

---

[j]References 29,41,94,95,114,115,128,165,224.

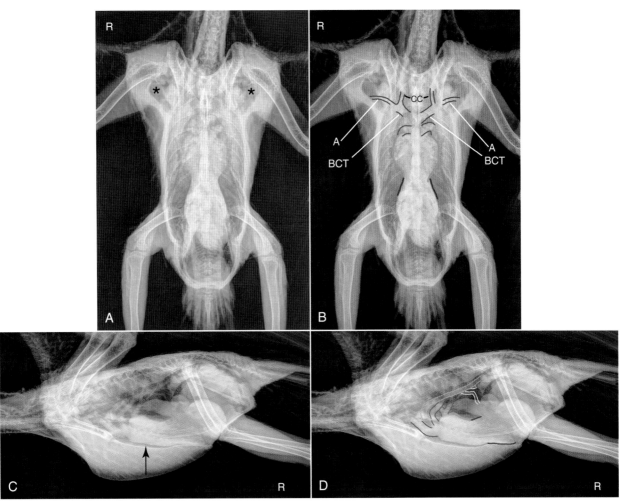

FIGURE 6-45 Digital radiographs of a hyacinth macaw *(Anodorhynchus hyacinthinus).* **A,** Ventrodorsal projection. Note: Intrathoracic diverticula of the clavicular air sac, appearing as radiolucent zones surrounding the heart base and great vessels, provide contrast for visibility of these structures; the axillary diverticula are among the extrathoracic diverticula of the clavicular air sac *(indicated by asterisks).* **B,** Ventrodorsal projection with outlined cardiac silhouette *(green),* hepatic silhouette *(purple),* brachiocephalic trunks (BCT), common carotid arteries (CC), and axillary arteries (A) *(red),* ascending aorta *(gold),* and pulmonary arteries *(blue).* **C,** Right lateral projection. Note: Intrathoracic diverticula of the clavicular air sac surround the heart base and great vessels and intervene between the heart and the sternum (sternal diverticulum, *indicated by the arrow).* **D,** Right lateral projection with outlined cardiac silhouette *(green),* hepatic silhouette *(purple),* superimposed brachiocephalic trunks *(red),* aorta *(gold),* pulmonary artery *(blue),* pulmonary veins *(magenta),* and coeliac and cranial mesenteric arteries *(yellow).*

Assessment of increased opacity is highly subjective and subject to variability in radiographic technique, although focal and linear mineralization associated with one or more vessels is highly suggestive of advanced, calcific lesions.[24] In psittacines, these lesions appear most often along the ascending and descending aorta, brachiocephalic trunks, and occasionally along smaller arteries, including the coeliac artery (Figure 6-47, *A* and *B*).

Other radiographic abnormalities

In addition to enlargement of the cardiac silhouette, radiographic abnormalities that may be seen in cases of congestive heart failure include an enlarged hepatic silhouette and caudodorsal displacement of the adjacent gastrointestinal tract, increased radiodensity of the pulmonary parenchyma, intracoelomic air sac compression, or loss of coelomic detail caused by ascites.[k]

Hepatic silhouette. The hepatic silhouette may appear enlarged (see Figure 6-46) as a result of hepatomegaly, perihepatic effusion (fluid accumulation in the hepatoperitoneal cavities),[29,264] or cardiomegaly or pericardial effusion, considering that the cardiac apex is positioned between the liver lobes.[165] Enlargement of the hepatic silhouette may also be

---

[k]References 41,94,95,114,123,128,224,263.

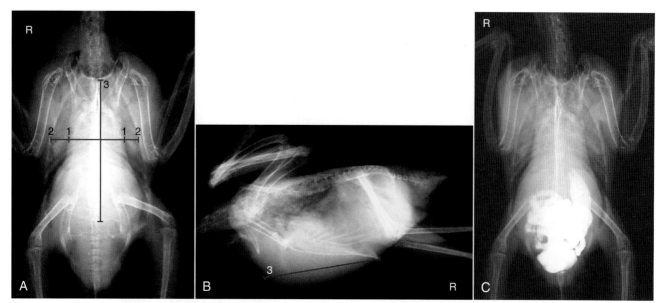

FIGURE 6-46 Radiographs of a jenday conure *(Aratinga jandaya)* demonstrating enlargement of the cardiac and hepatic silhouettes and compression of intracoelomic air sac space. Wings are not fully extended because of propatagial contracture. **A,** Ventrodorsal projection showing measurements of the width of the cardiac silhouette (1 to 1), thoracic width at the same level (2 to 2), and sternal length (3) used to calculate ratios of 64.7% (1:2) and 45.8% (1:3). **B,** Right lateral projection showing measurement of sternal length (3). **C,** Ventrodorsal projection, 75 minutes following gavage administration of barium sulfate into the ingluvies so that gastrointestinal dilatation could be ruled out as a cause of the enlarged hepatic silhouette. Note: Pericardial effusion and hepatomegaly were confirmed ultrasonographically in this individual.

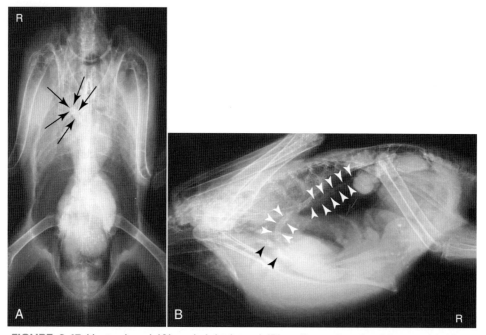

FIGURE 6-47 Ventrodorsal **(A)** and right lateral **(B)** radiographs of a 32-year-old, blue-fronted Amazon parrot *(Amazona aestiva)* with linear mineralization outlining the margins of the aorta *(black arrows,* VD projection; *white arrowheads,* right lateral projection) and focal mineral densities associated with the brachiocephalic trunk(s) and coeliac artery *(black arrowheads* and *red arrow,* respectively, right lateral projection). These findings are suggestive of advanced atherosclerotic disease. Note: Severe propatagial contracture in this individual prohibited complete extension of the thoracic limbs, resulting in superimposition of one wing tip over the coelom on the right lateral view and partial obscuration of the descending aorta.

seen with gastrointestinal dilatation, reproductive tract enlargement, splenomegaly, and midcoelomic masses as a result of summation or functional spreading of the liver lobes. Gastrointestinal contrast imaging, CT, or coelioscopy are often required to assist the practitioner in making many of these distinctions (see Figure 6-46, *C*).[263]

Contrast imaging. Soft tissue opacities within the coelom can be better delineated by effectively distinguishing the gastrointestinal tract from adjacent structures. Even so, pericardial or ascitic fluid cannot be conclusively differentiated from soft tissue without ultrasonography.[263] Barium sulfate or iohexol are the two most frequently used contrast media. Following administration, a series of radiographs can be obtained at regular intervals.[233,234] Fluoroscopy allows for real-time monitoring of contrast transit and evaluation of gastrointestinal motility and can be used as an alternative or supplement to radiographs.[234,265] Fluoroscopy offers an additional advantage in that it does not require patient restraint, sedation, or anesthesia,[265] thereby reducing the risk of aspiration and restraint-associated stress on the patient. However, it requires specialized equipment not readily available to most practitioners.[234]

Respiratory tract. Increased pulmonary density, particularly of the reticular pattern (Figure 6-48), may be seen with cardiogenic pulmonary edema or with primary disease of the pulmonary parenchyma (inflammatory or neoplastic infiltration, fibrosis).[94] Accurate interpretation of these changes requires the thoracic limbs be fully and symmetrically extended to minimize superimposition and obscuration of the pulmonary parenchyma.[234] However, this may be impossible in individuals with conditions that prevent normal wing extension, such as propatagial contracture or musculoskeletal disease. Varying degrees of compression of the cranial and caudal thoracic and abdominal air sacs are typically seen with ascites, organomegaly, or both (see Figure 6-46), and occasionally, compensatory hyperinflation of the axillary diverticula of the clavicular air sac is apparent (Figure 6-49). The intrathoracic diverticula of the clavicular air sac normally provide the contrast necessary to visualize the heart base and great vessels (see Figures 6-3 and 6-45). When this space is lost or diminished, as occurs with space-occupying masses or accumulation of exudate within the air sac, visibility of the great vessels is obscured (Figure 6-50).

Ultrasonography

Coelomic ultrasound is an essential diagnostic tool in avian medicine, and its clinical utility in the diagnosis of cardiovascular disease has been demonstrated in numerous species.[l] Ultrasonography allows for the identification of cardiac abnormalities, pericardial effusion, ascites,[m] and hepatic parenchymal changes that cannot be distinguished radiographically beyond enlargements of the cardiac and hepatic silhouettes. It can most often be performed in the awake[94,127,165] or sedated patient and represents a good option for those too compromised to withstand extended restraint or general anesthesia.[41]

---

[l]References 29,41,95,102,110,115,117,118,123,128,166.
[m]References 7,29,41,94,127,128,165,221.

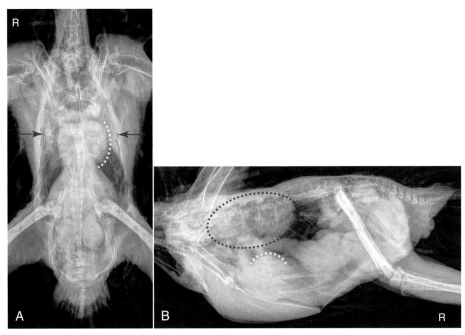

FIGURE 6-48 Ventrodorsal **(A)** and right lateral **(B)** digital radiographs showing increased pulmonary radiodensity *(indicated by red arrows and ellipse)* in a 26-year-old, female Moluccan cockatoo *(Cacatua moluccensis)* with left-sided congestive heart failure. Echocardiography confirmed cardiomegaly with marked left atrial dilatation (suggested radiographically, *yellow dotted line*), left ventricular dilatation and reduced myocardial contractility, and left atrioventricular valve insufficiency and regurgitation. Note: Mild oblique positioning on both projections was not considered a significant hindrance to radiographic interpretation.

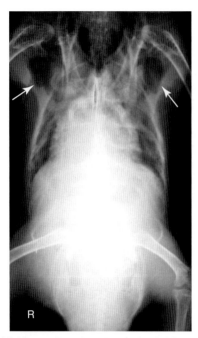

FIGURE 6-49 Ventrodorsal radiograph of a Grey parrot *(Psittacus erithacus)* diagnosed with congestive heart failure. Note enlargement of the cardiac silhouette (heart width-to-thoracic width ratio is 71%), loss of coelomic detail most suggestive of ascites, severe compression of intracoelomic air sac space, and hyperinflation of axillary diverticula of the clavicular air sac *(arrows).*

Birds can be allowed to stand or be held in an upright position to reduce positional respiratory or circulatory compromise[41,94,110] and should ideally by fasted prior to examination to reduce interference from the gastrointestinal tract. Even so, the presence of echogenic material (e.g., grit) within the ventriculus can hamper visibility.

Instrumentation and technique

Two-dimensional (B-mode) echocardiography is a well-established technique to assess morphologic and functional status in birds, but motion-mode (or M-mode) is not useful because only longitudinal and semitransverse views are attainable.[94,188,266] Minimal technical requirements of the ultrasound system include a frame rate of 100 frames per second, high-frequency probe ($\geq$7.5 megahertz [MHz]) with a small coupling surface (microconvex array, phased array, or one end of a linear array), Doppler function, and capability to record still images and video clips for later review.[94,188] Simultaneous ECG facilitates interpretation of images in relation to the cardiac cycle but is not essential because end-diastolic and end-systolic frames can be visually selected.

Anatomic limitations and approaches. Ultrasonographic examination is complicated by the unique anatomic features of birds, most notably the presence of a large sternal plate and air sacs, which substantially limit available acoustic windows.[188,266] Cardiac views, in particular, are constrained by the situation of the heart in an indentation of the sternum and surrounded by the clavicular and cranial thoracic air sacs. Given these limitations, two approaches are possible for transcoelomic ultrasonography—ventromedian and parasternal. The ventromedian approach is the most commonly used for psittacine and raptorial birds. The probe is placed just

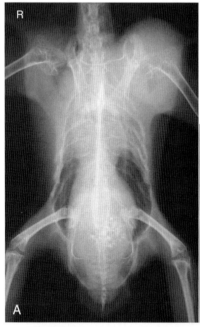

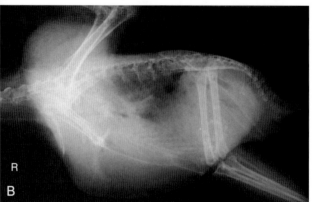

FIGURE 6-50 Ventrodorsal **(A)** and right lateral **(B)** radiographs of a 23-year-old, female blue-headed Pionus parrot *(Pionus menstruus)* with a soft tissue mass involving the left shoulder and obliterating the clavicular air sac space. Visibility of the great vessels is subsequently obscured. At postmortem examination, the mass was found to extend along the axillary diverticulum of the clavicular air sac to invade the cranial coelom and partially enclose the heart base (see Figure 6-33).

caudal to the sternum where a normally featherless area (apterium) lies along the ventral midline between adjacent feather tracts in most birds (excluding waterfowl) (Figure 6-51). The beam plane is directed craniodorsally, and the liver serves as an acoustic window, avoiding the air sacs laterally and the sternum ventrally (Figure 6-52).

The heart can be visualized in two longitudinal views—horizontal (four-chamber view) and vertical (two-chamber view)—the latter obtained by rotating the probe 90 degrees (see Figures 6-51, *B* and *C*; 6-52; 6-53; and 6-54). The horizontal view allows for visualization of the left and right ventricles, interventricular septum, left and right atria, left AV valve, muscular right AV valve, and aortic valve,[13,167,188] although it is difficult to distinguish the borders of the atria from the surrounding tissue.[167] The right ventricle appears triangular in shape, tapering toward the cardiac apex.[188,266,267] The vertical view permits visualization of the left atrium, left ventricle, and left AV valve; a marginal sliver of the right ventricle may also be visible adjacent to the sternum.[13,188,267] Reflection of the ultrasound beam off the sternum may produce a mirror artifact, in which a duplicated partial image of the heart appears on the opposite side of the sternum; this can create a false impression of chamber dilatation or aneurysm (Figure 6-55).[94]

The hepatic parenchyma should appear homogeneous and of moderate echogenicity, with a fine, granular texture. Hepatic vessels appear as anechoic channels passing through the parenchyma.[263,268] The parasternal approach can be used in birds whose ribs do not extend as far caudally, for example, pigeons and gallinaceous birds, allowing sufficient space to accommodate the probe on the lateral flank between the last rib and the pelvis. The right lateral approach is generally chosen to avoid the ventriculus, which often contains echogenic material that obstructs visibility of the heart. The leg is extended either cranially or caudally, and the probe is placed caudal to the last rib and dorsal to the lateral margin of the sternum, with the beam plane directed craniomedially. This approach provides longitudinal and semitransverse views of the heart.[94,188,266] Although views are limited for transcoelomic echocardiography, acoustic windows are greatly improved and visibility facilitated by cardiomegaly, hepatomegaly, ascitic fluid, and pericardial effusion, all frequently present in cases of congestive heart failure.

Transesophageal echocardiography, using human pediatric transesophageal probes, has been introduced as an alternative approach that offers improved resolution, five consistent views of cardiac structures, and the possibility of M-mode imaging. The probe is advanced down the esophagus and the heart imaged through the proventriculus. The method requires general anesthesia and patients large enough to accommodate the probe. It cannot be used in small psittacine birds because of a narrow thoracic inlet, and there is some risk of esophageal perforation.[269]

Color and spectral Doppler. Color Doppler provides a visual representation of blood flow velocity, wherein blood flow directed away from the probe is displayed in blue and blood flow toward the probe in red (Figure 6-56). It can be used to highlight hepatic venous congestion accompanying right-sided congestive heart failure and to detect turbulent flow associated with valvular insufficiency with regurgitation,

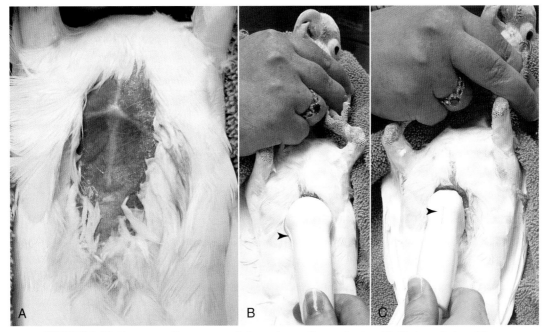

FIGURE 6-51 Ventromedian approach for echocardiography in a Goffin's cockatoo *(Cacatua goffiniana)* restrained in dorsal recumbency with pelvic limbs pulled cranially. **A,** The apterium along the ventral midline in this species eliminates the need to pluck feathers, which are instead wetted with alcohol and parted prior to application of standard, water-soluble acoustic gel. **B, C,** probe placement just caudal to the sternum for horizontal **(B)** and vertical **(C)** views. For the horizontal view, the index mark *(arrowhead)* is directed toward the bird's right and for the vertical view, the probe is rotated 90 degrees.

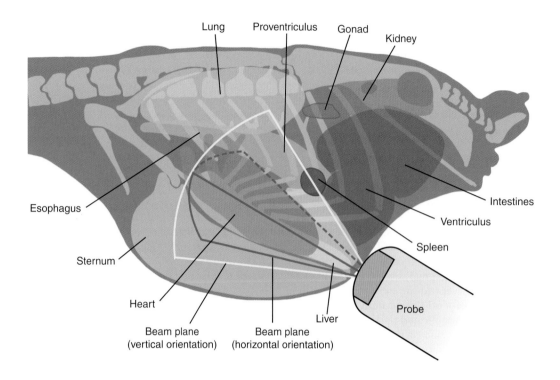

Lung   Proventriculus   Gonad   Kidney

Esophagus

Intestines

Ventriculus

Spleen

Sternum

Probe

Heart

Liver

Beam plane
(vertical orientation)

Beam plane
(horizontal orientation)

FIGURE 6-52 Echocardiography via the ventromedian approach, with the beam plane directed craniodorsally in horizontal *(blue)* versus vertical *(yellow)* orientation. (Modified from Pees M, Krautwald-Junghanns M: Avian echocardiography, *Semin Avian Exot Pets* 2005;14(1):14–21.)

septal defect, and aneurysm.[29,110,118] Unfortunately, use of this function decreases the frame rate and therefore temporal resolution, thus complicating assessment of blood flow.[94,188]

Spectral Doppler includes pulsed wave (PW) Doppler and continuous wave (CW) Doppler. The former allows measurement of blood flow velocity at a specific location of interest (selected by placement of the "gate") but is limited to velocities below 2 meters per second (m/s). It can be used via the ventromedian approach to measure diastolic inflow velocity into the left and right ventricles and systolic aortic outflow velocity (Figure 6-57), for which reference values for some species are available (Table 6-14).[94,188,267,270,271] Blood flow velocities have been shown to increase significantly with stress in raptors that are unaccustomed to being handled, so data should ideally be collected with these patients under anesthesia.[271]

CW Doppler can be used to measure higher blood flow velocities, but the measurement cannot be taken at a specific point, but only along a line.[94] No reference ranges are available, but the technique was used to measure regurgitant jet velocity through the incompetent right AV valve in a Grey parrot *(Psittacus erithacus)* with right-sided congestive heart failure. These data were used to estimate systolic pulmonary arterial pressure and make a diagnosis of cor pulmonale.[110]

Subjective assessments

Subjective assessments of chamber size, wall thickness, ventricular contractility, diastolic function, and valvular morphology and function can be made.[127,128,188] Chamber dilatation, myocardial hypertrophy, valvular insufficiency and anomalies (to include vegetations), cardiac masses, septal defects, some

aneurysms, pericardial effusion, ascites, and hepatic venous congestion can be identified with ultrasonography assisted by color Doppler (Figure 6-58).[29,110,118] Ascitic fluid can be collected via ultrasound-guided coelomocentesis and pericardial fluid by pericardiocentesis.[94,123,221] Hyperechogenicity of the walls of the ascending aorta is suggestive of mineralization that can accompany advanced atherosclerosis (see Figure 6-58, *L*).[24,228] In cases of right-sided congestive heart failure, the right ventricle is often demonstrably dilated such that it is of nearly equal size as the left ventricle. Thickening of the myocardium, to include the muscular right AV valve, is often appreciated (see Figure 6-58, *E* and *H*).[188] The right atrium may be dilated such that it is readily visible, and pericardial effusion, when present, appears as an anechoic area between the heart and the pericardium (see Figure 6-58, *F, I, J,* and *M*).[29,123,188,268] Dilatation of the hepatic veins and uniform hyperechogenicity of the hepatic parenchyma are consistent with passive congestion (see Figure 6-58, *F* to *H*).[110,114,188,267] Similarly, ventricular dilatation, myocardial thickening, and reduced myocardial contractility can be appreciated in cases of left-sided congestive heart failure, and a combination of these findings is seen with biventricular congestive heart failure.

Cardiac measurements and calculation of functional parameters

An adequate morphologic and functional assessment can often be made qualitatively in cases where disease is advanced and pathologic changes are readily apparent. However, quantitative evaluation may allow the practitioner greater sensitivity in

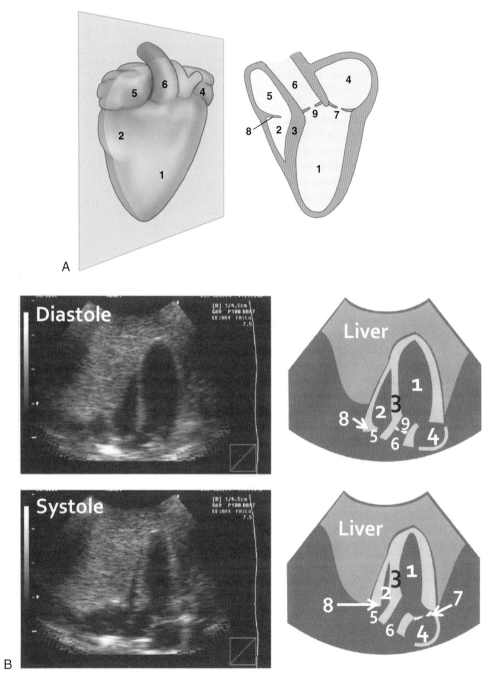

FIGURE 6-53 Horizontal (four-chamber) view of the heart obtained via the ventromedian approach. **A,** Illustration showing the beam plane *(blue)* oriented horizontally, allowing visualization of the left (1) and right (2) ventricles, interventricular septum (3), left (4) and right (5) atria, aorta (6), left (7) and right (8) atrioventricular valves, and aortic valve (9). **B,** These structures, as well as the surrounding liver parenchyma, as seen in a healthy Grey parrot *(Psittacus erithacus)*; diastole *(above)* and systole *(below)*. Note the indistinct margins of the atria. (Images courtesy Drs. Michael Pees and Maria-Elisabeth Krautwald-Junghanns, Clinic for Birds and Reptiles, University of Leipzig, Germany. Modified from Pees M, Krautwald-Junghanns M: Avian echocardiography, *Semin Avian Exot Pets* 14(1):14–21, 2005.)

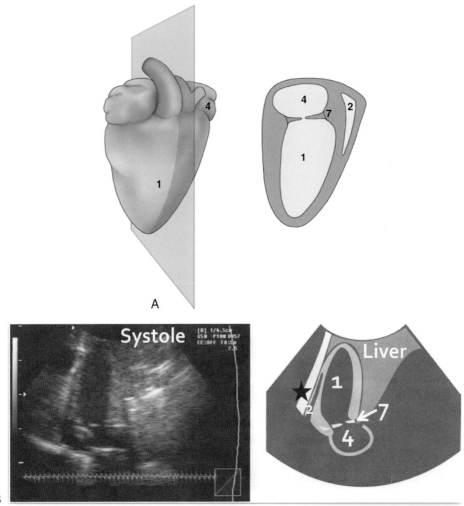

A

B

FIGURE 6-54 Vertical (two-chamber) view of the heart obtained via the ventromedian approach. **A,** Illustration showing the beam plane *(blue)* oriented vertically, allowing visualization of the left ventricle (1), left atrium (4), left atrioventricular valve (7), and inconsistently, a sliver of the right ventricle (2). **B,** These structures, as well as the adjacent sternum *(star)* and surrounding liver parenchyma, as seen in a healthy Grey parrot *(Psittacus erithacus)*; systole. Note the indistinct margins of the left atrium. (Images courtesy Drs. Michael Pees and Maria-Elisabeth Krautwald-Junghanns, Clinic for Birds and Reptiles, University of Leipzig, Germany. **A,** Modified from: Pees M, Krautwald-Junghanns M: Avian echocardiography, *Semin Avian Exot Pets* 14(1):14–21, 2005; and from: Pees M, Straub J, Krautwald-Junghanns M-E: Echocardiographic examinations of 60 African grey parrots and 30 other psittacine birds, *Vet Rec* 155(3):73–76, 2004; **B,** Modified from: Pees M, Krautwald-Junghanns M: Avian echocardiography, *Semin Avian Exot Pets* 14(1):14-21, 2005.)

FIGURE 6-55 Echocardiographic image, umbrella cockatoo *(Cacatua alba)* (ventromedian approach, horizontal view). Mirror artifact: duplication of the right and left ventricles at the left side of the image (2* and 1*, respectively) could lead to the mistaken impression of right ventricular dilatation. 1, Left ventricle; 2, right ventricle.

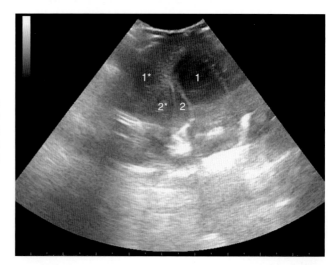

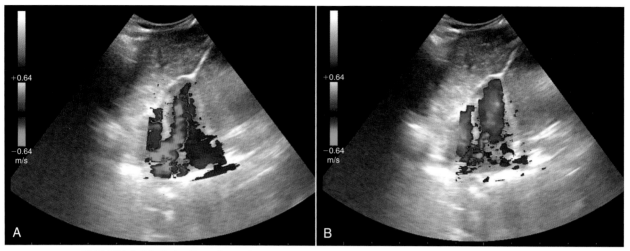

FIGURE 6-56 Color Doppler echocardiographic image, green-wing macaw *(Ara chloroptera)* (ventromedian approach, horizontal view). **A,** Systolic aortic outflow is blue (blood flow is directed away from the probe). **B,** Diastolic inflow into the ventricles is red (blood flow is directed toward the probe).

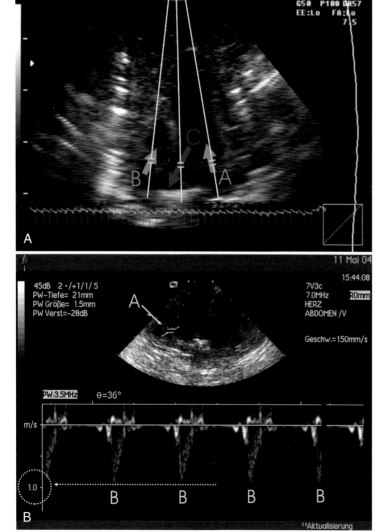

FIGURE 6-57 A, Spectral (pulsed wave) Doppler echocardiography (ventromedian approach, horizontal view) with gate placements shown for measurement of diastolic inflow velocities (left ventricle [A], right ventricle [B]) and systolic aortic outflow velocity (C). **B,** Placement of the gate (A) at the aortic root in a carrion crow *(Corvus corone),* allowing determination of maximum outflow velocity during systole of approximately 1 meter per second [m/s] (B). (Images courtesy Drs. Michael Pees and Maria-Elisabeth Krautwald-Junghanns, Clinic for Birds and Reptiles, University of Leipzig, Germany. **A** and **B,** From Pees M, Krautwald-Junghanns M: Avian echocardiography, *Semin Avian Exot Pets* 14(1):14–21, 2005.)

TABLE 6-14

Reference Intervals (in meters per second [m/s]) for Blood Flow Velocities Determined by Spectral Doppler Echocardiography (Ventromedian Approach, Horizontal View) in Selected Species[94,270,271]

Species	A/C	LV Diastolic Inflow	RV Diastolic Inflow	Systolic Aortic Outflow
Amazon parrots *(Amazona* spp.)	A	0.12–0.24	0.12–0.32	0.67–0.99
Greater sulfur-crested cockatoos *(Cacatua galerita)*	A	0.02–0.62		0.40–1.16
Grey parrots *(Psittacus erithacus)*	A	0.27–0.51		0.63–1.15
Macaws *(Ara* spp.)	A	0.40–0.68		0.55–1.07
Harris' hawks *(Parabuteo unicinctus)*	C	0.13–0.25	0.15–0.27	0.75–1.43
Falcons *(Falco* spp.)	C	0.15–0.27	0.13–0.29	0.81–1.09
	C(u)	0.18–0.38	0.17–0.37	1.07–1.43
Common buzzard *(Buteo buteo)*	A	0.12–0.16	0.10–0.18	1.08–1.28
	C	0.16–0.28	0.13–0.25	1.04–1.68
Barn owls *(Tyto alba)*	C	0.14–0.26	0.10–0.34	0.84–1.32

Note: To obtain a 95% reference interval, all published results in the form of mean ± SD were reported as mean ± 2SD.
A, Anesthetized; C, conscious (accustomed to handling); C(u), conscious (unaccustomed to handling); LV, left ventricle; RV, right ventricle.

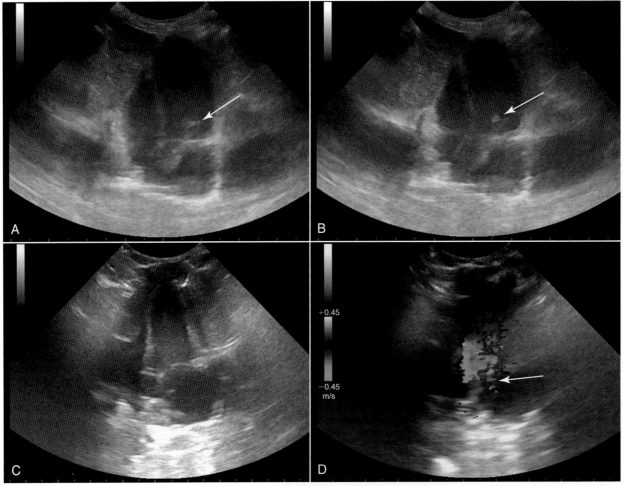

FIGURE 6-58 Coelomic ultrasonography and echocardiography (ventromedian approach, horizontal view) in psittacine birds with various pathologic findings. **A** and **B,** Biventricular congestive heart failure in a 32-year-old, male double-yellow-headed Amazon parrot *(Amazona ochrocephala)*; diastole **(A)**, systole **(B)**. There is marked dilatation of both atria and ventricles, thinning of the ventricular walls, no appreciable change in ventricular dimensions between diastole and systole (poor contractility), and insufficiency of the left atrioventricular (AV) valve (one thickened valve leaflet, indicated by the arrow, remains in an open position throughout the cardiac cycle). **C** and **D,** Marked left atrial dilatation associated with left AV valve regurgitation in a 37-year-old, male Moluccan cockatoo *(Cacatua moluccensis)*. Color Doppler reveals regurgitation of blood *(arrow)* into the left atrium during systole **(D)**.

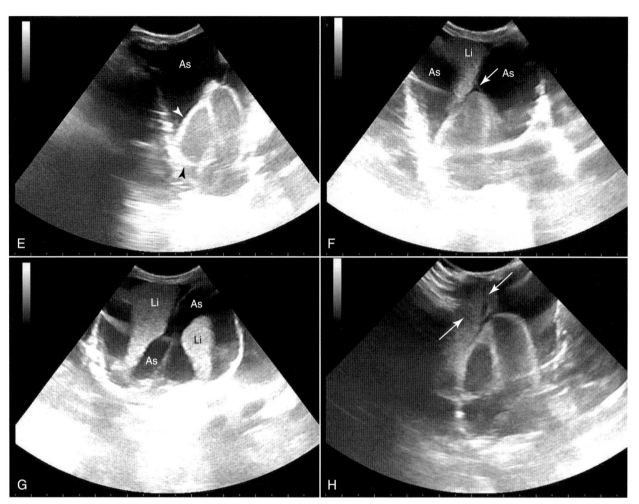

FIGURE 6-58, cont'd **E** to **G,** Biventricular congestive heart failure (predominantly right-sided) in a 35-year-old, male Grey parrot *(Psittacus erithacus)*. There is marked right ventricular dilatation such that it is larger than the left ventricle, concentric hypertrophy of the right ventricular wall and right AV valve *(arrowheads)* **(E)**; pericardial effusion and ascites (As) are present and the two can be distinguished in image **F** *(arrow* indicates pericardium); uniform hyperechogenicity of the hepatic parenchyma (Li, Liver) is consistent with passive congestion **(F** and **G)**. **H,** Right-sided congestive heart failure in a 24-year-old, female Grey parrot *(Psittacus erithacus)*. Findings are similar to the previous case, with dilatation of hepatic veins also demonstrable *(arrows)*. **I** and **J,** Biventricular congestive heart failure in a 32-year-old, male double-yellow-headed Amazon parrot *(Amazona ochrocephala)*;

Continued

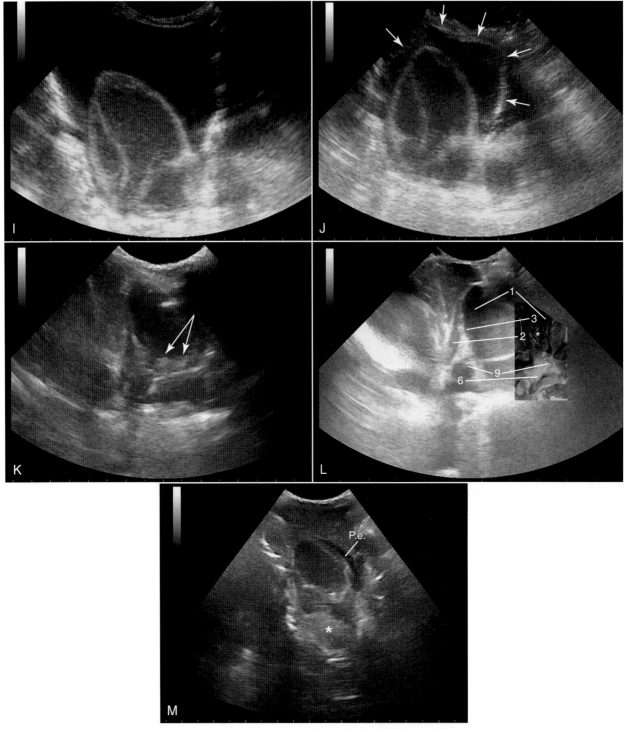

FIGURE 6-58, cont'd pre- **(I)** and post- **(J)** ultrasound-guided pericardiocentesis in which 20 milliliters (mL) of transparent, light yellow fluid was removed (characterized as a modified transudate). The thickened pericardium can be clearly seen following pericardiocentesis *(arrows)*. **K,** Vegetative lesions of the left AV valve *(arrows)* partially obstructing the left ventricular outflow tract in a 25-year-old, yellow-naped Amazon parrot *(Amazona auropalliata)* of unknown sex with a systolic murmur. **L,** Biventricular congestive heart failure (predominantly left-sided) in a 30-year-old, female military macaw *(Ara militaris)*. Note the hyperechogenicity of the interventricular septum, the left ventricular outflow tract, and the aortic walls. **Inset:** These structures were photographed after the bird's death (scaled and oriented for comparison with the echocardiographic image) (1, left ventricle; 2, right ventricle; 3, interventricular septum; 6, aorta; 9, aortic valve); atherosclerosis involving the aorta, aortic valve cusps, and an intramural coronary artery *(asterisk)* within the interventricular septum was confirmed at postmortem examination. **M,** Heart-based mass *(asterisk)* and biventricular congestive heart failure in a 34-year-old, female blue-front Amazon parrot *(Amazona aestiva)*. A large fibrotic mass was identified at postmortem examination, extending from the sternum to surround the heart base and invade the lungs. P.e., Pericardial effusion.

identifying more subtle changes and monitoring trends in a given patient over time. Ventricular and atrial dimensions, aortic diameter, and interventricular septum width can be measured in both systole and diastole, and some reference values are available for pigeons as well as for a few psittacine and raptorial species (Table 6-15).[94,188,266,267,272] The probe is positioned such that the cardiac chambers appear maximally expanded, and measurements are taken at their widest points using the inner edge method (Figure 6-59). It should be noted that accurate measurement of the atria (particularly the right atrium) can be hindered by indistinct borders and that of the right ventricle by its complex three-dimensional configuration and motion of the right AV valve. Measurements cannot be successfully taken in all individuals because of variations in image quality from one bird to the next.[267] Ventricular widths can be used to calculate fractional shortening:

$$(\text{Diastolic diameter} - \text{systolic diameter}) \times \frac{100}{\text{diastolic diameter}}$$

This is used for evaluation of ventricular contractility (reference values for some psittacine species are shown in Table 6-15).[94,188,267] Expected left ventricular length (LVL)

can be estimated from the sternal length (SL) in psittacines using the following equation[94]:

$$\text{LVL} = 0.5 + (0.33 \times \text{SL})$$

Accuracy and precision of echocardiographic measurements have been questioned by some authors, considering the small size of the structures imaged, the rapid heart rates of avian species, the current equipment resolution, and the fact that different observers can add up to 30% variability. Measurements should be taken from several cardiac cycles and averaged to obtain representative values. Follow-up measurements should be obtained by the same operator using the same equipment and technique, and only changes in measurements larger than 20% should be considered genuine. Transcoelomic echocardiography is also thought to underestimate the true fractional shortening of the highly efficient avian heart.[273]

Angiography

Angiography can provide an additional diagnostic modality to supplement echocardiographic findings and to identify vascular abnormalities.[29,94,95,235] Since flow-limiting stenosis is the main mechanism leading to clinical signs of atherosclerosis in

TABLE 6-15

Reference Intervals (in millimeters) for Echocardiographic Measurements in Selected Species*[94,267,272]

Parameter	Grey Parrots (*Psittacus erithacus*)	Amazon Parrots (*Amazona* spp.)	Cockatoos (*Cacatua* spp. and *Eolophus roseicapillus*)	Senegal Parrots (*Poicephalus senegalus*)	Diurnal Raptors‡	Pigeons (*Columba livia*) (Parasternal Approach)
LEFT VENTRICLE						
Length systole	18.4–26	16.5–25.7	16.4–21.6	12.0–16.8	9.1–20.3	15.9–19.9
Width systole	4.8–8.8	4.3–9.1	3.0–9.8	4.0–5.2	4.1–8.5	4.4–6.0
Length diastole	20.2–27.8	17.7–26.5	16.7–23.1	11.1–19.1	11.0–21.8	17.3–22.9
Width diastole	6.6–10.6	6.4–10.4	5.3–11.3	4.9–6.9	5.3–10.1	6.2–8.6
FS (%)	13.8–31.4	14.4–31.2	11.6–39.6	13.9–32.3		18.2–36.2
LEFT ATRIUM†						
Length systole	3.7–7.7	1.6–10	3.1–7.9	2.1–5.7		
Width systole	6.2–13.4	6.4–9.6	4.4–11.6	4.9–8.5		
Length diastole	2.4–7.2	0.2–9.4	4.3–5.9	2.4–4.4		
Width diastole	5.9–15.9	5.0–11.0	5.3–12.1	4.1–10.1		
RIGHT VENTRICLE						
Length systole	6.4–12.0	5.8–13.0	7.9–12.7	5.3–9.7	7.3–18.1	
Width systole	1.0–4.6	1.7–4.5	7.9–12.7	1.7–3.3	0.9–3.3	
Length diastole	7.7–15.3	7.7–12.9	6.7–15.9	7.2–8.0	8.9–18.9	8.3–11.5
Width diastole	2.6–7.0	2.6–7.8	2.5–4.5	2.7–3.9	0.9–4.1	3.0–5.0
FS (%)	17.0–64.6	26.7–41.5	12.7–53.9	16.8–62.4		
AORTA						
Diameter systole	2.8–4.4	2.0–4.0		1.9–3.1		
Diameter diastole	2.8–5.2	2.2–4.6		2.4	2.0–3.6	2.8–3.2
INTERVENTRICULAR SEPTUM						
Width systole	1.9–3.9	2.0–2.4	1.3–2.5	1.3–2.5	0.7–3.1	3.6–4.0
Width diastole	1.9–3.1	1.3–2.9	0.9–2.5	1.3–2.1	0.9–2.9	2.9–3.7

*Pigeons: parasternal approach, longitudinal view; others: ventromedian approach, horizontal view.
†Vertical view used for left atrial measurements.
‡European diurnal raptors included the common buzzard (*Buteo buteo*), Eurasian sparrowhawk (*Accipiter nisus*), northern goshawk (*Accipiter gentilis*), and red kite (*Milvus milvus*).
Note: To obtain a 95% reference interval, all published results in the form of mean ± SD were reported as mean ± 2SD.
FS, Fractional shortening (width).

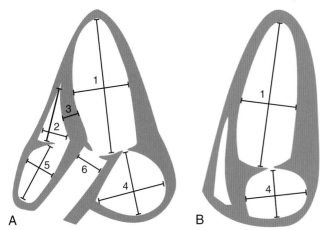

FIGURE 6-59 Points of echocardiographic measurement for the left ventricle (1), right ventricle (2), interventricular septum (3), left atrium (4), right atrium (5), and aorta (6) using the ventromedian approach (**A,** horizontal view; **B,** vertical view). (Diagrams courtesy Drs. Michael Pees and Maria-Elisabeth Krautwald-Junghanns, Clinic for Birds and Reptiles, University of Leipzig, Germany. Modified from Pees M, Straub J, Krautwald-Junghanns M-E: Echocardiographic examinations of 60 African grey parrots and 30 other psittacine birds, *Vet Rec* 155(3):73–76, 2004.)

psittacine birds, angiography can be applied to assess arterial luminal narrowing in these species. Angiography can be performed with the use of either fluoroscopy or CT. Since the circulation of intravenous contrast agents in birds is extremely fast, image acquisition should be performed during injection or shortly thereafter. Fluoroscopic angiography allows visualization of the heart and vascular tree in real time.

The anesthetized patient is initially positioned in left lateral recumbency on a fluoroscopy table. A bolus of nonionic iodinated contrast agent (2 milliliters per kilogram [mL/kg], intravenously [IV], iohexol 240 mg/mL; Omnipaque, GE Healthcare Inc., Princeton, NJ) is injected, at a rate of 1 to 2 mL/kg per second, through a catheter inserted into the cutaneous ulnar (basilic) vein or the medial metatarsal vein during video acquisition at a rate of 30 frames per second for the best resolution. The same bolus is repeated to obtain the ventrodorsal view, with the bird placed in dorsal recumbency. The brachiocephalic trunks, aorta, pulmonary arteries, pulmonary veins, and caudal vena cava can be visualized. The brachiocephalic trunks and aorta can be seen pulsating with the heartbeats, and marked lumen changes can be observed during the cardiac cycle. The procedure is easy and inexpensive and can be recorded for further analysis. Although fluoroscopic angiography is likely more useful for qualitative assessments, measurements can be taken, provided a calibrated marker is kept in the field during image acquisition to account for different degrees of magnification.[274] Ventricular hypertrophy, chamber dilatation, valvular or vascular stenosis, and aneurysms can be identified by using fluoroscopic angiography.[94] As yet, there are limited reports of its clinical use in birds. It was used in combination with echocardiography to identify an aneurysm of the right coronary artery in an umbrella cockatoo (*Cacatua alba*)[29] and to identify biventricular dilatation and stenosis of the brachiocephalic trunks and aorta

in a chestnut-fronted or severe macaw (*Ara severa*) with biventricular failure and severe atherosclerosis of these vessels.[95] It was also used to confirm cardiac functional impairment in a racing pigeon and to rule out a cardiovascular shunt in a dyspneic blue-and-gold macaw (*Ara ararauna*).[7,163]

Digital subtraction angiography is a fluoroscopic technique used in interventional radiology to clearly visualize blood vessels in a dense soft tissue or bone environment. The same bolus technique and a similar dose of contrast medium are used as in regular fluoroscopic angiography. A preliminary, nonenhanced fluoroscopic image is recorded before administering the contrast medium and is digitally subtracted during the angiography procedure, which results in visualization of the contrast-filled vessels only, without the background. It considerably enhances the outlines of the arteries and the detection of smaller arteries not seen with conventional angiography, specifically for extremities such as legs, wings, and head. However, images tend to be easily degraded by small motions and noise.

A CT examination provides an excellent assessment of all major arteries and their anatomy in psittacine and raptorial birds.[275,276] The addition of contrast media greatly enhances the visualization of the arteries and veins and their lumina. CT angiography (CTA) has shown great promise for identification of vascular disease, including arterial calcification and luminal stenosis related to atherosclerosis, aneurysms, and congenital vascular anomalies.[274] A CTA protocol for parrots has been standardized and published and was used to establish reference ranges for the diameters of the major arteries in healthy Hispaniolan Amazon parrots (*Amazona ventralis*).[276] In order to capture the CT images at the time of greatest intra-arterial contrast concentrations (enhancement peak), it is recommended to start the CTA scanning immediately after administration of contrast. Alternatively, a preliminary axial CT scan may be performed in order to determine the exact time to contrast enhancement peak.[274,276]

Advanced Imaging: Computed Tomography and Magnetic Resonance Imaging

CT and MRI are seldom used to image the avian heart because scans cannot be gated to the fast cardiac cycle in birds to reduce motion artifacts and improve diagnostic value. MRI was found to be of little diagnostic value with regard to the cardiovascular system in pigeons because of the fast circulation of contrast medium (gadolinium).[277] However, as discussed above, CT can be used to image the vasculature and can readily diagnose arterial calcification associated with advanced atherosclerosis (Figures 6-60 and 6-61), as well as cardiomegaly, ventricular dilatation, pericardial effusion, ascites, pulmonary edema, and venous congestion (see Chapter 14; Figure 6-62). Likewise, cerebral complications such as ischemic and hemorrhagic strokes can be diagnosed by using CT or MRI, although concurrent atherosclerosis cannot be detected unless lesion calcification is adequately severe.[28,226,278] MRI was used to identify cerebral infarction and hemorrhage secondary to a ruptured midbrain aneurysm in a blue-and-gold macaw (*Ara ararauna*)[28] and to identify two brain infarcts in a Grey parrot (*Psittacus erithacus*) consistent with an acute ischemic stroke.[226] There is ongoing research into the applications of micro-CT, including comprehensive mapping of

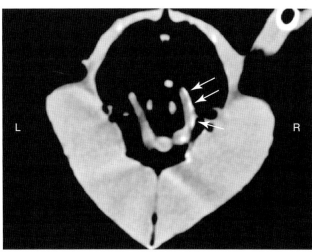

FIGURE 6-60 Computed tomography scan showing advanced aortic calcification of the ascending aorta *(arrows)* in a 35-year-old, female Grey parrot *(Psittacus erithacus)*. Mediastinal window. (Image courtesy Drs. Yvonne van Zeeland and Nico Shoemaker and the Division of Diagnostic Imaging, Faculty of Veterinary Medicine, Utrecht University, the Netherlands.)

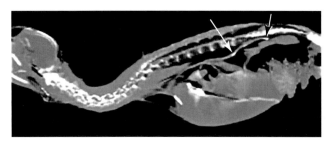

FIGURE 6-61 Computed tomography scan (sagittal view) showing advanced aortic calcification (two lesions, *arrows*) of the descending aorta in a 22-year-old, male Grey parrot *(Psittacus erithacus)*. (Image courtesy Drs. Yvonne van Zeeland and Nico Shoemaker and the Division of Diagnostic Imaging, Faculty of Veterinary Medicine, Utrecht University, the Netherlands.)

vascular anatomy, and micro-MRI, which can be utilized to evaluate blood flow, measure internal vascular diameter, and identify occlusions.[279]

Endoscopy

Endoscopy allows for both direct visual inspection of cardiovascular structures and targeted collection of diagnostic samples as appropriate.[7,280-283] Endoscopy can only detect gross abnormalities, including cardiomegaly, pericardial effusion, pericardial thickening or exudate, arterial discoloration (suggesting atherosclerotic disease) or gross structural changes, and neighboring masses or granulomas. Standard lateral approaches permit visualization of the heart, great vessels, lungs, and liver via the cranial and caudal thoracic air sacs and of the descending aorta and its major branches, caudal vena cava, and ischiatic veins via the abdominal air sacs.[238,283] The interclavicular approach (via the clavicular air sac) is the best means of visualizing the heart base, ascending aorta,

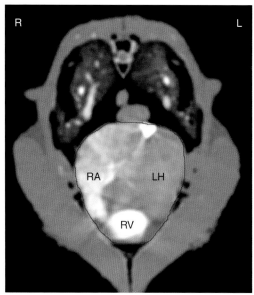

FIGURE 6-62 Computed tomography scan after injection of contrast in a Harris' hawk *(Parabuteo unicinctus)* with left-sided congestive heart failure and syncopal episodes, bone window. Cross-section cranially at the level of the enlarged heart *(outlined in red)*. The contrast agent *(white)* appears in the right atrium (RA) and right ventricle (RV) but fails to disseminate in the left heart (LH) because of impaired systolic function.

brachiocephalic trunks, carotid and subclavian arteries, pulmonary arteries, and jugular veins (Figures 6-63 and 6-64).[235]

The ventral midline approach, with entry into the ventral hepatoperitoneal cavities, permits evaluation of the liver, heart, and pericardium[283] and affords the opportunity for pericardiocentesis and pericardial biopsy with the use of an endoneedle and biopsy forceps advanced through the instrument channel.[7,127,189,284] The endoneedle should only be allowed to protrude by 1 to 2 mm to avoid puncturing the heart during the procedure, and tissue samples should be collected from the apex of the pericardium to avoid the great vessels and vagus nerve at the heart base.[189,284] The ventral midline approach is preferred for such a procedure and for patients with ascites because it does not require entry into the air sacs,[280,283] thereby minimizing risk of fluid leakage into the respiratory tract.[127,283]

Ancillary Diagnostics

Fluid analysis, cytology, culture, histopathology, and pathogen-specific testing of antemortem diagnostic samples can assist in determining the etiopathogenesis of cardiovascular disease, particularly when it involves infectious diseases or neoplasia. Certainly myocardial samples cannot realistically be obtained in the living bird, but pericardial and ascitic fluid, caseous exudates, and biopsies of the pericardium, other affected organs (e.g., liver, lung, and air sac), or tumors can be collected for analysis.

Fluid analysis and cytology

Pure transudates are typically clear and transparent, have low total solids (<2.5 grams per deciliter [g/dL]), and contain few

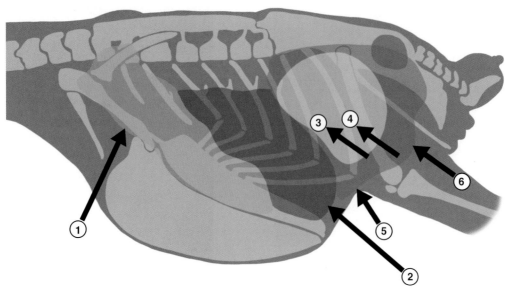

FIGURE 6-63 Endoscopic approaches to the coelom. The interclavicular approach, entering the clavicular air sac (1); ventral midline approach, entering the ventral hepatoperitoneal cavities (2); left and right lateral approaches *(left shown here)*, entering the caudal thoracic air sac (3, 4) and abdominal air sac (5, 6). (Modified from Lierz M: Diagnostic value of endoscopy and biopsy. In Harrison GJ, Lightfoot TL, editors: *Clinical avian medicine,* vol 2, Palm Beach, 2006, Spix Publishing, pp 631-652.)

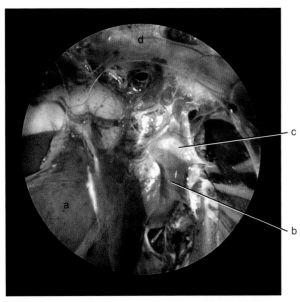

FIGURE 6-64 Endoscopic image, right lateral approach, showing the liver (a), heart and pericardium (b) with visible coronary fat (c), and lung (d). (Image courtesy Dr. Michael Lierz, Clinic for Birds, Reptiles, Amphibians, and Fish, University of Giessen, Germany.)

cells (<1500 cells per microliter [cells/μL]), primarily mesothelial cells and macrophages.[191,285,286] Modified transudates may appear slightly cloudy or serosanguineous and have relatively higher total solids (2.5 to 5.0 g/dL) and contain more cells (1000 to 7000 cells/μL), including mesothelial cells (often reactive), mononuclear cells, heterophils, and occasional

erythrocytes.[191,285,286] Congestive heart failure and toxin-related effusions are most frequently pure or modified transudates, appearing transparent and colorless to yellow.

Hemorrhagic effusions appear bloody and, unless acute or iatrogenic, should have a measurable hematocrit less than that of peripheral blood and no thrombocytes. Total solids are typically greater than 3.0 g/dL.[191] With chronicity, cytology may reveal erythrophagocytosis or hemosiderin engulfed by macrophages.[190,191,285,287] Exudates may appear cloudy, flocculent, or serosanguineous and have high total solids (>3.0 g/dL). They can be highly cellular (>5000 to 7000 cells/μL), and the types of cells present often reflect the underlying etiology, including inflammatory, infectious, or neoplastic disease.[190,191,286] Mesothelial cells, heterophils, lymphocytes, macrophages, plasma cells,[191,285] and erythrocytes may be present.[191] Septic effusions may contain causative microorganisms, either free or phagocytosed by macrophages.[191] Gram staining can be used to classify bacterial organisms,[285,287] in addition to Ziehl-Neelsen staining to identify acid-fast organisms including *Mycobacterium* spp., which are nonstaining with traditional stains,[10,190,192,207] and Giemsa, modified Gimenez, or Macchiavello staining to identify intracytoplasmic chlamydial inclusions.[285,287]

Malignant effusions in avian species are typically modified transudates or exudates and may contain neoplastic cells.[190,285] Cellular criteria suggestive of neoplasia include variations in cellular size, nuclear-to-cytoplasmic ratio, nuclear and nucleolar numbers, and increased frequency of mitotic figures.[287] However, reactive mesothelial cells are easily mistaken for malignant cells cytologically, as they may exhibit multinucleation, variation in nuclear size and shape, variation in nucleolar size and number, and high nuclear-to-cytoplasmic ratios.[191,285]

Standard microbiology

Tissue, exudate, and fluid samples can be submitted for bacterial and fungal culture,[218,288] including blood if sepsis or vegetative endocarditis is suspected.[7,29,103,218] Many reported bacterial and fungal pathogens causing cardiac and pericardial disease and effusion in birds can be isolated by using standard culture media under aerobic conditions.[10,288] Notable exceptions include anaerobic organisms, fastidious aerobic organisms, such as *Mycobacterium* spp.,[206,207,289,290] and obligate intracellular organisms such as *Chlamydia psittaci*.[218] Lack of microbial growth on standard aerobic culture may also occur with noninfectious or viral etiologies or as a result of errors in sample collection, handling, transportation, storage, and processing. Initiation of antimicrobial therapy prior to sample collection may also impair microbial isolation.[288]

Impression cytology and histopathology

Impression cytology of exudate and tissue samples can provide the clinician with immediate information to guide further diagnostic and treatment decisions pending culture and histopathology results.[287,291] Impression cytology of affected tissues may reveal inflammatory or neoplastic cells[287,291] or infective microorganisms.[218] Heterophils are most commonly seen with acute to subacute inflammation, whereas mononuclear cells predominate with chronic conditions.[190,193,218,287]

Histopathologic features of bacterial and fungal pericarditis include fibrin deposition, edema, and infiltration with heterophils, macrophages, lymphocytes, and plasma cells.[10,190,193,221] Causative organisms may be seen histologically, often within phagocytic cells.[10,207] Lesions associated with viral disease may include vasculitis and hemorrhage and are most often characterized by lymphoplasmacytic infiltrates.[190] Distinct histologic abnormalities of the pericardium may be lacking in cases of pericardial effusion resulting from hypoproteinemia, right-sided congestive heart failure, or toxic insult.[190]

Histologic lesions may be present in other organs, especially the liver and lungs. These lesions may reflect either a disease process causally related to cardiovascular disease or its secondary effects. Contributing systemic disease processes, including infectious, metabolic, and toxic etiologies are discussed in other portions of this text.

Severe hepatic fibrosis (cirrhosis), often accompanied by biliary hyperplasia and extramedullary hematopoiesis, may be identified as a contributing factor in the development of left-sided congestive heart failure. Likewise, hepatic fibrosis, necrosis, intracellular iron, and associated inflammation may be seen in cases of iron storage disease. Chronic noninfectious pulmonary disease relevant in cases of right-sided congestive heart failure can be characterized histologically. There may be liver or lung involvement with certain neoplastic diseases, including hemangiosarcoma and lymphosarcoma.[218,292] Passive congestion of the liver, which may occur secondary to right-sided congestive heart failure, results in dilation of the hepatic veins and congestion of the hepatic sinusoids. With chronicity, atrophy of the centrolobular hepatocytes, capsular thickening, and fibrosis occur.[193,218]

Pathogen-specific testing

If a particular infectious etiology is suspected on the basis of patient signalment, history, clinical signs, physical examination, and other diagnostic findings, specific pathogen testing

of fluid and tissue samples may be employed in an effort to confirm the diagnosis. This may include polymerase chain reaction (PCR) testing, use of specialized culture media, virus isolation, antigen detection methods, or serologic testing to demonstrate antibody titers.[241] Detection of etiologic agents by histopathology can be greatly facilitated by use of special staining, electron microscopy, immunohistochemistry, and in situ hybridization.[241,293,294]

THERAPEUTIC INTERVENTION

At the present time, therapeutic interventions for cardiovascular disease in companion birds are largely empirical and extrapolated, where possible, from small animal medicine and human medicine. Case reports of cardiovascular disease in which treatment was attempted are relatively few but include cases of atherosclerotic disease (stroke, peripheral arterial disease), of congestive heart failure, and of pericardial effusion.[n] There is a paucity of pharmacokinetic and pharmacodynamic data, and no clinical trials have been conducted in birds to study cardiovascular therapeutic agents used in mammals.[230] At present, the wide array of causative conditions, affected species, therapeutic interventions proposed or attempted, and outcomes precludes any conclusive association between therapeutic protocols and survival time.

The long-term prognosis for most cardiovascular diseases is guarded to poor, given that treatment is limited to management, rather than resolution of disease, in most cases. Prognosis is partly contingent on timely diagnosis, which proves challenging, given the absence or subtlety of clinical signs and the limited sensitivity of available diagnostic modalities before disease has become advanced. The primary goals are to identify and control risk factors, where possible, and to maintain quality of life and extend survival time after diagnosis of cardiovascular disease. The following section reviews treatment options that show promise for the management of clinical atherosclerotic disease, congestive heart failure and related conditions, and pericardial disease or effusion in birds. Medications that have been used empirically and those for which pharmacokinetic and pharmacodynamic data are available are presented in Table 6-16.

Atherosclerotic Disease

Treatment of atherosclerosis involves both controlling risk factors and managing sequelae, including peripheral hypoperfusion, ischemic stroke, and congestive heart failure (see following section).[24] Atherosclerotic lesions cannot be resolved, but diet, husbandry, and lifestyle changes may help prevent, slow the progression, or decrease the size of the lesions. Peripheral vasodilation may have symptomatic benefit by promoting improved peripheral perfusion and reducing afterload by decreasing vascular resistance.

Vasodilation

Isoxsuprine. Isoxsuprine is a peripheral vasodilator that causes vascular smooth muscle relaxation predominantly through α-adrenoreceptor blockade.[315,316] It has been used in veterinary medicine to increase peripheral blood flow in

---

[n]References 41,55,81,82,95,110,115-117,123,166,226,228,230,295.

TABLE 6-16
Selected Agents for Treatment of Cardiovascular Disease in Birds

Drug	Species	Dose / Frequency	Basis	Reference
DIURETIC DRUGS				
Furosemide	Parrots, raptors, mynah birds	0.1–2.2 mg/kg IM, PO q6-24h	EU	7, 94, 110, 115, 116, 296-300
	Parrots	1–5 mg/kg IM q2-12h (acute treatment)	EU	Author
		1–10 mg/kg PO q8-12h (maintenance)	EU	Author
	Chickens *(Gallus gallus domesticus)*	2.5 mg/kg IM	PD	301
		5 mg/kg PO	PD	301
Spironolactone	Chickens	1 mg/kg PO	PD	301
	Grey parrot *(Psittacus erithacus)*	1 mg/kg PO q12h	EU	110
VASODILATORS				
Isoxsuprine	Amazon parrot *(Amazona auropalliata)*	10 mg/kg PO q24h	EU	228
	Parrots	10 mg/kg PO q12h	EU	Author
Enalapril	Pigeons *(Columba livia)*	1.25 mg/kg PO q8-12h	PK	302
	Amazon parrots	1.25 mg/kg PO q8-12h	PK	302
	Parrots	2.5–5 mg/kg PO q12h	EU	123, 166, author
Benazepril	Grey parrot	0.5 mg/kg PO q24h	EU	110
POSITIVE INOTROPES				
Digoxin	Budgerigars *(Melopsittacus undulatus)*	0.02 mg/kg PO q24h	PK	303
	Quaker parrots *(Myiopsitta monachus)*	0.05 mg/kg PO q24h	PK	304
	Sparrows	0.02 mg/kg PO q24h	PK	303
	Indian ringneck parakeet *(Psittacula krameri)*	0.025 mg/kg PO q24h	EU	115
	Indian hill mynah *(Gracula religiosa)*	0.01 mg/kg PO q24h	EU	116
	Chickens	0.01 mg/kg PO q24h	EU	305
Pimobendan	Hispaniolan Amazon parrots *(Amazona ventralis)*	10 mg/kg PO q12h	PK	306
	Parrots	6–10 mg/kg PO q12h	EU	Author
	Harris' hawk *(Parabuteo unicinctus)*	0.25 mg/kg PO q12h	PK, EU	306
	Parrots	0.25 mg/kg PO q12h	EU	110,176
Dobutamine	Hispaniolan Amazon parrots	5–15 µg/kg/min (CRI)	PD	180
Dopamine	Hispaniolan Amazon parrots	5–10 µg/kg/min (CRI)	PD	180
NEGATIVE INOTROPES				
Carvedilol	Turkeys *(Meleagris gallopavo)**	1–20† mg/kg PO q24h	PD	307
Propranolol	Turkeys*	10 mg/kg PO q8h	PD	308
	Turkeys*	10–30 mg/kg PO q8h	PD	309
Atenolol	Most species	0.2 mg/kg IM, 0.04 mg/kg IV	EU	7
	Turkeys*	10–30 mg/kg PO q24h	PD	309
Carteolol	Turkeys*	0.01–10 mg/kg PO q12h	PD	310
Nifedipine	Turkeys*	10–50 mg/kg PO q8h	PD	309
Diltiazem	Most species	1–2 mg/kg PO q8-12h	EU	311
PARASYMPATHOLYTIC DRUGS				
Atropine	Most species	0.01–0.1 mg/kg IM, IV	EU	94
	Moluccan cockatoo *(Cacatua moluccensis)*	0.05 mg/kg IM	EU	176
Glycopyrrolate	Most species	0.01–0.02 mg/kg IM	EU	312
OTHER ANTIARRHYTHMIC DRUGS				
Lidocaine (preservative-free)	Chickens	6 mg/kg IV	PD	313
	Chickens	2.5 mg/kg IV	PK, PD	314
Propantheline	Moluccan cockatoo	0.3 mg/kg PO q8h	EU	176

*Broad-breasted white turkey poults.
†Some birds receiving carvedilol at 20 mg/kg had significantly decreased heart rate and blood pressure for up to 8 hours.
CRI, Continuous rate infusion; EU, empirical use; IM, intramuscularly; IV, intravenously; mg/kg, milligrams per kilogram; PD, pharmacodynamic study; PO, orally; PK, pharmacokinetic study; q8/12/24h, every 8/12/24 hours.

horses with vascular disorders of the lower limb and to address trauma-induced wing tip edema in raptors.[228,317] A 35-year-old yellow-naped Amazon (*Amazona auropalliata*) with presumptive atherosclerosis (based on clinical signs and suggestive radiographic findings) was treated with isoxsuprine (10 mg/kg, orally [PO] every 24 hours). Clinical signs of lethargy, weakness, hyporexia, weak grip, and ataxia resolved with treatment but recurred whenever the drug was discontinued and again resolved once it was reinstituted.[228] The author (BCF) has observed similar, apparent symptomatic improvement when using isoxsuprine (beginning at 10 mg/kg, PO every 12 to 24 hours) in numerous cases of presumed atherosclerosis (some of which were later confirmed at necropsy and with histopathology). Many of these patients have been treated and followed up for several months to several years, and during this time, the frequency and severity of strokelike events and other clinical signs appeared to decrease.

Angiotensin-converting enzyme inhibitors. Angiotensin-converting enzyme (ACE) inhibitors, including enalapril and benazepril, cause vasodilation by blocking the formation of AII.[318] AII promotes vasoconstriction and venoconstriction by mediating the release of catecholamines, which act on vascular smooth muscle via α-adrenergic receptors.[2] Although the relative vasodilatory effect of an ACE inhibitor compared with isoxsuprine in birds is not known, it is conceivable that the two used in combination would have synergistic effects: with the ACE inhibitor limiting α-adrenoreceptor stimulation and the isoxsuprine antagonizing α-adrenoreceptors. ACE inhibitors will be discussed in greater detail in the following section.

Other medical managements

Pentoxifylline. In mammals, pentoxifylline promotes passage of erythrocytes through damaged microvasculature by increasing their flexibility and has been used in human medicine for treatment of peripheral vascular and cerebrovascular disease.[319,320] In studies using small mammal models, tissue survival after frostbite was significantly improved by administration of pentoxifylline. It has therefore been suggested as an adjunct therapy for frostbite in birds and used empirically (15 mg/kg, PO, every 8 to 12 hours for 2 to 6 weeks) with no apparent adverse effects.[320] It may have value in improving peripheral perfusion in birds with atherosclerotic disease.

Statins. The statins are a group of lipid-lowering drugs used extensively in human medicine for their antiatherosclerotic effects through inhibition of cholesterol synthesis and other mechanisms. Statins reduce both plasma total cholesterol and LDL cholesterol concentrations and, to a lesser extent, increase HDL cholesterol concentration.[321] Several products are commercially available for human use: lovastatin, simvastatin, pravastatin, fluvastatin, atorvastatin, and rosuvastatin. Of these, only atorvastatin (Lipitor) and rosuvastatin (Crestor) have a long half-life in humans and are most commonly used.[321] Some statins have pharmacologic interactions, principally with drugs metabolized by the cytochrome P450 pathway, such as azole antifungals (e.g., itraconazole).[321,322]

Statins have been used in chickens (*Gallus gallus domesticus*) for research purposes; in one study, white leghorn hens fed a 0.03% or 0.06% atorvastatin or simvastatin diet had significantly lower plasma total cholesterol concentrations.[323]

Statins have been employed empirically in psittacine birds, but their use is controversial because no pharmacodynamic information is available for these species, and target levels of plasma total cholesterol and LDL cholesterol that would reduce atherosclerosis risk are unknown. A study investigating the pharmacokinetics of orally administered rosuvastatin (Crestor) in Hispaniolan Amazon parrots (*Amazona ventralis*) found that a dose of 10 mg/kg or 25 mg/kg (approximately 30 and 100 times the human dose, respectively) resulted in plasma concentrations below the limits of quantitation.[324]

Supportive care and husbandry considerations

Patients with signs of stroke may have marked neurologic deficits to include reduced mentation, limb paresis, and ataxia that prevent normal eating and drinking and impair mobility. They may experience seizures or suffer injuries from falls. Supportive care measures include fluid and nutritional support; analgesia; anticonvulsant therapy, when needed; and management of secondary conditions such as trauma and aspiration pneumonia. Exercise restriction should be part of the longer-term treatment plan, as well as appropriate housing modifications to accommodate and protect the birds with persistent deficits. Managements that may also have preventive value, particularly for at-risk species, include moderation of dietary calories and fat to prevent and resolve obesity, avoidance of dietary sources of cholesterol, and control of female reproductive activity.[23,24] Supplementation with omega-3 fatty acids, particularly α-linolenic acid (found in flaxseed oil), has been shown to improve lipid metabolism, reduce inflammation, and minimize the development of atherosclerosis in several avian species.[34,35,325] It is possible that increasing opportunities, early in life, for exercise, which is generally lacking for captive birds, may have some preventive value.[24] Physical activity can be promoted through training and by designing captive environments to facilitate locomotion and foraging behaviors. Operant learning methods should be employed to facilitate low-stress medication administration.

Congestive Heart Failure

Successful medical management of congestive heart failure is partly contingent on the earliest possible detection of disease. This can be enabled by teaching companion bird owners to identify clinical signs, even if subtle, by regular physical examinations on an annual or semiannual basis, by considering the option of baseline diagnostic imaging for at-risk individuals, and by heightened awareness in the clinical setting. For example, the author (BCF) has identified right-sided cardiac insufficiency in birds where the first premonitory sign was delayed absorption of subcutaneous fluids administered for a non-cardiovascular indication. Appropriate treatment also requires that known or hypothesized underlying cause(s) be addressed, if possible; some etiologies discussed in this chapter, such as bacterial and fungal infections and certain toxic insults, may carry a better prognosis for recovery. The mainstays of treatment of congestive heart failure in small animal medicine, namely diuretics, ACE inhibitors, and positive inotropes, can be applied to treatment of the condition in birds.[110] Beta-blockers, considered part of standard treatment in humans, may also have potential application.[307,326] The goal of initial treatment is to stabilize the patient presenting with acute or decompensated failure, followed by design of a longer-term management strategy. In the author's (BCF) experience, this has met with highly variable success, but some patients have been maintained in stable condition for up to 3 years.

Diuretics

Furosemide. Marked reduction of excessive circulating plasma volume (hypervolemia), edema, and effusion is an immediate treatment priority accomplished through the use of diuretics, principally furosemide. Parenteral administration of furosemide is an essential step in management of the acute crisis in dogs and cats. It is also the most effective agent for the management of chronic congestive heart failure in these species.[327,328]

Furosemide is a potent loop diuretic that inhibits the sodium, potassium, and chloride cotransporter in the ascending limb of the loop of Henle, thereby promoting diuresis and excretion of sodium and chloride.[328] It is efficacious and has a rapid onset of action in birds despite the presence of only 10% to 30% of looped nephrons in the avian kidney.[184]

Furosemide has been used for treatment of pericardial effusion, congestive heart failure, pulmonary edema, and ascites in birds[o] with a wide suggested dose range (0.1 to 2.2 mg/kg IM, IV, SC, or PO every 6 to 24 hours).[7,110,115,296-300] As in small animal medicine, the dose and administration interval are best determined by clinical response (i.e., normalization of respiratory rate and effort), the degree of which can be of diagnostic and prognostic value. In the author's (BCF) experience, a dose range of 1 to 5 mg/kg IM has been most efficacious when stabilizing psittacine patients with severely decompensated disease. An initial frequency of 2 hours is usually followed by a shift to 6- to 12-hour intervals. Once the patient has been stabilized, furosemide can be administered orally, with the dose increased at least twofold (presuming oral bioavailability is 60% to 75%, as in humans[329]) at a frequency of 8 to 12 hours. A study examining the diuretic effects of furosemide in chickens (adult laying hens) found that urine output significantly increased following parenteral administration (2.5 mg/kg) but did not in birds receiving the drug orally, even at twice the parenteral dose (5 mg/kg). In these birds, mean urine volume was 35% less than in those receiving parenteral furosemide, which suggests that there may be marked differences in bioavailability between the two routes of administration.[301] The ultimate goal for long-term management is to identify the lowest dose that controls the congestive signs.

With chronic use of furosemide, renal functional status (blood uric acid) and electrolytes should be monitored, given the potential for dehydration and hypokalemia.[94] It should be used with caution in patients with renal disease. Lories and lorikeets (subfamily Loriinae) have been reported to be extremely susceptible to the adverse effects of furosemide, namely, dehydration and electrolyte disturbances, so lower doses should be used in these species.[7] Diuretics should not be used alone in the long term because they further activate the RAAS.[330]

Spironolactone. Spironolactone is an aldosterone antagonist classified as a potassium-sparing diuretic that may be used concurrently with furosemide to offset potassium loss.[110,328,331] Its addition to the treatment regime might have merit in cases where congestive signs cannot be controlled with furosemide and an ACE inhibitor alone. However, spironolactone is not expected to be efficacious as a sole diuretic. Among its clinical benefits as an aldosterone antagonist, spironolactone is thought to prevent or decrease myocardial fibrosis in humans.[330]

Angiotensin-converting enzyme inhibitors

ACE inhibitors are an essential component of long-term medical management of congestive heart failure by blunting the effects of the RAAS. By interfering with AII formation and limiting aldosterone production, ACE inhibitors promote vasodilation and reduce sodium and water retention, thereby decreasing total peripheral resistance and pulmonary vascular resistance (afterload), and circulating volume (preload), allowing an increase in cardiac output.[94,302,318,332] Enalapril is thought to attenuate myocardial remodeling in humans and dogs.[333] Enalapril has been the most commonly used ACE inhibitor in birds, and empirical evidence suggests that it is both safe and efficacious.[302] It has been used, both alone and in combination with furosemide, to treat congestive heart failure and has achieved reduction in pericardial effusion, ascites, and hepatic congestion, as documented by echocardiography.[166,302] With inclusion of enalapril in the treatment regime, increased quality of life and longevity have been reported in birds with severe cardiac pathology.[302] Pharmacokinetic data support a dose of at least 1.25 mg/kg PO every 8 to 12 hours in pigeons and Amazon parrots. Enalapril has a shorter half-life and reaches a lower maximum plasma concentration in Amazon parrots compared with pigeons.[302] The author (BCF) has seen symptomatic benefit in psittacines with the use of this drug at a dose range of 1.25 to 5 mg/kg PO every 12 hours.

Potential adverse effects are hypotension, renal dysfunction, and hyperkalemia. The risk of hyperkalemia is likely diminished by concurrent use of furosemide but may be relatively greater if spironolactone is used as well.[318] Some authors have reported dehydration with long-term, higher-dose therapy (5 mg/kg daily). It is reasonable to consider similar biochemical and hematologic monitoring as for furosemide, but no significant changes in these parameters were found in pigeons receiving 10 mg/kg enalapril once daily for 3 weeks.[302] ACE inhibitors are rarely used alone; typically, they are combined with diuretics and positive or negative inotropes.

Positive inotropes

Positive inotropes are used to enhance myocardial contractility and are appropriate for the treatment of heart failure caused by systolic dysfunction. They are contraindicated in cases of hypertrophic cardiomyopathy (where diastolic dysfunction is the primary problem) and of outflow obstruction (e.g., aortic stenosis).[94,328,334] Likewise, it should be questioned whether their use is appropriate in birds with heart failure secondary to atherosclerotic disease and luminal stenosis of major arteries. In those cases with severe systolic dysfunction, however, it is fair to consider their inclusion in the treatment regime, at least in the short term, in an effort to stabilize the patient. Digoxin and pimobendan have been used or proposed for treatment of heart failure in avian

---

[o]References 7,29,41,94,95,166.

species, but pharmacodynamic data are lacking, and pharmacokinetic data and information as to their efficacy and margin of safety are extremely limited.[94,123,302,306]

Digoxin. Digoxin, a digitalis glycoside, increases myocardial contractility by directly inhibiting the sodium–potassium adenosine triphosphatase (Na^+/K^+ ATPase) pump, resulting in intracellular calcium accumulation through the activation of the sodium–calcium (Na^+/Ca^{2+}) exchanger. Other effects include mild diuresis, increased parasympathetic tone, and decreases in sympathetic tone and renin release. It is both a weak positive inotrope and a negative chronotrope, slowing the sinus rate and decreasing AV nodal conduction. It is useful for the treatment of heart failure complicated by supraventricular tachycardia (including atrial fibrillation) in mammals by slowing the ventricular rate.[335] It is also used in human patients with heart failure and left ventricular systolic dysfunction, whose symptoms are inadequately controlled with diuretics and ACE inhibitors.[336] However, the use of digoxin is becoming more controversial in small animal and human

cardiology because of its failure to reduce overall mortality and its proarrhythmic and gastrointestinal side effects.[335]

In birds, digoxin may have value in certain heart failure cases when used in combination with diuretics and ACE inhibitors, particularly when supraventricular tachyarrhythmia is a feature.[7] However, the narrow therapeutic index is a concern, and chronic, maintenance administration may prove problematic.[94,306] Some authors consider it most applicable to emergency situations.[94] The pharmacokinetics of digoxin have been investigated in several bird species.[303,304,337] In sparrows and budgerigars, a plasma concentration of 1.6 nanograms per milliliter (ng/mL) was achieved by administration of 0.02 mg/kg PO every 24 hours for 5 days,[303] and in Quaker parrots, a single oral dose of 0.05 mg/kg produced a maximum plasma concentration of 1.8 ± 0.36 ng/mL.[304] Use of digoxin, with monitoring of plasma levels, has been reported in several heart failure cases (Table 6-17).[7,81,115,116,338] In the case of an Indian hill mynah bird (*Gracula religiosa*) with biventricular congestive heart failure, marked clinical

TABLE 6-17

Survival Time After Diagnosis and Treatment for Selected Cases of Congestive Heart Failure (CHF) of Noninfectious Etiology*

Species	Ultimate Diagnosis	CHF	Treatment	Survival Time	Reference
Grey parrot (*Psittacus erithacus*)	Atherosclerosis Right atrioventricular (AV) valve insufficiency Cor pulmonale Myocardial fibrosis	Right	Coelomocentesis Furosemide Spironolactone Benazepril Pimobendan	35 days	110
Grey parrot (*Psittacus erithacus*)	Valve regurgitations, hyperechoic aorta	Biventricular	Furosemide Imidapril Pimobendan	30 days	295
Indian ringneck parakeet (*Psittacula krameri*)	Left and right AV valve insufficiency (myxomatous degeneration of left AV valve and hypertrophy of right AV valve) Myocardial degeneration and necrosis	Biventricular	Furosemide Digoxin	10 months	115
Blue-fronted Amazon parrot (*Amazona aestiva*)	Right AV valve insufficiency (congenital defect)	Right	Supportive Furosemide Digoxin	8 days	41
Yellow-crowned Amazon parrot (*Amazona ochrocephala*)	Cause undetermined	Right	Supportive Furosemide Enalapril	27 months	166
Severe macaw (*Ara severa*)	Atherosclerosis Diffuse fatty infiltration of the right ventricular myocardium	Biventricular	Furosemide	70 days	95
Grey-cheeked parakeet (*Brotogeris pyrrhopterus*)	Atherosclerosis Left and right AV valve insufficiency Myocardial degeneration and fibrosis	Biventricular	Supportive	3 days	128
Umbrella cockatoo (*Cacatua alba*)	Atherosclerosis Aneurysm of right coronary artery Myocardial fibrosis	Right	Supportive Furosemide	Euthanized at diagnosis	29
Umbrella cockatoo (*Cacatua alba*)	Atherosclerosis Left AV valve insufficiency (myxomatous degeneration and mineralization)	Left	Unspecified	Euthanized within 1 day of diagnosis	167

Continued

TABLE 6-17

Survival Time After Diagnosis and Treatment for Selected Cases of Congestive Heart Failure (CHF) of Noninfectious Etiology*—cont'd

Species	Ultimate Diagnosis	CHF	Treatment	Survival Time	Reference
Pukeko (*Porphyrio melanotus*)	Atherosclerosis Left AV valve insufficiency (endocardiosis) Left atrial thrombus Atrial fibrillation Myocardial degeneration	Biventricular	Supportive Digoxin	49 days	81
Red-tailed hawk (*Buteo jamaicensis*)	Dilated cardiomyopathy	Right	Supportive Furosemide	Euthanized 2 days after presentation	55
Indian hill mynah (*Gracula religiosa*)	Left AV valve insufficiency	Biventricular	Supportive Coelomocentesis Furosemide Digoxin	10 months	116
Greater hill mynah (*Gracula religiosa intermedia*)	Coronary mineralization	Right	Coelomocentesis	12 days	82
Mallard hybrid duck (*Anas* spp.)	Congenital left AV valve stenosis and subvalvular aortic stenosis	Biventricular	Supportive Coelomocentesis Furosemide	29 days	117
Grey parrot (*Psittacus erithacus*)	Dilated cardiomyopathy Atherosclerosis	Right	Supportive Furosemide Spironolactone Enalapril	30 days	Author
Grey parrot (*Psittacus erithacus*)	Atherosclerosis	Biventricular	Supportive Furosemide Spironolactone Enalapril Pimobendan	14 months	Author
Grey parrot (*Psittacus erithacus*)	Open	Right	Supportive Furosemide Enalapril Pimobendan	29 months to present	Author

*Cases managed by the author (unpublished) are highlighted in blue.

improvement was seen with digoxin (0.01 mg/kg PO every 24 hours) and furosemide (2.2 mg/kg PO every 12 hours), with trough serum digoxin concentration maintained at 1.6 ng/mL.[116] Administration of the drug to chickens with right-sided congestive heart failure (ascites syndrome) at a dose of 0.01 mg/kg PO every 24 hours over a 6-week period resulted in decreased ventricular size and ascites.[305]

Besides close monitoring of clinical status and biochemical and hematologic parameters, the risks posed by digoxin toxicity necessitate therapeutic drug monitoring and follow-up ECG.[94,339] Recommended therapeutic levels for digoxin in the dog are 0.8 to 1.2 ng/mL,[335] but anecdotal evidence from individual case reports suggests that the levels may range higher for some birds.[115,116] Digoxin toxicity can produce any type of arrhythmia (see Table 6-7), which may be further potentiated by hypokalemia resulting from diuretic use.[7] It is contraindicated in patients with SA nodal dysfunction or AV blocks and in those with ventricular arrhythmias, given the risk of ventricular fibrillation being induced.[7,127] In the case of the Indian hill mynah mentioned above, second-degree AV block developed when digoxin was used at 0.02 mg/kg PO

every 24 hours and trough serum digoxin concentration was 2.4 ng/mL.[116] Digoxin administered at a dose of 0.22 mg/kg PO every 24 hours produced arrhythmias in pigeons.[340]

Pimobendan. Pimobendan, a calcium sensitizer and phosphodiesterase inhibitor, is a positive inotrope and vasodilator (inodilator), as well as a positive lusitrope. It enhances myocardial contractility, primarily through calcium sensitization of cardiac myofibrils and by phosphodiesterase III inhibition, without increasing myocardial oxygen consumption.[306,335] Inhibition of phosphodiesterases III and V promotes systemic and pulmonary arterial and venous dilation, thereby reducing afterload and preload, respectively.[306] Pimobendan is commonly used in small animal cardiology and has been shown to increase both survival time and quality of life in dogs with dilated cardiomyopathy and heart failure secondary to mitral valve disease.[341] There are two reported cases where pimobendan (0.25 to 0.6 mg/kg every 12 hours) was used in conjunction with a diuretic and an ACE inhibitor to treat congestive heart failure in psittacines, with mixed results.[110,295] The apparent limited clinical effect may be explained by underdosing; there has since been a pharmacokinetic study in Hispaniolan

Amazon parrots (*Amazona ventralis*) demonstrating that a single oral dose of 10 mg/kg is required to achieve a peak plasma concentration of 8.26 ng/mL, comparable with levels considered therapeutic in dogs and humans.[306] An oral suspension formulated from commercially available tablets (crushed and combined with a suspending vehicle) produced six times greater plasma concentrations compared with a suspension made from the bulk chemical (powder). Extrapolation of the dose used in this study to other species groups should be done with caution. Plasma concentrations in a Harris' hawk (*Parabuteo unicinctus*) with congestive heart failure receiving 10 mg/kg pimobendan PO peaked at 25,196 ng/mL.[306]

Adverse effects reported in dogs are primarily gastrointestinal, and there may be some potential, although not confirmed, for proarrhythmic effects. A study in dogs with mitral regurgitation found that mitral valve disease worsened in dogs receiving pimobendan but did not in those receiving an ACE inhibitor alone.[334] Adverse effects have not been recognized in birds, but the safety and efficacy of this drug in avian species have not been established.

Sympathomimetic drugs. Dopamine and dobutamine are among the rapid-acting, intravenous positive inotropes used in small animal medicine for short-term (24 to 48 hours), life-saving intervention in cases of acute, profound myocardial failure. They are sympathomimetic drugs that act via β_1-adrenoreceptors to increase myocardial contractility and relaxation, as well as peripheral vasodilation. They can also promote vasoconstriction through their action at α-adrenoceptors. Both are short-lived and must be administered via constant rate infusion (CRI). They increase myocardial oxygen consumption, and their adverse effects include tachycardia and arrhythmia, requiring ECG monitoring during administration. Dopamine (a norepinephrine precursor) also has dopaminergic effects, which predominate at low infusion rates, promoting coronary, intracerebral, renal, and mesenteric vasodilation. The effects of adrenoreceptor stimulation follow as the rate is increased, until at high doses, α-mediated vasoconstriction overrides the desired effects. The risks of arrhythmia and tachycardia also increase with the infusion rate. Dobutamine (a synthetic dopamine analog) has the advantage of preferential binding of β_1-receptors over α-receptors and enhancement of contractility without marked heart rate elevation.[328,342]

The effects of these drugs on systolic function and cardiac output in birds is not known, but in Hispaniolan Amazon parrots anesthetized with isoflurane, dopamine (5, 7, and 10 μg/kg/min) and dobutamine (5, 10, and 15 μg/kg/min) CRIs significantly increased heart rate and arterial blood pressure (direct) in a dose-dependent manner (dopamine > dobutamine). Four study subjects developed second-degree AV block and hypotension while receiving dobutamine at 15 μg/kg/min.[180]

Negative inotropes

Beta-blockers. Beta-blockers are sympatholytic agents that block the binding of endogenous catecholamines to β-adrenoreceptors. They are negative inotropes, chronotropes, and lusitropes that also slow AV nodal conduction. First-generation, nonselective beta-blockers (e.g., propranolol, carteolol) block both β_1-adrenoreceptors and β_2-adrenoreceptors, whereas second-generation beta-blockers (e.g., atenolol,

metoprolol) are relatively β_1-selective. Carvedilol, a third-generation beta-blocker, is both a nonselective β-adrenoreceptor antagonist and selective α_1-adrenoreceptor antagonist such that it also has vasodilatory action to reduce afterload.[343-347] Beta-blockers are part of core therapy in humans for heart failure, both in early and advanced stages.[326,336,348] β-adrenoreceptor antagonism counters the increased sympathetic tone and RAAS activation characteristic of the neuroendocrine system that is central to the pathogenesis and progression of congestive heart failure.[328,349] By retarding its deleterious effects, beta-blockade is beneficial in treatment of heart failure in spite of the attendant negative inotropic effect. The antioxidant properties of some beta-blockers, including carvedilol, are also thought to contribute to their beneficial effects. Beta-blockers, in combination with diuretics and ACE inhibitors, are utilized in human cardiovascular medicine for treatment of chronic, stable congestive heart failure related to left ventricular systolic dysfunction. Multiple clinical trials have shown that second-generation and third-generation beta-blockers increase systolic performance and decrease mortality, at least in patients with stable congestive heart failure capable of tolerating the drugs' negative inotropic effects in the short term. Over time, these patients benefited from ultimate improvement in systolic function as a result of the drugs' longer-term actions: regression of myocardial hypertrophy, reversal of remodeling, and normalization of ventricular geometry.[326,328,336,349] Initiation of treatment is recommended in all patients with stable systolic heart failure as soon as a diagnosis is made in order to reduce risk of disease progression and death. Beta-blockers and ACE inhibitors are also used to prevent heart failure in cases with structural cardiac abnormalities (e.g., left ventricular hypertrophy, valvular disease) and systolic dysfunction that are as yet asymptomatic. In cases of acute, decompensated heart failure, addition of beta-blockers to the treatment regime is recommended as soon as the patient has been stabilized, volume has been controlled, and parenteral medications have been withdrawn.[326]

The beneficial effects of beta-blockers have also been documented in avian models of heart failure. Propranolol, carteolol, atenolol, metoprolol, and carvedilol have been investigated in the furazolidone-induced model of DCM in turkey poults as well as in spontaneously occurring, idiopathic DCM in these birds. The cardioprotective effects of these agents, both grossly and at the microscopic level, have been repeatedly demonstrated in birds concurrently receiving furazolidone. Propranolol has been found to prevent the gross morphologic changes (chamber dilatation, wall thinning) and microscopic changes (including cardiomyocyte hypertrophy) characteristic of the disease—benefits not seen with digoxin. Atenolol has similar, although lesser, cardioprotective effects, and both drugs have been shown to normalize myocardial contractility. Cardioprotective efficacy of beta-blockers is dose-dependent and greatest with nonselective beta-blockers; efficacy is ranked in descending order as: carteolol > propranolol > atenolol ≥ metoprolol.[107-110,350]

Some studies have focused on the treatment of established, advanced furazolidone-induced heart failure in turkeys, in which cardiac chamber dilatation and decreased systolic function were documented by echocardiography. All beta-blockers examined were found to improve systolic performance and decrease mortality. Treatment with carteolol, at a low dose

(0.01 mg/kg, PO every 12 hours) and a high dose (10 mg/kg, PO every 12 hours, uptitrated from 2.5 mg/kg over a period of 4 days), resulted in significant decreases in cardiac chamber sizes and wall thinning, improvement in systolic performance, reduction in myocardial fibrosis, and reversal of cardiomyocyte hypertrophy.[310] Birds receiving carvedilol for 4 weeks, at 1 mg/kg or 20 mg/kg, PO every 24 hours, showed significant improvements in left ventricular volume and fractional shortening (by 80% in some individuals) and had reduced apoptosis of cardiomyocytes (possibly as a result of the drug's antioxidant properties).[307]

In small animal medicine, carvedilol has garnered interest as adjunctive treatment for DCM in dogs, although its therapeutic value remains controversial.[328,346] A primary concern is that dogs may not live long enough to benefit from the long-term effects of beta-blockers and may be unable to tolerate initiation of treatment. One possible solution is concurrent administration of a low-dose positive inotrope such as pimobendan during the period of beta-blocker uptitration.[328]

Adverse effects of beta-blockers include bradycardia, hypotension, and precipitation or worsening of heart failure.[343–347] Beta-blockers are contraindicated in patients with decompensated heart failure, bradycardia, or greater than first-degree AV block.[344–347] In humans with heart failure, initiation of beta-blocker therapy may be accompanied by worsening of heart failure and congestion, but most patients stabilize with appropriate adjustments to their conventional therapy and go on to perform well with long-term treatment. Treatment should be initiated at a very low dose and gradually titrated upward. With this approach, the great majority of patients can tolerate treatment until the target dose is reached. Other adverse effects, including bradycardia, AV block, and hypotension can generally be managed by reducing the dose of the beta-blocker.[326]

In turkey poults with furazolidone-induced DCM, studies have indicated a maximum tolerated dose of 30 mg/kg propranolol PO every 8 hours and 30 mg/kg atenolol PO every 24 hours, each defined by the absence of adverse effects (sedation, persistent bradycardia, hypotension).[309] In the carteolol study, neither the low nor the high dose reduced blood pressure (as determined by indirect method), but heart rate acutely decreased (by less than 10%) for up to 4 hours in birds receiving the high dose.[310] Some individual birds receiving high-dose carvedilol (20 mg/kg) became moribund with significantly decreased heart rate and blood pressure for up to 8 hours. However, results of that study demonstrated that the beneficial effects of the drug do not require high enough doses to produce bradycardia and hypotension.[307]

We suggest that beta-blockers may have application in avian cardiology as adjunctive treatment of congestive heart failure, provided the condition is first stabilized using conventional management strategies. Close monitoring during initiation of treatment as well as regular follow-up over the long-term are essential.

Calcium channel blockers. Calcium channel blockers (CCBs) inhibit the influx of extracellular calcium ions across cardiomyocyte and vascular smooth muscle cell membranes, thereby inhibiting contraction. Effects are negative inotropy and chronotropy, slowing of the sinus rate and AV nodal conduction, and vasodilation.[172,311,351,352] CCBs are classified by their relative selectivity for the vasculature or for the myocardium; those that predominantly promote peripheral vasodilation and reduce total peripheral resistance (e.g., nifedipine and amlodipine) are indicated primarily for the treatment of hypertension, and those that influence conduction (e.g., verapamil and diltiazem) are indicated for the treatment of supraventricular tachyarrhythmias.[172,311,351,352] Adverse effects of CCBs include bradycardia, hypotension and reflex tachycardia, and AV block.[172,311,351,352] Contraindications include SA nodal dysfunction, second-degree or third-degree AV block, and decompensated heart failure.[311,351,352] In human patients with heart failure and systolic dysfunction, they confer no survival benefit and may exacerbate the condition.[326] They are mentioned here because their cardioprotective effects have been investigated in furazolidone-induced DCM in turkey poults and found to rival those of beta-blockers. Both nifedipine and verapamil are cardioprotective (nifedipine > verapamil), but the mechanisms by which these drugs confer their benefits are unknown.[309,350] A maximum tolerated dose of 50 mg/kg nifedipine PO every 8 hours was chosen for turkey poults based on the absence of adverse effects.[309]

Treatment of related conditions

Hypertrophic cardiomyopathy. Beta-blockers are utilized in human and small animal cardiology for the treatment of primary hypertrophic cardiomyopathy (HCM), including the obstructive type, which is characterized by systolic anterior motion (SAM) of the mitral valve. SAM results in dynamic, mechanical left ventricular outflow obstruction and mitral regurgitation. Because beta-blockers control heart rate, prolong and improve diastolic filling, and reduce outflow obstruction caused by SAM, they are among the treatment options recommended for both asymptomatic and symptomatic HCM in humans.[353,354] These drugs have similar effects in cats with HCM.[355] Verapamil and similar CCBs are suggested as alternative treatments for obstructive HCM in humans if beta-blocker therapy is inadequate or poorly tolerated.[353] Diltiazem has been employed to treat feline HCM, but its therapeutic value is doubtful.[311,355]

In contrast, HCM in birds is most often secondary, developing as a result of pressure overload states (such as aortic luminal stenosis caused by advanced atherosclerosis). Analogous conditions encountered in small animal medicine are ventricular outflow obstructions such as subvalvular aortic stenosis (SAS). In affected animals, beta-blockers are among the few medical management options; their potential benefit is based on reduction of heart rate and myocardial oxygen consumption, as well as improved diastolic coronary artery flow.[356] Hypothetically, beta-blockers may have merit for treatment of HCM in birds, but there are presently no reports of their use for this indication.

Systemic hypertension. Beta-blockers reduce arterial blood pressure by decreasing cardiac output and inhibiting RAAS activation. They are used to treat systemic hypertension in human and small animal medicine, often in conjunction with ACE inhibitors, CCBs, diuretics, or a combination of these agents.[326,357] In humans, such treatment markedly reduces the risk of developing heart failure, and combined therapy with a beta-blocker and ACE inhibitor is recommended in cases of diastolic heart failure with concurrent hypertension.[326] The CCB amlodipine is the treatment of choice for systemic hypertension in cats; it has been shown to significantly reduce blood pressure and, as shown in one study, resolved secondary ventricular hypertrophy in 50% of subjects.[357] At present, application of beta-blockers, CCBs, or other antihypertensive drugs for the treatment of systemic hypertension in birds is realistically precluded by the fact that there is no established definition of hypertension in avian species and no practical means to obtain accurate and repeatable arterial blood pressure measurements in the clinical setting.[231,249,257]

Arrhythmias. Before considering any antiarrhythmic therapy, factors underlying or contributing to the arrhythmia (e.g., hypoxia, electrolyte disturbances, intoxications) must be identified and addressed (see Table 6-7).[172,336] It is only appropriate to treat arrhythmias that are symptomatic, causing hemodynamic instability, and complicating or precipitating heart failure.[172,326,358] To date, reports of antiarrhythmic therapy in birds are extremely few.

Besides digoxin, beta-blockers and CCBs are used in small animal cardiology for treatment of supraventricular tachyarrhythmias, including atrial fibrillation, in order to slow the ventricular response rate.[172] These agents are generally contraindicated in patients with acute or decompensated congestive heart failure unless the arrhythmia is contributing to the condition such that conventional treatment alone has failed to stabilize the patient.[172,311,351,352] Even in this scenario, these drugs must be used with great caution, beginning at low dosages, with the aim of decreasing ventricular rate only marginally.[172]

Lidocaine is a parenteral antiarrhythmic agent used to control life-threatening ventricular tachyarrhythmias.[172,358] It reduces automaticity by blocking fast sodium channels, particularly in the damaged or ischemic portions of the myocardium. At usual doses, there is minimal effect on the cardiac conduction system or on myocardial contractility. Contraindications are SA or AV block. Adverse effects, that is, central nervous system (CNS) signs (reduced mentation, ataxia, or seizures), may be seen at high doses.[172,359] Studies using broiler chickens (*Gallus gallus domesticus*) have sought to determine the pharmacokinetics, the cardiovascular effects, and the safety of intravenous lidocaine in these birds. Transient bradycardia, with normal sinus rhythm, was noted following administration of 2.5 mg/kg lidocaine intravenously to isoflurane-anesthetized broilers.[156] In a similar experiment, infusion of 6 mg/kg lidocaine over 2 minutes was well tolerated, with only mild decreases in heart rate and mean arterial blood pressure. ED_{50} (dose at which 50% of test subjects would have mild cardiovascular depression) was determined to be 6.3 mg/kg.[313]

The antimuscarinic agents atropine and glycopyrrolate competitively inhibit binding of acetylcholine (and other cholinergic stimulants) to muscarinic receptors. They are used to treat bradycardias, including SA arrest and first-degree and second-degree AV block, and to determine whether these arrhythmias are related to increased vagal tone or other causes.[94,127,312,358,360] Another indication for their use is as antidotes for organophosphate and carbamate intoxication. These drugs are contraindicated in patients with tachycardia or tachyarrhythmias and must be used cautiously in patients with heart failure. Atropine crosses the blood-brain barrier and may cause adverse CNS effects. This is not true for glycopyrrolate or for propantheline, which is an oral antimuscarinic agent used in the treatment of anticholinergic-responsive bradycardias.[312,360,361] Heart rate and rhythm normalized in a 30-year-old Moluccan cockatoo (*Cacatua moluccensis*) with second-degree AV block (Mobitz type 2) following treatment with propantheline (0.3 mg/kg PO every 8 hours). Clinical signs of periodic dyspnea and syncopal episodes decreased, and the bird remained stable for at least 2 years.[176]

Supportive care and husbandry considerations

General supportive principles apply to the avian patient with heart failure, that is, rest; minimization of stress with judicious, limited handling and restraint; and provision of supplemental oxygen, when appropriate. Patients are typically dyspneic because of pulmonary edema, intracoelomic air sac compression by ascitic fluid, pericardial effusion, or a combination of these; oxygen supplementation is indicated for patients with pulmonary edema, whereas physical fluid removal is more efficacious to stabilize those with air sac compression and cardiac tamponade. Coelomocentesis will rapidly relieve air sac compression and can be performed periodically over the longer term, but it should not be used as a substitute for optimal pharmacologic management; pericardiocentesis is discussed in the following section. Care must be taken to avoid oxygen toxicity with excessive supplementation; repeated acute exposures (95% concentration for 3 hours on 3 consecutive days) and chronic exposure (95% concentration for 72 hours) resulted in pulmonary congestion, edema, inflammatory infiltrates, and thickening of the blood-gas barrier in budgerigars (*Melopsittacus undulatus*).[362]

As for stroke patients, weakness and ataxia may limit mobility and access to food and water and predispose the patients to falls. Patients may be presented in a severely debilitated state, with cachexia, dehydration, secondary renal dysfunction, and injuries. In-patient supportive care measures may include fluid and nutritional support, but parenteral fluid administration must be carefully considered. It is generally not indicated in the treatment of congestive heart failure when the primary, immediate goal is reduction of fluid overload. Furthermore, subcutaneous fluid absorption may fail in cases of right-sided congestive heart failure. Initial treatment of acute and decompensated congestive heart failure frequently results in some degree of dehydration and prerenal azotemia, but these abnormalities may resolve over a few days once food and water intake have normalized. For persistent, severe azotemia, it may be necessary to administer small volumes of parenteral fluids, but patients for which hemodynamic stability cannot be achieved without severe renal compromise have a poor prognosis. Maintaining the delicate balance between management of hypervolemia and concurrent dehydration and renal dysfunction is a profound clinical challenge, requiring close monitoring for changes in clinical status and adjustment of the treatment plan accordingly. This necessitates in-patient treatment until the patient has been stabilized to the extent that appetite and water intake are acceptable, hypervolemia is adequately controlled and hydration is adequate, oxygen supplementation is no longer needed, and parenteral medications have been withdrawn.

Longer-term husbandry considerations, including dietary changes (which should also entail sodium restriction), and lifestyle and housing modifications, mirror those discussed for atherosclerosis. Given that congestive heart failure often arises secondary to atherosclerotic disease in psittacine birds, preventive considerations may be applicable to both conditions.

Prognosis

A review of 14 published clinical cases of congestive heart failure in birds, employing a variety of treatments, shows a median survival time of 30 days (see Table 6-17). In small animals, long-term prognosis for congestive heart failure is also fair to poor, and, in dogs, reports indicate median survival times of 27 to 133 days for dilated cardiomyopathy and 588 days for preclinical mitral valve disease.[363-365] The shorter survival time reported in birds to date likely reflects the inherent challenges of treating a large variety of species for diseases for which there are a myriad of etiologies, limited understanding of pathophysiology, and often late-stage diagnosis. Pharmacologic information for cardiovascular therapeutic agents is extremely limited, and standardized treatment guidelines are lacking. Furthermore, it is daunting and potentially counterproductive to chronically medicate birds that may or may not be adequately socialized to such human interactions. Regular follow-up (with physical examination, repeat imaging, and biochemical monitoring) is essential, but it is dependent, at least in part, on owner compliance and financial constraints. Individually or combined, these variables complicate the treatment of cardiovascular disease and negatively impact survival time. However, the situation can be improved through preventive efforts, close scrutiny of patients for early clinical signs to achieve timely diagnosis, and formulation of treatment approaches that are customized to the individual, incorporating not only what limited information is available for birds but also therapeutic options in human and small animal cardiovascular medicine. Effective long-term management can be facilitated by thorough client education and communication, use of food vehicles and training techniques to enable stress-free medication administration, and consistent follow-up to re-evaluate patient status and the treatment regime.

Pericardial Effusion and Cardiac Tamponade

Treatment for pericardial effusion and cardiac tamponade is based first on removal of the fluid, and second on treatment of the underlying etiology of fluid accumulation.[7,94,189,194,284] Fluid removal can be accomplished either by ultrasound-guided pericardiocentesis (Figure 6-65)[94,123,221,302] or endoscopic pericardiocentesis or by endoscopic or surgical fenestration of the pericardium.[7,127,189,225,284] Diuretics are contraindicated in cardiac tamponade because they decrease the preload necessary to maintain ventricular filling pressure and cardiac output. However, furosemide with or without an ACE inhibitor may be useful to reduce pericardial fluid of low volume related to congestive heart failure.[7,41,94,166,302] Some authors have described successful resolution of high-volume pericardial effusion with the administration of enalapril (with or without furosemide) following pericardiocentesis.[302]

Ultrasound-guided pericardiocentesis in combination with furosemide (0.2 mg/kg, IM and PO every 12 hours) was used

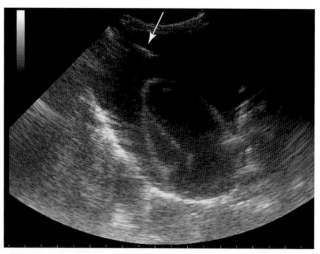

FIGURE 6-65 Ultrasound-guided pericardiocentesis (ventromedian approach, horizontal view) in a 32-year-old, male double-yellow-headed Amazon parrot (*Amazona ochrocephala*). The needle is visible penetrating the pericardium in the upper left of the image (*arrow*).

for management of profound idiopathic pericardial effusion in a Fischer's lovebird (*Agapornis fischeri*). Pericardiocentesis was repeated when effusion recurred 11 months following initial presentation, but the patient died 2 days later. At postmortem examination, pericarditis, myocarditis, and fibrosis, as well as hepatic and pulmonary fibrosis, were diagnosed through histopathology, but there was no evidence of infectious disease.[123] Furosemide has been used as a part of the combination medical management of congestive heart failure in a yellow-crowned Amazon parrot (*Amazona ochrocephala*) and in a blue-fronted Amazon parrot (*Amazona aestiva*) in which low-grade pericardial effusion was also a feature.[41,166] In the first case, furosemide was administered at a dose of 0.15 mg/kg, IM every 24 hours, in combination with enalapril, resulting in resolution of pericardial effusion.[166] In the second case, it was administered at a dose of 0.2 mg/kg, IM every 12 hours, in combination with a cardiac glycoside (digoxin), resulting in reduction, although not resolution, of pericardial effusion.[41] Endoscopic partial pericardiectomy was performed by the author (BCF) to relieve cardiac tamponade in a 14-year-old female jenday conure (*Aratinga jandaya*) with pericardial effusion and fibrinous pericarditis of undetermined primary cause. The bird has remained clinically healthy 6 years following this treatment.

REFERENCES

1. King AS, McLelland J: Cardiovascular system. In King AS, McLelland J, editors: *Birds—their structure and function*, ed 2, London, UK, 1984, Baillière Tindall, pp 214–228.
2. Smith FM, West NH, Jones DR: The cardiovascular system. In Whittow GC, editor: *Sturkie's avian physiology*, ed 5, San Diego, CA, 2000, Academic Press, pp 141–231.
3. Maina J: Perspectives on the structure and function in birds. In Rosskopf W, Woerpel R, editors: *Diseases of cage and aviary birds*, ed 3, Baltimore, MD, 1996, Williams & Wilkins, pp 163–217.

4. Baumel J: Systema cardiovasculare. In Baumel J, King A, Breazile J, et al, editors: *Handbook of avian anatomy: Nomina Anatomica Avium*, ed 2, Cambridge, MA, 1993, Nuttall Ornithological Club, pp 407–476.

5. West N, Langille B, Jones D: Cardiovascular system. In King A, McLelland J, editors: *Form and function in birds*, Vol 2, London, UK, 1981, Academic Press, pp 235–339.

6. Nickel R, Schummer A, Seiferle E, et al: Circulatory system. In Nickel R, Schummer A, Seiferle E, editors: *Anatomy of the domestic birds*, Berlin, Germany, 1977, Verlag Paul Parey – Springer Verlag, pp 85–107.

7. Lumeij J, Ritchie B: Cardiology. In Ritchie BW, Harrison GJ, Harrison LR, editors: *Avian medicine: principles and applications*, Lake Worth, FL, 1994, Wingers Publishing, pp 695–722.

8. King AS, McLelland J: Respiratory system. In King AS, McLelland J, editors: *Birds—their structure and function*, ed 2, London, UK, 1984, BaillièreTindall, pp 110–144.

9. Jaensch SM, Cullen L, Raidal SR: Air sac functional anatomy of the sulphur-crested cockatoo (*Cacatua galerita*) during isoflurane anesthesia, *J Avian Med Surg* 16(1):2–9, 2002.

10. Schmidt RE, Reavill DR, Phalen DN: Cardiovascular system. In Schmidt RE, Reavill DR, Phalen DN, editors: *Pathology of pet and aviary birds*, Ames, IA, 2003, Iowa State Press, pp 3–16.

11. Straub J, Valerius KP, Pees M, et al: Morphometry of the heart of budgerigars (*Melopsittacus undulatus*), Alisterus parrots (*Alisterus s scapularis*) and common buzzards (*Buteo buteo*), *Res Vet Sci* 72: 147–151, 2002.

12. Pees M, Zeh C, Filippich LJ, et al: Pathologisch-anatomische und morphometrische Untersuchungen am Herzen von wildlebenden Kakadus, *Tierärztliche Praxis Kleintiere* 6:390–396, 2014.

13. Krautwald-Junghanns ME, Braun S, Pees M, et al: Research on the anatomy and pathology of the psittacine heart, *J Avian Med Surg* 18:2–11, 2004.

14. McLelland J: Pericardium, pleura et peritoneum. In Baumel J, King A, Breazile J, et al, editors: *Handbook of avian anatomy: Nomina Anatomica Avium*, ed 2, Cambridge, MA, 1993, Nuttall Ornithological Club, pp 251–256.

15. Zandvliet MMJM: Electrocardiography in psittacine birds and ferrets, *J Exotic Pet Med* 14(1):34–51, 2005.

16. Duncker H: Coelomic cavities. In King A, McLelland J, editors: *Form and function in birds*, Vol 1, London, UK, 1979, Academic Press, pp 39–68.

17. Fletcher O, Abdul-Aziz T: Cardiovascular system. In Fletcher O, Abdul-Aziz T, editors: *Avian histopathology*, ed 3. Madison, WI, 2008, American Association of Avian Pathologists, Inc., pp 98–129.

18. de Morais HA, Schwartz DS: Pathophysiology of heart failure. In Ettinger SJ, Feldman EC, editors: *Textbook of veterinary internal medicine*, ed 5, St. Louis, MO, 2005, Saunders, pp 914–940.

19. Sturkie PD: Heart: contraction, conduction, and electrocardiography. In Sturkie PD, editor: *Avian physiology*, ed 4, New York, 1986, Springer-Verlag, pp 130–166.

20. Lang SA, Levy MN: Effects of vagus nerve on heart rate and ventricular contractility in chicken, *Am J Physiol* 256(5 Pt 2): H1295–H1302, 1989.

21. Wang H, Qiao J, Gao M, et al: Effects of endothelin A receptor antagonist BQ123 on femoral artery pressure and pulmonary artery pressure in broiler chickens, *Asian Australas J Anim Sci* 20(10):1503–1509, 2007.

22. Rosenthal K, Miller M: Cardiac disease. In Altman R, Clubb S, Dorrestein G, et al, editors: *Avian medicine and surgery*, Philadelphia, PA, 1997, W. B. Saunders Company, pp 491–500.

23. Beaufrere H: Atherosclerosis: comparative pathogenesis, lipoprotein metabolism, and avian and exotic companion mammal models, *J Exotic Pet Med* 22(4):320–335, 2013.

24. Beaufrere H: Avian atherosclerosis: parrots and beyond, *J Exotic Pet Med* 22(4):336–347, 2013.

25. Beaufrere H, Nevarez JG, Holder K, et al: Characterization and classification of psittacine atherosclerotic lesions by histopathology, digital image analysis, transmission and scanning electron microscopy, *Avian Pathol* 40(5):531–544, 2011.

26. Beaufrere H, Ammersbach M, Reavill DR, et al: Prevalence of and risk factors associated with atherosclerosis in psittacine birds, *J Am Vet Med Assoc* 242(12):1696–1704, 2013.

27. Walsh AL, Shivaprasad HL: Unusual lesions of atherosclerosis in psittacines, *J Exotic Pet Med* 22(4):366–374, 2013.

28. Grosset C, Guzman DS, Keating MK, et al: Central vestibular disease in a blue and gold macaw (*Ara ararauna*) with cerebral infarction and hemorrhage, *J Avian Med Surg* 28:132–142, 2014.

29. Vink-Nooteboom M, Schoemaker N, Kik M, et al: Clinical diagnosis of aneurysm of the right coronary artery in a white cockatoo (*Cacatua alba*), *J Small Anim Pract* 39(11):533–537, 1998.

30. Finlayson R: Spontaneous arterial disease in exotic animals, *J Zool* 147:239–343, 1965.

31. Beaufrere H, Cray C, Ammersbach M, et al: Association of plasma lipid levels with atherosclerosis prevalence in Psittaciformes, *J Avian Med Surg* 28(3):225–231, 2014.

32. Bavelaar FJJ, Beynen ACC: Plasma cholesterol concentrations in African grey parrots fed diets containing psyllium, *Int J Appl Res Vet Med* 1:1–8, 2003.

33. Stanford M: Significance of cholesterol assays in the investigation of hepatic lipidosis and atherosclerosis in psittacine birds, *Exotic DVM* 7(3):28–34, 2005.

34. Bavelaar FJ, Beynen AC: Severity of atherosclerosis in parrots in relation to the intake of alpha-linolenic acid, *Avian Dis* 47(3):566–577, 2003.

35. Petzinger C, Heatley JJ, Cornejo J, et al: Dietary modification of omega-3 fatty acids for birds with atherosclerosis, *J Am Vet Med Assoc* 236(5):523–528, 2010.

36. Dugan JP, Feuge RR, Burgess DS: Review of evidence for a connection between Chlamydia pneumoniae and atherosclerotic disease, *Clin Ther* 24(5):719–735, 2002.

37. Sessa R, Nicoletti M, Di Pietro M, et al: Chlamydia pneumoniae and atherosclerosis: current state and future prospects, *Int J Immunopathol Pharmacol* 22(1):9–14, 2009.

38. Hoymans VY, Bosmans JM, Ieven MM, et al: Chlamydia pneumoniae-based atherosclerosis: a smoking gun, *Acta Cardiol* 62(6): 565–571, 2007.

39. Pilny AA, Quesenberry KE, Bartick-Sedrish TE, et al: Evaluation of *Chlamydophila psittaci* infection and other risk factors for atherosclerosis in pet psittacine birds, *J Am Vet Med Assoc* 240(12):1474–1480, 2012.

40. Schenker OA, Hoop RK: Chlamydiae and atherosclerosis: can psittacine cases support the link? *Avian Dis* 51(1):8–13, 2007.

41. Pees M, Straub J, Krautwald-Junghanns ME: Insufficiency of the muscular atrioventricular valve in the heart of a blue-fronted Amazon (*Amazona aestiva aestiva*), *Vet Rec* 148:540–543, 2001.

42. Tappe JP, Andersen AA, Cheville NF: Respiratory and pericardial lesions in turkeys infected with avian or mammalian strains of *Chlamydia psittaci*, *Vet Pathol* 26:386–395, 1989.

43. Clippinger TL: Diseases of the lower respiratory tract of companion birds, *Semin Avian Exotic Pet Med* 6:201–208, 1997.

44. Kumar A, Jindal N, Shukla CL, et al: Pathological changes in broiler chickens fed ochratoxin A and inoculated with *Escherichia coli*, *Avian Pathol* 33:413–417, 2004.

45. Rubbenstroth D, Ryll M, Behr KP, et al: Pathogenesis of Riemerella anatipestifer in turkeys after experimental mono-infection via respiratory routes or dual infection together with the avian metapneumovirus, *Avian Pathol* 38:497–507, 2009.

46. Garner MM, Raymond JT: Retrospective study of atherosclerosis in birds, *Proc Annu Conf Assoc Avian Med* 59–66, 2003.

47. Finlayson R, Symons C, T-W-Fiennes RN: Atherosclerosis: a comparative study, *Br Med J* 502:501–507, 1962.

48. Griner LA: Birds. In Griner LA, editor: *Pathology of zoo animals*, San Diego, CA, 1983, Zoological Society of San Diego, pp 94–267.

49. Bohorquez F, Stout C: Aortic atherosclerosis in exotic avians, *Exp Mol Pathol* 17(3):50–60, 1972.

50. Al-Sadi HI, Abdullah AK: Spontaneous atherosclerosis in free-living pigeons in Mosul area, Iraq, *Pak Vet J* 31(2):166–168, 2011.

51. Jones MP: Vascular diseases in birds of prey, *J Exotic Pet Med* 22(4):348–357, 2013.

52. Keymer IF: Diseases of birds of prey, *Vet Rec* 90:579–594, 1972.

53. Cooper JE, Pomerance A: Cardiac lesions in birds of prey, *J Comp Pathol* 92(2):161–168, 1982.

54. Facon C, Beaufrere H, Gaborit C, et al: Cluster of atherosclerosis in a captive population of black kites (*Milvus migrans* subsp.) in France and effect of nutrition on the plasma lipid profile, *Avian Dis* 58(1):176–182, 2014.

55. Knafo SE, Rapoport G, Williams J, et al: Cardiomyopathy and right-sided congestive heart failure in a red-tailed hawk (*Buteo jamaicensis*), *J Avian Med Surg* 25(1):32–39, 2011.

56. Morishita TY, Fullerton AT, Lowenstine LJ, et al: Morbidity and mortality in free-living raptorial birds of Northern California: a retrospective study, 1983–1994, *J Avian Med Surg* 12(2):78–81, 1998.

57. Grunberg W, Kaiser E: Spontaneous arteriosclerosis in a population of free-living Egyptian vultures (*Neophron percnopterus*). II. Histochemistry of lesions and chemical analysis of aortic tissue and blood serum, *Acta Cardiol* 21(4):446–456, 1966.

58. Clair St. RW: The contribution of avian models to our understanding of atherosclerosis and their promise for the future, *Lab Anim Sci* 48(6):565–568, 1998.

59. Dauber DVV, Katz LNN: Experimental atherosclerosis in the chick, *Arch Pathol* 36(5):473–492, 1943.

60. Xiangdong L, Yuanwu L, Hua Z, et al: Animal models for the atherosclerosis research: a review, *Protein Cell* 2(3):189–201, 2011.

61. Bavelaar FJ, Beynen AC: The relation between diet, plasma cholesterol and atherosclerosis in pigeons, quails and chickens, *Int J Poult Sci* 3(11):671–684, 2004.

62. Toda T, Leszczynski D, Kummerow F: Vasculotoxic effects of dietary testosterone, estradiol, and cholesterol on chick artery, *J Pathol* 134(3):219–231, 1981.

63. Pick R, Stamler J, Rodbard S, et al: The inhibition of coronary atherosclerosis by estrogens in cholesterol-fed chicks, *Circulation* 6(2):276–280, 1952.

64. Fadly AM: Neoplastic diseases. In Saif Y, Fadly A, Glisson J, et al, editors: *Diseases of poultry*, ed 12, Ames, IA, 2008, Blackwell Publishing, pp 449–616.

65. Ojerio AD, Pucak GJ, Clarkson TB, et al: Diet-induced atherosclerosis and myocardial infarction in Japanese quail, *Lab Anim Sci* 22(1):33–39, 1972.

66. Bocan TM, Mazur MJ, Mueller SB, et al: Atherosclerotic lesion development in hypercholesterolemic Japanese quail following probucol treatment: a biochemical and morphologic evaluation, *Pharmacol Res* 29(1):65–76, 1994.

67. Chapman KP, Stafford WW, Day CE: Produced by selective breeding of Japanese quail animal model for experimental atherosclerosis, *Adv Exp Med Biol* 67:347–356, 1976.

68. Radcliffe JD, Liebsch KS: Dietary induction of hypercholesterolemia and atherosclerosis in Japanese quail of strain SEA, *J Nutr* 115(9):1154–1161, 1985.

69. Shih JCHHJ, Pullman EPPE, Kao KKJJ, et al: Genetic selection, general characterization, and histology of atherosclerosis-susceptible and -resistant Japanese quail, *Atherosclerosis* 49(1):41–53, 1983.

70. Gresham GA, Howard AN: Aortic rupture in the turkey, *J Athero Res* 1:75–80, 1961.

71. Crespo R, Shivaprasad H: Developmental, metabolic, and other noninfectious disorders. In Saif Y, Fadly A, Glisson J, et al, editors: *Diseases of poultry*, ed 12, Ames, IA, 2008, Blackwell Publishing, pp 1149–1195.

72. Krista L, McQuire J: Atherosclerosis in coronary, aortic, and sciatic arteries from wild male turkeys (*Meleagris gallopavo silvestris*), *Am J Vet Res* 49(9):1582–1588, 1988.

73. Anderson J, Smith S, Taylor R: Spontaneous atherosclerosis in pigeons: a good model for human disease. In Parthasarathy S, editor: *Atherogenesis*, Rijeka, Croatia, 2012, InTech Inc., pp 25–48.

74. Smith SC, Smith EC, Taylor RL: Susceptibility to spontaneous atherosclerosis in pigeons: an autosomal recessive trait, *J Hered* 92(5):439–442, 2001.

75. Clair St. RW: Metabolic changes in the arterial wall associated with atherosclerosis in the pigeon, *Federation Proc* 42(8):2480–2485, 1983.

76. Santerre RF, Wight TN, Smith SC, et al: Spontaneous atherosclerosis in pigeons. A model system for studying metabolic parameters associated with atherogenesis, *Am J Pathol* 67(1):1–22, 1972.

77. Prichard RW, Clarkson TB, Lofland HB, et al: Myocardial infarcts in pigeons, *Am J Pathol* 43:651–659, 1963.

78. Barakat St. HA, Clair RW: Characterization of plasma lipoproteins of grain- and cholesterol-fed white Carneau and show racer pigeons, *J Lipid Res* 26(10):1252–1268, 1985.

79. St. Leger J: Avian atherosclerosis. In Fowler ME, Miller RE, editors: *Zoo and wild animal medicine current therapy*, ed 6, St. Louis, MO, 2007, Saunders, pp 200–205.

80. St Leger JA: Acute aortic rupture in Antarctic penguins. In *Proceedings of the American Association of Zoo Veterinarians*, Minneapolis, MN, 2003, American Association of Zoo Veterinarians.

81. Beehler B, Montali R, Bush M: Mitral valve insufficiency with congestive heart failure in a Pukeko, *J Am Vet Med Assoc* 177:934–937, 1980.

82. Ensley PK, Hatkin J, Silverman S: Congestive heart failure in a greater hill mynah, *J Am Vet Med Assoc* 175(9):1010–1013, 1979.

83. Ruiz-Feria CA, Zhang D, Nishimura H: Age- and sex-dependent changes in pulse pressure in fowl aorta, *Comp Biochem Physiol A Mol Integr Physiol* 137(2):311–320, 2004.

84. Ferreras MC, González J, Pérez V, et al: Proximal aortic dissection (dissecting aortic aneurysm) in a mature ostrich, *Avian Dis* 45(1):251–256, 2001.

85. Baptiste KE, Pyle RL, Robertson JL, et al: Dissecting aortic aneurysm associated with a right ventricular arteriovenous shunt in a mature ostrich (*Struthio camelus*), *J Avian Med Surg* 11(3):194–200, 1997.

86. Courchesne S, Garner M: What is your diagnosis? *J Avian Med Surg* 23:69–73, 2009.

87. Vanhooser SL, Stair E, Edwards WC, et al: Aortic rupture in ostrich associated with copper deficiency, *Vet Hum Toxicol* 36(3):226–227, 1994.

88. Mitchinson MJ, Keymer IF: Aortic rupture in ostriches (*Struthio camelus*)—a comparative study, *J Comp Pathol* 87(1):27–33, 1997.

89. Gal A, Tabaran F, Taulescu M, et al: The first description of a congenital right ventricular cardiac aneurysm in a pigeon (*Columba livia domestica*, Cluj Blue Tumbler Pigeon), *Avian Dis* 56(4):778–780, 2012.

90. Julian R: Cardiovascular disease. In Jordan F, Pattison M, Alexander D, et al, editors: *Poultry diseases*, ed 5, London, UK, 2002, W. B. Saunders, pp 484–495.

91. Charlton B, Bermudez AJ, Boulianne M, et al: Cardiovascular diseases of chickens. In Charlton B, Bermudez AJ, Boulianne M, et al, editors: *Avian disease manual*, ed 6, Madison, WI, 2006, American Association of Avian Pathologists, Inc., pp 174–178.

92. Simpson CF, Kling JM, Palmer RF: Beta-aminopropionitrile-induced dissecting aneurysms of turkeys: treatment with propranolol, *Toxicol Appl Pharmacol* 16(1):143–153, 1970.

93. Oglesbee BL, Oglesbee MJ: Results of postmortem examination of psittacine birds with cardiac disease: 26 cases (1991–1995), *J Am Vet Med Assoc* 212:1737–1742, 1998.

94. Pees M, Krautwald-Junghanns ME, Straub J: Evaluating and treating the cardiovascular system. In Harrison GJ, Lightfoot TL, editors: *Clinical avian medicine*, Vol 1, Palm Beach, FL, 2006, Spix Publishing, pp 379–394.

95. Phalen DN, Hays HB, Filippich LJ, et al: Heart failure in a macaw with atherosclerosis of the aorta and brachiocephalic arteries, *J Am Vet Med Assoc* 209:1435–1440, 1996.

96. Fricke C, Schmidt V, Cramer K, et al: Characterization of atherosclerosis by histochemical and immunohistochemical methods in African grey parrots (*Psittacus erithacus*) and Amazon parrots (*Amazona* spp.), *Avian Dis* 53:466–472, 2009.

97. Zandvliet MMJM, Dorrestein GM, van der Hage M: Chronic pulmonary interstitial fibrosis in Amazon parrots, *Avian Pathol* 30: 517–524, 2001.

98. Fournier D, Luft FC, Bader M, et al: Emergence and evolution of the renin-angiotensin-aldosterone system, *J Mol Med* 90(5): 495–508, 2012.

99. Julian RJ: Rapid growth problems: ascites and skeletal deformities in broilers, *Poult Sci* 77(12):1773–1780, 1998.

100. Fischer I, Christen C, Scharf G, et al: Cardiomegaly in a whooper swan *(Cygnus cygnus)*, *Vet Rec* 156(6):178–182, 2005.

101. Pees M, Krautwald-Junghanns M-E: Cardiovascular physiology and diseases of pet birds, *Vet Clin North Am Exot Anim Pract* 12(1):81–97, vi, 2009.

102. Shrubsole-Cockwill A, Wojnarowicz C, Parker D: Atherosclerosis and ischemic cardiomyopathy in a captive, adult red-tailed hawk *(Buteo jamaicensis)*, *Avian Dis* 52(3):537–539, 2008.

103. Isaza R, Buergelt C, Kollias GV: Bacteremia and vegetative endocarditis associated with a heart murmur in a blue-and-gold macaw, *Avian Dis* 36(4):1112–1116, 1992.

104. Jessup D: Valvular endocarditis and bacteremia in a bald eagle, *Med Vet Pract* 61:49–51, 1980.

105. Burger WP, Naudé TW, Van Rensburg IB, et al: Cardiomyopathy in ostriches *(Struthio camelus)* due to avocado *(Persea americana* var. *guatemalensis)* intoxication, *J S Afr Vet Assoc* 65(3):113–118, 1994.

106. Fulton R: Other toxins and poisons. In Saif Y, Fadly A, Glisson J, et al, editors: *Diseases of poultry*, ed 12, Ames, IA, 2008, Blackwell Publishing, pp 1231–1258.

107. Czarnecki CM: Quantitative morphological alterations during the development of furazolidone-induced cardiomyopathy in turkeys, *J Comp Pathol* 96(1):63–75, 1986.

108. Hoerr F: Mycotoxicoses. In Saif Y, Fadly A, Glisson J, et al, editors: *Diseases of poultry*, Ames, IA, 2008, Blackwell Publishing, pp 1197–1229.

109. Dorrestein GM, Van Der Hage MH: Veterinary problems in mynah birds, *Proc Assoc Avian Vet* 263–274, 1988.

110. Sedacca CD, Campbell TW, Bright JM, et al: Chronic cor pulmonale secondary to pulmonary atherosclerosis in an African grey parrot, *J Am Vet Med Assoc* 234(8):1055–1059, 2009.

111. Currie RJ: Ascites in poultry: recent investigations, *Avian Pathol* 28(4):313–326, 1999.

112. Julian RJ: Ascites in poultry, *Avian Pathol* 22(3):419–454, 1993.

113. Olkowski AA: Pathophysiology of heart failure in broiler chickens: structural, biochemical, and molecular characteristics, *Poult Sci* 86(5): 999–1005, 2007.

114. Straub J, Pees M, Krautwald-Junghanns ME: Diagnosis of pericardial effusion in birds by ultrasound, *Vet Rec* 149:86–88, 2001.

115. Oglesbee BL, Lehmkuhl L: Congestive heart failure associated with myxomatous degeneration of the left atrioventricular valve in a parakeet, *J Am Vet Med Assoc* 218(3):360, 376–380, 2001.

116. Rosenthal K, Stamoulis M: Diagnosis of congestive heart failure in an Indian Hill Mynah Bird (Gracula religiosa), *J Assoc Avian Vet* 7(1):27–30, 1993.

117. Mitchell EB, Hawkins MG, Orvalho JS, et al: Congenital mitral stenosis, subvalvular aortic stenosis, and congestive heart failure in a duck, *J Vet Cardiol* 10(1):67–73, 2008.

118. Evans D, Tully T, Strickland K, et al: Congenital cardiovascular anomalies, including ventricular septal defects in 2 cockatoos, *J Avian Med Surg* 15(2):101–106, 2001.

119. Bailey T, Kinne J: Ventricular septal defect in a Houbara bustard *(Chlamydotis undulata macqueenii)*, *Avian Dis* 45:229–233, 2001.

120. Harari J, Miller D: Ventricular septal defect and bacterial endocarditis in a whistling swan, *Avian Pathol* 183:1296–1297, 1983.

121. Risi E, Testault I, Labrut S, et al: A case of congenital atrial communication and dilated cardiomyopathy on a griffon vulture *(Gyps fulvus)*, *Proc Annu Conf Eur Assoc Avian Vet* 244–249, 2011.

122. Olkowski AA, Classen HL: Progressive bradycardia, a possible factor in the pathogenesis of ascites in fast growing broiler chickens raised at low altitude, *Br Poult Sci* 39(1):139–146, 1998.

123. Straub J, Pees M, Enders F, et al: Pericardiocentesis and the use of enalapril in a Fischer's lovebird *(Agapornis fischeri)*, *Vet Rec* 152: 24–26, 2003.

124. Balamurugan V, Kataria JM: The hydropericardium syndrome in poultry—a current scenario, *Vet Res Commun* 28(2):127–148, 2004.

125. Jefferies JL, Towbin JA: Dilated cardiomyopathy, *Lancet* 375: 752–762, 2010.

126. Julian RJ: Production and growth related disorders and other metabolic diseases of poultry—a review, *Vet J* 169(3):350–369, 2005.

127. de Wit M, Schoemaker NJ: Clinical approach to avian cardiac disease, *Semin Avian Exotic Pet Med* 14:6–13, 2005.

128. Mans C, Brown CJ: Radiographic evidence of atherosclerosis of the descending aorta in a grey-cheeked parakeet *(Brotogeris pyrrhopterus)*, *J Avian Med Surg* 21(1):56–62, 2007.

129. Clarkson TB, King JS, Lofland HB, et al: Pathologic characteristics and composition of diet-aggravated atherosclerotic plaques during regression, *Exp Mol Pathol* 19(3):267–283, 1973.

130. Webb DM, DeNicola DB, Van Vleet JF: Serum chemistry alterations, including creatine kinase isoenzymes, in furazolidone toxicosis of ducklings: preliminary findings, *Avian Dis* 35:662–667, 1991.

131. Carrasco L, Gomez-Villamandos JC, Jensen HE: Systemic candidiasis and concomitant aspergillosis and zygomycosis in two Amazon parakeets *(Amazona aestiva)*, *Mycoses* 41(7-8):297–301, 1998.

132. Carrasco L, Bautista MJ, de las Mulas JM, et al: Application of enzyme-immunohistochemistry for the diagnosis of aspergillosis, candidiasis, and zygomycosis in three lovebirds, *Avian Dis* 37(3):923–927, 1993.

133. Staeheli P, Rinder M, Kaspers B: Avian bornavirus associated with fatal disease in psittacine birds, *J Virol* 84:6269–6275, 2010.

134. Vice CAC: Myocarditis as a component of psittacine proventricular dilatation syndrome in a Patagonian conure, *Avian Dis* 36:1117–1119, 1992.

135. Gancz A, Clubb S, Shivaprasad H: Advanced diagnostic approaches and current management of proventricular dilation disease, *Vet Clin North Am Exot Anim Pract* 13(3):471–494, 2012.

136. Palmieri C, Franca M, Uzall F, et al: Pathology and immunohistochemical findings of West Nile virus infection in psittaciformes, *Vet Pathol* 48(5):975–984, 2011.

137. Ellis AE, Mead DG, Allison AB, et al: Pathology and epidemiology of natural West Nile viral infection of raptors in Georgia, *J Wildl Dis* 43(2):214–223, 2007.

138. Saito EK, Sileo L, Green DE, et al: Raptor mortality due to West Nile virus in the United States, 2002, *J Wildl Dis* 43(2):206–213, 2007.

139. Page CD, Schmidt RE, English JH, et al: Antemortem diagnosis and treatment of sarcocystosis in two species of psittacines, *J Zoo Wildl Med* 23:77–85, 1992.

140. Page CD, Schmidt RE, Hubbard GB, et al: Sarcocystis myocarditis in a red lory *(Eos bornea)*, *J Zoo Wildl Med* 20:461–464, 1989.

141. Howerth EW, Rich G, Dubey JP, et al: Fatal toxoplasmosis in a red lory *(Eos bornea)*, *Avian Dis* 35(3):642–646, 1991.

142. Greenacre CB, Mann KA, Latimer KS, et al: Adult filarioid nematodes *(Chandlerella* sp.) from the right atrium and major veins of a Ducorps' cockatoo *(Cacatua ducorpsii)*, *J Assoc Avian Vet* 7(3):135–137, 1993.

143. Wu Y, Tobias AH, Bell K, et al: Cellular and molecular mechanisms of systolic and diastolic dysfunction in an avian model of dilated cardiomyopathy, *J Mol Cell Cardiol* 37(1):111–119, 2004.

144. Sileo L, Jones RN, Hatch RC: The effect of ingested lead shot on the electrocardiogram of Canada geese, *Avian Dis* 17(2):308–313, 1973.

145. Beyer WN, Spann JW, Sileo L, et al: Lead poisoning in six captive avian species, *Arch Environ Contam Toxicol* 17:121–130, 1988.

146. Hargis A, Stauber E, Casteel S, et al: Avocado *(Persea americana)* intoxication in caged birds, *J Am Vet Med Assoc* 194(1):64–66, 1989.

147. Lightfoot TL, Yeager JM: Pet bird toxicity and related environmental concerns, *Vet Clin N Am Exot Anim Pract* 11(2):229–59, vi, 2008.

148. Shropshire C, Stauber E, Arai M: Evaluation of selected plants for acute toxicosis in budgerigars, *J Am Vet Med Assoc* 7(1):936–939, 1992.

149. Dumonceaux G, Harrison G: Toxins. In Ritchie B, Harrison G, Harrison L, editors: *Avian medicine: principles and applications*, Lake Worth, FL, 1994, Wingers Publishing, pp 1030–1052.

150. Morris PJ, Avgeris SE, Baumgartner RE : Hemochromatosis in a greater Indian hill mynah *(Gracula religiosa)*, *J Assoc Avian Vet* 3(2):87–92, 1989.

151. Swenson J, Bradley GA: Suspected cholecalciferol rodenticide toxicosis in avian species at a zoological institution, *J Avian Med Surg* 27(2):136–147, 2013.

152. Degernes L: Waterfowl toxicology: a review, *Vet Clin North Am Exot Anim Pract* 11:283–300, 2008.

153. Redig P, Arent L: Raptor toxicology, *Vet Clin North Am Exot Anim Pract* 11:261–282, 2008.

154. Westerhof I, Van de Wal M, Lumeij J: Electrocardiographic changes in a galah *(Eolophus roseicapilla)* with lead poisoning, *Proc Annu Conf Europ Assoc Avian Vet* 59–60, 2011.

155. Martin, K: Psittacine behavioral pharmacotherapy. In Luescher A, editor: *Manual of parrot behavior*, Ames, IA, 2006, Blackwell Publishing, pp 267–279.

156. da Cunha AF, et al: Pharmacokinetics/pharmacodynamics of bupivacaine and lidocaine in chickens, *Proc Annu Conf Assoc Avian Vet* 313, 2011.

157. Gilbert CM, Filippich LJ, McGeary RP, et al: Toxicokinetics of the active doxorubicin metabolite, doxorubicinol, in sulphur-crested cockatoos *(Cacatua galerita)*, *Res Vet Sci* 83(1):123–129, 2007.

158. Hanley C, Wilson H, Latimer K, et al: Interclavicular hemangiosarcoma in a double yellow-headed Amazon parrot *(Amazona ochrocephala oratrix)*, *J Avian Med Surg* 19(2):130–137, 2005.

159. Buerkle M, Wust E: Bifid sternum in an African grey *(Psittacus erithacus)* and an orange-winged Amazon parrot *(Amazona amazonica)*, *Proc Annu Assoc Avian Med* 331, 2010.

160. Bennett RA, Gilson SD: Surgical management of bifid sternum in two African grey parrots, *J Am Vet Med Assoc* 214(3):352, 372–374, 1999.

161. Lichtenberger M: Determination of indirect blood pressure in the companion bird, *Semin Avian Exot Pet Med* 14(2):149–152, 2005.

162. Fudge AM, Reavill DR: Pulmonary artery aneurysm and polycythaemia with respiratory hypersensitivity in a blue and gold macaw *(Ara ararauna)*, *Proc Europ Conf Avian Med Surg* 382–387, 1993.

163. Taylor M: Polycythemia in the blue and gold macaw: a report of three cases, *Proc 1st Int Conf Zoo Avian Med* 95–104, 1987.

164. Taylor M, Hunter B: In my experience: a chronic obstructive pulmonary disease of blue and gold macaws, *J Assoc Avian Vet* 5(2):71, 1991.

165. McMillan MC: Imaging techniques. In Ritchie BW, Harrison GJ, Harrison LR, editors: *Avian medicine: principles and application*, Lake Worth, FL, 1994, Wingers Publishing, Inc., pp 246–326.

166. Pees M, Schmidt V, Coles B, et al: Diagnosis and long-term therapy of right-sided heart failure in a yellow-crowned amazon *(Amazona ochrocephala)*, *Vet Rec* 158(13):445–447, 2006.

167. Baine K: Atypical heart disease in an Umbrella cockatoo, *Proc Annu Conf Assoc Avian Vet* 285, 2012.

168. Murakami T, Uchida K, Naito H, et al: Ventricular septal defects in an ostrich *(Struthio camelus)* and a Chinese goose *(Cygnopsis cygnoid* var. *orientalis)*, *Adv Anim Cardiol* 1:33–37, 2000.

169. Olsen G, Gee G: Causes of Mississippi sandhill crane mortality in captivity, 1984-1993, *Proc North Am Crane Workshop* 249–252, 1997.

170. Siller W: Ventricular septal defects in the fowl, *J Pathol Bacteriol* 76:431–440, 1958.

171. Einzig S, Jankus E, Moller J: Ventricular septal defect in turkeys, *Am J Vet Res* 33:563–566, 1972.

172. Cote E, Ettinger S: Electrocardiography and cardiac arrhythmias. In Ettinger S, Feldman E, editors: *Textbook of veterinary internal medicine*, ed 6, St. Louis, MO, 2005, Saunders, pp 1040–1076.

173. Rembert MS, Smith JA, Strickland KN, et al: Intermittent bradyarrhythmia in a Hispaniolan Amazon parrot *(Amazona ventralis)*, *J Avian Med Surg* 22(1):31–40, 2008.

174. Kushner LI: ECG of the month. Atrioventricular block in a Muscovy duck, *J Am Vet Med Assoc* 214(1):33–36, 1999.

175. Nap AM, Lumeij JT, Stokhof AA: Electrocardiogram of the African grey *(Psittacus erithacus)* and Amazon *(Amazona spp.)* parrot, *Avian Pathol* 21(1):45–53, 1992.

176. Van Zeeland Y, Schoemaker N, Lumeij J: Syncopes associated with second degree atrioventricular block in a cockatoo, *Proc Annu Conf Assoc Avian Vet* 345–346, 2010.

177. Aguilar R, Smith V, Ogburn P, et al: Arrhythmias associated with isoflurane anesthesia in bald eagles *(Haliaeetus leucocephalus)*, *J Zoo Wildl Med* 26(4):508–516, 1995.

178. Martinez L, Jeffrey J, Odom T: Electrocardiographic diagnosis of cardiomyopathies in Aves, *Poul Av Biol Rev* 8(1):9–20, 1997.

179. Odom TW, Hargis BM, Lopez CC, et al: Use of electrocardiographic analysis for investigation of ascites syndrome in broiler chickens, *Avian Dis* 35(4):738–744, 1991.

180. Schnellbacher RW, da Cunha AF, Beaufrère H, et al: Effects of dopamine and dobutamine on isoflurane-induced hypotension in Hispaniolan Amazon parrots *(Amazona ventralis)*, *Am J Vet Res* 73(7):952–958, 2012.

181. Mukai S, Noboru M, Nishimura M, et al: Electrocardiographic observation on spontaneously occurring arrhythmias in chickens, *J Vet Med Sci* 58(10):953–961, 1996.

182. Scanes CG: Introduction to endocrinology: pituitary gland. In Whittow G, editor: *Sturkie's avian physiology*, ed 5, San Diego, CA, 2000, Academic Press, pp 437–460.

183. Carsia RV, Harvey S: Adrenals. In Whittow G, editor: *Sturkie's avian physiology*, ed 5, San Diego, CA, 2000, Academic Press, pp 489–537.

184. Goldstein D, Skadhauge E: Renal and extrarenal regulation of body fluid composition. In Whittow G, editor: *Sturkie's avian physiology*, ed 5, San Diego, CA, 2000, Academic Press, pp 265–297.

185. Cooper JE, Pomerance A: Cardiac lesions in birds of prey, *J Comp Pathol* 92(2): 161–168, 1982.

186. Naldo J, Samour J: Causes of morbidity and mortality in falcons in Saudi Arabia, *J Avian Med Surg* 18(4):229–241, 2004.

187. Kellin N: *Auswertung der sektions- und laborbefunde von 1780 vogeln der ordnung psittaciformes in einem zeitraum von vier jahren (2000 bis 2003)* [doctoral thesis], Giessen, Germany, 2009, University of Giessen, p 252.

188. Pees M, Krautwald-Junghanns ME: Avian echocardiography, *Semin Avian Exotic Pet Med* 14:14–21, 2005.

189. Echols S: Collecting diagnostic samples in avian patients, *Vet Clin North Am Exotic Anim Pract* 2:621–649, 1999.

190. Schmidt RE, Reavill DR, Phalen DN: Peritoneum and mesenteries. In Schmidt RE, Reavill DR, Phalen DN, editors: *Pathology of pet and aviary birds*, Ames, IA, 2003, Iowa State Press, pp 213–219.

191. Center SA: Fluid accumulation disorders. In Willard MD, Tvedten H, editors: *Small animal clinical diagnosis by laboratory methods*, ed 4, St. Louis, MO, 2004, Saunders, pp 247–269.

192. Lumeij JT: Gastroenterology. In Ritchie BW, Harrison GJ, Harrison LR, editors: *Avian medicine: principles and application*, Lake Worth. FL, 1994, Wingers Publishing, Inc., pp 482–521.

193. Barnes HJ, Nolan LK, Vaillancourt JP: Colibacillosis. In Saif YM, Fadly AM, Glisson JR, et al, editors: *Diseases of poultry*, ed 12, Ames, IA, 2008, Blackwell Publishing, pp 691–737.

194. Tobias AH: Pericardial disorders. In Ettinger SJ, Feldman EC, editors: *Textbook of veterinary internal medicine*, ed 6, St. Louis, MO, 2005, Saunders, pp 1104–1118.

195. Ozaki H, Murase T: Multiple routes of entry for Escherichia coli causing colibacillosis in commercial layer chickens, *J Vet Med Sci* 71:1685–1689, 2009.

196. Xi Y, Wood C, Lu B, et al: Prevalence of a septicemia disease in the crested ibis *(Nipponia nippon)* in China, *Avian Dis* 51:614–617, 2007.

197. Gerlach H: Bacteria. In Ritchie BW, Harrison GJ, Harrison LR, editors: *Avian medicine: principles and application*, Lake Worth, FL, 1994, Wingers Publishing, Inc., pp 949–983.

198. Akanbi OB, Breithaupt A, Polster U, et al: Systemic listeriosis in caged canaries *(Serinus canarius)*, *Avian Pathol* 37:329–332, 2008.

199. Cooper G, Charlton A, Bickford C, et al: Listeriosis in California broiler chickens, *J Vet Diagn Invest* 4:343–345, 1992.

200. Dhillon AS, Alisantosa B, Shivaprasad HL, et al: Pathogenicity of Salmonella enteritidis phage types 4, 8, and 23 in broiler chicks, *Avian Dis* 43:506–515, 1999.

201. Swan RA, Lidnsey MJ: Treatment and control by vaccination of erysipelas in farmed emus *(Dromaius novohollandiae)*, *Aust Vet J* 76:325–327, 1998.

202. Mohan R: Epidemiologic and laboratory observations of Chlamydia psittaci infection in pet birds, *J Am Vet Med Assoc* 184:1372–1374, 1984.

203. Mirandé LA, Howerth EW, Poston RP: Chlamydiosis in a red-tailed hawk *(Buteo jamaicensis)*, *J Wildlife Dis* 28:284–287, 1992.

204. Franson JC, Pearson JE: Probable epizootic chlamydiosis in wild California *(Larus californicus)* and ring-billed *(Larus delawarensis)* gulls in North Dakota, *J Wildlife Dis* 31:424–427, 1995.

205. Page LA, Derieux WT, Cutlip RC: An epornitic of fatal chlamydiosis *(ornithosis)* in South Carolina turkeys, *J Am Vet Med Assoc* 166:175–178, 1975.

206. Lennox AM: Mycobacteriosis in companion psittacine birds: a review, *J Avian Med Surg* 21:181–187, 2007.

207. Gelis S, Gill JH, Oldfield T, et al: Mycobacteriosis in gang gang cockatoos *(Callocephalon fimbriatum)*, *Vet Clin North Am Exot Anim Pract* 9:487–494, 2006.

208. Gough JF: Outbreaks of budgerigar fledgling disease in three aviaries in Ontario, *Can Vet J* 30:672–674, 1989.

209. Ritchie BW, Niagro FD, Latimer KS, et al: Avian polyomavirus: an overview, *J Assoc Avian Vet* 5:147–153, 1991.

210. Palya V, Ivanics E, Glávits R, et al: Epizootic occurrence of haemorrhagic nephritis enteritis virus infection of geese, *Avian Pathol* 33:244–250, 2004.

211. Lüschow D, Prusas C, Lierz M, et al: Adenovirus of psittacine birds: investigations on isolation and development of real-time polymerase chain reaction for specific detection, *Avian Pathol* 36:487–494, 2007.

212. Gerlach H: Viruses. In Ritchie BW, Harrison GJ, Harrison LR, editors: *Avian medicine: principles and application*, Lake Worth, FL, 1994, Wingers Publishing, Inc., pp 862–948.

213. Nakamura K, Mase M, Yamaguchi S, et al: Pathologic study of specific-pathogen-free chicks and hens inoculated with adenovirus isolated from hydropericardium syndrome, *Avian Dis* 43:414–423, 1999.

214. Nakamura K, Imada T, Imai K, et al: Pathology of specific-pathogen-free chickens inoculated with H5N1 avian influenza viruses isolated in Japan in 2004, *Avian Dis* 52:8–13, 2008.

215. Gough RE: Parvovirus infections. In Saif YM, Fadly AM, Glisson JR, et al, editors: *Diseases of poultry*, ed 12, Ames, IA, 2008, Blackwell Publishing, pp 397–404.

216. Ritchie BW, Carter K: Other avian viruses. In Ritchie BW, Carter K, editors: *Avian viruses: function and control*, Lake Worth, FL, 1995, Wingers Publishing, Inc., pp 413–438.

217. Ritchie BW, Carter K: Reoviridae. In Ritchie BW, Carter K, editors: *Avian viruses: function and control*, Lake Worth, FL, 1995, Wingers Publishing, Inc., pp 335–350.

218. Schmidt RE, Reavill DR, Phalen DN: Liver. In Schmidt RE, Reavill DR, Phalen DN, editors: *Pathology of pet and aviary birds*, Ames, IA, 2003, Iowa State Press, pp 67–93.

219. Greiner EC, Ritchie BW: Parasites. In Ritchie BW, Harrison GJ, Harrison LR, editors: *Avian medicine: principles and application*, Lake Worth, FL, 1994, Wingers Publishing, Inc., pp 1007–1029.

220. Latimer KS, Rakich PM: Necropsy examination. In Ritchie BW, Harrison GJ, Harrison LR, editors: *Avian medicine: principles and application*, Lake Worth, FL, 1994, Wingers Publishing, Inc., pp 355–379.

221. Mickley K, Buote M, Kiupel Matti, et al: Ovarian hemangiosarcoma in an orange-winged Amazon parrot *(Amazona amazonica)*, *J Avian Med Surg* 23:29–35, 2009.

222. Lightfoot TL: Overview of tumors: section I: clinical avian neoplasia and oncology. In Harrison GJ, Lightfoot TL, editors: *Clinical avian medicine*, Vol 2, Palm Beach, CA, 2006, Spix Publishing, pp 559–572.

223. Tully TN, Harrison GJ: Pneumonology. In Ritchie BW, Harrison GJ, Harrison LR, editors: *Avian medicine: principles and application*, Lake Worth, FL, 1994, Wingers Publishing, Inc., pp 556–581.

224. Steinmetz HW, Nitzl D, Curd S, et al: Ultrasonography in avian species: an underused diagnostic tool, *Exotic DVM* 8:66–77, 2006.

225. Hernandez-Divers SJ, McBride M, Hanley C: Minimally invasive endosurgery of the psittacine cranial coelom, *Exotic DVM* 6:33–37, 2004.

226. Beaufrere H, Nevarez J, Gaschen L, et al: Diagnosis of presumed acute ischemic stroke and associated seizure management in a Congo African grey parrot, *J Am Vet Med Assoc* 239(1):122–128, 2011.

227. Johnson JH, Phalen DN, Kondik VH, et al: Atherosclerosis in psittacine birds, *Proc Annu Conf Assoc Avian Vet* 87–93, 1992.

228. Simone-Freilicher E: Use of isoxsuprine for treatment of clinical signs associated with presumptive atherosclerosis in a yellow-naped Amazon parrot *(Amazona ochrocephala auropalliata)*, *J Avian Med Surg* 21(3):215–219, 2007.

229. Bennett RA: Neurology. In Ritchie BW, Harrison GJ, Harrison LR, editors: *Avian medicine: principles and applications*, Lake Worth, FL, 1994, Wingers Publishing, pp 723–747.

230. Beaufrere H, Holder KA, Bauer R, et al: Intermittent claudication-like syndrome secondary to atherosclerosis in a yellow-naped Amazon parrot *(Amazona ochrocephala auropalliata)*, *J Avian Med Surg* 25(4):266–276, 2011.

231. Acierno MJ, de Cunha A, Smith J, et al: Agreement between direct and indirect blood pressure measurements obtained from anesthetized Hispaniolan Amazon parrots, *J Am Vet Med Assoc* 233:1587–1590, 2008.

232. Lierz M: Diagnostic value of endoscopy and biopsy. In Harrison GJ, Lightfoot TL, editors: *Clinical avian medicine*, Vol 2, Palm Beach, CA, 2006, Spix Publishing, pp 631–652.

233. Helmer P: Advances in diagnostic imaging. In Harrison GJ, Lightfoot TL, editors: *Clinical avian medicine*, Vol 2, Palm Beach, CA, 2006, Spix Publishing, pp 653–659.

234. Silverman S, Tell LA: Radiology equipment and positioning techniques. In Silverman S, Tell LA, editors: *Radiology of birds: an atlas of normal anatomy and positioning*, St. Louis, MO, 2010, Saunders, pp 1–15.

235. Beaufrère H, Pariaut R, Rodriguez D, et al: Avian vascular imaging: a review, *J Avian Med Surg* 24:174–184, 2010.

236. Fudge AM: Avian liver and gastrointestinal testing. In Fudge AM, editor: *Laboratory medicine avian and exotic pets*, Philadelphia, PA, 2000, W. B. Saunders Company, pp 47–55.

237. Sharma S, Jackson PG, Makan J: Cardiac troponins, *J Clin Pathol* 57(10):1025–1026, 2004.

238. Briscoe JA, Rosenthal KL, Shofer FS: Selected complete blood cell count and plasma protein electrophoresis parameters in pet psittacine birds evaluated for illness, *J Avian Med Surg* 24:131–137, 2010.

239. Fudge AM: Avian complete blood count. In Fudge AM, editor: *Laboratory medicine avian and exotic pets*, Philadelphia, PA, 2000, W. B. Saunders Company, pp 9–18.

240. Fudge AM, Joseph V: Disorders of avian leukocytes. In Fudge AM, editor: *Laboratory medicine avian and exotic pets*, Philadelphia, PA, 2000, W.B. Saunders Company, pp 19–27.

241. Vanrompay D: Avian Chlamydial diagnostics. In Fudge AM, editor: *Laboratory medicine avian and exotic pets*, Philadelphia, PA, 2000, W. B. Saunders Company, pp 99–110.

242. Oglesbee BL, Avian A, Hamlindvm RL, et al: Electrocardiographic reference values for macaws (*Ara* species) and cockatoos (*Cacatua* species), *J Avian Med Surg* 15(1):17–22, 2001.

243. Mans C: Sedation of pet birds, *J Exotic Pet Med* 23(2):152–157, 2014.

244. Olkowski AA, Classen HL, Riddell C, et al: A study of electrocardiographic patterns in a population of commercial broiler chickens, *Vet Res Commun* 21(1):51–62, 1997.

245. Cinar A, Bagci C, Belge F, et al: The electrocardiogram of the Pekin duck, *Avian Dis* 40(4):919–923, 1996.

246. Lumeij JT, Stokhof AA: Electrocardiogram of the racing pigeon (*Columba livia domestica*), *Res Vet Sci* 38(3):275–278, 1985.

247. Burtnick N, Degernes L: Electrocardiography on fifty-nine anesthetized convalescing raptors. In Redig P, Cooper J, Remple J, Hunter D, editors: *Raptor biomedicine*, Minneapolis, MN, 1993, University of Minnesota Press, pp 111–121.

248. Czarnecki C, Good A: Electrocardiographic technique for identifying developing cardiomyopathies in young turkey poults, *Poult Sci* 59(7):1515–1520, 1980.

249. Zehnder AM, Hawkins MG, Pascoe PJ, et al: Evaluation of indirect blood pressure monitoring in awake and anesthetized red-tailed hawks (*Buteo jamaicensis*): effects of cuff size, cuff placement, and monitoring equipment, *Vet Anesth Analg* 36(5):464–479, 2009.

250. Joyner PH, Jones MP, Ward D, et al: Induction and recovery characteristics and cardiopulmonary effects of sevoflurane and isoflurane in bald eagles, *Am J Vet Res* 69(1):13–22, 2008.

251. Speckmann EW, Ringer RK: The cardiac output and carotid and tibial blood pressure of the turkey, *Can J Biochem Physiol* 41(11):2337–2341, 1963.

252. Zehnder AM, Hawkins MG, Pascoe PJ: Avian anatomy and physiology. In West G, Heard D, Caulkett N, editors: *Animal and wildlife immobilization and anesthesia*, ed 2, Ames, IA, 2014, Wiley-Blackwell, pp 391–398.

253. Touzot-Jourde G, Hernandez-Divers SJ, Trim CM: Cardiopulmonary effects of controlled versus spontaneous ventilation in pigeons anesthetized for coelioscopy, *J Am Vet Med Assoc* 227(9):1424–1428, 2005.

254. Hawkins MG, Wright BD, Pascoe PJ, et al: Pharmacokinetics and anesthetic and cardiopulmonary effects of propofol in red-tailed hawks (*Buteo jamaicensis*) and great horned owls (*Bubo virginianus*), *Am J Vet Res* 64(6):677–683, 2003.

255. Koch J, Buss EG, Lobaugh B, et al: Blood pressure of chickens selected for leanness or obesity, *Poult Sci* 62(5):904–907, 1983.

256. Langille BL, Jones DR: Central cardiovascular dynamics of ducks, *Am J Physiol* 228(6):1856–1861, 1975.

257. Johnston MS, Davidowski LA, Rao S, et al: Precision of repeated, Doppler-derived indirect blood pressure measurements in conscious psittacine birds, *J Avian Med Surg* 25(2):83–90, 2011.

258. Lichtenberger M, Ko J: Critical care monitoring, *Vet Clin North Am Exot Anim Pract* 10(2):317–344, 2007.

259. Straub J, Pees M, Krautwald-Junghanns ME: Measurement of the cardiac silhouette in psittacines, *J Am Vet Med Assoc* 221:76–79, 2002.

260. Barbon AR, Smith S, Forbes N: Radiographic evaluation of cardiac size in four falconiform species, *J Avian Med Surg* 24(3):222–226, 2010.

261. Lumeij JT, Shaik MAS, Ali M: Radiographic reference limits for cardiac width in peregrine falcons (*Falco peregrinus*), *J Am Vet Med Assoc* 238(11):1459–1463, 2011.

262. Hanley C, Murray H, Torrey S, et al: Establishing cardiac measurement standards in three avian species, *J Avian Med Surg* 11(1):15–19, 1997.

263. Gumpenberger M, Scope A: Diagnosis of abdominal diseases in birds by combined radiography and ultrasonography, *Eur J Comp Anim Pract* 12:153–162, 2002.

264. Wheler CL, Webber RA: Localized ascites in a cockatiel (*Nymphicus hollandicus*) with hepatic cirrhosis, *J Avian Med Surg* 16:300–305, 2002.

265. Vink-Nooteboom M, Lumeij JT, Wolvekamp WT: Radiography and image-intensified fluoroscopy of barium passage through the gastrointestinal tract in six healthy Amazon parrots (*Amazona aestiva*), *Vet Radiol Ultrasound* 44:43–48, 2003.

266. Krautwald-Junghanns ME, Schulz M, Hagner D, et al: Transcoelomic two-dimensional echocardiography in the avian patient, *J Avian Med Surg* 9:19–31, 1995.

267. Pees M, Straub J, Krautwald-Junghanns ME: Echocardiographic examinations of 60 African grey parrots and 30 other psittacine birds, *Vet Rec* 155:73–76, 2004.

268. Krautwald-Junghanns ME, Enders F: Ultrasonography in birds, *Semin Avian Exotic Pet Med* 3:140–146, 1994.

269. Beaufrère H, Pariaut R, Nevarez JG, et al: Feasibility of transesophageal echocardiography in birds without cardiac disease, *J Am Vet Med Assoc* 236:540–547, 2010.

270. Straub J, Forbes NA, Pees M, et al: Pulsed-wave Doppler-derived velocity of diastolic ventricular inflow and systolic aortic outflow in raptors, *Vet Rec* 154(5):145–147, 2004.

271. Straub J: Effect of handling-induced stress on the results of spectral Doppler echocardiography in falcons, *Res Vet Sci* 74(2):119–122, 2003.

272. Boskovic M, Krautwald-Junghanns M, Failing K, et al: Moglichkeiten und grenzen echokardiographischer untersuchungen bei tag-und nachgreivogeln (Accipitriformes, Falconiformes, Strigiformes), *Tierarztl Prax* 27:334–341, 1995.

273. Beaufrere H, Pariaut R, Rodriguez D, et al: Comparison of transcoelomic, contrast transcoelomic, and transesophageal echocardiography in anesthetized red-tailed hawks (*Buteo jamaicensis*), *Am J Vet Res* 73(10):1560–1568, 2012.

274. Beaufrere H, Pariaut R, Rodriguez D, et al: Avian vascular imaging: a review, *J Avian Med Surg* 24(3):174–184, 2010.

275. Krautwald-Junghanns M-E, Schloemer J, Pees M: Iodine-based contrast media in avian medicine, *J Exot Pet Med* 17(3):189, 2008.

276. Beaufrère H, Rodriguez D, Pariaut R, et al: Estimation of intrathoracic arterial diameter by means of computed tomographic angiography in Hispaniolan Amazon parrots, *Am J Vet Res* 72(2):210–218, 2011.

277. Romagnano A, Shiroma JT, Heard DJ, et al: Magnetic resonance imaging of the brain and coelomic cavity of the domestic pigeon (*Columba livia domestica*), *Vet Radiol Ultrasound* 37(6):431–440, 1996.

278. Jenkins JR: Use of computed tomography in pet bird practice, *Proc Annu Conf Assoc Avian Vet* 276–279, 1991.

279. Echols MS: African grey anatomy project, *Proc ICARE* 135–137, 2015.

280. Taylor M: Endoscopic techniques, *Semin Avian Exotic Pet Med* 3:126–132, 1994.

281. Murray M: Endoscopy, *Semin Avian Exotic Pet Med* 9:225–233, 2000.

282. Hernandez-Divers SJ: Endosurgical debridement and diode laser ablation of lung and air sac granulomas in psittacine birds, *J Avian Med Surg* 16:138–145, 2002.

283. Hernandez-Divers SJ, Hernandez-Divers SM: Avian diagnostic endoscopy, *Comp Cont Educ Pract Vet* 26:839–852, 2004.

284. Bennett RA: Thoracic and respiratory surgery in birds, Proc West Vet Conf, 2002. http://www.vin.com/Members/Proceedings/Proceedings.plx?CID=WVC2002&Category=&PID=1198&O=VIN. Accessed November 3, 2014.

285. Campbell TW: Cytology. In Ritchie BW, Harrison GJ, Harrison LR, editors: *Avian medicine: principles and application*, Lake Worth, FL, 1994, Wingers Publishing, Inc., pp 199–222.

286. Latimer KS: *Duncan and Prasse's veterinary laboratory medicine: clinical pathology*, ed 5, Ames, IA, 2011, Wiley-Blackwell.

287. Fudge AM: Avian cytodiagnosis. In Fudge AM, editor: *Laboratory medicine avian and exotic pets*, Philadelphia, PA, 2000, W. B. Saunders Company, pp 124–132.

288. Cooper JE: Avian microbiology. In Fudge AM, editor: *Laboratory medicine avian and exotic pets*, Philadelphia, PA, 2000, W. B. Saunders Company, pp 90–98.

289. Portaels F, Realini L, Bauwens L, et al: Mycobacteriosis caused by Mycobacterium genavense in birds kept in a zoo: 11-year survey, *J Clin Microbiol* 34:319–323, 1996.

290. Tell LA, Woods L, Foley J, et al: A model of avian mycobacteriosis: clinical and histopathologic findings in Japanese quail *(Coturnix coturnix japonica)* intravenously inoculated with Mycobacterium avium, *Avian Dis* 47:433–443, 2003.

291. Tvedten H, Cowell RL: Cytology of neoplastic and inflammatory masses. In Willard MD, Tvedten H, editors: *Small animal clinical diagnosis by laboratory methods*, ed 4, St. Louis, MO, 2004, Saunders, pp 356–380.

292. Schmidt RE, Reavill DR, Phalen DN: Respiratory system. In Schmidt RE, Reavill DR, Phalen DN, editors: *Pathology of pet and aviary birds*, Ames, IA, 2003, Iowa State Press, pp 17–40.

293. Phalen DN: Avian viral diagnostics. In Fudge AM, editor: *Laboratory medicine avian and exotic pets*, Philadelphia, PA, 2000, W. B. Saunders Company, pp 111–123.

294. Ritchie BW, Carter K: Diagnosing viral infections. In Ritchie BW, Carter K, editors: *Avian viruses: function and control*, Lake Worth, FL, 1995, Wingers Publishing, Inc., pp 83–104.

295. Beaufrere H, Aertsens A, Fouquet J: Un cas d'insuffisance cardiaque congestive chez un perroquet gris, *L'Hebdo Vet* 200:8–10, 2007.

296. Ritchie BW, Harrison GJ: Formulary. In Ritchie BW, Harrison GJ, Harrison LR, editors: *Avian medicine: principles and application*, Lake Worth, FL, 1994, Wingers Publishing, Inc., pp 457–478.

297. Tully TN: Psittacine therapeutics, *Vet Clin North Am Exot Anim Pract* 3:59–90, 2000.

298. Oglesbee B: Overview of avian cardiology, *Proc West Vet Conf*, 2003. http://www.vin.com/Members/Proceedings/Proceedings.plx?CID=WVC2003&Category=&PID=3384&O=VIN. Accessed November 3, 2014.

299. Krautwald-Junghanns ME, Straub J: Avian cardiology: part I, *Proc Annu Conf Assoc Avian Vet* 323–330, 2001.

300. Doneley B: Treating liver disease in the avian patient, *Semin Avian Exotic Pet Med* 13:8–15, 2004.

301. Esfandiary A, Rajaian H, Asasi K, et al: Diuretic effects of several chemical and herbal compounds in adult laying hens, *Int J Poult Sci* 9(3):247–253, 2010.

302. Pees M, Kuhring K, Demiraij F, et al: Bioavailability and compatibility of enalapril in birds, *Proc Annu Assoc Avian Med* 7–11, 2006.

303. Hamlin R, Stalnaker P: Basis for use of digoxin in small birds, *J Vet Pharmacol Ther* 10(4):354–356, 1987.

304. Wilson R, Zenoble R, Horton C, et al: Single dose digoxin pharmacokinetics in the Quaker conure *(Myiopsitta monachus)*, *J Zoo Wildl Med* 20(4):432–434, 1989.

305. Alvarez Maldonado MVZ: Reporte preeliminar: digitalizacion en pollos de engorda como metodo preventivo en el sindrome ascitico, *Proc 35th West Poult Dis Conf* 133, 1986.

306. Guzman DS, Beaufrere H, KuKanich B, et al: Pharmacokinetics of single oral dose of pimobendan in Hispaniolan Amazon parrots *(Amazona ventralis)*, *J Avian Med Surg* 28(2):95–101, 2014.

307. Okafor CC, Perreault-Micale C, Hajjar RJ, et al: Chronic treatment with carvedilol improves ventricular function and reduces myocyte apoptosis in an animal model of heart failure, *BMC Physiol* 3:6, 2003.

308. Gwathmey JK: Morphological changes associated with furazolidone-induced cardiomyopathy: effects of digoxin and propranolol, *J Comp Path* 104:33–45, 1991.

309. Glass MG, Fuleihan F, Liao R, et al: Differences in cardioprotective efficacy of adrenergic receptor antagonists and Ca2+ channel antagonists in an animal model of dilated cardiomyopathy, *Circ Res* 73(6):1077–1089, 1993.

310. Gwathmey JK, Kim CS, Hajjar RJ, et al: Cellular and molecular remodeling in a heart failure model treated with the β-blocker carteolol, *Am J Physiol* 276:H1678–H1690, 1999.

311. Plumb DC: Diltiazem. In Plumb DC, editor: *Plumb's veterinary drug handbook*, ed 6, Ames, IA, 2008, Blackwell Publishing, pp 396–398.

312. Plumb DC: Glycopyrrolate. In Plumb DC, editor: *Plumb's veterinary drug handbook*, ed 6, Ames, IA, 2008, Blackwell Publishing, pp 582–585.

313. Brandao J, da Cunha AF, Pypendop B, et al: Cardiovascular tolerance of intravenous lidocaine in broiler chickens *(Gallus gallus domesticus)* anesthetized with isoflurane, *Vet Anaesth Analg* 2014. doi: 10.1111/vaa.12226. [Epub ahead of print].

314. de Cunha AF, Stout R, Tully TN, et al: Pharmacokinetics/pharmacodynamics of bupivacaine and lidocaine in chickens, *Proc Annu Assoc Avian Med* 313, 2011.

315. Elliott J, Soydan J: Characterisation of beta-adrenoceptors in equine digital veins: implications of the modes of vasodilatory action of isoxsuprine, *Equine Vet J Suppl* 19:101–107, 1995.

316. Belloli C, Carcano R, Arioli F, et al: Affinity of isoxsuprine for adrenoreceptors in equine digital artery and implications for vasodilatory action, *Equine Vet J* 32(2):119–124, 2000.

317. Lewis JC, Storm J, Greenwood AG: Treatment of wing tip oedema in raptors, *Vet Rec* 133(13):328, 1993.

318. Bulmer B: Angiotensin converting enzyme inhibitors and vasodilators. In Ettinger S, Feldman E, editors: *Textbook of veterinary internal medicine*, ed 7, St. Louis, MO, 2010, Saunders, pp 1216–1223.

319. Plumb DC: Pentoxifylline. In Plumb DC, editor: *Plumb's veterinary drug handbook*, ed 6, Ames, IA, 2008, Blackwell Publishing, pp 959–961.

320. Wellehan JFX: Frostbite in birds: pathophysiology and treatment, *Compend Cont Edu Pract Vet* 25:776–781, 2003.

321. Paoletti R, Bolego C, Cignerella A: Lipid and non-lipid effects of statins. In von Eckarstein A, editor: *Atherosclerosis: diet and drugs*, Berlin, Germany, 2005, Springer Verlag, pp 365–388.

322. Pasternak RC, Smith SC Jr, Bairey-Merz CN, et al: ACC/AHA/NHLBI clinical advisory on the use and safety of statins, *J Am Coll Cardiol* 40(3):567–572, 2002.

323. Elkin RG, Yan Z, Zhong Y, et al: Select 3-hydroxy-3-methylglutaryl-coenzyme A reductase inhibitors vary in their ability to reduce egg yolk cholesterol levels in laying hens through alteration of hepatic cholesterol biosynthesis and plasma VLDL composition, *J Nutr* 129(5):1010–1019, 1999.

324. Beaufrere H, Papich MG, Nevarez J, et al: Pharmacokinetics of orally administered rosuvastatin in Hispaniolan Amazon parrots *(Amazona ventralis)*, *Proc Assoc Avian Vet* 25, 2014.

325. Bavelaar FJ, Beynen AC: Atherosclerosis in parrots. A review, *Vet Q* 26(2):50–60, 2004.

326. Yancy CW, Jessup M, Bozkurt B, et al: 2013 ACCF/AHA guideline for the management of heart failure: a report of the American College of Cardiology Foundation/American Heart Association Task Force on Practice Guidelines, *Circulation* 128:e240–e327, 2013.

327. Cote E: *Clinical veterinary advisor: dogs and cats*, St. Louis, MO, 2007, Mosby.

328. Bulmer BJ, Sisson DD: Therapy of heart failure. In Ettinger SJ, Feldman EC, editors: *Textbook of veterinary internal medicine*, ed 6, St. Louis, MO, 2005, Saunders, pp 948–972.

329. Plumb DC: Furosemide. In Plumb DC, editor: *Plumb's veterinary drug handbook*, ed 6, Ames, IA, 2008, Blackwell Publishing, pp 553–556.

330. Schroeder N: Diuretics. In Ettinger S, Feldman E, editors: *Textbook of veterinary internal medicine*, ed 7, St. Louis, MO, 2010, Saunders, pp 1212–1214.

331. Plumb DC: Spironolactone. In Plumb DC, editor: *Plumb's veterinary drug handbook*, ed 6, Ames, IA, 2008, Blackwell Publishing, pp 1116–1118.

332. Plumb DC: Enalapril maleate. In Plumb DC, editor: *Plumb's veterinary drug handbook*, ed 6, Ames, IA, 2008, Blackwell Publishing, pp 453–455.

333. Cohn JN: Structural basis for heart failure, *Circulation* 91:2504–2507, 1995.

334. Plumb DC: Pimobendan. In Plumb DC, editor: *Plumb's veterinary drug handbook*, ed 6, Ames, IA, 2008, Blackwell Publishing, pp 989–991.

335. Fuentes V. Inotropes: inodilators. In Ettinger S, Feldman E, editors: *Textbook of veterinary internal medicine*, ed 7, St. Louis, MO, 2010, Saunders, pp 1202–1207.

336. Gibbs CR, Davies MK, Lip GYH: ABC of heart failure. Management: digoxin and other inotropes, β blockers, and antiarrhythmic and antithrombotic treatment, *BMJ* 320(7233):495–498, 2000.

337. Pedersoli WM, Ravis WR, Lee HS, et al: Pharmacokinetics of single doses of digoxin administered intravenously to ducks, roosters, and turkeys, *Am J Vet Res* 51(11):1751–1755, 1990.

338. Wack RF, Kramer LW, Anderson NL: Cardiomegaly and endocardial fibrosis in a secretary bird (*Sagittarius serpentarius*), *J Assoc Avian Vet* 8(2):76–80, 1994.

339. Plumb DC: Digoxin. In Plumb DC, editor: *Plumb's veterinary drug handbook*, ed 6, Ames, IA, 2008, Blackwell Publishing, pp 388–393.

340. Miller MS: Electrocardiography. In Harrison GJ, Harrison LR, editors: *Clinical avian medicine and surgery*, Philadelphia, PA, 1986, Saunders, pp 286–292.

341. Summerfield NJ, Boswood A, O'Grady MR, et al: Efficacy of Pimobendan in the Prevention of Congestive Heart Failure or Sudden Death in Doberman Pinschers with Preclinical Dilated Cardiomyopathy (The PROTECT Study), *J Vet Intern Med* 26(6):1337–1349, 2012.

342. Plumb DC: Dobutamine. In Plumb DC, editor: *Plumb's veterinary drug handbook*, ed 6, Ames, IA, 2008, Blackwell Publishing, pp 422–424.

343. Gordon S: Beta blocking agents. In Ettinger S, Feldman E, editors: *Textbook of veterinary internal medicine*, ed 7, St. Louis, MO, 2010, Saunders, pp 1207–1212.

344. Plumb DC: Propranolol. In Plumb DC, editor: *Plumb's veterinary drug handbook*, ed 6, Ames, IA, 2008, Blackwell Publishing, pp 1048–1051.

345. Plumb DC: Atenolol. In Plumb DC, editor: *Plumb's veterinary drug handbook*, ed 6, Ames, IA, 2008, Blackwell Publishing, pp 104–106.

346. Plumb DC: Carvedilol. In Plumb DC, editor: *Plumb's veterinary drug handbook*, ed 6, Ames, IA, 2008, Blackwell Publishing, pp 186–188.

347. Plumb DC: Metoprolol. In Plumb DC, editor: *Plumb's veterinary drug handbook*, ed 6, Ames, IA, 2008, Blackwell Publishing, pp 817–819.

348. Klapholz M: Beta-blocker use for the stages of heart failure, *Mayo Clin Proc* 84(8):718–729, 2009.

349. Mann D, Bristow M: Mechanisms and models in heart failure: the biomechanical model and beyond, *Circulation* 111:2837–2849, 2005.

350. Liao R, Carles M, Gwathmey JK: Animal models of cardiovascular disease for pharmacologic drug development and testing: appropriateness of comparison to the human disease state and pharmacotherapeutics, *Am J Therapeutics* 4:149–158, 1997.

351. Plumb DC: Verapamil. In Plumb DC, editor: *Plumb's veterinary drug handbook*, ed 6, Ames, IA, 2008, Blackwell Publishing, pp 1236–1239.

352. Plumb DC: Amlodipine besylate. In Plumb DC, editor: *Plumb's veterinary drug handbook*, ed 6, Ames, IA, 2008, Blackwell Publishing, pp 59–61.

353. Prinz C, Farr M, Hering D, et al: The diagnosis and treatment of hypertrophic cardiomyopathy, *Dtsch Arztebl Int* 108(13):209–215, 2011.

354. Sherrid MV, Pearle G, Gunsburg DZ: Clinical investigation and reports. Mechanism of benefit of negative inotropes in obstructive hypertrophic cardiomyopathy, *Circulation* 97:41–47, 1998.

355. Kittleson M: Feline myocardial disease. In Ettinger SJ, Feldman EC, editors: *Textbook of veterinary internal medicine*, ed 6, St. Louis, MO, 2005, Saunders, pp 1082–1104.

356. Oyama MA, Sisson DD, Thomas WP, et al: Congenital heart disease. In Ettinger SJ, Feldman EC, editors: *Textbook of veterinary internal medicine*, ed 6, St. Louis, 2005, Elsevier Saunders, pp 972–1021.

357. Snyder PS, Cooke KL: Management of hypertension. In Ettinger SJ, Feldman EC, editors: *Textbook of veterinary internal medicine*, ed 6, St. Louis, MO, 2005, Saunders, pp 477–479.

358. Nieminen MS, Bohm M, Cowie MR, et al: Executive summary of the guidelines on the diagnosis and treatment of acute heart failure: a report of the task force on acute heart failure of the European Society of Cardiology, *Eur Heart J* 26:384–416, 2005.

359. Plumb DC: Lidocaine (systemic). In Plumb DC, editor: *Plumb's veterinary drug handbook*, ed 6, Ames, IA, 2008, Blackwell Publishing, pp 721–724.

360. Plumb DC: Atropine sulfate. In Plumb DC, editor: *Plumb's veterinary drug handbook*, ed 6, Ames, IA, 2008, Blackwell Publishing, pp 112–116.

361. Plumb DC: Propantheline bromide. In Plumb DC, editor: *Plumb's veterinary drug handbook*, ed 6, Ames, IA, 2008, Blackwell Publishing, pp 1040–1042.

362. Jaensch SM, Cullen L, Raidal SR: The pathology of normobaric oxygen toxicity in budgerigars (*Melopsittacus undulatus*), *Avian Pathol* 30:135–142, 2001.

363. Tidholm A, Svensson H, Sylvén C: Survival and prognostic factors in 189 dogs with dilated cardiomyopathy, *J Am Anim Hosp Assoc* 33(4):364–368, 1997.

364. Borgarelli M, Crosara S, Lamb K, et al: Survival characteristics and prognostic variables of dogs with preclinical chronic degenerative mitral valve disease attributable to myxomatous degeneration, *J Vet Intern Med* 26(1):69–75, 2012.

365. Martin MWS, Stafford Johnson MJ, Celona B: Canine dilated cardiomyopathy: a retrospective study of signalment, presentation and clinical findings in 369 cases, *J Small Anim Pract* 50(1):23–29, 2009.

CHAPTER 7

Clinical Significance of the Avian Cloaca: Interrelationships with the Kidneys and the Hindgut

W. Michael Taylor

The avian cloaca is a structure consisting of three chambers that receive the rectum, the ureters, and the left oviduct (in females) or paired ductus deferens (in males). It is also home to the cloacal bursa (bursa of Fabricius), a critical part of the developing immune system in juvenile birds (see Chapter 11). These statements have long been a part of comparative anatomy instruction and yet do little to explain the varied and interconnected roles of this terminal outlet shared by the gut and the renal, immune, and reproductive systems over the life of the bird. Challenging to examine or image in life, the cloaca is no easier to assess during dissection. The chambers are arranged linearly—from cranial to caudal—as coprodeum, urodeum, and proctodeum (CUP), but the separating folds are seldom distinct and become flattened when opened. The general anatomy of the cloaca of birds has been widely described and illustrated for over 100 years (Figure 7-1),[1-3] yet some of these depictions are incorrect or misleading.[4] There is also a surprising lack of information about the anatomy of the cloaca in most of the avian taxonomic orders that are of interest to the clinician.

The class Aves is very diverse, and as might be expected, there are many divergent and convergent adaptions of structure and function. This appears to be the case with the cloaca as well, although common trends prevail. The descriptions in this chapter are based upon the author's examinations of representatives of the taxonomic orders Psittaciformes, Strigiformes, Falconiformes, and Columbiformes and on the limited published descriptions of other orders.[2,5]

ANATOMY AND PHYSIOLOGY

Over the last 10 to 15 years, much work has been done on chicken and quail embryos to elegantly describe the embryonic development of the avian cloaca and its neural components.[6-10] These studies have been carried out to determine the origins of various anorectal defects in humans, such as persistent cloaca. When combined with the extensive work over the past 30 years to study the development of the enteric nervous system by using chick and quail models, we now have a better understanding of avian cloacal and rectal embryology. The author has listed a few of the key reviews for those wishing further information.[11-13]

The cloaca is composed of an endodermal component contributed by the hindgut and an outer (caudal) ectodermal component that forms the proctodeum and the bursa. How these components combine in embryologic development determines the morphology and function of the cloaca. Autonomic innervation is as important to the motility of the cloaca as it is for the rest of the intestinal tract. The colonization of the developing gut by migrating neural crest cells is one of the fascinating developmental events that will likely have increasing clinical importance as its secrets are unraveled. The cloaca and the rectum are innervated by the enteric nervous system (ENS), which is derived from vagal and sacral neural crest cells. These cells migrate from the dorsal regions of the embryonic neural tube ventrally to the forming gut.[6,7] The vagal neural crest cells comprise the largest population of neurons within the rectal and cloacal ENS and migrate caudally from their entrance into the cranial portions of the gut tube, making an incredible journey through the mesenchyme of the gut wall all the way to the cloaca. Colonization is facilitated and guided by various signaling peptides, with the submucosal plexus developing first, followed by the myenteric ganglia.[14] A smaller contribution of neurons comes from the sacral neural crest, as these neurons enter the cloacal region after the first wave of vagal neural crest cells. Entering from the pelvic plexus, the sacral cells colonize cranially, up to the level of the umbilicus.

The rectum of birds demonstrates the concentric, layered organization of a submucosal and myenteric plexus common to the rest of the intestinal tract. The cloacal myenteric plexus has a different, less organized appearance in comparison.[6] The sacral neural crest cells supply the majority of neurons for the intestinal nerve of Remak (INR), a structure found only in birds, which supplies autonomic innervation via a chain of ganglia to the intrinsic portions of the ENS within the wall of the hindgut. The INR runs parallel to the hindgut within the mesentery and the mesorectum, from the distal jejunum caudally to the cloaca. The pelvic plexus, also formed from sacral neural crest cells, develops to supply innervation to the cloaca and the bursa and becomes continuous with the distal end of the INR.[9] Motor innervation to the cloaca is supplied by the pudendal nerve and by the connexus caudalis, which branches ventrally from the caudal coxal nerve.[15]

Physiologic research has shown that the function of the cloaca is intimately tied to the kidneys and the hindgut so that homeostasis of electrolytes and body water is maintained.[16,17] These essential relationships allow birds to use uric acid as their primary nitrogenous waste while conserving water and nutrients and reducing overall body weight in aid of flight.

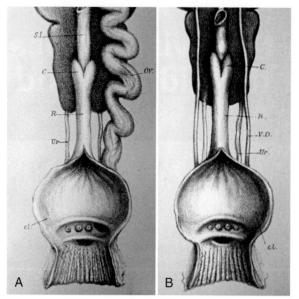

FIGURE 7-1 **A,** Penguin cloaca (female). **B,** Penguin cloaca (male). Photographs taken by the author of the original plates from drawings by the surgeon/anatomist Watson for the 1883 report of the scientific findings of the voyage of H.M.S. Challenger. The drawings are very detailed and accurate! (Photo courtesy W. Michael Taylor, DVM, 2014.)

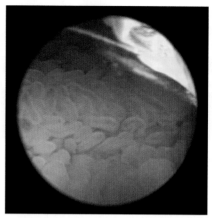

FIGURE 7-2 Papillae of the rectal mucosa in a great horned owl *(Bubo virginianus)*. (Photo courtesy W. Michael Taylor, DVM, 2014.)

Uricotelism also enables the oviparous method of reproduction by producing a virtually insoluble waste that can be safely stored in the allantois during development of the embryo. Uric acid has a very low solubility compared with urea, so it requires far less water for excretion and will not pass back through the chorioallantoic membranes of the egg.[17] The price paid for this insolubility is the large amount of protein required to provide a lubricating colloid and to bind the urates into a stable and safe format for excretion.[18,19]

Rectum

In Psittaciformes, the rectum enters the coprodeum from the left side at approximately an 80- to 90-degree angle, whereas in Columbiformes, the rectum attaches to the right side at a 60- to 90-degree angle.[20] In Strigiformes and Falconiformes, the rectum enters directly on or close to the cranial midline of the coprodeum. The rectal mucosa consists of tall, columnar epithelium with dense microvilli, interspersed with goblet cells.[21] Villi are a regular and prominent arrangement of the rectal epithelium of most birds such as the Great Horned Owl (Figure 7-2). It is difficult to view the rectal epithelium of the parrot or pigeon because of the sharp bend taken by the distal rectum as it enters the coprodeum.

A rectocoprodeal fold is present in the ostrich and is well developed.[2] A less dramatic rectocoprodeal sphincter is present at the junction of the rectum and the coprodeum in Strigiformes and Falconiformes (Figure 7-3). There is no rectocoprodeal fold or sphincter present in psittacines or pigeons.

Coprodeum

The coprodeum is the largest chamber of the psittacine cloaca. Its mucosa is a tall, columnar epithelium similar to that of the rectum, but it is vascular and free of villi in psittacines, Falconiformes, and some Columbiformes.[2,21] In the laughing dove *(Streptopelia senegalensis)*, the coprodeum has smaller villi than those of the rectum.[22]

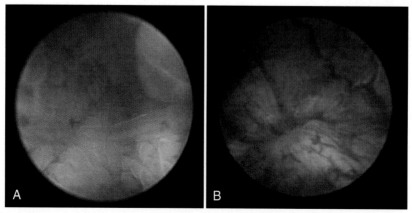

FIGURE 7-3 **A,** Rectocoprodeal sphincter of a great horned owl *(Bubo virginianus)*. **B,** Rectocoprodeal sphincter of an American kestrel *(Falco sparverius)*. (Photo courtesy W. Michael Taylor, DVM, 2014.)

The overall wall thickness is thinner and the epithelium is generally very smooth in most psittacines with a prominent, arborizing vascular pattern (Figure 7-4). The *coprourodeal fold* is a sphincterlike, 360-degree ridge that separates the coprodeum from the urodeum[22] (Figure 7-5). The coprodeum can be completely isolated from the urodeum and proctodeum by closure of this fold, which may become more developed just before oviposition in female birds.[2] This function is thought to help prevent soiling of the egg and the introduction of urofeces to the oviduct during egg laying.[2] The coprourodeal fold likely deflects or "cones" outwardly during the ejection of urofeces, preventing urofeces from touching the urodeum or the proctodeum.

Urodeum

The urodeum is the smallest chamber of the psittacine cloaca. It is demarcated cranially from the coprodeum by the coprourodeal fold and caudally from the proctodeum by the uroproctodeal fold (Figure 7-6). The mucosa of the urodeum is less vascular than the coprodeum and is covered by a similar columnar epithelium but with shorter microvilli.[21] Goblet cells and crypts are also present.

The ureters enter the urodeum via symmetric openings on either side of the dorsal midline. The ureteral orifice is a simple one in psittacines but is on a small papilla in Columbiformes and many Strigiformes (Figures 7-7 and 7-8, *A* and *B*).

In male birds, the left ductus deferens and the right ductus deferens enter the urodeum on symmetric, raised papillae located on the respective dorsolateral or ventrolateral walls of the urodeum.[2,20] The papillae are more prominent than the ureteral papillae (if present) and become further enlarged during periods of sexual activity (Figure 7-8, *C*). In many passerine birds, the distal ductus becomes very tortuous and enlarged for sperm storage and is called the *seminal glomus*.[2] This enlargement is noticeable externally as a

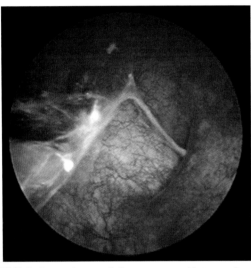

FIGURE 7-4 Coprodeum of *Amazona* sp. Note urofeces exiting the rectum, located on the left dorsolateral wall (patient in dorsal recumbency). (Photo courtesy W. Michael Taylor, DVM, 2014.)

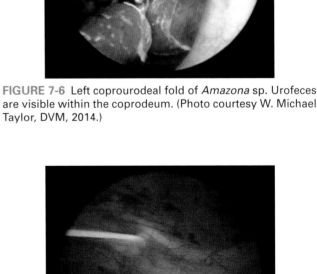

FIGURE 7-6 Left coprourodeal fold of *Amazona* sp. Urofeces are visible within the coprodeum. (Photo courtesy W. Michael Taylor, DVM, 2014.)

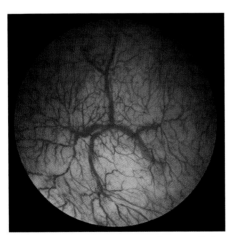

FIGURE 7-5 Coprodeal mucous membrane of *Amazona* sp. demonstrating the arborizing vascular pattern. (Photo courtesy W. Michael Taylor, DVM, 2014.)

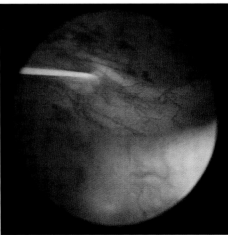

FIGURE 7-7 Dorsal wall of distended cloaca of *Amazona* sp. showing coprourodeal fold, left ureteral opening exuding urates and in the foreground, the uroproctodeal fold. (Photo courtesy W. Michael Taylor, DVM, 2014.)

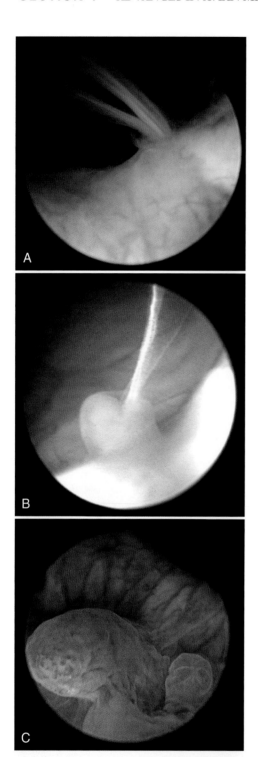

FIGURE 7-8 **A,** Left ureter of a green-winged macaw *(Ara chloroptera).* **B,** Left ureter of a great horned owl *(Bubo virginianus).* **C,** Papillae of the right ductus deferens and the right ureter of a rock pigeon *(Columba livia).* (Photo courtesy W. Michael Taylor, DVM, 2014.)

primarily dorsal enlargement of the cloaca, referred to as the *cloacal promontory* or *protuberance.*[23]

The oviductal opening has a prominent, rosettelike appearance in mature females that have oviposited and is located on the left dorsolateral wall near, or incorporated in, the uro-proctodeal fold.[21] As the oviduct of a female bird develops

in preparation for egg laying, the vaginal–urodeal junction broadens, encompassing most of the left lateral wall of the urodeum. The location for the oviductal opening is smaller and not patent in juveniles and therefore more difficult to visualize. Occasionally, a developed or retained right oviduct may be present but has been rarely encountered in the author's experience, although psittacines and chickens have been reported with this anomaly.[2,24-27]

The urodeum in some species contains tubular glands or crypts that may play a secondary role in sperm storage after coition with the male. These have been demonstrated in chickens and turkeys and are different in structure from the sperm storage tubules.[21,28] The distal oviduct (vagina) is lined by ciliated columnar epithelium, which changes to the columnar epithelium of the urodeum at their junction.[21] The utero-vaginal junction of the distal oviduct contains the sperm storage tubules that allow spermatozoa to reside so that fertilization can occur throughout the ovulatory cycle.

POSTRENAL MODIFICATION OF AVIAN URINE

Understanding avian fluid and electrolyte homeostasis requires re-evaluating many of the clinical truisms about renal function learned when evaluating the mammalian patient. Uric acid is a distinctly different chemical product from urea, and its handling by the avian kidney requires a different approach to excretion (Table 7-1). The avian kidney is only capable of concentrating urine to approximately 1.5 to 3 times the osmolality of plasma by the time it reaches the ureter.[17,19] This is in direct contrast to mammals, which can concentrate urine 10 to 20 times the plasma osmolality. As in other physiologic comparisons, birds can achieve a degree of water conservation similar to that by mammals but must use alternative methods to modify the urine *after* it has passed from the kidneys into the cloaca.

Retroperistalsis (antiperistalsis) of urates from the coprodeum takes place back into the rectum to the level of the cecae or to the anatomic region where cecae would be located if present.[29] Parrots lack a cecum, and in pigeons and Falconiformes, the location is marked by the paired cecal "tonsils" consisting primarily of lymphoid tissue (Figure 7-9). The author has documented waves of orad peristalsis to the cecal tonsil level in pigeons, geese, and swans, and to the equivalent level in psittacines. Strigiformes have well-developed cecae.

The movement of urine orad into the rectum is critical to the maintenance of water and solute balance in birds. It serves multiple purposes essential when uric acid is employed as the primary nitrogenous waste, as in birds.

TABLE 7-1	
Differences Between Uric Acid and Urea	
Uric Acid	**Urea**
Low solubility	Highly soluble
Can produce large and dangerous crystals	Noncrystalline under physiologic conditions
Must be stabilized using a protein matrix and delivered as a colloid	Stable in solution
Becomes very thick and pasty if concentrated	Remains liquid even when highly concentrated

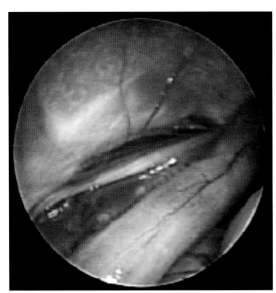

FIGURE 7-9 Rectal retroperistalsis in a rock pigeon *(Columba livia)*. In Columbiformes, the cecae are represented by elliptical swellings of lymphoid tissue, the cecal tonsils. (Photo courtesy W. Michael Taylor, DVM, 2014.)

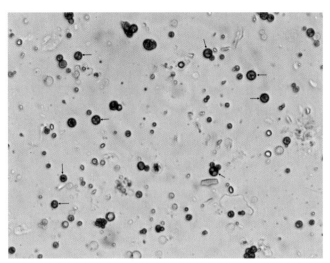

FIGURE 7-10 Fresh urates in saline solution, Grey parrot *(Psittacus erithacus)*. Uric acid spherules *(arrows)* vary in size but are all similarly round and refractile. (Photo courtesy W. Michael Taylor, DVM, 2014.)

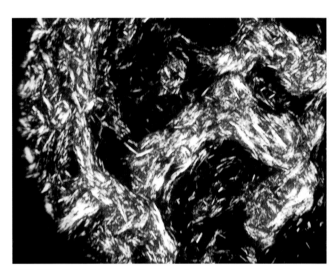

FIGURE 7-11 Monosodium urate crystals aspirated from periarticular deposition, viewed with polarized light. (Photo courtesy W. Michael Taylor, DVM, 2014.)

In most avian species studied, the ureters open into the urodeum, from where the typically hypo-osmolar urine rapidly moves orad into the coprodeum and from there into the rectum by small, coordinated, retroperistaltic smooth muscle waves of contraction.[17] If urine is sensed to have a higher osmotic potential compared with plasma after arrival in the coprodeum, it may not reflux into the rectum and, instead, may be excreted.

The rapid, small wave contractions do not impede fecal movement and yet propel urine back up the rectum, potentially as far as the cecae.[29] This thin layer of urine surrounds the fecal core and yet remains in close contact with the rectal mucosa. As water and solute are resorbed through the rectal wall, the urates become thicker and more closely applied to the outer surface of the tubular-shaped feces. It is clear that if the bird attempted to concentrate uric acid to this extent in the renal tubules, urine would cease to flow effectively. But the orad passage of urine into the rectum involves more than just water and solute conservation. The tubular secretion of urates and their subsequent passage along the collecting ducts to the ureters is dependent on the uric acid remaining stabilized in a colloidal suspension. The urates leave the ureter as small spherules ranging in size from 0.5 to 10 micrometers (μm). These spheres are composed of uric acid and protein bound in several concentric layers and linked by ionic potassium, sodium, or occasionally calcium.[30] The spherules are critical to the stabilization of the urates in an easily voided form and are readily detected in direct smears or saline wet mounts (Figure 7-10). Additional protein content in urine appears to be essential to prevent the spherules from aggregating and causing obstruction.[19] Uric acid circulates in plasma as monosodium urate, and if allowed to crystalize, it will assume a long, needlelike shape that irritates tissue and provokes inflammation (Figure 7-11).[31] These crystals are found deposited around joints (articular gout) or on serosal surfaces (visceral gout). In mammalian urine, anhydrous uric acid is known to form large platelike rectangular crystals that can accrete to form uroliths.[18,32] This perhaps happens to avian

urine when it is abnormally retained in the cloaca or rectum, leading to urolith formation.

Avian ureteral urine has a high protein content ranging from 20 to 50 grams per liter (g/L).[18] This large amount of protein, primarily albumin, is 80 to 100 times greater than amounts typically found in mammalian urine.[33] Mucopolysaccharides secreted by the distal tubules, collecting duct, and ureteral epithelium also form part of this protective and lubricating colloid, helping ensure safe urate transport with very little cost in water. The alternative cost lies in the large amount of protein required to complete this mission. The amount of energy in ureteral urine of white leghorn chickens over 24 hours was calculated to be 10% of the basal metabolic rate.[17] Retroperistalsis of urine into the rectum permits the recapture and digestion of much of this protein, preventing significant nutrient and energy losses. Another overlooked component of this postrenal modification of avian urine is the colonic and cecal breakdown of urate by uricolytic bacteria.[34]

Campbell and Braun demonstrated in Gambel's quail that 68% of the uric acid entering the lower gastrointestinal tract was degraded.[29] Much of the nitrogen can be reused by the bird in the form of other molecules such as glutamate or by the bacteria of the hindgut that produce fatty acids that the bird can absorb. Radiolabeled nitrogen in uric acid could be detected in glutamate molecules in the portal circulation of Gambel's quail.[29]

In summary, birds use uric acid, the least soluble of all protein breakdown products, as their primary nitrogenous waste to enable oviparity and avoid intoxication of the late-developing embryo. In so doing, birds engender savings in water demand but risk significant protein loss if the ureteral urine is not modified by time in the rectum, cecum, or both sites. In addition, bacteria in the hindgut of birds metabolize a large portion of the retrofluxed uric acid, thus providing useful compounds for absorption.

Proctodeum and Cloacal Bursa

The proctodeum is slightly larger than the urodeum in most species. It is separated from the urodeum by the uroproctodeal fold. The uroproctodeal fold is more prominent dorsally and gradually disappears ventrally (Figure 7-12). The epithelium of the proctodeum in chickens consists of tall, secretory cells with short microvilli; Dahm and Schramm reported finding variable numbers of mucus-secreting granules in the cells by using transmission electron microscopy.[21] The description of this secretory epithelium is at variance with other descriptions that suggest stratified squamous epithelium throughout the chamber.[2] As the columnar epithelium reaches the inner vent caudally, there is a change to stratified squamous epithelium that gradually becomes cornified squamous epithelium on the external vent lip. The proctodeum is the most frequent site of papilloma development in psittacines.[35]

The opening to the cloacal bursa (*bursa of Fabricius*) lies on the dorsal midline just caudal to the uroproctodeal fold. The bursa is the site of β-lymphocyte priming and production in the juvenile bird and is positioned over the dorsal wall of the cloaca (Figure 7-13). In the pigeon, the structure grows

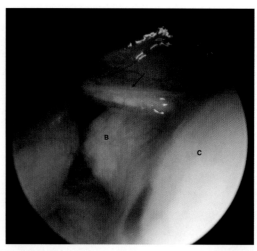

FIGURE 7-13 The cloacal bursa of a juvenile rock pigeon (*Columba livia*) as viewed from the left abdominal air sac. Arrow, Left ureter; B, bursa; C, coprodeum. (Photo courtesy W. Michael Taylor, DVM, 2014.)

slowly over the first 20 days after hatch but reaches its largest size (approximately 1.0 × 1.5 centimeters [cm]) by 60 days after hatching.[36] Internally, the structure has a pentagonal, honeycomb appearance, with lymphoid cells grouped in follicular arrays separated by epithelial septa. Antigens, drawn into the proctodeum, enter the bursa and are presented to the fundic openings of the follicles. Here, they can make direct contact with β-lymphocytes[36] (Figure 7-14).

Once matured and primed, the β-cells disperse via the bloodstream throughout the body, leading to the involution and disappearance of all lymphoid tissue in the bursa. The time of involution varies with the species but typically occurs between 2 and 6 months of age and certainly before sexual maturation.[2,36] Involution leaves behind the empty epithelial

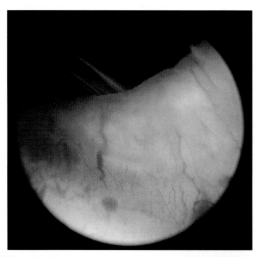

FIGURE 7-12 Uroproctodeal fold of a green-winged macaw (*Ara chloroptera*). Urates streaming from the left ureter are visible above the fold. (Photo courtesy W. Michael Taylor, DVM, 2014.)

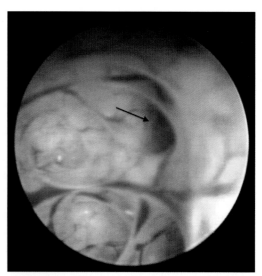

FIGURE 7-14 Interior view of the cloacal bursa of a juvenile rock pigeon (*Columba livia*) showing the reticulated appearance and ample vasculature as well as the opening to an individual follicle (*arrow*). (Photo courtesy W. Michael Taylor, DVM, 2014.)

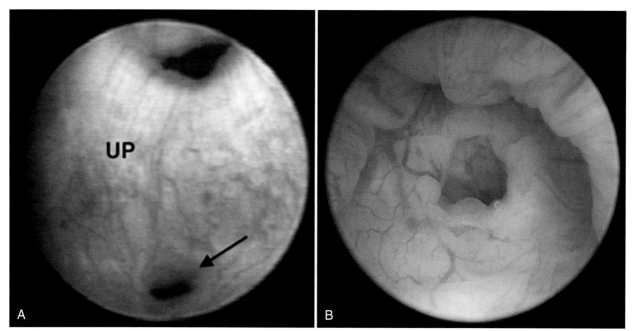

FIGURE 7-15 **A**, Remnant bursal opening of a mature American kestrel *Falco sparverius (arrow)*. **B**, Remnant bursal opening of a mature green winged macaw *Ara chloroptera*. UP, Uroproctodeal fold. (Photo courtesy W. Michael Taylor, DVM, 2014.)

"sac" of the structure, and the author's group has noted that the ostium of the bursa and its chamber frequently persist as reasonably sized chambers that can be located endoscopically (Figure 7-15). In birds with idiopathic cloacal prolapse, the structure can become dilated.[20]

Vent

The horizontal external opening of the cloaca is called the vent and is not completely analogous to the anus of mammals. The vent consists of dorsal and ventral lips with right and left commissures. Squamous epithelium extends onto the inner surface of the lip. The vent is supplied with a number of skeletal muscles and a rich nerve supply.[2,15] During the process of excretion in the parrot, the vent lips are first drawn dorsally and ventrally to open the pathway. Urofeces are then launched from the coprodeal chamber as the most cranial portion of the coprodeal wall is displaced caudally through the opened coprourodeal sphincter and the parted vent lips. In parrots (and most other species), this is performed cleanly and rapidly such that no waste material contacts the urodeum, the proctodeum, or the epithelium and the surrounding feathers of the vent or ventral tail. Figure 7-16 shows a complete, freshly excreted urofecal mass from an Amazon parrot in normal fluid and electrolyte balance. Note how the urates are arranged over the surface of the tubular feces, which are arranged in the shape of the coprodeum. Pigeons excrete feces similar to those of the parrot. The process of urofecal excretion does vary among species. Some Falconiformes evacuate a jet of urofeces.

It is well known that young chicks can make cloacal "sucking" or "drinking" movements that produce negative pressure and can draw fluids and small particulates into the proctodeum.[37,38] This is the mechanism the chick uses to expose the

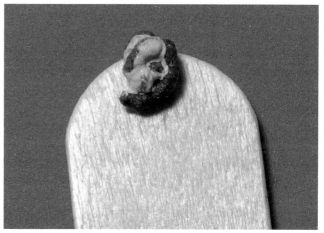

FIGURE 7-16 Normal urofeces of *Amazona* sp. (Photo courtesy W. Michael Taylor, DVM, 2014.)

β-lymphocytes of the cloacal bursa to environmental antigens. Labeled material has been shown to have been drawn into the proctodeum and deposited into the dorsally located bursa of chicks.[38] A similar cloacal technique has been documented in seasonally receptive breeding females of some species such as Strigiformes (Katherine Mckeever, 1984, personal communication) The female's ability to draw material into the cloaca may have significance for the breeding success of birds such as Psittacines and Columbiformes in which the male lacks an intromittent organ (phallus). The male places his vent against the females, allowing the negative pressure of her cloacal movements to draw spermatozoa into the urodeum and the oviduct.

Innervation and Vascular Supply

The afferent blood supply is from the pudendal artery. The cloaca is drained by the pudendal vein. The pudendal nerves follow the respective ureters to the left and right dorsolateral walls of the cloaca, supplying motor neuron function to the cloaca. They are also supplemented by the connexus caudalis of the caudal coxal nerve.[15] The ganglia of the cloacal plexus are located in the dorsal wall of cloaca.[2]

DIAGNOSTIC TECHNIQUES

Physical Examination

Examination should begin by visualizing the urofeces of the patient. Only in the ostrich are urine and feces expelled separately, so the appearance and consistency of the combined *urofecal* components can offer valuable insight into cloacal and hindgut health.[39] The author recommends starting from an understanding of the normal urofecal appearance for the species that are being examined. Frank blood may be present in small clots in urofeces or in larger volumes, perhaps diluted with the fluid portion of urine. The fecal component in many species should have a well-formed, cylindrical shape. The urates, under conditions of normal hydration, will be arranged around the surface of these fecal cylinders (see Figure 7-16). In conditions of water excess or other causes of polyuria, the urates will be less concentrated and form a pool around the feces.

The external morphology of the vent, the caudal abdomen, and the ventral tail region should always be examined and palpated during an avian physical examination. The lips of the vent and the ventral tail should not be soiled in the normal bird (Figure 7-17). Even with the aid of general anesthesia, only the vent lips and the proctodeum can be routinely visualized. It is important to look for inflammation, masses, or debris beyond the normal urofecal content. Modified nasal speculae have been used by many biologists and clinicians to enhance cloacal examinations.[40] Speculae are useful but require the aid of magnification and must be employed with care because iatrogenic trauma is possible, especially in manually restrained birds.

Radiography

Conventional radiography can provide some additional information about cloacal disease. Increased radiodensity because of the presence of uroliths, coprodeal dilation with air, filling defects, and abnormal vent lip morphology are all visible using standard techniques and high detail film or screen combinations (Figure 7-18). Barium or iohexol contrast, especially if combined with fluoroscopy, is an excellent way to detect lesions and observe rectal and coprodeal morphology and motility[17,41] (Figure 7-19).

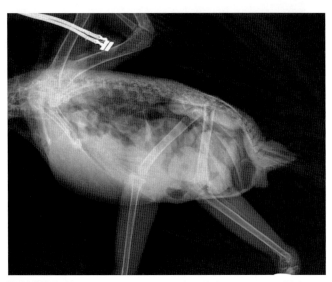

FIGURE 7-18 Lateral radiograph of an Eclectus parrot *(Eclectus roratus)* showing coprodeum filled with air. (Photo courtesy W. Michael Taylor, DVM, 2014.)

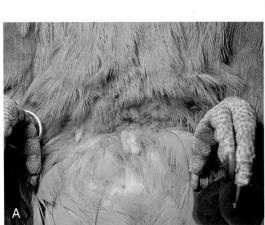
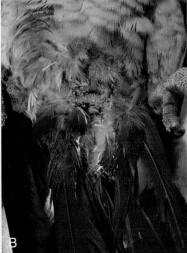

FIGURE 7-17 **A,** Normal pericloacal featheration and vent appearance in a yellow-crowned parrot *(Amazona ochrocephala).* **B,** Abnormal pericloacal and ventral tail appearance of a Grey parrot *(Psittacus erithacus)* with idiopathic cloacal prolapse. (Photo courtesy W. Michael Taylor, DVM, 2014.)

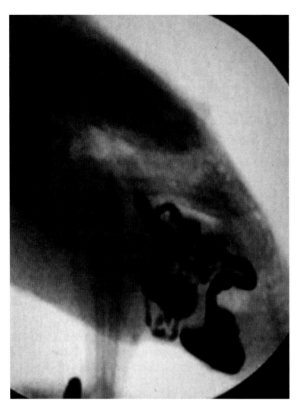

FIGURE 7-19 Fluoroscopic still image of a chestnut fronted macaw *(Ara severa)* demonstrating barium-labeled ingest in coprodeum. (Photo courtesy W. Michael Taylor, DVM, 2014.)

Magnetic resonance imaging (MRI) has the potential to define the cloaca and the caudal abdomen in some detail but remains a costly procedure. Smaller, laboratory animal magnets show promise for enhanced detail in smaller avian patients. More recently, a positron emission tomography (PET)

study using 18F-fluoro-D-glucose demonstrated cloacal reflux into the rectum of Hispaniolan parrots.[42]

Endoscopy

The use of saline infusion cloacoscopy using a high-quality rod lens endoscope with an instrumented sheath system has been described[43] (Storz Avian Diagnostic System, 2.7 mm, 30-degree telescope; and Taylor Sheath, Karl Storz Veterinary Endoscopy, www.ksvea.com). This is the only method currently available to examine the entire cloaca internally. The diagnostic sheath enables proper control of infusion of the cloaca and biopsy, and grasping and incising instruments are available for use with the system.

A constant rate infusion of warmed, sterile saline (0.9%) is administered through a pediatric microdrip administration set attached to the infusion port of the sheath (Figure 7-20). The fluids should be administered from a level approximately three to four feet above the patient. Fine control of the rate of infusion can be achieved by using the stopcock on the infusion port of the sheath. Absorbent towels or a mat are used to catch draining fluid. The tip of the sheath is gently inserted through the vent lips, with the saline infusion started and the supporting (non-dominant) hand used to close the vent lips around the telescopes sheath, as required. Initially, the clinician will likely want to "flush" any urofeces present from the coprodeum so that a clearer view of the mucosa is visible. Once the coprodeum is cleared, the examination can begin and should include the rectal entrance and the complete coprodeal mucosa. It is not possible to gain entrance to the rectum of Psittaciformes because of the acute angle present at the rectocoprodeal junction. It is occasionally possible to enter the rectum of large Columbiformes. In medium and large Strigiformes, the rectum can be examined and structures to the level of the cecae can be located (Figure 7-21).

Once examination of the coprodeum and rectum are completed, the sheath system is very slowly withdrawn over the

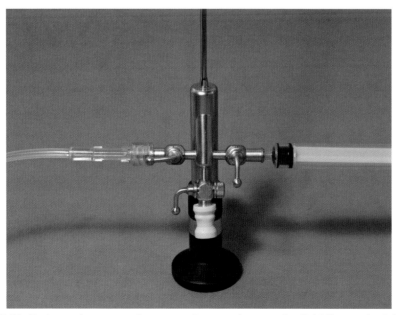

FIGURE 7-20 Endoscopic system demonstrating attachment of a fluid line to the left infusion port for installation of warmed saline. A syringe is attached to the right port for suction, if necessary. Note that the left port is in the open position, the right port is closed. (Photo courtesy W. Michael Taylor, DVM, 2014.)

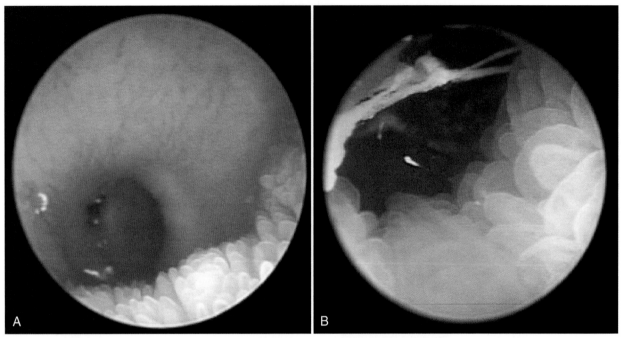

FIGURE 7-21 **A,** View of the ileocecal junction of a great horned owl *(Bubo virginianus).* In medium and large species, especially in those with straight egress of the rectum into the coprodeum, it is possible to insert the endoscopic system in a retrograde fashion to the level of the cecum. **B,** Urates in mucoid matrix remaining along the rectal wall after flushing of urofeces during examination of the rectum in a great horned owl *(Bubo virginianus).* (Photo courtesy W. Michael Taylor, DVM, 2014.)

coprourodeal fold and into the urodeum. The ureteral openings are located by scanning along the dorsal surface of the urodeum to the left and right of the midline. The papillae of the left and right ductus deferens in male birds are larger than the ureteral openings and located along the respective dorsolateral walls of the urodeum. The left oviductal opening varies in size, depending on the age and reproductive history of the hen. After examination of the urodeum is completed, the sheath system is again slowly withdrawn over the uroproctodeal fold and into the proctodeum. These movements are quite small but can be fully visualized by using a combination of an endoscopic camera and a monitor with saline infusion to maintain mild distention of the cloacal compartments.

Excessive infusion volume is to be avoided because of retrograde flow into the cranial gastrointestinal tract (and into the crop and out the mouth if care is not taken!). Lumeij[44] described a technique and rationale for cloacal infusion of rehydrating fluids in the pigeon, but volume overload could easily occur in anesthetized patients.

Insufflation of air is not as effective in revealing cloacal mucosal features as saline because it flattens the mucosal epithelium and can cause tissue vibration, markedly reducing detail (Figure 7-22). Delicate, precise control of the instruments is essential to avoid trauma to the cloaca. Care and practice in movement are critical because of the small working space, but the detail and diagnostic information achieved makes the learning curve well worth it. This is the *only method* currently available to image the fine detail of ureters, the ductus deferens, the oviductal opening, or the bursa.[43,45] Saline infusion cloacoscopy also enables close inspection and high magnification of the cloacal mucosa

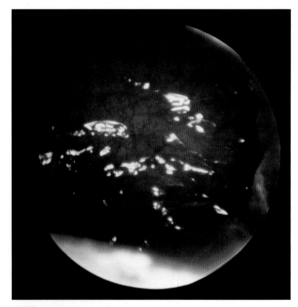

FIGURE 7-22 View of the coprodeum using air insufflation. (Photo courtesy W. Michael Taylor, DVM, 2014.)

without the structural flattening (or risk of emboli) that occurs using air insufflation (Figure 7-23).

Microbiology

Directly collected fresh cultures are often useful, but they may be difficult to interpret. A blindly collected sample from the cloaca will yield a portal culture that could represent bacteria

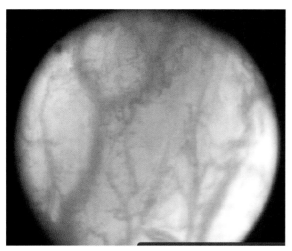

FIGURE 7-23 Demonstration of the magnification and resolution possible using a high-quality 2.7-mm rod lens endoscope. Blood cells can be seen flowing through the capillaries
of the proctodeal mucosa.

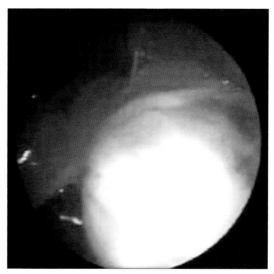

FIGURE 7-24 A diagnostic swab inserted into the cloaca of
a Moluccan cockatoo *(Cacatua moluccensis)* is viewed via
an endoscope placed into the left abdominal air sac. (Photo
courtesy W. Michael Taylor, DVM, 2014.)

excreted from the rectum, the ureters, the ductus deferens, or
even the oviduct. The yield from a cloacally inserted swab is
often small because of vent muscle tone and the timing of
cloacal filling with urofeces. Freshly voided urofeces may be
preferred if collectable from an appropriate surface. The identification of urine components is often easier in these samples.
To aid in the process, a sheet of waxed paper or plastic wrap
may be placed on the cage bottom before or as the patient
enters the examination room.

Cytology

Blindly collected samples represent only urofecal cytology
and must not be overinterpreted. These types of samples
are useful to obtain a feel for general fecal bacterial content
and morphology. Targeted sampling with visualization via
endoscopy is likely to be more valuable if cloacitis is suspected. The clinician is advised to remember that the coprodeal wall is quite thin in most species, and although it is
surprisingly flexible and resilient, perforation is possible
(Figure 7-24).

Biopsy

Biopsy of abnormal cloacal tissue is often the only method to
achieve a definitive diagnosis and is best achieved with endoscopic guidance.[43,45,46] Excessive depth in specimen collection,
especially near the coprourodeal sphincter, should be avoided
because this may cause iatrogenic fibrosis and scarring, which
can impede evacuation of the coprodeum. Cup biopsy size
should be selected relative to the size of the patient and the
nature of the lesion; 3-French (Fr), 5-Fr, and 7-Fr forceps
(equivalent to 1.0, 1.7, and 2.3 millimeters [mm], respectively)
in round or elliptical cup shapes allow for targeting of specific
lesions.[46] Aggressive, deep biopsies may lead to perforation of
the cloacal wall.

SURGICAL APPROACHES

A ventral midline incision is the only direct approach to the
cloaca. The incision may need to be extended between the

pubic bones to the level of the vent if the ventral cloaca is to
be entered (see Chapter 21). Once the intestinal peritoneal
cavity is entered, the distal portion of the left or right abdominal air sac may need to be retracted cranially and laterally. If the distal rectum and the rectocoprodeal junction are
to be examined externally, the midline incision need not
extend as far caudally; however, it will need to be extended
along the left pubis (in psittacines) or the right pubis (in
pigeons) for the best exposure.

Entry into the cloaca is best achieved via the ventral surface by using a midline incision to avoid the ureters and ductus deferens. The muscles of the vent must be transected to
approach the urodeum and the proctodeum and will need to
be closed with mattress sutures.[47] Gentle tissue handling and
use of magnification is essential to accurately assess, resect,
and reduce fibrosis and the risk of adhesions.

DISEASES AND PATHOPHYSIOLOGY

Neoplasia: Papillomatous Disease

Papillomatous disease is the most common cause of neoplasia
in the cloaca of New World psittacines. A herpesviral etiology
has been confirmed[48] (see Chapter 2). The papilliform hyperplasia of the epithelium is most commonly located in the proctodeum. Moderate to severe hyperplasia may lead to partial
obstruction of the proctodeum with mucosal proliferation that
extrudes through the vent lips (Figure 7-25). This usually leads
to irregular (and often noisy) ejection of urofeces with soiling
of the vent lips and the surrounding ventral tail feathers. The
affected tissue may bleed especially if exposed through the vent,
leading to drops of frank blood in urofeces. It has been the
author's experience that obstipation is surprisingly rare in uncomplicated papillomatous disease of the cloaca.[35] Concomitant epithelial lesions of the biliary and pancreatic ductular
systems are likely and are the cause of mortality in affected
birds followed long-term.[35] Although a wide range of New

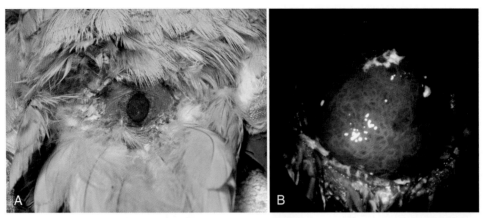

FIGURE 7-25 **A,** Papillomatous mucosa protruding from the vent of a yellow-headed Amazon parrot *(Amazona oratrix)*. **B,** Magnified view of similar mucosa showing papillomatous proliferation. (Photo courtesy W. Michael Taylor, DVM, 2014.)

World species is susceptible to this disease, *Amazona* sp. are particularly susceptible, with a high rate of mortality from biliary duct (and pancreatic duct) carcinoma.[49] Similar lesions caused by a herpesvirus have been confirmed in an Old World species, the Grey parrot *(Psittacus erithacus)*.[48] Garner makes a point of separating two possible phenotypes of cloacal papillomatosis, one involving epithelial proliferation and the second involving primarily mucous cells. The latter adenomatous polyps are more likely to become locally malignant in the form of adenocarcinomas.[49]

Apart from the changes seen in papillomatous disease, neoplasia of the avian cloaca is relatively rare. Adenocarcinomas, fibrosarcomas, and squamous cell carcinomas have been recorded.[49,50] The clinical effects caused by these changes in cell growth are variable, depending on location. Space occupation may lead to straining, obstipation, or painful defecation accompanied by abnormal vocalization. Tumor growth near the entrance of one (or both) of the ureters may cause obstructive hyperuricemia (Figure 7-26).

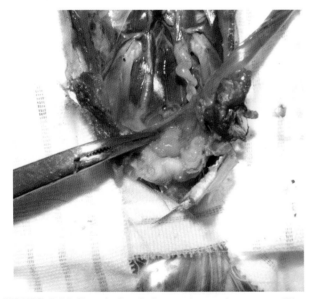

FIGURE 7-26 Neoplasia of cloaca obstructing ureter. (Photo courtesy Brian Speer.)

Prolapse

Idiopathic *coprodeal* prolapse in cockatoos *(Cacatua* sp.) and less commonly other psittacines (e.g., Grey parrots *[Psittacus erithacus]* and blue-and-yellow macaws *[Ara ararauna]*) is the most common form of prolapse in pet birds. The cause for this gradually progressive condition is still unconfirmed and is still being debated. In the population of birds in the study by the author's group, all affected individuals were single, intact pets, predominantly males, with similar behavioral profiles.[51] Each was very attached to a human member of its household, usually the person who had hand-reared it. Careful history collection revealed that these birds were usually raised without conspecifics and had a prolonged period of weaning or, indeed, were still being fed some warmed food material by their owners. The author's group noted that these birds usually began to exhibit this problem at around the time of sexual maturation, typically between 5 and 8 years in cockatoos, but did not show development of normal sexual behavior. Mild to moderate pushing and straining of the coprodeum progressed to partial prolapse and gradual reduction in vent sphincter tone with an increase in vent width.[51] Eventually, the coprodeum prolapses for longer periods (Figure 7-27). Owners often note urine dripping from the vent lips in these birds. Left untreated, the birds' condition progressively worsens and they become prone to opportunistic infections of the hindgut and die prematurely[51] (Taylor, unpublished).

Current surgical descriptions of therapy for this problem involve extensive suturing of the ventral coprodeal wall to the body wall often with attachment to the caudal ribs, in some form of cloacopexy (see Chapter 21). These patients often continue to strain even after cloacopexy. Work is now ongoing to examine the interrelationships of integrating behavioral interventional strategies (see Chapter 5), various hormones (see Chapter 12), chemical and surgical neutering (see Chapter 21), and ventplasty (see Chapter 21) as potential options for formulating more appropriate therapy for this problem in affected individuals. The author's group has noted the lack of normal behavioral development in these patients and offers the hypothesis of an abnormality in progressive maturation as has been recorded in primates. Prevention of the problem by rearing these intelligent, social birds with conspecifics and following normal fledging procedures is perhaps the most effective strategy (see Chapter 5).

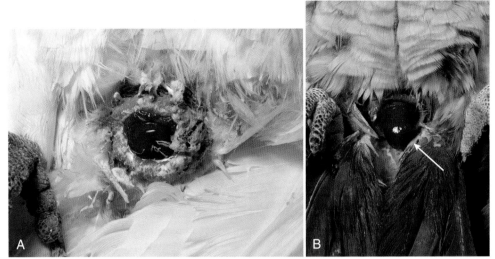

FIGURE 7-27 **A,** Idiopathic cloacal prolapse in an umbrella cockatoo *(Cacatua alba)*. Urofeces are visible exiting the rectocoprodeal junction. **B,** Idiopathic prolapse of the coprodeum in a Grey parrot *(Psittacus erithacus)*. Note the rectocoprodeal junction *(arrow)*. (Photo courtesy W. Michael Taylor, DVM, 2014.)

Oviductal prolapses may occur in egg-laying hens. These prolapses should be surgically investigated and replaced. Sometimes, salpingohysterectomy is required if there is severe exposure with or without avascular necrosis or trauma to the prolapsed oviduct.

Rectal prolapses are the least common form of prolapse from the cloaca but the most serious. Intussusception of the rectum through the coprodeum with prolapse from the vent lips is a surgical emergency. Endoscopy can be used to rapidly differentiate rectal prolapse from oviductal prolapse by identifying whether the tissue originates from the coprodeum or the urodeum. Surgical exploration, reduction, and possible resection are indicated. Resection of the rectum in most birds requires microsurgical techniques (8-0 to 10-0 suture, appropriate magnification) and is a challenging surgical procedure.[52]

Cloacitis

Bacterial cloacitis

Bacterial cloacitis is relatively uncommon but can create significant pathology. Bacteria may adhere abnormally to the coprodeal epithelium as a result of nutritional deficiencies, in the presence of the epithelial changes caused by papillomatous disease, or after trauma, as might occur during egg laying. Venereal transmission of pathogenic bacteria via natural and iatrogenic means (e.g., *Pasteurella multocida*, *Salmonella* sp., *Escherichia coli*, and *Staphylococcus*) has been reported.[53-55]

Fungal cloacitis

Fungal infections are primarily limited to pathogenic yeasts. A variety of *Candida* sp. has been isolated from the vent lips and proctodeum of birds but *C. albicans* remains the most common and clinically significant isolate at this site.[56,57] *C. parapsilosis*, *C. tropicalis*, and *C. glabrata* can occur less commonly. Immunosuppression and diets high in simple sugars have been proposed as reasons for the development of localized yeast infections. The opportunistic yeast *Trichosporon beigelii* has also been reported to cause similar lesions in an immunocompromised, hyperglycemic macaw.[58]

Parasitic cloacitis

Cloacotaenia megalops is a fairly common cestode with a worldwide occurrence in waterfowl and some marsh dwelling species. This tapeworm lives primarily within the coprodeum.[59,60] The intermediate host is typically an ostracod.

Brachylaimid trematodes (e.g., *Tinamutrema canoae* of tinamous) are frequently found in the cloaca and bursa of species that consume the snail, which is an intermediate host.[61]

Urogonimus macrostomus is another digenic trematode that inhabits the cloaca of temperate passerine birds.[62,63]

The first report in a nondomestic avian species of cryptosporidiosis was by Doster et al in two red-lored Amazons *(Amazona autumnalis)*.[64] *Cryptosporidium baileyi*, a small apicomplexan parasite of birds, often replicates in the cloaca and the bursa.[65] Other avian *Cryptosporidium* spp. that have been identified are more likely to be located in the intestine or respiratory tract.

Knemidocoptes pilae is most commonly seen as an infestation of the skin of the cere and feet but often causes similar crusty, perforated lesions in the epidermis surrounding the vent.[66]

Cloacoliths

Cloacoliths (coprodeoliths) are primarily composed of uric acid based upon composition analysis[67] (Taylor, unpublished). Although some feces can be present in the matrix, the primary component is a concretion of urates. Uroliths are relatively uncommon and poorly described, but recent reports and the experience of the author's group suggest a strong relationship to decreased or impaired coprodeal emptying, most often related to iatrogenic causes (Figure 7-28). Surgery of the cloaca for papilloma removal is the most commonly associated cause. Although the pathogenesis remains unclear, the author's group has noted that any impairment to coprodeal emptying, such as fibrosis in the region of the coprourodeal sphincter, leads to prolonged retention of urates within the coprodeum. Increased retention time is proposed to lead to digestion of the mucopolysaccharide and protein matrix of the excreted uric acid spherules by fecal bacteria and endogenous digestive enzymes.

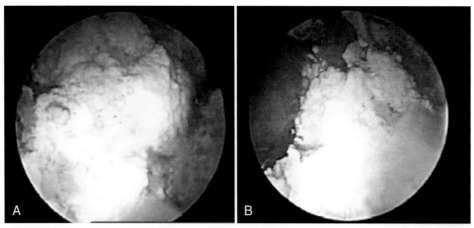

FIGURE 7-28 **A,** Coprodeolith from a blue-fronted Amazon parrot *(Amazona aestiva)*. The patient had developed a stricture at the coprourodeal fold after surgery for papilloma removal. **B,** Saline infusion cloacoscopy to examine a coprodeolith. (Photo courtesy W. Michael Taylor, DVM, 2014.)

This allows for chemical alteration of the urate composition, which facilitates uric acid crystallization and aggregation. Urates in mammalian urine form a platelike, rectangular crystal shape that can accrete to form kidney and bladder stones.[32]

Trauma

Injuries to the cloaca are surprisingly rare, considering how thin walled the structures are. Iatrogenic damage is a real possibility during blind insertion of swabs or instrumentation or during surgical approaches to the cloacal lining. Injury to the submucosa or muscularis can lead to fibrosis with stricture formation. Strictures frequently lead to problems with defecation and are the main cause of psittacine urolith formation. When performing surgery on the cloaca, the clinician should attempt to avoid stricture formation by ensuring careful and precise tissue handling that is aided by magnification.

Cloacopexy of the dilated coprodeum has been associated with colonic (rectal) entrapment, adhesion formation, and obstruction in cockatoos.[68] The colon of psittacines enters the coprodeum normally from the left side in a dorsolateral position. When the coprodeum is grossly dilated and atonic, as seen with idiopathic prolapse of the cloaca, the author has noted that the rectum is positioned more ventrally and that it is also possible to pull or deform the cloaca when performing a cloacopexy to the ventral abdominal wall, thus facilitating entrapment of the rectum (see Figure 7-28). For this reason, the author does not recommend cloacopexy until an attempt has been made to reduce the dilation and to improve coprodeal tone by using other measures. Careful attention to the anatomy is important.

The cloaca may also become traumatized during attempts to relieve dystocia. Assisted delivery of an egg can be performed with little to no trauma by using proper technique and general anesthesia with relevant pharmacologic assists such as calcium gluconate, prostaglandin E, and oxytocin (Figure 7-29). A vaginal approach to access the egg is less likely to cause iatrogenic problems, compared with a percutaneous approach, unless surgical removal is truly indicated. The author's group has had success relieving dystocia by drilling into the egg with a sterile 18-16-g needle via the cervix and aspirating the liquid content. The egg can then be carefully collapsed by breaking the shell, starting from the point of puncture. Careful technique and

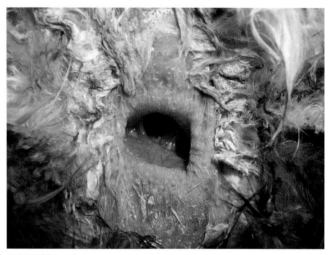

FIGURE 7-29 Cloaca of hen Harris' hawk *(Parabuteo unicinctus)* immediately after assisted delivery of an egg. The dilated oviductal–urodeal junction ("cervix") is visible to the right of image; the bird is in dorsal recumbency. (Photo courtesy W. Michael Taylor, DVM, 2014.)

sterile saline lubrication will prevent trauma to the oviduct. The author has had many hens return to full reproductive function after this type of delivery. Obviously, any nutritional and management issues must also be addressed after the procedure.

Unless an intact avian egg is pathologically thin shelled, any attempt to collapse it requires more force than recommended and may cause ureteral or oviductal tissue trauma. Iatrogenic rectal obstruction with rectal tearing occurred after relief of dystocia with the use of percutaneous collapse of the egg and removal of shell fragments in an Eclectus parrot. Repair of rectal and intestinal perforations requires magnification and very fine suture materials (e.g., 6-0 to 10-0). In the case described above, a serosal patch was also used to prevent leakage.[52]

Purse-string sutures are contraindicated in avian patients. If the vent is encircled with a suture, the normal dorsal and ventral movements of the lips during defecation are impeded, and the bird is more likely to become obstipated. The use of nonabsorbable *transverse sutures*, placed across the vent lips

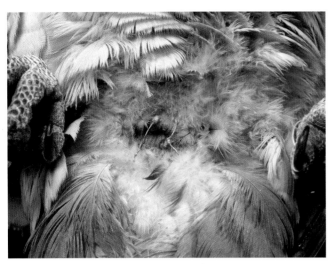

FIGURE 7-30 Transverse 2-0 monofilament, stainless steel sutures placed 30 days previously in this Grey parrot *(Psittacus erithacus)*. (Photo courtesy W. Michael Taylor, DVM, 2014.)

at intervals (usually two to three, depending on the size of the patient and the degree of vent dilation), are recommended as a better functional choice to prevent cloacal eversion[20] (Figure 7-30). The author prefers 2-0 monofilament surgical stainless steel sutures made with a swaged needle because of reduced tissue reactivity at this site. Occasionally, horizontal mattress sutures are required in patients that are aggressively straining. The suture must be applied with enough laxity to allow excretion without tissue prolapse. Potential complications that can occur from the use of transverse vent sutures include mechanical tearing and damage to the sphincter or vent lips through continued straining.

REFERENCES

1. Watson M: Report on the anatomy of the Spheniscidae collected during the voyage of H.M.S. Challenger. Report on the Scientific Results of the Voyage of the H.M.S. Challenger, *Zoology* Vol.7, 1883.
2. King AS: Cloaca. In King AS, McLelland J, editors: *Form and function in birds*, Vol 2, London and New York, 1981, Academic Press, pp 63–105.
3. Orosz S: Anatomy of the urogenital system. In Altman RB, Clubb SL, Dorrestein GM, et al, editors: *Avian medicine and surgery*, Philadelphia, PA, 1997, Saunders.
4. Ritchie BW, Harrison GJ, Harrison LR, editors: *Avian medicine: principles and application* [Figure 19], Lake Worth, FL, 1994, Wingers Publishing, pp 509.
5. Oliveira CA, Silva RM, Santos MM, et al: Location of the ureteral openings in the cloacas of tinamous, some ratite birds, and crocodilians: a primitive character, *J Morphol* 260:234–246, 2004.
6. Aisa J, Lahoz M, Serranno PJ, et al: Intrinsic innervation of the chicken lower digestive tract, *Neurochem Res* 22(12):1425–1435, 1997.
7. Doyle AM, Roberts DJ, Golstein AM: Enteric nervous system patterning in the avian hindgut, *Dev Dynam* 229:708–712, 2004.
8. Valasek P, Evans JRE, Maina F, et al: A dual fate of the hindlimb muscle mass: cloacal/perineal musculature develops from leg muscle cells, *Development* 132(3):447–458, 2005.
9. Nagy N, Brewer KC, Mwizerwa O, et al: Pelvic plexus contributes ganglion cells to the hindgut enteric nervous system, *Dev Dynam* 236:73–83, 2007.
10. Kluth D, Fiegel HC, Metzger R: Embryology of the hindgut, *Sem Ped Surg* 20(3):152–160, 2011.
11. Goldstein AM, Nagy N: A bird's eye view of enteric nervous system development: lessons from the avian embryo, *Pediatr Res* 64(4): 325–333, 2008.
12. O'Donnell AM, Puri P: Cholinergic innervation in the developing chick cloaca and colorectum, *J Ped Surg* 44:392–394, 2009.
13. Sasselli V, Pachnis V, Burns AJ: The enteric nervous system, *Dev Biol* 366:64–73, 2012.
14. Roberts DJ: Molecular mechanisms of development of the gastrointestinal tract, *Dev Dynam* 219:109–120, 2000.
15. Ohmori Y, Watanabe T: Location of motoneurons innervating the musculus sphincter cloacae in the domestic fowl, *Neurosci Lett* 101:1–5, 1989.
16. Skadhauge E: Cloacal absorption of urine in birds, *Comp Biochem Physiol* 55A:93–98, 1976.
17. Braun EJ: Integration of renal and gastrointestinal function, *J Exp Zool* 283:495–499, 1999.
18. Janes DN, Braun EJ: Urinary protein excretion in red jungle fowl (Gallus gallus), *Comp Biochem Physiol A* 118(5):1273–1275, 1997.
19. Braun EJ: Regulation of renal and lower gastrointestinal function: role in fluid and electrolyte balance, *Comp Biochem Physiol A* 136: 499–505, 2003.
20. Taylor WM, Murray MJ: The psittacine cloaca: a clinical review, *Proc Assoc Avian Vet* 410:265–269, 2002.
21. Dahm HH, Shcramm U, Lange W: Scanning and transmission electron microscopic observations of the cloacal epithelia of the domestic fowl, *Cell Tiss Res* 211:83–93, 1980.
22. Johnson OS, Skadhauge E: Structural-functional correlations in the kidneys and observations of colon and cloacal morphology in certain Australian birds, *J Anat* 120:495–505, 1974.
23. Schut E, Magrath MJL, van Oers K, et al: Volume of the cloacal protuberance as an indication of reproductive state in male blue tits (Cyanistes caeruleus), *Ardea* 100(2):202–205, 2012.
24. Nemetz L: Clinical pathology of a persistent right oviduct in psittacine birds, *Proc Assoc Avian Vet* 315:73–77, 2010.
25. Schmidt RE, Reavill DR, Phalen DN: Reproductive system. In *Pathology of pet and aviary birds*, Ames, IA, 2003, Blackwell Publishing Professional.
26. Hochleithner M, Lechner C: Egg binding in a budgerigar (Melopsittacus undulatus) caused by a cyst of the right oviduct, *AAV Today* 2(3):136–138, 1988.
27. Reece RL, Scott PC, Barr DA: Some unusual diseases in the birds of Victoria, Australia, *Vet Rec* 130:178–185, 1992.
28. Bakst MR, Akuffo V: Turkey sperm reside in the tubular glands in the urodeum following artificial insemination, *Poultry Sci* 87: 790–792, 2008.
29. Campbell CE, Braun EJ: Cecal degradation of uric acid in Gambel quail, *Am J Physiol* 251(RICP 20):R59–R62, 1986.
30. Cassoti G, Braun EJ: Ionic composition of urate-containing spheres in the urine of domestic fowl, *Comp Biochem Physiol A* 118(3): 585–588, 1997.
31. Martiullo MA, Nazal L, Critenden DB: The crystallization of monosodium urea, *Curr Rheumatol Rep* 16(400):1–8, 2014.
32. Presores JB, Swift JA: Adhesion properties of uric acid crystal surfaces, *Langmuir* 28:7401–7406, 2012.
33. Boykin SLB, Braun EJ: A role for serum albumin in the excretion of uric acid, *FASEB J* 10:A289, 1996.
34. Barnes EM, Impey CS: The occurrence and properties of uric acid decomposing anaerobic bacteria in the avian cecum, *J Appl Bact* 37:393–409, 1974.
35. Taylor M, Whiteside D, Smith DA: Long term effects of internal papillomatosis in *Amazona sp.*, *Proc of Euro Assoc Avian Vet* 122–123, 2001.
36. Abbate F, Pfarrer C, Jones CJP, et al: Age-dependent changes in the pigeon bursa of Fabricius vasculature: a comparative study using light microscopy and scanning electron microscopy of vessel casts, *J Anat* 211:387–398, 2007.

37. Sorvari R, Naukkarinen A, Sorvari TE: Anal sucking-like movements in the chicken and chick embryo followed by the transportation of environmental material to the bursa of Fabricius, caeca and caecal tonsils, *Poultry Sci* 56:1426–1429, 1977.

38. van der Sluis HJ, Dwars RM, Vernooij JCM, et al: Cloacal reflexes and uptake of fluorescein-labeled polystyrene beads in broiler chickens, *Poultry Sci* 88:1242–1249, 2009.

39. Duke GE: Mechanisms of excreta formation and elimination in turkeys and ostriches, *J Exper Zool* 283:478–479, 1999.

40. Miller WJ, Wagner FH: Sexing mature Columbiformes by cloacal characters, *Auk* 72(3):279–328, 1955.

41. Detweiler DA, Carpenter JW, Kraft SL, et al: Radiographic diagnosis: avian cloacal adenocarcinoma, *Vet Rad Ultrasound* 41(6):539–541, 2000.

42. Souza MJ, Wall JS, Stuckey A, et al: Static and dynamic FDG-PET in normal Hispaniolan Amazon parrots (Amazona ventralis), *Vet Rad Ultrasound* 52(3):340–344, 2011.

43. Taylor WM: Examining the avian cloaca using saline infusion cloacoscopy, *Exotic DVM* 3(3):77–79, 2001.

44. Lumeij JT, Ephocrti C: Theory and practice of rectal fluid therapy in birds, *Proc Europ Assoc Avian Vet* 101, 1997.

45. Hernandez-Divers SJ, Wilson GH, Lester VK, et al: Evaluation of coelioscopic splenic biopsy and cloacoscopic bursa of Fabricius biopsy techniques in pigeons (Columba livia), *J Avian Med Surg* 20(4):234–241, 2006.

46. Taylor M: Endoscopic examination and biopsy techniques. In Ritchie BW, Harrison GJ, Harrison LR, editors: *Avian medicine: principles and application*, Lake Worth, FL, 1994, Wingers Publishing, pp 327–354.

47. Dvorak L, Bennett RA, Cranor K: Cloacotomy for excision of cloacal papillomas in a Catalina macaw, *J Avian Med Surg* 12(1):11–15, 1998.

48. Styles DK, Tomaszewski EK, Jaeger LA, et al: Psittacid herpesviruses associated with mucosal papillomas in neotropical parrots, *Virology* 325: 24–35, 2004.

49. Garner MM: Overview of tumours: a retrospective study of submissions to a specialty diagnostic service. In Harrison GH, Lightfoot TL, editors: *Avian medicine*, Vol 2, Palm Beach, FL, 2006, Spix Publishing, pp 566–571.

50. Palmieri C, Cusinato I, Avallone G, et al: Cloacal fibrosarcoma in a canary (Serinus canaria), *J Avian Med Surg* 25(4):277–280, 2011.

51. Beaufrere H, Taylor WM: Case series: long-term management in five umbrella cockatoos with idiopathic cloacal prolapse syndrome, *Proc Eur Assoc Avian Vet* 163–169, 2009.

52. Briscoe JA, Bennett RA: Use of a duodenal serosal patch in the repair of a colon rupture in a female Solomon island Eclectus parrot, *J Am Vet Med Assoc* 238:922–926, 2011.

53. Keller LH, Benson CE, Krotec K, et al: Salmonella enteritidis colonization of the reproductive tract and forming and freshly laid eggs of chickens, *Infect Immun* 63(7):2443–2449, 1995.

54. Monleon R, Martin MP, Barnes HJ: Bacterial orchitis and epididymo-orchitis in broiler breeders, *Avian Pathol* 37(6):613–617, 2008.

55. Cariou N, Christensen H, Salandre O, et al: Genital form of pasteurellosis in breeding turkeys infected during artificial insemination and isolation of an unusual strain of Pasteurella multocida, *Avian Dis* 57(3):693–697, 2013.

56. Brihante RSN, Castello-Branco DSCM, Soares GDP, et al: Characterization of the gastrointestinal yeast microbiota of cockatiels (Nymphicus hollandicus): a potential hazard to human health, *J Med Microbiol* 59:718–723, 2010.

57. Costa Sidrim JJ, Collares Maia DC, Brilhante R, et al: Candida species isolated from the gastrointestinal tract of cockatiels (Nymphicus hollandicus): in vitro antifungal susceptibility profile and phospholipase activity, *Vet Microbiol* 145:324–328, 2010.

58. Taylor M: Systemic trichosporonosis in a green winged macaw with pancreatic atrophy, *Proc Assoc Avian Vet* 219–220, 1988.

59. Haukos DA, Neaville J: Spatial and temporal changes in prevalence of a cloacal cestode in wintering waterfowl along the Gulf coast of Texas, *J Wildl Dis* 39(1):152–160, 2003.

60. Nowak MR, Krolaczyk K, Kavetska K, et al: Morphological features of Cloacotaenia megalops (Nitzsch in Creplin, 1829) (Cestoda, Hymenolepididae) from different hosts, *Wiadomooeci Parazytologiczne* 57(1):31–36, 2011.

61. Zamparo D, Brooks D, Causey D: Tinamutrema canoae N. Gen. et N. Sp. (Trematoda: Digenea: Strigeiformes: Brachylaimidae) in Crypturellus cinnamomeus (Aves, Passeriformes, Tinamidae) from the area de conservacion Guancaste, Costa Rica, *J Parasitol* 89(4): 819–822, 2003.

62. Bakke TA: Urogonimus macrostomus (Rudolphi, 1803) (Digenea): its taxonomy and morphology as revealed by light and scanning electron microscopy, *Can J Zool* 56:2280–2291, 1978.

63. Iwaki T, Okamoto M, Nakamori J: Urogonimus macrostomus (Digenea: Leucochloridiidae) from the rustic bunting (Emberiza rustica) in Japan, *Parasitol Int* 58(3):303–305, 2009.

64. Doster AR, Mahaffey EA, McLearen JR: Cryptosporidia in the cloacal coprodeum of red-lored parrots (Amazona autumnalis), *Avian Dis* 23(3):654–661, 1979.

65. Egyed Z, Sreter T, Szell Z, et al: Polyphasic typing of Cryptosporidium baileyi: a suggested model for characterization of Cryptosporidia, *J Parasitol* 88(2):237–243, 2002.

66. Tsai SS, Hirai K, Itakura C: Histopathological survey of protozoa, helminths and ascarids of imported and local psittacine birds in Japan, *Jpn J Vet Res* 40:161–174, 1992.

67. Beaufrère H, Navarez J, Tully TN: Cloacolith in a blue-fronted Amazon parrot (Amazona aestiva), *J Avian Med Surg* 24(2):142–145, 2010.

68. Radlinsky MG, Carpenter JW, Mison MB, et al: Colonic entrapment after cloacopexy in two psittacine birds, *J Avian Med Surg* 18(3): 175–182, 2004.

CHAPTER 8

Pleura, Pericardium, and Peritoneum: The Coelomic Cavities of Birds and their Relationship to the Lung–Air Sac System

W. Michael Taylor

While the coelomic cavities of the bird have been well described in the anatomic literature for 40 years, the clinical significance of these structures has been largely ignored.[1-3] In 1993, we described these structures and their relevance to the endoscopist and acknowledged that a review of the avian clinical literature suggested a widespread lack of understanding of the existence of these structures as they relate to the unique and complex air sac system of the bird.[4,5] In the 20 years that have passed, problems have continued with the accurate description of clinical and diagnostic procedures such as surgery, endoscopy, imaging, and necropsy. In healthy birds, the air sac and mesothelial walls of these cavities are thin, transparent, and minimally vascularized. It cannot be overstated that the very process of removing the platelike sternum during dissection or necropsy tears many of these diaphanous membranes, disrupting orientation and adding to confusion (Figure 8-1). The potential spaces of the peritoneal cavities, especially the intestinal peritoneal cavity (IPC), are challenging to appreciate in healthy birds (Figure 8-2). But the fact remains that birds *do* have a peritoneal cavity that contains most of the gastrointestinal (GI) tract, the gonads, and the spleen. What perhaps is unusual for many clinicians is the concept that the right and left lobes of the liver are surrounded and contained within their own hepatic peritoneal cavities (HPCs).[3,6] The purpose of this chapter is to review the current knowledge regarding the eight coelomic cavities of birds and, more importantly, put this information into a context that is useful practically for the clinician or diagnostician. The embryonic coelom is rapidly divided into its component cavities by day 5 of incubation.[7] The coelomic cavities are, by definition, lined with mesothelium and produce lubricating serosal fluids.[3] In most vertebrates, the arrangement of the coelomic cavities is relatively simple, consisting of a pericardial sac and conjoined pleuroperitoneal or separate pleural and peritoneal cavities (Figure 8-3). Duncker, in his review,[6] noted that only some families of reptiles such as the Varanidae and Crocodilia demonstrate anything approaching the coelomic complexity of birds.

THE LUNG–AIR SAC SYSTEM

The expansion of air sacs during embryologic development in the bird partitions and complicates the arrangement of the peritoneum and, in fact, creates a new coelomic space unique to Aves. Correct anatomic description of these spaces is challenging. More than semantics, the ability to describe and accurately locate and orient specific organs, lesions, and other findings within the avian patient is essential to professional discourse and communication. The evolutionary development of the lung–air sac system in birds gave rise to rigid, tubular air exchange surfaces that are linked in a continuous flow pattern within lung parenchyma designed to remain fixed in volume and shape.[8-10] This is a completely different strategy than the bronchiolar–alveoli lung of mammals, where branching, treelike bronchi and bronchioles lead to terminal alveoli that must be emptied and refilled to achieve gas exchange. The lungs of birds are situated as far dorsally as possible within (and between) the dorsal curvature of the ribs, flanking the vertebral column. Ventilation of these rigid lungs is dependent upon large, compliant air sacs connected on several surfaces that expand and contract due to the bellows-like motion of the sternum at its cranial fulcrum.[8,10] Any evaluation of the coelomic cavities of birds must simultaneously assess the presence and role of the air sacs. An understanding of the regional and three-dimensional anatomy of the lung–air sac system can greatly enhance the clinician's ability to place the coelomic cavities in their proper location within the living bird (Figure 8-4). Correct anatomic location of observed gross and microscopic lesions in the avian patient is also an essential step to understanding the pathophysiology of disease (Box 8-1).

The class Aves is very diverse, and while we can expect much homology of the lung–air sac system for functional reasons, there are some differences between families.[2,8,10] Although the majority of air sac and coelomic cavity research conducted so far has been performed on chickens, pigeons, and ducks, Duncker thoroughly examined the lung–air sac systems of 155 species from 47 families of birds in a pivotal contribution, using exquisite latex air sac casts and fixed specimens.[2,8] Much of what we know about the early development of the lung and air sac systems has been gleaned from the study of Galliform embryos, primarily the chicken and the quail.[11] Jaensch et al looked at the air sac anatomy in cockatoos by using functional testing and air sac casts, and Krautwald-Junghanns described computed tomography (CT) findings in *Amazona* and *Psittacus*, comparing them with air sac casts.[12,13] Our endoscopic findings in Psittaciformes, Columbiformes, Falconiformes, Strigiformes, Anseriformes, and Passeriformes support the published findings[14] (Taylor unpublished). Endoscopy offers a number of benefits in birds for anatomic assessment such as in situ observation, without potential pressurization differences or cavity-filling artifacts inherent to injection casting techniques and the ability to observe processes such as respiratory muscle contractions in real time. This has proven valuable when evaluating internal air sac structures.[15]

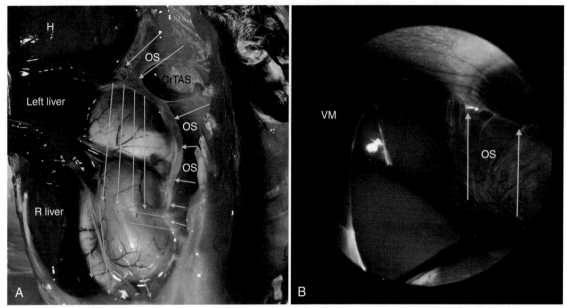

FIGURE 8-1 **A,** Left oblique septum and posthepatic septum of a Hahn's macaw *(Diopsittaca nobilis)* at post mortem examination. Note tear in posthepatic septum *(yellow arrows)* caused by pulling liver lobes to the right over the dilated proventriculus/ventriculus, after removing sternum. Blue arrows denote the extension of the posthepatic septum over the ventriculus and the area where it meets the oblique septum. (Yes, this bird had PDD.) **B,** Left VHPC of a pigeon *(Columbia livia).* OS, Left oblique septum reflection that attaches to ventral sternum, torn when sternum removed; VHPC, ventral hepatic peritoneal cavity; VM, ventral mesentery.

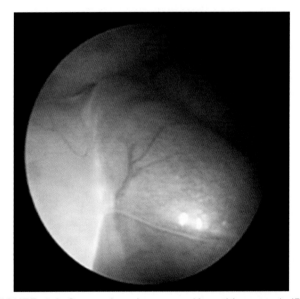

FIGURE 8-2 Green-winged macaw *(Ara chloroptera).* IPC viewed through the left AAS membrane. Note how the AAS separates from the IPC at the bottom of the frame. AAS, Abdominal air sac; IPC, intestinal peritoneal cavity.

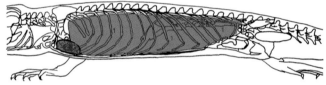

FIGURE 8-3 Line drawing of a generic lizard demonstrating the simplest form of coelomic cavity arrangement consisting of a cranial pericardial sac *(blue)* and a large combined pleuroperitoneal cavity *(red).*

Embryologic Development of the Body Cavities

To fully understand the coelomic cavity and its anatomic contortions that have plagued clinicians for so many years, we must begin with the embryologic development of the air sacs, which are primarily responsible for those changes. As the lung primordia develops during the first 5 days of incubation, small buds appear first on the caudal surfaces and then on the cranial and ventral surfaces. The abdominal air sac (AAS) buds develop from the terminus of the primary bronchus, where it ends on the caudal edge of the lung.[7,9] In the second week of incubation, the clavicular and cervical air sacs arise from the cranial aspect of the lung, with the cranial thoracic air sac (CrTAS) and caudal thoracic air sac (CaTAS) expanding from the ventromedial surface. The expansion of the CrTAS and CaTAS into the postpulmonary septum part and divide this structure as they expand ventrally and caudally away from each lung, creating an essentially extracoelomic cavity that is unique to birds.[3,6] The ventral surface of the lung is supported and strengthened by the development of the horizontal septum, which forms in concert with the attached walls of portions of the caudal thoracic and cranial thoracic air sacs. Around this time the visceral and parietal pleura on this surface of the lung fuse to the horizontal septum, serving to further strengthen the structure. The abdominal air sac pushes through the postpulmonary septum to expand within the IPC of all known birds except the Kiwi *(Apteryx* sp.).[6]

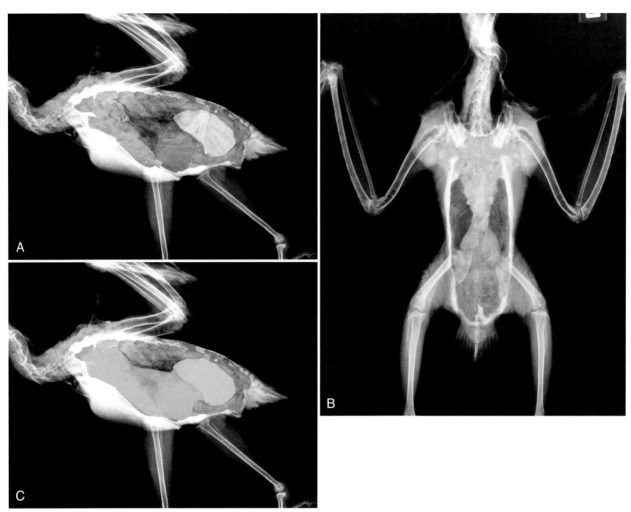

FIGURE 8-4 A, Lateral view of *Cacatua* sp. air sac latex casts superimposed upon a radiograph to demonstrate the location of the clavicular and cervical *(blue),* cranial thoracic *(brown),* caudal thoracic *(yellow)* and abdominal air sacs *(red).* Note the dorsal location of the lung *(green).* **B,** Ventrodorsal view of same cockatoo. Color coding is the same. **C,** Lateral view of the same cockatoo highlighting the extensive subpulmonary cavity *(green).*

BOX 8-1 THE COELOMIC CAVITIES BY DEFINITION

Coelom: the primordial body cavity, lined by mesoderm and formed by fusion of the lateral body folds early in embryonic development.[7]
Coelomic cavity: individual compartments, lined by mesothelium and producing serosal fluid. "Lower" reptiles have two cavities (pericardial, pleuroperitoneal), more highly developed reptiles have three (pericardial, pleural, peritoneal), mammals have a similar three, and birds have eight coelomic cavities.[6]

of the pericardial sac is attached dorsolaterally to the horizontal septum near the hilus of each lung (see Chapter 6). The ventral pericardium is attached to the inner surface of the sternum by numerous fibrous strands. The pericardium also lies in contact dorsally with the esophagus and primary bronchi. The outer layer of the sac is lined by parietal pericardium, but at the heart base where the great vessels issue, the pericardium reflects back on itself to produce the visceral pericardium, most commonly referred to as the "epicardium," which is adherent to the outer surface of the myocardium. The normal pericardial sac seldom contains more than 1 to 2 milliliters (mL) of free fluid in a large bird, less than 1 mL in a medium-sized parrot, and less than 0.5 mL in a small bird.

Pericardial Cavity

The pericardial cavity is situated ventrally on the midline, just dorsal to the sternum, and is restrained by a number of fibrous attachments to surrounding structures, most notably the sternum. The apex of the sac is intimately associated with, and positioned between, the two lobes of the liver. The base

Pleural Cavities

As previously mentioned, the lungs develop as dorsally as possible within and between the light but rigid ribs, parallel to the vertebral column. Contained within the visceral pleura, the lungs develop a unique, tubular architecture with fixed dimensions and bilateral symmetry. The parietal pleura that surrounds each lung and the mesothelial coating of the visceral pleura applied to the lung itself form a small, potential pleural cavity due to the fixed dimensions of the avian lung, however, in most species. The parietal and visceral pleura develop fibrous cross-connections starting along the ventromedial surface of the lung. The pleural cavity thus becomes limited to a small potential or nonexistent space, although along the lateral surface of the lung this space may be larger as noted in *Columbia livia*[14,16] (Taylor unpublished) (Figure 8-5). Further work in defining this arrangement in other species is needed, and the use of computed tomography is likely to be useful. The development of the horizontal septum in birds from the splitting of the postpulmonary septum is considered another

crucial step in helping maintain the rigidity of the lung during respiration. The septum is composed of a thick layer of connective tissue attached to the dorsal parietal pleura. Fan-shaped, striated muscle bundles *(m. costoseptalis)* run from the ribs of the lateral body wall and attach to the surface of the horizontal septum. These costoseptal muscles contract during expiration to help maintain the volume constancy of the lung (Figure 8-6). Of note also is the further support provided by the CrTAS and CaTAS walls that adhere to the horizontal septum where they contact. Cook et al[17] describe finding three layers of collagen as well as a variety of axons and secretory cells in their study of the chicken saccopleural membrane. King and McLelland had suggested this name for the complete multilayered structure of pleura, connective tissue (e.g., horizontal septum), and air sac.[3,17,18]

Subpulmonary Cavities

The right and left subpulmonary cavities are structures unique to birds and, strictly speaking, are not true coelomic cavities as they are not lined by mesothelium. They form when the CrTAS and CaTAS bud from the lung into the postpulmonary septum. As they enlarge, they split this connective tissue layer into the horizontal and oblique septa.[3,6] The clavicular and cervical air sacs develop cranially to the lung and laterally to the pericardial sac around the same time, expanding the left and right subpulmonary cavities cranially to the level of the thoracic inlet. The horizontal septa play an important role, forming the ventral walls of the pleural cavities. The bilateral horizontal septa are penetrated by a number of structures, most importantly the ostia of the cervical, clavicular, CrT, and CaT air sacs. The oblique septum is composed of the parietal peritoneum on its dorsal and medial surfaces and the air sac epithelium on the ventral and lateral surfaces. The oblique septa are also bilateral structures composed of the peritoneum and a connective tissue layer, and when including the air sac epithelium applied to the opposite side, they should be referred to as the left and right saccoperitoneal membranes.[17,18]

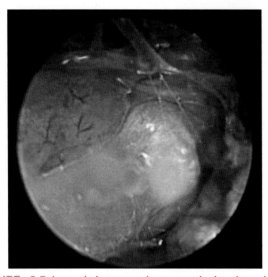

FIGURE 8-5 Lateral intercostal approach in the pigeon *(Columbia livia)*. Note lung tissue cranial and caudal to the rib and strands extending from the visceral pleura up to the parietal pleura (just out of frame).

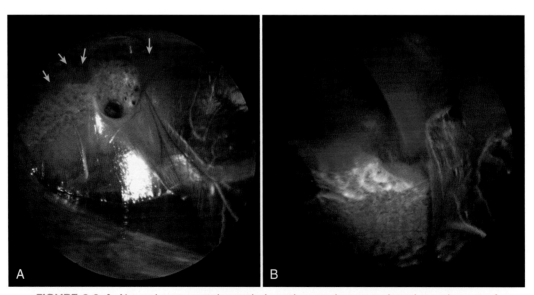

FIGURE 8-6 **A,** Normal costoseptal muscle insertion on the saccopleural membranes of the pigeon *(blue arrows)*. **B,** Moderate hypertrophy of costoseptal muscles in a blue-and-yellow macaw *(Ara ararauna)* due to chronic obstructive pulmonary disease.

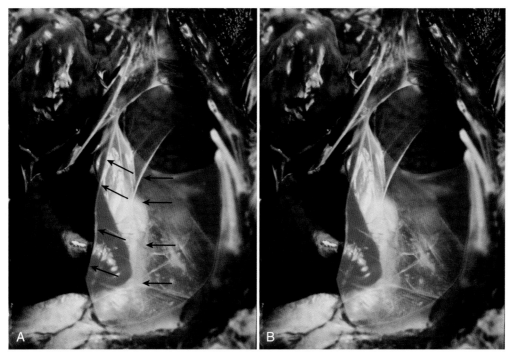

FIGURE 8-7 African Grey parrot *(Psittacus erithacus)* necropsy reveals the saccoperitoneal membrane *(black arrows).*

The author prefers to describe the complete structure for practical anatomic reasons, but there are times when it may be appropriate to refer to the component entities. The saccoperitoneal membranes run from the respective lateral body walls starting from where they split from the saccopleural membranes near the caudal border of the lungs. From here, they pass medially to the posthepatic septa, then reflect ventrally to attach to the sternum (Figure 8-7). This is the portion that is torn by removal of the sternum at necropsy (see Figure 8-1). The walls of the CrTAS and CaTAS are fixed to the horizontal and oblique septa so that their shapes are maintained. They are also fixed to each other where they contact, as will be noted during a routine endoscopic examination.[14] In all birds except the Kiwi, the abdominal air sac penetrates the unsplit oblique and horizontal septa near the caudolateral border of each lung to enter the IPC.[6] Only in the Kiwi are the abdominal air sacs within the subpulmonary cavities along with the CrTAS and the CaTAS.

Peritoneal Cavities

Birds have five distinct peritoneal cavities. Four HPCs surround the right and left liver lobes. The single, midline IPC contains most of the GI tract, the gall bladder (if present), the reproductive organs, and the spleen.

Hepatic peritoneal cavities

The HPCs are composed of two paired structures, the large left and right ventral HPCs (VHPCs) and the much smaller right and left dorsal HPCs (DHPCs) (Figure 8-8). In the chicken, the left DHPC communicates with the IPC via a small opening that is covered on the IPC side only by the AASs.[6,14,19] This connection is small and not easy to visualize, but it is likely present in most Aves. The author has been able to locate it in

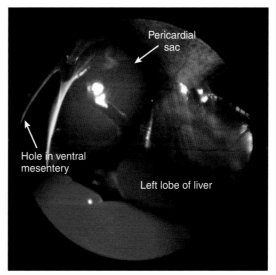

FIGURE 8-8 Normal left VHPC and view through puncture in the ventral mesentery to the right VHPC in the normal pigeon *(Columbia livia).* Note how the right lobe of the liver protrudes through the ventral mesentery. VHPC, Ventral hepatic peritoneal cavity.

very few patients, only when an effusion is present and when using the magnification of endoscopy (Figure 8-9).

The ventral wall of the VHPCs is the parietal peritoneum lining the sternum, the lateral walls are formed by the oblique septa (see Figure 8-1), and the dorsal wall is formed by the posthepatic septum. In passerine birds, the left and right oblique septa meet over the liver, and therefore form the

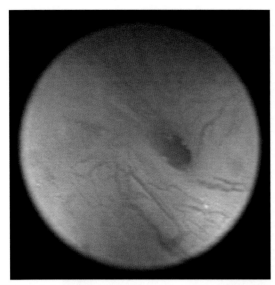

FIGURE 8-9 Left dorsal hepatic peritoneal cavity connection to the IPC in a pigeon with marked ascites. IPC, Intestinal peritoneal cavity.

ventral surface of the DHPCs[6] (Figure 8-10). HPCs are divided on the midline into right and left entities by the ventral mesentery.

The posthepatic septum separates the HPCs from the IPC and runs from a dorsal attachment at the vertebral column just caudal to the hilus of the lung and continues gradually in a caudoventral direction toward the caudal border of the sternum or the ventral body wall, depending on the species (see Figure 8-1). The HPCs are potential spaces under normal conditions with limited serosal fluid present. They are normally larger than the liver lobes, yet this is difficult to appreciate until there is significant pathology such as hepatic enlargement or an effusion expanding the cavities (Figure 8-11). In taxonomic orders with a

gall bladder such as members of the Falconiformes and Anseriformes, the gall bladder is located within the IPC but is attached to the posthepatic septum via the terminus of the ventral mesentery (Figure 8-12). At least one of the VHPCs must be entered in order to perform a hepatic biopsy.[14] This may be accomplished via an incision made at the caudal–sternal border and then penetrating the posthepatic septum into the caudal aspects of the VHPC or endoscopically from the left or right CaTAS (Figure 8-13). If the liver is abnormally enlarged, it may protrude well beyond the sternum, allowing a simpler percutaneous approach (Figure 8-14).

Intestinal peritoneal cavity

The single IPC is centrally located in the mid-to-caudal coelom and contains the proventriculus, ventriculus, gall bladder (if present), spleen, intestines, and male or female reproductive tracts.[3,6] The IPC is the only coelomic cavity containing air sacs (the left and right AASs), which enter the IPC through the small, unsplit portion of the horizontal and oblique septa and run dorsally and caudally toward the pelvic region of the bird. The AASs are the most variable in shape of all the air sacs because they are affected by the volume and relative location of the viscera, especially the proventriculus and the ventriculus. Only in the Kiwi are the CaTAS, CrTAS, and AASs all within the subpulmonary cavity.[6,18]

The complete GI system from the proventriculus to the rectum is suspended by the dorsal mesentery. The ovary is suspended dorsally by the mesovarium, the oviduct is suspended by the mesosalpinx, and the testicles are suspended dorsally by mesorchia. The ventral mesentery ends at or before the caudal wall of the ventriculus—that is, the IPC is a single chamber for most of its length, the exceptions being the right and left lateral "pockets" that run along the left proventricular–ventricular border and the right hepatic border. A ventral midline incision made caudal to the ventriculus leads directly and specifically into the IPC, not into the "coelom" or the "coelomic cavity." As such, the generic term

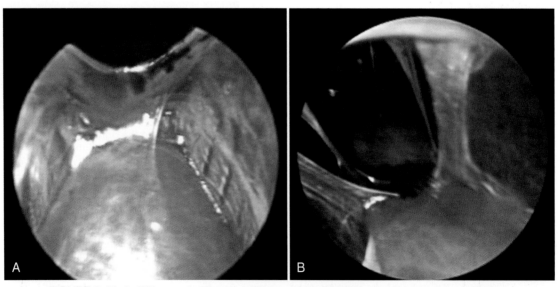

FIGURE 8-10 **A,** Hill mynah *(Gracula religiosa)* fused oblique septa over the ventral surface of the liver. **B,** Hill mynah showing fused oblique septa and attachments running from the oblique septum to the dorsal sternum.

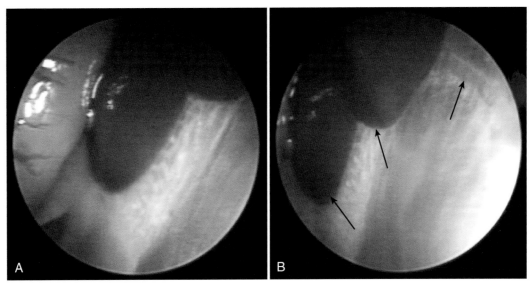

FIGURE 8-11 **A,** Caudodorsal portion of the posthepatic septum, viewed from the IPC in a pigeon. Note small intestine and liver lobes. **B,** Similar view to **A** taken even more to the left side of ventriculus. The septum is transparent in healthy birds. Note visible portions, especially at right arrow. IPC, Intestinal peritoneal cavity.

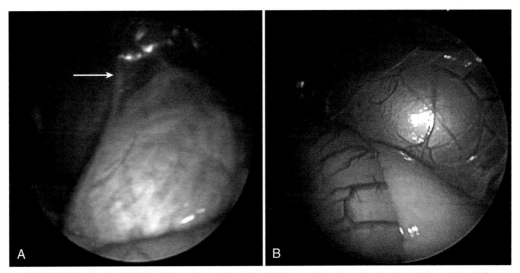

FIGURE 8-12 **A,** Gall bladder of a mallard duck *(Anas platyrhynchos)* viewed from the IPC. Note attachment to the terminal ventral mesentery *(arrow)*. **B,** Gall bladder of a red-tailed hawk *(Buteo jamaicensis)* viewed from the IPC. Duodenum and pancreas are visible in the foreground. IPC, Intestinal peritoneal cavity.

"coelomotomy" should not be used when referring to a specific anatomic space.

The IPC is a potential space in normal birds containing little visible fluid. The walls of the AAS and IPC are adherent in some areas, especially dorsally. The diaphanous, healthy air sac and peritoneal walls make some structures appear to lie within the AAS, but this is an illusion, facilitated by their transparency (Figure 8-15). Only where the AAS separates from the IPC, or when the IPC is filled with air or fluid is it possible to see this potential space more clearly (Figure 8-16).

In summary, birds have *eight coelomic cavities*: the single pericardial and intestinal peritoneal cavities, two pleural cavities, and four HPCs. Each cavity is lined with serous mesothelium,

which secretes small amounts of lubricating fluids. All of the visceral organs except the right and left liver lobes are contained within the IPC. Ascites due to portal hypertension or right heart failure will occur first in the HPCs, spilling over to the IPC only when a critical level is reached. An effusion, specifically of the IPC, may occur with internal ovulation; ovarian, testicular, and splenic disease processes; or lymphoid neoplasia.

Diagnostic Techniques

Physical examination

Look at the conformation of the bird as it perches and moves. Is the ventral body wall distended or irregular in appearance? Does the patient seem to favor the ventral body wall area or

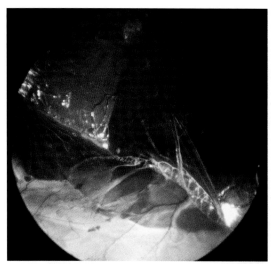

FIGURE 8-13 Left CaTAS in a pigeon *(Columbia livia)*. Note incision in the CaTAS–hepatic peritoneal wall so that a liver biopsy can be collected. CaTAS, Caudal thoracic air sac.

perch lower than normally? Abdominal neoplasia is frequently (but not always) painful (Figure 8-17). During your observation, note also the pattern of the bird's respiration. Peritoneal distension due to ascites causes a corresponding decrease in air sac volume, thereby reducing pulmonary reserve volume. Respiratory rate and depth are usually affected, with notable tachypnea, and may mimic clinical signs of respiratory disease.

Once the patient is restrained for examination, assess the patient's sternal border and ventral abdominal region, seeking evidence of a palpably enlarged liver (firm on palpation with well-defined borders) protruding beyond the sternum or peritoneal dilation with fluid (softer and fluctuant; sometimes a fluid wave can be detected) (Figure 8-18). The largest challenge at examination may be differentiating VHPC distension

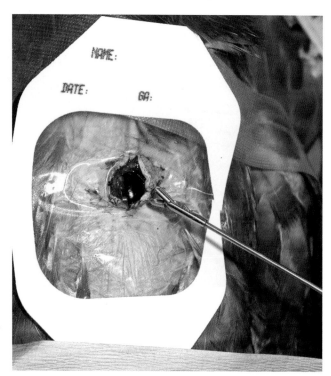

FIGURE 8-14 Open liver biopsy in a macaw with hepatomegaly.

from IPC distension, especially in smaller patients. If VHPC fluid accumulation begins slowly, a distinct dilation of the cavity may be detectable, creating a raised border at the caudal edge of the posthepatic septum. While this may resemble hepatic enlargement, it will feel appreciably different at palpation. If the fluid accumulation is rapid, filling the HPCs to capacity, overflow to the IPC occurs from the left DHPC (see Figure 8-9).

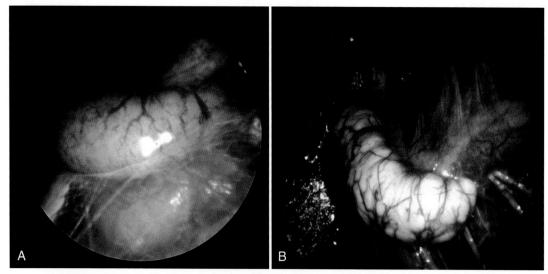

FIGURE 8-15 **A,** *Amazona* sp. testicles viewed from the left AAS. Note the right testicle visible through the dorsal mesentery. **B,** Left testicle of a trumpeter swan *(Cygnus buccinator)* viewed from the left AAS. Note how difficult it is to see the thin covering membranes of air sac and peritoneum. AAS, Abdominal air sac.

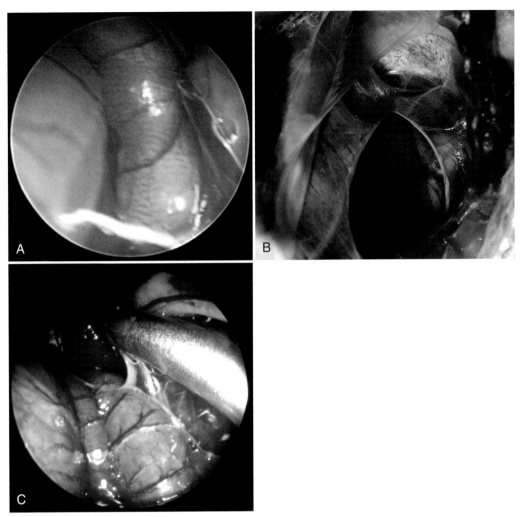

FIGURE 8-16 **A,** IPC visible from the caudal portion of the AAS in a pigeon. **B,** IPC distended with red-colored saline, bird in dorsal recumbency at necropsy. **C,** A 2.7-mm endoscope inserted into the IPC from the postischial approach in an orange-winged amazon *(Amazona amazonica)* is observed from another endoscope in the left AAS. Note the air sac and peritoneal membranes covering the endoscope within the IPC. AAS, Abdominal air sac; IPC, intestinal peritoneal cavity.

Paracentesis

Techniques for withdrawing a sample of fluid from the abdomen have been described and are relatively simple to perform.[20] However, understanding the regional anatomy of the poststernal coelom is important to minimize inadvertent organ trauma. The author recommends paracentesis as a diagnostic aid, with the caveat that aggressive peritoneal punctures may cause iatrogenic problems such as bowel perforation or hemorrhage from the liver or mesenteric vessels. Controlled puncture of the ventral body wall in a region of distension usually provides a usable fluid sample (Figure 8-19). Transillumination prior to and during paracentesis can greatly facilitate locating a site for puncture and can aid in helping the operator(s) avoid causing inadvertent trauma to underlying structures.

Imaging techniques

Traditional radiographic techniques remain one of the most cost-effective diagnostic procedures in avian medicine.

Improved digital radiographic systems have only enhanced the value of orthogonal right lateral and ventrodorsal images for detecting pulmonary, air sac, and visceral lesions. As always, proper positioning and good technique reward the clinician with highly diagnostic images. Under normal circumstances, the coelomic cavities have minimal serosal fluid content. The accumulation of effusion and debris, an increase in visceral size, or an increase in other intraperitoneal tissues (e.g., lipid) may increase the size of the peritoneal cavities on radiographs. The addition of nonionic iodinated contrast agents injected under endoscopic guidance or by using physical landmarks may be a useful adjunct to plain radiographs.[21] The author has used these products to aid in defining the normal HPCs and air sacs (Figure 8-20).

Fluoroscopy with barium contrast

Fluoroscopy using barium contrast can be a powerful tool for demonstrating GI contractions seen in the ventriculus and

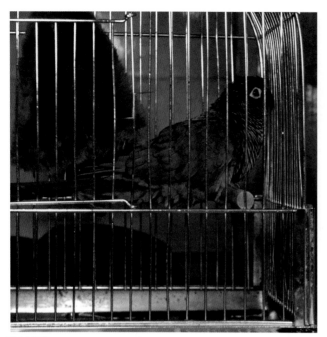

FIGURE 8-17 Green-cheeked conure *(Pyrrhura molinae)* with a pancreatic carcinoma, exhibiting abdominal pain through hunched posture and resting tail on perch.

duodenum of birds. Secondarily, it can be used to define, by subtraction of the GI elements, the shape of the HPCs and space-occupying structures within the IPC. The patients are fluoroscopically imaged in a standing or perching position, without the need for restraint, allowing the effects of gravity to be evident, compared with standard still contrast radiographs in which the patient is positioned in lateral or dorsal

recumbency (Figure 8-21). Although not often considered and used in avian private practice, used C-arm fluoroscopes can be relatively inexpensive to obtain.

Endoscopy

During the majority of avian endoscopic examinations, the air sac system is used to allow movement of the endoscope within the body so that structures can be examined through the thin, clear walls. For example, a recommended general approach is to enter directly into the CaTAS from the body wall on one side so that the associated CrTAS and AAS walls may be punctured and all three air sacs can be entered from a single body wall incision, which would allow a minimally traumatic, yet efficient unilateral examination.[14]

From the left version of the CaTAS endoscopic approach, the left AAS is entered by puncturing the saccoperitoneal membrane and the gonad, oviduct or ductus deferens, rectum, coprodeum, urodeum, spleen, and the left portions of the proventriculus and ventriculus, and some loops of the small intestine are visible suspended within the IPC. The adrenal gland; the cranial, middle, and caudal divisions of the left kidney, and the ureter are also clearly visible, but these structures are retroperitoneal and not within the IPC. Occasionally it is possible to actually see the components that make up the saccoperitoneal membrane as they separate after endoscopic puncture (Figure 8-22).

The IPC may be entered directly from the body wall without penetrating an air sac by using one of two approaches. A midline, paramedian, or transverse incision in the ventral body wall will enable one to enter the IPC when the incision is made caudal to the end of the posthepatic septum and medial to the distal limits of the CaTAS and AAS. This will vary somewhat between species but is equivalent to the red rectangular area depicted in Figure 8-23, a ventrodorsal radiograph

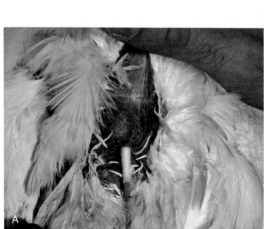

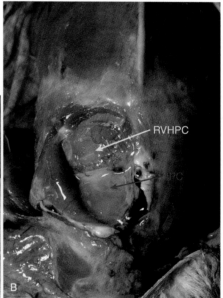

FIGURE 8-18 **A,** Goffin's cockatoo *(Cacatua goffini)* with marked hepatomegaly due to hepatic carcinoma. **B,** Green-winged macaw *(Ara chloroptera)* with distended HPCs and mildly distended IPC due to ascites. HPC, hepatic peritoneal cavity; IPC, intestinal peritoneal cavity; RVHPC, right ventral hepatic peritoneal cavity.

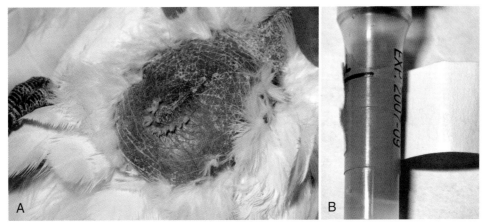

FIGURE 8-19 **A,** Distended IPC of an umbrella cockatoo *(Cacatua alba)* with egg-related peritonitis. Note rounded, full appearance caudal to the sternal border. **B,** Fluid aspirated via paracentesis from the intestinal peritoneal cavity (IPC) of the bird in **A**. Note the marked yellow appearance due to the presence of yolk lipids.

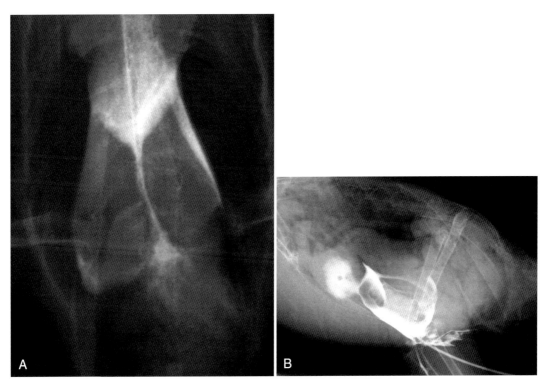

FIGURE 8-20 **A,** VHPCs of a cockatiel *(Nymphicus hollandicus)* demarcated by radiopaque dye. **B,** Lateral view of the left VHPC of an orange-winged amazon *(Amazona amazonica)* outlined with radiopaque dye. VHPC, Ventral hepatic peritoneal cavity.

of an *Amazona* sp. parrot (see Figure 8-23). The other site for direct entry from the body wall to the IPC is the left or right postischial approach.[14] A small skin incision dorsal to the pubis and just caudal to the ischium allows for a blunt puncture through the thin body wall dorsolateral to the coprodeum. The point of entry is shown on the lateral radiograph of the same *Amazona* sp. parrot (Figure 8-24, *A*). The tip of the endoscope first enters the lateral IPC (right or left), and the caudal wall of the respective AAS can be seen directly ahead of the telescope (see Figure 8-24, *B*). The IPC is a potential space and will need to be insufflated or the AAS otherwise manipulated to

reduce its size so that the peritoneal organs can be visualized and accessed.

DISEASES AND PATHOPHYSIOLOGY

Ascites

Ascites is the accumulation of excess fluid within the peritoneal cavities. This fluid may contain small, medium, or large amounts of protein and various inflammatory or neoplastic cells, and/or biochemical constituents, depending on the

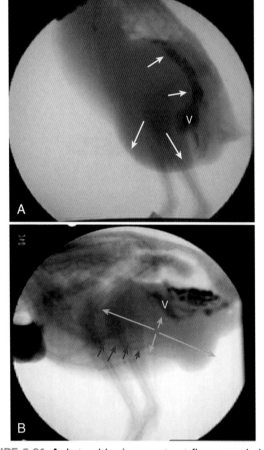

FIGURE 8-21 **A,** Lateral barium contrast fluoroscopic image of an Alexandrian parakeet *(Psittacula eupatria)* with marked hepatomegaly due to hepatic neoplasia. Note dorsal displacement of the proventriculus. **B,** Lateral barium contrast fluoroscopic image of a pigeon *(Columbia livia)* with hepatomegaly and ascites due to lymphosarcoma. Blue arrows, Hepatic expansion; red arrows, dorsal border of sternum; V, ventriculus.

cause of the effusion. Routine diagnostic testing of fluid should include an accurate determination of total protein (preferably using the biuret method) and cytology, including a total cell count. Under certain situations, measurement of biochemical constituents of the effusion such as triglycerides, cholesterol, and amylase may also be useful. If peritoneal

effusion is suspected based on clinical history, at necropsy, the pathologist should carefully enter the IPC first via a ventral midline incision to sample and measure the volume of fluid from the IPC. After examination and sampling from the IPC, the HPCs can then be examined for fluid, and sampling accomplished by incising the posthepatic septum while elevating the caudal edge of the sternum. Rapid removal of the sternum will disrupt the HPCs, making collection of fluid difficult and possibly confusing the location of the primary effusion. The author has also noted that many times at necropsy, the amount of fluid present in the cavities is ineffectively or crudely estimated. Accurate measurement of the fluid content will often yield more surprising volumes than anticipated.

Cardiac

Pericardial effusion

Pericardial effusion and active pericarditis are relatively common findings in birds (see Chapter 6). If the effusion occurs slowly and does not cause much fibrosis, the pericardial sac may greatly increase in size before cardiac deficits occur[22] (Figure 8-25). Many systemic bacterial infections cause pericardial inflammation as part of their pathogenesis, with *Chlamydia psittaci* being the most well known. Hydropericardium occurs frequently with pulmonary hypertension, with ascites of the HPCs.[22] Systemic viral infections, including polyomavirus infection in juvenile psittacines, will also often cause serous pericardial effusion.

Ascites secondary to cardiomyopathy and pulmonary hypertension

Ascites of the HPCs occurs in cases of slowly decompensating cardiomyopathy and pulmonary hypertension, leading to right heart failure that progresses slowly enough to lead to portal hypertension[23–26] (see Chapter 6). Much excellent work has been published on this problem in rapidly growing strains of broiler chickens.[23,24] Chronic interstitial fibrosis of the lung and the resulting hypoxemia lead to secondary polycythemia, gradual pulmonary hypertension, and eventually right heart failure.[27–29] This condition has been confirmed in *Ara* sp. macaws (predominantly *Ara ararauna*) and also *Amazona* sp. As the right heart begins to fail, increasing oncotic pressure within the hepatic portal system leads to the leakage of plasma from the liver sinusoids into the HPCs. The protein content of the fluid is high, and if a patient suffering from this type of

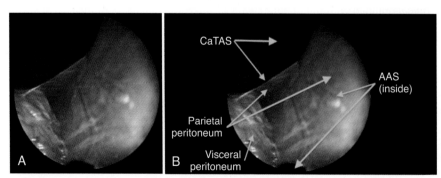

FIGURE 8-22 **A** and **B,** Components of the saccoperitoneal membrane in a green-winged macaw *(Ara chloroptera)*.

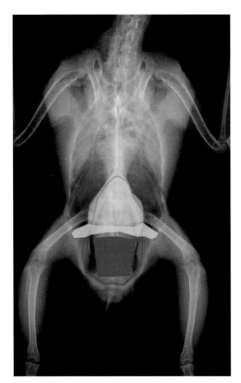

FIGURE 8-23 Ventrodorsal projection of a normal *Amazona* sp. with the HPCs *(yellow)*, caudal portion of the posthepatic septum *(blue)*, and IPC *(red line)* highlighted. The red box represents the area for direct surgical entry into the IPC using a ventral incision. HPC, Hepatic peritoneal cavity; IPC, intestinal peritoneal cavity.

effusion has been chilled before necropsy, the fluid often gels within the HPCs.[23] Fibrin clots are also frequently noted in the fluid. The four cavities can become very enlarged if the fluid accumulation occurs slowly enough; however, as the fluid pressure in the HPCs increases, overflow to the IPC will occur via the left dorsal HPC connection[23] (see Figure 8-9).

Hepatic cirrhosis

Chronic hepatic inflammation from various causes leads ultimately to fibrosis of the liver parenchyma as part of the healing response. Fibrosis can in turn lead to restriction of portal blood flow, creating portal hypertension. Chronic *Chlamydia* or *Coxiella* infections and excessive iron uptake (hemochromatosis) are common causes of hepatic fibrosis in pet birds. The amount of ascitic fluid present in the VHPCs due to fibrosis will vary with the degree of hepatic damage (Figure 8-26).

Neoplasia

Hepatic peritoneal cavities

Primary neoplasia of the liver and occasionally metastatic neoplasia to the liver can lead to ascites due to disruption of hepatic portal blood flow. Hepatic carcinoma, advanced biliary duct carcinoma, hemangiosarcoma of the liver, and lymphosarcoma have all been implicated in HPC ascites[30] (Taylor unpublished) (see Figures 8-21 and 8-27).

Intestinal peritoneal cavity

Neoplasia of the spleen, ovary, testes, and pancreas have been recorded and often lead to ascites of the IPC, most commonly by disrupting drainage of the lymphatic system.[19,31-35] Occasionally, tumors of the IPC may produce cystic structures as part of their neoplastic growth (e.g., some testicular and pancreatic tumors).[32]

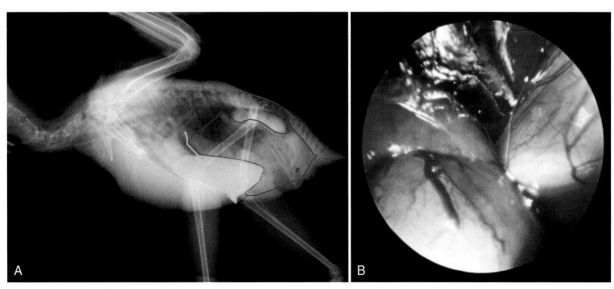

FIGURE 8-24 **A,** Lateral projection of the same bird in Figure 8-23, with the HPCs highlighted in yellow. The IPC is demarcated by the red line, and the posthepatic septum is colored orange. The red circle marks the site for the postischial insertion into the IPC. **B,** View looking cranially upon entering the IPC via a left postischial insertion in an *Amazona amazonica*. The caudal wall of the AAS is seen directly ahead of the endoscope. AAS, Abdominal air sac; HPC, hepatic peritoneal cavity; IPC, intestinal peritoneal cavity.

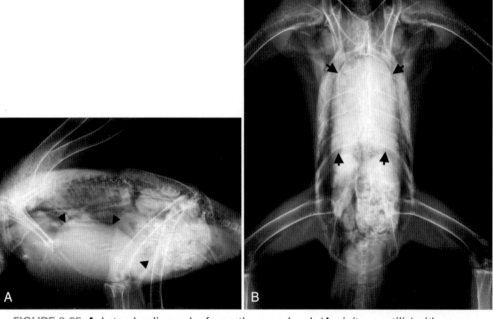

FIGURE 8-25 **A,** Lateral radiograph of a northern goshawk *(Accipiter gentilis)* with severe pericardial effusion. Black arrowheads denote perimeter of enlarged pericardial sac. **B,** Ventrodorsal view of the same bird showing extent of the pericardial effusion.

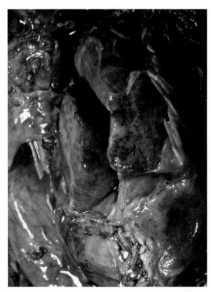

FIGURE 8-26 Green-winged macaw *(Ara chloroptera)* with ascites due to hepatic cirrhosis.

Peritonitis

Inflammation of the peritoneal mesothelium of mammals has, by convention, been called *peritonitis*. There is no indication why this should not be so in birds, even though they have more complex partitioning of their peritoneum into four HPCs and a single IPC. We noted in the preparation of this chapter that the term "coelomitis" has come into common use in the pet avian literature. Anatomically speaking, this term is too generalized and is no more useful in birds than it would

be in mammals. Birds have well-defined pleural, pericardial, and peritoneal cavities, and descriptive terminology should reflect this. The right and left lobes of the liver are surrounded by the parietal peritoneum of the HPCs. The spleen, ovary or testicles, ductus deferens or oviduct, gall bladder (if present), proventriculus, ventriculus, and intestines are all contained within the IPC. Inflammation within any or all of the four HPCs or the IPC will lead to peritonitis.

Egg related

Inflammation of the IPC may occur with the spillage of yolk at ovulation or the retropropulsion of an unfinished egg back into the cavity. It remains unclear why some spills of egg material clinically can cause marked effusions, whereas others do not. Although retrograde infection of the egg material is possible via the oviduct, many cases of "egg peritonitis" fail to yield an identifiable infectious agent or show cytologic evidence of host response to the presence of bacterial or fungal organisms. The effusion, once initiated, can produce considerable fluid, dilating the IPC and producing abdominal swelling (see Figure 8-19, *B*). Paracentesis will reveal a sample like that shown in Figure 8-19, *B*, which demonstrated triglyceride and cholesterol levels that were markedly elevated due to the spilled yolk content—200.8 mg/dL, 291.5 mg/dL, 3965.3 mg/dL, and 2203.9 mg/dL.

Bacterial

Bacterial peritonitis is relatively rare in pet birds but can occur following foreign body puncture of the GI tract, proventricular ulceration, ascending infection of the oviduct (usually with retropropulsion of egg material back into the IPC), or penetrating wounds. The usual suspects are implicated (e.g., *Escherichia coli*, *Pseudomonas aeruginosa*, *Klebsiella* sp.). Birds do

CHAPTER 8 • Pleura, Pericardium, and Peritoneum   359

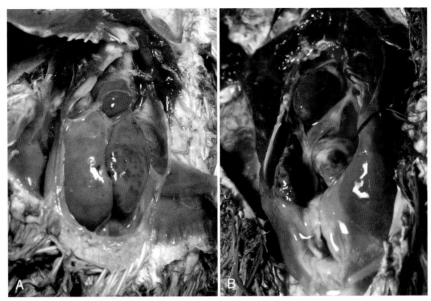

FIGURE 8-27 **A,** Hepatic lymphosarcoma with ascites in a pigeon *(Columbia livia).* **B,** Hemangiosarcoma of the liver with ascites in a blue-fronted amazon *(Amazona aestiva).*

not have a well-developed omentum, so the "patching" and adhesion formation so effective in mammals are unlikely to occur in avian GI perforations. Occasionally the liver or a fat pad may perform this role, but more often the perforation leads to ongoing IPC contamination, with high rates of morbidity and mortality.[36] Certain strains of *E. coli* are noted to cause marked effusion during hematogenous spread due to a toxin produced by the bacterium that damages the vascular endothelium.[37]

Viral

Viral serositis is the descriptive name for the generalized pathology caused by certain viruses that cause diffuse damage to the endothelium and the mesothelial surfaces, resulting in effusion into the pleural, pericardial, hepatic peritoneal, and intestinal peritoneal cavities. Eastern equine encephalitis virus and avian polyomavirus are known to cause lesions such as this in juvenile psittacine birds.[37]

Parasitic

Atoxoplasmosis is a disease caused by the tissue invasive forms of the apicomplexan protist *Atoxoplasma* genus and can cause widespread tissue damage in young passerine birds.[38,39] Much new work has been performed on the classification of these organisms by using molecular techniques[39] (see Chapter 2). The life cycle is direct, with oocytes shed in the urofeces, leading to infection if ingested by a susceptible bird. Peritoneal and pericardial effusions are not uncommon in response to the asexual reproduction of the organism in the liver, spleen, heart, lung, and intestine (Figure 8-28).

Eustrongylides sp. comprises a group of parasitic nematodes that migrate through the serosal surfaces of the ventriculus and proventriculus, leaving long tubelike tracts chronically and in severe infestations, causing peritonitis and visceral adhesions.[40] Heavy infestations in young birds are often fatal.[40,41] The intermediate host is usually a fish, and piscivorous birds are most commonly effected.

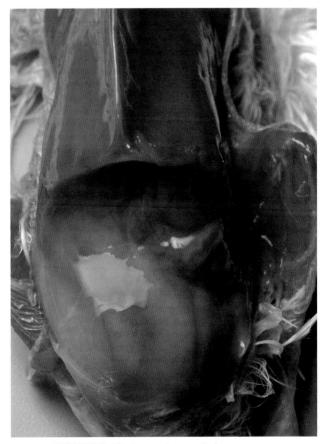

FIGURE 8-28 Atoxoplasmosis in a canary.

Other adult filarid worms have been observed occasionally in wild-caught psittacines, particularly cockatoos (*Cacatua* sp.), in which microfilaria were frequently noted in blood smears (Figure 8-29). Most of these species have yet to be identified due to the difficulty in linking microfilaria with

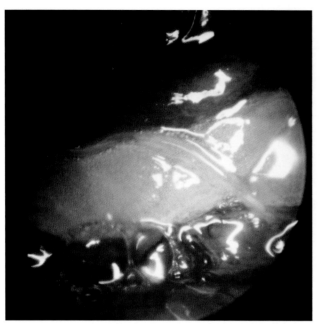

FIGURE 8-29 Adult filarid in the IPC of a Moluccan cockatoo *(Cacatua moluccensis)*. IPC, Intestinal peritoneal cavity.

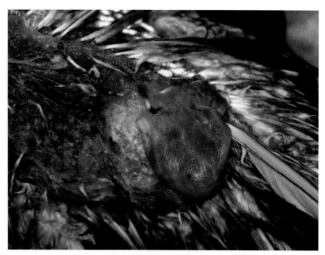

FIGURE 8-30 Herniation of the left IPC in a cockatiel *(Nymphicus hollandicus)*. IPC, Intestinal peritoneal cavity.

adult forms, although species of *Chandlerella*, *Cardiofilaria*, *Eulimdana*, *Lemdana*, and *Pelecitus* have been noted in a wide variety of birds.[42] The life cycle of these nematodes usually requires a biting arthropod for transmission.

Hernia Formation

Hernia of the abdominal wall

A hernia by definition represents the protrusion of a viscus, fat, or its fascial attachment through a defect in the body wall, creating a hernial sac. In birds this diagnosis may become challenging because of the tenuous nature of the normal ventral body wall. In certain conditions involving prolonged hyperestrogenism and abnormal abdominal fat accumulation, the ventral body wall from the caudal edge of the sternum to the cloaca may become grossly thinned and distended. This condition should not be considered true herniation, as the effect usually involves the entire body wall, although the term could be used if a more focal disruption could be shown in the thinned abdominal structure. The author has seen several cases of left lateral body wall and pericloacal herniation in female psittacines, where egg yolk, oviduct, or visceral fat (contents of the IPC) have passed through, creating a noticeable sac (Figure 8-30). The small defects without grossly increased abdominal fat are surgically reducible and do not recur if the excessive laying of the hen is dealt with. Those with excessive fat accumulation require a more complex approach to resolution. Many of these hens (often *Cacatua* sp.) exhibit abnormal ovarian cycling and potential multiendocrine abnormalities.

Hernia of hepatic peritoneal cavity, intestinal peritoneal cavity, or posthepatic septum

Internal herniation of loops of bowel or the mature oviduct caused by developmental or traumatic abnormalities has been reported rarely in the chicken.[43,44] Goodchild described a large number of cases of herniation of the duodenum into the right VHPC in several lines of inbred, adult White Leghorn chickens in England.[43] A smaller number of these birds had herniation of the oviduct into the left VHPC via the posthepatic septum. Some of these chickens even sustained bilateral hernias of the left and right VHPCs. No descriptions of related pathology were given (e.g., hepatic or pancreatic parenchymal changes, intestinal adhesions). The only other report is from Japan, and also involves a single juvenile SPF White Leghorn chicken.[44] The herniation in this young bird was of the duodenum into the right VHPC, which caused a noticeable depression in the surface and reduction in the length of the right lobe of the liver, suggesting entrapment from an early stage of development.

Postsurgical Causes

The unique design of the avian lung–air sac system and the effect this has on the development of the peritoneal cavities make it possible for iatrogenic causes of peritoneal herniation to occur. If surgical intervention leads to disruption of air sac and peritoneal integrity or traumatizes the posthepatic septum, it may be possible for intestinal loops or the oviduct of the female to herniate internally from the IPC into an air sac or the HPC. This appears to have been the case in an ostrich, in which surgical castration led to herniation and entrapment of the bowel within the large ostium of the caudal thoracic air sac.[45]

Traumatic Injuries

Although surprisingly rare, wild birds that collide with vehicles may suffer herniation. It is a testament to the design of the avian "airframe" that traumatic internal injuries are relatively uncommon. The author has most commonly recorded evidence of hemorrhage and fibrin in air sacs or peritoneal membranes without tearing; however, abdominal wall or peritoneal herniation is possible (Figure 8-31).

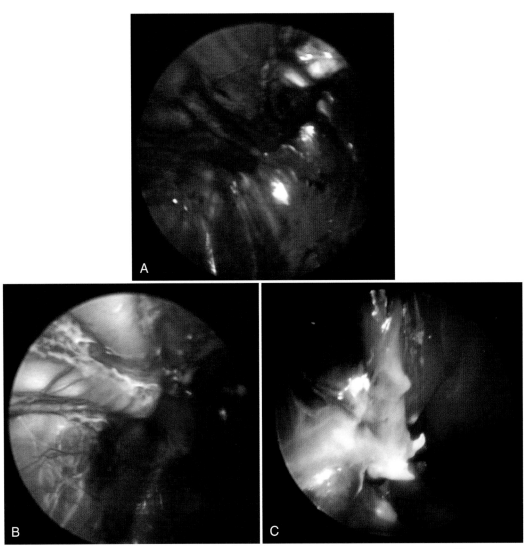

FIGURE 8-31 A, Trauma to the ribs, body wall, and air sac in a trumpeter swan *(Cygnus buccinator).* Note accumulation of fibrin and older hemorrhages. **B,** Another image from the same swan showing neovascularization and fibrin accumulation along ribs. **C,** Rib fracture with hematoma and fibrin accumulation in a red-tailed hawk *(Buteo jamaicensis).*

REFERENCES

1. Goodchild WM: Differentiation of the body cavities and air sacs of Gallus domesticus post mortem and their location in vivo, *Br Poultry Sci* 11:209–215, 1970.
2. Duncker HR: The lung air sac system: A contribution to the functional anatomy of the respiratory apparatus, *Adv Anat Embryol Cell Biol* 45:7–171, 1971.
3. McLelland J, King AS: Aves coelomic cavities and mesenteries. In Getty R, editor: *Sisson and Grossman's the anatomy of the domestic animals,* ed 5, Philadelphia, 1975, W. B. Saunders Co., pp. 1849–1856.
4. Taylor WM: Ventral hepatic and intestinal peritoneal cavities: An endoscopic perspective, *Proc Euro Assoc Avian Vet Utrecht* 132–136, 1993.
5. Taylor WM: Endoscopic examination and biopsy techniques. Sites of application: VHPC and IPC. In Ritchie BW, Harrison GJ, Harrison LR, editors: *Avian medicine: Principles and application,* Lake Worth, FL, 1994, Wingers Publishing, 343:346–347.
6. Duncker HR: Coelomic cavities. In King AS, McLelland J, editors: *Form and function in birds,* Vol 1, London, UK, 1979, Academic Press, pp. 39–67.
7. Bellairs R, Osmond R: *The atlas of chick development,* San Diego, CA, 2005, Elsevier Academic Press, p 77.
8. Duncker HR: Structure of the avian respiratory tract, *Resp Physio* 22:1–19, 1974.
9. Maina JN: What it takes to fly: The structural and functional respiratory refinements in birds and bats, *J Exp Bio* 203:3045–3064, 2000.
10. Maina JN: *The lung-air sac system of birds,* Berlin, Germany, 2005, Springer Verlag.
11. Stern CD: The chick: A great model system becomes even greater, *Dev Cell* 8:9–17, 2005.
12. Jaensch SM, Len Cullen L, Raidal SR: Air sac anatomy of the sulfur crested cockatoo (Cacatua galerita) during isoflurane anesthesia, *J Avian Med Surg* 16(1):2–9, 2002.
13. Krautwald-Junghanns ME, Valerius KP, Duncker HR: CT-assisted versus silicone rubber cast morphometry of the lower respiratory tract in healthy amazons (genus Amazona) and grey parrots (genus Psittacus), *Res Vet Sci* 65:17–22, 1998.
14. Taylor WM: Endoscopic examination and biopsy techniques. In Ritchie BW, Harrison GJ, Harrison LR, editors: *Avian medicine: Principles and application,* Lake Worth, FL, 1994, Wingers Publishing, pp 327–354.

15. Crespo R, Taylor M, Hunter DB: Endoscopic gross anatomy findings of the thoracic air sac of the turkey, *Avian Dis* 42(1):179–181, 1998.

16. Hunter DB, Taylor WM: Lung biopsy as a diagnostic technique in avian medicine, *Proc Assoc Avian Vet* 207–211, 1992.

17. Cook RD, Vaillant C, King AS: The structure and innervation of the saccopleural membrane of the domestic fowl, Gallus gallus: An ultrastructural and immunohistochemical study, *J Anat* 150:1–9, 1987.

18. McLelland J: Pleura, pericardia et peritoneum. In Bamuel JJ, editor: *Handbook of avian anatomy: Nomina anatomica avium*, ed 2, Cambridge, MA, 1993, The Nuttall Ornithological Club, pp 251–256.

19. Kajigaya H, Kamemura M, Tanahara N, et al: The Influence of celomic membranes and a tunnel between celomic cavities on cancer metastasis in poultry, *Avian Diseases* 31(1):176–186, 1987.

20. Campbell TW: Cytology. In Ritchie BW, Harrison GJ, Harrison LR, editors: *Avian medicine: Principles and application*, Lake Worth, FL, 1994, Wingers Publishing, pp 199–222.

21. Krautwald-Junghanns M-E, Schloemer J, Pees M: Iodine-based contrast media in avian medicine, *J Exotic Pet Med* 17(3):189–197, 2008.

22. Vink-Nooteboom M, Schoemaker NJ, Kik MJL, et al: Clinical diagnosis of aneurysm of the right coronary artery in a white cockatoo (Cacatua alba), *J Sm Anim Pract* 39:533–537, 1998.

23. Julian RJ: Ascites in poultry, *Avian Path* 22(3):419–454, 1993.

24. Julian RJ: The response of the heart and pulmonary arteries to hypoxia, pressure and volume. A short review, *Poul Sci* 85(6):1006–1011, 2007.

25. Sedacca CD, Campbell TW, Bright JM, et al: Chronic cor pulmonale secondary to pulmonary atherosclerosis in an African grey parrot, *J Am Vet Med Assoc* 234(8):1055–1059, 2009.

26. Knafo SE, Rapoport G, Williams J, et al: Cardiomyopathy and right-sided congestive heart failure in a red tailed hawk (Buteo jamaicensis), *J Avian Med Surg* 25(1):32–39, 2011.

27. Taylor M: *Polycythemia in the blue and golden macaw—a report of three cases.* Proceedings of the First International Conference of Zoological and Avian Medicine, Turtle Bay, HI, 1987, pp 95–104.

28. Fudge AM, Reavill DR: *Pulmonary artery aneurysm and polycythemia with respiratory hypersensitivity in a blue and gold macaw.* Proceedings of the European Conference of Avian Medicine and Surgery, Utrecht, NL, 1993, pp 382–387.

29. Amann O, Kik MJL, Passon-Vastenburg MH, et al: Chronic pulmonary interstitial fibrosis in a blue-fronted Amazon parrot (*Amazona aestiva aestiva*), *Avian Dis* 51(1):150–153, 2007.

30. Degernes LA, Trasti S, Healy LN, et al: Multicystic biliary adenocarcinoma in a blue and gold macaw (Ara ararauna), *J Avian Med Surg* 12(2):100–107, 1998.

31. Leach S, Heatley JJ, Ransom Pool R, et al: Bilateral testicular germ cell-sex chord-stromal tumor in a Peking duck (Anas platyrhynchos domesticus), *J Avian Med Surg* 22(4):315–319, 2008.

32. Mickley K, Buote M, Kiupel M, et al: Ovarian hemangiosarcoma in an orange-winged Amazon parrot (Amazona amazonica), *J Avian Med Surg* 23(1):29–35, 2009.

33. Strunk A, Imai DM, Osofsky A, et al: Dysgerminoma in an eastern rosella *(Platycercus eximius eximius)*, *Avian Dis* 55:133–138, 2011.

34. Saied A, Beaufrere H, Tully TN, et al: Bilateral seminoma with hepatic metastasis in a cockatiel (Nymphicus hollandicus), *J Avian Med Surg* 25(2):126–131, 2011.

35. Chen S, Bartrick T: Resection and use of a cyclooxygenase-2 inhibitor for treatment of pancreatic adenocarcinoma in a cockatiel, *J Am Vet Med Assoc* 228:69–73, 2006.

36. Hoefer H, Levitan D: Perforating foreign body in the ventriculus of an umbrella cockatoo (Cacatua alba), *J Avian Med Surg* 27(2):128–135, 2013.

37. Harcourt-Brown NH, Gough RE, Drury SE, et al: Serositis in two black-capped conures (Pyrrhura rupicola): A possible viral cause, *J Avian Med Surg* 12(3):178–183, 1998.

38. Cushing TL, Schat KA, States SL, et al: Characterization of the host response in systemic isosporosis (atoxoplasmosis) in a colony of captive American goldfinches (Spinus tristis) and house sparrows (Passer domesticus), *Vet Path* 48(5):985–992, 2011.

39. Hafeez MA, Stasiak I, Delnatte P, et al: Description of two new Isospora species causing visceral coccidiosis in captive superb glossy starlings, Lamprotornis superbus (Aves: Sturnidae), *Parasitol Res* 113(9):3287–3297, 2014.

40. Spalding MG, Forrester DJ: Pathogenesis of Eustrongyloides ignotus (Nematoda: Dioctophymatoidea) in Ciconiformes, *J Wild Dis* 29(2):250–260, 1993.

41. Ziegler AF, Welte SC, Miller EA, et al: Eustrongylidiasis in Eastern Great Blue Herons (Ardea herodias), *Avian Dis* 44(2):443–448, 2000.

42. Bartlett CM, Anderson RC: Lemdana wernaarti and other filarioid nematodes from Bubo virginianus and Asio Otus in Ontario, Canada, with a revision of Lemdana and a key to avian filarioid genera, *Can J Zool* 65:1100–1109, 1987.

43. Goodchild WM: Hernia of the posthepatic septum of Gallus domesticus, *Avian Path* 6:307–311, 1977.

44. Harady M, Sasaki J, Goryo M: Herniation of the duodenum into the right ventral hepatic peritoneal cavity with groove formation at the ventral hepatic surface in a 2-week-old chicken, *J Vet Med Sci* 75(10):1405–1407, 2013.

45. Pye GW: Intestinal entrapment in the right pulmonary ostium after castration in a juvenile ostrich (Struthio camelus), *J Avian Med Surg* 21(4):290–293, 2007.

CHAPTER 9

Clinical Avian Neurology and Neuroanatomy

Susan E. Orosz • Natalie Antinoff

A seizing, or neurologic, patient is a challenge for any veterinarian. Neurologic patients require rapid intervention, frequent assessment, and often, very intensive care. Although serial neurologic examinations may be the most important aspect of determining and modifying treatment and prognosis, the neurologic examination itself can be one of the most challenging aspects of this process. There are many variations in the avian nervous system compared with the mammalian nervous system, at both the anatomic and physiologic levels. We will begin with a discussion of the development and anatomy of the brain and spinal cord in birds, followed by an overview of the clinically relevant differences between birds and mammals as they pertain to the interpretation of the neurologic examination. We will conclude with current recommendations and practical therapeutics for the management of the neurologic or seizing avian patient.

CLINICAL NEUROANATOMY

The central nervous system (CNS) consists of the brain and the spinal cord (Figure 9-1). The peripheral nervous system (PNS) consists of the cranial nerves (CNs), the spinal nerves, and the visceral ganglia and plexi.

Central Nervous System

Brain development and anatomy

The brain of the bird, like those of mammals and reptiles, forms from a hollow tube of ectodermal tissue at the cephalic end of the embryo. This tube folds to form three divisions: the prosencephalon (forebrain), the mesencephalon (midbrain), and the rhombencephalon (hindbrain) (Figure 9-2).

The hindbrain and the midbrain retain homologous structures among the motor and sensory nuclei and the reticular formation. However, the forebrain, consisting of the telencephalon and the diencephalon, has followed a divergent line of evolution.

The telencephalon and diencephalon in birds are completely different from those in mammals. The telencephalon is composed of paired cerebral hemispheres with deep lateral ventricles that contain cerebrospinal fluid (CSF). The nuclei of the telencephalon are responsible for memory and behavior and for integration of motor and sensory information.

The lateral ventricles of the telencephalon come together in the midline to form a single third ventricle that is surrounded by the diencephalon. The diencephalon has a roof that has in the midline the pineal gland or the epiphysis. The majority of the diencephalon is composed of the thalamus and the hypothalamus. The thalamus receives retinal projections, auditory input, and some spinal somatic and visceral pathways. The choroid plexuses are evaginations of blood vessels and supporting cells into the ventricular system to secrete CSF.

The midbrain of the bird has a prominent feature, the optic tectum or the mesencephalic tectum, which surrounds it laterally. This optic tectum or optic lobe represents the superior or dorsal colliculus of mammals and carries visual reflex information. The caudal colliculus is buried beneath the optic lobe and carries sound reflexes. Dorsally and caudally, the midbrain is connected to the cerebellum by way of the superior or rostral cerebellar peduncle. In the dorsal midline is the cerebral aqueduct, which connects the third ventricle to the fourth ventricle of the hindbrain.

The rhombencephalon or the hindbrain contains the metencephalon and the myelencephalon. The metencephalon contains the cerebellum pons and the rostral portion of the fourth ventricle. In general, the cerebellum orchestrates willful motor movement. The myelencephalon becomes the medulla and the caudal portion of the fourth ventricle. The medulla contains the nuclei of a number of CN nuclei (VII to XII), is a reflex center for respiration, and is also a conduction pathway for numerous tracts carrying information to the higher centers and the spinal cord.

The outer surface of the cerebrum in birds has no neocortex. The corresponding structure is known as the *telencephalic complex*, which is located deeply within the cerebral hemispheres. The cerebral cortex of a bird or reptile brain is *lissencephalic*, which means that it is smooth and not punctuated by gyri and sulci (see Figure 9-1).

There is a subarachnoid space between the pia mater and the arachnoid mater, and there is a cistern between the cerebellum and the medulla. However, there are prominent venous sinuses in this region, and so collection of CSF poses a high risk of hemorrhage. There are no lateral foramina (mammalian structures that connect the fourth ventricle with the subarachnoid space). In birds, transfer of water and solutes occurs by diffusion through the roof of the fourth ventricle itself.

Brainstem

There is no obvious pons in the bird, but there are pontine fibers.

CNs V through XII arise from the medulla oblongata, and these nerves arise from two cell columns in the medulla and pons (Figure 9-3). CNs VI and XII arise ventromedially and are somatic motor nerves. CN III also arises ventromedially from the mesencephalon. CNs V and VII through XI arise ventrolaterally, are the equivalents of the dorsal roots of

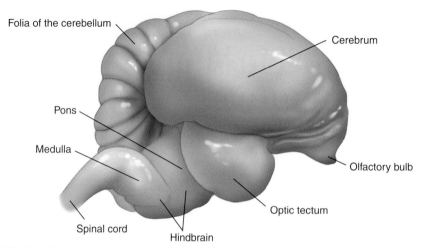

FIGURE 9-1 Side view of a zebra finch, demonstrating the physical external brain. (From Jarvis ED, Gunturkun O, Bruce L, et al: Perspectives. Avian brains and a new understanding of vertebrate brain evolution. The Avian Brain Nomenclature Consortium, *Nat Rev Neurosci* 6:151–159, 2005; with permission.)

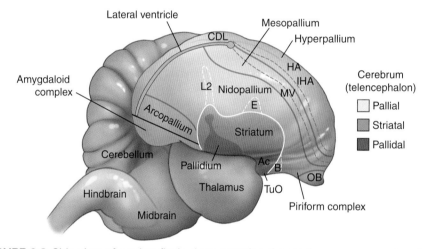

FIGURE 9-2 Side view of a zebra finch, demonstrating the modern consensus view for its structure from the Avian Brian Nomenclature Forum. Ac, Accumbens; B, basorostralis; CDL, dorsal lateral corticoid area; E, entopallium; HA, hyperpallium apicale; IHA, interstitial hyperpallium apicale; L2, field L2; MV, mesopallium ventrale; OB, olfactory bulb: Pt, putamen; TuO, olfactory tubercle. (From Jarvis ED, Gunturkun O, Bruce L, et al: Perspectives. Avian brains and a new understanding of vertebrate brain evolution. The Avian Brain Nomenclature Consortium, *Nat Rev Neurosci* 6:151–159, 2005, with permission.)

spinal nerves, and are primarily somatic afferent, visceral afferent and efferent, and special visceral efferent fibers. (VIII is a special somatic afferent and is the exception.)

Cerebellum

The cerebellum (Figure 9-4) consists of the vermis (center) and paired cerebellar hemispheres on either side of the vermis. The vermis is further subdivided into the rostral, caudal, and flocculonodular lobes. These three lobes are further divided transversely into 10 primary lobules or folia. As in mammals, the cerebellum regulates motor activities of posture and movement. Lesions of the cerebellum can cause tremors, nystagmus, and increases in muscle tone, all corresponding to alterations of posture and movement.

Optic lobe

Also known as the *optic tectum, mesencephalic colliculus,* and *mesencephalic tectum* (see Figure 9-4), the optic lobe lies ventrolaterally on the brainstem and is extremely well developed. It covers the mesencephalon laterally and dorsally. CNs III and IV emerge from the optic lobe. There are six main strata of the optic lobe, which subdivide into 15 layers. Associated with the optic lobe are the auditory and vestibular components that coordinate eye and head movements via the vestibular nuclei. In addition, the midbrain contains the *red nucleus* in the mesencephalon, which gives rise to the rubrospinal tract, and the *intercollicular nucleus* dorsally on the midline, which coordinates motor control of the respiratory and syringeal muscles.

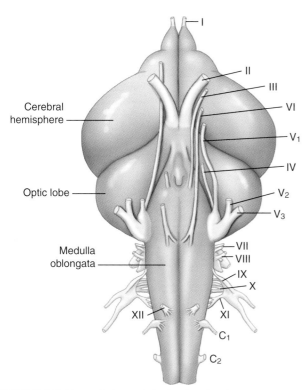

FIGURE 9-3 Ventral view of the brain of a domestic chicken. Cranial nerves (CNs) are represented by roman numerals. CN I and CN II are the first and second cervical spinal nerves. (From King AS, McClelland J: *Birds: their structure and function*, ed 2, Bath, U.K., 1984, Bailliere Tindall, pp 237–314.)

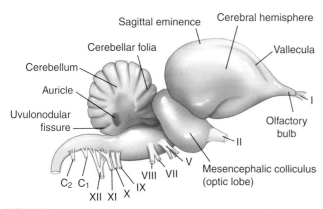

FIGURE 9-4 Lateral view of the brain of a domestic chicken, with cranial nerves indicated. (From King AS, McClelland J: *Birds: their structure and function*, ed 2, Bath, U.K., 1984, Bailliere Tindall, pp 237–314.)

Hypothalamus

The hypothalamus (see Figure 9-3) includes preoptic, paraventricular, supraoptic, and infundibular nuclei, all of which (except the preoptic nucleus) contribute to the hypothalamohypophyseal tract. The hypothalamohypophyseal tract controls autonomic function, thermoregulation, respiration, reproduction, eating and drinking, reproduction, and defensive reactions.

Epithalamus

The epithalamus is a region of the pineal gland involved in reproductive function, and it is strongly responsive to light, even after the eyes have been removed experimentally.

Olfactory lobe

The olfactory lobe (see Figure 9-4) of the cerebrum is smaller in birds compared with that in mammals. The hippocampus, which regulates emotional tone, is at the median fissure. The covering of the cerebrum is only one to two layers thick and forms the outer wall of the lateral ventricle. The hippocampus lies between the lateral ventricles. There is no neocortex in the avian cerebrum. There is a telencephalic complex in birds, a combination of elements in the avian cerebrum for which there is no comparative structure in the mammalian brain. Functionally, the avian telencephalic complex is similar to the mammalian neocortex. Both receive optic, retinal, and auditory projections, and both structures project motor pathways to the hindbrain and the spinal cord.

Spinal cord development

Formation of the spinal cord in chicks begins between 16 and 18 hours of incubation with a cell layer of ectoderm known as the *neural plate*. The cells of the neural plate invaginate to form the neural groove, and the lateral edges elevate to form neural folds. The folds then move together, eventually meeting to form the neural tube. This process begins in the region that will become the brain and continues caudally into the region that will become the spinal cord. Fusion of the neural tube is complete by hour 55 of incubation. The terminal aspect of the neural tube is known as the *rhomboid sinus*.

Before the neural groove closes completely, some cells from the lateral edges detach dorsally and bilaterally to form the neural crest. The neural crest cells begin to migrate ventrally and laterally, eventually developing into dorsal root ganglia and other dorsal and lateral parts of the spinal nerves, along with the sensory ganglia of the CNs, autonomic ganglia, and Schwann cells. These nerve roots begin to form by day 4 of embryonic development.

Dorsal nerve roots develop by medial growth of nerve fibers from the sensory neurons into the dorsolateral region of the spinal cord. This forms the central portion of the nerve, whereas fibers that grow distally from the sensory neurons develop into the peripheral portions of the nerve.

Ventral nerve roots develop from fibers growing outward (laterally) from the ventrolateral region of the spinal cord. These form the motor nerves that conduct motor impulses from the CNS to peripheral muscles. The dorsal and ventral roots fuse to form the spinal nerve.

Sympathetic ganglia develop from some of the neural crest cells and begin to develop on day 4 of embryonic development. Some of these cells become interconnected and continue to form the sympathetic ganglia. These sympathetic ganglia are aggregates of nerve cells along paired "cords" or trunks, which will become the paravertebral sympathetic trunks. Each sympathetic ganglion connects to the spinal cord by the ramus communicans, which eventually will contain both sensory and motor fibers.

Spinal cord anatomy

The spinal cord includes gray matter and white matter that are arranged in essentially the same pattern in birds as in mammals. There is a central region of gray matter that is "butterfly" shaped, although the "horns" or "wings" vary in size among birds. The ventral horn is larger than the dorsal horn, particularly in the cervical and lumbosacral enlargements. In addition, birds have marginal nuclei that surround the outer margins of the "butterfly" of gray matter. These nuclei appear to be ventral commissural neurons that project information from one side of the cord to the other. It is thought that they may represent multisynaptic neurons that transmit nonlocalizing pain fibers up and down the column.[1]

The *white matter* surrounds the gray matter. The white matter can be subdivided into the dorsal, lateral, and ventral columns, based on its anatomic location with relation to the horns of the gray matter. When compared with those in mammals, the ventral and lateral columns in birds are much larger, and the dorsal column is much smaller. This implies that the nerves in the dorsal column may be much shorter in birds than in mammals.

The spinal cord of birds is of the same length as the vertebral column.[2] Thus, the spinal cord segment is at the same level as the vertebral column segment. Spinal nerves pass laterally through the vertebral foramina rather than caudally as they do in mammals. There are generally two enlargements of the spinal cord, with most birds having a cervical enlargement and a lumbosacral enlargement. Birds that fly have a cervical enlargement that is more pronounced than their lumbosacral enlargement. The internal vertebral venous plexus of birds runs the entire length of the vertebral column.[2]

Birds have a unique structure in their lumbosacral cord.[2-4] The dorsal columns separate, and the space created contains a structure called the *glycogen body*. This consists of a collection of periependymal glycogen cells with nests of argentaffin cells. In addition, there are a number of nerve terminals that are basically of two anatomic types. These two types of nerve fibers may play a role in regulating vascular reflexes and are believed to have a neurosecretory role.[4]

The meninges consist of pia mater, arachnoid, and dura mater as in mammals.[2] However, in birds, the dura mater is separated from the periosteal lining, forming an epidural space in the cervical and thoracic regions. This space is filled with a gelatinous tissue that is believed to act as a shock absorber. Another unique feature of birds is that the internal vertebral venous plexus runs the entire length of the vertebral column. This venous plexus is connected to the venous drainage of the kidney and may transmit infectious agents or tumor cells to other parts of the body.

The Long Ascending Pathways

The *dorsal column* (fasciculus gracilis and fasciculus cuneatus of mammals) (Figure 9-5) consists of a collection of white matter fibers that originate from afferent neurons, whose cell bodies are in the dorsal root ganglion. The information transmitted from the body wall transmits touch, pressure, and kinesthesia or proprioception of the joints. These modalities are arranged somatotopically in the dorsal column. Information from the caudal region is carried medially in the column, whereas the more proximal areas are more lateral. Many of the axons are short or move to another location in the cord.

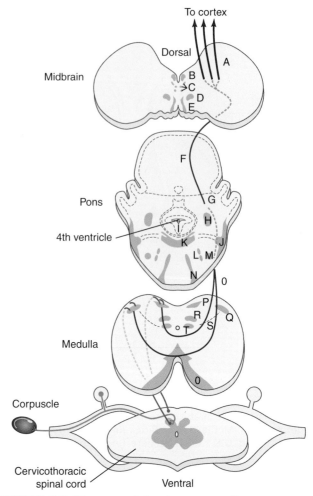

FIGURE 9-5 Diagram of the long ascending tracts concerned with conscious proprioception. These tracts (fasciculus gracilis and fasciculus cuneatus) comprise the dorsal column of the spinal cord. They are believed to carry information on discriminative touch and pressure and kinesthesia (sense of position and movement) to the nucleus gracilis and the nucleus cuneatus in the medulla. The secondary fibers form the medial lemniscus, which decussates in the medulla and ascends in the ventromedial brainstem. These fibers terminate primarily in the thalamus and secondarily in the mesencephalon and ventral hypothalamus. The thalamic nuclei (dorsolateral caudal nuclei) are relay nuclei that project to the telencephalon (hyperstriatum and neostriatum). It is here that the bird can perceive and discriminate touch, pressure, and sense of position and movement. **A,** Rostral cerebellar peduncle. **B,** Edinger-Westphal nucleus concerned with parasympathetic supply to the eye. **C,** Oculomotor nuclei. **D,** Red nucleus. **E,** Cranial nerve III (CN III), or oculomotor nerve. **F,** Cerebellum. **G,** Caudal cerebellar peduncle. **H,** Lateral vestibular nucleus. **I,** Lingual lobe, cerebellum. **J,** Medial lemniscus. **K,** CN abducens nucleus. **L,** CN VIII, facial nucleus. **M,** Superior olivary nucleus. **N,** CN VIII, or facial nerve; **O,** Medial lemniscus. **P,** Nucleus gracilis. **Q,** Nucleus cuneatus. **R,** Dorsal motor nucleus of the vagus. **S,** CN X, or vagus nerve. **T,** Hypoglossal nucleus. Cross-sectional slices were redrawn from a chicken.

These fibers end in the nucleus gracilis or the nucleus cuneatus in the distal end of the medulla. Axons ascend as the medial lemniscus and end in the thalamus. The thalamic projections ascend to the hyperstriatum and neostriatum of the telencephalon, where the bird can perceive touch and pressure and discriminate its location.

Fibers from the *dorsal ascending bundle* (dorsal spinocerebellar tract of mammals) (Figure 9-6) in birds send information from the muscle receptors to the cerebellum from the same side of the body (ipsilaterally). This information concerned with unconscious proprioception is confined to the wing.[2,3,5]

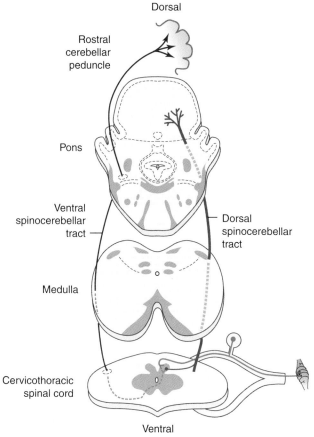

FIGURE 9-6 Diagram of the long ascending tracts transmitting unconscious proprioception to the cerebellum. The dorsolateral ascending bundle can be likened to the dorsal spinocerebellar tract. Information comes into the spinal cord from Golgi tendon organs and muscle spindles, where it synapses in a nucleus homologous to the Clarke column in mammals. The fibers of the tract ascend on the same side where the information was obtained. The tract enters the cerebellum through the caudal cerebellar peduncle on the ipsilateral side. It is believed that the information transmitted is confined to the wing. The other tract represents the ventrolateral ascending bundle or the ventral spinocerebellar tract of mammals. It is confined to information from the distal portion of the body, primarily the pelvic limb. This is a double-crossed system. The tract decussates once when it enters the spinal cord and again when it enters the cerebellum through the rostral cerebellar peduncle. The cross-sectional slices were redrawn from the spinal cord of a chicken.

The *ventrolateral ascending bundle* (ventral spinocerebellar tract of mammals) of fibers[1-3,6] (see Figure 9-6) comprises the activated muscle afferents of the hindlimb. The fibers decussate (or cross) to ascend as the ventrolateral ascending bundle. The fibers cross again in the rostral cerebellar peduncle. Like the dorsolateral system, the information concerning unconscious proprioception of the body is believed to be organized ipsilaterally with respect to the cerebellar hemispheres. The information that is transmitted to the cerebellum is then used to formulate a plan for motor activity of the body.[5]

The fibers in the *dorsolateral fasciculus* (tract of Lissauer or lateral spinothalamic tract), which are concerned with pain, temperature, and light touch, synapse in the substantia gelatinosa, decussate, and then ascend in the lateral column of the spinal cord and brainstem to the thalamus. In pigeons, this tract appears to transmit tactile information only.[7]

The *propriospinal system* (fasciculus proprius)[3,4,7] consists of short polysynaptic fibers that ascend up the spinal cord to the reticular formation. This system is concerned with vague sensations of pain that are nonlocalized.

The Long Descending Pathways

The long descending pathways of birds are not as well known as the long ascending pathways. Many of the tracts are long spinal–spinal pathways.

Lateral reticular tract (lateral reticulospinal tract of mammals)

This motor tract[1,2,6] (Figure 9-7) originates in the reticular formation of the brainstem and ends at the nucleus intermedius, which represents the preganglionic cell bodies of the autonomic motor system in mammals and is concerned with visceral motor function in birds.[5]

Rubrospinal tract (rubrospinal tract of mammals)

This motor tract[1-3,6] (Figure 9-8) originates in the red nucleus of the mesencephalon and ends near the α-motoneurons in the ventral horn of gray matter. These fibers enhance the flexor tone of skeletal muscles.[5]

Corticospinal tract (pyramidal tract of mammals)

This tract (see Figure 9-7) consists of a long tract from the archistriatum in the forebrain and decussates in the pyramids to provide upper motor neuron (UMN) input to the motoneurons within the ventral horn of the cervical region only.[5]

Vestibulospinal tract (vestibulospinal tracts of mammals)

The vestibulospinal tract[1,2,6] (see Figure 9-8) can be divided into two tracts: a medial tract and a lateral tract. These tracts stimulate the extensor tone of skeletal muscles. They arise, in part, from the medial longitudinal fasciculus, a tract that coordinates eye movement. Flight and the ability to move freely in three-dimensional space would require the bird to be able to coordinate eye and body movements quickly.[5]

Reticulospinal tract (medial reticulospinal tract of mammals)

The reticulospinal tract[1,2,6] arises from the pontine reticular nuclei and functions to alter somatic and visceral motor tone.

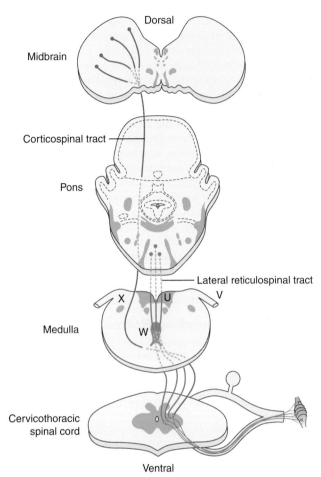

FIGURE 9-7 Motor pathways of the bird. The two tracts diagrammed are the cerebrospinal tract and the lateral reticulospinal tract. The former is concerned with willful movement and is believed to originate in the archistriatum of the telencephalon, where it descends in the ventral brainstem to decussate in the medulla. It then continues in the dorsal and ventral columns in the cervical region of the cord. It goes principally to segments concerned with the wing. It ends on the α-motoneurons in these segments. The lateral reticulospinal tract is not concerned with skeletal muscle but instead with smooth or visceral muscle. Fibers originate in the reticular formation to form the lateral reticulospinal tract. They end in the area of the nuclear intermedius, the preganglionic cell bodies of the autonomic nervous system. U, Medial vestibular nucleus; V, CN VIII; W, medial longitudinal fasciculus; X, descending vestibular nucleus. The cross-sectional slices were redrawn from a chicken.

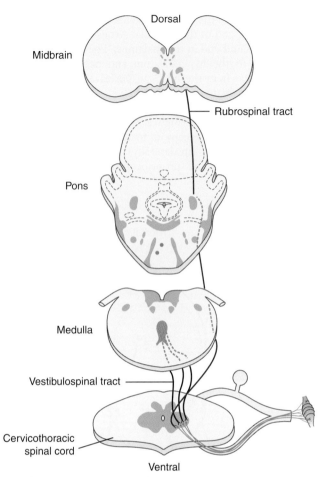

FIGURE 9-8 The motor pathways influencing tone of the skeletal muscles. In addition to the cerebrospinal tract concerned with willful movement, there are other tracts that affect tone. The rubrospinal tract enhances flexor tone. The tract originates in the red nucleus of the mesencephalon, where it decussates to descend in the lateral funiculus of the spinal cord. Fibers end in close proximity to the α-motoneurons. The vestibulospinal tract is subdivided into a ventral or medial tract and a lateral one. These tracts originate in the area of the vestibular nuclei of the medulla and run the length of the spinal column in the ventral funiculus. These two tracts enhance flexor tone. The cross-sectional slices were redrawn from a chicken.

Tectospinal tract (tectospinal tract of mammals)

This tract[1,2,6] originates in the optic tectum and coordinates reflex movements between the eyes and the upper body, particularly the neck.

Spinal nerves

Spinal nerves arise from the spinal cord. There is a ventral motor root and a dorsal sensory root for each nerve. Sensory ganglia are present in each dorsal root. The dorsal and ventral roots fuse and then exit the spinal canal, dividing into a dorsal ramus (branch) and a ventral ramus. The dorsal ramus supplies the muscles on the dorsal part of the body (back, dorsal muscles, and skin); and the ventral ramus supplies the ventral muscles and skin of the ventral body wall. The ventral ramus also communicates with the sympathetic portion of the autonomic nervous system. Spinal nerves (once they exit the spinal canal) are mixed sensory and motor nerves. Avian spinal nerves contain two types of sensory fibers and two types of motor fibers. The sensory fibers are the general somatic afferents (impulses to the CNS from the surface receptors and proprioceptors in muscles and tendons) and the general visceral afferents (from the visceral organs). The motor fibers are the general somatic efferents (from the CNS to skeletal muscle) and the general visceral efferents, which are autonomic fibers that conduct impulses to smooth muscle, cardiac muscle, and glands.

The number of spinal nerves varies among birds, but the spinal nerves exit laterally and supply the muscles and viscera in the immediately corresponding region of the body. This is in contrast to mammals, in which spinal nerves exit the spinal cord and then travel caudally through one to three vertebrae before supplying their corresponding muscles or organs. The chicken has 15 pairs of cervical nerves, 7 pairs of thoracic nerves, and 14 pairs of lumbosacral nerves. The spinal cord in birds extends the entire length of the vertebral column and has no cauda equina or filum terminale.

The numbering of spinal nerves in a bird depends on the number of vertebrae. For the cervical spinal nerves, the nerves exit the vertebral canal cranial to the correspondingly numbered vertebra, except for the last cervical nerve, which exits caudal to the last cervical vertebra. Therefore, there will always be one more cervical spinal nerve than the total number of cervical vertebra. The thoracic nerves then exit the vertebral canal caudal to the corresponding vertebra and rib, and the emerging intercostal nerves run along the caudal border of the rib.

THE AVIAN NEUROLOGIC EXAMINATION

The correct assessment of any neurologic patient is challenging, and the avian patient is certainly no exception. Perhaps the most challenging aspect in birds is adapting the standard tests used for mammals and finding an appropriate method or technique for performing these tests in birds. Once these diagnostics are performed, then the interpretation is also dependent on a thorough understanding of the nerves and their pathways of innervation.

There are six main features to assess in any neurologic examination: mentation, cranial nerves, posture and gait, postural reaction, spinal reflexes, and sensation (cutaneous sensation and deep pain).

Mentation

When assessing mentation, both the *level* and the *content* of consciousness, as well as the appropriateness for the surroundings, have to be considered. Changes may be manifested as personality, changes in awareness, or inappropriate behavioral responses. As an example, any bird, when in an examination room, should be alert and attempting to look aware; a bird that is fluffed and hiding its head and does not respond differently to the presence of a stranger has an altered *level* of consciousness. Delirium or lack of recognition of the owner represents an altered *content* of consciousness. In general, the level is mediated by the brainstem, and the content is affected by the cerebral cortex.[8] To further categorize mentation, it is necessary to define (or review) some of the basic neurologic terms.

Level of consciousness

Alert–demonstrates normal awareness of surroundings.
Lethargic–aware but slightly sluggish responses.
Depressed–decreased responses to environmental stimuli; sleeping when undisturbed.
Obtunded–decreased responses to environmental stimuli; sleeping even in strange surroundings, but easily roused.
Stuporous–requires noxious stimuli to elicit awareness of surroundings.

Comatose–no awareness of surroundings; voluntary responses cease; only reflex activity remains.
Note: Depression and lethargy are generally metabolically induced changes, whereas obtunded, stuporous, or comatose states indicate changes to the cerebrum or brainstem.[8]

Content of consciousness

Categories may be characterized as confusion, dementia, or delirium. *Dementia* is defined as having little awareness of or concern for surroundings (e.g., flying into walls). *Delirium* signifies overresponsiveness to stimuli, such as hyperexcitability in reaction to the owner or familiar situations. These states may indicate structural or metabolic damage to the cerebrum.[8]

The mental awareness of the patient can be determined, in part, from the historical answers of the owners. The state of awareness of the mammalian patient is affected primarily by the reticular activating system, the cerebral cortex, and the subcortical nuclei. These neuropathways that alter the state of awareness in mammals are likely similar to those in birds. Intracranial disease affecting these structures will result in mental depression. However, extracranial causes can secondarily affect the CNS. Examples include hypoglycemia and hepatoencephalopathy. Hyperexcitability is nonspecific but can occur with meningoencephalitis, which can be a consequence of avian bornavirus.

Cranial Nerve Examination

Examination of the cranial nerves is important to determine whether the brain and/or the brainstem are involved and to localize the lesion. Central pathways of CNs I and II travel through the telencephalon and diencephalon, whereas the remaining CNs have their respective nuclei in the brainstem. Because the examination relies primarily on reflexes, it is difficult to distinguish whether the lesion involves specific nuclei or the nerve. Often lesions within the brainstem affect the mental status of the patient because of involvement of the reticular activating system. In addition, motor tracts and/or sensory tracts are often involved. Patients with brainstem lesions commonly have abnormalities that affect proprioception, pain localization, and UMN signs. Lesions that affect only the CNs usually do not alter mental status.

CN I—Olfactory

Sensory for smell. The sense of smell is rarely assessed specifically in birds. The only way to determine function is to provide a noxious olfactory stimulus. Changes in appetite may suggest evaluation.[9]

CN II—Optic

Sensory for vision (Figure 9-9). Menace response: difficult to interpret in birds; blink is mediated by mandibular branch of CN V (*orbicularis oculi*) and CN VII. Try to assess vision or perception of object or avoidance of obstacles. Pupillary light response: also requires intact CN III for iris constriction. The papillary light response may be overridden in birds due to presence of striated muscle in iris and voluntary control of papillary constriction and dilation; however, it is possible to assess. Early in the exam, use a bright sudden focal light source aimed toward medial canthus. The consensual

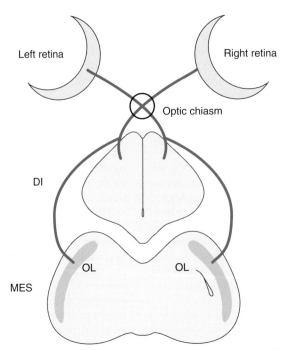

FIGURE 9-9 In the bird, all ganglion cell retinal fibers decussate, traveling to the contralateral side of either the diencephalon (DI) or the large optic lobe of the mesencephalon (MES). This arrangement is unique to birds. The fibers cross at the optic chiasm. OL, Optic lobe.

papillary light response is absent in birds due to complete decussation of optic nerves at the chiasm.[9]

CN III—Oculomotor

Motor and sensory innervation to upper eyelid muscle. Dysfunction: drooping of upper eyelid.

Motor innervation to extrinsic ocular muscle (dorsal). Dysfunction: ventrolateral deviation of globe. Parasympathetic to intrinsic ocular muscle (iris constriction). Involved in papillary light response; responsible for iris constriction; suspect dysfunction if patient seems visual but iris does not constrict. See also CN II (above) for papillary light response and evaluation.[2,9]

CN IV—Trochlear *(Figure 9-10)*

Motor and sensory to extrinsic ocular muscle (ventromedial). Dysfunction: dorsolateral deviation of globe.

CN V—Trigeminal

Trigeminal has three branches: ophthalmic, maxillary, and mandibular (see Figure 9-4). It provides mixed sensory (major sensory nerve for the head) (Figure 9-11) and motor innervation (muscles of mastication.

Ophthalmic—sensory to facial sensation around eye, upper eyelid, cornea, forehead, nares, and upper beak. Dysfunction: lack or loss of sensation to face or beak.

Maxillary—sensory to muscles of the face and mouth, both eyelids, hard palate, and nasal cavity. Dysfunction: lack or loss of sensation to face, beak, and mouth or palate.

Mandibular—motor: lower eyelid, chewing, commissures of beak (3M's: "motor to the muscles of mastication"). Dysfunction: inability to close eye, inability to close beak, diminished beak strength.

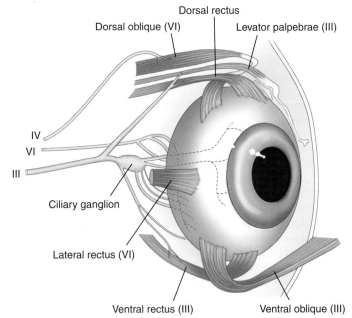

FIGURE 9-10 Schematic distribution of the oculomotor, trochlear, and abducent nerves. Cranial nerve (CN) III, or the oculomotor nerve, innervates the dorsal rectus, levator palpebrae superioris muscle of the upper lid, medial rectus, ventral rectus, and ventral oblique muscles. It also innervates the ciliary ganglion, which provides parasympathetic supply to the smooth muscles of the levator superioris muscle and the ciliary body. The ciliary body of a bird has both smooth muscle and skeletal muscle to control the size of the pupil. The trochlear nerve, CN IV, supplies the dorsal oblique muscle. The muscle is supplied by the contralateral motor nucleus. The abducent nerve (CN VI) supplies the lateral rectus muscle and the two muscles of the third eyelid, the quadratus and pyramidalis muscles.

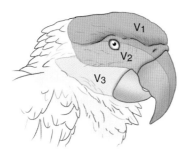

FIGURE 9-11 Regional representation of areas served by the trigeminal nerve, cranial nerve (CN) V. CN V forms three main branches. The ophthalmic nerve, CN V1, receives information from the upper eyelid, the skin of the forehead, and the rostral part of the nasal cavity. The maxillary division, CN V2, receives sensory information from the lower eyelid and the lateral margin of the upper bill. The mandibular division, CN V3, provides motor branches to the muscles of mastication and sensory branches to the skin and mucosa at the rictus and to the lower bill. It also receives sensory information from the sensitive tip of the lower bill.

CN VI—Abducens

Motor and sensory to lateral extrinsic ocular muscles and third eyelid (see Figure 9-10). Dysfunction: loss of function of third eyelid; medial deviation of globe. *Note:* third eyelid dysfunction or prolapse does not indicate Horner syndrome or loss of sympathetic innervation.[9]

CN VII—Facial

Mixed motor and sensory innervation (see Figures 9-3 and 9-4). Motor innervation to muscles of facial expression in mammals, not birds. Dysfunction: lack of response to skin touch/facial sensation; facial droop, or asymmetry. Sensory innervation to taste, which is also shared with CN IX; may be difficult to evaluate. Parasympathetic for many glands of the head (tears, mucous). Dysfunction: decreased secretions.

CN VIII—Vestibulocochlear

Provides special sensory innervation (see Figures 9-3 and 9-4). Sensory to hearing, balance, and coordination. Dysfunction: difficult to assess hearing in birds; a whistle in room may provide appropriate stimulus. Also provides sensory to vestibular system. Dysfunction: loss of equilibrium. Involved in oculocephalic reflex; normal physiologic nystagmus can be induced by moving the head side to side; fast phase is in the direction of movement. Dysfunction: spontaneous horizontal nystagmus, fast phase away from side of lesion. Dysfunction may also include head tilt and circling toward affected side.

CN IX—Glossopharyngeal

Provides mixed sensory and motor innervation (see Figures 9-3 and 9-4). Sensory to tongue, taste, and trachea. Dysfunction: decrease/loss of taste (unreliable to test); lack of tongue sensation. Also provides motor innervation to the pharynx, larynx, crop, and syrinx. Dysfunction: dysphagia, possible loss of voice, and gag reflex (difficult to assess). *Note:* Anastomoses with CN X; assess together.

CN X—Vagus

Provides mixed sensory and motor innervation (see Figures 9-3 and 9-4). Sensory to the larynx, pharynx, and viscera. Dysfunction causes regurgitation. Motor innervation to the larynx, pharynx, esophagus, and crop. Dysfunction: regurgitation, vocal dysphonia, possible loss of voice, and loss of the gag reflex (difficult to assess). Parasympathetic innervation to glands and viscera. Dysfunction: lack of rhythmic visceral or gastric contractions or increased heart rate. *Note:* Anastomoses with CN IX; assess together.

CN XI—Accessory

Provides motor innervation to the superficial neck muscles and the cranial scapula muscles (see Figures 9-3 and 9-4). Dysfunction: poor neck mobility and lateral deviation of the scapula (not generally clinically detectable).

CN XII—Hypoglossal

Provides motor innervation to the tongue, trachea, and syrinx. Dysfunction: deviation of the tongue, decreased tone of the tongue, change in or absence of song.

Clinical Notes on Cranial Nerve Examination

The visual system

The visual system includes CNs II, III, IV, and VI. To add the menace test, CN V has been included. Birds have voluntary control of pupillary constriction and dilation. It may be necessary to inhibit the skeletal muscles that constrict the iris with a skeletal muscle inhibitor such as tubocurarine to see the retina clearly. However, placing the bird in a darkened room may help. When Amazon parrots become excited, they will often alternately dilate and constrict their pupils. Pupillary constriction is controlled by both the voluntary motor and parasympathetic portions of CN III, whereas dilation is considered to be under voluntary and sympathetic control. Therefore, there may be no consensual or directed response when shining a light into each eye. Anisocoria may be the result of a lesion in the optic nerve or the oculomotor nerve. However, electrodiagnostic tests may be used in birds to determine whether CN II is intact.

In mammals, loss of sympathetic innervation to the face results in Horner syndrome. This is characterized by anisocoria, with miosis on the side of the lesion. In addition, there is ptosis, or drooping of the upper lid, as well as enophthalmos and protrusion of the third eyelid. In birds, there are smooth muscle fibers in the upper lid. However, it is unknown whether birds will develop clinically detectable signs of Horner syndrome if the sympathetic nerve supply to the facial area is damaged.

Cochlear function is tested by examining the patient's response to a sudden loud noise. Usually birds are less rousable. Electrodiagnostic testing would be helpful in determining a diagnosis.

With vestibular disease, it is important prognostically to determine whether the lesion is central or peripheral. Central disease involves the brainstem and carries a poorer prognosis than peripheral disease. Central lesions are often associated with changes in mental status, postural reaction deficits on the ipsilateral side of the lesions, and possibly other cranial nerve deficits. Vertical nystagmus is associated with brainstem lesions. Peripheral vestibular signs are often restricted to horizontal or rotatory nystagmus that does not change with changes in the position of the head. Most often, the slow component is ipsilateral to the side of the lesion. Postural reactions in mammals may appear to be affected because the patient may have ipsilateral hypotonia and contralateral hypertonia of the limbs. This most likely would occur in birds as well because they have similar neurocircuitry.

Posture and Gait

Postural responses are responsible for maintaining the body in an upright position and the use of the limbs in maintaining this position. The sensory and motor receptors in the PNS transmit information to and from the CNS, which interprets input and directs the appropriate response, translating impulses into actions. Interference in these pathways can occur in the lower motor neuron, the upper motor neuron, or in the brain itself. Generalized weakness or recumbency is nonspecific and may involve either the metabolic or the neurologic pathways.

The patient should be observed in its cage or at rest in a comfortable environment. In a normal posture, the perching bird species can stand on its perch appropriately with its head erect. The presence of a head tilt or a twisting of the body is considered abnormal. Postural changes may occur with vestibular or cerebellar disease or asymmetrical lesions of the cervical spinal cord.

Purposeful coordinated movement requires an intact extrapyramidal system. Birds rely heavily on the motor pathways outside the pyramidal system. Lesions from the brainstem caudally result in gait disturbances characterized by ataxia, paresis, or even paralysis.

Ataxia or lack of muscle coordination can result from lesions within the proprioceptive or sensory pathways, the vestibular system, or the cerebellum.[8] The proprioceptive pathways are either conscious pathways (fasciculus gracilis or cuneatus) or unconscious ones (dorsal and ventral spinocerebellar tracts). Lesions that affect those tracts are often described as producing sensory ataxia. For example, knuckling is considered to result from lesions in the conscious proprioceptive pathways. Lesions in the spinocerebellar tracts are associated with a greater degree of ataxia than those seen with the fasciculus gracilis or cuneatus. Often ataxia will not be observed when there are lesions affecting the motor systems. However, when there are selective lesions of the motor systems, the animal will exhibit paresis or paralysis without ataxia.

Lower motor neuron

Lesions affecting the nerve in the PNS, within the pathway connecting the muscle or limb to the CNS, will lead to loss of muscle power, decreased or absent reflexes, and flaccidity.

Upper motor neuron

Lesions in the CNS will cause increased muscle tone and rigidity in the muscles distal to the lesion. Lesions in the thoracic region of the spinal cord will cause hyperreflexia and rigidity in the pelvic limbs, but the wings will remain normal. Cervical lesions will cause these signs in all four limbs.

Brain

Opisthotonus is caused by an upper motor neuron lesion of the cerebellum or brainstem. *Decerebrate rigidity* involves extension of all four limbs and trunk, caused by a lesion of the rostral brainstem.

Vestibular system

The vestibular system also has central and peripheral components, which function in the same way as the peripheral nerves. The sensory and motor receptors are in the PNS, and the central vestibular system translates the inputs to enable the body, eyes, and limbs to respond. Abnormalities will manifest as nystagmus, head tilt, rolling, circling, and sometimes leaning to one side. A wide-based stance may also indicate vestibular disease.

Central vestibular system disease

Peripheral input is normal but the CNS is unable to respond or maintain appropriate eye, limb, or body position. Nystagmus is positional. Vertical or rotary nystagmus can only be present with central vestibular disease. (Horizontal nystagmus can exist with either central or peripheral lesions.) Proprioceptive deficits and sometimes changes in mentation are present.

Peripheral vestibular system disease

Horizontal nystagmus, fast phase away from the lesion, but no proprioceptive deficits or changes in mentation. Head tilt and circling may be present. Evaluation of gait involves assessment of both coordination and strength. Both voluntary and involuntary movements require the cerebral, cerebellar, vestibular, and proprioceptive pathways.

Cerebral lesion

Voluntary movement: lack of precise or finely tuned movement; may miss perches or be unable to move in certain directions. Involuntary movements: seizures, muscle tremors.

Cerebellar lesion

Voluntary movement: hypermetric or hypometric movements of limbs. Involuntary movements: intention tremors.

Vestibular lesion

Falling, loss of balance, circling.

Proprioceptive lesion

Paralysis or paraplegia of limbs.

Postural Reactions

These reactions have not been studied in birds, but generalities can be assumed. The placing reaction, for example, can be modified for birds. In this test in mammals, the patient is moved toward the edge of a horizontal surface and the thoracic limbs are brushed against it. Normal mammals will quickly lift their forelimbs and place them on top of the horizontal surface. This test is often performed on each of the forelimbs independently, with the patient's eyes first covered and then uncovered. Birds, particularly raptors, could be hooded and placed on a low perch. Another perch could be brought toward them, slightly higher so that the surface touches the feet. With psittacine birds, it would be very difficult to blindfold or hood the bird in order to perform this test. However, it could be easily performed observationally.

Another proprioceptive test that can be used to assess the thoracic limb would be the return of the wing to its normal flexed position after pulling it away from the body from different positions. This test would meet the requirements for a postural reaction.[9]

Spinal Reflexes

Spinal reflexes are used in conjunction with postural reactions to localize lesions to either the CNS or the PNS. Spinal reflexes are elicited by the sensory nerves transmitting impulses to the spinal cord and the motor nerves responding to the impulses. This reflex arc is independent of the brain, though the brain may modulate the response. The reflex response helps define whether the lesion represents a deficit of the UMN or the lower motor neuron (LMN) of the PNS. A LMN deficit results from a problem with the final common pathway or the ventral gray horn of the spinal cord. This pathway includes the motor root and the spinal nerve, the motor endplate, and the muscle fibers of the particular reflex being tested.

As discussed above, LMN lesions lead to hyporeflexia and diminished or absent responses, and UMN lesions lead to hyperreflexia. LMN lesions involve the reflex arc; UMN lesions involve the CNS proximal to the reflex arc. The standard scale of 0–4 used in companion animals is also used in birds, where 2 = normal, 3 = hyperreflexic, 4 = clonic, 1 = hyporeflexic, and 0 = absent.[8,9]

Clinical note: Muscle tone of each of the thoracic and pelvic limbs should be examined when the spinal reflex tests are performed. Each limb should be manipulated passively, and each of the muscle masses of the long bones palpated in order to detect atrophy. The limbs should be flexed and extended to determine differences in muscle tone. Rarely will the examiner be able to observe muscle fasciculations, but these abnormalities are important findings, if present. Differences in muscle tone are graded as increased, normal, or decreased for each limb.

There may be an increased resistance to manipulation of the limb. This can occur with lesions of the UMN system, increased facilitation of the efferent pathway, and alterations in muscle movement. It may be difficult to separate increased muscle tone from restriction of muscle movement from some mechanical cause. In addition to UMN disease causing increased tone, tone may be increased with muscle irritation or decreased inhibition of the intact LMN pathways. A perceived increase in tone may result from chronic LMN disease and muscle replacement with connective tissue. An example of a disease that results in increased muscle rigidity not of UMN origin is tetanus.

Muscle tone can be decreased with both UMN and LMN disease. However, decreased muscle tone is associated more commonly with LMN problems.

The standard myotactic reflex tests used in mammals are difficult to perform in birds. Extension of the wing and noxious stimulation of the distal wing should result in retraction. This wing withdrawal can be interpreted as a reflex of the thoracic limb. The pedal or pelvic limb withdrawal reflex is similar to that of mammals. Noxious stimulation of the digits should result in flexion of the pelvic limb. A crossed extensor reflex may occur when flexor reflexes are examined. This results in extension of the opposite limb when the one tested flexes because of a noxious stimulus. Crossed extensor reflexes occur with UMN lesions and are associated with severe lesions of the spinal cord.[8-10]

The cloacal reflex of birds is similar to the perineal reflex of mammals. A noxious or tactile stimulation of the area around the vent will result in contraction of the external sphincter muscles of the vent and ventral flexion of the tail.[10] This requires the pudendal nerves to be intact.

There are varying numbers of spinal nerves in different species of birds. There are small dorsal roots and large ventral roots and brachial and lumbosacral plexuses. In birds, the peripheral nerves emerge directly from the spinal cord segment, rather than several segments caudally, as is seen in mammals.[2] For spinal cord evaluation, the spinal cord can be divided into several anatomically evident regions: the cervical region, the brachial plexus, and the caudal region.

The *brachial plexus* innervates the wing.[2] Assessment includes wing withdrawal, which involves a pinch to a digit and replacement of the wing to the normal position.

The *distal spinal cord* includes the lumbosacral plexus, which includes the *lumbar plexus*, the *sacral plexus*, and the *pudendal plexus*.[2]

- *Lumbar plexus*—innervates leg; located in region of cranial renal division. Assessment: patellar reflex; gastrocnemius reflex (tibial branch).
- *Sacral plexus*—innervates leg; located in region of middle renal division. Assessment: withdrawal reflex in response to a toe pinch. LMN damage: decreased or absent withdrawal. UMN damage: crossed extensor reflex in contralateral limb.
- *Pudendal plexus*—innervates tail, vent sphincter, cloaca; located in region of caudal renal division. Assessment: vent sphincter reflex. LMN damage: flaccid sphincter and cloaca. UMN damage: hypertonic vent.

Sensory Examination

Evaluation of the sensory systems is important in localizing a lesion as well as in determining a prognosis. Unfortunately, it is difficult in birds to evaluate and localize temperature changes and light touch along the trunk. Information is transmitted by the spinothalamic tracts for the conscious perception of and ability to localize temperature, pain, and light touch.

The flexor response of the limb to a noxious stimulus is a reflex. It requires sensory input and a motor response. These flexor responses appear to be present in birds as well as in mammals. However, the conscious perception of pain is transmitted by the spinothalamic tracts to the thalamus and the telencephalon, where these centers localize the painful stimulus. In addition, deep pain that is nonlocalized is transmitted by a multisynaptic pathway of unmyelinated fibers. Therefore, loss of deep pain is associated with severe spinal cord disease. This most commonly occurs with compression. Compressive lesions, in general, cause loss of conscious and unconscious proprioception first, followed by loss of motor function and then superficial pain, and, last, deep pain. For

BOX 9-1 NEUROLOGIC EXAMINATION CHECKLIST FOR BIRDS

1. HISTORY
   a. When did the owner first notice clinical signs?
   b. What was the first sign? The next signs?
   c. What is the bird's mental status during an episode? Before? After?
   d. Were any treatments administered? What was the result?
   e. How long has the pet been in the current condition?
2. MENTATION
   a. Level of consciousness
      Alert (Normal)
      Lethargic (Slightly sluggish)
      Dull/depressed (Quiet, decreased responses; sleeping when undisturbed)
      Obtunded (Aware but not interested in the environment/ sleeping in strange surroundings; rousable only when stimulated)
      Stuporous (Only responds to noxious stimulation)
      Comatose (Unresponsive even to noxious stimulus; reflex activity only)
   b. Content of consciousness
      Confusion
      Dementia (Decreased awareness of surroundings)
      Delirium (Hyperexcitable or hyperresponsive to familiar things)
3. POSTURE AND GAIT/DESCRIPTION (Normal stance? Ambulatory, ataxia, paresis, what limbs affected?)
   General: _____
   Forelimbs (Wing position and strength): _____
   Hindlimbs: _____
4. CRANIAL NERVE EXAMINATION/DESCRIPTION (Normal or abnormal; describe if abnormal)
   Menace response: Right (R)_____ Left (L)_____ (Avoidance of obstacles, following a bright object) (CN II)
   Pupillary light reflex (+ or −): Direct only in birds: R___ L___ (CN II, III)
   Facial symmetry: _____

Facial sensation: Normal ____ Abnormal _____ (Eye, nares, upper beak, palate) (CN V)
Facial expression: Normal _____ Abnormal _____ (CN V)
Palpebral reflex: R_____ L_____ (CN V)
Ocular position: R_____ L_____
   Upper eyelid position: Normal _____ Abnormal _____ (CN III)
   Ventrolateral deviation: Y_____ N _____ (CN III)
   Dorsolateral deviation: Y_____ N _____ (CN IV)
   Medial deviation: Y_____ N _____ (CN VI)
   Nictitans function: Normal _____ Absent _____ (CN VI)
Ocular nystagmus (Physiologic present) Y_____ N _____
Ocular nystagmus (Pathologic, direction of fast phase) _____ (CN VII)
Head tilt present: Y_____ N _____ Direction/position _____
Gag reflex: Y_____ N _____ (CN IX, X, XII)
Tongue position: Normal _____ Abnormal _____ (CN XII)
5. PROPRIOCEPTION – scale: 0 (absent); 1 (decreased); 2 (normal)
   Conscious proprioception (Foot and digit placement): RH___ LH___
   Table top testing: RH___ LH___
   (Placement of limbs when brought to table edge)
   Hopping: RH_____ LH_____
   Wing strength: RF _____ LF _____
   Wing withdrawal: RF _____ LF_____
6. SPINAL REFLEXES – scale: 0 (absent); 1 (decreased); 2 (normal); 3 (increased); 4 (clonic)
   Withdrawal: RF___ RH___ LF___ LH___
   Patellar: RH___ LH___
   Cloacal: ___
7. SENSORY EVALUATION
   Sensation to all feet intact? Y _____ N _____
   Any pain on spinal palpation? Y _____ N _____
   Deep pain present? Y_____ N_____

this reason, loss of deep pain carries the poorest prognosis for return of function.[8,11]

In mammals, pain perception, the presence of hyperesthesia, and the panniculus reflex are used to localize a lesion of the spinal cord. The panniculus reflex may not be present in birds. However, pricking along the trunk and the bird responding by head movement or attempted flight away from a stimulus help localize a lesion along the thoracic and lumbar spinal cord.[10] Hyperesthesia occurs when there is a painful or increased response to a normal stimulation such as touching the area. When this occurs, it is important to distinguish a possible musculoskeletal problem from a nervous one. Non-localized pain can occur with diffuse inflammatory disease of the CNS or the PNS.

Cutaneous Sensation

Evaluation of cutaneous sensation can aid in assessment of the spinal cord as well as localization and severity of injury. Birds lack the panniculus response because of the absence of cutaneous trunci muscles. Instead, feather follicles can be used to assess sensation. The locations of avian dermatomes have not been described.

Deep Pain Sensation

Assessment of deep pain is necessary only when there are abnormalities of gait, spinal reflex, or proprioception. Of all sensory fibers, deep pain fibers are located the deepest in the spinal cord. When evaluating deep pain, there must be conscious awareness of the stimulus. Withdrawal alone is a reflex arc and does not indicate intact deep pain pathways. However, lack of withdrawal and presence of conscious awareness do indicate that deep pain neurons are intact and probably affords a better prognosis than simple withdrawal response.

A summary checklist for neurologic examinations is provided is Box 9-1.

SEIZURES

Seizures are composed of three phases. The phase immediately before the seizure is the *preictal phase*, or *aura*, and is typified by a change in behavior; this phase may not be evident in all patients. The *ictal phase*, or *seizure*, is often manifested by disorientation, with the bird undergoing tonic-clonic convulsions that are associated with extensor rigidity of its wings, legs, and neck. The *postictal phase* is characterized by some type of abnormal behavior. Birds may act lethargic, disoriented, depressed, and restless. This phase may last from seconds to hours, but it often lasts for several minutes.[12,13]

A diagnostic workup for seizures may include a number of tests based on history and physical examination, including a complete blood count; profile and radiography, including skull images; whole blood concentrations of lead; serum concentrations of zinc, acetyl cholinesterase activity, and insecticide residues; inhibition of δ-amino levulinic acid dehydratase (ALAD) activity and blood protoporphyrins; tests for chlamydiosis; *Aspergillus* serologic assays; avian bornavirus testing; electroencephalography; computed tomography; and magnetic resonance imaging.[10]

Acute Treatment for Status Epilepticus or Multiple Seizures in a Short Period

The treatment plan should be based on the diagnosis established and, hence, the underlying cause. The most important aspect to remember, regardless of species or etiology, is to *control the seizures* and *return the patient's body temperature to normal* (see Chapter 17). As in any animal, prolonged seizures may result in permanent changes or deficits, but the extent of these deficits cannot be assessed for several days. Supportive care may be required during that time, including fluid therapy, nutritional support, and sometimes even management of the sedated or debilitated patient, including turning the patient, lubricating the eyes, and physical therapy.

In any seizing patient, it is wise to check the blood glucose and administer a dextrose bolus of 1 to 2 mL/kg of 50% dextrose (dilute 1:1 with saline or lactated Ringer's solution [LRS] to decrease osmolarity) if necessary; however, hypoglycemia is very rare in adult birds. If vascular access is not readily available, or if the animal is actively seizuring, proceed as you would in any other species. Administer diazepam, 0.5 to 1.0 mg/kg.[12,14,15] Administer intravenously if possible, but venous access may be a challenge in seizuring patients. Instead, administer midazolam intramuscularly (same dose). The dose may be doubled if necessary. Diazepam or midazolam can also be absorbed across mucous membranes, so it can be administered cloacally—use double the IM dose for this route of administration.[12,15] This may be preferable to intramuscular administration in some species to enhance absorption.

If a single dose of a benzodiazepine is not effective, it may be repeated every 2 minutes up to three times.[12,13] Diazepam or midazolam can be administered via continuous intravenous (IV) or intraosseous (IO) infusion. Diazepam should be added to IV fluids and the infusion started at a rate of 0.5 to 1 milligram per kilogram per hour (mg/kg/hr).[12,14] If diazepam or midazolam does not control seizures, a constant rate infusion (CRI) of phenobarbital, 2 to 10 mg/kg/hr, is started.[12] This may be given in conjunction with the diazepam; the patient should be monitored closely for respiratory depression. Phenobarbital may also be given as a bolus of 2 to 5 mg/kg. In mammals, this can be repeated every 30 minutes up to a total dose of 20 mg/kg[12]; the author (NA) has used this dosing protocol successfully in avian patients. Intravenous propofol use is recommended in dogs and cats with uncontrolled cluster seizures or status epilepticus. The authors do not advocate its use in seizure management because of the significant risk of respiratory depression and apnea; however, it can be

considered if intubation and ventilation can be provided. The dosage for a bolus in companion animals is 4 to 6 mg/kg intravenously administered at 25% of the dose in increments to help prevent apnea.[12] Propofol can also be used as a CRI at 0.1 to 0.6 mg/kg.[12] If cerebral edema is suspected, mannitol 0.5 to 1.0 g/kg may be administered intravenously over 20 minutes.[14,15] Steroids should not be administered in birds, as they are highly susceptible to the immunosuppressive effects of steroids.

With any of the drugs mentioned, patients may become recumbent and nonresponsive; it is important to recognize that this is not a prognostic indicator. If patients are unresponsive, consider adding dextrose to the IV drip, as these patients may become hypoglycemic if not eating. Gavage feeding may be necessary but must be undertaken with caution because of the risk of passive regurgitation in recumbent patients. The head and neck should be elevated with pillows, towels, or any other means to keep the area above the level of the crop, and the patient should be positioned so there is no direct pressure on the crop after gavage feeding.

Once seizures have stopped for 6 to 12 hours, the CRI infusion is tapered slowly over another 12 to 24 hours. If multiple infusions have been used, it may be necessary to taper one agent at a time. In some instances, the clinician may wish to decrease the dose every 6 hours if close monitoring is available. It may take several days for the full sedative effects of these drugs to wear off enough to enable accurate assessment of the bird's neurologic status.

Long-Term Seizure Control

Once controlled, depending on etiology, phenobarbital can be used for long-term seizure management. Doses of 2 to 10 mg/kg every 12 hours have been used by the authors. Measurement of phenobarbital levels is recommended, although therapeutic levels in birds are not reported. The therapeutic level in dogs is 15 to 45 milligrams per milliliter (mg/mL); blood should be collected in a tube without a serum separator and should be evaluated 3 weeks from initiation of therapy or change of dose.[12] However, the authors have measured these levels in several birds undergoing therapy and have never seen a concentration above 5 mg/mL despite control of seizures, which suggests that lower levels in birds can be equally therapeutic. It is not necessary to increase the dose if seizures are well controlled.

Potassium bromide can be used as a single agent or in addition to other anticonvulsant therapy. A starting dose of 20 to 40 mg/kg every 24 hours can also be used for seizure control.[12,15] Loading dose of 400 to 600 mg/kg divided over several days may be beneficial. In the author's practice, a Grey parrot (*Psittacus erithacus*) received 150 mg/kg every 24 hours with no apparent adverse effects, and dosing of 100 mg/kg every 12 hours has been reported in one bird without apparent adverse effects.[16] In mammals, potassium bromide levels may not reach a steady state for 60 to 90 days, and serum levels of 100 to 300 milligrams per deciliter (mg/dL) are considered to be in the therapeutic range,[12] but these data are not known for birds. Dosages should be adjusted on the basis of blood levels if seizures are not well controlled or if toxicity is suspected.

Levetiracetam (Keppra), a newer drug, binds to a receptor in the brain that helps modulate neurotransmitter release and reuptake. Dosages in dogs and cats are 10 to 20 mg/kg every 8 hours.[12,15] The recommended starting dosage in birds is 10 mg/kg every 8 hours, and doses up to 100 mg/kg every 8 hours have been reported.[16]

Zonisamide (Zonegran) works by a variety of mechanisms for anticonvulsant activity and may also be neuroprotective. In dogs, the dosage is 10 mg/kg every 12 hours, and therapeutic levels are 10 to 40 micrograms per milliliter (μg/mL).[12] This drug has also been used in birds, and dosing up to 20 mg/kg every 8 hours is reported.[16]

Gabapentin and pregabalin (Neurontin, Lyrica) both work by blocking calcium channels and possibly increasing γ-aminobutyric acid (GABA) synthesis. Administration of gabapentin has been investigated in birds by both IV and oral routes, and 15 mg/kg every 8 hours has been proposed as a starting dose based on pharmacokinetic studies.[17] The therapeutic range in dogs is 4 to 16 mg/mL but is unknown for birds.[12] Side effects may include lethargy and sedation. Pregabalin has fewer side effects.

Potential Seizure Etiologies

Many causes have been suggested for seizures in birds. Causes suspected include heavy metal toxicosis, hepatic encephalopathy secondary to liver disease, other metabolic derangements, trauma, and hypocalcemia. Idiopathic epilepsy in red-lored Amazons (*Amazona autumnalis*) may be of genetic origin. Seizures have also been reported in greater Indian hill mynahs (*Gracula religiosa intermedia*), but the cause is unknown. Differentials for seizures in cockatiels include the following: chlamydiosis, heavy metal toxicosis, liver disease resulting in hepatic encephalopathy, and the secondary effects to yolk emboli. Raptors may seize as a result of concussive trauma, hypoglycemia, or systemic diseases, including exposure to neurotoxins.

Nutritional deficiencies have been suggested to cause seizures, particularly in young psittacine birds. Imbalances of calcium, phosphorus, and vitamin D_3, and deficiencies of the B vitamins (B_1 [thiamine], B_2 [riboflavin], B_6 [pyridoxine], and B_{12} [cyanocobalamin]), vitamin E, and selenium have all been implicated as causing seizures.[11]

Other potential etiologies to consider include infectious diseases such as chlamydiosis or proventricular dilatation disease, and paramyxoviral infections. Metabolic issues, including hepatic or renal failure, and vascular and hypoxic events, including atherosclerosis and hyperlipidemia, result in seizures.

Lead toxicosis: acute or chronic

Metal-dense particles may be radiographically evident, but their absence does not rule out nor confirm lead toxicosis. (Mineral densities in ventriculus should not be confused with metal density. Density should be compared with bone for mineral and with a radiopaque marker for metal.) Patients may be presented with clenched feet. Some species may have bloody urine (e.g., Amazon parrots, conures). Treatment includes fluids, supportive care, anticonvulsant drugs, chelation with CaEDTA (calcium–ethylenediaminetetraacetic acid, which can be given intramuscularly or subcutaneously), DMSA (dimercaptosuccinic acid, which is given orally), or D-penicillamine (orally; available at many regular pharmacies). Gavage with bulk feeding, peanut butter, and psyllium

helps eliminate metal from the gastrointestinal (GI) tract. Extreme caution should be used if the patient is regurgitating or vomiting (see Chapter 18).

Renal disease or failure

Renal disease or failure may result from dehydration (prerenal), true renal causes, or infectious agents. Urinary obstruction is extremely rare but may occur in severely egg-bound birds. The patient is treated, similar to other patients, with IV or IO fluids, histamine 2 (H_2) blockers, and supportive care, then it is reassessed. Omega-3 fatty acids and antiinflammatory drugs may be helpful in the management of chronic renal disease.

Hepatic disease

Whether or not hepatic encephalopathy truly occurs in birds is still being debated. Nitrogenous waste is not the end-product of hepatic metabolism in birds as it is in mammals, yet with severe hepatic disease, neurologic signs may be present. The underlying cause should be treated, and managed with supportive care; as with mammals, fluid therapy is vital in a bird with neurologic signs concurrent with hepatic disease or failure. Antimicrobials should be used, as well as B vitamins and lactulose, if infectious agents are suspected. Milk thistle (liquid alcohol-free formulation) and S-adenosylmethionine use may be considered in treatment (see Chapter 4).

Chlamydophila psittaci infection (psittacosis)

Psittacosis is an infectious disease that affects the liver, respiratory system, and CNS (see Chapter 2). Any or all body systems may be involved. The classic description is of a bird with ocular and nasal discharge, green urates, leukocytosis, and hepatic enzyme elevations. However, neurologic signs can occur alone. Seizures should be treated, as in other patients, with supportive care, fluid therapy, nutritional support, and anticonvulsant drugs. *Chlamydophila* infection is treated with doxycycline for 6 weeks or with azithromycin. Enrofloxacin may have partial efficacy in the treatment of this disease but is much less likely to eliminate the disease.

Proventricular dilatation disease

This is an immune-mediated inflammatory viral disease that affects ganglia and nerve fibers, with a predilection for the ganglia of the proximal GI tract, cerebellar nuclei, and other brain or brainstem components. Avian bornavirus (ABV) has been causally implicated (see Chapters 2 and 11). The classic disease form is intestinal, with whole seeds passing in droppings, weight loss, sometimes regurgitation, and enlarged proventriculus seen radiographically. However, the atypical form of the disease may have CNS manifestations, alone or in conjunction with GI signs. The proventriculus may or may not be enlarged, as seen radiographically. Diagnosis of proventricular dilatation disease (PDD) is histologically made by biopsy with classic lesions identified or at necropsy. A combination of serology, paired with polymerase chain reaction (PCR), may facilitate diagnosis of infection with ABV but may not necessarily correlate with diagnosis of PDD. Treatment is, as in other species, supportive care. Cyclo-oxygenase 2 (COX-2) inhibitors such as celecoxib or robenacoxib may be beneficial in treatment.

Atherosclerosis

As in humans, the cause of atherosclerosis is unknown, but the predisposing factors include obesity and a high-fat (all-seed) diet. It is most common in Amazon parrots and appears occasionally in macaws (*Ara ararauna*) and Grey parrots, but may exist in any species. Cholesterol and triglyceride elevations may or may not be present. Clinical signs are often cyclical, with waxing and waning focal or grand mal seizures that seem to respond to therapy but continue to recur intermittently. Mental dullness may persist (see Chapter 6). Diagnosis is often made at postmortem examination, but calcification of the great vessels (shown by radiography) and obstruction or dilation of the outflow tracts (shown by cardiac ultrasound) both indicate atherosclerosis.

Hyperlipidemic syndrome or lipid emboli

This syndrome is linked to hyperestrogenism in reproductively active females (see Chapter 12). Excessive lipid circulates in the bloodstream, causing vascular sludging and lipid emboli. The lay term is "yolk stroke," although it is not truly a yolk embolus. This syndrome can often be recognized at the time of blood collection; the blood is so saturated with lipid that the appearance has been described as "strawberry milkshake" or "creamy tomato soup," which is readily apparent. (Caution must be used when collecting blood, as these birds may have concurrent clotting disorders.) Cholesterol and triglycerides are consistently elevated in this disease. Treatment consists of dilution or diuresis with fluids, cholesterol-lowering statin drugs (human medicines such as gemfibrozil, simvastatin, and colestipol may be compounded for avian use), and diet modification (as needed). Niacin may be added as well. Treatment may be rewarding, but some manifestations such as head tilt may persist. Treatment should be continued for life. Lupron or deslorelin therapy may help decrease hormone levels in the acute stage.

Hypocalcemia

Hypocalcemia is most commonly identified in Grey parrots (genetic) or egg-laying hens of any species, as well as in pigeons or doves on poor diets. In addition to seizures, clinical signs include muscle fasciculation, pathologic fractures, ataxia, and posterior paresis. In reproductively active females, total body calcium may be normal. Ionized calcium levels are most useful for diagnosis. Treatment includes injectable and oral calcium, vitamin D, and supportive care, including nutritional support. Prognosis is good if the seizures can be controlled.

Hypoglycemia

Hypoglycemia is most common in juveniles that are weaning or rarely in debilitated, anorexic birds. Lack of food for 24 hours in any pet bird can be life threatening. Blood glucose values less than 150 mg/dL in a symptomatic bird warrant medical intervention. Treatment is with IV dextrose in slow boluses. An initial bolus of 50% dextrose (diluted 1:1 with LRS or saline to reduce osmolarity) should be given at a dose of 1 mL/kg and repeated after reassessment.[14] If necessary, it should be followed by IV infusion of 5% dextrose as a CRI until normoglycemia is achieved. Gavage feeding with 50% dextrose diluted 1:1 with lactated Ringer's solution or 0.9% sodium chloride may be performed. Adequate hydration should be ensured, as 50% dextrose is highly hypertonic. The underlying cause should be treated, seizures controlled, and regular gavage feeding of a highly digestible product started.

REFERENCES

1. Carpenter MB: *Core text of neuroanatomy*, ed 2, Baltimore, MD, 1978, Williams & Wilkin.
2. King AS, McClelland J: *Birds: their structure and function*, ed 2, Bath, U.K., 1984, Bailliere Tindall.
3. Sturkie PD, editor: *Avian physiology*, ed 4, New York, 1976, Springer Verlag. pp 1–73.
4. Pessacq Asenjo TP: The nerve endings of the glycogen body of embryonic and adult spinal cord: on the existence of two different varieties of nerve fibers, *Growth* 48(3):385–390, 1984.
5. Orosz SE: Principles of avian clinical neuroanatomy, *Semin Avian Exot Pet Med* 5(3):127–139, 1996.
6. De Lahunta A, editor: *Veterinary neuroanatomy and clinical neurology*, Philadelphia, PA, 1977, Saunders, pp 89–160.
7. Baumel JJ: Suspensory ligaments of nerves: an adaptation for protection of the avian spinal cord, *Zentralblatt fur Veterinarmedizin Reihe C: Anat Histol Embryol* 14(1):1–5, 1985.
8. Oliver JE, Lorenz MD: *Handbook of veterinary neurologic diagnosis*, ed 2, Philadelphia, 1993, WB Saunders.
9. Clippinger TL, Bennet RA, Platt SR: The avian neurologic examination and ancillary neurodiagnostic techniques, *J Avian Med Surg* 10: 221–247, 1996.
10. Clippinger TL, Bennett RA, Platt SR: The avian neurologic examination and ancillary neurodiagnostic tecchniques, *Vet Clin Exot Anim* 10:803–836, 2007.
11. Bennett RA: Neurology. In Ritchie BW, Harrison GJ, Harrison LR, editors: *Avian medicine: principles and application*, Lake Worth, FL, 1994, Wingers Publishing, pp 728–747.
12. Lorenz MD, Coates JR, Kent M: Seizures, narcolepsy, and cataplexy. In *Handbook of veterinary neurology*, ed 5, St. Louis, MO, 2011, Elsevier, pp 384–412.
13. Delk K: Clinical management of seizures in avian patients, *J Exot Pet Med* 21:132–139, 2012.
14. Kirk RW, Bistner SI, Ford RB: Metabolic emergencies. In *Handbook of veterinary procedures and emergency treatment*, ed 5, Philadelphia, 1990, WB Saunders, pp 133–145.
15. Plumb DC: *Veterinary drug handbook*, ed 8, Ames, Iowa, 2015, Iowa State University Press.
16. Beaufrere H, Nevarez J, Gaschen L, et al: Diagnosis of presumed acute ischemic stroke and associated seizure management in a Congo African Grey parrot, *J Am Vet Med Assoc* 239(1):122–128, 2011.
17. Baine K, Jones MP, Cox S, et al: Pharmacokinetics of gabapentin in hispanolan amazon parrots (*Amazona ventralis*), *Proc Annu Conf Assoc Avian Vet* 19–20, 2013.

CHAPTER 10

Clinical Endocrinology of the Protein Hormones

Susan E. Orosz • *Deborah Monks* • *Ricardo de Matos*

ANATOMY AND PHYSIOLOGY OF THE ENDOCRINE SYSTEM— PROTEIN HORMONES

Susan E. Orosz

The avian endocrine glands are similar to those of mammals. In general, each endocrine gland is ductless and produces hormones or chemical messengers that are released into the bloodstream. They act on distant tissues, cells, and organs, which are termed *target organs*, to produce an effect based on that particular hormone. The hormone binds to a receptor that may be on the cell surface (protein hormones) or in the cytoplasm and nuclei of the cells (steroid or thyroid hormones) of the target organ. The endocrine glands of birds that are comparable with those of mammals include the anterior pituitary gland, the hypothalamus, the posterior pituitary complex, the pancreatic islets, the adrenal gland, the thyroid gland, the parathyroid glands, the ultimobranchial bodies, the gonads, the pineal glands, and the gut-associated endocrine cells.

Although the traditional view of the endocrine system was that of only ductless glands that produce hormones that act downstream on other organs, recent developments suggest that this view is too restrictive. We now know that most, if not all, tissues produce biologically active proteins or peptides. Tissues that were construed as end organs for hormone action have been also found to produce hormones. These include adipose tissue (adiponectin and leptin), heart (natriuretic peptides), liver (insulin-like growth factor), and kidney (renin, followed by angiotensin I and II, 1,25 dihydroxy vitamin D_3 $(1,25\text{-}(OH)2\ D_3)$, and erythropoietin).[1]

The problem for avian veterinarians is that there are limited studies performed in traditional species—mainly psittacines—in practice. Most often, the chicken serves as the model for those that are cared for in a practice setting. Recent studies, however, suggest that extrapolation to other species from studies done with primarily chickens should be done with caution.[2] For example, the chicken was domesticated from jungle fowl about 10,000 years ago, but the thyrotropin-releasing hormone (TRH) receptor gene is constant in diverse breeds of domestic chickens but not present in that form in the jungle fowl.[3]

There are other peptides and other protein components that are classified on the basis of their origin, termination, and action in birds—these chemical messengers are often polypeptides (PPs) or neuropeptides, and most are associated with genomic research in chickens and zebra finches.[4,5] Additionally, some avian neuropeptides and their respective genes are not present in mammals. These include corticotropin-releasing factor (CRF) amide, c-type natriuretic peptide 1 precursor, renal natriuretic peptide,[4] and proteolipid protein.[6]

There are also some unique aspects of birds that have been addressed more recently. The salt gland of marine birds is unique and has its own mechanism of concentrating salt. The high rate of metabolism of birds is different, presumably for the intense activity of flight. Birds have a blood glucose that is twice that of mammals, and the value increases as the bird decreases in size. This is observed in hummingbirds that receive a high glucose meal without adverse effects.[7] Birds are also very different in terms of reproduction—from behaviors associated with nesting, laying, incubation, and post-hatching factors, to the very organs of reproduction, the internal testes, and the formation of an external egg. These will not be discussed in this chapter, and the remaining discussion will focus on the protein hormones and the traditional ductless glands associated with them.

HYPOTHALAMOPITUITARY COMPLEX

The pituitary gland is intimately associated with the hypothalamus both structurally and from an embryologic point of view (Figure 10-1). The hypothalamus is the ventral part of the thalamus of the brain and is derived from an ectodermal origin. The outgrowth from this area forms the neurohypophysis and consists of the pars nervosa (or the posterior pituitary), the infundibular stalk, and the median eminence.

In this area, the *Rathke pouch*, which is an outgrowth of the structures of the mouth, is also of ectodermal origin but of different tissue origin. This outpouching of tissue becomes the adenohypophysis. This tissue meets that of the downward-growing neurohypophysis to form this hypothalamopituitary complex. In mammals, the adenohypophysis becomes the pars tuberalis; pars intermedia, which sits next to the infundibular stalk; and the pars distalis. It is this pars distalis that forms the anterior pituitary. In birds, however, there is no pars intermedia.

The connection between the adenohypophysis and the neurohypophysis is physiologically important, and part of the reason is the blood vascular supply. A hypophyseal portal system takes blood, with the released hormones, from the median eminence to the adenohypophysis. There are also neurosecretory terminals that send information to the anterior pituitary.

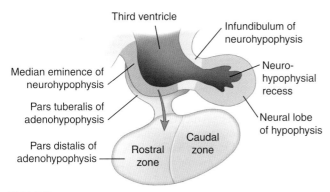

FIGURE 10-1 The pituitary gland, showing the neurohypophysis and the adenohypophysis lobes. The posterior pituitary, or neurohypophysis, is derived from the embryonic brain and is composed of the infundibulum and the neural lobe. The anterior pituitary, or adenohypophysis, contains secretory cells and folliculostellate cells.

The anterior pituitary is divided into two distinct lobes. The anterior pituitary gland is composed of secretory cells and folliculostellate cells together with extracellular colloid and fibrous material (Figure 10-2).[8] A large number of secretory cells of the anterior pituitary exist and include *corticotrophs*, which produce adrenocorticotropic hormone (ACTH); *gonadotrophs*, which produce either luteinizing hormone (LH) or follicle-stimulating hormone (FSH); *lactotrophs*, which produce prolactin; *somatotrophs*, which produce growth hormone (GH); and *thyrotrophs*, which produce thyroid-stimulating hormone (TSH). *Somatolactotrophs* produce both GH and prolactin in turkeys[9,10] and cells that coexpress both the large protein proopiomelanocortin (POMC) and the α-subunit of LH, FSH, and TSH in chickens.[11]

In addition to the secretory cells, folliculostellate cells are also present. Although there is little information on the function of these cells, it is presumed that they have paracrine-like activity. They most likely influence the response of the secretory cells surrounding them through their gap junctions. For example, they may influence thyrotropin function, as in a short-loop feedback system.

The pars tuberalis consists of the stalk of the adenohypophysis, which is just ventral to the median eminence. Secretory-specific cells from this portion of the adenohypophysis exist as well. The cells of the anterior lobe include gonadotrophs, thyrotrophs, corticotrophs, somatotrophs, and lactotrophs, as well as follicular cells and macrophages.

The posterior pituitary consists of neurosecretory terminals, which secrete arginine vasotocin (AVT) and mesotocin (MT). These hormones are produced in the hypothalamus of the supraoptic and paraventricular nuclei and transported by neurosecretory axons to the ends of these terminals in the posterior pituitary. From here, they will be transported by an additional portal system into the systemic circulation.

The gonadotropins from the anterior pituitary, LH and FSH, are glycoproteins that have a common α-subunit, which also includes TSH and a β-subunit that is hormone specific. Both subunits are required for biologic activity. LH in embryonic development causes an increase in the number of follicles as well as that of oocytes from oogonia, thus causing an increase in meiosis over mitosis to prepare the oocytes for ovulation.

In the mature bird, LH causes ovulation. Injection of LH will cause premature ovulation as well. In the mature follicle, it results in a series of anatomic events to cause the oocyte to be released into the infundibulum while causing other hormone changes to occur in the secondary and tertiary follicles. In the granulosa cells of mature follicles (F_1), with LH release, increased levels of progesterone and androstenedione are produced. In the theca cells from the next highest follicles (F_2), production of androstenedione takes place as well. In the theca cells from the small follicles (6 to 8 millimeters [mm]),

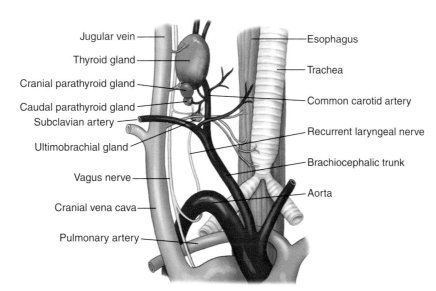

FIGURE 10-2 Location of the thyroid, parathyroid, and ultimobranchial glands, cranial to the junction of the subclavian and common carotid arteries of the domestic fowl.

progesterone, dehydroepiandrosterone (DHEA), androsterone, and estradiol are produced.

FSH acts to prime the ovary for reproduction and has more of an effect on the granulosa cells and the smaller follicles. It is involved in the rapid development of oocytes and yolk deposition. Under the influence of avidin, it, too, induces cell-specific differentiation markers that are important for fertilization of the mature chicken oocyte.[12]

As in male mammals, LH acts principally on the Leydig cells that are found within the stroma of the testicles to differentiate and produce testosterone. This has been confirmed to also occur in birds, with quails used as a model.[12] However, FSH in male quails stimulates spermatogenesis along with Sertoli cell differentiation.[13] It does not cause testosterone to be produced. Interestingly, it increases lipid production and metabolism in the chicken.[14]

The release of LH and FSH is under the stimulatory control of the hypothalamus; it is unclear if gonadotropin-releasing hormone (GnRH) 1 or 2 is the factor that causes the release from gonadotropins. LH and FSH are under the inhibiting control of gonadotropin-inhibiting hormone (GnIH), which was first isolated from the quail brain. The release of GnRH is under the control of a variety of chemical messengers that include norepinephrine and neuropeptide Y, whereas those that inhibit release include dopamine, β-endorphins, and GnIH.

In females, estradiol exerts a *negative feedback* effect on LH secretion. Progesterone can either stimulate or inhibit LH release, depending on the state of the bird, with the preovulatory LH surge in the hen induced by progesterone. Progesterone has a *positive feedback* effect on LH release in intact hens.

Increasing day length and temperature stimulates reproduction in temperate species. The presence of increased water supply has been shown to increase reproduction in song sparrows.

Avian TSH is a heterodimer that has both an α-subunit and a β-subunit; the molecule is a glycoprotein. TSH stimulates the release of thyroxine (T_4) from the thyroid gland, and there is rapid conversion in the peripheral circulation to triiodothyronine (T_3). In addition to activity in the thyroid gland, TSH acts on the brain, the pineal gland, and the retina. The release of TSH from the hypothalamus is under predominantly stimulatory control of two stimulatory releasing hormones (TRH and corticotropin-releasing hormone [CRH]) and also the inhibitory effects of somatostatin (SS or SRIF). T_3 causes a negative feedback to the pituitary for the release of TSH. Cold, along with fasting, evokes the release of TSH.[15]

PINEAL GLAND

The pineal gland is formed from the evagination of neuroepithelial tissue from the diencephalic roof. In fish and amphibians, it has both a secretory function and is photosensitive. In mammals, it is purely neuroendocrine, since it relays light information only indirectly through the neuronal pathways. There is a dichotomy in birds because diurnal birds have a well-developed pineal organ. Some of the nocturnal species examined have rudimentary organs.

The distal enlargement of the avian pineal glands is known as the pineal vesicle. This vesicle adheres to the dura mater and is exposed to the skull. Proximally, it has a slender stalk, which is connected to the wall of the third ventricle. The pineal glands in birds have three morphologic forms: *saccular* in passerines, *tubulofollicular* in pigeons and ducks, and *lobular* in chickens and quails. In birds, the gland contains photoreceptor-like cells, ependymal or interstitial cells, and neurons. The photoreceptor cells, when modified, have pinopsin in their outer segments, which is structurally related to rhodopsin. Melatonin that is produced in the gland is highly light dependent. The pinealocytes contain secretory granules. The nerve cells are mainly bipolar cells and connect with the brain.

Melatonin is produced in the pineal gland, although not exclusively. A characteristic feature of pineal melatonin is that it has a 24-hour secretion rhythm, with levels being high at night and low during daylight. It binds to high-affinity membrane-bound receptors in the retinal, tectofugal, thalamofugal, and accessory optic pathways in the brain. In the passerines examined, it has been found in the song nucleus of the brain and in the auditory relay nuclei and structures in the limbic system that are associated with arousal and vocalization. It appears that the pineal gland is a component of the circadian pacemaker.

THYROID GLAND

The avian thyroid glands are paired oval glands located ventrolateral to the trachea and caudal to the junction of the subclavian and the common carotid arteries. The architecture is like that in mammals, with spherically arranged follicles. The follicles are lined by an epithelium that secretes thyroglobulin, the storage form of thyroid hormone (Figure 10-3). This extracellular storage of a hormone is unique when compared with other endocrine glands and is thought to be caused by the scarcity of iodine.[16] The thyroid glands are well vascularized by the thyroid arteries, which branch off the carotids. Drainage occurs via the veins that drain into the jugular veins. Calcitonin (CT)-secreting cells, which are parafollicular cells in mammals, are not seen in avian species. Birds have

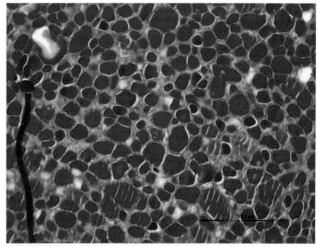

FIGURE 10-3 Normal histology of the thyroid gland; note the epithelium lined, colloid filled follicles. (Photo courtesy Dr. Helene Pendl.)

separate glands, the ultimobranchial glands, which contain CT-secreting cells. Thyroid growth is proportional to body growth in Galliformes both embryologically and posthatch. In precocial birds, the gland matures during the first half of embryonic life, and the hypothalamopituitary complex is established in the last half of embryonic development. In altricial birds, most histologic and functional development occurs following the hatch.[16,17]

As in mammals, birds have T_4, along with T_3. The numbers refer to the number of iodide groups on the structural formula of each. It appears that the mechanism for hormone synthesis and release by the glands is similar to that in mammals.[16] Endocytosis of droplets of colloid by the follicular cells with the subsequent digestion of thyroglobulin by lysosomal enzymes causes the release of T_3 and T_4 into the surrounding capillaries. Thyroid secretion rates (TSRs) range from 1 to 3 micrograms (μg) of T_4 per 100 grams (g) body weight (BW) per day in chickens, quails, and pigeons.[17] Cold temperatures increase the TSR, whereas iodine deficiency and aging tend to decrease it.

Iodide is transported from blood into the thyroid gland by a sodium-dependent iodide symporter, and pendrin, another transporter, plays a role in transporting iodide from the follicle cells into the colloid.[18] Concentrations of thyroid hormones and thyroid gland hormone are well regulated over a wide range of iodide intakes.

Thyroglobulin is a hormone storage protein found in the colloid and contains tyrosine residues, which are iodinated to initiate thyroid hormone synthesis. Iodination requires both thyroid peroxidase and an oxidized form of iodide to form both monoiodotyrosines and diiodotyrosines within the thyroglobulin; these are then converted to the hormonal thyronines T_3 and T_4 through additional thyroid peroxidase.

Concentrations of T_4 exceed those of T_3 several fold. Adult birds of many species had plasma or serum T_4 concentrations in the range of 5 to 15 nanograms (ng) of T_4 per milliliter (mL) (6 to 19 picomoles per milliliter [pmol/mL]) and T_3 levels in the range of 0.5 to 4 ng/mL (0.7 to 1.5 pmol/mL). In comparison with mammals, birds, in general, contain less T_4 but similar levels of T_3.[19] Factors that influence thyroid function include dietary iodine availability, food availability, food composition, seasonality, age, and time of day at the time of blood collection. Diurnal patterns of plasma thyroid hormone concentrations exist. Plasma T_4 concentrations rise and peak during the dark hours and T_3 levels rise and are highest during the light period. Extrathyroidal conversion of T_4 to T_3 is highest during the light period. Cold temperatures increase T_3 concentrations, whereas warm temperatures depress T_3 within the diurnal pattern.

With regard to the potency of T_4 versus T_3, early studies suggested that they are equipotent, but more recent studies of receptors have indicated that these thyroid receptors are T_3 receptors. The apparent T_4 effects are caused by its deiodination to T_3, and T_3 is responsible for most of the thyroid action in birds. The reason for the apparently greater potency of T_4 that triggers some physiologic actions is unknown.

Birds appear to possess deiodination pathways identical to those found in mammals. This also suggests that T_3 production is mostly extrathyroidal in birds as well as in mammals. T_3 levels measured in blood reflect the production and deiodination of T_4 in the peripheral tissues of the avian patient.

Most of the T_3 in the circulatory system and peripheral tissues derives from the deiodination of a single iodine from the phenolic outer ring of T_4.[20] Studies of avian and mammalian deiodinases have demonstrated similar homologies, revealing a strong conservation of iodothyronine deiodinases throughout the evolution of vertebrates.[21,22] In precocial birds, deiodinases influence circulating thyroid hormones during the perihatch period.

Deiodination enzymes are important to understand from a clinical perspective. Apparently, the brain is dependent on adequate levels of T_3. Iodothyronine type II 5'-deiodinase (5'D-II), a deiodination enzyme, plays an important role in protecting the T_3 supply to the central nervous system (CNS) when plasma levels of thyroid concentrations are low.[23,24]

Binding proteins transport circulating thyroid hormones to maintain extrathyroidal hormone stores and regulate hormone availability. These proteins include transthyretin (with high affinity and low capacity) and albumin (with low affinity but high capacity).

The avian thyroid gland is under the control of the *hypothalamic-pituitary-thyroid (HPT) axis*. The avian hypothalamus produces several hormones: TRH, CRH, and somatostatin. The first two stimulate and the latter inhibits TSH release in the anterior or cranial adenohypophysis. TSH, or thyrotropin, is the major controller of production and release of thyroid hormones of the thyroid gland. Negative feedback to the hypothalamus and pituitary is exerted by the levels of circulating thyroid hormones. TSH is a glycoprotein. The β-chain of avian TSH differs from that in mammals, but heterologous TSHs stimulate thyroid function in birds.

The HPT axis mediates the effects of temperature and food consumption on thyroid function. For example, in cold weather, the size of the thyroid gland increases, and thyroid secretion rates increase, showing increased pituitary TSH release. Hot weather has the opposite effect.

TRH, a tripeptide, appears to have an identical structure in mammals compared with that in birds, and it was shown that exogenous TRH could stimulate TSH release. However, recent studies have shown that CRH is more important as a hypothalamic stimulator of pituitary TSH than TRH in nonmammalian vertebrates.[25] In birds, TRH plays a role in stimulating GH release, which influences avian thyroid function by increasing circulating T_3.[25]

Thyroid hormones exert their actions through nuclear receptors that are members of the steroid superfamily.[26] They have one of two basic effects—metabolic or developmental. From a metabolic perspective, thyroid hormones are key controllers of heat production, necessary for maintaining body temperature. Administration of exogenous thyroid hormones causes an increase in oxygen production. Altered thyroid hormone concentrations influence metabolic energy supply. Storage of glycogen in the liver is facilitated by increases in thyroid hormone levels. With decreases in hormones, glycogen is depleted, and plasma glucose decreases. Thyroid hormones influence growth apparently indirectly.[27] Body growth stimulation appears to result from growth factors, including insulin-like growth factor-1 (IGF-1), which is under the control of GH. Thyroid hormones appear to be important for triggering tissue-specific differentiation and maturation. Thyroid hormones induce molt in birds and inhibition of reproductive activity because high concentrations have antigonadal effects. Estrogen decreases appear to initiate molt, whereas an increase in the thyroid hormone-to-estrogen ratio appears to be important for feather formation.[28] Thyroid hormones also are crucial in the development of the brain,[29] eye,[30] and ear[31] and in skeletal muscle differentiation and growth, although the latter also requires GH. Photoreceptors in the chicken retina are stimulated by thyroid hormones to maturity.[32] Behaviorally, thyroid hormones play a key role in early learning because they establish the beginning of the sensitive period for filial imprinting.[33]

PARATHYROID GLAND

Since birds need to mobilize calcium (Ca) at a rate much faster than in mammals, hormones that regulate calcium include parathyroid hormone (PTH), CT, and 1,25-$(OH)2$ D_3, along with prostaglandin (PGs)[34] and CT gene-related peptide (CGRP). The last two hormones affect avian Ca metabolism differently from that in mammals. This may, in part, be related to the laying of a shelled egg, which uses about 10% of the total body store of Ca.[35] Egg-laying hens possess a labile pool of calcium in medullary bone, which is uniquely avian. This bone develops in long bones as a response to gonadal steroids. It is influenced by the need for a skeleton that can respond to egg laying and that is rigid enough for flight. Ca metabolism is much faster in birds than in mammals. Ca uptake in the chick femur is less than 10 minutes, whereas that of dogs, rabbits, and rats is approximately 30 minutes.[36]

The number of parathyroid glands varies between two and four, depending on the species. These glands often sit caudal to the thyroid glands in birds and are encapsulated in connective tissue. The gland consists primarily of chief cells and does not contain oxyphil cells as in mammals. The low granular content of the organelles is consistent with the low levels of PTH that are secreted.

PTH is an 88-amino-acid PP in the chicken and is an 84-amino-acid PP in mammals. The first 34 amino acid sequence is similar between mammals and birds. Studies are extremely limited regarding circulating PTH levels in birds because normally the concentrations are thought to be lower, and pure avian PTH has not been available for study. Bioassay studies have shown that the levels increase during egg shell calcification and that a secondary but a lower spike occurs with oviposition. Levels of PTH were inversely related to plasma ionized Ca levels. PTH injections in Japanese quails caused Ca levels in the plasma to increase. The primary targets for PTH in birds are bones and kidneys.

The major stimulus for PTH release from the chief cells is a fall in Ca, whereas a rise in Ca will suppress its release. Since birds respond to PTH in less than 8 minutes, it seems unlikely that osteoclastic activity causes the response. Instead, it has been shown to be from the inhibition of Ca clearance from the plasma. In addition, there is an inhibition of Ca deposition into the skeleton as well. There are PTH receptors on the osteoblastic surfaces, but these may be absent in osteoclasts. The osteoclasts, if they have PTH receptors and blasts, may alter their size and shape and migrate to and from areas with high or low Ca-binding sites in order to regulate quick changes in plasma Ca levels. It appears that there is proton pumping of Ca and that the mechanism involves adenylate cyclase activity. Estradiol appears to block this enzyme activity at the micromolar levels, but not nanomolar levels. In the kidney, PTH causes increases in glomerular filtration, urine flow, and clearance of Ca and phosphorus.

ULTIMOBRANCHIAL GLAND

Birds have anatomically distinct, asymmetrically paired ultimobranchial glands that sit caudal to the parathyroid glands. In chickens, they are located caudodorsal to the base of the brachiocephalic artery and at the bifurcation of the common carotids and the subclavian arteries. The cells that secrete CT are C cells. These cells are derived from the sixth branchial pouch, but the cells that invade the pouch are ultimately of neural crest origin. CT is a PP hormone of 32 amino acids and has a seven-membered N terminal ring. The entire chain is required for biologic activity. Most often, CT levels are determined by bioassay because it is a protein hormone.

The role of CT in bone and Ca metabolism is not well understood. In mammals, CT has been shown to regulate plasma levels of Ca through its hypocalcemic action that inhibits osteoclastic bone resorption. CT is secreted primarily by rising plasma Ca levels. However, in submammalian species, including birds, plasma Ca levels are refractory to dosing with CT. High circulating CT concentrations are present in submammalian species, including birds. Studies have not shown a clear link to Ca metabolism, but they have suggested that CT receptors are downregulated under normal physiologic conditions, and this may be the reason that this direct link has not been determined. When long-term hypocalcemic chicks are injected with CT, Ca levels do rise abruptly, suggesting that under normal conditions, receptors are downregulated. In these studies, it is interesting to note that when CT of salmon origin was used, as bone formation proceeded, there was a proportional increase in alkaline phosphatase activity in the bones in culture.[37]

Studies across species lines to determine the location of renal binding sites for CT showed that there were no renal-binding sites in fish, amphibians, and reptiles. There were binding sites in the renal cortex and the medulla in rats, quails, and chickens.[38] Binding site patterns have suggested that CT receptors are associated with the glomeruli and the collecting tubules. Data from these studies suggested that CT receptors appear late in evolutionary development and that the regulation of renal function by CT is effective in only mammals and birds.

In egg-laying quail hens, the levels are highest immediately after ovulation and fall as egg shell calcification proceeds. Levels rise near the end of calcification. Steroid hormones, in particular androgens, appear to have the most influence on circulating CT levels. The levels of CT are influenced by the amount of Ca consumed. In chickens with high levels of Ca, there is a corresponding high level of circulating CT as well.

THE VITAMIN D SYSTEM

In 1931, Hou[39] reported that the removal of the preen gland from chicks resulted in rickets even when they were fed a normal diet and exposed to sunlight. He concluded that the preen gland produced a provitamin D_3 and that sunlight converted it to an active form. Much of the knowledge on vitamin

D metabolism is from studies in the ensuing years, in which the chicken was used as the model.

From this original work, it has been learned that sunlight converts the inactive provitamin D_3 to vitamin D_3, which is then ingested when the bird preens. Vitamin D_3 is metabolized to 25-(OH)-D_3 in the liver and then to 1,25-(OH)2 D_3 in the kidneys (Figure 10-4). The factors that stimulate the conversion of vitamin D_3 to the active form in the kidneys include PTH, prolactin, and 1,25-(OH)2 D_3 itself.[40] There are contradictory reports regarding the role of CT in vitamin D_3 production, but it most likely does not stimulate its production.

Birds are unable to use vitamin D_2, which is the major form of vitamin D used in dog and cat foods. Birds are able to discriminate between D_2 and D_3 because the protein that binds plasma vitamin D has a relatively low affinity for D_2 and so is more rapidly broken down.

There appears to be a cycle for the conversion of 25 vitamin D_3 to 1,25 during the egg shell calcification cycle in the hen. This was also described by Nys et al,[41] who demonstrated that hens that laid shell-less eggs did not show the cyclical fluctuations in 1,25-(OH)2 D_3 levels. Circulating levels of 1,25-(OH)2 D_3 increase in the prelaying period and again at the onset of egg production to prime Ca for the rapid drain in shell formation.

Intestinal absorption of Ca is regulated by 1,25-(OH)2 D_3 by inducing ribonucleic acid (RNA) transcription and the synthesis of proteins that promote the absorption of Ca. These proteins include three forms of calbindin D-28k. In vitamin D–deficient chicks, intestinal calbindin messenger RNA (mRNA) is barely detectable but increases dramatically with the addition of 1,25-(OH) D_3 injection. With the onset of ovulation, there is an increase in intestinal Ca absorption.

A calbindin, which is under the control of 1,25-(OH)2 D_3, is present in the uterus of the hen as well. The uterus or shell gland contains receptors for 1,25-(OH)2 D_3. Calbindin and its mRNA concentrations increase in immature pullets treated with estrogen. Interestingly, those hens that lay shell-less eggs have even higher levels of calbindin. It is thought that the sex steroids have an indirect effect on the oviduct because they affect its maturation and development, but not the levels of Ca directly.

Feeding a vitamin D–deficient diet to laying hens causes the resorption of medullary bone. This has also been observed clinically in seed cockatiel hens fed seed-only diets. In comparison, feeding a vitamin D–deficient diet to nonlaying hens causes osteodystrophy. Bone formation is facilitated by 1,25-(OH)2 D_3, which stimulates the biosynthesis of osteocalcin. Osteocalcin appears to bind Ca and has an affinity for hydroxyapatite, which suggests that it has a mineral dynamics function. It is released into the systemic circulation, where it may be a marker for new bone formation or an index for bone turnover, but not bone resorption.

About 30% to 40% of the calcium in the egg shell is derived from medullary bone. But medullary bone is induced by sex steroids and not by vitamin D levels. However, in order for the bone to be fully mineralized, both vitamin D and the sex steroids need to be present at normal levels. Cultures of medullary bone cells responded to increasing levels of 1,25-(OH)2 D_3. Renal functions of Ca metabolism are unaltered by a deficiency of vitamin D after Ca loading or PTH administration. When they are deficient in vitamin D, they do not increase phosphorus excretion in response to PTH stimulus.[42]

PROSTAGLANDINS AND CALCIUM METABOLISM

In birds, the effects of prostaglandins (PGs) are similar to those of PTH because prostaglandins stimulate cyclic adenosine monophosphate (cAMP) production, cause a transient increase in Ca influx, activate carbonic anhydrase, release lysosomal enzymes, and inhibit collagen synthesis. They affect osteoclasts and osteoblasts. For example, 16,16 dimethyl PGE_2 is hypercalcemic in chicks. PGE_2 and other eicosanoids have function and efficacy similar to both PTH and 1,25-(OH)2 D_3 in that they are powerful stimulators of bone resorption.[43]

Medullary bone of the bird is the most estrogen sensitive of all vertebrate bone types. It can form in male birds that are dosed with estrogens within a matter of days. It can be blocked from forming in these males with the addition of tamoxifen, which is antiestrogenic.[44] When estrogen is withdrawn,

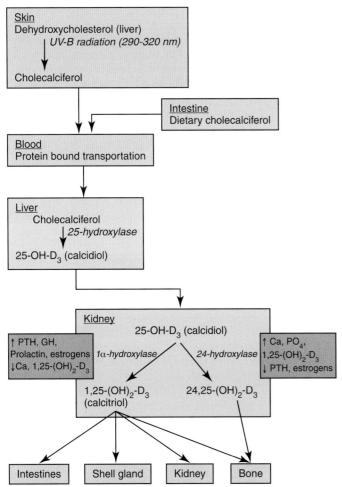

FIGURE 10-4 Vitamin D metabolism in birds. ↓, Downregulation; ↑, upregulation; Ca, calcium; GH, growth hormone; PO_4, phosphate; PTH, parathyroid hormone.

medullary bone rapidly resorbs, as can be observed clinically with injectable long-acting leuprolide acetate.

PANCREAS

The liver and the pancreas play a major role in the distribution and utilization of nutrients that are absorbed from the gastrointestinal (GI) tract. Both organs are strategically placed for glucoregulation. It is interesting to note that it is glucose, not protein or lipid metabolism, that is tightly regulated by the body in both mammals and birds. Several factors that allow glucose to trump proteins and lipids are involved. Glucose is the easiest substrate that cells utilize to release energy. It can be synthesized from noncarbohydrate sources. Some tissues, including the cells of the retina and adrenal medullary and neurons, require glucose as their only substrate to maintain normal function. Effective homeostatic regulation of glucose metabolism therefore adjusts protein and lipid metabolism to normalcy.

The avian liver, like that of mammals, plays a central role in the regulation of carbohydrate metabolism. Nutrients from the gut ascend to the liver, where they can be metabolized before moving through the caudal vena cava to be distributed systematically. The nutrients are transported by the portal veins to the hepatocytes. From there, the nutrients or their metabolites move through the hepatic veins to the vena cava and then to the right heart.

The histologic architecture of the liver in birds is similar to that in mammals. It does, however, receive blood from the renal portal system directly from the portal veins. This bypass of the caudal vena cava acts to dilute the nutrient-rich perfusate from the gut before entering the liver.

The liver of birds appears to have similar enzyme systems for the metabolism of nutrients. Unlike in mammals, most triglycerides are synthesized in the avian liver. High levels of glucose in the bloodstream of birds trigger the release of insulin from the B cells of the pancreas. Insulin aids the enzymatic machinery of the liver to carry out the anabolic processes in the liver and in muscle and adipose tissue to reduce the glucose load and maintain it in its narrow functional range.

During periods of fasting, nutrients must be retrieved from deposits in the body. During these periods, insulin levels are low, whereas glucagon levels are high, resulting in catabolism. The enzymatic machinery activated by glucagon during a catabolic state is directed toward producing glucose to be released into the systemic circulation for tissues that have an absolute requirement for glucose. These pathways include glycogenolysis, gluconeogenesis, the glucose 6 phosphatase system, and lipolytic pathways. Lipid degradation in adipose tissue and muscle protein and glycogen provides substrates for the liver to make glucose.

The avian pancreas is suspended by vascular components between the descending and ascending duodenum and the portal veins of the liver. It is lobulated and consists of dorsal, ventral, and splenic lobes. One of its major functions is to provide digestive enzymes to aid in digestion within the small intestine. The other role is its endocrine function. The endocrine portion of the pancreas occupies more tissue mass in birds than in mammals. The distribution of cell types that includes A, B, D, and F or PP cells appears more random.

A cells synthesize and release glucagon; B cells synthesize and release insulin; D cells synthesize and release somatostatin; and F cells make and release pancreatic PP.

Increasing blood glucose stimulates B-cell activity to release insulin, whereas decreasing blood glucose causes the release of glucagon. Absorbed nutrients stimulate D cells along with A cells. GI tract peptides, including cholecystokinin (CCK), secretin, gastrin, and absorbed amino acids stimulate F-cell release of somatostatin. The close anatomic and physiologic relationships among these cells in an islet allow them to share extracellular fluid. The A cells stimulate both B-cell and D-cell activities, thereby closing a short negative feedback loop. The D cells appear to inhibit all other islet cells and may regulate the proportion of insulin and glucagon simultaneously—thereby adjusting the insulin-to-glucagon (I/G) molar ratio on a moment-to-moment basis. The intraislet extracellular fluid link allows for communication with each of the islets in a more contiguous fashion than was previously thought. This would allow an easier and a finer control of glucose metabolism in the body.

Avian pancreatic insulin is many times more potent than equal concentrations of mammalian insulin to produce glycogenesis, hypoglycemia, and lipid formation. Glucagon differs by two amino acids in birds compared with mammals. It is a powerful catabolic hormone and circulates at levels six to eight times higher in birds than in mammals. Somatostatin concentrations in the pancreatic tissue of birds are 2 to 150 times greater than in mammalian tissue. Pancreatic PP hormones circulate at levels that are 20 to 40 times those in humans. It appears to inhibit GI tract mobility and secretion, inhibits gall bladder and exocrine pancreatic secretion, and induces a sense of satiety in the CNS.

All protein hormones are synthesized in a similar manner. Insulin and glucagon have been used as a model for hormone synthesis. Most are synthesized as giant molecules that lack biologic activity. After these are manufactured from the rough endoplasmic reticulum, each is conveyed as a prohormone in a membrane-lined vesicle to the Golgi apparatus. It is here that the cleaving, insertions, folding, and final conformational changes take place to form the biologically active hormone. This active hormone is packaged into secretory granules that move to the plasma membrane. The secretory vesicle membrane fuses with the plasma membrane, and the contents are extruded into the extracellular fluid and then into the adjacent blood vascular space for release into the systemic circulation.

Just as in mammals, the pancreatic islet hormones exert their effects on the actions of the cells of muscle, adipose tissue, liver, and, to a lesser extent, erythrocytes, chondrocytes, thymocytes, and other tissues.[45] Insulin is a powerful hypoglycemic agent in mammals but is less so in birds, although it varies among species. Doses that would be convulsive to a mammal were found to be moderately hypoglycemic in Aves. Chickens appear to be extremely resistant to insulin-induced convulsions, whereas pigeons are more sensitive to insulin. Fasting tends to increase the sensitivity to insulin in birds. With increased circulating insulin, there is uptake of glucose in the liver, muscle, and adipose tissue, primarily for the hypoglycemic effect of insulin. In addition to its effects on plasma glucose, insulin aids in the transport of metabolizable and nonmetabolizable amino acids into the cells of a wide variety of tissues—from myocardial cells to osteoblasts. Insulin can be thought of as an influx hormone because it causes glucose and amino acids to move into cells. It can reduce amino acid levels by about 30% to 40%, thereby inducing a positive nitrogen balance.[46] The reduction of free-circulating glucose in the blood after the release of insulin is corrected, but only after a time lag during which fatty acids are mobilized as an energy source. Glucagon appears to be responsible for the release of free fatty acids into the bloodstream. It appears that insulin directly removes glucose and amino acids from circulation and indirectly adds lipids to the plasma through glucagon release.[45]

The livers of mammals and birds do not depend on insulin to move glucose across the cell membrane. Instead, insulin exerts its major effect on the liver by increasing the activity of glucokinase, not hexokinase. Glucokinase phosphorylates glucose, thereby increasing the movement of free glucose from outside to inside the cell. This favors glycogen synthesis and storage by its influence on glycogen synthase. Insulin appears to exert its effect on the liver by shutting down glucose formation in favor of glycogenesis. However, glucagon favors the formation of glucose as it inhibits glycogen synthase and glucokinase activities. This promotes hyperglycemia by its action on the liver.

Insulin in mammals reduces gluconeogenesis, but it is not clear if it does so in birds; however, it is assumed that it does. It does increase the activity of liver phosphofructokinase. Glucagon decreases the flux through this pathway, thereby favoring the formation of glucose and releasing it into systemic circulation. It appears that in the liver of the bird, insulin induces lipogenic hormones and maintains lipogenesis. As expected, the opposite function can be ascribed to glucagon, since it controls lipolysis, especially after fasting. Glucagon blocks the synthesis of malic enzyme mRNA, whereas it activates hormone-sensitive lipase.[45]

The adipose tissue of birds is under extreme metabolic pressure to assist the liver to make lipids available as an energy substrate. With their high metabolic rate, birds also need energy for egg laying, migratory flight, and flight in general, along with fasting at the minimum overnight. Insulin appears to have only a mild stimulatory effect of lipogenesis, particularly compared with mammals. Epinephrine in mammals also has a major stimulatory role for lipolysis but is weakly lipolytic in birds. It appears that glucagon plays the main role in fat metabolism in birds, particularly during metabolic stress and irrespective of insulin levels. Prolonged flight releases free fatty acids, epinephrine, and norepinephrine, along with glucagon and GH.[47] The mobilized fatty acids are used as the energy source for flight, and because the catecholamines are not lipolytic in birds, their role may be to stimulate glucagon release. GH, as a stress hormone, would support the lipolytic action of glucagon as well.

Muscle metabolism is influenced by insulin levels, but the extent of involvement is not well known because of difficulties in experimental study. Insulin enhances the uptake of amino acids in the gut and is responsible for rapid myogenesis in the embryo and muscle structural protein formation in the adult. Protein synthesis is stimulated by insulin, whereas the degradation of protein is inhibited. Insulin at low concentrations has been shown to increase hepatic production of albumen, α_1-globulin, fibrinogen, and lipoproteins.

DISEASES OF THE ENDOCRINE SYSTEM—PROTEIN HORMONES

Ricardo de Matos, Deborah Monks

This section focuses on specific diseases involving the protein hormone–producing glands of avian species and the diagnosis and treatment of those diseases.

Antemortem diagnosis and treatment of endocrine disorders in birds remain a challenge, mainly because of the unknown pathophysiology of many of these conditions, lack of validated endocrine diagnostic tests, and limited to no information on the pharmacology and toxicity of the drugs recommended for the treatment of endocrine disorders in mammalian species. Considering the limited research in this field and the relatively low incidence of endocrine diseases in birds, most of the information available is from single case reports or relatively small case series.

HYPOTHALAMUS–HYPOPHYSIS

Despite the similarities between mammals and birds with regard to the hypothalamic–hypophyseal system (HHS) and the considerable number of diseases associated with this system in mammals, there are few case reports of HHS diseases in birds.[48]

Hypothalamus

Given the regulatory action of the hypothalamus, the clinical signs of primary hypothalamic endocrine dysfunction would likely be visible as secondary or tertiary gland malfunction. Hypothalamic pathology may simultaneously affect several endocrine systems, which would cause confusion and make accurate discrimination of individual hormone systems difficult. Lumeij[48] listed trauma, congenital abnormalities and lesions, granulomatous lesions, and neoplasia as possible hypothalamic pathologies. However, there are few or no records of primary hypothalamic pathologies that induce endocrine disturbance in avian species.

Pituitary

Pituitary endocrine dysfunction can occur via a number of pathways: a primary pituitary cell neoplasm causing oversecretion or undersecretion of a specific hormone (either adenohypophyseal or neurohypophyseal); pathologic stimulation or inhibition of adenohypophyseal cells by hypothalamic hormones (i.e., hypothalamic pathology causing certain effects on the adenohypophysis as a secondary gland); a mass effect preventing the passage of hypothalamic hormones to the adenohypophysis; and, finally, congenital, developmental, or granulomatous processes of surrounding tissue causing mass effects on pituitary cells and preventing hormone production as a result of atrophy or necrosis of adenohypophyseal and neurohypophyseal cells.

Specific pituitary diseases
Follicle-stimulating hormone (FSH) and luteinizing hormone (LH) are crucial for gonadal function and, at specific times, are significantly involved in other endocrine functions such as calcium regulation. In Japanese quails, embryonic exposure to endocrine-disrupting chemicals can cause alterations in

gonadotropin-releasing hormone (GnRH) production that may have lifelong ramifications. Intramuscular injection of a diesel exhaust derivative has caused decreases in LH and testosterone levels in the same species.[49,50]

Two acidophilic adenohypophyseal carcinomas in budgerigars demonstrated immunoreactivity with GH histologically, although there was no information available regarding clinical signs.[51] Langohr et al[52] described a series of 11 pituitary tumors in budgerigars, all of which stained positive for GH, justifying their being classified as somatotroph pituitary tumors. However, the clinical signs seemed to be more consistent with a space-occupying cranial mass or loss of function in other hormonal systems, rather than a pathologic increase in GH.

Pituitary dwarfism has been reported in chickens as a sex-linked recessive condition. In these birds, there are adequate levels of GH, but there appears to be impaired GH function, stemming from deletions in the GH protein coding.[53] Dwarfism has also been reported in a pheasant, a black-headed gull, and a great crested flycatcher.[48]

Diagnosis of dwarfism in birds is based mostly on clinical signs (delayed growth and obesity in chickens,[54] small size for age in other species[48]). In ducklings with short beaks and dwarfism syndrome secondary to goose parvovirus infection, diagnosis was based on clinical signs (including feathering disorders), serology, polymerase chain reaction (PCR), and postmortem examination (ascites, hydropericardium, serofibrinous perihepatitis, enteritis, and myocardial and muscular degeneration).[55] Other causes of stunted growth, such as nutritional deficiencies and primary hypothyroidism, need to be considered when investigating a dwarfism case. No treatment protocols have been described for dwarfism in birds.

Avian adrenocorticotropic hormone (ACTH) causes the release of corticosterone, aldosterone, and deoxycorticosterone from adrenal cortical cells.[56] Functional neoplasia of pituitary cells producing corticotrophin (ACTH) will result in clinical signs of hyperadrenocorticism, arising from bilateral adrenal hyperfunction. These signs include weight alteration, hepatic lipidosis, polyuria, polydipsia, polyphagia, delayed wound healing, muscular weakness and atrophy, hyperglycemia, hypophosphatemia, increased serum cholesterol and triglyceride levels, and glycosuria.[57]

A Moluccan cockatoo with a pituitary adenoma had bilateral adrenal hyperplasia and clinical signs suggestive of hyperadrenocorticism. Although antemortem diagnostic testing was not conclusive, the presence of ACTH immunoreactive tissue within the neoplasm was supportive of the authors' assertion that the most likely etiology was increased levels of ACTH arising from the pituitary adenoma.[58] Secondary hypoadrenocorticism is characterized by inadequate production and secretion of ACTH, leading to atrophy of the adrenal cortex and reduced secretion of glucocorticoids. Clinical signs may include dehydration, episodes of weakness, and vague gastrointestinal (GI) signs such as anorexia, periodic diarrhea, and generalized abdominal tenderness.[59]

Diabetes insipidus has been reported in a Grey parrot, chickens, Japanese quails, and a budgerigar.[60,61,63,64] In the Grey parrot, clinical signs included mild depression, bilateral mydriasis, decreased pupillary light reflexes bilaterally, and profound polyuria and polydipsia. The urine was

hyposthenuric. Unilateral mydriasis with reduced papillary light reflex, which was unresponsive to treatment (desmopressin), also developed. Although cranial imaging was not done, the authors postulated that an enlarging cranial neoplasm could have been the cause.[64] There are strains of chickens and quails with autosomal recessive nephrogenic diabetes insipidus.[60,63]

Diagnosis of central diabetes insipidus is based on clinical signs (marked polyuria and polydipsia), results of a water deprivation test, and measurement of blood levels of arginine vasotocin.[65] Routine diagnostic tests must first be performed to rule out other more frequent causes of polyuria and polydipsia in birds.

During the water deprivation test (in a fasted animal), water is withheld, and urine and plasma are collected every 1 to 2 hours for determination of osmolality. Body weight is determined at every time point. Once the body weight has dropped 3% to 5%, the test should be stopped. For both nephrogenic diabetes insipidus (NDI) and central diabetes insipidus (CDI), urine osmolality will remain low during the water deprivation test, whereas in normal individuals, urine osmolality will increase. Significant dehydration or weight loss and persistent polyuria and hypoosmolar urine or hyperosmolar plasma were noted during the 170-minute water deprivation test in the Grey parrot with CDI.[64] In healthy pigeons, a urine osmolality of 450 milliosmoles per kilogram (mOsm/kg) or higher is expected after 24 hours of water deprivation.[66] Once the water deprivation test is discontinued, a vasopressin analog is administered. This will help differentiate between CDI and NDI. Urine osmolality will increase significantly in cases of CDI but will not change significantly in cases of NDI.[65] For the Grey parrot with CDI described above, administration of desmopressin, a vasopressin analog, resulted in a 300% increase in urine osmolality and decrease in the frequency of urination compared with the period before desmopressin administration.[64]

In mammals, measurement of plasma vasopressin concentrations during osmotic stimulation by hypertonic saline infusion is considered a more direct and accurate diagnostic method for CDI.[65] A combination of this test and water deprivation test has been described in pigeons; in this test, blood levels of arginine vasotocin (AVT) (and not urine osmolality) were monitored during the water deprivation test. For this species, normal AVT release by the neurohypophysis is characterized by concentrations above 2.2 picograms per milliliter (pg/mL) after 24 hours of water deprivation.[48] In strains of chickens and quails with autosomal recessive nephrogenic diabetes insipidus, baseline levels of AVT are elevated compared with those of normal birds.[60,63] In addition, affected chickens also have very low urine osmolality.[60]

A simpler diagnostic test for the evaluation of polyuria in dogs consists of evaluating plasma or serum osmolality without water restrictions. Dogs with psychogenic polydipsia have low or low normal osmolality, whereas those with CDI or NDI usually have normal-to-high osmolality. Since NDI is very rare in dogs, CDI diagnosis can be made in animals with persistent low urine osmolality and high blood osmolality.[65]

Although polyuria and polydipsia are commonly reported in birds with intracranial neoplasia,[48] confirmation of CDI requires at least one of these specific tests.

The case of the Grey parrot with CDI is the only report of successful long-term management of CDI in an avian species. Injectable desmopressin (DDAVP, Aventis Pharmaceuticals, Bridgewater, NJ) was used, at a starting dose of 4.6 micrograms per kilogram (μg/kg) intramuscularly every 12 hours; the dose was adjusted on the basis of severity of clinical signs (polyuria and polydipsia) and was progressively increased to a maximum of 24 μg/kg 16 months after initial diagnosis.[64]

Generalized pituitary diseases

Although there are many reports of pituitary neoplasia in avian species, neoplasms have rarely been differentiated into cell types or classified according to hormone production. This makes it difficult to confidently ascribe clinical signs to one endocrinologic system alone. Additionally, many of the clinical signs of pituitary neoplasia (including blindness, depression, ataxia, seizures, convulsions, and exophthalmia) are referable to the space-occupying nature of a mass rather than to endocrinologic derangement.[57]

The most common clinical signs of functional pituitary neoplasm are polydipsia and polyuria. However, these signs could be caused by excess ACTH, excess GH, hyposecretion of AVT, or even cerebral compression alone.[58,67] Many birds with pituitary neoplasia show changes in plumage color and quality, cere color, and weight, which could relate to dysfunctional production of either thyroid or sex hormones.[57,67,68] Other signs of pituitary neoplasia include reproductive failure and hyperglycemia.[67] Unfortunately, none of these clinical signs is pathognomonic for a specific hormone system.

The most commonly diagnosed pituitary neoplasm is adenoma, although carcinomas are also diagnosed.[57] Both are diagnosed most frequently in budgerigars and can be associated with distant metastasis as well as local invasion.[48,52] A specific transmissible pituitary adenoma has been described in budgerigars.[67] A genetic predisposition has also been postulated.[52] Adenomas have been described in cockatiels, a Moluccan cockatoo, an Amazon parrot, a lovebird, a canary, and chickens.[48,58,67,69] A case report of a corticotroph adenocarcinoma in a budgerigar has been documented, although the clinical signs were related to blindness.[70] In one case series involving budgerigars with pituitary adenomas and carcinomas, all of the neoplastic cells were determined to be of somatotroph origin.[52]

A presumptive diagnosis of a pituitary tumor can be based on clinical signs (secondary to hormonal disturbances, compression of surrounding nervous system, or both), physical examination findings, a baseline blood test, and imaging (to rule out other systemic diseases). Hormone-specific assays and the water deprivation test may be performed, as suggested by the presenting signs and to possibly identify which pituitary hormones are being secreted in excess. Depending on the size of the bird and of the tumor, higher-resolution imaging techniques such as micro-computed tomography and higher-field-strength magnetic resonance imaging (MRI) may help visualize the tumor. Diagnosis can only be confirmed with postmortem evaluation of the pituitary gland. The gland normally lies in the sella turcica of the sphenoid bone, just posterior to the optic chiasm; tumors frequently extend beyond the sella turcica. Metastases are rarely described.[52,71,72] There are no reports of surgical, radiation, or medical therapy of pituitary tumors in birds.

PINEAL GLAND

There are sparse reports of pineal neoplasia. A cockatiel with unilateral head tilt, loss of grip, depression, and polydipsia was diagnosed with a pineoblastoma, and two chickens and a dove were incidentally diagnosed with pinealoma.[69,73,74]

THYROID GLAND

Diseases of the thyroid gland are characterized by enlargement (goiter), hypofunction, or hyperfunction. As in the case of other glands, disorders can be classified as primary, secondary, or tertiary, depending on the origin of the problem (thyroid gland, pituitary, or hypothalamus, respectively). There are few documented cases of hyperthyroidism or hypothyroidism in avian species and absolutely none in which the dysfunction was proven to be caused by hypothalamic or pituitary dysfunction. Thyroid gland pathology includes hyperplasia, neoplasia, infection, inflammation, and atrophy. In nonfunctional enlargement—the etiologies of which include cystic changes, plant goitrogens, toxins, congenital abnormalities, amyloidosis, and some neoplasia—the clinical signs often relate to those of a space-occupying mass.[48] Signs of hyperthyroidism include polydipsia, polyuria, regurgitation, tachycardia, weight loss, plumage changes, convulsions, and death.[75] Clinical signs of hypothyroidism can include feather loss, epidermal atrophy, and noninflammatory skin changes, hypercholesterolemia, nonregenerative anemia, and obesity.[76,77]

Goiter

Thyroid gland hyperplasia and enlargement (goiter) is most often caused by iodine deficiency. Although most commonly reported in budgerigars, this species rarely appears to suffer from thyroid endocrinopathy.[48,78] At necropsy, an increased prevalence of hyperplastic goiter has been seen in blue-and-gold macaws, although concomitant thyroid dysfunction has not been described in that species.[78]

In certain strains of pigeons, hyperplastic goiter can be functional, leading to clinical signs of hypothyroidism, including lethargy, obesity, reduced reproductive parameters, myxoedema, and feather abnormalities. The birds are usually on fat-rich, iodine-deficient diets.[48] In captive-reared black stilts, an iodine-responsive goiter has been reported to cause decreased survivability after release.[79] This syndrome responded to prerelease iodine supplementation.

A diagnosis of goiter in birds can be achieved on the basis of information obtained from the history (diet deficient in iodine), clinical signs (regurgitation, dyspnea, inspiratory squeak), and response to treatment (iodine supplementation). Despite the considerable increase in the size of the gland in some cases, the enlarged gland cannot be palpated because of the location in the thoracic inlet (Figures 10-5 and 10-6).[48,80] Radiographically, the trachea may be dorsally or ventrally displaced by the enlarged gland.[48] Clinical hypothyroidism does not occur in psittacines with goiter, so thyroid function tests are not valuable for diagnosis.

Pigeons with goiter have a different clinical presentation, with clinical signs characteristic of hypothyroidism and palpable mass (gland) at the thoracic inlet. Dyspnea and respiratory stridor are only seen in severe cases. No thyroid function

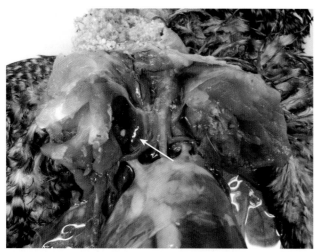

FIGURE 10-5 Postmortem image of bilateral goiter in a domestic chicken; note the in situ remaining enlarged right thyroid gland *(arrow)*. (Photo courtesy Dr. Jarra Jagne.)

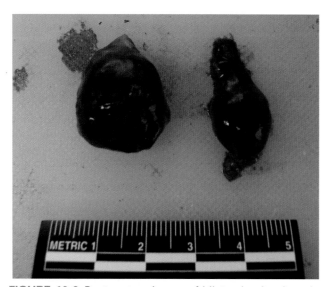

FIGURE 10-6 Postmortem image of bilateral goiter in a domestic chicken; ex situ image of the glands in the case in Figure 10-5. (Photo courtesy Dr. Jarra Jagne.)

tests have been performed in pigeons with goiter to confirm hypothyroidism.[48]

Treatment consists of oral iodine supplementation through iodized seed or iodine in the water (one drop of 0.3% Lugol solution per 20 mL of water—daily for the first week; three times a week for the second week; then once weekly).[48,80] More severe cases of goiter may require oxygen supplementation and daily intramuscular injections of 60 milligrams per kilogram (mg/kg) of 20% sodium iodine.[81] Goiter can be prevented by feeding a completely formulated diet.[80]

Hypothyroidism

Histiocytic thyroiditis has been described in passerines with atypical, disseminated mycobacteriosis, although there was no clinical evidence of hypothyroidism.[75] Thyroiditis can also be caused by infection by viruses and pyogenic bacteria.[48]

In chickens with spontaneous autoimmune thyroiditis, classic signs of hypothyroidism first develop 2 to 3 weeks after the hatch, although histologic evidence of thyroid pathology is present earlier.[77,82] The clinical signs, which can be reversed by supplementation with thyroxine, include small body size and comb size, cold sensitivity, low fertility, poor hatchability, lipemia, and weight gain.[82] Histologically, there appears to be a similar condition in Grey parrots.[77] Japanese quails with chemically induced hypothyroidism exhibit gonadal and adrenal disturbances.[83] Thyroidectomized ducks become hypoglycemic, with large hepatic glycogen stores.[84] Thyroid dysplasia was reported in a hyacinth macaw with ulcerative dermatitis and valvular endocarditis. Although hypothyroidism was suspected as a possible cause of the dermatitis and self-mutilation, no antemortem testing was performed to confirm the diagnosis.[85]

There has been a confirmed case of hypothyroidism in a scarlet macaw, which presented with feather loss, obesity, hypercholesterolemia, and nonregenerative anemia.[76] No thyroid biopsy was done, and the precise etiology was not elucidated. Schmidt and Reavill[77] briefly described a case of hypothyroidism, but with no specific details. Clinical signs included severe feather loss, epidermal atrophy, and noninflammatory skin changes. Rae[75] also attested to several cases in older, obese Amazon parrots, in which histologic findings were consistent with hypothyroidism, and the cause of death was attributed to secondary complications from hypothyroidism (infarction and atherosclerosis).

Diagnosis of hypothyroidism in birds should be based on manifestation of characteristic clinical signs and lack of response to the thyroid-stimulating hormone (TSH) stimulation test. Clinical signs, low basal thyroxine (T_4) concentration, and response to L-thyroxine therapy can be suggestive of hypothyroidism, but the TSH stimulation test is required for an accurate diagnosis. The clinical signs of hypothyroidism are not specific to this condition and can be seen with other diseases. Birds have lower T_4 and similar (low) triiodothyronine (T_3) plasma concentrations compared with mammals. In addition, T_4 levels can vary from species to species, depending on the assay used and several internal and external factors.[48,80,86] For this reason, hypothyroidism cannot be diagnosed by comparing single T_4 values with the published reference interval for the species.[48,80] In addition, hypothyroid-like clinical signs may improve with L-thyroxine therapy even in birds with normal thyroid function.[80] Scintigraphy has been shown to be capable of detecting thyroid hypofunction in an experimental model of hypothyroidism in cockatiels.[87] This diagnostic technique is not readily available, and there are no reports of its use for the diagnosis of spontaneously occurring hypothyroidism in birds.

Protocols for TSH testing in chickens, pigeons, and psittacines have been described, with different doses of TSH and time for post-TSH T_4 level determination listed in Table 10-1. The initial studies with TSH stimulation test in birds were done using bovine TSH, which proved to be both safe and effective. Since this product is no longer available, the use of human synthetic TSH for the TSH stimulation test in birds was investigated. The product was also found to be safe and effective in raising total T_4 levels in euthyroid birds. Doses used and magnitude of response obtained were similar to what was described for bovine TSH.[88,89] The main

TABLE 10-1

Thyroid-Stimulating Hormone Testing Protocols Published for Different Bird Species

Species	TSH Type and Dose	Normal T_4 Increase after TSH Administration	Reference
Psittacines*	Bovine; 1 IU/bird IM	Twofold or higher at 4 hours	92
Psittacines†	Bovine; 1–2 IU/bird IM	Twofold or higher at 4–6 hours	91
Blue-and-gold macaw	Human; 0.2 IU/kg IM	Twofold at 4 hours after	88
Blue-fronted Amazon parrot, Hispaniolan parrot	Human; 1 IU/kg IM	Twofold at 6 hours after	88
Psittacines‡	Human; 1 IU/kg IM	Twofold at 6 hours after	94, 95
Cockatiel	Bovine; 0.1 IU/bird	Threefold to 24-fold at 6 hours after	96
Pigeon	Bovine TSH 0.1, 0.3, or 1 unit/bird	2.5-fold between 4 and 24 hours (up to 36 hours with 1 IU/bird dose)	97
Chicken	Bovine; 0.25 IU/kg IM	Fivefold at 4 hours after	93
	Bovine; 0.1 IU/kg IM	Threefold between 3 and 8 hours	93

*Red-lored Amazon parrot, blue-fronted Amazon parrot, Grey parrot; healthy parrots.
†Amazon parrot, cockatoo, scarlet macaw, blue-and-gold macaw, Grey parrot, conure, and cockatiel.
‡Blue-and-gold macaw, Moluccan cockatoo, Goffin's cockatoo, rose-breasted cockatoo, Eclectus parrot, blue-fronted Amazon parrot, red-lored Amazon parrot, Tucuman Amazon parrot, budgerigar; all birds presented abnormal feathers and were being investigated for evidence of hypothyroidism.
IM, Intramuscularly; IU/kg, international unit per kilogram; TSH, thyroid-stimulating hormone.

limitation for the use of human synthetic TSH is its cost (approximately $2500 [€1900] or $300 [€220] per kilogram body weight of bird to be tested). Recombinant canine TSH appears safe and effective in stimulating T_4 production in chickens.[90] However, recombinant canine TSH is not readily available. Despite the multitude of TSH doses and time points published, normal thyroid response to TSH stimulation in birds is characterized by an increase of T_4 levels of at least twofold over the baseline value.[48,80,88,91-93]

Several techniques have been used for determining total T_4 levels in birds, including protein-bound iodine tests, isotope dilution mass spectrometric tests, enzyme immunoassay, and radioimmunoassay (RIA). Despite being recommended as a reference method, the isotope dilution–mass spectrometric assay is rarely used because of its complexity. Enzymatic methods are, in general, considered accurate and precise and are available for use in bench top models (IDEXX, Abaxis). Woerpel and Rosskopf determined baseline T_4 concentrations for several avian species by using a commercially available enzyme immunoassay.[98] Enzymatic methods have not been validated for use in birds, and T_4 levels obtained with this method are usually lower compared with values obtained with RIA. Enzymatic tests are also not linear when T_4 levels are below 0.5 microgram per deciliter (μg/dL).[89] RIA is the most accurate, most sensitive, and most commonly used assay for determining avian thyroid hormone levels.[86] Many of the published reference intervals for total T_4 in avian species were established by using RIA. The most commonly used test for determining total T_4 levels in birds is a canine solid-phase RIA (Coat-a-Count Canine T4 Kit, Diagnostic Products Corporation, Los Angeles, CA), which has not been validated for use in birds and has a relatively high limit of detection (0.5 μg/dL; 6.4 nanomoles per liter [nmol/L]).[99,100] In two studies investigating TSH testing in healthy psittacines, the authors validated two commercial kits (human T_4 RIA kit [GammaCoat Free/Total T4 RIA Kit, Clinical Assays, Cambridge, MA] and canine T_4 double-antibody kit [Double-Antibody Canine T4, Diagnostic Products Corporation, Los Angeles, CA; no longer commercially available]) for

determining total T_4 levels in serum samples. The limits of detection for these assays were 0.13 μg/dL (1.67 nmol/L) and 0.15 μg/dL (1.93 nmol/L), respectively.[91,92] More recently, a high-sensitivity RIA was developed and validated for use in psittacines birds.[100] The test was based on a free T_4 RIA kit (Free T_4 Kit, Nichols Institute Diagnostics, San Juan Capistrano, CA), with protocol adjustment allowing accurate determination of total T_4 concentrations as low as 0.02 μg/dL (0.24 nmol/L). This test is no longer available.[89]

Reference interval values for baseline total T_4 concentration have been published for several species. Considering the marked variations in these reference intervals between species and in some cases within the same species and the different assays used for each study, reference interval values should be used carefully, and more relevance should be given to the pre-TSH and post-TSH injection values obtained for the patient under investigation.

As for mammals, baseline value and the post-TSH administration total T_3 value vary significantly, rendering the diagnosis of hypothyroidism with this method inaccurate in birds.[91-93]

Since thyroxine-binding globulin is absent in birds[86] and free T_4 (fT_4) blood levels are less affected by protein concentrations and concurrent diseases,[101] the use of fT_4 for diagnosis of thyroid disease in birds has been proposed and investigated. fT_4 appears to be present in higher concentrations in avian samples compared with those of mammals when measured with equilibrium dialysis (ED) and column chromatography. However, fT_4 and fT_3 concentrations were similar to those in mammals when measured by using RIA.[86] Normal blood levels of total (RIA) and free (ED) T_4 and T_3 were recently reported for Hispaniolan Amazon parrots. Total and fT_4 reference intervals were 1.7 to 8.2 nmol/L and 0.6 to 7 pmol/L, respectively, whereas total and fT_3 values were 0.72 to 1.43 nmol/L and 6.64 to 15.14 pmol/L, respectively.[102] Determination of blood levels of fT_4 with ED (and of total T_4 with RIA) was used to support the diagnosis of hyperthyroidism secondary to a thyroid carcinoma in a barred owl.[103]

Secondary and tertiary hypothyroidism can be diagnosed by performing the thyrotropin-releasing hormone (TRH) stimulation test and measuring pre-TRH and post-TRH TSH levels (secondary) or by determining blood levels of TRH (tertiary).[48] The assays for determining TRH and TSH blood levels have not been validated for use in birds, and there are no published normal values.[89]

Pharmacologic and toxicity studies of thyroid hormone replacement therapy in avian species are not available. Suggested treatment protocols, mostly adapted from mammalian protocols, are described in Table 10-2.[104] Birds under treatment should be monitored closely and the dose adjusted on the basis of clinical response, evidence of toxicity (GI, cardiac) and total T_4 concentrations (in comparison with pretreatment levels). It is expected that birds will become more active, molt, and lose weight during treatment. Considering the potential for life-threatening complications with L-thyroxine treatment (including the risk of iatrogenic hyperthyroidism), initiation of treatment is not recommended until a TSH stimulation test has been performed and hypothyroidism confirmed.[48,105]

There is a single case report of confirmed hypothyroidism in a scarlet macaw.[76] Diagnosis was supported by clinical signs (feather loss with no molting, skin thickening, excessive subcutaneous fat), blood tests (anemia, hypercholesterolemia), and decreased response to the TSH stimulation test (50% increase in serum total T_4 concentration after TSH stimulation test using 1 international unit [IU] of bovine TSH). Baseline total T_4 concentration was within the published reference interval for the species. The bird was treated with L-thyroxine at 0.02 mg (0.015 mg/kg) orally twice daily for 5 months and once a day thereafter. Adjustments in dosage were based on resolution of clinical signs and hypercholesterolemia and determination of T_4 concentration at 4 and 12 hours after treatment. The medication was well tolerated by the bird, with yellow discoloration of normally red contour feathers in the nape and back being the only abnormality reported. It was not clear from the report if lifelong treatment was required to control the clinical signs or if the bird was eventually weaned off the medication. This information would be necessary to understand if the hypothyroid state was permanent or reversible.

The relationship between hypothyroidism and feather abnormalities (nonpruritic feather loss, feather-damaging behavior) and other skin conditions has been proposed by several authors and practitioners but has not been well documented in several of these reports. One author performed TSH testing using human synthetic TSH in several parrots presenting with signs of obesity, poor feather condition, or

elevated cholesterol. Eleven of a total of 13 birds showed at least a twofold increase of total T_4 concentration 6 hours after TSH administration, and 2 birds (a scarlet macaw and a caique) did not, which suggested hypothyroidism.[89] No further information was provided regarding the treatment and outcome of the suspected hypothyroid cases. In another study by the same author, white Carneaux pigeons failed to respond to low (0.2 IU/kg intramuscularly [IM]) or high (1 IU/kg IM) doses of synthetic human TSH. Approximately 50% of the pigeons also had baseline total T_4 concentrations below normal. On postmortem examination, all pigeons presented lymphocytic thyroiditis, with antemortem test results suggesting a relationship between thyroiditis and hypothyroidism.[88] In a more recent study in Grey parrots, the results of several diagnostic tests (including TSH stimulation test) in birds with normal plumage and birds with feather damaging behavior were compared.[106] Despite the authors' conclusion that the results of the study supported the association of feather-damaging behavior and altered thyroid function, both groups presented a higher than 2.5-fold increase in T_4 levels in response to bovine TSH administration (0.5 IU/bird) and were determined to be euthyroid. Several older case reports of presumptive hypothyroidism in birds were based on clinical signs, low levels of total T_4, and significant clinical improvement with thyroxin treatment. In one report, a budgerigar was diagnosed with hypothyroidism resulting from low baseline total T_4 levels and complete remission of lipomatous growths with L-thyroxine administration.[107] Three Amazon parrots with self-mutilation lesions on the feet received L-thyroxine (0.08 mg/kg, orally daily) for treatment of "low circulating levels of T_4" (low levels based on in-house reference interval of 2.4 to 5.5 µg/dL; normal levels based on the published reference intervals for the species[91,98]). The skin lesions resolved in 3 weeks with the daily use of thyroxin and a topical antiseptic; T_4 levels after treatment were normal (based on in-house reference interval). In one bird, lesions recurred after discontinuing treatment and resolved again once treatment was reinstituted. Thyrotropin stimulation test was performed in one of these three birds, and the response was considered normal.[108]

Hyperthyroidism

Thyroid tumors are relatively rare in birds, with the majority of thyroid enlargement cases being thyroid hyperplasia secondary to iodine deficiency.[48] Thyroid tumors in birds, unlike in mammals, do not appear to be functional, and clinical signs are related to compression of the surrounding tissues, as in the case of goiter.[105] For this reason, histologic diagnosis is necessary to differentiate thyroid neoplasia from goiter. Brandão et al[103] described a case of productive follicular thyroid carcinoma in a wild barred owl that was presented as a trauma case.

There are reports of hyperthyroidism attributed to overdose of exogenous thyroxine.[75] Broiler breeder hens had exogenous T_4 added to the drinking water to produce transient hyperthyroidism. No clinical signs were recorded, although the offspring were more resistant to cold-induced ascites.[109]

As described above, histologic diagnosis is necessary to differentiate thyroid neoplasia from goiter. Surgical excision, with adjuvant radiation and chemotherapy treatment, is often recommended in human and small animal medicine. There

TABLE 10-2

Levothyroxine (L-Thyroxine) Treatment Protocols in Birds[104]

5–200 µg/kg PO q12h	Amazon parrots
20 µg/kg PO q12h-24h	Most species, including psittacines
20–100 µg/kg PO q12h	Psittacines
280–830 µg/L drinking water for 5–10 days	Most species

µg/kg, Microgram per kilogram; µg/L, microgram per liter; PO, orally; q12h, every 12 hours; q12h-24h, every 12 hours to every 24 hours.

are no peer-reviewed reports of treatment of thyroid tumors in birds.

In the case report of thyroid carcinoma in an owl,[102] a unilateral soft tissue opacity cranial to the syrinx was noted on radiographic images. The bird died soon after being presented before any clinical signs referable to hyperthyroidism could be observed. Diagnosis was based on elevated levels of total and fT$_4$ and postmortem findings (mass in the region of the right thyroid gland identified with histopathology and special stains as a functional thyroid carcinoma).

PARATHYROID GLAND

Hyperparathyroidism can be classified as primary, secondary, or tertiary. Primary hyperparathyroidism occurs as a result of excessive production of parathyroid hormone (PTH) caused by a genetic abnormality or neoplasia.[110] Primary hyperparathyroidism has not been diagnosed in avian species.

Secondary hyperparathyroidism occurs when there are elevated levels of PTH, associated with normal or decreased ionized calcium levels. Calcium is an essential nutrient, which is used in the protection of the embryo (egg shell), the maintenance of body structure and capacity for movement (bones), and many critical biochemical processes (e.g., muscle contraction, blood coagulation, nerve conduction). Hyperparathyroidism is thus a normal parathyroid response to abnormal calcium levels, and can be caused by chronic renal failure and nutritional deficiencies (Figure 10-7).[110,111] Ultrastructurally, the parathyroid is hypertrophic or hyperplastic.[75]

To date, all reports of hyperparathyroidism in birds have been secondary and represent appropriate physiologic responses to other conditions.

Parathyroid hyperplasia secondary to nutritional deficiencies (involving calcium, phosphorus, and/or vitamin D$_3$), also known as *nutritional secondary hyperparathyroidism*, is the most commonly reported disorder of the parathyroid gland in birds. Renal secondary hyperparathyroidism has not been reported in avian species.[94,105]

Grey parrots, in particular, seem predisposed to hypocalcemia, which causes muscular weakness, ataxia, seizures, osteodystrophy, poor reproductive performance, and even death.[112] It is thought that from an ecologic viewpoint, this species may depend more on ultraviolet light for calcium metabolism compared with other species.[112] However, in cases of severe enough calcium or vitamin D deficiency, even "hardier" species such as Amazon parrots can develop clinical hypocalcemia.[113]

Nutritional secondary hyperparathyroidism is often suspected in the context of dietary history, clinical signs, physical examination findings, blood tests, and radiographic abnormalities. Clinical signs of calcium deficiency vary, depending on species, age, sex, reproductive status, and severity of deficiency. In the early stages of disease, hens commonly present with abnormal eggs, egg binding, and poor reproductive performance (mainly because of increased embryo mortality); osteomalacia with pathologic fractures, and "cage paralysis" will develop with persistent calcium deficiency. Adult birds can also present with bone deformities and poor feather condition or feather picking. Growing birds can present with abnormal growth and skeletal deformities or fractures of the long bones and spinal column (Figure 10-8). Weakness, ataxia, or even seizures can occur in the more advanced stages of the disease when blood calcium levels are low; these neurologic signs are more commonly seen in Grey parrots.[112,114,115] In most cases, alkaline phosphatase levels are elevated, and total blood calcium levels are normal or elevated, both as a result of increased PTH activity in response to low bioavailability of calcium.[114] Determination of ionized calcium and blood levels of PTH and vitamin D$_3$ can potentially aid the diagnosis of disorders of calcium metabolism. Blood calcium levels must be interpreted carefully since (1) it is common to

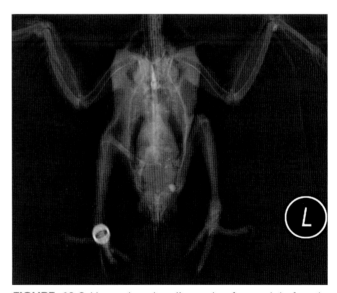

FIGURE 10-8 Ventrodorsal radiograph of an adult female cockatiel with a 7-day history of anorexia, lethargy, and lameness. This bird was offered an all-seed diet. The overall bone density is reduced and the right radius and ulna and left tarsometatarsus present pathologic fractures. The plasma total calcium levels in this bird were within the reference range for the species.

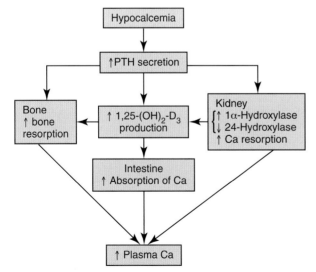

FIGURE 10-7 The control of hypocalcemia. Calcium blood concentrations are restored mainly by the actions of parathyroid hormone (PTH) and 1,25-(OH)2 D$_3$ in the bone, kidneys, and intestinal tract. ↓, Downregulation; ↑, upregulation; Ca, calcium.

find normal total calcium concentrations within the reference interval for the species even when history, physical examination findings, and imaging suggest a calcium disorder and (2) hypercalcemia or hypocalcemia can be caused by many conditions not directly related to parathyroid disease. Determination of ionized calcium levels provides a more precise estimate of an individual's calcium status, especially in cases of abnormal protein concentration and metabolite or electrolyte imbalances.[116] The authors recommend that normal values of ionized calcium be established for each laboratory on the basis of species, type of sample, and analyzer used. Measurements of PTH and vitamin D_3 blood levels could potentially aid in the diagnosis of nutritional secondary hyperparathyroidism, as described in American crows[117] and Grey parrots.[118] In mammals, PTH assays are used for differentiation of primary and secondary hyperparathyroidism and malignant hypercalcemia. Parathyroid hormone concentrations must be interpreted in comparison with total or ionized calcium levels. With normal parathyroid function, hypercalcemia should be associated with low PTH concentration, whereas a high PTH concentration should occur during hypocalcemia.[119] Further investigation of PTH levels and validation of assays are needed before the usefulness of this test for diagnosis of parathyroid disorders in birds can be determined.

Radiography of affected birds can reveal poor bone mineralization, pathologic fractures, and bone deformities.[114,120] Quantitative computed tomography has been used in wild gray herons with metabolic bone disease for objective evaluation of bone mineral density.[121]

Hypocalcemic seizures occur frequently in Grey parrots. The syndrome could potentially be classified as nutritional secondary hyperparathyroidism, since most of the affected birds are offered diets deficient in calcium and vitamin D, and parathyroid hyperplasia is observed on necropsy.[94,105]

Treatment of severe hypocalcemia consists of injectable calcium gluconate (10 to 100 mg/kg IM) and supportive care. Exercise restriction and careful handling and restraint are necessary to prevent pathologic fractures. More stable cases are managed with oral calcium supplements and diet modification. Prognosis for nutritional secondary hyperparathyroidism in birds depends on the severity of bone abnormalities and other clinical conditions that may develop.

Tertiary hyperparathyroidism occurs in humans when functional adenomas develop within chronically hyperplastic parathyroid glands and is associated with elevated PTH, calcium, and phosphorous levels.[75] This condition has not yet been diagnosed in birds. Environmental pollutants such as chlorinated hydrocarbons can exert effects on parathyroid function, although these may differ with the dose and affected species.[122] Some drugs such as omeprazole appear to cause hypertrophy and hyperplasia of the parathyroid gland.[123]

Nonphysiologic hypercalcemia in birds is most commonly secondary to marked and prolonged excessive dietary calcium and vitamin D_3. Presumptive cholecalciferol rodenticide toxicity was recently described in several avian species at a zoologic institution.[124] Other causes of hypercalcemia in mammals, such as primary hyperparathyroidism and pseudohyperparathyroidism (hypercalcemia associated with neoplasia), have not been reported in birds.

Primary hypoparathyroidism and pseudohypoparathyroidism have also not been reported in avian species.[94,105]

ULTIMOBRANCHIAL GLAND

In mammals, ultimobranchial bodies produce CT, which induces hypocalcemia and hypophosphatemia.[125] No diseases involving ultimobranchial gland dysfunction have been documented in birds.[56]

PANCREAS

It has been said that the normal bird resembles a mammal with uncontrolled diabetes in that the basal blood levels of glucose, glucagon, and somatostatin are much higher than in a mammal, as are pancreatic somatostatin levels.[126] However, it appears that the ratio of insulin to glucagon, regulated in part by somatostatin, is the crucial component of blood glucose regulation, rather than any one hormone in isolation.[127]

Endocrine pancreatic dysfunction manifests as either hyperglycemia or hypoglycemia. The most common syndrome in birds is diabetes mellitus (DM)—the failure to adequately constrain blood glucose levels. Sitbon[127] defined DM as a "pathological or experimental dysfunction of the islets of Langerhans as a whole." This definition takes into account the differing etiologies, involving any or all of the hormones insulin, glucagon, and somatostatin, all of which could lead to hyperglycemia. One of the difficulties in the avian literature is that many cases of DM have not had hormone analyses performed but have been diagnosed clinically, leaving the pathophysiology unclear.

In mammalian species, DM is divided into type 1 (insulin dependent) and type 2 (non–insulin dependent). Type 1 DM is associated with destruction of pancreatic B cells, whereas type 2 DM is caused by either a relative insulin deficiency or a peripheral cellular resistance to the effects of insulin.[45,75] This classification system is not entirely useful in birds, in which the insulin-to-glucagon ratio is important. In fact, even in humans, the Expert Committee for the Diagnosis and Classification of Diabetes Mellitus[128] has stated that it is more important to understand the pathogenesis of hyperglycemia in the particular individual than it is to classify it.

Histologically, visible destruction of B cells within the pancreatic islets (which would be consistent with human type 1 DM) has been documented in avian species.[129] Etiologies include diseases that only afflict the pancreas, such as chronic lymphocytic pancreatitis and those affecting multiple organs but also causing pancreatic inflammation or destruction, including iron storage disease, peritonitis (especially reproductively related in hen birds), paramyxovirus infection, and herpesvirus infection.[45,129,130] Ultimately, any pathologic process causing widespread pancreatic inflammation or destruction could progress to involve the pancreatic islets.[131] It is not uncommon to see nonspecific islet cell degeneration at necropsy.[132] However, this does not necessarily correlate with clinical signs of glucose dysfunction.

Causes of peripheral insulin resistance (consistent with human type 2 DM) have been identified, including obesity; high circulating levels of endogenous or exogenous corticosteroids; high circulating levels of diabetogenic hormones such as glucagon, growth hormone, or epinephrine; and high levels of circulating iron.[129,130,133]

There is also some confusion regarding the differential effects of glucagon and insulin within the class Aves. For example, there is the belief that carnivorous birds are more predisposed to insulin-dependent DM, whereas granivorous birds are more glucagon dependent. Regardless of the species, after a complete pancreatectomy, any bird will die from severe hypoglycemia unless given glucagon or glucose infusions. Given the difficulty of total pancreatectomy in some avian species, it is likely that several studies have reported the results of inadvertent subtotal pancreatectomy. Responses to subtotal pancreatectomy vary. For instance, ducks will become transiently diabetic, but geese will become permanently diabetic.[45] It is assumed that these differences relate to a difference in the distribution and proportion of islet cell types in the remaining pancreas.

Schmidt and Reavill[134] described cases of islet cell hypertrophy and hyperplasia, which were grossly unapparent but most of which immunohistochemically were A cells, producing glucagon.

Neoplasia affecting the pancreatic islet cells has been seen, although rarely.[132,135] There has been one reported case of pancreatic islet carcinoma associated with DM in a budgerigar.[135] To the authors' knowledge, there are no documented reports of insulinoma in avian species.

A presumptive diagnosis of DM in birds is based on clinical signs (polyuria, polydipsia, polyphagia with weight loss, and possibly other nonspecific clinical signs), persistent hyperglycemia, and glycosuria. Blood glucose in birds is significantly higher than in mammals, with numbers between 9.9 mmol/L and 19.4 mmol/L (180 and 350 mg/dL) being normal for several bird species. Since birds can develop transient stress-related hyperglycemia, diagnosis of DM in birds should not be based exclusively on a single hyperglycemia occurrence.[80,129] Blood glucose levels above 44.4 mmol/L (800 mg/dL) are usually diagnostic, with values above 55.5 mmol/L (1000 mg/dL) frequently reported. With this severe hyperglycemia, renal glucose threshold is surpassed, and glucose can be detected with urine reagent test strips.[129] Normal avian urine is reported to be negative or trace positive on the reagent urine strip.[136] To avoid readings of false elevation of glucose with urine dip strips because of fecal contamination, the liquid portion of the droppings should be aspirated soon after they are passed. Glycosuria with hyperglycemia allows differentiation between DM and primary renal glycosuria.[80] Healthy bird urine is free of ketones.[136] Ketonuria in the presence of hyperglycemia and glycosuria is

strongly supportive of a diagnosis of DM.[129] Ketonuria is not a consistent finding, and one author questions the link between ketonuria and DM, considering that ketone metabolism is different in birds.[80] It is also important to consider that standard mammalian urine dipstick tests are not designed or validated for use in birds, so the results should be interpreted with caution. The use of other mammalian DM-specific diagnostic tests in avian species has been proposed by a few authors, including determination of blood levels of insulin, glucagon, fructosamine, and β-hydroxybutyric acid (BHBA).

Published reference interval values for serum insulin and plasma glucagon are summarized in Table 10-3.[137-141] The variability of the results of insulin and glucagon blood levels in birds with DM suggests that the pathogenesis of this disease varies significantly among the different species and even within the same species. This variability also creates problems with standardizing these assays for the diagnosis of DM in birds. Despite this, determining blood levels of insulin and glucagon may be useful when establishing a treatment plan, mainly with regard to the use of insulin versus other hypoglycemia medications.[104]

Fructosamines are proteins that result from irreversible, nonenzymatic and insulin-independent binding of glucose to serum proteins. Their concentration is directly related to the blood glucose concentration over the lifespan of the circulating protein (1 to 3 weeks in dogs and cats), making it a good indicator of mean blood glucose concentration over that period. Fructosamine concentration is not affected by acute and temporary increases in blood glucose but can be affected by low albumin.[142] In small animal medicine, fructosamine levels are often used for monitoring response to treatment,[142] with a similar application proposed in cases of DM in avian species. Considering that the half-life of avian serum proteins is much shorter than for domestic mammals (approximately 3 days for albumin in chickens[143]), fructosamines will likely reflect the blood glucose levels in diabetic birds over a shorter period compared with those in mammals. One report described normal fructosamine levels in psittacine birds to be between 113 and 238 micromoles per liter (μmol/L) in comparison with a diabetic macaw that had levels above 300 μmol/L. The levels were later brought within normal limits after initiation of insulin treatment and resolution of clinical signs.[130] In another case report, a fructosamine level of 87 μmol/L obtained 4 days after initiation of treatment suggested response to

TABLE 10-3
Reference Interval Values for Serum Insulin and Plasma Glucagon in Birds

Species	Sample Size	Serum Insulin (Microunit per Milliliter [µU/mL])	Plasma glucagon (Picogram per milliliter [pg/mL])	Reference
Amazon parrot	10	5.9–12.3		137
Amazon parrot	1	7.7	604	138
Bald eagle	13 animals/27 samples	1.42–5.44	229–1239	139
Cockatiel	2 (insulin); 4 (glucagon)	5.8–8.6[‡]	780–964[‡] (*)	138
Macaw	19	4.18–12.4*[‡]	299–1801[†‡]	140
Sulfur-breasted toucan	2		758–1327[†‡]	141
Toco toucan	1 (insulin); 4 (glucagon)	2.4	577–1378	138

*Microparticle enzyme immunoassay or radioimmunoassay (RIA).
[†]RIA assay.
[‡]Reference interval based on highest and lowest values reported.

insulin administration.[144] Determination of blood levels of BHBA, a ketone, is routinely performed in human emergency medicine to distinguish simple hyperglycemia from life-threatening ketoacidosis.[145] Reference interval for BHBA levels in normal psittacine birds have been reported to be between 450 and 1422 μmol/L, and this assay was used for diagnosis and management of DM in two macaws. In both cases, reduction of BHBA and fructosamine to normal levels, together with resolution of clinical signs and hyperglycemia, were used to demonstrate successful treatment with insulin.[130] As for other mammalian-specific tests, commercial assays for measuring insulin, glucagon, fructosamine, and BHBA have not been validated for use with avian samples, so the results should be interpreted with caution. For insulin, the commercially available mammalian assays may not be able to detect the suggested normal low blood insulin levels of granivorous birds.[105] Further work is required before blood levels of these parameters can be used objectively for diagnostic, therapeutic, and prognostic purposes in birds with DM.

Although elevation of amylase and lipase may be suggestive of pancreatic disease in birds, DM can be associated with nonpancreatic disease, and normal levels of these enzymes have been described in a bird with DM secondary to pancreatitis.[144]

Since several cases of DM in birds appear to be secondary to other diseases, a thorough diagnostic medical workup is recommended for birds with hyperglycemia, including complete blood count, chemistry panel, survey radiography, infectious disease testing (*Chlamydophila psittaci*, polyomavirus, paramyxovirus-3, psittacine herpesvirus, adenovirus), and blood levels of zinc, among other tests. Pancreatic biopsy and possibly liver and kidney biopsies may be required in some cases for a definitive diagnosis. When pathology of the pancreas is identified on routine hematoxylin and eosin staining, immunohistochemistry should be performed to determine which cell type is primarily affected. Antemortem characterization of the dysfunction of specific islet cell types can be difficult, considering that the various types of islet cells may not be uniformly distributed throughout the avian pancreas.[105]

Recommended treatment protocols for DM in domestic animals include insulin or oral hypoglycemic agent(s), dietary changes, weight management, and cessation of treatment with diabetogenic drugs. Successful management of DM requires identification and treatment of the underlying inflammatory, infectious, neoplastic, or endocrine disorder.[142]

Several case reports have described the successful use of insulin for the treatment of DM in birds (Table 10-4). Protocols for insulin treatment of DM in birds are extrapolated from domestic animals, with smaller birds usually requiring relatively higher doses compared with larger birds. Short-acting insulin preparations are recommended for the management of patients with unstable DM, whereas intermediate-acting and long-acting preparations are used for the long-term management of uncomplicated diabetes.[142] Insulin type availability and names differ significantly among countries. The new human recombinant insulin analogs provide longer and more predictable effects in mammals[142] and may be a good alternative for use in birds.

Birds presenting with depression, dehydration, anorexia, and vomiting require hospitalization for supportive care,

initiation of insulin therapy, and glucose monitoring. Therapy is initiated with regular insulin at 0.1 to 0.2 units/kg (subcutaneously [SC] or IM). Blood glucose should be monitored every 2 to 3 hours for at least 12 to 24 hours.[80,129] Urine reagent strips can be used as an alternative in smaller birds, in which repeated blood sampling is not possible.[129] Blood glucose curves are extremely important in birds, since response to insulin treatment can be erratic, and peak and duration of effect of insulin preparations in avian species are unknown. These curves are used to adjust the dose and frequency of insulin administration required to maintain blood glucose close to the normal interval. The importance of initial monitoring following insulin administration is highlighted by two cases of birds with presumptive DM that developed life-threatening hypoglycemia within 1 hour of administration of a very low dose of insulin.[129] When the bird's clinical condition has improved, treatment with long-acting insulin such as neutral protamine Hagedorn (NPH) or protamine zinc insulin (PZI) is initiated. Birds with uncomplicated DM on initial presentation are immediately started on longer-acting insulin formulations. Effective dosages vary significantly from bird to bird (0.002 to 3.3 IU/kg IM every 12 to 48 hours). Birds with uncomplicated DM should still be initially hospitalized for blood glucose curve studies to determine the effective insulin protocol. For smaller birds and when using very low doses, insulin may have to be diluted with sterile water. Diluted insulin remains stable under refrigeration for 30 days.[80] Variation of duration of effects with dilution is to be expected, since the vehicle is also diluted.

Treatment with injectable insulin is continued at home, with twice-a-day, once-a-day, or once-every-other-day protocols described.[80,129] Goals for the long-term management of DM in birds are to improve body condition and to reduce or resolve clinical signs. Response to treatment at home is often based on resolution of the clinical signs of DM and monitoring of urine glucose two to three times per day. Since hypoglycemia can be life-threatening, strict regulation of blood glucose within the reference interval is not recommended. Birds should be maintained at a slightly hyperglycemic state, with some associated polyuria and slight positive or trace level of urine glucose. The insulin dose must be carefully adjusted on the basis of these findings. Blood glucose curves should be repeated 1 week after initiation of insulin treatment (since it takes several days to achieve glucose homeostasis), and every 2 to 3 months after in patients with well-controlled DM. If hypoglycemia occurs or signs of DM recur, glucose curve studies should be repeated for readjustment of insulin dosage.[80]

The variety of responses to insulin therapy in birds described in the literature is well correlated with the variety of underlying causes and the fact that in a few of these cases, the DM or hyperglycemia was transient and resolved when the primary disease process was addressed. The variability in the types of insulin used, doses, and frequency of administration also makes comparison of protocols difficult. Theoretically, birds with low levels of insulin are more likely to respond to insulin treatment, but birds with elevated glucagon may also respond, as insulin regulates glucagon's secretion and action. No initial response, excessive initial response, good initial response, recurrence of disease, and complete resolution of clinical signs without requiring insulin treatment for life have all been reported in birds.

TABLE 10-4

Summary of Diabetes Mellitus Cases in the Literature

Species	Clinical Signs	Relevant Diagnostic Test Results	Treatment	Outcome	Final Diagnosis	Reference
Blue-and-gold macaw (*Ara ararauna*)	Polyuria Polydipsia Weight loss	Hyperglycemia Glycosuria Low insulin/ normal glucagon levels	Insulin (no further information)	Seizures and death 4 days after presentation	Pancreas: hyperplasia and hypertrophy A cells; decrease size of islets and number of B cells Liver: hemosiderosis Kidney: glomerulosclerosis	149
Blue-and-gold macaw (*Ara ararauna*)	Polyuria Polydipsia	Hyperglycemia Elevated cholesterol and triglycerides Glycosuria Elevated glucagon/ normal insulin levels	Change in diet→ no effect→ somatostatin 3 microgram per kilogram (μg/kg) subcutaneously (SC) twice daily and up to 10 μg/kg SC twice daily→ no effect→ neutral protamine Hagedorn (NPH) insulin (Iletin) 0.2 units/kg SC twice daily	Successfully managed for 7 months Glucagon levels returned to normal		140
Military macaw (*Ara militaris*)	Polyuria Polydipsia Polyphagia Weight loss	Hyperglycemia Elevated cholesterol Glycosuria Ketonuria Ketonemia Elevated fructosamine levels	Bovine protamine zinc insulin (PZI) 0.5 units/kg AM to 0.3 units/kg PM→ 0.15 units/kg AM to 0.1 units/kg PM Low iron diet Phlebotomy	Successfully managed 29 months Insulin demand reduced with phlebotomy Fructosamine and β-hydroxybutyric acid (BHBA) normal 4 weeks after initiating insulin Diet and phlebotomy→ reduced iron in liver biopsy at 12 months	Biopsy: hemosiderosis liver and pancreas (no endocrine pancreas on sample)	130
Chestnut-fronted macaw (*Ara severus*)	Polyuria Polydipsia Lethargy	Hyperglycemia Glycosuria Ketonuria Ketonemia	Porcine PZI (Caninsulin) 0.5– 0.67 international units per kilogram (IU/ kg) twice daily; changed to bovine PZI needed after 22 months Low iron diet Deferoxamine treatment	Successfully managed for 22 months Insulin demand reduced during deferoxamine treatment Diet and deferoxamine resulted in reduced iron in liver biopsy at 20 months	Biopsy: hemosiderosis liver and pancreas; nodular hyperplasia of the exocrine pancreas (no endocrine pancreas sampled) Postmortem: hepatic and renal hemosiderosis; atherosclerosis (endocrine/ exocrine pancreas normal)	130
Chestnut-fronted macaw (*Ara severus*)	Polyuria Polydipsia Weight loss	Hyperglycemia Glycosuria Ketonuria	NPH insulin 1 unit twice daily; increased dose by 0.5 unit daily for 5 days Supportive care	No response to insulin therapy (clinical signs or hyperglycemia persisted); died 5 days after initiating insulin treatment	Type 1 diabetes mellitus Pancreas: marked islet cell vacuolar degeneration, multifocal lymphocytic pancreatitis; exocrine pancreas hyperplasia; immunohistochemical stain with no A or B cells on islets; perivascular fungal meningoencephalitis, presumptive zygomycosis; hepatic hemosiderosis	150

Glipizide, an oral hypoglycemic drug used for treatment of type 2 DM in humans and cats, has been used in the management of diabetic birds with variable to no success.[129] Since its primary effect is to stimulate insulin secretion by B cells, some cell function is required for the drug to be effective. In cats, the drug is only used for uncomplicated and mild to moderate cases of DM.[142] Published treatment protocols for glipizide in birds include 0.3 to 0.5 mg/kg, orally (PO) twice daily,[146] 1 mg/kg, PO twice daily,[147] or a 10-mg tablet dissolved in the bird's drinking water.[129] The treatment goals for glipizide are the same as those described for insulin. There are no peer-reviewed case reports of use of other oral hypoglycemic drugs in birds with DM. Based on the proposed mechanism of DM in granivorous birds (excessive glucagon secretion with normal insulin secretion) and the physiologic effect of somatostatin in suppressing glucagon production and release by pancreatic A cells, one author used a synthetically derived analog of somatostatin (Sandostatin; 3 μg/kg, SC twice daily) for the treatment of DM in a sulfur-breasted toucan. Although the clinical signs improved, blood glucose and glucagon levels remained elevated.[141] The same drug was used in a blue-and-gold macaw with DM. The treatment was not effective in resolving clinical signs, hyperglycemia, or glycosuria, even when the drug was given at a dose of 10 μg/kg, SC twice daily.[140]

As for domestic mammals, birds with DM should be offered a high-fiber, low-sugar, and low-fat diet because of its benefits in achieving weight loss and reducing postprandial variations in blood glucose.[80,129] A change to a low-iron diet seemed to result in reducing the insulin requirements in one diabetic toucan[148] and two diabetic macaws.[130] Diet modifications should be made gradually and only when the bird is clinically stable.

Birds with DM should be monitored closely for the occurrence of bacterial or fungal infection because of the risk of impaired immunity, as described for mammals with DM.

Excellent client education, communication, and compliance are important for successful long-term management of DM in birds.

Case reports of DM in birds are summarized in Table 10-4.[130,140,149,150] The majority of the cases presented involve macaws, budgerigars, and toucans. It has been stated that toucans are overrepresented with regard to DM, but the link between DM and iron storage disease needs to be further elucidated.[130,148]

REFERENCES

1. Scanes CG: Avian endocrine system. In Whittow GC, editor: *Sturkie's avian physiology*, ed 6, St. Louis, MO, 2015, Elsevier, pp 489–496.
2. Sawai H, Kim HL, Kuno K, et al: The origin and genetic variation of domestic chickens with special reference to jungle fowls *Gallus g. gallus* and *G. varius*, *PLoS One* 5:e10639, 2010.
3. Rubin CJ, Zody MC, Eriksson J, et al: Whole-genome resequencing reveals loci under selection during chicken domestication, *Nature* 464:587–591, 2010.
4. Delfino KR, Southey BR, Sweedler JV, et al: Genome-wide census and expression profiling of chicken neuropeptide and prohormone convertase genes, *Neuropeptides* 44:31–44, 2010.
5. Xie F, London SE, Southey BR, et al: The zebra finch neuropeptidome: prediction, detection and expression, *BMC Biol* 8:28, 2010.
6. Wang Y, Li J, Yan Kwok AH, et al: A novel prolactin-like protein (PRL-L) gene in chickens and zebrafish: cloning and characterization of its tissue expression, *Gen Comp Endocrinol* 166:200–210, 2010.
7. Beuchat CA, Chong CR: Hyperglycemia in hummingbirds and its consequences for hemoglobin glycation, *Comp Biochem Physiol A Mol Integr Physiol* 120:409–416, 1998.
8. Mohanty B: Extracellular accumulations in the avian pituitary gland: histochemical analysis in two species of Indian wild birds, *Cells Tissues Organs* 183:99–106, 2006.
9. Ramesh R, Solow R, Proudman JA, et al: Identification of mammosomatotrophs in the turkey hen pituitary: increased abundance during hyperprolactinemia, *Endocrinology* 139:781–786, 1998.
10. Ramesh R, Kuenzel WJ, Proudman JA: Increased proliferative activity and programmed cellular death in the turkey hen pituitary gland following interruption of incubation behavior, *Biol Reprod* 64:611–618, 2001.
11. Pals K, Boussemaere M, Swinnen E, et al: A pituitary cell type coexpressing messenger ribonucleic acid of proopiomelanocortin and the glycoprotein hormone alpha-subunit in neonatal rat and chicken: rapid decline with age and reappearance in vitro under regulatory pressure of corticotropin-releasing hormone in the rat, *Endocrinology* 147:4738–4752, 2006.
12. Maung ZW, Follett BK: Effects of chicken and ovine luteinizing hormone on androgen release and cyclic AMP production by isolated cells from the quail testis, *Gen Comp Endocrinol* 33:242–253, 1977.
13. Brown N, Bayle J, Scanes C, et al: The actions of avian LH and FSH on the testes of hypophysectomized quail, *Cell Tissue Res* 156:499–520, 1975.
14. Cui H, Zhao G, Liu R, et al: FSH stimulates lipid biosynthesis in chicken adipose tissue by upregulating the expression of its receptor FSHR, *J Lipid Res* 53:909–917, 2012.
15. Scanes CG: Pituitary gland. In Whittow GC, editor: *Sturkie's avian physiology*, ed 6, St. Louis, MO, 2015, Elsevier, pp 497–533.
16. McNabb FMA: *Thyroid hormones*, Englewood Cliffs, NJ, 1992, Prentice Hall.
17. Wentworth BC, Ringer RK: Thyroids. In Sturkie PD, editor: *Avian physiology*, New York, 1986, Springer-Verlag, pp 452–465.
18. Bizhanova A, Kopp P: Minireview: the sodium-iodide symporter NIS and pendrin in iodide homeostasis of the thyroid, *Endocrinology* 150:1084–1090, 2009.
19. McNabb FMA: Thyroids. In Whittow GC, editor: *Sturkie's avian physiology*, ed 5, San Diego, CA, 2000, Academic Press, pp 461–471.
20. McNabb FMA, Darras VM: Thyroids. In Whittow GC, editor: *Sturkie's avian physiology*, ed 6, St. Louis, MO, 2015, Elsevier, pp 535–547.
21. Darras VM, Van Herck SL: Iodothyronine deiodinase structure and function: from ascidians to humans, *J Endocrinol* 215:189–206, 2012.
22. Orozco A, Valverde-R C, Olvera A, et al: Iodothyronine deiodinases: a functional and evolutionary perspective, *J Endocrinol* 215:207–219, 2012.
23. Rudas P, Bartha T, Frenyo VL: Elimination and metabolism of triiodothyronine depend on the thyroid status in the brain of young chickens, *Acta Vet Hung* 42:465–476, 1994.
24. Rudas P, Bartha T, Frenyo LV: Thyroid hormone deiodination in the brain of young chickens acutely adapts to changes in thyroid status, *Acta Vet Hung* 41:381–393, 1993.
25. De Groef B, Van der Geyten S, Darras VM, et al: Role of corticotropin-releasing hormone as a thyrotropin-releasing factor in non-mammalian vertebrates, *Gen Comp Endocrinol* 146:62–68, 2006.
26. Lazar MA: Thyroid hormone receptors: multiple forms, multiple possibilities, *Endocr Rev* 14:184–193, 1993.
27. McNabb FMA, King DB: Thyroid hormone effects on growth, development and metabolism. In Schreibman MP, Scanes CG, Pang PKT, editors: *The endocrinology of growth, development, and metabolism of vertebrates*, New York, 1993, Academic Press, pp 393–417.
28. Decuypere E, Verheyen G: Physiological basis of induced moulting and tissue regeneration in fowls, *Worlds Poult Sci J* 42:56–68, 1986.

29. Bernal J: Thyroid hormone receptors in brain development and function, *Nat Clin Pract Endocrinol Metab* 3:249–259, 2007.

30. Forrest D, Swaroop A: Minireview: the role of nuclear receptors in photoreceptor differentiation and disease. *Mol Endocrinol* 26:905–915, 2012.

31. Rusch A, Ng L, Goodyear R, et al: Retardation of cochlear maturation and impaired hair cell function caused by deletion of all known thyroid hormone receptors, *J Neurosci* 21:9792–9800, 2001.

32. Fischer AJ, Bongini R, Bastaki N, et al: The maturation of photoreceptors in the avian retina is stimulated by thyroid hormone, *Neuroscience* 178:250–260, 2011.

33. Yamaguchi S, Aoki N, Kitajima T, et al: Thyroid hormone determines the start of the sensitive period of imprinting and primes later learning, *Nat Commun* 3:1081, 2012.

34. Dacke CG: *Calcium regulation in submammalian vertebrates*, London, UK, 1979, Academic Press.

35. Kenny AD: Parathyroid and ultimobranchial glands. In Sturkie PD, editor: *Avian physiology*, ed 4, New York, 1986, Springer-Verlag, pp 466–478.

36. Shaw AJ, Whittaker G, Dacke CG: Kinetics of rapid 45Ca uptake into chick skeleton in vivo: effects of microwave fixation, *Q J Exp Physiol* 74:907–915, 1989.

37. Farley JR, Tarbaux NM, Hall SL, et al: The anti-bone-resorptive agent calcitonin also acts in vitro to directly increase bone formation and bone cell proliferation, *Endocrinology* 123:159–167, 1988.

38. Bouizar Z, Khattab M, Taboulet J, et al: Distribution of renal calcitonin binding sites in mammalian and nonmammalian vertebrates, *Gen Comp Endocrinol* 76:364–370, 1989.

39. Hou HC: Relation of the preen gland of birds to rickets. III. Site of activation during irradiation, *Chin J Physiol* 5:11–18, 1931.

40. Henry HL, Norman AW: Vitamin D: metabolism and biological actions, *Annu Rev Nutr* 4:493–520, 1984.

41. Nys Y, N'Guyen TM, Williams J, et al: Blood levels of ionized calcium, inorganic phosphorus, 1,25-dihydroxycholecalciferol and gonadal hormones in hens laying hard-shelled or shell-less eggs, *J Endocrinol* 111:151–157, 1986.

42. Clark NB: Renal clearance of phosphate and calcium in vitamin D-deficient chicks: effect of calcium loading, parathyroidectomy, and parathyroid hormone administration, *J Exp Zool* 259:188–195, 1991.

43. Dacke CG: Eicosanoids, steroids and miscellaneous hormones. In Pang PKT, Schreibman MP, editors: *Vertebrate endocrinology: fundamentals and biomedical implications*, New York, 1989, Academic Press, pp 171–210.

44. Williams DC, Paul DC, Herring JR: Effects of antiestrogenic compounds on avian medullary bone formation, *J Bone Miner Res* 6:1249–1256, 1991.

45. Hazelwood RL: Pancreas. In Whittow GC, editor: *Sturkie's avian physiology*, ed 5, San Diego, CA, 2000, Academic Press, pp 539–556.

46. Simon J: Chicken as a useful species for the comprehension of insulin action, *Crit Rev Poult Biol* 2:121–148, 1989.

47. George JC, John TM, Mitchell MA: Flight effects on plasma levels of lipid, glucagon and thyroid hormones in homing pigeons, *Horm Metab Res* 21:542–545, 1989.

48. Lumeij JT: Endocrinology. In Ritchie BW, Harrison GJ, Harrison LR, editors: *Avian medicine: principles and application*, Lake Worth, FL, 1994, Wingers, pp 582–606.

49. Li C, Takahashi S, Taneda S, et al: Impairment of testicular function in adult male Japanese quail (*Coturnix japonica*) after a single administration of 3-methyl-4-nitrophenol in diesel exhaust particles, *J Endocrinol* 189:555–564, 2006.

50. Ottinger MA, Lavoie ET, Thompson N, et al: Is the gonadotropin releasing hormone system vulnerable to endocrine disruption in birds? *Gen Comp Endocrinol* 163:104–108, 2009.

51. Suchy A, Weissenböck H, Schmidt P: Intracranial tumours in budgerigars, *Avian Pathol* 28:125–130, 1999.

52. Langohr IM, Garner MM, Kiupel M: Somatotroph pituitary tumors in budgerigars (*Melopsittacus undulatus*), *Vet Pathol* 49:503–507, 2012.

53. Hull KL, Marsh JA, Harvey S: A missense mutation in the GHR gene of Cornell sex-linked dwarf chickens does not abolish serum GH binding, *J Endocrinol* 161:495–501, 1999.

54. Cogburn LA, Burnside J, Scanes CG: Physiology of growth and development. In Whittow GC, editor: *Sturkie's avian physiology*, ed 5, San Diego, CA, 2000, Academic Press, pp 635–656.

55. Palya V, Zolnai A, Benyeda Z, et al: Short beak and dwarfism syndrome of mule duck is caused by a distinct lineage of goose parvovirus, *Avian Pathol* 38:175–180, 2009.

56. Ritchie M, Pilny AA: The anatomy and physiology of the avian endocrine system, *Vet Clin North Am Exot Anim Pract* 11:1–14, v, 2008.

57. de Matos R: Adrenal steroid metabolism in birds: anatomy, physiology, and clinical considerations, *Vet Clin North Am Exot Anim Pract* 11:35–57, vi, 2008.

58. Starkey SR, Morrisey JK, Stewart JE, et al: Pituitary-dependent hyperadrenocorticism in a cockatoo, *J Am Vet Med Assoc* 232:394–398, 2008.

59. Ritchie M: Neuroanatomy and physiology of the avian hypothalamic/pituitary axis: clinical aspects, *Vet Clin North Am Exot Anim Pract* 17:13–22, 2014.

60. Braun EJ, Stallone JN: The occurrence of nephrogenic diabetes insipidus in domestic fowl, *Am J Physiol Renal Physiol* 256:F639–F645, 1989.

61. Brummermann M, Braun EJ: Renal response of roosters with diabetes insipidus to infusions of arginine vasotocin, *Am J Physiol* 269:R57–R63, 1995.

62. Reference deleted in pages.

63. Minvielle F, Grossmann R, Gourichon D: Development and performances of a Japanese quail line homozygous for the diabetes insipidus (di) mutation, *Poult Sci* 86:249–254, 2007.

64. Starkey SR, Wood C, de Matos R, et al: Central diabetes insipidus in an African grey parrot, *J Am Vet Med Assoc* 237:415–419, 2010.

65. Rijnberk A: Diabetes insipidus. In Ettinger SJ, Feldman EC, editors: *Textbook of veterinary internal medicine*, ed 7, St. Louis, MO, 2010, Saunders, pp 1716–1722.

66. Alberts H, Halsema WB, de Bruijne JJ, et al: A water deprivation test for the differentiation of polyuric disorders in birds, *Avian Pathol* 17:385–389, 1988.

67. Romagnano A, Mashima TY, Barnes HJ, et al: Pituitary adenoma in an Amazon parrot, *J Avian Med Surg* 9:263–270, 1995.

68. Schlumberger HG: Neoplasia in the parakeet. I. Spontaneous chromophobe pituitary tumors, *Cancer Res* 14:237–245, 1954.

69. Latimer K: Oncology. In Ritchie B, Harrison G, Harrison L, editors: *Avian medicine: principles and application*, Lake Worth, FL, 1994, Wingers Publishing, pp 640–672.

70. Dezfoulian O, Abbasi M, Azarabad H, et al: Cerebral neuroblastoma and pituitary adenocarcinoma in two budgerigars (*Melopsittacus undulatus*), *Avian Dis* 55:704–708, 2011.

71. Wheler C: Pituitary tumors in cockatiels, *J Assoc Avian Vet* 6:92, 1992.

72. Schmidt RE, Reavill DR, Phalen DN: Endocrine system. In *Pathology of pet and aviary birds*, Ames, IA, 2003, Blackwell Publishing, pp 121–130.

73. Swayne DE, Rowland GN, Fletcher OJ: Pinealoma in a broiler breeder, *Avian Dis* 30:853–855, 1986.

74. Wilson RB, Holscher MA, Fullerton JR, et al: Pineoblastoma in a cockatiel, *Avian Dis* 32:591–593, 1988.

75. Rae M: Endocrine disease in pet birds, *Semin Avian Exot Pet Med* 4:32–38, 1995.

76. Oglesbee BL: Hypothyroidism in a scarlet macaw, *J Am Vet Med Assoc* 201:1599–1601, 1992.

77. Schmidt RE, Reavill DR: The avian thyroid gland, *Vet Clin North Am Exot Anim Pract* 11:15–23, v, 2008.

78. Schmidt RE: Avian thyroid metabolism and diseases, *Semin Avian Exot Pet Med* 11:80–83, 2002.

79. Alley MR, Twentyman CM, Sancha SE, et al: Hyperplastic goitre and mortality in captive-reared black stilts (*Himantopus novaezelandiae*), *N Z Vet J* 56:139–144, 2008.

80. Oglesbee BL: Diseases of the endocrine system. In Altman RB, Clubb SL, Dorrestein GM, et al, editors: *Avian medicine and surgery*, Philadelphia, PA, 1997, Saunders, pp 482–488.

81. Hawkins M, Barron HW, Speer B, et al: Birds. In Carpenter JW, Marion CJ, editors: *Exotic animal formulary*, ed 4, St. Louis, MO, 2013, Elsevier, pp 184–438.

82. Wick G, Andersson L, Hala K, et al: Avian models with spontaneous autoimmune diseases, *Adv Immunol* 92:71–117, 2006.

83. Weng Q, Saita E, Watanabe G, et al: Effect of methimazole-induced hypothyroidism on adrenal and gonadal functions in male Japanese quail (*Coturnix japonica*), *J Reprod Dev* 53:1335–1341, 2007.

84. Merryman JI, Buckles EL: The avian thyroid gland. Part Two: A review of function and pathophysiology, *J Avian Med Surg* 12:238–242, 1998.

85. Huynh M, Carnaccini S, Driggers T, et al: Ulcerative dermatitis and valvular endocarditis associated with Staphylococcus aureus in a hyacinth macaw (*Anodorhynchus hyacinthinus*), *Avian Dis* 58:223–227, 2014.

86. McNabb FMA, Darras VM: Thyroids. In Scanes CG, editor: *Sturkie's avian physiology*, ed 6, San Diego, CA, 2015, Academic Press, pp 535–547.

87. Harms CA, Hoskinson JJ, Bruyette DS, et al: Technetium-99m and iodine-131 thyroid scintigraphy in normal and radiothyroidectomized cockatiels (*Nymphicus hollandicus*), *Vet Radiol Ultrasound* 35:473–478, 1994.

88. Greenacre CB, Olsen JH, Wilson GH, et al: The use of synthetic TSH to evaluate the thyroid gland, *Proc Assoc Avian Vet Annu Conf* 13, 2002.

89. Greenacre CB: Diagnostic testing in the field: the researcher's prospective on thyroid testing in psittacine birds, *Proc Assoc Avian Vet Annu Conf* 89–94, 2009.

90. Greenacre CB, Jaques J: TSH testing in birds using canine, bovine or human TSH, *Proc Assoc Avian Vet Annu Conf* 49, 2011.

91. Lothrop CD Jr, Loomis MR, Olsen JH: Thyrotropin stimulation test for evaluation of thyroid function in psittacine birds, *J Am Vet Med Assoc* 186:47–48, 1985.

92. Zenoble RD, Kemppainen RJ, Young DW, et al: Endocrine responses of healthy parrots to ACTH and thyroid stimulating hormone, *J Am Vet Med Assoc* 187:1116–1118, 1985.

93. Williamson RA, Davison TF: The effect of a single injection of thyrotrophin on serum concentrations of thyroxine, triiodothyronine, and reverse triiodothyronine in the immature chicken (*Gallus domesticus*), *Gen Comp Endocrinol* 58:109–113, 1985.

94. de Matos R: Calcium metabolism in birds, *Vet Clin North Am Exot Anim Pract* 11:59–82, vi, 2008.

95. Greenacre CB: Thyrogen for use in TSH testing of healthy and suspected hypothyroid parrots, *Proc Eur Assoc Avian Vet* 125–126, 2009.

96. Harms CA, Hoskinson JJ, Bruyette DS, et al: Development of an experimental model of hypothyroidism in cockatiels (*Nymphicus hollandicus*), *Am J Vet Res* 55:399–404, 1994.

97. Lumeij JT, Westerhof I: Clinical evaluation of thyroid function in racing pigeons (*Columba livia domestica*), *Avian Pathol* 17:63–70, 1988.

98. Woerpel RW, Rosskopf WJ Jr: Clinical experience with avian laboratory diagnostics, *Vet Clin North Am Small Anim Pract* 14:249–286, 1984.

99. Rosskopf WJ, Woerpel RW, Rosskopf G, et al: Normal thyroid values for common pet birds, *VM SAC* 77:409–412, 1982.

100. Greenacre CB, Young DW, Behrend EN, et al: Validation of a novel high-sensitivity radioimmunoassay procedure for measurement of total thyroxine concentration in psittacine birds and snakes, *Am J Vet Res* 62:1750–1754, 2001.

101. Scott-Moncrieff JC: Hypothyroidism. In Ettinger SJ, Feldman EC, editors: *Textbook of Veterinary internal medicine*, ed 7, St. Louis, MO, 2010, Saunders, pp 1751–1761.

102. Brandao J, Rick M, Beaufrere H, et al: Free and total thyroid hormones reference interval in the Hispaniolan Amazon parrot, *Proc Assoc Avian Vet Annu Conf* 29, 2014.

103. Brandão J, Manickam B, Blas-Machado U, et al: Productive thyroid follicular carcinoma in a wild barred owl (*Strix varia*), *J Vet Diagn Invest* 24:1145–1150, 2012.

104. Pollock C, Carpenter JW, Antinoff N: Birds. In Carpenter JW, editor: *Exotic animal formulary*, ed 3, St. Louis, MO, 2005, Elsevier, pp 135–346.

105. Rae M: Avian endocrine disorders. In Fudge A, editor: *Laboratory medicine avian and exotic pets*, Philadelphia, PA, 2000, Saunders, pp 76–89.

106. Clubb SL, Cray C, Arheart KL, et al: Comparison of selected diagnostic parameters in African grey parrots (*Psittacus erithacus*) with normal plumage and those exhibiting feather damaging behavior, *J Avian Med Surg* 21:259–264, 2007.

107. Rosskopf WJ, Woerpel RW: Remission of lipomatous growths in a hypothyroid budgerigar in response to L-thyroxine therapy, *Vet Med Sm Anim Clin* 9:1415–1418, 1983.

108. Parrott T: Pododermatitis in three amazon parrots and treatment with L-thyroxine, *Proc Assoc Avian Vet Annu Conf* 1–2, 1991.

109. Akhlaghi A, Zamiri MJ, Zare Shahneh A, et al: Maternal hyperthyroidism is associated with a decreased incidence of cold-induced ascites in broiler chickens, *Poult Sci* 91:1165–1172, 2012.

110. Blackburn M, Diamond T: Primary hyperparathyroidism and familial hyperparathyroid syndromes, *Aust Fam Physician* 36:1029–1033, 2007.

111. Phalen DN, Drew ML, Contreras C, et al: Naturally occurring secondary nutritional hyperparathyroidism in cattle egrets (*Bubulcus ibis*) from central Texas, *J Wildl Dis* 41:401–415, 2005.

112. Stanford M: Calcium metabolism. In Harrison GJ, Lightfoot TL, editors: *Clinical avian medicine*, Palm Beach, FL, 2006, Spix Publishing, pp 141–151.

113. Randell MG: Nutritionally induced hypocalcemic tetany in an Amazon parrot, *J Am Vet Med Assoc* 179:1277–1278, 1981.

114. Wallach JD, Flieg GM: Nutritional secondary hyperparathyroidism in captive birds, *J Am Vet Med Assoc* 155:1046–1051, 1969.

115. Yagil R, van Creveld C, Levy A: Ostrich endocrinology II: PTH and calcium, *Int J Anim Sci* 8:5–8, 1993.

116. Norman AW: Studies of the vitamin D endocrine system in the avian, *J Nutr* 117:797–807, 1987.

117. Tangredi BP, Krook LP: Nutritional secondary hyperparathyroidism in free-living fledgling American crows (*Corvus brachyrhynchos brachyrhynchos*), *J Zoo Wildl Med* 30:94–99, 1999.

118. Stanford M: Calcium metabolism in grey parrots: the effects of husbandry [Diploma of Fellowship thesis], London, UK, 2005, Royal College of Veterinary Surgeons.

119. Rosol TJ, Chew DJ, Nagode LA, et al: Disorders of calcium: hypercalcemia and hypocalcemia. In DiBartola SP, editor: *Fluid therapy in small animal practice*, ed 2, Philadelphia, PA, 2000, Saunders, pp 108–161.

120. Smith JM, Roudybush TE: Nutritional disorders. In Altman RB, Clubb SL, Dorrestein GD, et al, editors: *Avian medicine and surgery*, Philadelphia, PA, 1996, Saunders, pp 501–515.

121. Feltrer Y, Draper ER, Perkins M, et al: Skeletal deformities and mortality in grey herons (*Ardea cinerea*) at Besthorpe heronry, Nottinghamshire, *Vet Rec* 159:514–521, 2006.

122. Rattner BA, Eroschenko VP, Fox GA, et al: Avian endocrine responses to environmental pollutants, *J Exp Zool* 232(3):683–689, 1984.

123. Gagnemo-Persson R, Samuelsson A, Hakanson R, et al: Chicken parathyroid hormone gene expression in response to gastrin, omeprazole, ergocalciferol, and restricted food intake, *Calcif Tissue Int* 61(3):210–215, 1997.

124. Swenson J, Bradley GA: Suspected cholecalciferol rodenticide toxicosis in avian species at a zoological institution, *J Avian Med Surg* 27(2):136–147, 2013.

125. Johnston MS, Ivey ES: Parathyroid and ultimobranchial glands: calcium metabolism in birds, *Semin Avian Exot Pet* 11(2):84–93, 2002.

126. Hazelwood RL: Pancreatic hormones, insulin/glucagon molar ratios, and somatostatin as determinants of avian carbohydrate metabolism, *J Exp Zool* 232(3):647–652, 1984.

127. Sitbon G, Laurent F, Mialhe A, et al: Diabetes in birds, *Horm Metab Res* 12(1):1–9, 1980.

128. Expert Committee for the Diagnosis and Classification of Diabetes Mellitus: Diagnosis and classification of diabetes mellitus, 2011 <http://care.diabetesjournals.org/content/34/Supplement_1/S62.full>. (Accessed June 28, 2014.)

129. Pilny AA: The avian pancreas in health and disease, *Vet Clin North Am Exot Anim Pract* 11(1):25–34, 2008.

130. Gancz AY, Wellehan JF, Boutette J, et al: Diabetes mellitus concurrent with hepatic haemosiderosis in two macaws (*Ara severa, Ara militaris*), *Avian Pathol* 36(4):331–336, 2007.

131. American Diabetes Association: Diagnosis and classification of diabetes mellitus, *Diabetes Care* 36(Suppl 1):S67–S74, 2013.

132. Schmidt R, Reavill D: Endocrine lesions in psittacine birds, *Proc Assoc Avian Vet Conf* 27–29, 2006.

133. Candeletta SC, Homer BL, Garner MM, et al: Diabetes mellitus associated with chronic lymphocytic pancreatitis in an African grey parrot, *J Assoc Avian Vet* 7(1):39–43, 1993.

134. Schmidt RE, Reavill DR: Lesions of the avian pancreas, *Vet Clin North Am Exot Anim Pract* 17(1):1–11, 2014.

135. Ryan CP, Walder EJ, Howard EB: Diabetes mellitus and islet cell carcinoma in a parakeet, *J Am Anim Hosp Assoc* 18:139–142, 1982.

136. Pollock C: Diagnosis and treatment of avian renal disease, *Vet Clin North Am Exot Anim Pract* 9(1):107–128, 2006.

137. Zenoble RD, Kemppainen RJ: Endocrinology of birds. In Kirk RW, editor: *Current veterinary therapy small animal practice*, ed 9, Philadelphia, PA, 1986, Saunders, pp 702–705.

138. Lothrop CD, Harrison GJ, Schultz D, et al: Miscellaneous diseases. In Harrison GJ, Harrison LR, editors: *Clinical avian medicine and surgery*, Philadelphia, PA, 1986, Saunders, pp 525–536.

139. Minick MC, Duke GE: Simultaneous determinations of plasma insulin, glucose and glucagon levels in fasting, previously stressed but convalescing bald eagles, *Haliaeetus leucocephalus* Linnaeus, *Comp Biochem Phys A* 99(3):307–311, 1991.

140. Bonda M: Plasma glucagon, serum insulin and serum amylase levels in normal and hyperglycemic macaw, *Proc Assoc Avian Vet Conf* 77–88, 1996.

141. Kahler J: Sandostatin (synthetic somatostatin) treatment for diabetes mellitus in a sulfur breasted toucan (*Rhamphastos sulfuratus sulfuratus*), *Proc Assoc Avian Vet Conf* 269–273, 1994.

142. Reusch C: Feline diabetes mellitus. In Ettinger SJ, Feldman EC, editors: *Textbook of veterinary internal medicine*, ed 7, St. Louis, MO, 2010, Saunders, pp 1796–1816.

143. Patterson R, Youngner JS, Weigle WO, et al: The metabolism of serum proteins in the hen and chick and secretion of serum proteins by the ovary of the hen, *J Gen Physiol* 45:501–513, 1962.

144. Desmarchelier M, Langlois I: Diabetes mellitus in a nanday conure (*Nandayus nenday*), *J Avian Med Surg* 22(3):246–254, 2008.

145. Charles RA, Bee YM, Eng PH, et al: Point-of-care blood ketone testing: screening for diabetic ketoacidosis at the emergency department, *Singap Med J* 48(11):986–989, 2007.

146. Pollock CG, Pledger T: Diabetes mellitus in avian species, *Proc Assoc Avian Vet Conf* 151–154, 2001.

147. Hudelson KS, Hudelson PM: Endocrine considerations. In Harrison GJ, Lightfoot TL, editors: *Clinical avian medicine*, Palm Beach, FL, 2006, Spix Publishing, pp 541–557.

148. Murphy J: Diabetes in toucans, *Proc Assoc Avian Vet Conf* 165–170, 1992.

149. Shivaprasad HL, Bonda M: Diabetes mellitus in an adult blue and gold macaw (*Ara ararauna*), *Proc Assoc Avian Vet Conf* 341–342, 2009.

150. Pilny A, Luong R: Diabetes mellitus in a chestnut-fronted macaw (*Ara severa*), *J Avian Med Surg* 19(4):297–302, 2005.

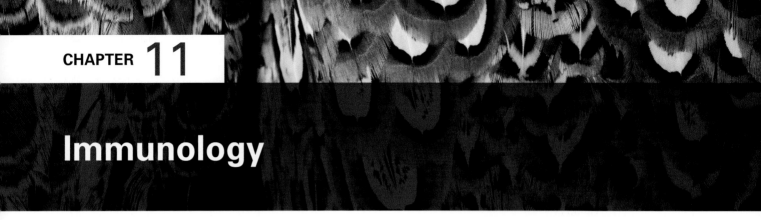

CHAPTER 11

Immunology

Helene Pendl • Ian Tizard

The purpose of immunologic defenses in birds is not only to protect each individual against external pathogens but also to eliminate abnormal body cells, even those with minor deviations, that is, aged, virus-infected, and neoplastic cells. To achieve this, vertebrates have developed multiple defensive mechanisms that collectively ensure that they survive and thrive in the presence of large numbers of microbes, many of which take every opportunity to invade the body. The avian immune system has developed diverse modules that rapidly eliminate invaders, as well as cells with specific receptor systems for detecting microbial antigens and cellular abnormalities. It has to be emphasized that not only recognition itself but also the appropriate response to these threats is essential for a physiologic immune reaction. Thus, not all microbial agents present a threat to the body. The bacteria of the normal gut flora, for example, are beneficial commensals and need not trigger a potent defensive response. Thus, the immune system must not simply differentiate "self" from "nonself" but also assess the nature of any threat and mount a proportional response. Failure to recognize and destroy an infectious agent can lead to fatal disease, as is the case in overwhelming septicemia. Adding to the complexity of this picture, different phases of an individual's life result in different demands and influences on the immune system. Thus, immune responses are subject to continuous alterations and adaptations throughout life as microbial challenges change and the bird migrates and ages.

THE IMMUNE SYSTEM

Most studies on the avian immune system have focused on chickens. Thus, the statements to follow, although generally true of chickens, may not necessarily apply to all bird species. In fact, as data accumulate, it is clear that the immune systems of birds are just as diverse as those of mammals. There is information regarding immunity in other domestic species, including the turkey, the domestic (graylag) goose, and the domestic duck (mallards and muscovies), and there is evidence that similar defense mechanisms are present in exotic avian species. Nevertheless, there are differences in the details.

Birds diverged from mammalian precursors about 300 million years ago, a time span that has provided ample opportunity for the evolution of major differences in the immune systems of mammals and birds. Notwithstanding these long evolutionary time scales, the overall structure of the avian immune system is identical to that of mammals. Thus, the three major layers of protection—physical barriers, innate immunity, and adaptive immunity—are present in both. Likewise, the major division of

the adaptive immune system into a humoral component, in which antibodies protect against extracellular organisms, and cell-mediated components, which protect against intracellular invaders, is retained.

Analysis of the draft chicken genome has provided some interesting insights into the evolution of the immune system in this species. For example, it has been proven possible to identify chicken orthologs of immune-related genes that were previously believed to be restricted to mammals. It is also of interest to note that some immune gene families are found in chickens to a greater extent than in humans. They include some immunoglobulin receptors, major histocompatibility complex (MHC) class I molecules, natural killer (NK) cell receptors, and T cell antigens. The significance of this expansion is unclear, but it may simply reflect the different histories of exposure to infectious agents encountered by birds and primates.

Birds have a smaller repertoire of immune system genes compared with mammals, and some key genes appear to be missing. For example, they lack TLR8 as well as RIG-1, both detectors of single-stranded ribonucleic acid (RNA). Birds have only three immunoglobulin (Ig) isotypes and do not make IgD. Ducks, but not chickens, make a truncated form of IgY. Chickens have an expanded family of leukocyte immunoglobulin-like receptor (LILR) genes with hundreds of members, including many IgY receptor genes. Some, but not all, birds have a very small MHC, and the presentation of peptides to the MHC appears to be constrained. The absence of lymphotoxins α and β in birds may be linked to the absence of formed lymph nodes.[1]

Lymphoid Organs

The avian immune system consists of primary and secondary lymphoid organs (Figure 11-1). The primary lymphoid organs include the bone marrow, thymus, bursa of Fabricius, and yolk sac. The secondary organs are the spleen and disseminated or mucosal-associated lymphoid tissue (MALT). Within this category are the nasal-associated lymphoid tissue (NALT), bronchial-associated lymphoid tissue (BALT), and gut-associated lymphoid tissue (GALT). In some species of birds there are also a few structures resembling lymph nodes.[2]

Lymphoid Development

In the chicken embryo, the first hematopoietic cells come from the yolk sac. The bursa of Fabricius appears as an epithelial infolding of the cloacal wall. It eventually extends away from the cloaca as it is colonized by hematopoietic cells. The thymus originates with the parathyroid gland from the third

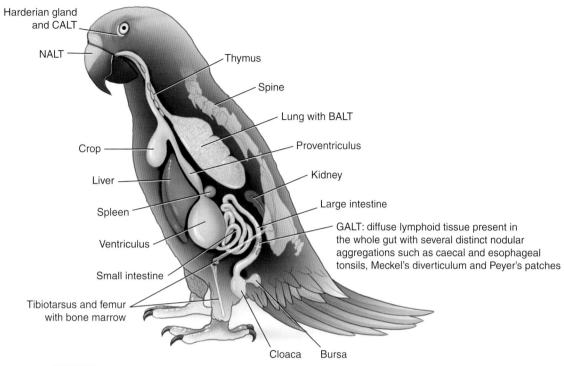

FIGURE 11-1 Primary and secondary lymphoid organs of the avian immune system.

and fourth pharyngeal pouches. The lymphoid cells in the thymus are derived from immigrant bloodborne stem cells. The splenic anlage originates as a slight swelling of mesenchymal tissue in the dorsal mesentery near the dorsal pancreas. During the late phase of embryonic development, T and B lymphocytes migrate to the spleen. T and B lymphocytes originate shortly after the tenth day of incubation.[2]

Bursa of Fabricius

The bursa of Fabricius is found only in birds. It is a round sac located just above the cloaca (Figure 11-2). Like the thymus, the bursa reaches its greatest size in the chick about 1 to 2 weeks

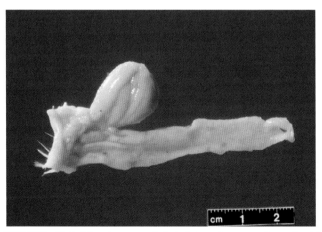

FIGURE 11-2 The bursa of Fabricius from a 1-week-old chicken. The bursal sac has been cut open to reveal the tissue folds inside.

after hatching and then shrinks as the bird ages. It is difficult to identify in mature birds. The bursa consists of lymphocytes embedded in epithelial tissue. This epithelial tissue lines a hollow sac connected to the cloaca by a duct. Inside the sac, folds of epithelium extend into the lumen, and scattered through the folds are lymphoid follicles (Figure 11-3). Each follicle is divided into a cortex and a medulla. The cortex contains lymphocytes, plasma cells, and macrophages. At the corticomedullary junction there is a basement membrane and capillary network, on the inside of which are epithelial cells. These medullary epithelial cells are replaced by lymphoblasts and lymphocytes in the center of the follicle. Specialized neuroendocrine dendritic cells of unknown function surround each follicle. The bursa may be destroyed either surgically or by infecting newborn chicks with infectious bursal disease virus. Since the bursa shrinks when chicks become sexually mature, bursal atrophy can also be provoked by administration of testosterone. Bursectomized birds have very low levels of antibodies in their blood, and antibody-producing cells disappear from lymphoid organs.

However, they still possess circulating lymphocytes, can defend against viruses, and can reject foreign skin grafts.[3] Thus, bursectomy has little effect on the cell-mediated immune response. Bursectomized birds are more susceptible than normal to leptospirosis and salmonellosis but not to intracellular bacteria such as *Mycobacterium avium*.[4,5] Thus, the bursa functions as a maturation and differentiation site for the cells of the antibody-forming system. Lymphocytes originating in the bursa are therefore called B cells. Lymphoid stem cells produced in the yolk sac migrate to the bursa. These cells then proliferate rapidly, but 90% to 95% of these eventually die by apoptosis—the negative selection of self-reactive

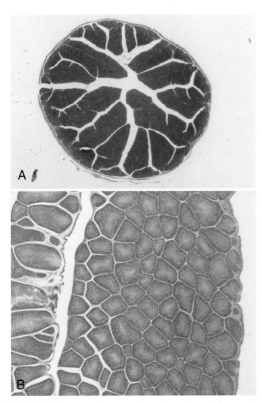

FIGURE 11-3 Photomicrographs showing the structure of the bursa of Fabricius. **A,** Low-power micrograph showing the bursa of a 13-day-old chick. Original magnification ×5. **B,** A high-power view. Original magnification ×360. (Courtesy specimen provided by Drs. N.H. McArthur and L.C. Abbott.)

B cells. Once their maturation is completed, the surviving B cells emigrate to secondary lymphoid organs. Close examination shows that the bursa can also trap antigens and undertake some antibody synthesis.

In effect, the establishment of the bursa means that B-cell lymphopoiesis is physically separated from that of other hematopoietic lineages. The bone marrow plays no role in B-cell development, perhaps for weight distribution reasons.

The relative size of the bursa reflects a bird's current health and its ability to respond to an infection. Selection of birds for increased antibody responses to antigens such as sheep red blood cells (RBCs) also selects for increased bursal size. Relative bursal size is also associated with hole nesting habits, migration, and coloniality.[6,7]

Thymus

The thymus in birds and in primitive mammals is present in the neck region. There may be multiple thymic lobules in a chain stretching from the angle of the jaw to the thoracic inlet. It consists of lobules covered by a connective tissue capsule. Each lobule has a cortex and medulla.[2]

Spleen

The spleen is present in the adult on the right side between the proventriculus and ventriculus. Its size and shape vary from species to species.[2]

Surface lymphoid tissues

The Harderian glands are located within the eye sockets medioventrally to the eyeball, and their secretory duct opens onto the surface of the nictitating membrane.[2] In birds, the conjunctiva-associated lymphoid tissue (CALT) and the Harderian glands are important in mounting responses to aerosolized antigens They contain B cells, γδ and αβ T cells, and both T-helper (Th) and cytotoxic T cells. On appropriate immunization, they produce antibodies as well as cytokines such as interferon (IFN)-γ.[8]

Disseminated lymphoid tissue (MALT) includes sites in the upper (NALT) and lower (BALT) respiratory system, the gastrointestinal (GI) system (GALT), and the Harderian gland.[2]

Lymph nodes

True primitive lymph nodes only occur in some waterfowl, including ducks and geese. There is a pair near the thyroid gland and another near the kidneys.[2]

Although other birds are commonly considered not to possess lymph nodes, they do possess structures that can be considered their functional equivalent. These avian lymph nodes consist of a central sinus that is the main lumen of a lymphatic vessel. The sinus is surrounded by a sheath of lymphoid tissue that contains germinal centers. Avian lymph nodes have no external capsule.

Functional Elements

Physical barriers, innate immunity modules and adaptive immune mechanisms encompassing both humoral immunity, and antigen-responsive cells form the basic functional elements of the avian immune system.

Physical barriers

As in mammals, preventing microbial invasion through body surfaces such as the GI, respiratory, and urogenital tracts represents the first line of defense against invading pathogens. Thus, continuous epithelia are additionally strengthened with local defense mechanisms such as a low pH and the secretion of soluble antimicrobial molecules (e.g., lysozyme) and peptides (e.g., defensins and cathelicidins). In addition, the natural microbiota found on all body surfaces, especially the intestine, is of particular importance. The microbiota consists of microorganisms with low pathogenicity that are best adapted to the local environment. Their protective effect against pathogenic microorganisms is based on competitive occupation of space and receptors, production of inhibitory metabolic products, bacteriocins, and induction of both low pH and low oxygen tension. The microflora is largely species-specific. It colonizes surfaces in the first 3 to 4 weeks after the hatch and serves as a source of continuous antigenic stimulation for the development of the immune system. It should be noted, therefore, that prolonged antibiotic therapy during this sensitive phase will have a major impact on the immune system development in the growing bird.

Cells of the immune system

Heterophils. Heterophils, the avian equivalents of mammalian neutrophils, are critical to the immune defense of birds. They bind and detect invading pathogens through the use of Toll-like receptors (TLRs), Fc receptors, and complement receptors. Once triggered, they respond by activating a network of signaling pathways and activate a multitude of microbial killing mechanisms, including an oxidative burst, cellular degranulation, and the production of extracellular nets.[9] Phagocytosis of opsonized particles involves antibody and complement receptors, whereas unopsonized bacteria require dectin 1, mannose, and scavenger receptors. Ingestion is immediately followed by degranulation and an oxidative burst. The granules contain multiple enzymes and some antimicrobial peptides. The granules are released into tissues. In addition, the production of extracellular nets is also associated with degranulation, serving to trap and kill microbes. Avian heterophils lack myeloperoxidase, so they mount a fairly weak respiratory burst and rely mainly on nonoxidative killing mechanisms.

Eosinophils. The function of avian eosinophils differs substantially from those in mammals. Molecules similar to mammalian eotaxins or eotaxin receptors have not been detected in birds. Automated methods for cell differentiation based on fluorescence-activated cell sorting have failed to distinguish between eosinophils and basophils in chickens.[10] Experiments that trigger eosinophilia in mammals produce inconsistent results in birds, making eosinophils an unreliable indicator for intestinal parasitism and hypersensitivity reactions in birds.[11,12] Clinical and experimental findings suggest that avian eosinophils participate in delayed rather than in immediate hypersensitivity reactions.[13] Empirically, a correlation between eosinophilia and tissue trauma, especially of the respiratory tract and the skin, has been observed. Related conditions include smoke inhalation, feather picking, self-mutilation, cannibalism, flying accidents, carnivore attacks, drug injections, and postsurgical recovery.[12] Blood eosinophilia can occur in various infectious diseases such as mycoplasmosis, West Nile virus (WNV) infection, mycobacteriosis, streptococcosis, staphylococcosis, listeriosis, and erysipeloid.

Lymphocytes. Bird lymphocytes originate in the yolk sac and migrate either to the bursa or to the thymus. Immature lymphocytes that enter the thymus mature under the influence of molecules produced by thymic epithelial cells and mature T cells emigrate from the thymus. These T cells constitute between 60% and 70% of blood lymphocytes. Chicken T cells can participate in delayed hypersensitivity reactions, graft-versus-host disease, and graft rejection. They possess specific antigen receptors (TCRs). Avian homologs of mammalian γ/δ TCR (TCR-1) and α/β TCR (TCR-2 and TCR-3) have been identified. TCR-2 and TCR-3 are subsets of α/β TCRs. As in mammals, these cells use a signaling complex involving CD3 to communicate from the TCR to the cell. The structure of the chicken CD3 signaling complex differs in its details from that in mammals. In addition to the presence of lymphocytes in lymphoid organs, birds also have large numbers of lymphocytes in the cecal tonsils and in the skin. The intestinal and reproductive tracts have large numbers of γδ T cells.

The third major lymphocyte population, NK cells, shares surface antigens with T cells. They are probably large granular lymphocytes. NK cells are found in the thymus, bursa, spleen, and intestinal epithelium. They attack human cancer

cells, lymphoid leukosis, leukemia virus, and Marek disease virus–infected cells.[11,12] The chicken leukocyte receptor complex contains molecules that appear to function as NK cell receptors. Likewise, NK cells employ C-type lectins, members of the signaling lymphocyte activation molecule family and receptors that interact with nectins as well as adhesion molecules.[14] Both inhibitory and activating receptors are present on their surface.

Innate Immunity

Activation of innate immune mechanisms recruits heterophils and macrophages to sites of microbial invasion (Figure 11-4). Unlike in mammals, avian heterophils do not depend on an oxidative burst to kill bacteria. Antibacterial peptides appear to be especially important in birds. Macrophages play a similar role in birds and mammals. The nucleated platelets of birds are not only important in hemostasis, but they also can phagocytose bacteria and kill them in an oxidative response.

Pattern-recognition receptors

The hardwired innate immune system is designed to detect and respond to invaders. The presence of these invaders is first detected by cellular receptors that recognize and respond to common microbial structures or patterns. Birds possess multiple pattern-recognition receptors such as the TLRs. These bind to highly conserved microbial structures, also called *pathogen-associated molecular patterns*. Once bound, inflammatory and other defensive responses are triggered. As a result, birds mount inflammatory responses that serve to localize invaders.[15]

Ten TLRs have been identified in chickens. Six of these, TLRs 2a, 2b, 3, 4, 5, and 7, are orthologs of mammalian TLRs. In addition TLR21 and TLR15 are unique to birds. TLR 2a and 2b both recognize peptidoglycans, TLR4 binds lipopolysaccharides, TLR5 recognizes flagellin, and TLR21 recognizes unmethylated CpG motifs in bacterial DNA. TLR21 is a functional homolog of mammalian TLR9 in that it recognizes CpG oligodeoxynucleotides.[16,17]

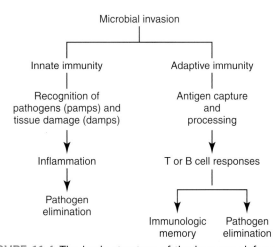

FIGURE 11-4 The basic structure of the immune defenses of the bird. Innate immunity is triggered by pathogen-associated molecular patterns and damage-associated molecular patterns.

As might be anticipated, TLR expression varies among birds. Thus, they show a pattern of gene duplication and gene loss, as seen in both the chicken and the zebra finch. Both species show duplication of TLR1 and TLR2. In the zebra finch, duplication of TLR7 has been identified recently. Studies of TLR gene sequences in wild bird populations such as red jungle fowl also indicate that TLRs are selected within the populations based on pathogen challenge within their environment.[18]

Antimicrobial molecules

Host defense peptides[19] are broad-spectrum antimicrobial proteins that play a key role in avian innate immunity. Birds, like mammals, have two broad classes: defensins and cathelicidins. Birds have only β-defensins and lack the α- and θ-defensins found in mammals. Over 25 β-defensins have been identified in birds. Defensins can kill both gram-positive and gram-negative bacteria, mainly by causing pore formation. Cathelicidins are shorter antibacterial peptides. These peptides are produced by a wide variety of tissues, including leukocytes, lymphoid organs, the respiratory and digestive tracts, and the reproductive tracts in males and females. Fowlicidin-1 is an avian cathelicidin with potent antibacterial activities in vitro and in vivo.[20] It also promotes adaptive immunity.

There are significant differences in the zebra finch repertoire of antimicrobial peptides compared with that of the chicken. There are no cathelicidins in the zebra finch genome, but they have 12 novel defensins.[21] IFNs, especially IFN-γ, induced in response to virus recognition by TLRs are critical to antiviral immunity.

Adaptive Immunity

Polarization of the adaptive immune system

The microorganisms that pose a threat to the health of birds can in a broad sense be divided into two major categories: (1) intracellular organisms such as viruses and some bacteria, which must be attacked through cell-mediated mechanisms; and (2) extracellular organisms such as many bacteria and parasites, which must be combatted by soluble molecules such as antibodies. Thus, when a bird is invaded by a microorganism, the adaptive immune system must make a decision as to which of these two mechanisms to activate. It is likely that this initial decision is made on the basis of which pattern-recognition receptors are first activated. This, in turn, determines which Th cell populations are activated and subsequently polarizes the immune reaction into a Th1 pathway promoting cell-mediated responses and a Th2 pathway promoting antibody-mediated responses. Antigen-specific stimulation of Th1 cells induces the synthesis of interleukins (ILs)[12,18] and subsequently IFN-γ. The typical Th2 cytokine cascade consists of an initial synthesis of IL4 and IL13, followed by an additional production of IL5, IL9, and IL19. A third helper cell population, comprising Th17 cells, regulates and promotes innate immunity and inflammation.[22,23] For a long time, it was not clear whether the Th1–Th2 paradigm exists in avian species, since the avian immune system shows some fundamental differences compared with that of mammals. Birds have a different pattern of immunoglobulins (see below); typical Th2-associated allergies have not been reported, since functional eosinophils, eotaxins, and eotaxin receptors appear to be absent and IL5 is not expressed in

avian T cells. Nevertheless, recent studies on cytokine profiles after challenge with intracellular and extracellular pathogens strongly indicate the existence of this polarization of adaptive immune reactions in chickens. Immune responses to Newcastle disease virus (NDV) and infectious bursal disease virus (IBDV) were dominated by IFN-γ (Th1), whereas responses to *Ascaridia galli* and *Histomonas meleagridis* were dominated by IL4, IL13, and IL19 (Th2).[23] Figure 11-5 summarizes the current roles of Th-cell subsets in birds.

The Th1 response and cell-mediated immunity

In general, cell-mediated immune responses are mediated by T cells. These T cells consist of many different specialized subpopulations with different functions. For example, the major subpopulation has antigen receptors (TCRs) consisting of α and β chains and hence are called TCRαβ. A minor subpopulation has TCRs consisting of γ and δ chains. These four TCR chains, αβ, γδ are found in all jawed vertebrates. The TCRs act as signaling receptors for T cells (B cells use immunoglobulins as their signaling receptors). Immunoglobulins are secreted by B cells, whereas the TCRs remain cell bound. Immunoglobulins bind native antigens directly, and TCRs bind only processed antigens presented when attached to the MHC molecules. The γδ TCRs can bind free antigens as well as MHC-presented antigens. In birds, there are two forms of γδ TCR expressed in chickens and turkeys but only one in the zebra finch.[24]

The Th2 responses and antibody-mediated immunity

Immunoglobulins are produced by B cells. B cells are activated by the presence of antigens in association with Th2 cells. There are three principal immunoglobulin classes produced in birds (chickens): IgY, IgM, and IgA. Birds lack the IgD genes found in mammals. The principal immunoglobulin in chicken serum is called *IgY*. Although somewhat similar to mammalian IgG, it has sufficient molecular differences to warrant a different designation (Figure 11-6). Like the immunoglobulins of mammals, IgY consists of two heavy chains and two light chains. The heavy chains, called *upsilon (υ) chains*, usually consist of one variable and four constant domains, and the complete molecule is about 180 kilodaltons (kDa). However, some birds have a truncated isoform that has only two constant domains (lacking the third and fourth constant domains). This isoform is about 120 kDa. Some birds such as ducks and geese have both full-sized and truncated IgY. Others such as chickens have only full-sized molecules. The truncated isoform of IgY is produced as a result of alternative splicing of heavy-chain messenger ribonucleic acid (mRNA). Its correct name is, therefore, *IgY(ΔFc)*. Because the molecule lacks an Fc region, it cannot activate complement or bind to Fc receptors, and its function is unclear. There has, however, been a tendency during evolution to make low-molecular-weight immunoglobulins. These low-molecular-weight molecules may offer some selective advantage. For example, it has been suggested that these molecules will not trigger potentially lethal hypersensitivity reactions. Evidence from mallards (*Anas platyrhynchos*) suggests that the ratio of truncated IgY to intact IgY affects the efficiency of phagocytosis and determines whether immune complexes are phagocytosed in the spleen or in the liver. Both forms of IgY lack a

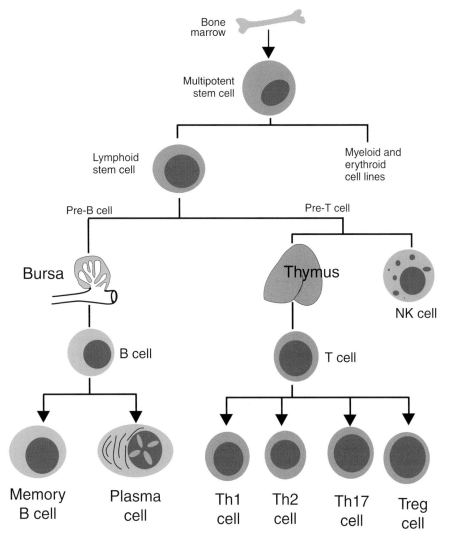

FIGURE 11-5 Development of T and B lymphocytes. Both arise from bone marrow precursors. B cells develop in the bursa and Peyer patches. T cells develop in the thymus. Natural killer cells are a third population of lymphocytes that are distinct from T and B cells. Treg, regulatory T-cell

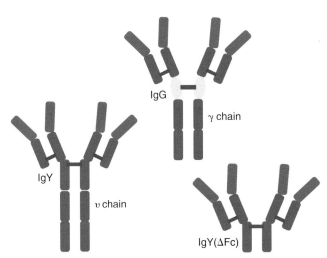

FIGURE 11-6 The structure of avian IgY and IgY(δFc) compared with mammalian IgG. Ig, Immunoglobulin.

hinge region and, as a result, are somewhat inflexible and only cause precipitation or agglutination in the presence of high salt concentrations. Studies on the interrelationships of the vertebrate immunoglobulins clearly show that IgY is related to both IgG and IgE in mammals. In fact, it may have arisen from an evolutionary precursor of these two classes.

Immunoglobulin A

The structure of chicken IgA is similar to mammalian IgA. The only significant difference is that chicken IgA has four heavy-chain C domains, whereas mammalian IgA has only three. Chicken serum IgA exists in both dimeric (340 kDa) and monomeric (170 kDa) forms. Intestinal IgA is associated with a secretory component, a protein produced by epithelial cells that protects IgA from proteolytic digestion. IgA production and immunity in the intestine is regulated by a balance between Th17 and regulatory T cells. Thus, in older chickens, infection with *Salmonella* does not result in significant pathology. This is probably a result of the activities of

T-reg cells releasing the suppressive cytokines transforming growth factor (TGF)-β and IL10.[25]

Antibody diversity

Chickens generate antibody diversity in a manner that is quite unlike that seen in mammals. Chickens have only one functional *V* gene and one *J* gene for both light chains and heavy chains, although they do have 16 different *D* genes. Chicken immunoglobulin diversity is, therefore, generated by inserting gene sequences from nonfunctional pseudogenes in a process called *gene conversion*. Although they have only one functional *V* gene, chickens have a large number of *V* pseudogenes that serve as sequence donors. During recombination of the *V* and *J* genes, single bases are also added to each gene (N-region addition), and joining occurs at random. Chicken immunoglobulins are further diversified by somatic hypermutation and imprecise V–J joining. A second major difference involves the timing of this process. In mammals, rearrangement of immunoglobulin genes occurs throughout life. In chickens, however, immunoglobulin genes are rearranged as a single wave between 10 and 15 days of embryogenesis, when there is clonal expansion of B cells in the bursa of Fabricius. During that 5-day period, birds generate all the antibody specificities they will need for the rest of their lives. After the bursa degenerates at puberty, the chicken must largely make do with the B cell diversity generated in early life. However, once a mature chicken B cell is stimulated by exposure to an antigen, it can generate additional V-region diversity by further gene conversion. The chicken can generate about 10^6 different immunoglobulin molecules. This is approximately one order of magnitude less than in the mouse.

Primary and secondary responses

Birds produce primary and secondary responses in a manner similar to that in mammals. After antigenic challenge, the initial synthesis of specific IgM is switched to the production of increasing amounts of IgY. The predominance of IgM production in the primary immune response and of IgY in the secondary response is less marked than in mammals. A monomeric IgM can be detected in chicken eggs and in 1-day-old chicks. It is thought to be derived from oviduct secretions in the hen.

Genetics of the Immune System

Like all other body systems, the development and functioning of the avian immune system is determined by the genes that code for the production of the key molecules involved in innate and adaptive immunity. Although these include the genes coding for such obvious immune proteins as immunoglobulins or T-cell antigen receptors, the most critical genetically regulated components of the avian immune system are those molecules that bind antigens and present them to T cells and B cells. These molecules belong to the MHC and are thus called *MHC molecules* (Figure 11-7). They fall into two broad categories. MHC class I molecules recognize antigens produced by the body's own cells. These include proteins synthesized by virus-infected cells and are classified as endogenous antigens. Endogenous antigens tend to promote Th1 responses, especially the production of cytotoxic T cells. MHC class II molecules bind the antigens that are released when foreign antigens are destroyed by antigen-presenting

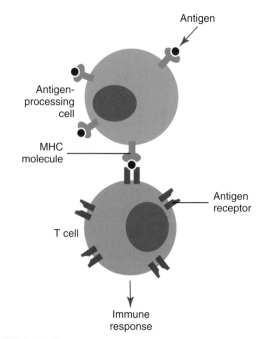

FIGURE 11-7 The key initial step in any immune response is the presentation of antigens by antigen-processing cells to antigen-sensitive cells. This step is mediated by major histocompatibility complex molecules located on the surface of antigen-processing cells.

cells such as the molecules present in invading bacteria (Figure 11-8). These exogenous antigens tend to promote Th2 responses.

Birds, as exemplified by chickens, recognize and process antigens by a somewhat different process compared with mammals. Mammals possess a huge number of polymorphic MHC class I molecules that bind to a diverse array of antigens such as those found in infectious agents. Once bound, the antigens are all processed through what is, in effect, a common antigen-processing pathway. As a result, mammals show broad resistance to a multitude of infectious agents, and it is difficult to show a direct genetic association with infectious disease resistance. Birds, in contrast to mammals, have multiple polymorphic antigen-processing molecules. As a result, birds are either resistant or susceptible to specific infectious agents, and it is not difficult to show inherited resistance to specific infectious agents. When birds are exposed to infectious agents, the optimal antigen-processing pathways are selected for each agent. It is likely that this pattern adopted by birds is the primitive pattern also seen in fish, amphibians, and reptiles.

In chickens, for example, there are only two class I genes, and only one is expressed at a high level. As a result, this can show strong associations between the MHC molecules and resistance to specific pathogens. In the common chicken haplotypes, only one class I and one class II molecule are dominantly expressed. Since viruses contain relatively few proteins, MHC-dependent disease susceptibility depends on virus antigens binding to the dominant MHC class I molecule. As a result, possession of specific haplotypes determines viral disease susceptibility. For example, the haplotype B21 is

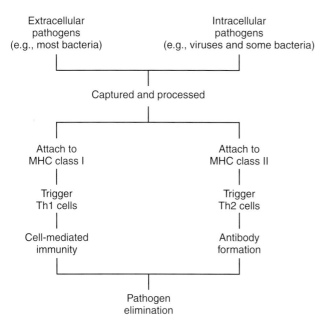

FIGURE 11-8 The body responds to intracellular and extracellular pathogens quite differently. Thus, antigens from intracellular invaders such as viruses bind to major histocompatibility complex (MHC) class II molecules and trigger cell-mediated immunity. Conversely, antigens from extracellular bacteria bind to MHC class I molecules and trigger antibody responses.

independent regions designated MHC-B and MHC-Y (Figure 11-9). Both are located on microchromosome 16, but they are separated by the nucleolar organizer region. The B region contains three gene clusters. Cluster 1, or the B-F/B-L region, contains a two class I α-chain genes (*B-F*), a *C4* gene, and two class II β-chain genes (*B-L*). There is a single class II α-chain gene located about 5 centimorgans from the β-chain gene. Two clusters (V and VI) form the *B-G* or class IV region. The *B-G* gene products are membrane proteins ranging from 40 to 48 kDa. These molecules can form monomers, homodimers, and heterodimers and are mainly found on RBCs and thrombocytes. Related *B-G* molecules are found at low levels on lymphocytes. Their function is unknown. The Y region consists of two clusters containing two MHC class I and two MHC class II loci. They differ from the B region loci in that their products are not expressed on RBCs. Genes within the Y region also regulate NK cell recognition. The B locus of the turkey is very similar to that of the chicken.[26] It is a small, constricted locus with 34 genes in near-perfect synteny with that of the chicken MHC-B. In house sparrows, a single MHC class I allele appears to regulate the response to sheep erythrocytes and phytohemagglutinin.[27]

Chickens, turkeys, and sparrows are not typical of the entire species of birds. Passerine birds, for example, have a complex MHC structure with multiple duplicated copies of each class of gene, pseudogenes, and longer introns and intergenic regions. Good examples of this are Darwin's finches.[28] Even the kiwi (*Apteryx owenii*), a very primitive bird, has at least five MHC class II genes, three of which are expressed and are functional.[29] Likewise, in red knots (*Calidris canutus*), the MHC complex is very diverse, with at least 36 alleles in 8 individuals and evidence for six functional and expressed MHC 1 genes in a single bird. This is not surprising, since these birds will encounter multiple diverse pathogens during the course of their long-distance migration.[30] In the scarlet rosefinch (*Carpodacus erythrinus*), another long-distance migrant, MHC class I variation is also extremely high.[31] There were 82 different variants in one rosefinch population nesting site. They have at least 5 expressed class I genes. In many such cases, the high diversity of the MHC is related to extreme migration and presumably reflects the need for migrating birds to counter the diverse pathogens they encounter in the course of their journey.

Wild birds are also under considerable pressure to adapt rapidly to environmental changes. For example, house finches

associated with resistance to Marek disease, whereas the B19 haplotype is associated with susceptibility. Chickens homozygous for B1 generally have high adult mortality, are highly susceptible to Marek disease, and respond poorly to *Salmonella pullorum* or to human serum albumin. Birds homozygous for B5 are able to mount a better antibody response and develop less severe lesions in response to infection with *Eimeria tenella* compared with B2 homozygous birds. Certain MHC genotypes (BA4/A4 and BA12/A12) are significantly overrepresented in birds suffering from bacterial arthritis and osteomyelitis caused by *Staphylococcus aureus*.

On the basis of the situation observed in chickens, it has been widely assumed that the avian MHC is small and simple. For example, the chicken MHC occupies only 92 kilo base (kb) and contains only 19 genes. It is divided into two

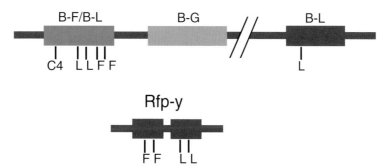

FIGURE 11-9 The major histocompatibility complex of the chicken is relatively simple compared with that of mammals. It consists of two gene regions: B region *(top)* and the Y region *(bottom)*. F genes are class II genes, and L genes are class I genes.

(Carpodacus mexicanus) in the eastern United States have been severely affected by conjunctivitis caused by *Mycoplasma gallisepticum*. When finches from the eastern United States and from western populations with no prior exposure to *M. gallisepticum* are exposed to this agent, the eastern finches had 33% lower *M. gallisepticum* loads in the conjunctiva compared with the western birds. This difference appears to be associated with differences in the immune genes expressed in the spleen.

Blood Group Systems

Chickens have at least 12 different blood group systems with multiple alleles. The RBC B system is also the MHC in the chicken.

VARIATIONS IN IMMUNOCOMPETENCE DURING LIFE HISTORY

The phenotype of a bird consists of morphologic, physiologic, and behavioral traits. To ensure optimal survivability, performance trade-offs are necessary, especially between those traits supporting individual survival and those that support successful reproduction. Equilibration and adjustment of available energy resources between the two are carried out by a complex network of neuronal and hormonal signal cascades that is subject to continuous adjustments.[32] Consequently, the immunocompetence of birds varies at different stages of life. Increased investment in other life-history traits may decrease immunocompetence and increase susceptibility to disease. For example, the responses of wild birds to infectious challenge is affected by the significance of the challenge.[33] Thus, if an infection is genuinely threatening to a species, birds with strong immune responses to the pathogen are positively selected and will survive. In contrast, should a pathogen not pose a severe threat, the costs of any immune response may outweigh any benefits. In such cases, a strong immune response may confer no advantage in terms of conservation of energy resources and depend on the type of pathogen, its immunoevasive mechanisms, and host hypersensitivity reactions to infection. There may be even detrimental effects to the host.

r- and K-Strategists

To achieve optimal life-history performance, animals may resort to two completely different reproductive strategies, called *r-strategy* and *K-strategy*. In species using an r-strategy, reproductive activity maximizes population growth without regard to space, food, or other resources. These species rely on low numbers of reproductive cycles with high clutch sizes without regard to the expense of self-maintenance. The term *r* simply refers to the growth rate of the population. Examples of r-strategists would include the house sparrow, zebra finch, and the common pigeon. Species that apply a K-strategy adjust their reproductive behavior based on the availability of resources. The term *K* refers to the carrying capacity of the environment. Compared with r-strategists, K-strategists tend to be slower-growing species with smaller clutch sizes, longer life expectancies, and more robust immune responses. Their behavior increases the number of reproductive cycles by favoring a greater investment in both parent and offspring survival. Examples of K-strategists would be large psittacines, birds of prey, and large marine birds.

Signs of Immunologic Fitness—Plumage Quality and Song Complexity

When seeking a mate, it is always best to select the healthiest. Birds do this by checking prospective mates for signs of immunologic health such as plumage quality. Of course, unhealthy birds also want to find a mate and seek to cover up any inadequacies. When selecting a mate, one should look for signals that reflect the "true" condition of a potential partner. For example, the sexually selected forehead patch of the collared flycatcher *(Ficedula albicollis)* seems to be an "honest" badge of status that indicates the quality of the immune response. Antibody responses correlate strongly with badge expression during the mating period.[34] In general, plumage quality is seen by potential mates as the best guide to selecting a healthy mate. Song complexity is another indirect measure of immune competence. In adult passerine birds, T-cell responses as assessed by phytohemagglutinin (PHA) skin test and the size of the bursa were positively correlated with bird song complexity. Nestling T-cell responses were not related to song complexity, reflecting age-dependent selective pressures.[35]

Stress as a Key Factor

In general, changes of the immune status reflect an animal's reaction to a stressful stimulus.[36] Some authors even consider the possibility of the immune system itself being the long-term result of the host's response to the stress of pathogen challenge.[37] *Stress* is defined as an adaptive response to threats to an animal's health and survival. The type and intensity of the response to a stress stimulus depend on its novelty, severity, duration, and the current physiologic status of the animal itself. Stress stimuli could be of internal or external origin. Internal stressors include genetic disposition (inbreeding), age (immature versus adult individuals), gender, and body conditions in normal life history, such as development, growth, reproduction, molting, and migration. External, environmental stressors include temperature, light (duration and composition), air quality (ammonia, ozone), infectious agents, environmental contaminants (mycotoxins, pesticides), diet, housing, social interactions, noise, and even geographic location. Impacts on the immune system are thought to be primarily induced by hormones, but direct neural modulation and dietary effects may also be of importance.[32]

Stress hormones

As in mammals, stress reactions in chicken are mainly mediated by catecholamines and glucocorticoids. Peracute and severe stress triggers the so-called "fight or flight" response, where the release of catecholamines such as epinephrine, norepinephrine, and dopamine rapidly increase heart rate and cardiovascular and neuromuscular functions in the bird to ensure rapid exit from the stressful situation.[32]

Acute and chronic stress reactions are mediated additionally by glucocorticoids, which are released in the course of the activation of the hypothalamic–pituitary–adrenal (HPA) axis. The hypothalamic corticotrophin-releasing factor (CRF) and vasopressin trigger the secretion of adrenocorticotropic hormone (ACTH) in the cephalic lobe of the anterior pituitary gland.[38] ACTH stimulates the adrenal cortex to secrete glucocorticoid and mineralocorticoid hormones (Figure 11-10).[39]

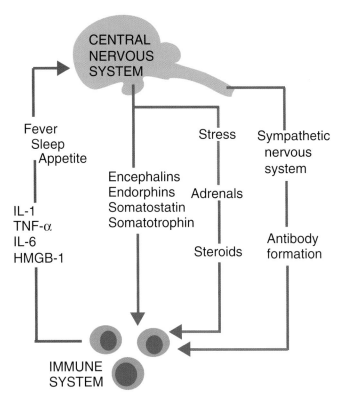

FIGURE 11-10 Some of the many ways in which the central nervous system and the immune system interact. TNF, tumor necrosis factor, HMGB-1, high motility group protein B 1

differential count. The effect of corticosterone may even be selective for certain lymphocyte subpopulations. It has been shown that in rats, stress-induced reduction of peripheral blood lymphocytes was primarily based on a decrease in numbers of B cells, NK cells, and Th cells.[43]

Prolonged exposure to a stressful situation or experimental overdose results in immunosuppression, which affects both the humoral and cellular components of the immune system. With regard to cellular defense mechanisms, chronic corticosterone administration reduces bursal, thymic, and splenic mass by inducing apoptosis in immature T cells and B cells. As for humoral immunity, experimental activation of the ACTH–glucocorticoid axis suppresses primary and secondary antibody responses, reduces cutaneous responses to PHA, impairs IL2 and IFN-γ production, and decreases phagocytosis and prostaglandin E_2 (PGE_2) production in adherent blood monocytic cells. The overall benefit of chronic stress–induced immunosuppression has been hypothesized to be either a self-protection against possible overreactions of the immune system during prolonged stimulation or downregulation resulting from shortage of energy and nutrient supplies, which are needed to maintain other important life traits such as growth, reproduction, or predator avoidance.[32]

In conclusion, it can be stated that the effects of corticosteroids on the immune system do not follow a stereotypical reaction pattern but are modulated by various intrinsic and extrinsic factors. Responses are affected by the level of corticosterone, the time of exposure (e.g., short-term or long-term exposure) and the immune parameter measured[32] and may enhance or suppress or have no effect on immunologic variables.[44] Besides their impact on the immune system, glucocorticoids have a major influence on a bird's metabolism, in general, as well as its social behavior in reproduction (courtship, mating, fostering), cognitive and learning abilities, hunting, and migration.[45] All these aspects have a direct or indirect influence on the current immune status of the individual.

Maternal modulation of immune function in chicks
Epigenetic maternal influences on the immune function of chicks have been extensively revised by Hasselquist et al[46] and are mainly based on the transfer of three major components into the egg—immunoglobulins, steroid hormones, and antioxidants.

The development and stress responsiveness of chicks are related to the level of deposition of corticosterone into the egg. Male chicks hatched from eggs with elevated corticosterone levels have slower growth rates, whereas female chicks display a reduced response to corticosterone.[47] Gull chicks that hatched from eggs inoculated with corticosterone displayed a reduced response to phytohemagglutinin and a lower begging rate.[45] Another stress factor is predation risk. Eggs that were taken from flycatcher nests in the vicinity of a predator (Pygmy owl, *Glaucidium passerinum*) or exposed to the urine of a mammalian predator (least weasel, *Mustela nivalis*) contained higher immunoglobulin levels compared with eggs from appropriate control nests.[48] It is suggested that this may compensate for the hazards by increasing the probability of offspring survival. In contrast, female great tits that experience high predation risk during egg formation have offspring that carry higher flea loads and might reflect a lower immune capacity as a result of maternal stress.[49]

Both catecholamines and glucocorticoids have direct effects on the immune system.[40] Lymphoid tissue is directly innervated by the sympathetic and parasympathetic nervous systems, whose neurotransmitters are catecholamines. Lymphocytes have high-affinity receptors for ACTH and glucocorticoids that are upregulated by immune stimulation. This immune stimulation is fine-tuned by a negative feedback mechanism of corticosteroid blood levels on ACTH secretion in the pituitary gland. Lymphocytes themselves contribute to this regulation, as they synthesize ACTH, corticosterone, and other neuroendocrine mediators.[41,42]

Hence, in contrast to traditional consensus in the avian veterinary community, it has to be emphasized that corticosteroids can both enhance or suppress avian immune reactions, depending on the level and the duration of the stressful situation (reviewed by Koutsos and Klasing[32]). Short-term influence of corticosteroids enhances immunoreactivity, and long-term influence suppresses immunoreactivity. Early responses to corticosteroids result in an increased expression of mRNA for proinflammatory cytokines and chemokines in both heterophils and lymphocytes, whereas chronic corticosteroid exposure results in downregulation of cytokine and chemokine expression and a transition to a noninflammatory phenotype in both cell populations. Moreover, early response to corticosterone results in a shift of intravascular lymphocytes to extravascular spaces such as lymphoid tissue or sites of immune reaction and a reverse shift of heterophils from bone marrow into the peripheral bloodstream. This results in an increase of the heterophil-to-lymphocyte ratio in the

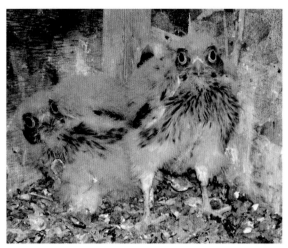

FIGURE 11-11 Nestlings do have a different immunoreactivity from that of adult birds and it even differs between siblings. (Photo courtesy F. Hauska, Regensburg.)

The mixture of maternal immunomodulating components varies even within the eggs of one clutch (Figure 11-11): Late eggs in the laying order of black-headed gulls tend to have decreased amounts of immunoenhancing yolk antioxidants and immunoglobulins but higher amounts of testosterone compared with previously laid eggs. This suggests that the deposition of higher amounts of testosterone in late eggs compensates for reduced egg quality, enabling the hatchlings to overcome the deficits with testosterone-dependent increased growth and competitive skills.[50] In contrast, in zebra finches, both yolk testosterone and antioxidant levels decrease over the laying order. Interestingly, females mated to an attractive male transferred higher androgen and lower antioxidant levels to early eggs and higher antioxidant levels in late eggs compared with females paired with unattractive males. In other words, eggs of females paired with an attractive male contain higher testosterone levels at the beginning of egg deposition and maintain more even antioxidant levels throughout the whole clutch of eggs.[46]

Newly hatched chicks are exposed to a high risk of oxidative damage. The sudden change to pulmonary respiration and rapid growth is likely to cause an increased formation of reactive oxygen species (ROS). Additionally, because of their underdeveloped adaptive immune system, their defense mechanisms are mainly based on innate macrophage–phagocyte functions with an increased production of free radicals during oxidative burst in microbial killing. Supplementation of antioxidants such as carotenoids, vitamin E, and selenium to the diet of chicks has been shown to exert a positive effect on the development of lymphoid organs and cell-mediated and humoral immune responses in both commercial and noncommercial bird species. Dietary supplementation of these antioxidants to females prior to oviposition increases their levels in the egg. This protects the embryo, the egg yolk, and maternal antibodies from lipid peroxidation deposited therein and may even contribute, for some time in the newly hatched chick, toward protection against ROS-related damage.[46]

Social stress

Social interactions play a vital role in the life of birds and influence the immune system and susceptibility to disease.

Dominant individuals in a flock usually have higher glucocorticoid levels compared with subordinates. In winter, however, the opposite is the case, which may be related to the stress of competition for scarce food resources.[51] The degree of social stress–induced immunosuppression varies significantly among chicken strains selected for high versus low corticosterone blood levels. Chickens exposed to Marek disease virus (MDV) that were kept in a socially stressful environment had a higher prevalence of tumors compared with the MDV-infected chickens kept in a low-stress environment. The effects were more prominent in birds selected for high plasma corticosterone concentrations. Pharmacologic blockage of the conversion of deoxycorticosterone to the biologically active corticosterone in the adrenal glands resulted in a reduction of these effects, which suggested that the impact of social stress on Marek disease is mediated by activation of the HPA axis.[44]

Immunosuppressive Effect of Reproductive Effort and Sexual Ornamentation

Reproductive effort or sexual ornamentation generally reduces immune responsiveness and as a result increases the prevalence of parasites.[52] In female collared flycatchers (*Ficedula albicollis*), increased reproductive effort resulted in a decreased antibody immune response to vaccination against NDV and an increased intensity of *Haemoproteus* infections, with decreased bird survival to the next season.[53] In breeding zebra finches, all nonbreeding birds produced antibodies when injected with sheep RBCs but less than half of the breeding birds did so.[54] In female eiders (*Somateria mollissima*), responses to PHA skin test and immunoglobulin levels during incubation dropped by about 40% and 25%, respectively. This observation was independent of the number of eggs laid by the females. Corticosterone did not vary significantly during incubation, irrespective of clutch size. During incubation, eiders do not eat, and these results were interpreted as a response to limited energy supplies possibly mediated by hormonal changes.[55] Similar results were observed with phytohemagglutinin (PHA) skin testing in mature turkey breeder hens: Laying hens had a dermal response to PHA that was about 69% of the response in nonlaying hens.[56] In domestic poultry, birds selected for high antibody responses to sheep erythrocytes had poorer sexual ornaments (comb size) compared with the birds selected for low antibody responses.[57] Likewise, the ability of roosters to respond to sheep erythrocytes is inversely correlated with the size of their tail plumage. In another example, epaulet size in red-winged blackbirds is negatively correlated with the bactericidal activity of blood heterophils but not with the PHA swelling response.[50] Likewise, excessive investment in ornamentation such as the tail streamers of barn swallows can also be immunosuppressive. Thus, male swallows with longer streamers are more likely to breed successfully and early. However, they have lower blood γ-globulin levels.[58] All these effects may simply be the result of the immunosuppressive effects of testosterone.

Density effects, genetic bottlenecks, inbreeding for color mutations

Møller et al showed that there is a density-dependent increase in immune competence in altricial birds. This appears to reflect T-cell competence, especially in adults. This may be related to the increased chances of parasitism in dense flocks.[59]

Hale and Briskie looked at leukocyte counts and external and blood parasites in two populations of the New Zealand robin (*Petroica australis*). They compared a genetically restricted population with a genetically enriched one. The two populations had similar parasite loads, but the bottlenecked group had lower responses to PHA and lower total leukocyte counts.[60]

Inbreeding for specific color mutations has a negative impact on immunocompetence. Cockatiels with color mutations have a reduced lifespan and an increased susceptibility to infectious disease.[61] The underlying pathways have not been investigated in exotic bird species so far. In chicken, however, both autosomal-related albinism and gonadal-related albinism affect immunocompetence in newly hatched chicks. Albino chicks show an impaired ability to absorb and utilize yolk sac material, including maternal antibodies, resulting in an increased risk of developing "starve-out syndrome": Impaired nutrient supply from the yolk sac will cause retardation of growth rate and organ development. Subsequent insufficient activation of the digestive system and ongoing endogenous lipolysis will further exacerbate the situation. In the worst case, the chicks will die of starvation.[62,63] If they survive, it is likely that these chicks will suffer from a lifetime of reduced immunocompetence.

Bird migration, survival, and diet

Migrating birds are immunocompromised. Owen and Moore investigated three thrush species during spring migration, breeding season, and fall migration. Migrating birds had lower leukocyte and lymphocyte counts, lower hematocrit, lower fat stores, and higher heterophil-to-lymphocyte (H/L) ratios relative to nonmigrating birds. This immunosuppression was especially significant during spring migration.[64] This is, of course, another example of selective resource allocation. If a bird stops to rest and replenish its immune function during migration, it may arrive too late to find a mate or a good nesting site.

As might be anticipated, immunocompetence is associated also with survival. Thus, Saino et al showed that male barn swallows that survived to a subsequent breeding season had higher antibody levels compared with those that did not survive.[58]

Barn swallows provided with a protein-rich food at intervals after the hatch had better PHA responses compared with unsupplemented control birds.[65]

Comparing multiple paired species across the main avian genera, carcass scavengers had larger spleens or body size and higher blood leukocyte counts compared with nonscavengers. Presumably, this was a result of parasite selective pressure on their immune defenses. Their H/L ratios were higher, however, suggesting a greater reliance on innate defenses rather than adaptive defenses. Following inoculation with sheep RBCs or PHA, scavengers mount greater humoral responses compared with nonscavengers but not their cell-mediated responses.[66]

Age

Immunocompetence of the newly hatched chick. Newly hatched birds emerge from the sterile environment of the egg and, like mammals, require temporary immunologic assistance. Serum immunoglobulins are actively transported from the hen's serum to the yolk while the egg is still in the ovary. IgY in the fluid phase of egg yolk is, therefore, found at levels equal to or greater than those in hen serum. In addition, as the fertilized ovum passes down the oviduct, IgM and IgA from oviduct secretions are acquired with the albumin. As the chick embryo develops in ovo, it absorbs the yolk IgY, which then appears in its circulation. At the same time, the IgM and IgA from the albumin diffuse into the amniotic fluid and are swallowed by the embryo (Figure 11-12). Thus, when a chick hatches, it possesses IgY in its serum and IgM and IgA in its intestine. The newly hatched chick does not absorb all of its yolk sac antibodies until about 24 hours after the hatch. These maternal antibodies effectively prevent successful vaccination until they disappear between 10 and 20 days after the hatch. Although the development of proper defense mechanisms starts during embryonic life, immunocompetence only appears a few days after the hatch. The post-hatch period is crucial, since the chick is confronted by a wide variety of antigens and maternal immunity ceases. Possibly because of immature secondary lymphoid tissues, the inoculation of bovine serum albumin does not trigger antibody production in 1-day-old neonates, whereas a clear humoral response with specific antibody production can be seen in 1-week-old chicks. However, gut-associated lymphoid tissue, which provides an important enteric protection in the absence of oral maternal antibodies, is functional as early as 4 days after the hatch, but the secretory IgA response against enteric antigens develops only gradually, maturing toward the end of the second week of life.[67] Natural IgA production begins about day 3 in the bursa and day 7 in the gut and lung.[68]

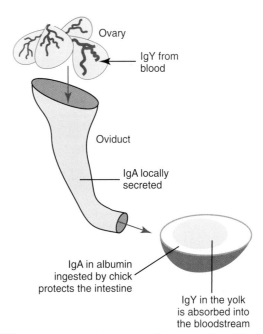

FIGURE 11-12 The mechanisms of the transfer of immunity from a hen to her chick. Egg yolk contains concentrated serum antibodies, primarily IgY. Egg albumen contains antibodies derived from the oviduct and uterine walls, primarily IgA. Ig, Immunoglobulin.

Because of increased needs during the fetal and post-hatch periods of growth, additional sites of hematopoiesis outside the bone marrow, bursa, thymus, and spleen are seen in normal chicks. These include the erythropoiesis and granulopoiesis and can be observed in the liver, kidney, vertebrae, cranial nerves, spinal ganglia, heart, pancreas, pharynx, subcutaneous tissue, muscles, and gonads. According to studies in domestic pigeons (*Columba livia* var. *domestica*), quail (*Coturnix coturnix*) and budgerigars (*Melopsittacus undulatus*), erythropoietic tissue starts to decrease to adult values once the chick has reached adult body mass.[69] In psittacine chicks, extramedullary erythropoiesis is mostly seen in the liver, whereas granulopoiesis predominantly takes place in the kidney, the liver, and, to a lesser degree, the spleen. Based on literature citations and histologic comparisons between nestlings of the same species at the same age, Ollé[69] estimated the physiologic maturity of the hematopoietic system in psittacines. As small species develop more quickly compared with large species, the assessments were correlated with the size of adult birds (Figure 11-13). This estimation does not rule out the possibility that some species may require longer periods for development. For birds other than psittacines, periods ranging from weeks to months have been suggested.[70] Renal extramedullary granulopoiesis in king penguins (*Aptenodytes patagonicus*) may persist until the age of 1½ years.[71] Delayed hematopoiesis as a pathologic condition has been observed histologically, mainly in small psittacine species such as *Psittacula* sp., *Poicephalus rufiventris*, and *Aratinga solstitialis*, as well as in a medium-sized species *Primolius couloni*.[69]

Ongoing maturation and proliferation of the immune system during the first months of life are reflected by higher total white blood cell (WBC) counts in chicks compared with adults and an increase of lymphocytes in the peripheral bloodstream.[72] This is of practical importance because differential counts in chicks show a physiologic shift from a predominantly heterophilic pattern to a more lymphocytic pattern. This is most prominent in species with a predominantly lymphocytic mature differential count, such as in galliform species. The H/L ratio changes from over 2.0 to less than 0.5 within the first weeks after the hatch. To a lesser extent, this can also be observed in species with a predominantly heterophilic adult differential count. H/L ratios in certain psittacine species decrease from approximately 2.0 to 1.0 during the first 6 months of life.[72,73]

Immunosenescence. The immune function of animals declines with age. Key cell populations are not fully replenished, and eventually this impacts immune function. In mammals, T cell "shortage" tends to have the greatest effect on immunosenescence, with a consequent decline in cell-mediated responses. In birds, the supply of T cells from the thymus and B cells from the bursa declines once those organs atrophy. Age-related declines in humoral immune responses have been reported in collared flycatchers (*Ficedula albicollis*) and barn swallows (*Hirundo rustica*).[74] The rate of decline seems to be inversely correlated to longevity. Fast-paced species with shorter lifespans show a higher rate of cell-mediated immunosenescence compared with slow-paced species with a longer lifespan.[75] When comparing both humoral and cellular immunoreactivity, studies in Japanese Quail (*Coturnix japonica*) and tree swallows (*Tachycineta bicolor*) show a shift toward humoral immune responses in aged birds compared with younger individuals. From these results, it has been hypothesized that reallocation of energy and nutrient supplies to the less costly humoral immune responses may save resources to maintain overall biologic fitness in older birds.[74]

	Size of parrots		
	Small	Medium	Large
	Average time (days of life)		
Well-colonized thymus	3	5	7
Well-colonized cloacal bursa	5	7	9
Well-colonized spleen	7	7	7
Well-colonized bone marrow	−1	1	2
End of extramedullary erythropoiesis	7	9	9
End of extramedullary granulopoiesis in the spleen	1	2	2
End of extramedullary granulopoiesis in the kidney	7	9	9
End of extramedullary granulopoiesis in the liver	7	9	9
End of extramedullary granulopoiesis in the cloacal bursa	1	2	2

FIGURE 11-13 Estimated physiologic development of the hematopoietic system in psittacines after the hatch. (From Ollé RD: The glycogen body in neonate birds of the order psittaciformes and its role in neonate mortality [doctoral thesis]. Giessen, Germany, 2006, Justus-Liebig-Universität Giessen.)

DISORDERS OF THE IMMUNE SYSTEM

Malfunctions of the immune system are characterized by an inappropriate immune response to a pathogenic threat. Both excessive and insufficient reactions can occur. Immune-mediated disease will result from the first and immunodeficiencies will cause the latter. Underlying causes could be of infectious, noninfectious, or neoplastic origin. As outlined at the beginning of this section, a physiologic immune reaction consists of not only correct recognition of the pathogen but also an appropriate and controlled response. Controlled collateral tissue damage during inflammation is acceptable if it eliminates or compartmentalizes (granuloma formation) a pathogen.

Loss of Control—Septicemic Shock

Septicemic shock is an example of collateral tissue damage getting out of control. It occurs predominantly in infections with gram-negative bacteria, which contain lipopolysaccharides (LPSs) in their cell wall, also referred to as *endotoxins*. Gram-positive bacteria and fungi with analogous molecules in their cell walls may also lead to this condition. When bacteria die, free LPSs attach to a circulating binding protein. The complex binds to TLR4 on monocytes, macrophages, and heterophils. This triggers the production of effector cytokines such as IL1, IL-6, and tumor necrosis factor (TNF) in mononuclear cells.[76] These cytokines have a variety of effects on endothelial cells, which, in combination with the acute-phase proteins synthesized by the liver, contribute to an efficient eradication of the pathogen by the innate immune system. At high levels of LPSs, the production of the same cytokines and secondary mediators is massively increased and results in systemic, instead of local, vasodilation (hypotension); diminished myocardial contractility; widespread endothelial injury; and increased vascular permeability. In poultry, colisepticemia is frequently associated with pericarditis and myocarditis. Marked electrocardiographic changes can be detected often before the onset of gross lesions.[76] In cases with fatal outcomes, the hypoperfusion resulting from the combined effects of widespread vasodilation, increased permeability, and myocardial pump failure causes multiorgan system failure. It has been debated whether disseminated intravascular coagulation, a prominent feature in septicemia in mammals, also occurs in birds.

Immune-Mediated Disease

In *immune-mediated disease*, the protective immunologic reaction against a pathogen results in the clinical symptoms of the disease itself, and these symptoms may persist beyond the elimination of the pathogen. In this context, *hypersensitivity* is defined as the altered reactivity to a specific antigen that results in pathologic reactions upon exposure of a presensitized host to that specific antigen. The prefix "hyper" erroneously implies that these responses are generally greater than *normal* immune reactions. In fact, these responses are better characterized as "inappropriate" or "misdirected." In contrast to immunity being a beneficial immune response, hypersensitivity is a harmful response, with damaging, uncomfortable, and sometimes fatal effects. Historically, hypersensitivity has been classified into types I to IV, depending on the onset and the pathophysiologic mechanisms involved. Today, it is recognized that the majority of immune-mediated diseases result from a mixture of types of hypersensitivity.

Autoimmune diseases are a subset of immune-mediated diseases characterized by a breakdown of self-tolerance and immune responses to self-antigens, causing tissue damage. Autoimmune disease is mediated by hypersensitivity reactions types II to IV. Reactions can be triggered by structural changes on the surface antibodies or receptors of autologous cells (type II), by immune complex formation (type III), or by antigen-dependent T-cell stimulation (type IV).[77] For convenience, two basic types—organ-specific and systemic autoimmune diseases—can be distinguished. Most of the current information on immune-mediated disease in birds has come from studies on chickens. Examples of organ-specific autoimmune diseases in the chicken include Hashimoto thyroiditis, vitiligo, and scleroderma.[78] There are several syndromes and conditions in pet bird species, and their pathologies are assumed to be at least partially driven by hypersensitivity or immune-mediated reactions. Examples of suspected immune-mediated pathophysiologies include allergic dermatitis and food allergy (type I), immune-mediated hemolytic anemia (type II), chronic proventricular dilatation disease (combination of receptor-dependent type IIb and type IV), polyomavirus infection (type II to IV), aspergillosis, mycobacteriosis, erysipeloid, listeriosis, streptococcosis, staphylococcosis, bumble foot (T cell–mediated type IV), and respiratory syndrome resembling human interstitial lung disease (type IV) in macaws and Amazon parrots.

Type I—hypersensitivity: considerations on feather-picking behaviors

Allergies—immediate hypersensitivity. Immediate hypersensitivity (IH) in humans is characterized by a short response time ranging from a few seconds to 30 minutes after antigen exposure in a presensitized patient. This immune reaction is mediated in mammals by IgE, with subsequent mast cell degranulation as the central pathway. Clinical signs of local swelling and reddening are common. Histologically, eosinophilic and basophilic inflammation is usually encountered. Examples of immediate hypersensitivity reactions in mammals include skin urticaria and eczema, anaphylaxis, conjunctivitis, rhinorrhea and rhinitis, asthma, and gastroenteritis.[77] Many feather-picking birds are believed to be pruritic, and their behavior is thus presumed to be analogous to scratching and self-mutilation in mammals with itchiness. Because of this, it has been suggested that feather picking may be an expression of an underlying hypersensitivity reaction.[79,80] To date, however, the clinical conditions studied have not been conclusively linked to a Th2 pathway. The pathophysiology is not fully understood, since birds lack IgE. They produce IgY, which is believed to be an evolutionary precursor of mammalian IgE and seems to have similar biologic properties. After antigenic challenge, the initial synthesis of specific IgM is switched to the production of increasing amounts of IgY. Isotype switching occurs in the germinal centers where B cell memory develops. Hypermutation also occurs in these germinal centers. This is necessary for the affinity maturation of the antibodies involved in the secondary immune response.[67] Birds do possess mast cells, which are the source of inflammatory and purinergic molecules in mammals. Large numbers are present in the thymus, which does not become fully involuted. Mast cell degranulation may be an integral part of suspected IH, cutaneous basophil hypersensitivity (CBH), and anaphylactic and neurogenic reactions in birds, since these can be blocked by antihistamines. A possible pathway would be initiated by antigen binding to a mast cell–bound antibody. The subsequent release of vasoactive and inflammatory molecules, including histamine, causes an immediate local inflammation.[81] Experimental proof of these hypotheses, however, is still lacking. Intradermal skin testing widely employed in mammals as a method of identifying allergic individuals has failed to produce reliable results in avian patients. This may be, in part, the result of the mechanical challenges of intradermal skin testing on the very thin epidermis of a bird. The reactions tend to be weak and strongly influenced by the amount of fluid injected and by endogenous cortisone production. The response to histamine is highly inconsistent, and a wheal does not always develop in normal skin. Given the stress of the testing procedure, the consequent release of endogenous corticosteroids may also suppress histamine responses. Heatley et al have shown that corticosteroid levels rise rapidly in healthy birds during clinical examination.[82] Even if positive skin test results do develop, it is clear that the inflamed skin of feather-picking birds may be more prone to irritation and thus respond more strongly to intradermal injections. The site normally selected for intradermal skin testing is the sternal region adjacent to the keel. The most suitable positive control substance is codeine phosphate 1:100,000 weight per volume (wt/vol) in 0.02 mL. Sites should be read at 5 minutes.[83] In chickens, intradermal inoculation of histamine results in an increase in local permeability. This can be revealed by intravenous administration of fluorescein and subsequent examination under an ultraviolet lamp. Studies on psittacines, however, have suggested that differences between positive and negative controls are subjective and inconsistent.[84] Similar difficulties apply to the histopathologic evaluation of skin biopsies. In routine histopathology, eosinophils are hardly distinguishable from heterophils, and degranulated mast cells are difficult to detect in general. Instead of eosinophilia and basophilia, a predominantly mononuclear infiltration with few suspected eosinophils is observed in birds. Moreover, cases of suspected dermal hypersensitivity are usually aggravated by signs of self-mutilation and secondary infection, producing a high variety of clinical and histopathologic signs. Erythema of the skin and angiocentric mononuclear dermatitis may be the features most likely related to hypersensitivity (Figure 11-14).[85]

Neuronal degranulation of mast cells—psychogenic stressors. Besides immunogenic mechanisms, mast cell degranulation can be triggered by neuronal overstimulation in cases of physical exhaustion or severe emotional stress. In humans, it is known that mast cells connect neurogenic and immunologic inflammation and can be activated by psychological stress. Consequently, psychological stress has important modulative impact on the onset and degree of inflammatory diseases in the skin, joints, and the cardiopulmonary, urinary, and nervous systems. In emotional excitement, autonomic nerves transmit stimuli to the primary afferent sensory nerves, resulting in the antidromic release of neuropeptides from sensory nerve endings and degranulation of mast cells. Immobilization and isolation stress in rats has been shown to cause mast cell degranulation in the skin, dura mater, gut, and urinary

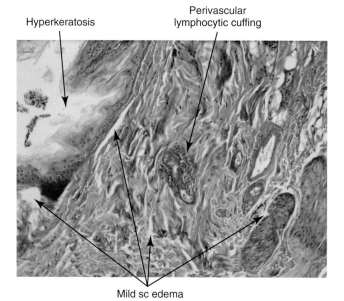

Hyperkeratosis

Perivascular lymphocytic cuffing

Mild sc edema

FIGURE 11-14 Skin biopsy from a feather-plucking orange-winged Amazon *(Amazona amazonica)*. Mild angiocentric mononuclear dermatitis, mild subcutaneous edema, hyperkeratosis, and hyperemia *(not depicted here)* are the most consistent features in suspected dermal hypersensitivity. H&E stain. Original magnification ×100.

bladder. In case of isolation stress, skin reaction was mediated by the inflammatory neuropeptides substance P (SP) of anaphylaxis, CRF, and neurotensin, which are mediators known to induce neurogenic inflammation.[86] It is not known if these factors are present in suspected cases of psychogenic feather picking in avian patients. However, comparing the mechanisms of the roles of stressors and immunologically mediated inflammation, some correlates could be applied in birds. Clinical selection of least intrusive treatment modalities for birds with inflammatory skin disease or feather-damaging disorders may require selection not only on an ethical and behavioral basis but also on a neurobiologic basis.[87]

Pseudohypersensitivity—anaphylaxis. Anaphylactic, pseudohypersensitive reactions result from mast cell degranulation without preceding IgE involvement. They develop in response to a large variety of substances and conditions and need to be distinguished from IH reactions. Anaphylatoxic effects are known to be caused by many drugs, chemicals, and toxins. It is not difficult to induce an experimental anaphylaxis-like reaction in chickens by using a foreign protein such as bovine serum albumin, but the relevance of this response to actual clinical disease is unclear.

The signs of acute anaphylaxis in chickens and other birds are similar to those in mammals, although the anaphylaxis is likely mediated by IgY. Increased salivation, defecation, ruffling of feathers, dyspnea, convulsions, cyanosis, collapse, and death are seen in the chickens. The major target organ is probably the lung, and death results from pulmonary arterial hypotension, right-sided heart dilation, and cardiac arrest. The mediating pharmacologic agents involved in pseudohypersensitivity include histamine, serotonin, kinins, and leukotrienes.

Type II—cytotoxic hypersensitivity

Type II reactions result from the destruction of cells either by cytotoxic cells or antibodies that activate complement. Type II reactions can be subclassified into an antibody-dependent type IIa and receptor-dependent type IIb reactions. Heterophils, macrophages, and some lymphocytes have receptors for immunoglobulin Fc fragments and can lyse target cells that are coated with immune complexes. Biologically active substances from the destroyed cells may contribute to inflammation. Graft rejection and many autoimmune diseases result from cytotoxic hypersensitivity reactions.[81] Examples of type IIa reactions include autoimmune skin disease, autoimmune hemolytic anemia, and Hashimoto-like thyroiditis. Myasthenia gravis is an example of a receptor-dependent type IIb reaction.

Autoimmune skin disease. Autoimmune skin disease has been suspected in some birds with intraepidermal pustule formation and acantholysis (Figures 11-15 and 11-16).[85]

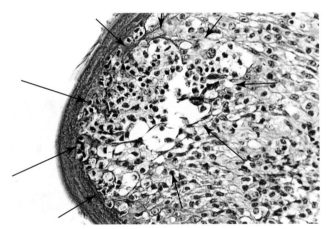

FIGURE 11-15 Suspected type II cytotoxic autoimmune skin disease with intraepidermal pustule formation (Photo courtesy Dr. Robert Schmidt, Zoo/Exotic pathology service.)

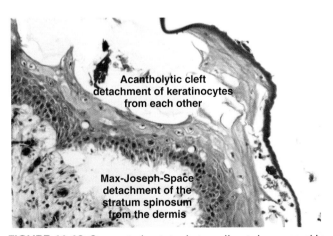

FIGURE 11-16 Suspected cytotoxic type II autoimmune skin disease in a macaw with acantholysis (cleft formation within the stratum corneum as a result of loss of cohesion between keratinocytes), and Max Joseph's spaces (cleft formation between stratum spinosum and dermis as a result of weakening of epithelial connective tissue interphase). (Photo courtesy Dr. Robert Schmidt, Zoo/Exotic pathology service.)

Birds reject skin allografts in about 7 to 14 days. Histologic examination shows massive infiltration of the grafted tissue by lymphocytes. These cells are believed to be T cells, since neonatal thymectomy results in a failure to reject grafts.

Autoimmune hemolytic anemia. Immune-mediated hemolytic anemia was the presumptive diagnosis in a blue-crowned conure *(Aratinga acuticaudata)*[88] and an Eclectus parrot *(Eclectus roratus)*[89] Common clinicopathologic signs, in both cases, included biliverdinuria and a marked regenerative anemia with increased amounts of spherocyte-like erythrocytes. Prednisolone treatment in the conure resulted in temporary resolution of the symptoms, whereas in the Eclectus parrot, treatment with immunosuppressive doses of cyclosporine did not have any positive effect.

Nonsuppurative myocarditis. Infection with *Chlamydia* sp. in mice has been shown to lead to immune-mediated nonsuppurative myocarditis. The autoimmune reaction is triggered by chlamydial peptides, which mimic murine heart muscle–specific α-myosin heavy chains. As infection with *Chlamydia* is a common feature in pet birds, a similar mechanism may be the underlying cause of idiopathic nonsuppurative myocarditis occasionally seen in avian patients.[85]

Autoimmune thyroiditis. The inbred obese chicken strain (OS) develops a spontaneous autoimmune thyroiditis similar to Hashimoto disease in humans. It is mediated by the production of antithyroglobulin and other antithyroid antibodies. Depletion of CD4+ or CD8+ cell populations indicated that CD4+ cells are required for the development of autoimmune thyroiditis, whereas CD8+ cells were only marginally involved.[90] Morphologically similar lesions have been reported in young Grey parrots *(Psittacus erithacus).*[85,91]

Type III—immune complex reactions

Type III reactions are mediated by immune complex formation. An immune complex is defined as the binding of an antibody to a soluble antigen. The soluble antigen can be of external (mainly viral, parasitic, bacterial) or internal (e.g., non–organ-specific antigen as in systemic lupus erythematosus [SLE]) origin and usually has been present in high levels for a prolonged time. With the bound antigen acting as epitope, immune complexes can be subject to subsequent innate responses such as complement deposition (C3a, C4a, and C5a), opsonization, phagocytosis, or processing by proteases. Besides SLE, immune complex deposition is a prominent feature in rheumatoid arthritis and scleroderma.[77,92]

Glomerulonephritis. In mammals, glomerulonephritis most often develops as an immune-mediated late sequel of a variety of conditions that lead to high antigen–antibody titers, with subsequent deposition of immune complexes in the mesangial stroma or the capillary basal membranes of the glomerulus. Depending on the etiology, the immunoglobulin involved, and the location of the lesion, different subtypes can be classified. Subsequent impairment of glomerular filtration leads to clinical disease. In case of a secondary immune reaction directed against the altered structures, autoimmune disease such as lupus nephritis develops. In birds, deposition of immune complexes in the basal membranes of the capillary loops is considered the cause of membranous glomerulopathy in chronic infections such as avian polyoma

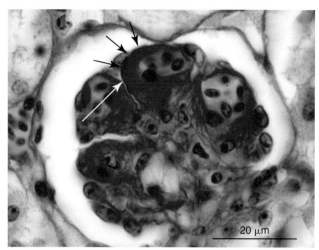

FIGURE 11-17 Membranous glomerulopathy in an APV-positive orange-winged Amazon parrot (*Amazona amazonica*). PAS stain. Original magnification ×1000.

virus (APV) infection (Figure 11-17). Clinical glomerular-related disease should be expected to occur later in birds than it does in humans, as the tubular function of birds is comparatively much higher. As a result, birds should be capable of coping with a much higher degree of glomerular damage, compared with humans, prior to the advent of clinical signs.

Type IV—delayed hypersensitivity

Delayed hypersensitivity (DH) reactions are characterized by a localized inflammatory response more than 24 hours after contact with antigen. The reaction is antibody independent and mediated by sensitized T cells. The resulting immune response is either mediated by direct cytotoxicity or by the release of cytokines that primarily act through macrophages. Based on reaction time, clinical appearance, histology, antigen, and site, DH reactions can be classified into three subtypes: contact dermatitis, tuberculin reaction, and granuloma-fibrosis reaction. Contact dermatitis and tuberculin reaction develop within 48 to 72 after antigen contact. In contact dermatitis, epidermal antigens such as organic chemicals, plant toxins (poison ivy), and heavy metals trigger an edematous swelling with lymphocytic infiltration, followed by macrophages. Tuberculin-type reactions are triggered by intradermal antigens such as tuberculin or lepromin and result in a local induration characterized histologically by a mononuclear infiltration of lymphocytes, monocytes, and macrophages. A granuloma–fibrosis type of reaction develops much later (21 to 28 days after antigen challenge). Clinically, a hardening of the affected areas with fibrosis, macrophages, and epithelioid, giant cells is noticed as histologic key features. A granuloma-type reaction develops in case of failure to eliminate the pathogen. As a replacement, it is compartmentalized by granuloma formation. Typical examples for type IV DH reactions include tuberculosis, leprosy, Johne disease, rheumatoid arthritis, multiple sclerosis, equine recurrent uveitis, and chronic allograft rejection.[77,92]

Cutaneous basophil hypersensitivity. Some clinical presentations of DH reactions have been shown to follow a different pathophysiologic pathway. They are characterized macroscopically by less prominent induration and erythema than in DH and are additionally accompanied by signs of a typical IH reaction such as reddening, hyperemia, and pain. The reaction is related to a T cell–dependent mast cell degranulation, the so-called CBH. CBH is a distinct form of hypersensitivity reaction with a delayed time course. It differs from both classic DH and IH reactions, as it requires both T-cell and B-cell involvement. A basophil chemotactic factor as a mediator of the reaction has been identified. First detected in guinea pigs, it is now known to occur in humans and many other mammals. Histologically, basophilia in the papillary dermis can be observed, in addition to mononuclear infiltrations. CBH seems to be an important pathway in hypersensitivity reactions associated with natural infections. It has been induced experimentally in several mammalian species by sensitization with a variety of antigens such as viruses, allografts, parasites, and fungal antigens and challenge with the specific antigen a week later by skin testing.[93] Today, this pathway is assumed to be also valid for birds.[32] The local inflammatory response is caused by vasoactive lymphokines and substances released from mast cells.[81] DH reactions are age dependent. When injected with human γ-globulin, 6- to 12-week-old chickens exhibited a significantly greater DH reaction compared with 3-week-old birds.[67]

Cutaneous DH studies such as tuberculin reactions have been described in poultry. Avian diseases whose pathology is suspected to be governed by T cell–mediated DH reactions include aspergillosis, mycobacteriosis, streptococcosis, staphylococcosis, listeriosis, erysipeloid, foreign body reactions, and bumblefoot. As a general rule, some granuloma formation is dependent on T cells. Consequently, histologic absence of expected granuloma formation suggests a compromised immune reaction not only on the level of heterophils and macrophages but also that of T lymphocytes.[71] T-cell suppression is a common immunoevasive strategy of many pathogens, including the *Mycobacterium* and *Mycoplasma* species. Their histopathologic features are characterized by the absence of granuloma formation but prominent mononuclear pleomorphic infiltrates with lymphocytes, macrophages, epithelioid cells, and multinucleated giant cells.

Inflammatory lung disease in psittacines. A respiratory syndrome resembling human inflammatory lung disease (ILD) has been reported in psittacines, specifically in blue-and-yellow macaws (*Ara ararauna*)[94-96] and Amazon parrots.[97,98]

ILDs in human medicine are defined as a group of more than 200 lung diseases characterized by chronic inflammation and progressive fibrosis of the lung tissue. According to their etiologies, they are classified in three main categories: (1) ILDs with a known extrinsic etiology such as environmental hazards, exposure to allergens, professional risks, drugs, and infections; (2) ILDs with a known intrinsic etiology such as systemic disorders and genetic predisposition; and (3) rare miscellaneous or idiopathic interstitial pneumonias of unknown etiology. Idiopathic pulmonary fibrosis (IPF) belongs to the last group and is characterized by progressive and lethal pulmonary fibrosis unresponsive to treatment.[97] Although the etiology of IPF is still unknown, there seem to be several predisposing conditions and risk factors for disease outbreak, such as genetic predisposition, cigarette smoking, organic dusts, or environmental contamination with heavy metals (see Toxin-Induced and Drug-Induced Immunosuppression, later in this section of the chapter). The antigenicity of certain avian fecal proteins and their role in human pulmonary disease (e.g., pigeon fancier's lung) is well documented. In a recently conducted case-cohort study on human patients with confirmed IPF, almost half the patients were found to suffer from chronic hypersensitivity pneumonitis, most of them associated with exposure to occult avian antigens from commonly used feather bedding.[99,100]

In affected birds, clinical signs include respiratory difficulty, exercise intolerance, signs of right heart failure, and detectable cyanosis of the facial skin. Sudden occasional coughing may be caused by hyperresponsiveness. Airway hyperresponsiveness is a well-known clinical feature in human patients following a transient and often subclinical viral infection of the lower respiratory tract. Coughing results from exaggerated bronchoconstriction following exposure to mild stimuli such as cold air.[101] Clinical pathology may reveal hypoxia or hypercapnia with polycythemia or hyperchromic normocythemia. Characteristic for the latter are total erythrocyte numbers with an increase in cell size (mean corpuscular volume >200 femtoliters [fl]) resulting in an increase in packed cell volume, sometimes up to more than 70%. The hemoglobin content may exceed 20 grams per liter (g/L) and the RBC cytomorphology in the blood film appears to be rounded as a result of prominent expansion of the cytoplasm, which is packed with hemoglobin.[95,96,98,102] Pulmonary biopsy is required for definitive diagnosis intra vitam (during life).[97] The lung lesions are generally advanced when polycythemia occurs. Postmortem findings include a loss of functional lung tissue, pulmonary interstitial fibrosis, right heart failure, hyperemia, ascites, and congestion of vessels and liver tissue.[98] Histopathologic findings are restricted to the lower respiratory tract, with perivascular edema and thickening of the atrial and parabronchiolar walls being key findings. The thickening is caused by smooth muscle hypertrophy and edematous, fibroblastic to fibrotic changes of the atrial and interparabronchial septae. This results in a decreased number of air capillaries and partial or complete obliteration of the parabronchial lumina. In severe cases, complete obstruction of airways and concurrent emphysema caused by the destruction of alveolar walls is seen. Cellular inflammatory infiltrates are often lacking; if present, they usually consist of diffuse, mild to moderate lymphocytic infiltrates and few macrophages in the fibrotic areas. Granulocytic infiltration, proliferation of parabronchial lymphoid tissue, and formation of lymphoid nodules may occur in various degrees, depending on the stage of disease and the secondary infections involved. Additionally, goblet cell hyperplasia, cuboidal appearance of the atrial epithelium with edematous fluid accumulation within the aerated spaces can be seen. These findings suggest the involvement of more than one type of inflammatory reaction, with possible involvement of hypersensitivity mechanisms.

As with human ILDs, the primary cause for the lung damage often remains undetected. Environmental allergens, toxins, and preceding microbial infections have been suggested to play a causative role, including powder-down from other parrots.[94-96] Certain psittacines produce prodigious quantities of fine epithelial debris. In two cases, the affected macaws

were housed in a mixed collection with cockatoos in poor conditions of ventilation. It was postulated that high particulate levels in the air and poor ventilation may predispose certain species to chronic respiratory distress and consecutive disease. Treatment is primarily symptomatic and includes a strict separation of the birds from suspected sources of inhaled antigen, nonsteroidal antiinflammatory drugs, bronchodilators, occasionally corticosteroids, and exercise restriction. Most birds with confirmed ILD should not be expected to have a normal life expectancy.

Bornavirus-related neuropathy. Based on the histopathology of the lesions in affected nervous tissues and on previous studies in laboratory animals, immune-mediated mechanisms have long been suspected to contribute to the pathogenesis of proventricular dilatation disease (PDD).[103] The lesions seemed to be triggered by an infectious agent as the disease spreads through bird collections. At present, avian bornavirus (ABV) is the only known etiologic agent (see Chapter 2).[104] Its causal association with PDD has been demonstrated with several successful experimental infections.[105-110] PDD, however, does not develop in every ABV-infected parrot. Despite the remarkably common detection of ABV, many infected birds remain clinically healthy for an indefinite period. It seems that several factors besides the infection of the host with ABV are necessary for the development of clinical PDD.[104-111] Although different from mammalian Borna disease virus (BDV) in many ways, ABV has some features in common with BDV. Both ABV and BDV infect the central nervous system (CNS) and the peripheral nervous system (PNS) and induce viral encephalitis and polyneuritis with selective destruction of Purkinje cells, lymphocyte infiltration, and dysfunction of the CNS, PNS, and the autonomic nervous system.[106] Direct viral cytopathic effects are unlikely to be important for clinical outbreak of disease, since ABV, like BDV, is noncytopathic.[104]

As for BDV, experimental infection causes a persistent infection of the CNS. BDV is noncytolytic, and development of BDV encephalomyelitis is based on virus-induced autoimmune reactions. The infiltrating immune cells in infected brains have been characterized as CD4+, CD8+ T cells, macrophages, and B cells. Of these, CD8+ T cells, which exhibit antigen specificity for the p40 nucleoprotein, seem to predominately represent the effector cell population. Their presence appears to be obligatory for development of neurologic symptoms and inflammation. Treatment of experimentally infected rats with anti-CD8 antibodies results in a decrease of MHC class I expression with subsequent inhibition of inflammation and prevention of neuronal degeneration in spite of the persistent presence of CD4+ T cells and macrophages. These findings suggest that CD4+ T cells and macrophages need to be triggered by antigen specific CD8+ T cells to provoke an inflammatory reaction of DH. In addition to their trigger function, CD8+ T cells seem to be directly involved in tissue destruction. In contrast to CD4+ T cells and macrophages, which mainly accumulate perivascularly, CD8+ T cells are found predominantly in the brain parenchyma close to the degenerating neurons. Proinflammatory humoral factors may play an additional role in clinical onset. Levels of the mRNA of several cytokines directly correlate with the degree of inflammation and neurologic symptoms. Cytokine patterns indicate a switch from a Th1 cellular immune response to a Th2 humoral immune response, which suggests an additional antibody-dependent pathway. Numerous B cells are present in encephalitis lesions and a prominent humoral immune response can be seen in BDV-infected animals. Several studies, however, have indicated that antiviral antibodies do not play a significant role in the immunopathogenesis of BDV.[112]

In a recent study carried out by Fluck et al[113] ABV antibody titers and viral RNA shedding in clinically healthy birds, birds with feather-damaging behaviors, and birds with clinically manifested neurologic disease were compared. Birds with neurologic symptoms showed the highest values in both tests, followed by birds with feather-damaging behaviors showing lower values and the clinically healthy but ABV-positive birds showing the lowest values. These findings suggest a possible role of ABV antibodies in the clinical course of PDD. The difference in antibody titers between neurologically affected birds and clinically healthy birds was significant. Conversely, there was no significant difference in antibody titers seen in birds with feather-damaging behaviors and clinically healthy birds, providing no evidence in support of causality between ABV infection and feather-damaging behaviors. Further studies are needed to substantiate this hypothesis.

Although phenotyping of inflammatory infiltrates and evaluation of cytokine profiles have not been undertaken for ABV infections so far, it is believed that cytotoxic T cell–mediated inflammation in terms of a DH reaction is likely to be the key autoimmune pathway also for ABV-related neurologic disorders.[114] Long-term survival and clinical remission of chronic PDD in a Grey parrot (*Psittacus erithacus*) under cyclosporine A (CsA) treatment, a selective T-cell immunosuppressant, seems to support this hypothesis.[115] The positive effect of CsA in this single case report, however, could not be confirmed in cockatiels (*Nymphicus hollandicus*) experimentally infected with the pathogenic M24 strain of ABV 4, which may be a result of the different pharmacodynamics in other bird species or natural infections.[104,116]

Recently, antiganglioside antibodies have been claimed to significantly contribute to the clinical manifestation of PDD. Rossi et al had challenged cockatiels experimentally with a mixture of purified gangliosides from the PNS of parrots.[117-119] On the basis of their findings, they concluded that gangliosides, if not the only cause of PDD, were, at least, involved in its induction, by acting as antigens to evoke an autoimmune reaction at ganglioside receptors. Hence the authors stated that PDD shared similarities with certain human inflammatory neuropathies such as the Guillain-Barré syndrome (GBS) and suggested that PDD in parrots is a useful model for human GBS.[119] It has to be emphasized that, to date, other research groups or even the same authors could not successfully repeat and confirm these results, even in proven cases of PDD.[120] Nevertheless, autoantibodies to myelin basic protein and other neural autoantigens have been detected in PDD cases. Their clinical and diagnostic relevance and their relationship to ABV infections remain to be investigated.[106,121]

Other avian polyneuropathies. The histologic finding of a lymphoplasmacytic infiltrate in peripheral nerve tissue at a single location is not diagnostic for PDD. In fact, it depicts a non–pathogen-specific inflammatory reaction, which can be

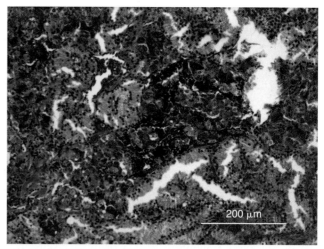

FIGURE 11-18 Lymphoplasmacytic infiltration of the medullary–chromaffin portion of the adrenal gland in a blue-fronted Amazon parrot *(Amazona aestiva)*. Similar infiltrates were found in the ganglia of the crop and the gizzard, suggesting bornavirus infection as the etiology. H&E stain. Original magnification ×100.

found in other conditions such as in gastroenteric ganglia of birds with WNV infection. Careful evaluation of multiple sites to assess distribution patterns and consideration of other findings such as affected bird species are necessary for differentiation (Figure 11-18).[85]

Guillain-Barré syndrome (GBS) is an umbrella term for several variants of polyneuropathies, which, among other criteria, differ from each other by the characteristic distribution of the individual target ganglioside. GBS in the vast majority of cases exclusively affects the PNS, whereas PDD frequently affects both the PNS and the CNS. This fundamental difference makes PDD an inadequate model for human GBS and has been a problem also for the currently most frequently employed model, the experimental autoimmune neuritis (EAN) in Lewis rats.[121]

A possibly adequate avian model for GBS has been thoroughly investigated recently. Spontaneous paresis, now termed *avian acute inflammatory demyelinating polyneuropathy* (AvIDP) in juvenile white leghorn chickens immunobiologically resembles the late-acute stages of the GBS variant *acute inflammatory demyelinating polyneuropathy* (AIDP). It primarily affects the craniospinal nerve roots and associated ganglia with a clear border of inflammation at the CNS–PNS transition without any inflammatory signs in the CNS.[122] The reason for this clear-cut restriction of inflammation to the PNS is unknown but may be associated with the distribution of the—still to be determined—target molecule for immuno-aggression, most likely a specific type of ganglioside. Clinical manifestation is correlated with a Th1-to-Th2 shift with lymphoplasmacytic and macrophageal infiltration of the endoneurium, deposition of myelin-bound IgG, and antibody-dependent reaction of macrophages against myelin sheaths. Macrophage recruitment seems to be triggered both by auto-reactive Th cells and opsonization of myelin epitopes by autoantibodies. Macrophage processes subsequently invade myelin spirals, which leads to centripetal delamination of myelin lamellae from morphologically intact axons. Interestingly, a clinical outbreak in chickens was significantly linked to a genetic susceptibility factor at the avian MHC, the B-complex, proposing an increased risk of disease development or certain genotypes.[122]

Amyloidosis

Amyloidosis is caused by systemic or organ-specific deposition of malformed proteins, which results in cell toxicity and organ dysfunction. Misfolding of protein fragments is a common feature in the course of protein metabolism. Usually, these fragments are eliminated by enzymatic proteolysis. Sometimes, the misfolding results in a β-pleated secondary protein structure. As this form is hydrophobic, the fragments cannot be removed by normal proteolysis. In the hydrophilic environment, the hydrophobic fragments tend to aggregate to oligomers and finally to fibrils. Amyloidosis can be of inherited origin, such as with the production of abnormal protein precursors in Siamese and Abyssinian cats or Shar Pei dogs. Amyloidosis is also associated with acquired high protein production such as overproduction of immunoglobulin light chains in multiple myeloma in dogs (AL amyloid), or with continuous overproduction of acute-phase proteins in chronic inflammation (AA amyloid), as in serum production and chronic parasitoses of horses.[77,123] In birds, the most frequent form of amyloidosis is AA amyloid, deposited in cases with chronic inflammatory conditions such as aspergillosis, mycobacteriosis, and bumblefoot. It is particularly seen in waterfowl and shore birds but also frequently observed in passerine birds and Falconiformes (especially *Falco rusticolus*). Amyloid deposition leads to functional impairment of the enclosed cells (Figure 11-19). In case of hepatic and renal–glomerular involvement, ascites and peripheral edema caused by hypoglobulinemia can be a prominent clinical feature.[124]

Immunodeficiencies

As in mammals, some avian viruses can evade the consequences of immune activation. Thus, they may be immunosuppressive, destroy the immune system, or simply hide within intracellular locations. *Immunosuppression* is defined as

a state of temporary or permanent dysfunction of the immune response resulting from insults to the immune system and leading to increased nonspecific susceptibility to disease and often a suboptimal antibody response. In contrast, *immunoevasion* is defined as pathogen-initiated responses counteracting the immune responses to the specific pathogen.[44] The major difference between immunosuppression and immunoevasion is that immunosuppression increases the overall susceptibility to pathogens in a nonspecific manner, whereas immunoevasion is achieved by pathogen-specific mechanisms, primarily favoring replication of this pathogen. This may not result necessarily in increased susceptibility to other pathogens. Today, it is assumed that most, if not all, viruses need to employ immunoevasive mechanisms to survive even the innate immune responses of the host. Viruses causing a persistent infection additionally need to be able to counteract adaptive immune responses. In some instances, infections can result both in immunosuppression and immunoevasion, such as in Marek disease. Immunoevasive mechanisms are known from avian herpesvirus, poxvirus, orthomyxovirus, paramyxovirus, and reovirus. Economically important viruses that induce immunosuppression in poultry include IBDV, chicken infectious anemia virus, reovirus, and tumor-causing viruses such as MDV, avian leukosis virus (ALV), and reticuloendotheliosis virus.

Premature atrophy of the bursa of Fabricius

Given the key role played by the bursa in the development of the immune system, it is clear that bursal destruction will lead to an immunodeficiency primarily affecting the antibody-forming B cells. The bursa normally involutes spontaneously as birds develop sexual maturity, leaving few bursal remnants in the mature bird. Clearly, however, this bursal atrophy can occur prematurely and thus prevent the complete maturation of the immune system. The most significant cause of premature bursal atrophy is severe nonspecific stress mediated through increased blood levels of corticosteroids. This stress can induce bursal cell necrosis. Thus, poor nutrition, chronic infections, poor management, and environmental stressors, including inappropriate temperature and humidity, can lead to psychological stress and bursal atrophy. As pointed out above, premature bursal atrophy, if it prevents maximum expansion of the B cell repertoire, will not only result in decreased antibody levels, but the diversity of these immunoglobulins will also be reduced. As a result of this premature atrophy, birds may show increased susceptibility to secondary infections.

Therefore, in cases involving bacterial, fungal, or protozoal infections of the bursa, a possible primary immunosuppression always has to be considered. Bacterial infections appear to result from ascending infections from the cloaca. The bursal lumen may contain necrotic or caseous material. Alternatively, the bursal tissues may contain typical microabscesses surrounded by macrophages and giant cells. In extreme cases, the entire bursa may be invaded. Occasional bursal lesions are seen in cases of chlamydiosis. *Salmonella enteritidis* may localize within the bursa. Yeast infections of the bursa have been recognized in young cockatiels and goslings. The follicles are severely depleted of cells. Foci of necrosis with yeasts and pseudohyphae are present together with a complex of mixed inflammatory reactions and granuloma formation.[125]

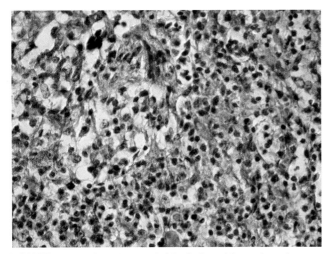

FIGURE 11-19 Splenic amyloidosis in a blue-winged parrot (*Neophema chrysostoma*). Congo red stain under polarized light. Original magnification ×400.

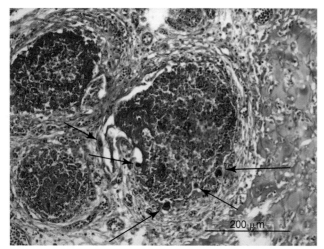

FIGURE 11-20 Bursal necrosis with adenovirus inclusion bodies, *Amazon* sp., 6w. H&E stain. Original magnification ×100.

Virus-induced immunosuppression

Many of the common viral diseases of pet birds will result in bursal lesions and in damage to bursal lymphocytes. The list includes Pacheco disease, parvovirus of ducks and geese, avian influenza[126,127] and adenovirus infections (Figure 11-20).[128] However, it is important to point out that this virus-induced immunosuppression may simply be secondary to stress, rather than a direct effect of the invading virus.

Circovirus. In exotic avian medicine, the most prominent example of virus-induced immunosuppression is infection with viruses of the family Circoviridae. Infection with subsequent disease has been reported in species of the order Psittaciformes, Anseriformes, and Columbiformes,[129] Passeriformes,[130,131] Charadriiformes,[131] and Struthioniformes.[132] All avian circoviruses such as psittacine beak and feather disease virus (PBFDV), pigeon circovirus (PiCV), and goose circovirus (GoCV) are associated with immunosuppression accompanied by wasting.[129] These viruses infect both T and B cells, and depletion of both cell types is therefore common. As a result, affected birds exhibit ill-thrift and a predisposition to secondary infections. It is interesting to note that another avian circovirus, the chicken anemia virus (CAV), in contrast, infects only T cells, and this induces a pure T-cell deficiency.

Psittacine beak and feather disease virus. In Psittaciformes, all species are considered to be susceptible to infection with PBFDV, but disease is predominantly seen in parrots of African and Australasian origins and is most common in birds less than 3 years of age (see Chapter 2). Its portals of entry appear to be the lymphoid tissues of the avian GI tract, including the bursa of Fabricius. Primary replication of the virus occurs in these intestinal lymphoid organs before the virus spreads secondarily to the liver, thymus, epidermis, and other tissues. As a result of this virus infection, both the bursa and the thymus atrophy. In addition, destruction of bone marrow cells may leave it pale and yellowish, and birds may be severely anemic and leukopenic.[133] Depending on the time of infection, feather dystrophies, liver necrosis and atrophy, and necrosis of lymphoid tissue of varying severity are the main histopathologic features. Immunosuppression with subsequent fatal secondary infection is seen in juvenile birds

infected before bursal regression. In this age group, young Grey parrots show a specific clinical picture without feather abnormalities predominated by massive leukopenia, anemia, and liver necrosis.[85,133] Heteropenia to agranulocytosis, seen in the peripheral blood films of these birds, is caused by atrophy and necrosis of the granulopoietic stem cells in bone marrow (Figure 11-21). Because this virus attacks and kills B cells, it can cause extensive necrosis of bursal follicles and lymphocytolysis. These areas of necrosis can, in turn, develop into cysts containing proteinaceous fluid and cell debris. Blood vessel disruption may also lead to bursal hemorrhage. Functionally, affected birds are profoundly immunosuppressed. Circoviral inclusion bodies are restricted to the bursal follicles only, which makes direct viral attacks of granulocytic precursors in the bone marrow rather unlikely (Figure 11-22). A possible cause could be viral affection of lymphoid or epithelioid supporting tissue in the bone marrow, resulting in a

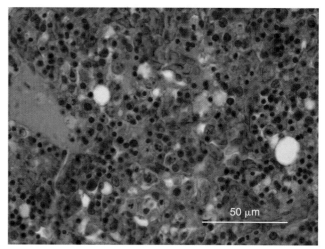

FIGURE 11-21 Atrophy and necrosis of granulopoietic stem cells in the extrasinusoidal compartment of the bone marrow caused by circovirus infection in a juvenile Grey parrot. H&E stain. Original magnification ×400.

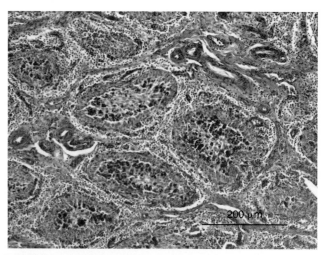

FIGURE 11-22 Medullary necrosis of bursal follicles with circovirus inclusion bodies in a juvenile Grey parrot. H&E stain. Original magnification ×100.

change of microenvironment detrimental to myelopoiesis. Secondary infections could be of bacterial, fungal, and protozoal origins. Among protozoal infections, bursal cryptosporidiosis seems to be specifically related to PBFDV infection.[134] Bursal cryptosporidiosis has also been reported as a consequence of Marek disease in chickens.[135]

Pigeon circovirus. Immunosuppression is also induced by PiCV infections. Circovirus infections have been diagnosed in pigeons in Europe, North America, and Australia.[136,137] The pigeon circovirus is distinct from PBFDV. Nevertheless, like the psittacine virus, it is profoundly immunosuppressive. The presence of circovirus inclusions in the bursa of pigeons is associated with lymphoid depletion in the bursa, spleen, and bone marrow.[138] Viral inclusions have been identified in splenic, bursal, gut-associated, and bronchus-associated lymphoid tissue. The lesions in the bursa ranged from mild lymphocellular necrosis to severe cystic bursal atrophy. These lesions were accompanied by concurrent bacterial, viral, fungal, and parasitic infections.[139]

Avian polyomavirus

APV is a DNA virus that primarily affects budgerigars and other psittacines. The disease is highly lethal. Affected birds suffer from generalized viral invasion, with dermal edema and necrosis and significant hepatomegaly. Splenomegaly and ascites are common. The primary lesion is virus-induced cellular necrosis often accompanied by hemorrhage. One feature of nestlings dying as a result of APV infection is swelling and hemorrhage of the bursa. The nestlings may also show necrosis and a resulting depletion of bursal medullary lymphocytes. Basophilic intranuclear inclusion bodies may be detected in bursal lymphocytes from APV-infected birds. Because so few birds survive this infection, it is not common to see birds with a secondary immunodeficiency as a result of APV infections.

Infectious bursal disease virus

In poultry, IBDV, a birnavirus, will kill immature B cells, leading to extensive necrosis, bursal swelling, and B-cell destruction. As a result of B-cell depletion, affected birds are often severely immunocompromised. Secondary splenic hypoplasia may result. This virus may also affect ostriches. This loss of bursal function can lead to increased susceptibility to bacterial and fungal infections, not only as a result of decreased antibody levels but also as a result of what appear to be reduced inflammatory responses.

Reovirus

Reovirus infections in young Grey parrots can also affect the bursa.[140] The virus was found in the large mononuclear cells within the bursa, and affected birds show significant lymphoid depletion. Birds suffer from secondary mycotic infections with *Aspergillus* spp. and Zygomycetes.

Duck enteritis virus

Duck enteritis virus, a herpesvirus, causes massive depletion of bursal and thymic lymphocytes, resulting in profound bursal and thymic atrophy and multiple secondary bacterial infections.[141] In commercial white Pekin ducks (mallards), the thymic atrophy was temporary, but the bursal atrophy appeared to be irreversible. Lymphoid depletion occurs not only in the thymus and the bursa but also in the spleen and the harderian gland.

Avian influenza virus

When this virus infects dendritic cells, it dysregulates cytokine production, which, in turn, contributes to the pathology of the disease.[142] Depending on the influenza virus strain, there may be induced massive increases in IFN-α and IFN-β as well as IL8 and TLR1. This flood of new molecules may trigger dysregulation of the immune response, as seen in some cases of avian flu (see Chapter 2).

Toxin-induced and drug-induced immunosuppression

Several environmental toxins can cause severe lymphocyte depletion as a result of lymphoid cell destruction. These can include crude oil, selenium, mycotoxins, and some organochlorides, including pesticides, disinfectants, and anthelmintic drugs.

Effects of crude oil in seabirds. Oiled seabirds suffer from severe and prolonged immunosuppression. Recent studies on birds released from cleaning facilities revealed that affected birds suffer from higher than expected mortality rates and fail to breed for 1 or more years.[143] These long-term effects cannot be explained by the immunosuppressive effects of handling stress during treatment alone. Instead, results from clinical and experimental studies as reviewed by Briggs et al[143,144] suggested that both handling stress and the toxic effects of petrochemical components contribute to a compromised immune status, resulting in reduced disease resistance, survival, behavior, and breeding success. Initially, ingestion of oil components causes GI inflammation with impairment of GI barrier functions, local immunity, and nutrient absorption, all of which affect systemic immunoreactivity. Furthermore, ingestion of crude oil shifts myelopoiesis toward erythropoiesis to compensate for lead-induced anemia and depresses leukocyte numbers, particularly T lymphocytes. As a consequence, not only cell-mediated immune responses but also secondary antibody responses that depend on T-cell stimulation are affected. Petrochemical ingestion in poultry resulted in greater mortality and depressed ability to kill or phagocytose bacterial pathogens.

Lead. The major mechanism of lead toxicity results from its ability to bind to proteins such as enzymes with subsequent alteration of their biologic function. Among other documented toxic effects, impairment of immune function has been reported in humans, other mammals,[145] and birds poisoned with sublethal dosages of lead.[146] In red-tailed hawks, short-term exposure to sublethal levels of lead acetate did not affect antibody titers to foreign RBCs or the mitogenic stimulation of T lymphocytes. Increased exposure time, however, resulted in a significant decrease in T-cell mitogenic responses.[147] Recent studies in humans and mammals suggest that long-term environmental exposure to low doses of lead has a major impact by skewing the adaptive immune response toward type-2 immunity. This, as a consequence, may elevate the risk of chronic immune-related disease (Th2) and decrease host resistance to infectious agents and cancer (Th1).[145] The main cause of this enhancement of type-2-related immunity appears to be a lead-induced functional modulation of bone marrow (BM)–derived dendritic cells (DCs) rather than a direct effect on T cells. Under the influence of lead, the DCs preferentially polarize antigen-specific T cells to Th2 cells in vitro and inhibit Th1 effects on humoral and cell-mediated immunity in vivo.[148] These findings correspond to the fact that lead is relatively noncytotoxic. As a result, it produces only modest changes to immune cell populations and lymphoid organs, which makes this immunotoxic hazard extremely difficult to identify.[145]

Mycotoxins. Mycotoxins are secondary metabolites of filamentous fungi. Clinical syndromes can develop, when moldy food is ingested or in cases of systemic fungal infections with toxin-producing strains. Apart from causing the frequently encountered hepatotoxicity and nephrotoxicity, mycotoxins also suppress immune responses, decrease host resistance to infectious disease, and act as immunomodulators.[32,149] Clinical symptoms depend on the type, amount, duration, and combination of mycotoxins ingested and can range from acute death to growth retardation, reduced reproduction, and immunosuppression. Impaired immunity is usually seen with intake of low to moderate amounts of toxins. The immunosuppressive effect of many mycotoxins is based on their inhibition of DNA, RNA, and protein biosynthesis. Depending on the mechanisms involved, this can result in impaired B-cell, T-cell, and macrophage functions, decreased synthesis of immunoglobulins, and reduced activity of IFNs and complement.[149]

Aflatoxin and T-2. Aflatoxin B1 induces gross and microscopic lesions in the bursa and thymus. These include depletion of lymphocytes, cystic degeneration, and fibrous tissue proliferation. Thus, it suppresses both humoral and cell-mediated adaptive immune responses. Moreover, it impairs chemotaxis, phagocytosis, and intracellular killing of heterophils and macrophages. T-2 belongs to the group of trichothecene mycotoxins, which are considered the most potent small molecule toxins to inhibit protein synthesis in eukaryotic cells. It strongly inhibits peptidyl-transferase activity, which indirectly affects DNA and RNA synthesis, resulting in cytotoxic radiomimetic-like lesions in tissues with a high cell turnover. In chickens and turkeys, severe necrosis and depletion of lymphocytes in the spleen, thymus, and bursa of Fabricius have been reported. Additionally, impaired macrophage and neutrophil functions, similar to those caused by aflatoxin, have been observed in mammals. In vitro studies in chicken macrophages showed that T-2 impairs the antifungal properties of macrophages against *A. fumigatus conidia* but upregulates the expression of proinflammatory cytokines, chemokines, and Th1 cytokines.[150] The apparent paradoxical enhancement of macrophage activity under T-2 treatment may represent the result of a normal macrophage response to reduced control by T suppressor cells depleted by the toxin.[149]

Aspergillus-related toxins. Ochratoxin A (OTA), cyclopiazonic acid (CPA), gliotoxin, and patulin are mycotoxins produced by several *Aspergillus* species. Lymphoid depletion of the thymus, bursa, and spleen, resulting in leukopenia and lymphopenia, have been reported in poultry for both OTA[151] and CPA.[152] OTA is hepatotoxic and nephrotoxic and inhibits phenylalanyl-transfer RNA synthetase activity by binding competitively at the site for phenylalanine.[149] Feed supplementation with l-phenylalanine in OTA-exposed laying hens[151] and broiler chicks[153,154] revealed a protective effect

against the toxic effects of OTA. Similar positive effects may be seen with aqueous extracts of artichokes and sesame seed as food additives in laying hens.[151] Patulin impairs the function of alveolar macrophages in rats in vitro[155,156] and, like gliotoxin, may predispose to allergies in humans. Human T-cell exposure to citrinin, gliotoxin, and patulin in vitro resulted in a selective inhibition of IFN-γ–producing Th1 cells.[157,158] This supports the hypothesis that mycotoxins are responsible for the Th1 lymphopenia observed in children exposed to molds. These children have a higher risk for the development of allergic diseases,[159] possibly caused by a shift of T-cell polarization toward the Th2 type under the influence of the mycotoxins.[157] Similar pathophysiologic mechanisms caused by secondary toxins may also apply to aspergillosis in noncommercial avian species. Infections with *Aspergillus* sp. are frequently associated with signs of liver and kidney disease and lymphopenia. To date, however, corresponding data for birds other than poultry are not available.

Benzimidazoles. A breakdown of myelopoiesis has been reported in cases of intoxication with benzimidazole anthelminthic drugs. Clinical signs are usually seen within 48 hours after treatment and include acute death, secondary septicemia, heteropenia to agranulocytosis, and sometimes anemia. Additionally, marked atrophy and necrosis of the intestinal villi with dilation and loss of crypts are noted histologically. The mode of action of benzimidazoles is based on their affinity for tubulin, compromising cellular division. This primarily affects tissues with a high cell turnover, that is, bone marrow and intestines. As the drug binds to both mammalian and parasitic tubulin, its relative efficacy against parasites and safety for the host is a question of drug dosage and species susceptibility. Fenbendazole has been used safely in many different avian species. Bone marrow toxicosis has been reported in Columbiformes, Psittaciformes, painted storks (*Mycteria leucocephala*), vultures (*Cathartes* sp.), and Marabou storks (*Leptoptilos crumeniferus*). Toxicity is assumed to be associated with species or individual variations in liver enzyme systems of the cytochrome P-450 cascade resulting in increased toxic metabolites or reduced metabolism and clearance.[160]

Malnutrition and energy deficiency

Deficiencies in nutrition both in terms of absolute quantities and relative composition can have a negative impact on immunoreactivity.[32] The nutritional needs for leukocyte function are relatively small compared with those necessary for maintenance of the antimicrobial properties of natural body surfaces or the production of acute-phase proteins by the liver. Additionally, when stimulated, leukocytes are able to activate membrane-bound accumulation systems for nutrients such as zinc, lysine, arginine, and glucose, endowing them with a priority of nutrient uptake relative to other tissues. Calorie deprivation as well as hypovitaminosis A will result in premature bursal atrophy, mediated both by direct nutritional influences and indirect hormonal influences caused by the stress of feed restriction. Metaplastic changes in epithelial cells, resulting from vitamin A deficiency, cause severe impairment of their barrier functions against microbial invaders in the GI, respiratory, and urogenital tracts. In chicken, thymic involution occurs in severe deficiencies of branched-chain amino acids such as leucine, isoleucine, and valine. The subsequent lymphopenia is often compensated for by increased innate immune responses with enhanced inflammatory reactions and may culminate in immunopathologic conditions. Some nutrients such as long-chain polyunsaturated fatty acids (PUFA) and vitamins A, D, and E show immunomodulatory properties when fed at levels above the nutritional requirements. Similar effects have been observed for several nonessential nutrients such as carotenoids, phytonutrients, and vitamin C. It has to be emphasized that beneficial effects are frequently achieved with moderate amounts of supplementation and that higher levels may cause adverse effects. In mammals, fatty acids, vitamin A, lutein, and antioxidants dampen inflammatory responses by decreasing the expression of proinflammatory cytokines through a down regulation of NF kappa B activity. Additionally, many of these nutrients seem to shift the Th1/Th2 balance from a cell-mediated (Th1) reaction to a humoral (Th2) reaction, which may be either an advantage or disadvantage. Assessment in avian species is complicated by the fact that responses to immunomodulating nutrients are often species-specific and may even vary between individuals of the same species.[32]

Tumors of the Immune System

Neoplastic diseases of the immune system in birds can be of infectious and noninfectious etiology. In contrast to the sporadically occurring noninfectious tumors, infectious neoplastic diseases caused by oncogenic viruses are widespread and of major economic importance in poultry. The three neoplastic diseases mainly affecting the poultry immune system are (1) Marek disease–associated T-cell lymphomas, (2) ALV-induced tumors of B cells and other hematopoietic cells, and (3) Reticuloendotheliosis virus–induced tumors. Additionally, lymphoproliferative disease in turkeys has been reported as an infectious neoplasm involving the lymphoid organs.[161] Both lymphatic and myeloid neoplasms are occasionally seen in exotic pet birds. Egg transmission of a retrovirus has been suspected in one case of myelocytomatosis in an 18-day-old orange-winged Amazon parrot (*Amazona amazonica*[69]). Primary tumors of the bursa are rare. There is one record of an undifferentiated sarcoma arising in the bursa of a budgerigar. Lymphosarcomas may arise in the bursa of chickens as a result of viral infections.

ASSESSMENT OF IMMUNOCOMPETENCE

Under some circumstances, it may be desirable to determine a bird's overall immune status. As a result, a panel of tests that can provide an index of immune activity has been developed. These tests often require minimal sampling from the bird, provide fairly rapid results, and thus allow for measurements even in field situations. Many immunologic tests are designed for use in poultry that are a precocial species and hence are more developmentally mature at the hatch. Many wild species, however, are developmentally immature (altricial) and are blind, naked, and totally dependent on their parents for survival. In wild birds, one may either monitor immunocompetence generally as a reflection of a bird's overall health or one can look at specific features of the immune response. Figure 11-23 outlines examples of methods, which have been used both in poultry and nonpoultry species.

The most common assay applied in a clinical setting is a complete WBC count with the determination of the total count (TWBC) and the differential count. The counts not only provide absolute and relative numbers but also serve as a basis for determining the H/L ratio. It must be emphasized that the WBC count only provides information on the circulating cellular immunity[74]; that is, it represents a gross numerical measure of one part of the immune system at a single time point without giving information on its functionality.[162] To capture the complexity of immune competence,[162] however, various measures of immunity are necessary. Therefore, WBC counts are increasingly performed in combination with other measures of innate and adaptive immunity,[162] such as concentrations of plasma proteins,[163-167] especially blood levels of acute phase proteins (innate response) or humoral mediators such as cytokines (innate and acquired response) and immunoglobulins (acquired responses). Functionality can be assessed by challenging with an infectious or noninfectious immunogenic agent and measuring cellular and humoral immune components after the challenge.[168-172] Experimentally, these challenge tests are frequently used to assess the immunomodulatory effects of specific stressors. Poultry immunologists recommend a panel of tests, including enzyme-linked immunosorbent assay (ELISA) for antiviral antibodies, CD4 and CD8 numbers, nitric oxide production, and NK activity for the innate immune response; a PHA skin test for the adaptive immune response (see below); and the H/L ratio for both.[173]

Few studies exist on combined measures for assessment of immune function in nonpoultry species. Olias et al compared mRNA expression of certain cytokines, histologic inflammatory patterns, immunohistochemistry, and nested polymerase chain reaction (PCR) in the brains of experimentally infected pigeons to explore the immunomodulative effects of *Sarcocystis calchasi* in pigeon protozoal encephalitis.[174] Millet et al determined immune competence by measuring serum bactericidal activity, heterophil phagocytosis, and bioassays for mannan-binding protein and lysozyme (both of which are acute-phase proteins). They used *Staphylococcus aureus* and *Escherichia coli* as target bacteria and showed species differences between captive and free-living birds. Birds stressed by capture and prolonged handling had diminished phagocytic and antibacterial activity. All these tests could be done with as little as 10 microliter (µL) of blood or plasma.[175] Matson et al used a hemolysis–hemagglutination assay in bird samples. This test measures natural antibody-mediated complement activation and RBC agglutination. They found that lysis and agglutination increase with age in chickens and that the results varied between species.[170]

A widely used functional test in many bird species is the PHA skin test.[176] PHA, like concanavalin A (ConA) is a plant lectin obtained from legumes (Leguminosae). Both PHA and ConA have mitogenic properties and are used to trigger T-lymphocyte mitosis. Their ability to stimulate various subsets of T cells makes them useful in the study of cell-mediated immune responses in vivo (PHA) and in vitro (ConA). An in vitro whole blood lymphocyte stimulation test based on PHA and ConA has been developed for bald eagles (*Haliaeetus leucocephalus*), red-tailed hawks (*Buteo jamaicensis*), and great horned owls (*Bubo virginianus*).[177] As for the in vivo skin test, PHA is injected unilaterally into the wing web or the

Type of test	Method	Assessment of	Information on	Ref.
Quantitative	CBC (TWBC and diff. count)	Leukocyte numbers in the intravascular space	Amount of circulating immune cells of the innate and adaptive immune system	(1)
	Protein electrophoresis	Blood levels of plasma proteins	Circulating innate and adaptive humoral factors (rough estimate)	(2-6)
Quantitative and functional	Cytokine expression profiles	Detection and quantification of mRNA expression levels of cytokines within affected tissue with PCR techniques with or without preceding antigen challenge	Type of immune reaction *in situ*	(7)
Functional	Bacteria killing and phagocytosis assays	Capacity of whole blood to kill or phagocytize microorganisms or non-vital structures, evaluation of complement, natural antibodies (NAbs), acute phase proteins, and phagocytes	Innate humoral and cellular response	(8-10)
	Lipopolysaccharide (LPS)	Acute phase proteins and sickness behavior mediated by pro-inflammatory cytokines	Innate humoral and cellular response	(10-12)
	Hemolysis-hemagglutination assay	NAbs and NAb-mediated complement activation, ability of complement to lyse foreign blood cells	Innate humoral immune response (complement); approximation for specific antibody response (NAbs)	(13)
	Phytohaemagglutinin (PHA); concanavalin (ConA)	T-cell activity and production of inflammatory cytokines	Cell-mediated adaptive immunity and innate humoral immunity	(14-16)
	Challenge tests with highly immunogenic antigens	T-cell activity and antibody response to key-hole limped hemocyanin (KLH), newcastle disease virus (NDV), diphtheria-tetanus vaccine, *mycobacterium butyricum*	Cell-mediated and humoral adaptive immunity	(8, 9)

1. O'Neal DM, Ketterson ED. Life-history evolution, hormones, and avian immune function. In: Demas GE, Nelson RJ, editors. Ecoimmunology. New York: Oxford University Press; 2012. p. 8-44.
2. Briscoe JA, Rosenthal KL, Shofer FS. Selected complete blood cell count and plasma protein electrophoresis parameters in pet psittacine birds evaluated for illness. Journal of avian medicine and surgery. 2010;24(2):131-7.
3. Cray C, King E, Rodriguez M, Decker LS, Arheart KL. Differences in protein fractions of avian plasma among three commercial electrophoresis systems. Journal of avian medicine and surgery. 2011;25(2):102-10.
4. Cray C, Reavill D, Romagnano A, Van Sant F, Champagne D, Stevenson R, et al. Galactomannan assay and plasma protein electrophoresis findings in psittacine birds with aspergillosis. Journal of avian medicine and surgery. 2009;23(2):125-35.
5. Cray C, Rodriguez M, Zaias J. Protein electrophoresis of psittacine plasma. Veterinary clinical pathology / American Society for Veterinary Clinical Pathology. 2007;36(1):64-72.
6. Jones MP, Arheart KL, Cray C. Reference intervals, longitudinal analyses, and index of individuality of commonly measured laboratory variables in captive bald eagles (Haliaeetus leucocephalus). Journal of avian medicine and surgery. 2014;28(2):118-26.
7. Olias P, Meyer A, Klopfleisch R, Lierz M, Kaspers B, Gruber AD. Modulation of the host Th1 immune response in pigeon protozoal encephalitis caused by Sarcocystis calchasi. Veterinary research. 2013;44:10.
8. Minozzi G, Parmentier HK, Bed'hom B, Minvielle F, Gourichon D, Pinard-van der Laan MH. Delayed-type hypersensitivity response to KLH in F2 and backcrosses of two immune selected chicken lines: effect of immunisation and selection. Developments in biologicals. 2008;132:267-70.
9. Minozzi G, Parmentier HK, Mignon-Grasteau S, Nieuwland MG, Bed'hom B, Gourichon D, et al. Correlated effects of selection for immunity in White Leghorn chicken lines on natural antibodies and specific antibody responses to KLH and M. butyricum. BMC genetics. 2008;9:5.
10. Millet S, Bennett J, Lee KA, Hau M, Klasing KC. Quantifying and comparing constitutive immunity across avian species. Developmental and comparative immunology. 2007;31(2):188-201.
11. Owen-Ashley NT, Turner M, Hahn TP, Wingfield JC. Hormonal, behavioral, and thermoregulatory responses to bacterial lipopolysaccharide in captive and free-living white-crowned sparrows (Zonotrichia leucophrys gambelii). Hormones and behavior. 2006;49(1):15-29.
12. Owen-Ashley NT, Wingfield JC. Seasonal modulation of sickness behavior in free-living northwestern song sparrows (Melospiza melodia morphna). The Journal of experimental biology. 2006;209(Pt 16):3062-70.
13. Matson KD, Ricklefs RE, Klasing KC. A hemolysis-hemagglutination assay for characterizing constitutive innate humoral immunity in wild and domestic birds. Developmental and comparative immunology. 2005;29(3):275-86.
14. Redig PT, Dunnette JL, Sivanandan V. Use of whole blood lymphocyte stimulation test for immunocompetency studies in bald eagles, red-tailed hawks, and great horned owls. American journal of veterinary research. 1984;45(11):2342-6.
15. Smits JEB, G. R.; Tella J.L. Simplifying the phystohaemagglutinin skin-testing technique in studies of avian immunocompetence. Funct Ecol. 1999;13:567-72.
16. Collette JC, Millam JR, Klasing KC, Wakenell PS. Neonatal handling of Amazon parrots alters the stress response and immune function. Applied animal behaviour science. 2000;66(4):335-49.

FIGURE 11-23 Selected methods for assessment of immunocompetence in birds.

interdigital web. Differences of swelling between the injected site and the control contralateral side (native or injected with phosphate buffered saline) 24 hours after injection are measured and compared with reference values.[178] Histologic evaluation of skin challenged with 75 micrograms (µg) of PHA revealed a transient heterophilia between 3 and 6 hours after challenge followed by a prominent perivascular lymphocytic infiltration at 6 to 12 hours, with additional macrophage appearance peaking 24 hours after injection. By 48 hours after the challenge, the PHA-induced hypercellularity had disappeared. As PHA fails to evoke a lymphocytic reaction in thymectomized chickens, the type of lymphocytic infiltration is believed to be of T-cell origin. PHA binds to T cells and triggers them to respond by dividing and releasing a mixture of cytokines. The most important of these are IL1β, IL6 and TGF-β. Since these are critical to inflammation, it appears that the PHA test measures a component of the innate response rather than T-cell responses, a measure of adaptive immunity. Variations in the injection site swelling depend on the number of responding cells and correlate well with cytokine release. The PHA response has been correlated with such factors as the signaling value of colorful plumage, the health of selected populations, the heritability of immune defenses, or the influence of neonatal handling on immune function in psittacine chicks.[179]

THERAPEUTIC CONSIDERATIONS FOR MODULATION OF THE IMMUNE SYSTEM

Immunoenhancing Therapy

Necessity of new strategies of disease control in poultry

With an average of 50 billion chickens produced per year globally, the poultry industry plays an important part in worldwide livestock production. Food safety can only be achieved by rigorous disease control and is of political importance, as it has a major impact on economic and social prosperity. For over 50 years, antibiotic growth promoters and therapeutic antimicrobials have been used in food animals. Public concern over the risk of chemical contamination of food, the environment, and the emergence of antibiotic-resistant bacteria has resulted in a ban of in-feed antibiotics by several countries. Studies on MDV have shown that vaccination with live attenuated vaccines selects for hypervirulent strains in the pathogenic virus. Animal welfare considerations have led to a shift from intensive indoor housing to more extensive outdoor rearing, which comes with a different spectrum of pathogenic challenges. In addition, effective disease control is complicated by increasing numbers of poultry kept in private collections. Increased awareness of zoonotic threats such as avian influenza virus, *Salmonella*, and *Campylobacter* has added to the pressure to develop effective novel intervention strategies. These political, medical, and economic pressures have considerably advanced research in poultry immunology, resulting in an enormous increase of knowledge in understanding both host mechanisms of infection resistance and the mechanisms for determining pathogen virulence. The goal of all these efforts is to find safe, effective, and environmentally friendly tools to improve resistance against infectious disease; these tools should be compatible with animal welfare regulations and meet the needs of the poultry industry for easy and cost-effective administration. New strategies in breeding, vaccination, and the development of immunostimulant therapeutics are the three major approaches to achieve this goal.[11,180-182]

Breeding for disease resistance

The availablity of the genome sequence of the chicken, zebra finch, turkey, scarlet macaw, bobwhite quail, and mallard has substantially contributed to the recent advances in avian immunology. It has provided the molecular tools to develop postgenomic technologies to identify genes or markers associated with improved disease resistance. Current research in defined inbred lines of chicken has focused on the identification of markers or genes associated with resistance to particular viral and bacterial diseases. Future areas include breeding of disease-resistance genes into commercial chicken lines and the development of vaccines tailored to chicken lines genetically selected for increased reactivity to a specific vaccine.[22]

New-generation vaccines

Recombinant vectored subunit vaccines represent the solution of choice to counteract the potential threat of generating hypervirulent pathogen strains by using traditional live attenuated vaccines. In addition, the technique of vector transfection offers the possibility of delivering protective antigens from multiple pathogens at once. Currently marketed recombinant poultry vaccines use viral or bacterial vectors.[22] Future vaccines may even use transfected anticoccidial live vaccines to mount resistance against nonprotozoal pathogens.[183]

Research in immunology of nonpoultry avian species is hampered by the poor cross-reactivity of most of the chicken molecular tools and the small size of the market, resulting in the reluctance of vaccine manufacturers to invest substantial sums for products of limited profitability. In the face of current epizootic threats, however, increased efforts are undertaken to investigate the cross-species reactivity of commercially available vaccines such as those against avian influenza,[184,185] Newcastle disease,[186] and WNV.[187] Additionally, there are ongoing experimental trials on recombinant subunit vaccines for nondomestic species, as exemplified by studies carried out on vaccines against PBFD[188,189] and *Chlamydophila psittaci*[190] in psittacines, and against WNV in wild and zoo bird species.[191-194]

To achieve immunogenic properties similar to those induced by live attenuated vaccines, subunit vaccines need to be combined with vaccine adjuvants. Traditional adjuvants are gradually being withdrawn from use because of ineffectiveness or induction of side effects such as hypersensitivity reactions and ulcerative inflammation at the site of injection.[182] Subsequent searches for alternatives suggest the use of cytokines[181,182,195-199] as *natural adjuvants*[22] delivered as proteins, DNA plasmids, or expressed in recombinant viruses. However, the costs of such products are prohibitive at the present time.

Cytokines as immunotherapeutics

Apart from their properties as possible vaccine adjuvants, avian cytokines have been intensively investigated for their potential use as immunoenhancing therapeutics in stages of immunosuppression.[180,181,195,197,198] It must, however, be pointed out that at the present time, the cost of such products is uneconomical in the poultry industry.

In human medicine, colony-stimulating factors (CSFs) have been widely used for the prevention and treatment of leukopenia-related pathologies, especially associated with cancer chemotherapy.[200] Recent considerations include the application of CSFs and IFN-γ in systemic fungal disease as reviewed by Safdar.[201] In summary, both granulocyte colony-stimulating factor (G-CSF) and granulocyte macrophage colony-stimulating factor (GM-CSF) stimulate the proliferation of myeloid cells, enhance antimicrobial function of mature neutrophils and monocytes against fungal targets, and reverse steroid-induced suppression of neutrophil and macrophage function in vitro. Clinical experience of the use of CSFs in patients with established mycosis is still limited but encouraging, especially in combination with IFN-γ, which has a direct damaging effect on *Aspergillus* hyphae. Concerns about CSFs include the risk of de novo stimulation of myelodysplastic syndromes or transformation into acute myeloid leukemia and in the case of IFN-γ, exacerbation of tissue inflammation, ischemia, necrosis, and graft rejection, all of which have been hypothetical or rarely seen in practice so far.

These findings are of avian medical interest as both CSFs and IFN-γ have been cloned and engineered in avian species and show biologic functions similar to their mammalian counterparts.

Inoculation of 1-day-old chicks with live recombinant fowlpox virus expressing chicken myelomonocytic growth factor resulted in a sustained increase of blood monocytes, both in number and state of activation during the first 2 weeks of life. During this time span, chicks are immunosuppressed because of their immature immune system and decreasing maternal antibody protection, which make them highly susceptible to opportunistic infections.[197]

Multiple injections of human recombinant G-CSF (filgrastim, Neupogen, AMGEN) in a circovirus-positive, leukopenic young Grey parrot raised leukocyte counts, suggesting a mammalian–avian cross-species reactivity of this cytokine. The initial WBC count was below 700 cells/μL and could be raised to around 7000 cells/μL within a week under therapy. In follow-up health checks during the next 2 years, the bird maintained a normal WBC count but was, interestingly, always PCR positive for circovirus and developed circovirus feather lesions.[202]

Intraperitoneal injection of recombinant chicken IFN-γ (ChIFN-γ) in 1-day-old chicks reduced the weight loss and enhanced the rate of weight gain after natural recovery from challenge with *Eimeria acervulina*.[197] In ovo administration of ChIFN-γ alleviates the depletion of T-cell precursors caused by infection with CAV. As T-cell depletion is a fundamental mechanism of many immunosuppressive states, these findings indicate that ChIFN-γ may have a *booster* effect in immunocompromised states in general.[195] Cross-species reactivity of IFN-γ has been reported for Galliformes, Columbiformes, and Anseriformes[203-205] and seems to be also valid for psittacine species, as exemplified by the successful treatment of circovirus infection in Grey parrots (*Psittacus erithacus*) with ChIFN-γ.[206]

Another candidate for cross-species application in immunosuppressed bird patients could be the B-cell activating factor (BAFF). BAFF is a member of the TNF family and is essential for B-cell survival and maturation. In vitro studies showed that goose BAFF is critical for the proliferation and survival of goose B cells and that functional cross-reactivity exists among chicken, duck, and goose BAFFs.[207]

In summary, although most of these in vitro studies show a positive effect, detailed analysis of the in vivo biologic function of these cytokines is usually not available. High production costs and safety concerns such as uncontrolled toxic cytokine effects in the host, or even the inadvertent creation of highly virulent viruses that could potentially be used as biologic weapons, as discussed for the IL4 recombinant ectromelia virus, are potential undesired consequences.[208] Finally, the receptivity of the public to genetically modified food is a significant concern. Careful investigations and clinical trials need to be undertaken to prove the safety and efficacy of cytokine-enriched vaccines and therapeutics in a commercial setting.

Immunosuppressive Therapy
Calcineurin inhibitors

Treatment of type II to IV hypersensitivity reactions consists of immunosuppressive and antiinflammatory drugs. Calcineurin inhibitors such as CsA and FK506 are potent T-cell selective immunosuppressants, which are widely used in human medicine. CsA is routinely applied in the chicken to inhibit T-cell activity in experimental settings to elucidate the role of cellular immunity against infectious pathogens.[209] Both CsA and FK506 block the Ca2+/calmodulin-dependent serine phosphatase calcineurin in the cytoplasm of activated T lymphocytes. This results in the inhibition of gene transcription synthesis of several lymphokines such as IL2, IL3, TNF-α, and IFNγ. Studies on BDV-infected laboratory rodents indicated that disease is mediated by cytotoxic T cells[210,211] and that treatment with CsA prevents the clinical outbreak of neurologic disease.[212] Long-term survival and clinical remission of chronic PDD in a Grey parrot under CsA treatment suggested that the pathophysiology of PDD follows a similar pattern.[115] The positive effect of CsA, however, could not be confirmed in cockatiels (*Nymphicus hollandicus*) experimentally infected with the pathogenic M24 strain of ABV 4, which may be attributed to the differences in pharmacodynamics in different bird species.[104,116] Chronic nephrotoxicity of CsA and FK506 is one of the major side effects in humans.[213] Furthermore, under certain circumstances, CsA paradoxically aggravates autoimmune reactions after withdrawal. A hyperreactive rebound effect of primed T cells has been hypothesized as the underlying pathway. CsA only inhibits lymphokine production at a pretranscriptional level but does not interfere with the antigen-specific priming of T cells.[214] This has also been reported for the Smyth delayed-amelanotic chicken line, an avian model for human vitiligo, which develops a spontaneous autoimmune posterior uveitis. After successful remission under CsA treatment, a rebound enhancement of symptoms occurred 4 to 8 weeks after withdrawal of CsA.[215] These side effects have to be taken into consideration in further exploration of the use of calcineurin inhibitors in exotic avian patients.

Corticosteroids

Corticosteroids have been a longstanding treatment to suppress the host's immune system and to control inflammation.

Common corticosteroids that are used in avian practice for the purpose of immunosuppression include prednisolone and dexamethasone. Treatment benefits, however, must be carefully weighed against the risks of opportunistic infections. It is known that the function of respiratory macrophages is severely impaired following exposure to systemic corticosteroids because of disruption of the translocation and activation of nuclear factor (NF)–κB.[201] As respiratory macrophages mediate the early immune defense against *Aspergillus fumigatus* infection in birds, corticosteroid treatment predisposes the patient to fungal respiratory disease. Therefore, the benefits of corticosteroid use have to be evaluated on an individual case basis, and treatment should be accompanied by close monitoring of the patient.

Gonadotropin-releasing hormone agonists

It has been anecdotally claimed that some birds with inflammatory dermatopathies or that show feather-damaging behaviors may clinically improve when treated with leuprolide acetate, deslorelin, or both. Both leuprolide acetate/leuprorelin and deslorelin are agonists at pituitary GnRH receptors. Their chemical properties protect them from proteolysis and enhance their receptor-binding affinity, resulting in prolonged binding. This interrupts the normal pulsatile stimulation and the desensitization of GnRH receptors. As a consequence of indirect downregulation of luteinizing hormone (LH) and follicle-stimulating hormone (FSH) secretion, hypogonadism and a decrease of progesterone, androstenedione, dehydroepiandrosterone, and estradiol levels in both sexes is seen. In mammals, β-estradiol reduces DH responses and production of IL2 and IFN-γ while increasing the levels of IL4 and IL10, which suggests that estrogen can shift the immune reaction from a Th1 to Th2 type of response. In other words, suppression of estrogen production may have a positive effect on exaggerated Th2 type responses, that is, hypersensitivity reactions.[32,216] In birds, as mentioned previously, immunosuppression with decreased reactivity to PHA skin testing occurs naturally during phases of low LH/FSH levels such as during incubation.[55,56] To summarize the findings, it is tempting to conclude that low LH/FSH levels in birds treated with leuprorelin and deslorelin may result in decreased immunoreactivity, which, as a side effect, could relieve signs of dermal hypersensitivity. However, the direct effect of low GnRH agonist-induced suppression of LH/FSH levels still lacks experimental proof.

REFERENCES

1. Magor KE, Miranzo Navarro D, et al: Defense genes missing from the flight division, *Dev Comp Immunol* 41(3):377–388, 2013.
2. Schmidt RE, Pendl H: The avian immune system. In *Proceedings of the First International Conference on Avian, Herpetological, and Exotic Mammal Medicine*, Wiesbaden, Germany, 2013, pp 11–14.
3. Cook JK, Davison TF, Huggins MB, et al: Effect of in ovo bursectomy on the course of an infectious bronchitis virus infection in line C white leghorn chickens, *Arch Virol* 118(3-4):225–234, 1991.
4. Wigley P: Immunity to bacterial infection in the chicken, *Dev Comp Immunol* 41(3):413–417, 2013.
5. Wigley P, Hulme S, Powers C, et al: Oral infection with the Salmonella enterica serovar Gallinarum 9R attenuated live vaccine as a model to characterise immunity to fowl typhoid in the chicken, *BMC Vet Res* 1:2, 2005.
6. Møller AP, Erritzoe J: Parasite virulence and host immune defence: host immune response is related to nest re-use in birds, *Evolution Int J Organic Evolution* 50(5):2066–2072, 1996.
7. Møller AP, Erritzoe J: Host immune defence and migration in birds, *Evol Ecol* 12:945–953, 1998.
8. van Ginkel FW, Gulley A, Lammers FJ, et al: Conjunctiva-associated lymphoid tissue in avian ocular immunity, *Dev Comp Immunol* 36:289–297, 2012.
9. Genovese KJ, He H, Swaggerty CL, et al: The avian heterophil, *D Dev Comp Immunol* 41(3):334–340, 2013.
10. Seliger C, Schaerer B, Kohn M, et al: A rapid high-precision flow cytometry based technique for total white blood cell counting in chickens, *Vet Immunol Immunopathol* 145(1-2):86–99, 2012.
11. Campbell TW: *Avian Hematology and cytology*, ed 2, Ames, IA, 1995, Iowa State University Press.
12. Fudge AM, Joseph V: Disorders of avian leukocytes. In Fudge AM, editor: *Laboratory medicine avian and exotic pets*, Philadelphia, 2000, Saunders, pp 19–25.
13. Maxwell MH: The avian eosinophil—a review, *World Poult Sci* 43:190–207, 1987.
14. Straub C, Neulen ML, Sperling B, et al: Chicken NK cell receptors, *Dev Comp Immunol* 41(3):324–333, 2013.
15. St. Paul M, Brisbin JT, Abdul-Careem MF, et al: Immunostimulatory properties of toll-like receptor ligands in chickens, *Vet Immunol Immunopathol* 152(3-4):191–199, 2013.
16. Keestra AM, de Zoete MR, Bouwman LI, et al: Chicken TLR21 is an innate CpG DNA receptor distinct from mammalian TLR9, *J Immunol* 185(1):460–467, 2010.
17. Brownlie R, Zhu J, Allan B, et al: Chicken TLR21 acts as a functional homologue to mammalian TLR9 in the recognition of CpG oligodeoxynucleotides, *Mol Immunol* 46(15):3163–3170.
18. Downing T, Lloyd AT, O'Farrelly C, et al: The differential evolutionary dynamics of avian cytokine and TLR gene classes, *J Immunol* 184(12):6993–7000, 2010.
19. Cuperus T, Coorens M, van Dijk A, et al: Avian host defense peptides, *Dev Comp Immunol* 41(3):352–369, 2013.
20. Bommineni YR, Pham GH, Sunkara LT, et al: Immune regulatory activities of fowlicidin-1, a cathelicidin host defense peptide, *Mol Immunol* 59(1):55–63, 2014.
21. Cormican P, Lloyd AT, Downing T, et al: The avian Toll-Like receptor pathway—subtle differences amidst general conformity, *Dev Comp Immunol* 33(9):967–973, 2009.
22. Kaiser P: Advances in avian immunology—prospects for disease control: a review, *Avian Pathol* 39(5):309–324, 2010.
23. Kaiser P, Staeheli P: Avian cytokines and chemokines. In Schat KA, Kaspers B, Kaiser P, editors: *Avian Immunology*, ed 2, New York, 2014, Academic Press, pp 189–204.
24. Parra ZE, Miller RD: Comparative analysis of the chicken TCRalpha/delta locus, *Immunogenetics* 64(8):641–645, 2012.
25. Withanage GS, Wigley P, Kaiser P, et al: Cytokine and chemokine responses associated with clearance of a primary Salmonella enterica serovar Typhimurium infection in the chicken and in protective immunity to rechallenge, *Infect Immun* 73(8):5173–5182, 2005.
26. Chaves LD, Krueth SB, Reed KM: Defining the turkey MHC: sequence and genes of the B locus, *J Immunol* 183(10):6530–6537, 2009.
27. Bonneaud C, Richard M, Faivre B, et al: An MHC class I allele associated to the expression of T-dependent immune response in the house sparrow, *Immunogenetics* 57(10):782–789, 2005.
28. Sato A, Tichy H, Grant PR, et al: Spectrum of MHC class II variability in Darwin's finches and their close relatives, *Mol Biol Evolution* 28(6):1943–1956, 2011.
29. Miller HC, Bowker-Wright G, Kharkrang M, et al: Characterisation of class II B MHC genes from a ratite bird, the little spotted kiwi (*Apteryx owenii*), *Immunogenetics* 63(4):223–233, 2011.

30. Buehler DM, Verkuil YI, Tavares ES, et al: Characterization of MHC class I in a long-distance migrant shorebird suggests multiple transcribed genes and intergenic recombination, *Immunogenetics* 65(3):211–225, 2013.

31. Promerova M, Albrecht T, Bryja J: Extremely high MHC class I variation in a population of a long-distance migrant, the scarlet rose-finch *(Carpodacus erythrinus)*, *Immunogenetics* 61(6):451–461, 2009.

32. Koutsos EA, Klasing KC: Factors modulating the avian immune system. In Schat KA, Kaspers B, Kaiser P, editors: *Avian immunology*, ed 2, New York, 2014, Academic Press, pp 299–313.

33. Raberg L, Stjernman M: Natural selection on immune responsiveness in blue tits Parus caeruleus, *Evolution Int J Organic Evolution* 57(7):1670–1678, 2003.

34. Andersson MS, Ödeen A, Håstad O: A partly coverable badge signalling avian virus resistance, *Acta Zoologica* 87(1):71–76, 2006.

35. Garamszegi LZ, Møller AP, Erritzoe J: The evolution of immune defense and song complexity in birds, *Evolution Int J Organic Evolution* 57(4):905–912, 2003.

36. Dohms JE, Metz A: Stress—mechanisms of immunosuppression, *Vet Immunol Immunopathol* 30(1):89–109, 1991.

37. Blecha F: Immune system response to stress. In Moberg GP, Bench JA, editors: *The biology of animal stress*, Wallingford, U.K., 2000, CAB International, pp 111–121.

38. Hayashi H, Imai K, Imai K: Characterization of chicken ACTH and alpha-MSH: the primary sequence of chicken ACTH is more similar to Xenopus ACTH than to other avian ACTH, *Gen Comp Endocrinol* 82(3):434–443, 1991.

39. Collie MA, Holmes WN, Cronshaw J: A comparison of the responses of dispersed steroidogenic cells derived from embryonic adrenal tissue from the domestic chicken *(Gallus domesticus)*, the domestic Pekin duck and the wild mallard duck *(Anas platyrhynchos)*, and the domestic muscovy duck *(Cairina moschata)*, *Gen Comp Endocrinol* 88(3):375–387, 1992.

40. Mumma JO, Thaxton JP, Vizzier-Thaxton Y, Dodson WL: Physiological stress in laying hens, *Poult Sci* 85(4):761–769, 2006.

41. Smith EM, Morrill AC, Meyer WJ, 3rd, et al: Corticotropin releasing factor induction of leukocyte-derived immunoreactive ACTH and endorphins, *Nature* 321(6073):881–882, 1986.

42. Mashaly MM, Trout JM, Hendricks GL, 3rd: The endocrine function of the immune cells in the initiation of humoral immunity, *Poult Sci* 72(7):1289–1293, 1993.

43. Dhabhar FS, Miller AH, Stein M, et al: Diurnal and acute stress-induced changes in distribution of peripheral blood leukocyte subpopulations, *Brain behavior Immun* 8(1):66–79, 1994.

44. Schat KA, Skinner MA: Avian immunosuppressive diseases and immune evasion. In Schat KA, Kaspers B, Kaiser P, editors: *Avian immunology*, ed 2, New York, 2014, Academic Press, pp 275–299.

45. Rubolini D, Romano M, Boncoraglio G, et al: Effects of elevated egg corticosterone levels on behavior, growth, and immunity of yellow-legged gull *(Larus michahellis)* chicks, *Hormones Behav* 47(5):592–605, 2005.

46. Hasselquist D, Tobler N, et al: Maternal modulation of offspring immune function in vertebrates. In Demas GE, Nelson RJ, editors: *Ecoimmunology*, New York, 2012, Oxford University Press, pp 165–224.

47. Hayward LS, Wingfield JC: Maternal corticosterone is transferred to avian yolk and may alter offspring growth and adult phenotype, *Gen Comp Endocrinol* 135(3):365–371, 2004.

48. Morosinotto C, Ruuskanen S, Thomson RL, et al: Predation risk affects the levels of maternal immune factors in avian eggs, *J Avian Biol* 44:427–436, 2013.

49. Coslovsky M, Richner H: Predation risk affects offspring growth via maternal effects, *Function Ecol* 25:878–888, 2011.

50. Groothuis TG, Eising CM, Blount JD, et al: Multiple pathways of maternal effects in black-headed gull eggs: constraint and adaptive compensatory adjustment, *J Evol Biol* 19(4):1304–1313, 2006.

51. Lindstrom KM, Hasselquist D, Wikelski M: House sparrows *(Passer domesticus)* adjust their social status position to their physiological costs, *Hormones Behav* 48(3):311–320, 2005.

52. Norris KE, et al: Ecological immunology: life history trade-offs and immune defense in birds, *Behav Ecol* 11(1):19–26, 1999.

53. Nordling DA, Zohari S, Gustafsson L: Reproductive effort reduces specific immune response and parasite resistance, *Proc Biol Sci Royal Soc* 265(1403):1291–1298, 1998.

54. Deerenberg CA, Daan S, Bos N: Reproductive effort decreases antibody responsiveness, *Proc Biol Sci Royal Soc* 264(1384):1021–1029, 1997.

55. Bourgeon S, Criscuolo F, Le Maho Y, et al: Phytohemagglutinin response and immunoglobulin index decrease during incubation fasting in female common eiders, *Physiol Biochem Zool PBZ* 79(4):793–800, 2006.

56. Scott RP, Siopes TD: Evaluation of cell-mediated immunocompetence in mature turkey breeder hens using a dewlap skin test, *Avian Dis* 38(1):161–164, 1994.

57. Verhulst S, Dieleman SJ, Parmentier HK: A tradeoff between immunocompetence and sexual ornamentation in domestic fowl, *Proc Natl Acad Sci U S A* 96(8):4478–4481, 1999.

58. Saino N, Bolzern AM, Møller AP: Immunocompetence, ornamentation, and viability of male barn swallows *(Hirundo rustica)*, *Proc Natl Acad Sci U S A* 94(2):549–552, 1997.

59. Møller AP, Martin-Vivaldi M, Merino S, et al: Density-dependent and geographical variation in bird immune response, *Oikos* 115:463–474, 2006.

60. Hale KA, Briskie JV: Decreased immunocompetence in a severely bottlenecked population of an endemic New Zealand bird, *Anim Conservation* 10(1):2–10, 2007.

61. Gerlach H: Defense mechanisms of the avian host. In Ritchie BW, Harrison GJ, Harrison LR, editors: *Avian medicine: principles and application*, Lake Worth, FL, 1994, Wingers Publishing Inc, pp 109–120.

62. Santos GA, Silversides FG: Utilization of the sex-linked gene for imperfect albinism (S*ALS). 1. Effect of early weight loss on chick metabolism, *Poult Sci* 75(11):1321–1329, 1996.

63. Pardue SL, Ring NM, Smyth JR Jr: Autosomal albinism affects immunocompetence in the chicken, *Dev Comp Immunol* 14(1):105–112, 1990.

64. Owen JCM, et al: Seasonal differences in immunological condition of three species of thrushes, *Condor* 108(2):389–398, 2006.

65. Saino NC, Møller AP: Immunocompetence of nestling barn swallows in relation to brood size and parental effort, *J Anim Ecol* 66(6):827–836, 1997.

66. Blount JD, Houston DC, Møller AP, et al: Do individual branches of immune defence correlate? A comparative case study of scavenging and non-scavenging birds, *Oikos* 102:340–350, 2003.

67. Fellah JS, Jaffredo T, Dunon D: Development of the avian immune system. In Davison FK, Schat KA, editors: *Avian immunology*, New York, 2008, Academic Press, p 61.

68. Bar-Shira E, Cohen I, Elad O, et al: Role of goblet cells and mucin layer in protecting maternal IgA in precocious birds, *Dev Comp Immunol* 44(1):186–194, 2014.

69. Ollé RD: *The glycogen body in neonate birds of the order psittaciformes and its role in neonate mortality [doctoral thesis]*, Giessen, Germany, 2006, Justus-Liebig-Universität Giessen.

70. Schmidt RE: The avian liver in health and disease, *Proc Ass Avian Vet* 273, 1999.

71. Gerlach H: *personal communication*, 2005.

72. Joyner KL, Swanson J, Hanson JT: Psittacine pediatric diagnostics, *Proc Ass Avian Vet* 60–82, 1990.

73. Clubb SL, Schubot RM, Joyner K, et al: Hematologic and serum biochemical reference intervals in juvenile macaws *(Ara sp)*, *J Assoc Avian Vet* 5(3):154–162, 1991.

74. O'Neal DM, Ketterson ED: Life-history evolution, hormones, and avian immune function. In Demas GE, Nelson RJ, editors: *Ecoimmunology*, New York, 2012, Oxford University Press, pp 8–44.

75. Tella JL, Scheuerlein A, Ricklefs RE: Is cell-mediated immunity related to the evolution of life-history strategies in birds? *Proc Biol Sci Royal Soc* 269(1495):1059–1066, 2002.

76. Barnes HJ, Vaillancourt JP, Gross WB: Colibacillosis. In Saif YM, editor: *Diseases of poultry*, ed 11, Ames, IA, 2003, Iowa State Press, pp 636–639.

77. Snyder PW: Diseases of immunity. In McGavin MD, Zachary JF, editors: *Pathologic basis of veterinary disease*, ed 4, St. Louis, MO, 2007, Mosby, pp 193–251.

78. Erf GF: Autoimmune diseases of poultry. In Davison FK, Schat KA, editors: *Avian immunology*, New York, 2008, Academic Press, pp 339–358.

79. Tully TN, Foil CS, et al: Status of intradermal skin testing in avian species, *Proc Ass Avian Vet* 33, 2006.

80. Nett CS, Hodgin EC, Foil CS, et al: A modified biopsy technique to improve histopathological evaluation of avian skin, *Vet Dermatol* 14(3):147–151, 2003.

81. Gerlach H, Kaspers B: *Avian defense mechanisms*, 2005 (unpublished material).

82. Heatley JJ, Oliver JW, Hoosgood G, et al: Serum Corticosterone Concentrations in response to restraint, anesthesia, and skin testing in Hispaniolan Amazon parrots (*Amazona ventralis*), *J Avian Med Surg* 14(3):172–176, 2000.

83. Colombini SF, Hoosgod G, Tully TN: Intradermal skin testing in Hispaniolan parrots (*Amazona ventralis*), *Vet Dermatol* 11(4):271–276, 2008.

84. Nett CS, Hosgood G, Heatley JJ, et al: Evaluation of intravenous fluorescein in intradermal allergy testing in psittacines, *Vet Dermatol* 14(6):323–332, 2003.

85. Schmidt RE, Reavill DR, Phalen DN: *Pathology of pet and aviary birds*, Ames, IA, 2003, Iowa State Press, p 33.

86. Woiciechowsky C: Neurogenic inflammation and the "inflammatory reflex": two pathways of immunoregulation by the nervous system. In Berczi I, editor: *New insights into neuroimmune biology*, Toronto, Canada, 2010, Elsevier, pp 163–176.

87. Pendl H, Speer BL, et al: Immune Mediated disease in avian species: hypersensitivity and autoimmune disease, *Proc Ass Avian Vet* 169–180, 2012.

88. Jones JS, Thomas JS, Bahr A, Phalen DN: Presumed immune-mediated hemolytic anemia in a blue-crowned conure (*Aratinga acuticaudata*), *J Avian Med Surg* 16(3):223–229, 2002.

89. Johnston MS, Son TT, Rosenthal KL: Immune-mediated hemolytic anemia in an eclectus parrot, *J Am Vet Med Assoc* 230(7):1028–1031, 2007.

90. Cihak J, Hoffmann-Fezer G, Wasl M, et al: Inhibition of the development of spontaneous autoimmune thyroiditis in the obese strain (OS) chickens by in vivo treatment with anti-CD4 or anti-CD8 antibodies, *J Autoimmun* 11(2):119–126, 1998.

91. Juan-Salles C, Soto S, Garner MM, et al: Congestive heart failure in 6 African grey parrots (*Psittacus e erithacus*), *Vet Pathol* 48(3):691–697, 2011.

92. Ghaffar A: Immunology. In *Hypersensitivity reactions, University of South Carolina School of Medicine*, 2010. http://pathmicro.med.sc.edu/ghaffar/hyper00.htm. Accessed August 22, 2010.

93. Mahapatro D, Mahapatro RC: Cutaneous basophil hypersensitivity, *Am J Dermatopathol* 6(5):483–489, 1984.

94. Fudge AM, Reavill DR: Pulmonary artery aneurysm and polycythaemia with respiratory hypersensitivity in a blue and gold macaw (*Ara ararauna*), *Proc Europ Conf Avian Med Surg* 382–387, 1993.

95. Taylor M: Polycythaemia in the blue and gold macaw, *Proc 1st Int Conf Zoo Avian Med* 95–104, 1987.

96. Taylor M, Hunter B: A chronic obstructive pulmonary disease of blue and gold macaws, *J Assoc Avian Vet* 5(2):71, 1991.

97. Amann O, Kik MJ, Passon-Vastenburg MH, et al: Chronic pulmonary interstitial fibrosis in a blue-fronted Amazon parrot (*Amazona aestiva aestiva*), *Avian Dis* 51(1):150–153, 2007.

98. Zandvliet MM, Dorrestein GM, Van Der Hage M: Chronic pulmonary interstitial fibrosis in Amazon parrots, *Avian Pathol* 30(5):517–524, 2001.

99. Allen JT, Spiteri MA: Pigeon breeder's disease, *J Lab Clin Med* 127(1):10–12, 1996.

100. Morell F, Villar A, Montero MA, et al: Chronic hypersensitivity pneumonitis in patients diagnosed with idiopathic pulmonary fibrosis: a prospective case-cohort study, *Lancet Respir Med* 1(9):685–694, 2013.

101. Lopez A: Respiratory system. In McGavin MD, Zachary JF, editors: *Pathologic basis of veterinary disease*, ed 4, St. Louis, MO, 2007, Mosby, p 504.

102. Pendl H, Reball H: Hyperchrome Normämien bei Amazonen—hämatologisches Bild. XVI Tagung über Vogelkrankheiten, Deutsche Veterinärmedizinische Gesellschaft, Fachgruppe Geflügelkrankheiten (WVPA); 4.-6.3.2004; Institut für Geflügelkrankheiten der Ludwig-Maximilians-Universität München, 2004. pp 14–24.

103. Graham DM: An update on selected pet virus infections, *Proc Assoc Avian Vet* 267–280, 1984.

104. Hoppes SM, Tizard I, Shivaprasad HL: Avian bornavirus and proventricular dilatation disease: diagnostics, pathology, prevalence, and control, *Vet Clin North Am Exot Anim Pract* 16(2):339–355, 2013.

105. Piepenbring AK, Enderlein D, Herzog S, et al: Pathogenesis of avian bornavirus in experimentally infected cockatiels, *Emerg Infect Dis* 18(2):234–241, 2012.

106. Gray P, Hoppes S, Suchodolski P, et al: Use of avian bornavirus isolates to induce proventricular dilatation disease in conures, *Emerg Infect Dis* 16(3):473–479, 2010.

107. Gancz AY, Kistler AL, Greninger AL, et al: Experimental induction of proventricular dilatation disease in cockatiels (*Nymphicus hollandicus*) inoculated with brain homogenates containing avian bornavirus 4, *Virol J* 6:100, 2009.

108. Lierz M, Piepenbring A, Heffels-Redmann U: Experimental infection of cockatiels with different avian bornavirus genotypes, *Proc Annu Conf Assoc Avian Vet* 9–10, 2012.

109. Mirhosseini N, Gray PL, Hoppes S, et al: Proventricular dilatation disease in cockatiels (*Nymphicus hollandicus*) after infection with a genotype 2 avian bornavirus, *J Avian Med Surg* 25(3):199–204, 2011.

110. Payne S, Shivaprasad HL, Mirhosseini N, et al: Unusual and severe lesions of proventricular dilatation disease in cockatiels (*Nymphicus hollandicus*) acting as healthy carriers of avian bornavirus (ABV) and subsequently infected with a virulent strain of ABV, *Avian Pathol* 40(1):15–22, 2011.

111. Villanueva ID: *Selected studies on avian RNA viruses*, College Station, TX, 2010, Texas A&M University.

112. Stitz L, Bilzer T, Planz O: The immunopathogenesis of borna disease virus infection, *Frontiers Biosci* 7:d541–d555, 2002.

113. Fluck A, Enderlein D, Piepenbring A, et al: Avian bornavirus infection in psittacine birds with neurological signs and feather plucking, *1st Int Conf Avian Herpetol Exot Mammal Med* 388, 2013.

114. Payne SL, Delnatte P, Guo J, et al: Birds and bornaviruses. *Anim Health Res Rev* 13(2):145–156, 2012.

115. Gancz AY, Elbaz D, Farnoushi Y, et al: Clinical recovery from proventricular dilatation disease following treatment with cyclosporine A in an African grey parrot (*Psittacus erithacus*), *Proc 17 DVG Tagung über Vogelkrankheiten Giessen*, Germany, 2012, Deutsche Veterinärmedizinische Gesellschaft (DVG) Service GmbH, pp 130–133.

116. Hoppes SM, Tizard IR, Shivaprasad HL, et al: Treatment of avian bornavirus-infected cockatiels (*Nymphicus hollandicus*) with oral meloxicam and cyclosporine, *Proc Ann Conf Assoc Avian Vet* 27, 2012.

117. Rossi GC, Checcherelli R, Pesaro S: New evidence in PDD pathogenesis: can ganglioside sensitization satisfy Koch's postulates. *Proc Europ Committee Ass Avian Vet* 155, 2009.

118. Pesaro SC, Bertoni P, Ceccherelli R, et al: Anti-ganglioside antibodies production like a theory for PDD's pathogenesis, *Proc Europ Committee Assoc Avian Vet* 89, 2009.

119. Rossi GC, Pesaro S: Parrot proventricular dilatation disease: a possible model of Guillain-Barré syndrome? *Nature Preceedings*, hdl:10101/npre.2008.2590.1, Dec 2, 2008. Accessed August 3, 2014.

120. Rossi G, Enderlein D, Herzog S, et al: *Comparison of anti-ganglioside antibodies and anti-ABV antibodies in psittacines*, 11th European AAV conference, 1st Scientific ECZM Meeting, Madrid, 2011, p 187.

121. Tizard IR, Villanueva I, Gray P, et al: Update on avian borna virus and proventricular dilatation disease, *Proc Austr Assoc Avian Vet* 93–100, 2009.

122. Bader SR, Kothlow S, Trapp S, et al: Acute paretic syndrome in juvenile white leghorn chickens resembles late stages of acute inflammatory demyelinating polyneuropathies in humans, *J Neuroinflamm* 7:7, 2010.

123. Wohlsein P: Pathohistologie der Organsysteme. In Baumgärtner W, editor: *Pathohistologie für die Tiermedizin*, Stuttgart, Germany, 2007, Enke Verlag, pp 174–175.

124. Lumeij JT: Hepatology. In Ritchie BW, Harrison GJ, Harrison LR, editors: *Avian medicine: principles and application*, Lake Worth, FL, 1994, Wingers Publishing Inc. p 536.

125. Beytut E, Ozcan K, Erginsoy S: Immunohistochemical detection of fungal elements in the tissues of goslings with pulmonary and systemic aspergillosis, *Acta veterinaria Hungarica* 52(1):71–84, 2004.

126. Silvano FD, Kanata Y, Takeuchi M, et al: Avian influenza A virus induced stunting syndrome-like disease in chicks, *J Vet Med Sci* 59(3):205–207, 1997.

127. Bano S, Naeem K, Malik SA: Evaluation of pathogenic potential of avian influenza virus serotype H9N2 in chickens, *Avian Dis* 47 (Suppl 3):817–822, 2003.

128. Naeem K, Niazi T, Malik SA, et al: Immunosuppressive potential and pathogenicity of an avian adenovirus isolate involved in hydropericardium syndrome in broilers, *Avian Dis* 39(4):723–728, 1995.

129. Todd D: Avian circovirus diseases: lessons for the study of PMWS, *Vet microbiol* 98(2):169–174, 2004.

130. Shivaprasad HL, Hill D, Todd D, et al: Circovirus infection in a Gouldian finch (*Chloebia gouldiae*), *Avian Pathol* 33(5):525–529, 2004.

131. Todd D, Scott AN, Fringuelli E, et al: Molecular characterization of novel circoviruses from finch and gull, *Avian Pathol* 36(1):75–81, 2007.

132. Eisenberg SW, van Asten AJ, van Ederen AM, et al: Detection of circovirus with a polymerase chain reaction in the ostrich (*Struthio camelus*) on a farm in The Netherlands, *Vet Microbiol* 95(1-2):27–38, 2003.

133. Schoemaker NJ, Dorrestein GM, Latimer KS, et al: Severe leukopenia and liver necrosis in young African grey parrots (*Psittacus erithacus erithacus*) infected with psittacine circovirus, *Avian Dis* 44(2):470–478, 2000.

134. Latimer KS, Steffens WL 3rd, Rakich PM, et al: Cryptosporidiosis in four cockatoos with psittacine beak and feather disease, *J Am Vet Med Assoc* 200(5):707–710, 1992.

135. Abbassi H, Dambrine G, Cherel Y, et al: Interaction of Marek's disease virus and Cryptosporidium baileyi in experimentally infected chickens, *Avian Dis* 44(4):776–789, 2000.

136. Woods LW, Latimer KS, Niagro FD, et al: A retrospective study of circovirus infection in pigeons: nine cases (1986-1993), *J Vet Diag Invest* 6(2):156–164, 1994.

137. Coletti M, Franciosini MP, Asdrubali G, et al: Atrophy of the primary lymphoid organs of meat pigeons in Italy associated with circoviruslike particles in the bursa of Fabricius, *Avian Dis* 44(2):454–459, 2000.

138. Shivaprasad HL, Chin RP, Jeffrey JS, et al: Particles resembling circovirus in the bursa of Fabricius of pigeons, *Avian Dis* 38(3):635–641, 1994.

139. Roy P, Dhillon AS, Lauerman L, et al: Detection of pigeon circovirus by polymerase chain reaction, *Avian Dis* 47(1):218–222, 2003.

140. Sanchez-Cordon PJ, Hervas J, Chacon de Lara F, et al: Reovirus infection in psittacine birds (*Psittacus erithacus*): morphologic and immunohistochemical study, *Avian Dis* 46(2):485–492, 2002.

141. Shawky S, Sandhu T, Shivaprasad HL: Pathogenicity of a low-virulence duck virus enteritis isolate with apparent immunosuppressive ability, *Avian Dis* 44(3):590–599, 2000.

142. Vervelde L, Reemers SS, van Haarlem DA, et al: Chicken dendritic cells are susceptible to highly pathogenic avian influenza viruses which induce strong cytokine responses, *Dev Comp Immunol* 39(3):198–206, 2013.

143. Briggs KT, Gershwin ME, Anderson DW: Consequences of petrochemical ingestion and stress on the immune system of seabirds, *ICES J Marine Sci* 54:718–725, 1997.

144. Briggs KT, Yoshida SH, Gershwin ME: The influence of petrochemicals and stress on the immune system of seabirds, *Regulat Toxicol Pharmacol* 23(2):145–155, 1996.

145. Dietert RR, Piepenbrink MS: Lead and immune function, *Crit Rev Toxicol* 36(4):359–385, 2006.

146. Kendall RJ, Lacher TE, Bunck C, et al: An ecological risk assessment of lead shot exposure in non-waterfowl avian species: upland game birds and raptors, *Environ Toxicol Chem* 15(1):4–20, 1996.

147. Redig PT, Lawler EM, Schwartz S, et al: Effects of chronic exposure to sublethal concentrations of lead acetate on heme synthesis and immune function in red-tailed hawks, *Arch Environ Contam Toxicol* 21(1):72–77, 1991.

148. Gao D, Mondal TK, Lawrence DA: Lead effects on development and function of bone marrow-derived dendritic cells promote Th2 immune responses, *Toxicol Appl Pharmacol* 222(1):69–79, 2007.

149. Corrier DE: Mycotoxicosis: mechanisms of immunosuppression, *Vet Immunol Immunopathol* 30(1):73–87, 1991.

150. Li SJ, Pasmans F, Croubels S, et al: T-2 toxin impairs antifungal activities of chicken macrophages against Aspergillus fumigatus conidia but promotes the pro-inflammatory responses, *Avian Pathol* 42(5):457–463, 2013.

151. Stoev SD: Studies on some feed additives and materials giving partial protection against the suppressive effect of ochratoxin A on egg production of laying hens, *Res Vet Sci* 88(3):486–491, 2010.

152. Kamalavenkatesh P, Vairamuthu S, Balachandran C, et al: Immunopathological effect of the mycotoxins cyclopiazonic acid and T-2 toxin on broiler chicken, *Mycopathologia* 159(2):273–279, 2005.

153. Gibson RM, Bailey CA, Kubena LF, et al: Impact of L-phenylalanine supplementation on the performance of three-week-old broilers fed diets containing ochratoxin A. 1. Effects on body weight, feed conversion, relative organ weight, and mortality, *Poult Sci* 69(3):414–419, 1990.

154. Bailey CA, Gibson RM, Kubena LF, et al: Impact of L-phenylalanine supplementation on the performance of three-week-old broilers fed diets containing ochratoxin A. 2. Effects on hematology and clinical chemistry, *Poult Sci* 69(3):420–425, 1990.

155. Sorenson WG, Simpson J, Castranova V: Toxicity of the mycotoxin patulin for rat alveolar macrophages, *Environ Res* 38(2):407–416, 1985.

156. Sorenson WG, Gerberick GF, Lewis DM, et al: Toxicity of mycotoxins for the rat pulmonary macrophage in vitro, *Environ Health Perspect* 66:45–53, 1986.

157. Wichmann G, Herbarth O, Lehmann I: The mycotoxins citrinin, gliotoxin, and patulin affect interferon-gamma rather than interleukin-4 production in human blood cells, *Environ Toxicol* 17(3):211–218, 2002.

158. Luft P, Oostingh GJ, Gruijthuijsen Y, et al: Patulin influences the expression of Th1/Th2 cytokines by activated peripheral blood mononuclear cells and T cells through depletion of intracellular glutathione, *Environ Toxicol* 23(1):84–95, 2008.

159. Muller A, Lehmann I, Seiffart A, et al: Increased incidence of allergic sensitisation and respiratory diseases due to mould exposure: results of the Leipzig Allergy Risk children Study (LARS), *Int J Hyg Environ Health* 204(5-6):363–365, 2002.

160. Wiley JL, Whittington JK, Wilmes CM, et al: Chronic myelogeneous leukemia in a great horned owl (*Bubo virginianus*), *J Assoc Avian Vet* 23(1):36–43, 2009.

161. Nair V: Tumours of the avian immune system. In Davison FK, Schat KA, editors: *Avian immunology*, New York, 2008, Academic Press, pp 359–372.

162. Demas GE, Zysling DA, Beechler BR, et al: Beyond phytohaemagglutinin: assessing vertebrate immune function across ecological contexts, *J Anim Ecol* 80(4):710–730, 2011.

163. Briscoe JA, Rosenthal KL, Shofer FS: Selected complete blood cell count and plasma protein electrophoresis parameters in pet psittacine birds evaluated for illness, *J Avian Med Surg* 24(2):131–137, 2010.

164. Jones MP, Arheart KL, Cray C: Reference intervals, longitudinal analyses, and index of individuality of commonly measured laboratory variables in captive bald eagles (*Haliaeetus leucocephalus*), *J Avian Med Surg* 28(2):118–126, 2014.

165. Cray C, King E, Rodriguez M, et al: Differences in protein fractions of avian plasma among three commercial electrophoresis systems, *J Avian Med Surg* 25(2):102–110, 2011.

166. Cray C, Reavill D, Romagnano A, et al: Galactomannan assay and plasma protein electrophoresis findings in psittacine birds with aspergillosis, *J Avian Med Surg* 23(2):125–135, 2009.

167. Cray C, Rodriguez M, Zaias J: Protein electrophoresis of psittacine plasma, *Vet Clin Pathol* 36(1):64–72, 2007.

168. Minozzi G, Parmentier HK, Bed'hom B, et al: Delayed-type hypersensitivity response to KLH in F2 and backcrosses of two immune selected chicken lines: effect of immunisation and selection, *Dev Biologicals* 132:267–270, 2008.

169. Minozzi G, Parmentier HK, Mignon-Grasteau S, et al: Correlated effects of selection for immunity in white leghorn chicken lines on natural antibodies and specific antibody responses to KLH and M. butyricum, *BMC Genet* 9:5, 2008.

170. Matson KD, Ricklefs RE, Klasing KC: A hemolysis-hemagglutination assay for characterizing constitutive innate humoral immunity in wild and domestic birds, *Dev Comp Immunol* 29(3):275–286, 2005.

171. Owen-Ashley NT, Turner M, Hahn TP, et al: Hormonal, behavioral, and thermoregulatory responses to bacterial lipopolysaccharide in captive and free-living white-crowned sparrows (*Zonotrichia leucophrys gambelii*), *Hormones Behav* 49(1):15–29, 2006.

172. Owen-Ashley NT, Wingfield JC: Seasonal modulation of sickness behavior in free-living northwestern song sparrows (*Melospiza melodia morphna*), *J Exp Biol* 209(Pt 16):3062–3070, 2006.

173. Dietert RR, Golemboski KA, Austic RE: Environment-immune interactions, *Poult Sci* 73(7):1062–1076, 1994.

174. Olias P, Meyer A, Klopfleisch R, et al: Modulation of the host Th1 immune response in pigeon protozoal encephalitis caused by Sarcocystis calchasi, *Vet Res* 44:10, 2013.

175. Millet S, Bennett J, Lee KA, et al: Quantifying and comparing constitutive immunity across avian species, *Dev Comp Immunol* 31(2):188–201, 2007.

176. Vinkler M S J, Munclingera P, Albrechta T: Phytohaemagglutinin skin-swelling test in scarlet rosefinch males: low-quality birds respond more strongly, *Anim Behav* 83(1):17–23, 2012.

177. Redig PT, Dunnette JL, Sivanandan V: Use of whole blood lymphocyte stimulation test for immunocompetency studies in bald eagles, red-tailed hawks, and great horned owls, *Am J Vet Res* 45(11):2342–2346, 1984.

178. Smits JE, Bortolotti GR, Tella JL: Simplifying the phytohaemagglutinin skin-testing technique in studies of avian immunocompetence, *Funct Ecol* 13:567–572, 1999.

179. Collette JC, Millam JR, Klasing KC, et al: Neonatal handling of Amazon parrots alters the stress response and immune function, *Appl Anim Behav Sci* 66(4):335–349, 2000.

180. Hilton LS, Bean AG, Lowenthal JW: The emerging role of avian cytokines as immunotherapeutics and vaccine adjuvants, *Vet Immunol Immunopathol* 85(3–4):119–128, 2002.

181. Lowenthal JW, O'Neil TE, David A, et al: Cytokine therapy: a natural alternative for disease control, *Vet Immunol Immunopathol* 72(1–2):183–188, 1999.

182. Asif M, Jenkins KA, Hilton LS, et al: Cytokines as adjuvants for avian vaccines, *Immunol Cell Biol* 82(6):638–643, 2004.

183. Clark JD, Oakes RD, Redhead K, et al: Eimeria species parasites as novel vaccine delivery vectors: anti-Campylobacter jejuni protective immunity induced by Eimeria tenella-delivered CjaA, *Vaccine* 30(16):2683–2688, 2012.

184. Vergara-Alert J, Fernandez-Bellon H, Busquets N, et al: Comprehensive serological analysis of two successive heterologous vaccines against H5N1 avian influenza virus in exotic birds in zoos, *Clin Vaccine Immunol* 18(5):697–706, 2011.

185. Lierz M, Hafez HM, Klopfleisch R, et al: Protection and virus shedding of falcons vaccinated against highly pathogenic avian influenza A virus (H5N1), *Emerg Infect Dis* 13(11):1667–1674, 2007.

186. Lloyd C, Wernery U: Humoral response of hybrid falcons inoculated with inactivated paramyxovirus-1 vaccine, *J Avian Med Surg* 22(3):213–217, 2008.

187. Angenvoort J, Fischer D, Fast C, et al: Limited efficacy of West Nile virus vaccines in large falcons (*Falco* spp.), *Vet Res* 45:41, 2014.

188. Bonne N, Shearer P, Sharp M, et al: Assessment of recombinant beak and feather disease virus capsid protein as a vaccine for psittacine beak and feather disease, *J Gen Virol* 90(Pt 3):640–647, 2009.

189. Duvenage L, Hitzeroth II, Meyers AE, et al: Expression in tobacco and purification of beak and feather disease virus capsid protein fused to elastin-like polypeptides, *J Virol Methods* 191(1):55–62, 2013.

190. Harkinezhad T, Schauttet K, Vanrompay D: Protection of budgerigars (*Melopsittacus undulatus*) against Chlamydophila psittaci challenge by DNA vaccination, *Vet Res* 40(6):61, 2009.

191. Redig PT, Tully TN, Ritchie BW, et al: Effect of West Nile virus DNA-plasmid vaccination on response to live virus challenge in red-tailed hawks (*Buteo jamaicensis*), *Am J Vet Res* 72(8):1065–1070, 2011.

192. Escribano-Romero E, Gamino V, Merino-Ramos T, et al: Protection of red-legged partridges (*Alectoris rufa*) against West Nile virus (WNV) infection after immunization with WNV recombinant envelope protein E (rE), *Vaccine* 31(41):4523–4527, 2013.

193. Young JA, Jefferies W: Towards the conservation of endangered avian species: a recombinant West Nile Virus vaccine results in increased humoral and cellular immune responses in Japanese Quail (*Coturnix japonica*), *PloS One* 8(6):e67137, 2013.

194. Davis MR, Langan JN, Johnson YJ, et al: West Nile virus seroconversion in penguins after vaccination with a killed virus vaccine or a DNA vaccine, *J Zoo Wildl Med* 39(4):582–589, 2008.

195. Guo P, Thomas JD, Bruce MP, et al: The chicken TH1 response: potential therapeutic applications of ChIFN-gamma, *Dev Comp Immunol* 41(3):389–396, 2013.

196. Rahman MM, Eo SK: Prospects and challenges of using chicken cytokines in disease prevention, *Vaccine* 30(50):7165–7173, 2012.

197. Lowenthal JW, York JJ, O'Neil TE, et al: Potential use of cytokine therapy in poultry, *Vet Immunol Immunopathol* 63(1–2):191–198, 1998.

198. Lowenthal JW, Lambrecht B, van den Berg TP, et al: Avian cytokines—the natural approach to therapeutics, *Dev Comp Immunol* 24(2–3):355–365, 2000.

199. Su BS, Shen PC, Hung LH, et al: Potentiation of cell-mediated immune responses against recombinant HN protein of Newcastle disease virus by recombinant chicken IL-18, *Vet Immunol Immunopathol* 141(3–4):283–292, 2011.

200. Fernandez-Varon E, Villamayor L: Granulocyte and granulocyte macrophage colony-stimulating factors as therapy in human and veterinary medicine, *Vet J* 174(1):33–41, 2007.

201. Safdar A: Immunotherapy for invasive mold disease in severely immunosuppressed patients, *Clin Infect Dis* 57(1):94–100, 2013.

202. Rosenthal KL: Filgrastim treatment in a circovirus-positive young African grey parrot, *personal communication*, 1994.

203. Kaiser P, Sonnemans D, Smith LM: Avian IFN-gamma genes: sequence analysis suggests probable cross-species reactivity among galliforms, *J Interferon Cytokine Res* 18(9):711–719, 1998.

204. Fringuelli E, Urbanelli L, Tharuni O, et al: Cloning and expression of pigeon IFN-gamma gene, *Res Vet Sci* 89(3):367–372, 2010.

205. Huang A, Scougall CA, Lowenthal JW, et al: Structural and functional homology between duck and chicken interferon-gamma, *Dev Comp Immunol* 25(1):55–68, 2001.

206. Stanford M: Interferon treatment of circovirus infection in grey parrots *(Psittacus erithacus)*, *Vet Rec* 154(14):435–436, 2004.

207. Dan WB, Guan ZB, Zhang C, et al: Molecular cloning, in vitro expression and bioactivity of goose B-cell activating factor, *Vet Immunol Immunopathol* 118(1–2):113–120, 2007.

208. Mullbacher A, Lobigs M: Creation of killer poxvirus could have been predicted, *J Virol* 75(18):8353–8355, 2001.

209. Ganapathy K, Bradbury JM: Effects of cyclosporin A on the immune responses and pathogenesis of a virulent strain of Mycoplasma gallisepticum in chickens, *Avian Pathol* 32(5):495–502, 2003.

210. Rott R, Herzog S, Richt J, et al: Immune-mediated pathogenesis of borna disease, *Med Microbiol Infect Dis Virol Parasitol* 270(1–2):295–301, 1988.

211. Hallensleben W, Schwemmle M, Hausmann J, et al: Borna disease virus-induced neurological disorder in mice: infection of neonates results in immunopathology, *J Virol* 72(5):4379–4386, 1998.

212. Stitz L, Soeder D, Deschl U, et al: Inhibition of immune-mediated meningoencephalitis in persistently borna disease virus-infected rats by cyclosporine A, *J Immunol* 143(12):4250–4256, 1989.

213. Naesens M, Kuypers DR, Sarwal M: Calcineurin inhibitor nephrotoxicity, *Clin J Am Soc Nephrol* 4(2):481–508, 2009.

214. Prud'homme GJ, Parfrey NA, Vanier LE: Cyclosporine-induced autoimmunity and immune hyperreactivity, *Autoimmunity* 9(4):345–356, 1991.

215. Fite KV, Pardue S, Bengston L, et al: Effects of cyclosporine in spontaneous, posterior uveitis, *Curr Eye Res* 5(10):787–796, 1986.

216. Whittlow GC, editor: *Sturkie's avian physiology*, ed 5, San Diego, CA, 2000, Academic Press.

CHAPTER 12

Reproduction

Michael Lierz • Olivia A. Petritz • Jaime Samour

ADVANCEMENTS IN METHODS FOR IMPROVING REPRODUCTIVE SUCCESS

Michael Lierz

Birds are bred in captivity for various reasons. Owners' desire to have the offspring of their own pet or aviary birds, commercial interests for production of offspring for the pet trade, and conservation efforts for endangered species are the most common indications. Different approaches to attain successful reproduction may be required, in part dependent on the specifics of what ultimate outcome is desired and what problems in goal attainment may be present. Most bird species reproduce in bonded pairs or groups, which necessitates a strategy to include control of both sexes. This represents usually the first and main problem if owners are aiming to produce offspring from a single kept pet bird. In typical pet mammals, a relatively short amount of appropriately timed male–female contact is required for successful reproduction. Birds, however, require considerably more general and species-specific display behaviors between the sexes, and stimulation of the female by the male is usually required. In commercial breeding setups, the aviculturist often works to maximize the number of offspring per species to increase commercial success. This might lead to pairing of different subspecies if matching partners are not available or for the purpose of producing color mutations or even cross-species hybrids. In breeding efforts for the purpose of species conservation, usually rare species are maintained, so adequate or ideal partners are not regularly available, and pairing of different subspecies is not recommended. Common problems in endangered species breeding programs include surplus animals of one sex, partner incompatibility issues, and infertility. Because breeding birds are usually rare in those programs, replacement of such birds is usually difficult.

With domestic mammals, veterinarians are often requested to help with increasing reproductive success, but this same request is rarely the case in birds. Most often, breeders try to solve problems on their own, and pair or re-pair birds. A detailed analysis of the reasons for reproductive failure is usually not performed. Veterinary examination and evaluation methods can play a vital role in increasing reproductive success and should be included in the process.

EVALUATION OF BREEDING FITNESS

Evaluation of Breeding Setups

Usually the veterinarian is consulted when reproduction success is not as high as expected or desired by the breeder. As a first step, the veterinarian needs to investigate the complete breeding facility and its management.[1] First of all, the species being bred and their biologic needs must be considered. Management failures, even by experienced breeders, are the most common reason for reproductive failure. These managerial problems include deficits in breeding group setups, including, but not limited to, male-to-female ratios, contact or no contact with conspecifics, permanent or temporary pairings, and other variables. In addition, details about food supply, in particular food quality, quantity, and feeding intervals, are important. The enclosure, nest construction, enclosure furniture, and so on might be key factors. Depending on the taxonomic details, more ethologic sources of information should be consulted.[2]

Evaluation of Systemic Health of Breeding Birds

As the second step, the breeding birds must be examined. Are the birds already sexually mature? This should be followed by a general physical examination of the birds. Hematology and blood chemistry should be done. In cases of questionable nutritional status, assessment of blood vitamin levels may be helpful. Inadequate vitamin E, selenium, vitamins B_1 and B_{12} are common reasons for decrease in reproductive success.[2] Common infectious disease agents should be screened for. Depending on susceptibility and prevalence or risk factors, some common pathogens that may be screened include, but are not limited to, circovirus and polyomavirus (psittacines), *Chlamydia* spp. (all), *Salmonella* spp. (all), herpesvirus (e.g., psittacines, falcons, cranes, storks), which are known to affect the reproductive success of their respective species hosts. In all cases, repeated parasite control measures are required. This list is far from being complete, and the reader is directed to more specific literature according to the taxa of concern.

These steps are followed by a complete evaluation of the reproductive health of the birds. A detailed examination of the reproductive tract includes complete endoscopic evaluation of the gonads, oviduct, or deferent duct. Here, the anatomic normal appearance must be monitored and assessed, identifying all necessary structures. In females, in addition to inspection of the ovary, the oviduct and, more importantly, the supporting ligament crossing the cranial division of the kidney must be seen to ensure that eggs can be laid and females are not anatomically rendered sterile. The same applies for the assessment for a complete and uninterrupted deferent duct in males, which should be followed from the epididymis to the cloaca (see section on Endosurgical Methods for Reducing Reproductive Success). In case of abnormal findings, in particular in the gonads, biopsy specimens should be taken for further investigation. If the bird is considered systemically and anatomically healthy, a more detailed examination of reproductive functionality should be done. Females that have previously laid eggs have established the potential to successfully produce eggs and, therefore, offspring. Those hens that have not laid eggs, however, may not necessarily do so. Behavioral observation and assessments should help clarify if pairing and display behaviors seem to be normal or altered. In male birds, this assessment is far more difficult because the male display is more difficult to judge, especially if the male seems to demonstrate successful copulation behavior. However, in suspect males, the veterinarian has the option of investigating semen quality to evaluate if infertile eggs occur because of male infertility or other reasons.

Semen Collection

For semen analysis and evaluation of male fertility, semen must first be collected. Considering the high diversity of avian species, this is one of the most problematic tasks. Semen collection in birds was first described in 1935[3] and is mainly used in poultry, in particular turkeys,[4] as a routine technique. It is also well described in birds of prey,[2] cranes,[5] pigeons,[6] and passerines,[7] as well as in a few other species. Usually, semen collection is accomplished by using a massage technique (Figures 12-1 and 12-2), or trained birds may provide semen voluntarily, particularly in the case of falcons.[2] The success of those techniques is dependent on the species, and semen collection methods have not been described for many

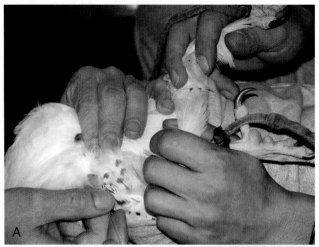
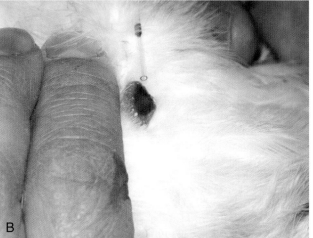

FIGURE 12-2 **A** and **B**, Massage technique for semen collection in a falcon. Here, the back is not massaged, only pressure is applied on the abdominal wall and semen collected directly in a capillary tube. (Photo courtesy Falcon Center, Helvesiek, Germany.)

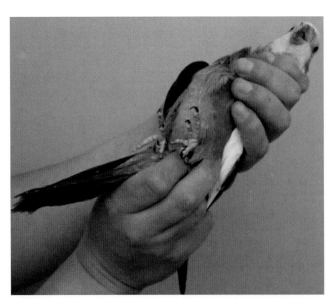

FIGURE 12-1 Massage technique for semen collection in a cockatiel. Massaging the back seems to be important.

species. Even within one taxon, the success rate of semen collection varies. In small psittacine species, successful semen collection by using the massage method has been described.[8-12] In a more recently described technique in the cockatiel (*Nymphicus hollandicus*), the thumb and forefinger are positioned lateral to the cloaca, and the middle finger massages the synsacrum of the bird[8] (see Figure 12-1).

Semen collection in larger psittacine species by using a massage technique has been described anecdotally,[13-17] but this method has never been described as being successful in a larger set of different species or individuals. The recent development of a novel semen collection method based on electrostimulation has led to successful semen collection in 109 different species or subspecies of large psittacines,[18] including highly endangered species such as Spix's macaw (*Cyanopsitta spixii*) or the St. Vincent amazon (*Amazona guildingii*). The technique is based on the use of a bipolar probe that is inserted into the cloaca of the male. The size of the probe is appropriate to the birds' size (Figure 12-3), and it is ensured that the probe has full contact with the mucosa of the cloaca. The technique is used in nonanesthetized birds,

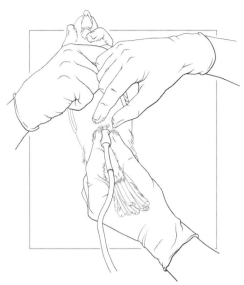

FIGURE 12-3 The bird is ideally held by an assistant, who restrains the bird by holding the head and wings gently. The bird is in dorsal recumbency, with the head up, legs pulled cranially, and the complete body lifted so that the person collecting semen has the cloaca at shoulder height. (Drawing courtesy Ankat Hermanns, http://www.ankatsart.com/.)

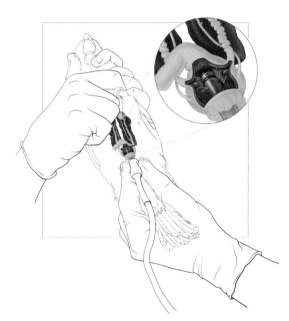

FIGURE 12-4 Placement of the electric probe within the cloaca of the male. The current stimulates muscle contraction and ejaculation of the semen. (Drawing courtesy Ankat Hermanns, http://www.ankatsart.com/.)

immediately after they have been restrained and placed in dorsal recumbency. The probe is then passed into the urodeum (Figure 12-4). It must be ensured that the probe is not inserted into the rectum to reduce the risk of fecal contamination of the semen sample. An electric current (varying between 1 and 14 volts [V]) is applied in 1- to 2-second intervals (interrupted by 2- to 5-second breaks), with the voltage increased after every interval. When contractions of the cloaca

and the muscles of the tail are observed, ejaculation has occurred and the procedure is terminated. Semen, after being gently massaged out of the cloaca, is either collected indirectly by using a capillary tube or is directly collected by using a capillary tube that is inserted into a channel of the probe (Figures 12-5 and 12-6). The required voltage and number of intervals varies between species and should be adjusted according to experience.[18,19] No more than 10 intervals should be applied. In total, the complete procedure requires approximately 3 to 5 minutes. This technique has been proven to be successful in a large amount of different species,[18] including highly endangered species such as Spix's Macaw[18,19] and the St. Vincent amazon[20] and also in nonpsittacine species such as the sharp-tailed grouse.[21] The quality of semen collected by methods based on electrostimulation may be adversely affected by the current, reducing fertility. Studies evaluating the specific effects of electrostimulation on avian semen quality are lacking. Lierz et al[18] were able to clearly demonstrate that semen collected by this technique could fertilize eggs after the females had been artificially inseminated with such semen. At present time, there seems to be no other options for collecting semen from large psittacine species.

As described above, studies on success rates of different semen collection techniques and their influence on semen parameters are uncommon. Bublat et al[22] investigated the success rate of the electrostimulation method and the variation of semen parameters in large psittacines in an entire year. Amazons and macaws were shown to be seasonal, and semen production ceased during September to November. In cockatoos and Eclectus parrots, the success rate also varied during the year, but semen was available from males in those groups

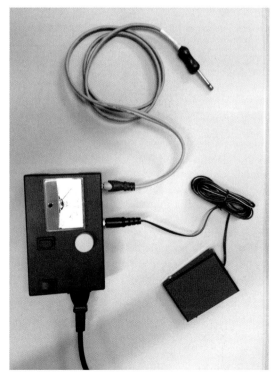

FIGURE 12-5 Electrostimulation device for semen collection in psittacines, according to Lierz et al.[18]

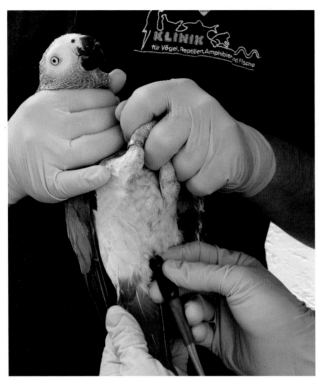

FIGURE 12-6 Correct restraint of a Grey parrot for semen collection using an electrostimulation device.

during the entire year, and a strict seasonality was not observable. In that study, it was shown that individual Amazon males stopped semen production shortly after their female partner completed clutching. Semen quality parameters were not significantly affected during the year. In case semen is provided, the quality is more or less constant in the individual male.[22] This information is important when evaluating the semen quality of individual males, as it seems that those parameters are not significantly influenced by the time point of semen collection for the most part. It remains unclear if and how sexual stimulation prior to semen collection has an influence on semen quality. Bublat et al[22] demonstrated only minor differences in the semen collection success rate of singly kept large psittacine males and paired males. Semen quality between those groups did not vary significantly. The authors also demonstrated that semen collection was always successful in paired males that fathered offspring, whereas failures of semen collection occurred only in males that were paired with hens laying infertile eggs and in single unpaired males. Further work is needed to investigate the influence of reproductive stimulation of the male on semen production and quality with respect to the different species and taxonomic groups of birds. It is fair to assume that the findings from one taxonomic or specifically managed group cannot be extended to another. Even more important, findings from one species might not be extended to another species. Individual species' ethology, natural biology, and geographic origin seem to be major factors influencing semen donation and semen parameters.

The veterinarian collecting semen to evaluate the fertility of males should consider that even in fertile males, individual semen collection attempts can be unsuccessful. Therefore, the failure to collect semen should not result in assessing such a male infertile. The male might not be stimulated, might be out of season, or might have just recently ejaculated (copulation with hen, masturbation), making semen not available at the time of the collection attempt. After repeated collection failures, further diagnostics should be applied.[23] In those cases and in situations where very poor semen quality or an increased amount of morphologically altered spermatozoa are seen, endoscopic testicular biopsy should be considered.

Semen Evaluation

Semen evaluation of breeding males cannot be overestimated. It allows a more detailed examination of the reasons for infertile clutches and for males to be rated according to their semen quality. Infertile males can be identified and removed from the breeding flock, thereby preventing pair bonding of valuable females in pairings less likely to succeed. These infertile males might be used as stimulation partners to help encourage females to lay, and then those females can be artificially inseminated (see below). Semen evaluation is also important when case-assisted reproduction techniques such as artificial insemination are considered. In artificial insemination, only semen of good quality should be used. Semen of excellent quality and volume can also be divided, resulting in more samples for multiple inseminations.[18]

Generally, semen evaluation in birds is comparable with those described techniques in humans and mammals.[24-26] The amount of semen collected is very low compared with mammals, making complete evaluation of all parameters challenging. In such cases, semen can be diluted with 1% glucose solution, but the results must then be calculated according to the dilution used. General evaluation parameters are spermatozoa concentration, volume, total number of spermatozoa, color, consistency, pH, and contaminations (by feces, urine, blood).[19,27] Motility parameters (e.g., total motility, progressive motility) and the live-to-dead ratio of spermatozoa (vitality) are the most important parameters. A first evaluation of sperm density and motility is done in the capillary tube used to collect the semen ($\times$100 magnification). If scaled capillary tubes are used, the volume can also be measured immediately. A drop of semen is placed on commercial indicator paper to assess pH. This is followed by a more detailed microscopic examination on a prewarmed slide (36° C, $\times$400 magnification), where motility is assessed within five fields of view. Concentration and total sperm count can be assessed by using a Neubauer's counting chamber. Eosin-B stains (2%) seem to be sufficient to detect the live-to-dead ratio and color dead spermatozoa red and leaving live ones unstained (Figure 12-7). SYBR green stains (Figure 12-8) seem to be very effective in raptors and psittacines, but experience in many other non-domestic bird species is limited. The morphology of the spermatozoa needs to be evaluated with special attention to abnormally formed structures. Modern techniques include computer-assisted semen analysis (CASA), which provides additional information[28-30] (e.g., viscosity, single spermatozoa movements), but this sophisticated equipment is less commonly available in a typical practice setting. In certain cases where the basic parameters are insufficient to achieve the required result and adequately explain reproductive failure or in situations with very valuable single males, such techniques should be employed. Using CASA requires that the software be adapted to the species to be examined, as spermatozoa size and other factors differ.[30] In some species such as raptors,

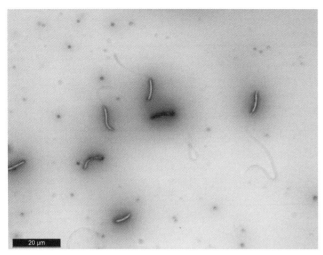

FIGURE 12-7 Eosin red staining of psittacine semen. Dead spermatozoa stain red, and live are unstained.

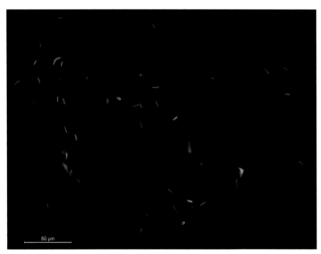

FIGURE 12-8 SYBR green stain of psittacine semen: dead spermatozoa stain red, whereas live stain green.

CASA has limitations. Semen structures (e.g., round bodies) interfere with the system and are incorrectly calculated,[27] whereas in other taxonomic groups, CASA seems to work well.[30,31] Usually, there is a good correlation between semen values (spermatozoa concentration, progressive motility) and fertility. Figure 12-9 shows an example of an examination sheet for avian semen for orientation.

However, semen evaluated as good might still be unable to fertilize eggs. In such cases, spermatozoa functionality tests are performed. In nonpoultry avian species, these types of tests have only recently been established. One of those tests is the perivitelline membrane penetration test.[32] The inner perivitelline membrane of a fresh infertile egg is separated and incubated with a semen sample to be examined. Following the allocated period, the membrane is then stained and evaluated microscopically. Identification of holes in the membrane indicates that the spermatozoa were able to penetrate it, which is a basic requirement for fertilization (Figure 12-10). This works well if the membrane and the tested semen originate from the same species. Cross-species testing may fail. Cockatiel semen

could not be tested with chicken perivitelline membrane, compared with falcon semen, which showed minor success.[32] Therefore, this test is limited at present, and an evaluation should be done first to determine which species can serve as a membrane donor for the semen to be tested. Spermatozoa can be examined using electron microscopy, which might demonstrate in which part of the spermatozoa the alteration is located (Figure 12-11).

In many species, apart from poultry, reference values are rarely published. Therefore, estimations and evaluations should be based on closely related species. However, large differences in semen parameters have even been detected within one taxonomic group, potentially related to the different breeding behaviors of the individual species.[18] As an example, macaws showed an average spermatozoa concentration of 70,068/μL compared to Eclectus parrots having an average of 3,781,285 spermatozoa/μL. Eclectus females copulate with several males at the same time, so sperm competition to fertilize an egg is very high. Therefore the evolutionary pressure on each male to have a high amount of spermatozoa in the semen is high, resulting in increased chances to successfully father offspring. Macaws, being strictly monogamous, do not have this pressure, and males with lower spermatozoa concentrations and quality will be able to father offspring in a viable pair bonded setting.[18] Table 12-1 provides a short overview of some published semen parameters for orientation. The table is far from being complete and should be used as a guideline. In recent years, more and more semen values are being published, and the reader should screen the literature when looking for semen parameters of specific species.

Artificial Insemination

Artificial insemination has been successfully performed in several different avian species and is becoming an increasingly used tool in reproductive management with the advent of improved availability of semen. The most recent successful progress has been made in psittacines. As semen was available in small psittacines for some time, successful inseminations were consequently described for a few small psittacine species or single cases.[8,14,33,34] As semen from large parrots has only recently more routinely become available, successful inseminations and the production of offspring in those groups are the latest and more dramatic developments. Confirmed by paternity testing, Lierz et al[18] described the first offspring in a macaw (*Ara chloropterus*) as well as *Pionopsitta pileata*, *Cacatua haematuropygia*, and species of Psittaculinae by assisted reproduction techniques. These successful procedures were then applied to highly endangered species such as the St. Vincent amazon[20] and the Spix's macaw.[19]

Usually, artificial insemination is requested if breeding pairs produce infertile eggs or if single females are laying eggs. In species conservation breeding efforts, artificial insemination is also considered as a means to manage genetic diversity, especially when only a limited amount of breeding birds are available. Genetic representation of previously underrepresented genetically valuable males can be expedited, as semen of such a male can be inseminated into several females at the same time, whereas in natural pair settings only one female may produce offspring of this particular male. Additionally, single housed, or imprinted, aggressive or injured males which are not able to copulate naturally can

---

Spermatological examination

	Time:

Species: _____   Date: _____
Identification: _____   Temperature: _____
General condition: _____   Sample-Nr.: _____
Nutrition status: _____   Miscellaneous: _____

Pre-Exam

Volume: _____ µl   Contamination: O Erythrocytes O Uric acid O Feces

Color: _____   Consistency: O Creamy O Wheylike O Milky
                                        O Watery

Examination Capillary
	Time:

Amount sperm: Motility: Distribution:
O -   O 0   O Single
O (+)   O 1   O Front (wax)
O +   O 2   O Rear (FAB)   pH: _____
O ++   O 3
O +++   O 4   Occupancy of FAB: _____ %
O ++++

Motility
	Time:

Semen volume: _____ µl   Diluter: _____
Dilution: 1 : _____

Field of view 1:   T _____   P _____   L _____   C _____
Field of view 2:   T _____   P _____   L _____   C _____
Field of view 3:   T _____   P _____   L _____   C _____
Field of view 4:   T _____   P _____   L _____   C _____
Field of view 5:   T _____   P _____   L _____   C _____
Total: **P** _____   **L** _____   **C** _____

T _____   **P+L+C =** _____   **Motility =** _____ %
                                    $(P+L+C)/T \times 100$

Live/Dead-Stain
	Time:

Live _____ %   Dead _____ %

Density

Dilution: 1 : _____   Dilution factor: _____

Spermatozoa   **Spermatozoa concentration [c]:**
Field of view 1: _____ $n \times \text{Dilution factor} / 0.02 =$ _____ [c] in n/µl
Field of view 2: _____   _____ x _____ / 0.02 = _____ / µl
Field of view 3: _____
Field of view 4: _____   **Total number spermatozoa [N]:**
Field of view 5: _____   [c] x x Semen volume = [N]
Total: _____ (=n)   _____ / µl x _____ µl = _____

Remarks
_____
_____

FAB, Fluid-air-border; P, progressive-motility; L, local motility; C, circle motility; T, total.

FIGURE 12-9 Example of an evaluation sheet for semen analysis, used in the Clinic for Birds, Reptiles, Amphibians and Fish, Justus-Liebig-University of Giessen, Germany.

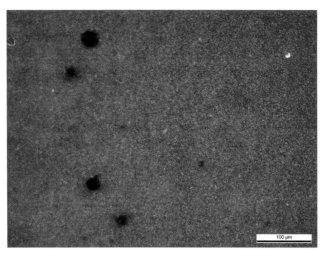

FIGURE 12-10 Stained perivitelline membrane after incubation with semen; penetration holes are clearly visible. (Photo courtesy J. Krohn and A. Wehrend.)

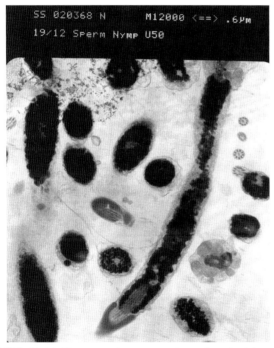

FIGURE 12-11 Electron microscopy view of cockatiel semen. (Courtesy M. Bergmann and H. Schneider.)

potentially father offspring through artificial insemination methods, thereby including their genetics in the breeding pool.[20] However, even surplus females of conservation breeding project can now be included, pairing those females with males of a different but related species which has been sterilized (see the section on Endosurgical Methods for Reducing Reproductive Success). This allows for that hen to be inseminated with semen of its own species. In some species, surplus females can be human-imprinted to stimulate them to lay eggs and inseminate them. This technique is routinely used in falcons and other birds of prey[2] and may be considered for other taxa as well. However, it must be ensured that

imprinted females lay and that those females are capable of raising their offspring naturally, to have nonimprinted offspring for further breeding or release. In raptors, this works very well.

Before artificial insemination is employed in a breeding flock, a complete assessment of the circumstances, in particular, reasons for the production of infertile eggs, is required. It is important to adequately judge if the inclusion of assisted reproduction techniques offers viable potential to overcome the specific problem. First of all, eggs need to be laid before artificial insemination is employed, which seems not clear to some breeders. Second, semen of sufficient quality needs to be available at a specific time point. This time point may be very short, as the potential time span for insemination to fertilize an egg is very short (see below). Therefore, semen donors should be nearby, and ideally more than one potential semen donor should be available in case semen collection in one male fails when semen is needed. In many avian species, fresh semen is used for artificial insemination, but preservation of semen for longer times would be incredibly helpful (see below).

The insemination of females does represent a stressful event, as the birds need to be caught and restrained. Therefore, the number of insemination procedures should be kept to a minimum. Alternatively, birds should be trained or, in some species such as raptors, human-imprinted, so inseminations are well tolerated. It is always discussed that such an intervention interrupts to a varying degree the breeding cycle of the female and therefore is contraindicated. This, however, is not the case in trained or imprinted birds—so inseminations can be performed at any time during the reproductive cycle. In nontrained birds, often the case in several conservation projects, particularly Psittacines, the first egg should be laid before insemination is started. This approach usually does not lead to an interruption of further oviposition and completion of a clutch. In species that lay only one egg, insemination must be started approximately 5 days prior to oviposition, which, in turn, can result in cessation of lay as a result of disturbance of the hen in the process.

The timing of each insemination is very important. The ovulated ovum has only a limited time span when it is able to merge with spermatozoa because once the egg-white and membranes are produced in the oviduct, spermatozoa are not able to penetrate into the germ cell. This means that the spermatozoa should be already in the infundibulum once the ovum is ovulated. However, spermatozoa have only a limited lifespan in the female reproductive tract. This lifespan varies among the different species and may reach several days, as sperm storage in the female reproductive tract is common in avian species. The particular duration of spermatozoal life expectancy in the female reproductive tract is unknown in most nondomestic species, whereas in domestic species such as chickens, turkey, quails, and ducks it may reach 2 to 15 weeks, according to the species.[35] As a general rule, the first insemination should be done daily from 3 to 5 days before the first egg of a clutch is expected. This time frame is judged by behavior, the presence of abdominal distension and previous records of laying dates, as many birds lay around the same time each year. Following inseminations are performed immediately (up to 5 hours) after the next egg is laid. In nontrained or nonimprinted females, inseminations should start

TABLE 12-1

Selected Spermatologic Values of Fresh Semen from Different Avian Species

Species	Number of Birds [n]	Volume [µl]	Sperm Concentration [n/µl]	Total Sperm Count [n/ejaculate]	pH	Osmolality [mOsm/kg]	Total Motility [%]
Northern pintail (Anas acuta)	20	66.0 ± 14.1	5,700,000 ± 4,300,000	Not specified	8.5 ± 0.1	275 ± 8.2	57.4 ± 6.1
Quaker parakeet (Myiopsitta monachus)	8	1.96 ± 0.26 (0.5–4.8)	346,600 ± 64,600 (4000–688,000)	0.71 ± 0.16 (×10'6) (<0.1–2.8)	8.05–8.5	Not specified	Not specified
Cockatoos	21	12.4 (1.8–54)	427,704 (850–4,500,000)	5,183,354 (10,540–69,300,000)	Not specified	Not specified	77.9 (40–5)
Macaws	6	7.4 (3–19.5)	70,068 (27,500–150,000)	435,750 (41,300–806,664)	Not specified	Not specified	75.8 (70–85)
Amazons	11	8.5 (12.8–18.4)	77,532 (8750–231,000)	675,050 (101,050–2,263,800)	Not specified	Not specified	80 (all 80)
Eclectus ssp./ Tanygnathus sp. Lories	26	11.4 (1–29)	3,781,285 (187,000–16,000,000)	35,828,804 (550,000–157,200,000)	Not specified	Not specified	87.3 (60–95)
	12	6.3 (1.3–2.6)	1,534,965 (29,583–5,050,000)	9,806,674 (82 823–41,265,000)	Not specified	Not specified	86.8 (70–95)
Cockatiels (Nymphicus hollandicus)	30	3.15 ± 3.07 (0.1–19.4)	872,325 (30,000–5,950,000)	Not specified	7.42 ± 0.42 (6.4–8.0)	298.62 ± 9.56 (290–320)	77.31 ± 7.01 (67.32–90.16)
Cockatiels (conventional)	15	Not specified	305,300	Not specified	Not specified	Not specified	55
Cockatiels (CASA)	9	Not specified	241,800	Not specified	Not specified	Not specified	50.89 ± 18.06 (6.66–100)
Spix's Macaw (Cyanopsitta spixii)	13	6.9 ± 5.9 (0.5–22.2)	24,857 ± 23,509 (500–97,500)	183,429 ± 238,366 (7,500–877,500)	7.4 ± 0.4 (6.4–8)	Not specified	29 ± 11 (5–42)
St. Vincent Amazon (Amazona guildingii)		5.9 (0.1–62)	21,252 (100–110,500)	Not specified	Not specified	Not specified	Not specified
Budgerigar (Melopsittacus undulatus)	10	5.4 ± 1.2	3,723,300 ± 92,900	Not specified	Not specified	Not specified	68.7 ± 8.9
Rosy-faced lovebird (Agapornis roseicollis)	34	1.6 ± 0.6	7,194,000 ± 6,735,100	Not specified	Not specified	Not specified	48.4 ± 28.1
Large falcons	115	72.4 ± 40.64 (2–222)	73,500 ± 40,520	5,260,000 ± 4,999,000	6.4–8	Not specified	Not specified
Domestic fowl (Ross broiler)	15	Not specified	6,600,000 ± 530,000	Not specified	Not specified	Not specified	78 ± 1.7
Indian white-backed vulture (Gyps bengalensis)	4	340 ± 260	58,400 ± 33,200	Not specified	7.1 ± 0.21	Not specified	46.8 ± 16.5
Blue rock pigeon (Columbia livia)	10	10.5 ± 2.6 (5.0–20)	3,200,000 ± 460,000 (500,000–14,000,000)	Not specified	6.8 ± 0.2 (6–7.3)	340 ± 1.2 (338–352)	71.9 ± 3.1 (25–95)
Bronze turkey (Meleagris gallopavo)	10	290	8,500,000	2,450,000,000	Not specified	Not specified	Not specified
Sharp-tail sandgrouse (Tympanuchus phasianellus columbianus)	21	Dec-72	12,375	Not specified	Not specified	Not specified	33.1
Magellanic penguin (Spheniscus magellanicus)	13	35.6 ± 12.1	608,00000 ± 10,120,000	11,400,000 ± 3,200,000	7.4 ± 0.03	415.3 ± 6.4	59.2 ± 3.9
Ostrich (Struthio camelus australis)	56	640 ± 220	16,400,000 ± 5,200,000	Not specified	7.3 ± 0.1	Not specified	78 ± 4

CASA, Computer-assisted semen analysis; LIN, linearity; VSL, straight line velocity; VAP, average path velocity; VCL, curvilinear velocity.

Progressive Motility [%]	Viability [%]	Morphologic Normal Spermatozoa [%]	Structurally Abnormal Spermatozoa [%]	CASA VAP [μm/s]	CASA VCL [μm/s]	CASA VSL [μm/s]	CASA LIN [%]	Reference
2.7 ± 0.2	Not specified	85.6 ± 1.7	Not specified	Not specified	Not specified	Not specified	Not specified	41
Not specified	Not specified	Not specified	Not specified	Not specified	Not specified	Not specified	Not specified	9
71.5 (30–80)	90.3 (71–6.5)	Not specified	Not specified	Not specified	Not specified	Not specified	Not specified	18
70 (60–80)	87.1 (81–2.5)	Not specified	Not specified	Not specified	Not specified	Not specified	Not specified	18
75 (all 75)	87.9 (83.5–91)	Not specified	Not specified	Not specified	Not specified	Not specified	Not specified	18
82.3 (55–90)	94.6 (87–99)	Not specified	Not specified	Not specified	Not specified	Not specified	Not specified	18
81.4 (60–95)	95.9 (92–99.5)	Not specified	Not specified	Not specified	Not specified	Not specified	Not specified	18
70.74 ± 7.82 (57.6–82.59)	84.45 ± 4.42(94–80)	49.5	Not specified	Not specified	Not specified	Not specified	Not specified	28
50	91	Not specified	Not specified					30
43.74 ± 19.69 (3.48–100)	94.7 (90.2–97.8)	Not specified	Not specified	29.23 ± 8.66 (4.92–69.34)	46.16 ± 12.25 (14.06–103.49)	21.67 ± 8.10 (1.23–62.11)	0.46 ± 0.08 (0.04–0.94)	30
16 ± 7 (3–30)	50.5 ± 20.5 (5–87)	21.95	Not specified	Not specified	Not specified	Not specified	Not specified	19
Not specified	Not specified	Not specified	Not specified	Not specified	Not specified	Not specified	Not specified	20
54 ± 15.9	64.4 ± 9.7	Not specified	Not specified	78.1 ± 5.1	111.1 ± 9.5	69 ± 4.9	62 ± 6	58
44.4 ± 26.3	Not specified	Not specified	Not specified	42.9 ± 10.1	67.6 ± 17.8	34.1 ± 8.1	54.0 ± 7.7	59
Not specified	Not specified	Not specified	Not specified	Not specified	Not specified	Not specified	Not specified	27
Not specified	82.25 ± 2.04	Not specified	10.13 ± 0.4	Not specified	Not specified	Not specified	Not specified	60
Not specified	Not specified	82.2 ± 10.2	Not specified	81.64 ± 16.50 (48–146)	98.34 ± 22.80 (60–197)	79.62 ± 16.20 (46–146)	81.70 ± 7.50 (48–94)	61
3.9 ± 0.6 (3–4.5) [0–5 scale]	Not specified	75.2 ± 0.2	Not specified	114.1 ± 23.7 (70–199)	153.5 ± 26.0 (89.8–226.2)	109.3 ± 24.8 (64.5–196))	71.4 ± 10.9 (40–89)	42
Not specified	83.2	Not specified	Not specified	Not specified	Not specified	Not specified	Not specified	62
Not specified	Not specified	40.1	37 tail abnormalities	Not specified	Not specified	Not specified	Not specified	21
2.8 ± 0.1	83.5 ± 2.3	76.6 ± 3.0	24.4 ± not specified	Not specified	Not specified	Not specified	Not specified	63
Not specified	80		17 ± 3.7	Not specified	Not specified	Not specified	Not specified	64

after the first egg is laid. In poultry, it is known that one insemination is suitable to fertilize several following eggs, in raptors usually about two consecutive eggs,[2] whereas this is unknown in most of the other species. A fair recommendation is to repeat inseminations after each egg has been laid.

Inseminations can be accomplished via cloacal (Figure 12-12) or oviductal procedures (Figure 12-13). Insemination directly into the oviduct is recommended, as the success rate is higher and a lower number of spermatozoa are needed for fertilization.[30] Oviductal insemination procedures require more restraint of the birds, even in imprinted females. It also carries a higher risk of oviduct infection, as contaminated semen can be directly introduced in the oviduct. Therefore, special care must be taken not to use such semen in oviduct insemination. In trained or imprinted birds, and if enough semen is available, cloacal inseminations are sufficient, which is a method regularly used in raptor reproduction. For direct oviductal insemination, the female is placed in dorsal recumbency and ideally wrapped in a towel. The cloaca is spread by a rabbit mouth spreader, and the oviduct is usually visible as a prominent rosette in laying birds at the left lateral wall of the urodeum (see Figure 12-13). Semen is introduced through a small flexible tube such as an intravenous catheter (Figure 12-14). Introduction of the glass capillary tube into the oviduct should be avoided, as the risk of injury is too high. In cloacal insemination methods, semen is placed in the cloaca directly near the oviductal opening (Figure 12-15). Some of the first indicators of a problematic insemination (e.g., increased stress [procedure took too long], contaminated semen, oviduct infections) include eggs that are laid with poor quality or depigmented shells. Additionally, it should be considered that semen samples may contain different viral[36,37] and bacterial[38,39] pathogens. It is also for these reasons that it is recommended that the health status of the semen donor be properly investigated prior to collection.

The amount and quality of semen used for insemination are very important to consider in providing the highest potential to fertilize eggs. The minimal doses required are nearly unknown and proper studies to investigate this are rare. In Houbara bustards 10×10^6 spermatozoa,[40] in the Northern pintailed-duck[41] 310×10^6 spermatozoa, in the blue rock pigeons 250×10^6 to 300×10^6 spermatozoa,[42] and in falcons 0.9×10^6 spermatozoa[27] were needed for egg fertilization. Similar ranges are described for poultry varying between

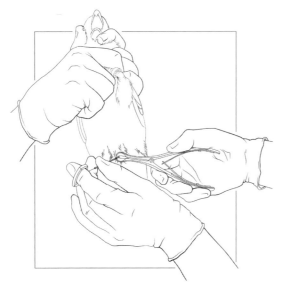

FIGURE 12-12 For insemination, the female bird is restrained by holding the head and wings gently. The bird is placed in dorsal recumbency, with the head up, legs pulled cranially, and the complete body lifted so that the person inseminating the bird has the cloaca at shoulder height. The cloaca is spread by a speculum to visualize the oviductal opening, where the semen is placed. (Drawing courtesy Ankat Hermanns, http://www.ankatsart.com/.)

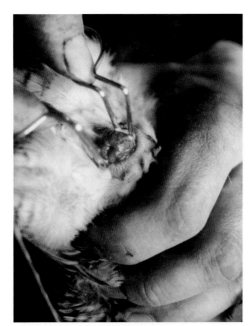

FIGURE 12-13 Oviductal opening is clearly visible in birds during clutching. (Photo courtesy Falcon Center, Helvesiek, Germany.)

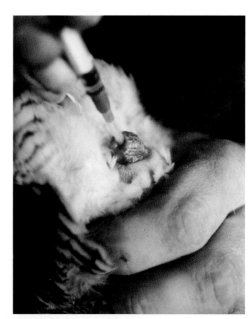

FIGURE 12-14 Insemination of a falcon by placing a small rubber tube directly into the oviduct. (Photo courtesy Falcon center, Helvesiek, Germany.)

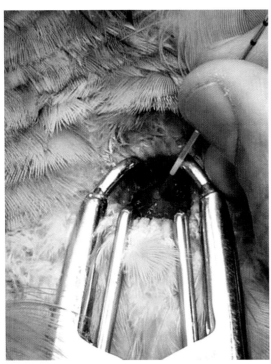

FIGURE 12-15 Cloacal insemination of a St. Vincent Amazon parrot near the oviductal opening according to Fischer et al.[20]

30×10^6 spermatozoa in chickens[43] and 75 to 150 $\times 10^6$ spermatozoa in turkeys.[44]

In psittacines such values have been described anecdotally by Lierz et al.[18] The insemination of 19.2 μL semen (concentration of 9,000 sperm/μL and a total sperm number of 172,800) prior to first oviposition, and 18.2 μL semen [containing sporadic sperm cells (+)] after the first egg lead to a fertile egg (second of clutch) in a green-winged macaw *(Ara chloropterus)*. A sample of 17.1 μL (1,590,000 sperm/μL) divided in three aliquots (two 5 μL and one 6.5 μL) fertilized the eggs of three different females of red-sided Eclectus parrot *(Eclectus roratus polychloros)*. This type of multihen insemination from a single semen sample is important to consider in species conservation projects when semen donors are limited or genetic representation of single males should be increased. A preliminary study to investigate minimal semen concentration for egg fertilization after artificial insemination in Psittacines was done by Fischer et al[30] in cockatiels. The authors described a minimum number of 232,500 spermatozoa (PMOT >70%) in a volume of 5 μL by intracloacal insemination to fertilize an egg. 250,000 spermatozoa in 5 μL resulted in the fertilization of two consecutive eggs. Intracloacal inseminations using a lower volume were unsuccessful, whereas intravaginal insemination with 2 μL containing 250,000 sperm resulted in a fertile egg.[30] It needs to be kept in mind that failure of artificial insemination might not only be related to insufficient semen quality. Defecation of the female after insemination might be another reason, especially after cloacal inseminations. Inadequate insemination timing, subclinical diseases of the female reproductive tract (inflammation and pH-alterations of the oviduct) or genetic mismatching of female and male might be additional reasons, the last in particular if the species is genetically compromised.

Even considering the above, fertility rates of at least 69.4% could be reached in psittacines,[8,18] only slightly lower than those rates reached through natural copulation in the same species.[8]

Semen Storage and Cryopreservation

In avian reproduction, usually fresh semen is used for artificial insemination. However, because of the short time frame in which insemination is promising, the availability of matching semen, especially in rare species, is not always ensured. This is in particular true if long distances must be overcome. Short-term storage of semen seems possible by cool storage of semen around 2° to 4° C (35.6° to 39.2° F) and diluting it with a semen extender (see below) or 1% glucose solution. With this approach, storage for 12 to 24 hours is usually possible, and in rare cases, storage may be successful even longer. The duration of time for successful storage may depend, at least in part, on the individual male, as differences in storage time were also observed between males of one species. Cryopreservation would ensure availability of semen, technically at any time point at any place in the world and therefore should remain a longer-term goal.[28,33,45] Cryopreservation of semen, in this light, would help to enable the establishment of genetic databases. Cryopreservation has been used in mammals for decades, and some studies in commercial poultry are available.[46,47] Experiences in other avian species are limited to some anecdotal reports, such as in peregrine falcons *(Falco peregrinus)*,[48,49] golden eagles *(Aquila chrysaetos)*,[50] and budgerigars *(Melopsittacus undulatus)* with a fertility rate of 66%.[33] However, species-specific differences in spermatozoa morphology and semen parameters (physiology), especially in osmolality, metabolism, and osmotolerance, hinder the transfer of a cryopreservation protocols from one species to another.[51,52] The first step of a cryopreservation protocol is to find a semen extender. This provides energy to the spermatozoa, maintains the pH value despite spermatozoal metabolism, and preserves the osmolality of the semen. Common semen extenders for poultry semen are Lake's diluent[53] and Beltsville Poultry Semen Extender (BPSE).[54] It has, however, been clearly demonstrated that semen extenders have different effects on the semen of different species, and therefore these products need to be adjusted to the particular species that they are to be used in.[28] As an example, when 0.1 M betaine hydrochloride and 30 mM adenosine triphosphate (ATP) were added to BPSE, a positive influence on the survival and motility of crane and turkey spermatozoa was noted.[55] Therefore, the intensive investigation of the basic parameters of semen of a particular species, such as osmolality must be known before starting to create a cryopreservation protocol. A motility rate of more than 70% should be maintained after adding the adjusted semen extenders to proceed with the second step of a cryopreservation protocol.[28]

As a second step for cryopreservation, a cryoprotectant needs to be added for spermatozoal survival at a storage temperature of −196° C (−320° F) in liquid nitrogen. So far, mainly glycerol is used in different avian species, but it has been shown that this cryoprotectant had the least benefit in cockatiel semen.[56] Alternatives are dimethylacetamide (DMA) or dimethylsulfoxide (DMSO), but statistically significant studies comparing those protectants are lacking, especially if it is considered that those studies should be applied specifically for a species or at least an avian family.[56,57] The same appears to be the case for the cooling rate, which is the last step of a cryopreservation protocol. Further studies, especially for endangered avian species, are needed. The reader is directed to screen the literature for recent developments in this field.

CONCLUSIONS

Assisted reproduction techniques represent a very important tool in species conservation projects but can also be helpful for pet bird owners who desire offspring from their single pet or aviary birds. Commercial advantages are also present with the appropriate use of assisted reproduction techniques. For many species, those techniques are relatively new and are more often attempted and described anecdotally, and it appears to be difficult to transfer experiences and basic data of one species, family, or other taxonomic group to another. Regardless, these techniques are already used in a number of different species and recent significant progress has been made, particularly with larger Psittacines.

The introduction of such techniques into the operation of a breeding collection requires preparation. First, the flock needs to be investigated to identify potential problems and other reasons for low reproductive success rates. Low numbers of eggs laid cannot be overcome with assisted reproduction techniques. Second, males must be investigated for the semen quality and potential semen donors should be identified prior to the time of planned insemination of the hen in order to have semen available at the time of imminent oviposition. If potential males are not in the collection, others need to be contacted, and logistical means for speedy and efficient semen transport determined. Structural preparations need to be made in the aviary in order to ensure that the birds can be caught for semen collection and artificial insemination in a speedy, efficient, and minimally stressful manner. The amount and locations of perches may require strategic location consideration, and operant conditioning may help facilitate the use of capture cages. Additional aviary preparations can include the installation of nest cameras to identify the time of oviposition more precisely. Imprinting or training of some individuals might be considered, according to the species. In most cases where assisted reproduction techniques fail, organization and procedural or facility preparations were insufficient, client compliance was poor, or expectations for outcome were inappropriate. Therefore those techniques, the requirements, and the consequences should be discussed, and no unjustified promises should be made.

REFERENCES

1. Echols MS, Speer BL: A comprehensive approach for the management of flock reproductive performance. In Fudge AM, Speer BL, editors: *Obstetrical and reproductive medicine, seminars in avian and exotic pet medicine*, Philadelphia, PA, 1996, WB Saunders.
2. Lierz M: Reproductive disease, incubation and artificial insemination. In Chitty J, Lierz M, editors: *Manual of raptors, pigeons and passerine birds*, Gloucestershire, U.K., 2008, BSAVA Publisher, pp 235–249.
3. Burrows WH, Quinn JP: A method of obtaining spermatozoa from the domestic fowl, *Poult Sci* 14:251–254, 1935.
4. Christensen VL, Bagley LG: Efficacy of fertilization in artificially inseminated turkey hens, *Poult Sci* 68(5):724–729, 1989.
5. Bourne D: Use and limitations of artificial insemination in cranes (Gruidae), *European Association of Zoo and Wildlife Veterinarians (EAZWV) Second scientific meeting*, Chester, U.K., 1998.
6. Berens von Rautenfeld D, Bley G, Hickel EM: Zur Technik der künstlichen Besamung und Sterilisation bei der Taube (*Columbia livia*), *Prakt Tierarzt* 12(1):103–105, 1979.
7. Birkhead TR, Fletcher F: Depletion determines sperm numbers in male zebra finches, *Anim Behav* 49:451, 1995.
8. Neumann D, Kaleta EF, Lierz M: Semen collection and artificial insemination in cockatiels (*Nymphicus hollandicus*)—a potential model for Psittacines, *Tierärztl Prax (K)* 41:101–105, 2013.
9. Anderson SJ, Bird DM, Hagen MD: Semen characteristics of the Quaker parakeet (*Myiopsitta monachus*), *Zoo Biol* 21:507–512, 2002.
10. Behncke H: Spermagewinnung und–untersuchung sowie endoskopische Beurteilung des Geschlechtsapparats in Abhängigkeit von der Spermaproduktion bei Psittaziden am Beispiel des Wellensittichs (*Melopsittacus undulatus*) [dissertation], Leipzig, Germany, 2002, Veterinärmedizinische Fakultät Universität Leipzig.
11. Samour JH, Smith CA, Moore HD, et al: Semen collection and spermatozoa characteristics in budgerigars (*Melopsittacus undulatus*), *Vet Rec* 118:397–399, 1986.
12. Stelzer G, Crosta L, Bürkle M, et al: Attempted semen collection using the massage technique and semen analysis in various psittacine species, *J Avian Med Surg* 19:7–13, 2005.
13. Harrison GJ, Wasmut D: Preliminary studies of electrostimulation to facilitate manual semen collection in psittacines, *Proc Conf AAV* 2:207–213, 1983.
14. Brock M: Semen collection and artificial insemination in the Hispaniolan parrot (*Amazona ventralis*), *J Zoo Wildl Med* 22(1):107–114, 1991.
15. Joyner KL: Theriogenology. In Ritchie BW, Harrison GJ, Harrison LR, editors: *Avian medicine: principles and application*, Lake Worth, FL, 1994, Wingers Publishing Inc., pp 748–804.
16. Behncke H, Stelzer G: Case report: semen collection, analysis and first attempt of artificial insemination (AI) in red-tailed cockatoos (*Calyptorhynchus magnificus*). In *Proceedings of the 7th EAAV Conference and 5th ECAMS Scientific Meeting*, Litografia Romero Puerto de la Cruz, Teneriffa, Spanien, 2003, pp 367–369.
17. DellaVolpe A, Volker S, Krautwald-Junghanns M-E: Attempted semen collection using the massage technique in blue-fronted amazon parrots (Amazona aestiva aestiva), *J Avian Med Surg* 25:1–7, 2011.
18. Lierz M, Reinschmidt M, Müller H, et al: A novel method for semen collection and artificial insemination in large parrots (Psittaciformes), *Sci Rep* 3:2066, 2013.
19. Fischer D, Neumann D, Purchase C, et al: The use of semen evaluation and assisted reproduction in Spix's macaws in terms of species conservation, *Zoo Biol* 33(3):234–244, 2014.
20. Fischer D, Neumann D, Schneider H, et al: Assisted reproduction in two rare psittacine species—the Spix's macaw and the St. Vincent amazon. In: *Proceedings of the 1st International Conference on Avian, Herpetological and Exotic mammal Medicine*, Wiesbaden, Germany, 2013, VVB Laufersweiler Verlag, pp 295–296.
21. Fischer D, Schneider H, Mathews S, et al: Assisted reproduction in Columbian sharp-tailed grouse as part of a species conservation project. In *Proceedings of the 2nd International Conference on Avian, Herpetological and Exotic mammal Medicine*, Paris, France, April 18-23, 2015.
22. Bublat A, Fischer D, Bruslund S, et al: Species-specific and seasonal variations in semen availability and semen characteristics in large parrots. In *Proceedings of the 2nd International Conference on Avian, Herpetological and Exotic mammal Medicine*, Paris, France, April 18-23, 2015.

23. Crosta L, Bürkle M, Gerlach H, et al: Testicular biopsy in psittacine birds: technique and histological findings, *Proc Conf Eur Assoc Avian Vet* 113–116, 2003.

24. Weitze K-F: Prinzipien der andrologischen Untersuchung, Spermatologische Untersuchung. In: Busch W, Holzmann A, editors: *Veterinärmedizinische Andrologie*, Stuttgart, Germany, 2001, Schattauer GmbH.

25. Waberski D, Petrunkina AM: Spermatologie. In Busch W, Waberski D, editors: *Künstliche Besamung bei Haus- und Nutztieren*, Stuttgart, Germany, 2007, Schattauer GmbH.

26. World Health Organization: *WHO laboratory manual for the examination and processing of human semen*, Geneva, Switzerland, 2010, World Health Organization Press.

27. Fischer D, Garcia de la Fuente J, Wehrend A, et al: Semen quality and semen characteristics of large falcons with special emphasis on fertility rate after artificial insemination, *Reprod Domest Anim* 46:14, 2011.

28. Schneider H, Fischer D, Bergmann M, et al: Investigations on cryopreservation of psittacine semen. In *Proceedings of the 1st International Conference on Avian, Herpetological and Exotic Mammal Medicine*, Wiesbaden, Germany, 2013, VVB Laufersweiler Verlag, pp 386–387.

29. Fischer D, Lierz M: *Assistierte Reproduktion beim Vogel - Neue Chancen für den Artenschutz*. Tagungsband der 34, Ehlscheid, 2013, Tagung über tropische Vögel der Gesellschaft für Tropenornithologie und der Estrilda.

30. Fischer D, Neumann D, Wehrend A, et al: Conventional and computer-assisted semen analysis in cockatiels (*Nymphicus hollandicus*) and evaluation of minimum sperm concentration for artificial insemination, *Theriogenology* 83:613–620, 2014.

31. Klimowicz M, Nizanski W, Batkowski F, et al: The comparison of assessment of pigeon semen motility and sperm concentration by conventional methods and the CASA system (HTM IVOS), *Theriogenology* 70:77–82, 2008.

32. Krohn J, Meinecke-Tillmann S, Schneider H, et al: Technical note: Investigations on the accomplishment of the avian perivitelline membrane penetration assay, *Reprod Domest Anim* 33, 2012.

33. Samour JH: The reproductive biology of the Budgerigar (*Melopsittacus undulatus*): semen preservation techniques and artificial insemination procedures, *J Avian Med Surg* 16(1):39–49, 2002.

34. Department of Conservation (DOC) kakapo recovery team: *Successful artificial insemination a world first*, 2009. http://www.KAKAPORECOVERY.ORG.NZ. Accessed October 28, 2009.

35. Sasanami T, Matsuzaki M, Mizushima S, et al: Sperm storage in the female reproductive tract in birds, *J Reprod Dev* 59(4):334–338, 2013.

36. Hoop RK: Transmission of chicken anaemia virus with semen, *Vet Rec* 27(133):551–552, 1993.

37. Metz AL, Hatcher L, Newman JA, et al: Venereal pox in breeder turkeys in Minnesota, *Avian Dis* 29:850–853, 1993.

38. Lierz M, Hafez HM: Occurrence of mycoplasmas in semen samples of birds of prey, *Avian Pathol* 37(5):495–497, 2008.

39. Blanco JM, Höfle U: Bacterial and fungal contaminants in raptor ejaculates and their survival to sperm cryopreservation protocols. In *Proceedings 6th conference of the European Wildlife Disease Association*, 2004.

40. Saint Jalme M, Gaucher P, Paillat P: Artificial insemination in Houbara bustards (*Chlamydotis undulata*): influence of the number of spermatozoa and insemination frequency on fertility and ability to hatch, *J Reprod Fertil* 100:93–103, 1994.

41. Penfold L, Harnal V, Lynch W, et al: Characterization of northern pintail (*Anas acuta*) ejaculate and the effect of sperm preservation on fertility, *Reprod* 121:267–275, 2001.

42. Sontakke SD, Umapathy G, Sivaram V, et al: Semen characteristics, cryopreservation, and successful artificial insemination in the blue rock pigeon (*Columba livia*), *Theriogenology* 62:139–153, 2004.

43. Bandyopadhyay UK, Chaudhuri D, Johari DC, et al: Determination of minimum insemination dose of spermatozoa for optimum fertility and profitability in White Leghorn chicken using artificial insemination, *Indian J Poultry Sci* 41:95–97, 2006.

44. Donoghue AM, Holsberger DR, Evenson DP, et al: Semen donor selection by in vitro sperm mobility increases fertility and semen storage in the turkey hen, *J Androl* 19:295–301, 1998.

45. Blanco J, Wildt D, Hofle U, et al: Implementing artificial insemination as an effective tool for ex situ conservation of endangered avian species, *Theriogenology* 71:200–213, 2009.

46. Sexton TJ, Buckland RB, Lopez R: Comparison of two procedures for freezing semen from cocks of high and low fertility with frozen semen, *Poult Sci* 57(2):550–552, 1978.

47. Tselutin K, Narubina L, Mavrodina T, et al: Cryopreservation of poultry semen. *Br Poult Sci* 36(5):805–811, 1995.

48. Parks JE, Heck WR, Hardaswick V: Cryopreservation of peregrine falcon semen and post-thaw dialysis to remove glycerol, *Raptor Res* 20(1):16–20, 1986.

49. Blanco JM, Gee GF, Wildt DE, et al: Producing progeny from endangered birds of prey, urine contamination, intramagnal insemination, *J Zoo Wildlife Med* 33:1–7, 2002.

50. Knowles-Brown A, Wishart G: Progeny from cryopreserved golden eagle spermatozoa, *Avian Poult Biol Rev* 12:201, 2001.

51. Blanco J M, Höfle U, Moorhouse R, et al: Improved avian sperm cryopreservation through comparative studies, *Cryobiology* 55(3):2, 2007.

52. Siudzinska A, Lukaszewicz E: Effect of semen extenders and storage time on sperm morphology of four chicken breeds, *J Appl Poult Res* 17(1):101–108, 2008.

53. Lake PE, Stewart JM: Preservation of fowl semen in liquid nitrogen—an improved method, *Br Poult Sci* 19(2):187–194, 1978.

54. Sexton TJ: A new poultry semen extender. 1. Effects of extension on the fertility of chicken semen, *Poult Sci* 56(5):1443–1446, 1977.

55. Blanco JM, Long JA, Gee G, et al: Comparative cryopreservation of avian spermatozoa: benefits of non-permeating osmoprotectants and ATP on turkey and crane sperm cryosurvival, *Anim Reprod Sci* 123(3-4):242–248, 2011.

56. Schneider HD, Fischer M, Bergmann C, et al: Untersuchungen zur Kryokonservierung von Psittazidensperma. In *Proceedings der 1. Jahrestagung der DVG-Fachgruppe Vögel-und Reptilien*, München, Germany, March 6-8, 2013, pp 3–5.

57. Lierz M: Assisted reproduction techniques in psittacines–Recent developments. In *Proceedings of the 35th Annual Conference of the Association of Avian Veterinarians*, New Orleans, USA, August 2-8, 2014, p 399.

58. Gloria A, Contri A, Carluccio A, et al: The breeding management affects fresh and cryopreserved semen characteristics in *Melopsittacus undulates*, *Anim Reprod Sci* 144(1–2):48–53, 2014.

59. Dogliero A, Rota A, von Degerfeld MM, et al: Use of computer-assisted semen analysis for evaluation of Rosy-faced lovebird (*Agapornis roseicollis*) semen collected in different periods of the year, *Theriogenology* 83(1):103–106, 2015.

60. Tabatabaei S, Batavani R, Talebi A: Comparison of semen quality in indigenous and Ross broiler breeder roosters, *J Anim Vet Adv* 8(1):90–93, 2009.

61. Umapathy G, Sontakke S, Reddy A, et al: Semen characteristics of the captive Indian white-backed vulture (*Gyps bengalensis*), *Biol Reprod* 73(5):1039–1045, 2005.

62. Kamar GA, Rizik MA: Semen characteristics of two breeds of turkeys, *J Reprod Fertil* 29(3):317–325, 1972.

63. O'Brien JK, Oehler DA, Malowski SP, et al: Semen collection, characterization and cryopreservation in a Magellanic penguin (*Spheniscus magellanicus*), *Zoo Biol* 18:199–214, 1999.

64. Hemberger M, Hosper R, Bostedt H: Semen collection, examination and spermiogram in ostriches, *Reprod Domest Anim* 36:241–243, 2001.

ADVANCEMENTS IN METHODS FOR DECREASING REPRODUCTIVE SUCCESS

Olivia A. Petritz, Michael Lierz, Jaime Samour

CLINICAL APPLICATIONS AND CONSIDERATIONS FOR THE USE OF GnRH AGONISTS

Olivia A. Petritz

Overview of Female Reproductive Physiology

Diseases of the female reproductive tract, including egg binding, dystocia, oviductal and ovarian disease, yolk coelomitis, and cloacal prolapse, are commonly seen in avian medicine. Surgical removal of the reproductive tract is a common treatment for mammals with reproductive disease. In avian species, the only portion of the female reproductive tract that is routinely surgically removed is the oviduct, as the ovary is supplied by multiple, short ovarian arteries, which are challenging to ligate and in close proximity to the aorta. Therefore, continued ovarian activity is not uncommonly encountered. Problems that may be seen include internal ovulation, cystic ovarian disease, estrogenically mediated physiologic changes, and reproductively associated problem behaviors (aggression, feather-destructive behavior, masturbation), which may still occur following salpingohysterectomy. Many of these reproductive disorders are, in part, managed medically with the use of a variety of drugs designed to decrease plasma sex hormones such as gonadotropin-releasing hormone (GnRH) agonists. To determine the best course of treatment for the individual patient, it is imperative that a clinician must have an understanding of avian reproductive physiology. Extensive reviews on this subject have been published elsewhere[1-5]; therefore, this section serves only as a brief overview of the subject, with emphasis on clinically relevant information.

Environmental factors

One of the most important environmental factors to stimulate reproductive activity is photoperiod in many avian species. More equatorial species should overall be anticipated to be less responsive to photoperiod changes compared with those that originate from habitats further away from the equator with greater seasonal day length variations. Photoreceptors in the retina and pineal gland become sensitized, and this stimulates the release of GnRH from the hypothalamus.[4] Most species respond to increasing day length, with the Emperor penguin (*Aptenodytes forsteri*) being one of the few avian species that shows increased reproductive activity during decreased day length.[4] Maximum stimulation occurs with 12 to 14 hours of light, but there is a variable onset of when a bird is most sensitive to the effects of light, termed the *photosensitive phase*.[5] This phase is species dependent and typically occurs 13 to 17 hours after the onset of dawn. As long as there is light exposure during this phase, reproductive activity can be stimulated without a need for continuous long day lengths.[4,6,7]

Rainfall stimulates reproductive activity in species native to both tropical and desert environments, such as zebra finches (*Taeniopygia guttata*) and cockatiels (*Nymphicus hollandicus*).[5] For wild species, rainfall also increases the available food supply, which often coincides with reproduction. Certain species, such as the white-crowned sparrow (*Zonotrichia leucophrys*) can override the inhibitory effects of shortened day length if provided with adequate food.[7] The presence of a mate, or a perceived mate (mirror or human caregiver), is another powerful reproductive stimulus in many avian species. While birds with physical contact with a mate will have the most stimulation,[1] auditory contact with a male conspecific has also been shown to induce cycling in females of certain species such as budgerigars (*Melopsittacus undulatus*) and ring-necked doves (*Streptopelia capicola*).[2,7] Nesting material and the presence of a nesting box have also been shown to stimulate egg-laying and plasma luteinizing hormone (LH) secretion in cockatiels and other cavity-nesting species.[1,8]

Neuroendocrine control

The hypothalamic–pituitary–gonadal (HPG) axis controls avian reproduction, similar to most other vertebrates. The initiating factor in this hormonal cascade are the GnRHs. These peptide hormones are transported to the anterior pituitary gland, which, in turn, stimulates the release of LH. The ability of GnRH to stimulate follicle-stimulating hormone (FSH) in avian species is unclear; therefore, some references use the term luteinizing hormone–releasing hormone (LHRH) rather than GnRH for birds.[7,9] GnRH is released in a pulsatile fashion in response to environmental and tactile cues (i.e., photoperiod, food availability, rainfall, presence of a mate). LH stimulates the production of androgens, estrogens, and progestins; FSH appears to also be involved with steroidogenesis and ovarian folliculogenesis, but its role in avian species is still not completely clear.[7]

Most vertebrates, including birds, possess multiple forms of GnRH, which can be classified into three major forms—GnRH-I, GnRH-II, GnRH-III. GnRH-I is considered an "ancient" form that is conserved across species.[9] In fact, avian GnRH-I differs from its mammalian counterpart by only one amino acid.[9] Avian GnRH-II and GnRH-III have a greater number of genetic differences compared with the mammalian peptide hormones. Their ability to stimulate LH, and possibly FSH release from the anterior pituitary, is variable, depending on the species, sex, and reproductive status of the bird. In addition, multiple types of GnRH receptors have been identified and are subdivided into mammalian and non-mammalian receptors.[10] The incongruities between avian and mammalian GnRH peptides and their receptors may explain the reduced efficacy of synthetic GnRH-agonists, including leuprolide acetate and deslorelin acetate in avian species.

Endogenously, avian reproduction is controlled by the HPG axis. However, there are numerous exogenous elements that have a considerable influence on reproduction. The exogenous and endogenous mechanisms of activation or suppression of the HPG axis and their roles in some common reproductive or reproductively associated problems are displayed in Figures 12-16 and 12-17. As such, any treatment that affects only the endogenous reproductive hormone cascade, including the use of GnRH agonists, will be rendered less effective if the environmental factors are not also addressed simultaneously. Therefore, GnRH agonist therapy should not be used as a sole therapy for suppression

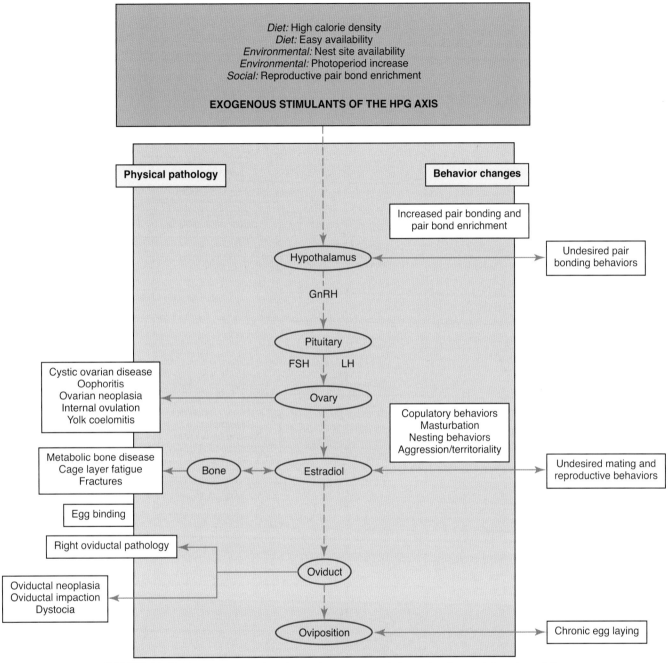

FIGURE 12-16 Exogenous and endogenous aspects of the activation and function of the hypothalamic–pituitary–gonadal (HPG) axis. The pink background represents normal physiologic and behavioral activities. Exogenous stimuli are included in the dark green box, and endogenous mechanisms are represented by the dotted green arrows. The dark green double-ended arrows represent cyclical and physiologically normal influences, and the dark green one-way arrows represent the development of pathologic changes. Behavior changes are depicted on the right and physical pathology on the left. The further outside of the normal range of physiologic parameters a problem is identified, the greater is the probable need for medical, surgical, or behavioral intervention.

of reproductive activity in any avian species. Behavioral modification, for both the patient and the owner, is often one, if not the largest, component of most aspects of treatment and prevention. Figure 12-18 displays the level of influence on the HPG axis of antecedent arrangement and behavior-change strategies, GnRH agonist therapy, ovarian surgery, and oviductal surgery. Treatment options for common reproductive and reproductively associated problems are further compared with regard to therapy and prevention, in relation to outcome expectations, in Tables 12-2 and 12-3.

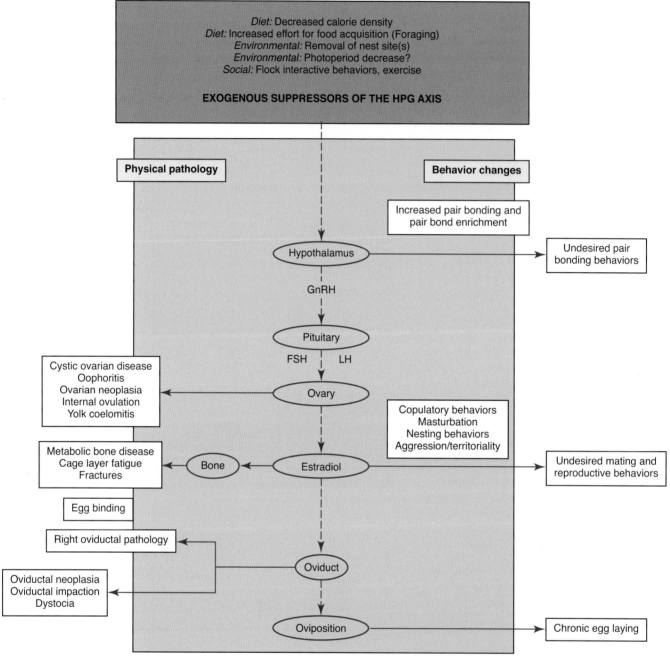

FIGURE 12-17 Exogenous and endogenous aspects of suppression of function of the hypothalamic–pituitary–gonadal (HPG) axis. The pink background represents normal physiologic and behavioral activities. Exogenous suppressors are included in the dark red box, and endogenous mechanisms are represented by the dotted red arrows. The dark red arrows represent the resultant negative influence on probability of HPG activity–associated problems. As noted in Figure 12-16 the further outside of the normal range of physiologic parameters a problem is identified, the greater is the probable need for medical, surgical, or behavioral intervention.

Overview of GnRH Agonists

Synthetic GnRH agonists, also termed *super-agonists*, have a long half-life and reportedly higher affinity for GnRH receptors compared with endogenous GnRH in mammals.[11] Like the naturally occurring hypothalamic decapeptide GnRH, these super-agonists stimulate the secretion of LH and FSH from the pituitary gland. Lecirelin, a short-acting GnRH agonist, increased the onset of reproductive activity in breeding pairs of canaries *(Serinus canaria)* after topical application compared with control birds.[12] A similar GnRH agonist,

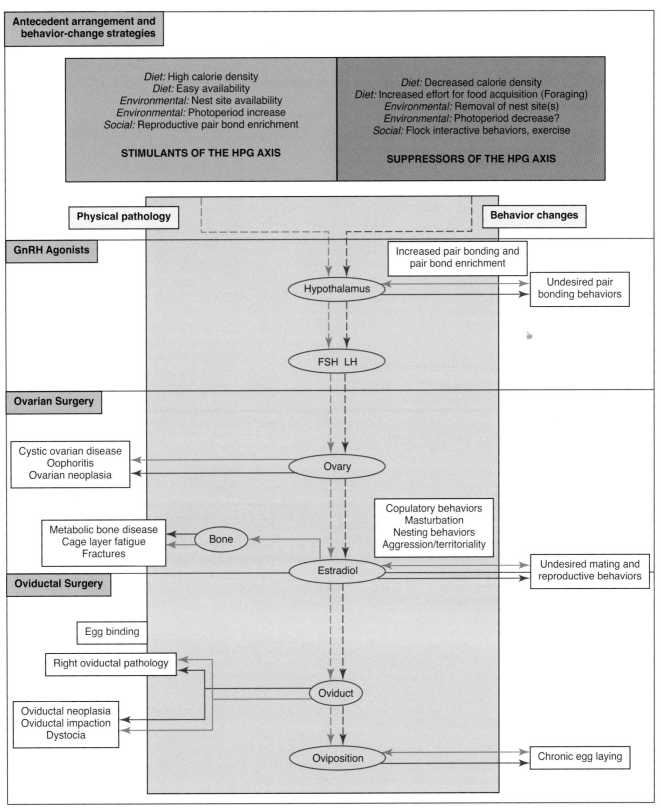

FIGURE 12-18 Combined exogenous and endogenous aspects of the activation and suppression of function of the hypothalamic–pituitary–gonadal (HPG) axis. The level of influence on the HPG axis and associated problems by antecedent arrangement and behavior-change strategies, gonadotropin-releasing hormone (GnRH) agonist therapy, ovarian surgery, and oviductal surgery are depicted by their respectively identified overlaid boxes *(blue)*. The complexities of selecting the most appropriate management and treatment intervention strategies are more apparent when viewing the complexity of the figure. The pink background again represents normal physiologic and behavioral activities. Exogenous stimuli are included in the dark green box, and endogenous mechanisms are represented by the dotted green arrows. Exogenous suppressors are included in the dark red box, and endogenous mechanisms are represented by the dotted red arrows. The dark green double-ended arrows represent cyclical and physiologically normal influences, and the dark green one-way arrows represent the development of pathologic changes. The dark red arrows represent the resultant negative influence on probability of HPG activity–associated problems. As noted in Figures 12-16 and 12-17, the further outside of the normal range of physiologic parameters a problem is identified, the greater is the probable need for medical, surgical, or behavioral intervention.

TABLE 12-2

Comparison of Treatment Method Options for Specifically Identified Reproductive Problems

Treatments	Behavior-Change and Antecedent Arrangement Strategies	GnRH Agonists	Complete Ovariectomy	Partial Ovariectomy	Salpingotomy	Salpingohysterectomy
Cystic ovarian disease	−	−	+	+/−	−	−
Oophoritis	−	−	+	+/−	−	−
Ovarian neoplasia	−	+	+	+/−	−	−
Metabolic bone disease	−	+/−	+	−	−	−
Yolk coelomitis	−	−	−	−	−	−
Egg binding	−	−	−	−	−	+
Right oviductal pathology	−	−	−	−	−	+
Oviductal neoplasia	−	+	−	−	+/−	+
Oviductal impaction	−	−	−	−	+	+
Dystocia	−	−	−	−	+	+
Increased pair-bonding behaviors	+	+/−	+/−	+/−	−	−
Undesired pair-bonding behaviors	+	+/−	+/−	+/−	−	−
Aggression/territoriality	+	+/−	+/−	+/−	−	−
Undesired mating and reproductive behaviors	+	+/−	+/−	+/−	−	−
Chronic egg laying	+	+	+	+/−	−	+

Treatment or intervention options are displayed at the top as they should influence the problems listed in the left column.
(−) No effect should be anticipated when the problem is present.
(+/−) No effect or partial effect or palliation should be anticipated, with eventual need for additional intervention(s).
(+) A favorable effect should be anticipated.
GnRH, Gonadotropin-releasing hormone.

TABLE 12-3

Comparison of Treatments When Used as Preventative Methods and Their Anticipated Effect Against Risk or Probability of Specific Reproductive or Associated Problems

Preventions (Reduce or Remove Risk of Problems)	Behavior-Change and Antecedent Arrangement strategies	GnRH Agonists	Complete Ovariectomy	Partial Ovariectomy	Salpingotomy	Salpingohysterectomy
Cystic ovarian disease	+	+	+	+/−	−	−
Oophoritis	+	+	+	+/−	−	−
Ovarian neoplasia	+	+/−	+	+/−	−	−
Metabolic bone disease	+	+	+	+/−	−	−
Yolk coelomitis	+	+	+	+/−	−	−
Egg binding	+	+	+	+	−	+
Right oviductal pathology	+	+	+	−	−	+/−
Oviductal neoplasia	+	+/−	+	−	−	+
Oviductal impaction	+	+	+	+	−	+
Dystocia	+	+	+	+	−	+
Increased pair bonding behaviors	+	+/−	+/−	−	−	−
Undesired pair bonding behaviors	+	+/−	+/−	−	−	−
Aggression/territoriality	+	+/−	+/−	−	−	−
Undesired mating and reproductive behaviors	+	+/−	+/−	−	−	−
Chronic egg laying	+	+/−	+	+	−	+

Treatment or intervention options are displayed at the top as they should influence the problems listed in the left column.
(−) No effect should be anticipated when the problem is present.
(+/−) No effect or partial effect or palliation should be anticipated, with eventual need for additional intervention(s).
(+) A favorable effect should be anticipated.

buserelin, increased circulating testosterone after a single intramuscular (IM) injection in cockatiels and sulfur-crested cockatoos (*Cacatua galerita*).[13] A single injection of buserelin administered intramuscularly to budgerigars also increased reproductive activity and egg laying in that species.[14] However, if synthetic GnRH agonists are administered repeatedly or in a sustained-release form, these agonists will ultimately lead to the downregulation of GnRH receptors via negative-feedback mechanisms.[15,16] The two long-acting GnRH agonists used most commonly in avian medicine are leuprolide acetate and deslorelin acetate.

Leuprolide acetate

Leuprolide acetate (Lupron, TAP Pharmaceuticals Inc., Lake Forest, IL) is a synthetic, GnRH agonist available as a depot formulation to provide long-term treatment for various reproductive diseases in humans, including prostatic hyperplasia and precocious puberty.[11] The parent compound, leuprorelin, is released over a predefined period from a lipophilic synthetic polymer in the long-acting formulation after subcutaneous injection.[17] Leuprolide acetate was originally developed for use in humans, but it has been used in several exotic species, particularly in ferrets for treatment of adrenal cortical disease and in psittacines for treatment of reproductive disorders. In avian species, it is used most commonly for treatment of excessive egg laying and to decrease undesired reproductively associated problem behaviors. In addition, there are several published reports that describe its use for management of ovarian neoplasia in cockatiels along with periodic coelomocentesis.[18,19]

Although leuprolide acetate has been used extensively in many avian species, there are few controlled clinical trials that examine the efficacy of this drug. Leuprolide acetate was found to reversibly prevent egg laying in cockatiels after a single IM injection. Specifically, the treated cockatiels had a 12- to 19-day delay in egg laying compared with a control group.[20] Racing pigeons (*Columbia livia domestica*) administered 500 and 1000 μg/kg IM of leuprolide acetate had no alterations in plasma sex hormones nor egg production.[21] A single injection of leuprolide acetate administered to non-breeding adult Hispaniolan Amazon parrots (*Amazona ventralis*) at a dose of 800 μg/kg IM reduced plasma sex hormone levels for less than 21 days.

In addition to unknown efficacy in most avian species, the published dose range is wide, from 100 to 1200 μg/kg IM.[22] The recommended dose range and treatment interval for most psittacines is 400 to 1000 μg/kg IM every 2 to 3 weeks.[23,24] This may not be financially feasible for all clients, as long-term treatment is usually required. Also, anecdotally, the efficacy of leuprolide acetate decreases after long-term repeated administration. Despite its widespread use, there is only one published report of a suspected anaphylactic reaction and death following administration of leuprolide acetate in two female elf owls (*Micrathene whitneyi*).[25] Both birds had been treated intermittently with the drug for 2 to 4 years without complication prior to the two fatalities. Fatal reactions to leuprolide acetate are also rarely reported in humans and are suggested to be caused by impurities in the formulations.[26]

Deslorelin acetate

Deslorelin acetate (Suprelorin, Peptech Animal Health, Macquarie Park, New South Wales, Australia) is another GnRH agonist that is formulated into a subcutaneous, controlled-release implant designed for use in dogs for reversible suppression of testosterone production, and thus contraception, for 6 to 12 months, depending on implant size.[16] It is currently commercially available as a 4.7-mg or 9.4-mg implant and is considerably less expensive than repeated treatments with leuprolide acetate. Recently, the 4.7-mg deslorelin implants have become available in the United States as an FDA-Indexed Minor Use/Minor Species product for management of adrenal cortical disease in domestic ferrets. At the time of this writing, the 4.7-mg deslorelin implant is not FDA approved for use in any other species in the United States, nor has a withdrawal period in animals intended for human consumption been established.

The implants come from the manufacturer in a preloaded needle with a separate applicator syringe, similar to a microchip (see Figure 12-19). The 4.7-mg deslorelin implants are cylindrical, approximately 2.3 mm wide by 12.5 mm long, and weigh 50 mg. An in vivo study demonstrated that the elution rate from the 4.7-mg deslorelin implant was approximately 20 μg/day in mice, and this considerably decreased after 25 to 30 days.[27] In addition, 90% of the drug is released in vitro within 3 to 4 weeks from the 4.7-mg deslorelin implant versus 6 weeks from the 9.4-mg implant.[27] This has been attributed to discrepancies between the matrix compositions of the implants, which is proprietary knowledge of the manufacturer. To the author's knowledge, no studies have been performed to determine the elution rate from either size of deslorelin implant in any avian species.

Similar to leuprolide acetate, deslorelin acetate is primarily used to decrease reproductively associated problem behaviors and egg laying in avian species. It has also been used successfully for long-term management of nonresectable ovarian neoplasia in cockatiels[19,28] and Sertoli cell tumors in budgerigars.[29] In the last, it is used as treatment to decrease the size of the tumor to expand the lifespan of the patient or to allow surgical removal of the affected testicle. In addition to treatment of ovarian neoplasia, there is evidence that GnRH agonists such as deslorelin acetate have chemopreventive effects in domestic chickens against development of ovarian neoplasia.[30] There are several published case reports and retrospective studies describing the use of deslorelin acetate in psittacines;[19,28,29,31,32] however, the only prospective controlled studies to date on deslorelin acetate in birds are in chickens,[33] quail,[34-36] and pigeons.[37]

Chickens treated with a 4.7-mg deslorelin acetate implant had reduced egg production for a mean of 180 days, whereas a 9.4-mg implant inhibited egg production for 319 days.[33] In Japanese quails (*Coturnix coturnix japonica*), a single 4.7-mg deslorelin acetate implant reversibly decreased egg production in 6 out of 10 birds for 70 days.[34] Plasma sex hormones, specifically 17β-estradiol and androstenedione, were significantly lower in the treatment group than in the control group on day 29, but at no other time points. A similar study treated Japanese quails with a single 4.7-mg deslorelin implant and reported decreased egg production, plasma corticosterone, and 17β-estradiol concentrations in 89% of the birds for 7 to 18 weeks.[36] In 55% of the female quails, the effects of deslorelin lasted more than 14 weeks, and in 70% of male quails, the duration of action was longer than 9 weeks. Pigeons (*Columba livia*) implanted with a single 4.7-mg deslorelin implant had reduced egg production for 5 to 7 weeks and reduced serum LH concentrations for 84 days compared with control birds.[37]

Determining an effective dose to prevent contraception for deslorelin acetate has proven challenging across several species, even those of similar weight and taxonomy.[38,39] Despite dramatically higher doses administered to Japanese quails compared with dogs[40] (31.5 to 37.3 mg/kg versus 0.15 to 0.76 mg/kg, respectively), the efficacy and duration were both less in quails. This discrepancy may have resulted from the differences in GnRH or GnRH receptors in birds,[9] an inherent difference in drug metabolism in this or all avian species, or both. A single 4.7-mg implant had a longer period of effect in chickens than in quails, both of which are galliformes. This suggests that there is also a substantial interspecies variation, in addition to individual variation with deslorelin acetate implants. Based on this information, extrapolation of these results to other avian species such as psittacines should be done with caution.

Because of the reduced efficacy and shorter duration of deslorelin in Japanese quails, a recent study examined the effects of two 4.7-mg deslorelin acetate implants versus one 9.4-mg implant on egg production and plasma progesterone concentrations in this species.[35] Seven out of 10 birds treated with two 4.7-mg implants ceased egg laying 1 week after implantation and remained nonovulatory for approximately 100 days. Cessation of egg laying in the 9.4-mg treatment group occurred in 7 out of 10 birds, onset was variable (weeks 5 to 12), and continued for the remainder of the study period. Plasma progesterone concentrations for the deslorelin treatment groups were not significantly different from those of the placebo group at any time point. These results indicated that doubling the dose of deslorelin acetate in Japanese quails did not increase the efficacy of the drug but did prolong its duration of action. Interestingly, the single 9.4-mg deslorelin implant, which is not yet commercially available in the United States, had a slower onset but longer duration of action compared with the two 4.7-mg implants. In vitro studies have shown that deslorelin released on a daily basis from a single 9.4-mg implant is only 1.5 times, rather than two times, that of one 4.7-mg implant as the milligram concentration would imply.[27]

In addition to selecting an effective dose, another challenge that clinicians face with long-acting GnRH agonists is selecting an appropriate dosing interval. Return of reproductive behaviors, egg laying, or both have been used as the best indicators for reimplantation. In the prospective studies mentioned previously, egg laying was the most consistent sign of cessation of efficacy for deslorelin implants because the plasma hormone measurements were often highly variable and did not accurately reflect the reproductive status of the bird. A recent retrospective case series in the non–peer-reviewed literature reviewed the use of 4.7-mg deslorelin acetate implants in 96 psittacine patients.[31] Thirty-two of those birds were females, which received a single 4.7-mg deslorelin implant to prevent chronic egg laying. The most common interval between implants for that group of birds was 3 months with a range of 2 to 5 months. In addition to behavioral and environmental modifications, treatment with repeated implantation of a single 4.7-mg deslorelin implant consecutively over a period of 6 to 9 months led to a successful resolution of chronic egg laying. As with leuprolide acetate, there is anecdotal evidence of decreased efficacy over time after repeated administration of deslorelin implants in several avian species.[39]

Deep sedation or general anesthesia is recommended for placement of the implant because of the large size of the needle relative to the small size of most psittacine patients (Figure 12-19). The recommended implantation site is subcutaneously in the midscapular region (Figure 12-20). Other authors have placed implants subcutaneously in the knee fold

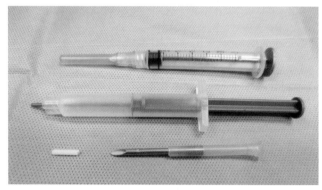

FIGURE 12-19 A 4.7-mg deslorelin acetate implant (Suprelorin) with application syringe and needle. The implant normally is preloaded in the application needle, as provided by the manufacturer. A 3-mL syringe with an attached 22-gauge needle is included for size comparison.

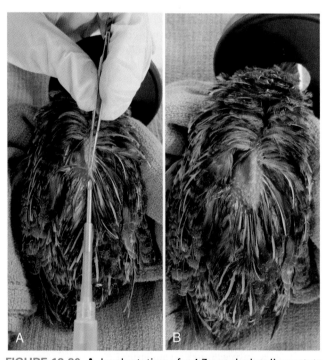

FIGURE 12-20 A, Implantation of a 4.7-mg deslorelin acetate implant (Suprelorin) subcutaneously between the scapulae of an anesthetized Japanese quail *(Coturnix coturnix japonica)*. **B,** The same site following implantation, with the deslorelin acetate implant visible subcutaneously.

in budgerigars.[29] The applicator syringe is nonsterile and can be used repeatedly as it does not come into contact with the sterile implant. Plucking of the feathers and sterile preparation of the site is recommended prior to implant placement. A small amount of tissue adhesive can be used on the skin defect created by the application needle to prevent loss of the implant. In the author's experience, the dissolution rate for both sizes of deslorelin implants is variable and unrelated to clinical efficacy. Ninety days after implantation into Japanese quails, some 4.7-mg implants were almost completely dissolved, whereas others remained visibly intact.[35] Removal of the implants can be performed but is not usually necessary in avian patients. Self-mutilation of the implant site and implant removal by the patient has been reported in several psittacine birds;[31] therefore, close monitoring of the site for several days after placement is recommended. In the author's experience, the most common side effect of placement is treatment failure.

REFERENCES

1. Shields KM, Yamamoto JT, Millam JR: Reproductive behavior and LH levels of cockatiels (*Nymphicus hollandicus*) associated with photostimulation, nest-box presentation, and degree of mate access, *Hormones Behav* 23:68–82, 1989.
2. Hudelson KS: A review of the mechanisms of avian reproduction and their clinical applications, *Semin Avian Exot Pet Med* 5:189–198, 1996.
3. Ottinger MA, Wu J, Pelican K: Neuroendocrine regulation of reproduction in birds and clinical applications of GnRH analogues in birds and mammals, *Semin Avian Exot Pet Med* 11:71–79, 2006.
4. Millam JR: Reproductive physiology. In Altman RB, Clubb SL, Dorrestein GM, et al, editors: *Avian medicine and surgery*, Philadelphia, PA, 1997, WB Saunders, pp 12–28.
5. Joyner K: Theriogenology. In Ritchie B, Harrison G, Harrison L, editors: *Avian medicine: principles and application*, Lake Worth, FL, 1994, Wingers Publishing Inc., pp 748–773.
6. Cunningham F: Ovulation in the hen: neuroendocrine control. In Clark J, editor: *Oxford reviews of reproductive biology*, vol 9, Oxford, 1987, Clarendon Press, pp 96–136.
7. Pollock CG, Orosz SE: Avian reproductive anatomy, physiology and endocrinology, *Vet Clin North Am Exot Anim Pract* 5:441–474, 2002.
8. Millam JR, Roudybush TE, Grau CR: Influence of environmental manipulation and nest-box availability on reproductive success of captive cockatiels (*Nymphicus hollandicus*), *Zoo Biol* 7:25–34, 1988.
9. Bedecarrats G, Shimizu M, Guemene D: Gonadotropin releasing hormones and their receptors in avian species, *J Poult Sci* 43:199–214, 2006.
10. Pawson A, Katz A, Sun Y, et al: Contrasting internalization kinetics of human and chicken gonadotropin-releasing hormone receptors mediated by C-terminal tail, *J Endocrinol* 156:R9–R12, 1998.
11. Plosker GL, Brogden RN: Leuprorelin: a review of its pharmacology and therapeutic use in prostatic cancer, endometriosis and other sex hormone-related disorders, *Drugs* 48:930–967, 1994.
12. Robbe D, Todisco G, Giammarino A, et al: Use of a synthetic GnRH analog to induce reproductive activity in canaries (*Serinus canaria*), *J Avian Med Surg* 22:123–126, 2008.
13. Lovas EM, Johnston SD, Filippich LJ: Using a GnRH agonist to obtain an index of testosterone secretory capacity in the cockatiel (*Nymphicus hollandicus*) and sulphur-crested cockatoo (*Cacatua galerita*)., *Aust Vet J* 88:52–56, 2010.
14. Costantini V, Carraro C, Bucci FA, et al: Influence of a new slow-release GnRH analogue implant on reproduction in the Budgerigar (*Melopsittacus undulatus*, Shaw 1805), *Anim Reprod Sci* 111:289–301, 2009.
15. Romagnoli S, Stelletta C, Milani C, et al: Clinical use of deslorelin for the control of reproduction in the bitch, *Reprod Domest Anim* 44(Suppl 2):36–39, 2009.
16. Trigg TE, Wright PJ, Armour AF, et al: Use of a GnRH analogue implant to produce reversible long-term suppression of reproductive function in male and female domestic dogs, *J Reprod Fertil Suppl* 57:255–261, 2001.
17. Periti P, Mazzei T, Mini E: Clinical pharmacokinetics of depot leuprorelin. *Clin Pharmacokinet* 41:485–504, 2002.
18. Nemetz L: Leuprolide acetate control of ovarian carcinoma in a cockatiel (*Nymphicus hollandicus*.. In *Proceedings of the 31st Annual Association of Avian Veterinarians Conference*, 2010, pp 333–338.
19. Keller KA, Beaufrère H, Brandão J, et al: Long-term management of ovarian neoplasia in two cockatiels (*Nymphicus hollandicus*), *J Avian Med Surg* 27:44–52, 2013.
20. Millam J, Finney H: Leuprolide acetate can reversibly prevent egg laying in cockatiels (*Nymphicus hollandicus*), *Zoo Biol* 13:149–155, 1994.
21. De Wit M, Westerhof I, Pefold L: Effect of leuprolide acetate on avian reproduction. In *Proceedings of the 25th Annual Association of Avian Veterinarians*, 2004, pp 73–74.
22. Hawkins M, Barron HW, Speer B: Birds. In Carpenter JW, editor: *Exotic animal formulary*, ed 4, St. Louis, MO, 2012, Saunders, p 284.
23. Mans C, Pilny A: Use of GnRH-agonists for medical management of reproductive disorders in birds, *Vet Clin North Am Exot Anim Pract* 17:23–33, 2014.
24. Mitchell MA: Leuprolide acetate, *Semin Avian Exot Pet Med* 14:153–155, 2005.
25. Stringer EM, De Voe RS, Loomis MR: Suspected anaphylaxis to leuprolide acetate depot in two Elf owls (*Micrathene whitneyi*), *J Zoo Wildl Med* 42:166–168, 2011.
26. Biffoni M, Battaglia A, Borrelli F, et al: Immunology. Allergenic potential of gonadotrophic preparations in experimental animals: relevance of purity, *Hum Reprod* 9:1845–1848, 1994.
27. Navarro C, Schober P, et al: Pharmacodynamics and pharmacokinetics of a sustained-release implant of deslorelin in companion animals. In *Proceedings of the 7th International Symposium on Canine and Feline Reproduction in a Joint Meeting with the European Veterinary Society for Small Animal Reproduction*, 2012.
28. Nemetz L: Deslorelin acetate long-term suppression of ovarian carcinoma in a cockatiel (*Nymphicus hollandicus*). In *Proceedings of the 33rd Annual Association of Avian Veterinarians Conference and Expo*, 2012, pp 37–42.
29. Straub J, Zenker I: First experience in hormonal treatment of sertoli cell tumors in budgerigars (*Melopsittacus undulatus*) with absorbable extended-release GnRH chips (Suprelorin®). In *Proceedings of the 1st International Conference on Avian, Herpetological & Exotic Mammal Medicine*, 2013, pp 299–300.
30. de Matos R: Investigation of the chemopreventative effects of deslorelin in domestic chickens with a high prevalence of ovarian cancer. In *Proceedings of the 1st International Conference on Avian, Herpetological & Exotic Mammal Medicine*, 2013, p 90.
31. Van Sant F, Sundaram A: Retrospective study of deslorelin acetate implants in clinical practice. In *Proceedings of the 34th Annual Conference Association of Avian Veterinarians*, 2013, pp 211–220.
32. Cook K, Riggs G: Clinical report: gonadotropic releasing hormone agonist implants. In *Proceedings of the 28th American Association of Avian Veterinarians Annual Conference*, 2007, pp 309–315.
33. Noonan B, Johnson P, de Matos R: Evaluation of egg-laying suppression effects of the GnRH agonist deslorelin in domestic chickens. In *Proceedings of the 33rd Annual Association of Avian Veterinarians Conference and Expo*, 2012, p 321.
34. Petritz OA, Sanchez-Migallon Guzman D, Paul-Murphy J, et al: Evaluation of the efficacy and safety of single administration of 4.7-mg deslorelin acetate implants on egg production and plasma sex hormones in Japanese quail (*Coturnix coturnix japonica*), *Am J Vet Res* 74:316–323, 2013.

35. Petritz O, Guzman DS, Hawkins M, et al: Evaluation of deslorelin acetate implant dosage on egg production and plasma progesterone in Japanese quail (*Coturnix coturnix japonica*). In *Proceedings of the 34th Annual Conference of the Association of Avian Veterinarians*, 2013, p 17.

36. Schmidt F, Legler M, Einspanier A, et al: Influence of the GnRH-slow release agonist deslorelin on the gonadal activity of Japanese quail (*Coturnix coturnix japonica*). In *Proceedings of the 1st International Conference on Avian, Herpetological and Exotic Mammal Medicine*, 2013, pp 501–502.

37. Cowan ML, Martin GB, Monks DJ, et al: Inhibition of the reproductive system by deslorelin in male and female pigeons (*Columba livia*), *J Avian Med Surg* 28:102–108, 2014.

38. Asa C, Porton IJ: *Wildlife contraception: issues, methods, and applications*, Baltimore, MD, 2005, The Johns Hopkins University Press.

39. Asa C, Boutelle S: Contraception. In Miller R, Fowler M, editors: *Fowler's zoo and wild animal medicine current therapy*, vol 7, St. Louis, MO, 2011, Elsevier, pp 8–14.

40. Trigg TE, Doyle AG, Walsh JD, et al: A review of advances in the use of the GnRH agonist deslorelin in control of reproduction, *Theriogenology* 66:1507–1512, 2006.

ENDOSURGICAL METHODS FOR REDUCING REPRODUCTIVE SUCCESS

Michael Lierz

Whereas any hormonal treatment is reversible, surgical interaction with the reproductive tract is permanent. In general, surgical interventions do initially carry anesthetic and procedural risks but usually do not require re-treatment. The following section focuses on the surgical techniques to decrease reproductive success prophylactically in avian patients.

Decreasing reproductive success is usually reached by sterilization or castration of males or females. Both are a routine procedure in veterinary medicine. Beside improvement of meat quality, modification of behavior, control of feral pet populations, or adaptation to the owner for an easier keeping are reasons for such interventions. In domestic bird species, male chickens are castrated in some countries to improve their meat quality. However, the owners of nondomestic bird species may, at times, also require or request such interventions for some of the following reasons:

◆ Castration of male and ovariectomy of female birds as an effort to reduce sexually related aggression
◆ Ovariectomy and sterilization of female pet birds to prevent chronic egg laying
◆ Castration and sterilization to control free-ranging populations (feral pigeons, geese)[1,2]
◆ Sterilization of male birds to stimulate female partners, especially for assisted reproduction techniques[3,4]
◆ Legal requirements to castrate or sterilize species hybrids to avoid introduction of foreign genetic material in free-ranging native populations[5,6]

Surgical techniques should overall be as minimally invasive as possible, and endoscopy-guided surgical procedures seem to offer a great advantage in this regard. Besides being minimally invasive, the gonads that are located at the cranial division of the kidney are far easier to reach by endoscopic guided techniques compared with open surgical methods. Magnification that is provided by the endoscope can be used to improve visibility of the structures of the reproductive tract, particularly in juvenile birds. The basic requirements

and basic techniques for endoscopic guided surgery are described in more detail elsewhere.[5-8]

Different endoscopic techniques are described, and the use of a single-entry technique is the most common. In this method, a single instrument is directed through the working channel of the endoscope into the visual field. This means that the instrument cannot be manipulated independently from the endoscope. When using a double entry technique, an additional cannula (working channel) with trocar is inserted into the bird, enabling the surgeon to work with two different instruments. By using the triple entry technique, two cannulas are placed in addition to the endoscope, which is placed centrally. As with all surgical procedures, hemostasis must be maintained. Therefore, laser or radiosurgical units may be necessary augmentations of the experienced endosurgeon's skillset. For most bird species, 2-mm to 3-mm human pediatric laparoscopy equipment (Karl Storz Inc., Tuttlingen, Germany) is used for endosurgery.[8] For the purpose of endocastration and sterilization, the basic endoscopic equipment (2.7-mm 30-degree telescope within working channel, flexible biopsy and grasping forceps, endoscissors) should have monopolar parts that are connectable to the radiosurgery unit. Bipolar forceps and a monopolar sling are necessary in addition to this basic endoscopic equipment for some endosterilization procedures.

The surgery starts with the preparation of the surgical field, as in a normal endoscopic examination. The anesthetized patient is placed in right lateral recumbency, and the left pelvic limb is pulled caudally, with the approach caudal to the last rib.[5] Additional cannulas are placed cranioventrally to the endoscope between the last two ribs (double entry) and ventrocaudally to the endoscope (triple entry). This enables a perfect triangulation of the two cannulas with the endoscope central, which is important (Figures 12-21 and 12-22). Alternatively, the left pelvic limb can be pulled cranially.[6,7]

Endoscopic Ovariectomy

The ovary is closely attached to the cranial division of the kidney, and is well vascularized and fragile. Therefore,

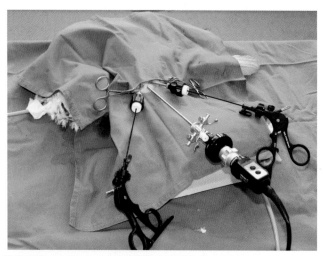

FIGURE 12-21 Endosurgical setup using a triple entry technique. The endoscope needs to be placed in the center of the additional working channels for an optimal view and handling.

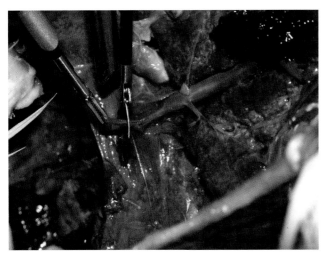

FIGURE 12-22 Triangulation of the endoscope and working channels containing the instruments is most important when using endoscopy-guided surgical techniques.

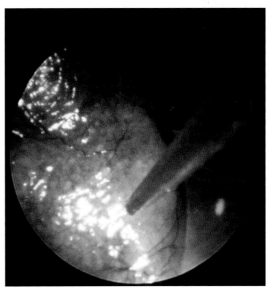

FIGURE 12-23 A diode laser is forwarded toward the ovarian tissue through the working channel of the endoscope. First, the diode laser is used in contact mode because adsorption of laser light by gonadal tissue is not optimal until the first vaporization has occurred.

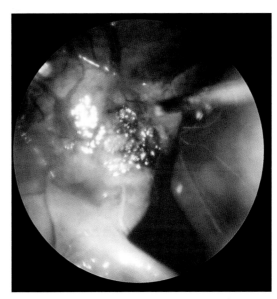

FIGURE 12-24 After starting vaporization of the ovarian tissue in contact mode, the procedure is continued in the noncontact mode of the light fiber until the complete ovarian tissue is vaporized.

complete removal is generally considered very risky and often is incomplete, leaving hormone-producing ovarian tissue inside. Therefore, ovariectomy in adult birds is not recommended. However, removal of ovarian tissue in juvenile birds was demonstrated by laser vaporization in falcons with success, whereas it failed in 6-week-old chickens.[9] Therefore, this method is recommended in birds with small inactive juvenile ovaries. The advantage of this technique is that only the endoscope in a working channel is introduced into the bird and the light fiber of the diode laser is inserted through the working channel directly to the ovary. The power of 1 watt was efficient enough to vaporize the ovarian tissue. Increasing the power of the laser resulted in a faster rate of tissue vaporization but increased the amount of smoke and vapor produced, which, in turn, caused severe respiratory distress in the anesthetized birds—even death. For this reason, care should be taken to ensure that only minor, nearly nonvisible amounts of smoke and vapor are produced during this procedure. The diode laser has to be used first in contact mode until the ovarian capsule is damaged, followed by the noncontact mode as light absorption by the tissue is sufficient (Figures 12-23 through 12-25). Care should be taken to only vaporize ovarian tissue and not too deeply beneath the ovary, since its arterial and venous supplies are located below the ovary and a risk of hemorrhage exists. It is advantageous to first vaporize the border of the ovary and then work toward the middle to avoid collateral tissue damage. Smaller hemorrhages can usually be controlled by the laser; however, damage of large vessels may lead to uncontrollable blood loss.

Endoscopic Salpingohysterectomy

In juvenile birds, a grasping forceps can be introduced through the endoscope working channel (single-entry technique). The infundibulum can be grasped and the oviduct removed from underlying tissue by gentle pulling. By this way it is possible to remove nearly the entire oviduct without significant hemorrhage[10] (Figure 12-26). Obliteration of the oviduct by electrocautery or laser is not recommended, since

oviductal cysts have been described to occur later.[10] In the author's experience, the ovary develops with the age and overall maturity of the bird. In a study in juvenile female cockatiels ranging in age from 3 to 11 months, no external complications were observed 4 to 10 months following endoscopic salpingohysterectomy, in the absence of repeat endoscopic examinations.[11] However, as the ovary remains after this procedure, further studies are needed to investigate the longer-term effects of endoscopic salpingohysterectomy in juvenile birds with regard to the benefits in the prevention of

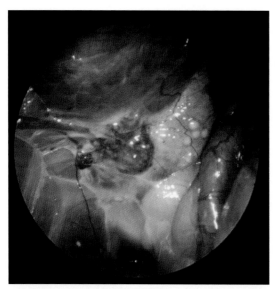

FIGURE 12-25 The juvenile ovary is vaporized, leaving only minor amounts of charred tissue.

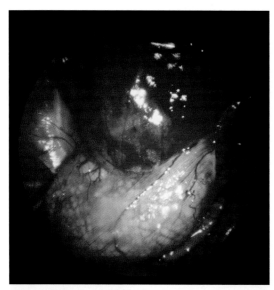

FIGURE 12-26 Endoscopic view on the cranial division of the kidney with the ovary in front. Note that the suspensory ligament of the oviduct and parts of the oviduct are lacking because of its removal by endoscopic sterilization.

ovulation and other reproductively associated problems. In adult birds, the oviduct should be endoscopically removed using a double-entry or triple-entry technique. The oviduct is held by a grasping forceps and obliterated as far cranially as possible by using a monopolar or bipolar grasping forceps through a second entry port. A second obliteration is placed slightly behind the first one, followed by a cut of the oviduct between both obliterations by using a monopolar scissor. The same procedure is then repeated at the most caudal part of the oviduct that can be accessed, and the oviduct can be removed. As in juvenile birds, long-term studies are necessary to assess the benefits and risks of further ovulations occurring.

Endoscopic Castration of Male Birds

Castration of males should ideally be performed when they are juveniles, as the testicles are small, with low and controllable blood supply. In juvenile birds, single-entry or, ideally, double-entry techniques are used. The testicle is grasped and removed by a radiosurgical sling, obliterating the testicular vessels when closing the sling. In very young birds, the testicle can be grasped by a forceps and taken out after monopolar coagulation with a radiosurgical probe touching the tip of the forceps or even without any coagulation if there is poorly developed vasculature.

Successful vaporization of the juvenile testicles has been described in 6-week-old chickens and juvenile falcons[9]. Testicular tissue was completely removed by minor collateral damage of surrounding tissue, with only mild side effects during surgery, demonstrated by histologic evaluation of the surgical field. In falcons only 0.5 watts were necessary to achieve this complete removal.[9] Parallel to the ovarian tissue, the organ is vaporized first in contact mode followed by the noncontact mode (Figures 12-27 and 12-28). As described with this equivalent procedure in females, care should be taken to avoid increased smoke and vapor production. Laser vaporization is highly advantageous in juvenile birds, in which the small testes are closely attached to the kidney (e.g., falcons) and cannot be separated from underlying tissue, especially large vessels. In other bird species such as chickens the juvenile testicles are already solid organs, completely detached from the cranial pole of the kidney. In those species, grasping the testicles would be preferred rather than laser vaporization.

The castration of adult male birds seems only possible using a double-entry or triple-entry technique. Especially the triple-entry technique allows a better view into the surgical field (Figure 12-29). First, the testicle is elevated from the kidney by using a grasping forceps through the working channel of the endoscope (double-entry technique) or an extra

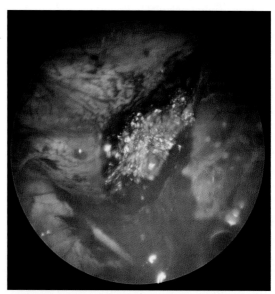

FIGURE 12-27 Endoscopic view of the surgical field of a vaporized testicle of a juvenile gyr-saker hybrid falcon. Only a minor amount of the remaining charred tissue is visible.

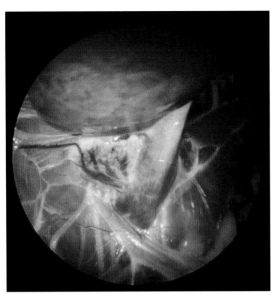

FIGURE 12-28 The same bird as in Figure 12-27 8 weeks later. The lack of testicular tissue is clearly visible, and only very scant charred tissue remains.

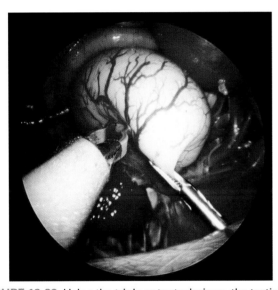

FIGURE 12-29 Using the triple entry technique, the testicle of an adult bird is lifted for better access to the deferent duct or to cauterize the supplying blood vessels in order to remove the testicle completely.

entry port (triple-entry technique). The mesorchium is then cut by using monopolar coagulation scissors. Larger blood vessels should be separately coagulated by using a bipolar forceps followed by removal of the organ. Laser vaporization of the testicles of adult males is usually impossible, as tissue material is too much for complete vaporization without significant risk of adverse side effects. With increasing activation of the hypothalamic–pituitary–gonadal (HPG) axis, the blood supply to this organ is increased. Therefore, sexually active males should not be castrated as the potential risk of fatal hemorrhage is higher. Castration of adult birds should always be performed in phases of reproductive inactivity. Conversely,

endoscopic vasectomy (see below) is more readily accomplished during phases of reproductive activity.

It needs to be kept in mind that laser (electrosurgery to some point as well) applies a high amount of power onto a very focal point. Usually, birds are anesthetized with volatile anesthetics, using pure oxygen as a carrier gas. This results in risk that the laser may cause fire in the oxygen-saturated environment.[12] Therefore, pure oxygen should be avoided as carrier gas in case laser intervention is planned, and pressurized air can be added to lower the delivered oxygen concentrations.

Sterilization of Male Birds—Vasectomy

Sterilization of male birds has been described using a laparotomy.[12] In general, the endosurgical technique and approach employed are similar to those used in juvenile female birds for salpingohysterectomy (single portal of entry, left flank approach). In juvenile males, the ductus deferens can be grasped and removed by a pulling action, using a grasping forceps through the endoscope working channel[10] (Figure 12-30). By using this method in Japanese quails, it was demonstrated that the testicles continued to develop uneventfully and that the testosterone blood levels increase with sexual maturity as in unsterilized males. In addition, the reproductive behaviors of vasectomized males were unaltered.[6] It is advantageous to first use a biopsy forceps to open the serosa and then grasping the deferent duct with a grasping forceps. This method minimizes the primary risk of damaging the ureter, which often parallels the deferent duct. As an alternative, the deferent duct can also be obliterated by electrosurgery. Cystic development, as was observed with radiosurgical obliteration of the oviduct of females, has not been observed with this equivalent procedure on the ductus of males. Radiosurgical obliteration, however, can be very difficult in the inactive or juvenile bird, as the risk of collateral damage to the ureter might occur.

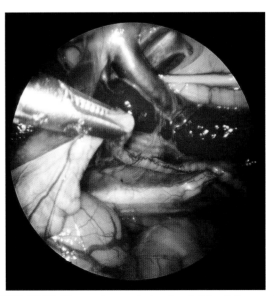

FIGURE 12-30 The active and clearly visible deferent duct (note the garlandlike appearance) is already detached from the underlying tissue and can now be more easily removed.

In adults, particularly reproductively active individuals, sterilization via vasectomy is more easily accomplished by endoscopically teasing away the deferent duct from the ureter. The deferent duct is very prominent with a garlandlike appearance (see Figure 12-30). The differentiation from the ureter is also more straightforward. As in juvenile birds, the serosa should be cut, allowing the deferent duct to be grasped and pulled out (see Figure 12-30). The duct will usually rupture, and the ends should be regrasped so that the surgeon can remove as much of the duct as possible. Gently pulling to allow the duct to detach from the serosa is highly recommended. In rare cases, active testicles might obscure the cranial parts of the deferent duct. In these situations, a double-entry or triple-entry technique is required, which enables manipulation of the testicle to the side, which results in an elevation of the deferent duct. This, in turn, makes it easier to reach the duct before it attaches to the surface of the kidney. Usually, the best location to reach the deferent duct is directly adjacent to the testicle. It is highly recommended to remove at least 1 cm of the duct to avoid re-establishment of functional patency if both ends reunify. This complication has been described in the past.[5,10] Procedural risk of endoscopy-guided surgical sterilization of males is very low, and anesthesia-associated risks are only slightly increased. Unwanted tissue damage (e.g., ureter, kidney, adrenal gland) might rarely occur, and the risk is certainly reduced with increasing experience of the surgeon. A large study in which male feral city pigeons were sterilized for population control by using the above-described method clearly demonstrated that the technique is highly effective, has a low risk, and is quick once experience is gained.[1]

REFERENCES

1. Heiderich L, Schildger B, Lierz M: Endoscopic vasectomy of male feral pigeons (*Columba livia*) as a possible method of population control, *J Avian Med Surg* 29(1):9–17, 2015.
2. Converse KA, Kenelly JJ: Evaluation of Canada goose sterilisation for population control, *Wildl Soc Bull* 22:112–117, 1994.
3. Lierz M: Raptors: reproductive disease, incubation and artificial insemination. In Chitty, J, Lierz M, editors: *BSAVA manual of raptors, pigeons and passerine birds*, Gloucester, U.K., 2008, British Small Animal Veterinary Association, pp 235–249.
4. Lierz M, Reinschmidt M, Müller H, et al: A novel method for semen collection and artificial insemination in large parrots (Psittaciformes), *Sci Rep* 3:2066, 2013.
5. Lierz M: Endoscopy, biopsy and endosurgery. In Chitty J, Lierz M, editors: *BSAVA manual of raptors, pigeons and passerine birds*, Gloucester, U.K., 2008, British Small Animal Veterinary Association, pp 128–142.
6. Jones R, Redig PT: Endoscopy guided vasectomy in the immature Japanese quail (*Coturnix coturnix japonica*). In *Proceedings of the 7th Conference of the European Association of Avian Veterinarians and the 5th Scientific meeting of the European College of Avian Medicine and Surgery*, Spain, April 22–26, 2003, pp 117–123.
7. Hernandez-Divers SJ, Stahl SJ, Wilson GH, et al: Endoscopic orchidectomy and salpingohysterectomy of pigeons (*Columba livia*): an avian model for minimally invasive endosurgery, *J Avian Med Surg* 21:22–37, 2007.
8. Lierz M: Endoskopie. In Pees M, editor: *Leitsymptome bei Papageien und Sittichen*, Stuttgart, Germany, 2004, Enke Verlag, pp 185–194.
9. Lierz M, Gruber AD, Wittschen P, et al: Endoscopic castration of male and female falcons. In *Proceedings of the 10th Conference of the European Association of Avian Veterinarians and 8th Scientific Meeting of the European College of Avian Medicine and Surgery*, Antwerp, Belgium, March 17–21, 2009, pp 75–77.
10. Lierz M, Hafez HM: Endoscopy guided multiple entry surgery in birds. In *Proceedings of the Conference of the European Association of Avian Medicine and the European College of Avian Medicine and Surgery*, Arles, France, 2005, pp 184–189.
11. Pye GW, Bennett RA, Plunske R, et al: Endoscopic salpingohysterectomy of juvenile cockatiels (*Nymphicus hollandicus*), *J Avian Med Surg* 15:90–94, 2001.
12. Lierz P, Lierz M, Gustorff B, et al: Management of intratracheal fire during laser surgery in veterinary medicine, *Internet J Vet Med* 2:2, 2006.

ADVANCEMENTS IN METHODS FOR DECREASING REPRODUCTIVE SUCCESS

Jaime Samour

External Vasectomy

External vasectomy is the surgical removal of a portion of the ductus deferens on either side of the cloaca with the objective to induce infertility. This procedure has been carried out to prepare teaser budgerigar (*Melopsittacus undulatus*) males for an artificial insemination program[1] and for studies on the fertile period of zebra finches (*Taeniopygia guttata*) and society finches (*Lonchura striata domestica*).[2]

Anatomic considerations

The ductus deferens is a tortuous tubule originated from the epididymis, on the dorsal aspect of the testis, running alongside the ureter, across the dorsal aspect of the coelom, and penetrating the dorsal wall of the urodeum, where it forms the short papilla of the ductus deferens. In seasonal species, its diameter increases significantly during the culmination phase of the breeding cycle.[3]

In many species of passerine birds studied, to date,[3] and the budgerigar,[1,4] the caudal portion of the ductus deferens forms a paired convoluted structure denominated the *seminal glomera*, located on the lateral lower section of the coelomic cavity. During the culmination phase of the breeding cycle, the seminal glomera increases in size and volume, forming small rounded swellings that bulge on either side of the cloaca. These swellings are commonly referred to as *cloacal promontory*. These structures can be used to determine the sex of passerine birds during the breeding season. In these species, the seminal glomera is used as a storage site maintaining the spermatozoa at approximately 3.9° C (39° F) lower than the deep rectal temperature.[3]

Anesthesia and surgical considerations

General anesthesia is induced and maintained using isoflurane (Forane, Abbott Laboratories, Queenborough, England) delivered through a custom-made face mask adequate for the size of the species. In small species such as budgerigars or finches, a small operating table made of acrylic top and aluminum sides measuring 20 cm long, 12 cm wide, and 10 cm high was used to ease the surgical procedure. The acrylic top was molded to accommodate the shape of the small birds. A heating mat was placed underneath the table in order to provide temperature by conduction of approximately 27.7° to 29.4° C

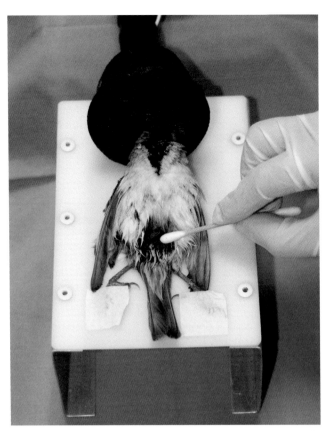

FIGURE 12-31 General anesthesia is induced and maintained using isoflurane delivered through a custom-made face mask adequate for the size of the species. A small operating table with an acrylic top and aluminum sides measuring 20 cm long, 12 cm wide, and 10 cm high is used to facilitate handling of the surgical procedure. The acrylic top is molded to accommodate the shape of small birds. A heating mat is placed underneath the table in order to provide temperature by conduction of approximately 27.7° to 29.4° C (82° to 85° F) to the table top.

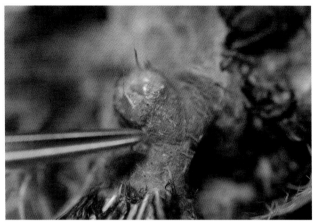

FIGURE 12-32 The seminal glomus in a common house sparrow *(Passer domesticus)* is identified as a mass immediately below the skin beside the cloaca. During the culmination phase of the breeding cycle, the seminal glomera increases in size and volume, forming small, rounded swellings bulging on either side of the cloaca. These swellings are commonly termed *cloacal promontory* and can be used to determine the sex of passerine birds during the breeding season.

(82° to 85° F) to the operating tabletop (Figure 12-31). The use of this operating table greatly enhanced the ability of the attending veterinarian to conduct the surgery.[1]

Surgical technique

External vasectomy is indicated in those species that possess seminal glomera.[1,5] After anesthesia, the bird is placed on the dorsal position and the legs secured caudally by using masking tape. The lower abdominal wall beside the cloaca is plucked and prepared for surgery. A small surgical incision (3 to 5 mm) is made midway on the straight line between the cloaca and the pubic bone. The use of magnification is highly recommended. In previous studies with budgerigars, and zebra and society finches,[1,2,5] all external vasectomies were carried out under a ×10 operating microscope. In a more recent study, using common house sparrows *(Passer domesticus)*, vasectomies were carried out with the aid of a ×6 surgical binocular loupe (Heine Optotechnik, Herrsching, Germany) and was found to be adequate.[6] The use of a fine-tipped, blunted probe eases the debriding and differentiating of the ductus deferens within the subcutaneous space (Figures 12-32 and

12-33). After identification, the ductus deferens is grasped by using a pair of fine-tip dissecting forceps, and a small section (5 to 8 mm) is severed by using a pair of fine-tip microsurgery scissors (Figure 12-34). The same procedure is carried out on the opposite side while maintaining the bird in the same position. No ligature or hemoclip placement is considered necessary. The skin is sutured by using one or two interrupted stitches with 5/0 absorbable suturing material (Surgicryl, smi AG, Hünningen, Belgium).[1,6] Correct placement of the stitches is essential to avoid exerting tension on the cloaca because tenesmus has been previously reported in budgerigars during the postoperative period.[1]

Postoperative fertility assessment

After vasectomy, it is essential to assess the effectiveness of the procedure by using a functional assay. Different techniques

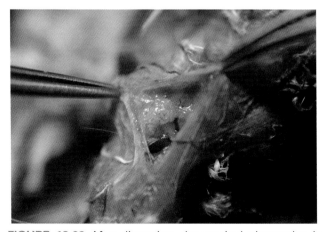

FIGURE 12-33 After dissection, the seminal glomerulus is identified as a relatively large round mass formed by the convoluted ductus deferens.

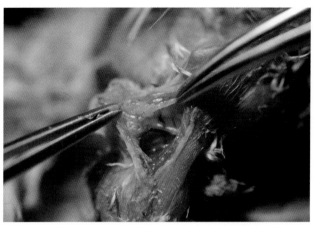

FIGURE 12-34 The ductus deferens is grasped by using a pair of fine-tip dissecting forceps, and a small section (5 mm to 8 mm) is severed by using a pair of fine-tip microsurgery scissors. The same procedure is carried out on the opposite side while maintaining the bird in the same position.

have been used in previous studies. In this respect, semen collection was attempted in vasectomized male budgerigars at monthly intervals, followed by examination of any fluid obtained during the process by using standard light microscopy techniques.[1,7] Conversely, vasectomized male zebra finches and male society finches were all paired up with females and allowed copulation and egg laying. Following oviposition and natural incubation, or artificial incubation, fertility was assessed through candling, or by opening up and examining the internal content of the eggs in order to assess fertility.[2]

External vasectomy in passerine birds and the budgerigar can be carried out by following the surgical procedure described above. However, vasectomy does not arrest courtship and copulatory behavior, and orchidectomy should be considered instead as an alternative method to eliminate sexual behavior and to produce permanent infertility in birds.

REFERENCES

1. Samour J, Markham JA: Vasectomy in budgerigars, *Vet Rec* 120:115, 1987.
2. Birkhead TR: Sperm storage and the fertile period in the Bengalese finch, *Auk* 109(3):620–625, 1992.
3. King AS, McLelland J: Male reproductive system. In King AS, McLelland J, editors: *Birds: their structure and function*, London, U.K., 1984, Baillière Tindall, pp 166–174.
4. Samour J, Spratt DMJ, Holt WV, et al: Ultrastructure and secretory nature of the seminal glomus in budgerigars (*Melopsittacus undulatus*), *Res Vet Sci* 45:194–197, 1988.
5. Birkhead TR, Pellatt JE: Vasectomy in small passerine birds, *Vet Rec* 125:646, 1989.
6. Samour J: Vasectomy in birds: a review, *J Avian Med Surg* 24(3): 169–173, 2010.
7. Samour J: Semen collection, spermatozoa cryopreservation and artificial insemination in non-domesticated birds, *J Avian Med Surg* 18(4):219–223, 2004.

CHAPTER 13

Advances in Clinical Pathology and Diagnostic Medicine

Elizabeth Marie Rush • Morena Wernick • Hugues Beaufrère • Mélanie Ammersbach • Claire Vergneau-Grosset • Nicole Stacy • Helene Pendl • James F.X. Wellehan Jr • Kristin Warren • Anna Le Souef • Crissa Cooey • Hillar Klandorf

FOUNDATIONS IN CLINICAL PATHOLOGY

Elizabeth Marie Rush, Morena Wernick

Clinical pathology is the diagnosis of disease based on laboratory analysis of body fluids through hematology, chemistry, microbiology, and molecular pathology. These may include blood, urine, and tissue extracts or homogenates. In the avian patient, hematology and biochemistry are commonly used in conjunction with clinical examination of a patient to evaluate overall health. This chapter will discuss the methods in clinical pathology that are available and useful in the evaluation of avian patients in clinical practice.

Physical examination is important when considering assessment of health status with the assistance of clinical pathology samples. Up to 10% of the blood volume (approximately 1% of the body weight in grams) can typically be collected from a healthy bird.[1] However, in the ill or unthrifty patient, the clinician should consider the possible detrimental effect of sample collection on the patient versus the anticipated benefit of the results that may be obtained from laboratory diagnostic evaluations.

The right jugular vein is convenient and generally used for obtaining blood samples in most of the avian species. Pressure may be applied to the site after venipuncture to avoid hemorrhage into the cervical subcutaneous space or cervicocephalic air sacs. The right jugular vein is generally larger than the left jugular vein, and in many species, there are apteria, or a featherless tract, present over the right jugular furrow. Easy visualization of the vessel is achieved by light air application to the surrounding feathers or dampening with water, isopropyl alcohol, or saline and dividing surrounding feathers. Some Columbiformes and Anseriformes lack apteria, which complicates the direct visualization of the vessel. In these species, blood sample collection via the jugular is best accomplished through restraint, with the bird's neck extended and head stabilized, and by applying pressure to the distal jugular near the thoracic inlet to distend and stabilize the mobile vessel. The cutaneous ulnar wing vein, or basilic vein is a common site for blood collection in medium to large birds. This vessel crosses the ventral surface of the humeroradioulnar joint and is typically readily visible in the healthy patient. Appropriate stabilization of the wing is necessary for venipuncture at this site, and blood can be collected via needle and syringe or with a capillary tube. The medial metatarsal vein is also an acceptable site for venipuncture in many bird species. This vein (caudal tibial) courses down the medial aspect of the tibiotarsus and crosses over the medial aspect of the hock (tibiotarsus–tarsometatarsal joint). With the leg stabilized, the needle is also introduced at a shallow angle into the vein for blood collection. As with the blood collection from the jugular vein, after collection from the wing or leg, apply pressure at the site of collection, as needed, to prevent hemorrhage.[2] The toenail clip method of blood sample collection has been described in the literature for blood collection in smaller birds. The collected capillary blood often contains cellular debris and macrophages and cells such as osteoblasts and osteoclasts, which are not normally found in peripheral blood.[3] This method is generally not recommended because of the questionable accuracy of the results as well as for the comfort of the bird.

Blood smears are still of tremendous importance in avian clinical pathology. Several preanalytical errors could occur in the preparation of the smears. The blood cells of birds are generally much more fragile than those of mammals. Some of the slide-to-slide techniques used in mammalian medicine may lead to cellular artifacts such as formation of smudge cells. Smudge cells most often represent ruptured leukocytes and interfere with appropriate quantitation and differentiation of cells.[1] Blood smears should always be made at the time of blood collection, since smears from aging whole blood will show a considerable decrease in cell quality. Serial collection methods should remain consistent to avoid misinterpretation of artifact.[1-14]

Care must be exercised when handling blood specimens and in packing for shipment, since sample vials can be broken or improper application of tops may lead to leaks. Hematology samples exposed to formalin fumes show marked degradation in cell morphology, decreasing the accuracy of differential counts.[1] Prior to filling a tube with the collected blood sample, the date and the identification of the bird should be written on the printed label of the collection tube in order to avoid any confusion. This is particularly important when several samples are collected from different patients at the same time. Ensure that the correct test has been ordered for the correct patient.

REFERENCE RANGES AND STATISTICAL ANALYSIS METHODS

Reference ranges have been established for many of the avian species. These ranges are determined through original studies of healthy species. Data are contributed by the cooperating institutions to central databases for cataloguing of complete blood count (CBC) and biochemical values. Databases are used to develop normal reference values for individual species and related groups.[15-20] These reference values can be used by the veterinary clinician to assess health in patients.

Reference ranges should be established for each species because there are often differences in ranges between, and within, subgroups of a species.[21-49] These differences between and within the subgroups may be related to health, gender, age, reproductive status, breed, and environmental or husbandry conditions (e.g., temperature, humidity, diet).[50-85] Values within the database, influenced by these factors, limited the populations of some species, and the expense of establishing values may also decrease the statistical significance of some of the reference ranges of some species. The minimum number of animals acceptable for establishment of a normal reference range is 40; however, it is ideal to have 120 animals sampled to establish a more statistically reliable reference range.[86-90]

Statistical methods are applied to the values obtained from these studies, and various methods may be used to establish reference ranges. The method used depends on the distribution of values from the sample population. If the values are plotted on the basis of frequency of occurrence and form a bell-shaped, or Gaussian, curve, they are considered normal. Parametric tests can be applied to normal values. However, if the curve is not bell shaped, then these methods are not reliable, and other statistical methods to produce a more Gaussian curve may be applied, or nonparametric statistics may be used. It is not accurate to merely visually evaluate the curve, and statistical methods should be used to determine if distribution is normal. Often, it is best to consider that results are not parametric and apply statistics accordingly, and this will lead to reliable results that are comparable with those that would have been found using parametric methods, if applicable.[86-90]

Even with normal distribution of values, there will be values that fall outside of the curve. These are called *outliers*, and they are typically markedly higher or lower than the other values. Inclusion of outliers in the final reference range calculations will widen the range, which decreases the sensitivity of the test for unhealthy animals being compared with the reference values. However, removal of these outliers will narrow the range and increase the sensitivity but may exclude some healthy animals that are valuable references. There are different methods of exclusion for some of these outliers to allow for the most accurate establishment of a reference range, and these are commonly applied when interpreting results of prospective laboratory studies. Ultimately, the range typically includes 95% of the study population, with 5% of the study animals falling outside the normal range and thus those values discarded.[89]

In some cases, especially with respect to reference values, there is a limit below or above which there is no clinical significance to an individual's level. When this is the case, the reference range will often end at a value that represents that limit. This is the cutoff value, or threshold value.[89]

Sensitivity and Specificity

Sensitivity, specificity, and predictive values must be considered when interpreting clinical pathology results and potential laboratory abnormalities in a patient. Sensitivity and specificity are statistical measures of a binary classification test, also known as *classification function*. Sensitivity is sometimes called the "true-positive rate" because it measures the proportion of actual positives identified correctly by a research method. For example, in a study of people who have a certain condition, the number of sick people who are identified correctly by the testing method as having the condition is the true-positive rate. The true-positive rate is complementary to the false-negative rate. A positive result on a test with high sensitivity does not help to rule in disease because it does not take into account false positives. A test with high sensitivity is reliable when its test result is negative because it rarely misdiagnoses individuals with disease. This is the characteristic that makes a test with high sensitivity a good choice for an initial screening test in a population. A clinician can be confident that a negative result is true, whereas a positive result will require confirmation, likely using a test with a high specificity.[89,90] The specificity is also called the true-negative rate and identifies the percentage of negatives that are correctly identified in a sampled population. So, in the same study, this would be the group of healthy individuals who are correctly identified by the testing method as not having the disease. This is complementary to the false-positive rate. Specificity indicates the ability of a test to accurately exclude a condition. A test with a high specificity is very useful for ruling in disease and rarely gives positive results for healthy individuals. If a test has 100% specificity, it will read negative for 100% to exclude disease from all healthy individuals. However, a positive result indicates a high probability of disease presence in an individual. Ideally, a predictor would be perfect and have 100% sensitivity and specificity. The predictive value, or precision, of a test is the ratio of true positives to combined true and false positives.[90]

Prevalence and Incidence

When working with larger groups of individuals or samples, the proportion of animals found to have a condition (usually a risk factor or disease) is known as the prevalence of the condition within that population. Prevalence is expressed as a proportion and usually describes something that is widespread or evenly distributed throughout a group, that is, the routine burden of a disease among a given population. Prevalence is often contrasted with incidence, which is a measure of new cases that arise in a group over a given amount of time. This is important when looking at flocks or breeding groups of birds and evaluating them for rate of new cases of infection with a disease, genetic abnormalities, or other conditions. The prevalence of a condition among the population may be considered normal; however, an increase in the incidence of the condition could be indicative of a problem.[90] An example of a disease where prevalence and incidence were used to indicate a disease introduction is the introduction of West Nile virus (WNV) in the United States in 1999. WNV quickly spread across North America and had a high prevalence among raptor species. In 2013 and 2014, there were several incidences of WNV, which were noted in specific locations throughout the United States and caused severe disease in bald eagles and hawks. This increase in incidence, or unexpected cases, in these two populations was significant, but the incidences appear to have been localized and limited in their time of occurrence, thus not altering the overall prevalence of WNV in those populations.

Precision and Accuracy

In an ideal setting, a test would be both precise and accurate, where accuracy represents how well a test correctly identifies or excludes a condition or disease, and precision represents the ratio of true positives to combined true and false positives. Accuracy is therefore the proportion of true positives and true negatives in the population. When a test has an accuracy of 100%, it means that the measured values are the same as the given values.[87-90]

LABORATORY TESTING AND SELECTION OF OPTIONS

Clinicians routinely decide between using in-house laboratory analysis or sending blood samples out to commercial laboratories. The decision will depend on many variables, including patient condition, test expense, turnaround time, and reliability of test results with respect to various testing methods. Specific samples may be required for diagnosis of some pathologic processes or conditions.[91-104] In-house analyzers give rapid diagnostics but may yield variable results when compared with each other. It is best to consistently use the same analyzer for chemistry analysis for an individual or group. Reagents used in bench-top analyzers should be consistent over time so that reference ranges are developed in-house. Altering reagents or analyzer manufacturers can yield variability in results and make long-term in-house reference ranges less reliable.[105-107] Some analytes may not be reliable if measured using in-house chemistry analyzers or using methods that have been developed for other nonavian species,[8,108] whereas others may correlate well in some species but not in others.[109-112] Point-of-care analyzers come with standard calibration and testing methods and schedules to ensure quality control. All manufacturer guidelines for use of the instrument should be followed regularly to ensure that uniformity is maintained for sample testing.[105-107] Consistency in sample collection, handling, and laboratory analysis will allow for the accurate comparison of results over time and the establishment of more reliable reference ranges for a greater number of avian species using in-house or point-of-care analyzers.

When choosing a commercial laboratory, it is important to consider cost benefits and turnaround time for results, as well as the variety of testing offered for avian patients. Although many laboratories may offer laboratory services for avian species, few have long-term experience with avian samples, so it is important for the clinician to choose a company that has reliable reference ranges for avian species and uses precise, species-specific instrumentation for animal specimens. It is recommended that clinicians consider requesting a copy of quality control measures and standards for calibration of instrumentation, including reagents used for avian samples. Consultation with specialists and pathologists is available with some larger laboratories, and this can be an advantage for the submitting clinician, especially at commercial laboratories that routinely handle avian samples. Human laboratories may have the capability to run samples but lack adequate quality control for avian samples. This may result in variability of results and a decrease in reliability.

CONSIDERATIONS FOR INDIVIDUAL BIRD TESTING

Introduction of new birds to an existing collection can be an anxious time for both owners and attending veterinarians. Biosecurity is crucial to successful avian collection management and requires both a vigilant owner and an engaged veterinarian. At a minimum, each bird should receive a physical examination and evaluation of history prior to introduction into an existing facility. Owners should be offered not only the physical examination for their bird but also should be provided with informed options for some commonly performed laboratory evaluations, including complete blood counts, disease testing, blood chemistry, and gender determination, where applicable. The details of specific analyses that may be considered are further discussed in this section. Basic physical evaluation and laboratory testing may be a limiting financial factor for some owners. In the case where financial limitations are a factor, discussions between the owner and the veterinarian will help establish what diagnostics and or procedures offer the greatest benefit for the individual bird or population of concern. Case-based laboratory diagnostic selection can significantly decrease expense for the owner but may limit critical information for future comparison with other samples. Quarantine is always recommended when introducing a bird into a multiple-bird facility. A common quarantine of 30 to 45 days is recommended in many, but not all, situations. Specific details of the duration of quarantine period and diagnostic procedures implemented are dependent on species and disease of concern, among other variables.[113] The clinician should also recognize the limitations of analysis performed on samples, as some may have limited ability to predict disease or the presence of some pathogens.

LABORATORY ERRORS

Laboratories play a major role in patient care and diagnosis of disease. Automation is standard in most veterinary diagnostic laboratories dealing with clinical pathology submissions; however, variables may still result in false results. The more common variables resulting in errors can be divided into three major categories: preanalytical errors, analytical errors, and postanalytical errors. Management and recording of errors are mandatory to improve the quality and accuracy of avian laboratory results.

Preanalytical errors may occur any time before processing a sample in the laboratory. In contrast to the common assumption, errors are most likely to occur in this phase and not in the analytical phase, as most laboratories follow strict quality control programs and comply with government regulations to improve their analytical work. In human medicine, preanalytical errors represent up to 68.2% of the total laboratory errors, whereas analytical errors only represent 13.3% and postanalytical errors only 18.5% of total errors.[114] Preanalytical errors are the most common errors made by clinicians and often are easy to prevent or to rectify.

Examples for common preanalytical errors in avian clinical pathology include incorrect sampling methods, sample site collection, choice of anticoagulant, anticoagulant-to-blood ratio; improper packaging, processing or labeling of samples, and incorrect choice of laboratory test to be performed.

ANALYTICAL ERRORS

Especially in avian medicine, collected blood samples have to be quickly processed for cell counting or should be transferred into a collection tube for hematology or blood chemistry in order to prevent hemolysis and clotting.[3] Care must be taken not to forcefully squirt samples through a needle, as this may produce disruption of the fragile blood cells. Chemistry samples should be immediately centrifuged to harvest plasma.[1]

Blood can be collected from various sites. The species, the health of the patient, and the size of the sample needed for testing often influence the choice of collection site. Venous blood is preferred for hematologic studies. For most avian species, ethylenediaminetetraacetic acid (EDTA) is the anticoagulant of choice for hematology samples, since heparin may interfere with staining techniques and alter cytology results. Although EDTA is considered a reliable anticoagulant in avian hematology, blood from several avian groups (e.g., crows, jays, ravens, magpies, and ostriches) and some species of ducks, cranes, and hornbills may show partial hemolysis when collected in EDTA. Most avian blood samples are collected into tubes containing EDTA, heparin, or sodium citrate as anticoagulants. Heparin may then be used as an alternative but may result in clumping of leukocytes and thrombocytes, which makes cell counting inaccurate. The use of heparin may also lead to improper staining of cells, provoking false leukocyte counts.[3] Storing blood samples in sodium citrate is recommended for samples designated for laser flow cytometry. The amount of anticoagulant must be appropriate in comparison with the volume of the blood sample, as an excessive volume will dilute the sample and artificially decrease hematocrit and total cell concentrations.[3] Anesthesia and sample handling may also alter results of clinical pathology sample values in some species.

In the last years, standardization, automation, and technical progresses have significantly improved the analytical reliability of laboratory results in avian medicine.

To prevent analytical errors (errors which occur during laboratory testing), internal laboratory monitoring is of major importance and will significantly decrease the likelihood of analytical errors.

EXAMPLES FOR ANALYTICAL ERRORS IN AVIAN CLINICAL PATHOLOGY

Monitoring and Preparation of Reagents in Avian Hematology

Errors may occur in preparation of cell counting diluent for avian hematology (wrong dilution or diluent not filtered before use, as, for example, necessary for the Natt and Herrick solution).

Improper storage of cell counting diluent (e.g., temperature too low, too high) may allow for degradation. Formol-citrate solution, used with phase contrast microscopy, for example, has to be refrigerated at 8° to 12° C.[115] Overfilling or underfilling of hemocytometer chambers (red blood cell [RBC] counts, white blood cell [WBC] counts) may also lead to errors during manual cell counts. Failure in timely counting (regarding hematocytometer methods) results in overstaining of cells.[5]

Laboratory Equipment

Examples of laboratory equipment not being accurately maintained include failure to annually calibrate balances and pipettes.

Method Validation

Not all methods for automated cell counting or biochemistry analysis used in mammalian medicine are applicable for avian hematology or biochemistry. As avian species have nucleated erythrocytes, impedance counters, for example, are precluded for leukocyte counts in birds.[5]

Thrombocyte counts can be performed by laser flow cytometry, but leukocyte degeneration and swelling can falsely elevate these counts.[5] Results of biochemistry analyzers may vary significantly, depending on the methodology used (e.g., point-of-care-analyzers, bench-top analyzers; see section on Variability and Limitations in Clinical Avian Hematology for further information). Particular measurement techniques may not be reliable in avian medicine, for example, dye-binding methods for protein measurement. Reference intervals used for avian hematology and biochemistry must be species (and analyzer) specific.

Quality Control

Repetition of measurements may be needed if results are outside of expected or acceptable ranges. Performance of test analyses on a regular basis is necessary.

Personnel Requirements

Laboratory analysts must be proficient in avian cell identification—further education and thorough training are mandatory.

POSTANALYTICAL ERRORS

The postanalytical phase can be divided into one phase performed within the laboratory (verifying and communicating laboratory results, insertion of data in the laboratory information system) and a second phase in which the clinician receives and interprets laboratory results. Errors may occur in both phases and generally represent approximately 18.5% of the total laboratory errors.[114]

Examples of Postanalytical Errors
Recording
Results or data may be incorrectly recorded or communicated. This includes transcription errors.

Interpretation
All laboratory tests must be interpreted considering the clinical situation of the patient. This is subjective, and results may vary between interpreters. Reference intervals used must be appropriate for the species and age of the bird.

Turnaround time

Results should be reported in a timely manner. "Critical results" may indicate a life-threatening situation.

CONCLUSION

This chapter is the product of a collaboration of specialists and clinicians in the field of avian medicine and provides information about the logistics, techniques, collection methods, provision of diagnostic tests, and interpretation of clinical pathology tests and laboratory data in the avian species.

REFERENCES

1. Fudge A: Avian blood sampling and artifacts considerations. In Fudge A, editor: *Laboratory medicine: avian and exotic pets*, Philadelphia, PA, 2000, W.B. Saunders Company, pp 1–8.
2. Samour J, Howlett JC: Clinical and diagnostic procedures. In Samour J, editor: *Avian medicine*, ed 2, Philadelphia, PA, 2008, Mosby.
3. Campbell T, Ellis C: Hematology of birds. In Campbell T, Ellis C, editors: *Avian and exotic animal hematology and cytology*, ed 3, Oxford, UK, 2007, Wiley-Blackwell, pp 3–50.
4. Clark P, Boardman W, Raidal S: Atlas of clinical avian hematology, Chichester, UK, 2009, John Wiley & Sons, pp 200.
5. Fudge A: Avian complete blood count. In Fudge A, editor: *Laboratory medicine: avian and exotic pets*, Philadelphia, PA, 2000, W.B. Saunders Company, pp 9–18.
6. Walberg J: White blood cell counting techniques in birds, *Semin Avian Exot Pets* 10(2):72–76, 2001.
7. Natt MP, Herrick CA: A new blood diluent for counting the erythrocytes and leucocytes of the chicken, *Poult Sci* 31(4):735–738, 1952.
8. Cray C, Wack A, Arheart KL: Invalid measurement of plasma albumin using bromcresol green methodology in penguins (*Spheniscus species*), *J Avian Med Surg* 25:14–22, 2011.
9. Guzman DS-M, Mitchell MA, Gaunt SD, et al: Comparison of hematologic values in blood samples with lithium heparin or dipotassium ethylenediaminetetraacetic acid anticoagulants in Hispaniolan Amazon parrots (*Amazona ventralis*), *J Avian Med Surg* 22(2):108–113, 2008.
10. Harr KE, Raskin RE, Heard DJ: Temporal effects of 3 commonly used anticoagulants on hematologic and biochemical variables in blood samples from macaws and Burmese pythons, *Vet Clin Pathol* 34(4):383–388, 2005.
11. Hrubec T, Whichard JD, Larsen CT, et al: Plasma versus serum: specific differences in biochemical analyte values, *J Avian Med Surg* 16:101–105, 2002.
12. Waldoch J, Wack R, Christopher M: Avian plasma chemistry analysis using diluted samples, *J Zoo Wildl Med* 40:667–674, 2009.
13. Pond J, Thompson S, Hennen M, et al: Effects of ultracentrifugation on plasma biochemical values of prefledged wild peregrine falcons (*Falco peregrinus*) in northeastern Illinois, *J Avian Med Surg* 26:140–143, 2012.
14. Dressen P, Wimsatt J, Burkhard M: The effects of isoflurane anesthesia on hematologic and plasma biochemical values of American kestrels (*Falco sparverius*), *J Avian Med Surg* 13(3):173–179, 1999.
15. Geffré A, Friedrichs K, Harr K, et al: Reference values: a review, *Vet Clin Pathol* 38(3):288–298, 2009.
16. Tang F, Messinger S, Cray C: Use of an indirect sampling method to produce reference intervals for hematologic and biochemical analyses in psittaciform species, *J Avian Med Surg* 27(3):194–203, 2013.
17. Teare J: *International Species Information System-physiological data reference values*, Apple Valley, MN, 2002, International Species Information System.
18. Virtanen A, Kairisto V, Uusipaikka E: Regression-based reference limits: determination of sufficient sample size, *Clin Chem* 44(11):2353–2358, 1998.
19. Fudge A: Laboratory reference ranges for selected avian, mammalian, and reptilian species. In Fudge A, editor: *Laboratory medicine: avian and exotic pets*, Philadelphia, PA, 2000, WB Saunders, pp 375–400.
20. Geffré A, Braun JP, Trumel C, et al: Estimation of reference intervals from small samples: an example using canine plasma creatinine, *Vet Clin Pathol* 38(4):477–484, 2009.
21. Meredith A, Surguine K, Handel I, et al: Hematologic and biochemical reference intervals for wild osprey nestlings (*Pandion haliaetus*), *J Zoo Wildl Med* 43(3):459–465, 2012.
22. Montesinos A, Sainz A, Pablos MV, et al: Hematological and plasma biochemical reference intervals in young white storks, *J Wildl Dis* 33(3):405–412, 1997.
23. Puerta ML, Munõz Pulido R, Huecas V, et al: Hematology and blood chemistry of chicks of white and black storks (*Ciconia ciconia and Ciconia nigra*), *Comp Biochem Physiol A Comp Physiol* 94(2):201–204, 1989.
24. Hollamby S, Afema-Azikuru J, Sikarskie JG, et al: Clinical pathology of nestling marabou storks in Uganda, *J Wildl Dis* 40(3):594–599, 2004.
25. Le Souëf AT, Holyoake CS, Vitali SD, et al: Hematologic and plasma biochemical reference values for three species of black cockatoos (*Calyptorhynchus species*), *J Avian Med Surg* 1:14–22, 2013.
26. Clubb S, Schubot R, Joyner K: Hematologic and serum biochemical reference intervals in juvenile cockatoos, *J Assoc Avian Vet* 5:16–26, 1991.
27. Clubb S, Schubot R, Joyner K: Hematologic and serum biochemical reference intervals in juvenile macaws (*Ara sp.*), *J Assoc Avian Vet* 5:154–162, 1991.
28. Clubb S, Schubot R, Joyner K: Hematologic and serum chemistry reference intervals in juvenile Eclectus parrots, *J Assoc Avian Vet* 4:218–225, 1991.
29. Lanzarot MP, Barahona MV, Andrés MIS, et al: Hematologic, protein electrophoresis, biochemistry, and cholinesterase values of free-living black stork nestlings (*Ciconia nigra*), *J Wildl Dis* 41(2):379–386, 2005.
30. Wakenell P: Hematology of chickens and turkeys. In Weiss D, Wardrop K, editors: *Schalm's veterinary hematology*, ed 6, Ames, IA, 2010, Wiley-Blackwell, pp 958–967.
31. Spagnolo V, Crippa V, Marzia A, et al: Reference intervals for hematologic and biochemical constituents and protein electrophoretic fractions in captive common buzzards (*Buteo buteo*), *Vet Clin Pathol* 35:82–87, 2006.
32. Deem SL, Ladwig E, Cray C, et al: Health assessment of the ex situ population of St Vincent parrots (*Amazona guildingii*) in St Vincent and the Grenadines, *J Avian Med Surg* 22:114–122, 2008.
33. Hernández M, Margalida A: Hematology and blood chemistry reference values and age-related changes in wild bearded vultures (*Gypaetus barbatus*), *J Wildl Dis* 46(2):390–400, 2010.
34. Naidoo V, Diekmann M, Wolters K, et al: Establishment of selected baseline blood chemistry and hematologic parameters in captive and wild-caught African white-backed vultures (*Gyps africanus*), *J Wildl Dis* 44(3):649–654, 2008.
35. Work TM: Weights, hematology, and serum chemistry of seven species of free-ranging tropical pelagic seabirds, *J Wildl Dis* 32(4):643–657, 1996.
36. Szabó Z, Beregi A, Vajdovich P, et al: Hematologic and plasma biochemistry values in white storks (*Ciconia ciconia*), *J Zoo Wildl Med* 41(1):17–21, 2010.
37. Haefele HJ, Sidor I, Evers DC, et al: Hematologic and physiologic reference ranges for free-ranging adult and young common loons (*Gavia immer*), *J Zoo Wildl Med* 36(3):385–390, 2005.
38. Dujowich M, Mazet JK, Zuba JR: Hematologic and biochemical reference ranges for captive California condors (*Gymnogyps californianus*), *J Zoo Wildl Med* 36(4):590–597, 2005.

39. Allgayer MC, Guedes NMR, Chiminazzo C, et al: Clinical pathology and parasitologic evaluation of free-living nestlings of the hyacinth macaw (*Anodorhynchus hyacinthinus*), *J Wildl Dis* 45(4):972–981, 2009.

40. Samour JH, Naldo JL, John SK: Normal haematological values in gyr falcons (*Falco rusticolus*), *Vet Rec* 157(26):844–847, 2005.

41. Samour J, Naldo J, Rahman H, et al: Hematologic and plasma biochemical reference values in Indian peafowl (*Pavo cristatus*), *J Avian Med Surg* 24: 99–106, 2010.

42. Fudge A: Laboratory reference ranges for selected avian, mammalian, and reptilian species. In Fudge A, editor: *Laboratory medicine: avian and exotic pets*, Philadelphia, PA, 2000, W.B. Saunders Company, pp 375–400.

43. Dutton CJ, Allchurch AF, Cooper JE: Comparison of hematologic and biochemical reference ranges between captive populations of northern bald ibises (*Geronticus eremita*), *J Wildl Dis* 38(3):583–538, 2002.

44. Padrtova R, Lloyd CG: Hematologic values in healthy gyr x peregrine falcons (*Falco rusticolus x Falco peregrinus*), *J Avian Med Surg* 23(2):108–113, 2009.

45. Zaias J, Fox WP, Cray C, et al: Hematologic, plasma protein, and biochemical profiles of brown pelicans (*Pelecanus occidentalis*), *Am J Vet Res* 61:771–774, 2000.

46. Garcia-Montijano M, Garcia A, Lemus JA, et al: Blood chemistry, protein electrophoresis, and hematologic values of captive Spanish imperial eagles (*Aquila adalberti*), *J Zoo Wildl Med* 33:112–117, 2002.

47. Black PA, Macek M, Tieber A, et al: Reference values for hematology, plasma biochemical analysis, plasma protein electrophoresis, and Aspergillus serology in elegant-crested tinamous (*Eudromia elegans*), *J Avian Med Surg* 27:1–6, 2013.

48. Jones MP, Arheart KL, Cray C: Reference intervals, longitudinal analyses, and index of individuality of commonly measured laboratory variables in captive bald eagles (*Haliaeetus leucocephalus*), *J Avian Med Surg* 28:118–126, 2014.

49. Gelli D, Ferrari V, Franceschini F, et al: Serum biochemistry and electrophoretic patterns in the Eurasian buzzard (*Buteo buteo*): reference values, *J Wildl Dis* 45:828–833, 2009.

50. Charles-Smith LE, Rutledge ME, Meek CJ, et al: Hematologic parameters and hemoparasites of nonmigratory Canada geese (*Branta canadensis*) from Greensboro, North Carolina, USA, *J Avian Med Surg* 28(1):16–23, 2014.

51. Hawkins M, Barron H, Speer B, et al: Birds. In Carpenter J, Marion C, editors: *Exotic animal formulary*, ed 4, St. Louis, MO, 2013, Elsevier, pp 332–376.

52. Jones MP, Arheart KL, Cray C: Reference intervals, longitudinal analyses, and index of individuality of commonly measured laboratory variables in captive bald eagles (Haliaeetus leucocephalus), *J Avian Med Surg* 28(2):118–126, 2014.

53. Roman Y, Bomsel-Demontoy MC, Levrier J, et al: Influence of molt on plasma protein electrophoretic patterns in bar-headed geese (*Anser indicus*), *J Wildl Dis* 45:661–671, 2009.

54. Franson JC, Hoffman DJ, Schmutz JA: Plasma biochemistry values in emperor geese (*Chen canagica*) in Alaska: comparisons among age, sex, incubation, and molt, *J Zoo Wildl Med* 40:321–327, 2009.

55. Hawkey C, Hart MG, Samour HJ: Age-related haematological changes and haemopathological responses in Chilean flamingos (*Phoenicopterus chilensis*), *Avian Pathol* 13(2):223–229, 1984.

56. Kocan R, Pitts S: Blood values of the canvasback duck by age, sex, and season, *J Wildl Dis* 12(3):341–346, 1976.

57. McDonald DL, Jaensch S, Harrison GJ, et al: Health and nutritional status of wild Australian psittacine birds: an evaluation of plasma and hepatic mineral levels, plasma biochemical values, and fecal microflora, *J Avian Med Surg* 24:288–298, 2010.

58. Lumeij JT, Meidam M, Wolfswinkel J, et al: Changes in plasma chemistry after drug-induced liver disease or muscle necrosis in racing pigeons (*Columba livia domestica*), *Avian Pathol* 17:865–874, 1988.

59. Howlett J, Samour J, Bailey T, et al: Age-related haematology changes in captive-reared kori bustards (*Ardeotis kori*), *Comp Haematol Int* 8:26–30, 1998.

60. Harper EJ, Lowe B: Hematology values in a colony of budgerigars (*Melopsittacus undulatus*) and changes associated with aging, *J Nutr* 128(Suppl 12):2639S–2640S, 1998.

61. Nalubamba KS, Mudenda NB, Bwalya EC, et al: Seasonal variations in health indices of free-ranging asymptomatic guinea fowls (*Numida meleagris*) in Zambia, *Asian Pac J Trop Med* 7S1:S143–S149, 2014.

62. Schmidt EM, dos S, Lange RR, et al: Hematology of the red-capped parrot (Pionopsitta pileata) and Vinaceous Amazon parrot (Amazona vinacea) in captivity, *J Zoo Wildl Med* 40(1):15–17, 2009.

63. Rehder NB, Bird DM: Annual profiles of blood packed cell volumes of captive American kestrels, *Can J Zool* 61(11):2550–2555, 1983.

64. Dolka B, Włodarczyk R, Zbikowski A, et al: Hematological parameters in relation to age, sex and biochemical values for mute swans (*Cygnus olor*), *Vet Res Commun* 38(2):93–100, 2014.

65. Kasprzak M, Hetmański T, Kulczykowska E: Changes in hematological parameters in free-living pigeons (*Columba livia f.* urbana) during the breeding cycle, *J Ornithol* 147(4):599–604, 2006.

66. Mazzaro LM, Meegan J, Sarran D, et al: Molt-associated changes in hematologic and plasma biochemical values and stress hormone levels in African penguins (*Spheniscus demersus*), *J Avian Med Surg* 27(4):285–293, 2013.

67. Cray C, Stremme DW, Arheart KL: Postprandial biochemistry changes in penguins (*Spheniscus demersus*) including hyperuricemia, *J Zoo Wildl Med* 41:325–326, 2010.

68. Parga ML, Pendl H, Forbes NA: The effect of transport on hematologic parameters in trained and untrained Harris's hawks (Parabuteo unicinctus) and peregrine falcons (*Falco peregrinus*), *J Avian Med Surg* 15(3):162–169, 2001.

69. Gray HG, Paradis TJ, Chang PW: Research note: physiological effects of adrenocorticotropic hormone and hydrocortisone in laying hens, *Poult Sci* 68(12):1710–1713, 1989.

70. Speer B, Kass P: The influence of travel on hematologic parameters in hyacinth macaws, *Proc Annu Assoc Avian Med* 1–6, 1995.

71. Black P, Mcruer D, Horne L: Hematologic parameters in raptor species in a rehabilitation setting before release, *J Avian Med Surg* 25(3):192–198, 2011.

72. Polo FJ, Peinado VI, Viscor G, et al: Hematologic and plasma chemistry values in captive psittacine birds, *Avian Dis* 42(3):523–535, 1998.

73. Fischer I, Christen C, Lutz H, et al: Effects of two diets on the haematology, plasma chemistry and intestinal flora of budgerigars (*Melopsittacus undulatus*), *Vet Rec* 159(15):480–484, 2006.

74. Candido MV, Silva LCC, Moura J, et al: Comparison of clinical parameters in captive Cracidae fed traditional and extruded diets, *J Zoo Wildl Med* 42(3):437–443, 2011.

75. Dyer KJ, Perryman BL, Holcombe DW: Site and age class variation of hematologic parameters for female greater sage grouse (*Centrocercus urophasianus*) of Northern Nevada, *J Wildl Dis* 46(1):1–12, 2010.

76. Dyer KJ, Perryman BL, Holcombe DW: Fitness and nutritional assessment of greater sage grouse (*Centrocercus urophasianus*) using hematologic and serum chemistry parameters through a cycle of seasonal habitats in northern Nevada, *J Zoo Wildl Med* 40(1):18–28, 2009.

77. Le Maho Y, Karmann H, Briot D, et al: Stress in birds due to routine handling and a technique to avoid it, *Am J Physiol* 263(4 Pt 2):R775–R781, 1992.

78. Mans C, Guzman DS-M, Lahner LL, et al: Sedation and physiologic response to manual restraint after intranasal administration of midazolam in Hispaniolan Amazon parrots (*Amazona ventralis*), *J Avian Med Surg* 26(3):130–139, 2012.

79. Small M, Baccus J, Mink J, et al: Hematologic responses in captive white-winged doves (*Zenaida asiatica*), induced by various radiotransmitter attachments, *J Wildl Dis* 41(2):387–394, 2005.

80. Sinclair KM, Church ME, Farver TB, et al: Effects of meloxicam on hematologic and plasma biochemical analysis variables and results of histologic examination of tissue specimens of Japanese quail (*Coturnix japonica*), *Am J Vet Res* 73(11):1720–1727, 2012.

81. Karesh W, del Campo A, Braselton E, et al: Health evaluation of free-ranging and hand-reared macaws (*Ara spp.*) in Peru, *J Zoo Wildl Med* 28(4):268–377, 1997.

82. Katavolos P, Staempfli S, Sears W, et al: The effect of lead poisoning on hematologic and biochemical values in trumpeter swans and Canada geese, *Vet Clin Pathol* 36:341–347, 2007.

83. Stanford M: Effects of UVB radiation on calcium metabolism in psittacine birds, *Vet Rec* 159: 236–241, 2006.

84. Norambuena MC, Bozinovic F: Effect of malnutrition on iron homeostasis in black-necked swans (*Cygnus melanocoryphus*), *J Zoo Wildl Med* 40:624–631, 2009.

85. Burgdorf-Moisuk A, Wack R, Ziccardi M, et al: Validation of lactate measurement in American flamingo (*Phoenicopterus ruber*) plasma and correlation with duration and difficulty of capture, *J Zoo Wildl Med* 43:450–458, 2012.

86. Petersen P, Jensen E, Brandslund I: Analytical performance, reference values and decision limits. A need to differentiate between reference intervals and decision limits and to define analytical quality specifications, *Clin Chem Lab Med* 50(5):819–831, 2011.

87. Freund R, Wilson W: Statistical methods. ed 2, San Diego, CA, 2003, Academic Press, p 673.

88. Walton RM: Subject-based reference values: biological variation, individuality, and reference change values, *Vet Clin Pathol* 41(2): 175–181, 2012.

89. Lassen ED: Perspectives in data interpretation. In Thrall MA, editor: *Veterinary hematology and clinical chemistry*, Baltimore, MD, 2004, Lippincott, Williams & Wilkins, pp 45–54.

90. Steinberg DM: Sample size for positive and negative predictive value in diagnostic research using case-control designs, *Biostatistics* 10(1):94–105, 2009.

91. Kummrow M, Silvanose C, Di Somma A, et al: Serum protein electrophoresis by using high-resolution agarose gel in clinically healthy and Aspergillus species-infected falcons, *J Avian Med Surg* 26:213–220, 2012.

92. Cray C, Gautier D, Harris DJ, et al: Changes in clinical enzyme activity and bile acid levels in psittacine birds with altered liver function and disease, *J Avian Med Surg* 22:17–24, 2008.

93. Kolmstetter CM, Ramsa EC: Effects of feeding on plasma uric acid and urea concentrations in blackfooted penguins (*Spheniscus demersus*), *J Avian Med Surg* 14:177–179, 2000.

94. Desmarchelier M, Langlois I: Diabetes mellitus in a nanday conure (*Nandayus nenday*), *J Avian Med Surg* 22:246–254, 2008.

95. Stanford M: The Significance of serum ionized calcium and 25–hydroxycholecalciferol (*vitamin D3*) assays in African Grey parrots, *Exotic DVM* 5:1–6, 2003.

96. Kirchgessner MS, Tully TN Jr, Nevarez J, et al: Magnesium therapy in a hypocalcemic African Grey parrot (*Psittacus erithacus*), *J Avian Med Surg* 26:17–21, 2012.

97. Starkey SR, Wood C, de Matos R, et al: Central diabetes insipidus in an African Grey parrot, *J Am Vet Med Assoc* 237:415–419, 2010.

98. Cray C, Watson T, Rodriguez M, et al: Application of galactomannan analysis and protein electrophoresis in the diagnosis of aspergillosis in avian species, *J Zoo Wildl Med* 40:64–70, 2009.

99. Briscoe JA, Rosenthal KL, Shofer FS: Selected complete blood cell count and plasma protein electrophoresis parameters in pet psittacine birds evaluated for illness, *J Avian Med Surg* 24: 131–137, 2010.

100. Villar D, Kramer M, Howard L, et al: Clinical presentation and pathology of sarcocystosis in psittaciform birds: 11 cases, *Avian Dis* 52:187–194, 2008.

101. Lennox A, Clubb S, Romagnano A, et al: Monoclonal hyperglobulinemia in lymphosarcoma in a cockatiel (*Nymphicus hollandicus*) and a blue and gold macaw (*Ara ararauna*), *Avian Dis* 58:326–329, 2014.

102. Tatum LM, Zaias J, Mealey BK, et al: Protein electrophoresis as a diagnostic and prognostic tool in raptor medicine, *J Zoo Wildl Med* 31:497–502, 2000.

103. Caliendo V, McKinney P, Bailey T, et al: Serum amyloid A as an indicator of health status in falcons, *J Avian Med Surg* 27(2):83–89, 2013.

104. Potier R: Lipid blood profile in captive Brahminy kite (*Haliastur indus*) as a possible indication of increased susceptibility to atherosclerosis, *J Zoo Wildl Med* 44:549–554, 2013.

105. Walton RM: Validation of laboratory tests and methods, *Semin Avian Exotic Pet Med* 10:59–65, 2001.

106. Bell R, Harr K, Rishniw M, et al: Survey of point-of-care instrumentation, analysis, and quality assurance in veterinary practice, *Vet Clin Pathol* 43:185–192, 2014.

107. Flatland B, Vap LM: Quality management recommendations for automated and manual in-house hematology of domestic animals, *Vet Clin North Am Small Anim Pract* 42(1):11–22, 2012.

108. Acierno MJ, Schnellbacher R, Tully TN Jr: Measuring the level of agreement between a veterinary and a human point-of-care glucometer and a laboratory blood analyzer in Hispaniolan Amazon parrots (*Amazona ventralis*), *J Avian Med Surg* 26: 221–224, 2012.

109. Greenacre CB, Flatland B, Souza MJ, et al: Comparison of avian biochemical test results with Abaxis VetScan and Hitachi 911 analyzers, *J Avian Med Surg* 22:291–299, 2008.

110. Rettenmund CL, Heatley JJ, Russell KE: Comparison of two analyzers to determine selected venous blood analytes of Quaker parrots (*Myiopsitta monachus*), *J Zoo Wildl Med* 45:256–262, 2014.

111. Acierno MJ, Mitchell MA, Schuster PJ, et al: Evaluation of the agreement among three handheld blood glucose meters and a laboratory blood analyzer for measurement of blood glucose concentration in Hispaniolan Amazon parrots (*Amazona ventralis*), *Am J Vet Res* 70:172–175, 2009.

112. Lieske CL, Ziccardi MH, Mazet J, et al: Evaluation of 4 handheld blood glucose monitors for use in seabird rehabilitation, *J Avian Med Surg* 16(4):277–285, 2002.

113. Ritchie B, Harrison G, Harrison L, editors: *Avian medicine: principles and application*, Lake Worth, FL, 1994, Wingers, pp 33–34, 48–59.

114. Plebani M: Errors in clinical laboratories or errors in laboratory medicine, *Clin Chem Lab Med* 44(6):750–759, 2006.

115. Samour J, Howlett JC: Hematology analyses. In Samour J, editor: *Avian medicine*, ed 2, Philadelphia, PA, 2008, Mosby.

VARIABILITY AND LIMITATIONS IN CLINICAL AVIAN HEMATOLOGY

Hugues Beaufrère, Mélanie Ammersbach

THE CORE OF THE PROBLEM

The complete blood cell count (CBC) is often the first line of diagnostic tests performed in clinical situations and is regularly used for health assessment and in quarantine protocols in many bird species. Indeed, the CBC has been shown to be one of the most sensitive tests to detect illnesses in avian patients.[1] However, the interpretation of the avian hemogram is flawed with many problems that must be understood and considered in the clinical decision-making process. Practitioners and diagnosticians will be better served with a thorough understanding of all potential sources of variability in the hematology results obtained and of their importance across clinical situations. This knowledge will ultimately lead to improved techniques and improved interpretation of the hemogram, maximizing the chances of appropriate clinical decisions and positive patient outcomes.

All laboratory hematology techniques for nonpoultry bird species are currently manual, which practically translates into a lack of standardization across laboratories or veterinary hospitals, automatization, and greater variability. Automated hematology analyzers used to generate mammalian CBCs employ techniques that vary greatly from one analyzer to another, but in reference laboratories, they are regularly calibrated. Most analyzers classically provide cell counts for erythrocytes, leukocytes (nucleated cells), and platelets based on a high number of counted cells. Additionally, certain cell parameters are directly measured (e.g., mean cell volume [MCV]) and the differentiation of leukocytes is performed by using various direct measurements (cell size, complexity, peroxidase content) and indirect methods (e.g., differential cell lysis). On the other hand, manual hematology techniques rely on hematocytometers, chemical stains, and mathematical formulas, and hematology results are only based on a few hundred counted cells or less. In addition, techniques are highly variable between laboratories and personnel. These major drawbacks come from the fact that all avian blood cells are nucleated, so automated analyzers cannot distinguish leukocytes from erythrocytes and thrombocytes, as in mammals. Bare nuclei from lysed cells, nucleated thrombocytes, and lymphocytes are of similar sizes and are difficult to distinguish by impedance or light scatter properties. There are differences in the contents of the leukocyte granules compared with those in mammals. For instance, the lack of peroxidase enzymes in the heterophils of birds hinders differentiation by peroxidase staining. The size, shape, dimensions, fragility, and staining characteristics of blood cells vary in avian groups and pose further challenges to the potential for automatization and add to the overall variability of the manual techniques.[2,3] In addition, this limits the use of centrifugal hematology analyzer such as the quantitative buffy coat analysis, impedance, and laser cytometry tools to differentiate all types of cells.[2,4-7] Overall, these differences make the development of species-specific protocols applicable to the majority of patients difficult.

Baseline data are scarcely available or nonexistent for many species of birds. Most of the older literature is also flawed, with poor representation of the target populations, poorly disclosed hematologic methodology, and inadequate statistical determination of reference intervals. In practice, clinicians also frequently extrapolate reference values from other species, sometimes belonging to different taxonomic groups with dramatic ecologic differences in lifestyle. Biologic variability within individuals and populations and high frequency of laboratory errors inherent to manual counting techniques further add to the problem. Finally, the hematologic response to disease may also vary, depending on species and disease, as is seen in different mammal species.

A substantial part of most clinical decisions is based on the interpretation of the hemogram. The magnitude of hematologic changes observed must be weighed against the multiple sources of variability inherent to hematologic techniques, including biological variability (interindividual and intraindividual) and laboratory variability (preanalytical, analytical, and postanalytical). If these sources of variability are not considered, gross misinterpretation may ensue and confound

diagnostic, therapeutic, and follow-up assessments of patients. A high variability coupled with a low magnitude of changes in cell counts may substantially decrease the sensitivity and value of hematology in many circumstances.

The hematologic techniques used in birds to obtain a CBC have changed minimally for over 50 years[2,8]; the absolute white blood cell (WBC) count is still obtained using hemocytometers and various stains, including phloxine B, Natt and Herrick solution, Rees-Ecker solution, eosin, or other colorants; and the differential count is still obtained by using a microscope and a human observer.[2,8-11] The packed cell volume is still obtained using a microhematocrit tube and centrifugation. However, since red blood cells (RBCs) outnumber WBCs by a factor of 1,000, the RBC count can be obtained by using standard laboratory instruments; the hemoglobin may also be obtained by using similar analytical machines. Over this 50-year time frame, significant progress has been made in our understanding of biologic variabilities and laboratory variabilities in clinical hematology, laboratory quality control, and methods of comparison of statistical assessment and reference values. There also have been a high number of publications of articles on reference values in birds.

Several thorough references are available on avian hematology, but not much attention has been paid to its limitations and their impact on clinical interpretation. This chapter intends to review and discuss the plethora of factors and concepts that may affect the interpretation of the CBC in avian medicine and that may add uncertainty to the clinical decision-making process. It will also introduce potential measures and future directions to minimize sources of variability in avian hematology and promote quality assurance and standardization. This chapter will not describe current hematologic techniques in detail, since it is outside its scope. The main techniques used in practice are summarized in several inserted boxes in this manuscript, as the knowledge of basic laboratory techniques is a prerequisite to understanding their limitations.[2]

BIOLOGIC VARIABILITY

General Concepts

Biologic variability reflects the normal intraindividual and interindividual variability associated with various factors. Living organisms constantly adapt to changing environments and some of these adaptations or responses may lead to fluctuations in hematologic parameters. Furthermore, animals' physiologic response changes with age, sex, ecology, and other uncontrolled factors. Variability associated with normal biologic processes must be assessed and quantified because it may confound the interpretation of the CBC and overlap with the hematologic response to disease. Factors influencing biologic variability are usually not controllable, and thus comparatively little action can be undertaken to minimize this source of variability. As such, there is a complex interplay of covariables and confounding factors responsible for the biologic variability in hematological values and reports. In addition, avian blood cells have shorter lifespans compared with those of mammals, which may result in more dynamic changes and biologic variability.[12] This section merely serves to alert the avian clinicians on the many biologic factors that may affect blood values at multiple levels and is not exhaustive.

Variability Associated with Physiologic Processes

Hematologic parameters may change over time with aging. Packed cell volume (PCV) is generally lower in young birds, and the WBC is higher than in adults.[2,13] For instance, from 30-day-old to 60-day-old Eclectus parrots (*Eclectus roratus*), blue-and-gold macaws (*Ara ararauna*), and Amazon parrots (*Amazona* spp.), the WBC decreased by 2 to 10 × 10^9/L.[14-16] Likewise, PCV increased by as much as 20%.[14-16] Other species from a variety of taxonomic orders showed similar trends with an increase in PCV, a decrease in WBC, or both at adulthood.[13,17-25] These higher WBC counts in nestling birds are of the same magnitude that could be expected in sick birds exhibiting leukocytosis. However, in kori bustards (*Ardeotis kori*), whereas a similar trend was seen for PCV, an opposite trend was observed for the WBCs, which was steadily increasing from 1 month to 15 months.[26] Several other species also showed an increase in WBC count at adulthood rather than a decrease.[18,27] In all species studied, PCV in fledglings was either lower than or the same as adult birds.[13] In some species, age-related or sex-related changes are not seen on the WBC count or PCV. Nevertheless, since reference values may differ for the same species between published sources, depending on the demographics of the sample population and techniques employed, these trends may be inconsistently represented across the scientific literature.

The gender may also have some influence on PCV, which is usually slightly lower in female birds than males. These changes tend to appear or become exacerbated during the breeding season. This pattern was found in several published reference intervals in multiple species from various orders.[8,12,28,29] However, a meta-analysis on 36 studies on wild birds did not find any difference in hematocrit between sexes in selected species, and other peer-reviewed reports on various avian species also failed to find differences.[13,29,30] In most birds, PCV is found to decrease during breeding in females even when no prebreeding differences between sexes are seen.[13] In several species of ducks, females may have higher PCV and RBC indices compared with males in the prenesting period.[31,32] Occasionally, a slightly higher WBC count is also found in laying females than in males in some reports.[27,33]

Molting may also be associated with a decrease or an increase in hematocrit, depending on the species, but a decrease is more frequent.[13,29,34-36] This decrease is particularly well documented in Sphenisciformes, during which they stop feeding and remain on land, and in Anseriformes, which molt all their flight feathers at once.[23,37-39] These changes may be caused by an expansion in body plasma volume with extensive wing feather replacement, as it has been demonstrated in passerines.[13,36,40] Species with a continuous molt throughout the year should not be expected to demonstrate such changes.

Some species, such as birds of prey, penguins, and others, experience significant periods of fasting during winter and migration or due to fluctuations in food availability. In these wild situations, fasting may be considered physiologic, as part of the species' survival strategy. Fasting may induce a lower hematocrit and shifting of the heterophil-to-lymphocyte (H/L) ratio.[13,41,42] Refeeding after a period of fasting may also

decrease PCV.[13] The MCV also fluctuates with body condition in many species.[2]

Migration may result in hematologic changes (increase or decrease in PCV, changes in RBC indices) as a result of prolonged fasting that may accompany migration, higher energy expenditure, and increased altitude and oxygen demand.[13,25,43,44] Some of these changes may occur in captive birds, which are unable to migrate, but may also be caused by confounding factors occurring at the same time of the year. Interestingly, bar-headed geese flying at high altitudes over the Himalayan mountains do not have a higher hematocrit but have a hemoglobin with higher oxygen affinity instead.[43] This shows that physiologic responses to similar ecologic constraints are different across species and this likely depends on the level of adaptations and specialization to specific ecologic niches.

The effects of stress on avian hematologic variables (stress leukogram) has been investigated in a variety of species, including, at least, hawks, falcons, pigeons, ratites, passerines, macaws, and chickens.[12,45-51] The types and degrees of changes observed may vary with the species and the conditions but could include an increase in the H/L ratio, leukocytosis or leukopenia, heterophilia, lymphopenia, eosinopenia, and monocytosis. The H/L ratio, heterophil count, and lymphocyte count seemed to be the parameters with the most stress-induced consistent changes overall. In falcons and hawks, the level of falconry training affected the hematologic response to transport-induced stress, but changes remained within published reference intervals.[45] In that study, both untrained groups showed a significant increase in the H/L ratio. Peregrine falcons showed no other significant change, but untrained Harris's hawks had additional significant leukopenia, lymphopenia, and eosinopenia. Trained Harris's hawks showed significant monocytosis, whereas trained peregrines showed no significant change. Hyacinth macaws (*Anodorhynchus hyacinthinus*) were also found to exhibit hematologic changes with transport, with birds travelling less than 1 hour having lower WBC counts and lower H/L ratios than those travelling more than 1 hour.[51] In a study in chickens, stress was mimicked by adrenocorticotropic hormone (ACTH) administration and corticosteroid treatment and resulted in heterophilia, monocytosis, eosinophilia, basophilia, and lymphopenia.[50] Handling, even when minimal, may induce substantial stress in birds (see later). The effects of stress on blood parameters are mediated by increased production of corticosterone and epinephrine.[52]

Variability Associated with Taxonomy and Ecologic Niches

Since many bird species have adapted to specific ecologic niches, the biologic variability resulting from interspecies differences needs to be discussed in concert with their specific biology. These differences are less of concern if species-specific reference values are used but should be known when extrapolating data across taxonomic groups. Domestic birds such as chickens and turkeys present some hematologic differences between breeds or genetic lines.[53] It may be similar in the various color morphs produced through inbreeding in pet psittacine species, hybrids, or subspecies.

Most birds have relatively similar hematologic values, with PCV usually being around 45 to 55 and the WBC count in the range of 5 to 15 × 10³/μL (5 to 15 × 10⁹/L). However, adopting a "one size fits all" approach is not optimal and certainly not supported by evidence-based medicine. Extrapolating the interpretation of the hemogram from Psittaciformes, Falconiformes, and Accipitriformes to less-well-characterized bird groups may also prove problematic.

For instance, the WBC counts of multiple species of the orders Strigiformes, Procellariiformes, Pelecaniformes, domestic Galliformes, and many others normally exhibit high upper reference limits of 30 × 10³/μL (30 × 10⁹/L) or even higher.[19,53-55] Clark et al recently published a hematologic text organized by avian taxon, which may help pinpoint species-specific differences.[3] Other species of the more commonly encountered taxonomic orders may also show unique differences within their respective taxonomic order. For instance, some macaws tend to show higher WBC counts than other psittacine species, arctic owls tend to show lower WBC counts than temperate owls, and some vultures and marabou storks tend to show higher WBC counts than other accipitrid and ciconiid species, respectively.[22,54,56-58] Some of these changes may be caused by species-specific adaptations to ecologic niches, such as higher WBC counts seen in birds more exposed to pathogens (e.g., scavengers) or lower WBC counts in birds less exposed to pathogens (e.g., arctic species). Indeed, some of these trends were confirmed at a larger scale. A study on a broad group of birds confirmed that scavenger birds have significantly higher WBC counts and lower lymphocyte percentage (because of stronger innate than adaptive immunity) than nonscavenging birds.[59] It is important to note that these general trends may not hold true at the individual species level as, for instance, in gyrfalcons (*Falco rusticolus*), the most arctic Falconiforme species, has similar WBC counts as other falcons, and some vulture species have WBC counts comparable with those of hawks and eagles.[18,58,60] As a consequence, leukocytosis, anemia, and other hematologic abnormalities may be wrongly diagnosed in some species if species-specific criteria are not applied.

The H/L ratio also varies across species. Most Accipitriformes are predominately heterophilic, and most Passeriformes are predominately lymphocytic.[12] However, variations within orders and families may also be encountered, as is found in Strigiformes or Psittaciformes, for instance.[54,57] Different species may also exhibit variations in cell morphology. Eosinophils tend to be the cells with the most variability in cell morphology across species.[54,61] For instance, birds of prey tend to have eosinophils with bright pink granules, whereas parrots have eosinophils with blue granules (Figure 13-1).

With regard to PCV and erythrocyte counts, similar changes may be observed but may be caused by different factors. Chickens tend to show lower PCV and erythrocyte counts compared with other birds.[53] PCV, erythrocyte counts, and RBC indices may be linked to metabolism in animals.[13] At least PCV does not seem to differ dramatically between birds of higher metabolism (e.g., Trochiliiformes, mean of 0.56), medium metabolism, and lower metabolism (Struthioniformes, mean of 0.48).[62-64] However, erythrocyte counts and MCV may differ dramatically; for instance, hummingbirds have the highest erythrocyte counts (mean of 6.5 × 10⁶/μL [6.5 × 10¹²/L]) of any bird with very low MCV (mean of 86 fL/cell, 86 μm³/cell) and ostriches have a fairly low RBC (mean of 2.4 × 10⁶/μL [2.4 × 10¹²/L]) with high MCV (mean of 201 fL/cell, 201 μm³/cell).[58,63-65] Penguins have relatively low RBC counts (around 1.8 × 10⁶/μL, 1.8 × 10¹²/L) and high MCV (around 250 fL/cell, 250 μm³/cell) compared with most birds.[58] Overall, the MCV tends to increase with species body size and decrease with metabolism.

Variability Associated with Environmental and Temporal Factors

Seasonal variations in hematologic values have been documented and can be of great magnitude. For instance, in

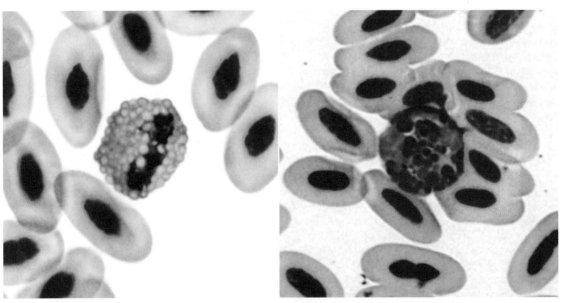

FIGURE 13-1 *Left panel,* Eosinophil of a spectacled owl *(Pulsatrix perspicillata)* illustrating a species with brightly eosinophilic granules. *Right panel,* Eosinophil of a Quaker parrot *(Myiopsitta monachus)* illustrating a species with basophilic granules.

American kestrels (*Falco sparverius*), the total PCV change was about 20% in absolute values throughout the year.[29] In wintering ducks, PCV and RBC counts may be higher than during other seasons.[66,67] Other reports have mentioned higher PCV in winter, but some studies showed no variation between seasons.[13] These associated seasonal changes are caused by differing physiology across the year (e.g., breeding, molting), changes in environmental temperatures, and changes in activity and state of nutrition of wild birds.[13] Captive birds may not experience the same degree of seasonal hematologic changes as their wild counterparts do.

Captivity may affect the hemogram, depending on species and husbandry conditions. In addition, captivity itself demands some physiologic adaptations that may be reflected on the blood values. For instance, some species showed higher WBC counts, lymphopenia, and lower PCV in captivity.[12,68,69] This observation may result from factors associated with captivity, including failure to meet the species' nutritional needs and the levels of stress being perceived by the birds. Reverse trends are also observed in different situations and are hypothesized to depend on the length of time in captivity, the individual species' response to captivity, and the origin of the birds (wild caught vs. captive-bred).[70-72] For example, blue-fronted Amazon parrots (*Amazona aestiva*) were found to have markedly lower heterophil counts (an approximately 70% decrease) in captivity, but PCV was the same compared with their wild counterparts.[72] The overall variability of hematologic parameters may be lower in captive populations than in their wild counterparts, most likely because of the homogeneity of captive conditions and consistent access to food and water.[70] Captive diets may also differ, and several hematologic changes have been observed depending on the quality of captive diets in birds.[73,74] Group housing versus single housing in captivity may also affect the hematologic variables.[75]

In most birds, the PCV tends to increase with altitude, particularly in birds with broad geographic distribution, but may also be independent because of other adaptations to enhance oxygen uptake.[12,13,43,44] In chickens, the increase in PCV with altitude is well documented as a factor in the development of the ascites syndrome.[76]

Geographic locations may also have profound effects on multiple hematologic variables and most likely depend on various cofactors such as habitat quality, nutrition, infectious pressure, and climate. At a larger geographic scale, species living in the different ecozones (Palearctic, Nearctic, Afrotropic, Neotropic, Australasia, Indo-Malaya, Oceania, and Antarctic) may have various adaptations to their habitats and climates. Birds living in urban environments may show hematologic alterations, which may be caused by increased exposure to environmental toxins and dietary adaptations.[77-79]

Finally, it is expected that global anthropogenic alterations of the natural world through increasing environmental pollutants, climate change, habitat loss and fragmentation, and increasing urbanization may promote further changes in wild bird ecology that will be reflected in hematologic values and their variability.

Variability Associated with Subclinical Conditions, Chronic Stable Illnesses, and Iatrogenic Effects

Changes associated with subclinical, stable chronic but unrelated, and iatrogenic conditions may confound the diagnostic effort to detect and identify other concurrent clinical entities. Some of these overlapping conditions may be associated with aging, such as atherosclerosis or other degenerative changes, whereas others can be associated with captivity, such as chronic egg laying. Others may include parasitism, such as with gastrointestinal nematodes, hematozoans, or blood-sucking arthropods. There is a plethora of scientific articles on the cost of parasitism to the avian hosts; the parasitism may either remain hematologically silent, since most parasites do not cause clinical disease, or may result in decrease in PCV and increase in WBC counts.[13] In pet Psittaciformes, chronic feather-damaging behaviors or self-mutilation may lead to a mild anemia, with or without mild leukocytosis or monocytosis. Birds with chronic reproductive issues, including chronic egg laying, and some reproductive disorders may exhibit mild anemia and leukocytosis.

Furthermore, some medical procedures and drugs may induce anticipated or unanticipated hematologic responses that are not directly related to the current health status. First, handling and restraint may cause an acute stress response leading to hematologic changes.[46,49,80] Even in calm birds which are accustomed to being handled and that show no outwardly apparent signs of stress, a marked stress response may be encountered with routine handling.[81] In house finches (*Carpodacus mexicanus*), a predominantly lymphocytic species, the time of handling caused a decrease, not an increase, in WBC within 1 hour after capture.[82] Consequently, blood sampling should ideally be done as soon as possible in a patient and before other medical procedures are performed, especially knowing that corticosterone production typically shows a 2- to 3-minute delay after an acute stressor.[83] The use of sedation may also decrease the stress response.[84] Recurrent blood sampling, in which excessive volumes are taken, may also induce alterations of RBC parameters. Current recommendations are to collect no more than 1% of a bird's body mass per venipuncture and no more than 2% of a bird's body mass over a 14-day period.[85-87] Transfusion of avian patients may increase PCV transiently and erythrocyte morphologic differences should be expected. PCV may not significantly increase in heterologous transfusions because of hemolysis of donor cells.[88] Intramuscular injections, especially when repeated, may lead to local muscular necrosis and inflammation, which, in turn, can result in mild leukocytosis. Several drugs may have some unwanted effects on blood parameters. The most notable is fenbendazole, which has been shown to exhibit bone marrow toxicosis in several bird species.[89-91] Meloxicam does not appear to have any effect on blood variables.[92] Parenteral fluid administration may induce mild hemodilution even in birds with normal hydration and can worsen preexisting anemia. Isoflurane gas anesthesia has been reported to decrease PCV and basophil counts in American kestrels. In that study, PCV changes may have been caused by RBC sequestration or decrease in vascular hydrostatic pressures.[93] WBCs are also reported to increase in anesthetized patients compared with rapid collection in conscious birds.[94]

Finally, hematologic response to clinical disease varies, depending on the species, etiologic agent involved, and disease state. Some species and individuals may respond with variable magnitude of changes in WBC count and PCV in what appears to be the same disease condition. In addition, response to infectious agents may be more lymphocytic or heterophilic depending on the species.

LABORATORY VARIABILITY

General Concepts

Laboratory variability reflects the uncertainties associated with blood sampling, storage, shipping, processing, blood analysis, observer variability, equipment variability, interlaboratory differences, and the reporting of results. Since laboratory variability is associated with techniques, it can be minimized with improvements and standardization of the details of the techniques employed. Laboratory variability includes preanalytical, analytical, and postanalytical variability. Some preanalytical and postanalytical issues may be identifiable by the clinician, but analytical errors usually cannot readily be detected. Since most avian WBC techniques are manual, laboratory error is expected to be high.

Preanalytical Variability

A variety of factors may affect hematologic values and techniques at a later stage. First, venipuncture techniques may be associated with unwanted or unanticipated effects. Prolonged periods of restraint and medical procedures performed prior to blood sampling may exacerbate hematologic stress responses.[46,49,80,90]

The venipuncture sites used may also influence hematologic variables. For instance, a study in Japanese quails (*Coturnix japonica*) found differences in PCV between blood samples obtained from the medial metatarsal vein, jugular vein, brachial vein, and heart. PCV was the highest from the medial metatarsal vein, and the variability was the lowest from the jugular vein.[95] Applying excessive suction during sampling or expelling blood in collection tubes through small needles may lead to hemolysis.[94] As coagulation in birds is extremely fast, collected blood should be transferred quickly into collection tubes to minimize clotting, which may subsequently reduce cell counts. Insufficient mixing between coagulants and blood may also cause small clots. Obtaining blood through a nail clip is not recommended and may induce several artifacts such as bacterial contamination, cellular debris, and cell distortion, and it is painful[2] (Figure 13-2).

Anticoagulants may lead to hematologic artifacts. Heparin does not prevent thrombocyte aggregation and may lead to cell morphologic changes and staining artifacts.[2,94] In one study, it was found that heparin had deleterious effects on avian erythrocytes, but the heparin concentrations used were much higher than what is typically used clinically.[96] The effects of lower concentrations of heparin were not examined. Ethylenediaminetetraacetic acid (EDTA) is generally the anticoagulant of choice for use in hematology, but its use has been associated with hemolysis in certain species, including ostriches (*Struthio camelus*), crowned cranes (*Balearica* spp.), and some species of hornbills, curassows, ducks, Megapodidae, and Corvidae.[2,94] In a study in Amazon parrots, the hematocrit was slightly lower and lymphocytes slightly greater in heparin than in EDTA, but other cell counts were similar.[97] In another study in macaws (*Ara* spp.), citrate was found to cause increased cell lysis compared with heparin and EDTA.[98] Citrate has also been found to decrease PCV in chickens compared with other anticoagulants.[99] Heparin was found to be the most suitable anticoagulant for hematocrit determination in pigeons (*Columba livia*) in one study, but EDTA was

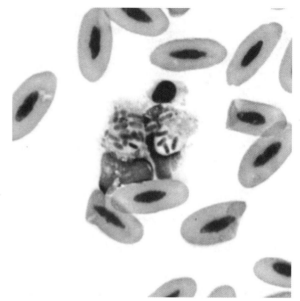

FIGURE 13-2 Intracellular bacteria in the heterophils in a cockatoo initially diagnosed with bacteremia. It was later found that blood was collected using a toenail clip during a routine health check. Bacterial contamination of the blood sample with subsequent phagocytosis of bacteria by heterophils occurred in vitro prior to processing.

found to be superior in another study of the same species.[100,] Preheparinized syringes are not recommended (and seldom needed) because of the large amount of heparin that can be present, leading to sample dilution and staining artifacts.[2,94,101]

The time and conditions of sample storage greatly influence the presence of artifacts in blood samples. Delayed processing can be caused by a lag between sample collection and transportation, the duration of transportation itself, and a lag between sample reception at the laboratory and blood analysis. For instance, it was found in macaws that WBCs started to decrease at 12 hours in all anticoagulants, but the differences were only statistically significant at 24 hours at 4° C.[98] Prolonged storage may also result in problems from bacterial contamination if the sample was not collected sterilely (e.g., toenail clip), extraerythrocytic translocation of some *Haemoproteus* spp. gametocytes may occur, and this may complicate and confuse identification of those blood parasites.[2,94] Sample labeling errors can lead to data that are generated but assigned to the wrong patient.

Analytical Variability

Precision and accuracy

The considerable advances in hematology instrumentation have mainly benefited mammalian patients, but very little of this progress has translated into clinical applications for birds. As such, the analytical variability is expected to be high in birds, as total and differential cell counts are typically determined manually. When performing laboratory assays, their precision and accuracy must be known. Precision (or consistency) is the degree of repeatability of the techniques and is measured by variance, standard deviation, or coefficient of variation of the technique (random error) repeated over the same sample. Reported coefficients of variation for

TABLE 13-1
Selected Manual Techniques and Their Approximate Reported Coefficient of Variation for White Blood Cells

Technique	Taxon	CV (%)	Ref
Estimation from the smear	Galliformes	11	126
Lymphocytes		15	
Heterophils		16	
Monocytes		19	
Eosinophils		38	
Basophils		25	
Estimation from the smear	Psittaciformes	28	124
Phloxine B	Various	10	123
Phloxine B	Psittaciformes	12	124
Eosin	Psittaciformes	13	9
Natt and Herrick	Various	15	123

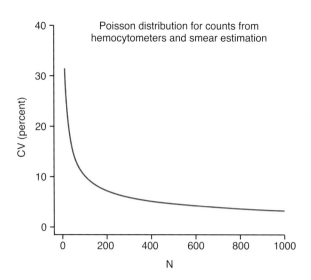

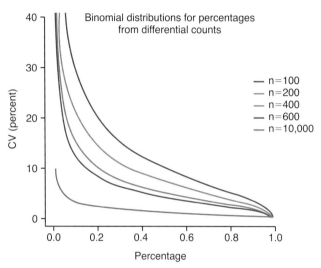

FIGURE 13-3 *Top panel,* Poisson distribution for counts, graph of the coefficient of variation (CV) over the number of counted cells (N). *Bottom panel,* Binomial distribution for percentages, graph of the coefficient of variation (CV) over percentages in a differential count (the bottom orange curve represents the numbers of counted cells most associated with hemocytometer-based techniques; the upper four curves represent the number of counted cells most associated with automated techniques).

selected counting methods are reported in Table 13-1. The accuracy of a laboratory assay is the degree of closeness to the true values and is measured by agreement statistics such as biases (systematic error) against highly accurate techniques referred to as "gold standards" for those tests. "Reliability" refers to the degree to which accurate results can be obtained on a consistent basis, thus it is a combination of both accuracy and precision. In companion and zoologic birds, there is no gold standard in hematology because no manual technique is sufficiently accurate and precise to warrant such appellation.

The total number of cells counted is generally lower when using manual methods compared with what is seen with automated analyzers in mammalian species. We can reasonably assume that counting random events, such as individual cells, follows the Poisson distribution. Graphing this function over the number of counted cells is shown in Figure 13-3. Thus, the variation of counting about 100 blood cells in a smear estimation (about 10 cells per microscope field for 10 fields) is about 10%. Likewise, the coefficient of variation for hemocytometer counting of WBCs is expected to be about 5% to 10% (if counting 100 to 400 cells), whereas it is expected to be approximately 1% for automated cell counters that count about 10,000 cells. Table 13-1 shows these statistical estimations from published reports.

Similarly, the differential counts on a blood smear use a low number of counted cells to assess relative distribution. We can assume that the percentages of blood cells follow a binomial distribution (they actually follow a multinomial distribution). Graphing this function over the probability (percentages) across several sample sizes is shown in Figure 13-3. Thus, the variation of counting common cells such as heterophils and lymphocytes is about 5% to 15%, but it gets very high and close to 25% to 40% for less common cell types such as eosinophils or monocytes. Table 13-1 shows these statistical estimations from published reports.

All variabilities from different sources are cumulative, and if known, the overall coefficient of variation may be calculated as below as an example:

$$CV_{total} = \sqrt{(CV_{hemocytometer}^2 + CV_{differential}^2 + CV_{observer}^2 + CV_{blood\ smear}^2 + \ldots)}$$

It can be easily realized that variability becomes rapidly enormous for manual hematology and that its magnitude would likely be considered unacceptable in human and domestic mammalian patients for diagnostic purposes, compared with using automated methods.[102,103]

Blood smear techniques and staining

Blood smears are made in order to produce a monolayer of blood cells that is used for calculating estimated cell counts, providing differential cell counts, and assessing cell morphology. Blood smears are subject to numerous potential artifacts, depending on the techniques employed.[2,94,104–106] Unfortunately, no studies have looked precisely at all sources of variation in blood smear preparation and the magnitude of their influence on results obtained. Factors that may affect the quality of blood smears performed by the wedge technique include, among others, the time lapse between collection and smear preparation, delayed fixation, operator performing the smear, the amount of pressure applied, the velocity of the smear procedure, the angle of the slides during smear procedure, the speed of drying and fixation, environmental humidity and temperature, and the viscosity of the blood.[2,94,104,105] Blowing on smears may cause artifacts by increasing moisture. Water or drying artifacts, which are associated with high humidity, are common and lead to morphologic changes in the RBCs. Avian cells are particularly prone to lysis (smudged cells), and this is more common in Psittaciformes than in other taxonomic orders (Beaufrère, personal observation).[94] In order to decrease the percentage of smudged cells, different procedures such as performing a squash preparation instead of a smear using the wedge technique (Figure 13-4), using the coverslip method with two coverslips, and adding bovine albumin to the blood prior to performing the smear have been implemented.[2,94] The use of the same spreader slide to make blood smears for multiple patients may lead to carryover of blood cells, which may be significant in case of hemoparasites or leukemic cells.[105] Depending on the technique used, a large degree of variation may be seen between techniques, which may add additional uncertainty to the CBC or subsequently affect comparisons between laboratories using different techniques

The stains used and the staining process may also affect cytologic assessment of the hemogram. Quick in-house stains are typically not as consistent and frequently result in low quality staining. They are also frequently contaminated with debris. Manual staining methods result in much variability, so automatic slide stainers are recommended (e.g., Hema-tek). Smears made with coverslip techniques cannot be stained by using an automated slide stainer and require manual staining methods instead.

The cell distribution on the smear may vary with the techniques used. With the wedge method, large leukocytes such as monocytes tend to be pushed to the feathered edge and to the edges of the slide, which may lead to inaccurate estimated and differential counts.[105,106] With the coverslip or the squash preparation techniques, the WBCs have a better distribution, which may lend itself to more accurate WBC.[104]

Manual cell counting

Different methods have been described for WBC determination, including estimation from the blood smear (Box 13-1), semidirect techniques such as using phloxine B or eosin and hemacytometer (Box 13-2 and Figures 13-5 to 13-7), or direct techniques such as Natt and Herrick solution or the Rees-Ecker solution (Box 13-3 and Figure 13-8). The latter techniques may also be used to obtain the RBC count (Box 13-4).

The WBC count obtained from the smear is heavily influenced by the blood smear technique and can only provide an estimate, since the leukocytes are not quantitated in a set volume of blood. In addition, since most leukocytes are present near the feather edge, the WBCs obtained from the smear may be artificially altered. If a large number of cells are lysed during the blood smear preparation, the WBCs may be artificially decreased. Consequently, WBC estimates from the smear are likely the least reproducible and accurate techniques and may be subject to large intraobserver and interobserver variability. Nevertheless, the differential count has to be performed on a stained blood smear. It is usually calculated per 100 cells, but hematologic studies in various species have shown that by increasing the number of counted cells, there is an increase in the precision and accuracy of the technique (see earlier, and Figure 13-3).[106] Furthermore, the estimated WBC count from the smear is frequently based on a single formula (see Box 13-1). However, since WBCs are counted in a monolayer area with a certain spread of the RBCs, failure to correct for too low or too high a PCV may artificially modify the count. The fields of view that are examined vary with the microscope, and formulas may have to be adapted to the specific microscope used. This may

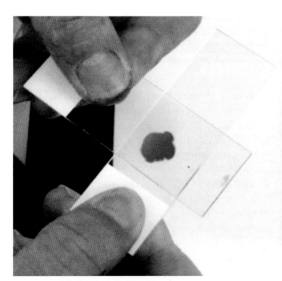
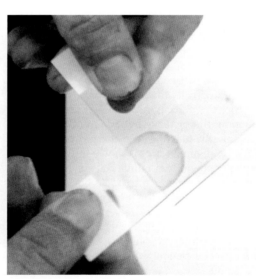

FIGURE 13-4 Blood smear being performed using a squash preparation. This technique is recommended to avoid cell lysis common in avian blood samples while processing the slide in an automated slide stainer.

BOX 13-1 ESTIMATION FROM THE SMEAR

At 400 magnification (×40 objectives and ×10 eyepiece), all leukocytes in 10 fields are counted in the monolayer area.

Formula: WBC (× 10⁹/L)= N/10·1.5

→ for a microscope with a field of view of 0.24 mm² at ×400 magnification with an eyepiece of 22 mm.
→ The area of field of view can be easily calculated by taking a picture of the field of view using a stage micrometer scale. This formula may then be adapted based on specific fields of view.

Corrective factor in anemic birds: WBC · PCV/45

BOX 13-2 WHITE BLOOD CELL COUNT— PHLOXINE B AND EOSIN TECHNIQUES

Phloxine B technique: Using a micropipette, mix 25 μL of blood with 775 μL of 0.1% phloxine B (Vetlab supply, Palmetto Bay, FL) to obtain a 1:32 dilution. Incubate for 5 minutes at room temperature on a rocker. Transfer on hemocytometer, and allow 5 minutes for cell settling in chambers. Read at the ×10 objective. All red-staining cells are counted in 5 square millimeters (four corner squares and the central large square) of both chambers (see Figures 13-5 and 13-6) using the *L* rule (see Figure 13-7). The phloxine only stains heterophils and eosinophils.

Eosin technique: Identical except that the stain is the eosin stain of a quick stain (e.g., J-322-3, Jorgensen Laboratories Inc. Loveland, CO) diluted at 1:10 using distilled water (optimal dilution factor to reduce erythrocytes staining).

WBC (× 10⁹/L) = N·32·100/(10·0.1·1000· Percentage heterophils+eosinophils)

Simplified formula: WBC (× 10⁹/L) = N·3.2/ Percentage heterophils+eosinophils

be accomplished by performing a small in-house study comparing with a quantitative method. Also, different observers are likely to select different fields and areas of the slides for performing their differential counts.

Misidentification of blood cell types may also increase laboratory error and depends on the level of experience and competency of the operators involved (Figure 13-9).

The estimation of the percentage of band heterophils may be complicated in birds by their granules that tend to obscure the nucleus and the lower degree of segmentation of the nucleus. An early study in chickens reported a high interobserver variability in the differential cell counts.[107] Also, polychromatophils and erythrocytes with abnormal shapes are usually reported using semiquantitative scales (1+ to 4+) (decreased, normal, increased) that may lead to great variation among observers and over serial CBCs. The experience and qualification of the observer (trained clinical pathologists) are also of paramount importance, and a higher degree of experience and skill may decrease the variability in interpretation and the accuracy of hematologic diagnostics.

Several studies have investigated the precision of manual cell counting methods (see Table 13-1). Overall, the technique employing phloxine B seems superior. This technique is indirect because phloxine B only stains granules from heterophils and eosinophils, thus requiring the differential counts to still be used to mathematically obtain the WBCs (see Box 13-2). Nevertheless, it seems more precise than direct techniques such as the Natt and Herrick method probably because of the difficulties in differentiating some WBCs from thrombocytes with the latter.[8,54,106,108,109] The Rees-Ecker technique is another direct method and seems superior to the Natt and Herrick technique, at least in chickens.[8,110] All these techniques have some limitations in common. Protocols for cell staining need to be followed, as each stain has an optimal incubation time at which identification of positively stained cells is the most accurate. For instance, phloxine tends to start staining other cells after some time, thus artificially increasing cell counts if excessive staining time has been used

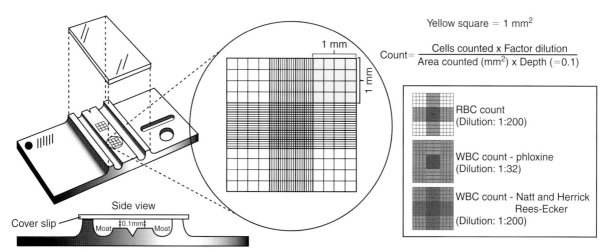

Yellow square = 1 mm²

$$\text{Count} = \frac{\text{Cells counted} \times \text{Factor dilution}}{\text{Area counted (mm}^2\text{)} \times \text{Depth (=0.1)}}$$

RBC count (Dilution: 1:200)

WBC count - phloxine (Dilution: 1:32)

WBC count - Natt and Herrick Rees-Ecker (Dilution: 1:200)

FIGURE 13-5 Hemocytometer and a close-up view of the counting areas as seen under the microscope. The *red insert box* shows the different counting areas, depending on the technique with the dilution factor. The general formula for hemocytometer-based cell count is also given. (Modified from Hippel T: Routine testing in hematology. In Rodak B, Fritsma G, Doig K, editors: *Hematology: clinical principles and applications,* ed 3, St Louis, MO, 2007, Saunders, pp 160–174.)

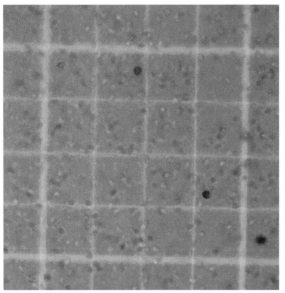

FIGURE 13-6 Phloxine B method. Three red-staining cells are positive.

BOX 13-3 WHITE BLOOD CELL COUNT: NATT AND HERRICK/REES AND ECKER TECHNIQUES

NH technique: Using a micropipette, mix 10 μL of blood with 2 mL of Natt and Herrick solution (Vetlab supply, Palmetto Bay, FL) to obtain a 1:200 dilution. The stain is based on methyl violet 2B. Incubate for 5 minutes at room temperature on a rocker. Transfer on hemocytometer and allow 5 minutes for cell settling in chambers. Read at the 10× objective. All dark purple–staining cells (see Figure 13-8) are counted in 9 square millimeters (all large squares [see Figure 13-5]) of one chamber using the L rule (see Figure 13-7). Caution must be taken not to count thrombocytes (they should not be larger than the RBC nucleus width, unlike leukocytes).

Rees and Ecker technique: Identical except that the stain is the Rees and Ecker solution (RICCA chemical, Arlington, TX). The stain is based on brilliant cresyl blue.

$$WBC\ (\times 10^9/L) = N \times 200/(9 \cdot 0.1 \cdot 1000)$$

$$\text{Simplified Formula: } WBC\ (\times 10^9/L) = N/4.5$$

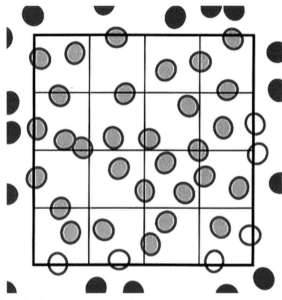

FIGURE 13-7 One square of hemocytometer indicating which cells to count. Cells touching the left and top lines are counted *(solid circles)*. Cells touching bottom and right are not counted *(open circles)*. (From Hippel T: Routine testing in hematology. In Rodak B, Fritsma G, Doig K, editors: *Hematology: clinical principles and applications*, ed 3, St Louis, 2007, Saunders, pp 160–174.)

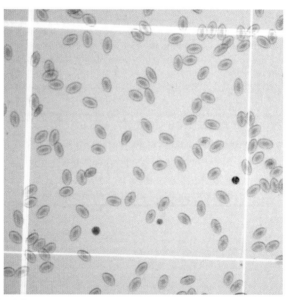

FIGURE 13-8 Natt and Herrick method. Two dark purple staining cells are positive. The smaller lighter cell is probably a thrombocyte and should not be counted. However, it is difficult to differentiate small lymphocytes from thrombocytes with this technique.

(Figure 13-10).[4] Other factors that may add to the analytical error of hemocytometer-based techniques include lack of proper settling of cells in the hemocytometer chambers, the presence of small clots, uneven charging of the hemocytometer chambers, improper use of the microscope (e.g., condenser position), observer variability, and the presence of a large number of hypogranular heterophils that may remain unstained (see Figure 13-10). Some parrots also have deeply basophilic eosinophil granules (see Figure 13-1), and it is not certain that they stain positively with phloxine B in all species. Moreover, the different manual cell counting techniques show poor agreement with each other in birds, and this variation has been demonstrated in chickens, macaws, and owls.[54,109,110] In owls, estimated WBC counts from the smear tended to be higher than hemocytometer-phloxine B counts and the WBC count obtained through the Natt and Herrick method was lower. The disagreement increased with the increasing absolute counts, suggesting that methods become

BOX 13-4 RED BLOOD CELL COUNT USING NATT AND HERRICK SOLUTION

Using a micropipette, mix 10 μL of blood with 2 mL of Natt and Herrick solution (Vetlab supply, Palmetto Bay, FL) to obtain a 1:200 dilution. The stain is based on methyl violet 2B. Incubate for 5 minutes at room temperature on a rocker. Transfer on hemocytometer, and allow 5 minutes for cell settling in chambers. Read at the ×40 objective. All erythrocytes are counted in five small squares (four corner squares and the central small square = 5/25 small squares [see Figures 13-5 and 13-8]) of the central square millimeter of one chamber using the *L* rule (see Figure 13-7).

Formula: RBC (× 10^{12}/L) = N·200·5/(0.1·1,000,000)

Simplified formula: RBC (× 10^{12}/L) = N/100

less and less comparable as the true number of WBCs increases. It was also shown that different owl species exhibited different staining properties of their leukocytes with hemocytomer-based stains. This was notably translated into variable difficulties in differentiating thrombocytes from lymphocytes with the Natt and Herrick stain.[54] A similar trend was found in macaws, in which WBC estimations from the smear were higher than the hemocytometer–phloxine B counts.[109] In mammals, a study found wide discrepancies between estimated WBC and automated analyzers for dogs and cats that were presented on emergency, with also a tendency to overestimate.[111] As reported in owls, these discrepancies increased as the cell counts increased.

Postanalytical Variability

This type of variability pertains to the reporting and communication of results. Nonstandardized methods with improper storage of hematologic data may lead to subsequent mistakes.

Minimizing the Impact of Laboratory Errors

Different steps and procedures commonly known as "quality assurance measures" should be followed in order to minimize laboratory errors and their impact. There are no regulations in veterinary medicine regarding quality assurance of laboratory test performance. As such, the various stakeholders should demonstrate and share a commitment for optimal maintenance, correct calibration, self-monitoring, and appropriate quality assurance.[112] The American Society for Veterinary Clinical Pathology (ASVCP) has released quality assurance guidelines in order to minimize preanalytical and analytical factors in veterinary hematology, with special attention given to nonmammalian species.[112] Unfortunately, no commercially prepared control materials are available for nonmammalian cell counting, which prevents a thorough evaluation of the accuracy and variability of manual cell counting techniques in birds as well as performing quality control in the laboratory.[112]

A variety of techniques are used for CBCs and both in-clinic and reference laboratories should select the least variable, most accurate, and most reproducible analytical techniques. Considering experiments performed on manual cell counting in birds, it appears that under the present circumstances, these prerogatives are best met by hemocytometer techniques that either employ semidirect counting with the phloxine B stain or direct

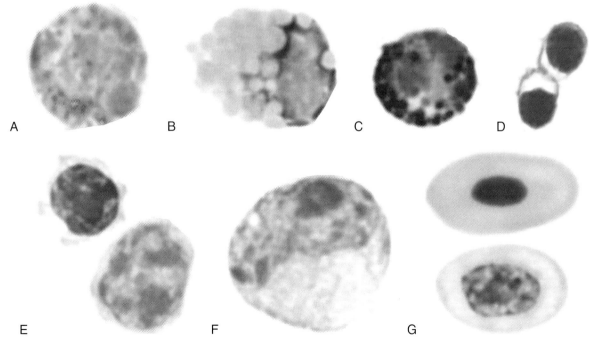

FIGURE 13-9 Morphology of white blood cells, example in Psittaciformes stained with a modified Wright stain in an automated slide stainer. **A,** Heterophil. **B,** Eosinophil. **C,** Basophil. **D,** Two thrombocytes. **E,** A small and a large lymphocyte. **F,** Monocyte. **G,** Erythrocyte and polychromatophil *(bottom cell).*

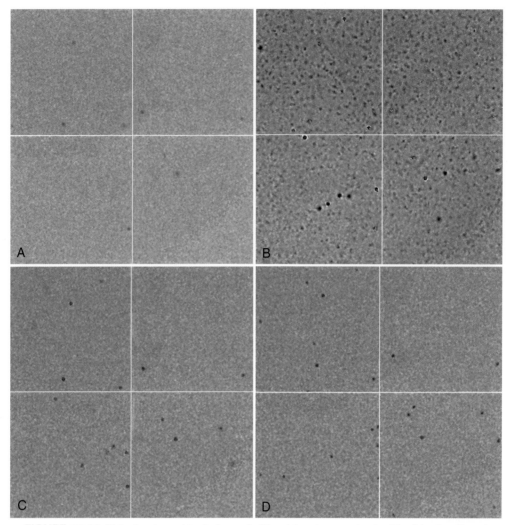

FIGURE 13-10 Phloxine-based technique. **A,** Blood has been mixed with phloxine B and transferred to a hemocytometer, but cells have not yet settled. **B,** The condenser is raised too close to the slide, which may complicate differentiation of positive cells. **C,** This shows positive cells after 15 minutes of incubation in the hemocytometer. **D,** This shows positive cells after 1 hour of incubation in the hemocytometer. Compared with *C,* there is an increase in positive cells likely caused by overstaining on cells other than heterophils and eosinophils.

counting using the Rees-Ecker stain. Other stains and techniques add much more uncertainty to hematologic results and should be used only when these techniques are not available, or if used, rigorous standardization must be implemented to minimize all controllable sources of variation (e.g., same observer, same microscope). For differential counts, smears made using a squash preparation limit both the amount of morphologic and cell distribution artifacts and allow staining using an automated slide stainer. Counting the highest number of cells possible will decrease random error (see Figure 13-3). Since variability associated with the blood smear method is likely responsible for a large proportion of the total variability in results obtained in avian hematology, consistent ability to make excellent quality blood smears as early as possible after blood sampling cannot be overemphasized. When hematology samples are being submitted to reference laboratories, it is advised to select those with a good reputation in zoologic species hematology, specifically avian species. There should be known high-quality assurance standards, and there should be trained clinical pathologists with experience in avian species.

REFERENCE INTERVALS AND THEIR APPLICATIONS IN AVIAN MEDICINE

General Concepts and Limitations in Avian Clinical Pathology

Reference intervals are statistically determined numerical intervals, based on the 95% of values of a healthy representative sample of a population. This is classically the interval between the 2.5% and the 97.5% percentiles. They include a point estimate for the lower limit and for the upper limit and typically a 90% confidence interval around the point estimates. These reference intervals represent the spread of values within a healthy population, and include all sources of variability (biologic and laboratory), except when stratified.

Reference limits are merely statistical estimations of the true reference limits of a population of animals, which are not realistically obtainable. Therefore, only a relatively small but hopefully representative sample can be used. Since these reference limits are estimations, a measure of precision must be given, which is the confidence interval. When assessing the clinical usefulness and precision of reported reference limits for a given hematologic parameter in a given species, it is crucial to look at these confidence intervals. This is especially true in uncommon bird species, where the chances for imprecision are the greatest.

In order to make an optimal inference of these reference intervals (to get a better idea of the true reference limits), several criteria must be met on the sample used for the approximation. The higher the sample size, the higher the precision of the reference limits and the narrower the confidence intervals around the limits will be. The sample used should also be representative of the population under study, or the statistical inferences will not be correct. Practically, using a sample of laboratory birds under controlled conditions to make an inference on reference limits in a population of pet birds under variable captive conditions may not be the best strategy because the sample will not be representative. Likewise, using a sample of wild birds that are being treated in a rehabilitation center to make inferences on captive-bred birds in a zoologic institution accustomed to captivity may not be representative. In theory, samples must be a random subset of the target population in order to limit the possibility of selection bias.

The American Society for Veterinary Clinical Pathology (ASVCP) has released comprehensive guidelines for the establishments of reference intervals.[113] Unfortunately, in most situations, it is improbable that these guidelines would be met in avian reference intervals studies. First, samples are rarely representative of target populations because they are often convenience samples obtained on available research colonies of birds, populations of birds under different captivity situations, or as add-on studies on other research projects using birds. For instance, laboratory colonies of animals are usually very homogeneous in age distribution and husbandry conditions, which leads to tighter reference intervals that may translate into a high rate of false-positive results when applied to the target population (loss in specificity). Stress levels may also be different, depending on captive and sampling conditions and may impact several hematologic parameters.[45,46] The wide application of reference intervals is based on the assumption of the homogeneity of the population, which may not be the case in most avian species groups. Second, accurate determination of health status may be problematic in species that frequently conceal clinical signs, when there is less familiarity with the species in question, when the CBC is the purpose of the research, and when medical diagnostics are not available under field conditions.

Perhaps the most significant limitation in avian reference intervals determination is low sample size. Although researchers may strive to sample as many individuals of a species or population as possible, for less common species, they often are restricted by what is available, and reference intervals will have greater uncertainties as a result.[114] Indirect sampling, which is sampling from medical databases, may be used to increase sample sizes but adds to the uncertainty of

the techniques used, since the health status of the subjects is uncertain. However, a study in Psittaciformes using this method showed poor results and wide reference intervals.[115] Multicenter studies may also allow an increase in sample sizes, but all laboratories should have identical analytical techniques. In zoological medicine, the International Species Information System (ISIS) has made available hematologic reference values for a large number of avian species, but various selection criteria, heterogeneity of hematologic techniques, lack of statistical analysis, and other confounding variables may lower the usefulness of such a resource.[116] Specifically, the ASVCP recommends a sample size of 120 individuals, which can be challenging to meet in many bird species. Estimation of reference intervals from sample sizes lower than 20 individuals should not be performed. For sample sizes lower than 10 individuals, reference values should not be reported. These small sample sizes also preclude other refinement processes such as stratification and partitioning by age, sex, season, or subspecies. For reference intervals that are refined over a continuous variable (covariate), regression-based reference limits are the method of choice.[117] It has been estimated by statistical simulation that a minimum sample size of 70 would be needed for a covariate such as age.[117] Examples of reference intervals focused on an age group can be found for juvenile Psittaciformes, bustards, ciconiid species, and accipitrid species.[a] Overall, the more the sources of variability can be identified and accounted for, the more sensitive the reference values will be. Nevertheless, reference intervals tend to be broader in birds than in domestic mammals because of the considerable biologic and laboratory variations inherently encountered.

The ASVCP guidelines also expand on analytical procedures and statistical analysis.[113] There are different types of statistics that can be performed, depending on the sample size and data distribution. Recommendations are to use nonparametric techniques for sample sizes higher than 120 subjects, robust or parametric methods for sample sizes between 40 and 120, and robust methods for sample sizes less than 40 individuals. In all cases, confidence intervals of the reference limits should be obtained as a measure of uncertainty. A study on a canine analyte with a heavily skewed distribution showed that for small sample sizes (n = 27), reference limits estimated were highly variable, confidence intervals of the limits could not be meaningfully calculated, and none of the available statistical methods was satisfactory for estimating reference intervals.[119] The authors also suggested reporting all individual values for small samples. Nevertheless, robust methods are recommended when dealing with small sample sizes over other statistical methods but a minimum sample size of 40 is ideal.[113,120,121] Most hematologic variables are not normally distributed, and nonparametric or robust statistics should be used whenever possible.[122] An example in birds is the distribution of the WBCs in Strigiformes, which showed that despite large samples sizes, the distribution was not normal, which likely reflects the true underlying nonnormal distribution of these hematologic parameters (Figure 13-11).[54] Detection of outliers that may confound statistical calculations should also be implemented. Specific software products are available to

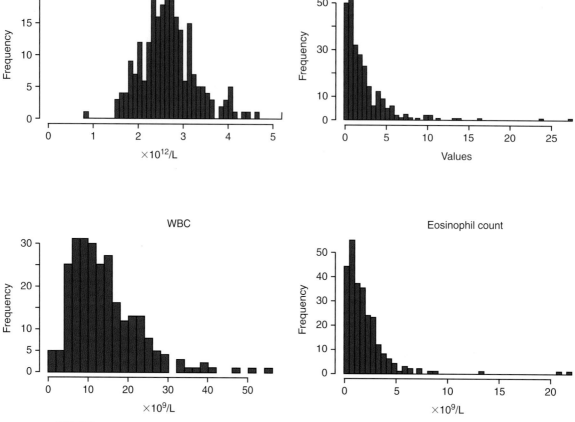

FIGURE 13-11 Frequency distribution of blood cells in a large population of captive owls. Although the erythrocyte count tends to show a normal distribution, the heterophil-to-lymphocyte (H/L) ratio, the white blood cell, and the eosinophil counts are examples of cells that have significant right skewness.

calculate reference intervals. Some of these software products such as Reference Value Advisor or the R-package "referenceIntervals," are free of charge.[123,124] Both these free software products are based on ASVCP guidelines.

In addition, the transfer of reference intervals determined by one technique to another should be properly evaluated by agreement studies.[113,125] There is a wide array of techniques used for manual cell counting in birds, and several studies have shown large disagreement between the techniques.[54,109,110,126] Consequently, the transference of reference intervals in avian hematology from one technique to another is unlikely to be feasible.

In order to increase the sensitivity of reference intervals when interindividual variability is higher than intraindividual variability, subject-based reference intervals may be used instead (see above).[127] The usefulness of subject-based reference intervals may be based on the calculation of the index of individuality (IoI). The IoI is equal to $\sqrt{(CV_{individual}^2 + CV_{analytical}^2)}/CV_{group}$ and the lower it is, the greater is the individuality of the analyte.[113,127] In automated assays, the $CV_{analytical}$ is frequently omitted because the $CV_{individual}$ and the CV_{group} are so much higher.[113,127] However, because of large analytical errors in avian hematology, this simplification cannot be justified. Subject-based reference intervals are recommended when IoI

is less than 0.6 and population-based reference intervals are recommended when IoI is greater than 1.4.[113,127] Few studies have been performed on the index of individuality of avian hematologic parameters, but it appears to be low overall for avian blood analytes except PCV, which supports the use of subject-based reference intervals (recalculated for Jones et al to account for $CV_{analytical}$).[28,128] Subject-based reference intervals can be obtained during routine health checks over several years before the patient actually presents with a clinical condition. Such reference intervals have been especially recommended in zoological medicine, where the generation of population-based reference intervals is problematic.[127]

Published Reference Intervals and their Use in the Clinical Decision-Making Process

The use of published reference values in peer-reviewed or non-peer-reviewed (e.g., ISIS, books, web-based) sources depends on the validity and appropriateness of the criteria used to obtain them. However, most reference intervals published in avian hematology are derived from samples with low number of animals, poorly representative of the population of interest, and obtained without randomized sampling and by using variable hematologic and counting techniques.

Furthermore, statistical analysis and proper reporting may be lacking, especially on the precision of the reference limits. Indeed, a survey of the avian medical literature between 2007 and 2011 reported that approximately 93% of statistical reference interval studies failed to either properly determine or report reference limits.[129] In addition, the high number of avian species precludes the determination of adequate reference intervals in all species, so some extrapolation is anticipated. To complicate the issue, reference intervals may show large differences between sources for the same species, probably because the demographics of the population and the techniques were different (see above for biologic and laboratory variability). For instance, the WBC reference values from blue-and-gold macaws (*Ara ararauna*) varies by as much as 100% with the following means reported: 8.5, 16.6, 12.75, 14 ×10⁹/L.[56,58,130,131]

Although it is best for laboratories to establish their own reference intervals, this is seldom done for most species of birds, and hematologic techniques and demographic data may not be disclosed. Nevertheless, laboratories may try to validate and transfer published reference intervals with a subset of their database providing that preanalytical and analytical criteria are similar. Before using published reference intervals for clinical interpretation, one should assess scientific papers for approximate compliance with the ASVCP guidelines. The reference intervals should be somewhat representative of the demographics of the population they are used on, and analytical techniques need to be similar to those used to obtain the patient's results. However, some references may not provide enough information to assess the quality of the reference values.[113]

Under the assumption that some information is better than none, clinicians must learn how to deal with poorly determined reference intervals when nothing else is available. First, when reported data are insufficient, a 95% reference interval may be approximated. If the mean, median, and standard deviation (SD) are available, then normality could be roughly assumed if the mean is equal to the median. Then, according to the empirical rule, the mean ± 2 SD approximately encompasses 95.4% of the data and thus can be used as an alternative reference intervals (mean ± 1 SD only encompasses 68.3% of the data). If only the mean and standard error of the mean (SEM) are reported, then, provided that data are normally distributed, an approximate 95% reference interval is: mean ± 2√(n)SEM. The clinician may also have to consider the extra variability associated with the poor reporting and the lack of proper statistical determination. If the raw data are available, then repeating the statistical analysis may be warranted. If the technique used in the manuscript is different from the technique used for the patient, then an extra 20% to 30% variability must be added, which roughly corresponds to the variability of most manual counting techniques.

Furthermore, clinicians must acknowledge the fact that most published reference intervals only constitute rough estimates of hematologic values and should not think in terms of absolute numbers. If 90% confidence intervals of the reference limits are present, the interval between the lower confidence limit of the lower reference limit and the upper confidence limit of the upper reference limit may be used as the reference interval to decrease the false-positive rate.

Conversely, clinicians must acknowledge that the false-negative rate may be high with wide reference intervals, and patient values close to the upper or lower reference limits in a bird with clinical signs may still bear some significance.

Blood counts must differ greatly from reference limits to have diagnostic significance. Also, although the numbers are useful, it must be realized that cell morphology on the blood smear may provide tremendous information such as the presence of a left shift, erythrocyte regeneration, cell toxicity, the presence of blood parasites, and other cytologic changes. In any case, once a diagnosis is obtained, initial hematologic values can be used for follow-up. It should also be recognized that, by definition, 2.5% of the normal population will have higher values and 2.5% lower values than the reference intervals.

In some fields and for some analytes, clinical decision threshold and cutoff values have been used. Ideally, these values should be based on prospective diagnostic accuracy studies and epidemiologic outcome analysis aiming at finding decision limits that maximize sensitivity and specificity (typically using receiver-operating characteristic curves).[113,132] To the authors' knowledge, such studies have not yet been performed in avian hematology. Alternatively, decision threshold may be based on expert opinion or a consensus of clinicians.

Extrapolation and Alternatives to Reference Intervals in Birds

In zoological medicine and a fortiori in avian medicine, one of the unique challenges seldom encountered in domestic animal medicine is the complete lack of reference intervals. To overcome this limitation, individualized reference intervals should be established prior to the development of clinical conditions in these animals. However, this may not always be possible or available.

Comparison of values of a sick bird to several healthy control individuals of the same species, if available, may be used for interpretation, but it will give an incomplete picture of the different sources and the degree of biologic variations. However, control subjects are usually kept under somewhat similar husbandry and nutritional conditions, thus minimizing most sources of environmental variations.

Reference intervals at a higher taxonomic level, such as genus, family, or order, may be a reasonable alternative to consider. The reporting of hematologic values at a higher taxonomic level than species has been used multiple times in avian medicine for groups of birds considered taxonomically, ecologically, or morphologically homogeneous, such as some Psittaciformes genera or raptorial groups.[14,15,54,130,133] This approach may increase sample size, allowing the use of better statistical techniques through better assessment of the underlying statistical distributions. Higher-level taxonomic groupings may be a starting point to assess species-specific differences within a specific group. Obviously, there will be more uncertainty and less sensitivity than with species-specific reference intervals, but they may prove useful in some circumstances such as when hematologic responses to disease are of great magnitude.

Direct extrapolation from other avian species is also frequently employed in practice and is probably the least recommendable option. No rules govern interspecies extrapolation, but using the phylogenetically closest species seems logical.

However, phylogenetically close species may display drastic morphologic, ecologic, and geographic differences that undoubtedly impact hematologic variables. For instance, within the order Strigiformes, great horned owls (*Bubo virginianus*) and snowy owls (*Bubo scandiacus*) have markedly different hematologic reference intervals while being remarkably close phylogenetically.[54] Furthermore, it was shown that scavenging ethology was a strong predictor for a higher WBC count regardless of phylogenetic relationships.[59] If interspecies extrapolation is performed, a species that is close not only phylogenetically but also ecologically must be selected. Nevertheless, there are tremendous uncertainties associated with such a practice.

Serial sampling to obtain consecutive hematologic values may also be performed in an attempt to identify trends toward pathophysiologic states, dynamic hematologic responses to disease, or response to treatment. In the absence of reference values, this strategy may prove to be clinically valuable. Significant changes between consecutive measurements are called "reference change value" or "critical differences." This is different from subject-based reference intervals because it is usually determined from a small population of individuals sampled serially rather than in the same individual and the focus is more on detecting changes in a monitoring situation for diseased animals, not the development of a reference interval per se.[127] The other difference is that the $CV_{individual}$ is ideally taken from sick animals rather than healthy animals as it is expected to be higher in the former, leading to less false-positive results. However, to assess critical differences among consecutive measurements, biologic (individual and group) and laboratory variability must be known for each hematologic parameter (see above).[113,134] The critical difference is typically defined as $z_{0.05} \sqrt{(SD_{analytical}^2 + SD_{individual}^2)}$ for a probability of 95% to find differences, thus SD_{group} is excluded (representing interindividual biologic variation).[135] In automated assays, the critical difference formula simplifies when considering that $SD_{analytical}$ is considerably lower than $SD_{individual}$ to $1.96 \times \sqrt{(2)} \times SD_{individual}$, which further simplifies as $2.8SD_{individual}$.[113,134,135] One may also use coefficient of variation (CV) in place of SD. However, since avian hematologic techniques have much larger variability than automated techniques, in the range of $CV_{analytical} = 10\%$ to 20%, such simplification should not be done. The $CV_{individual}$ has not often been reported in birds but 10% to 15% may be a reasonable estimation for leukocyte counts, for instance.[28] Consequently, it is to be expected that critical differences in birds for leukocyte counts are in the range of $1.96 \times \sqrt{[2(0.1 + 0.1)^2]}$ to $1.96 \times \sqrt{[2(0.2 + 0.15)^2]}$, simplifying to 55% to 97% for individuals' serial measurements. These differences may appear large, but some hematologic variables such as the WBC count appear to show greater variation in birds than other analytes such as the PCV (with critical differences expected to be around 14% in birds). These variations may mask changes attributed to disease effects and dynamics. A critical difference of 34% for leukocyte counts has also been reported for humans.[135] Critical differences as high as 50% have even been reported for canine biochemistry analytes.[134] In addition, this is a rough approximation that could be refined if bird individual variability for analytes (through serial measurements in health) and laboratory errors of specific reference or in-house laboratories were measured.

FUTURE DIRECTIONS

Back to Basics

There is a critical lack of scientific investigations into the reliability and accuracy of the different hematologic techniques for birds and on the quantification of the various sources of variability (see Table 13-1). In addition, there are few reports that looked at intermethod agreement.[54,109,110] It would be beneficial to have a systematic approach comparing the different techniques and quantifying the different sources of variability in different species. Except for an early study in chickens, we could not find reports documenting intraobserver and interobserver variability of these techniques despite the fact that they are highly observer dependent.[107] Likewise, more artifacts and challenges occur with blood smear techniques in birds, yet no experiment has quantified the different sources of variability and how to minimize them. These sources of variability include blood smear techniques, operators, microscope field of views, staining, cytologist, and so on. Studies aimed at determining critical differences for hematologic parameters over serial measurements would be useful to differentiate between the dynamics of the response being seen and normal intraindividual day-to-day variation.

Although the guidelines on reference intervals released by the ASVCP has promoted better quality reports in avian hematology, proper reference intervals are still lacking for most species. Establishing multicenter-based reference intervals and values with adequate statistical presentation, based on collaborative work and shared hematologic information, would address both the problem of low sample size and representation of the population. The data presented by the ISIS give an insight into what may be achievable, but reporting the distribution of the data, sources of the samples, and hematologic techniques used and presenting statistically calculated reference intervals would be ideal.

Ultimately, even if all sources of variability are known and controlled as much as possible, manual cell counting will still remain grossly imprecise and inaccurate because of the inherent imprecision associated with a low number of counted cells and inconsistency of manual procedures. If avian hematology is to improve and become a better and more sensitive tool for diagnostic purposes, automated techniques will have to be developed. The two main areas that we think may have potential applications in avian CBC automatization are image and flow cytometry. It has been shown that the precision of these techniques in birds is high, close to 2%.[136,137]

Image Cytometry

Image cytometry consists of measuring various parameters including size, shape, color, and texture on cells from captured images of biologic materials using computer software. Automated hematology analyzers using image cytometry for mammals are commercially available, for example, the CellaVision DM96 (CellaVision AB, Sysmex America, Mundelein, IL), but we could not find reports of this technique having been used to generate avian CBCs. This machine uses blood smears, machine learning, and iterative feedback and is able to detect abnormal cell types such as neoplastic cells.[138,139] It would be valuable to test the performance of such machines in avian hematology, where all blood cells are nucleated. Image cytometry has been investigated in Psittaciformes by using a high-resolution slide scanner and open-source software, such as Cellprofiler (Broad institute, www.cellprofiler.org) and Cellprofiler Analyst.[136] Hemoparasite detection and quantification of parasitemia in birds were performed successfully in a study using the ImageJ software (ImageJ, NIH, http://imagej.nih.gov/ij).[140] Furthermore, image cytometry has already been applied to nucleated cells in human bone marrow samples.[141,142] Image cytometry algorithms and machine-learning processes are constantly refined and perfected, computing power is ever increasing, and image recognition is now being used in a variety of real-life processes. Therefore, clinical applications in the field of nonmammalian hematology are possible in the near future. Automated microscopy, in which blood smears are automatically performed in a standardized manner and image acquisition is digital, may also provide enhanced precision for avian hematologic samples.

Flow Cytometry

Flow cytometry consists of counting and sorting cells based on a variety of parameters, including light scattering at various angles, fluorescent characteristics, immunophenotyping by using antibodies, and other dye-labelling processes. The development of more specific techniques such as flow cytometric immunophenotyping using a panel of blood cell antibodies is currently difficult because of the wide diversity of avian species, which means that antibodies may recognize antigens on only one or a few species. This technique is also labor intensive, and the reagent costs are prohibitive. Hematologic analyses by immunophenotyping have been reported in several studies of commercial poultry for leukocytes, lymphocytes, and thrombocytes, but is unlikely to be applicable at a wider scale in avian medicine.[137,143-145] Other flow cytometric analyses that do not use antibodies have been used with variable success in quails, chickens, and geese.[146,147] These studies used a fluorescent lipophilic dye, the 3, 3-dihexyloxacarbocyanine ($DiOC_6(3)$), which preferentially stains leukocytes and thrombocytes. In an initial study in quails, the method could not differentiate between lymphocytes and thrombocytes or between heterophils and eosinophils.[146] Further refinement of the study using $DiOC_5(3)$ instead of $DiOC_6(3)$ led to adequate differentiation between lymphocytes and thrombocytes in quails, chickens, and geese.[147] The successful application of the latter technique to different avian species is promising for wider application in avian hematology. Overall, with the constant improvement in the technology and cost, flow cytometric techniques may offer real possibilities for performing automated avian CBC that could be applied to a variety of avian species in the future.

REFERENCES

1. Briscoe JA, Rosenthal KL, Shofer FS: Selected complete blood cell count and plasma protein electrophoresis parameters in pet psittacine birds evaluated for illness, *J Avian Med Surg* 24(2):131–137, 2010.
2. Campbell T, Ellis C: Hematology of birds. In Campbell T, Ellis C, editors: *Avian and exotic animal hematology and cytology*, ed 3, Oxford, UK, 2007, Wiley-Blackwell, pp 3–50.
3. Clark P, Boardman W, Raidal S: *Atlas of Clinical avian hematology*, Chichester, UK, 2009, Wiley-Blackwell, p 200.
4. Fudge A: Avian complete blood count. In Fudge A, editor: *Laboratory medicine: avian and exotic pets*, Philadelphia, PA, 2000, W.B. Saunders Company, pp 9–18.
5. Lilliehöök I, Wall H, Tauson R, et al: Differential leukocyte counts determined in chicken blood using the Cell-Dyn 3500, *Vet Clin Pathol* 33(3):133–138, 2004.
6. Walberg J: White blood cell counting techniques in birds, *Semin Avian Exot Pets* 10(2):72–76, 2001.
7. Leclerc A, Roman Y, Berthet M, et al: Comparison between manual and electrical impedance measurement automated total and differential blood counts in the African Grey parrot (*Psittacus erithacus*), *Proc Eur Assoc Avian Vet* 256–263, 2007.
8. Lucas A, Jamroz C: *Atlas of avian hematology*, Washington DC, 1961, Agriculture monograph 25, United States Department of Agriculture, p 271.
9. Aroch I, Targan N, Gancz A: A novel modified semi-direct method for total leukocyte count in birds, *Isr J Vet Med* 68(2):111–118, 2013.
10. Natt MP, Herrick CA: A new blood diluent for counting the erythrocytes and leucocytes of the chicken, *Poult Sci* 31(4):735–738, 1952.
11. Wiseman BK: An improved direct method for obtaining the total white cell count in avian blood, *Exp Biol Med* 28(9):1030–1033, 1931.
12. Scanes C: Blood. In Scanes C, editor: *Sturkie's avian physiology*, ed 6, San Diego, CA, 2015, Academic Press, pp 167–192.
13. Fair J, Whitaker S, Pearson B: Sources of variation in haematocrit in birds, *Ibis (Lond 1859)* 149(3):535–552, 2007.
14. Clubb S, RM S, Joyner K: Hematologic and serum biochemical reference intervals in juvenile cockatoos, *J Assoc Avian Vet* 5:16–26, 1991.
15. Clubb S, Schubot R, Joyner K: Hematologic and serum biochemical reference intervals in juvenile macaws (*Ara sp.*), *J Assoc Avian Vet* 5:154–162, 1991.
16. Clubb S, Schubot R, Joyner K: Hematologic and serum chemistry reference intervals in juvenile Eclectus parrots, *J Assoc Avian Vet* 4:218–225, 1990.
17. Lanzarot MP, Barahona MV, Andrés MIS, et al: Hematologic, protein electrophoresis, biochemistry, and cholinesterase values of free-living black stork nestlings (*Ciconia nigra*), *J Wildl Dis* 41(2):379–386, 2005.
18. Hernández M, Margalida A: Hematology and blood chemistry reference values and age-related changes in wild bearded vultures (*Gypaetus barbatus*), *J Wildl Dis* 46(2):390–400, 2010.
19. Work TM: Weights, hematology, and serum chemistry of seven species of free-ranging tropical pelagic seabirds, *J Wildl Dis* 32(4):643–657, 1996.
20. Haefele HJ, Sidor I, Evers DC, et al: Hematologic and physiologic reference ranges for free-ranging adult and young common loons (*Gavia immer*), *J Zoo Wildl Med* 36(3):385–390, 2005.
21. Allgayer MC, Guedes NMR, Chiminazzo C, et al: Clinical pathology and parasitologic evaluation of free-living nestlings of the hyacinth macaw (*Anodorhynchus hyacinthinus*), *J Wildl Dis* 45(4):972–981, 2009.
22. Van Wyk E, van der Bank H, Verdoorn GH: Dynamics of haematology and blood biochemistry in free-living African whitebacked vulture (*Pseudogyps africanus*) nestlings, *Comp Biochem Physiol A Mol Integr Physiol* 120(3):495–508, 1998.
23. Merino S, Barbosa A: Haematocrit values in chinstrap penguins (*Pygoscelis antarctica*): variation with age and reproductive status, *Polar Biol* 17(1):14–16, 2014.
24. Amat JA, Rendón MA, Ramírez JM, et al: Hematocrit is related to age but not to nutritional condition in greater flamingo chicks, *Eur J Wildl Res* 55(2):179–182, 2008.
25. Kocan R, Pitts S: Blood values of the canvasback duck by age, sex, and season, *J Wildl Dis* 12(3):341–346, 1976.
26. Howlett J, Samour J, Bailey T, et al: Age-related haematology changes in captive-reared kori bustards (*Ardeotis kori*), *Comp Haematol Int* 8:26–30, 1998.
27. Charles-Smith LE, Rutledge ME, Meek CJ, et al: Hematologic parameters and hemoparasites of nonmigratory Canada geese (*Branta canadensis*) from Greensboro, North Carolina, USA, *J Avian Med Surg* 28(1):16–23, 2014.

28. Jones MP, Arheart KL, Cray C: Reference intervals, longitudinal analyses, and index of individuality of commonly measured laboratory variables in captive bald eagles (*Haliaeetus leucocephalus*), *J Avian Med Surg* 28(2):118–126, 2014.

29. Rehder NB, Bird DM: Annual profiles of blood packed cell volumes of captive American kestrels, *Can J Zool* 61(11):2550–2555, 1983.

30. Dolka B, Włodarczyk R, Zbikowski A, et al: Hematological parameters in relation to age, sex and biochemical values for mute swans (*Cygnus olor*), *Vet Res Commun* 38(2):93–100, 2014.

31. Mulley RC: Haematology and blood chemistry of the black duck Anas superciliosa, *J Wildl Dis* 15(3):437–441, 1979.

32. Mulley RC: Haematology of the wood duck, Chenonetta jubata, *J Wildl Dis* 16(2):271–273, 1980.

33. Joyner KL: Theriogenology. In Ritchie BW, Harrison GJ, Harrison LR, editors: *Avian medicine: principles and applications*, Lake Worth, FL, 1994, Wingers Publishing, pp 748–804.

34. Berry WD, Gildersleeve RP, Brake J: Characterization of different hematological responses during molts induced by zinc or fasting, *Poult Sci* 66(11):1841–1845, 1987.

35. Cleaver WT, Christensen VL, Ort JF: Physiological characteristics of a molt and second cycle of egg laying in turkey breeder hens, *Poult Sci* 65(12):2335–2342, 1986.

36. Chilgren J, Degraw W: Some blood characteristics of white-crowned sparrows during molt, *Auk* 94(1):169–171, 1977.

37. Driver E: Hematological and blood chemical values of mallard, Anas platyrhynchos, drakes before, during and after remige moult, *J Wildl Dis* 17(3):413–421, 1981.

38. Mazzaro LM, Meegan J, Sarran D, et al: Molt-associated changes in hematologic and plasma biochemical values and stress hormone levels in African penguins (*Spheniscus demersus*), *J Avian Med Surg* 27(4):285–293, 2013.

39. Sergent N, Rogers T, Cunningham M: Influence of biological and ecological factors on hematological values in wild little penguins, Eudyptula minor, *Comp Biochem Physiol A Mol Integr Physiol* 138(3):333–339, 2004.

40. deGraw WA, Kern MD: Changes in the blood and plasma volume of Harris' sparrows during postnuptial molt, *Comp Biochem Physiol A Comp Physiol* 81(4):889–893, 1985.

41. Totzke U, Fenske M, Hüppop O, et al: The influence of fasting on blood and plasma composition of herring gulls (*Larus argentatus*), *Physiol Biochem Zool* 72(4):426–437, 2010.

42. Hazelwood RL, Wilson WO: Comparison of hematological alterations induced in the pigeon and rat by fasting and heat stress, *Comp Biochem Physiol* 7(3):211–219, 1962.

43. Fedde M: High-altitude bird flight: exercise in a hostile environment, *Physiology* 5(5):191–193, 1990.

44. Prats M, Palacios L, Gallego S, et al: Blood oxygen transport properties during migration to higher altitude of wild quails (*Coturnix coturnix*), *Physiol Zool* 69(4):912–929, 1996.

45. Parga ML, Pendl H, Forbes NA: The effect of transport on hematologic parameters in trained and untrained Harris's hawks (*Parabuteo unicinctus*) and peregrine falcons (*Falco peregrinus*), *J Avian Med Surg* 15(3):162–169, 2001.

46. Scope A, Filip T, Gabler C, et al: The influence of stress from transport and handling on hematologic and clinical chemistry blood parameters of racing pigeons (*Columba livia domestica*), *Avian Dis* 46(1):224 229, 2002.

47. Bejaei M, Cheng KM: Effects of pretransport handling stress on physiological and behavioral response of ostriches, *Poult Sci* 93(5):1137–1148, 2014.

48. Menon DG, Bennett DC, Schaefer AL, et al: Transportation stress and the incidence of exertional rhabdomyolysis in emus (*Dromaius novaehollandiae*), *Poult Sci* 93(2):273–284, 2014.

49. C rule D, Krama T, Vrublevska J, et al: A rapid effect of handling on counts of white blood cells in a wintering passerine bird: a more practical measure of stress. *J Ornithol* 153(1):161–166, 2011.

50. Gray HG, Paradis TJ, Chang PW: Research note: physiological effects of adrenocorticotropic hormone and hydrocortisone in laying hens, *Poult Sci* 68(12):1710–1713, 1989.

51. Speer B, Kass P: The influence of travel on hematologic parameters in hyacinth macaws, *Proc Annu Assoc Avian Med* 1–6, 1995.

52. Blas J: Stress in birds. In Scanes C, editor: *Sturkie's avian physiology*, ed 6, San Diego, CA, 2015, Academic Press, pp 769–810.

53. Wakenell P: Hematology of chickens and turkeys. In Weiss D, Wardrop K, editors: *Schalm's veterinary hematology*, ed 6, Ames, IA, 2010, Wiley-Blackwell, pp 958–967.

54. Ammersbach M, Beaufrere H, Tully T: Laboratory Blood analysis in strigiformes-Part I: hematologic reference intervals and agreement between manual blood cell counting techniques, *Vet Clin Pathol* 44(1):94–108, 2015.

55. Black P, Mcruer D, Horne L: Hematologic parameters in raptor species in a rehabilitation setting before release, *J Avian Med Surg* 25(3):192–198, 2011.

56. Polo FJ, Peinado VI, Viscor G, et al: Hematologic and plasma chemistry values in captive psittacine birds, *Avian Dis* 42(3):523–535, 1998.

57. Hawkins M, Barron H, Speer B, et al: Birds. In Carpenter J, Marion C, editors: *Exotic animal formulary*, ed 4, St Louis, MO, 2013, Elsevier, pp 184–438.

58. Apo M: Hematology reference values. In Samour J, editor: *Avian medicine*, ed 2, Philadelphia, PA, 2008, Mosby Elsevier, pp 420–436.

59. Blount JD, Houston DC, Moller AP, et al: Do individual branches of immune defence correlate? A comparative case study of scavenging and non-scavenging birds, *Oikos* 102(2):340–350, 2003.

60. Samour JH, Naldo JL, John SK: Normal haematological values in gyr falcons (*Falco rusticolus*), *Vet Rec* 157(26):844–847, 2005.

61. Lind PJ, Wolff PL, Petrini KR, et al: Morphology of the eosinophil in raptors, *J Assoc Avian Vet* 4(1):33–38, 1990.

62. Hawkey CM, Bennett PM, Gascoyne SC, et al: Erythrocyte size, number and haemoglobin content in vertebrates, *Br J Haematol* 77(3):392–397, 1991.

63. Gregory TR, Andrews CB, McGuire JA, et al: The smallest avian genomes are found in hummingbirds, *Proc Biol Sci* 276(1674):3753–3757, 2009.

64. Palomeque J, Pintó D, Viscor G: Hematologic and blood chemistry values of the Masai ostrich (*Struthio camelus*), *J Wildl Dis* 27(1):34–40, 1991.

65. Ketz-Riley C, Sanchez C: Trochiliformes (*hummingbirds*). In Miller R, Fowler M, editors: *Fowler's zoo and wild animal medicine: current therapy*, vol 8, St. Louis, MO, 2015, Elsevier, pp 209–213.

66. Shave HJ, Howard V: A hematologic survey of captive waterfowl, *J Wildl Dis* 12(2):195–201, 1976.

67. Olayemi F, Arowolo R: Seasonal variations in the haematological values of the Nigerian duck (*Anas platyrhynchos*), *Int J Poult Sci* 8(8):813–815, 2009.

68. Puerta ML, Campo ALG Del, Abelenda M, et al: Hematological trends in flamingos, Phoenicopterus ruber, *Comp Biochem Physiol Part A Physiol* 102(4):683–686, 1992.

69. Dutton CJ, Allchurch AF, Cooper JE: Comparison of hematologic and biochemical reference ranges between captive populations of northern bald ibises (*Geronticus eremita*), *J Wildl Dis* 38(3):583–588, 2002.

70. Sepp T, Sild E, Hõrak P: Hematological condition indexes in greenfinches: effects of captivity and diurnal variation, *Physiol Biochem Zool* 83(2):276–282, 2010.

71. Mason GJ: Species differences in responses to captivity: stress, welfare and the comparative method, *Trends Ecol Evol* 25(12):713–721, 2010.

72. Deem SL, Noss AJ, Cuéllar RL, et al: Health evaluation of free-ranging and captive blue-fronted Amazon parrots (*Amazona aestiva*) in the Gran Chaco, Bolivia, *J Zoo Wildl Med* 36(4):598–605, 2005.

73. Fischer I, Christen C, Lutz H, et al: Effects of two diets on the haematology, plasma chemistry and intestinal flora of budgerigars (*Melopsittacus undulatus*), *Vet Rec* 159(15):480–484, 2006.

74. Candido MV, Silva LCC, Moura J, et al: Comparison of clinical parameters in captive Cracidae fed traditional and extruded diets, *J Zoo Wildl Med* 42(3):437–443, 2011.

75. Snyder J, Bird D, Lague P: Variations in selected parameters in the blood of captive American kestrels, *Proc Intern Symp Dis Birds Prey*, London, UK, 1980, Chiron pp 113–115.

76. Julian RJ: Ascites in poultry, *Avian Pathol* 22(3):419–454, 1993.

77. Ruiz G, Rosenmann M, Novoa FF, et al: Hematological parameters and stress index in rufous-collared sparrows dwelling in urban environments, *Condor* 104(1):162, 2002.

78. Llacuna S, Gorriz A, Riera M, et al: Effects of air pollution on hematological parameters in passerine birds, *Arch Environ Contam Toxicol* 31(1):148–152, 1996.

79. Bobby Fokidis H, Greiner EC, Deviche P: Interspecific variation in avian blood parasites and haematology associated with urbanization in a desert habitat, *J Avian Biol* 39(3):300–310, 2008.

80. Collette J, Millam J, Klasing K, et al: Neonatal handling of Amazon parrots alters the stress response and immune function, *Appl Anim Behav Sci* 66(4):335–349, 2000.

81. Le Maho Y, Karmann H, Briot D, et al: Stress in birds due to routine handling and a technique to avoid it, *Am J Physiol* 263(4 Pt 2):R775–R781, 1992.

82. Davis AK: Effect of handling time and repeated sampling on avian white blood cell counts, *J F Ornithol* 76(4):334–338, 2005.

83. Romero LM, Reed JM: Collecting baseline corticosterone samples in the field: is under 3 min good enough? *Comp Biochem Physiol A Mol Integr Physiol* 140(1):73–79, 2005.

84. Mans C, Guzman DS-M, Lahner LL, et al: Sedation and physiologic response to manual restraint after intranasal administration of midazolam in Hispaniolan Amazon parrots (*Amazona ventralis*), *J Avian Med Surg* 26(3):130–139, 2012.

85. Fair J, Paul E, Jones J: *Guidelines to the use of wild birds in research*, Washington, DC, 2010, The Ornithological Council.

86. McGuill M, Rowan A: Biological effects of blood loss: implications for sampling volumes and techniques, *ILAR J* 31:5–18, 1989.

87. Owen JC: Collecting, processing, and storing avian blood: a review, *J F Ornithol* 82(4):339–354, 2011.

88. Degernes L, Harrison L, Smith D, et al: Autologous, homologous, and heterologous red blood cell transfusions in conures of the genus Aratinga, *J Avian Med Surg* 13(1):10–14, 1999.

89. Wiley JLJ, Whittington JKJ, Wilmes CM, et al: Chronic myelogenous leukemia in a great horned owl (*Bubo virginianus*), *J Avian Med Surg* 23(1):36–43, 2009.

90. Bonar CJ, Lewandowski AH, Schaul J: Suspected fenbendazole toxicosis in 2 vulture species (*Gyps africanus*, Torgos tracheliotus) and Marabou storks (*Leptoptilos crumeniferus*), *J Avian Med Surg* 17(1):16–19, 2003.

91. Weber MA, Terrell SP, Neiffer DL, et al: Bone marrow hypoplasia and intestinal crypt cell necrosis associated with fenbendazole administration in five painted storks, *J Am Vet Med Assoc* 221(3):369, 417–419, 2002.

92. Sinclair KM, Church ME, Farver TB, et al: Effects of meloxicam on hematologic and plasma biochemical analysis variables and results of histologic examination of tissue specimens of Japanese quail (*Coturnix japonica*), *Am J Vet Res* 73(11):1720–1727, 2012.

93. Dressen P, Wimsatt J, Burkhard M: The effects of isoflurane anesthesia on hematologic and plasma biochemical values of American kestrels (*Falco sparverius*), *J Avian Med Surg* 13(3):173–179, 1999.

94. Fudge A: Avian blood sampling and artifacts considerations. In Fudge A, editor: *Laboratory medicine: avian and exotic pets*, Philadelphia, PA, 2000, W.B. Saunders Company, pp 1–8.

95. Arora K: Differences in hemoglobin and packed cell volume in blood collected from different sites in Japanese quail (*Coturnix japonica*), *Int J Poult Sci* 9(9):828–830, 2010.

96. Freidlin PJ: Destructive effect of heparin on avian erythrocytes, *Avian Pathol* 14(4):531–536.

97. Guzman DS-M, Mitchell M, Gaunt SD, et al: Comparison of hematologic values in blood samples with lithium heparin or dipotassium ethylenediaminetetraacetic acid anticoagulants in Hispaniolan Amazon parrots (*Amazona ventralis*), *J Avian Med Surg* 22(2):108–113, 2008.

98. Harr KE, Raskin RE, Heard DJ: Temporal effects of 3 commonly used anticoagulants on hematologic and biochemical variables in blood samples from macaws and Burmese pythons, *Vet Clin Pathol* 34(4):383–388, 2005.

99. Uko OJ, Ataja AM: Effects of anticoagulants and storage (4 degrees C) on packed cell volume (PCV) of Nigerian domestic fowl (*Gallus domesticus*) and guinea fowl (Numida meleagris), *Br Poult Sci* 37(5):997–1002, 1996.

100. Fourie F: Effects of anticoagulants on the haematocrit, osmolarity and pH of avian blood, *Poult Sci* 56:1842–1846, 1977.

101. Johnson JG, Nevarez JG, Beaufrère H: Effect of manually preheparinized syringes on packed cell volume and total solids in blood samples collected from American alligators (*Alligator mississippiensis*), *J Exot Pet Med* 23(2):142–146, 2014.

102. Pierre RV: Peripheral blood film review. The demise of the eye-count leukocyte differential, *Clin Lab Med* 22(1):279–297, 2002.

103. Kjelgaard-Hansen M, Jensen AL: Is the inherent imprecision of manual leukocyte differential counts acceptable for quantitative purposes? *Vet Clin Pathol* 35(3):268–270, 2006.

104. Maedel L, Doig K: Examination of the peripheral blood smear and correlation with the complete blood count. In Rodak B, Fritsma G, Doig K, editors: *Hematology: clinical principles and applications*, ed 3, St Louis, MO, 2007, Saunders, pp 175–192.

105. Houwen B: Blood film preparation and staining procedures, *Clin Lab Med* 22(1):1–14, 2002.

106. Latimer K, Bienzle D: Determination and interpretation of the avian leukogram. In Weiss D, Wardrop K, editors: *Schalm's veterinary hematology*, ed 6, Ames, IA, 2010, Wiley-Blackwell, pp 345–357.

107. Chubb LG, Rowell JG: Counting blood cells of chickens, *J Agric Sci* 52(02):263, 1959.

108. Dein F, Wilson A, Fischer D, et al: Avian leucyte counting using the hemocytometer, *J Zoo Wildl Med* 25(3):432–437, 1994.

109. Russo EA, McEntee L, Applegate L, et al: Comparison of two methods for determination of white blood cell counts in macaws, *J Am Vet Med Assoc* 189(9):1013–1016, 1986.

110. Denington EM, Lucas AM: Blood technics for chickens, *Poult Sci* 34(2):360–368, 1955.

111. Lanaux TM, Rozanski EA, Simoni RS, et al: Interpretation of canine and feline blood smears by emergency room personnel, *Vet Clin Pathol* 40(1):18–23, 2011.

112. Vap LM, Harr KE, Arnold JE, et al: ASVCP quality assurance guidelines: control of preanalytical and analytical factors for hematology for mammalian and nonmammalian species, hemostasis, and crossmatching in veterinary laboratories, *Vet Clin Pathol* 41(1):8–17, 2012.

113. Friedrichs K, Harr K, Freeman K, et al: ASVCP reference interval guidelines: determination of de novo reference intervals in veterinary species and other related topics, *Vet Clin Pathol* 41(4):441–453, 2012.

114. Geffré A, Friedrichs K, Harr K, et al: Reference values: a review, *Vet Clin Pathol* 38(3):288–298, 2009.

115. Tang F, Messinger S, Cray C: Use of an indirect sampling method to produce reference intervals for hematologic and biochemical analyses in psittaciform species, *J Avian Med Surg* 27(3):194–203, 2013.

116. Teare J: International Species Information System-physiological data reference values, Apple Valley, MN, 2002, International Species Information System.

117. Virtanen A, Kairisto V, Uusipaikka E: Regression-based reference limits: determination of sufficient sample size, *Clin Chem* 44(11):2353–2358, 1998.

118. Puerta ML, Munõz Pulido R, Huecas V, et al: Hematology and blood chemistry of chicks of white and black storks (*Ciconia ciconia and Ciconia nigra*), *Comp Biochem Physiol A Comp Physiol* 94(2):201–204, 1989.

119. Geffré a, Braun JP, Trumel C, et al: Estimation of reference intervals from small samples: an example using canine plasma creatinine, *Vet Clin Pathol* 38(4):477–484, 2009.

120. Siest G, Henny J, Gräsbeck R, et al: The theory of reference values: an unfinished symphony, *Clin Chem Lab Med* 51(1):47–64, 2013.

121. Clinical and Laboratory Standards Institute: *Defining, establishing, and verifying reference intervals in the clinical laboratory; approved guideline*, ed 3, Wayne, PA, 2008, CLSI.

122. Pavlov IY, Wilson AR, Delgado JC: Reference interval computation: which method (not) to choose. *Clin Chim Acta* 413(13–14):1107–1114, 2012.

123. Geffré A, Concordet D, Braun J-P, et al: Reference Value Advisor: a new freeware set of macroinstructions to calculate reference intervals with Microsoft Excel, *Vet Clin Pathol* 40(1):107–112, 2011.

124. Finnegan D: *Reference intervals: reference intervals, R Package version 111*, http://CRAN.R-project.org/package=referenceIntervals. 2014.

125. Jensen AL, Kjelgaard-Hansen M: Method comparison in the clinical laboratory, *Vet Clin Pathol* 35:276–286, 2006.

126. Dein FJ, Wilson A, Fischer D, et al: Avian leucocyte counting using the hemocytometer, *J Zoo Wildl Med* 25(3):432–437, 1994.

127. Walton RM: Subject-based reference values: biological variation, individuality, and reference change values, *Vet Clin Pathol* 41(2):175–181, 2012.

128. Scope A, Schwendenwein I, Gabler C: Short-term variations of biochemical parameters in racing pigeons (*Columba livia*), *J Avian Med Surg* 16(1):10–15, 2002.

129. Beaufrere H, Kearney M, Tully T: Can we trust the avian medical literature. *Proc Annu Conf Assoc Avian Vet* 35, 2012.

130. Fudge A: Laboratory reference ranges for selected avian, mammalian, and reptilian species. In Fudge A, editor: *Laboratory medicine: avian and exotic pets*, Philadelphia, PA, 2000, WB Saunders, pp 375–400.

131. Karesh W, del Campo A, Braselton E, et al: Health evaluation of free-ranging and hand-reared macaws (Ara spp.) in Peru, *J Zoo Wildl Med* 28(4):268–377, 1997.

132. Petersen P, Jensen E, Brandslund I: Analytical performance, reference values and decision limits. A need to differentiate between reference intervals and decision limits and to define analytical quality specifications, *Clin Chem Lab Med* 50(5):819–831, 2011.

133. Woerpel R, Rosskopf P: Clinical experience with avian laboratory diagnostics, *Vet Clin North Am Exot Anim Pract* 14:254, 1984.

134. Jensen AL, Aaes H: Critical differences of clinical chemical parameters in blood from dogs, *Res Vet Sci* 54(1):10–14, 1993.

135. Ricós C, Cava F, García-Lario J V, et al: The reference change value: a proposal to interpret laboratory reports in serial testing based on biological variation, *Scand J Clin Lab Invest* 64(3):175–184, 2004.

136. Beaufrère H, Ammersbach M, Tully Jr TN: Complete blood cell count in psittaciformes by using high-throughput image cytometry: a pilot study, *J Avian Med Surg* 27(3):211–217, 2013.

137. Seliger C, Schaerer B, Kohn M, et al: A rapid high-precision flow cytometry based technique for total white blood cell counting in chickens, *Vet Immunol Immunopathol* 145(1–2):86–99, 2012.

138. Kratz A, Bengtsson H-I, Casey JE, et al: Performance evaluation of the cellavision DM96 system: WBC differentials by automated digital image analysis supported by an artificial neural network, *Am J Clin Pathol* 124(5):770–781, 2005.

139. Tvedten HW, Lilliehöök IE: Canine differential leukocyte counting with the CellaVision DM96Vision, Sysmex XT-2000iV, and Advia 2120 hematology analyzers and a manual method, *Vet Clin Pathol* 40(3):324–339, 2011.

140. Degroote LW, Rodewald PG: An improved method for quantifying hematozoa by digital microscopy, *J Wildl Dis* 44(2):446–450, 2008.

141. Feng Q, Yu S, Wang H: A new automatic nucleated cell counting method with Improved Cellular Neural Networks (ICNN). In *2006 10th International Workshop on Cellular Neural Networks and Their Applications*, 2006, IEEE, pp 1–4.

142. Bauer KD, Jose de la Torre-Bueno, Diel IJ, et al: Reliable and sensitive analysis of occult bone marrow metastases using automated cellular imaging, *Clin Cancer Res* 6(9):3552–3559, 2000.

143. De Boever S, Croubels S, Demeyere K, et al: Flow cytometric differentiation of avian leukocytes and analysis of their intracellular cytokine expression, *Avian Pathol* 39(1):41–46, 2010.

144. Bohls RL, Smith R, Ferro PJ, et al: The use of flow cytometry to discriminate avian lymphocytes from contaminating thrombocytes, *Dev Comp Immunol* 30(9):843–850, 2006.

145. Burgess S, Davison T: Counting absolute numbers of specific leukocyte subpopulations in avian whole blood using a single-step flow cytometric technique: comparison of two inbred lines of chickens, *J Immunol Methods* 227(1–2):169–176, 1999.

146. Moritomo T, Minami A, Inoue Y, et al: A new method for counting of quail leukocytes by flow cytometry, *J Vet Med Sci* 64(12):1149–1151, 2002.

147. Uchiyama R, Moritomo T, Kai O, et al: Counting absolute number of lymphocytes in quail whole blood by flow cytometry, *J Vet Med Sci* 67(4):441–444, 2005.

CLINICAL BIOCHEMISTRY

Claire Vergneau-Grosset, Hugues Beaufrère, Mélanie Ammersbach

Biochemistry is one of the diagnostic tools most commonly available for the evaluation of avian patients, and this implies a need for understanding its limitations and the many differences compared with mammals in order to reach an appropriate assessment.[1] Reference intervals for selected avian species are available in Appendix 2 of this book; the reader should confirm whether these have been established with similar techniques as the ones used in his or her laboratory and the methods in accordance with the American Society for Veterinary Clinical Pathology (ASVCP) guidelines on reference intervals.[2] This chapter's objective is to guide clinicians in their choice of selection of the biochemistry panel best suited to investigate their clinical suspicions or for general health screening purposes. As part of this chapter, the database of the William R. Pritchard Veterinary Medical Teaching Hospital of the University of California, Davis (VMTH-UCD), was reviewed between 2000 and 2014 to estimate the sensitivity of biochemical parameters in association with renal and hepatic conditions in psittacine birds. Histopathologic evaluations of liver and kidney tissues obtained by biopsy or postmortem examinations were assessed in conjunction with serum or plasma biochemistry data obtained within the week prior to tissue collection. Retrospective data illustrate the limited sensitivity of currently available biochemistry panels. Our understanding of avian biochemistry is improving, but progress is slow, and many aspects still need to be refined to more reliably detect organ damage and dysfunction processes. In addition, the usefulness of most biochemical analytes has not been correlated with clinical conditions in birds other than in experimentally induced organ impairment, and scientific reports have only involved a limited number of species. Biochemical abnormalities may be different in spontaneously occurring diseases. It must be acknowledged that as in mammals, different avian species with the same disease may have different biochemical abnormalities, depending on various factors such as the magnitude of enzyme activities per organ, the presence of isoenzymes of the measured enzymes, and other physiologic differences such as electrolyte concentrations and corporal temperatures at which optimal enzyme activities occur compared with the constant temperatures of incubation in automated analyzers. For an extensive discussion of critical thinking in clinical test interpretation, the reader should refer to the section on Variability and Limitations in Clinical Avian Hematology and also Chapter 1.

CHOICE OF BIOCHEMISTRY ANALYZER, SAMPLE QUALITY, AND BIOCHEMISTRY PANEL

Choice of Biochemistry Analyzer

Choosing an appropriate biochemistry analyzer for veterinary patients includes an evaluation of the analyzer's accuracy and precision, the availability of basic and more comprehensive biochemical panels with avian-specific parameters, including uric acid, the costs of the analyzer and of consumables, the turnaround time for routine as well as STAT results (including in-house versus reference laboratories), and the volume of whole blood, serum, and plasma needed. Blood volume may range between 6% and 13% of a bird's body weight, depending on the species[3] and on the physiologic status of each individual.[4] Another major consideration when choosing a biochemical analyzer is its validation in the target species, including precision of the assay.[5] Veterinary diagnostic laboratories and clinical laboratories are not required to conform to the Clinical Laboratory Improvements Amendments (CLIA) standards, so avian veterinarians should have a self-commitment to investigate analyzer performances.[5]

Several tabletop analyzers such as the VetScan VS2 Chemistry Analyzer (Abaxis Inc., Union City, CA) and IDEXX VetTest 8008 Chemistry Analyzer (IDEXX Laboratories Inc. Westbrook, ME), among others, are available to veterinary clinics.[6] Many require a low volume of blood; for instance, only 0.1 mL of serum, plasma, or whole blood is needed to perform a chemistry panel on a 12-parameter avian and reptile rotor (Avian/Reptilian Profile Plus, Abaxis Inc., Union City, CA). However, a larger biochemistry panel is needed in many clinical situations (Table 13-2). Bile acid values are not determined below 35 micromoles per liter (μmol/L) with the VetScan VS2 Chemistry Analyzer, which can lower the sensitivity of this parameter.[7] In addition, single parameters cannot be rechecked separately with a rotor system, which can be cost prohibitive. Finally, although the analysis is fast in tabletop analyzers (e.g., 12 minutes for the VetScan), only one analysis can be performed at a time; each needs to be manually started, so performing multiple blood analysis is time consuming compared with the larger, more fully automated analyzers, in which batches of sample can be run simultaneously (e.g., Roche Cobas 501). Finally and most importantly, accuracy and precision of point-of-care analyzers have been established only rarely in avian species to date.[8-10] Some veterinary diagnostic laboratory analyzers used in human medicine have been evaluated and shown to comply with

standards of reliability and accuracy established in human laboratory medicine in the CLIA established by the National Committee for Clinical Laboratory Standards.[5] As expected, results for many analytes are significantly different when comparing the results obtained from point-of-care analyzers and veterinary diagnostic laboratory analyzers.[7,10-12] These differences can be attributed to different methodologies. Results among veterinary diagnostic laboratory analyzers have been reported to be more consistent compared with benchtop

TABLE 13-2

Examples of Comprehensive Avian Chemistry Panels*

Chemistry Panel UCD-VMTH[1] Analyzer: Roche Cobas c501 Plasma Volume Required: 0.2 mL	Chemistry Panel OVC-UoGuelph[2] Analyzer: Roche Cobas c501 Plasma Volume Required: 0.2 mL	Vet-Scan Plasma Volume Required: 0.1 mL (may be performed on whole blood)
Glucose	Glucose	Glucose
Uric acid	Uric acid	Uric acid
Urea	Urea	
Total protein	Total protein	Total protein
Albumin	Albumin	Albumin
Globulin (calculated)	Globulin (calculated)	Globulin
	A/G ratio (calculated)	
AST	AST	AST
GLDH	GLDH	
	GGT	
	LDH	
Alkaline phosphate		
Bile acids	Bile acids	Bile acids
Creatine kinase	Creatine kinase	Creatine kinase
Cholesterol	Cholesterol	
	Amylase	
	Lipase	
Anion gap (calculated)	Anion gap (calculated)	
Sodium	Sodium	Sodium
Potassium	Potassium	Potassium
Chloride	Chloride	
Phosphorus	Phosphorus	Phosphorus
Calcium	Calcium	Calcium
Bicarbonate		
	Carbon dioxide	
Hemolysis index	Hemolysis index	
Icteric index	Icteric index	
Lipemic index	Lipemic index	

*Offered by two veterinary medical teaching hospitals, from the University of California, Davis, and the Animal Health Laboratory University of Guelph, Ontario, and basic avian/reptile panel obtained from a benchtop analyzer.
A/G, Albumin-to-globulin ratio; *AST*, aspartate aminotransferase; *BUN*, blood urea nitrogen; *GLDH*, glutamate dehydrogenase, *GGT*, γ-glutamyl transferase; *LDH*, lactate dehydrogenase.
[1]University of California–Davis: William M. Pritchard Veterinary Medical Teaching Hospital.
[2]Animal Health Laboratory, Ontario Veterinary College, University of Guelph.
[3]Vet-Scan Avian/Reptilian Panel.

analyzers.[11] In veterinary medicine, the ASVCP released some guidelines on allowable total errors in clinics.[13] A study in Amazon parrots found that four analytes of the Vetscan rotor—aspartate aminotransferase (AST), calcium, glucose, and uric acid—were in good agreement with a reference analyzer.[10] A larger study in Strigiformes found that no Vetscan analyte was in analytical agreement with a reference analyzer, and four analytes (glucose, AST, creatine kinase [CK], and total protein) were in acceptable clinical agreement.[12] Studies of some reptilian species have also shown some significant discrepancies.[7,11,14] Therefore, analyzer-specific reference intervals are needed in most species, and different analyzers may not be considered clinically equivalent. Likewise, hand-held glucose meters have also been shown to be unreliable to measure blood glucose in psittacine birds compared with reference biochemistry analyzers, since they have a tendency to underestimate actual glycemia.[15,16] The use of point-of-care testing in birds must comply with the ASVCP guidelines on veterinary patients.[17]

Also, classically used protein measurement techniques (dye-binding methods) are usually not reliable in birds and appropriate analytical techniques such as electrophoresis must be chosen in birds for protein determination. Evaluation of coagulation parameters is beyond the scope of this chapter because this is rarely performed clinically and requires specialized equipment.[18] Reviews about avian coagulation and the appropriateness of various techniques are available.[19]

Sample Quality

Sample collection requires restraint of the patient, choice of the most appropriate sample type, and evaluation of the volume needed. Some patients may require sedation or anesthesia for venipuncture. Effects of anesthesia on biochemistry results have been evaluated in birds.[20] In the American kestrel, anesthesia with isoflurane has been shown to decrease uric acid and increase potassium concentration; although these variations were statistically significant, they had minimal clinical relevance.[20]

Studies comparing the use of serum and plasma for biochemistry have been published in various avian species.[21-23] The use of plasma, rather than serum, for protein electrophoresis has been advocated in avian species to allow fibrinogen analysis, which migrates in the beta-globulin fraction,[1,24,25] although some studies using serum have also been published.[26]

When the volume of the blood sample is limited by the size of the patient, dilution of plasma with sterile water or ultracentrifugation in microhematocrit tubes has been reported.[27,28] In juvenile peregrine falcons, plasma collected after ultracentrifugation (5079 g for 3 minutes) has shown no significant difference for any biochemical parameters when compared with classic centrifugation at 1411 g for 5 minutes in microcentrifuge tubes.[28] However, dilution of plasma with sterile water should be evaluated critically because many parameters do not give reliable results, as demonstrated in thick-billed parrots.[27] Significant differences were observed in clinical chemistry results obtained from diluted plasma samples for all analytes except AST, CK, and glucose. Uric acid concentration was not significantly different at dilutions of up to 1:3.[27] Although diluting plasma samples is intuitively appealing, the resulting decrease in analyte accuracy values may be more than expected with dilution alone. For instance,

enzyme activities may depend on many factors, including electrolyte concentrations and pH, which may change with diluents.

Suboptimal blood samples, hemolyzed or lipemic, are sometimes obtained from small patients, and it is important to know the consequences of substances interfering with various biochemical parameters when making an interpretation. Similar to what is seen in mammals, hemolysis increases the concentration of analytes that are present in higher concentrations within the red blood cells (RBCs) compared with plasma or serum. Hemolysis or lipemia both artifactually increase certain parameters measured via spectrophotometry if there is overlap in the absorbance spectra of hemoglobin and the measured reaction product[28]; these include potassium, calcium, albumin, amylase, lactate dehydrogenase (LDH), CK, creatinine phosphokinase (CPK), alanine aminotransferase (ALT), and AST, whereas triglycerides are often artifactually decreased.[29] When using a colorimetric assay to measure bile acids, hemolysis can artifactually decrease bile acid value, whereas the result is unaffected if a radioimmunoassay technique is used.[29] The effect of hemolysis on other parameters such as glucose, phosphorus, magnesium, alkaline phosphatase (ALP), and lipase depends on the methodology used.[29] When a hemolyzed sample is used for electrophoresis, the resulting pattern can mimic chronic inflammation in some species, with an increase of the γ-globulin fraction in bar-headed geese and an increase of the γ-globulin and β-globulin fractions in black kites. In comparison, hemolysis in mammalian samples typically causes an increase in the α_2- and β-globulin fractions.[30] The reason for this difference in comparison with mammals is thought to be the absence haptoglobin in some birds,[31] which migrates to the α_2-globulin fraction in mammals.[30]

Lipemic samples can mimic an increase of hepatocellular leakage enzymes, bile acids, calcium, phosphorus, glucose, and some proteins when analytes are determined via refractometry and via many spectrophotometric methods by increasing the turbidity of samples.[29,32] Ultracentrifugation or precipitation of the lipids prior to sample analysis can also result in artifacts (Figure 13-12).[29]

Several species groups such as flamingoes (Phoenicopteriformes) may have colored plasma (because of dietary pigments), which may cause spectrophotometric interference.

Choice of Biochemistry Panel

Selected avian biochemistry panels should maximize information in a reasonable volume of plasma and should include a variety of analytes related to various organs and metabolic processes. The choice of the panel and its components should take into consideration the sensitivity and specificity of each analyte, as well as the temporal changes in plasma in accordance with disease dynamics. The goal is to screen for major homeostatic abnormalities, metabolic disturbances, organ damage, and dysfunction. The authors recommend that the standard biochemistry panel include at least electrolytes; total protein; those analytes associated with major organs such as liver, pancreas, kidney, and muscle; and metabolic parameters, including glucose, cholesterol, and uric acid (see Table 13-2). For electrolytes, the minimum is to include sodium, chlorides, and potassium to be able to calculate the anion gap and

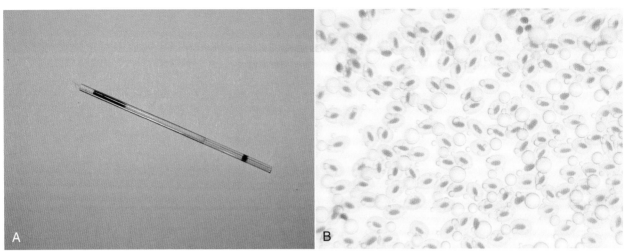

FIGURE 13-12 Severely lipemic sample from a Quaker parrot *(Myiopsitta monachus).*
A, Microhematocrit. **B,** Blood smear from the same patient.

the strong ion difference. Combinations of analytes that measure different aspects of organ integrity (function, leakage enzymes) are valuable to maximize the sensitivity of biochemical assessment. Panels of reduced size may be offered by some laboratories, including (but not limited to) liver or renal profiles. Furthermore, some biochemical values of clinical significance may be calculated, such as anion gap, sodium-to-potassium (Na:K) ratio, strong ion difference, and calculated osmolality.

Once the standard panel has been performed and an initial differential diagnostic list has been narrowed, other analytes may be subsequently obtained to further assess organ and metabolic functions. These include blood gases analysis, other electrolytes such as ionized calcium and magnesium, glucose metabolism parameters such as beta-hydroxybutyric acid and fructosamine,[33] toxicologic tests,[34] other hepatic enzymes such as sorbitol dehydrogenase (SDH),[35] lipid metabolism parameters such as lipoproteins and fatty acids, myocardial injury markers (troponins), inflammatory markers such as protein electrophoresis and fibrinogen, or iron metabolism analytes such as total iron or total iron-binding capacity (TIBC).[36]

There is a trade-off in using point-of-care biochemical analyzers in that they are typically less accurate and the panel is limited compared with reference laboratories. They should be reserved for situations of low sample volume, limited access to reference laboratories with avian biochemical panels, or emergency situations when the analyzer is available in-house.

When receiving the results of a biochemical panel, the clinician faces the challenge of finding appropriate reference values: for a more in-depth discussion of this point, the reader should refer to the section on Foundations in Clinical Pathology and the section on Variability and Limitations in Clinical Avian Hematology. Biochemistry results should be interpreted according to reference intervals established for the species, for the biochemistry analyzer used for the patient, and ideally following the ASVCP guidelines for the determination of the reference intervals in veterinary species.[2] In many situations, this is not practically possible, and clinicians

should keep in mind the limitations to interpretation when trying to make appropriate decisions for their patients. Alternatively, subject-based reference intervals or changes observed over serial measurements may be used.

CLINICAL SIGNIFICANCE OF BIOCHEMICAL PARAMETERS

Organ Evaluation

Tissue enzyme activities have been determined in chickens, mallard ducks, turkeys,[19] pigeons,[37,38] Grey parrots,[19] cockatiels,[39] and budgerigars[19,40] among others (Table 13-3). Presence of an enzyme in a tissue does not necessarily equal a measurable plasma increase of this enzyme in case of tissue damage. For instance, although glutamate dehydrogenase (GLDH) is present in the kidney, the plasma concentration of GLDH will not rise with renal disease because of urinary excretion of the renal isoform.[41,42] Also, some enzymes of low cytosolic concentrations such as γ-glutamyl transferase (GGT) may exhibit induction of new enzyme activities during certain states. Normal enzyme levels in most avian patients tend to be higher than in mammals, and specific reference intervals established with the same methodology are critical for confident interpretation of a panel.[41]

Liver evaluation

Hepatocellular leakage is associated with increases in cytosolic enzymes such as AST, LDH, and ALT, whereas hepatic necrosis and more significant hepatic damage can cause increases in mitochondrial enzymes such as GLDH,[19,41] and biliary tract damage can cause GGT and ALP increase.[19,29,35] Including CK as part of a biochemistry panel to evaluate the liver is important to differentiate between hepatic and muscle injuries, since this cytosolic and mitochondrial enzyme is present in skeletal, cardiac, and smooth muscles, as well as in the brain.[29] ALP is of very limited value in the evaluation of the liver because marked elevations have only been reported in cases of enhanced osteoblastic activity[29] and egg laying,[43] and very low concentrations are detectable in hepatic tissue.[41]

TABLE 13-3

Simplified Tissue Distribution of Commonly Used Enzymes in Avian Biochemistry[19,38,39]

	Hepatic Tissue			Muscular Tissue			Other Tissues
	Detection	Sensitivity	Specificity	Detection	Sensitivity	Specificity	Detection
AST	++	+++	−	++	+++	−	-
GLDH	+++	+	+++	+	−	−	+++ (kidney but excreted in urine)
GGT	+	+	+++	−	−	−	+++ (kidney)
LDH	++	+	−	++	+	−	+
ALT	++	++	−	++	+++	−	+
ALP	+	−	−	++	−	−	+ (duodenum, bone, kidney)
CK	−	−	−	+++	+++	+++	-
NAG	+	−	−	−	−	−	+++ (6 times higher in kidneys)

For detection: −, absence; +, presence in low quantity; ++, presence in substantial quantity compared with other tissues, but less than twice the quantity within other tissues; +++, presence in more than twice the quantity in other tissue.
For test specificity and sensitivity: + to +++, indicating a graduation in sensitivity and specificity.
ALP, alkaline phosphatase; *ALT,* alanine aminotransferase; *AST,* aspartate aminotransferase; *CK,* creatine kinase; *GLDH,* glutamate dehydrogenase; *GGT,* γ-glutamyl transferase; *LDH,* lactate dehydrogenase; *NAG,* N-acetyl-β-d-glucosaminidase.

ALT should probably not be included in biochemistry panels because this enzyme has a very low hepatic specificity and is present in only low concentrations.[29,41] When using serum or plasma biochemistry information to evaluate for the presence of liver disease, one must remember that liver injury, cholestasis, and decreased liver function can occur independently of one another or concurrently.

Enzymes. Because of the variable half-lives of hepatic enzymes, the degree of enzyme elevation observed does not correlate to the severity of the lesion or the degree of liver functional impairment, especially for limited enzyme increases.[41] The half-lives of hepatic enzymes have been studied in racing pigeons,[37] and it is unknown if these data can be extrapolated to other avian species. In pigeons, GLDH declines most rapidly, followed, in order, by LDH, CK, AST, and ALT.[37] A common recommendation to interpret increased enzymes is to compare the values for CK with values obtained for AST[44]; however, CK has a shorter half-life compared with AST; thus, chronic muscle damage can result in elevated AST, with a normal CK after return to baseline.[37] This situation should be kept in mind when evaluating and interpreting elevations in these enzymes (see Table 13-3). The main advantage of including LDH in a biochemistry panel is to differentiate muscle damage from liver damage. Because LDH half-life is shorter than CK half-life, a persistently elevated LDH concomitant with a decreasing CK and increased AST points toward hepatic disease (specifically cellular damage);[41] however, hemolysis also leads to LDH elevation. Overall, persistent LDH elevation in the absence of hemolysis points to persistent cellular damage. The reported values of these hepatic enzymes must be much greater than the upper reference limit (at least threefold to fourfold) to be considered clinically significant. Also, following chronic liver injury, liver enzymes may decrease to within the normal reference intervals despite continued cell damage or necrosis when the number of hepatocytes present in the liver is markedly decreased, for example, in a cirrhotic liver.[44]

In an experimental study involving Indian ring-necked parakeets (*Psittacula krameri*) subjected to induced traumatic acute liver damage, SDH was shown to be the most specific indicator of endoscopically induced hepatic damage, compared with bile acids, GLDH, GGT, ALP, ALT, AST, and LDH.[35] Marked SDH increase was noticed 12 hours after acute liver injury followed by rapid return to baseline because of its short half-life. In another study involving various psittacine birds with a variety of hepatic diseases, SDH correlated poorly with the presence of hepatic lesions. In that study, however, the highest end of the reference interval used, which was established in only 20 individuals, was more than four times higher than the one used in Indian ring-necked parakeets.[44] More studies are needed to evaluate the clinical benefit of this enzyme, and it should be acknowledged that experimentally induced liver damage may not adequately reproduce naturally occurring lesions.

GLDH is a mitochondrial enzyme that is considered liver specific in humans[45] but has a low sensitivity in many species.[41] GLDH reference values have been published in a limited number of species, including the cockatiel,[39] peregrine falcon,[46] ostrich,[47] Canada geese,[48] domestic chicken,[49] various species of owls,[12] and three species of cockatoos.[50] Compared with humans, a similar organ distribution has been described in the cockatiel,[39] pigeon,[37] and domestic chicken,[51] and this enzyme activity is highest in the liver, followed by the kidney and muscle. Most renal GLDH is located in the cells of the proximal tubules and is excreted in urine in cases of tubular cell injury, rather than into the blood circulation.[39] Hepatocellular necrosis that is experimentally induced by using ethylene glycol or d-galactosamine has been correlated with elevated plasma GLDH in pigeons.[52] Since the enzyme is mitochondrial, significant cell lysis must occur before plasmatic elevation is observed, as with hepatic necrosis and hepatic tumors.

CK is frequently elevated because of a variety of factors, including intramuscular injections, striated and smooth muscle diseases, seizures, prolonged recumbency, and extreme muscular activity during restraint.[19] The magnitude of change may also be meaningful, especially in case of severe increases. It appears that, clinically, the severity and extent of tissue injury may be correlated with CK blood activity but because of the extremely short half-life of this enzyme, elevations may not be consistent over time. For instance, injections or restraint usually cause mild increase in CK around a few thousand units per liter, whereas capture myopathy induces change of a few hundred thousand units per liter. The magnitude of CK elevation may also have prognostic indications in certain situations, especially when CK elevation is associated with tissue necrosis from neoplasms.

Bile acids and functional tests. Bile acids are the principal pathway for cholesterol catabolism,[53] which contains cholesteryl ester and triglycerides in birds.[54] In case of liver disease, plasmatic concentrations of bile acids can be increased because of an impaired enterohepatic cycle, as in cholestasis, obstruction, or impaired intestinal absorption; alternatively, it can be decreased with decreased liver function.[29,53] Bile acids also tend to increase with hepatic congestion caused by congestive heart failure. Decreased bile acid concentrations are not a specific indicator of liver disease and can also be observed in physiologic situations. Clinicians should also be aware that bile acid values obtained via radioimmunoassay are typically lower than those via colorimetry[29]; therefore, only method-specific reference intervals should be used.[55] Measurement of bile acids by radioimmunoassay has been described as the most sensitive indicator of hepatic disease among clinically available biochemical parameters in a retrospective study involving psittacine birds.[44] A retrospective study evaluated the association between histologically confirmed hepatic lesions and biochemistry results: a statistical association was established in Psittacidae by using 20 cases with hepatic lesions and 92 controls, including healthy and ill birds with no suspected hepatic disease. The results obtained indicated a stronger statistical correlation between the presence of liver disease and elevated bile acid or α_2-globulin levels than for AST and LDH.[44] This study concluded that relying only on increased AST concomitant with low CK to diagnose the presence of hepatic disease would be a very insensitive test.[44] Possible limitations of this study were the low number of cases; the fact that only birds with a 1.5-fold or more AST increase were included, which may have artifactually decreased the sensitivity of AST measurement; and the lack of hepatic biopsy performed in the control group, potentially including birds with hepatic lesions among control birds. Hepatic enzymes and bile acids also test different aspects of liver disease, so the magnitude of changes may not correlate well and depend on the type of hepatic disease. Finally, the combined interpretation of AST, CK, and LDH is complex and may not lend itself to statistical analysis of indirect data well. Regardless, it is key to include measurement of bile acids as part of any biochemistry panel when liver function is to be evaluated.

Overall biochemistry parameters sensitivity most likely depends on the type and chronicity of liver injury being investigated. In experimentally induced acute hepatic injury with aflatoxin, a study showed no increases in serum bile acids, in contrast to observed elevations in AST and LDH.[56] This type of observation is expected, as an acute injury is likely to result in elevated hepatic leakage enzymes, whereas liver function may not be impacted. Elevated AST indicates acute liver damage, whereas bile acids may remain elevated after AST levels have returned to baseline in case of chronic liver disease with impaired liver function.[44]

Bilirubin occurs in scant quantities in avian plasma because of the lack of biliverdin reductase.[41] Bilirubin assays have been reported to provide limited clinical information,[41] although increased bilirubin has been reported in ducks after experimental infection with duck virus hepatitis[57] and in Canada geese intoxicated with lead.[48] More information regarding the clinical relevance of bilirubinemia in birds may need to be collected, but one author (HB) has observed elevated bilirubin with severe liver disease on a consistent basis.

Currently, plasma ammonia measurements do not have common applications in avian biochemistry evaluations, since hepatic encephalopathy has not been thoroughly documented in birds[19] despite anecdotal suspicions.[29] Fasted ammonia values in healthy psittacine birds are much higher than in dogs and could be mistaken for an increased value.[19]

Evaluation of hepatic function also includes protein metabolism, which is discussed below. As in mammals, other liver metabolites such as glucose, cholesterol, coagulation factors, albumin, and uric acid may also be decreased with liver failure.

Retrospective study. Records from psittacine patients presented to VMTH-UCD between 2000 and 2014, with histopathologic diagnosis of a liver biopsy or a complete necropsy, were reviewed. The VMTH-UCD computerized pathology database was searched using the keywords "liver," "hepatic," and "avian/reptile panel." Necropsy reports were reviewed, and all lesions classified as "mild" or "minimal" were excluded to avoid underestimating the sensitivity of biochemical hepatic parameters. All biochemistry panels were performed with the Roche Cobas C501 Chemistry Analyzer (Roche Diagnostics, Indianapolis, IN), but the liver parameters evaluated varied across patients, depending on specific parameters requested by clinicians and because parameters offered in the basic avian or reptile panel evolved over time. Biochemistry panel results were analyzed on the basis of references included in Appendix 2 of this book and specific VMTH-UCD laboratory references, when available. Sixty-three psittacine birds were found to have had biochemistry panels performed within a week before hepatic lesions were diagnosed histologically. Lesions included a combination of the following: hepatitis (n = 24), hepatic necrosis (n = 15), hepatic fibrosis (n = 12), primary and secondary hepatic neoplasms (n = 9), hepatic lipidosis (n = 9), hepatocellular degeneration (n = 2), and other hepatic lesions (n = 13). Those with abnormal biochemistry results among these cases and corresponding test sensitivity are included in Table 13-4. Similar to previous findings,[44] bile acids were found to have a high sensitivity to detect hepatic lesions relative to other parameters. However, bile acid sensitivity, including decreased or increased values, was only 64% in this retrospective study, whereas a 74% sensitivity had been reported previously in 20 psittacine cases.[44] When taking into account only increased bile acids, AST and bile acid sensitivity was similar, as has been suggested by some authors.[19] It is expected that the sensitivity of each parameter will depend on the type of hepatic lesion and timing of biochemical testing after injury and may also vary among avian species until proven otherwise. When evaluating an individual patient, it is challenging to determine a single best parameter to evaluate the liver, which is why a well-designed and most complete biochemistry panel is needed. Liver wedge-biopsy, endoscopy-guided liver biopsy,[58] and ultrasound-guided aspiration[59] may have a higher sensitivity and do not always correlate with biochemistry results.[35]

TABLE 13-4

Number of Abnormal Biochemical Results in a Population of Psittacine Birds with Hepatic Histologic Lesions and Sensitivity of Some Hepatic Biochemical Parameters*

	Number of Birds with Abnormal Results	Sensitivity	95% Binomial Confidence Interval
Complete hepatic panel	56 of 63	74%	62-86
Increased AST	36 of 63	58%	46-70
Increased AST and CK within normal limits	5 of 63	8%	1-15
Increased GLDH	14 of 45	32%	18-46
Increased bile acids	18 of 38	47%	31-63
Increased or decreased bile acids	23 of 38	61%	45-77
Increased ALP	1 of 24	4%	0-12
Increased LDH	7 of 18	39%	16-62

*Obtained from the Roche Cobas C501 Chemistry Analyzer (Roche Diagnostics, Indianapolis, IN), and analyzed on the basis of references included in Appendix 2 of this book and specific laboratory references intervals when available.

ALP, Alkaline phosphatase; AST, aspartate aminotransferase; CK, creatine kinase; GLDH, glutamate dehydrogenase; LDH, lactate dehydrogenase.

It is also noteworthy that about one out of four cases of advanced hepatic disease in the VMTH-UCD database did not seem to show any abnormalities in the biochemical panel.

Kidney evaluation

Renal function can be evaluated by measuring plasma uric acid, blood urea nitrogen (BUN), and N-acetyl-β-d-glucosaminidase (NAG) concentrations and via urinalysis. Ammonia represents a minimal part of nitrogenous waste, except in some nectarivorous birds.[60,61] Creatinine is not a relevant parameter of the biochemistry panel for clinical evaluation of renal function.[62,63] Creatinine is continuously formed from creatine phosphate and is excreted via urine, for the most part, before it is converted to creatinine.[62] Only a minimal amount of plasma creatinine is detectable, and this has been used in experimental settings to evaluate water restriction effects in poultry in relation to muscle mass.[64,65] As a side note, exogenous creatinine has been used to evaluate glomerular filtration rate (GFR) in healthy pigeons, although the technique remains to be validated in patients with decreased renal function.[66] In mammals, GFR is maintained except in case of dehydration or renal disease, whereas in birds a constant GFR is not maintained,[66] so GFR markers must be interpreted in this context.

Uric acid and urea. Urea is 100% filtered by glomerular filtration, whereas 90% of uric acid is secreted at the level of the tubules, and only 10% is filtered.[62,63] Azotemia and hyperuricemia are neither sensitive[67] nor specific markers of renal disease, since elevation of urea and uric acid are influenced by the diet, particularly in carnivorous birds.[38] In case of severe dehydration, urea demonstrates a more pronounced increase[64]

compared with uric acid. The reason for this is impaired glomerular filtration by dehydration to a wider extent than tubular secretion, which is largely independent of urine flow rate.[62] In pigeons, experimental water restriction for 4 days led to an 85% increase in uric acid, but overall values remained within the reference interval, whereas urea increased 5.3-fold to 15.6-fold and above the reference interval. Thus, urea was considered a more sensitive measurement for dehydration.[62] Numerous reports have stated that uric acid does not increase in association with dehydration because of the active tubular secretion and vascularization of the tubules by the renal portal system.[67,68] However, other authors have reported that hyperuricemia above specific reference intervals can be observed clinically with severe dehydration without persistent renal lesions, although the causative physiologic mechanism remains to be investigated.[63,69] The authors have also frequently observed hyperuricemia concurrent with dehydration in Psittaciformes, with return to normal levels with fluid replacement therapy in most cases. Uric acid frequently increases postprandially in carnivorous and piscivorous birds, with levels similar to those observed in renal diseases (see below, levels around 30.26 mg/dL [1800 μmol/L] in peregrine falcons[70] and around 20.17 mg/dL [1200 μmol/L] in blackfooted penguins,[71] for instance). Thus, these bird species should ideally be fasted for 24 hours to reduce this effect. Gastrointestinal (GI) bleeding has not been shown to result in an increase in uric acid or urea in birds.[72] Because of the low sensitivity[38] and specificity of urea and uric acid to detect renal lesions, clinicians should be critical of biochemistry results and assess renal function through rehydration and the possible utilization of additional tests, including imaging, urinalysis, and histopathology, among other methods.[73]

Tubular markers. Another parameter evaluated more recently in birds is NAG, which is a marker of tubular dysfunction found both in plasma and urine.[38] As markers of decreased renal function (urea and uric acid) may require at least a two-thirds decrease of renal function in mammals to be elevated, markers of injury such as NAG may be useful adjuncts to the renal biochemistry panel to increase the sensitivity of detection of kidney injury. NAG is a parameter used in human medicine; artifactual increase can occur with dehydration or sample freezing.[38] Normal NAG ranges have been evaluated in a limited number of pigeons (n = 22 birds)[38] and Hispaniolan amazon parrots (n = 12 birds, 36 samples).[74] NAG has been evaluated as a marker of acute renal injury induced by gentamycin in pigeons[38] but needs to be evaluated in a higher number of cases to determine its clinical relevance. Moreover, because many renal diseases are chronic, the usefulness of acute injury markers, including NAG, Kim-1,[75] and cystatin C[76] may be low.

Retrospective study. Medical records of birds with a histologic diagnosis (biopsy or postmortem examination) or renal disease were reviewed from the VMTH-UCD between 2000 and 2014. The VMTH-UCD computerized pathology database was searched using the keywords "kidney," "renal," and "avian/reptile panel." All biochemistry panels were performed with the Roche Cobas C501 Chemistry Analyzer (Roche Diagnostics, Indianapolis, IN). Biochemistry panel results were analyzed on the basis of specific VMTH-UCD laboratory references. Sixty psittacine birds were found to have had a biochemistry panel performed within a week before renal lesions were diagnosed histologically. Lesions included a combination of the following: nephritis (n = 19), renal neoplasm (n = 8), glomerulosclerosis (n = 7), interstitial fibrosis (n = 6), tubular necrosis (n = 5), tubulonephrosis (n = 3), tubular cysts (n = 2), and other renal lesions (n = 17). Those with abnormal biochemistry results among these cases and corresponding test sensitivity are included in Table 13-5. It is remarkable that birds with renal lesions would have been undetected when relying only on biochemical evaluation (Figure 13-13) because of the relatively low test sensitivity. In addition, the calcium-to-phosphorus ratio was confirmed to have a very poor sensitivity to detect renal disease, in contrast to what is noted in reptiles, in which it is considered the most sensitive indicator of renal disease. As recommended in reptiles, renal assessment in birds may include biochemistry in addition to other diagnostic modalities to reach the best sensitivity.[77]

Pancreas evaluation

Glycemia values are typically higher in birds than in mammals.[19] Regulation mechanisms are similar to those in mammals, although glucagon concentration is typically higher and insulin concentration typically lower in the pancreas of granivorous birds compared with mammalian pancreas.[19] Hyperglycemia can be associated with stress, pancreatitis, steroid administration, and diabetes mellitus, reported in numerous avian species.[33,78-82] Hypoglycemia can be associated with septicemia, liver failure, neoplasia, and, rarely, starvation.[29] Fructosamine has been used in birds to confirm the chronicity of hyperglycemia.[33] However, it is unknown if its interpretation is similar to that in mammals, and it is likely that elevated fructosamine is associated with a shorter duration of hyperglycemia.[33]

No specific marker for evaluation of the exocrine pancreas has been described in birds. Both plasma amylase and lipase can increase in case of pancreatic disease, enteritis, and renal disease, causing a decrease in their excretion.[29] However, the value of these tests to diagnose pancreatic disease is unknown. Amylase activity values obtained depend on the reagents and methods used; therefore, a reference interval specific to the assay should be used.[19]

Electrolytes

Calcium, magnesium, and phosphorus. Calcium and phosphorus are key parameters of the biochemistry panel and should be included in any basic panel. Total calcium includes ionized calcium, protein-bound calcium, and calcium complexed with a variety of anions such as citrate.[32,83] Calcium regulation and metabolism in birds have been reviewed in detail elsewhere.[32,84] Evaluation of both total calcium and ionized calcium is recommended to obtain an accurate assessment, as ionized calcium is the active calcium fraction. Ionized calcium does not increase during egg laying in poultry, in contrast to total calcium.[32] If ionized calcium is not available, formulas that enable calculation of adjusted total calcium in function of albumin and total proteins have been established for peregrine falcons[85] and ostriches.[19] These formulas are inherently approximations, as they do not take into account complexed calcium.[19,86,87] In Grey parrots, conflicting studies have been published,[83,88] whereas in Amazon parrots, no correlation could be established between calcium and albumin or total proteins.[88] Therefore, direct measurement of ionized calcium is recommended as it is in dogs and cats.[86,87] Ionized calcium reference intervals have been established in Grey parrots, thick-billed parrots,[89] and *Pionus* sp. parrots, among other species,[43,90] and was shown to vary significantly with diet[19] and ultraviolet B (UVB) exposure in Grey parrots.[84] Differential diagnoses for hypercalcemia include physiologic causes of increased total calcium, such as hyperproteinemia and reproductive activity in female birds, hypervitaminosis D, and calciferol rodenticides;[91] spurious

---

TABLE 13-5

Number of Abnormal Results in a Population of Psittacine Birds with Renal Histologic Lesions and Sensitivity of Some Renal Biochemical Parameters*

	Number of Birds with Abnormal Results	Sensitivity	95% Binomial Confidence Interval
Increased uric acid	35 of 60	58%	46–70
Increased urea	26 of 60	43%	31–56
Decreased Ca:P (<1)	6 of 60	10%	2–18

*Obtained from the Roche Cobas C501 Chemistry Analyzer (Roche Diagnostics, Indianapolis, IN), and analyzed on the basis of specific laboratory reference intervals.
Ca:P, Calcium-to-phosphorus ratio.

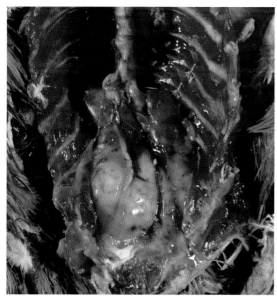

FIGURE 13-13 Gross necropsy picture from a 50-year-old male red-lored Amazon parrot *(Amazona autumnalis)* diagnosed with a multifocal lymphoma involving the kidneys, liver, lung, and spleen; an invasive renal mass is visible in the caudal coelom. On this patient's biochemistry panel, only a moderate hyperuricemia was noted (22.6 mg/dL), and liver parameters, including bile acids, were within normal limits. This case illustrates that other diagnostic tests should complete the biochemistry panel to improve sensitivity. (Courtesy the UC Davis School of Veterinary Medicine.)

results such as a lipemic sample;[32] osteolytic lesions; and nutritional secondary hyperparathyroidism.[92] Primary hyperparathyroidism has yet to be reported in birds.[19,32] The occurrence of paraneoplastic hypercalcemia in birds is controversial and has not been thoroughly demonstrated.[19,32,93] Hypocalcemia can result from nutritional causes, including low dietary calcium or vitamin D and increased consumption associated with chronic egg laying and has been commonly reported in Grey parrots, manifesting as seizures despite appropriate bone structure.[19] Magnesium should also be measured in case of suspected hypocalcemia in Grey parrots, since magnesium complexes with parathyroid hormone receptors and hypomagnesaemia result in impaired response to parathyroid hormone.[94] Renal disease and hypocalcemia have not been correlated in birds, and renal secondary hyperparathyroidism has not been confirmed in birds.[32]

Iron. Iron storage disease is a common problem in many bird species, including lories, lorikeets, mynahs,[95] toucans, hornbills,[96] starlings, tanagers, birds of paradise,[97] and many others.[98] Attempts have been made to correlate hemosiderosis to blood parameters, including total iron, TIBC, and transferrin saturation.[97,99] TIBC has been shown to decrease when an iron-deficient diet is offered to birds of paradise,[97] whereas TIBC increases in mammals as a result of decreased iron intake.[100,101] This may be caused by transferrin being a positive acute-phase protein in birds, whereas it is a negative acute-phase protein in mammals.[102] As the iron overload and inflammation resolve, it is possible that transferrin also decreases in birds, resulting in overall lower TIBC. Some drugs, including chloramphenicol, can also artifactually increase TIBC.[96] Overall, serum total iron, transferrin, and TIBC have been shown to correlate poorly with hemosiderosis in many birds.[96,103] Of note, hematocrit is also not a reliable indicator to investigate iron storage disease because hematocrit can decrease with chronic inflammation, which can itself be associated with hemosiderosis.[97] Blood hepcidin and ferritin concentrations have not been evaluated in birds with iron storage disease,[104] and the presence of hepcidin in birds is controversial.[97,105,106] These parameters require species-specific antibodies, which remain to be developed for birds,[29] but they have been shown to be more reliable parameters to investigate iron storage disease in some mammalian species and warrant further studies.[97,100,107,108] Detailed reviews of iron homeostasis and iron storage disease across taxa are available.[97,98] At this time, liver biopsy for liver iron determination, histopathology,[19] and magnetic resonance imaging (MRI) are more reliable testing modalities than blood parameters to investigate iron storage disease in birds.[96,109]

Other electrolytes. Potassium, chloride, sodium, and bicarbonate concentrations are also important and mostly pertain to assessment of critical and dehydrated patients, certain intoxications such as salt intoxication, and acid-base disorders as in the case of some forms of endocrine disease[110,111] and possibly to monitor renal disease, although the latter is controversial.[67] The carbon dioxide parameter of biochemistry panel is an indirect measure of bicarbonates. Results of electrolyte measurement should guide the choice of fluid replacement therapy. The pattern of electrolytic disorders should be interpreted with acid-base disorders by using the standard approach, the strong ion difference approach, or both.[112,113] Although the principles applied in mammals may be extrapolated to birds to a certain extent,[45] the pattern of association between calcium, phosphorus, potassium, chloride, sodium, or magnesium and renal disease has not been well established in birds.[32,67,114,115] Other than bicarbonates, lactates can also help define the origin of acid-base disorders. Measurement of lactates has been used to compare restraint techniques in avian medicine.[116,117] The anion gap ($Na^+ + K^+ - Cl^- - HCO_3^-$) and strong ion differences (modified: $Na^+ - Cl^-$) are calculated with the same formula as in mammals, and the interpretation is similar.[29] If a blood gas machine is not available, information gathered from the standard biochemical panel may be used instead. For instance, a low chloride level coupled with an increased carbon dioxide level is highly suggestive of hypochloremic metabolic alkalosis typically caused by vomiting or GI third spacing (e.g., GI obstruction). Likewise, metabolic acidosis may also be characterized partially. These parameters and the calculation of the anion gap and the strong ion difference should not be overlooked because they may prove to be critical through the correct implementation of a fluid replacement therapy plan.

Osmolality. Plasma osmolality reference intervals have been established in some psittacine species[118,119]; the best approximation to calculating plasma osmolality in Hispaniolan Amazon parrots is (in SI units), $Osm = 2(Na^+ + K^+) +$ uric acid/16.8 + glucose/18 or $Osm = 2(Na^+ + K^+) +$ glucose/18.[118] Unlike in mammals, in birds plasma osmolality gradually increases in response to water deprivation to conserve water as protein catabolic wastes are eliminated through tubular secretion.[63,120] Plasma osmolality is particularly useful when investigating marked polyuria–polydipsia. For instance, marked polydipsia associated with high plasma osmolality is almost pathognomonic for diabetes insipidus, whereas low plasma osmolality is typical of psychogenic polydipsia.[121] Both disorders have been seen several times in Grey parrots by the authors and are also reported in the literature in this same species[122] as well as in chickens.[123]

Proteins

Among protein measurement techniques, electrophoresis and the Biuret technique can be used, but the dye-binding methods with bromocresol are unreliable[19,24,124]; in birds, bromocresol green typically results in lower total protein values compared with bromocresol purple because of a weaker binding to avian albumin, although both are considered unreliable.[23] To date, no veterinary biochemistry analyzer has the ability to perform automated albumin measurement by electrophoresis despite routine reporting of albumin as part of the biochemistry panel. However, all common biochemistry evaluations use the Biuret technique for total protein measurement.[1] Refractometry is used to measure total solids, the value of which is consistently higher than the total protein value in birds and should not be interpreted as an evaluation of total proteins, as the correlation between the two is weak.[19] Different types of equipment are available to perform plasma protein electrophoresis, including semiautomated agarose gel systems,[125] high-resolution agarose gel,[26] and an automated capillary system.[126] Compared with the traditional semiautomated agarose gel system, the automated capillary system has been shown to have superior repeatability and reproducibility but requires a much higher sample volume (e.g., 14 times larger volume). This higher volume requirement makes it impractical for use in many species. Reference intervals need to be established for this technique, since some proteins detected in the α-globulin fraction with traditional technique migrate to the prealbumin fraction.[126] Protein electrophoresis facilitates evaluation of the patient's inflammatory patterns and provides a base for objective monitoring.[127,128] In birds, proteins from the α-globulin and β-globulin fractions are acute-phase proteins, whereas γ-globulins are typically raised in case of chronic inflammation.[19,25] α-Lipoprotein, α_1-antitrypsin, haptoglobin when present, and α-macroglobulin, migrate with the α-globulin fractions, whereas fibronectin, transferrin, and fibrinogen migrate with the β-globulin fraction.[129] Often a prealbumin fraction is observed in birds,[19] which can be more prominent than albumin in some avian species such as budgerigars and monk parakeets.[25] Whether or not prealbumin should be included in the albumin fraction when calculating the albumin-to-globulin (A/G) ratio is controversial.[25] β-Globulins are the major globulin fraction in birds, whereas γ-globulins are lower than in mammals.[25] Transferrin, which migrates in the β-globulin fraction, is a positive major acute-phase protein in birds, whereas it is a negative acute-phase protein in mammals.[102] As a result, acute inflammation in birds causes an increase of the beta-globulin fraction, whereas the beta-globulin fraction is mainly elevated with chronic inflammation in mammals.[25] Protein migration patterns vary among species; therefore, specific reference intervals are necessary.[24,130-139] As an example, a prealbumin peak is normally absent in Grey parrots (Figure 13-14), chickens,[25] and ostriches,[138] among others. The A/G ratio is typically higher than 1.0 in healthy birds. Inflammation may raise the globulin fractions with or without hypoalbuminemia, resulting in a decrease of the A/G ratio.[19] Prolonged refrigeration, repeated freeze-thawing, hemolysis, and lipemia can alter the electrophoresis results.[24] Although some studies have investigated the link between electrophoretic pattern and specific diseases,[26] protein electrophoresis is a nonspecific test.[128] In studies attempting to establish a correlation between a certain disease and an electrophoretic pattern, control groups are often omitted to focus on case series, and thus protein electrophoresis specificity is seldom evaluated.[129,131,140] The main drawback of this technique is low specificity. A statistical association between decreased prealbumin concentration and aspergillosis has been shown in Falconidae in a study that included a control group.[26] Increase of α_2-globulin has been statistically correlated with hepatobiliary disease, although the control group was only recruited on the basis of history and physical examination performed by the veterinarians submitting the samples.[44] Monoclonal gammopathy has been described in a limited number of psittacine birds with lymphoproliferative disease.[141] In a population of psittacine birds presented with various illnesses, recruited according to the history provided by the owners or physical examination findings, electrophoresis, and complete blood cell count (CBC), respective sensitivities were compared.[129] Overall, a higher sensitivity was found for the CBC compared with electrophoresis to detect illness.[129] This result, however, was expected given the design of the study, which could have included noninflammatory diseases. In addition, some abnormal hematologic results could have been attributed to stress leukograms.[129] Further studies including only birds affected by inflammatory conditions confirmed histologically may be relevant to compare electrophoresis with other testing modalities. Review articles about electrophoresis in birds are available.[24,25,142] Because inflammatory patterns are similar in numerous diseases, electrophoresis can confirm a clinical suspicion, but confirmation of the type of lesion through the use of other testing modalities is mandatory for accurate diagnosis. Although protein electrophoresis is useful as a screening test for health status in quarantine situations, for example, the authors do not consider it useful in individual patients other than to provide further characterization of dysproteinemia.

Positive acute-phase proteins in birds include ovotransferrin, which is a major acute phase protein in chickens,[143] serum amyloid A,[144,145] haptoglobin,[102] α_1-acid glycoprotein, transferrin,[102,144,146] and ceruloplasmin.[147,148] Haptoglobin is not present in all avian species: chicken plasma is devoid of haptoglobin, whereas it is present in ostriches.[31] These proteins are nonspecific markers of inflammation, which are part of the innate immune system.[102] A correlation has been shown between inflammatory diseases and serum amyloid A in Falconidae[145] and ceruloplasmin in quail.[147] No correlation was detected between serum amyloid A and amyloidosis in Falconidae.[145] Overall, measurement of acute-phase proteins is a promising tool in avian medicine, but further studies are needed to establish its clinical significance.[102]

Butyrylcholinesterase is a glycoprotein enzyme found in plasma and in various compartments within the body.[19] This enzyme, which is used in the diagnosis of cholinesterase-inhibitor agent intoxications including organophosphates and carbamates, decreases in case of intoxication. The values reported vary also with the health status of birds and overall increases in sick birds.[34] Reference intervals have been established in birds of prey,[149] psittacine birds,[34,150] and others.[151] Potential clinical applications need to be investigated for this enzyme, although variations associated with age, diet, and seasonality in some species can make interpretation more complex.[34,151]

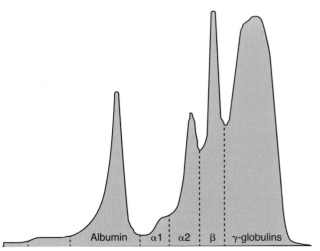

FIGURE 13-14 Serum protein electrophoresis from a 10-year-old Grey parrot *(Psittacus erithacus)* diagnosed with a plasma cell dyscrasia. This electrophoretogram is characterized by a mildly decreased albumin, mildly increased β globulins, and marked polyclonal gammopathy.

Lipoprotein panel

The lipid components of a typical lipoprotein panel are cholesterol, triglycerides, and the lipoproteins high-density lipoprotein (HDL), low-density lipoprotein (LDL), and very-low-density lipoprotein (VLDL).[152]

Hypercholesterolemia has been associated with reproductive activity, reproductive disorders, cholestasis, endocrine diseases[33,153] and has been seen postprandially.[29] Nephrotic syndrome has also been suggested as a cause of hypercholesterolemia,[29] although this has not been thoroughly documented in birds. In psittacine birds, hypercholesterolemia has been shown to have an association with atherosclerosis.[154,155] However, hypercholesterolemia itself is not diagnostic of atherosclerosis, and birds with normal cholesterolemia may have lesions of atherosclerosis.[156] Hypocholesterolemia can be associated with liver failure, intestinal malabsorption, and starvation.[29] As a side note, among markers of cardiac injury, troponin T has been evaluated in chickens,[157-163] whereas troponin I has not been validated in birds, and the protein sequence homology with mammals is variable (typically around 70% and higher[164]); values obtained from different assays may vary.[165]

Lipoproteins are micellar conglomerations of proteins, phospholipids, cholesterol, and triglycerides, primarily formed in the liver and the small intestine.[166] HDL is the predominant lipoprotein in most birds, as opposed to humans and most companion mammals, in which it is LDL.[54] Data about lipoprotein profiles have been published for captive Amazon parrots,[152] Grey parrots,[167] cockatiels,[155] cockatoos of the genus *Cacatua*,[155] macaws of the genus *Ara*,[155] monk parakeets,[168-170] geese,[171] pigeons and chickens,[172] among others.[173] VLDL and LDL concentrations are typically calculated by using the Friedewald formula[174] by analogy to mammals,[152,168] although this formula has not been thoroughly validated in birds.[155] Surprisingly, a positive correlation at the population level has been noted between prevalence of atherosclerosis in psittacine species and HDL values in the same species, although the significance of this finding at the individual level remains to be determined.[155] The ratio LDL/HDL also seems to be higher in species with higher atherosclerosis prevalence.[155] In a model of experimental atherosclerosis in monk parakeets (*Myiopsitta monachus*), a significant increase of LDL has been noted concomitantly with the development of atherosclerotic lesions, whereas HDL did not vary significantly.[168] Although a correlation between lipoprotein concentration and atherosclerosis in psittacine birds needs to be further investigated at the patient level, applications of lipoprotein panels include investigations of gonadal diseases,[175] endocrine diseases,[153] monitoring of the effects of nutrition transitions,[168,170] exercise,[176] or statin therapy.[177]

PHYSIOLOGIC VARIATIONS IN BIOCHEMICAL PARAMETERS

Variations Associated with Molt

Other resources are available about hormonal changes associated with molting.[178] Molt is associated with a decrease of total protein concentration, albumin, and most globulin fractions except α_1-globulin.[179] This decrease in most globulin fractions has been attributed to thyroid hormones' immunosuppressive effect.[179] Total protein decrease may be caused by increased plasma volume associated with the follicle vascularization, particularly in Passeriformes.[4] Significant elevations of prealbumin and α_1-globulin during molt have been attributed to the migration of transthyretin hormone in these fractions.[179,180] These biochemical changes should be kept in mind when sampling birds in molt.[181]

Variations Associated with the Postprandial Period

Postprandial changes include elevated uric acid for at least 12 hours associated with high-protein meals in carnivorous birds, which can increase more than threefold, similar to levels observed in renal disease.[71,182] In birds of prey, BUN also increases postprandially.[19] When measuring uric acid and BUN in birds of prey, a 24-hour fasting period has been recommended.[19] Significant postprandial bile acids increase has been reported in blackfooted penguins,[182] mallard ducks,[183] Falconidae,[184] ostriches, and pigeons,[183] among others. Contrary to previous assumptions, observed postprandial bile acids increases are, therefore, independent of the presence of a gall bladder, with only ostriches and pigeons lacking a gall bladder. These changes are also independent of the presence of a crop, since only penguins, ostriches, and ducks lack a crop.[184] Overall, the magnitude of postprandial increase remains lower in healthy birds than in some cases of hepatobiliary disease.[19] In some psittacine species, postprandial decrease of bile acids have been documented,[185] although a single-point bile assay still provides useful information.[41] In psittacine species, there is no need to measure preprandial and postprandial bile acid concentrations because both remain within the same reference interval.[41] In blackfooted penguins, postprandial triglyceride increase has also been demonstrated, whereas glycemia and BUN did not change significantly.[71,182] Postprandial lipemia does not typically occur in birds.[186]

Variations Associated with the Reproductive Status

In female birds, egg-laying is associated with an increase in globulins and total calcium as a result of estradiol secretion,[32] phosphorus, cholesterol,[19] and ALP.[43] Albumin has also been shown to rise by up to 100% in chickens in relation to egg laying,[187] which is expected because total calcium increases but ionized calcium remains stable.[188] Overall the A/G ratio decreases during egg laying because of hyperglobulinemia associated with egg formation.[19,186] Lipemia is a common finding in ovulating birds.[186] Nesting may also be associated with biochemical changes in female birds, which vary depending on the avian species.[181,189] Egg-bound females with calcium metabolism disorders often retain normal total blood calcium values.[32]

CONCLUSIONS

Many aspects of biochemistry evaluations in birds still require further investigation, and biochemical markers used in other species may find future applications in avian practice. Regardless, critical selection of biochemistry tests to be performed, combined with critical interpretive assessments of the results obtained, can optimize and improve the immediate diagnostic value of the use of plasma biochemistry in birds.

ACKNOWLEDGEMENTS

The authors wish to thank Dr. Joanne Paul-Murphy, Dr. Michelle Hawkins, and Dr. David Guzman, as well as the Companion Avian and Exotic Pet Medicine residents of the VMTH-UCD, for their clinical contributions to the cases included in this review and the Clinical Pathology laboratory of the VMTH-UCD.

REFERENCES

1. Fudge A, Speer BL: Selected Controversial topics in avian diagnostic testing, *Semin Avian Exotic Pet Med* 10: 96–101, 2001.
2. Friedrichs KR, Harr KE, Freeman KP, et al: ASVCP reference interval guidelines: determination of de novo reference intervals in veterinary species and other related topics, *Vet Clin Pathol* 41:441–453, 2012.
3. Bond CF, Gilbert PW: Comparative study of blood volume in representative aquatic and nonaquatic birds, *Am J Physiol* 194:519–521, 1958.
4. deGraw WA, Kern MD: Changes in the blood and plasma volume of Harris' sparrows during postnuptial molt, *Comp Biochem Physiol A Comp Physiol* 81:889–893, 1985.
5. Walton RM: Validation of laboratory tests and methods, *Semin Avian Exotic Pet Med* 10:59–65, 2001.
6. Zender AM, Hawkins MG, Pascoe PJ: Cagebirds. In West G, Heard D, Caulkett N, editors: *Zoo Animal and wildlife immobilization and anesthesia*, Ames, IA, 2014, Wiley Blackwell, pp 399–434.
7. Atkins A, Jacobson E, Hernandez J, et al: Use of a portable point-of-care (Vetscan VS2) biochemical analyzer for measuring plasma biochemical levels in free-living loggerhead sea turtles (*Caretta caretta*), *J Zoo Wildl Med* 41:585–593, 2010.
8. Steinmetz HW, Vogt R, Kastner S, et al: Evaluation of the i-STAT portable clinical analyzer in chickens (Gallus gallus), *J Vet Diagn Invest* 19:382–388, 2007.
9. Rettenmund CL, Heatley JJ, Russell KE: Comparison of two analyzers to determine selected venous blood analytes of Quaker parrots (*Myiopsitta monachus*), *J Zoo Wildl Med* 45:256–262, 2014.
10. Greenacre CB, Flatland B, Souza MJ, et al: Comparison of avian biochemical test results with Abaxis VetScan and Hitachi 911 analyzers, *J Avian Med Surg* 22:291–299, 2008.
11. Wolf KN, Harms CA, Beasley JF: Evaluation of five clinical chemistry analyzers for use in health assessment in sea turtles, *J Am Vet Med Assoc* 233:470–475, 2008.
12. Ammersbach M, Beaufrere H, et al: Laboratory blood analysis in Strigiformes-Part II: Plasma biochemistry reference intervals and agreement between the Abaxis Vetscan V2 and the Roche Cobas c501, *Vet Clin Path* 44(1):128–140, 2015.
13. Harr KE, Flatland B, Nabity M, et al: ASVCP guidelines: allowable total error guidelines for biochemistry, *Vet Clin Pathol* 42:424–436, 2013.
14. McCain SL, Flatland B, Schumacher JP, et al: Comparison of chemistry analytes between 2 portable, commercially available analyzers and a conventional laboratory analyzer in reptiles, *Vet Clin Pathol* 39:474–479, 2010.
15. Acierno MJ, Schnellbacher R, Tully TN Jr: Measuring the level of agreement between a veterinary and a human point-of-care glucometer and a laboratory blood analyzer in Hispaniolan Amazon parrots (*Amazona ventralis*), *J Avian Med Surg* 26:221–224, 2012.
16. Acierno MJ, Mitchell MA, Schuster PJ, et al: Evaluation of the agreement among three handheld blood glucose meters and a laboratory blood analyzer for measurement of blood glucose concentration in Hispaniolan Amazon parrots (*Amazona ventralis*), *Am J Vet Res* 70:172–175, 2009.
17. Bell R, Harr K, Rishniw M, et al: Survey of point-of-care instrumentation, analysis, and quality assurance in veterinary practice, *Vet Clin Pathol* 43:185–192, 2014.
18. Keller KA, Acierno MJ, Beaufrere H, et al: *Thromboelastography reference values in healthy Hispaniolan Amazon parrots (Amazona ventralis)*, Seattle, Annual Conference of Association of Avian Veterinarian, 2011, 37.
19. Lumeij JT: Avian clinical biochemistry. In Kaneko JJ, Bruss ML, editors: *Clinical biochemistry of domestic animals*, San Diego, CA, 2008, Academic Press, pp 839–872.
20. Dressen P, Wimsatt J, Burkhard MJ: The effects of isoflurane anesthesia on hematologic and plasma biochemical values of American kestrels (*Falco sparverius*), *J Avian Med Surg* 13:173–179, 1999.
21. Hrubec T, Whichard JD, Larsen CT, et al: Plasma versus serum: specific differences in biochemical analyte values, *J Avian Med Surg* 16:101–105, 2002.
22. Hawkins MG, Kass PH, Zinkl JG, et al: Comparison of biochemical values in serum and plasma, fresh and frozen plasma, and hemolyzed samples from orange-winged Amazon parrots (*Amazona amazonica*), *Vet Clin Pathol* 35:219–225, 2006.
23. Franco K, Hoover JP, Backues KA, et al: Comparison of biochemical values of paired serum and plasma samples from American flamingos (*Phoenicopterus ruber*), Indian runner ducks (*Anas platyrhynchos*), and hyacinth macaws (*Anodorhynchus hyacinthinus*), *J Exot Pet Med* 19:169–176, 2010.
24. Cray C, Rodriguez M, Zaias J: Protein electrophoresis of psittacine plasma, *Vet Clin Pathol* 36: 64–72, 2007.
25. Melillo A: Applications of serum protein electrophoresis in exotic pet medicine, *Vet Clin North Am Exot Anim Pract* 16:211–225, 2013.
26. Kummrow M, Silvanose C, Di Somma A, et al: Serum protein electrophoresis by using high-resolution agarose gel in clinically healthy and Aspergillus species-infected falcons, *J Avian Med Surg* 26: 213–220, 2012.
27. Waldoch J, Wack R, Christopher M: Avian plasma chemistry analysis using diluted samples, *J Zoo Wildl Med* 40:667–674, 2009.
28. Pond J, Thompson S, Hennen M, et al: Effects of ultracentrifugation on plasma biochemical values of prefledged wild peregrine falcons (Falco peregrinus) in northeastern Illinois, *J Avian Med Surg* 26: 140–143, 2012.
29. Harr EH: Diagnostic value of biochemistry. In Harrison GJ, Lightfoot TL, editors: *Avian medicine: principles and application*, Palm Beach, FL, 2006, Spix Publishing, pp 611–631.
30. Roman Y, Bomsel-Demontoy MC, Levrier J, et al: Effect of hemolysis on plasma protein levels and plasma electrophoresis in birds, *J Wildl Dis* 45:73–80, 2009.
31. Wicher KB, Fries E: Haptoglobin, a hemoglobin-binding plasma protein, is present in bony fish and mammals but not in frog and chicken, *Proc Natl Acad Sci USA* 103:4168–4173, 2006.
32. De Matos R: Calcium metabolism in birds, *Vet Clin North Am Exot Anim Pract* 11:59–82, 2008.
33. Gancz AY, Wellehan JF, Boutette J, et al: Diabetes mellitus concurrent with hepatic haemosiderosis in two macaws (*Ara severa*, Ara militaris), *Avian Pathol* 36:331–336, 2007.
34. Grosset C, Bougerol C, Sanchez-Migallon Guzman D: Plasma butyrylcholinesterase concentrations in psittacine birds: reference values, factors of variation, and association with feather-damaging behavior, *J Avian Med Surg* 28:6–15, 2014.
35. Williams SM, Holthaus L, Barron HW, et al: Improved clinicopathologic assessments of acute liver damage due to trauma in Indian ring-necked parakeets (*Psittacula krameri manillensis*), *J Avian Med Surg* 26:67–75, 2012.
36. Helmick KE, Kendrick EL, Dierenfeld ES: Diet manipulation as treatment for elevated serum iron parameters in captive raggiana bird of paradise (*Paradisaea raggiana*), *J Zoo Wildl Med* 42:460–467, 2011.
37. Lumeij JT, De Bruijne JJ, Slob A, et al: Enzyme activities in tissues and elimination half-lives of homologous muscle and liver enzymes in the racing pigeon (*Columba livia domestica*), *Avian Pathol* 17:851–864, 1988.
38. Wimsatt J, Canon N, Pearce RD, et al: Assessment of novel avian renal disease markers for the detection of experimental nephrotoxicosis in pigeons (*Columba livia*), *J Zoo Wildl Med* 40:487–494, 2009.

39. Battison AL, Buczkowski S, Archer FJ: The potential use of plasma glutamate dehydrogenase activity for the evaluation of hepatic disease in the cockatiel (*Nymphicus hollandicus*), *Vet Clin Pathol* 25: 43–47, 1996.

40. Sulakhe SJ, Lautt WW: The activity of hepatic gamma-glutamyl-transpeptidase in various animal species, *Comp Biochem Physiol Part B Comp Biochemistry* 82:263–264, 1985.

41. Fudge A: Avian liver and gastrointestinal testing. In Fudge A, editor: *Laboratory medicine, avian and exotic pets*, Philadelphia, PA, 2000, Saunders.

42. Tschopp R, Bailey T, Di Somma A, et al: Urinalysis as a noninvasive health screening procedure in Falconidae, *J Avian Med Surg* 21:8–12, 2007.

43. Harr KE: Clinical chemistry of companion avian species: a review, *Vet Clin Pathol* 31:140–151, 2002.

44. Cray C, Gautier D, Harris DJ, et al: Changes in clinical enzyme activity and bile acid levels in psittacine birds with altered liver function and disease, *J Avian Med Surg* 22:17–24, 2008.

45. Fudge A: Avian clinical pathology-hematology and chemistry. In Altman NH, Clubb S, Dorrestein GM, et al: editors: *Avian medicine and surgery*, Philadelphia, PA, 1997, WB Saunders, pp 142–157.

46. Lumeij JT, Remple JD, Remple CJ, et al: Plasma chemistry in peregrine falcons (*Falco peregrinus*): reference values and physiological variations of importance for interpretation, *Avian Pathol* 27:129–132, 1998.

47. Verstappen FA, Lumeij JT, Bronneberg RG: Plasma chemistry reference values in ostriches, *J Wildl Dis* 38:154–159, 2002.

48. Katavolos P, Staempfli S, Sears W, et al: The effect of lead poisoning on hematologic and biochemical values in trumpeter swans and Canada geese, *Vet Clin Pathol* 36:341–347, 2007.

49. Diaz GJ, Squires EJ, Julian RJ: The use of selected plasma enzyme activities for the diagnosis of fatty liver-hemorrhagic syndrome in laying hens, *Avian Dis* 43:768–773, 1999.

50. McDonald DL, Jaensch S, Harrison GJ, et al: Health and nutritional status of wild Australian psittacine birds: an evaluation of plasma and hepatic mineral levels, plasma biochemical values, and fecal microflora, *J Avian Med Surg* 24:288–298, 2010.

51. Clarkson MJ, Richards TG: The liver with special reference to bile acid formation. In Bell DJ, Freeman MB, editors: *Physiology and biochemistry of the domestic fowl*, New York, NY, 1971, Academic Press, pp 1085–1114.

52. Lumeij JT, Meidam M, Wolfswinkel J, et al: Changes in plasma chemistry after drug-induced liver disease or muscle necrosis in racing pigeons (Columba livia domestica), *Avian Pathol* 17:865–874, 1988.

53. Tennant BC: Hepatic function. In Kaneko JJ, Bruss ML, editors: *Clinical Biochemistry of domestic animals*, San Diego, CA, 2008, Academic Press, pp 379–412.

54. Petzinger C, Heatley JJ, Cornejo J, et al: Dietary modification of omega-3 fatty acids for birds with atherosclerosis, *J Am Vet Med Assoc* 236:523–528, 2010.

55. Hawkins MG, Barron HW, Speer BL, et al: Birds. In Carpenter JW, editor: *Exotic animal formulary*, St. Louis, MO, 2013, Saunders, pp 183–437.

56. Hadley TL, Grizzle J, Rotstein DS, et al: Determination of an oral aflatoxin dose that acutely impairs hepatic function in domestic pigeons (Columba livia), *J Avian Med Surg* 24:210–221, 2010.

57. Ahmed AA, El-Abdin YZ, Hamza S, et al: Effect of experimental duck virus hepatitis infection on some biochemical constituents and enzymes in the serum of white Pekin ducklings, *Avian Dis* 19: 305–310, 1975.

58. Taylor M: Endoscopic examination and biopsy techniques. In Ritchie BW, Harrison GJ, Harrison LR, editors: *Avian medicine: principles and application*, Lake Worth, FL, 1994, Wingers Publishing, pp 327–354.

59. Nordberg C, O'Brien RT, Hawley B, et al: Ultrasound examination and guided fine-needle aspiration of the liver in Amazon parrots (*Amazone species*), *J Avian Med Surg* 14:180–184, 2000.

60. McWhorter TJ, Powers DR, Martinez Del Rio C: Are hummingbirds facultatively ammonotelic? Nitrogen excretion and requirements as a function of body size, *Physiol Biochem Zool* 76:731–743, 2003.

61. Braun EJ: Osmoregulatory systems of birds. In Scanes CG, editor: *Sturkie's avian physiology*, San Diego, CA, 2015, Elsevier, pp 285–300.

62. Lumeij JT: Plasma urea, creatinine and uric acid concentrations in response to dehydration in racing pigeons (*Columba livia domestica*), *Avian Pathol* 16:377–382, 1987.

63. Phalen D: Avian renal disorders. In Fudge AM, editor: *Laboratory medicine: avian and exotic pets*, Philadelphia, PA, 2000, Saunders, pp 61–68.

64. Alamer MA, Ahmed AS: Effect of short-term water restriction in hot season on some blood parameters and immune response to Newcastle disease vaccine of local and commercial layers in the late phase of production, *J Anim Physiol Anim Nutr* 96:717–724, 2012.

65. Chikumba N, Swatson H, Chimonyo M: Haematological and serum biochemical responses of chickens to hydric stress, *Animal* 7: 1517–1522, 2013.

66. Scope A, Schwendenwein I, Schauberger G: Plasma exogenous creatinine excretion for the assessment of renal function in avian medicine—pharmacokinetic modeling in racing pigeons (*Columba livia*), *J Avian Med Surg* 27:173–179, 2013.

67. Echols MS: Evaluating and treating the kidneys. In Ritchie BW, Harrison GJ, Harrison LR, editors: *Avian medicine: principles and application*, Palm Beach, FL, 2006, Spix Publishing, pp 451–493.

68. Lumeij JT: Nephrology. In Ritchie BW, Harrison GJ, Harrison LR, editors: *Avian medicine: principles and application*, Lake Worth, FL, 1994, Wingers Publishing Inc, pp 538–555.

69. Pollock C: Diagnosis and treatment of avian renal disease, *Vet Clin North Am Exot Anim Pract* 9:107–128, 2006.

70. Lumeij JT, Remple JD: Plasma urea, creatinine and uric acid concentrations in relation to feeding in peregrine falcons (*Falco peregrinus*), *Avian Pathol* 20:79–83, 1991.

71. Kolmstetter CM, Ramsa EC: Effects of Feeding on plasma uric acid and urea concentrations in blackfooted penguins (*Spheniscus demersus*), *J Avian Med Surg* 14:177–179, 2000.

72. Sheldon J, Hoover JP, Payton ME: Plasma uric acid, creatinine, and urea nitrogen concentrations after whole blood administration via the gastrointestinal tract in domestic pigeons (*Columba livia*), *J Avian Med Surg* 21:130–134, 2007.

73. Murray MJ, Taylor M: Avian renal disease: endoscopic applications, *Semin Avian Exot Pet Med* 8:115–121, 1999.

74. Dijkstra B, Sanchez-Migallon Guzman D, Gustavson K, et al: Renal, gastrointestinal and hemostatic effects of oral meloxicam administration in Hispaniolan Amazon parrots (*Amazona ventralis*), *J Am Vet Med Assoc* 76(4):308–317, 2015.

75. Rouse R, Min M, Francke S, et al: Impact of pathologists and evaluation methods on performance assessment of the kidney injury biomarker, Kim-1, *Toxicol Pathol* 43(5):662–674, 2015.

76. Konopska B, Gburek J, Golab K, et al: Influence of aminoglycoside antibiotics on chicken cystatin binding to renal brush-border membranes, *J Pharm Pharmacol* 65:988–994, 2013.

77. Hernandez-Divers SJ, Stahl SJ, Stedman NL, et al: Renal evaluation in the healthy green iguana (*Iguana iguana*): assessment of plasma biochemistry, glomerular filtration rate, and endoscopic biopsy, *J Zoo Wildl Med* 36:155–168, 2005.

78. Murphy J: Diabetes in toucans, *Proc Annu conf Assoc Avian Vet* 165–170, 1992.

79. Candeletta SC, Homer BL, Garner MM, et al: Diabetes mellitus associated with chronic lymphocytic pancreatitis in an African Grey parrot (*Psittacus erithacus erithacus*), *J Assoc Avian Vet* 7:39–43, 1993.

80. Wallner-Pendleton EA, Rogers D, Epple A: Diabetes mellitus in a red-tailed hawk (*Buteo jamaicensis*), *Avian Pathol* 22:631–635, 1993.

81. Kahler J: Sandostatin (synthetic somatostatin) treatment for diabetes ellitus in a sulfur breasted toucan (*Ramphastus sulfuratus sulfuratus*), *Proc Annu Conf Assoc Avian Vet* 269–272, 1994.

82. Desmarchelier M, Langlois I: Diabetes mellitus in a nanday conure (*Nandayus nenday*), *J Avian Med Surg* 22:246–254, 2008.

83. Stanford M: The Significance of serum ionized calcium and 25-hydroxycholecalciferol (vitamin D3) assays in African Grey parrots, *Exotic DVM* 5:1–6, 2003.

84. Stanford M: Effects of UVB radiation on calcium metabolism in psittacine birds, *Vet Rec* 159:236–241, 2006.

85. Lumeij JT, Remple JD, Riddle KE: Relationship of plasma total protein and albumin to total calcium in peregrine falcons (*Falco peregrinus*), *Avian Pathol* 22:183–188, 1993.

86. Schenck PA, Chew DJ: Prediction of serum ionized calcium concentration by use of serum total calcium concentration in dogs, *Am J Vet Res* 66:1330–1336, 2005.

87. Schenck PA, Chew DJ: Prediction of serum ionized calcium concentration by serum total calcium measurement in cats, *Can J Vet Res* 74:209–213, 2010.

88. Lumeij JT: Relation of plasma calcium to total protein and albumin in African Grey (*Psittacus erithacus*) and Amazon (*Amazona spp.*) parrots, *Avian Pathol* 19:661–667, 1990.

89. Howard LL, Kass PH, Lamberski N, et al: Serum concentrations of ionized calcium, vitamin D3, and parathyroid hormone in captive thick-billed parrots (*Rhynchopsitta pachyrhyncha*), *J Zoo Wildl Med* 35:147–153, 2004.

90. Adkesson MJ, Langan JN: Metabolic bone disease in juvenile Humboldt penguins (*Spheniscus humboldti*): investigation of ionized calcium, parathyroid hormone, and vitamin D3 as diagnostic parameters, *J Zoo Wildl Med* 38:85–92, 2007.

91. Tarrant KA, Westlake GE: Histological technique for the identification of poisoning in wildlife by the rodenticide calciferol, *Bull Environ Contam Toxicol* 32:175–178, 1984.

92. Phalen DN, Drew ML, Contreras C, et al: Naturally occurring secondary nutritional hyperparathyroidism in cattle egrets (Bubulcus ibis) from central Texas, *J Wildl Dis* 41:401–415, 2005.

93. de Wit M, Schoemaker NJ, Kik MJ, et al: Hypercalcemia in two Amazon parrots with malignant lymphoma, *Avian Dis* 47:223–228, 2003.

94. Kirchgessner MS, Tully TN Jr, Nevarez J, et al: Magnesium therapy in a hypocalcemic African Grey parrot (*Psittacus erithacus*), *J Avian Med Surg* 26:17–21, 2012.

95. Mete A, Hendriks HG, Klaren PH, et al: Iron metabolism in mynah birds (*Gracula religiosa*) resembles human hereditary haemochromatosis, *Avian Pathol* 32:625–632, 2003.

96. Sandmeier P, Clauss M, Donati OF, et al: Use of deferiprone for the treatment of hepatic iron storage disease in three hornbills, *J Am Vet Med Assoc* 240:75–81, 2012.

97. Ganz T, Nemeth E: Iron homeostasis and its disorders in mice and men: potential lessons for rhinos, *J Zoo Wildl Med* 43:S19–S26, 2012.

98. Lowenstine LJ, Stasiak IM: Update on iron overload in zoological species. In Miller RE, editor: *Fowler's zoo and wild animal medicine*, St. Louis, MO, 2014, Saunders, pp 674–681.

99. Norambuena MC, Bozinovic F: Effect of malnutrition on iron homeostasis in black-necked swans (*Cygnus melanocoryphus*), *J Zoo Wildl Med* 40:624–631, 2009.

100. Williams CV, Junge RE, Stalis IH: Evaluation of iron status in lemurs by analysis of serum iron and ferritin concentrations, total iron-binding capacity, and transferrin saturation, *J Am Vet Med Assoc* 232:578–585, 2008.

101. Helmick KE, Milne VE: Iron deficiency anemia in captive aalayan tapir calves (*Tapirus indicus*), *J Zoo Wildl Med* 43:876–884, 2012.

102. Cray C: Biomarkers of inflammation in exotic pets, *J Exot Pet Med* 22:245–250, 2013.

103. Worell AB: Further investigation in Ramphastids concerning hemochromatosis, *Proc Assoc Avian Vet* 98–107, 1993.

104. Klasing KC, Dierenfeld ES, Koutsos EA: Avian iron storage disease: variations on a common theme. *J Zoo Wildl Med* 43: S27–S34, 2012.

105. Fu YM, Li SP, Wu YF, et al: Identification and expression analysis of hepcidin-like cDNAs from pigeon (*Columba livia*), *Mol Cell Biochem* 305:191–197, 2007.

106. Hilton KB, Lambert LA: Molecular evolution and characterization of hepcidin gene products in vertebrates, *Gene* 415:40–48, 2008.

107. Peters A, Raidal SR, Blake AH, et al: Haemochromatosis in a Brazilian tapir (*Tapirus terrestris*) in an Australian zoo, *Aust Vet J* 90:29–33, 2012.

108. Stasiak IM, Smith DA, Crawshaw GJ, et al: Characterization of the hepcidin gene in eight species of bats, *Res Veterinary Sci* 96:111–117, 2014.

109. Matheson JS, Paul-Murphy J, O'Brien RT, et al: Quantitative ultrasound, magnetic resonance imaging, and histologic image analysis of hepatic iron accumulation in pigeons (*Columbia livia*), *J Zoo Wildl Med* 38:222–230, 2007.

110. Rosskopf WJ: Pathogenesis, diagnosis, and treatment of adrenal insufficiency in psittacine birds, *Calif Vet* 5:26–30, 1982.

111. Ritchie M: Neuroanatomy and physiology of the avian hypothalamic/pituitary axis: clinical aspects, *Vet Clin North Am Exot Anim Pract* 17:13–22, 2013.

112. Carlson GP, Bruss M: Fluid, electrolyte and acid-base balance. In Kaneko JJ, Harvey JW, Bruss ML, editors: *Clinical Biochemistry of domestic animals*, San Diego, CA, 2008, Academic Press, pp 529–559.

113. Silverstein D, Hopper K: *Small animal critical care medicine*, St. Louis, MO, 2008, Saunders.

114. Blaxland JD, Borland ED, Siller WG, et al: An investigation of urolithiasis in two flocks of laying fowls, *Avian Pathol* 9:5–19, 1980.

115. Wideman RF, Mallinson ET, Rothenbacher H: Kidney function of pullets and laying hens during outbreaks of urolithiasis, *Poult Sci* 62:1954–1970, 1983.

116. Burgdorf-Moisuk A, Wack R, Ziccardi M, et al: Validation of lactate measurement in American flamingo (*Phoenicopterus ruber*) plasma and correlation with duration and difficulty of capture, *J Zoo Wildl Med* 43:450–458, 2012.

117. Harms CA, Harms RV: Venous blood gas and lactate values of mourning doves (Zenaida macroura), boat-tailed grackles (*Quiscalus major*), and house sparrows (*Passer domesticus*) after capture by mist net, banding, and venipuncture, *J Zoo Wildl Med* 43:77–84, 2012.

118. Acierno MJ, Mitchell MA, Freeman DM, et al: Determinination of plasma osmolality and agreement between measured and calculated values in healthy adult Hispaniolan Amazon parrots (*Amazona ventralis*), *Am J Vet Res* 70:1151–1154, 2009.

119. Beaufrere H, Acierno M, Mitchell M, et al: Plasma osmolality reference values in African Grey parrots (Psittacus erithacus erithacus), Hispaniolan Amazon parrots (Amazona ventralis), and red-fronted macaws (Ara rubrogenys), *J Avian Med Surg* 25:91–96, 2011.

120. Saito N, Grossmann R: Effects of short-term dehydration on plasma osmolality, levels of arginine vasotocin and its hypothalamic gene expression in the laying hen, *Comp Biochem Physiol Part A Mol Integr Physiol* 121:235–239, 1998.

121. Lumeij JT, Westerhof I: The use of the water deprivation test for the diagnosis of apparent psychogenic polydipsia in a socially deprived African Grey parrot (*Psittacus erithacus erithacus*), *Avian Pathol* 17:875–878, 1988.

122. Starkey SR, Wood C, de Matos R, et al: Central diabetes insipidus in an African Grey parrot, *J Am Vet Med Assoc* 237: 415–419, 2010.

123. Braun EJ, Stallone JN: The occurrence of nephrogenic diabetes insipidus in domestic fowl, *Am J Physiol* 256:F639–F645, 1989.

124. Cray C, Wack A, Arheart KL: Invalid measurement of plasma albumin using bromcresol green methodology in penguins (*Spheniscus species*), *J Avian Med Surg* 25:14–22, 2011.

125. Cray C, King E, Rodriguez M, et al: Differences in protein fractions of avian plasma among three commercial electrophoresis systems, *J Avian Med Surg* 25:102–110, 2011.

126. Roman Y, Bomsel-Demontoy MC, Levrier J, et al: Plasma protein electrophoresis in birds: comparison of a semiautomated agarose

gel system with an automated capillary system, *J Avian Med Surg* 27:99–108, 2013.

127. Eckersall PD: Proteins, proteomics, and the dysproteinemias. In Kaneko JJ, Harvey JW, Bruss ML, editors: *Clinical biochemistry of domestic animals*, San Diego, CA, 2008, Academic Press, pp 117–156.

128. Cray C, Watson T, Rodriguez M, et al: Application of galactomannan analysis and protein electrophoresis in the diagnosis of aspergillosis in avian species, *J Zoo Wildl Med* 40:64–70, 2009.

129. Briscoe JA, Rosenthal KL, Shofer FS: Selected complete blood cell count and plasma protein electrophoresis parameters in pet psittacine birds evaluated for illness, *J Avian Med Surg* 24:131–137, 2010.

130. Zaias J, Fox WP, Cray C, et al: Hematologic, plasma protein, and biochemical profiles of brown pelicans (*Pelecanus occidentalis*), *Am J Vet Res* 61:771–774, 2000.

131. Lanzarot MP, Montesinos A, San Andres MI, et al: Hematological, protein electrophoresis and cholinesterase values of free-living nestling peregrine falcons in Spain, *J Wildl Dis* 37:172–177, 2001.

132. Garcia-Montijano M, Garcia A, Lemus JA, et al: Blood chemistry, protein electrophoresis, and hematologic values of captive Spanish imperial eagles (*Aquila adalberti*), *J Zoo Wildl Med* 33:112–117, 2002.

133. Lanzarot MP, Barahona MV, Andres MI, et al: Hematologic, protein electrophoresis, biochemistry, and cholinesterase values of free-living black stork nestlings (*Ciconia nigra*), *J Wildl Dis* 41:379–386, 2005.

134. Spagnolo V, Crippa V, Marzia A, et al: Reference intervals for hematologic and biochemical constituents and protein electrophoretic fractions in captive common buzzards (*Buteo buteo*), *Vet Clin Pathol* 35:82–87, 2006.

135. Deem SL, Ladwig E, Cray C, et al: Health assessment of the ex situ population of St Vincent parrots (*Amazona guildingii*) in St Vincent and the Grenadines, *J Avian Med Surg* 22:114–122, 2008.

136. Gelli D, Ferrari V, Franceschini F, et al: Serum biochemistry and electrophoretic patterns in the Eurasian buzzard (*Buteo buteo*): reference values, *J Wildl Dis* 45:828–833, 2009.

137. Samour J, Naldo J, Rahman H, et al: Hematologic and plasma biochemical reference values in Indian peafowl (*Pavo cristatus*), *J Avian Med Surg* 24:99–106, 2010.

138. Black PA, Macek M, Tieber A, et al: Reference values for hematology, plasma biochemical analysis, plasma protein electrophoresis, and Aspergillus serology in elegant-crested tinamou (*Eudromia elegans*), *J Avian Med Surg* 27:1–6, 2013.

139. Jones MP, Arheart KL, Cray C: Reference intervals, longitudinal analyses, and index of individuality of commonly measured laboratory variables in captive bald eagles (*Haliaeetus leucocephalus*), *J Avian Med Surg* 28:118–126, 2014.

140. Villar D, Kramer M, Howard L, et al: Clinical presentation and pathology of sarcocystosis in psittaciform birds: 11 cases, *Avian Dis* 52:187–194, 2008.

141. Lennox A, Clubb S, Romagnano A, et al: Monoclonal hyperglobulinemia in lymphosarcoma in a cockatiel (*Nymphicus hollandicus*) and a blue and gold macaw (*Ara ararauna*), *Avian Dis* 58:326–329, 2014.

142. Tatum LM, Zaias J, Mealey BK, et al: Protein electrophoresis as a diagnostic and prognostic tool in raptor medicine, *J Zoo Wildl Med* 31:497–502, 2000.

143. Xie H, Huff GR, Huff WE, et al: Identification of ovotransferrin as an acute phase protein in chickens, *Poult Sci* 81:112–120, 2002.

144. Chamanza R, Toussaint MJ, van Ederen AM, et al: Serum amyloid A and transferrin in chicken. A preliminary investigation of using acute-phase variables to assess diseases in chickens, *Vet Quarter* 21:158–162, 1999.

145. Caliendo V, McKinney P, Bailey T, et al: Serum amyloid A as an indicator of health status in falcons, *J Avian Med Surg* 27:83–89, 2013.

146. Roy K, Kjelgaard-Hansen M, Pors SE, et al: Performance of a commercial Chicken-Ovo-transferrin-ELISA on the serum of brown layer chickens infected with Gallibacterium anatis and Streptococcus zooepidemicus, *Avian Pathol* 43:57–61, 2014.

147. Goetting V, Lee KA, Woods L, et al: Inflammatory marker profiles in an avian experimental model of aspergillosis, *Med Mycol* 51:696–703, 2013.

148. Zulkifli I, Najafi P, Nurfarahin AJ, et al: Acute phase proteins, interleukin 6, and heat shock protein 70 in broiler chickens administered with corticosterone, *Poult Sci* 93:3112–3118, 2014.

149. Roy C, Grolleau G, Chamoulaud S, et al: Plasma B-esterase activities in European raptors, *J Wildl Dis* 41:184–208, 2005.

150. Tully TN Jr, Osofsky A, Jowett PL, et al: Acetylcholinesterase concentrations in heparinized blood of Hispaniolan Amazon parrots (*Amazona ventralis*), *J Zoo Wildl Med* 34:411–413, 2003.

151. Hill EF, Murray HC: Seasonal variation in diagnostic enzymes and biochemical constituents of captive northern bobwhites and passerines, *Comp Biochem Physiol Part B Comp Biochemistry* 87:933–940, 1987.

152. Ravich M, Cray C, Hess L, et al: Lipid panel reference intervals for Amazon Parrots (*Amazona species*), *J Avian Med Surg* 28:209–215, 2014.

153. Oglesbee BL: Hypothyroidism in a scarlet macaw, *J Am Vet Med Assoc* 201:1599–1601, 1992.

154. Pilny AA, Quesenberry KE, Bartick-Sedrish TE, et al: Evaluation of Chlamydophila psittaci infection and other risk factors for atherosclerosis in pet psittacine birds, *J Am Vet Med Assoc* 240:1474–1480, 2012.

155. Beaufrere H, Cray C, Ammersbach M, et al: Association of plasma lipid levels with atherosclerosis prevalence in psittaciformes, *J Avian Med Surg* 28:225–231, 2014.

156. Grosset C, Guzman DS, Keating MK, et al: Central vestibular disease in a blue and gold macaw (*Ara ararauna*) with cerebral infarction and hemorrhage, *J Avian Med Surg* 28:132–142, 2014.

157. Maxwell MH, Robertson GW, Moseley D: Potential role of serum troponin T in cardiomyocyte injury in the broiler ascites syndrome, *Br Poult Sci* 35:663–667, 1994.

158. Maxwell MH, Robertson GW, Moseley D: Serum troponin T values in 7-day-old hypoxia-and hyperoxia-treated, and 10-day-old ascitic and debilitated, commercial broiler chicks, *Avian Pathol* 24:333–346, 1995.

159. Maxwell MH, Robertson GW, Moseley D: Serum troponin T concentrations in two strains of commercial broiler chickens aged one to 56 days, *Res Vet Sci* 58:244–247, 1995.

160. Maxwell MH, Robertson GW, Moseley D, et al: Characterisation of embryonic cardiac-derived troponin T in broiler chicks bled one to 168 hours after hatching, *Res Vet Sci* 62:127–130, 1997.

161. Maxwell MH, Robertson GW, Bautista-Ortega J, et al: A preliminary estimate of the heritability of plasma troponin T in broiler chickens, *Br Poult Sci* 39:16–19, 1998.

162. Sribhen C, Choothesa A, Songserm T, et al: Sex-based differences in plasma chemistry and cardiac marker test results in Siamese fighting fowl, *Vet Clin Pathol* 35:291–294, 2006.

163. Shao JJ, Yao HD, Zhang ZW, et al: The disruption of mitochondrial metabolism and ion homeostasis in chicken hearts exposed to manganese, *Toxicol Lett* 214:99–108, 2012.

164. Biesiadecki BJ, Schneider KL, Yu ZB, et al: An R111C polymorphism in wild turkey cardiac troponin I accompanying the dilated cardiomyopathy-related abnormal splicing variant of cardiac troponin T with potentially compensatory effects, *J Biol Chem* 279:13825–13832, 2004.

165. Knafo SE, Rapoport G, Williams J, et al: Cardiomyopathy and right-sided congestive heart failure in a red-tailed hawk (*Buteo jamaicensis*), *J Avian Med Surg* 25:32–39, 2011.

166. Bruss ML: Lipids and ketones. In Kaneko JJ Harvey JW, Bruss ML, editors: *Clinical biochemistry of domestic animals*, San Diego, CA, 2008, Academic Press, pp 81–115.

167. Bavelaar FJ, Beynen AC: Atherosclerosis in parrots. A review, *Vet Quarter* 26:50–60, 2004.

168. Beaufrere H, Nevarez JG, Wakamatsu N, et al: Experimental diet-induced atherosclerosis in Quaker parrots (*Myiopsitta monachus*), *Vet Pathol* 50:1116–1126, 2013.

169. Belcher CJ, Heatley J, Petzinger C, et al: Evaluation of plasma cholesterol, triglyceride, and lipid density profiles in captive monk parakeets (*Myiopsitta monachus*), *J Exot Pet Med* 23:71–78, 2014.

170. Petzinger C, Larner C, Heatley JJ, et al: Conversion of alpha-linolenic acid to long-chain omega-3 fatty acid derivatives and alterations of HDL density subfractions and plasma lipids with dietary polyunsaturated fatty acids in monk parrots (*Myiopsitta monachus*), *J Anim Physiol Anim Nutr* 98:262–270, 2014.

171. Hermier D, Saadoun A, Salichon MR, et al: Plasma lipoproteins and liver lipids in two breeds of geese with different susceptibility to hepatic steatosis: changes induced by development and force-feeding, *Lipids* 26:331–339, 1991.

172. Lizenko MV, Regerand TI, Bakhirev AM, et al: [Content of the main lipid components in blood serum lipoproteins of human and of various animal species], *Zhurnal evoliutsionnoi biokhimii i fiziologii* 43:155–161, 2007.

173. Potier R: Lipid blood profile in captive Brahminy kite (*Haliastur indus*) as a possible indication of increased susceptibility to atherosclerosis, *J Zoo Wildl Med* 44:549–554, 2013.

174. Friedewald WT, Levy RI, Fredrickson DS: Estimation of the concentration of low-density lipoprotein cholesterol in plasma, without use of the preparative ultracentrifuge, *Clin Chem* 18:499–502, 1972.

175. Nemetz L: The relevance of plasma triglyceride determination and hypertriglyceridemia in birds, *Int Conf Avian Herpetol Exot Mammal Med* 419–420, 2013.

176. Gustavsen K, Stanhope K, Lin A, et al: Effects of exercise on lipid metabolism in Hispaniolan Amazon parrots (*Amazona ventralis*) with hypercholesterolemia, Orlando, Florida, 2014, Conference of the American Association of Zoo Veterinarians.

177. Qureshi AA, Peterson DM: The combined effects of novel tocotrienols and lovastatin on lipid metabolism in chickens, *Atherosclerosis* 156:39–47, 2001.

178. Dawson A: Avian molting. In Scanes CG, editor: *Sturkie's avian physiology*, San Diego, CA, 2015, Elsevier, pp 907–917.

179. Roman Y, Bomsel-Demontoy MC, Levrier J, et al: Influence of molt on plasma protein electrophoretic patterns in bar-headed geese (*Anser indicus*), *J Wildl Dis* 45:661–671, 2009.

180. Cookson EJ, Hall MR, Glover J: The transport of plasma thyroxine in white storks (*Ciconia ciconia*) and the association of high levels of plasma transthyretin (thyroxine-binding prealbumin) with moult, *J Endocrinol* 117:75–84, 1988.

181. Franson JC, Hoffman DJ, Schmutz JA: Plasma biochemistry values in emperor geese (*Chen canagica*) in Alaska: comparisons among age, sex, incubation, and molt, *J Zoo Wildl Med* 40:321–327, 2009.

182. Cray C, Stremme DW, Arheart KL: Postprandial biochemistry changes in penguins (*Spheniscus demersus*) including hyperuricemia, *J Zoo Wildl Med* 41:325–326, 2010.

183. Lumeij JT: Fasting and postprandial plasma bile acid concentrations in racing pigeons (*Columba livia domestica*) and mallards (*Anas platyrhynchos*), *J Assoc Avian Vet* 5:197–200, 1991.

184. Lumeij JT, Remple JD: Plasma bile acid concentrations in response to feeding in peregrine falcons (Falco peregrinus), *Avian Dis* 36:1060–1062, 1992.

185. Flammer K: Serum bile acids in psittacine birds, *Proc Ann Conf Assoc Avian Vet* 9–12, 1994.

186. Capitelli R, Crosta L: Overview of psittacine blood analysis and comparative retrospective study of clinical diagnosis, hematology and blood chemistry in selected psittacine species, *Vet Clin North Am Exot Anim Pract* 16:71–120, 2013.

187. Williams TD, Reed WL, Walzem RL: Egg size variation: mechanisms and hormonal control. In Dawson A, Chaturvedi CM, editors: *Avian endocrinology*, Pangbourne, UK, 2001, Alpha Science International Ltd), pp 205–213.

188. Stanford DM: *Calcium metabolism in grey parrots: the effects of husbandry [thesis]*, London, UK, 2005, The Royal College of Veterinary Surgeons.

189. Alonso-Alvarez C: Age-dependent changes in plasma biochemistry of yellow-legged gulls (*Larus cachinnans*), *Comp Biochem Physiol Part A Mol Integr Physiol* 140:512–518, 2005.

CYTOLOGY

Nicole Stacy, Helene Pendl

Cytologic evaluation of tissue aspirates, tissue imprints, or peritoneal fluids or effusions has become a clinically valuable diagnostic tool in daily avian medical practice. Cytology is minimally invasive and comparatively inexpensive and requires minimal equipment. In context with clinical pathology and diagnostic imaging findings, cytology can deliver rapid information and guidance for additional diagnostic testing, thus being an essential tool for optimization of resources. In cases of inconclusive results of cytologic interpretation, need for information on tissue architecture, poorly cellular or non-representative specimens, or presence of a mixed cell population (mixture of inflammatory cells and tissue cells with features of cellular atypia), histopathology may be elected for further or definitive diagnostic information. Such examples include differentiation of granulomatous inflammation or granulation tissue from fibrosarcoma, or the presence of vascular invasion of a malignant tumor as a criterion for its biologic behavior.

SAMPLE COLLECTION, SLIDE PREPARATION TECHNIQUES, AND STAINING

The choice of cytologic specimen type depends on the lesion to be sampled and is dependent upon its accessibility and character. For example, epithelia that exfoliate cells require less aggressive sampling methods compared with connective tissue, which typically does not exfoliate well. Fine-needle aspirates, scrapings, swabs, washes, and tissue imprints are the most commonly used samples and sampling techniques to obtain cytologic samples in avian patients. Table 13-6 provides a list of commonly presented lesions with options for sample types and processing for best diagnostic quality. Cytologic preparations on glass slides need to be prepared and air-dried immediately after collection, since delay in sample processing can result in cell degeneration or microbial overgrowth. Preparation of two to four smears per collection site provides a sufficient number of slides for regular stains (e.g., Romanowsky type-based stains), special stains (see below), and archiving at the clinic, if desired. Fixation of slides with high-quality, acetone-free, absolute methanol for 5 minutes will provide optimal sample preservation for submission to the diagnostic laboratory or for in-house filing. Best preservation of cytologic samples is achieved by avoiding any exposure to heat, sunlight, humidity, or formalin fumes. Procedures such as heat fixation and storage in the refrigerator or the freezer will inevitably destroy the sample.

TABLE 13-6

Commonly Presented Lesions by Organ System and Appropriate Types of Cytologic Specimens in Avian Medicine and Surgery

Organ System	Lesion	Cytology Specimen
Skin	Soft tissue mass	Fine-needle aspirate (FNA)
	Ulcerative lesion	Scraping, swab, and/or FNA
	Suspicion for ectoparasites	Swab (wet or dry)
		Scraping (deep and under pressure for intradermal parasites)
		Scotch tape imprint
Feathers	Full feather	Direct microscopy under low magnification (parasites, anatomical abnormalities)
	Calamus/pulp/follicle	Squash preparation, imprint, swab
Peritoneal cavity	Peritoneal fluid, cystic structures	FNA of fluid; aliquots in EDTA (cell counts, cytology) and tube without anticoagulant (culture) or culturette; direct and sediment smear/cytospin preparation; total solids by refractometer, color of fluid
	Caseous material, tissue mass	FNA; direct and, if applicable, squash preparation
	If tissue obtained during surgery or biopsy taken	Tissue imprints after blotting
Skeletal	Synovial fluid	Direct smear, total solids, viscosity, color
	Mass	FNA, tissue imprint
Respiratory	Nasal/tracheal flushes	Swab; flushes into EDTA for preparation of direct and sediment smear/cytospin
	External lesion on nares	Moistened swab
Gastrointestinal	Crop	Wash or swab
	Fecal	Voided sample or cloacal swab: wet mount, direct smear, parasitology, Gram stain
Gross lesions during necropsy	External or internal lesions	Tissue imprints, swabs, fluid collection

Fine-Needle Aspirates

Fine-needle aspiration (FNA) of solid masses is performed with or without maintaining negative pressure during sample collection. Using the least amount of negative pressure is of benefit in highly vascularized tissue. Retrieval from the lesion is best performed without vacuum to avoid aspiration of the material from the needle lumen into the syringe. The sample is then expelled onto a slide and spread gently with a second slide. The pressure applied should be as low as possible to ensure sufficient cell separation with minimal cell destruction. A multidirectional aspiration within the lesion will enhance the probability of a representative sample. Ultrasound-guided aspiration is recommended for internal masses.

Imprints, Scrapings, and Swabs

Imprint smears from biopsies or postmortem tissue samples provide the best cytologic quality if excess blood on the freshly cut surface is removed by gentle blotting of the tissue on lint-free paper. Excellent sample quality can be obtained by imprinting the slide onto the tissue rather than the tissue onto the slide. Hemodilution can hinder the evaluation of cellular detail (Figure 13-15). Scrapings performed with a scalpel blade perpendicular to the surface of the lesion will remove sufficient material from firm, nonexfoliative tissue such as solid connective tissue masses. The material can also be processed with squash preparations (Figure 13-16). In case of dry superficial lesions, scraping until appearance of some blood or serum will support sticking of the material onto the slide. The use of moistened swabs (with isotonic saline) on mucosal surfaces is gentle on the patient and facilitates

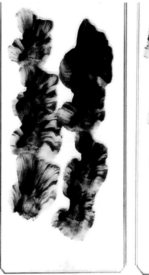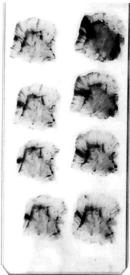

FIGURE 13-15 Liver tissue imprint before *(left)* and after *(right)* blotting.

adhesion of collected cellular material to the swab. Swabs need to be carefully rolled rather than smeared on the slide to avoid cell damage.

Washes and Fluids

Fine-needle aspirates of fluids need to be processed in different ways, depending on their physical properties. Opaque

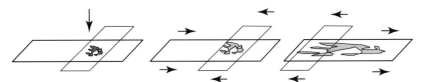

FIGURE 13-16 Cytologic evaluation of nonexfoliative tissue samples—squash preparation technique. (From BSAVA: Pendl H, Kreyenbuehl K: Clinical pathology. In Poland G, Raftery A, editors: *BSAVA manual of backyard poultry*, Gloucester, UK, in press, BSAVA Publications.)

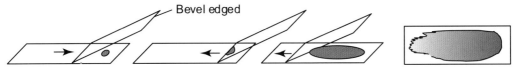

FIGURE 13-17 Cytologic evaluation of opaque fluids—wedge smear technique. (From BSAVA: Pendl H, Kreyenbuehl K: Clinical pathology. In Poland G, Raftery A, editors: *BSAVA manual of backyard poultry*, Gloucester, UK, in press, BSAVA Publications.)

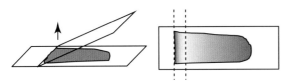

FIGURE 13-18 Cytologic evaluation of translucent fluids—line smear concentration technique (From BSAVA: Pendl H, Kreyenbuehl K: Clinical pathology. In Poland G, Raftery A, editors: *BSAVA manual of backyard poultry*, Gloucester, UK, in press, BSAVA Publications.)

TABLE 13-7
Wright-Giemsa Stain

Stain	Staining
3 g Wright stain powder[1]	Flood smear, allow to stand for 3 min
	Add equal amount of buffer 6.8[4]
0.3 g Giemsa stain powder[2]	Mix gently by blowing using a pipette or a straw until metallic green sheen forms on the surface
5 ml glycerol	
1000 ml absolute methanol (acetone free)[3]	Allow to stand for 6 min
	Rinse with buffer allowing to stand for 1 min for differentiation
Filtered and stored	Wash copiously with buffer
	Prop in rack until dry or use hair dryer
	Wipe the back of the smear to remove excess stain
	Mount with Entellan[5] and cover glass

Protocol from JH Samour, 2002, personal communication.
[1]Merck No 1.09278.0025.
[2]Merck No 1.09203.0025.
[3]Merck No 1.06009.1000.
[4]Merck No 1.11374.0100.
[5]Merck No 1.07961.0100.

fluids are spread onto the slide similar to blood films by using the wedge smear technique (Figure 13-17). Application of a bevel edged slide for smearing reduces rupture of cellular material. The drop of fluid should be completely distributed on the slide and result in a monolayer with a feathered edge. For translucent fluids with low cellularity, direct smears for evaluation of the cellularity of the sample and concentrated preparations for additional qualitative assessment are helpful for best diagnostic information. Concentration techniques of fluids (peritoneal fluid, nasal or crop washes) include the line smear concentration technique, cytospin, and sediment smears. The line smear concentration technique concentrates cells at the end of the smear (Figure 13-18). For a sediment smear preparation, the fluid is centrifuged for 5 minutes, and after removal of the supernatant, a direct smear is prepared from the cellular sediment. Evaluation of body cavity effusions and synovial fluid for color, transparency, specific gravity, and white and red blood cell counts, will provide additional characterization of the specimen. Evaluation of viscosity is useful for evaluation of synovial fluid specimens. A detailed description of fluid analysis and cytology is outlined in Chapter 6.

Staining

A Wright-Giemsa Staining (WGS) protocol developed by J.H. Samour (personal communication, 2002) and outlined in Table 13-7 has been demonstrated to be of superior value in terms of quality and demonstration of cellular details. Quick stains (e.g., Diff-Quik, Hema-Color) are extremely useful for daily routine because they are easy and rapid to perform. However, because of their aggressive nature in quickly penetrating the cellular membranes, they tend to cause loss of granular structure and staining in granulocytes, which may interfere with the diagnosis of subtle pathologic changes in cell morphology.

Special stains can be very useful for additional diagnostic information. Useful complementary stains include Gram stain for differentiation of gram-positive and gram-negative microorganisms (Figure 13-19), periodic acid-Schiff (PAS) stain and Gomori methenamine silver stain for yeast and fungi (Figure 13-20), acid-fast stain for *Cryptosporidia* oocysts and acid-fast-positive bacteria (including mycobacteria; Figure 13-21), and modified

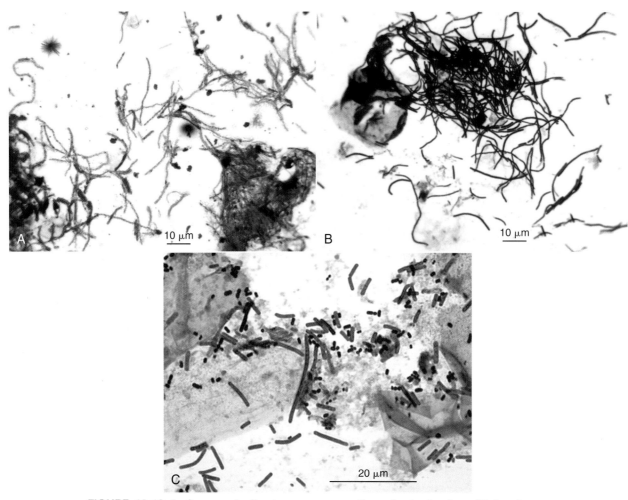

FIGURE 13-19 **A,** Crop swab direct smear preparation of a budgerigar *(Melopsittacus undulatus)* with proventricular dilation: large rodlike structures of *Macrorhabdus ornithogaster.* Wright-Giemsa stain. **B,** Gram stain of specimen shown in *A.* The organisms stain gram positive. **C,** Fecal direct smear of a Grey parrot *(Psittacus erithacus):* predominance of gram-negative-staining rod-shaped bacteria suggestive of abnormal colonic microflora.

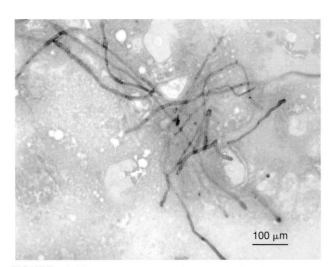

FIGURE 13-20 Tissue imprint of a lung lesion in a chicken *(Gallus gallus):* positive-staining fungal hyphae. GMS stain.

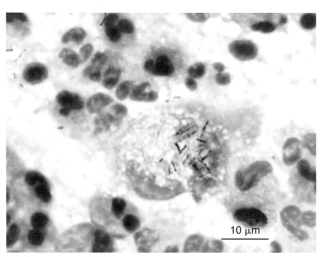

FIGURE 13-21 Synovial fluid direct smear of a great horned owl *(Bubo virginianus):* multinucleate macrophage with acid-fast-positive-staining rod-shaped bacteria suggestive of *Mycobacterium* spp. Ziehl-Neelsen acid-fast stain.

Giménez stain for Chlamydiae. Gram staining of specimens can be very helpful for rapid selection of proper antimicrobial treatment in cases with clinically and cytologically (phagocytosis of bacteria by leukocytes) suspected bacterial infection.

CYTOLOGIC EVALUATION

Assessment of cytologic specimens provides the best diagnostic results if approached systemically, as shown in Figure 13-22 and by using a standard protocol as outlined in Figure 13-23.

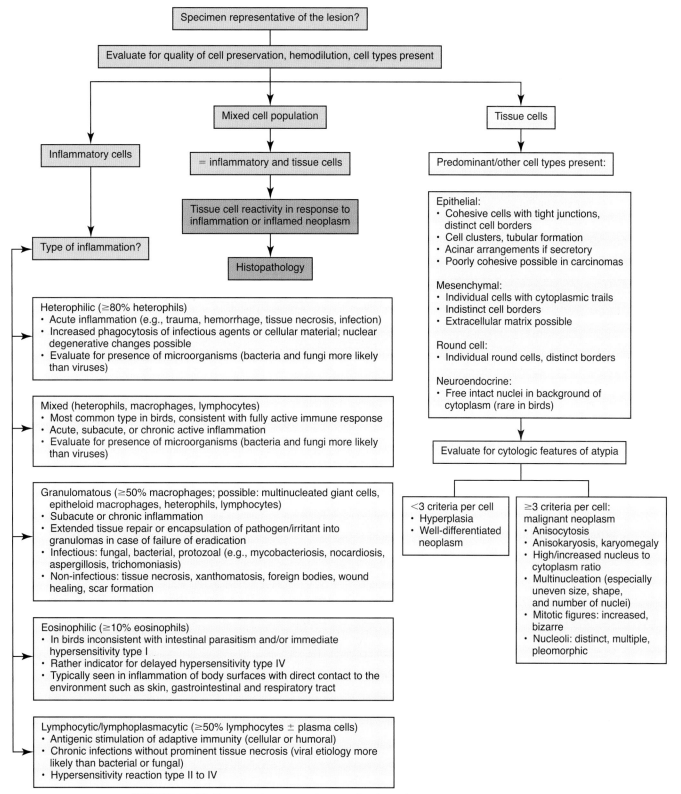

FIGURE 13-22 Systematic approach to evaluation of avian cytologic specimens.

EVALUATION PROTOCOL FOR CYTOLOGIC SPECIMENS

Date of sample collection: _____ Date of analysis: _____

Patient ID/Name: _____ Species: _____

History: _____

_____

_____

Specimen/Location: _____

Fluid samples-Color/Transparency: _____ TS (g/dL): _____ WBC estimate/count: _____

Preparation technique: _____ Stain: _____

LOW MAGNIFICATION (x4 to x20):

Sample quality (semiquantitative scale from 1=unacceptable to 5=excellent):

Representative cellular material:		☐ Yes	☐ No
Cellularity	☐ Mild	☐ Moderate	☐ High
Cell preservation	☐ Poor	☐ Fairly well	☐ Adequate
Hemodilution	☐ Mild	☐ Moderate	☐ Marked
Cell distribution	☐ Individual	☐ Aggregates	☐ Sheets

HIGH MAGNIFICATION (x40 to x100):

Cell types present (%) Epithelial _____ Mesenchymal _____

Round cell_____ Other _____

Cytologic description (including cytologic features of atypia):

> 3 criteria of malignancy per cell	☐ Yes	☐ No
Inflammation	☐ Yes	☐ No
Type of inflammation	☐ Heterophilic ☐ Mixed ☐ Lymphoplasmacytic	☐ Granulomatous ☐ Lymphocytic ☐ Eosinophilic
Microbes	☐ Yes	☐ No
If yes, please specify	☐ Bacterial ☐ Viral ☐ Other parasites	☐ Fungal ☐ Protozoal
Endogenous material	☐ Yes	☐ No
If yes, please specify	☐ Crystalloid material	☐ Other
Hemorrhage	☐ Yes	☐ No
If yes, please specify	☐ Acute	☐ Chronic

CYTOLOGIC INTERPRETATION

Further diagnostic tests recommended	☐ yes	☐ No
If yes, please specify	☐ Culture ☐ Molecular ☐ Histochemical stains	☐ Histopathology ☐ Parasitology ☐ Other

Additional comments

Signature

FIGURE 13-23 Evaluation protocol for cytologic specimens.

The objective of cytologic evaluation is the classification of the lesion into one or more of the following cytologic categories: inflammation, neoplasia, mixed cell population, cyst, and hemorrhagic lesion, as one or more of these categories may be present within the same lesion. We refer to other resources for in-depth description of these cytologic categories.[1-3] The most frequently encountered cytologic categories in avian medicine are inflammation, neoplasia, and mixed cell population.

Cytologic samples are initially scanned at low power for evaluation of overall quality (representative of the lesion, hemodilution, cell preservation) and sufficient cellularity. Evaluation in areas of even cell distribution at higher magnification is initiated by assessment of the cellularity and determination of tissue types present, including proportions of all cell types within the sample. Depending on the tissue of origin of the collected sample, pertaining tissue cells are expected, for example, columnar ciliated respiratory epithelial cells in tracheal washes, squamous epithelial cells in swabs from the oral cavity or crop, and mesothelial cells in peritoneal fluid.

Inflammation

Inflammation is characterized by the predominance of leukocytes in a higher concentration than from what would be expected from hemodilution. Hemogram results can be helpful in the assessment of hemodiluted samples. Identification of the type of inflammation may provide indication of the underlying etiology (see Figure 13-22), because it can be caused by microorganisms (bacteria, fungi, viruses, parasites), and nonvital (traumatic, chemical, thermal) or neoplastic processes. Acute inflammatory reactions in birds are characterized by a rapid heterophil infiltrate within hours, followed by a perivascular infiltrate of lymphocytes, and then tissue infiltration by macrophages 24 hours after injection of phytohemagglutinin (PHA).[4] Based on the experiments with PHA injections in birds, a mixed inflammatory reaction is observed in acute inflammatory lesions and consistent with an active immune response. Etiologic agents, including bacteria (Figure 13-24), parasites, or nonvital structures such as cholesterol or urate crystals (Figure 13-25), may be identified

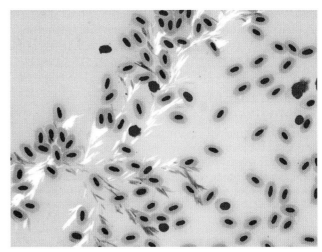

FIGURE 13-25 Synovial fluid of Grey parrot *(Psittacus erithacus):* urate crystals. Wright-Giemsa stain, original magnification ×400.

upon cytologic evaluation. The cytologic identification of microorganisms may be hindered by recent or current antimicrobial administration. Following the acute phase of inflammation (Figure 13-26), granuloma formation may develop if the pathogen cannot be eliminated in the acute phase of the inflammatory response. Granulomas are characterized by greater than 50% macrophages and frequently associated with multinucleated giant cells[5] Information on additional types of inflammation and potential etiologies is given in Table 13-8.

Viral inclusions are rarely diagnosed in cytologic specimens. Examples where diagnoses may be established include poxvirus infections with ballooning degeneration (Bollinger

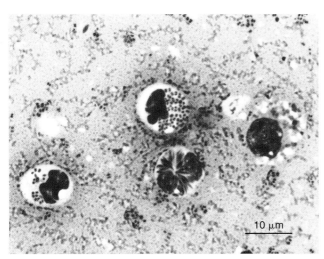

FIGURE 13-24 Corneal scraping of the left eye of a Peregrine falcon *(Falco peregrinus):* three heterophils and a macrophage (position 3). Cocci and diplococci are observed within the cytoplasm of two heterophils and in the background. Culture revealed *Micrococcus* spp. Wright-Giemsa stain.

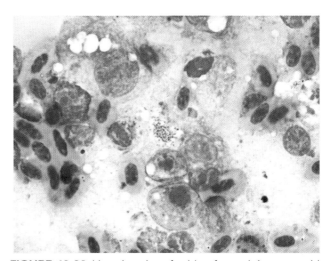

FIGURE 13-26 Liver imprint of a blue-fronted Amazon with fibrinoid hemorrhagic polyserositis, enteritis, and peritoneal and pericardial effusion at necropsy; positions 5 and 6: hepatocellular hyperplasia in response to inflammation (anisocytosis, anisokaryosis, and nucleolysis), position 12-1 (the cell is at the position between 12 and 1 on the face of a clock) macrophage with phagocytized erythrocytes and bacteria *(center),* suggesting bacterial hepatitis and septicemia as underlying causes. Wright-Giemsa stain, original magnification ×1000.

bodies) within the cytoplasm of epithelial cells of the eyelid or conjunctiva, or intranuclear adenoviral inclusions[1,2] (Figure 13-27). Molecular techniques such as fluorescent antibody staining or polymerase chain reaction (PCR) are more sensitive than cytology for identification of viral pathogens.

Tissue Cells: Malignancy versus Reactivity

Characteristics of epithelial, mesenchymal, round cell, or neuroendocrine tissue are briefly summarized in Figure 13-22. The cellular population is then evaluated for cytologic criteria of atypia to determine whether there is increased cell reactivity or immaturity, or malignancy (Figures 13-28 through 13-31). Atypical cytologic features (e.g., anisocytosis, anisokaryosis,

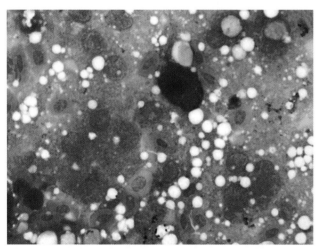

FIGURE 13-27 Liver imprint from a chicken *(Gallus gallus)* with intranuclear, basophilic, polymorphic inclusion bodies suggestive of adenoviral inclusion body hepatitis (IBH), confirmed by histology. Wright-Giemsa stain, original magnification ×400.

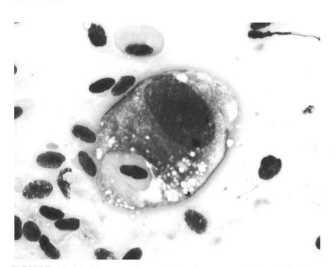

FIGURE 13-28 Fine-needle aspirate from a pathologic fracture of the right wing in a cockatiel; mesenchymal cell with more than three cellular features of malignancy: karyomegaly (> 3 erythrocytes), macrocytosis, distinct nucleolus, coarse chromatin, increased nuclear-to-cytoplasmic ratio, erythrophagocytosis, fine irregular cytoplasmic vacuolation, and increased cytoplasmic basophilia. Wright-Giemsa stain, original magnification ×1000.

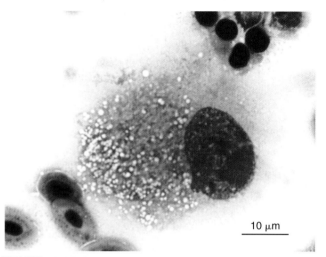

FIGURE 13-29 Malignant mesenchymal cell in a sarcoma of the wing of a rose-ringed parakeet *(Psittacula krameri)* showing karyomegaly, nuclear budding (position 7), prominent and pleomorphic nucleolus, coarse chromatin, increased nuclear-to-cytoplasmic ratio, fine irregular cytoplasmic vacuolation. Wright-Giemsa stain.

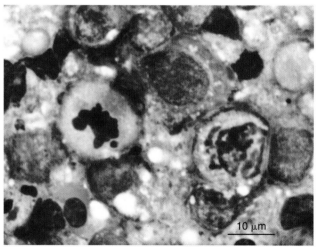

FIGURE 13-30 Tissue aspirate of cutaneous lesion on head: squamous cell carcinoma in a Grey parrot *(Psittacus erithacus)*; cluster of variably cohesive cells with anisocytosis, anisokaryosis, high nuclear-to-cytoplasmic ratio, coarse chromatin, cytoplasmic basophilia, fine perinuclear cytoplasmic vacuolation (position 1), and atypical mitotic figures suggesting a high rate of proliferation. Wright-Giemsa stain.

karyomegaly, and pleomorphism) can be observed in tissue cells as a reactive response to irritation and inflammation (e.g., reactive fibroplasia with inflammation) (Figure 13-32). Malignancy is suspected in cases in which three or more criteria of malignancy can be consistently identified in cells of the same tissue origin, especially in the absence of inflammation (Figure 13-33).

Mixed Cell Population

If inflammatory and tissue cells are observed concurrently, the cytologic category of mixed cell population applies. The diagnostic challenge in specimens of mixed cell populations is

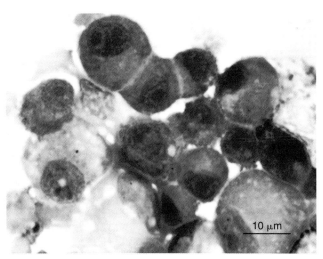

FIGURE 13-31 Fine-needle aspirate of fluid in subcutaneous swelling in a nanday conure *(Aratinga nenday)*. Poorly cohesive epithelial cells of low grade of differentiation, with acinar architecture indicated at position 12 suggestive of adenocarcinoma. Wright-Giemsa stain.

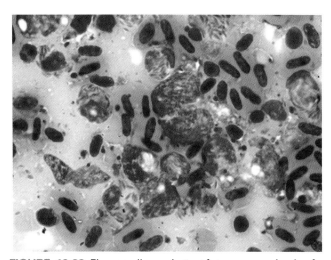

FIGURE 13-32 Fine-needle aspirate of a mass on beak of a budgerigar *(Melopsittacus undulatus)*: the sample revealed multiple atypical mesenchymal cells *(center)* admixed with inflammatory cells (heterophils and vacuolated macrophages), consistent with mixed cell population. Bacterial culture was positive, and antibiotic therapy resulted in complete remission of the mass. Wright-Giemsa stain, original magnification ×1000.

the differentiation of a reactive from a neoplastic process, that is, cytologic differentiation of tissue cell reactivity in response to inflammation from an inflamed neoplasm. This often cannot be accomplished by cytology, and histopathology is needed for additional diagnostic information, since it allows for evaluation of tissue architecture. A classic example are atypical mesenchymal cells admixed with inflammatory cells, a lesion which may represent granulation tissue or scar formation, or an inflamed sarcoma (see Figure 13-32).

Cyst

Although mainly encountered in mammalian cytology, a rare but reported presentation in birds are epidermal cysts

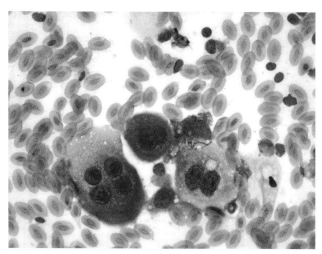

FIGURE 13-33 Fine-needle aspirate from a firm mass in the left kneefold in a Eurasian eagle owl *(Bubo bubo)*: several clusters of mesenchymal cells with multinucleation and various nuclear features of malignancy suggestive of osteoclastoma or malignant fibrous histiocytoma. Wright-Giemsa stain, original magnification ×1000

associated with the feather follicle.[1] Cyst formation is cytologically identified by the presence of uniform squamous epithelial cells, amorphous cellular debris, cholesterol crystals, keratin bars, and possibly the presence of hemorrhage in the early stages[1] (Figure 13-34).

Hemorrhage

Hemorrhage can be present as a sequel of other cytologic categories, or it may be the primary cause of the lesion, for example, hematoma and hemoperitoneum. Cytologic features indicative of hemorrhage include erythrophagocytosis, and presence of phagocytized amorphous greenish-basophilic material suggestive of hemosiderin, or hematoidin crystals (Figure 13-35). Hemosiderin can be visualized by Prussian blue reaction.

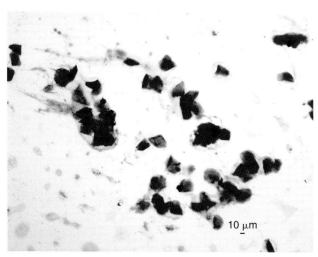

FIGURE 13-34 Fine-needle aspirate of left periorbital area of a parakeet *(Melopsittacus undulatus)*: presence of well-differentiated squamous epithelial cells suggestive of an epidermal cyst. Wright-Giemsa stain.

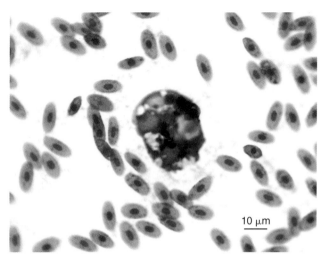

FIGURE 13-35 Direct smear of peritoneal effusion in a helmeted guineafowl *(Numida meleagris)* with mesothelioma (confirmed by histopathology): macrophage with phagocytized erythrocytes, dark blue-black globular pigment suggestive of hemosiderin, and refractile rhomboid golden hematoidin crystals. The effusion with a packed cell volume of 7% was consistent with a hemoperitoneum. Wright-Giemsa stain.

CYTOLOGY OF FREQUENTLY EVALUATED ORGAN SYSTEMS IN AVIAN CLINICAL PRACTICE

Each organ system is composed of tissue-specific cells and their cytologic features (i.e., background material). The most common lesions and abnormalities are presented in Table 13-8 with reference to additional images (Figures 13-36 through 13-43). The reader is referred to in-depth references[1,2] if further information is desired.

CYTOLOGY AS IN-HOUSE DIAGNOSTIC TOOL

In-house evaluation of cytologic samples can provide rapid diagnostic information to the clinician. In cases of questionable interpretation, the specimen should be submitted to a diagnostic laboratory for additional evaluation by an experienced pathologist. An in-house case archive with filed reports and a searchable database can be helpful for learning and training opportunities. Slides stained with Romanowsky type-based stains and coverslips preserve well over many years. For archiving unstained slides, the authors recommend fixation in 95% high-quality, acetone-free methanol for 5 minutes.

TABLE 13-8

Most Common Lesions and Abnormalities Found in Avian Patients by Organ System and Their Cytologic Features[1,2]

Organ System/ Lesion	Cytologic Findings	Interpretation	Options for Additional Diagnostics
Skin	Well-differentiated squamous epithelial cells Possible mixed bacilli population (contaminants)	Normal	N/A
Skin lesions, mass or ulceration	Inflammatory cells (see Figure 13-22) Infectious organisms (bacteria, esp. cocci, fungal hyphae, yeast, parasites, viral inclusions)	Inflammation Infection (see Figure 13-22)	Cultures (bacterial, fungal) depending on type of inflammation; parasitology (see Figure 13-22)
	Granulomatous inflammation, lipid material, cholesterol crystals	Xanthomatosis	Evaluate history (e.g., diet, metabolic derangements), plasma biochemistry, histopathology
	Squamous epithelial cells, keratin bars, cellular debris (see Figure 13-34)	Cyst	N/A
	Phagocytosis of erythrocytes and/or hemosiderin; ± hematoidin crystals	Hematoma	Evaluate history
Skin, masses	Tissue cells of same tissue of origin (see Figure 13-22)	Neoplasia *Most common in birds:*	Histopathology, special stains if applicable
	Well-differentiated adipocytes	Lipoma	
	Free lipid, cholesterol crystals, vacuolated macrophages, multinucleated giant cells	Xanthoma	*Note: For any mass, always consider reactive changes vs. malignancy (see Figure 13-22)*
	Uniform mesenchymal cells	Fibroma, hemangioma, granulation tissue, scar formation	
	Predominance of lymphoblasts (see Figure 13-42)	Lymphoid neoplasia	
	Atypical squamous epithelial cells ± inflammation (see Figure 13-30)	Squamous cell carcinoma	

TABLE 13-8

Most Common Lesions and Abnormalities Found in Avian Patients by Organ System and Their Cytologic Features—cont'd

Organ System/ Lesion	Cytologic Findings	Interpretation	Options for Additional Diagnostics
Conjunctiva, normal	Atypical mesenchymal cells Fibrosarcoma: extracellular matrix Hemangiosarcoma: possible presence of acute and/or chronic hemorrhage Uniform adipocytes and hematopoietic cells Squamous and/or columnar epithelial cells	Sarcoma (see Figure 13-29) Fibrosarcoma, hemangiosarcoma Myelolipoma Normal	N/A
	Inflammatory cells (see Figure 13-22) Infectious organisms (bacteria, esp. cocci, yeast, fungal hyphae) *C. psittaci* elementary bodies in epithelial cells, macrophages	Inflammation Infection (see Figure 13-24) Chlamydiosis	Cultures (bacterial, fungal) depending on type of inflammation PCR
Respiratory tract	Low cellularity: squamous epithelial cells (sample contaminants from oral cavity), ciliated columnar epithelial cells, goblet cells, small amount of mucus	Normal	N/A
Upper respiratory tract	Inflammatory cells (see Figure 13-22) Infectious organisms (*C. psittaci, M. gallisepticum,* fungal hyphae, yeast, parasites such as mites, *Cryptococcus* spp. [see Figure 13-41], *C. baileyi*) Numerous uniform squamous epithelial cells	Inflammation Infection Squamous cell metaplasia	Cultures (bacterial, fungal) depending on type of inflammation; parasitology (see Figure 13-22) Differential diagnoses: hypovitaminosis A, mechanical irritation, inflammation
Air sacs	Branching, septate fungal hyphae (possible microconidia/macroconidia) Inflammatory cells (see Figure 13-22) Mites, microfilaria, *C. psittaci* elementary bodies, *Mycobacterium avium*	Fungal infection/ suspicion for aspergillosis Inflammation Infection	GMS stain, culture, PCR Cultures (bacterial, fungal) depending on type of inflammation; parasitology (see Figure 13-22); special stains (*Chlamydia* spp: Gimenez or Macchiavello, *Mycobacterium* spp: acid fast (see Figure 13-43)
Upper gastrointestinal tract	Low cellularity: squamous epithelial cells, normal microflora (mixed bacilli, commensal *Alysiella filiformis* (see Figure 13-26) ± plant and seed material; rare yeast), mucus Inflammatory cells (see Figure 13-22) Infectious organisms (bacterial, yeast, parasites such as trichomonads, *Capillaria ova*)	Normal Inflammation Infection Trauma	N/A Cultures (bacterial, fungal) depending on type of inflammation; parasitology (see Figure 13-22); wet mount for trichomonads
Crop	Squamous epithelial cell hyperplasia and metaplasia Low cellularity: squamous epithelial cells (keratinized and/or intermediate stages); mixed bacilli; rare yeast Inflammatory cells (see Figure 13-22) Infectious organisms (abnormal bacterial flora, yeast, fungus, parasites such as trichomonads, *Capillaria ova*)	Hypovitaminosis A Normal Inflammation Infection (see Figure 13-39) Trauma	 N/A Cultures (bacterial, fungal) depending on type of inflammation; parasitology (see Figure 13-22)
Colon, cloaca, vent	Columnar epithelial cells, goblet cells, vent: squamous epithelial cells; plant/food material, mixed bacilli, mucus; urates possible Inflammatory cells (see Figure 13-22) Infectious organisms (spore-formers, yeast, fungus *Macrorhabdus ornithogaster,* parasites)	Normal Inflammation Infection	N/A Cultures (bacterial, fungal) depending on type of inflammation; parasitology (see Figure 13-22); Gram stain
Fecal	Highly cellular, heterogenous bacilli population If urinary excretions present: urates in variable amounts	Normal (see Figure 13-37)	N/A

Continued

TABLE 13-8

Most Common Lesions and Abnormalities Found in Avian Patients by Organ System and Their Cytologic Features—cont'd

Organ System/ Lesion	Cytologic Findings	Interpretation	Options for Additional Diagnostics
	Predominance of one type of bacterium	Abnormal colonic microflora	Gram stain (see Figure 13-19C) and/or culture
	Low number of mixed bacilli	Abnormal colonic microflora	Evaluate clinical history as this can be seen with recent or current antimicrobial administration
	Increased/predominance of spore-formers	Abnormal microflora	Anaerobic culture and/or *Clostridium* spp. toxin ELISA
	Cryptosporidium spp. oocysts	Cryptosporidiosis	Acid-fast stain, PCR for species ID (host vs. prey species)
Liver	Additional findings as for "colon, cloaca, vent" Well-differentiated hepatocytes ± biliary epithelial cells	Normal	N/A
	Distinct vacuolation in hepatocytes	Hepatic lipidosis Normal in very young birds	Oil red O stain, Sudan III or IV, New Methylene blue
	Macrophages and/or hepatocytes with hemosiderin	Excess iron	Prussian blue, Perl's stain
	Inflammatory cells (see Figure 13-22)	Inflammation (see Figure 13-27)	Cultures (bacterial, fungal) depending on type of inflammation; parasitology (see Figure 13-22); buffy coat: *Atoxoplasma* spp.
	Infectious organisms (mycobacteriosis, *Plasmodium* spp., *Atoxoplasma* spp.)	Infection	
	Bright pink extracellular material in liver, spleen, and/or joints	Amyloidosis	Congo red stain and polarizer
	Myeloid and/or erythroid precursors	Extramedullary hematopoiesis	CBC
	Uniform adipocytes and hematopoietic cells	Myelolipoma	Histopathology
Peritoneal fluid/ effusion	Low cellularity fluid	Normal	N/A
	Mononuclear phagocytes (macrophages, mesothelial cells, ± ciliated cuboidal cells from air sacs) *If possible, differentiate IPC from HPC fluid (see Chapter 8)*		
	Inflammatory cells (see Figure 13-22)	Peritonitis	Cultures (bacterial, fungal) depending on type of inflammation
	Bacteria, fungi	Infection	
	Effusions due to right heart failure related to hepatic neoplasia	*Mainly HPC*	
	Variably intense yellow-colored fluid	Yolk peritonitis (see Figure 13-38)	Culture
	Macrophages, heterophils, mesothelial cells, multinucleated giant cells, yolk	*Mainly IPC*	
	Moderately to markedly atypical epithelial cells	Carcinoma *Mainly IPC: gonadal, splenic, pancreatic neoplasm origin vs. mesothelial hyperplasia*	Histopathology
	Phagocytosis of erythrocytes ± hemosiderin, PCV >3%	Hemoperitoneum (see Figure 13-35)	Consider differential diagnoses: Trauma, hemostasis defects, neoplasia
Synovial fluid	Mononuclear cells, pink granular background	Normal	N/A
	Increased mononuclear or other inflammatory cells	Synovitis (see Figure 13-21)	Cultures (bacterial, fungal) depending on type of inflammation
	Bacteria	Infection	
	Uric acid crystals	Gout (see Figure 13-25)	Evaluation under polarized light

Please note that this table provides a basic overview; cytology samples may contain one or more pathologic processes and may not exactly fit textbook definitions.

N/A, Not applicable; GMS, Gomori methenamine silver stain; IPC, intestinal peritoneal cavity; HPC, hepatic peritoneal cavities.

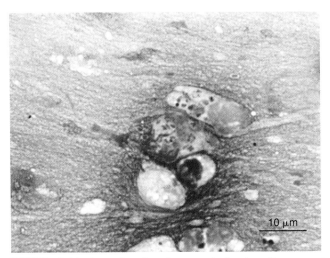

FIGURE 13-36 Tissue imprint of tongue lesion in a Grey parrot *(Psittacus erithacus)*: highly proteinaceous background, and mixed inflammatory cells with phagocytized bacteria suggestive of bacterial infection. An underlying primary cause of different etiology for the lesion cannot be excluded. Wright-Giemsa stain.

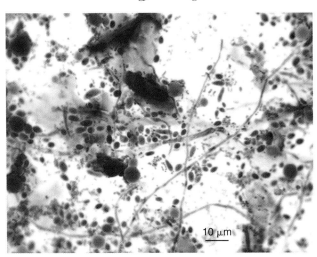

FIGURE 13-39 Direct smear of crop swab of a red-and-green macaw: mixed bacterial population and numerous yeast organisms with formation of pseudohyphae consistent with spp. Wright-Giemsa stain.

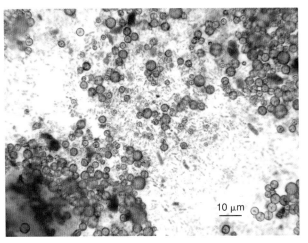

FIGURE 13-37 Direct fecal smear from a bald eagle *(Haliaeetus leucocephalus)*: presence of frequent mixed rod-shaped bacteria suggestive of normal colonic microflora, and urate crystals. Wright-Giemsa stain.

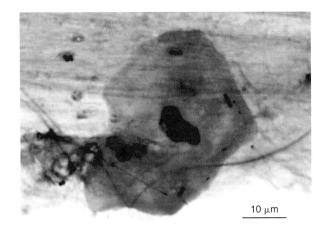

FIGURE 13-40 Direct smear of mucus from oral cavity in a red-tailed hawk *(Buteo jamaicensis)*: mature squamous epithelial cell with three adhered, plump, rod-shaped bacteria consistent with commensal *Alysiella filiformis*. Wright-Giemsa stain.

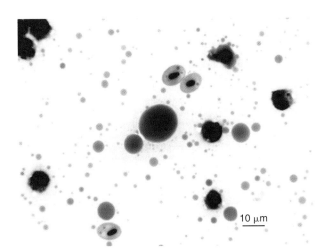

FIGURE 13-38 Direct smear of a peritoneal effusion in a cockatiel *(Nymphicus hollandicus)*: globular proteinaceous material and dense heterophils consistent with yolk peritonitis. Wright-Giemsa stain.

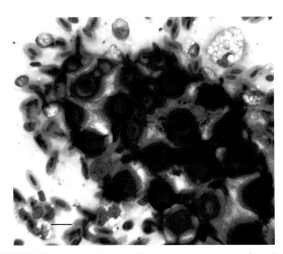

FIGURE 13-41 Lung imprint from a salmon-crested cockatoo *(Cacatua moluccensis)* with yeast organisms exhibiting narrow-based budding and a thick capsule consistent with *Cryptococcus* spp. and granulomatous and heterophilic inflammation. Wright-Giemsa stain. (Image courtesy Dr. Amy Weeden.)

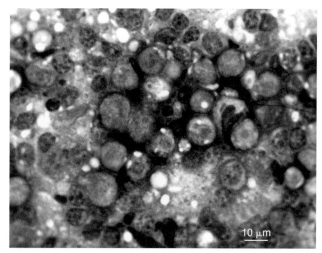

FIGURE 13-42 Fine-needle aspirate of a mass in the nostrils of a Grey parrot *(Psittacus erithacus)*: neoplastic round cells consistent with lymphoma. Wright-Giemsa stain.

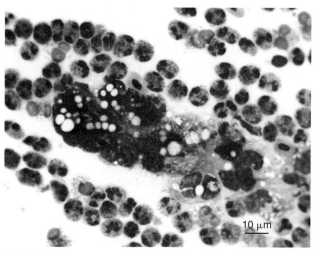

FIGURE 13-43 Synovial fluid direct smear of a great horned owl *(Bubo virginianus;* same patient as Figure 13-21): marked heterophilic and granulomatous synovitis with multinucleated giant cells exhibiting phagocytized, negative-staining, rod-shaped bacteria suggestive of *Mycobacterium* spp. and a low number of dark-staining, refractile structures consistent with urate crystals (systemic mycobacterial infection and articular gout was confirmed by histopathology).

If slides need to be transported or may be exposed to humid air conditions, desiccating granule packets can be very helpful. Fecal cytology samples should be stained in a separate stain set to avoid bacterial contamination by nonfecal samples. In-house stains need to be maintained, filtered, and changed per manufacturer's recommendations and used stain properly disposed according to environmental regulations. These in-house stains can be very helpful for the clinician to facilitate rapid selection of proper antimicrobial treatment if clinically indicated.

CYTOLOGY USED WITH PARASITOLOGIC SPECIMENS AND GENERAL PARASITOLOGIC EVALUATION OF AVIAN PATIENTS

Some cytologic techniques are useful to search for parasites. These include swabs, imprints, flushes, skin scrapings, scotch tape preparations, and direct cotton tip wet mounts.[11] Blood films may contain hemoparasites. Fecal samples may be evaluated by various means for adult parasites or their developmental stages. Experience is required to distinguish between true parasites, transient nonparasitic organisms, and pseudoparasitic structures. Diagnostic challenges may be posed by artifacts such as air bubbles, plant material, pollen, contaminant fungal hyphae or spores, parasites from prey, and accidentally swallowed eggs and larvae from free-living nematodes.

Ectoparasites

Deep skin scrapings from dermal crusts can be useful to detect skin mites, which in birds most commonly belong to the genus *Knemidocoptes* (Figure 13-44). Microscopic evaluation at low power will reveal the adult females in epidermal burrows (Figure 13-45). The affected skin area is squeezed between the thumb and the forefinger of one hand and the surface scraped bluntly with a scalpel blade until bleeding occurs. Visibility of the parasite is improved when the sample is boiled or stored overnight in 10% potassium hydroxide. Ectoparasites on the skin surface, such as lice (Figures 13-46 through 13-48), mites, and flat flies are often already seen with careful clinical examination. Small specimens, larval stages, and eggs may be viewed with a scotch tape imprint (Figure 13-49). The tape is gently pressed onto the skin and then stuck onto a glass slide for microscopic examination at low power and dropped condensor. Surfaces of the housing can be examined this way when an infestation with arthropods not permanently living on the host, for example, the red poultry mite *(Dermanyssus gallinae)*, is suspected (Figures 13-50 and 13-51).

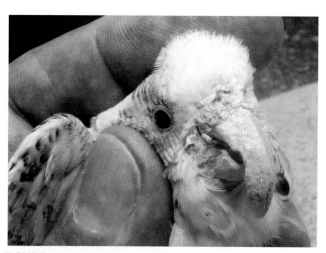

FIGURE 13-44 Budgerigar *(Melopsittacus undulatus)* with beak mange caused by infestation with *Knemidocoptes* sp. (Photo courtesy Neil Forbes.)

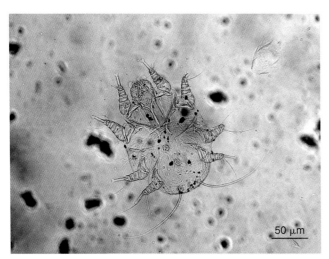

FIGURE 13-45 *Knemidokoptes pilae*, macaw (*Ara* sp.), original magnification ×160. (Photo courtesy Dr. Heather Walden, University of Florida.)

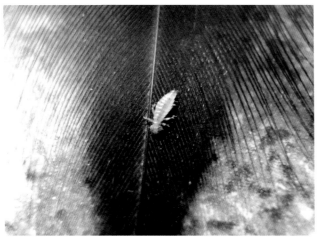

FIGURE 13-46 Feather louse, Harris hawk *(Parabuteo unicinctus)*. (Photo courtesy Neil Forbes.)

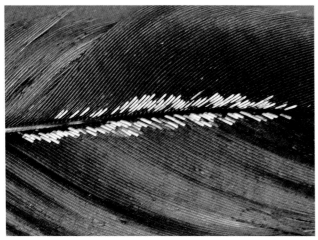

FIGURE 13-47 Louse eggs at the base of the feather barbs, Harris hawk *(Parabuteo unicinctus)*. (Photo courtesy Neil Forbes.)

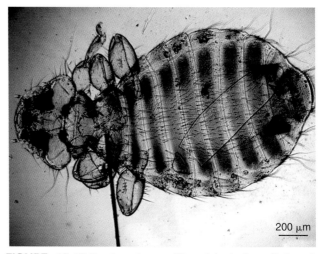

FIGURE 13-48 Feather louse *(Kurodaia* haliaeeti*)* female with nit from an osprey *(Pandion haliaetus)*. Original magnification ×40. (Photo courtesy Dr. Heather Walden, University of Florida.)

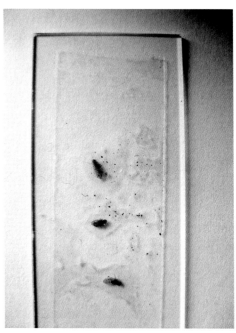

FIGURE 13-49 Scotch tape imprint with feather lice from a domestic chicken *(Gallus gallus* var. *dom)*.

Parasites of the Upper Respiratory Tract and Upper Gastrointestinal Tract

Tracheal and nasal flushes may contain upper respiratory parasites such as gapeworms (*Syngamus* spp., *Cyathostoma* spp., *Serratospiculum* sp.), mites (*Sternostoma tracheacolum*; Figure 13-52), and flukes (*Tracheophilus* spp.). Cryptosporidia are quite firmly attached to the epithelium (both respiratory and gastrointestinal). Vigorous swabbing of the surface with a wet cotton tip may be necessary to detach the small round organisms from the brush border. Cryptosporidial oocysts are characterized by their small size (2 to 6 μm) and their clear to

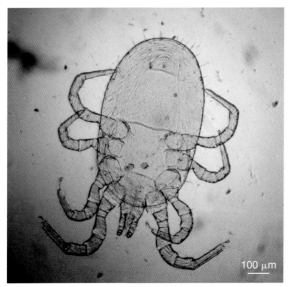

FIGURE 13-50 Red chicken mite *(Dermanyssus gallinae)*. (Photo courtesy Dr. Heather Walden, University of Florida.)

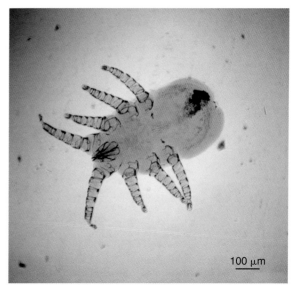

FIGURE 13-52 *Sternostoma tracheacolum* from an airsac of a finch. (Photo courtesy Dr. Heather Walden, University of Florida.)

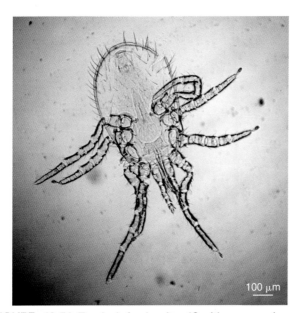

FIGURE 13-51 Tropical fowl mite *(Ornithonyssus bursa)*, American kestrel *(Falco sparverius)*: in contrast to *Dermanyssus* spp., *Ornithonyssus* spp. live permanently on the host and present with more pointed caudal ends of the dorsal and anal plates and readily visible chelicerae. (Photo courtesy Dr. Heather Walden, University of Florida.)

(Trichomonas spp.), and from cecal *(Histomonas* spp.) or duodenal contents *(Hexamita* spp.). A warm drop of fluid, or a small heat-producing light bulb will ensure a warm environment during microscopy, which is necessary to maintain motility. Phase contrast or special stains are necessary to visualize subcellular structures. *Trichomonas* spp. (5 to 9 μm in length, 2 to 9 μm in width) are characterized by their pearlike shape with an undulating membrane at one side, and four flagella protruding from the anterior pole of the body (Figures 13-53 through 13-55). *Histomonas meleagridis*, the etiologic agent of infectious enterohepatitis or blackhead disease (Figure 13-56), shows high morphologic variability, with occasionally one single flagellum present in its intraluminal stage. The nonamoeboid round tissue stage is difficult to distinguish from macrophages and varies in size (3 to 16 μm). The relatively long (6 to 12 μm) and thin (2 to 5 μm) *Hexamita* spp. are characterized by eight prominent flagella symmetrically emerging from different parts of the body. Their rapid movements display a typical twitching pattern.

Fecal Samples

Sample collection

The minimum amount of feces necessary for a parasitologic examination is about 5 grams. Samples are best collected immediately after voiding has occurred. Ideally, collection is performed at different times of the day, as shedding intensity follows a circadian rhythm in many parasites. Deposition of paper under the perches reduces environmental contamination. Fecal samples should be examined as soon as possible after collection. In case of a delay of sample processing, samples need to be wrapped safely and stored in the refrigerator. If the sample has to be stored for more than 24 hours, dilution with 10% formalin after collection is recommended to prevent embryonation. Some parasites are visible macroscopically, such as tapeworms, their proglottids, or large nematodes. Typical size, shape, and color even may allow for a species diagnosis ("redworms" for *Syngamus* spp.). Visibility is facilitated by filtering the sample through a finely

light blue staining in direct smear preparations.[6] Evaluation is ideally performed under high power with phase contrast. Romanowsky type-based stains such as Wright-Giemsa stain reveal a dark blue granulation. Their bright pink appearance in acid-fast stains allows for differentiation from morphologically similar structures such as yeast.

Flagellates

Fresh, direct wet smears are the method of choice to detect motile protozoans from the crop or the oral cavity

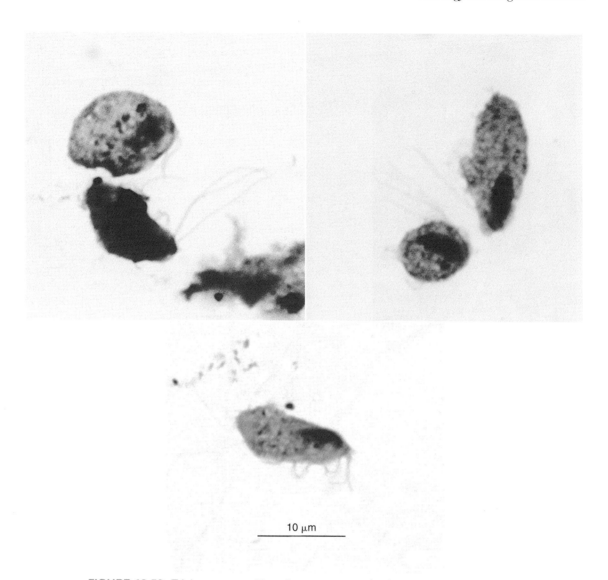

FIGURE 13-53 *Trichomonas gallinae* from a crop swab of a pigeon *(Columba livia).*

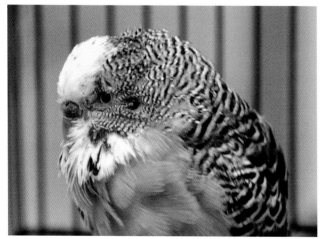

FIGURE 13-54 Trichomoniasis in a budgerigar *(Melopsittacus undulatus)*; head plumage covered with clots of saliva from regurgitation and head shaking. (Photo courtesy Neil Forbes.)

meshed sieve. The remnants are allowed to sediment for 10 minutes in a petri dish. Examination against a monochrome light or dark background will help to detect small and thin nematodes.

Direct wet mounts

For direct microscopic evaluation, a small amount of feces is placed in the center of a microscopic glass slide. The specimen is then diluted with a drop of tap water or physiologic saline solution and covered with a coverglass. Addition of diluted iodine solution (Betadine) will selectively stain protozoal cysts and eggshells of *Ornithobilharzia* sp. Watery 1% methylene blue solution simplifies differentiation of yellow brown parasitic eggs from blue-staining plant material and dust. Examination under the microscope is performed at low magnification with an almost closed aperture and a dropped condensor. All areas of the specimen should be systematically scanned for small worms, larvae, eggs, and oocysts. Direct mounts are not very sensitive; thus detection

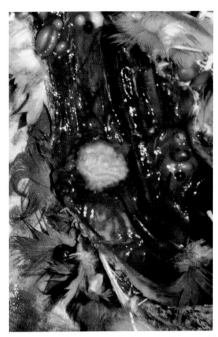

FIGURE 13-55 Granulomatous inflammation and hyperemia in the crop of a common pigeon *(Columba livia)* with trichomoniasis. (Photo courtesy Neil Forbes.)

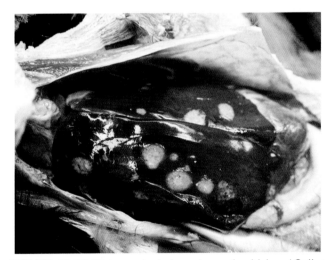

FIGURE 13-56 Histomoniasis in a domestic chicken (*Gallus gallus* var. *dom*). (Photo courtesy Neil Forbes.)

of stages of one or more parasite species indicates a moderate to high infestation. False-negative results may occur with low-grade infestations or in cases of only sporadic shedding of ova and oocysts.

Flotation

Flotation as concentration technique is based on the fact that worm eggs will float to the surface in solutions that have a higher specific gravity (SG) than them. Nematode eggs will float at an SG of more than 1.15. Eggs from trematodes and

cestodes will float at an SG from 1.35 and higher. However, high SGs of parasite ova bear some disadvantages. The higher the SG of the solution, the sooner the deformation of parasites and their ova will occur and the more pseudoparasitic structures will also float. Hence, additional steps of washing and filtration of the feces prior to flotation may be necessary. Concentrated solutions with stable SGs are commercially available. Self-made watery saturated solutions can be prepared from salt or sugar with saline solutions being superior to sugar in terms of stability. A useful combination for daily practice is saturated saline (sodium chloride [NaCl], SG = 1.2 at 20°C [68°F]) for nematodes and most cestodes, and zinc chloride (zinc chloride [$ZnCl_2$], SG = 1.50 at 20°C [68°F]) for trematodes and some cestodes. The fecal sample is homogeneously mixed with the fluid, and the solution is allowed to stand for 10 to 15 minutes. The egg-containing surface is then gently removed and transferred onto a glass slide either by a fine wire loop or by a coverglass. In case of the latter, the glass is left on the surface for about 1 minute, lifted in a perpendicular manner, and then placed directly onto the slide. Systematic scanning of the slide is again performed as described for direct wet mounts (see above). Parasitic load is reported semiquantitatively from + (low, 1 parasitic structure per sample) to +++ (more than 10 structures per sample). Worm eggs are classified by their sizes, shapes, poles, contents, and specific appendages. For further details, the reader is referred to parasitology textbooks.[7] Examples of the most common types of eggs in avian patients are depicted in Figures 13-57 through 13-65. Eggs of *Ascaridia* sp. can be differentiated from *Heterakis* sp. by their smaller size and their unbowed length sides (Figures 13-57 through 13-59). All cestode eggs (onchospheres) contain a hexacanth embryo (Figures 13-60 and 13-61), whereas the eggs of *Capillaria* sp. exhibit a typical lemon shape with asymmetric sides and prominent pole plugs (Figure 13-62). The clinical presentation can be quite similar to infection with trichomonads or

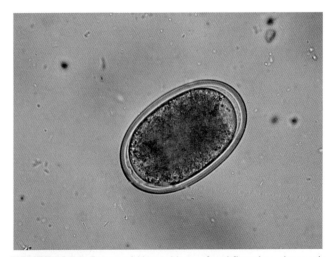

FIGURE 13-57 Ovum of *Heterakis* sp., fecal flotation, domestic chicken (*Gallus gallus* var. *dom*). (From Pendl H, Kreyenbuehl K: Clinical pathology. In Poland G, Raftery A, editors: *BSAVA manual of backyard poultry*, Gloucester, UK, in press, BSAVA Publications.)

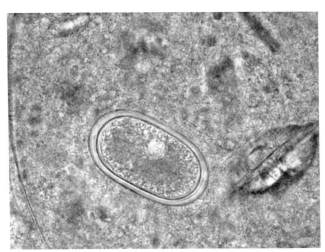

FIGURE 13-58 Ovum of *Ascaridia* sp., fecal direct wet mount, domestic chicken (*Gallus gallus* var. *dom*). (From Pendl H, Kreyenbuehl K: Clinical pathology. In Poland G, Raftery A, editors: *BSAVA manual of backyard poultry*, Gloucester, UK, in press, BSAVA Publications.)

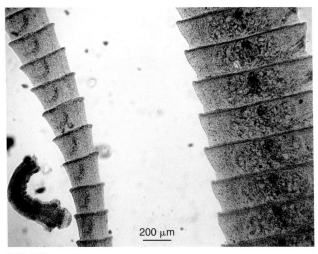

FIGURE 13-60 Tapeworm of the genus *Raillietina. From left to right:* scolex, immature and mature proglottids; great horned owl *(Bubo virginianus).* Original magnification ×40. (Photo courtesy Dr. Heather Walden, University of Florida.)

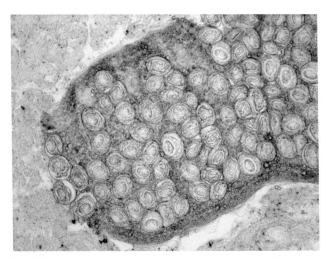

FIGURE 13-61 *Cestode* sp., gravid proglottid with oncospheres, domestic chicken (*Gallus galls* var. *dom*). Original magnification ×40.

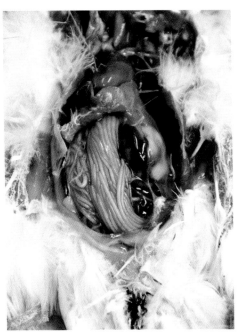

FIGURE 13-59 Ileus caused by massive infestation with *Ascarids*, Bourke parakeet *(Neopsephotus bourkii).* (Photo courtesy Neil Forbes.)

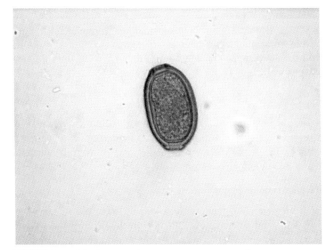

FIGURE 13-62 Ovum of *Capillaria* sp.; fecal flotation, goose *(Anser anser).*

yeast (Figure 13-63). The oval, thin-walled eggs of trematodes are relatively large compared with nematode eggs. They are dark colored and have a single operculum at one pole (Figure 13-64). Coccidial oocysts are usually small (15 to 30 µm), translucent, round to oval structures. In contrast to air bubbles, they show light refraction at different depths of focus (Figure 13-65). Their detection in living birds is inconsistent because shedding follows a circadian rhythm. More reliable results can be obtained at necropsy of fresh carcasses

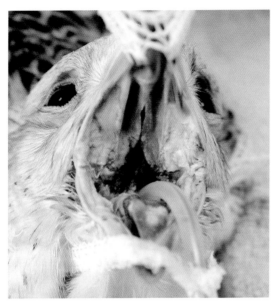

FIGURE 13-63 Capillariasis with granulomatous–diphtheroid inflammation of the oropharynx aggravated by secondary bacterial infection, Saker falcon *(Falco cherrug)*. (Photo courtesy Neil Forbes.)

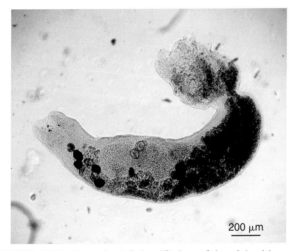

FIGURE 13-64 Intestinal fluke *(Strigea falconis)* with eggs visible, red-tailed hawk *(Buteo jamaicensis)*. Original magnification ×40. (Photo courtesy Dr. Heather Walden, University of Florida.)

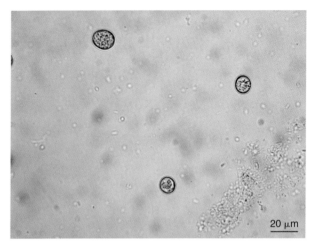

FIGURE 13-65 Coccidial oocysts, sandhill crane *(Grus canadensis)*. Original magnification ×400. (Photo courtesy Dr. Heather Walden, University of Florida.)

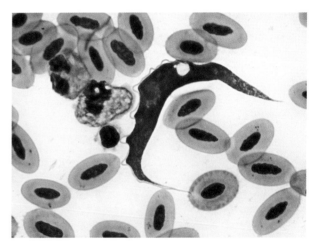

FIGURE 13-66 *Trypanosoma* sp., buffy coat preparation, Toco toucan *(Ramphastos toco)*. Wright-Giemsa stain, original magnification 31,000. (From Samour J: *Avian medicine*, St. Louis, MO, 2015, Elsevier.)

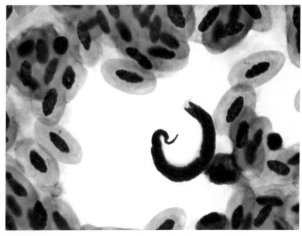

FIGURE 13-67 Same sample as in Figure 13-66, concurrent infection with microfilaria, buffy coat preparation, Toco toucan *(Ramphastos toco)*. Wright-Giemsa stain, original magnification ×1000.

by swabbing several areas of the intestinal tract and—in anseriformes—the kidney *(Eimeria truncata)*. The same is valid for intestinal cryptosporidia because of their attachment to the epithelial surface (see above).

Hemoparasites

Hemoparasites are frequently found in avian blood. *Trypanosoma* spp. and microfilaria concentrate in the buffy coat and are best viewed with direct buffy coat smear preparations from the spun capillary tube (Figures 13-66 and 13-67). In blood films, gametocytes of the genera *Haemoproteus*, *Plasmodium*,

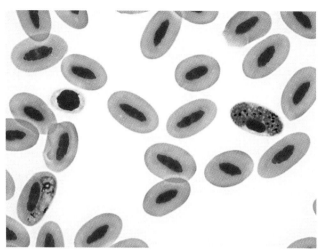

FIGURE 13-68 Gametocyte of *Haemoproteus* sp. with horseshoe-like encircling of the host cell nucleus, Ural owl *(Strix uralensis)*, blood film. Wright-Giemsa stain, original magnification ×1000.

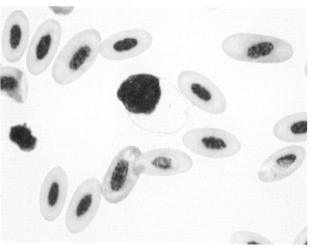

FIGURE 13-70 Intensively stained and granulated macrogametocyte of *Leucozytozoon toddi* surrounding the host cell nucleus; the cytoplasmic membrane of the host cell is visible as fine, bowed line directed to the lower right corner of the image; Harris hawk *(Parabuteo unicinctus)*, blood film. Wright-Giemsa stain, original magnification ×1000. (Specimen courtesy of Neil Forbes.)

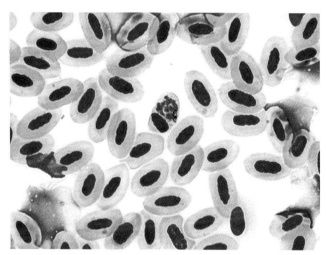

FIGURE 13-69 Gametocyte of *Plasmodium* sp. with lateral displacement of the host cell nucleus, great tit *(Parus major)*, blood film. Wright-Giemsa stain, original magnification ×1000.

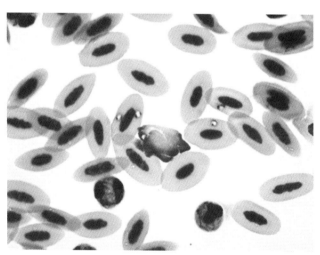

FIGURE 13-71 Trophozoites of *Babesia shortti* in a Saker falcon *(Falco cherrug)*, blood film. Wright-Giemsa stain, original magnification ×1000. (Specimen courtesy J.H. Samour.)

and *Leucozytozoon* spp. display as fine granular structures in the cytoplasm of erythrocytes (Figures 13-68 through 13-70). *Plasmodium* and *Leucozytozoon* typically displace the nucleus of the host cell to the side. In contrast, *Hemoproteus* tends to envelop the centrally remaining nucleus in a more or less horseshoe-like pattern. The intensively stained macrogametocytes of *Leucozytozoon* can be misinterpreted as dark, granulated cytoplasm of an unknown type of blood cell. Trophozoites of *Babesia shortti*, which cause severe hemolytic anemia in falcons,[8,9] may be mistaken for cytoplasmic vacuoles or artifacts (Figure 13-71). Detailed analysis of blood parasites for species identification should be left to specialized laboratories. For transport, fresh blood films are best fixed in absolute, acetone-free absolute methanol for 10 minutes and stored in a dust-free, dry environment.

In the majority of cases, hematozoa are consistent with an incidental finding, since parasite and host are well adapted to each other. This is especially true for strongly host-specific genera such as *Hemoproteus* and *Leucozytozoon*. Clinical manifestation, however, may develop in otherwise debilitated or chronically stressed patients and juvenile birds, with concurrent infections with several hemoparasites, or in case of a host switch to a new naïve species. Such a switch has been proposed for *Hemoproteus* spp. adapted to European songbirds, which caused fatal outbreaks of malaria in captive collections of psittacines.[10] Malaria is more frequently seen in infections with *Plasmodium* spp. because they have a broad host spectrum and therefore tend to switch more easily. The grade of hemoproteus parasitemia has been used as an index for the grade of recovery in wild birds. Gametocyte numbers are typically present in higher concentrations in diseased patients compared with healthy animals, and the numbers decrease when the bird recovers.[1] *Atoxoplasma* spp. cause systemic coccidiosis predominantly in juvenile passerines. The common name "black spot disease" refers to the transdermally visible enlarged liver protruding well beyond the sternum into the abdominal cavity. Intrahepatic hemorrhages and necrosis cause the typical reddish black coloration. The parasites are most frequently found in imprints from the liver, spleen, lung, and heart. In Romanowsky-type stained samples they present as pink staining, round, intracellular structures in monocytes and macrophages (Figure 13-72). The nucleus of the host cell is displaced to the side and deformed to a crescent shape. Buffy coat preparations as mentioned above may help to identify low-grade infections in mononuclear cells of live birds (Figure 13-73).

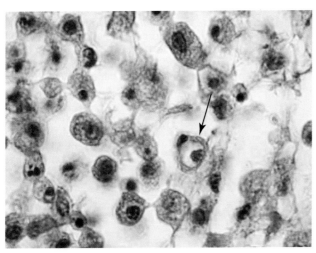

FIGURE 13-72 *Atoxoplasma* sp. in a macrophage of an inflamed pericardium in a Sunda laughing thrush *(Garrulax palliatus)*; the parasite appears as light pink round structure displacing the host nucleus laterally; histologic section. Hematoxylin and eosin stain, original magnification ×400.

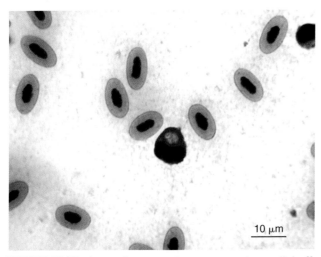

FIGURE 13-73 *Atoxoplasma* sp. in a mononuclear cell, buffy coat preparation, Bulbul. Giemsa stain, original magnification ×1000. (Photo courtesy Dr. Heather Walden, University of Florida.)

REFERENCES

1. Campbell TW, Ellis CK: Avian and exotic animal hematology and cytology, ed 3, Ames, IA, 2007, Blackwell Publishing Professional.
2. Latimer KS, Rakich PM: Avian cytology, *Vet Clin North Am Exot Anim Pract* 10:131–154, 2007.
3. Valenciano AC, Cowell AC: Cowell and Tyler's diagnostic cytology and hematology of the dog and cat, ed 4, St. Louis, MO, 2013, Mosby.
4. Goto N, Kodama H, Okada K, et al: Suppression of phytohemagglutinin skin response in thymectomised chickens, *Poult Sci* 57:246–250, 1978.
5. Mischke R: Zytologisches Praktikum für die Veterinärmedizin (Cytological practical training for veterinary medicine), Hannover, Germany, 2005, Schlütersche Verlagsgesellschaft.
6. Michael HT, Willette M, Sharkey L: What is your diagnosis? Choanal swab from a young Gyrfalcon, *Vet Clin Pathol* 39:571–572, 2010.
7. Ritchie BW, Harrison GJ, Harrison LR: *Avian medicine: principles and Application*, Lake Worth, FL, 1994, Wingers Publishing.
8. Muñoz E, Molina R, Ferrer D: *Babesia shortti* infection in a common kestrel (*Falco tinnunculus*) in Catalonia (northeastern Spain), *Avian Pathol* 28(2):207–209, 1999.
9. Samour JH, Peirce MA: *Babesia shortti* infection in a saker falcon (*Falco cherrug*), *Vet Rec* 139(7):167–168, 1996.
10. Olias P, Wegelin M, Zenker W, et al: Avian malaria deaths in parrots, Europe, *Emerg Infect Dis* 17(5):950–952, 2011.
11. Arends JJ, McDougald LR, Norton RA, et al: Section IV: Parasitic diseases. In Saif YM, Barnes HJ, Glisson JR, et al, editors: *Diseases of poultry*, ed 11, Ames, IA, 2003, Iowa State Press/Blackwell Publishing Company.

MOLECULAR DIAGNOSTIC TESTING

James F.X. Wellehan Jr.

Molecular diagnostic testing has resulted in a revolution both in our knowledge of the diversity of avian pathogens as well as in our ability to diagnose them. It has brought a more nuanced understanding of the complex interactions among host, pathogen, co-infections, and environment in causing disease. However, these techniques may not be understood by the practitioner and can lead to misinterpretation of results and bad clinical decisions. It is important for clinicians to understand the basics of molecular diagnostic testing, potential problems, common errors, and the clinical implications of results obtained. First, it is important to understand the differences between nucleic acid–based testing and other methods of testing.

IMMUNOLOGICALLY BASED TESTING

Immunologic testing involves looking for a host immune response to a pathogen. There are two branches of the acquired immune system: cellular immunity and humoral immunity. A humoral immune response produces antibodies that specifically recognize extracellular pathogens, whereas a cellular immune response centers around T-cell receptor recognition of a specific intracellular pathogen presented by a major histocompatibility complex, which is present on all host cells (see Chapter 11). A cellular immune response is typically most protective for intracellular pathogens such as viruses. Cellular and humoral immune responses are often found together, but not always. An animal may have a cellular immune response without a significant humoral immune response, and vice versa. Virtually all immunologic testing available for birds looks for a humoral immune response. Antibodies may be present long after an infection is cleared, and the presence of an antibody titer does not mean that an infectious agent is currently present.

Especially in avian species in which pathogen diversity has not been well studied, there is concern of nonspecific cross-reactivity of antibodies against as-yet unstudied but antigenically related species. Although antibody cross-reactivity does correlate with genetic distance,[1] small genetic distances may be highly clinically significant. For example, in the family Herpesviridae, genus *Mardivirus*, the species *Gallid herpesvirus 2* (GaHV2) causes Marek disease in chickens. Turkeys carry the closely related *Meleagrid herpesvirus 1* (MeHV1), which is not known to cause disease. However, the two viruses are closely enough related that the immune response to MeHV1 in chickens is cross-protective against GaHV2, and MeHV1 is commonly used as a Marek disease vaccine. This illustrates a corollary diagnostic conundrum; an immune response to one pathogen will detect closely related pathogens. Although two known pathogens can be tested to determine where they differ antigenically, outside of commercial poultry, little of avian pathogen diversity is currently known, and so an assay for a known pathogen may or may not detect a related agent of vastly different clinical significance, thus confusing interpretation.

CULTURE

Culture of a pathogen from a diseased bird has traditionally been utilized for direct identification of infectious agents. Appropriate sample selection for culture is more difficult than selection of immunodiagnostic samples; the sample must contain viable organism, and a negative result does not mean the agent is not present elsewhere in the bird. Although culture is still important, for some highly significant avian pathogens such as *Chlamydia psittaci* or *Mycobacterium genavense*, standard culture conditions will not support growth. Successful culture conditions have yet to be determined for the vast majority of microbes. Typically, around 10% of bacterial species can be cultured in a given ecologic niche,[2] and success at culturing viruses or protozoa is even lower. Even if an agent has been cultured, it is still necessary to identify it. Biochemical methods for bacterial identification have been the standard for the past century. These methods have been best developed for two phyla of bacteria: Proteobacteria, the "typical" gram-negatives, and Firmicutes, the "typical" gram-positives. However, as examples, the two previously mentioned clinically significant bacteria in birds, *Mycobacterium* spp. (phylum Actinobacterium) and *Chlamydia* (phylum Chlamydiae), fall outside of these phyla. Even within the better studied phyla, there is a bias toward human pathogens; *Bordetella avium*, in the phylum Proteobacteria, is a common etiologic agent of upper respiratory tract disease and sinusitis in birds. Uncommon as a human pathogen, it is often misidentified by standard biochemical identification as *Alcaligenes faecalis*.[3] Molecular methods involving nucleic acid sequencing are superior at identification.[4] The contrast is even more stark in molecular versus classic fungal identification, where

identification has been morphologic, missing significant cryptic diversity. Sequence-based identification methods should be used to identify any agent when there is reason to question identification by conventional means.

MOLECULAR DIAGNOSTICS

The most commonly used molecular methods are based on polymerase chain reaction (PCR). Other techniques such as rolling circle amplification and next generation sequencing have primarily been utilized for virus discovery rather than routine clinical use, but as next generation sequencing becomes less expensive and methods of interpretation are improved, it may enter clinical use. These methods directly test for the presence of nucleic acid from an infectious agent (pathogen). Like pathogen isolation techniques, this requires that the clinician submit an appropriate sample that contains the actual pathogen. A negative test result does not mean that the pathogen is not present elsewhere in the patient. Unlike pathogen isolation, with PCR, the suspected agent does not need to be viable, but the nucleic acid needs to be intact. Formalin degrades nucleic acids significantly.[5] The first step in sample processing is nucleic acid extraction. If an RNA template (typically an RNA virus) is the target, the RNA will typically have to be transcribed into DNA, a process known as reverse transcription.

Polymerase Chain Reaction

PCR directly tests for the presence of a specific nucleic acid, in this context from an infectious agent (pathogen). DNA is composed of two complementary strands oriented in opposite directions (Figure 13-74, *A*). Primers (short, single-stranded segments of DNA) are designed to match the sequence of the two strands of pathogen DNA in a manner such that they face one another. The DNA is heated so that the two strands separate (see Figure 13-74, *B*). The temperature is then decreased to an appropriate temperature for the primers to anneal (bind) with the DNA (see Figure 13-74, *C*). If the primers do not

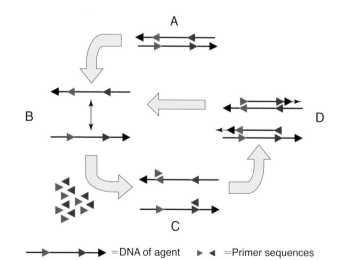

FIGURE 13-74 Polymerase chain reaction. **A,** Double-stranded template DNA. **B,** Heating to separate DNA strands. **C,** Binding of complementary primers. **D,** New strand synthesis starting from primers by DNA polymerase.

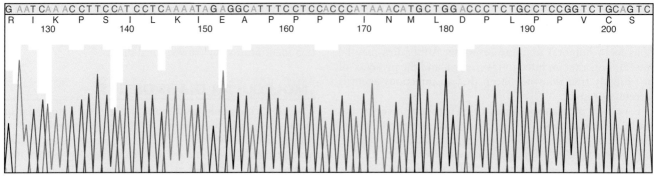

G AAT CAA AC CT TC CAT C CT C AAA ATA G AGG CAT T TC CT C CAC C CAT AA ACA TG C TGG ACC C TC TGC C TC CGG TC T GC AG TC
R I K P S I L K I E A P P P I N M L D P L P P V C S
   130   140   150   160   170   180   190   200

FIGURE 13-75 Sequence chromatogram of an adenoviral polymerase chain reaction product from a brown pelican showing novel aviadenovirus sequence. Note the clean traces, as compared to the mixed peaks seen in Figure 13-78.

match with the DNA sequence, they will not anneal, and no product will be formed. The temperature is then increased to an appropriate temperature for thermostable DNA polymerase to extend the primer, making a matching strand for the DNA (see Figure 13-74, D). The amount of DNA between the primers present is thus doubled. The cycle starts over again as the DNA is reheated to separate the strands. The cycle is repeated many times, and the amount of DNA increases geometrically.

The PCR product must then be validated—that is, it must be determined to be the appropriate product and not an accidental binding of the primers to an unexpected site on a different DNA template. This is absolutely crucial for clinical use. Formerly, older validation methods may have been limited to measurement of the size of the product by gel electrophoresis or restriction fragment length polymorphism (RFLP). These methods are significantly less accurate than modern methods such as sequencing or probe hybridization, will result in a high false-positive rate, and should no longer be considered acceptable.

The most definitive way to determine the identity of the PCR product is to sequence it (Figure 13-75). To validate a product by sequencing, the PCR reaction must be confirmed as a single product by gel electrophoresis; appropriate bands must be cut out and purified from the gel; sequencing reactions must be run, electrophoresed, and edited; and then the sequence data must be analyzed. Although this was once relatively expensive, rapid improvements in sequencing technology have taken place, and costs are now minimal. This provides not only the possibility of identifying known organisms but also characterization of novel organisms by comparison with reference sequences and subsequent phylogenetic analysis. Although capable of identifying novel organisms, it is slower and more labor intensive than probe hybridization quantitative PCR (qPCR).

Probe Hybridization Quantitative PCR

Probe hybridization quantitative PCR (qPCR), also known as real-time PCR, is a PCR variant. Similar to standard PCR, primers (short, single-stranded segments of DNA) are designed to match the sequence of the two strands of pathogen DNA in such a manner that they face one another. The difference is the addition of a dye-labeled probe that matches and binds to sequence between the two primers. Two dyes—a reporter dye, to be detected by a spectrophotometer during

the reaction, and a quencher dye, which absorbs the spectrum emitted by the reporter dye—are bound to the probe (Figure 13-76, A). As before, the DNA is heated so that the two strands separate (see Figure 13-76, B). The temperature is then decreased to an appropriate temperature for the primers and probe to anneal (bind) with the DNA (see Figure 13-76, C). If the primers do not match with the DNA sequence, they will not anneal, and no product will be formed. The temperature is then increased to an appropriate temperature for thermostable DNA polymerase to extend the primer, making a matching strand for the DNA (see Figure 13-76, D). DNA polymerase, in addition to extending the primer to match the template DNA, also has exonuclease activity, which means that it will chew up any DNA in front of it that gets in the way as it is extending the primer. If the probe is bound to the template in front of the primer, the polymerase will chew through the probe, releasing the labeled dye. This separates the reporter dye from the quencher dye, and the released reporter dye can be measured with a spectrophotometer. This has two distinct advantages. First, the validation of the PCR product is rapid. Validation in probe hybridization qPCR is

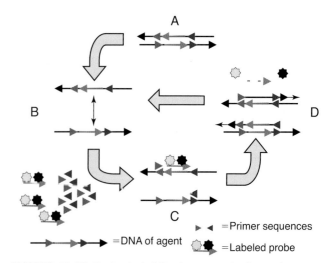

A

B

D

C

▶ ▸ = Primer sequences

⟶ ▸▸ = DNA of agent

⬡ ✶ = Labeled probe

FIGURE 13-76 Probe hybridization quantitative polymerase chain reaction. A, Double-stranded template DNA. B, Heating to separate DNA strands. C, Binding of complementary primers and dye-labeled probe. D, New strand synthesis starting from primers by DNA polymerase, which digests probe bound in front of it, freeing dyes.

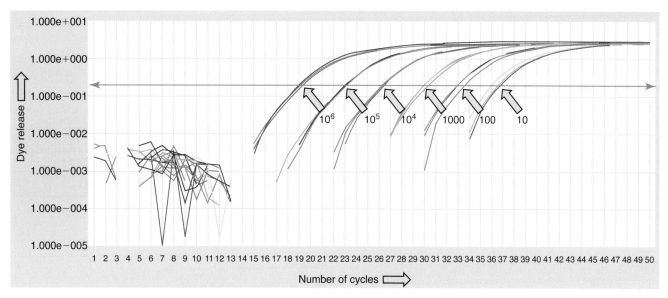

FIGURE 13-77 Measurement of dye release in probe hybridization quantitative polymerase chain reaction enables quantitation of the amount of starting template. Larger amounts take fewer cycles to reach a threshold level of dye release.

done during the reaction, data output is simple, and no further steps are necessary. Second, the release of dye depends on the amount of template present, providing quantitative information. In Figure 13-77, a qPCR standard curve is shown. The horizontal axis is the number of cycles, and the vertical axis is fluorescence. The arrows drawn on the figure indicate the number of template copies present in the initial reaction. When there are only 10 copies initially present, it takes approximately 37 cycles for the reaction to release enough dye to cross the threshold (green) line. When there are 1,000,000 copies initially present, the threshold is crossed after approximately 19 cycles. This provides a standard to compare samples with and also provides a control to ensure that reactions are working well and efficiently. Quantitative information can be clinically useful to determine whether loads are sufficient to consider as a disease etiology and to follow trends over time to assess response to therapy. A well-designed qPCR is a highly useful tool for specific identification of a known agent. When well designed and properly validated to ensure the assay specifically identifies only the target DNA, probe hybridization qPCR can be a sensitive, specific, rapid, quantitative, and relatively inexpensive test. Proper validation is critical, and laboratories should provide a peer-reviewed publication on validation of a given probe hybridization qPCR assay for diagnostic use to clinicians for evaluation. There are established guidelines for validation of a qPCR assay.[6]

It is important to realize that there are other assays, commonly called "real-time PCR," that do not involve validation by probe hybridization. The most common of these utilizes the SYBR green dye, which is incorporated into DNA as it is synthesized. This methodology does not provide any data on the size or sequence of the PCR amplicon, making it even more prone to false positives than gel electrophoresis. Especially when dealing with diverse host species, as is commonly done in avian medicine, this methodology should not be utilized.

Consensus PCR Techniques

Validation of primers is critical, and laboratories should provide a peer-reviewed publication on validation of a given primer set for diagnostic use to clinicians for evaluation. Before primers can be designed, the nucleic acid sequence must be known. Some nucleic acid sequences are specific to a given species or even strain. Other nucleic acid sequences have stayed the same through evolution and are found across groups of related organisms. These are known as "consensus sequences." Genes that are conserved throughout evolution are typically essential for the function of the organism, such as ribosomal RNAs (rRNA) or viral polymerases. Primers may be designed to be very specific for a given organism or may be designed to regions conserved across a wider taxonomic group. When dealing with a consensus PCR technique, it is critical to always validate the identity of the PCR product by sequencing. This is illustrated by the earlier MeHV1/GaHV2 example, with very different clinical significance of two closely related herpesviruses in two different species. Pan-herpesviral consensus PCR protocols are available,[7] but without sequence data, they will not distinguish these two viruses and are clinically uninterpretable. This same technique can be used to discover novel agents in a given group, an important advantage, given the lack of knowledge of avian pathogen diversity.[8] Diverse published assays are available for a wide variety of taxonomic levels, ranging from the entire domain of Prokaryotes,[9] the class Coccidia,[10] the family Adenoviridae,[11] the genus *Orthoreovirus*,[12], to even more specific. The ability to detect a broader group of agents can reduce the number of tests needed; however, caution is needed. When more than one member of a clade is present in a sample, direct sequencing of a PCR product will result in mixed sequence that is unreadable (Figure 13-78). Protocols such as pan-bacterial or pan-fungal PCR are highly useful for identification of isolated bacteria or fungi, respectively, when identification by conventional methods is questionable.

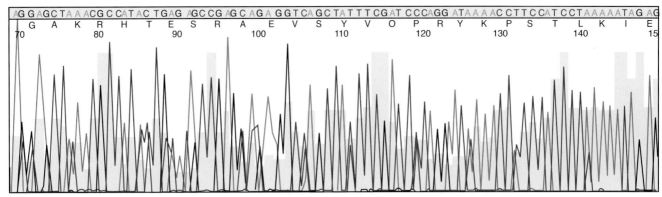

FIGURE 13-78 Sequence chromatogram of an adenoviral polymerase chain reaction product from a brown pelican showing mixed adenoviruses. Note the presence of several mixed peaks, as compared to the clean traces seen in Figure 13-75.

However, application of these methods directly to clinical samples that are likely to have diverse bacterial or fungal flora present, such as oral samples or fecal samples, is unlikely to result in a product that can be directly sequenced and interpreted. More narrowly targeted assays should therefore be used on such samples (e.g., genus *Mycobacterium*-specific PCR, if that is an important differential) to detect more specific agents of possible concern. It is important to know what a given set of primers are expected to amplify; for example, many labs offer tests labeled as "avian polyomavirus," which actually utilize primers that specifically amplify the species *Budgerigar fledgling disease polyomavirus*, rather than the genus *Avipolyomavirus* or the family Polyomaviridae. There is significant diversity present in the polyomaviruses of birds, and the details of primer selection and amplification are important in order to optimize the clinical merits of their use in practice.

Rolling Circle Amplification

Rolling circle amplification (RCA) is a technique for amplification of small circular DNA genomes, as are found in several families of viruses, including papillomaviruses, polyomaviruses, anelloviruses, hepadnaviruses, and circoviruses. It does not require knowledge of any sequence from the agent. The technique involves a polymerase that moves around the circle as it synthesizes a complementary strand. When the beginning of the circle is reached, the polymerase continues around again, and the new strand is a long series of repeated copies of the circle. This strand is then cut with a restriction enzyme, which recognizes specific short four to six base-pair sequences. Since these sequences will be in the same place every time the circle is repeated, the restriction enzymes cut the circle into a set of pieces of specific size. These pieces can then be cloned and used as sequencing template. Because it does not require any known sequence, RCA has proven useful for obtaining sequence template of divergent agents and has found significant use in avian virology.[13] However, this technique requires a significant amount of cloning and sequencing and is therefore labor intensive and costly.

High-Throughput Sequencing

Recent years have seen amazing advances in sequencing technology. Costs have been reduced by several orders of magnitude. New techniques, including pyrosequencing, Illumina sequencing, and SOLiD sequencing are capable of producing millions of sequences in a single run. This has enabled the development of metagenomics, in which nucleic acid representing an entire sample is sequenced, rather than targeted amplification of a specific region. This enables an understanding of the diversity of complex and diverse environments such as the avian gastrointestinal tract.[14] The ability to obtain such datasets is a bioinformatic challenge; although it provides the ability to obtain sequence from previously unknown and divergent pathogens, it requires the ability to recognize and sift these sequences out of literally millions of nontarget sequences. It has resulted in significant advances in avian infectious disease. Diverse avian bornaviruses were first identified using metagenomic techniques.[15,16] The costs for metagenomic methods are still considerable, but they are decreasing rapidly, and what was a $100,000 project a few years ago is a $1000 project now. It is only a matter of time before these techniques become clinically affordable.

Sample Collection for Nucleic Acid–Based Diagnostics

The first thing the practitioner needs to do is talk with the diagnostic laboratory. It is important first to understand what methodologies are offered, and peer-reviewed references describing testing methodologies should be provided to the clinician. Common problems and pitfalls should be discussed in advance, as well as limitations of diagnostic testing.

Histologic evaluation of a necropsy is often one indication that an agent requiring molecular testing is present. It is important to collect a complete set of tissues in formalin for histologic evaluation as well as another set without formalin to be kept frozen for further diagnostics as indicated by histology. Tissues should be routinely kept at least until histologic results are back.

Sample choice is critical for nucleic acid–based diagnostics; the agent must be in the sample. This requires an understanding of the common distribution of the agent in the animal. Although plasma has historically been a common sample collected for infectious disease diagnostics because of the use of serodiagnostics, relatively few infectious agents are themselves commonly found in plasma, making it a suboptimal sample choice for testing for most avian pathogens. A laboratory with significant clinical experience with a given avian pathogen may be able to most accurately advise on sample choice.

PCR is a highly sensitive technique, and the potential for false positives from slight contamination anywhere from collection to laboratory is high. As such, it is crucial that measures be taken to avoid contamination during sample collection and transport and that appropriate controls are run.

Transport needs to be discussed in advance with the laboratory. Agents such as enveloped RNA viruses tend to be significantly less environmentally stable. Media such as RNAlater can be used to preserve the viability of nucleic acids. Shipping on ice or even dry ice is often preferable. When same-day transport is not available, overnight shipping is indicated. The laboratory should be notified in advance so that potential problems can be identified and brought up with the shipping service on the same day if a delivery does not arrive.

These are exciting times in avian medicine. Molecular techniques are enabling us to begin to understand the diversity of pathogens in birds and detect them in a clinically applicable fashion. An understanding of molecular diagnostic options and proper clinical interpretation of testing is essential in modern avian practice.

REFERENCES

1. Nollens HH, Ruiz C, Walsh MT, et al: Cross-reactivity of immunoglobulin G of whales and dolphins correlates with evolutionary distance of cytochrome B genes, *Clin Vaccine Immunol* 15:1547–1554, 2008.
2. Safaee S, Weiser GC, Cassirer EF, et al: Microbial diversity in bighorn sheep revealed by culture-independent methods, *J Wildl Dis* 42:545–555, 2006.
3. Savelkoul PH, de Groot LE, Boersma C, et al: Identification of Bordetella avium using the polymerase chain reaction, *Microb Pathol* 15:207–215, 1993.
4. Petti CA, Polage CR, Schreckenberger P: The role of 16S rRNA gene sequencing in identification of microorganisms misidentified by conventional methods, *J Clin Microbiol* 43:6123–6125, 2005.
5. Tokuda Y, Nakanure T, Satonaka K, et al: Fundamental study on the mechanisms of DNA degradation in tissues fixed in formaldehyde, *J Clin Pathol* 43:748–751, 1990.
6. Bustin SA, Benes V, Garson JA, et al: The MIQE guidelines: minimum information for publication of quantitative real-time PCR experiments, *Clin Chem* 55:611–622, 2009.
7. VanDevanter DR, Warrener P, Bennett L, et al: Detection and analysis of diverse herpesviral species by consensus primer PCR, *J Clin Microbiol* 34:1666–1671, 1996.
8. Quesada RJ, Heard DJ, Aitken-Palmer C, et al: Detection and phylogenetic characterization of a novel herpesvirus from the trachea of two stranded common loons, *J Wildl Dis* 47:233–239, 2011.
9. Schuurman T, de Boer RF, Kooistra-Smid AM, et al: Prospective study of use of PCR amplification and sequencing of 16S ribosomal DNA from cerebrospinal fluid for diagnosis of bacterial meningitis in a clinical setting, *J Clin Microbiol* 42:734–740, 2004.
10. Garner MM, Gardiner CH, Wellehan JFX, et al: Intranuclear coccidiosis in tortoises, nine cases, *Vet Pathol* 43(3):311–320, 2006.
11. Wellehan JF, Johnson AJ, Harrach B, et al: Detection and analysis of six lizard adenoviruses by consensus primer PCR provides further evidence of a reptilian origin for the adenoviruses, *J Virol* 78(23):13366–13369, 2004.
12. Wellehan JF Jr, Childress AL, Marschang RE, et al: Consensus nested PCR amplification and sequencing of diverse reptilian, avian, and mammalian orthoreoviruses, *Vet Microbiol* 133(1–2):34–42, 2009.
13. Johne R, Wittig W, Fernández-de-Luco D, et al: Characterization of two novel polyomaviruses of birds by using multiply primed rolling-circle amplification of their genomes, *J Virol* 80:3523–3531, 2006.
14. Koskey AM, Fisher JC, Traudt MF, et al: Analysis of the gull fecal microbial community reveals the dominance of Catellicoccus marimammalium in relation to culturable enterococci, *Appl Environ Microbiol* 80:757–765, 2014.
15. Honkavuori KS, Shivaprasad HL, Williams BL, et al: Novel borna virus in psittacine birds with proventricular dilatation disease, *Emerg Infect Dis* 14(12):1883–1886, 2008.
16. Kistler AL, Gancz A, Clubb S, et al: Recovery of divergent avian bornaviruses from cases of proventricular dilatation disease: identification of a candidate etiologic agent, *Virol J* 5:88, 2008.

DIAGNOSTIC TESTING OF AGE OF BIRDS AND ITS APPLICATIONS

Kristin Warren, Anna Le Souef, Crissa Cooey, Hillar Klandorf

AGING BIRDS AND THE SCIENCE BEHIND PENTOSIDINE ANALYSIS

The ability to age birds is of importance, as age can play a critical role in survival rates, reproductive success, and disease susceptibility and is of relevance at an individual level for captive birds and population level for wild birds. However, until recently, given the lack of external signs of senescence in most birds, a practical method for the accurate estimation of age in birds past sexual maturity has proven elusive for most avian species. Traditionally, studies of wild bird populations have involved banding and other methods of permanent identification, which are restrictively time consuming, with generally limited numbers of band retrieval or sightings.

Research has recently shown that pentosidine, a biomarker that is associated with nonenzymatic glycation and found in skin collagen,[1] correlates with chronologic age in mammals[2] and birds.[3-7] Pentosidine can be extracted from skin samples of birds of known age,[7] and the concentration of this biomarker can be measured to establish age curves, which can then be used to estimate the age of conspecifics or closely related species for which the life histories are not known.

METHODOLOGY OF SAMPLE COLLECTION

The technique has been proven for use in several bird species, including psittacids.[8] Skin biopsy sampling methods for this technique are also attractively straightforward; since the method is minimally invasive and can be performed simply on birds under anesthesia or on conscious, easily handled birds with local anesthesia.[8]

The biopsy skin sample should be collected from the medial patagium in an area where there are as few blood vessels and tendons as possible (Figure 13-79).

The skin should be disinfected with a 70% alcohol solution. Depending on the species, there is usually little need to pluck feathers, as there are minimal feathers in this area and the disinfectant solution wets the feathers, thus exposing the skin. A subcutaneous injection of lidocaine (diluted 50:50 with saline) should be administered to anesthetize the local area at the sampling site (Figure 13-80). This should still be done, even in cases where birds are anesthetized, since the injected liquid bolus has the effect of lifting the skin away

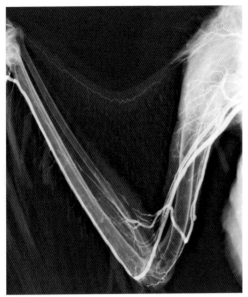

FIGURE 13-79 Golden eagle *(Aquila chrysaetos)* arteriovenogram injected with BriteVu. (Courtesy Dr. Scott Echols, Scarlet Imaging, LLC, Salt Lake City, Utah, USA.)

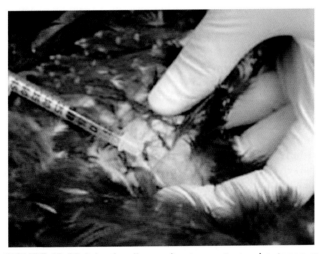

FIGURE 13-80 Injecting lignocaine to create a subcutaneous bleb.

from the underlying layers, facilitating biopsy collection. The skin should be stretched such that it is taut, and a 6-mm diameter disposable biopsy punch should be used to take the skin sample (Figure 13-81). If the bird is smaller than 200 g, then a smaller 4-mm biopsy punch may be used, but a 6-mm sample is recommended to be collected, if possible, for easier handling and processing. Likewise, if the bird is large enough, an 8-mm or 10-mm punch may be used. The punch biopsy is gently rotated in a clockwise and counter-clockwise direction so that it only penetrates one layer of skin. Care should be taken when rotating the biopsy punch to ensure that only one dermal layer is penetrated, since application of excessive force can result in deeper tissue or full-thickness damage to the wing. The biopsy can be grasped with forceps or a clamp and lifted from the subdermal layers. Small sharp scissors are then

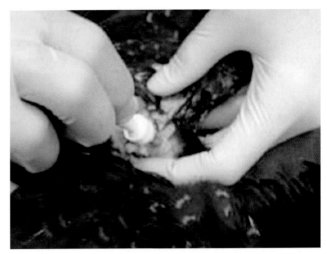

FIGURE 13-81 Collection of skin biopsy sample.

used to carefully remove the skin biopsy. A 4- or 6-mm diameter biopsy punch provides a sufficient tissue sample and has been used on live birds ranging in size from bridled terns (110 to 180 g) to black cockatoos (520 to 790 g) and whooping cranes (6.0 to 7.8 kg) (unpublished data).

A gauze swab should be used to apply gentle pressure and prevent or stop any bleeding at the biopsy site. The biopsy site can then be closed by using tissue glue (quickly pressing the wound shut with sterile forceps, immediately after apply the glue, to ensure closure) or a single interrupted suture (Figure 13-82 and 13-83).

The skin sample should be placed in a small screw-lid container with distilled water. The sample stored should then be frozen at −20° C until analyses. Previous studies have shown that samples can be stored frozen for many months, without affecting the results of analyses (unpublished data). Samples have also been successfully collected from museum specimens stored in alcohol and as dried skins by the authors and in a previous study.[5]

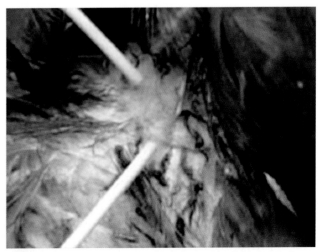

FIGURE 13-82 Closing the biopsy site with Vetbond tissue adhesive.

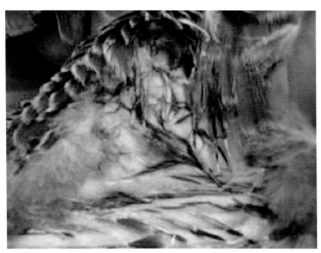

FIGURE 13-83 The glued incision site being held open to enable the glue to dry.

METHODOLOGY OF PENTOSIDINE ANALYSIS

Skin samples are prepared for pentosidine analysis by using the technique described by Cooey et al (2010) (adapted from the procedure discussed in Iqbal et al, 1997).[11] This involves removal of feathers, feather shafts, dead skin cells and other debris, and the fat and epidermal layer, mincing, delipidation (by adding 5 mL of a 2:1 chloroform–methanol solution and agitating at 4° C for 18 hours) and rehydration (by adding 2 to 3 mL of a 1:1 methanol–distilled water solution and standing for 2 hours at 20° C). Acid hydrolysis is then performed, by adding 1 mL nitrogen flushed 6N hydrochloric acid per 10 mg of tissue and incubating for 18 hours at 110° C, followed by acid evaporation in a Speed-Vac centrifuge dryer (Savant Instruments, Farmingdale, New York, NY). A second rehydration is then required, by adding 500 μL of filtered distilled water and vortexing until all solid particles have dissolved. The sample is then filtered using a Costar Spin-X centrifuge tube filter (Corning Costar, Cambridge, MA) and, finally, centrifuged in an Eppendorf 5415 microcentrifuge (Eppendorf, Hauppauge, New York, NY) at 10,000 rpm for 10 minutes.

The collagen content of the sample is determined through spectrophotometric hydroxyproline analysis, at a 564-nm wavelength, with a DU 640 spectrophotometer (Beckman Coulter, Fullerton, CA). In determining the collagen content, it is generally assumed that 14% of collagen by weight is hydroxyproline.[12]

Pentosidine concentration is measured from a 200-μL sample by using reverse-phase high-performance liquid chromatography. Duplicate samples are spiked with a pentosidine standard (150-μL sample to 50-μL pentosidine standard) to determine elution time. The final pentosidine concentration of a sample is determined by comparing the pentosidine peak of the 200-μL sample to the pentosidine peak of the spiked sample. Once the pentosidine peak is properly identified on the original sample's chromatograph, then the pentosidine value is identified from the peak integration data. The software package Empower 2 (Waters Corporation, Milford, MA) is used for integration of the peaks.

Analyzed samples from birds of unknown age can be determined through the prior establishment of a species or genus-specific curve by using samples collected from birds of known age or through the use of a general wild bird curve established by Chaney et al (2003).

AGING ENDANGERED BLACK COCKATOOS BY USING PENTOSIDINE ANALYSIS: A CASE STUDY

The three species of black cockatoo (*Calyptorhynchus* spp.) endemic to Western Australia are threatened with extinction, primarily because of habitat loss and fragmentation, as well as poaching, shooting, and competition with other species.[13-16] Conservation efforts to save these threatened black cockatoos are hampered by a lack of ecologic and age demographic data. Conservationists concerned about population declines hypothesized that suboptimal rates of juvenile recruitment among black cockatoo populations may have occurred because of the loss of large areas of breeding habitat following clearing of inland regions in the last century[15]; this could lead to senescent flocks of wild black cockatoos, consisting primarily of postreproductive-age birds, resulting in a rapid reduction in numbers after these older birds die. Additionally, the capacity to estimate age of sick and injured black cockatoos could also provide valuable information on the life histories of cockatoos in rehabilitation programs and would be helpful when determining suitable candidates for captive breeding.

Prior to the current demographic research study on black cockatoos undertaken by the authors of this chapter, data on maximum and reproductive ages of wild black cockatoos resulted from re-sightings of stainless steel patagial tags or leg bands.[17,18] Pentosidine analysis is currently being used to develop a genus-specific age curve for black cockatoo (*Calyptorhynchus*) species, which involves plotting age against pentosidine levels for individual birds of known age and fitting a trend line to determine the relationships among the variables, which can then be used in reverse to estimate the age of a bird of unknown age using its pentosidine level. This age curve is being developed using samples collected from 53 black cockatoos of known age ranging from 6 weeks to 33 years, which is 1 year less than the oldest reported age for a wild black cockatoo[18] and will provide the most comprehensive avian age estimation curve using pentosidine analysis. The opportunity to sample such a large number of endangered birds is rare and was possible because of the popularity of black cockatoos as part of captive collections, as well as the existence of established rehabilitation programs in Western Australia. The findings from this study provide a tool for age estimation in black cockatoos, which will have useful applications for recovery efforts of these endangered birds.

The research findings from the ongoing black cockatoo demographic research will enable the estimation of age of black cockatoos entering rehabilitation programs, providing valuable data on the life histories of injured and debilitated wild birds. Age estimation in black cockatoos using pentosidine analysis may lead to a better understanding of the reproductive history of these endangered birds and can also be applied to captive breeding programs, since pairing birds of a similar age can increase breeding success.[19] Further, the technique may be applied to determine the ages of black cockatoos that are found during mass mortality events such as the heat stress event in 2010,[20] which may provide data on the age demographics of local wild populations. Data collected on the age of wild birds can provide insights into age structure demographics of wild populations, which can inform the development of population viability models and species recovery efforts for black cockatoos. It can also be used to apply estimated ages to population demographics, such as clutch size, hatching rate, fledging rate, predation events, and overall reproductive success, and to compare age demographics between managed and unmanaged environments to determine the effect on age structure of local management efforts.

BROADER APPLICATIONS OF PENTOSIDINE ANALYSIS FOR AVIAN AGING

Pentosidine analysis has great potential for use in aging birds involved in captive breeding and reintroduction programs, associated with recovery efforts to save threatened avian species, as exemplified by the black cockatoo research discussed above. There is also the potential for pentosidine analysis to be used to enable aging of pet birds of commonly kept species, which would be of great assistance to the medical management and care of avian patients, and for aging museum specimens.

One of the difficulties in using the pentosidine aging technique is finding a large enough sample of known-aged birds from different ages of the study species.[7,21] However, for species that are commonly kept in captivity as pets or bred in captivity for endangered species recovery programs, obtaining sufficient individuals to establish a species or genus-specific age curve may be possible. In cases where it is difficult to obtain samples from known age individuals, samples may be collected from closely related species or can be assessed by using the more general wild bird curve.

Although pentosidine analysis is currently not commercially available, the technique is currently being applied by research groups at Murdoch University and West Virginia University and has also been applied by the United States Department of Agriculture (USDA), Animal and Plant Health Inspection Service (APHIS), Wildlife Services (WS), and National Wildlife Research Center (NWRC). However, the laboratory methodology outlined above uses relatively standard laboratory equipment that should be available in laboratories in major cities in most parts of the world. Therefore, it should be possible for interested clinicians and researchers to discuss the possibility of local laboratories, particularly those that are zoo or research based, developing capability to undertake pentosidine analyses to enable establishment of age curves and aging analyses of the specific bird species of interest.

REFERENCES

1. Suji G, Sivakami S: Glucose, glycation and aging, *Biogerontology* 5(6):365–373, 2004.
2. Sell DR, Lane MA, Johnson WA, et al: Longevity and the genetic determination of collagen glycoxidation kinetics in mammalian senescence, *Proc Natl Acad Sci* 93(1):485–490, 1996.
3. Iqbal M, Probert LL, Alhumadi NH, et al: Protein glycosylation and advanced glycosylated endproducts (AGEs) accumulation: an avian solution. *J Gerontol Series A Biol Sci Med Sci* 54(4):B171–B176, 1999.
4. Chaney R, Blemings K, Bonner J, et al: Pentosidine as a measure of chronological age in wild birds, *Auk* 120(2):394–399, 2003.
5. Fallon J, Cochrane R, Dorr B, et al: Interspecies comparison of pentosidine accumulation and its correlation with age in birds, *Auk* 123(3):870–876, 2006.
6. Cooey CK: *Development and evaluation of a minimally invasive sampling technique to estimate the age of living birds [masters thesis]*, West Virginia University, 2008.
7. Cooey CK, Fallon JA, Avery ML, et al: Refinement of biomarker pentosidine methodology for use on aging birds, *Hum Wildl Interactions* 4(2):304–314, 2010.
8. Klandorf H, Iqbal M, Bonner J: Estimation of age in wild birds, *Br Poult Sci* 41(3):50–51, 2000.
9. Higgins PJ, Davies SJJF, editors: Handbook of Australian, New Zealand and Antarctic birds, vol 3: *Snipe to pigeons*, Melbourne, Australia, 1996, Oxford University Press.
10. Johnstone RE, Storr GM, Taylor DL: Handbook of Western Australian birds, vol 1: *Non-passerines (emu to dollarbird)*, Perth, Australia, 1998, Western Australian Museum.
11. Iqbal M, Probert LL, Klandorf H: Effect of aminoguanidine on tissue pentosidine and reproductive performance in broiler breeders, *Poult Sci* 76:1574–1579, 1997.
12. Maekawa T, Rathinasamy TK, Altman KI, et al: Changes in collagen with age. I. The extraction of acid soluble collagens from the skin of mice, *Exp Gerontol* 5:177–186, 1970.
13. Saunders DA: Problems of survival in an extensively cultivated landscape: the case of Carnaby's cockatoo (*Calyptorhynchus funereus latirostris*), *Biol Conservation* 54(3):277–290, 1990.
14. Mawson P: A captive breeding program for Carnaby's cockatoo (*Calyptorhynchus latirostris*), *Eclectus* 3:21–23, 1997.
15. Mawson P, Johnstone RE: Conservation status of parrots and cockatoos in Western Australia, *Eclectus* 2:4–9, 1997.
16. Saunders DA, Ingram JA: Twenty-eight years of monitoring a breeding population of Carnaby's cockatoo, *Pacific Conservation Biol* 4: 261–270, 1997.
17. Saunders DA: The breeding behaviour and biology of the short-billed form of the white-tailed black cockatoo Calyptorhynchus funereus, *Br Ornithologists' Union* 422–455, 1982.
18. Saunders DA, Dawson R: Update on longevity and movements of Carnaby's black cockatoo, *Pacific Conservation Biol* 15:72–74, 2009.
19. Fulai L, Bin L, Seming S, et al: First captive breeding of the oriental crested ibis (*Nipponia nippon*), *Colonial Waterbirds* 18:23–29, 1995.
20. Saunders DA, Mawson P, Dawson R: The impact of two extreme weather events and other causes of death on Carnaby's Black Cockatoo: a promise of things to come for a threatened species. *Pacific Conservation Biol* 17:141–148, 2011.
21. Fallon J, Klandorf H: A new technique for avian age estimation. In Proceedings of the Association of Avian Veterinarians, Milwaukee, WI, 2009, Milwaukee's Best: 30th Annual Conference and Expo, pp 21–24.

CHAPTER 14

Advances in Diagnostic Imaging

Yvonne R.A. van Zeeland • Nico J. Schoemaker • Edward W. Hsu

Diagnostic imaging has revolutionized the practice of medicine by making noninvasive visualization of the body's anatomy and physiology feasible. Applications of these imaging technologies in avian medicine, although slow in the start, appear to have gained momentum in recent years. Among the various imaging techniques that are currently available, conventional or projection radiography is one of the most popular and commonly used techniques. In recent years, ultrasonography has become recognized as an important tool for diagnosing internal disease in birds. Of the more advanced diagnostic imaging modalities, computed tomography (CT) is a technique increasingly used to achieve more detailed and precise information. CT has already proven its value with many potential applications in the field of avian medicine. Magnetic resonance imaging (MRI) and nuclear imaging (e.g., scintigraphy or positron emission tomography [PET]), on the other hand, are still comparatively new in avian medicine. There is, however, great potential for the use of these techniques in avian medicine, once their resolution increases and the cost of an examination decreases. This chapter explores these advanced imaging modalities to help foster a foundational understanding of what they have to offer and when they may be considered or applied in diagnosing birds.

TOMOGRAPHY

CT and MRI display objects in multiple images or pictures, with every image representing one slice of the object. The word *tomos* is Greek for slice, hence, the word tomography. Each two-dimensional (2D) image is built out of picture elements (pixels). When the thickness of the slice is taken into account, these pixels then have three dimensions and should be referred to as volume elements (voxels).[1]

Computed Tomography

CT is a diagnostic imaging technique that uses x rays to obtain cross-sectional images of the body. Previously, this technique was called computed axial tomography. With modern CT scanners, however, axial, coronal, and sagittal images can be made, which subsequently can be digitally processed with a computer to obtain three-dimensional (3D) views and allow for reconstruction of data into alternate planes.[1] Since the introduction of the first CT scanner in the 1970s, this technique rapidly made its way into human medicine[1] and later into veterinary medicine. In both fields, CT has become a valuable tool for diagnosing disease,

trauma, or organ abnormalities, and is also useful for planning, guiding, and monitoring therapy. In the field of avian medicine and surgery, CT is currently an established technique used in a variety of different bird species, including psittacines, raptors, waterfowl, and pigeons.[2-7]

The main advantage of CT imaging compared with conventional radiography is that there is no interference from superimposition. Thus, despite their lower resolution, the serial transverse images obtained through CT imaging enable better visualization of various tissues and structures, including those that would otherwise have remained undetected with conventional radiographs (Figure 14-1). When comparing the use of CT imaging with MRI, CT imaging is mostly used for imaging bony structures, whereas MRI is superior for imaging soft tissues. CT imaging, however, has a much shorter investigation time; therefore, it is currently preferred over MRI in avian patients.

Technique

The CT scanner consists of a moving table on which the patient is placed and a gantry in which the rotating x-ray tube and a ring of x-ray detectors are placed (Figure 14-2). Alternatively, some CT scanners also have a moving gantry. During each rotation an image is created. With the modern CT scanners more than 200 images per second can be created.[1] Specific software enables reconstruction of these images so that a 3D view of the organs/tissues can be created.

In each image different values of gray are seen representing different anatomic tissues and fluids. Depending on the composition and nature of the tissue, more or less radiation will be attenuated, thereby resulting in brighter or darker colored areas. Quantification of the gray values is possible using a standardized CT attenuation coefficient, referred to as Hounsfield units (HUs). The HUs have been defined such that HU of air and water are −1000 and 0, respectively.[1] Darker (hypoattenuating) areas in the image, representing, for example, air (HU: −1000) and fat (HU: −50 to −100), thus have a negative HU value whereas lighter (hyperattenuating) areas, representing, for example, soft tissues (HU ~ +100) and mineralized structures (HU up to +3000) have a positive HU value.

Since 1989, scanning times first decreased with the introduction of helical (spiral) CT scanners in which the x-ray tube circles around the patient in a continuous movement combined with simultaneous movement of the table. A couple of years later multislice CT scanners were introduced, in which multiple images (slices) are created per rotation of the x-ray tube,

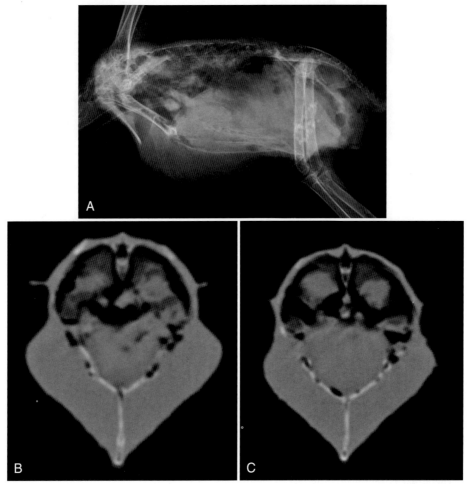

FIGURE 14-1 A lateral radiograph **(A)** taken by the referring practitioner of a 30-year-old Grey parrot *(Psittacus erithacus)*, which presented with labored breathing for less than 3 weeks. The peribroncheal structures are irregularly whitened, but the extent of the lesions could not be assessed. Transverse CT images at two levels of the lungs **(B** and **C)** show severe consolidation of the lungs. Postmortem examination determined it to be a chronic, active pneumonia of undetermined cause. (**B** and **C**, Courtesy the Division of Diagnostic Imaging, Faculty of Veterinary Medicine, Utrecht University, the Netherlands.)

further decreasing scanning times.[1] With a helical CT scanner investigation times as short as 1 or 2 minutes were easily achieved for a bird. This time can be further shortened when the bird is placed transverse to the gantry opening of the CT scanner, allowing the collection of longitudinal rather than sagittal slices.[8] With the current high scanning times, however, longitudinal scanning seems the preferred method for birds because it is also the standard for dogs, cats, rabbits, and humans. This allows the radiologist to view the anatomy in a similar plane, which makes interpretation more consistent.

Procedure

Although the length of the procedure is short, either sedation[8] or general anesthesia[9,10] is required to reduce the stress experienced by the bird during the procedure, achieve appropriate positioning, and prevent movement between scans, resulting in less distortion and artifacts and thus producing better quality images. The choice between conscious sedation and general anesthesia is largely dependent on the goal of the procedure, health status, and stress sensitivity of the patient.[8]

Birds are best placed in ventral recumbency, to allow the bird to breathe more easily during the procedure, and perpendicular to the gantry, to allow scanning in a transverse plane (Figure 14-2). The latter is also the routine mode of placement for dogs and cats, which allows the images to be interpreted by the radiologist in a similar fashion. With modern rendering and reconstruction software it is possible to recreate a symmetric image. However, because the anatomical structures are very small it is best that the patient is positioned as symmetrically and as straight as possible within the scanner to enable the most reliable interpretation of the images. Various materials can be used to aid in positioning, such as towels, foam pads, or intravenous fluid bags. Sandbags are not recommended because they may interfere with the images.[11] Tape or a special restraint board may be used to prevent the bird from moving during the exam.[8,11]

Contrast media may be used to increase the radiodensity of tissues, organs, and/or vascular systems, which helps depict lesions or abnormalities (Figures 14-3 through 14-5). Soft

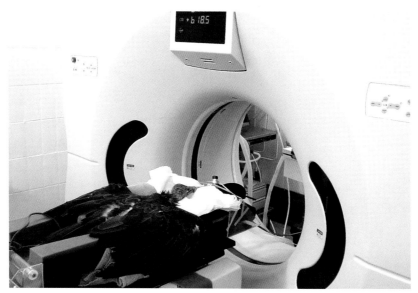

FIGURE 14-2 A 4-year-old male hooded vulture (*Necrosyrtes monachus*) is anesthetized with isoflurane and placed on a sliding table that moves into the gantry of a helical CT scanner to obtain a series of 195 images within 2 minutes.

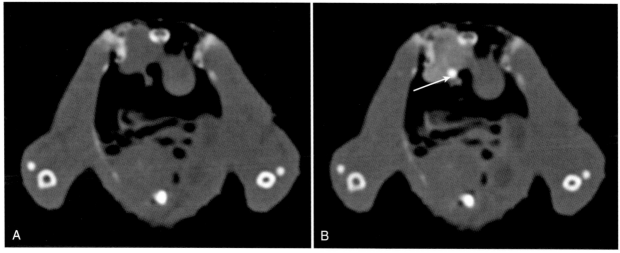

FIGURE 14-3 Transverse CT images of a 31-year-old female, blue-fronted Amazon parrot (*Amazona aestiva*), which presented with fresh blood in the feces. **A,** No difference in radiolucency can be seen between the left and right kidney. **B,** Exemplifies the benefit of intravenous administration of contrast medium, because in this image the contrast medium is clearly visible in the right ureter *(arrow)* and not in left ureter. In addition, the right kidney is also more radiolucent compared with the left kidney. (Photos courtesy the Division of Diagnostic Imaging, Faculty of Veterinary Medicine, Utrecht University, the Netherlands.)

tissue structures with abnormal vascularization caused by disease (e.g., neoplasia, inflammation) will show increased uptake of contrast medium, differentiating it from normal tissue. To use contrast media in CT imaging, intravenous access should be obtained and maintained throughout the procedure without having to move the patient between the precontrast and postcontrast scan. Both iodinated and noniodinated contrast media may be administered.[11] Iodinated compounds containing 250 to 300 mg iodine/mL can be given intravenously in a dose of 2 mL/kg. In birds, intravenous administration may pose practical challenges, since the relatively fast circulation and thereby quick elimination of contrast render it necessary to keep the time between administration of the contrast and scanning as short as possible (~1 to 2 minutes) in order to enable visualization of contrast uptake.

CT technology also allows the accurate placement of needles or biopsy instruments to collect tissue or fluids for diagnostic tests. For such procedures the slice of interest is selected, after which the position of this slice is indicated by a thin light or laser beam. Placement of the needle or biopsy instrument can subsequently be verified before collecting the desired material (Figure 14-6).[10]

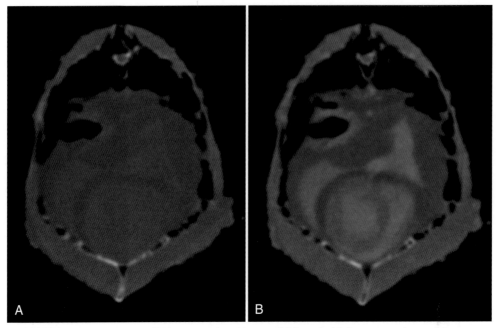

FIGURE 14-4 Transverse CT images of a 17-year-old female Moluccan cockatoo (*Cacatua moluccensis*), which presented with lethargy and a distended coelom. **A,** The contours of the heart and liver can vaguely be distinguished. **B,** After intravenous administration of a contrast medium, the liver, proventricular wall, and heart can more easily be distinguished from the ascites. An extensive amount of contrast-rich blood is present in the right ventricle, indicating right-sided cardiomyopathy. The contrast-poor areas around the liver are an indication of ascites (or fat). Postmortem examination confirmed the right-sided heart failure in combination with ascites. (Photos courtesy the Division of Diagnostic Imaging, Faculty of Veterinary Medicine, Utrecht University, the Netherlands.)

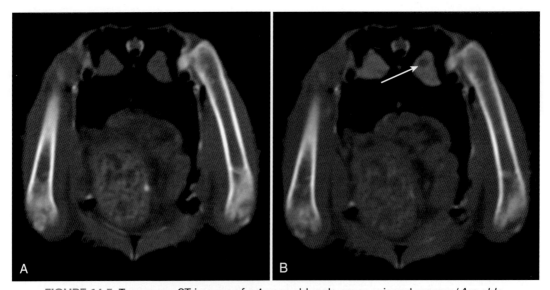

FIGURE 14-5 Transverse CT images of a 4-year-old male green-winged macaw (*Ara chloroptera*), which presented for CT evaluation of the heart and lungs. As a coincidental finding a kidney cyst *(arrow)* was detected after intravenous administration of contrast medium **(B),** while this cyst was not visible on the image obtained without contrast medium **(A).** (Photos courtesy the Division of Diagnostic Imaging, Faculty of Veterinary Medicine, Utrecht University, the Netherlands.)

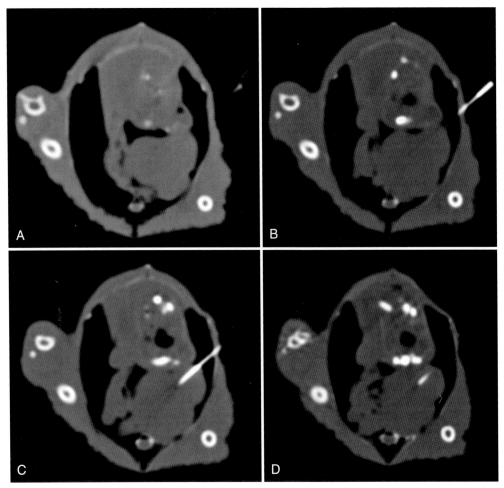

FIGURE 14-6 **A** to **D,** A series of four consecutive, transverse CT images of a 14-year-old female Grey parrot that underwent CT scanning because of seizures. As an incidental finding, a mass with a diameter of 2.4 cm was found in the left caudal thoracic air sac. A CT-guided, fine-needle aspiration biopsy was taken, confirming this mass to be an ovarian tumor. (Photos courtesy the Division of Diagnostic Imaging, Faculty of Veterinary Medicine, Utrecht University, the Netherlands.)

Applications

After scanning the patient, the obtained CT images can be evaluated with advanced software programs. With these programs multiplanar reconstructions (MPRs) and (3D) image reconstructions and renderings are possible. With MPR the organs and structures can be reviewed in three different planes (e.g., sagittal, longitudinal, transverse; Figure 14-7). Although all images are 2D, the combination of the three planes shows a 3D reconstruction. These software programs also allow different types of measurements (e.g., size, volume, density).

A CT image may be composed of up to 4200 gray (Gy) values, while a person can only distinguish up to 256 values at a time. "Windowing" and "leveling," therefore, may be used to adjust the range of values seen at certain times. This is perceived as adjusting the contrast and brightness levels of the image, allowing for optimal display of the tissue of interest. Aside from specific presets (e.g., bone, lung, abdomen) the settings may also be adjusted on screen.

CT can be used to evaluate a wide variety of different organ systems. In birds, the main clinical indications for CT imaging are currently for assessment of known or suspected abnormalities in the skeletal structures and respiratory tract.[8] Micro-CT imaging has recently become popular among anatomists because this technique provides high-quality visualization of the musculature without the need for time-consuming and difficult dissections.[12,13] Staining of the anatomical specimen with an iodine solution greatly enhances differentiation between the different muscles.[12] The technique, however, typically involves specialized hardware and requires longer scanning times than conventional CT, thereby making it less applicable to clinical avian cases in current times.

For many years, CT has been considered the most reliable and sensitive method for diagnosing lower respiratory tract disease in birds.[8,14] Although large abnormalities in the respiratory tract may be identified by conventional radiographs, many early and smaller lesions may be missed or misinterpreted.[4,15,16] CT images allow for cross-sectional evaluation of the homogenous "honeycomb like" lungs, providing detailed information about alterations of the respiratory tract in birds such as increased (multi)focal radiopacity (e.g., mycotic or

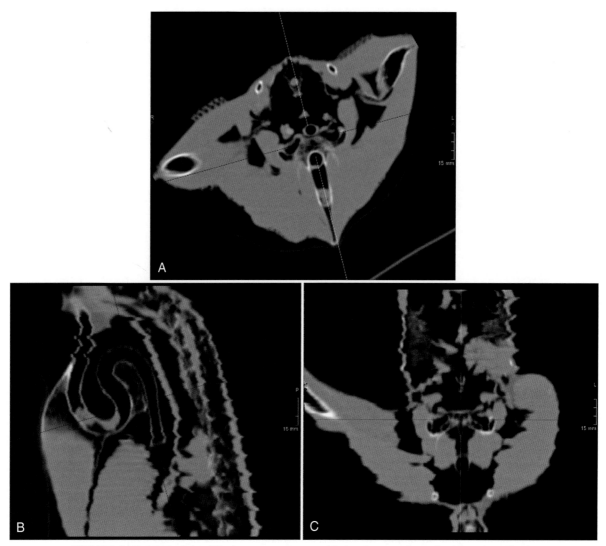

FIGURE 14-7 MPR of the CT of a crowned crane (*Balearica regulorum*) with aspergillosis in the trachea and lung. The green line in **(A)** and **(C)** represents the location of the plane displayed in **(B)**. The blue line in **(A)** and **(B)** represents the location of the plane displayed in **(B)**, and the red line in **(B)** and **(C)** represents the location of the plane displayed in **(A)**. (Photos courtesy the Division of Diagnostic Imaging, Faculty of Veterinary Medicine, Utrecht University, the Netherlands.)

mycobacterial pneumonia) or decreased volume of the lung parenchyma (typical for lung fibrosis) (Figure 14-8).[4,14-17] In addition to imaging abnormalities in the lung parenchyma, CT also enables visualization of abnormalities of the trachea (e.g., intraluminal or extraluminal masses, strictures, stenosis or displacement), syrinx, bronchi, and air sacs (e.g., overinfla-tion, airsacculitis, empyema, compression by ascites, egg or intracoelomic masses) (Figure 14-9).[4,8,14]

In areas with significant bone superimposition CT imag-ing has been found especially useful. CT has a large range of relevant and practical applications, particularly for the head. CT is considered superior to radiographs for evaluating the nasal cavity, conchae, and sinuses, allowing detailed studies of the various anatomic structures. Furthermore, calculation of the volume of pneumatized areas and establishing the location and extent of pathological changes in birds with (chronic) sinusitis or rhinitis can be done using CT.[5] Recently, a

fluid-filled quadrate bone was found in a goose with vestibular disease by using CT and MRI. By finding this abnormality a further diagnostic and therapeutic approach could be per-formed by drilling a hole in the bone, collecting a sample for culture, and flushing the cavity.[18] CT may also provide infor-mation about the shape and size of the eye, lens, and scleral rings, but is not able to differentiate intraocular structures such as the pectin oculi.[19] In birds with neurologic disease resulting from hydrocephalus, other congenital malforma-tions (e.g., meningoencephaloceles in crested ducks), trauma, large intracranial masses, or hemorrhage, CT examination may be used for a quick diagnosis (Figure 14-10),[2,9,20] whereas for other brain diseases additional techniques, such as MRI, may be necessary.

Conventional radiographs are usually adequate for diagnos-ing the majority of cases that affect the skeletal system (e.g., fractures). Spinal fractures are an important exception and are

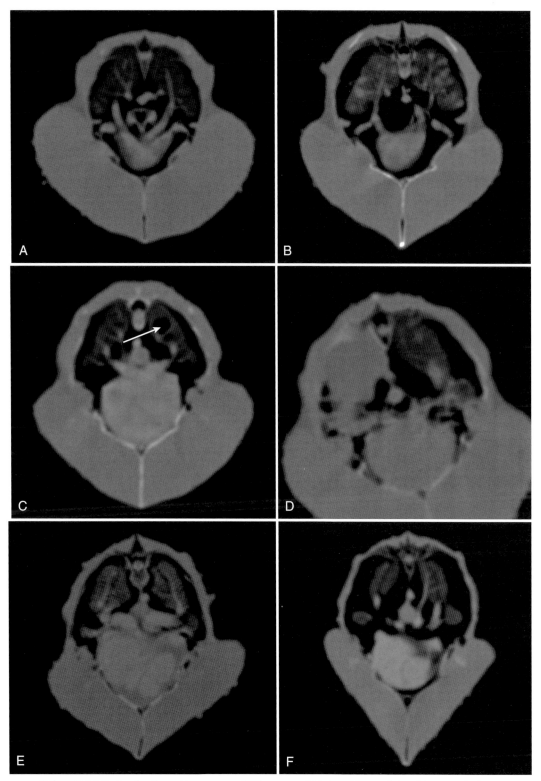

FIGURE 14-8 A selection of transverse CT images of birds with a variety of lung pathology. The following diagnoses were made: normal lung **(A)**, multifocal mycotic pneumonia **(B)**, pulmonary cyst *(arrow)* **(C)**, lung tumor **(D)**, lung edema **(E)**, and lung fibrosis **(F)**. (Photos courtesy the Division of Diagnostic Imaging, Faculty of Veterinary Medicine, Utrecht University, the Netherlands.)

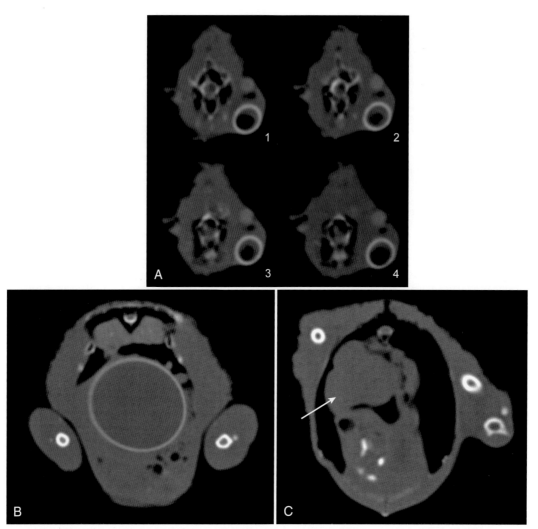

FIGURE 14-9 A selection of abnormalities that can be diagnosed with the aid of CT imaging. **A,** A series a four consecutive CT images shows a partial tracheal obstruction. **B,** The lining of an egg is seen. This would also have been visible on a regular radiograph. **C,** A mass in the left dorsal part of the coelom was found (arrow). With a fine-needle aspiration (see Figure 14-6 where the bird was place in dorsal recumbency) this mass was confirmed to be an ovarian tumor. (Photos courtesy the Division of Diagnostic Imaging, Faculty of Veterinary Medicine, Utrecht University, the Netherlands.)

missed in more than half of the cases.[21] For these type of fractures, CT offers increased sensitivity for visualization and identification.[21] Other examples of areas where CT shows superior imaging quality over conventional radiographs are the shoulder joint (Figure 14-11), pelvis (where a great deal of superimposition of overlying soft tissue structures and wings or legs is present; Figure 14-12), and skull (in particular the hyoid bone and beak apparatus).[3,8,22,23] Along with fractures or fissures, luxations and/or focal bony changes (e.g., infections, lysis) may be visualized and assessed, but the bones may also be judged regarding their radiodensity and cortical thickness.[24-26]

Enlargement of various intracoelomic organs, such as liver, kidney, and spleen, may easily be detected with CT imaging, especially when contrast medium is used.[3] The gastrointestinal tract can also be visualized, especially the gas-filled proventriculus and grit-containing ventriculus. Recognizing pathology in the intestinal tract is, however, often more difficult without the use of an intraluminal contrast medium such as

barium sulfate.[3] CT also may be useful in determining the size and extent of masses of various origins and locations, which also helps to determine and plan the possibilities for therapeutic intervention and associated prognoses (Figure 14-6).[22,27-29]

Computed tomographic angiography (CTA), in which contrast media are administered intravenously, allows the visualization and assessment of the larger veins and arteries in larger psittacines and raptorial birds. It provides new insights and methods for diagnosing cardiovascular diseases such as cardiomyopathy (Figure 14-4), atherosclerosis, aneurysms, or congenital vascular anomalies.[30,31] Because of the rapid circulation in birds, CTA scans are performed immediately after administration of contrast.[31]

Current limitations
In clinical practice, the limitations of CT for imaging structures and organs are mainly dependent on the spatial resolution of the CT scanner and size of the patient. Particularly in

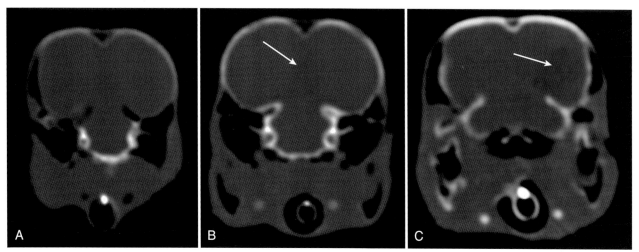

FIGURE 14-10 Transverse sections of the skull/brain of three different Grey parrots (*Psittacus erithacus*). **A,** No abnormalities in the brain can be seen. **B,** A slightly darker area is seen around the hemispheres *(arrow)*. On postmortem examination this proved to be the result of meningitis. **C,** A darker irregular area can be seen in the right hemisphere *(arrow)*. Differential diagnoses included tumor or granuloma. (Photos courtesy the Division of Diagnostic Imaging, Faculty of Veterinary Medicine, Utrecht University, the Netherlands.)

smaller-sized patients, such as budgerigars, resolution of the regularly used CT scanners may be poor, limiting its diagnostic value for evaluating the presence of abnormalities. For these patients, however, the more modern (helical) multislice CT scanners may produce images of high enough resolution to depict the different structures with sufficient detail and allow for identification of abnormalities. Similarly, micro-CTs may provide a good alternative for use in small-sized birds once they become available for use in patients in the future. Additionally, factors such as differences in density between the object of interest and its surrounding structures and size of the object may play a role.[8]

Magnetic Resonance Imaging

MRI is one of the latest cross-sectional imaging modalities to gain wide acceptance, particularly in the area of soft tissue and neurologic imaging, because with this technique distinction between the different types of soft tissue can be visualized easily. This imaging modality has also been considered safe because the images are generated by a powerful magnetic field.[1] Recent studies, however, have shown that attention and concentration on detail are negatively affected in personnel that are exposed to movement-induced time-varying magnetic fields within a static magnetic field of a 7 T MRI scanner.[32] Compared with CT, during which patients are subject to and personnel can risk exposure to ionizing radiation, these side-effects are nonetheless small. The strength of the magnetic field, which is also called magnetic flux density *B*, is expressed in Tesla (T). For comparison, the earth's magnetic field is 0.05 mT. MR scanners used for research purposes can have magnets producing up to 14 T. In clinical veterinary medicine, however, they typically range from 0.2 to 3 T.[32a]

Technique

Unlike CT scans or traditional radiographs, which use x-rays, MRI uses a powerful magnetic field (for signal strength) in combination with high-frequency radio waves to align and spin protons (nuclei of hydrogen atoms) in the body and obtain signals resulting from the spinning protons.[33] Because most of the hydrogen atoms are trapped in water molecules, the MR image produced is mainly a representation of the different types, distributions, and volumes of water in the various tissues.[32] Although the speed and resolution of MRI do not compare with those of conventional radiography and CT, a key advantage of MRI is its unique ability to differentiate soft tissues and the wide variety of ways in which image contrast, referred to as "weighting" in the field, can by generated for visualizing the body's anatomy and physiology. By changing the settings of the MRI scanner (e.g., pulse repetition time, echo time) different tissue weightings are obtained, which are subsequently used to analyze the tissue composition. The three types of weightings commonly used are as follows:

- *T1-weighted images*, increasingly known as longitudinal relaxation or simply T1, relate to the rate of recovery of the proton spins after each perturbation (called excitation) required to elicit an observable signal. Therefore, tissues with long T1 (e.g., water) appear hypo-intense (Table 14-1).
- *T2-weighted images*, increasingly known as transverse relaxation or simply T2, relate to the rate of decay of the observable signal. Therefore, in contrast to T1, tissues with long T2 appear hyper-intense (Table 14-2).
- *Proton–density–weighted or spin–density–weighted images (PDW)*: Contrast between tissues is primarily dependent on the amount of available spins (protons) (i.e., brightness is highest in tissues with a high-protein density); these images minimize the T1 and T2 effects, therefore resulting in less contrast than T1 or T2 images; although these images may be useful for depicting normal anatomy, they are used less often.[33,34]

Because each type of tissue has its own characteristics for T1, T2, and PDW, the images obtained from these three

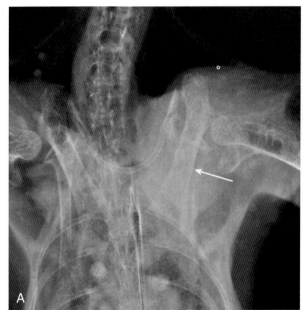

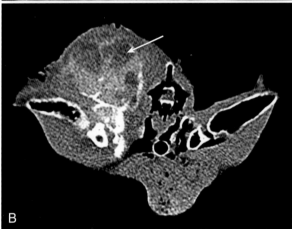

FIGURE 14-11 A ventrodorsal radiograph **(A)** and a transverse CT image **(B)** at the level of the scapula of a 6-month-old, female scarlet macaw (*Ara macao*) with a giant cell tumor of the left scapula. On the radiograph bone lysis of the left scapula can be seen *(arrow)*, although the superposition of the coracoid bone makes it easy to overlook this abnormality. On the CT, however, the magnitude of the swelling and bone lysis *(arrow)* cannot be overlooked. (Photos courtesy the Division of Diagnostic Imaging, Faculty of Veterinary Medicine, Utrecht University, the Netherlands.)

weighting types can be combined to identify the origin of the tissue involved.

Procedure

Magnetic imaging requires general anesthesia. This in turn warrants the use of special anesthetic machines and monitoring equipment, because nothing magnetic may be taken into the scanner room and radio waves emitted by electric devices may interfere with the procedure, resulting in nondiagnostic images. To facilitate breathing, the patient should be placed in a semi-upright position with the use of MRI-compatible materials (e.g., pillows, sandbags). Prior to starting the procedure it is also important to check for the presence of metal implants

or objects present in the body, which may result in large-scale signal extinction and/or movement of the metal within the body, potentially causing damage to internal organs. Some experts recommend screening birds for the presence of metal in their gastrointestinal tract with a radiograph prior to performing an MRI.[35] Most microtransponders, which are commonly used to identify birds, contain metal and result in signal extinction in MR scanners of 0.2 T. Luckily most foot bands are made of aluminum, which does not result in artifacts. There is so little metal in microtransponders that no artifacts are produced in the MR scanners with a magnet of 1.5 T.

Besides the intrinsic relaxation or density-based contrast mechanisms of tissues, exogenous agents that alter the intrinsic relaxation can be used to enhance the MRI signal for special purposes like highlighting microcirculation in the tissue. Gadolinium, a paramagnetic intravenous contrast agent, is one of the agents that can be used as a contrast medium for MRI studies (dose 0.25 mmol/kg IV). After administration of the compound via an intravenous catheter the gadolinium is distributed throughout the body. It changes the local magnetic field in tissues in which it is present in high concentrations (i.e., highly vascularized tissues), causing delineation from the surrounding structures. The contrast-enhanced images subsequently obtained may be particularly useful in detecting whether an active inflammation or neoplasm is present.[11,34] Unfortunately, scientific studies on the use of gadolinium in birds are lacking.

Applications

Thus far, MRI has been used in various bird species (e.g., pigeons, poultry, pet birds) for anatomical studies of various organ systems,[35-37] and it is used in various scientific studies such as the analysis of the topographical relationship between brain structures and singing ability in songbirds.[38]

MRI has also been used with some success in avian patients. Because of its characteristics, it is primarily used to diagnose soft tissue changes. Thus it has been mainly applied in birds for diagnosing neurologic disease (e.g., brain abnormalities) and/or internal disease (e.g., sinusitis).[35,36] It is very useful for visualizing and evaluating various parts of the central nervous system (CNS), including the cerebral hemispheres (Figure 14-13), cerebellum, optic chiasm, brainstem, and spinal cord.[35] Its application in the diagnosis of a variety of different CNS diseases has also been demonstrated by various researchers. Among the diseases that have been diagnosed on MRI examination are (viral) encephalitis, lead poisoning, vestibular disease, hydrocephalus, ischemic stroke, spinal cord trauma, and a peripheral nerve sheath tumor.[18,21,35,39-44] MRI is also an excellent diagnostic tool for evaluating the eye, orbit, and sinuses; identifying, localizing, and characterizing lesions in these tissues; and planning the proper therapeutic approach.[45,46]

Furthermore, MRI has potential value in visualizing the gastrointestinal tract, liver, spleen, and urogenital tract,[34-36] whereas it is found to be less useful for imaging the heart and lungs of birds because cardiac motion creates artifacts obscuring the heart and adjacent lungs.[35] Pancreas and adrenal glands also are not identified on MRI.[35]

Current limitations

Although MRI has many potential uses in avian medicine it is not frequently used. The most important reason for its

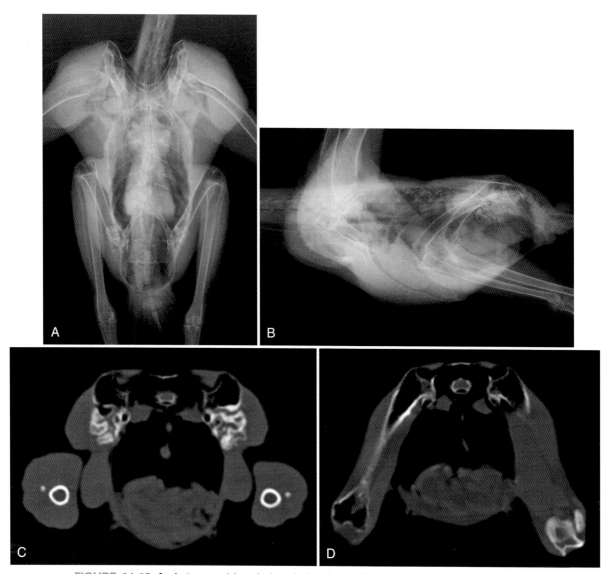

FIGURE 14-12 **A,** A 4-year-old male hooded vulture (*Necrosyrtes monachus*) presented with bilateral lameness. On radiographs no clear abnormalities could be noticed, aside from the fact that the legs could not be extended to allow for correct positioning (**A** and **B**). On the transverse CT images it became clear that a significant amount of bone formation was present around the hip joints (**C**). For comparison a CT scan was performed from another hooded vulture from the same owners, which clearly demonstrated a normal hip joint (**D**). (Photos courtesy the Division of Diagnostic Imaging, Faculty of Veterinary Medicine, Utrecht University, the Netherlands.)

limited use is the prolonged period of time needed to perform the MRI scan. In combination with the need for multiple sequences, this results in prolonged anesthesia times (a full investigation may take at least 45 minutes), which may be detrimental to the patient, especially since access to the patient for the anesthesiologist is limited during the procedure. Additionally, the small size of most birds in combination with the relative low spatial resolution of most systems (less than 0.5 T) limits the diagnostic value that MRI has in avian patients, especially since the minimal slice thickness needs to be 1 to 3 mm to achieve a usable signal-to-noise ratio with these machines. Imaging may further be hindered by the high respiratory and heart rates or by the presence of artifacts caused by the presence of air sacs and/or a microtransponder.[11,34,36]

Cost may also be an issue because MRI is usually much more expensive than CT. With the increased availability of higher resolution systems, the use and practical implication of MRI in avian medicine is likely to become more prevalent.

MR angiography
Along with unmatched versatility in differentiating soft tissues for anatomical visualization, MRI can use mechanisms to generate signal contrast beyond the standard T1, T2, and proton density for capturing the physiology of the body, including the circulatory system. The ability to study the vascular anatomy and function is critical for avian veterinary care, since cardiovascular diseases such as atherosclerosis, stroke, and ventricular and atrial disorders are common in

TABLE 14-1

Signal Intensity of Various Tissues at T1-Weighted MRI

T1W1	Dark	Air, mineral-rich tissue (cortical bone and stones), fast-flowing blood
	Low	Collagenous tissue (ligaments, tendons, and scars) High free-water tissue (kidneys, gonads, edema, fluids [urine, bile], simple cysts, bladder, gallbladder, spleen, and cerebrospinal fluid) High bound water tissues (liver, pancreas, adrenals, hyaline cartilage, and muscle)
	Intermediate	Proteinaceous tissue (abscess, complex cysts, and synovial fluid)
	Bright	Fatty bone marrow, blood products (methemoglobin [metHb]), slow-flowing blood, radiation change, and paramagnetic contrast agent

Note: It should be taken into consideration that the signal characteristics of proteinaceous tissues vary according to the amount of protein content. Tissues with high concentrations of protein may have a high signal intensity on T1-weighted images (T1W1).
Adapted from Wallack S: Basic magnetic resonance imaging principles used for evaluating animal patients with neurologic disease, *Vet Clin North Am Exotic Pet Pract* 10:909–925, 2007.

TABLE 14-2

Signal Intensity of Various Tissues at T2-Weighted MRI

T2W1	Dark	Air, mineral-rich tissue (cortical bone and stones), fast-flowing blood
	Low	Collagenous tissue (ligaments, tendons, and scars), bone islands High bound water tissues (liver, pancreas, adrenals, hyaline cartilage, and muscle)
	Intermediate	High bound water tissues (liver, pancreas, adrenals, hyaline cartilage, and muscle) Fat and fatty bone marrow
	Bright	Fat and fatty bone marrow High free water tissue (kidneys, gonads, odema, fluids [urine, bile], simple cysts, bladder, gallbladder, spleen, and cerebrospinal fluid), proteinaceous tissue, and blood products (oxyhemoglobin, and extracellular methemoglobin [metHb])

Note: Signal characteristics of proteinaceous tissues vary according to the amount of protein content: Tissues with high concentrations of protein may have low signal intensity on T2-weighted images (T2W1).
Adapted from Wallack S: Basic magnetic resonance imaging principles used for evaluating animal patients with neurologic disease, *Vet Clin North Am Exotic Pet Pract* 10:909–925, 2007.

avian species but currently poorly understood. Although CT provides faster scan speed and better spatial resolution, the main reason for using MRI for vascular visualization is that it does not require the use of exogenous agents to generate the desirable vessel-to-tissue contrast. This can be highly desirable because circulation in avian species can make contrast agent administration and subsequent imaging rather challenging. Examples of MRI techniques particularly suited and being applied to avian angiographic imaging include phase-contrast (PC) and time-of-flight (TOF) imaging.

In general, the MRI signal is dependent on both the concentration and motion of water molecules. PC MRI utilizes the latter to generate images whose intensities are essentially rotating vector entities with coherent motion of water molecules encoded as the vector's angular displacement, or phase. The most commonly used PC MRI makes the signal phase directly proportional to the velocity of the water molecules along the direction of observation, and by measuring the velocities in perpendicular directions 3D motion of the tissue or blood flow can be reconstructed. Because an underlying assumption is that water molecular motion is uniform with the image voxel, PC MRI is suitable for evaluating bulk motion that occurs in large organs (e.g., cardiac left ventricular myocardium) and laminar flow in large blood vessels.

Time-of-flight MRI is based on the fact that the observed MRI intensity is also dependent on the balance between depletion and recovery of the signal between successive excitations. By bringing nondepleted signal into the imaged volume, blood flow can make the vessel appear brighter, as if the signal has recovered faster, compared with surrounding stationary tissues. Using appropriate combinations of the image volume, orientation, location and excitation repetition time, and subsequent digital concatenation of the individual image volumes, the vasculatures of specific organs or even the entire vascular system of the body can be mapped, despite the wide variability in the blood-flow direction and speed. Figure 14-14 shows an example of whole-body MRI TOF angiographic images obtained in a healthy pigeon (*Columba livia domestica*). Figure 14-15 describes a clinical case study where MRI TOF angiography was used to guide the surgical removal of an abnormal caudal vertebral mass in a Moluccan cockatoo (*Cacatua moluccensis*).

Functional MRI

To study brain activity during different tasks, functional MRI (fMRI) has become an important neuroimaging technique in cognitive neuroscience. This technique relies on blood oxygen level-dependent contrast, which reflects a local change in the ratio between oxygenated and deoxygenated hemoglobin in the blood induced by a local increase in oxygen consumption during neuronal activation. Only one research center is currently using this technique in birds (i.e., zebra finches and pigeons) with the aid of a 7 T scanner.[47,48] Results of these studies will give insight into the complex sensorimotor and cognitive processes underlying vocal communication in zebra finches and lateralization of the brain in pigeons.

Histological imaging

In many areas of clinical practice, light microscopy of specimen sections remains the gold standard for detailed examination of the normal and pathological anatomy at whole-organ

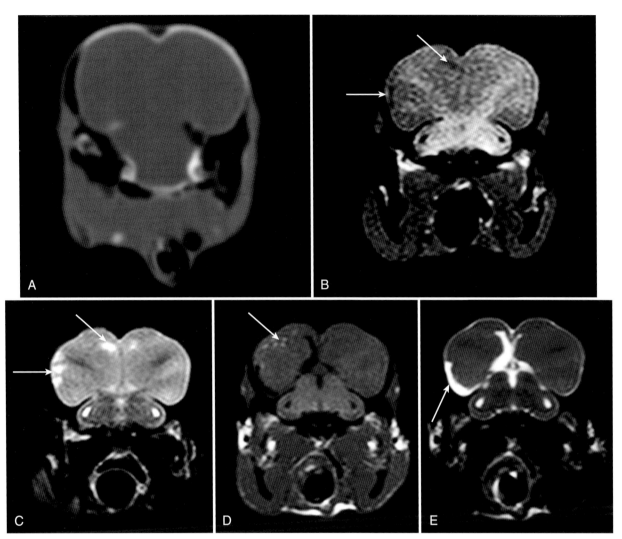

FIGURE 14-13 Advanced diagnostic imaging of a 22-year-old male Grey parrot (*Psittacus erithacus*) that presented with weakness in the legs, falling off the perch, and signs of aphasia. On the transverse CT image of the brain (**A**) no abnormalities can be seen. On the MR images, however, multiple focal reactions in the right hemisphere can be seen (*arrows*: black on T1 [**B**] and white on T2 [**C**]). Although the parrot improved during the following 11 weeks, it continued to have episodes of weakness. On the T1-weighted MR image, signs of recent hemorrhages could be seen (**D**, *arrow*), while on the T2-weighted image an accumulation of fluid around the right hemisphere could be detected (**E**, *arrow*). (Photos courtesy the Division of Diagnostic Imaging, Faculty of Veterinary Medicine, Utrecht University, the Netherlands.)

and tissue levels. Although their spatial resolutions do not and likely will not match that of light microscopy, diagnostic imaging technologies such as CT and MRI offer the benefits of relative speed, convenience, and a nondestructive nature, which are beginning to be recognized and exploited for virtual dissection via histological imaging. Similar to conventional histology, CT and MRI can be performed on freshly excised or prepared (e.g., fixed) specimens, using one of a variety of intrinsic mechanisms (e.g., T1, T2 contrast for MRI) or modality-specific exogenous agents to generate the tissue contrast serving the equivalent role of staining. Unlike histology, the image data obtained by CT and MRI are inherently digital and

3D, which allow them to be readily used by recent advances in image processing and analysis for unprecedented visualization of the anatomy without the labor-intensive and error-prone 2D-to-3D reconstruction.

Because the animals are typically scanned postmortem, histological imaging permits wider options for specimen preparation and scanning protocols, which can provide more detailed visualization of the anatomy than standard CT and MRI. Two particularly promising recent advances in histological imaging are the use of iodine staining and vascular casting in CT. By taking advantage of the molecular-binding affinity and x-ray-attenuating capability of iodine, pretreating

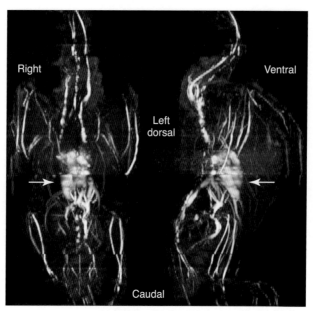

FIGURE 14-14 Whole-body MRI TOF angiography of a healthy pigeon (*Columba livia domestica*). The images are shown as ventral view *(left)* and lateral view *(right)* maximum-intensity projections of the 3D volume reconstructed from separately scanned axial subvolumes. The anatomical orientations are as indicated, and the solid arrows point to the heart. Minor discontinuities of the vessels are a result of motion during the scans and stitching artifact. (Images courtesy Drs. M. Scott Echols and Edward Hsu.)

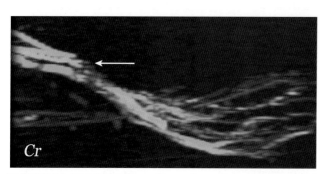

FIGURE 14-15 MRI TOF maximum-intensity projection angiography of a Moluccan cockatoo's (*Cacatua moluccensis*) lower spinal region showing blood vessels through the caudal synsacrum and tail. *Cr*, direction to the cranium. Compared with vessels that normally are continuous and run ventrolateral to and through the caudal vertebrae, the arrow points to vessels that leave the caudal aspect of the synsacrum and steeply dive ventral to the caudal vertebrae. The blood flow disruption was later determined to be associated with an abnormal synsacral-caudal junction caused by septic osteomyelitis. Guided by the MRI angiographic regional vascular map, the vertebral mass was removed in a near bloodless procedure. (Image courtesy Drs. M. Scott Echols and Edward Hsu.)

specimens with iodine solutions (e.g., immersion in Lugol's solutions) allows them to be imaged with the speed and resolution benefits of CT and soft tissue contrast that rivals MRI. This technology, which was originally developed for high-throughput phenotype screening of embryos, has been extended to whole birds.[49] Similarly, by filling the vascular space with x-ray-attenuating solutions that subsequently solidify, casting can be combined with digital subtraction CT to allow the vascular network to be visualized in unprecedented detail. Figure 14-16 demonstrates the benefits of the technique on a Grey parrot head obtained using a novel, easy-to-use casting agent (BriteVu, Scarlet Imaging, Salt Lake City, UT).

NUCLEAR-IMAGING TECHNIQUES

Nuclear-imaging techniques use radiopharmaceuticals, which are intravenously administered or taken orally. The radiation, emitted following the decay of these compounds, is captured by gamma cameras and used to form images. There are several techniques available within the field of nuclear imaging, such as scintigraphy, single-photon emission computed tomography (SPECT), and PET.

In contrast to MRI and CT, which both focus on a particular section of the body (e.g., head, chest, extremity), nuclear-imaging techniques generally target a specific organ or tissue (e.g., lungs, heart, bone, brain). Additionally, they are primarily intended to show physiological/pathological function of the investigated organ system rather than displaying an anatomical image. Nuclear-imaging modalities may visualize the presence of pathologic processes because a change in function resulting from these processes can be demonstrated by a concurrent change in uptake of the radionuclide tracer. Diseases associated with an increase in physiological function often lead to increased concentrations of the radionuclide tracer in the tissue, resulting in the appearance of a "hot spot"

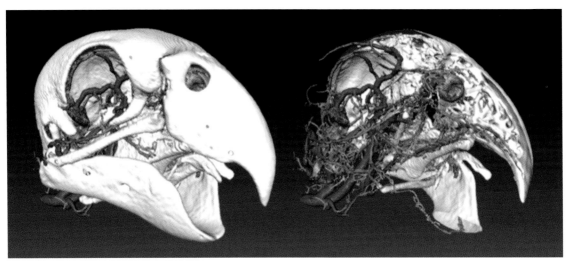

FIGURE 14-16 CT of a Grey parrot (*Psittacus erithacus erithacus*). CT was performed on the whole animal postmortem before and after BriteVu injection into the vascular space. The bony anatomy and vascular network of the head were separated via digital subtraction; colored in gray and orange-red, respectively; and visualized using 3D surface rendering. *Left,* Shows the vasculature within the intact skeletal anatomy. *Right,* Right half of the bony structure digitally removed to expose the interior vascular network. By analyzing these and other images, one can readily see the intense vascular supply to the nares and location of the blood supply along the ventral aspect of the upper mandible and periocular vessels contained within the bony orbit. The unique information revealed is expected to help guide medical and surgical decisions and open up new possibilities in the field of avian research. (Images courtesy Drs. M. Scott Echols and Edward Hsu.)

(i.e., focal increase) or generalized accumulation throughout the tissue. Other disease processes may result from a decrease in physiological function, which results in the appearance of a "cold spot" (i.e., focal decrease) because of exclusion or decreased uptake of the tracer.

Technique

A variety of different radionuclides or radioisotopes are available for use in nuclear-imaging studies. The most commonly used radionuclides are technetium (^{99m}Tc), iodine (^{123}I and ^{131}I), thallium (^{201}Tl), gallium (^{67}Ga), fluorine-18 fluorodeoxyglucose (^{18}F FDG), xenon (^{133}Xe), and krypton (^{81m}Kr), which may be intravenously administered (e.g., iodine) or inhaled (e.g., xenon).[50] The choice for a specific radionuclide largely depends on the type of tissue investigated. For example, iodine (which has a long half-life) may be used for imaging the thyroid gland, whereas technetium (with a very short half-life) may be used for bone scans.

In contrast to x-rays, which are transmitted in a radial path, gamma rays from the radioisotope within a patient are emitted equally in all directions. Collimators are, therefore, needed in nuclear-imaging devices to permit only photons following certain trajectories to reach the detector while absorbing most of the remaining photons. Unfortunately, this results in wasting most of the emitted photons (over 99.9%). The loss of photons during a PET scan is much less, because this technique forms images in a different way.[1]

The radiation emitted by the radioisotopes is detected with a scintillation camera. The camera head consists of a lead-containing parallel hole collimator, followed by a thallium-activated sodium iodide [NaI(Tl)] crystal, which emits visible or ultraviolet light after interaction with the ionized radiation. This is then followed by multiple photomultiplier tubes (PMTs), which convert the light from the crystal into an electrical signal further amplified by the PMT and preamplifiers.[1] The obtained data may be comprised out of one or more images. Multi-image datasets may be "dynamic" (i.e., represent a time sequence) or "spatial" (i.e., represent a sequence where the gamma camera has been moved relative to the patient).

Scintigraphy

Scintigraphy is a nuclear-imaging technique that uses internal radionuclides to create 2D images, in contrast to PET and SPECT, which form 3D images. Scintigraphy has many applications, both in human and veterinary medicine. Main indications can be found in the field of internal medicine, such as lung scintigraphy or ventilation-perfusion scans to diagnose pulmonary embolism, hepatobiliary scintigraphy to diagnose liver shunts or bile duct obstruction, renal scintigraphy to assess kidney function (glomerular filtration rate [GFR]), or thyroid scintigraphy to diagnose hyperthyroidism or hypothyroidism or thyroid neoplasia.[51] Bone scintigraphy is further used in orthopedic patients to diagnose the presence of neoplasia, including metastasis (e.g., osteosarcoma), or identify the cause for lameness in cases where other imaging techniques have failed.[51]

In avian medicine, scintigraphy is a technique mainly used for research purposes. This includes the study of normal function (e.g., GFR or hepatic clearance) and organ failure (i.e., liver, kidney) after exposure to various toxic substances (e.g., ethylene glycol, aflatoxin, gentamycin).[52-56] Scintigraphy has also been performed in normal and radiothyroidectomized cockatiels, which demonstrated to be a helpful technique in detecting hypofunction of the thyroid gland.[57] In a clinical setting scintigraphy is certainly feasible for evaluating the thyroid gland in psittacines (Figure 14-17) and diagnosing an osteosarcoma in a goose.[58]

Furthermore, scintigraphy has demonstrated its potential use in avian patients with a variety of orthopedic problems[59] and its usefulness in the therapeutic monitoring of patients with various types of neoplasia, including diagnosing the presence of metastasis.[60-62]

Procedure

Scintigraphy is generally performed under general anesthesia with the animal placed in dorsal recumbency. An intravenous catheter is placed to administer the radioisotopes. The dose needed is dependent on the type of radioisotope used and size of the animal. Scans are usually obtained at regular time intervals, which are mostly determined by the type of study and tissue examined, and may take up to 1 hour. Although some research protocols are available, no systematic studies have been performed on the use of scintigraphy in avian patients.

Single-photon emission computed tomography

SPECT is a technique that is essentially similar to conventional scintigraphy. It does, however, use a rotating gamma camera, which enables the object to be examined from a variety of different positions. The obtained images form a stack of slices of the body that can be reconstructed into a 3D image, representing the distribution of the radionuclide within the patient. The information is typically presented as cross-sectional slices, but reconstructions can be made in different planes by manipulating the data. In human medicine, SPECT can be useful for functional imaging of heart and brain and imaging bone, thyroid tissue, neoplasia, and/or infection. Although its use has also been described in veterinary medicine,[63,64] no applications have been reported in avian medicine.

Positron emission tomography

PET is similar to SPECT and scintigraphy in its use of radioactive tracer materials and detection of gamma rays. In contrast to SPECT, in which the emitted gamma radiation is measured directly, PET tracers emit positrons that annihilate with adjacent electrons, causing two gamma rays to be emitted in opposite directions. A PET scanner subsequently detects the emissions of these "coincident pairs," thus providing more accurate information about the localization of the radiation event.[65] The localization accuracy is even further enhanced by the fact that most commercially available PET systems are now sold integrated with an x-ray CT scanner enabling the exact localization of the lesion seen with the PET system.[1]

The most commonly used radiopharmaceutical agent in PET imaging is FDG. This sugar-based tracer is mainly distributed to organs or tissues with a high blood flow or metabolic rate (e.g., brain, liver, heart, kidney, neoplasia, inflamed tissue) and may be used as an indicator for altered tissue function. The characteristics of this specific tracer make the technique particularly important in the diagnosis of brain disease and monitoring of cancer treatments. Depending on the definition of the problem and diagnostic/research question (i.e., blood flow, metabolism, enzyme or receptor function), other radioisotopes may be used.

PET typically involves the use of short-lived isotopes, for example, carbon (^{11}C), nitrogen (^{13}N), oxygen (^{15}O), and fluorine (^{18}F), which may be incorporated into various compounds used in the body (e.g., glucose, water, ammonia) or into molecules that bind to receptors or other sites of drug action. Because of the short longevity (half-lives of less than 20 minutes), the radioisotopes should be prepared in close proximity to the PET-imaging facility, warranting the need for on-site cyclotrons (i.e., the apparatus that produces the radioisotopes).[1]

Over the last few years there have been some studies performed with PET imaging in birds. These include studies into the functioning of the parrot brain, in particular regarding its function in the perception of pain and use of analgesics.[66-68] A study of brain activity in crows, using PET scan images, demonstrated that this bird species is capable of discriminating human faces and associating them with an emotional significance for that person.[69] A number of applications in clinical cases have also been described that include the use of PET for planning and monitoring cancer therapy and determining the "activity" of lesions/nodules and the diagnosis of fractures of the skull and/or luxations of facial bones.[70-72] To enable comparison of these findings with those found in normal birds, PET scans were performed in 10 healthy Hispaniolan parrots (*Amazona ventralis*)[73] and eight healthy bald eagles (*Haliaeetus leucocephalus*).[74] Results of scans performed

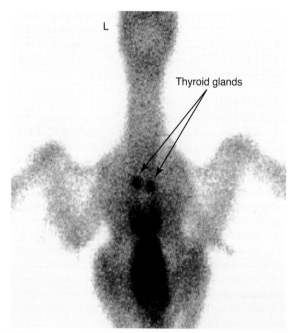

FIGURE 14-17 Scintigraphy scan of a Grey parrot (*Psittacus e. erithacus*) that was suspected of hypothyroidism. On the scan, however, both thyroid glands are equally visible.

60 minutes post-[18]FDG injection showed a high variability in the intestinal radioactivity, which could be largely attributed to reflux of the compound into the cloaca. This finding should be taken into account when performing PET imaging of birds, particularly in cases where the gastrointestinal tract is the main object of interest, and may warrant the performance of "dynamic" rather than "static" studies.[73] Aside from a high uptake in the cloaca in the bald eagles, these birds showed an even higher uptake in the kidneys, which was attributed to the higher plasma glucose concentrations found in birds and the gluconeogenic capabilities of avian kidneys.[74]

Despite the growing number of studies conducted, PET imaging is currently not expected to gain widespread use in the field of veterinary medicine. The main factors responsible for its limited use in clinical cases are the need for special equipment and associated higher expenses. Therefore, it is expected that for now PET imaging will remain a technique that is mostly accessible for universities and in research settings.

CONCLUSION

Diagnostic imaging should be considered an integral part of the medical and surgical management of avian patients. With the emergence of new imaging modalities the possibilities for diagnosing disease have increased drastically. Particularly in the last decade, advanced imaging modalities are used more often in avian medicine, both for research purposes and clinical evaluation of patients. Each technique has its own advantages and limitations, which largely determine its potential applications in the diagnostic and therapeutic plan. Dependent on the goal of the procedure, availability and type of equipment, associated costs, and experience of the examiner in performing the technique and interpreting the images, a well-thought out choice can be made between the various available modalities (Tables 14-3 and 14-4).

TABLE 14-3
Recommendations, Indications, and Limitations for CT Scanning in Clinical Practice

Minimal requirements for scanner type	Helical single slice
Minimal requirements for scanning sequence	A slice thickness of 2 mm with reconstruction to 1 mm is recommended
Indications	• Respiratory system • Bone structures that are less well visualized with radiographs (spinal column, skull, and hip joints) • Internal organs with the use of (intravenous) contrast medium
Limitations	• Resolution (preferably birds >100 to 150 grams) • Soft tissue structures (such as the brain) are better visualized with MRI • Cost of the CT scanning

TABLE 14-4
Recommendations, Indications, and Limitations for MRI Scanning in Clinical Practice

Minimal requirements for scanner type	Preferable 1.5 Tesla and up (resolution is too poor and scanning times are too great with 0.2 Tesla MRI scanners)
Indications	• Soft tissue structures (such as the brain and sinuses)
Limitations	• Resolution (preferably birds >100 to 150 grams) • Scanning time in combination with respiration rate limits usability for intracoelomic (soft tissue) structures • Cost of the MRI scanning (even greater compared with CT)

REFERENCES

1. Bushberg JT, Seibert JA, Leidholdt EM Jr, et al: *The essential physics of medical imaging*, Philadelphia, 2012, Wolters Kluwer Health/Lippincott Williams & Wilkins.
2. Bartels T, Krautwald-Junghanns ME, Portmann S, et al: The use of conventional radiography and computer-assisted tomography as instruments for demonstration of gross pathological lesions in the cranium and cerebrum in the crested breed of the domestic duck (Anas platyrhynchos f. dom.), *Avian Pathol* 29:101–108, 2000.
3. Gumpenberger M, Henninger W: The use of computed tomography in avian and reptile medicine, *Semin Av Exotic Pet Med* 10:174–180, 2001.
4. Krautwald-Junghanns ME, Schuhmacher F, Tellehlm B: Evaluation of the lower respiratory tract in psittacines using radiology and computed tomography, *Vet Radiol Ultrasound* 34:382–390, 1993.
5. Krautwald-Junghanns ME, Kostka VM, Dörsch B: Comparative studies on the diagnostic value of conventional radiography and computed tomography in evaluating the heads of psittacine and raptorial birds, *J Avian Med Surg* 12:149–157, 1998.
6. Martel A, van Caelenberg A, Gielen I, et al: *Computed tomographic (ct) anatomy of the pigeon (Columba livia)*. Proceedings of the 26th Annual Conference of the Association of Avian Veterinarians, 2005, pp 373–374.
7. Orosz SE, Toal RL: Tomographic anatomy of the golden eagle (Aquila chrysaetos), *J Zoo Wildl Med* 23:39–46, 1992.
8. Krautwald-Junghanns ME, Pees M: Computed tomography (CT). In Krautwald-Junghanns ME, Pees M, Reese S, Tully T, editors: *Diagnostic imaging of exotic pets*, Hannover, Germany, 2010, Schlütersche, pp 54–63.
9. Jenkins J: *Use of computed tomography (CT) in pet bird practice*. Proceedings of the 12th Annual Conference of the Association of Avian Veterinarians, 1991, pp 276–279.
10. Mackey EB, Hernandez-Divers SJ, Holland M, et al: Clinical technique: application of computed tomography in zoological medicine, *J Exotic Pet Med* 17:198–209, 2008.
11. Silverman S, Dennison S: *Imaging in special species*. Proceedings of the 31st Annual Conference of the Association of Avian Veterinarians, 2010, pp 237–246.
12. Lautenschlager S, Bright JA, Rayfield EJ: Digital dissection—using contrast-enhanced computed tomography scanning to elucidate hard- and soft-tissue anatomy in the common buzzard (Buteo buteo), *J Anat* 224:412–431, 2014.

13. Quayle MR, Barnes DG, Kaluza OL, et al: An interactive three dimensional approach to anatomical description—the jaw musculature of the Australian laughing kookaburra (Dacelo novaeguineae), *Peer J* 2:e355, 2014, doi 10.7717/peerj.355.

14. Romagnano A, Krautwald-Junghanns ME: *Respiratory radiology and imaging*. Proceedings of the 18th Annual Conference of the Association of Avian Veterinarians, 1997, pp 17–21.

15. Krautwald-Junghanns ME: *Computertomographie des aviären Respirationstraktes. Reihe: Akademisches Forum*, Berlin, 1997, Blackwell Wissenschafts-Verlag.

16. Westerhof I, Schoemaker NJ, Barthez P, et al: *Spiral computed tomography in respiratory diseases birds*. Proceedings of the 8th Biannual Conference of the European Association of Avian Veterinarians, 2005, pp 27–28.

17. Amann O, Kik MJL, Passon-Vastenburg MHAC, et al: Chronic pulmonary interstitial fibrosis in a blue-fronted amazon parrot (Amazona aestiva aestiva), *Avian Dis* 51:150–153, 2007.

18. Delk KW, Mejia-Fava J, Jiménez DA, et al: Diagnostic imaging of peripheral vestibular disease in a Chinese goose (Anser cygnoides), *J Avian Med Surg* 28:31–37, 2014.

19. Gumpenberger M, Kolm G: Ultrasonic and computed tomographic examinations of the avian eye: physiologic appearance, pathologic findings, and comparative biometric measurement, *Vet Radiol Ultrasound* 47:492–502, 2006.

20. Rosenthal K, Stefanacci J, Quesenberry K, et al: *Computerized tomography in 10 cases of avian intracranial disease*. Proceedings of the 16th Annual Conference of the Association of Avian Veterinarians, 1995, p 305.

21. Whittington JK, Osterbur KA, O'Dell-Anderson K: *Imaging modalities and limitations in diagnosing spinal fractures of birds*. Proceedings of the 29th Annual Conference of the Association of Avian Veterinarians, 2008, pp 353–359.

22. Amann O, Meij BP, Westerhof I, et al: Giant cell tumor of the bone in a scarlet macaw (Ara macao), *Avian Dis* 51:146–149, 2007.

23. van Zeeland YRA, Schoemaker NJ, Veraa S, et al: *Femoral head resection in a hooded vulture (Necrosyrtus monachus)*. Proceedings of the 30th Annual Conference of the Association of Avian Veterinarians, 2009, pp 349–350.

24. Fischer I, Liesegang A, Hatt J-M, et al: *Quantitative computed tomography for the assessment of bone density in budgerigars: a pilot study*. Proceedings of the 8th Biannual Conference of the European Association of Avian Veterinarians, 2005, pp 307–309.

25. Streubel R, Bartels T, Krautwald-Junghanns ME, et al: Computertomographische, chemische und biomechanische Untersuchungen zur Knochendichte und Knochenbruchfestigkeit von Legehennen, *Archiv für Geflügelkunde* 69:206–212, 2005.

26. Bergen DJ, Gartrell BD: Discospondylitis in a yellow-eyed penguin (Megadyptes antipodes), *J Avian Med Surg* 24:58–63, 2010.

27. Graham JE, Werner JA, Lowenstine LJ, et al: Periorbital liposarcoma in an African grey parrot (Psittacus erithacus), *J Avian Med Surg* 17:147–153, 2003.

28. Spaulding K, Loomis M: Principles and applications of computed tomography and magnetic resonance imaging in zoo and wildlife medicine. In Fowler M, Miller R, editors: *Zoo and wild animal medicine: current therapy 4*, Philadelphia, 1999, WB Saunders, pp 83–88.

29. Beaufrère H, Castillo-Alcala F, Holmberg DL, et al: Branchial cysts in two Amazon parrots (Amazona species), *J Avian Med Surg* 24:46–57, 2010.

30. Beaufrère H, Pariaut R, Rodriguez D, et al: Avian vascular imaging: a review, *J Avian Med Surg* 24:174–184, 2010.

31. Beaufrère H, Rodriguez D, Pariaut R, et al: Estimating intrathoracic arterial diameter using CT angiography in Hispaniolan Amazon parrots (Amazona ventralis), *Am J Vet Res* 72:210–218, 2011.

32. van Nierop LE, Slottje P, van Zandvoort MJE, et al: Effects of magnetic stray fields from a 7 Tesla MRI scanner on neurocognition: a double-blind randomised crossover study, *Occup Environ Med* 69:759–766, 2012.

32a. Cao Z, Park J, Cho ZH, Collins CM: Numerical evaluation of image homogeneity, signal-to-noise ratio, and specific absorption rate for human brain imaging at 1.5, 3, 7, 10.5, and 14T in an 8-channel transmit/receive array, *J Magn Reson Imaging* 41(5):1432–1439, 2015. doi: 10.1002/jmri.24689. Epub 2014 Jun 27

33. Wallack S: Basic magnetic resonance imaging principles used for evaluating animal patients with neurologic disease, *Vet Clin North Am Exotic Pet Pract* 10:909–925, 2007.

34. Ludewig E, Krautwald-Junghanns ME: Magnetic Resonance Imaging (MRI). In Krautwald-Junghanns ME, Pees M, Reese S, Tully T, editors: *Diagnostic imaging of exotic pets*, Hannover, Germany, 2010, Schlütersche, pp 64–69.

35. Romagnano A, Shiroma JT, Heard DJ, et al: Magnetic Resonance Imaging of the brain and coelomic cavity of the domestic pigeon (Columba livia domestica), *Vet Radiol Ultrasound* 37:431–440, 1996.

36. Enders F, Jurina K, Straub J, et al: Magnetic resonance imaging in birds. In *Proceedings of the 6th biannual conference of the European association of avian veterinarians*, 2001, pp 87–91.

37. Janzen EG, Leeson S, Partlow GD, et al: *Cross-sectional anatomy of chickens: an atlas for magnetic resonance imaging*, Ontario, Canada, 1989, University of Guelph.

38. de Groof G, Verhoye M, van Meir V, et al: In vivo diffusion tensor imaging (DTI) of brain subdivisions and vocal pathways in songbirds, *Neuroimage* 29:754–763, 2006.

39. Fleming GJ, Lester NV, Stevenson R, et al: High field strength (4.7T) magnetic resonance imaging of hydrocephalus in an African grey parrot (Psittacus erithacus), *Vet Radiol Ultrasound* 44:542–545, 2003.

40. Keller KA, Guzman DSM, Muthuswamy A, et al: Hydrocephalus in a yellow-headed amazon parrot (Amazona ochrocephala oratrix), *J Avian Med Surg* 25:216–224, 2011.

41. Redig PT, Nicolas de Francisco O, Armién AG, et al: *Use of MRI and histological methods for detection of lead-induced lesions in the CNS of bald eagles*. Proceedings of the 31st Annual Conference of the Association of Avian Veterinarians, 2010, pp 33–34.

42. Stauber E, Holmes S, Deghetto DL, et al: Magnetic Resonance Imaging is superior to radiography in evaluating spinal cord trauma in three bald eagles (Haliaeetus leucocephalus), *J Avian Med Surg* 21:196–200, 2007.

43. Beaufrère H, Nevarez J, Gaschen L, et al: Diagnosis of presumed acute ischemic stroke and associated seizure management in a Congo African grey parrot, *J Am Vet Med Assoc* 239:122–128, 2011.

44. Wernick MB, Dennler M, Beckmann K, et al: Peripheral nerve sheath tumor in a subadult golden eagle (Aquila chrysaetos), *J Avian Med Surg* 28:57–63, 2014.

45. Morgan RV, Donnell RL, Daniel GB, et al: Magnetic resonance imaging of the normal eye and orbit of a screech owl (Otus asio), *Vet Radiol Ultrasound* 35:362–367, 1994.

46. Pye GW, Bennet RA, Newell SM, et al: Magnetic resonance imaging in psittacine birds with chronic sinusitis, *J Avian Med Surg* 14:243–256, 2000.

47. van Ruijssevelt L, van der Kant A, de Groof G, et al: Current state-of-the-art of auditory functional MRI (fMRI) on zebra finches: technique and scientific achievements, *J Physiol Paris* 107:156–169, 2013.

48. de Groof G, Jonckers E, Güntürkün O, et al: Functional MRI and functional connectivity of the visual system of awake pigeons, *Behav Brain Res* 239:43–50, 2013.

49. Lautenschlager S, Bright JA, Rayfield EJ: Digital dissection—using contrast-enhanced computed tomography scanning to elucidate hard- and soft-tissue anatomy in the common buzzard Buteo buteo, *J Anat* 224:412–431, 2014.

50. Barber D, Roberts R. Imaging: nuclear, *Vet Radiol Ultrasound* 24:50–57, 1983.

51. Balogh L, Andocs G, Thuroczy J, et al: Veterinary nuclear medicine: scintigraphical examinations—a review, *Acta Vet Brno* 68:231–239, 1999.

52. Degernes LA, Fisher PE, Trogdon M, et al: *Gastrointestinal scintigraphy in psittacines*. Proceedings of the 20th Annual Conference of the Association of Avian Veterinarians, 1999, pp 93–94.

53. Grizzle J, Hadley TL, Rotstein DS, et al: Effects of dietary milk thistle on blood parameters, liver pathology and hepatobiliary scintigraphy in white Carneaux pigeons (Columba livia) challenges with B1 aflatoxin, *J Avian Med Surg* 23:114–124, 2009.

54. Hadley TL, Daniel GB, Rotstein DS, et al: Evaluation of hepatobiliary scintigraphy as an indicator of hepatic function in domestic pigeons (Columba livia domestica) before and after exposure to ethylene glycol, *Vet Radiol Ultrasound* 48:155–162, 2007.

55. Marshall KL, Craig LE, Jones MP, et al: Quantitative renal scintigraphy in domestic pigeons (Columba livia domestica) exposed to toxic doses of gentamicin, *Am J Vet Res* 4:453–462, 2003.

56. Radin MJ, Hoepf TM, Swayne DE, et al: Use of a single injection solute-clearance method for determination of glomerular filtration rate and effective renal plasma flow in chickens, *Lab Anim Sci* 43:594–596, 1993.

57. Harms CA, Hoskinson JJ, Bruyette DS, et al: Technetium-99m and iodine-131 thyroid scintigraphy in normal and radiothyroidectomized cockatiels (Nymphicus hollandicus), *Vet Radiol Ultrasound* 35:473–478, 1994.

58. Mayer J, DeCubellis J, Rau S, et al: *Management of osteosarcoma in a grey goose*. Proceedings of the 30th Annual Conference of the Association of Avian Veterinarians, 2009, pp 335–336.

59. Goggin JM, Hoskinson JJ, Carpenter JW, et al: Scintigraphic assessment of digital extremity perfusion in 17 patients, *Vet Radiol Ultrasound* 38:211–220, 2005.

60. Jones MP, Orosz SE, Richman LK, et al: Pulmonary carcinoma with metastasis in a Moluccan cockatoo (Cacatua moluccensis), *J Avian Med Surg* 15:107–113, 2001.

61. Lung N, Ackerman N: *Scintigraphy as a tool in avian orthopedic diagnosis*. Proceedings of the 14th Annual Conference of the Association of Avian Veterinarians, 1993, p 45.

62. Wiley JL, Whittington JK, Wilmes CM, et al: Chronic myelogenous leukemia in a great horned owl (Bubo virginianus), *J Avian Med Surg* 23:36–43, 2009.

63. Martlé V, Peremans K, van Ham L, et al: High-resolution micro-SPECT to evaluate the regional brain perfusion in the adult Beagle dog, *Res Vet Sci* 94:701–706, 2013.

64. LeBlanc AK, Peremans K: PET and SPECT imaging in veterinary medicine, *Semin Nucl Med* 44:47–56, 2014.

65. Myers R, Hume S: Small animal PET, *Eur Neuropsychopharmacol* 12:545–555, 2002.

66. Converse AK, McCutcheon RA, Sladky KK, et al: 2-Deoxy-2-[18F]fluoro-d-glucose positron emission tomography imaging of parrot brain, *Mol Imaging Biol* 7:1536–1632, 2005.

67. Paul-Murphy J, Converse AK, Sladky KK, et al: *Using positron emission tomography imaging of the parrot brain to understand response to painful arthritis*, 2005, Association of Zoo Veterinarians. Association of Wildlife Veterinarians and Nutritional Advisory Group Annual Conference, pp 140–141.

68. Paul-Murphy J, McCutcheon RA, Standing B, et al: *Functional imaging of the avian brain during pain*. Proceedings of the 28th Annual Conference of the Association of Avian Veterinarians, 2007, pp 3–5.

69. Marzluff JM, Miyaoka R, Minoshima S, et al: Brain imaging reveals neuronal circuitry underlying the crow's perception of human faces, *Proc Natl Acad Sci USA* 19:15912–15917, 2012.

70. Grunkemeyer VL, Jones MP, Greenacre CB, et al: *Humeral air sac cystadenocarcinoma in a Moluccan cockatoo (Cacatua moluccensis) monitored via serial 18F-fluorodeoxyglucose integrated positron emission tomography—computed tomography scans*. Proceedings of the 31st Annual Conference of the Association of Avian Veterinarians, 2010, pp 343–344.

71. Souza MJ, Greenacre CB, Jones MP, et al: *Clinical use of Micro PET and CT imaging in birds*. Proceedings of the 27th Annual Conference of the Association of Avian Veterinarians, 2006, pp 13–16.

72. Souza MJ, Newman SJ, Greenacre CB, et al: Diffuse intestinal T-cell lymphosarcoma in a yellow-naped Amazon parrot (Amazona ochrocephala auropalliata), *J Vet Diagn Invest* 20:656–660, 2008.

73. Souza MJ, Wall JS, Stuckey A, et al: Static and dynamic 18FDG-PET in normal Hispaniolan Amazon parrots (Amazona ventralis), *Vet Radiol Ultrasound* 52:340–344, 2011.

74. Jones MP, Morandi F, Wall JS, et al: Distribution of 2-deoxy-2-fluoro-d-glucose in the coelom of healthy bald eagles (Haliaeetus leucocephalus), *Am J Vet Res* 74:426–432, 2013.

CHAPTER 15

Management and Medicine of Backyard Poultry

Patricia Wakenell

The term "poultry" includes all species of birds that can be consumed for food. Traditional poultry species are the chicken, turkey, duck, and goose. Other species such as pheasants, quail, chukar partridges, pigeons, guinea fowl, and ratites have variable popularity dependent on cultural tradition, geographic location, and availability. "Backyard" or "pet" poultry loosely refers to any of the above species of birds that are maintained for pleasure and/or small-scale sale of birds, meat, or eggs. Often included are those birds owned by breeders and exhibitors of fancy poultry and small commercial operators selling to niche markets (e.g., live bird markets, range eggs, local production). In contrast, the commercial poultry industry is a billion dollar business involving large numbers of birds worldwide. The industry is split into meat (broiler chickens, turkeys, ducks, and geese) and egg-laying (table-egg and breeder) types of birds. Large meat-bird operations are generally vertically integrated—the company controls all aspects of production from hatch to processing. Chicken farms maintained for table-egg production are often individually owned, but may market their eggs cooperatively. Breeding is centralized with only a few primary breeders controlling the pedigreed genetic stock. Commercial companies often employ contract farms that are owned by an individual farmer; however, the birds belong to the larger commercial entity.

CHICKEN-RELATED TERMINOLOGY

Young female chicks are called pullets, young males are called cockerels, adult males are called cocks or roosters, and adult females are called hens. A genetic female chicken with a male phenotype is called a pollard. Broiler is a meat chicken approximately 2.27 kg (5 pounds) live weight at slaughter and a roaster is a meat chicken 2.72 to 3.63 kg (6 to 8 pounds) live weight at slaughter. Chooks are the popular Australian term for chickens. A capon is a castrated male. Alektorophobia is the fear of chickens. The pecking order is a descriptive term for the dominance hierarchical system of the social organization in chickens. Chickens that have no feathers growing from their shanks are referred to as clean legged, whereas feather-legged breeds, such as Cochins or Brahmas, do have feathers. The crest refers to the puff of feathers on the heads of breeds such as Houdan, Silkie, or Polish, and is also called a "topknot."

Feathers that curl rather than lay flat are referred to as frizzle feathers, and this term is also a common show category. The saddle is the part of a chicken's back just before the tail. The shank is the part of a chicken's leg between the foot and ankle, called the tarsometatarsus. A sex feather is a hackle, saddle, or tail feather that is rounded in a hen but usually pointed in a rooster. Sickles are the long, curved tail feathers of some roosters. Turkeys have a snood, which is a long fleshy appendage attached to the face behind the nares. The snood has no known use but can be raised and lowered at will.

Cannibalism is the general term used to describe chickens eating each other's flesh, feathers, or eggs. A pickout or peckout specifically describes cannibalism at the vent. Hatch refers to either the process by which a chick comes out of the egg or a group of chicks that come out of their shells at approximately the same time. A batch of eggs that are hatched together, either in a nest or in an incubator, is termed a clutch. A nest egg is an artificial egg placed in a nest to encourage hens to lay there. A straight run refers to a clutch of newly hatched chicks that have not been sexed. A hen that is no longer laying well is referred to as spent. Tiny eggs that have been quickly passed through the oviduct without reaching full size may be referred to as fart eggs, rooster eggs, or oops eggs.

MANAGEMENT
Housing

Poultry are adaptable to a wide variety of housing, and there are many designs to the buildings mostly because of aesthetic reasons rather than a specific need. Generally, the variables that should drive the choice of housing are climate, bird type, number of different species owned, and neighbors. Housing that has an outdoor component will require protection from predators with a fenced roof and fenced siding and side fences set into the ground at least 1 foot (30.5 cm).[1-3]

Most adult poultry are able to withstand climate changes, with the exception of extremely hot or cold regions. If birds are not ill and are completely feathered (not in molt), heating of buildings is not required (certain breeds can be more cold resistant than others). In fact, housing is often sealed too tightly to retain heat, resulting in lack of adequate ventilation, which causes the onset of respiratory disease. Ventilation is crucially important in all climates.[2] If bird density is high, then better ventilation and more frequent cleaning are necessary. Lack of proper ventilation will result in the buildup of ammonia. High levels of ammonia destroy the cilia on the trachea and allow viruses and bacteria free entry into the lower respiratory tract. In hot climates, forced ventilation (fans) and misters may be necessary to reduce heat. Swamp coolers that cool air by forcing the air over cold water can be inexpensive and beneficial.

In cold climates, often the combined body heat of the birds will be sufficient to keep them warm. Additional heat can be provided by a red heat lamp often used for the posthatch period or heated floor mats (Figure 15-1). For both types of heating, extra caution must be taken to not overheat the birds or cause a fire hazard from flammable materials (shavings and wood) touching a heat source. The flock behavior will be evidence of overheating. If the heat is a point source, birds will crowd away from the source. With central heat, the birds will crowd near exits, windows, and outside walls. If birds are housed entirely outside, a source of shade is necessary. If birds are raised for show, sun exposure can cause the feathers to change color and result in disqualification. All housing should be predator proof. This may require sinking walls 12 or more inches (30.5 cm) in the ground, using concrete aprons surrounding the buildings, or raised wire floors.

Bird type will help determine the type of housing required. Most breeds of chickens are hardy although meat-type birds are usually sturdier than egg layers. Show breeds often do not have hybrid vigor and require heated or cooled housing. Be sure to check the normal space requirements for the birds—these may not be exclusively determined by the size of the bird but also by activity levels. Commercial breeds of turkeys often will be frightened by loud and unusual noises, sometimes causing them to pile in corners and suffocate. Heavier breeds can damage their feet jumping down from perches that are too high and smaller birds can become trapped in corners and small spaces.

For all perching birds, perches need to be round, rough, and placed so that when the birds jump down they will not land on hard surfaces or sharp objects. Covering wooden dowels with artificial turf helps provide the roughness for removing extra keratin on the surfaces of the feet (Figure 15-2). If birds are nesting, at least two nest boxes for flocks of three to five hens and one additional nest box for every two to three hens will help reduce fighting for nest space.

Mixing species of birds is a common, but risky, practice in backyard operations. Certain species are more aggressive and "lifestyles" may not be compatible (ducks and geese water play, creating an environment that is too moist for chickens). Some species can carry diseases that do not affect them but will be harmful to other species (e.g., histomoniasis). It is best to have individual housing units for each species. If this is not possible, keep the most valuable (economically or emotionally) species in separate housing.

In highly populated areas, both poultry and human neighbors are a concern. Poultry create a tremendous amount of dust and feather debris and are a magnet for flies and other insects. Indoor housing reduces these problems and noise concerns. Many communities ban ownership of roosters and peafowl. Neighboring poultry are a disease risk, and housing should be placed as far away as possible and upwind from these areas. Chickens will destroy all vegetation, so the outside area is often either dusty or muddy. Absorbent material, such as wood shavings, can be helpful for controlling wet ground.

Choosing Stock: Hatch or Buy?

It is always a good practice for clients to use the same degree of care in choosing the species and/or breed of poultry as they would exercise in choosing any other companion animal.[2,4] Commercial types of birds are genetically selected to optimize their function, meat or egg production, and should not be recommended for the average backyard operation. A commercial broiler is genetically selected to reach market weight in 6 to 7 weeks and will continue to grow if not processed at that time. Without significant feed restriction, "old" broilers will rapidly outgrow the ability of their legs and cardiopulmonary systems to support their weight. Most noncommercial chicken breeds are dual-purpose breeds that offer both good egg production and adequate meat. Generally, laying-type breeds are more active and lighter weight but can be more aggressive. Meat breeds are less commonly kept in backyard

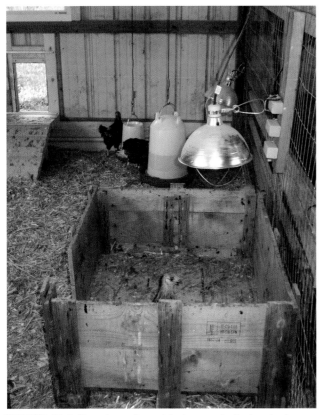

FIGURE 15-1 Heat lamp for added warmth during inclement weather.

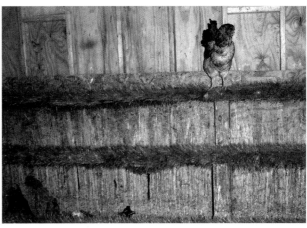

FIGURE 15-2 Artificial turf on perch.

settings but are usually calmer and less aggressive. Dual-purpose breeds offer a happy medium between the two.

Probably the largest determinant to the decision of buying hatched chicks or hatching your own is the size of the flock that is desired. For small flocks, inexpensive incubator/hatchers that are easy to operate are available either at farm stores or through mail-order catalogs. When first starting out, as many as 50% of the eggs may not hatch, making egg space a concern if a large hatch is needed. Most inexpensive incubators have good temperature control but inadequate control of humidity.[5] Chicken eggs can withstand shifts in humidity during incubation. Other species such as turkeys, however, are much more sensitive to fluctuations in humidity during incubation. In the commercial industry, chicken eggs are switched from the incubator to the hatcher at 18 days of embryonation (incubation to hatch = 21 days). This is done primarily to keep down and egg debris from contaminating the incubators, to prevent chicks from falling to the bottom of the incubator, and to change temperature and humidity requirements between incubation and hatching.

These changes are not necessarily required for hatching, but optimize the hatch for commercial companies. With home incubators, temperatures should be regulated for at least 2 to 3 days before the eggs are placed. During incubation, the temperature should be checked twice daily (fluctuations between 98° F [36.7° C] and 101° F [38.3° C] are fine for chicken eggs, but temperature requirements for other species should be researched before incubation) and the water pan kept full. Eggs (except dark shelled) should be candled at least once during incubation. Candling consists of shining a light through the egg to determine embryo viability by detecting movement of the embryo and presence of blood vessels. Dead eggs can then be removed before possibly exploding. Eggs need to be turned approximately four times a day until the last few days before hatch (embryonation Day 18 for chicken eggs). If eggs do not hatch, examination of the dead embryos can yield some clues to the cause.

Common problems with the hatch include (1) early deaths (infertile eggs, too long or improper storage of eggs prior to incubation, and extreme temperature fluctuation), (2) late deaths but not pipped (extreme temperature fluctuation and poor humidity), (3) pipped but dried and stuck to the egg shell (generally poor humidity in late incubation and hatching period, and can also be due to weakened embryos from temperature fluctuations), and (4) pipped but drowned in egg fluids or malpositioned embryos (turning malfunction during incubation).[6] Once chicks are hatched, they should not be moved until dry and fluffed (Figure 15-3). Occasionally chicks will hatch that have not completely absorbed their yolk sac and/or intestines. These chicks should be euthanized. Euthanizing newly hatched chicks to 10 days of age can be accomplished by cervical dislocation. One practical method is to take a scissors handle (ones that close completely opposed to each other), place directly behind the skull, and squeeze together to cervically dislocate. Embryonated eggs are best euthanized by chilling (as discussed in Chapter 22). If possible, all chicken chicks should be vaccinated for Marek's disease within 24 hours post hatch (see Disease Prevention and Control).

If chicks are obtained from an outside source, efforts should be made to receive them as soon as possible after hatch (unless they are raised at the hatchery). Chicks can withstand

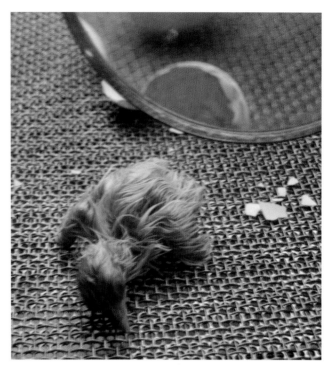

FIGURE 15-3 Newly hatched, wet baby chick.

a period of 24 to 48 hours post hatch without food or water if they are kept warm. Longer periods will result in weakened and immunocompromised birds. Chickens acquired from the hatchery should be vaccinated for Marek's disease and, for all species, it is recommended to inquire about which vaccinations the hens have received (chicks get their antibodies from the hens via the yolk). This information can be important when making decisions in some flock management situations. Chicks need to be shipped without feed or water and in a container labeled prominently "do not feed or water," because they can drown in very small amounts of liquid.

For commercial flocks, chicks and poults are sexed at hatch by manual inspection of the vent or feathering. As the birds grow, it is difficult to determine sex until secondary sex characteristics become apparent. In some strains, sex can be visually determined by using sex-linked traits such as color or feathering. Two common varieties are the black sex link and the red sex link. Blacks are a cross between a Rhode Island Red or New Hampshire rooster and a Barred Rock hen. Black sex-linked males have white natal down on their heads, whereas hens do not. Red sex links are a cross between a Rhode Island Red or New Hampshire rooster and a White Rock, Silver Laced Wyandotte, Rhode Island White, or Delaware hen. Red sex-linked hens have red natal down, whereas the males are white/yellow. With adult birds, the phallus can be observed by eversion of the vent (all that is needed in waterfowl where the organ is easily visible) and manual stimulation (chickens and turkeys). Male chickens and turkeys do not have an actual phallus but have two dorsal papillae that can be observed after eversion of the vent.[7]

Rearing and Feeding

All young poultry need a source of heat until fully feathered.[8,9] The least expensive option is to arrange a screen-covered heat lamp so that the distance from floor to lamp is 18 inches (45.72 cm) to 2½ feet (76.2 cm) depending on the lamp wattage. The lamp should be red rather than white to discourage cannibalism in older chicks. Floor temperature should be approximately 100° F (37.8° C) directly under the lamp. A round, 1- to 2-foot-high (30.4 to 60.1 cm) brooder ring is placed under the lamp to keep chicks from straying too far from the heat source (Figure 15-4). It is unwise to use a square enclosure because some species will pile in corners and suffocate or suffer from hypothermia. This ring can be removed after the first week. The best rule of thumb for achieving the proper temperature is observing the distribution of the chicks at rest under the lamp. Chicks should be in an even and fanned pattern outward from the lamp. If they are piled under the lamp, the temperature is too cold; if they are pressed against the brooder ring, the temperature is too hot.

Most young poultry species need some introduction to feed and water. If the flock size is large, about 25% of the flock can have "formal instruction" and those can be counted on to "teach" the rest. Instruction consists of dipping the beak into the water and then the feed. The appearance of the shiny drop of water and/or feed on the beak will also encourage exploration of these new objects by other chicks. It is best to place the feed into egg trays or flat low-sided dishes for the first week. Chicks continually peck at objects around their toes and will become familiar with the feed by this method. Feeding trays can be kept in the ring at the same time, and they will learn to eat from these gradually. Feeder trays are covered to keep the older chicks from scratching out feed and wasting it. In addition, older birds need feeders and waterers raised from ground level to be approximately equal to the thoracic inlet to help prevent fecal contamination. Waterers must have a small lip for the chicks to drink from, and it should be smaller if the species has tiny chicks. Generally waterers are bell shaped, allowing water from the center holder to refill the lip as needed. Water sources that are big enough for the chicks to fall into should be avoided. Newly hatched chicks are unstable on their feet and have trouble righting themselves if flipped over. This can result in mass drowning if waterers consist of open dishes. If this is a concern, placing brightly colored marbles or stones in the waterers reduces the depth of the water and the possibility of entrapment. Gradually, the feeders and waterers can be replaced with larger units to accommodate the growing birds.

The number of different feed types can be overwhelming for the novice, and veterinarians should familiarize themselves with what is available in their area.[9] Generally, feed falls into three growth-related categories: starter, finisher, or meat builder and laying/breeding ration. It is extremely important to buy the right feed for the right growth stage, particularly for breeder/layer hens. When in doubt, it is best to choose a name brand feed supplied in a labeled bag. When purchasing bulk feed from a feed mill or farm store, it is recommended to see the label (or nutrient list) from the feed mix and/or obtain a copy. Often problems occur when inexperienced store clerks sell feed that is different from what the consumer expects. Scratch or single-source feeds (corn only) are not advisable unless used only as a supplement to the complete feed. Birds will preferentially eat the scratch, so it should not be offered until the nutritionally balanced feed is consumed. Laying birds must have calcium supplementation and layer ration. Another feed option is medicated feed. This is a general term used to describe feeds that have either anticoccidials or antibiotics added or both. For pet poultry, the addition of anticoccidials is recommended because of the prevalence of coccidiosis in backyard flocks. Feed containing antibiotics will need to be prescribed by a veterinarian, but these additives can be useful in situations where posthatch mortality is high from bacterial infections.

Adulthood

Management changes during the adult stage need to address adequacy of housing and feed adjustment, as described earlier. For laying hens, nest boxes that are just large enough to fit one "seated" hen are desirable (Figure 15-5).[6] If eggs are to be collected only for consumption, then efforts need to be made to curb broodiness in the hens. The term "broody" refers to a hen that stops laying eggs to sit on the eggs, even when there are none in the nest box. As soon as this behavior is noticed, the hen should be moved to a wire cage. Broody hens can be aggressive, so caution must be taken during handling.

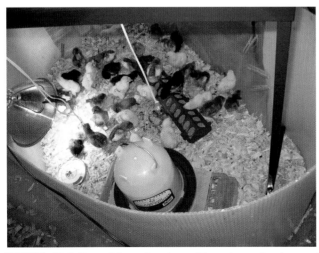

FIGURE 15-4 Round brooder ring with waterer, feeder, and heat lamp.

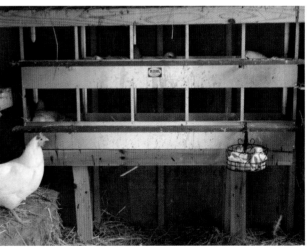

FIGURE 15-5 Nest boxes appropriate for a single laying hen.

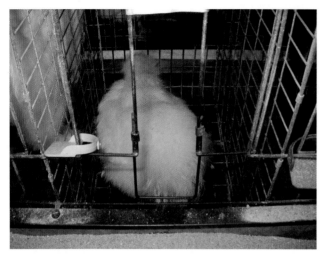

FIGURE 15-6 Broody Silkie hen placed in a cage to discourage broodiness.

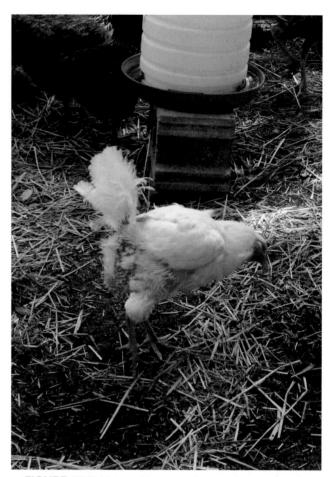

FIGURE 15-7 Unusual but not abnormal natural molt.

Most hens treated this way will recover from their broodiness in 2 to 3 days. Without intervention, hens may remain broody for 3 to 4 weeks. Broodiness is breed dependent, with Silkies having the highest incidence (Figure 15-6). Artificial lighting will increase the number of eggs laid during the winter months, but will not increase the total number of eggs laid by the hen.[10] Light schedules for laying hens are usually 13-hour days or lights are kept on all night. Supplemented lighting will increase the risk of cannibalism in birds that are not individually caged. In general, light is progressively decreased throughout the growing period and is changed to a progressive increase at sexual maturity. The average targets for the start of increased lighting are 20 weeks for layer pullets and 23 weeks for meat pullets. These can vary depending on the season and the breed. Commercial chickens used for table-egg production are kept in lay for approximately 1 year and then are usually force molted. Broiler breeders rarely are kept in production longer than 44 weeks (layer breeders generally 52 weeks). Pullets used for table-egg production are usually caged and those used for production of hatching eggs are usually floor maintained with nest box access. Breeder pullets must be taught to use the nest box to prevent floor eggs.

In commercial laying operations, hens are force molted by reducing light and providing low nutrition feed to bring the whole flock into molt at the same time.[10] This way commercial farmers provide a needed rest for the birds and can concurrently be sure that all hens are fed appropriately. Often backyard flocks will undergo a 3- to 4-month or longer molt period. As long as feather loss is not associated with ectoparasite infestation, reddened or abraded skin, poor nutrition, or open wounds, an "unusual molt" can be assumed for lengthy or bizarre-appearing feather loss (Figure 15-7). All hens need to be molted after approximately a year in lay. Hens need this rest period to rebuild calcium and energy stores. If hens do not molt naturally, then reduction of light will usually stimulate them to do so. If desired, this is also the time period that hens can be culled from the flock. In general, even the best hens will only approach about 70% of their former production level in their subsequent production period. Chickens that are fed xanthophyll-containing feeds will continually

blanch (skin, shanks, and beak) throughout lay. The vent in a laying hen will be larger, moist, and pliable compared with a small, hard, and puckered vent in a nonlayer. The easiest way to determine lay on farm is to palpate the pubic bones. The bones in a nonlayer almost meet just below the vent, whereas the layer will have a "2 to 3 finger spread." The comb and wattles will be large, smooth, and firm in a layer and shriveled in nonlayers. When a hen lays an egg, her vent will evert to allow passage of the egg without contamination by feces. Once the egg is laid, her vent will usually return to the normal position quickly.

Breeding

Most backyard flock clients will be satisfied with random, natural mating in their flocks. With chickens and turkeys, the phallus does not actually penetrate the vagina; rather, the female cloaca everts exposing the vaginal opening and the male deposits the semen at the opening via gravity. If specific breeding is needed for breed maintenance, artificial insemination can be used. Turkey breeders virtually require artificial insemination because their size makes natural mating difficult. Artificial insemination is also used by many meat chicken primary breeders. The male is stimulated either by rubbing the back at the base of the tail and gently squeezing behind the tail or by massaging the soft part of the abdomen toward the vent. Semen quantity will be approximately 0.75 mL from the rooster and a little less from the tom. The semen needs to be used immediately because semen storage does not maintain adequate quality for most avian species.

NATIONAL POULTRY IMPROVEMENT PLAN

The National Poultry Improvement Plan (NPIP) is a voluntary cooperative plan involving State and Federal governments and the poultry industry.[11] It was started in 1935 to coordinate State control of *Salmonella pullorum* and it is aimed at reducing/eliminating predominantly vertically transmitted diseases in breeder flocks. Since its inception, the incidence of *S. pullorum* and *Salmonella gallinarum* has been significantly reduced. States may require that chickens/turkeys entering the state be from NPIP participants, or be proven free of certain diseases. NPIP is primarily aimed at preventing vertically transmitted diseases, but it does have a provision for monitoring low pathogenicity avian influenza (LPAI). The plan is administered by the United States Department of Agriculture (USDA) Animal and Plant Health Inspection Service and "Official State Agencies" (usually the poultry association in the State or the State Veterinarian). Producers sign onto state participation plans and the rules are outlined in the #9CFR Sections 145 and 147. Producers with farms in multiple states can establish cooperative agreements between the states. Backyard poultry owners who have breeding birds can become NPIP participants through Section E for exhibition birds. In addition to providing assurances of a commitment to health and disease prevention to customers purchasing chicks or eggs, NPIP is an amazing source of information on biosecurity, disease prevention, maintenance of flock health, and management.

MANAGEMENT-RELATED ILLNESS

Cannibalism

Pecking or cannibalism is one of the most frustrating and difficult problems to control in floor-reared birds. Certain species such as pheasants and quail are notorious for cannibalism, often leading to the use of individual cages as the only housing option. Even within a species, certain breeds can be more aggressive than others. Cannibalism usually does not begin in earnest under 2 to 3 weeks of age. If observed in young chicks, it is generally the result of insufficient feed or diarrhea (soiled vents can be attractive pecking sites). In older birds, methods of controlling pecking and cannibalism include reduction of lighting, reduction of bird density, increased numbers of feeders, and trimming the beaks. If a bird has been pecked, spraying the affected area with pruning tar (used for trees) is a good, practical at-home solution. The tar protects the skinless area from fluid loss, is nontoxic even when used on open wounds, and has the advantage of "identifying" the perpetrators by staining their beaks black. Pruning tar can be used for large areas as long as the deeper body cavities have not been penetrated. More severe wounds may be treated with a variety of bandages, appropriate pain management, supportive care, and surgical closure. If small numbers of birds are the aggressors, these birds can be given red spectacles that attach to their nares or be fitted with red contact lenses (available at most poultry supply stores).

Trauma

This is the most common "disease" condition of pet poultry and includes predator injury, entrapment of limbs in cages or other equipment, cannibalism, crushing injuries (e.g., stepped on, trapped in doors), and self-trauma (from spurs, beak, and nails). Most adult poultry are highly resilient and seem to recover from extensive injuries. Supportive therapy that can be accomplished at home includes providing warmth (via brooder lamp), providing adequate hydration (powdered milk at half-concentration provides extra protein), and force-feeding warm molasses-sweetened feed. If a pet bird owner is force-feeding, he should select a soft, flexible feeding tube and place it into the esophagus just past the laryngeal opening. Since most poultry have a crop, the food will enter the crop first, allowing for a slower filling of the proventriculus. The tube should not be forced because lacerations of the cervical esophagus or crop and subsequent fungal/yeast infections can result (Figure 15-8). Aspiration and regurgitation are also risks associated with force-feeding procedures. Wounds that are not penetrating into the respiratory or abdominal cavities can typically be treated with topicals and basic wound care and management procedures. Parenteral antibiotics may not be required for treatment of many wounds. Most poultry will show evidence of recovery in 2 to 3 days. After this period of time, the prognosis for full recovery is generally poor, without more intensive veterinary care.

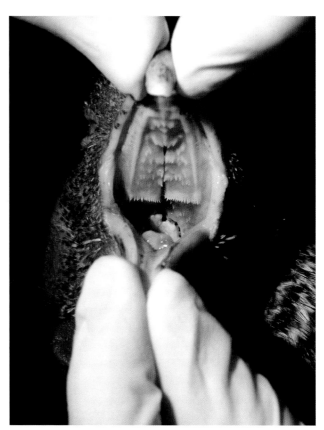

FIGURE 15-8 Fungal plaque resulting from injury caused by feeding tube at the caudal oropharynx.

Bumblefoot

Bumblefoot is an inflammatory condition of the foot characterized by swelling, ulceration, and erythema.[12] It is commonly localized to the plantar metatarsal pad or plantar digital pads. Primary foot trauma at the weight-bearing aspects of the foot is followed by secondary bacterial infections (Figure 15-9). *Staphylococcus* sp. and *Escherichia coli* are the more commonly identified infectants. Heavy-bodied species are at the greatest risk, and trauma can be from puncture (direct inoculation) or from pressure necrosis. There is no age predisposition for bumblefoot, but common contributors to the condition include poor perch design, untrimmed claws, hypovitaminosis A, and poor weight management of birds. The epidermis is thicker in areas of pressure and plantar scabs inhibit healing and cause pressure ischemia. Heterophils can ingest *Staphylococcus*, but the enzymatic degradation is not efficient because of their lack of a specific lysozyme and dependence on other enzymes to kill bacteria. Acute infections are more often associated with caseous necrosis rather than purulent and liquefied exudate. Soaking the foot in magnesium sulfate (Epsom salts) twice a day for 10 minutes can help remove the scabs. Topical antibacterials and bandaging are usually sufficient for most poultry. Appropriate analgesia should be a part of most treatment regimes. Pressure and weight-deferring bandages can add great benefit by functionally removing any further pressure on the lesions as they are treated and given time to heal. There is a direct venous return from the foot to the kidney in birds and oral antibiotics may be needed to prevent systemic infection. The prognosis for successful treatment declines when there is osteomyelitis.

Fatty Liver

Although all laying birds retain more fat in their livers than nonlayers or males, this condition is characterized by extreme fat deposition, sudden drop in egg production, and increased mortality.[7] The hens are often obese, have pale combs, and wattles and combs may be covered with dandruff. The etiology is thought to be a combination of fatty feed consumption and decreased exercise. Birds that are kept as house pets and are fed table scraps are at high risk for this condition. Mortality is a result of liver rupture and hemorrhaging with large blood clots found in the abdomen on postmortem examination (Figure 15-10). Treatment is by prevention—most backyard birds have adequate access to exercise but diet needs to be controlled. Lipotropic agents and dietary supplements (alfalfa, wheat bran, fish meal, dried brewer's yeast, soybean mill feed, vitamin E, and torula yeast) have been used with sporadic results.

Caged-Layer Fatigue (Osteoporosis)

Caged-layer fatigue is similar to milk fever in mammals.[7] It is common in chickens, coturnix quail, and khaki Campbell ducks. Birds are unable to stand and have brittle bones. The ribs are often caved in or fractured at the junction of the sternal and vertebral components. Paralyzed birds are alert and responsive unless dehydrated from inability to access water. The probable causes are vitamin D_3, calcium, and phosphorus deficiencies and/or imbalances. Birds may die acutely (often from fractured spinal vertebrae and severed spinal cords) or can rapidly recover (4 to 7 days) after placement on the floor with easy access to food and water. With backyard poultry, treatment with intramuscular vitamin D_3 or intravenous calcium gluconate can be helpful. Where indicated, appropriate analgesia should be a part of the treatment plan. Oyster shell can be added to the diet *ad libitum* to prevent this condition. The oyster shell must not be ground so small that it passes through the intestinal tract because it needs to be retained in the gizzard. The strain of bird and type of housing also affect the incidence of the condition. The key is to ensure good nutrition (and good cortical bone formation) prior to onset of lay. However, increased calcium in the diet for too long prior to production can result in urolithiasis and/or a permanent cessation of parathyroid gland activity.

"Vent Blow-Out" or Cloacal Prolapse

Normally the vent will prolapse during delivery of the egg. However, slow retraction due to obesity or in poorly developed hens (those that came into lay too early) will attract cannibalism, trauma, and edema formation, which will often

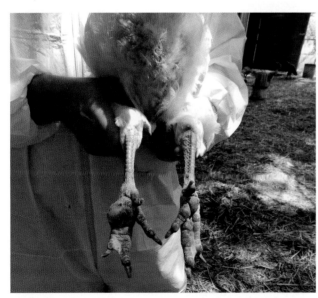

FIGURE 15-9 Bumblefoot caused by poor perch design.

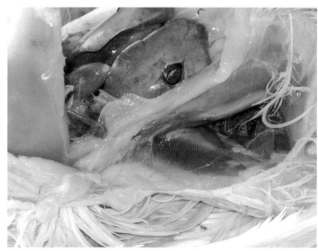

FIGURE 15-10 Fatty liver with previous healed intrahepatic hemorrhage.

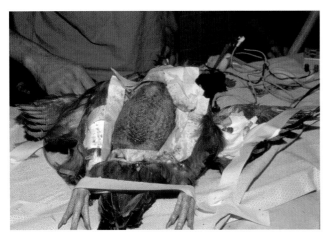

FIGURE 15-11 Hen being prepped for a midventral approach for surgical address of oviductal impaction with an infected egg.

prevent retraction.[7] Normally, these chickens are culled and prevention is practiced by controlling obesity, stocking density of cages, lighting, precocious onset of lay, and proper beak trimming. For pet poultry, stopping lay (reduced light and sharp reduction in feed), isolation, and keeping the vent clean until retracted will sometimes be effective in mild cases. In more severe cases of cloacal prolapse, medical and surgical options may be pursued. If chicks are hatched in the fall, an increase of light in the early spring can induce them to come into lay when they are physically immature, predisposing those young hens to prolapse. Controlling light is extremely important in this circumstance.

Egg Binding and Dystocia

Again, this is seen most commonly in pullets that are brought into production too early or in hens that are obese.[7] Ranges of this condition can be from a temporary binding observed in pullets that lay large eggs to complete obstruction of the oviduct. There can be eggs in the abdominal cavity (refluxed); single or multiple eggs in the oviduct; or shell membranes, shells, and yolk/albumin concretions in the oviduct. Egg binding and dystocia can be seen concurrently with other reproductive tract disease. The impaction can generally be identified upon abdominal palpation, ultrasound, and/or radiographic examination. Commercial hens are culled. Medical and surgical management methods vary from the conservative provision of warmth and massaging the abdomen, to using analgesia, parenteral fluids, manual obstetrical delivery methods, salpingotomy, and salpingohysterectomy (Figure 15-11). After removal of the oviduct, other reproductive problems can be seen because the hypothalamic-pituitary-gonadal axis remains intact. Internally ovulated ova may be absorbed or can lead to egg-yolk coelomitis. Cystic ovarian disease may be seen and ovarian neoplasia still can ultimately be encountered. Some salpingo-hysterectomized hens will assume male characteristics (crowing, aggression, and spurs) after surgery and these birds are called pollards.

BIOSECURITY

Losses from disease can be reduced substantially if good biosecurity practices are followed.[13] The biggest single source of

pathogen entry is the introduction of other birds both from the same species and from different species. No person or animal should be allowed to visit the flock if they have recently been around other birds. Frequent transgressors are domestic animals (dogs and cats) and rodents. These animals can mechanically transmit disease or function as biological vectors. Attractants that bring animals to the area where birds are housed need to be removed. Feed must be kept in rodent-proof containers and spilled feed rapidly cleaned up. Carcasses should be removed immediately and disposed of appropriately (local regulations are important). If burial is chosen, carcasses can be covered with lime to reduce the likelihood of being dug up by animals or exploding out of the ground during the summer. Good rodenticide and insecticide programs, including monthly rotation of chemicals, are essential. Waterers and feeders must be cleaned daily and disinfected at least every 2 to 3 days and houses should be cleaned when litter becomes moist. Store feed in containers that are not exposed to the sun, which can cause condensation when the containers cool at night, resulting in subsequent mold growth. Use feed rapidly and store no more than a 1-week supply. Foot pans filled with a dilute iodine solution or diluted bleach can reduce the risk of carrying in infectious organisms on boots. When the iodinated water becomes clear, it needs to be replaced. Bleach water needs to be changed every 24 hours. All equipment must be thoroughly cleaned and disinfected before use. Organic matter left on equipment can render even the best disinfectant useless. Again, species should not be mixed and, in best conditions, ages should not be mixed as well.

All birds leaving the premises and encountering other birds (i.e., shows) and newly purchased birds should be quarantined for 6 weeks in a separate facility. Be sure not to use medicated feed during quarantine. Any equipment used at shows such as cages, feeders, waterers, and egg flats needs to be disinfected before storage or reuse. Be sure to check and service quarantined birds last.

Birds should never be purchased from auctions or sale barns. These birds are often sold because of "deficiencies," and they are housed with numerous other species, increasing the potential for infectious disease. Ideally, birds are purchased from a reputable supplier and preferably NPIP certified. A visit to the farm of origin, prior to purchase, can be helpful. NPIP breeders can be found through the USDA website http://poultryimprovement.org/statesContent.cfm. A good source of information is your state's poultry association.

DISEASE PREVENTION AND CONTROL
General Aspects

Most pet poultry, unless used for show, rarely encounter the same intensity of disease exposure as commercial poultry. Many "disease" conditions are actually the result of environmental or feed mismanagement or are unusual presentations of normal events (molt). Vaccinations, with a few exceptions, are unnecessary for resident birds and can be difficult to obtain in the proper dose size. Most vaccines are sold in bottles of 500 to 10,000 doses and mixing errors can be devastating. In addition, waterborne and foodborne medication is also frequently tailored for commercial flock sizes and dilution errors for small flocks are common. Be sure to document all dilution calculations in case of possible overdosing. In general, when using medications off-label, the dosage recommendations for cats work well for poultry. Poultry are considered food animals *even when they are pets*, and medications banned for use in food animals (e.g., enrofloxacin) must not be used in backyard poultry, even off-label. The following list of diseases is not meant to be comprehensive, but includes some of the more common conditions that are encountered in backyard poultry practice.

Parasitism

As in other species, the common poultry parasites are mites, lice, ticks, worms, and protozoa. Some parasites can present a public health concern and/or be transmissible to other food animals and pets (bed bugs). Regular monthly examinations by owners for external parasites are recommended. Parasites, both internal and external, can also be carriers of other disease agents.

Mites

Two common mites of poultry are the northern fowl mite (*Ornithonyssus sylviarum*) and the red mite (*Dermanyssus gallinae*).[14] The northern fowl mite lives on its host and is most commonly found around the vent, tail, and breast of the bird (Figure 15-12). They are easily observed and are a reddish brown color. The red mite does not live on its host and only feeds at night, making daytime diagnosis difficult. They can be found in cracks and seams near the bedding areas and appear as white fuzz balls or salt-and-pepper–like deposits. Red mites will cause feather loss, irritation, and anemia. Insecticides are available over the counter (OTC) in both powder and spray application for treatment of both mites. Do not use carbaryl powder (Sevin) either on the bird or on the premises. Either oral or injectable (200 µg/kg) ivermectin may be used off-label. Treatment with ivermectin should be monthly for at least 3 months even if mites are not observed. In flocks with a chronic or persistent problem with mites, monthly preventive treatment with OTC insecticides is recommended. Be sure to rotate the type of insecticide used to prevent resistance. Although poultry mites prefer to feed on poultry, they can

move onto humans and will bite if trapped by tight clothing or other binding objects such as casts.

Lice

There are several species of lice that live on poultry and lice or nits can be observed at the base of the feathers (see Figure 15-12).[14] With severe infestations, growth and egg production can be affected because the birds will become anemic. The previously mentioned insecticides used for mites are available for treatment and the same prevention methods for mites can be used for lice. Lice are obligate parasites of poultry and will not transfer to other species for any length of time.

Ticks

Fowl ticks comprise a group of soft ticks that parasitize many species of poultry and wild birds.[14] Ticks are easily missed because they spend relatively little time on the bird. Heavy infestations can cause anemia or tick paralysis and ticks can be vectors for *Borrelia anserina* (spirochetosis) among other diseases. Spraying of buildings with insecticide (not Sevin) is the treatment of choice. Chlorpyrifos, pyrethroids, or chlorpyrifos and dichlorvos combined can be used for houses that are not occupied. Professional pest control may be needed for frequently infested flocks.

Bed bugs

Bed bug (*Cimex lectularius*) infestation of commercial poultry houses is a sporadic condition but is of concern both because of public health aspects and difficulty in controlling the problem.[14,15] Bed bugs are reddish brown and approximately the size of ticks. Heavy infestations can cause a reduction in egg production, cloacal irritation, feather loss, and anemia. As with ticks, relatively little time is spent on the bird. Treatment of the house can be as described for ticks but pyrethroids generally do not work well for bed bugs. As with ticks, professional pest control treatment may be required.

Internal parasites

Large roundworms and tapeworms are the most common poultry worms and are generally the result of soil contamination and poor management.[16] Unless infestations are heavy, clinical disease is usually not evident (Figure 15-13). Piperazine

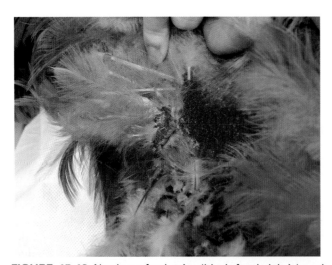

FIGURE 15-12 Northern fowl mite (black fecal debris) and lice nits (white nits at the base of the barbs at the rachis) with feather loss.

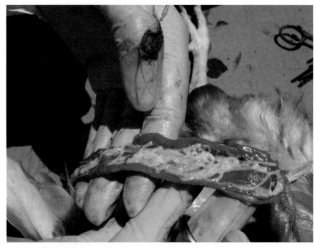

FIGURE 15-13 Tapeworms in the small intestine.

can be used for roundworms and dibutyltin dilaurate for tapes. Do not use these compounds in laying hens. Resistance to piperazine is common, and fenbendazole (10 to 50 mg/kg) may be used off-label and needs to be repeated 7 to 10 days later. Piperazine may stun tapeworms without killing them and whole, live worms may be found in the litter. Proper litter management will reduce parasite loads and reinfection. Yearly fecal examination is recommended to ascertain the endoparasite status of flocks.

Coccidia

Control of coccidia is one of the more costly problems of raising commercial and backyard poultry.[17] Coccidia are found primarily in the intestinal tract of most poultry, but occur in the kidney in geese. Coccidiosis is generally observed in young birds between the ages of 1 and 4 months. Birds under 1 week of age do not have chymotrypsin and bile salts for breaking apart oocysts and are not susceptible to disease. Coccidia are species specific. The disease causes diarrhea that is often bloody and frequently leads to death if not treated. Lesions in the intestinal tract vary with the species of coccidia involved, but the same treatment/preventive regimens can be used. Coccidia thrive in moist, heavily soiled litter and disease is often a result of too high a population density of birds. The kind of crowded housing found more often in winter months is an example of when population density may increase from acceptable to excessive. Poultry yards should be rototilled monthly after treatment with dilute bleach or lime to reduce oocysts available to birds. Prevention can be obtained by supplying coccidiostats in the feed. Coccidiostats are not included in organic feed, and these flocks must be monitored closely for coccidia. Outbreaks of disease can be treated with amprolium or with sulfadimethoxine (Albon) off-label. Sulfa drugs should not be used in laying hens. Amprolium has a very narrow margin for error and overdoses can lead to hemorrhagic diathesis and death. Vaccines are available but are generally only used in commercial birds *in ovo* or at hatch. It is recommended to submit a pooled fecal sample once a year for routine parasite screening and more often for problem flocks.

Histomonas

The disease caused by *Histomonas meleagridis* is commonly known as blackhead and was first described in turkeys in 1895.[17] When it was determined that a milder form occurred in chickens who became carriers, the poultry producers stopped rearing turkeys on land previously used for chickens. The chicken cecal worm, *Heterakis gallinarum*, and earthworms are accessory hosts. Turkeys become infected by eating infected *Heterakis* eggs or earthworms containing juvenile heterakids. Direct transmission through feces is uncommon because of low survivability of histomonads when unprotected by *Heterakis* eggs. Losses are greatest in turkeys (especially under 3 months of age) but *Histomonas* can infect chickens, pheasants, chukars, ruffed grouse, peafowl, guinea fowl, bobwhite quail, and pheasants. The natural incubation period is 7 to 12 days and mortality in turkeys can approach 100% and morbidity is 80% to 90%. Recovered birds may continue to harbor histomonads in their ceca. Affected turkeys have sulfur-colored feces; depressed, drooping wings; and a stilted gait. Although the disease is called blackhead, not all turkeys will have a cyanotic head. Chickens often have an unapparent infection without

sulfur-colored feces but can have blood in the feces. Leukocytosis, decreased uric acid and hemoglobin, transient rise in blood sugar, and increased aspartate aminotransferase (AST) and lactate dehydrogenase (LDH) are usually seen. The gross lesions are primarily in the ceca and liver. Lesions in the ceca include enlargement, thickened hyperemic walls, caseous luminal cores, and ulceration of the mucosa. Lesions in the liver commonly have circular, depressed areas of necrosis circumscribed by a raised ring (targets). Diagnosis is generally based on clinical signs and gross lesions. Demonstration of histomonads in ceca from freshly killed birds is difficult because the histomonads die quickly and are harder to identify. The best prevention is not to place turkeys on ranges inhabited previously by chickens or other game birds and to control earthworms. Range rotation is not practical as histomonads have tremendous survivability in heterakid eggs (4 years or more). There are no vaccinations or treatments available in the United States, since the use of imidazoles has been banned in all food-producing animals.

Viral Diseases

Marek's disease

Marek's disease (MD) is a common viral disease of chickens caused by a herpesvirus. MD is one of the top two diseases (along with coccidia) found in backyard chickens in the United States The primary lesions are tumors of the viscera, muscle, skin, and peripheral nerves.[18] Nerve lesions can be an early indicator of the disease resulting in a condition termed *range paralysis*. Birds with visceral tumors will often have only cachexia as a clinical sign. Tumors of the muscles and skin are frequently palpable. In a small percentage of birds, tumors of the iris can be observed antemortem, producing a grayish discoloration to the iris. Backyard chickens often present with enlarged crops from paralysis of the vagus nerve. Secondary impactions with ingesta are not uncommon, and, as such, MD should remain on the differential diagnosis when treating crop impactions. The crop can be manually or surgically emptied, but the prognosis is grave as morbidity caused by MD ultimately equals mortality (Figure 15-14).

The virus is shed by the feather follicles and therefore is found in feathers and dander. In this form, MD virus is quite

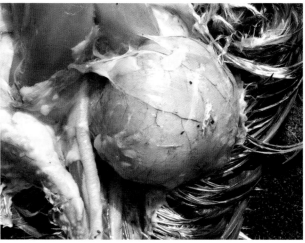

FIGURE 15-14 Enlarged crop due to involvement of the vagus nerve in Marek's disease.

hardy and can last for many months, making control by disinfection and biosecurity difficult. MD cannot be treated, but is preventable by vaccination at hatch. The vaccine is either applied via the *in ovo* route (at the hatchery) or subcutaneous in the skin of the neck after hatch. The vaccine cannot be overdosed even if all 1000 doses were applied to one bird, making it safe for clients to apply. The efficacy of vaccinations applied to birds older than 1 to 2 weeks of age is unknown. Vaccination does not prevent infection or shedding of the virulent virus but it prevents clinical disease. Clinical MD typically affects birds between 4 and 14 weeks of age; however, it is not uncommon in older birds. Outbreaks with high mortality are generally seen in younger birds, and older birds will usually succumb sporadically and often subsequently to an immunosuppressive event. If tumors are found in the viscera of deceased birds, carcasses should be submitted to a diagnostic laboratory for differential diagnosis between MD and another common lymphoid tumor disease, avian leukosis. Avian leukosis is more often found in birds older than 14 weeks and tumors are very similar to those found with MD. Avian leukosis also has no treatment or vaccination but is only a sporadic problem in backyard flocks. If MD virus is diagnosed in a flock of mature birds, depopulation is not necessary as mortality is generally sporadic. However, all incoming birds must be vaccinated, regardless of age.

Infectious bronchitis

Infectious bronchitis virus (IBV) causes a rapidly spreading respiratory disease in young chicks.[19] Laying hens experience reduced production, egg shell abnormalities, and decreased internal egg quality. Certain strains of IBV will also cause kidney disease. The disease is caused by a coronavirus and IBV can be easily killed by disinfectants as long as it is not in organic matter. Chicks that are infected early in life may have permanent damage to the oviduct, which will prevent them from laying eggs (false layers). Although IBV is highly transmissible, most birds will recover with supportive treatment including increased housing temperature and half-normal concentration of powdered milk instead of water. Antibiotics can be applied to the water to prevent secondary infection. Vaccines are available; however, backyard chickens are usually not vaccinated unless they come in contact with other chickens (neighbors and shows). Live vaccines are applied in the water, by spray or via eye drops, and killed vaccines are applied intramuscularly.

Newcastle disease

Newcastle disease virus (NDV) affects numerous species of birds and was the reason quarantine regulations for birds entering the United States were established.[20] Both velogenic (exotic) NDV and highly pathogenic avian influenza (HPAI) are on the United States select agent list, making them a national security concern. Exotic ND is highly fatal and does not exist in the United States at this time. However, in any incidence of acute mortality involving large numbers of birds or more than 50% of the flock over a 24- to 48-hour period, velogenic NDV and HPAI must be considered. Outbreaks in the United States have occurred in the past, resulting in the slaughter of thousands of birds and export bans.

Birds with NDV die acutely with no gross lesions. Common lesions for both HPAI and velogenic NDV include blue discoloration of the shanks, wattles, and comb; skin hemorrhages; torticollis; ataxia; and piling. NDV does exist in milder forms in the United States, and they are primarily characterized by respiratory disease and a drop in egg production. Mortality is variable and depends upon the strain of the virus. As with IBV, vaccination is available (same routes of application) but is generally only given to pet poultry exposed to other birds. Vaccination is not used for prevention of exotic NDV but for prevention of infection by pathogenic endemic strains.

Poxvirus

Fowl poxvirus causes nodular lesions primarily on the unfeathered portions of the bird (Figure 15-15).[21] Occasionally, it can cause lesions in the mouth and trachea, causing death from suffocation (wet form). Once the bird recovers from the disease, immunity is generally lifelong. Not all pox outbreaks are caused by fowl poxvirus; they can be caused by related strains such as turkey pox, psittacine pox, and quail pox. Strains are somewhat species specific but can occasionally affect other species. One strain may not cross-protect with another. Vaccination is available and should be applied to flocks on premises with a previous history of pox or with presence of pox in nearby birds. The poxvirus vaccine is not attenuated, but is applied in a location that pox does not occur. For this reason, it is important to follow the label directions for vaccine application. The most common application is using a "stab stick," which is dipped into the vaccine and then passed through the wing web. The cups in the two sticks deposit the vaccine into the thin tissue of the wing web. Approximately 7 to 10 days post vaccination the area is checked for two small bumps at the inoculation site called "takes." With turkeys and other birds that sleep with their heads under their wings, the vaccine should be applied to the drumstick after parting the feathers. Turkeys can actually get pox infection of the head transferred from the vaccine takes, which is the reason for the alternate location for application. Poxvirus is transmitted through contact of infected lesions with open wounds and by insect bites (mosquitoes). Elimination of standing water and other mosquito sources is important for prevention. Preventing cannibalism during an outbreak and keeping

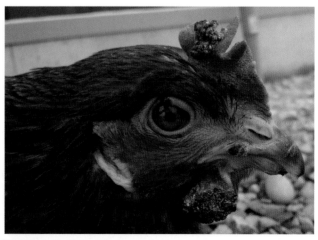

FIGURE 15-15 Pox lesions on the comb, wattles, and eyelid.

lesions clean and free of insects can decrease recovery time for affected birds.

Avian encephalomyelitis

Avian encephalomyelitis (AE) occurs in chickens, turkeys, pheasants, and quail and primarily affects young chicks 1 to 3 weeks old.[22] Nearly all commercial flocks are infected, but clinical disease is low due to the passage of maternal antibodies. AE can be transmitted vertically in eggs laid between 5 and 13 days post infection, and it is an enteric infection under natural conditions. The spread is more rapid in floor-raised birds than in cage-raised birds. Clinical signs include central nervous system deficits such as spinning, seizure-like activity, and torticollis. Mortality can be 50% or more and recovered chicks may be permanently blind in one or both eyes. Chicks hatched from recovered birds may also have blindness for unknown reasons, so keeping recovered birds for breeding is not recommended. There is no treatment. Vaccination of the breeders (both chicken and turkey) provides maternal antibodies for the young that are critical for prevention of infection. Since many specialty breeders, particularly those that sell stock to feed stores or other secondary distributers, do not vaccinate, AE is a fairly common viral disease in backyard birds. Vaccination should be given after 8 weeks of age but by at least 4 weeks prior to production. The vaccine can be co-applied with the pox vaccine using the stab-stick method.

Avian influenza

Avian influenza (AI) is worldwide in distribution and occurs in multiple species.[23] Migratory waterfowl yield the most viruses but disease is primarily in chickens and turkeys. Waterfowl can shed for long periods and often do not have detectable seroconversion whereas chickens and turkeys generally stop shedding after seroconversion. Transmission occurs via the respiratory tract and feces, and the incubation period is from a few hours to 3 days. Influenza is caused by an orthomyxovirus with three antigenically distinct types: A, B, and C. It is typed by the antigenic nature of the nucleoprotein and matrix antigens. Type A is classified into subtypes based upon the hemagglutination and neuraminidase types and B and C occur only in humans. The standard nomenclature is name = type of host (except human), geographic origin, strain number, year of isolation, and hemagglutinin-neuraminidase (HN) category. As with velogenic NDV, HPAI should be considered in any cases of acute mortality involving many birds. However, screening for LPAI is of national importance for HPAI prevention in both commercial and backyard flocks. The NPIP has an LPAI program and individual states often have monitoring programs for both resident and imported birds. Testing is done either by a direct antigen test or polymerase chain reaction (PCR) on swabs from the choanal cleft (gallinaceous birds) or cloaca (waterfowl) or an agar gel immunodiffusion test conducted on either serum or egg fluid. Serology and direct antigen tests are generally used for screening and PCR is used for confirmation. Flocks positive by screening tests must have samples sent to an accredited laboratory for PCR confirmation. If it is H7 or H5, the samples are sent by the laboratory to the National Veterinary Services Laboratories (NVSL). All flocks confirmed positive for either LPAI or HPAI will be depopulated. No vaccination for AI is permitted in the United States without permission from the USDA.

Bacterial Infections

Salmonellosis

There are many different species in the bacterial genus of *Salmonella*, not all of which carry the same pathogenicity.[24,25] Generally speaking, *S. pullorum* and *S. gallinarum* cause the greatest problem for poultry while *Salmonella typhimurium* and *Salmonella enteritidis* (SE) are important from a public health aspect. *S. pullorum* is egg transmitted and causes a diarrheal disease in young chicks and poults resulting in high mortality. Adult birds are asymptomatic carriers. Diagnosis is based upon disease history and isolation of the bacteria. Prevention is achieved by purchasing birds from disease-free flocks. Treatment is not recommended because it can cause birds to become carriers. Fowl typhoid (*S. gallinarum*) occurs in chickens and turkeys and many other game and wild birds. Fowl typhoid is similar in disease presentation and diagnosis to pullorum, although mature birds can show clinical signs of fowl typhoid. Prevention is again achieved by obtaining disease-free stock (NPIP certified). As with LPAI, small flock owners can participate in NPIP and have birds tested for pullorum/typhoid (PT) for show and breeding purposes. PT testing can be conducted by certified trained individuals or veterinarians, and consists of taking a small blood drop from the wing vein and conducting a plate agglutination test right on the farm (Figure 15-16). Commercial PT antigen and equipment are available for purchase by the public, and the USDA provides a training DVD (Figure 15-17). Any birds that test positive by the plate test must have serum tested by an accredited veterinary diagnostic laboratory for confirmation.

Clinical signs are infrequently observed in poultry infected with SE and *S. typhimurium*. Flocks can be monitored by obtaining egg samples and environmental samples for culturing the organism. In the United States, owners of

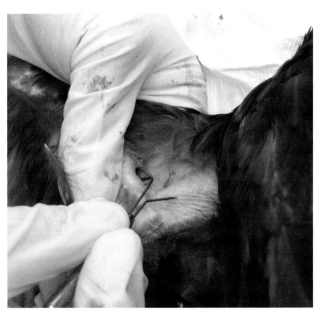

FIGURE 15-16 Needle placement for PT testing.

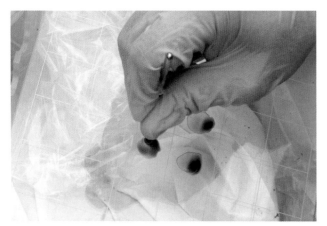

FIGURE 15-17 Mixing of antigen and blood for PT testing.

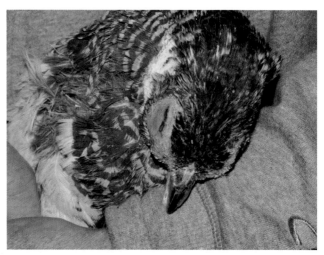

FIGURE 15-18 Pheasant with swollen sinuses due to *Myco-plasma gallisepticum.*

flocks over 3000 birds that sell eggs must participate in the Food and Drug Administration (FDA) SE clean certification program. Even small flock owners that sell eggs for human consumption should be tested at least yearly. Contact the state or provincial veterinary laboratory for sample testing requirements.

Colibacillosis

Colibacillosis is caused by the organism *E. coli* and is usually secondary to other infections such as IBV and mycoplasmosis.[26] A wide variety of clinical signs, both respiratory and enteric, can be observed and the organism occurs in most species and age groups. Vigorous adherence to biosecurity and sanitation programs will effectively prevent the organism from causing disease. Many antibiotics can be used for treatment and sensitivity to the antibiotic should be obtained. Treatment is usually successful if the disease is caught in the early stages.

Mycoplasmosis (chronic respiratory disease)

Chronic respiratory disease in poultry (primarily chickens and turkeys) is generally caused by *Mycoplasma gallisepticum* (MG) infection.[27] Pathogenicity of the organism is enhanced by infection with other organisms. Clinical signs of respiratory disease develop slowly in a flock, and feed consumption drops (Figure 15-18). Infection of the sinuses is common in turkeys. Since there are no certified MG-clean noncommercial breeders, it is crucial that clients only purchase birds from a reputable supplier or to visit the farm before purchase to be sure the birds are free of respiratory diseases. Serology, PCR, and isolation and identification of the organism can be used for diagnosis. An on-farm plate test, similar to that for PT, is available for screening purposes. Both live and killed vaccines are available, but the use of live vaccines may need State or Provincial approval. Killed vaccines can be effective for preventing/reducing clinical signs but will not prevent the birds from transmitting the disease vertically or horizontally. Depopulation and restocking is advised for breeding flocks. Treatment is expensive and the disease often recurs after cessation of treatment. Either injectable or feed/water-based Tylosin is the best approved treatment. It can be used for up to 1 month but egg and meat withdrawal times must be observed. MG is a reportable disease in turkeys in some states and provinces, and depopulation may be required. Other important mycoplasmas in poultry include *Mycoplasma synoviae* (infectious synovitis) and *Mycoplasma meleagridis* (venereal infection and airsacculitis), but are not commonly seen in backyard poultry.

Pasteurella multocida (fowl cholera)

In the 1850s it was discovered that fowl cholera (FC) could be transmitted both by cohabitation of infected birds with naive birds and via inoculation.[28] This discovery stimulated the first attempts to prevent the disease. FC is one of the four diseases for which the veterinary division of the USDA was created. It is more prevalent in the late summer, fall, and winter and occurs both sporadically and enzootically. FC is primarily a problem in chickens, turkeys, ducks, and geese but it is probable that all types of birds are susceptible.

Turkeys are the most severely affected and it is most common in young mature birds, but all ages are susceptible. Mortality is variable but can approach 80% or more depending upon the virulence of the strain and the environmental conditions (in turkeys). Laying chickens are more commonly affected than broilers because of their older age; chickens less than 16 weeks old are very resistant. FC occurs primarily in ducks over 4 weeks of age and mortality ranges up to 50%. *P. multocida* from avian species will kill rabbits and mice, but other mammals are fairly resistant to clinical signs. Chronically infected birds are the major sources of infection and birds are essentially infected for life. There is no relationship between FC and human cholera but humans can transmit FC to poultry or become infected from poultry via excretions from the nose or mouth.

Clinical signs of FC include both acute and chronic forms. The acute form is very rapid and signs may only be present for a few hours before death including fever, anorexia, ruffled feathers, mucous discharge from the beak, diarrhea, increased respiratory rate, and cyanosis just prior to death. Geese may just die acutely with no premonitory signs. The chronic form can occur following an acute stage or be from low-virulence organisms. It consists of localized infections whose site(s) determine the type of clinical signs, which include swollen wattles, sinuses, joints, foot pads, and sternal bursae; exudative conjunctivitis and pharyngitis; torticollis; tracheal rales; dyspnea; and roup and bloody discharge from the beak.

P. multocida can be isolated from viscera of acutely infected birds and from lesions from chronic cases, and the bacteria can be tentatively identified by observing bipolar organisms in liver imprints stained with Wright's stain. The organism is gram-negative on Gram stains. For live birds, the nasal cleft can be swabbed. Serology is primarily used to evaluate efficacy of vaccination. Antibiotics have variable success depending on the sensitivity of the strain and the duration of the disease before treatment. Sulfonamides are only bacteriostatic and usually cannot be used to cure localized abscesses or the effect of toxins. Sulfamethazine doses are 0.5% to 1% in food or 0.1% in the water for at least 5 days and often the FC will recur after treatment is discontinued. Streptomycin, penicillin, and chlortetracycline administered intramuscularly can also be used. If tetracyclines are used, the addition of citric acid to the drinking water and reduction of calcium use will increase the efficacy of the antibiotic. Biosecurity is very important especially since this is not a disease of the hatchery. There are vaccinations including both live and killed products, but these would be only advisable for flocks with a history of FC or at risk for FC in their immediate area and the causative serotypes need to be ascertained to select the best vaccine.

Avian tuberculosis

Mycobacterium avium and *Mycobacterium intracellulare* are called *M. avium* complex (MAC), which affects both mammals (miniature schnauzers, Siamese cats, Bassett hounds, various ruminants [deer], pigs, and rabbits) and birds.[29] Food animals and rarely humans are infected with an *M. avium* subsp. Paratuberculosis, which causes an infectious inflammatory bowel disease. Mycobacteriosis in chickens was first recognized as a separate disease around 1884 but is seldom observed in commercial poultry. It is more common in small flock operations that maintain older chickens and in game birds. Mycobacterial disease has a prolonged clinical course with high total morbidity and mortality. MAC in birds is a chronic wasting disease and is a World Organization for Animal Health (OIE) list B disease. All species of birds are susceptible but it is rare in turkeys. Mycobacteriosis usually occurs after 3 weeks of age and clinical signs include biliverdinuria, lameness, and diarrhea. The liver and spleen are enlarged grossly and may rupture. In addition, granulomas are seen in the spleen, liver, intestine, and rarely lungs. Transmission is from ingestion of materials contaminated with bird feces, which contain large numbers of bacilli. *Mycobacterium* persists in the environment for long periods. Importation of live poultry into countries free of MAC may require tuberculum testing. There is no treatment because of the associated public health aspects, and depopulation and destruction of equipment and housing through burning and application of cresylic compounds to the ground is advised.

Fungal Diseases

Aspergillosis (brooder pneumonia)

Brooder pneumonia occurs in many poultry and nonpoultry species of birds.[30] Birds under 3 weeks of age are most commonly affected and infection is obtained from hatchers or brooders that are contaminated with fungal spores. Older birds can be chronically affected and lesions can occur in virtually any tissue. Voice changes and ocular infection are common in chronic infections. Morbidity is variable and mortality can be high in clinically affected birds. Gross lesions include white caseous nodules scattered throughout lungs, air sacs, trachea, tongue, syrinx, and bronchi, and the nodules eventually become yellow or green (fungal mats) and caseated. Aspergillosis is generally observed in birds that are already immunosuppressed for other reasons. Antibody responses to infection are not well defined because of difficulty with testing methods. Antemortem diagnosis is often difficult because of nonspecific clinical signs. Culturing of the fungus, demonstration of typical fungal hyphae, or PCR from fresh preparations from lesions is used for diagnosis. Prevention is obtained by thoroughly cleaning hatchers, incubators, waterers, feeders, and ventilation fans and keeping litter clean and dry. Alternating wet and dry conditions encourage fungal growth. Treatment is expensive and may not be effective. Ketoconazole has been used with variable success, and itraconazole and voriconazole offer greater success as the systemic component of a treatment strategy. For prevention of spread within a flock, a 1:2000 aqueous solution of copper sulfate is provided in place of drinking water and the ground can be sprayed with either nystatin or copper sulfate.

Mycotoxins

The essential mechanism of action for all mycotoxins is interference with protein synthesis and destruction of rapidly dividing cells.[31] The target organs can vary among the different mycotoxins. There is no treatment and identification of the mycotoxin and removal of the source is crucial. Where there is concern for the potential for foodborne mycotoxicosis, for every new batch of feed used, a small Ziploc bag sample should be held back for possible future testing.

Aflatoxin

Aflatoxin includes aflatoxins B1, B2, G1, and G2. Aflatoxin B1 is most common in grains but all are toxic and carcinogenic. Aflatoxin primarily affects the liver and can be found in virtually all kinds of feed and many types of litter. Clinical signs include decreased appetite and growth, decreased carcass pigmentation, abnormal crying, picking at feathers, purple discoloration of legs and feet, lameness, ataxia, convulsions, death, decreased semen volume, and decreased hatchability of eggs. The major gross lesions are enlarged and pale liver and kidneys. In chronic cases, the liver may be shrunken and the gallbladder enlarged.

Ergotism

Ergotism is caused by *Claviceps* in cereal grains (rye) and is the oldest known mycotoxin. Mold in the feed replaces grain with a hard black mass called an ergot. Ergotism killed thousands in the middle ages (St. Anthony's fire) and it produces alkaloids. Toxins affect the nervous, vascular (vasoconstriction and resultant gangrene), and endocrine systems. Clinical signs include decreased food intake and growth; necrosis of beak, comb, and toes; distorted feather development; and enteritis. Ergotism primarily affects leghorns and other laying breeds and only trace amounts remain in the meat.

Trichothecenes

Trichothecenes have both caustic and radiomimetic effects and are primarily caused by *Fusarium*. They were first observed in Russia in the early twentieth century. Overwintering of grains in the field promoted mold growth and caused "alimentary toxic aleukia" with morbidity and mortality often greater than 50%. Trichothecenes are found in numerous feedstuffs and usually cause feed refusal. Clinical signs include necrosis of oral mucosa and skin, acute gastrointestinal signs, severe depression, and skin lesions on feet and legs. Necrosis of oral mucosa, reddening of gastrointestinal mucosa, mottled liver, distended gallbladder, visceral hemorrhages, and splenic atrophy are the most common gross lesions. The bone marrow is altered and there is a decrease in egg production. Birds generally recover when given new feed.

Nutritional Diseases

Nutrition is the process of furnishing cells inside the animal with that portion of the external environment for optimum functioning of the many metabolic chemical reactions.[32] It involves procurement, ingestion, digestion, and absorption. Water is also considered an important "nutrient." Poor nutrition can result from inappropriate diet for the bird type, lack of important nutrients, inability to ingest or digest the offered food, and loss of nutrients in the feed from improper storage, among other causes. It is extremely important to have a trustworthy and reliable source of feed. Since backyard flocks are such small consumers of feed, often large feed mills will sell their lower quality feed for noncommercial flocks. In addition, feed mills dedicated to specialty food animal herds or flocks may be mixing different feeds on the same day and residual ingredients can be problematic. Be sure always to save a copy of the feed label for later examination.

Dehydration

Water intake should be double the feed intake. Drop in water intake may be observed 24 hours before other clinical signs in a flock. Dehydration can be identified by increased skin turgidity and shriveled shanks. Some of the causes of dehydration are prolonged hatch, prolonged shipping time, dry brooders, drinkers at the wrong height or water pressure, and water refusal.

Vitamin A deficiency

Vitamin A is associated with depleted feed corn due to improper storage, no alfalfa added to the feed, or hatchlings from vitamin A-deficient hens. Xerophthalmia (dry eye), anorexia, retarded growth, and ataxia are usually observed from 1 to 7 weeks of age. Chicks often die before xerophthalmia develops. Gross lesions include pustules in the upper gastrointestinal tract, exudate in the conjunctiva and nasal cavity, opaque and dry cornea, scales surrounding the choanal cleft, and hyperkeratosis of the plantar surfaces. Feed samples should have 5000 IU/lb, liver samples 60 to 300 ppm, and serum 0.3 to 1.7 ppm of vitamin A. Treatment consists of water-dispersible vitamin A.

Rickets/osteomalacia

Rickets is the term used for younger birds and osteomalacia for mature birds. In poultry, the etiology is a deficiency or imbalance of calcium, phosphorus, and vitamin D_3. Lesions include a soft and pliable beak, claws, and keel; beading of the ribs; enlarged epiphysis; fractures of the long bones and spine; and enlarged parathyroid glands. Vitamin D_3 deficiency can be treated with three times the normal levels of vitamin D_3 provided in the feed or liquid vitamin D_3 in the water for 2 to 3 weeks. Calcium and phosphorus levels need to be adjusted for the species, breed, reproduction status, and age levels of the birds.

Exudative diathesis/muscular dystrophy

The etiology of this condition is vitamin E/selenium deficiency and most commonly occurs in chickens, quail, turkeys, and ducks. Gross lesions include subcutaneous green-tinged fluid and pale streaks in the skeletal muscles, gizzard, and heart; degeneration of the skeletal muscle and cardiac muscle; and pancreatic acinar necrosis. Encephalomalacia can be prevented by providing synthetic antioxidants in the feed but there is no treatment. Muscular dystrophy can be treated by adding cysteine to the feed and exudative diathesis is treated by adding selenium to the feed. For individual birds, a single oral dose of 300 IU of vitamin E is effective.

MEDICATIONS/DRUGS

It is crucial to know what drugs are banned for use in food animals versus those that are not labeled for poultry. Pet, show, and backyard poultry are still considered food animals by the FDA. There are few drugs labeled for use for hens in lay. Most commercial poultry veterinarians will be able to give advice concerning drug withdrawal times and approved drugs. For information contact aaap.info or the local State or Provincial Veterinarian. The *Avian Disease Manual* (aaap.info) has

TABLE 15-1

Drugs Banned from Use in Poultry in the United States

Drug Group (Examples)	Reason for Prohibition
Neuraminidase inhibitors (amantadine)	Concerns about creation of resistant AI strains
Chloramphenicol (prohibited since 1984)	Potential development of an idiosyncratic, non–dose-dependent, irreversible, aplastic anemia that may develop in humans
Fluoroquinolones (enrofloxacin, ciprofloxacin, sarafloxacin) (FDA banned extra-label use of fluoroquinolones in poultry in 1997 and all use in 2005)	Resistant *Campylobacter* spp. in poultry linked to an increased incidence of infection with resistant *Campylobacter* spp in humans
Gentian violet	
Nitrofurans	
Vancomycin	Must avoid development of resistant human pathogens
Nitroimidazoles (metronidazole, dimetridazole, ipronidazole, ronidazole, and tinidazole)	Have in vitro and in vivo potential for carcinogenesis

TABLE 15-2

Drug Groups and Specific Examples that May be Used in Poultry in the United States

Drug Group	Examples
Macrolides	Tylosin, erythromycin
Tetracyclines	Oxytetracycline, chlortetracycline, doxycycline (extra-label)
Lincosamides	Lincomycin, clindamycin (extra-label)
Sulfonamides	Trimethoprim sulfa (extra-label)
Aminoglycosides	Gentamycin, novobiocin, streptomycin
Penicillins	
Spectinomycin	
Novobiocin	
Bacitracin	

Note: Prior to use, seek specific guidance on egg and meat withdrawal times.

a table of approved drugs and withdrawal times that is updated every 5 years. The Food Animal Residue Avoidance Databank (FARAD) also is an excellent source to consult prior to using any drugs. FARAD can be contacted through their website: http://www.farad.org/. The Canadian equivalent can be contacted through their website: https://cgfarad.usask.ca/home.html. You will need to provide FARAD with your contact information, species of poultry, number of animals, average body weight, food product in question, number and name of drugs to be used, route of administration, and number of doses or you can search Vetgram for the withdrawal time for the intended drug, should it be an approved drug for poultry. Table 15-1 lists the drugs banned from use in poultry in the United States, and Table 15-2 offers the groups of drugs that can be considered for treatment of poultry species.

REFERENCES

1. *Backyard Poultry and Pigeon Houses*, Penn State Extension Bulletin No. IP727-25. http://www.abe.psu.edu. 1997.
2. *Poultry Tips*, University of Georgia Extension. http://www.poultry.uga.edu/extension/tips/index.htm. 2014.
3. Damerow G: *Building chicken coops*, North Adams, MA, 1999, Storey Publishing Co.
4. Batty J: *Breeds of poultry and their characteristics*, ed 6, West Sussex, UK, 2010, Beech Publishing House.
5. Stromberg J: *A guide to better hatching*, ed 2, Fort Dodge, IA, 2001, Stromberg Publishing Co.
6. North MO, Bell DD: *Commercial chicken production manual*, ed 4, New York, 1990, Chapman and Hall.
7. Wakenell PS: Obstetrics and reproduction of backyard poultry, *Semin Avian Exot Pet Med* 5(4):199–204, 1996.
8. Drowns G: *Storey's guide to raising poultry*, ed 3, North Adams, MA, 2013, Storey Publishing Co.
9. Leeson S, Summers JD: *Scott's nutrition of the chicken*, ed 4, Guelph, Ontario, 2001, University Books.
10. Etches RJ: *Reproduction in poultry*, Wallingford, UK, 1996, CAB International.
11. *National Poultry Improvement Plan (NPIP)*. http://www.poultry-improvement.org. 2015.
12. Wilcox CS, Patterson J, Cheng HW: Use of thermography to screen for subclinical bumblefoot in poultry, *Poult Sci* 88(6):1176–1180, 2009.
13. Wakenell PS: *Biosecurity, cleaning and disinfection, California egg quality assurance plan*. http://www.pacificegg.org. 2015.
14. Hinkle NC, Hickle L: External parasites and poultry pests. In Saif YM, Fadly AM, et al, editors: *Diseases of poultry*, ed 12, Ames, IA, 2008, Blackwell Publishing, pp 1011–1024.
15. Goddard J, Edwards K: *What to do about bed bugs in poultry houses*, Mississippi State University Information Sheet 1945, 2012.
16. McDougald LR: Internal parasites. In Saif YM, Fadly AM, et al, editors: *Diseases of poultry*, ed 12, Ames, IA, 2008, Blackwell Publishing, pp 1025–1066.
17. McDougald LR: Protozoal infections. In Saif YM, Fadly AM, et al, editors: *Diseases of poultry*, ed 12, Ames, IA, 2008, Blackwell Publishing, pp 1067–1117.
18. Schat KA, Nair V: Marek's disease. In Saif YM, Fadly AM, et al, editors: *Diseases of poultry*, ed 12, Ames, IA, 2008, Blackwell Publishing, pp 452–514.
19. Cavanagh D, Gelb J: Infectious bronchitis. In Saif YM, Fadly AM, et al, editors: *Diseases of poultry*, ed 12, Ames, IA, 2008, Blackwell Publishing, pp 117–137.
20. Alexander DJ, Senne DJ: Newcastle disease. In Saif YM, Fadly AM, et al, editors: *Diseases of poultry*, ed 12, Ames, IA, 2008, Blackwell Publishing, pp 75–100.
21. Tripathy DN, Reed WM: Pox. In Saif YM, Fadly AM, et al, editors: *Diseases of poultry*, ed 12, Ames, IA, 2008, Blackwell Publishing, pp 291–309.
22. Calnek BW: Avian encephalomyelitis. In Saif YM, Fadly AM, et al, editors: *Diseases of poultry*, ed 12, Ames, IA, 2008, Blackwell Publishing, pp 430–441.
23. Swayne DE, Halvorson DA: Influenza. In Saif YM, Fadly AM, et al, editors: *Diseases of poultry*, ed 12, Ames, IA, 2008, Blackwell Publishing, pp 153–185.
24. Shivaprasad HL, Barrow PA: Pullorum disease and fowl typhoid. In Saif YM, Fadly AM, et al, editors: *Diseases of poultry*, ed 12, Ames, IA, 2008, Blackwell Publishing, pp 620–636.
25. Gast RK: Paratyphoid infections. In Saif YM, Fadly AM, et al, editors: *Diseases of poultry*, ed 12, Ames, IA, 2008, Blackwell Publishing, pp 637–665.
26. Barnes HJ, Nolan LK, Vaillancourt J-P: Colibacillosis. In Saif YM, Fadly AM, et al, editors: *Diseases of poultry*, ed 12, Ames, IA, 2008, Blackwell Publishing, pp 691–738.
27. Ley DH: Mycoplasma gallisepticum infection. In Saif YM, Fadly AM, et al, editors: *Diseases of poultry*, ed 12, Ames, IA, 2008, Blackwell Publishing, pp 807–834.
28. Glisson JR, Hofacre CL, Christensen JP: Fowl Cholera. In Saif YM, Fadly AM, et al, editors: *Diseases of poultry*, ed 12, Ames, IA, 2008, Blackwell Publishing, pp 739–758.
29. Fulton RM, Sanchez S: Tuberculosis. In Saif YM, Fadly AM, et al, editors: *Diseases of poultry*, ed 12, Ames, IA, 2008, Blackwell Publishing, pp 940–951.
30. Charlton BR, Chin RP, Barnes HJ: Fungal Infections. In Saif YM, Fadly AM, et al, editors: *Diseases of poultry*, ed 12, Ames, IA, 2008, Blackwell Publishing, pp 989–1010.
31. Hoerr FJ: Mycotoxicosis. In Saif YM, Fadly AM, et al, editors: *Diseases of poultry*, ed 12, Ames, IA, 2008, Blackwell Publishing, pp 1197–1230.
32. Klasing KC: Nutritional Disease. In Saif YM, Fadly AM, et al, editors: *Diseases of poultry*, ed 12, Ames, IA, 2008, Blackwell Publishing, pp 1121–1148.

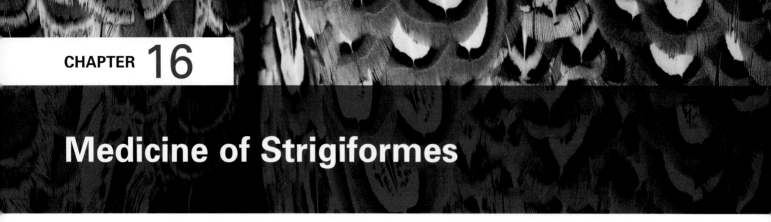

CHAPTER 16

Medicine of Strigiformes

Hugues Beaufrère • Delphine Laniesse

Owls are classified within the order Strigiformes, which is further divided into two families: Tytonidae and Strigidae. Tytonidae includes 19 species of barn owls (*Tyto* spp.) and bay owls (*Phodilus* spp.) and Strigidae includes approximately 200 species of typical owls.[1] Strigiformes are not phylogenetically close to other nocturnal birds such as Caprimulgiformes nor are they related to other birds of prey taxa such as the Falconiformes or Accipitriformes. While owls are not phylogenetically close to any other bird orders, they are closer to Coraciiformes, Piciformes, and Trogoniformes than to other avian orders.[2,3]

Owls are distributed worldwide and approximately 10% to 15% of the species are threatened with extinction, and most species are experiencing a decrease in population number. The barn owl *(Tyto alba)* is one of the most widely dispersed land birds in the world. The smallest owl is the elf owl (*Micrathene whitneyi*) and the largest is the Eurasian eagle owl (*Bubo bubo*). Female owls are generally larger (except in the burrowing owl; differences may be mild), darker, and more heavily marked than males. In general, owls show low sexual dimorphism with the exception of snowy owls in which males are almost pure white and females are barred with dark brown.[4,5]

Owls are mainly crepuscular or nocturnal species but some arctic species are mainly diurnal, such as the snowy owl (*Bubo scandiacus)*, the Northern hawk-owl (*Surnia ulula)*, and some pygmy owls (*Glaucidium* spp.).

Unfortunately, Strigiformes have not benefited from the same degree of veterinary investigation as Falconiformes and Accipitriformes, and despite distant phylogenetic relationships and drastically different natural biology, they have frequently been lumped together with other raptors in scientific studies. Hence the veterinary scientific literature is relatively reduced, especially for Strigiformes-specific articles, and reference values are often and regretfully lacking for most owl species. While the practicing avian veterinarian is more commonly exposed to trauma-related disorders in Strigiformes,[6,7] the collection of scientific information from these species has great value for advancing our awareness of clinically relevant topics. Less commonly discussed health aspects of owl medicine still remain relatively rare in the literature, and there is a need for development of an organized synthesis of data and literature review in a more accessible format. Consequently, this chapter will mainly deal with the internal medicine disorders and diseases of owls; captive management, rehabilitation, wound management, ophthalmology, and traumatology will not be discussed because they have been thoroughly reviewed in other references.

SPECIFIC ANATOMY AND PHYSIOLOGY

Tytonidae are characterized by heart-shaped, sound-reflective facial disks (divided in bay owls), no ear tufts, and a pectinate middle claw used for grooming (Figure 16-1), whereas the Strigidae are characterized by a round-shaped facial disk and often harbor distinctive ear tufts (which are not ear coverts but regular body coverts). The skull and beak of barn owls are also more elongated than those of typical owls.

The Auditory Apparatus

Hearing is highly developed in owls, particularly in nocturnal species. In both families, the external ear opening is asymmetrical, with the left higher than the right in Tytonidae and varying in Strigidae (right usually higher), allowing the birds to determine the exact location of sounds and hunting in the complete dark or for concealed prey.[4,5,8] This asymmetry is either restricted to the soft tissue part (e.g., in most species feathers, aural flaps, dermal septum in long-eared owls) of the ears or may involve the bony structure of the external ears (e.g., Ural owl, great gray owl, boreal owl, northern saw-whet owl, barn owls).[8] Aural asymmetry does not extend to the middle and inner ears. In owls, the feathers of the orbital region form a circular concave surface called the facial disk, which directs the sounds toward the ear openings. Its shape is adjustable to focus hearing. The facial disk is particularly well developed in great gray and barn owls. The posterolateral aspect of the facial disk bears modified covert feathers called the ear coverts (as in other birds over the external ear). Cranial and caudal to the auditory meatus are the preaural (also known as the operculum) and postaural folds, which can be erected and the shape of the opening (normally closed) altered by the muscles that insert onto the skull.[8,9] The facial disk feathers insert caudally to the ear opening on the postaural skin flap.[8] The auditory meatus is located in the orbital region unlike most other birds, where it is located in the postorbital region. The stape (bony part of the middle ear columella) in Tytonidae is shaped differently than the stape in Strigidae.[10]

The Eye

Owls have relatively large, tubular forward-directed eyes with a more spherical lens and well-developed scleral ossicles. The large eyes are typical of nocturnal animal species. The owl *fundus oculi* is characterized by an avascular retina with a thin or absent external retinal pigment epithelium, which allows visualization of choroidal vascularization (the so-called

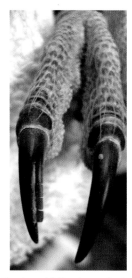

FIGURE 16-1 Pectinate middle claw of a barn owl *(Tyto alba)*.

tigroid fundus), and a single temporal fovea. They do not possess a *tapetum lucidum* unlike nocturnal mammals or the nocturnal order of the Caprimulgiformes.[11,12] Tytonidae do not appear to have a fovea,[13] and their *pecten oculi* is more compact than other birds of prey.[11] Unlike most birds, the owl retina has many more rods than cones, which are more sensitive to low light.[5] Owls have a Harderian gland but lack the lacrimal gland. Tytonidae have a thick and complete interorbital septum contrary to strigids and most other birds.[14] They have binocular vision and are able to swivel their head as much as 270 degrees without moving their body, which compensates for their ocular immobility. To avoid impeding blood flow in the vessels coursing through the neck, owls have several vascular adaptations including a high number of cervical vertebrae, large vertebral transverse foramina for their vertebral arteries, carotid arteries running close to the center of rotation within a ventral cervical groove (canal carotidus), a large intercarotid anastomosis at the base of the skull, and multiple collateral arterial vascularizations and anastomoses.[15,16]

Flight, Plumage, and the Thoracic Limbs

Owls have the ability to fly silently. This occurs because of the reduction of air turbulence over the wing surfaces and the reduction of feather friction during extension and flexion of the wings and during wingbeats. Specific feather adaptations reduce noise, such as the serrated leading edge of the outer primary feathers, which maintains a laminar flow over the airfoil's extrados; the downy trailing edge of most flight feathers and contour feathers; the long pennula of the distal barbules at overlapping zones (friction zones) of wing feathers; and the fluffy down feathers of the wings and legs.[9,17,18] Silent flight also permits owls to hear sounds that would normally be obscured by flying noises.

Tytonidae molt over a 2-year cycle, except for tropical species, which molt all their feathers each year.[4] Strigidae molt once a year and frequently shed all their tail feathers nearly simultaneously, which may leave them tailless for a short period.[5] The tarsi and toes of the snowy owls *(B. scandiacus)* have dense feathering that creates a covering over the plantar surface. Several other owl species have feathers on

the tarsi and digits as well but not to the extent of the snowy owl. Owls also possess thick bristles pointing forward around the beak and face.

Owl wing anatomy is roughly similar to other birds but they have relatively low wing loading. A large and long radial sesamoid (also called *os prominens*) is associated with the tendon of the propatagialis muscle pars longus as it bends over the distal radius to insert on the extensor process of the carpometacarpus (Figure 16-2).[14,19] Strigidae also possess a small humeroscapular bone in the area of the deltoid muscle that may be visible on a craniocaudal radiographic view of the shoulder joint.[14,20] The radial sesamoid and the humeroscapular bone are absent in Tytonidae. Some tendons of the flexor or extensor muscles of the manus may also appear calcified on wing radiographs, but these calcifications are usually less marked than those for the pelvic limbs (Figure 16-3).[14] The distal clavicles of Tytonidae are fused to the cranial edge of the sternum but are free in Strigidae.[5,14]

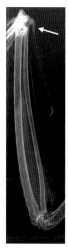

FIGURE 16-2 Ventrodorsal radiographs of the antebrachium of a snowy owl *(Bubo scandiacus)*. *Arrow,* radial sesamoid. Calcified tendons are also visible in the interosseous area.

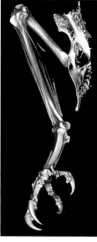

FIGURE 16-3 High-resolution computed tomography of the pelvic limb of a great horned owl *(Bubo virginianus)*. The calcified tendons are clearly visible around the tibiotarsus and tarsometatarsus. (Courtesy M. Scott Echols.)

The Pelvic Limb

The feet of owls have a semi-zygodactyl arrangement. They are able to shift positions from mainly zygodactyl when perching and grasping to anisodactyl when flying or for some other activities. The fourth digit rotates cranially or caudally. In fish-eating species such as *Ketupa* spp. and *Scotopelia* spp., the scales on the plantar surface harbor spicules that assist in holding slippery fish similar to the osprey. The femur is not pneumatized in at least the long-eared owl *(Asio otus)*, the Eurasian scops owl *(Otus scops)*, the Indian scops owl *(Otus bakkamoena)*, and the Ural owl *(Strix uralensis)* and possibly most strigid species.[21] Digits in owls and the tarsal trochlea are larger and the tarsometatarsus is shorter than in diurnal raptors.[22] Owls generate more force than hawks and falcons when closing their talons, which anatomically translates into stronger digit flexor muscles, more robust bones, and stronger tendons with ossification. For instance, the great horned owl *(Bubo virginianus)* generates approximately twice as much force than the red-tailed hawk *(Buteo jamaicensis)*, a similar sized diurnal raptor.[22] The tendons of the flexor and extensor muscles located around the tibiotarsus and tarsometatarsus are calcified in most owls, with the exception of the Tytonidae (see Figure 16-2).[23] The talons are usually longer and less curved than those of diurnal birds of prey.[24]

Gastrointestinal System

Owls lack a crop; often swallow their prey whole; and do not digest bones, feathers, and arthropod cuticles, which they egest as a pellet. This is probably because they have a higher gastric pH than diurnal birds of prey (six times less acidic than hawks).[5,25] Strigiformes have well-developed elongated ceca (4 to 11 cm), and may show apical dilations (e.g., bay owls), whereas the ceca is small or vestigial in diurnal birds of prey.[26] Owls periodically evacuate the cecal content by producing a dark fetid "cecal mute."[16] The gastrointestinal motility of the great horned owl has been studied in detail by fluoroscopy.[27,28] Three successive phases were observed corresponding to different phases of meal digestion: mechanical, chemical, and pellet egestion. Contractions of the ventriculus are simpler than in granivorous birds with simple peristaltic contractions from the isthmus to the pylorus.[28,29]

SPECIFICITIES IN DIAGNOSTICS

The physical examination and sample collection methods for owls are relatively similar to other avian species. Some owls may "freeze," feign death, stretch out vertically to "blend in," or adopt a threat posture.[5] In addition, some owls, such as the great gray owl *(Strix nebulosa)*, may lose large tufts of feathers during restraint, probably as a defense mechanism (Figure 16-4).

A complete ophthalmologic examination must be performed on all owls because of the frequency of traumatic lesions and fundic manifestations of systemic diseases.[12] The posterior aspect of the eye can be seen through the operculum. Because of the shape of the owl's eyes, the peripheral area of the fundus that is visible by ophthalmoscopy is smaller than in other birds of prey. Strigiformes have a lower intraocular pressure (approximately 10 mmHg) and tear production (approximately 5 to 10 mm on Schirmer's tear test, but seems higher in large owls) than diurnal raptors. A large body

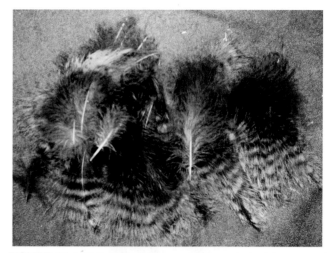

FIGURE 16-4 Tuft of feathers spontaneously lost by a great gray owl *(Strix nebulosa)* during restraint.

of the Strigiformes veterinary literature has focused on ophthalmology and the reader is referred to these publications for further details.

Blood Pressure

The systemic blood pressure of the great horned owl appears to be higher than that of most other birds. For instance, the direct systolic blood pressure of awake and anesthetized great horned owls was determined to be 232 and 243 mmHg, respectively.[30] However, this needs to be confirmed in other Strigiformes species and in further studies.

Clinical Pathology

Venipuncture is typically performed from the right jugular vein or ulnar (basilic) vein. Jugular venipuncture is more challenging in owls than in other bird species because of their wide skull base and short neck (Figure 16-5). The medial metatarsal vein is less ideal than in most species as a result of the feather covering.

The total white blood cell count of most Strigiformes is normally high when compared with most other bird species and should not be misinterpreted for leukocytosis (20 to 30,000 × 10^6/L may be normal in some species/individuals).[25,31] Eosinophil morphology varies markedly between owl species.[31,32] Hematologic reference intervals have been published for several species of owls.[31,33-35] As a general rule, arctic species have lower white blood cell counts than temperate and tropical species.[31] Furthermore, some species are predominantly heterophilic (e.g., barn owl, great horned owl), whereas others are lymphocytic (e.g., long-eared owl, eastern screech owl, barred owl).[31]

Biochemistry reference intervals are similar to other species for most analytes. Barn owls tend to have lower blood glucose than strigid species and lower blood electrolyte concentrations have been observed in healthy northern saw-whet owls *(Aegolius acadicus)*.[36] Most owl species also show higher glutamate dehydrogenase (GLDH) plasma activity (a very specific liver enzyme) than other studied avian species.[36] Postprandial effects are similar to other carnivorous birds and include elevations in uric acid and bile acids. Some northern

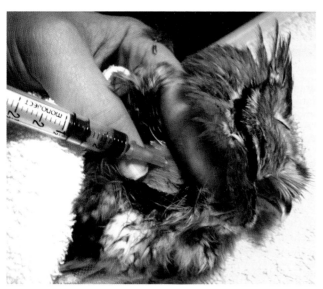

FIGURE 16-5 Venipuncture from the right jugular vein in an eastern screech owl *(Megascops asio)*. Venipuncture is more difficult in these strigids because of their small size, the seemingly short neck, and wide skull base.

species may hide their food in their flight cage during the winter, which must be taken into account during fasting. Trauma and intramuscular injections may result in aspartate transaminase (AST) and creatine kinase (CK) elevations lasting several days. It is likely that other currently unidentified, species-specific biochemical peculiarities may impair the interpretation of the biochemical panel in an unfamiliar Strigiformes. Specifically, there is a scarcity of clinical pathologic data on African, Asian, and South American owl species, which may live in very different ecological niches than North American and European owls. The Abaxis Vetscan showed relatively good reliability for clinical purposes in Strigiformes.[36] Fecal steroid testing to monitor the reproductive cycle has been developed for some species.[37]

Diagnostic Imaging, Electrocardiogram, and Electromyogram

The radiographic anatomy of owls is similar to other birds, but some osteological peculiarities should be known that could lead to misinterpretation. External acoustic meati are asymmetrical in some owl species and should not be mistaken as a deformity on skull radiographs.[14] The small humeroscapular bone should not be mistaken for a fracture fragment on craniocaudal views of the shoulder joint.[14] Tendon calcifications are also common in the limbs and readily apparent on radiographs or computed tomography (CT) scan, especially for the pelvic limbs (see Figure 16-3). The trochlea of the distal tarsometatarsus may look radiographically different from other birds of prey because it is slightly more lateral because of the fourth digit and the semi-zygodactyl foot.[14] Perching joint angles have been determined for the barred owl *(Strix varia)* to be 34, 34, and 90 degrees for the hip, stifle, and intertarsal joints, respectively.[38]

Radiographic cardiac sizes (regression based) only have been determined for a single owl species, the eastern screech owl.[39] Specific reports on advanced imaging (CT scan and magnetic resonance imaging) other than single case reports or functional imaging have not been found in owls. Electromyographic parameters were reported for barred owls.[40] Electrocardiography has been reported in several species of owls and did not show any specific differences from other birds of prey overall, except for maybe a tendency for Strigiformes to have lower QRS amplitude than other raptors.[41,42] Angiography of peripheral arteries has been reported in barred owls using iohexol with specific mention of intracranial vessels.[43] Transcoelomic echocardiographic examination has been reported in owls and the procedure is similar to other birds. Reference intervals for some parameters were reported.[44] Transesophageal echocardiography was successfully performed in three barred owls and was facilitated by the lack of a crop.[45] Coelioscopic examination is similar to other birds.

THERAPEUTICS

In terms of supportive care and classic medical procedures, few differences have been outlined specifically for owls. Reported species-specific iatrogenic toxicoses are scarce. Intravenous enrofloxacin in great horned owls induced weakness and bradycardia in some individuals.[46] A high dose of gentamicin resulted in renal failure and death in great horned owls after 2 to 3 days.[47] Fenbendazole treatment resulted in bone marrow toxicosis, affecting both the erythroid and myeloid lines in a great horned owl with concurrent leukemia.[48] Like most birds, owls are a corticoid-sensitive species. For instance, a single administration of dexamethasone suppressed endogenous corticosterone production for 24 hours in barred owls (longer than in hawks).[49]

Few pharmacologic studies have been performed in owls, and most pharmacodynamics studies have focused on anesthetics and analgesics. Meloxicam at 0.5 mg/kg had an extremely short half-life of under an hour in great horned owls (versus about 15 hours in Amazon parrots) and a higher dose and frequency may be needed to achieve therapeutic effects.[50] Butorphanol administered at 0.5 mg/kg intramuscularly in great horned owls was metabolized quickly as in most birds but the plasma concentration was higher than in red-tailed hawks.[51] The butorphanol plasma concentration was also higher than in parrots receiving 10 times the studied dose, suggesting that lower dosages but similar administration frequency are advisable in owls. The authors have noticed that owls often appear sedated with doses of butorphanol in the range of 1 mg/kg. No analgesimetry study has been performed in Strigiformes thus far. The use of inhalant anesthetics has not proved to be different from other raptors. Ketamine-α-2 agonist combinations have been extensively used in owls before halogenate inhalants became widely available and their use is not currently recommended.[52] Tiletamine-zolazepam has also been used successfully in two species of owls.[53] Constant rate infusions of propofol were investigated in great horned owls and showed respiratory depression, prolonged recovery, and neurologic excitation on recovery.[30]

Very few pharmacokinetic studies are available for antimicrobials in Strigiformes and most have been performed on the great horned owl (Table 16-1). Most other dosages are extrapolated from other bird species.

TABLE 16-1

Selected Antimicrobial Doses in Strigiformes as Determined by Pharmacokinetic Studies

Antibiotic	Species	Dose	Reference
Piperacillin	*Bubo virginianus*	100 mg/kg intramuscularly every 4-6 hours	54
Long-acting oxytetracycline	*B. virginianus*	16 mg/kg intramuscularly every 24 hours	55
Enrofloxacin	*B. virginianus*	15 mg/kg by mouth every 24 hours	46
Marbofloxacin	*Bubo Bubo*	2 (or higher) mg/kg intravenously every day 12-24 hours	56
Gentamicin	*B. virginianus*	2.5 mg/kg IM every 8 hours	57
Amphotericin B	*B. virginianus*	1.5 mg/kg intravenously	58

INFECTIOUS DISEASES

Viral Diseases

West Nile virus

In North America, West Nile Virus (flavivirus) is the most significant viral disease of owls. West Nile virus is transmitted by mosquitoes, primarily of the *Culex* genus, but other mechanical vectors have been reported in owls, such as *Icosta americana* (hippoboscid fly), in an outbreak in captive owls in Ontario, Canada.[59] Clinical signs are mainly neurological, weakness, or depression. Pinched off feathers may also be noted in owls. In one study, great horned owls were shown to be more likely to show neurological signs with West Nile virus infection than American kestrels (*Falco sparverius*) and Swainson's hawks (*Buteo swainsonii*).[60] Chorioretinal lesions are common in diurnal birds of prey but they are considerably less prevalent in Strigiformes.[25,61,62] Along with neurological lesions (lymphoplasmacytic encephalitis and meningitis), frequent postmortem findings also include cachexia, myocardial lesions, hepatomegaly, and splenomegaly.[62,63] Lymphoplasmacytic myocarditis was the most prevalent lesion on postmortem examination in owls in one study.[64] Kidneys, heart, and cerebellum contained the most viral antigens in owls in decreasing order.[62,63] Northern owl species, in particular the great gray owl (*S. nebulosa*), the snowy owl (*B. scandiacus*), the boreal owl (*Aegolius funereus*), the northern saw-whet owl (*A. acadicus*), and the northern hawk-owl (*Surnia ulula*), experience acute deaths. At necropsy, disease is characterized by a disseminated form of the infection, high viremia at time of death, hepatic and splenic necrosis, and an overall higher mortality rate than temperate species, as was determined in a 2002 outbreak at The Owl Foundation, Ontario.[59,62,65] Conversely, eastern screech owl (*Megascops asio*) and barn owl (*T. alba*) were found to be resistant to the disease.[59] An experimental infection trial was also conducted on the eastern screech owl.[66] Seven of nine infected owls did not display any clinical signs despite the development of high viremia, but significant histologic lesions were found.[66]

Diagnosis is mainly based on presumptive clinical signs and time of the year. Paired serology (2 to 4 weeks apart) demonstrating a rising titer is valuable, but early diagnosis is not possible with this technique. Owls readily seroconvert following West Nile virus infection.[59,64,67] PCR on blood is usually not considered useful because of the short viremia (3 to 7 days) that occurs prior to the onset of clinical signs. Northern species have been shown to be viremic when clinical but the rapid course of the disease may preclude antemortem diagnosis.

As viral shedding in oral secretions persists longer than the viremia, an antigen capture test (Vectest) has been used extensively on oropharyngeal swabs as a screening test in multiple avian species. However, it was only shown to provide reliable results in northern species of owls.[68] Splenomegaly may be noted on radiographs.[25]

Moderately susceptible species may recover with supportive care and anti-inflammatory treatment (e.g., meloxicam).[25,60] Vaccination with a killed vaccine or a recombinant vaccine has been used without adverse effects in owls, but immunogenicity is unknown and generally low in birds. Passive transfer of immunity has been recorded in eastern screech owls.[69] Owls may shed large quantities of virus, which could be a source of infection for human handlers.[70] Setting up mosquito-proof screening around flight cages may be recommended for northern owls.

Herpesvirus

Herpesvirus has been recognized to cause inclusion body hepatitis and splenitis in owls for some time.[71-75] It has recently been demonstrated that the previously known Strigid herpesvirus 1 (also known as owl hepatosplenitis and hepatosplenitis infectiosa strigum) and Falconid herpesvirus 1 are indeed identical to the Columbid herpesvirus 1.[76-79] Owls, as other raptors, are aberrant hosts for this alphaherpesvirus, hence the severity of clinical signs. Infection occurs via consumption of contaminated columbids, of which a large percentage of adults are subclinically infected. The herpesvirus infection has been reported mainly as a naturally acquired infection in great horned owl, Eurasian eagle owl (*B. bubo*), long-eared owl (*A. otus*), snowy owls, eastern screech owls, barking owls (*Ninox connivens*), and powerful owls (*Ninox strenua*).[71,72,75,78] Infection has been reported in other strigid species following experimental infection.[74] Tawny owls, barred owls, and barn owls were resistant to experimental infection.[71,72,74] Necrosis of the liver, spleen, and bone marrow with eosinophilic intranuclear inclusion bodies were the main lesions reported.[71,72,78] Pharyngeal ulceration and necrosis have been commonly encountered in the great horned owl, snowy owl, and Eurasian eagle owl. These lesions may be observed during a physical examination as white plaques in the throat, which could be confused with trichomoniasis, but do not seem frequent in other raptors.[73,74,77,80] Unilateral keratitis and conjunctivitis may develop in surviving owls.[74] Diagnosis is obtained by molecular diagnostics of the affected lesions or histopathology. Preventatively, pigeons should not be fed to captive owls. Acyclovir treatment may be attempted.

Rabies

Rabies (rhabdovirus) infection and shedding for short periods is recognized in great horned owls, probably because they frequently feed on skunks, a common North American rabies reservoir.[16] Seropositivity to rabies is rare but low titers have been reported in great horned and barred owls.[81] Another study in California failed to find neutralizing antibodies in great horned owls.[82] In another experiment, a great horned owl was experimentally infected with rabies by eating an inoculated skunk carcass.[83] The owl subsequently seroconverted and shed the rabies virus in oropharyngeal secretion. Immunosuppression induced with dexamethasone failed to induce disease. There is no report of clinical signs in owls naturally or experimentally infected with rabies. It is wise that persons handling great horned owls be vaccinated against rabies, especially in skunk rabies-endemic areas.

Avipoxvirus

Owl poxviruses belong to the fowlpox clade of avipoxviruses.[84] Cutaneous pox lesions have been described in several species of owls and are similar to other raptors but appear to be uncommon.[85,86] Pox lesions have been recorded in barn owls, eastern screech owls, long-eared owls, Eurasian eagle owls, great horned owls, and barred owls.[85-88] An isolate from a long-eared owl was infectious to chickens and caused cutaneous lesions.[88] Intracytoplasmic epidermal inclusions (Bollinger bodies) or PCR on tissue are diagnostics.

Other viral infections

Most other viral diseases of owls are described predominantly as single reports. A great horned owl was suspected of developing Marek disease in an early report.[89] Lesions were characterized by lymphoid tumors in viscera and enlarged sciatic nerves infiltrated with lymphocytes, but definitive evidence of Marek herpesvirus presence was not provided. Interestingly, there are also several recent reports of lymphoproliferative disorders specifically in great horned owls (see Noninfectious Diseases) but specific tests for Marek disease, including PCR, were not performed.

An adenovirus caused the death of a Verreaux's eagle owl (*Bubo lacteus*) and a Bengal owl (*Bubo bengalensis*) with hepatomegaly and necrosis, splenomegaly and necrosis, renomegaly, and intranuclear inclusion bodies.[90] Strigiformes appear to be resistant to infection by paramyxovirus I (Newcastle disease).[91] Single velogenic cases included a barn owl, a tawny owl, and two Eurasian scops owls.[92,93] Avian influenza virus (Orthomyxoviridae) has been detected in several owl species in Europe, but is not very prevalent and Strigiformes do not significantly contribute to its epidemiology.[94-97] Owls most likely are contaminated with influenza virus when feeding on infected ducks. Avian influenza surveillance in the European Union in 2006 detected the H5N1 highly pathogenic avian influenza virus in 0.43% of 924 owls sampled.[94] In vaccination studies across avian orders, Strigiformes were part of the groups exhibiting the lowest titers after vaccination with a killed H5N2 vaccine but showed good seroconversion rate in a subsequent study using a killed H5N9 vaccine.[98,99]

Bacterial Diseases

Strigiformes are expected to be susceptible to a variety of bacterial infectious diseases that also affect other birds. Wild Strigiformes have been documented with a variety of bacterial infections most often acquired through hunting or scavenging contaminated prey, especially during wild bird die-offs (e.g., avian cholera and short-eared owls).

As in other raptorial species, *Mycoplasma* spp. may be a normal inhabitant of the upper respiratory system of some species of owls, but it is less prevalent in owls than in Accipitriformes and Falconiformes.[100,101] Strigiformes have been reported as susceptible to chlamydiosis but the prevalence is low. *Chlamydia psittaci* infection has been recorded in at least 9% of all Strigiformes species.[102] *Mycobacterium* spp. have been isolated in different owl species with disease presentations similar to other raptors.[6,103-107] Outbreaks of *Salmonella typhimurium* have been reported in children after dissection of pellets from barred owls.[108] Owlets may also be susceptible to salmonellosis.[109,110] *Salmonella* infection in captive owls is often associated with the feeding of poultry meat, rodents, or day-old chicks. Strigiformes also appear to have a lower prevalence of *Campylobacter* spp. in their gastrointestinal tract compared with diurnal raptors.[111]

Infectious pododermatitis may be seen in captive Strigiformes and is similar to that described in other birds of prey. Lesions are often associated with suboptimal captive conditions such as a deficient diet, obesity, inappropriate perching surface, poor hygiene of perching surfaces, lack of flying activity, and stressful environment. Trauma to the foot, self-puncture of the plantar surface with a talon, or bite wound from prey may also lead to bacterial pododermatitis. A retrospective survey on pododermatitis lesion development in rehabilitated raptors found owls (including great horned owls, burrowing owls, and screech owls) to be the least susceptible to pododermatitis.[112] The snowy owl seems particularly predisposed to pododermatitis as a result of captivity.[25] Several factors may partly explain this susceptibility such as their heavy weight, their different perching behavior (they do not typically perch on branches and stay on the ground), and the temperature in warmer periods of the year. Snowy owls also seem to have decreased foot feathering, hence plantar padding, during warmer seasons. Bacterial infection is usually secondary and a variety of bacteria have been isolated. The authors have seen several pododermatitis lesions in snowy owls in which liquid pus was found, contrary to what is typically observed in other avian species. *Staphylococcus aureus* is reported as the most frequent bacterial pathogen involved in diurnal raptor pododermatitis.[113] Whether it is also true in owls is unknown, but the authors have frequently isolated more than one bacterial species from the same lesion, most often other than *S. aureus*. A case of bilateral severe pododermatitis with osteomyelitis associated with *Fusobacterium necrophorum* was reported in a great horned owl.[114]

Classification systems established for other raptors are applicable to owls. Radiographs of the feet are recommended to assess bony structures and articulations. Treatments are similar to other raptors and usually consist of local debridement of devitalized and necrotic tissue (if necessary), local sustained release antimicrobials (e.g., PMMA beads, poloxamer 407 gel mixed with injectable antibiotics), systemic antibiotics, topical ointment and/or dressing, and protective bandages. The bandages protect the wound, hold the dressing, and relieve the pressure from the affected plantar surfaces. Depending on the severity of the lesions, incorporating a custom-fitted silicone shoe (or other materials) may be necessary (Figure 16-6).[115] Bandages need to be changed frequently and the overall treatment may take several months. The particular anatomy of the foot must be also taken into consideration when applying bandages, especially since some species may prefer to have their feet in a zygodactyl position while perching.

Fungal Diseases

Aspergillosis has been diagnosed in several species of Strigiformes but overall case reports are limited. Several case reports have been published in great horned owls.[116-118] Many northern raptor species show increased susceptibility to aspergillosis and within Strigiformes the snowy owl appears to be particularly susceptible.[25,119] This species is the most arctic in range of any Strigiformes and lives in open space (e.g., tundra), which may translate into a low exposure to fungal spores and poorly developed immunity against this fungal infection. Snowy owls are frequently kept in captivity in more temperate climates where the higher temperature most of the year may predispose these birds to multiple health issues. Some other species of Strigiformes living in the arctic may also show increased susceptibility to infection as well, including the arctic subspecies of the great horned owls (*Bubo virginianus subarcticus*) and Eurasian eagle owls (*Bubo bubo sibiricus*). Risk factors for aspergillosis may be similar to other birds and include a high environmental spore load, hay or straw substrates, stress, concurrent diseases (e.g., a great horned owl developed aspergillosis concurrent to a lymphoproliferative disorder),[117] the use of antibiotics and corticosteroids, and respiratory irritants. Clinical signs, diagnosis, and treatment are similar to those described for other avian species. Coelioscopy with the demonstration of fungal lesions is the only reliable tool to confirm diagnosis and should ideally be performed before initiating an antifungal treatment that frequently lasts several months.

Reports on other fungal diseases are scarce in owls. In a snowy owlet, meningoencephalitis was caused by *Dactylaria constricta* var. *gallopava* (an agent of encephalitis in poultry).[120] Oral candidiasis is also seen on occasion.

Parasitic Diseases

A wide variety of parasites infest Strigiformes, most without causing any clinical signs. Only the most clinically important information will be reviewed as a large number of articles have been published on avian parasites.

The most common hemoparasites encountered in owls are similar to other raptors and include *Haemoproteus* spp., *Plasmodium* spp., and *Leucocytozoon* spp. The arthropod vectors are hippoboscid flies and *Culicoides* spp., *Culex* spp., and Simuliidae, respectively. The prevalence in the wild owl population may be high, especially for *Leucocytozoon* and *Haemoproteus*, but clinical infection is rare.[121,122] The life cycle is relatively similar for these three hemoparasites and consists of merogony in the reticuloendothelial system, capillary endothelium, and some other tissue (e.g., muscle, liver); gametocytes in circulating blood cells; and sexual cycle within an arthropod.[123]

Plasmodium differs from *Haemoproteus* and *Leucocytozoon* in that merogony also occurs and is visible in circulating blood cells.[124] Hemoparasite infections may be clinical in certain situations or species and the parasitemia may increase in debilitated or immunocompromised owls. The main *Leucocytozoon* species found in Strigiformes is *L. danilewskyi* and the main Haemoproteus species are *H. noctuae* and *H. syrnii*.[123,125] Various species of *Plasmodium* have been found in owls. Snowy owls (*B. scandiacus*) appear to be more susceptible to

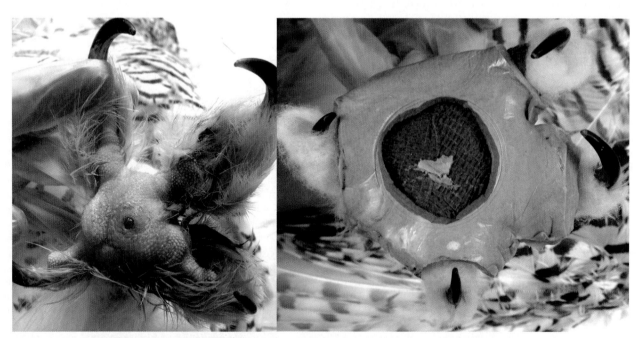

FIGURE 16-6 *Left,* Infectious pododermatitis with gross swelling of the foot in a snowy owl. The central scab was removed and a large amount of liquid pus was present within the foot. *Right,* After application of topical ointment and dressing, an interdigital bandage was applied as well as a custom-fitted silicone shoe.

the clinical effects of hemoparasites.[126] Severe regenerative anemia has been documented in snowy owls with *H. noctuae*, *H. syrnii*, and *L. ziemanni* (=*L. danilewskyi*) infestations.[123,127] Another report suggested concurrent pathogenic effects of hemoparasites with West Nile virus infection in a group of snowy owls.[128] Clinical *Plasmodium* spp. infections have also been recorded in snowy owls.[104] They may be immunologically naive to several hemoparasites not typically encountered in the arctic, which may explain the pathogenicity of *Haemoproteus* spp. usually not associated with clinical disease in other raptor species.[126] Great horned owls and tawny owls were also reported with anemia consecutive to *H. syrnii* infestation in the United Kingdom.[123] Clinical *P. supraecox* infection was observed in an eastern screech owl at a rehabilitation center that received corticosteroid.[129] *Leucocytozoon* infections appear to be potentially pathogenic in fledgling great horned owls as demonstrated in the wild (concurrently to severe black flies feeding) and according to occasional deaths observed at The Owl Foundation, Canada (H. Beaufrère, personal observation).[130] A *Babesia* spp. was also diagnosed in a great horned owl with anemia and biliverdinuria.[131] Other hematozoa infections reported in owls but in the absence of clinical signs include *Atoxoplasma* spp. and *Trypanosoma* spp. Treatment of hematozoa is as described for other avian species.

Other systemic protozoosis occurs sporadically in owls. Strigiformes are definitive hosts for a variety of *Sarcocystis* spp., which usually do not cause disease, such as *Sarcocystis rauschorum* in snowy owls, *S. scotti* and *sebeki* in tawny owls, and *S. dispersa* in long-eared (*A. otus*) and barn owls.[132-134] Intermediate hosts are rodents. Enteral coccidian load may be high and have a clinical impact in juveniles or debilitated owls.[135] In rare cases, owls may be aberrant intermediate hosts for other *Sarcocystis* spp. for which they are not normally part of the life cycle.[136,137] For instance, a great horned owl with neurological signs was diagnosed with *S. falcatula* (Virginia opossum is the definitive host) schizonts in the central nervous system and muscles.[136] Strigiformes have been shown to be infected by *Toxoplasma gondii* through multiple serologic surveys, but clinical disease is rare despite the isolation of the organism in multiple tissues.[138] Seroprevalence of *Toxoplasma* infection is usually high in birds of prey from exposure through their prey. Owls seem relatively resistant to clinical toxoplasmosis as experimental infection of great horned owls, barred owls, and eastern screech owls failed to cause clinical signs.[139] Serological tests were validated in these three strigid species during this study. In a rare case, *T. gondii* was found to be the cause of severe hepatitis with necrosis in a barred owl.[140] Chorioretinal lesions associated with toxoplasmosis have also been described.[12]

Cryptosporidium baileyi infection causes upper respiratory signs and conjunctivitis in raptors and is most often found in Falconiformes. However, an outbreak of *C. baileyi* was described in a group of owlets of Eurasian scops owls (*O. scops*).[141] Signs reported in the owlets included conjunctivitis, epiphora, corneal edema, and rhinitis. Azithromycin (40 mg/kg every 24 hours) was effective in treating the infection. Enteral coccidiosis is common in captive owls and the species involved are typically *Caryospora* spp. and *Eimeria* spp. (Table 16-2). Clinical disease seems rare but occasionally occurs in juvenile and debilitated owls.[135,142,143] Since most coccidia have a direct life cycle, infection can rapidly escalate in the confines of an aviary.

TABLE 16-2

Selected Coccidia and Their Strigiformes Hosts[135,142,144–147]

Coccidia	Strigiformes
Caryospora bubonis	*Bubo virginianus*
Caryospora henryae	*Bubo bubo*
Caryospora strigis	*Tyto alba*
Eimeria atheni	*Athene brama*
Eimeria bubonis	*B. virginianus*
Eimeria megabubonis	*B. bubo*
Eimeria spectytoi	*B. virginianus*
Eimeria strigis	*Athene cunicularia*
Eimeria varia	*Strix aluco*
Eimeria bemricki	*Strix varia*
Eimeria nycteae	*Strix nebulosa*
	Bubo scandiacus

Caryospora spp. have a facultative heteroxenous life cycle in which rodents may act as intermediate hosts.[135] Treatment is as described for other raptors.

Trichomoniasis caused by *Trichomonas gallinae* is a frequent disease of several species of owls but has not been as well characterized as in diurnal birds of prey. The species often recorded as infected include the barn owl, the European scops owl, the eastern screech owl, the great horned owl, the Eurasian eagle owl, the spotted eagle owl (*Bubo africanus*), the tawny owl, the barred owl, and the little owl (*Athene noctua*).[148-150] The disease seems most prevalent in barred and barn owls. They are infected by consuming infected birds such as pigeons or passerines (e.g., domestic sparrows). The disease is similar in its appearance to other raptors and causes white necrotic plaques in the oropharyngeal cavity, which may expand into adjacent tissues, especially the choanae.[149] Treatment is identical to other species.

Many species of helminths parasitize Strigiformes but most do not cause clinical disease, except occasionally in owlets. The most clinically important helminths in owls are the tracheal, filarioid, and capillarid nematodes. *Cyathostoma* spp. have been reported in the trachea of barred owls, snowy owls, eastern screech owls, northern saw-whet owls, burrowing owls, and Eurasian eagle owls.[151,152] Lesions may be especially severe in air sacs and lungs.[152] Earthworms are important intermediate hosts and controlling for earthworms was successful in the management of cyathostomiasis in a captive owl collection in Canada.[152] Various filarioid nematode species have been recovered from owls and the life cycle typically includes an adult stage living in body cavities (mainly vascular and respiratory systems), microfilariae in the blood, and an arthropod vector. Filarioids of the genera *Pelecitus*, *Aproctella*, *Cardiofilaria*, *Splendidofilaria*, and *Lemdana* have been reported in owls. Most are not pathogenic.[153] However, a high microfilaria burden (unidentified species) was recently described in wild, emaciated boreal owls (*A. funereus*) and suggested that they played a role in the deaths of some individuals.[154] Capillarid nematodes most frequently found in owls include *Capillaria tenuissima* and *Baruscapillaria falconis*, which parasitize the small intestine and esophagus.[155] Earthworms may serve as intermediate hosts and rodents as

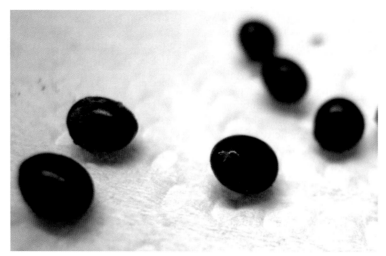

FIGURE 16-7 Pupae of hippoboscid flies *(Icosta americana)* collected in a great gray owl *(Strix nebulosa)* aviary.

paratenic hosts. Trematodes are also seen with various frequencies on fecal examination.

A large number of external parasites may feed on Strigiformes. In addition, some may be vectors of infectious diseases (see above). Hippoboscid flies are particularly prevalent in North American owls and can be found in great numbers in debilitated individuals, owlets, and in aviaries (Figure 16-7). Other common ectoparasites are similar to other avian orders and include ticks, chewing lice, mites, and simuliids.

NONINFECTIOUS DISEASES
Neoplasia

A broad range of neoplastic diseases has been described in Strigiformes, and most of them published as individual case reports. Great horned owls are over-represented in Strigiformes oncology cases and this may be from either the commonality of the species or a true predisposition.

Among neoplastic diseases identified in owls, lymphoid tumors are preponderant and seem to be affecting *Bubo* spp. in general and great horned owls in particular.[89,117,156,157] A lymphoma of presumptive T-cell origin was diagnosed in a great horned owl and was associated with multiple masses, either palpable or noted on whole-body radiographs.[156] Only a mild leukocytosis with monocytosis was noted. The tumor involved the oropharynx, subcutaneous tissues, spleen, liver, air sacs, thyroid, and parathyroid glands. Chemotherapy with chlorambucil was attempted without success. Another lymphoid proliferative disease was described in a great horned owl with a homogenous population of large lymphocytes infiltrating the liver, spleen, and kidneys.[117] In this case, however, a severe leukocytosis with lymphocytosis was evidenced. Another lymphoproliferative disease in a great horned owl was described in 1971, which the author qualified as compatible with Marek disease, but viral testing was not performed.[89] A severe leukocytosis was also noted in another great horned owl, which was heterophilic, however, and a diagnosis of myelogenous leukemia was confirmed at the postmortem examination.[48] Interestingly, self-mutilation of the wing was one of the clinical signs. Other anecdotal cases included lymphoma

in a snowy owl, lymphoid leukosis in a Eurasian eagle owl, and visceral lymphomatosis, here again mentioned as compatible with Marek disease, in a little owl.[157] A thymoma was also diagnosed after surgical resection in a burrowing owl.[158] The only clinical sign reported was weight loss, and the mass could be palpated at examination. Surgical resection is described as a possible treatment for thymomas in other animals, although associated with high risks, and in this particular case the bird died six days after surgery from secondary lesions to the esophagus.

Myelocytomatosis was identified on postmortem examination in an eastern screech owl, responsible for multiple small nodules in the liver and spleen, which consisted in aggregates of neoplastic myelocytic cells. Results of virus isolation and West Nile virus PCR were negative.[159]

Several gastrointestinal tissue neoplasms have been described in owls, including a mucinous adenocarcinoma of the tongue in a great horned owl and a proventricular adenocarcinoma in another great horned owl that showed weakness but no specific digestive signs.[160,161] Reported tumors of the eyes include a histiocytic sarcoma that was responsible for periocular swelling and metastasis in one of the digits and an iridal melanoma, both in great horned owls.[162,163] Mast cell tumors have been reported several times in owls. Two cutaneous mast cell tumors were diagnosed on the head in a single great horned owl, an oral mast cell tumor in a burrowing owl, and an eyelid mast cell tumor in a pueo *(Asio flammeus sandwichensis)*.[164,165] All mast cell tumors reported in Strigiformes have been on the head and one author suggested that owls were over-represented in cases of mast cell tumors in nondomestic birds.[164] Other tumors diagnosed in great horned owls include a lipoma (J. Brandão, personal communication), an astrocytoma, and a pulmonary carcinoma.[157,166] Concerning the latter, the bird presented with weakness, dyspnea, and hematochezia. Severe extensive lesions were identified in the air sacs upon radiographic examination.

Other anecdotal cases of neoplasia in owls include an osteoma on the left proximal radius of a barred owl, responsible for impaired flight; secondary muscle atrophy and local skin ulceration; an osteoma in a Ural owl; a chondroma in a tawny owl; fibrosarcomas in a tawny owl, a burrowing owl, and a snowy owl; adenocarcinomas in little owls; a feather folliculoma in a barn owl responsible for a proliferative cutaneous mass; and a squamous cell carcinoma and a presumptive testicular tumor in Eurasian eagle owls.[157,167,168] A thyroid follicular carcinoma in a barred owl also was recently described associated with higher total and free thyroxin values compared with four control healthy barred owls.[169]

Synovial Chondromatosis

Synovial chondromatosis (SC) has been widely described in great horned owls, mainly affecting the scapulohumeral joints, usually bilaterally, and in most cases at least another joint.[25,170-172] Synovial chondromatosis is a disease of the synovium, which, in human medicine, is divided into two categories: primary SC and secondary SC.[173] In primary SC, multiple nodules of metaplastic hyaline cartilage develop in the tissues of the joint. Although occasional mitoses may be found upon histopathology, SC is not a neoplastic disease; however, in humans at least, it does have a potential to transform into a chondrosarcoma. Secondary SC develops when fragments of bone or hyaline cartilage break free into the joint cavity, usually secondary to osteonecrosis, fractures, or other articular diseases. In owls, the clinical signs include weakness, emaciation, reduced amplitude in the extension of the wings, poor ability to perch, pain upon manipulation of the affected joints, and swollen joints. Radiographs may show multiple mineralized foci in the affected joints. The cause of SC in strigids remains unknown (Figure 16-8).

Cardiovascular Diseases

Atherosclerosis is the most commonly reported vascular disease in birds of prey, but is infrequent in Strigiformes. Two retrospective studies reported a prevalence of atherosclerosis in Strigiformes of 2.9% (N = 136) and 1.1% (N = 87).[174-176] In a review of 45 postmortem examinations of Strigiformes, a higher prevalence of 15.6% (7/45) was noted.[177] In these studies, the following species were affected: two spotted eagle owls (*B. africanus*), a Cape eagle owl (*Bubo capensis*), a great horned owl, an Indian scops owl (*O. bakkamoena*), a laughing owl (*Sceloglaux albifacies*), a tawny owl, a Woodford's owl (*Strix woodfordii*), a Fraser's eagle owl (*Bubo poensis*), a Javan

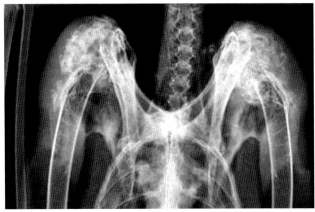

FIGURE 16-8 Ventrodorsal view of the shoulders of a great horned owl *(Bubo virginianus)* with synovial chondromatosis. (Courtesy J. Ponder, The Raptor Center.)

fish owl (*Scotopelia* spp.), an Aharoni's eagle owl (*Bubo bubo interpositus*), and a snowy owl.

Cardiac diseases have rarely been described in owls. Among nine owl hearts examined histologically in a retrospective study, only one had cardiac lesions compatible with myofiber degeneration.[178] Rupture of the left auricle and hemopericardium were also identified postmortem in a Javan fish owl kept in a zoological park; the etiology was unknown but another Javan fish owl was diagnosed with atherosclerosis and myocardial infarction a few years later in this same facility.[179]

Gastrointestinal Diseases

A mucocele, originating from the esophageal mucosal gland, has been described in a spectacled owl (*Pulsatrix perspicillata*) and was characterized by a soft fluid-filled mass in the cervical region of the bird.[180] A fine-needle aspirate of the mass revealed a clear to yellow mucoid fluid with low cellularity and staining positively with periodic acid fast. Surgical excision was performed successfully with no recurrence at the 6-month follow-up.

Gastrointestinal diseases with no evidence of infectious cause were identified in several species of owls kept in zoological parks: a barn owl died of intestinal hemorrhage secondary to a 5-mm ulcer situated just below the pylorus; a spotted eagle owl had ventriculitis associated with intestinal hemorrhage; and ventriculus impactions were identified in a Magellan eagle owl (*Bubo virginianus nacurutu*), an Indian scops owl, and a barn owl.[177,181] A cloacolith with secondary intestinal obstruction was diagnosed on postmortem examination in a barn owl.[181]

Hepatic Diseases

Hepatic lipidosis has recently been described in two barred owls, an elf owl (*Micrathene whitneyi*), and fatty degeneration had previously been reported in a little owl and a spotted eagle owl.[177,182,183] Although the etiology has not been clearly demonstrated in owls, overfeeding energy-dense food is the most probable cause. Clinical signs may include lethargy, dysorexia or anorexia, obesity, and distension of the coelomic cavity due to hepatomegaly. The latter can be confirmed by imaging. In a recent case report, hepatic lipidosis was associated with elevated AST, LDH, cholesterol, and bile acids on the biochemistry panel. The diagnosis can be confirmed on liver biopsy. Supportive care including force feeding, fluids, and vitamin E supplementation has been associated with good clinical results.

Other hepatic diseases reported in owls included fibrosis and parenchymatous degeneration in two older owls of unknown origin, cholecystitis and hepatitis in a Javan fish owl, and hepatitis in a barn owl.[177]

Renal Diseases

A cross-sectional study reported a prevalence of 20% (9/45) renal diseases in Strigiformes.[177] Nephritis and visceral gout were identified in a little owl and in a brown hawk owl (*Ninox scutulata*) and nephrosis was diagnosed in two little owls, a snowy owl, a Cape eagle owl, a Eurasian eagle owl, a barn owl, and an Indian scops owl.

Endocrine Diseases

Hyperthyroidism was discovered in a barred owl associated with a thyroid follicular carcinoma (see above). Both total and free thyroxine values were significantly higher in this bird compared with four healthy barred owls. The owl had been found on the ground unable to fly, with an unrelated wing injury, and died shortly after of unknown cause.

Reproductive Diseases

A 10-year retrospective study performed at the London Zoo (1966 to 1975) identified a prevalence of 10.5% of reproductive diseases in female owls (4/38).[184] These diseases included obstruction of the oviduct, salpingitis, and a case of functional right ovary in an Aharoni's eagle owl. Other anecdotal reproductive diseases reported in owls included egg peritonitis in a tawny owl and egg binding in an eagle owl.[177] A great gray owl with a ruptured oviduct and ectopic egg and a snowy owl with cystic ovaries were also diagnosed at The Owl Foundation, Canada.

Respiratory Diseases

Several cases of acute and chronic pneumonia have been reported in a survey in owls (tawny, laughing, barn, Magellan eagle, and scops owls) with no evident infectious cause. It is worth pointing out, however, that at the time of this survey (1956 to 1971) methods to identify infectious pathogens were not as sensitive as those today.[177]

Tracheal stenosis may occur in owls as in other species and has been described in a barn owl[185] and an eastern screech owl (H. Beaufrère, personal observation). Tracheal resection and anastomosis was performed with success in the first case.

Toxins

Strigiformes are susceptible to both biological toxins and pesticides and are exposed to toxins similarly to other raptorial orders. Owls usually are contaminated by biotoxins when feeding on intoxicated animals (see Chapter 18). Botulism appears to be exceedingly rare in Strigiformes but has still been described in great horned owls, snowy owls, and short-eared owls.[186] Avian vacuolar myelinopathy, a disease of the southeastern United States caused by a cyanobacterial toxin, has been reported in great horned owls (see Chapter 18).[187] The owls showed severe neurological signs with inability to perch and opisthotonus. A case of lethal toxicosis caused by the consumption of a California newt (*Taricha torosa*) was reported in a great horned owl.[188] These salamanders synthetize tetrodotoxins, a neurotoxin that can kill an avian predator within 2 minutes.

A wide variety of pesticides may affect Strigiformes but the most problematic currently are the anticoagulant rodenticides (see Chapter 18). Recent surveys in North America have found residues in most of the common owl species and the prevalence is generally higher than in Falconiformes or Accipitriformes.[25,189] In a study from Massachusetts, 100% of great horned owls, 87% of eastern screech owls, and 75% of barred owls that presented to a wildlife center were positive for anticoagulant residues.[189] Brodifacoum, a second-generation rodenticide, is the main chemical found in 99% of cases. Other studies confirmed the high exposure of great horned owls to these types of toxins.[190-192] One study from Western Canada found a 70% prevalence of anticoagulant rodenticide residues in the liver, but the highest prevalence was found in barred owls (92%) at this location. Subclinical intoxication is most common, but prolonged bleeding, anemia, and spontaneous or exacerbated hemorrhages are not uncommon.[189,191] An antemortem suspicion of intoxication is based on compatible clinical signs, increased prothrombin time, and increased whole-blood clotting time.[25] Tissue levels are necessary for a confirmatory diagnosis. The treatment is parenteral vitamin K1 at 2.5 mg/kg/day and homologous blood transfusion if indicated. If recent exposure is suspected, the stomach may be emptied and lavaged and activated charcoal may be prescribed. Because of the commonality of the intoxication, it may be wise to give vitamin K to owls in rehabilitation regardless of the presenting complaints.

Toxicoses from acetylcholinesterase inhibitors and heavy metals are also reported in Strigiformes, but seem less prevalent than those seen in diurnal raptors. Studies of normal brain and plasma acetylcholinesterase activity in great horned owls, eastern screech owls, and tawny owls have been published and may help with the diagnosis of organophosphate and carbamate poisoning.[192] Carbofuran is the most prevalent acetylcholinesterase toxin present in the environment. Famphur, an insecticide used topically in cattle, has been responsible for avian toxicities and death. It seems mostly to affect magpies and, secondarily, hawks, but there is one case that reports the death of a great horned owl by tertiary poisoning. This occurred because it had indeed preyed on a red-tailed hawk that was intoxicated from eating a magpie.[193] Secondary poisoning by Famphur has also been experimentally replicated in barn owls.[194] Clinical lead poisoning seems uncommon in owls overall.

Nutritional Diseases

Osteomalacia has been diagnosed in hand-reared tawny owls on several occasions.[177] Moreover, a survey looking at mortality causes in 45 owls showed a prevalence of 24.4% (11/45) owls displaying signs compatible with nutritional and metabolic disorders.

Miscellaneous Diseases

Two elf owls that had been treated for several years with leuprolide acetate died immediately after a subsequent administration, suggestive of an anaphylactic reaction.[183] Ancillary tests failed to find another explanation for these deaths. A case of pulmonary oxalosis concurrent with aspergillosis was documented in a great horned owl.[116] Xanthogranulomatosis was reported in a fledging great horned owl, with an atypical presentation, as the xanthoma involved periosseous tissues of both tibiotarsi, and, to a lesser extent, femur, humerus, radius and ulna.[195] Clinical signs include poor ability to fly, firm swelling of the affected bones, and pain upon palpation of the affected bones. The periosseous proliferations could be identified on radiographs, and the definitive diagnosis was made with a biopsy of an affected area. The lesions became smaller with time, but never resolved completely. The owl lived for at least 5 years after diagnosis. Horner syndrome has been described several times in owls, such as in an African spotted eagle owl and an eastern screech owl.[196,197] It is usually associated with a ptosis of the upper eyelid and an asymmetry in the position and movements of the ear-tuft feathers. Unlike mammals, birds do not typically present with miosis, which may be due to the dominance of striated muscle fibers in the iridal muscle in avian species. As Horner syndrome is caused by a loss of sympathetic innervation of the eye, a drop of phenylephrine in the eye will reverse the clinical signs. The cause of the syndrome was unidentified in a case and suspected to be secondary to a head trauma in the second. No treatment is recommended and the clinical signs usually resolve on their own after a few days to a few weeks (26 days for the screech owl).

Skunks constitute a major prey item for the great horned owl in some areas of North America and it is not uncommon that they are present to wildlife centers after having been sprayed by a skunk. The content of the liquid expressed by the anal scent glands of skunks when under attack may cause skin and ocular irritation. In addition, skunk musk causes methemoglobin and Heinz body formation that may result in anemia in mammals.[198,199] A small review identified five great horned owls received in wildlife centers in California between 1976 and 1978 that had been sprayed by a skunk. The report described that the birds were emaciated, their eyes had a clouded appearance, and they had discoloration of some of the feathers of the face and chest.[200] In addition, it is not uncommon to receive great horned owls in rehabilitation smelling like skunks but with no other detectable abnormalities.

REFERENCES

1. Clements J, Chulenberg T, Iliff M, et al: The eBird/Clements checklist of birds of the world, version 6.7, 2012. http//www.birds.cornell.edu/clements/downloadable-clements-checklist. Accessed Nov. 1, 2014.
2. Jetz W, Thomas GH, Joy JB, et al: The global diversity of birds in space and time, *Nature* 491(7424):444–448, 2012.
3. Hackett SJ, Kimball RT, Reddy S, et al: A phylogenomic study of birds reveals their evolutionary history, *Science* 320(5884):1763–1768, 2008.
4. Bruce M: Family Tytonidae (barn owls). In del Hoyo J, Elliott A, Sargatal J, editors: *Handbook of the birds of the world*, vol 5, Barcelona, Spain, 1999, Lynx Edicions, pp 34–75.
5. Marks J, Cannings R, Mikkola H: Family strigidae (typical owls). In del Hoyo J, Elliott A, Sargatal J, editors: *Handbook of the birds of the world*, vol 5, Barcelona, Spain, 1999, Lynx Edicions, pp 76–243.
6. Franson J, Little S: Diagnostic findings in 132 great horned owls, *J Raptor Res* 30(1):1–6, 1996.
7. Morishita T, Fullerton A: Morbidity and mortality in free-living raptorial birds of northern California: a retrospective study, 1983–1994, *J Avian Med Surg* 12(2):78–81, 1998.
8. Kuhne R, Lewis B: External and middle ears. In King A, McLelland J, editors: *Form and function in birds*, vol 5, London, UK, 1985, Academic Press, pp 227–271.
9. Lucas A, Stettenheim P: In Lucas A, Stettenheim P, editors: *Avian anatomy: integument, Part I. Agriculture*, Washington DC, 1972, Agricultural Research Service, U.S. Department of Agriculture, p 340.
10. Feduccia A, Ferree CE: Morphology of the bony stapes columella in owls evolutionary implications, *Proceedings of the Biological Society of Washington* 91:431–438, 1978.
11. Wood C: *The fundus oculi of birds*, Chicago, IL, 1917, The Lakeside Press, p 180.
12. Korbel RT: Disorders of the posterior eye segment in raptors–examination procedures and findings. In Lumeij JT, Remple D, Redig PT, Lierz M, Cooper JE, editors: *Raptor biomedicine III*, Lake Worth, FL, 2000, Zoological Education Network, pp 179–194.
13. Lisney TJ, Iwaniuk AN, Bandet MV, et al: Eye shape and retinal topography in owls (Aves: strigiformes), *Brain Behav Evol* 79(4):218–236, 2012.
14. Smith SAS, Smith BJB: Normal xeroradiographic and radiographic anatomy of the great horned owl (*Bubo virginianus*), with special reference to the barn owl (*Tyto alba*), *Vet Radiol Ultrasound* 32(1):6–16, 1991.
15. De Kok-Mercado F, Habib M, Phelps R, et al: Adaptations of the owl's cervical and cephalic arteries in relation to extreme neck rotation, *Poster*. https://nsf-scivis.skild.com/skild2/nsf2012/viewEntryDetail.action?pid=40747.
16. Aguilar R: Strigiformes (owls). In Fowler M, Miller R, editors: *Zoo and wild animal medicine*, ed 5, St Louis, MO, 2003, Saunders Elsevier, pp 213–223.
17. Lilley G: *A study of the silent flight of the owl*, 4th AIAA/CEAS Aero-acoustics Conference, Toulouse, France, 1998, pp 2004–2186.
18. Sarradj E, Fritzsche C, Geyer T: Silent owl flight: bird flyover noise measurements, *AIAA J* 49(4):769–779, 2012.
19. Bock W, McEvey A: The radius and relationship of owls, *Wilson Bull* 81(1):55–58, 1969.
20. Smith BJ, Smith SA: The humeroscapular bone of the great horned owl (*Bubo virginianus*) and other raptors, *Anat Histol Embryol J Vet Med Ser C* 21(1):32–39, 1992.
21. Kadosaki M: Lung and air-sac system of the strigidae, *Jpn J Ornithol* 26:87–92, 1977.
22. Ward AB, Weigl PD, Conroy RM: Functional morphology of raptor hindlimbs: implications for resource partitioning, *Auk* 119(4):1052, 2002.
23. Berge JC Vanden, Storer RW: Intratendinous ossification in birds: a review, *J Morphol* 226(1):47–77, 1995.
24. Fowler DW, Freedman EA, Scannella JB: Predatory functional morphology in raptors: interdigital variation in talon size is related to prey restraint and immobilisation technique, *PLoS One* 4(11):e7999, 2009.
25. Ponder J, Willette M: Strigiformes. In Miller R, Fowler M, editors: *Fowler's zoo and wild animal medicine current therapy*, vol 8, St Louis, MO, 2015, Elsevier, pp 189–198.
26. Clench M, Mathias J: The avian cecum: a review, *Wilson Bull* 107(1):93–121, 1995.
27. Rhoades D, Duke G: Cineradiographic studies of gastric motility in the great horned owl (*Bubo virginianus*), *Condor* 79(3):328–334, 1977.
28. Kostuch TE, Duke GE: Gastric motility in great horned owls (*Bubo virginianus*), *Comp Biochem Physiol A* 51(1):201–205, 1975.
29. Beaufrère H, Nevarez J, Taylor WM, et al: Fluoroscopic study of the normal gastrointestinal motility and measurements in the Hispaniolan Amazon parrot (*Amazona ventralis*), *Vet Radiol Ultrasound* 51(4):441–446, 2010.
30. Hawkins MG, Wright BD, Pascoe PJ, et al: Pharmacokinetics and anesthetic and cardiopulmonary effects of propofol in red-tailed hawks (*Buteo jamaicensis*) and great horned owls (*Bubo virginianus*), *Am J Vet Res* 64(6):677–683, 2003.
31. Ammersbach M, Beaufrere H, Tully T: Laboratory blood analysis in Strigiformes–Part I: hematologic reference intervals and agreement between manual blood cell counting techniques, *Vet Clin Pathol* 44(1):94–100, 2015.
32. Lind PJ, Wolff PL, Petrini KR, et al: Morphology of the eosinophil in raptors, *J Assoc Avian Vet* 4(1):33–38, 1990.
33. Smith E, Bush M: Haematologic parameters on various species of strigiformes and falconiformes, *J Wildl Dis* 14:447–450, 1978.
34. Black PA, McRuer DL, Horne L-A: Hematologic parameters in raptor species in a rehabilitation setting before release, *J Avian Med Surg* 25(3):192–198, 2011.
35. Spagnolo V, Crippa V, Marzia A, et al: Hematologic, biochemical, and protein electrophoretic values in captive tawny owls (*Strix aluco*), *Vet Clin Pathol* 37(2):225–228, 2008.
36. Ammersbach M, Beaufrere H, Tully T: Laboratory blood analysis in Strigiformes–Part II: Plasma biochemistry reference intervals and agreement between the Abaxis Vetscan V2 and the Roche Cobas c501, *Vet Clin Pathol* 44(1):128–140, 2015.
37. Wasser SK, Hunt KE: Noninvasive measures of reproductive function and disturbance in the barred owl, great horned owl, and northern spotted owl, *Ann NY Acad Sci* 1046:109–137, 2005.
38. Bonin G, Lauer SK, Guzman DS-M, et al: Radiographic evaluation of perching-joint angles in cockatiels (*Nymphicus hollandicus*), Hispaniolan Amazon parrots (*Amazona ventralis*), and barred owls (*Strix varia*), *J Avian Med Surg* 23(2):91–100, 2009.

39. Hanley C, Murray H, Torrey S, et al: Establishing cardiac measurement standards in three avian species, *J Avian Med Surg* 11(1):15–19, 1997.

40. Clippinger TL, Platt SR, Bennett RA, et al: Electrodiagnostic evaluation of peripheral nerve function in rheas and barred owls, *Am J Vet Res* 61(4):469–472, 2000.

41. Burtnick N, Degernes L: Electrocardiography on fifty-nine anesthetized convalescing raptors. In Redig P, Cooper J, Remple J, Hunter D, editors: *Raptor biomedicine*, Minneapolis, MN, 1993, University of Minnesota Press, pp 111–121.

42. Talavera J, Guzmán MJ, del Palacio MJF, et al: The normal electrocardiogram of four species of conscious raptors, *Res Vet Sci* 84(1):119–125, 2008.

43. Beaufrère H, Pariaut R, Rodriguez D, et al: Avian vascular imaging: a review, *J Avian Med Surg* 24(3):174–184, 2010.

44. Pees M, Krautwald-Junghanns ME, Straub J: Evaluating and treating the cardiovascular system. In Harrison GJ, Lightfoot TL, editors: *Clinical avian medicine*, Palm Beach, FL, 2006, Spix Publishing, pp 379–394.

45. Beaufrere H, Pariaut R, Nevarez JG, et al: Feasibility of transesophageal echocardiography in birds without cardiac disease, *J Am Vet Med Assoc* 236(5):540–547, 2010.

46. Harrenstien LA, Tell LA, Vulliet R, et al: Disposition of enrofloxacin in red-tailed hawks (*Buteo jamaicensis*) and great horned owls (*Bubo virginianus*) after a single oral, intramuscular, or intravenous dose, *J Avian Med Surg* 14(4):228–236, 2000.

47. Bauck L, Haigh J, et al: Toxicity of gentamicin in great horned owls (*Bubo virginianus*), *J Zoo Wildl Med* 15(2):62–66, 1984.

48. Wiley JLJ, Whittington JKJ, Wilmes CM, et al: Chronic myelogenous leukemia in a great horned owl (*Bubo virginianus*), *J Avian Med Surg* 23(1):36–43, 2009.

49. Quesenberry K, Hillyer E, et al: Supportive care and emergency therapy. In Ritchie B, Harrison L, Harrison G, editors: *Avian medicine: principles and applications*, Lake Worth, FL, 1994, Wingers Publishing, pp 382–415.

50. Lacasse C, Gamble KC, Boothe DM, et al: Pharmacokinetics of a single dose of intravenous and oral meloxicam in red-tailed hawks (*Buteo jamaicensis*) and great horned owls (*Bubo virginianus*), *J Avian Med Surg* 27(3):204–210, 2013.

51. Riggs SM, Hawkins MG, Craigmill AL, et al: Pharmacokinetics of butorphanol tartrate in red-tailed hawks (*Buteo jamaicensis*) and great horned owls (*Bubo virginianus*), *Am J Vet Res* 69(5):596–603, 2008.

52. Raffe M, Mammel M, Gordon M: Cardiorespiratory effects of ketamine-xylazine in the great horned owl, *Raptor biomedicine*, Minneapolis, MN, 1993, University of Minnesota Press.

53. Kreeger T, Degernes L, Kreeger J, et al: Immobilization of raptors with tiletamine and zolazepam. In Redig P, Cooper J, Remple J, Hunter D, editors: *Raptor biomedicine*, Minneapolis, MN, 1993, University of Minnesota Press, pp 141–144.

54. Robbins PK, Tell LA, Needham ML, et al: Pharmacokinetics of piperacillin after intramuscular injection in red-tailed hawks (*Buteo jamaicensis*) and great horned owls (*Bubo virginianus*), *J Zoo Wildl Med* 31(1):47–51, 2000.

55. Teare JA, Schwark WS, Shin SJ, et al: Pharmacokinetics of a long-acting oxytetracycline preparation in ring-necked pheasants, great horned owls, and Amazon parrots, *Am J Vet Res* 46(12):2639–2643, 1985.

56. Garcia-Montijano M, Waxman S, San Andres M, et al: Pharmacokinetics behaviour of intravenous marbofloxacin in Eurasian griffons and eagle owls. In *Proceedings of the Annual Conference of the European Association of Avian Veterinarians*, 2007, pp 217–222.

57. Bird JE, Miller KW, Larson AA, et al: Pharmacokinetics of gentamicin in birds of prey, *Am J Vet Res* 44(7):1245–1247, 1983.

58. Redig PT, Duke GE, et al: Comparative pharmacokinetics of antifungal drugs in domestic turkeys, red-tailed hawks, broad-winged hawks, and great-horned owls, *Avian Dis* 29(3):649–661, 1985.

59. Gancz AY, Barker IK, Lindsay R, et al: West Nile virus outbreak in North American owls, Ontario, 2002, *Emerg Infect Dis* 10(12):2135–2142, 2004.

60. Nemeth NM, Kratz GE, Bates R, et al: Clinical evaluation and outcomes of naturally acquired West Nile virus infection in raptors, *J Zoo Wildl Med* 40(1):51–63, 2009.

61. Pauli AM, Cruz-Martinez LA, Ponder JB, et al: Ophthalmologic and oculopathologic findings in red-tailed hawks and Cooper's hawks with naturally acquired West Nile virus infection, *J Am Vet Med Assoc* 231(8):1240–1248, 2007.

62. Gancz AY, Smith DA, Barker IK, et al: Pathology and tissue distribution of West Nile virus in North American owls (family: Strigidae), *Avian Pathol* 35(1):17–29, 2006.

63. Wünschmann A, Shivers J, Bender J, et al: Pathologic and immunohistochemical findings in goshawks (*Accipiter gentilis*) and great horned owls (*Bubo virginianus*) naturally infected with West Nile virus, *Avian Dis* 49(2):252–259, 2005.

64. Fitzgerald SD, Patterson JS, Kiupel M, et al: Clinical and pathologic features of West Nile virus infection in native North American owls (Family strigidae), *Avian Dis* 47(3):602–610, 2003.

65. Lopes H, Redig P, Glaser A, et al: Clinical findings, lesions, and viral antigen distribution in great gray owls (*Strix nebulosa*) and barred owls (Strix varia) with spontaneous West Nile virus infection, *Avian Dis* 51(1):140–145, 2007.

66. Nemeth NM, Hahn DC, Gould DH, et al: Experimental West Nile virus infection in Eastern screech owls (*Megascops asio*), *Avian Dis* 50(2):252–258, 2006.

67. Nemeth NM, Kratz GE, Bates R, et al: Naturally induced humoral immunity to West Nile virus infection in raptors, *Ecohealth* 5(3):298–304, 2008.

68. Gancz AY, Campbell DG, Barker IK, et al: Detecting West Nile virus in owls and raptors by an antigen-capture assay, *Emerg Infect Dis* 10(12):2204–2206, 2004.

69. Hahn DC, Nemeth NM, Edwards E, et al: Passive West Nile virus antibody transfer from maternal Eastern screech-owls (*Megascops asio*) to progeny, *Avian Dis* 50(3):454–455, 2006.

70. Komar N: West Nile virus: epidemiology and ecology in North America, *Adv Virus Res* 61:185–234, 2003.

71. Burtscher H, Sibalin M: Herpesvirus strigis: host spectrum and distribution in infected owl, *J Wildl Dis* 11(2):164–169, 1975.

72. Green RG, Shillinger JE: A virus disease of owls, *Am J Pathol* 12(3):405–410.1, 1936.

73. Sileo L, Carlson H, Crumley S: Inclusion body disease in a great horned owl, *J Wildl Dis* 11(1):92–96, 1975.

74. Kaleta E, Docherty D: Avian herpesviruses. In Thomas N, Hunter D, Atkinson C, editors: *Infectious diseases of wild birds*, Ames, IA, 2007, Blackwell Publishing, pp 63–86.

75. Gough R, Capua I, Wernery U: Herpesvirus infections in raptors. In Lumeij J, Remple J, Redig P, Lierz M, Cooper J, editors: *Raptor biomedicine III*, Lake Worth, FL, 2000, Zoological Education Network, pp 9–11.

76. Gailbreath KL, Oaks JL: Herpesviral inclusion body disease in owls and falcons is caused by the pigeon herpesvirus (Columbid herpesvirus 1), *J Wildl Dis* 44(2):427–433, 2008.

77. Rose N, Warren AL, Whiteside D, et al: Columbid herpesvirus-1 mortality in great horned owls (Bubo virginianus) from Calgary, Alberta, *Can Vet J* 53(3):265–268, 2012.

78. Phalen DN, Holz P, Rasmussen L, et al: Fatal columbid herpesvirus-1 infections in three species of Australian birds of prey, *Aust Vet J* 89(5):193–196, 2011.

79. Woźniakowski GJ, Samorek-Salamonowicz E, Szymański P, et al: Phylogenetic analysis of Columbid herpesvirus-1 in rock pigeons, birds of prey and non-raptorial birds in Poland, *BMC Vet Res* 9:52, 2013.

80. Gough RE, Drury SE, Higgins RJ, et al: Isolation of a herpesvirus from a snowy owl (*Nyctea scandiaca*), *Vet Rec* 136(21):541–542, 1995.

81. Gough PM, Jorgenson RD, et al: Rabies antibodies in sera of wild birds, *J Wildl Dis* 12(3):392–395, 1976.

82. Shannon LM, Poulton JL, Emmons RW, et al: Serological survey for rabies antibodies in raptors from California, *J Wildl Dis* 24(2):264–267, 1988.

83. Jorgenson R, Gough PM, Graham DL: Experimental rabies in a great horned owl, *J Wildl Dis* 12(3):444–447, 1976.
84. Gyuranecz M, Foster JT, Dán Á, et al: Worldwide phylogenetic relationship of avian poxviruses, *J Virol* 87(9):4938–4951, 2013.
85. Van Riper III C, Forrester D: Avian pox. In Thomas N, Hunter D, Atkinson C, editors: *Infectious diseases of wild birds*, Ames, IA, 2007, Blackwell Publishing, pp 131–176.
86. Deem S, Heard D, Fox J: Avian pox in Eastern screech owls and barred owls from Florida, *J Wildl Dis* 33(2):323–327, 1977.
87. Vargas G, Albano A, Fischer G: Avian pox virus infection in a common barn owl (*Tyto alba*) in southern Brazil, *Pesqui Veterin Brasil* 31(7):620–622, 2011.
88. Chiocco D: Owl pox virus: isolation and cross challenge studies in fowls, *Acta Med Vet (Napoli)* 38(3/4):261–266, 1992.
89. Halliwell W: Lesions of Marek's disease in a great horned owl, *Avian Dis* 15(1):49–55, 1971.
90. Zsivanovits P, Monks DDJ, Forbes NAN, et al: Presumptive identification of a novel adenovirus in a Harris hawk (*Parabuteo unicinctus*), a Bengal eagle owl (*Bubo bengalensis*), and a Verreaux's eagle owl (*Bubo*), *J Avian Med Surg* 20(2):105–112, 2006.
91. Jones MP: Selected infectious diseases of birds of prey, *J Exot Pet Med* 15(1):5–17, 2006.
92. Manvell R, Wernery U, Alexander D, et al: Newcastle disease (Avian PMV-1) viruses in raptors. In Lumeij J, Remple J, Redig P, Lierz M, Cooper J, editors: *Raptor biomedicine III*, Lake Worth, FL, 2000, Zoological Education Network, pp 3–8.
93. Choi K-S, Lee E-K, Jeon W-J, et al: Isolation of a recent Korean epizootic strain of Newcastle disease virus from Eurasian scops owls affected with severe diarrhea, *J Wildl Dis* 44(1):193–198, 2008.
94. Hesterberg U, Harris K, Stroud D, et al: Avian influenza surveillance in wild birds in the European Union in 2006, *Influenza Other Respi Viruses* 3(1):1–14, 2009.
95. Yasue M, Feare CJ, Benun L, et al: The epidemiology of H5N1 avian influenza in wild birds: why we need better ecological data, *Bioscience* 56(11):923, 2006.
96. Globig A, Staubach C, Beer M, et al: Epidemiological and ornithological aspects of outbreaks of highly pathogenic avian influenza virus H5N1 of Asian lineage in wild birds in Germany, 2006 and 2007, *Transbound Emerg Dis* 56(3):57–72, 2009.
97. Choi J-G, Kang H-M, Jeon W-J, et al: Characterization of clade 2.3.2.1 H5N1 highly pathogenic avian influenza viruses isolated from wild birds (mandarin duck and Eurasian eagle owl) in 2010 in Korea, *Viruses* 5(4):1153–1174, 2013.
98. Lécu A, De Langhe C, Petit T, et al: Serologic response and safety to vaccination against avian influenza using inactivated H5N2 vaccine in zoo birds, *J Zoo Wildl Med* 40(4):731–743, 2009.
99. Bertelsen MF, Klausen J, Holm E, et al: Serological response to vaccination against avian influenza in zoo-birds using an inactivated H5N9 vaccine, *Vaccine* 25(22):4345–4349, 2007.
100. Lierz M, Schmidt R, Brunnberg L, et al: Isolation of Mycoplasma meleagridis from free-ranging birds of prey in Germany, *J Vet Med B* 47(1):63–67, 2000.
101. Lierz M, Hagen N, Hernandez-Divers SJ, Hafez HM: Occurrence of mycoplasmas in free-ranging birds of prey in Germany, *J Wildl Dis* 44(4):845–850, 2008.
102. Kaleta EF, Taday EMA: Avian host range of *Chlamydophila* spp. based on isolation, antigen detection and serology, *Avian Pathol* 32(5):435–461, 2003. doi:10.1080/03079450310001593613.
103. Tell L, Ferrell S, Gibbons P: Avian mycobacteriosis in free-living raptors in California: 6 cases (1997–2001), *J Avian Med Surg* 18(1):30–40, 2004.
104. Willette M, Ponder J, Cruz-Martinez L, et al: Management of select bacterial and parasitic conditions of raptors, *Vet Clin North Am Exot Anim Pract* 12(3):491–517, table of contents, 2009.
105. Bucke D, Mawdesley-Thomas LE, Mawdesly-Thomas L: Tuberculosis in a barn owl, *Vet Rec* 95(16):373, 1974.
106. Rooke KB: Tuberculosis in wild birds. Fatal cases in a barn-owl and a chaffinch, *Ibis (Lond 1859)* 88(3):394–397, 2008.
107. Mollhoff W: Avian tuberculosis in a saw-whet owl, *Wilson Bull* 88(3):505, 1976.
108. Smith KE, Anderson F, Medus C, et al: Outbreaks of salmonellosis at elementary schools associated with dissection of owl pellets, *Vector Borne Zoonotic Dis* 5(2):133–136, 2005.
109. Battisti A, Di Guardo G, Agrimi U, et al: Embryonic and neonatal mortality from salmonellosis in captive bred raptors, *J Wildl Dis* 34(1):64–72, 1998.
110. Kirkpatrick C, Colvin B: Salmonella spp. in nestling common barn owls (*Tyto alba*) from southwestern New Jersey, *J Wildl Dis* 22(3):340–343, 1986.
111. Dipineto L, Bossa LMDL, Cutino EA, et al: Campylobacter spp. and birds of prey, *Avian Dis* 58(2):303–305, 2014.
112. Rodriguez-Lainz AJ, Hird DW, Kass PH, et al: Incidence and risk factors for bumblefoot (pododermatitis) in rehabilitated raptors, *Prev Vet Med* 31(3-4):175–184, 1997.
113. Remple J: Raptor bumblefoot: a new treatment technique. In Redig P, Cooper J, Remple J, Hunter D, editors: *Raptor biomedicine*, Minneapolis, MN, 1993, University of Minnesota Press, pp 173–179.
114. Gentz E: Fusobacterium necrophorum associated with bumblefoot in a wild great horned owl, *J Avian Med Surg* 10(4):258–261, 1996.
115. Remple D: A multifaceted approach to the treatment of bumblefoot in raptors, *J Exot Pet Med* 15(1):49–55, 2006.
116. Wobeser G, Saunders J: Pulmonary oxalosis in association with Aspergillus niger infection in a great horned owl (*Bubo virginianus*), *Avian Dis* 19(2):388–392, 1975.
117. Kelly TTR, Vennen KKM, Duncan R, et al: Lymphoproliferative disorder in a great horned owl (*Bubo virginianus*), *J Avian Med Surg* 18(4):263–268, 2004.
118. Clark F, Chinnag A, Garner S, et al: Aspergillosis in a great horned owl (*Bubo virginianus*): a case report, *Southwest Vet* 37:11–12, 1986.
119. Redig PT: Fungal diseases–aspergillosis. In Samour J, editor: *Avian medicine*, ed 2, Philadelphia, PA, 2008, Mosby Elsevier, pp 373–387.
120. Salkin I, Dixon D: Fatal encephalitis caused by Dactylaria constricta var. gallopava in a snowy owl chick (*Nyctea scandiaca*), *J Clin Microbiol* 28(12):2845–2847, 1990.
121. Ishak HD, Dumbacher JP, Anderson NL, et al: Blood parasites in owls with conservation implications for the spotted owl (*Strix occidentalis*), *PLoS One* 3(5):e2304, 2008.
122. Leppert LL, Dufty AM, Stock S, et al: Survey of blood parasites in two forest owls, northern saw-whet owls and flammulated owls, of western North America, *J Wildl Dis* 44(2):475–479, 2008.
123. Atkinson C: Haemoproteus. In Atkinson C, Thomas N, Hunter D, editors: *Parasitic diseases of wild birds*, Ames, IA, 2008, Wiley-Blackwell, pp 13–34.
124. Atkinson C: Avian malaria. In Atkinson C, Thomas N, Hunter D, editors: *Parasitic diseases of wild birds*, Ames, IA, 2008, Wiley-Blackwell, pp 35–53.
125. Forrester D, Greiner E, et al: Leucocytozoonosis. In Atkinson C, Thomas N, Hunter D, editors: *Parasitic diseases of wild birds*, Ames, IA, 2008, Wiley-Blackwell, pp 54–107.
126. Remple JD: Intracellular hematozoa of raptors: a review and update, *J Avian Med Surg* 18(2):75–88, 2004.
127. Evans M, Otter A, et al: Fatal combined infection with Haemoproteus noctuae and Leucocytozoon ziemanni in juvenile snowy owls (*Nyctea scandiaca*), *Vet Rec* 143(3):72–76, 1998.
128. Harasym CA: West Nile virus and hemoparasites in captive snowy owls (*Bubo scandiacus*)–management strategies to optimize survival, *Can Vet J* 49(11):1136–1138, 2008.
129. Tavernier P, Sagesse M, Wettere A Van, et al: Malaria in an eastern screech owl (*Otus asio*), *Avian Dis* 49(3):433–435, 2009.
130. Hunter DB, Rohner C, Currie DC, et al: Mortality in fledgling great horned owls from black fly hematophaga and leucocytozoonosis, *J Wildl Dis* 33(3):486–491, 1997.

131. Beaufrere H, Cruz-martinez L, Redig PT: Diagnostic challenge–babesiosis in a great horned owl, *J Exot Pet Med* 16(1):55–57, 2007.

132. Greiner E: Isospora, atoxoplasma, and sarcocystis. In Atkinson C, Thomas N, Hunter D, editors: *Parasitic diseases of wild birds*, Ames, IA, 2008, Wiley-Blackwell, pp 108–119.

133. Cawthorn RJ, Gajadhar AA, Brooks RJ: Description of Sarcocystis rauschorum sp. n. (Protozoa: Sarcocystidae) with experimental cyclic transmission between varying lemmings (*Dicrostonyx richardsoni*) and snowy owls (*Nyctea scandiaca*), *Can J Zool* 62(2):217–225, 1984.

134. Vorísek P, Votýpka J, Zvára K, et al: Heteroxenous coccidia increase the predation risk of parasitized rodents, *Parasitology* 117(Pt 6):521–524, 1998.

135. Cawthron R: Cyst forming coccidia of raptors: significant pathogens or not? In Redig P, Cooper J, Remple J, Hunter D, editors: *Raptor biomedicine*, Minneapolis, MN, 1993, University of Minnesota Press, pp 14–20.

136. Wünschmann A, Rejmanek D, Cruz-Martinez L, et al: Sarcocystis falcatula—associated encephalitis in a free-ranging great horned owl (*Bubo virginianus*), *J Vet Diagn Invest* 21(2):283–287, 2009.

137. Krone O, Rudolph M, Jakob W: Protozoa in the breast muscle of raptors in Germany, *Acta Protozool* 39(1):35–42, 2000.

138. Dubey J: Toxoplasma. In Atkinson C, Thomas N, Hunter D, editors: *Parasitic diseases of wild birds*, Ames, IA, 2008, Wiley-Blackwell, pp 204–222.

139. Dubey J, Porter S, Tseng F, et al: Induced toxoplasmosis in owls, *J Zoo Wildl Med* 23(1):98–102, 1992.

140. Mikaelian I, Dubey JP, Martineau D: Severe hepatitis resulting from toxoplasmosis in a barred owl (*Strix varia*) from Québec, Canada, *Avian Dis* 41(3):738–740, 1997.

141. Molina-Lopez RA, Ramis A, Martin-Vazquez S, et al: Cryptosporidium baileyi infection associated with an outbreak of ocular and respiratory disease in otus owls (*Otus scops*) in a rehabilitation centre, *Avian Pathol* 39(3):171–176, 2010.

142. Papazahariadou M, Georgiades GK, Komnenou, et al: Caryospora species in a snowy owl (*Nyctea scandiaca*), *Vet Rec* 148(2):54–55, 2001.

143. Forbes NA: Raptors: parasitic disease. In Chitty J, Lierz M, editors: *BSAVA manual of raptors, pigeons and passerine birds*, Gloucester, UK, 2008, BSAVA, pp 202–211.

144. Averbeck G, Cooney J: Exogenous stages of Eimeria bemricki n. sp. (Apicomplexa: Eimeriidae) from the great gray owl, Strix nebulosa (Foster), *J Parasitol* 84(5):976–977, 1998.

145. Upton SJ, Campbell TW, Weigel M, et al: The Eimeriidae (Apicomplexa) of raptors: review of the literature and description of new species of the genera Caryospora and Eimeria, *Can J Zool* 68(6):1256–1265, 1990.

146. Volf J, Koudela B, Modrý D: Eimeria nycteae sp. n. (Apicomplexa: Eimeriidae), a new parasite species from the snowy owl, Nyctea scandiaca, *Folia Parasitol (Praha)* 46(3):168–170, 2013.

147. Cawthorn RJ, Stockdale PHG: The developmental cycle of Caryospora bubonis Cawthorn and Stockdale 1981 (Protozoa: Eimeriidae) in the great horned owl, Bubo virginianus (Gmelin), *Can J Zool* 60(2):152–157, 1982.

148. Forrester D, Foster G: Trichomonosis. In Atkinson C, Thomas N, Hunter D, editors: *Parasitic diseases of wild birds*, Ames, IA, 2008, Wiley-Blackwell, pp 120–153.

149. Pokras M, Wheeldon E, Sedwick C: Trichomoniasis in owls: report on a number of clinical cases and a survey of the literature. In Redig P, Cooper J, Remple J, Hunter D, editors: *Raptor biomedicine*, Minneapolis, MN, 1993, University of Minnesota Press, pp 88–91.

150. Ueblacker S: Trichomoniasis in American kestrels (*Falco sparverius*) and Eastern screech owls (*Otus asio*). In Lumeij J, Remple J, Redig P, Lierz M, Cooper J, editors: *Raptor biomedicine III*, Lake Worth, FL, 2000, Zoological Education Network, pp 59–63.

151. Fernando M, Barta J: Tracheal worms. In Atkinson C, Thomas N, Hunter C, editors: *Parasitic diseases of wild birds*, Ames, IA, 2008, Wiley-Blackwell, pp 343–354.

152. Hunter D, McKeever K, Bartlett C: Cyathostoma infections in screech owls, saw-whet owls, and burrowing owls in Southern Ontario. In Redig P, Cooper J, Remple J, Hunter D, editors: *Raptor biomedicine*, Minneapolis, MN, 1993, University of Minnesota Press, pp 54–56.

153. Bartlett C: Filarioid nematodes. In Atkinson C, Thomas N, Hunter D, editors: *Parasitic diseases of wild birds*, Ames, IA, 2008, Wiley-Blackwell, pp 439–462.

154. Larrat S, Dallaire AD, Lair S: Emaciation and larval filarioid nematode infection in boreal owls (*Aegolius funereus*), *Avian Pathol* 41(4):345–349, 2012.

155. Yabsley M: Capillarid nematodes. In Atkinson C, Thomas N, Hunter D, editors: *Parasitic diseases of wild birds*, Ames, IA, 2008, Wiley-Blackwell, pp 463–497.

156. Malka S, Crabbs T, Mitchell EEB, et al: Disseminated lymphoma of presumptive T-cell origin in a great horned owl (*Bubo virginianus*), *J Avian Med Surg* 22(3):226–233, 2008.

157. Forbes N, Cooper J, Higgins R: Neoplasms of birds of prey. In Lumeij J, Remple J, Redig P, Lierz M, Cooper J, editors: *Raptor biomedicine III*, Lake Worth, FL, 2000, Zoological Education Network.

158. Kinney ME, Hanley CS, Aczm D, et al: Surgical removal of a thymoma in a burrowing owl (*Athene cunicularia*), *J Avian Med Surg* 26(2):85–90, 2012.

159. Shrader SM, Ellis AE, Howerth EW: Pathology in practice, *J Am Vet Med Assoc* 244(12):1393–1395, 2014.

160. Dillehay D: Mucinous adenocarcinoma of the tongue in a great horned owl, *Vet Pathol* 22(5):520–521, 1985.

161. Yonemaru K, Sakai H, Asaoka Y, et al: Proventricular adenocarcinoma in a Humboldt penguin (*Spheniscus humboldti*) and a great horned owl (*Bubo virginianus*); identification of origin by mucin histochemistry, *Avian Pathol* 33(1):77–81, 2004.

162. Sacré BJ, Oppenheim YC, Steinberg H, et al: Presumptive histiocytic sarcoma in a great horned owl (*Bubo virginianus*), *J Zoo Wildl Med* 23(1):113–121, 2014.

163. Rodriguez-Ramos Fernandez J, Dubielzig RR: Ocular and eyelid neoplasia in birds: 15 cases (1982–2011), *Vet Ophthalmol* 18(Suppl 1):113–118, 2015.

164. Schmidt R, Okimoto B: Mast cell tumors in two owls, *J Assoc Avian Vet* 6(1):23–24, 1992.

165. Swayne D, Weisbrode S: Cutaneous mast cell tumor in a great horned owl (*Bubo virginianus*), *Vet Pathol* 27(2):124–126, 1990.

166. Rettenmund C, Sladky KK, Rodriguez D, et al: Pulmonary carcinoma in a great horned owl (*Bubo virginianus*), *J Zoo Wildl Med* 41(1):77–82, 2010.

167. Hahn K, Jones M: Clinical and pathological characterization of an osteoma in a barred owl, *Avian Pathol* 27(3):306–308, 1998.

168. Frasca S, Schwartz DR, Moiseff A, et al: Case report–feather folliculoma in a captive-bred barn owl (*Tyto alba*), *Avian Dis* 43(3):616–621, 2014.

169. Brandão J, Manickam B: Productive thyroid follicular carcinoma in a wild barred owl (*Strix varia*), *J Vet Diagn Invest* 24(6):1145–1150, 2012.

170. Stone EG, Walser MM, Redig PT, et al: Synovial chondromatosis in raptors, *J Wildl Dis* 35(1):137–140, 1999.

171. State I: Synovial chondromatosis in a great horned owl (*Bubo virginianus*), *J Wildl Dis* 32(2):370–372, 1996.

172. Xie S, Nevis J, Lezmi S, et al: Pathology in practice, *J Am Vet Med Assoc* 245(7):767–769, 2014.

173. Connell JXO: Pathology of the synovium, *Am J Clin Pathol* 114:773–784, 2000.

174. Beaufrère H: Avian atherosclerosis: parrots and beyond, *J Exot Pet Med* 22(4):336–347, 2013.

175. Griner LA: Birds. In Griner LA, editor: *Pathology of zoo animals*, San Diego, CA, 1983, Zoological Society of San Diego, pp 94–267.

176. Garner MM, Raymond JT: A retrospective study of atherosclerosis in birds. In *Proceedings of the Annual Conference of the Association of Avian Veterinarians*, 2003, pp 59–66.

177. Keymer IF: diseases of birds of prey, *Vet Rec* 90:579–594, 1972.

178. Cooper JE, Pomerance A: Cardiac lesions in birds of prey, *J Comp Pathol* 92(2):161–168, 1982.

179. Hamerton AE: Report on the deaths occurring in the society's gardens during the years 1939–1940, *Proceedings of the Zoological Society of London* B111(1–2):151–185, 1941.

180. Huynh M, Brandão J, Sabater M, et al: Mucocele in a spectacled owl (*Pusilatrix perspicillata*), *J Avian Med Surg* 28(1):45–149, 2014.

181. Hamerton AE: Report on deaths occurring in the society's gardens during the year 1933–1934, *Proceedings of the Zoological Society of London* 104(2):389–428, 1934.

182. James SB, Raphael BL, Clippinger T: Diagnosis and treatment of hepatic lipidosis in a barred owl (*Strix varia*), *J Avian Med Surg* 14(4):268–272, 2000.

183. Stringer EM, De Voe RS, Loomis MR: Suspected anaphylaxis to leuprolide acetate depot in two elf owls (*Micrathene whitneyi*), *J Zoo Wildl Med* 42(1):166–168, 2011.

184. Keymer IF: Disorders of the avian female reproductive system, *Avian Pathol* 9(3):405–419, 1980.

185. Mama KKR, Phillips L, Pascoe P: Use of propofol for induction and maintenance of anesthesia in a barn owl (*Tyto alba*) undergoing tracheal resection, *J Zoo Wildl Med* 27(3):397–401, 2014.

186. Rocke T, Bollinger T: Avian botulism. In Thomas N, Hunter D, Atkinson C, editors: *Infectious diseases of wild birds*, Ames, IA, 2007, Wiley-Blackwell, pp 377–416.

187. Fischer J, Lewis-Weis L, Tate C, et al: Avian vacuolar myelinopathy outbreaks at a southeastern reservoir, *J Wildl Dis* 42(3):201–210, 2006.

188. Mobley JA, Stidham TA: Great horned owl death from predation of a toxic California newt, *Wilson Bull* 112(4):563–564, 2000.

189. Murray M: Anticoagulant rodenticide exposure and toxicosis in four species of birds of prey presented to a wildlife clinic in Massachusetts, 2006–2010, *J Zoo Wildl Med* 42(1):88–97, 2011.

190. Stone WB, Okoniewski JC, Stedelin JR: Anticoagulant rodenticides and raptors: recent findings from New York, 1998–2001, *Bull Environ Contam Toxicol* 70(1):34–40, 2003.

191. Albert C, Wilson L, Mineau P: Anticoagulant rodenticides in three owl species from western Canada, 1988–2003, *Arch Environ Contam Toxicol* 58(2):451–459, 2010.

192. Redig P, Arent L: Raptor toxicology, *Vet Clin North Am Exot Anim Pract* 11:261–282, 2008.

193. Henny CJ, Kolbe EJ, Hill EF, et al: Case histories of bald eagles and other raptors killed by organophosphorus insecticides topically applied to livestock, *J Wildl Dis* 23(2):292–295, 1987.

194. Hill EF, Mendenhall VM: Secondary poisoning of barn owls with famphur, an organophosphate insecticide, *J Wildl Manage* 44(3):676–681, 1980.

195. Raynor PL, Kollias GV, Krook L, et al: Periosseous xanthogranulomatosis in a fledgling great horned owl (*Bubo virginianus*), *J Avian Med Surg* 13(4):269–274, 2014.

196. Williams DL, Cooper JE: Horner's syndrome in an African spotted eagle owl (*Bubo africanus*), *Vet Rec* 134(3):64–66, 1994.

197. Gancz AY, Lee S, Higginson G, et al: Horner's syndrome in an eastern screech owl (*Megascops asio*), *J Avian Med Surg* 159(10):320–322, 2006.

198. Fierro BR, Agnew DW, Duncan AE, et al: Skunk musk causes methemoglobin and Heinz body formation in vitro, *Vet Clin Pathol* 42(3):291–300, 2013. doi:10.1111/vcp.12074.

199. Zaks KL, Tan EO, Thrall MA, et al: Heinz body anemia in a dog that had been sprayed with skunk musk, *J Am Vet Med Assoc* 226(9):1516–1518, 2005.

200. Garcelon D, et al: Mortality of great horned owls associated with skunks, *Murrelet* 62(1):26, 1981.

CHAPTER 17

Critical Care

Marla Lichtenberger • *Angela Lennox*

INTRODUCTION AND INITIAL ASSESSMENT

Like other exotic species, birds are masters at hiding signs of illness; therefore many birds presenting for what appears to be acute illness are actually suffering from a chronic disease process. Treatment of the critical bird is complicated by relatively small patient size, species diversity, and lack of clinical research and data on response to therapy.

Veterinary staff must be trained to recognize the potentially critical bird from an over-the-phone description, and urge the owner to seek care immediately. Front office staff should be able to identify the critical bird upon arrival to the clinic, and be instructed to bring these patients back to the hospital for immediate care (Table 17-1). While the bird is brought back for evaluation, another team member should obtain a thorough history from the owner.

In general, the healthy bird tolerates skilled handling, diagnostic sampling, and treatment well; this tolerance can be greatly diminished in the critically ill bird. The practitioner should understand that both a failure to intervene and the intervention itself could worsen clinical condition and result in death. Quick assessment and placement of the patient into condition categories (discussed in the following) can help drive diagnostic and treatment decisions.

Before handling the bird, perform a brief visual examination of the bird from a slight distance. An exception is the bird that has collapsed, which should be evaluated immediately for cardiopulmonary arrest. Look for visual clues such as decreased attention to novel surroundings or increased respiratory rate and effort, the latter often identified by the presence of a tail bob with each breath. With experience, avian veterinarians begin to develop a "gut feeling" for those birds that are sicker than they appear, based on subtle clues. Familiarity with the behavior of normal birds in the clinical setting helps to quickly identify birds not completely "in tune" to their surroundings (Figure 17-1).

Before beginning physical examination, be mindful of indications that the bird should be released at once and the examination postponed. These include worsening dyspnea, excessive struggling, inability to grasp, and the presence of marked coelomic swelling. In these cases, the bird should be released at once, and emergency stabilization planned. For the ill bird that tolerates handling, physical examination should be thorough.

TABLE 17-1

Symptoms and Signs Indicating the Need for Immediate Care in Birds

Over-the-Phone Description	Upon Presentation to the Hospital
No longer perching	Mentally dull, poorly responsive to novel environment
Mentally dull, lethargic	
Uncontrolled bleeding	Actively bleeding
Seizures	Seizures
Breathing harder and faster	Dyspnea
Decreased appetite to anorexia, especially presence of small, dark, tarry stools	Overall pallor, pale nares, and vent
Vent prolapse	
Tissue protruding from the vent	

It is often helpful to categorize the critical bird to plan diagnostic testing and treatment. In general, the authors find the following categories helpful:

Quiet but Responsive: Although ill, these birds are still alert and responding to the environment. For this category of birds, continued handling and diagnostic testing may or may not worsen clinical condition. If handling worsens the patient's clinical condition, discontinue and administer warmth, oxygen if indicated, and subcutaneous (SC) fluids. Observe condition carefully for 1 to 2 hours, then reevaluate. Consider using a low-dose sedation with midazolam 0.25 to 0.5 mg/kg and butorphanol 1 to 2 mg/kg administered intramuscularly (IM).[1] The authors have found that these doses typically reduce the risk of struggling during handling, without worsening clinical condition in the ill bird.

If handling does not worsen clinical condition, diagnostic sampling and treatment can likely proceed, watching carefully for any change in condition.

Depressed and Minimally Responsive: Birds in this category are lethargic and uninterested in their surroundings. Clinical signs including ataxia or dyspnea may be exhibited. For these birds, diagnostic testing is delayed until after 1 to 2 hours of stabilization, which typically includes warmth, oxygen, and fluids administered SC. It should be noted that for this group of birds, more aggressive therapeutics such as placement of intravenous (IV) or intraosseous (IO) catheters

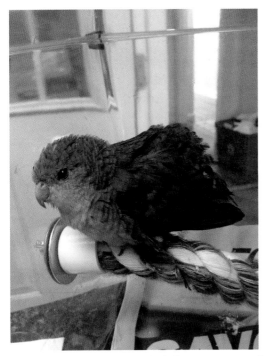

FIGURE 17-1 Appearance of an ill bird upon presentation for examination. Notice the drooped wing appearance. The bird appears "tuned out" to the novel situation of the veterinary examination room.

TABLE 17-2

Flow Chart for Cardiopulmonary Resuscitation in Birds

No respirations (respiratory arrest), but pulse and heartbeat present
- Turn off anesthesia if applicable
- Intubate or apply tight-fitting mask and ventilate with 100% oxygen at 40-50 BPM
- Place air sac cannula in case of upper airway obstruction
- Administer doxapram at 1-2 mg/kg IM, IV, IO
- If bradycardic, administer atropine at 0.02 mg/kg IV, IO
- If successful, check blood pressure and correct fluid deficits
- Check temperature and correct if necessary
- Begin diagnostic workup
- Treat underlying disorders

No respirations (respiratory arrest), and no pulse or heartbeat (cardiac arrest)
- Turn off anesthesia if applicable
- Intubate or apply tight-fitting mask and ventilate with 100% oxygen at 40-50 BPM
- Place air sac cannula in case of upper upper-airway obstruction
- Administer doxapram at 1-2 mg/kg IV, IO, IM
- Begin chest compressions 100-120/min (efficacy is uncertain)
- Use vasopressin 0.8 U/kg IV, IO; double dose if used via endotracheal tube
- If no response in 1 minute, consider epinephrine 0.01 mg/kg IV, IO; double dose if used via endotracheal tube
- If successful, check blood pressure and correct fluid deficits
- Check temperature and correct if necessary
- Begin diagnostic workup
- Treat underlying disorders

often results in stress and struggling, which can lead to death. Once patient condition improves, proceed with caution, and strongly consider low-dose sedation as above.

Nonresponsive: The patient in this category should be evaluated immediately for cardiopulmonary arrest, and resuscitation should be initiated, including therapy for shock as outlined in the following.

CARDIOPULMONARY RESUSCITATION

Mammalian principles of cardiopulmonary resuscitation (CPR) have been applied to avian patients with some reported success.[2] The goal of CPR is restoration of spontaneous breathing and circulation.[3] All supplies for CPR should be readily available in a designated "crash cart" or specifically stocked area of the hospital. Supplies should be inspected and restocked regularly. Post a resuscitation flow chart and a chart with suggested emergency drug dosages based on patient weight for easy reference (Tables 17-2 and 17-3).

Respiratory Arrest

Treatment for respiratory arrest is immediate endotracheal intubation and ventilation. Ideal ventilatory rate for birds has not been determined; however, based upon normal respirations and high metabolic rate, it may be as high as 40 to 50 breaths per minute. An alternative to intubation is forced high-flow 100% oxygen ventilation using a very-tight-fitting mask over the beak or bill and face. Success depends upon the ability to achieve a tight seal. In cases of complete or suspected marked upper-airway obstruction, perform immediate air sac cannulation. Doxapram is given IV, IO, or at twice the dose via the endotracheal (ET) tube (see Table 17-2).

Cardiac Arrest

Patients in cardiac arrest should be intubated and ventilated with 100% oxygen or, alternatively, should have forced high-flow oxygen delivered as described in the previous paragraph. As in other species, another team member performs chest compression simultaneously.[3] However, there is concern that chest compression may not be effective in birds because of the presence of the bony keel and the rapid compression rate likely required for effective resuscitation. For this reason, some experts do not recommend chest compression. Both epinephrine and vasopressin have been used anecdotally in birds. These agents may be given IV, IO, or via the ET tube (see Table 17-2).[3]

Shock and Fluid Therapy

Shock is caused by low or uneven blood flow or unevenly distributed blood flow, resulting in poor tissue blood perfusion and oxygen delivery. In other species, three phases of shock have been recognized: early compensatory, early decompensatory, and decompensatory.[4] It is unclear which phases actually occur in birds. Birds in shock should receive fluids via direct vascular access (IV or IO), which can proceed immediately in birds in cardiopulmonary arrest or who are minimally responsive and unlikely to struggle.[3]

TABLE 17-3
Suggested Drug Dosages Useful for Resuscitation in the Critical Bird*

Drug (Concentration)	Dose	mL/50 g	mL/100 g	mL/kg	mL/2 kg
Epinephrine (1:1000) (1 mg/mL)	0.01 mg/kg	0.0005	0.001	0.01	0.02
Atropine (0.54 mg/mL)	0.02 mg/kg	0.002	0.004	0.037	0.074
50% Dextrose (diluted 50% w/saline)	0.25 ml/kg	0.05	0.1	1.0	2.0
Calcium gluconate (100 mg/mL)	50 mg/kg	0.025	0.05	0.5	1.0
Doxapram (20 mg/mL)	2.0 mg/kg	0.005	0.01	0.1	0.2
Vasopressin (20 U/mL)	0.8 U/kg	0.002	0.004	0.04	0.08

*Note these have been extrapolated from other species and have not been thoroughly investigated in birds.

Vascular Access

Vascular access in birds can be performed via two routes: IV and IO; the choice of which route to employ depends on patient size and condition and the practitioner's personal preference.[5] Catheters may sometimes be placed successfully using manual restraint and local anesthetic only in very calm or minimally responsive patients. Patients judged to be at risk because of struggling during the procedure benefit from low-dose sedation as described previously, with infusion of local lidocaine at 1 to 2 mg/kg at the catheter insertion site. Roll the skin away from the vein and inject lidocaine buffered with sodium bicarbonate (1 part sodium bicarbonate to 10 parts lidocaine); allow the skin to roll back over the venipuncture site. Allow a few minutes for the drug to dissipate from the site. General anesthesia is seldom required for intravenous catheterization, and it may represent increased risk for the critical patient.

IV catheters are routinely placed in cockatiel and larger-sized birds, using 24- to 26-g catheters. Site choices include the right jugular, basilic (or ulnar), and medial metatarsal veins[5]; however, sites other than the jugular vein are only useful for larger birds. The smallest IV catheters that the authors routinely place are 25- to 26-g catheters into the jugular vein of a cockatiel or small conure. A potential complication of jugular catheterization in birds is inadvertent infusion of fluid or leakage of blood into the adjacent air sacs, which in large enough volumes could be fatal.

The medial metatarsal catheter can be secured using tape only. Basilic and jugular catheters are commonly sutured in place. No bird should be left unattended with an IV catheter in place because of the risk of fatal hemorrhage should the bird disrupt the catheter.

IO catheterization is well described in birds and can be performed in patients as small as a finch (8 to 18 g) (Figures 17-2 and 17-3). Sites include the proximal tibiotarsus at the cnemial crest, and the distal ulna.[5] The relatively soft bone cortex of most birds allows the use of standard injection needles as IO catheters, and commonly used needle size in pet birds ranges from 22 to 27 g. See also Chapter 19, where specific procedure is described for IO catheter placement.

Correct IO catheter placement is best confirmed with two orthogonal radiographic views (single views are notoriously misleading). As the needle can pass in and out of both bone

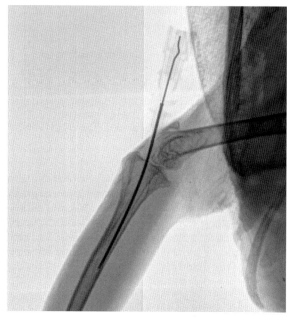

FIGURE 17-2 Gray-scale reverse radiographic image of a 22-gauge spinal needle placed in the ulna of a military macaw *(Ara militaris)*. The needle is inserted into the medullary space distal to the condyle of the dorsal ulna, avoiding the joint. (Photo courtesy Brian Speer.)

cortices, firm seating of the needle is not always indicative of success. Fluids injected into an incorrectly placed catheter often can be detected accumulating into soft tissue spaces. However, it should be kept in mind that too much "wobble" during placement might result in a large entrance point in the bone from which fluids may leak during infusion. Proper placement of an ulnar catheter may enable visualizing a blanching of the basilic vein during fluid administration. The IO catheter can be capped with a standard IV injection cap and secured by taping to the limb.

Use of IO catheters in pet birds is mostly anecdotal. Studies in human patients and some animal models indicate that IO vascular access can be considered equivalent to IV access in terms of onset of action of therapeutic agents and time to establishment of peak drug levels.[6] Recommendations for physicians include maintenance of the catheter no more than

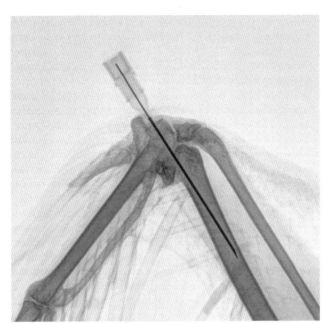

FIGURE 17-3 Gray-scale reverse radiographic image of a 22-gauge spinal needle placed into the proximal tibiotarsus of a military macaw *(Ara militaris)*. The needle is inserted to the side of, or through, the patellar tendon into the medullary space. (Photo courtesy Brian Speer.)

72 hours. Complications in humans are uncommon and include displacement of the catheter and extravasation of fluids into soft tissue. Serious complications such as compartment syndrome and osteomyelitis were rare, at less than 1%.[7] The authors have not experienced any complications after more than 10 years of use of this technique in clinical practice;

however, the authors are aware of a single report of infection at the placement site, and fatal hemorrhage after self-removal of the catheter (N. Schoemaker, personal communication, 2012). It should be noted that successful placement of a functional IO catheter in female birds with hyperostotic endostosis of long bones is difficult if not impossible.

All catheters that are to be maintained in a conscious patient should be secured carefully by wrapping with elastic-style tape. Wing catheters are protected by wrapping the wing using a typical figure 8–style bandage with or without wrapping the wing to the body (Figure 17-4, *A*).

Fluids used successfully in birds for resuscitation include crystalloids (lactated Ringer's solution, normal saline, and hypertonic saline), synthetic colloids such as hydroxyethyl starch (HES) (hetastarch 6%, Hospira, Illinois) and natural colloids (whole blood, plasma, and albumin).[2] Hypertonic saline rapidly draws fluid into the intravascular space from other body compartments, helping to raise blood pressure. All fluids should be warmed to body temperature; all fluids mentioned earlier can be warmed to 102° to 103° F (39° C).[2]

Even though hypoglycemia appears to be uncommon in birds, dextrose solutions may be added to crystalloid solutions when indicated. Hypoglycemia should be confirmed via measurement of blood glucose. An initial bolus of 50% dextrose diluted 1:4 with saline can be used; blood glucose should be monitored frequently after administration.

FLUID RATES AND VOLUMES FOR RESUSCITATION

As in all species, the lowest effective volume for restoration of normal endpoints should be used. For correction of hypovolemia, the endpoint of fluid administration is the successful restoration of normal blood pressure.[6]

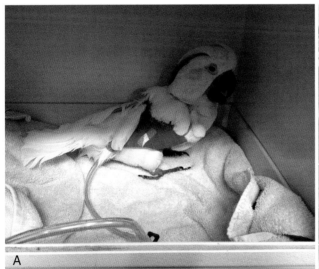
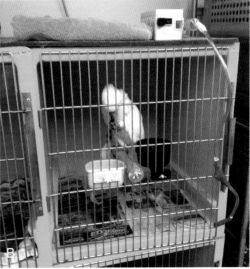

FIGURE 17-4 **A,** A cockatoo in renal failure receiving fluid diuresis via a basilic catheter sutured into place. The wing has been taped to the body. The infusion line is protected with aquarium tubing slit down the side and placed over the infusion line. The syringe pump is in the incubator under several layers of towels. **B,** The same bird 24 hours later. The bird is stable and much brighter, and had begun to eat and investigate the incubator. The bird was moved to a larger cage, and the syringe pump was placed out of reach on top of the cage. The bird was unable to disrupt the fluid line through the aquarium tubing.

Measurement of blood pressure can be challenging in birds, but is possible, especially in birds larger than cockatiels (75 to 100 g). Indirect blood pressure measurements can be obtained with a sphygmomanometer placed around the humerus, and an ultrasonic Doppler placed over the basilic vessels (ventral elbow) or, in larger birds, with oscillometric methods.[2] Although reference ranges for blood pressure have not been established for all species and there is limited ability of indirect blood pressure measurements to accurately reflect actual central blood pressure, these indirect blood pressure measurements are an extremely useful monitoring tool during resuscitation efforts. Other less specific indications of a favorable response to therapy include restoration of superficial vein turgor and improved mentation.

The authors regularly use the following protocol for treatment of hypovolemic shock in birds (Box 17-1):

BOX 17-1 FLOW CHART FOR CORRECTION OF PERFUSION DEFICITS IN BIRDS*

Decompensatory Phase of Shock (Bradycardia, Hypotension, and Hypothermia)

Slow IV or IO bolus over 10 minutes hypertonic saline 7.2% to 7.5% (3 mL/kg) + hetastarch (3 mL/kg)
↓
Begin external and core body temperature warming over 1 to 2 hours
Begin crystalloids at maintenance rate (3 to 4 mL/kg per hour)
↓
When patient is warmed to 98° F (36.6° C), begin correction of hypovolemia to indirect systolic blood pressure >90 mm Hg (recheck pressure after each bolus)
Repeat boluses 3 to 4 times until blood pressure is normal:
  1. Crystalloids (LRS, Normosol, and PlasmaLyte) at 10 mL/kg
  2. Colloids (HES) at 3 to 5 mL/kg
↓
Positive response: indirect systolic blood pressure >90 mm Hg:
Crystalloids to correct dehydration plus ongoing losses
↓
Add maintenance fluids (3 to 4 mL/kg per hour)
Negative response: indirect systolic blood pressure <90 mm Hg:
Repeat above
↓
No response:
Check blood glucose, electrolytes, PCV and total protein, ECG
↓
If hypoglycemic:
Give 50% dextrose diluted 50:50 with saline at 0.25 mg/kg
If PCV < 12% to 15% and low total protein:
Consider whole blood transfusion
If abnormal cardiac function:
Correct contractility (nitroglycerin ⅛ inches/2.5 kg)
↓
No response:
Consider vasopressor at small animal dose

*Note many of these have been extrapolated from other species and have not been thoroughly investigated in birds.

1. Administer a bolus infusion of warmed 7.2% to 7.5% hypertonic saline (3 mL/kg IV/IO) slowly over a period of 10 minutes).
2. Administer a bolus infusion of warmed HES (5 mL/kg IV/IO) over a period of 5 to 10 minutes.
3. Measure blood pressure and observe other clinical markers; once improved, administer maintenance isotonic crystalloids (2 to 3 mL/kg/h) while rewarming the patient.
4. If no improvement in clinical markers, repeat steps 1 and 2. Patients with hypoproteinemia can be given a constant rate infusion (CRI) of HES at 0.8 mL/kg per hour, which will help prevent further dilution of protein and help maintain oncotic pressures in the intravascular space.[2]

Patients who do not respond to shock therapy should be evaluated further. In other species, causes of nonresponsive shock can include severe anemia, hypoglycemia, electrolyte imbalances, acid-base disorders, cardiac dysfunction, and hypoxemia.[3] Many of these may be challenging to quickly or definitively identify in birds. Some conditions, however, can be addressed directly: for example, blood transfusion in the severely anemic bird (see the discussion in the following).

Fluid Therapy for Dehydration

Once hypovolemia is corrected, the immediate hydration deficits are addressed. Some traditional parameters for determination of hydration status, such as assessment of skin turgor, are less useful in avian patients. Hydration deficits can be inferred by history and supported by blood analysis parameters, such as elevated albumin, total protein, and in some cases uric acid. The authors determine volume of fluids for deficit correction using the following formula:

$$\% \text{ dehydration} \times \text{kg} \times 1000 \text{ mL}$$

Replace fluid deficits over 12 to 24 hours. If fluid loss is rapid, replacement can be performed over 4 to 5 hours. Add maintenance fluid requirements as well, adjusting these for continued excessive losses, for example, diarrhea and polyuria. Although maintenance rates have not been established for bird species, the authors use 3 mg/kg per hour.

Constant Rate Infusion of Fluids

Fluids for resuscitation are given as boluses. Once shock has been resolved, fluids for maintenance and correction of dehydration are given as a constant infusion, using a pediatric infusion pump or a syringe pump (Figure 17-5). Another option is periodic IV bolus, which is less than ideal. Infusion and syringe pumps are available from human and veterinary sources, and can often be found in the second-hand equipment market, as well. Critically ill birds usually tolerate the presence of the catheter and infusion line well. However, as birds recover, many will attempt to investigate and disrupt the catheter, infusion line, and pump if left in the patient's enclosure. Infusion lines can be covered with various-sized aquarium pump tubing, which has been slit completely down one side. The infusion line is inserted into the tubing via the slit (see Figure 17-4). Some birds may benefit from the placement of an Elizabethan or cervical restraint collar; however, these can be extremely stressful to some patients and can adversely affect patient condition. The ability to tolerate the collar should be determined for each patient. Another temporary option is the use of low-dose sedation.

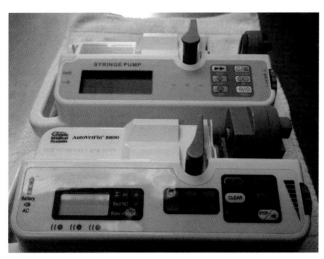

FIGURE 17-5 Two types of syringe pumps useful for birds and other exotic animals.

BLOOD TRANSFUSION

Birds tolerate blood loss surprisingly well. In a study using ducks, hypovolemic shock secondary to acute blood loss did not appear until removal of approximately 60% of the blood volume.[8] The authors have regularly encountered birds with chronic blood loss producing packed cell volume (PCV) as low as 6% to 7%. Transfusion should be considered for the following: ongoing blood loss, PCV below 12% to 15% with signs of weakness likely attributed to anemia, presence of a coagulopathy, or contemplated surgery in the presence of preexisting and significant anemia.

Sourcing whole blood for transfusion in birds can be challenging. Several studies have shown that erythrocyte lifespan is significantly longer in birds receiving transfusion from a homologous species (e.g., cockatiel to cockatiel).[9] When a homologous species is not available, consider transfusion from as closely related a species as possible. The authors maintain a list of local exotic bird rescues and other clients willing to bring in patients for blood donation in exchange for clinic credit. Cross matching would be ideal; however, its use has not been fully investigated in birds.[10]

Blood collection is performed in the carefully restrained, sedated, or anesthetized healthy donor via the jugular vein. Sodium citrate, heparin, acid-citrate dextrose (ACD), and other anticoagulants have been described for use in birds.[11] Use heparin at 0.25 mL/10 mL blood, or other products at the manufacturer's suggestion. Most authors recommend the use of a filter to remove aggregated debris. Collect no more than 10% of the donor's blood volume.

Administer donor blood by slow bolus over 10 minutes or by infusion with a syringe pump into IV or IO catheter. In cases of massive hemorrhage, administer blood more rapidly, within minutes. Administer all whole blood within 4 hours of collection to prevent the growth of bacteria, according to standards set by the American Association of Blood Banks.[12]

RESTORATION OF NORMOTHERMIA

Hypothermia is a common clinical feature in moderately to severely ill birds. Accurate measurement of body temperature is challenging in the bird, but it can be performed in unconscious birds with a flexible temperature probe inserted into the crop and proximal proventriculus. Normal reference ranges for body temperatures may not be available for all avian species.

Externally delivered warming methods include heated incubators, warming pads, radiant heat lamps, circulating warm water or air blankets, and administration of warmed SC fluids.[13] Core body temperature warmth is delivered through the administration of warmed IV or IO fluids.

DIAGNOSTIC WORKUP

For the critical patient, initial rapid in-house testing is ideal to help guide treatment decisions immediately. The avian practitioner should be able to manually evaluate the hemogram in an attempt to identify conditions requiring immediate intervention, such as anemia and leukocyte changes suggestive of sepsis. For biochemistry analysis, one bench-top analyzer offers an avian panel requiring only 0.13 mL of high quality whole blood (VetScan, Abaxis, Union City, California).

Diagnostic imaging can be useful in terms of diagnostic yield in the critically ill avian patient, and it may help identify specific conditions such as the presence of metal, and organ displacement or enlargement. Conscious sedation may facilitate the safe acquisition of diagnostic radiographic images, without the absolute necessity of general anesthesia.

TREATMENT OF THE CRITICAL PATIENT

Ideal treatment is based upon information gleaned from history, physical examination, and diagnostic testing. Some treatments can be delayed during the stabilization phase; examples may include primary wound care and fracture stabilization. Analgesics and antibacterial drugs are appropriate when indicated (e.g., the presence of open wounds, history of exposure to predators [even without identification of puncture wounds], history of exposure to other birds with likely bacterial infections, and evidence of infection noted on evaluation of the hemogram). "Shot gun" administration of antibiotics should be avoided. Antifungal drugs may be indicated in sick birds as well, especially those with marked elevations in leukocyte counts and evidence of respiratory disease.

Sick birds with evidence of gastrointestinal (GI) densities consistent with metal and compatible clinical signs of toxicosis should undergo chelation therapy while awaiting laboratory confirmation.

Fluid Support

Fluid therapy for the critical patient is described in detail already. Once the patient is stable, fluid needs may be met via SC administration and via the alimentary tract (tube feeding, if the patient is not drinking adequately on its own).[2]

Nutritional Support

Most ill birds do not take in enough food to meet their caloric needs. Adequate food consumption should not be gauged by the disappearance or disruption of food from the bowl, because many sick birds eat less than is actually required or manipulate food without actually eating enough of it. The best gauge of adequate food consumption is the appearance of normal-appearing, formed brown to green stool in the bird's enclosure, and maintenance of body weight. As GI transit time is normally rapid, fecal production should be monitored continuously during hospitalization. Pectoral muscle mass should subjectively be maintained, if caloric needs are being effectively met.

Supportive force-feeding is accomplished with the use of various-sized curved metal-ball-tipped feeding tubes manufactured specifically for this purpose. Rubber feeding tubes may be adequate for smaller birds and for many non-parrot species. These rubber feeding tubes are less applicable for most parrots, with their more powerful beaks, which may be capable of biting off and swallowing the feeding tube. Nutritional products used for hand feeding include commercial baby bird hand-feeding formula, and products specifically designed for ill birds (Emeraid, Lafeber Company, Cornell, Illinois). Tube feeding is stressful for most birds, and it should be accomplished quickly and competently. The metal-ball tip is introduced into the oral cavity, past the glottis and into the crop. Proper positioning can be confirmed by palpating the presence of a separate tube and the trachea. Food is delivered into the crop, and the tube is removed while maintaining a semifirm seal around the neck to prevent regurgitation of hand-feeding solution.

SEDATION AND ANESTHESIA

Anesthesia should be avoided where appropriate in the critically ill patient; however, some of the needed diagnostic testing and procedures can produce discomfort and stress, and thus affect patient survival negatively. The risks of sedation and/or anesthesia should be weighed against the risks of foregoing diagnostics and treatments or of attempting procedures in the conscious patient. Historically, avian practitioners have favored isoflurane induction via face mask or quickly performing many diagnostic procedures without anesthesia at all. Even though isoflurane and sevoflurane have a wider margin of safety compared with many older anesthetic agents, they are not benign. Volatile anesthesia can produce apnea and hypotension, especially at the higher concentrations required when used as sole agents. For many procedures, sedation is a superior option for the critical patient, especially at the low dosages suggested previously.[1]

REFERENCES

1. Lennox AM: Sedation as an alternative to general anesthesia in pet birds. In *Proceedings of the Association of Avian Veterinarians*, Seattle, 2001, pp 289–292.
2. Lennox AM, Lichtenberger M: Advanced fluid support for birds. In *Proceedings of the Association of Avian Veterinarians*, Seattle, 2011, pp 185–190.
3. American Heart Association: American Heart Association guidelines for cardiopulmonary resuscitation and emergency cardiovascular care, *Circulation* 112(Suppl 24):IVI–203, 2005.
4. Astiz ME: Pathophysiology and classification of shock states. In Fink MP, Abraham EA, Vincent J-L, Kochanek PM, editors: *Textbook of critical care*, Philadelphia, 2005, Elsevier Saunders, pp 897–997.
5. Bowles H, Lichtenberger M, Lennox A: Emergency and critical care of pet birds, *Vet Clin Exot Anim* 10:345–394, 2007.
6. Anderson NL: Intraosseous fluid therapy in small exotic animals. In Kirk RW, Bonagura JD, editors: *Current veterinary therapy XII: small animal practice*, Philadelphia, 2005, Saunders, pp 1331–1335.
7. Hallas P, Brabrand M, Fokestad L: Complication with intraosseous access: Scandinavian user's experience, *West J Emerg Med* 14(5):440–443, 2013.
8. Lichtenberger M, Orcutt C, Cray C, et al: Comparison of fluid types for resuscitation after acute blood loss in mallard ducks (*Anas platyrhynchos*), *J Vet Emerg Crit Care* 19(5):467–472, 2009.
9. Yagi K, Holowaychuk M, editors: *Manual of veterinary transfusion medicine and blood banking*, Wiley, in press.
10. Degernes LA, Crosier ML, Harrison LD, et al: Autologous, homologous and heterologous red blood cell transfusions in cockatiels (*Nymphicus hollandicus*), *J Avian Med Surg* 13(1):2–9, 1999.
11. Morrisey JK, Hohenhaus AE, Rosenthal KL: Comparison of three media for the storage of avian whole blood. In *Proceedings of the Association of Avian Veterinarians*, 1997, pp 279–290.
12. American Association of Blood Banks: http://www.aabb.org. Accessed July 26, 2014.
13. Rembert MS, Smith JA, Hosgood G, et al: Comparison of traditional thermal support devices with the forced air warmer system in anesthetized Hispaniolan Amazon parrots (*Amazona ventralis*), *J Avian Med Surg* 15(3):187–193, 2001.

Advancements in Diagnosis and Management of Toxicologic Problems

Tina Wismer

Whether they are wild, caged, or farmed, birds can be exposed to a myriad of household and environmental toxins. Most decontamination techniques transfer easily from one species to another; however, some techniques may vary due to the uniqueness of the birds' physiology. Birds readily chew on or ingest foreign material in their environments. Birds have a fast gastrointestinal transit time, quick absorption rates, and a high metabolic rate compared with mammals. Their respiratory system is extremely sensitive to gases and smoke. There is variation between species in their response to different toxins.

Diagnosis of most toxicoses is based on history and clinical signs, as specific tests are uncommon and oftentimes limited in availability. Management for most suspected toxicities consists of stabilizing the patient, preventing further exposure, decreasing further absorption, administering an antidote (if available), increasing the removal of absorbed toxicants, and supportive therapy.

In most cases, supportive care includes parenteral fluids and a warm cage environment capable of providing enriched oxygen. Stress needs to be minimized, as it has profound adverse effects on the well-being of ill birds. Moving more slowly and allowing the patient downtime can help reduce stress during assessments and treatments. The strategic use of sedatives and anesthesia can make the management of many toxicoses much easier for you and the patient. If possible, take a complete history while the patient is being stabilized. The history for owned birds should include information such as whether the animal has been exposed to infectious disease, the animal's environment, diet, reproductive status, and previous illnesses. Environmental history includes information about caging, flight capabilities, and exposure to toxins. With wildlife, the information should include where the bird was found and what the clinical signs were at the time.

DECONTAMINATION

For birds with a recent history of exposure to a toxin, decontamination may help decrease the severity of the clinical signs. Decontamination can be performed for ocular, dermal, and oral exposures. Veterinary staff should wear proper protective clothing, including gloves or mask, to prevent personal injury. Ocular exposures in birds can be irritating or even corrosive to the cornea, depending on the substance, the concentration, and the exposure time. With any ocular exposure, the eyes should be flushed repeatedly with tepid water or a saline solution for a minimum of 20 to 30 minutes.[1] An eyedropper can be used for smaller birds. With larger birds, a flexible, nonbreakable cup can be used to slowly pour fluids over the ocular area. A mild sedative before flushing may make this procedure easier, if the health of the patient will allow. If no sedation is used, the patient should be allowed to rest at regular intervals during the flushing to minimize stress. Fluorescein-stain the eye after flushing to check for corneal ulceration. Lubricant ointments should be used following staining.

Dermal exposures to a large variety of substances can occur, including petroleum distillates, pesticides, corrosives, and adherent substances (tar, asphalt, sap, and glue). Once again, removal of dermal substances may be less stressful for the patient and safer for the handler if the patient is sedated. If not sedated, the patient should be allowed to rest at regular intervals during bathing to minimize stress. Depending on what the substance is and the amount, dermal substances may be removed from birds by misting with room-temperature water in a warm environment. The bird should be misted until you can no longer smell or feel the product on the bird's feathers. If misting alone does not remove the product and soap is needed, a liquid hand dishwashing detergent should be diluted and applied. After removal of the substance, the bird should be rinsed with plain water until all soap is removed. After misting or bathing, the bird should be wiped with a dry towel and kept in a warm environment away from drafts until completely dry.[1] When removing sticky substances from feathers, do not use solvents, which may be irritating, corrosive, or destructive to normal feather architecture. Work a small amount of vegetable oil, olive oil, corn oil, mayonnaise, or peanut butter through the substance until it breaks down into "gummy balls." Afterward, wash with liquid dishwashing detergent as described above. Do not use mineral oil, as it is very hard to remove from feathers.

Dilution with water or juicy fruits or vegetables is recommended in cases of corrosive ingestion. Dilution is not recommended in patients who are at an increased risk of aspiration.[1] While birds can regurgitate, inducing emesis is not recommended. A crop or proventriculus lavage is used in birds to remove recently ingested toxicants (1 to 3 hours postingestion). An endotracheal tube should be placed under anesthesia to prevent aspiration.[2] The crop should be flushed gently with warm saline or tap water and aspirated. This should be repeated three to four times or as needed until material is no longer being removed. Crop lavages should not be performed in cases of caustic or petroleum distillate ingestion.

Activated charcoal adsorbs toxicants and facilitates their excretion via the feces. Activated charcoal can be given orally with a gavage tube. The recommended dose of activated

TABLE 18-1

Crop Volume

Species	Crop Volume (ml)
Finch	0.1–0.5
Canary	0.25–0.5
Budgie	1
Lovebird	1–4
Cockatiel	2–4
Small Parrot	3–6
Medium Parrot	10–15
Large Parrot	20–30

charcoal for all species of animals is 1 to 3 g/kg (or 1 to 3 mg/g) body weight.[3] See Table 18-1 for estimated crop volumes in selected species. Many birds can regurgitate a portion of the activated charcoal dose given. Activated charcoal should not be given to birds that have ingested caustic materials. Other materials that are not effectively absorbed by activated charcoal include heavy metals, ethanol, methanol, fertilizer, fluoride, petroleum distillates, iodides, nitrates, nitrites, and chlorates.

Bulk and osmotic cathartics can be used in birds. Cathartics enhance the elimination of substances, including activated charcoal, by decreasing gastrointestinal transit time. Without cathartics, the toxicant bound by activated charcoal may eventually be released and reabsorbed.

Bulk cathartics such as psyllium (0.5 tsp with 60 mL baby food), diluted peanut butter, fruit, or vegetables can help move heavy items through the digestive tract. Osmotic cathartics pull electrolyte-free water into the gastrointestinal tract.[4] Sorbitol, an osmotic cathartic, is commonly combined with activated charcoal in prepared products, and its dosage is 3 mL/kg. Oil-based cathartics are not recommended due to the risk of aspiration.[2] Enemas are also not recommended for birds.

LEAD

Lead toxicosis, or "plumbism," has been recognized in both humans and domestic animals for thousands of years. Historically it has been one of the most common toxicoses described in birds.[2] All species of birds are susceptible to lead toxicosis, but it has been most commonly associated with waterfowl. Since the ban on lead shot was implemented (1991 in the United States), studies that compared the prevalence of lead poisoning in waterfowl before and after the ban showed a 44% to 64% reduction in lead poisoning.[5] Wildlife may still be exposed to lead from lead shot deposited before the ban or used to hunt upland game, from ingestion of tissue from prey containing lead shot or bullets, from ingestion of lead sinkers or jigs lost by fishermen, or from environmental contamination from lead smelters or sewage sludge. Captive and household birds may ingest lead from leaded paints, caulking, solder, or linoleum.[6]

Once ingested, lead is solubilized in the acidic environment of the proventriculus and ventriculus and absorbed in the small intestine.[7] The lower the pH in the digestive tract (raptors = pH 1), the more rapid the absorption is, compared with higher-pH environments (psittacines, granivorous birds =

pH 2 to 4).[8,9] Organolead is most readily absorbed, followed by lead salts and then metallic lead.[10] The degree of absorption of lead from the gut can also be affected by diet; cracked corn diets were shown to increase the absorption of lead when compared to "soft" diets in ducks and geese.[11] High-fiber diets have been associated with more severe clinical signs and elevated levels of blood and tissue lead concentration in mallard ducks.[12] Diets higher in calcium reduced morbidity and mortality in experimentally lead-poisoned ducks.[13] The casting mechanism present in raptors may provide a means of shortening exposure as well as eliminating lead fragments from the stomach. Lead may also be inhaled if the dust is in a fine particulate state (sanded lead paint). Once deposited in the lungs, lead is almost completely absorbed.[14] Lead shot that is embedded in soft tissues, such as muscle, is not appreciably absorbed unless inflammation is present, while lead shot in joint cavities (acidic environment) can be absorbed.[10]

Once absorbed, more than 90% of lead is bound to red blood cells and is then distributed to the body. Lead is distributed to all tissues. The blood, parenchymal organs, nervous system, and soft tissues will store about 6% of the total body burden of lead, and approximately 94% of the burden will be in bone. Lead distribution is in three compartments, and it can move from one to another. The rapid exchange compartment, composed largely of blood and highly perfused organs, comprises about 4% of the total body burden. The intermediate rate of exchange compartment is soft tissue, including the nervous system, and holds only about 2% of the body burden. The third compartment is bone, which has a slow rate of exchange and may hold 94% of the body burden.[15] Hydroxyapatite crystals in bone have a high affinity for lead, and therefore most of the body burden of lead is stored there. Due to this storage in the bone, blood-lead values represent only a small amount of the total body burden.[15] Remodeling bone or chelation can release stored lead, resulting in clinical signs long after the original lead exposure.[6] Ingestion of lead by poultry can also lead to human health concerns. Eggs accumulate lead in their shells, yolk, and albumen, with the highest concentration occurring in the shells.[16] The lowest concentration of lead is found in skeletal muscle.[16]

Lead is excreted from the body in various ways. The majority of ingested lead is excreted in the feces without being absorbed.[17] Absorbed lead is filtered across the glomeruli and can accumulate in the renal tubular epithelium. Chelating agents will enhance the urinary excretion of lead.

Lead interferes with multiple processes within the body. It affects various cell types, enzymes, tissues, and organ systems (vascular, nervous, renal, immune, reproductive, hematological, and behavioral).[18,19] Anemia is common in chronic lead toxicosis in humans and animals. By binding with –SH (sulfhydryl) groups of enzyme systems, lead interferes with enzymes involved in heme synthesis, such as δ-aminolevulinic acid dehydratase (ALAD) (also known as porphobilinogen synthase) and ferrochelatase. The effects of δ-ALAD inhibition in birds may be more severe than in mammals, since they have more metabolically active nucleated red blood cells that require porphyrin synthesis not only for hemoglobin production, but also for respiratory heme-containing enzymes.[20,21] These alterations cause an accumulation of hemoglobin precursors (delta amino levulinic acid, protoporphyrins [free and zinc-bound]).[22,23] These hemoglobin precursors cause red blood cell abnormalities.[6] Damage to membrane-associated enzymes and sodium-potassium pumps results in red blood cell fragility and a shortened lifespan. Basophilic stippling of red blood cells occurs due to accumulated ribosomal RNA aggregates. RNA cannot be degraded or dephosphorylated by pyrimidine-5′-nucleotidase (P5NT), as lead inhibits the activity of P5NT.[24] Accumulation of ALA causes a neuropathogenic effect, most likely by acting as a γ-aminobutyric acid (GABA) receptor agonist in the nervous system; it also stimulates reactive oxygen species (ROS) and lipid peroxidation, contributing to hemolysis and anemia.[25] The membrane-associated damage also causes an increase in biliverdinuria and fibrinoid vascular necrosis in multiple organs that manifests as perivascular hemorrhage.[26]

Lead impairs gastroenteric motility by altering synaptic transmission at the neuromuscular junction of visceral smooth muscle, leading to impactions and lead colic.[27] Lead colic is from spasmodic contractions of the smooth muscles of the intestinal wall.[28] In pigeons, lead causes a cyclic adenosine monophosphate (AMP)–induced relaxation of smooth muscle in the crop.[29,30]

Lead not only competes with calcium ions, resulting in substitution for calcium in bone, it also mimics or inhibits many cellular actions of calcium and alters calcium flux across membranes. This increases levels of cytoplasmic calcium in many cell types, leading to calcium-mediated cell death and chronic impairment in neuronal differentiation and synaptogenesis.[31-33] Rising levels of intracellular calcium in the cerebrovascular endothelium disturb microfilaments and/or other cellular components responsible for the integrity of tight junctions and contributes to the development of cerebral edema.[34] Lead's inhibition of calcium flux is responsible for some of its effects on central and peripheral neurotransmission.[32] Lead interferes with cellular energy and metabolism in mitochondria. It can also lead to inhibition of cytochrome P-450, which in turn results in aberrant neurotransmission of serotonergic pathways.[6] This may explain some of the changes in behavior seen in birds. Other nervous system–related effects include progressive demyelination of peripheral nerves.[35-37]

Lead binds to sulfhydryl groups in proteins and breaks disulfide bonds that are important for maintaining proper conformation for biological activity.[15,38] It can alter many enzymes via its competing effects with other cations, such as ferrous iron and zinc. Lead also interrupts zinc-dependent enzyme processes interfering with GABA production or activity in the central nervous system.[10]

The clinical signs of lead toxicosis will vary depending on whether the exposure is acute or chronic. The onset of clinical signs can vary with the amount and rate of lead ingestion and dietary factors. Turkey vultures *(Cathartes aura)* and red-tailed hawks *(Buteo jamaicensis)* tolerate higher lead levels than other raptors, such as bald eagles *(Haliaeetus leucocephalus).*[9] Death may occur within a few days to several months, depending on the degree of exposure (e.g., number of shot ingested). Experimentally poisoned Canada geese given a large number of pellets (n = 25) developed rapid elevations of blood-lead levels, acute clinical signs of lead poisoning, and death within 10 days.[39] Geese dosed with 10 pellets had a slower increase in blood-lead levels, exhibited signs of chronic lead poisoning, and lived longer (up to 72 days).[39] In orally dosed bald eagles (4 to 5 kg bird), uptake of 19 to 40 mg of lead was lethal in 10 to 12 days.[40] A chip of lead-based paint the size of a thumbnail may contain 50 to 200 mg of lead.

Acute lead toxicosis in birds generally results in anorexia, lethargy, bile-green diarrhea, discolored urates, altered voice (dysphonia), respiratory distress, blindness, muscle weakness that progresses to paresis/paralysis, seizures, coma, and death.[41] Among caged birds, the larger parrot species are more likely to show hematuria than parakeets or cockatiels.[41] Chronically, birds have weight loss with atrophy of the breast muscles, resulting in a "razor keel" appearance. Impaction of the gizzard and/or proventriculus with food, sand, or other ingesta may occur due to impaired motility of the ventriculus.[42] Impaction of the distal esophagus and proventriculus is reported more often in lead-poisoned waterfowl than in other avian species.[36,43] These birds are depressed and biliverdinuric, but do not typically exhibit neurologic signs other than depression.[9] Lead-induced immunosuppression may result in secondary infections.

Clinical pathology abnormalities include heterophilia, hypochromic regenerative anemia, cytoplasmic vacuolization of red cells, hypoproteinemia, elevations in lactic dehydrogenase, aspartate transaminase, creatine phosphokinase, and uric acid.[15] On gross necropsy, an engorged gall bladder (bile stasis, raptors), pale streaks on the myocardium, hydropericardium, cephalic edema in geese and swans, and submandibular edema (Canada and snow geese) may be noted.[44-46] Histopathologic lesions are seen in various tissues. Hepatic lesions include degeneration, necrosis and atrophy of the hepatocytes, and hemosiderin accumulation in the Kupffer cells and hepatocytes.[12] Renal lesions include proximal tubular necrosis and degeneration, visceral gout, hemosiderosis, and acid-fast intranuclear inclusion bodies (not present in every lead-poisoned bird).[39,47] Myocardial degeneration and necrosis may be secondary to fibrinoid vascular necrosis of arterioles in the heart and other organ locations.[39,45] Neurologic lesions consist of brain and meningeal edema and demyelination of the peripheral nerves, including the vagus, brachial, and sciatic nerves.[36] In birds with proventricular impaction, atrophy of the plica and glands in the proventriculus may be present.[10]

The initial diagnosis of lead toxicosis may be difficult, as the clinical signs and gross lesions are nonspecific in nature. A diagnosis of lead poisoning is based on history of exposure, clinical signs, clinical pathology findings, blood-lead concentrations, and radiographic evidence of metallic densities in the gastrointestinal tract. Radiographs can detect the presence of radiopaque metallic pellets in the ventriculus, but nontoxic shot (copper, steel, tungsten, tin, bismuth) and lead cannot be differentiated radiographically. Also, the absence of metal particles does not rule out heavy metal toxicosis. Blood-lead concentration is the definitive test for confirmation.[9]

Heparinized whole blood is the preferred sample, as more than 90% of circulating lead is bound to erythrocytes. Unfortunately, reference values are not available for all species of birds, but some generalizations can be made. Blood-lead concentrations less than 0.5 mg/kg (ppm) are generally not associated with clinical signs.[42] Birds with blood-lead concentrations between 0.5 and 1.0 mg/kg are usually mildly to moderately symptomatic. Clinical signs worsen when blood-lead concentrations exceed 1.0 mg/kg.

Blood-lead concentration, measured by atomic absorption spectrophotometry, is the most sensitive method for assessment.

Unfortunately, a delay of 1 to 3 days may ensue before results are known. A portable blood-lead analyzer may be useful in field studies for rapid identification of lead intoxication.[48]

δ-ALAD activity is another biomarker for lead exposure in birds.[49] It is useful to determine chronicity and prognosis. Postmortem lead levels in the liver and kidney are used to make a diagnosis of lead poisoning. Liver-lead concentrations greater than 6.0 mg/kg wet weight are generally considered diagnostic.[46]

Treatment of lead toxicosis includes eliminating the metal from the gastrointestinal tract to stop further absorption, chelation therapy to reduce blood-lead levels, and general supportive care. Animals should be stabilized as needed before other therapies are instituted. Removal of lead objects from the gastrointestinal tract is necessary before chelation, as most chelators will enhance lead absorption.[50,51] Removal of the lead can be achieved with cathartics, gavage, endoscopy, or surgery.[52] Various lead chelation agents have been used off-label in avian species. CaEDTA (calcium disodium ethylenediaminetetraacetic acid), BAL (British-Anti-Lewisite), D-penicillamine (cuprimine), and succimer (DMSA, Chemet) all have advantages and disadvantages to their use.

The calcium disodium salt of ethylenediaminetetraacetic acid, $CaNa_2EDTA$ or CaEDTA, has been the principal chelator for lead poisoning in birds. It forms stable complexes with lead and increases urinary excretion. CaEDTA is more effective in removing lead stored in bone than in removing lead from soft tissues.[53] CaEDTA must be administered parenterally as absorption from the gastrointestinal tract is poor. Administration of oral CaEDTA with lead still in the digestive tract has been shown to increase systemic absorption of lead in mammals.[54] The established dose for CaEDTA is 35 to 50 mg/kg given every 8 to 12 hours by intramuscular or subcutaneous routes.[29,42] Higher doses, up to 100 mg/kg, have been used in birds without observed ill effect.[52,55] In mammals, incidental chelation of zinc and nephrosis are common, but none of these are described in birds even with high levels of CaEDTA and prolonged courses of therapy.[52] Classical treatment schedules are three days on, two days off to allow for replenishment of any divalent cations that were chelated by the CaEDTA and to allow any developing nephrosis to subside.[56] In birds, clinicians have deviated considerably from this regimen. It is recommended to recheck blood-lead levels 3 to 4 days after stopping parenteral CaEDTA. The removal of lead from bone can increase blood-lead levels and precipitate clinical signs during chelation.

D-penicillamine is an oral lead chelator. Reports of its use in avian species are few.[15] The dose is 55 mg/kg PO every 12 hours for 5 days, and repeat after 5 days if needed. D-penicillamine can be tube-fed to birds (suspend a 125 mg capsule in 15 mL lactulose: 1 drop/100 g PO).[4] Keep the bird hydrated during therapy.

BAL was originally used as an antidote to arsenic-based weaponized gas (Lewisite), and later it was found to be effective in chelating lead. An advantage of BAL compared with CaEDTA is its ability to cross the blood-brain barrier. It adsorbs lead from the erythrocytes, removes lead from parenchymatous tissues (especially the brain), and increases both urinary and biliary excretion of lead.[50] However, BAL is nephrotoxic and very painful on injection.[56] It can be used alone or in conjunction with CaEDTA.

Meso 2,3-dimercaptosuccinic acid (DMSA, succimer) is a water-soluble derivative of BAL used to treat lead poisoning. It is an oral chelator that is capable of chelating lead from the brain and other soft tissues, but it does not chelate lead from bone.[56] Unlike CaEDTA or penicillamine, succimer does not chelate essential minerals such as zinc. DMSA has a narrow therapeutic index, so accurate dosing is important. While 30 mg/kg/day PO is recommended, it has been shown that in cockatiels DMSA could be safely administered at 40 mg/kg twice daily for at least 21 days; however, doses as low as 15 mg/kg have been reported effective.[57-59] The dose can be sprinkled onto food. DMSA produces a more rapid rate of reduction of blood-lead levels in cockatiels when compared with CaEDTA.[59] However, it has a narrow therapeutic index (less than twofold), and considerable regurgitation was observed among treated birds. Survival rates among lead-poisoned cockatiels were similar between DMSA and CaEDTA-treated birds. Other studies with CaEDTA and DMSA combinations have yielded more favorable results. Degernes et al[42] used CaEDTA alone or in combination with DMSA in lead-poisoned trumpeter swans (*Cygnus buccinator*). The survival rate was 35% with EDTA alone and 50% with combination therapy. Combining DMSA with taurine (50 to 100 mg/kg) in rats increases depleted blood glutathione (GSH) levels, increases the activity of ALAD, and reduces the blood zinc protoporphyrin ZPP levels to near normal.[60]

Other adjuncts to chelation therapy include fluid therapy, nutritional support, and supportive care (blood transfusions, prokinetics). Antioxidative therapies with supplemental vitamin C and zinc may be instituted, as lead is an inducer of free radicals. Vitamin B complex may aid the recovery of injury to the nervous system.[61] Species that are susceptible to aspergillosis (e.g., swans, sea ducks) should be prophylactically treated with antifungals (itraconazole, voriconazole) for the first 7 to 10 days of therapy.[42,62]

Different species of birds have different tolerances of lead. For example, the upper limit of "treatable" lead poisoning in bald eagles is a blood level of 1.2 ppm, while condors have been treated successfully up to 6 ppm.[9] Above this threshold limit, death or permanent impairment is likely, and humane euthanasia is recommended. However, since the kinetics of lead are dynamic, there are some birds that present with levels well above the upper limit that appear to be only mildly affected. Permanent impairments can range from visual impairment to lack of stamina. There are no data about long-term survivability and productivity for lead-poisoned birds.[9]

ZINC

Zinc toxicosis has been reported in captive birds and free-flying waterfowl.[63-65] Most commonly, animals may be exposed through ingestion of zinc from objects such as carpentry hardware (nuts and bolts), U.S. pennies minted after 1982, and galvanized items (fence clips).[63]

Zinc-containing objects in the stomach or gizzard are corroded by the low pH. The zinc is ionized and readily absorbed into the bloodstream. Zinc is directly damaging to red blood cells, resulting in hemolysis and renal failure secondary to hemoglobinuria. Zinc is irritating to the gastrointestinal tract, and regurgitation may be noted for a few days before the onset of more severe signs. Nonspecific clinical signs of

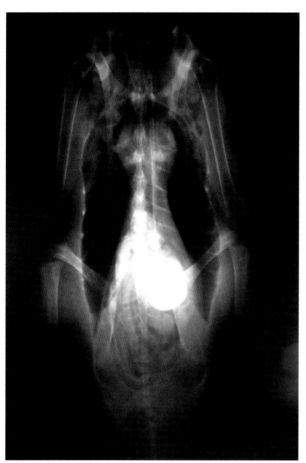

FIGURE 18-1 Ventrodorsal radiographic image of a mallard duck with acute-onset clinical signs consistent with zinc intoxication. The silhouettes of multiple coins were apparent in the ventriculus. (Photo courtesy Brian Speer.)

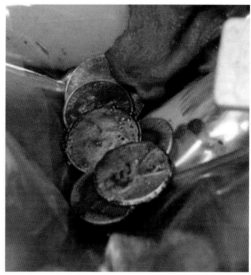

FIGURE 18-2 Intraoperative photo of some of the coins removed from the ventriculus of the duck. Note that there is corrosion of the edges of the pennies, but not the dime or quarter. US pennies minted after 1982 can be a rich source of excessive zinc exposure in ground-feeding bird species. (Photo courtesy Brian Speer.)

zinc toxicosis include pallor, weakness, ataxia, paresis or paralysis of the legs, anemia, diarrhea, weight loss, and death.[63-65]

Diagnosis is based on history, clinical signs, radiology, pathologic findings, and elevated serum or tissue (liver, pancreas, or kidney) zinc concentrations. Radiographic identification of metallic foreign bodies in the stomach or gizzard may help in narrowing the diagnosis; however, these findings do not confirm or deny diagnosis (Figure 18-1). Serum zinc levels may help confirm the diagnosis, but turnaround times

may be too long for acute cases. Normal plasma or serum zinc levels vary depending on the species (Table 18-2).[66,67] Toxic levels described in case reports typically have exceeded 10 mg/kg.[63,64,66] Postmortem, the pancreas is the tissue of choice for assessment of zinc toxicosis in birds, but liver and kidney levels are also useful. Mean tissue levels of 530 (pancreas), 440 (liver), and 210 (kidney) mg/kg dry weight were reported in one group of zinc-poisoned waterfowl.[65] Histopathologic changes include necrotizing ventriculitis, pancreatic necrosis and degeneration, and focal mononuclear degeneration of liver and kidney.[15]

Treatment of zinc toxicosis entails stabilizing the patient with fluids and blood transfusions if needed. Any metal found in the gastrointestinal tract should be removed (Figure 18-2). Many times, zinc levels will rapidly drop following removal of the foreign object, and chelation will not be needed. Parenteral CaEDTA is the chelator of choice for zinc in avian species.

POLYTETRAFLUOROETHYLENE

Polytetrafluoroethylene (PTFE, Teflon) is an inert nonstick coating used on cookware and heat bulbs. Pyrolysis of PTFE releases highly toxic carbonyl fluoride, hydrogen fluoride, and perfluoroisobutylene.[68] Pyrolysis of PTFE occurs at temperatures greater than 260° C (536° F), but reported cases of toxicosis have occurred at lower temperatures (Table 18-3).[68-70] Both Forbes[71] and Boucher et al[70] reported deaths with birds under PTFE-coated heat bulbs. Some brands of heat bulbs are coated with PTFE to protect them and make them easy to clean. PTFE-coated drip pans should not be used in households with birds. The pans, located under burners, will reach over 315° C (600° F) or higher within minutes during normal use because of their close proximity to the heating element of the burner.

TABLE 18-2

Normal Zn Levels[66,67]

Genus	Serum/plasma ppm
Macaw	0.23–2.38
Cockatoo	0.25–3.41
Cockatiel	0.70–2.34
Conure	0.35–1.91
Amazon	0.38–2.56
Hispaniolan amazon	1.25–2.29
Eclectus parrot	0.41–2.63
African Grey	0.15–2.46

TABLE 18-3

Temperatures Relevant to PTFE Toxicosis

Temperature (F)	Common Cooking Temperatures
325	Birds died from preheated oven[69]
350	Common baking temperature
396	Temperature of PTFE-coated lightbulbs under which Missouri birds died[70]
500	Searing temp for meat in oven or grill
536	Birds killed in DuPont lab experiments
700	Preheated grill
750	Surface of PTFE-coated pan after heating for 8 minutes on conventional stove[68]
1000	Drip pans (gas range)
1500	Broiling temperature for high-end ovens

Birds are extremely sensitive to chlorofluorocarbon fumes. These fumes sensitize the myocardium, causing arrhythmias, pulmonary congestion, and cardiac failure. On necropsy, hemorrhagic and edematous lungs are the most common findings. Most birds will develop respiratory signs and die immediately, but environmental conditions and ventilation can be vastly different between rooms and homes. Birds affected by PTFE are often off their perch, uncoordinated, open mouth breathing, have respiratory rales, and will tail bob with each respiratory effort.[72] If a bird only has a mild exposure, treatment includes humidified oxygen, diuretics to reduce pulmonary edema, nonsteroidal antiinflammatory drugs, broad-spectrum antibiotics, and supportive care.[72]

CARBON MONOXIDE (CO)

Carbon monoxide (CO) is produced by inefficient combustion of carbon-based fuels (wood, coal, petroleum, natural gas). CO is toxic to all species of domestic animals, birds, and humans. Birds with high respiratory and metabolic rates are more susceptible than mammals to CO poisoning. CO has a similar density to air, so it does not segregate or stratify readily. It will accumulate in garages, homes, closed trailers, livestock housing units, and operating vehicles with poor ventilation or leaks in the exhaust system.[73]

CO competes with oxygen for binding to hemoglobin. Hemoglobin has 240 times more affinity for CO than oxygen and will selectively bind CO. This higher affinity results in production of carboxyhemoglobin (COHb). Acute CO toxicosis results when COHb concentration in blood exceeds 30%.[74] COHb is detectable in blood for several days, and the test is available at many clinical laboratories, in hospitals, and some veterinary diagnostic laboratories.

Acute CO toxicosis causes initial dyspnea, ataxia, rapid depression, coma, respiratory paralysis, and death. The blood is bright red due to the color of COHb. Anoxia leads to necrosis of the cerebral cortex and white matter, globus pallidus, and brainstem. Recovered animals can have permanent brain damage and locomotor impairment.[75] COHb is very stable and can remain in the bloodstream when CO exposure ceases. If hyperbaric oxygen is available, it is the treatment of choice. If not, place the animal in an oxygen cage, or intubate and ventilate as needed with 100% oxygen. Carbon monoxide prognosis is guarded. Poisonings can be prevented in homes

and animal confinement units with alarmed CO detectors. Even low levels of CO can affect hatchery situations. Exposure to 100 ppm reduces hatchability by 21% and 200 ppm by 83%.[73]

ANTICOAGULANTS

Anticoagulant rodenticides are widely used to control rodent populations in both urban and rural areas. They are especially toxic to raptors. Anticoagulants work by inhibiting 1,2,3-vitamin K epoxide reductase, causing a loss of vitamin K regeneration. This results in depletion of active vitamin K, which leads to the inhibition of coagulation synthesis. The vitamin K–dependent factors are II, VII, IX, and X. Birds lack factors XI and XII; however, both the tissue factor pathway (extrinsic) and the amplification or contact pathway (intrinsic) function in avian coagulation are affected.[76]

There are both first- and second-generation anticoagulants. The first-generation anticoagulants (coumarin, warfarin, and indandione) require frequent, multiple feedings by rodents to produce toxicosis. The second-generation anticoagulants (SGARs) (brodifacoum, bromadiolone) have a much longer biological half-life. SGARs are slowly metabolized by the liver and allow predators to accumulate lethal doses by ingesting multiple intoxicated rodents. The rodents can survive for several days after consuming a lethal dose and may continue feeding on the bait, increasing the possibility that the body burden in poisoned rodents may significantly exceed the LD_{50} or even LD_{100} dose.[77] These rodents may exhibit an altered state of behavior, such as spending more time in open areas in a lethargic state, predisposing them to predation.[77] Once ingested by the bird, SGARs persist for at least 6 months in liver and tissues.[78]

Toxicosis in birds is dependent on the dose and the susceptibility of the species (Table 18-4).[79-81] Toxicity is possible when a dose is ingested greater than or equal to 1/10 of the LD_{50}. Birds that have ingested anticoagulants often present with pale mucous membranes and anemia. They are weak, lethargic, and frequently have subcutaneous ecchymoses and bleed profusely from superficial wounds.[82]

For free-ranging birds, diagnosis is often made based on clinical signs at the time of presentation. For avian species, there is little available information regarding clotting profiles.[82] Intoxication due to rodenticides is often discovered postmortem. On gross necropsy, massive internal hemorrhage and a lack of a postmortem heart blood clot are generally present. Plasma, stomach contents, or liver may be used to check for the presence of anticoagulants.[83] Great horned owls can develop subcutaneous hemorrhaging with liver concentrations of brodifacoum as low as 0.01 μg/g.[78]

Decontamination can be attempted to decrease the absorption of consumed bait itself or from poisoned rodents. Gavage and activated charcoal can both be used. When treating anticoagulant rodenticides, both clotting factors and oxygen-carrying capacity (blood) must be replaced. Vitamin K_1 (2.2 mg/kg q4 to 8 h) should be administered IM until the bird is stable, then dosed PO every 24 hours for at least 3 weeks.[62] If a bird presents with a packed cell volume (PCV) less than 20% and has clinical signs suggesting need, a whole blood transfusion should be attempted. A healthy, conspecific individual can donate 1% of its body weight. Whole blood

TABLE 18-4

Reported Oral LD₅₀ for Some Anticoagulants

Species	Brodifacoum	Defethialone	Bromadiolone	Chlorphacinone	Diphacinone
Canada Goose	< 0.75 mg/kg[79]				
Blackbird	> 3 mg/kg[79]			430 mg/kg[80]	
California quail	3.3 mg/kg[79]				
Ring-necked pheasant	10 mg/kg[79]			> 100 mg/kg[80]	
Mallard Duck	0.26–4.6 mg/kg[79,81]				3158 mg/kg[81]
Bobwhite Quail		0.264 mg/kg[81]	138–170 mg/kg[81]	258 mg/kg[81]	400–2000 mg/kg[81]

should be collected in heparin, citrate phosphate dextrose, sodium citrate, or citrate dextrose.[84] The donor should receive replacement fluids, and the whole blood should be administered either IV or IO to the recipient at 2 mL/min shortly after collection using a blood filter.[84] Due to the risk of hemorrhage, gentle handling must be used to prevent self-inflicted trauma and subsequent hemorrhage. Oxygen, cage rest, and nutritional support are also needed.

HYDROCARBONS/PETROLEUM DISTILLATES

Petroleum distillates are hydrocarbons. Hydrocarbons can range from volatile compounds like gasoline and mineral spirits to solid waxes. Both wild and household birds have the opportunity to be exposed to several types of petroleum distillates (Table 18-5).[85] Hydrocarbons can be absorbed by inhalation, by ingestion, or dermally. The rate of absorption is determined

by the substance: Volatile compounds are absorbed quickly, while oils are more slowly absorbed. Preferential distribution to fatty tissues occurs, and neurotoxicity is thought to occur when lipophilic hydrocarbons dissolve in nerve cell membranes and disrupt membrane protein function. Adverse effects in birds are related to the type of hydrocarbon, the amounts of exposure, and the duration of exposure. Morbidity from oral hydrocarbon exposures is primarily due to complications of aspiration.[86]

Marine and shore birds are often most severely affected by oil spills.[87] When covered with petroleum products, the normal interlocking structures of the barbicels of intact feathers are disrupted, destroying their ability to provide waterproofing and insulation. Thus, oiled birds may be unable to fly and can die from hypothermia or drowning. Unable to forage normally, affected birds can become progressively more dehydrated, debilitated, and susceptible to predation.[88] Oil ingestions in birds have also been shown to increase mixed-function

TABLE 18-5

Hydrocarbon Classes and Examples of Common Substances[85]

Petroleum distillates	Diesel fuel and exhaust Gasoline Naphtha (lighter fluid) VM&P naphthas (varnish, dry cleaning products) Stoddard solvent (dry cleaning solvent, general cleaner/degreaser, paint thinners, photocopier toners, printing inks, adhesives) Mineral spirits Mineral seal oil (furniture polish) Kerosene (No. 1 fuel oil)* Jet fuel Fuel oil (No. 2 fuel oil, gas oil, diesel oil) Lubricating oils (motor oil, grease) Petroleum jelly/petrolatum jelly Paraffin wax Asphalt	Aromatic hydrocarbons	Benzene Toluene Xylene
		Selected terpenes	Turpentine Pine oil (pine oil cleaner)
		Chlorinated (halogenated) hydrocarbons	Carbon tetrachloride Chlorinated hydrocarbon insecticides Chloroform Methyl chloride Methylene chloride Tetrachloroethylene Trichloroethane Vinyl chloride Trichloroethylene
		Other hydrocarbons	Automatic transmission fluid Coal pitch and coal tar pitch volatiles Naphthalene Machining fluids Pressurized paints Thermoplastic road paint Waste oils
Other aliphatic hydrocarbons (alkanes, alkenes, alkynes)	Butane Ethane Hexane Methane Propane		

*Note: Kerosene is often called paraffin in the United Kingdom and other countries. This confusion is thought to be responsible for some human poisonings, particularly in children.

oxidase activity in the liver and to have reproductive, endocrine, and hematopoietic effects and osmoregulatory alterations.[88] Amounts as low as 1 to 10 µl on eggshells can cause deformities of eye, brain, and beak and embryonic death.[73]

Dermal decontamination consists of washing with a general liquid hand dishwashing detergent. When bathing diving birds, make sure to assess the hardness of the water used for both washing and rinsing. Excessive mineral salts in hard water can deposit onto feathers and prevent the restoration of normal waterproofing. Detergent residues left over from incomplete rinsing after bathing can also produce the same effect.[88] With volatile hydrocarbons, birds should be bathed until the product can no longer be smelled on the feathers. If the bird is too stressed for a detergent bath, corn starch can be used to absorb oils until the bird is well enough for a bath.[89] Eyes should be flushed with a sterile saline solution. Lavages are not recommended in animals exposed to hydrocarbons due to the risk of aspiration. Radiographs of the respiratory system are indicated in any cases involving respiratory signs, and serial radiography may be needed.[87] Oxygen, assisted ventilation (positive end-expiratory pressure), antibiotics, and bronchodilators should be initiated as appropriate.[90]

When treating oiled birds, swabs from oil-contaminated feathers and legs can be wrapped in aluminum foil (shiny side in) and frozen. These samples may be useful later to verify specific sources of oil contamination.[88] There are no gross or microscopic lesions considered characteristic for the toxic effects of oil in animals.[87]

BARBITURATES

Barbiturate compounds are often used for euthanasia of animals. Carcasses that are not disposed of correctly or buried deep enough can become a source of barbiturate exposure for scavengers. Barbiturates are lipophilic and stable compounds and can persist in the dead carcass for up to several weeks or longer. The onset of intoxication occurs within a few hours after ingestion of these contaminated carcasses or entrails. The bird becomes weak and has difficulty flying, walking, or standing and often collapses. Respiratory efforts are affected, and the animal may become comatose and die.[91]

Intoxicated animals can receive successful treatment if the patient is still breathing. Maintaining a patent airway, adequate respiration, and oxygenation is critical. Assisted or mechanical respiration may be necessary by using a placed, cuffed endotracheal tube and positive pressure mechanical ventilation as needed. Barbiturates have a long half-life, and repeated administration of activated charcoal by stomach tube can reduce the body burden and achieve quicker recovery time.[92] Prevention of inadvertent secondary poisoning can be achieved by proper burial or incineration of barbiturate-contaminated carcasses.

DICLOFENAC AND VULTURES

In the late 1990s, scientists realized that three species of Gyps vultures (*Gyps bengalensis*, Oriental white-backed vulture; *Gyps indicus*, long-billed vulture; and *Gyps tenuirostris*, slender-billed vulture) were in a serious state of decline, with populations across the Indian subcontinent reduced by 95% to 100%.[93] The nonsteroidal drug diclofenac was determined to

TABLE 18-6

Half-life of Diclofenac in Selected Species of Birds

Species	Oral half-life (hours)
Chicken (*Gallus gallus*)	0.89[95]
Pied crow (*Corvus albus*)	2.33[94]
Turkey vulture (*Cathartes aura*)	6.29–6.43[96]
Cape griffon vulture (*Gyps coprotheres*)	12.24[97]
African white-backed vulture (*Gyps africanus*)	16.78[95]

be a major cause of this population decline. Diclofenac is widely used to provide immediate but short-term pain relief to livestock in South Asia.

Vultures, being obligate scavengers, were feeding upon carcasses of domesticated ungulates treated shortly before death with diclofenac. The vultures became severely depressed about 24 hours postexposure, became comatose, and died around 48 hours postexposure.[94] These vultures were dying from acute renal failure. At necropsy, there were large urate aggregates obscuring renal architecture and urate precipitation on the surface and within organ parenchyma (visceral gout).[94]

Compared with other species of birds, vultures appear to be extremely sensitive to diclofenac. Pied crows (*Corvus albus*) given 10 mg/kg of diclofenac showed no signs of toxicity, while Cape griffon vultures (*Gyps coprotheres*) died at 0.8 mg/kg.[94] The half-life of diclofenac is much longer in vultures than in other species of birds (Table 18-6).[94-97] It has been recommended that diclofenac use in ruminants be replaced with meloxicam (ketoprofen is also renal toxic to vultures).[98]

Vultures are long-lived and have some of the lowest reproductive rates among birds. A large die-off could be devastating to the population, and extinction would have far-reaching economic, ecological, and public health implications. Vultures play a central role in the control of human and animal diseases such as anthrax, tuberculosis, and brucellosis by their rapid disposal of infected animals and inactivation of pathogens. They also play a role in the control of other highly contagious animal diseases such as foot-and-mouth disease, rinderpest, and others. In areas where the vulture population has decreased, there has been an increase in the rat population and in the incidence of rabies in feral dogs.[93]

AVIAN VACUOLAR MYELINOPATHY

Avian vacuolar myelinopathy is a neurologic disease linked to cyanobacteria. It has caused mortality in bald eagles, great horned owls, American coots, killdeer, and waterfowl (mallards, ring-necked ducks, buffleheads, and Canada geese) in the southeast United States since the early 1990s.[99-101] Feeding studies have implicated the flowering plant species *Hydrilla verticillata* (Hydrocharitaceae) and an associated epiphytic cyanobacterial species (order Stigonematales) as the cause of the clinical signs.[99] The cyanobacteria produces the neurotoxic amino acid β-N-methylamino-L-alanine (BMAA). BMAA is thought to injure neurons via mechanisms involving overactivation of neuroexcitatory glutamate receptors.[102]

Birds are ataxic and unable to walk, swim, or fly.[103,104] Signs begin less than 1 week after exposure and are typically seen in the late fall to early winter.[105] There are no grossly visible lesions in the nervous system. On histopathology, diffuse spongy symmetrical vacuolation and degeneration are found throughout the white matter of the brain and spinal cord, with the optic tectum most severely affected.[103] There are no known treatments for this disease, but some birds will recover with supportive care.[104]

AVOCADO (PERSEA AMERICANA)

Avocado ingestion has been associated with myocardial necrosis in birds. The R antimere of persin isolated from avocados has caused lesions similar to those reported in field cases. Persin is found in the fruits, leaves, and seeds. The leaves appear to be the most toxic part. Myocardial insufficiency may develop within 24 to 96 hours after ingestion and is characterized by lethargy, respiratory distress, edema, cyanosis, cough, and death. Birds can also exhibit agitation and feather pulling.[106] Some controversy exists about the toxicity of different strains of avocados and species susceptibility. The Hass and Fuerte cultivars were lethal to budgerigars at 50 to 100 g/kg, whereas Hass caused mortality at 100 g/kg in canaries.[106] Caged birds appear more sensitive to the effects of avocado, while chickens and turkeys appear more resistant.

Diagnosis of avocado poisoning relies on history of exposure and clinical signs. No specific tests are readily available to confirm diagnosis. On gross necropsy there may be congestion of lungs and liver, pulmonary edema, subcutaneous edema, and free fluid within the abdominal cavity, pericardial sac, and thoracic cavity. Histopathologic lesions include myocardial degeneration and necrosis of myocardial fibers with a marked infiltration of heterophils and possible interstitial hemorrhage and/or edema.[107] Treatment should consist of oxygen, diuretics, and antiarrhythmic drugs as needed. Recovery has been reported in field cases.[107]

CONCLUSION

Birds, with their differences in physiology, can present a challenge. However, the adage remains: Treat the patient, not the poison.

REFERENCES

1. Rosendale ME: Decontamination strategies, *Vet Clin North Am Small Anim Pract* 32:311–321, 2002.
2. Frazier DL: Avian toxicology. In Olsen GH, Orosz SE, editors: *Manual of avian medicine*, St. Louis, 2000, Mosby.
3. Buck WB, Bratich PM: Activated charcoal: preventing unnecessary death by poisoning, *Vet Med* 81:73–77, 1986.
4. Richardson JA, Murphy LA, Khan SA, et al: Managing pet bird toxicoses, *Exotic DVM* 3(1):23–27, 2001.
5. Needleman H: Lead poisoning, *Annu Rev Med* 55:209–222, 2004.
6. ATSDR, US Public Health Service, Agency for Toxic Substances and Disease Registry: *Toxicological Profile for Lead*, Atlanta, GA, USA, 2011, Agency for Toxic Substances and Disease Registry, US Dept of Health and Human Services. http://www.atsdr.cdc.gov/substances/toxsubstance.asp?toxid=22. Accessed November 11, 2014.
7. Fisher IJ, Pain DJ, Thomas VG: A review of lead poisoning from ammunition sources in terrestrial birds, *Biol Conserv* 131:421–432, 2006.
8. Duke GE: Alimentary canal: secretion and digestion, special digestive functions, and absorption. In Sturkie PD, editor: *Avian physiology*, ed 4, New York, 1986, Springer-Verlag, pp 289–302.
9. Redig PT, Arent LR: Raptor toxicology, *Vet Clin North Am Exot Anim Pract* 11(2):261–282, 2008.
10. Gwaltney-Brant SM: Heavy metals. In Hascheck-Hock W, et al, editors: *Handbook of toxicologic pathology*, ed 2, San Diego, 2002, Academic Press.
11. Mahaffey KR: Nutritional factors in lead poisoning, *Nutr Rev* 39:353–365, 1981.
12. Clemens ET, Krook L, Aronson AL, et al: Pathogenesis of lead shot poisoning in the mallard duck, *Cornell Vet* 65:248–285, 1975.
13. Carlson BL, Nielsen SW: Influence of dietary calcium on lead poisoning in mallard ducks (*Anas platyrhynchos*), *Am J Vet Res* 46:276–282, 1985.
14. Harbison RM: *Hamilton and Hardy's industrial toxicology*, ed 5, St. Louis, MO, 1998, Mosby.
15. Mautino M: Lead and zinc intoxication in zoological medicine: a review, *J Zoo Wildl Med* 28:28–35, 1997.
16. Bakalli RI, Pesti GM, Ragland WL: The magnitude of lead toxicity in broiler chickens, *Vet Hum Toxicol* 37:15–19, 1995.
17. Lewis RJ: *Hawley's condensed chemical dictionary*, ed 14, New York, 2001, John Wiley & Sons, Inc.
18. Burger J: A risk assessment for lead in birds, *J Toxicol Environ Health* 45(4):369–396, 1995.
19. Eisler R: *Handbook of chemical risk assessment*, Vol 1, Metals, Boca Raton, 2000, Lewis.
20. Brace K, Altland PD: Life span of the duck and chicken erythrocytes as determined with C14, *Proc Soc Exp Biol Med* 92:615–617, 1956.
21. Allen RL: *Physiology and biochemistry of the domestic fowl*, New York, 1971, Academic.
22. Lumeij S: Clinicopathologic aspects of lead poisoning in birds: a review, *VetQ* 7:133–138, 1985.
23. Hoffman DJ, Patee OH, Wiemeyer SN, et al: Effects of lead shot ingestion on deltaaminolevulinic acid dehydratase activity, hemoglobin concentration, and serum chemistry in bald eagles, *J Wildl Dis* 17(3):423–431, 1981.
24. George JW, Duncan JR: Pyrimidine-specific 5′ nucleotidase activity in bovine erythrocytes: effect of phlebotomy and lead poisoning, *Am J Vet Res* 43:17, 1982.
25. Brennan MJ, Cantrill RC: Delta-aminolaevulinic acid is a potent agonist for GABA autoreceptors, *Nature* 280:514–515, 1979.
26. Ochiai IK, Jin K, Itakura C, et al: Pathological study of lead poisoning in Whooper Swans (*Cygnus cygnus*) in Japan, *Avian Dis* 36:313–323, 1992.
27. Janin Y, Couinuad C, Stone A, et al: The "lead-induced colic" syndrome in lead intoxication, *Surg Ann* 17:287–307, 1985.
28. Anzelmo V, Bianco P: Gastrointestinal and hepatic effect of lead exposure. In Castellino N, Castellino P, Sannolo N, editors: *Inorganic lead exposure*, Boca Raton, FL, 1995, Lewis Publishers, CRC Press Inc.
29. Corey-Slechta DA, Garman RH, Seidman D: Lead induced crop dysfunction in the pigeon, *Toxicol Appl Pharm* 52:426–427, 1980.
30. Boyer IJ, DiStefano V: An investigation of the mechanism of lead-induced relaxation of pigeon crop smooth muscle, *J Pharmacol Exp Ther* 234:616–623, 1985.
31. Shanne FAX, Kane AB, Young FE, et al: Calcium dependence of toxic cell death: a final common pathway, *Science* 206:700, 1979.
32. Bressler JP, Goldstein GW: Mechanism of lead neurotoxicity, *Biochem Pharmacol* 41:479–484, 1991.
33. Simmons TJB: Lead-calcium interactions in cellular lead toxicity, *Neurotoxicology* 14:77–86, 1993.
34. Hariri RJ: Cerebral edema, *Neurosurg Clin North Am* 5:687–706, 1994.

35. Hunter B, Haigh JC: Demyelinating peripheral neuropathy in a guinea hen associated with subacute lead intoxication, *Avian Dis* 22:344–349, 1978.

36. Hunter B, Wobeser G: Encephalopathy and peripheral neuropathy in lead-poisoned mallard ducks, *Avian Dis* 24:169–178, 1980.

37. Platt SR, Helmick KE, Graham J, et al: Peripheral neuropathy in a turkey vulture with lead toxicosis, *J Am Vet Med Assoc* 214:1218–1220, 1999.

38. Redig PT, Lawler EM, Schwartz S, et al: Effects of chronic exposure to sublethal concentrations of lead acetate on heme synthesis and immune function in red-tailed hawks, *Arch Environ Contam Toxicol* 21:72–77, 1991.

39. Cook RS, Trainer DO: Experimental lead poisoning of Canada geese, *J Wildl Manage* 30:1–8, 1966.

40. Pattee O, Wiemeyer SN, Mulhern BM, et al: Experimental lead-shot poisoning in bald eagles, *J Wildl Manage* 45:806–810, 1981.

41. Morgan RV, Moore FM, Pearce LK, et al: Clinical and laboratory finding in small companion animals with lead poisoning: 347 cases (1977–1986), *J Am Vet Med Assoc* 199(1):93–102, 1991.

42. Degernes LA, Frank RK, Freeman ML, et al: Lead poisoning in trumpeter swans. In *Proceedings of the Annual Meeting of the Association of Avian Veterinarians*, Seattle, WA, 1989, pp 144–155.

43. Sanderson GC, Anderson WL, Foley GL, et al: Effects of lead, iron, and bismuth alloy shot embedded in the breast muscles of game-farm mallards, *J Wildl Dis* 34:688–697, 1998.

44. Bagley GE, Locke LN, Nightingale GT: Lead poisoning in Canada geese in Delaware, *Avian Dis* 11:601–608, 1967.

45. Karstad L: Angiopathy and cardiopathy in wild waterfowl from ingestion of lead shot, *Conn Med* 35:355–360, 1971.

46. Beyer WN, Franson JC, Locke LN, et al: Retrospective study of the diagnostic criteria in a lead-poisoning survey of waterfowl, *Arch Environ Contam Toxicol* 35:506–512, 1998.

47. Simpson VR, Hunt AE, French MC: Chronic lead poisoning in a herd of mute swans, *Environ Pollut* 18(3):187–202, 1979.

48. Brown CS, Luebbert J, Mulcahy D, et al: Blood lead levels of wild Steller's eiders (*Polysticta stelleri*) and black scoters (*Melanitta nigra*) in Alaska using a portable blood lead analyzer, *J Zoo Wildl Med* 37:361–365, 2006.

49. Gomez-Ramirez P, Martinez-Lopez E, Maria-Mojica P, et al: Blood lead levels and δ-ALAD inhibition in nestlings of Eurasian Eagle Owl (*Bubo bubo*) to assess lead exposure associated to an abandoned mining area, *Ecotoxicology* 20:131–138, 2011.

50. Kowalczyk DF: Clinical management of lead poisoning, *J Am Vet Med Assoc* 184:858–860, 1984.

51. Shannon M: Lead. In Shannon MW, Borron SW, Burns MJ, editors: *Haddad and Winchester's clinical management of poisonings and drug overdosage*, ed 4, Philadelphia, PA, 2007, WB Saunders.

52. Samour JH, Naldo J: Diagnosis and therapeutic management of lead toxicosis in falcons in Saudi Arabia, *J Avian Med Surg* 16(1):16–20, 2002.

53. Hammond PB, Aronson AL, Olson WC: The mechanism of mobilization of lead by ethylenediaminetetraacetate, *J Pharmacol Exp Ther* 157:196–206, 1967.

54. Jugo S, Maljkovic T, Kostial K: Influence of chelating agents on the gastrointestinal absorption of lead, *Toxicol Appl Pharm* 34(2):259–263, 1975.

55. Corey-Slechta DA, Weiss B, Cox C: Mobilization and redistribution of lead over the course of calcium disodium ethylenediamine tetraacetate chelation therapy, *J Pharmacol Exp Ther* 243:804–813, 1987.

56. Andersen O: Principles and recent developments in chelation treatment of metal intoxication, *Chem Rev* 99:2683–2710, 1999.

57. Hoogesteijn AL, Raphael BL, Calle P, et al: Oral treatment of avian lead intoxication with meso-2,3dimercaptosuccinic acid, *J Zoo Wildl Med* 34:82–87, 2003.

58. Corey-Slechta DA: Mobilization of lead over the course of DMSA chelation therapy and long-term efficacy, *J Pharmacol Exp Ther* 246:84–91, 1988.

59. Denver MC, Tell LA, Galey FD, et al: Comparison of two heavy metal chelators for treatment of lead toxicosis in cockatiels, *Am J Vet Res* 61:935–940, 2000.

60. Flora SJS, Pande M, Bhadauria S, et al: Combined administration of taurine and meso 2,3-dimercaptosuccinic acid in the treatment of chronic lead intoxication in rats, *Human Exper Toxicol* 23:157–166, 2004.

61. Gurer H, Ercal N: Can antioxidants be beneficial in the treatment of lead poisoning? *Free Radic Biol Med* 29:927–945, 2000.

62. Carpenter JW: *Exotic animal formulary*, ed 3, St. Louis, MO, 2005, Elsevier Saunders.

63. Zdziarski JM, Mattix M, Bush RM, et al: Zinc toxicosis in diving ducks, *J Zoo Wildl Med* 25:438–445, 1994.

64. Carpenter JW, Andrews GA, Beyer WN: Zinc toxicosis in a free-flying trumpeter swan (*Cygnus buccinator*), *J Wildl Dis* 40:769–774, 2004.

65. Beyer WN, Dalgarn J, Dudding S, et al: Zinc and lead poisoning in wild birds in the Tri-state Mining District (Oklahoma, Kansas, and Missouri), *Arch Environ Con Tox* 48:108–117, 2005.

66. Puschner B, St. Judy L, Galey FD: Normal and toxic zinc concentrations in serum/plasma and liver of psittacines with respect to genus differences, *J Vet Diagn Invest* 11:522–527, 1999.

67. Osofsky A, Jowett P, Hosgood G, et al: Determination of normal blood concentration of lead, zinc, copper and iron in Hispaniolan Amazon (*Amazona vetralis*), *J Avian Med Surg* 15(1):31–36, 2001.

68. Wells RE, Slocombe RF, Trapp AL: Acute toxicosis in budgerigars (*Melopsittacus undulatus*) caused by pyrolysis products from heated polytetrafluoroethylene: clinical study, *Am J Vet Res* 43:1238–1242, 1982.

69. Stewart B: *Personal communication with Dr. Jennifer Klein*, May 9, 2002, Environmental Working Group.

70. Boucher M, Ehmler TJ, Bermudez AJ: Polytetrafluoroethylene gas intoxication in broiler chickens, *Avian Diseases* 44(2):449–453, 2000.

71. Forbes NA: PTFE toxicity in birds, *Vet Rec* 140:512, 1997.

72. Ritchie BW: Emergency care of avian patients, *Vet Med Report* 2:230–245, 1990.

73. Olsen GH: Embryologic considerations. In Olsen GH, Orosz SE, editors: *Manual of avian medicine*, St. Louis, MO, 2000, Mosby, p 206.

74. Burrell GA: *The use of mice and birds for detecting carbon monoxide after mine fires and explosions*, Technical Paper 11, 1912, Department of the Interior, Bureau of Mines.

75. Fan HC, Wang AC, Lo CP, et al: Damage of cerebellar white matter due to carbon monoxide poisoning: a case report, *Am J Emerg Med* 27(6):757, 2009.

76. Thomson AE, Squires EJ, Gentry PA: Assessment of factor V, VII and X activities, the key coagulant proteins of the tissue factor pathway in poultry plasma, *Br Poult Sci* 43(2):313–321, 2002.

77. Cox P, Smith RH: Rodenticide ecotoxicology: pre-lethal effects of anticoagulants on rat behavior. In Borreco JE, Marsh RE, editors: *Proc 15th Vert Pest Conf*, Davis, CA, 1992, University of California, pp 165–170.

78. Stone WB, Okoniewski JC, Stedelin JR: Poisoning of wildlife with anticoagulant rodenticides in New York, *J Wildl Dis* 35:187–193, 1999.

79. Godfrey MER: An evaluation of the acute-oral toxicity of brodifacoum to birds, *Proc Vert Pest Conf* 12:78–81, 1986.

80. Clark JP: *Vertebrate pest control handbook*, ed 4, Sacramento, California, Dept. Food and Agriculture, 1994, p 803.

81. EPA, Reregistration Eligibility Decision (RED): *Rodenticide Cluster*, EPA738-R-98-007. pp 307, 1998. http://www.epa.gov/pesticides/reregistration/status.htm. Accessed November 11, 2014.

82. Ritchie RW, Harrison GJ, Harrison LR: *Avian medicine: principles and applications*, Lake Worth (FL), 1994, Wingers Publishing, pp 1051.

83. Kuijpers EPA, den Hartigh J, Savelkoul TJF, et al: A method for the simultaneous identification and quantitation of five superwarfin rodenticides in human serum, *J Anal Toxicol* 19:557–562, 1995.

84. Jenkins JRA: Avian critical care and emergency medicine. In Altmann RB, Clubb SL, Dorenstein GM, et al, editors: *Avian Medicine and Surgery*, Philadelphia, 1997, W.B. Saunders Co, pp 839–864.

85. Poisindex editorial staff: *Hydrocarbons*, expires 2014, Poisindex System Truven Health Analytics.

86. Geehr EC, Salluzzo RF: Dermal injuries and burns from hazardous materials. In Sullivan JB Jr, Krieger GR, editors: *Hazardous Materials Toxicology: Clinical Principles of Environmental Health*, Baltimore, 1992, Williams & Wilkins, pp 420–421.

87. Jessup DA, Leighton FA: Oil pollution and petroleum toxicity to wildlife. In Fairbrother A, Locke LN, Hoff GL, editors: *Noninfectious diseases of wildlife*, Ames, 1996, Iowa State University Press, pp 141–156.

88. Miller EA, Welte SC: Caring for oiled birds. In Fowler ME, Miller RE, editors: *Zoo & wild animal medicine: current therapy 4*, Philadelphia, PA, 1999, WB Saunders Company, pp 300–309.

89. LaBonde JJ: Poisoning in the avian patient. In Peterson ME, Talcott TA, editors: *Small animal toxicology*, ed 3, St. Louis, MO, 2013, Elsevier, pp 259–273.

90. Snodgrass WR: Clinical toxicology. In Klaassen CD, editor: *Casarett & Doull's toxicology: The basic science of poisons*, ed 5, New York, 1996, McGraw-Hill, p 978.

91. Hayes B: British Columbia: Deaths caused by barbiturate poisoning in bald eagles and other wildlife, *Can Vet J* 29(2):173–174, 1998.

92. Langelier KM: Barbiturate poisoning in twenty-nine bald eagles. In Redit PT, Cooper JE, Remple D, et al, editors: *Raptor biomedicine*, Minneapolis, MN, 1993, University of Minnesota Press, pp 231–232.

93. Ogada DL, Kessing F, Virani MZ: Dropping dead: causes and consequences of vulture population declines worldwide, *Ann NY Acad Sci* 1249:57–71, 2012.

94. Naidoo V, Monpati KF, Duncan N, et al: The Pied Crow (*Corvus albus*) is insensitive to diclofenac at concentrations present in carrion, *J Wildl Dis* 47(4):936–944, 2011.

95. Naidoo V, Duncan N, Bekker L, et al: Validating the domestic fowl as a model to investigate the pathophysiology of diclofenac in *Gyps* vultures, *Environ Toxicol Pharmacol* 24(3):260–266, 2007.

96. Rattner BA, Whitehead MA, Gasper G, et al: Apparent tolerance of turkey vultures (*Cathartes aura*) to the non-steroidal anti-inflammatory drug diclofenac, *Environ Toxicol Chem* 27:2341–2345, 2008.

97. Naidoo V, Swan GE: Diclofenac toxicity in *Gyps* vulture is associated with decreased uric acid excretion and not renal portal vasoconstriction, *Comp Biochem Physiol C Toxicol Pharmacol* 149(3):269–274, 2009.

98. Naidoo V, Wolter K, Cromarty D, et al: Toxicity of non-steroidal anti-inflammatory drugs to Gyps vultures: a new threat from ketoprofen, *Biol Lett* 6(3):339–341, 2010.

99. Wilde SB, Murphy TM, Hope CP, et al: Avian vacuolar myelinopathy linked to exotic aquatic plants and a novel cyanobacterial species, *Environ Tox* 20:348–353, 2005.

100. Fischer JR, Lewis-Weis LA, Tate CM, et al: Avian vacuolar myelinopathy outbreaks at a southeastern reservoir, *J Wildl Dis* 42:501–510, 2006.

101. Wiley FE, Wilde SB, Birrenkott AH, et al: Investigation of the link between avian vacuolar myelinopathy and a novel species of cyanobacteria through laboratory feeding trials, *J Wildl Dis* 43:337–344, 2007.

102. Vyas KJ, Weiss JH: BMAA – an unusual cyanobacterial neurotoxin, *Amyotroph Lateral Sc* 10(Suppl 2):50–55, 2009.

103. Thomas NJ, Meteyer CU, Sileo L: Epizootic vacuolar myelinopathy of the central nervous system of bald eagles (*Haliaeetus leucocephalus*) and American coots (*Fulica americana*), *Vet Pathol* 35:479–487, 1998.

104. Larsen RS, Nutter FB, Augspurger T, et al: Clinical features of avian vacuolar myelinopathy in American coots, *J Am Vet Med Assoc* 221:80–85, 2002.

105. Rocke TE, Thomas NJ, Augspurger T, et al: Epizootiologic studies of avian vacuolar myelinopathy in waterbirds, *J Wildl Dis* 38:678–684, 2002.

106. Hargis AM, Stauber E, Castell S, et al: Avocado (*Persea americana*) intoxication in caged birds, *JAVMA* 194:61–66, 1989.

107. Burger WP, Naude TW, Van Rensburg IBJ, et al: Cardiomyopathy in ostriches (*Struthio camelus*) due to avocado (*Persea Americana* var. *guatemalensis*) intoxication, *J S Afr Vet Ass* 65(3):113–118, 1994.

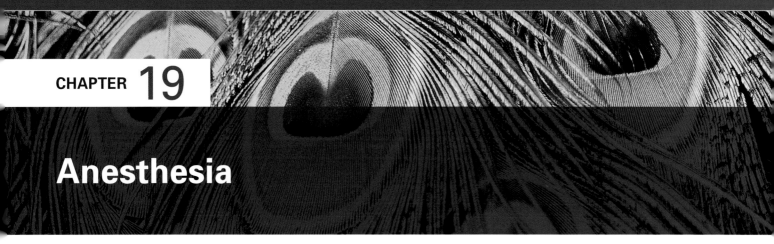

CHAPTER 19

Anesthesia

Darryl Heard

Avian anesthesia remains a clinical challenge despite many years of experience and research. Although poorly documented, it appears to have a greater morbidity and mortality than in domestic mammals. This may be due in part to the physiology and diversity of species encountered by the avian veterinarian. Additionally, birds are more often presented in the latter stages of disease. These patients obviously represent a greater risk due to impaired cardiopulmonary, hepatic, and renal function and marked metabolic imbalances. Most companion and aviary birds are also not domesticated and likely to be more stressed during handling in the perianesthetic period. This results in greater sympathetic tone and catecholamine levels, perhaps leading to a greater frequency of fatal arrhythmias.

This chapter emphasizes those areas in which clinicians can have the greatest effect on reducing perianesthetic morbidity and mortality. In the recent past, clinical anesthesia was based around an inhalant anesthetic, with no additional drugs and minimal supportive care. This was done to minimize recovery time and the potential adverse effects of additional drugs, including analgesics. Unfortunately, modern inhalants (i.e., isoflurane and sevoflurane) provide little to no antinociception despite inducing unconsciousness. In recent years, the importance of analgesia in the perianesthetic period has become widely accepted due both to a welfare requirement and to increased understanding of the long-term effects of subacute to chronic nociception (see Chapter 20). Consequently, the addition of analgesics, sedatives, tranquilizers, and low-dose dissociative anesthetics as part of a balanced anesthetic regimen is making a resurgence.[1]

ANATOMY AND PHYSIOLOGY

An understanding of normal anatomy and physiology, especially cardiopulmonary, is essential for any anesthesia. These are well described in the definitive guides to avian physiology and anatomy by Whittow[2] and Baumel,[3] respectively.

Upper Airway

Most birds breathe through paired openings or nares at the base of the beak. In kiwis, the nares are located at the end of the beak. Several diving birds (e.g., Pelecaniformes) do not have nares and breathe through spaces at the angle of mouth. Others breathe through tubular extensions (e.g., Procellariiformes, or albatrosses and petrels). The nasal cavity communicates with the paired infraorbital sinuses. These ramify throughout the head including the beak, behind the eyes, and around the back of the head. The sinuses may also communicate with cervicocephalic air sacs not connected to the lower respiratory system. In some *Leptoptilos* spp. (e.g., marabou stork) there are major connections between the nasal cavity and the air pouches of the neck.

The larynx is simple and does not participate in vocalization. The glottal opening approximates the choana or common opening in the palate to the nasal cavity. These openings close during swallowing and drinking. The glottal opening is larger than the middle to lower tracheal diameter (Figure 19-1). Pressing too large an endotracheal tube against this narrowing is a common cause of mucosal trauma. The penguin trachea is bifurcated almost to the larynx by a median septum containing cartilaginous bars continuous with the tracheal rings. To overcome this barrier to intubation, clinicians can use two endotracheal tubes, cut the endotracheal tube very short, or maintain the birds on a mask. A septum is also present in some Procellariiformes.

The trachea is mobile and extensible, and the rings are complete. The tracheal diameters are greater than those of comparable-sized mammals. In emus, there is a ventral tracheal opening into a ventricle that may inflate with positive pressure ventilation. Wrapping the lower neck prevents this. The trachea of cranes and some galliformes (e.g., guans, curassows) is very long and tortuous and may extend into the keel. Its shape predisposes it to trapping inhaled fluids or inflammatory secretions due to tracheal trauma.

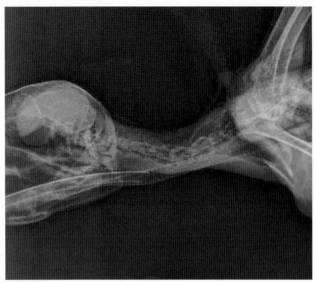

FIGURE 19-1 Lateral radiograph of a 14-week-old blue and gold macaw *(Ara ararauna)* showing how the trachea narrows in birds. If the endotracheal tube is pushed into this narrowing, the potential exists for mucosal trauma and subsequent stenosis formation. Note also the complete tracheal rings.

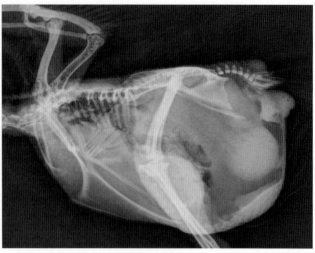

FIGURE 19-2 Lateral radiograph of a domestic chicken with egg yolk peritonitis and egg binding. This bird would be at high risk during anesthesia for hypoventilation leading to hypercapnia and hypoxemia. Although domestic poultry are easy to restrain, they are often an anesthetic risk due to obesity that reduces air sac volume, as in this diseased bird.

The syrinx is located at the tracheal bifurcation into the two major bronchi. It is clinically important because it is where inhaled foreign bodies are most likely to lodge. The syrinx can make noise on both exhalation and inhalation; this sometimes occurs during assisted ventilation. The thyroids lie close to the syrinx in budgerigars; goiter due to malnutrition can cause partial occlusion of the syrinx, altered vocalization, and potential hypoventilation. As in other vertebrates, the tracheal mucosa includes cilia for transporting mucus toward the glottis. When this material reaches the endotracheal tube, it can cause partial or complete obstruction. Some species groups (e.g., pigeons and doves) appear to produce more mucus during anesthesia, necessitating frequent assessment of patency of the endotracheal tube.

Lung and Air Sacs

Birds do not possess a diaphragm separating a thoracic and abdominal cavity (see Chapter 8). The lungs are small, do not change volume, and are located dorsolateral within the coelomic cavity. The sites of gas exchange are the small air capillaries, which are at right angles to blood flow, resulting in very rapid and efficient gas exchange. In most birds the flow of air through the lungs is unidirectional. Although inhaled air may take two respiratory cycles to move completely through, it is not necessary to ventilate birds with closely paired breaths. Efficient respiration promotes rapid uptake and removal of inhalant anesthetics, making overdosage more likely.

The air sacs ramify throughout the coelomic cavities and into the appendicular skeleton but do not participate in gas exchange. Open fractures in pneumatic bones will allow leakage of inhalant anesthetic. In addition to contamination of the environment, increased vaporizer and flowmeter settings may be required to maintain adequate surgical depth. Blood or lavage fluids can also move into the respiratory system from

the fracture site. In some species (e.g., pelicans, California condors) the pneumatic bones include the ulna, precluding the placement of intraosseous catheters in the ulna, which is a commonly utilized location in most birds.

Any material or fluid accumulation within the coelomic cavities reduces air sac volume and ventilatory efficiency. Obesity is common in many birds maintained in captivity; the resulting hypoventilation in spontaneously breathing patients may be one cause of increased mortality (Figure 19-2). Other causes of reduced air sac volume include organomegaly, fluid accumulation, neoplasia, and granulomas. Assisted ventilation can ameliorate some, but not all, of these effects.

Renal Portal System

The avian renal portal system theoretically could affect drug elimination. Some portion of the blood returning to the heart from the caudal body and legs passes through the kidneys (see Chapter 6).[4] This could decrease availability of drugs excreted predominantly through the kidneys and cause damage from renal-damaging drugs (e.g., aminoglycosides). Pharmacokinetic studies and observation, however, suggest the renal portal system does not clinically affect drug administration. This is fortunate because intramuscular (IM) and intravenous (IV) administration of anesthetics into the legs is preferable for some large birds, including ratites and waterfowl.

PREANESTHETIC PREPARATION

Examination and physiologic stabilization preferably occur before induction, but this may not be feasible for stressed and aggressive patients. Examination should focus on mentation and cardiopulmonary function (see Chapter 17).

Many clues to potential anesthetic complications are obtained by first examining the bird in its cage or at rest. Altered mentation may reflect increased intracranial pressure that can be exacerbated by inhalant anesthetics and other drugs.

Hypoglycemia is not an uncommon cause of depression in anorectic small bird species. In anesthetized birds, unrecognized hypoglycemia can cause bradycardia and peripheral vasodilation, leading to hypotension and possible circulatory collapse. Respiratory distress at rest is an important indicator of increased risk since it suggests physiologic reserve has been exceeded. Open-mouth breathing, however, may simply indicate obstructed nares and not marked compromise. Tail bobbing, due to recruitment of abdominal wall muscles associated with increased respiratory effort, should not last longer than 15 minutes after handling. Alterations in skin and mucous membrane color can indicate altered oxygen delivery due to anemia, hypoxemia, impaired circulation, hypotension, or hypovolemia. The droppings passed by the bird may be a guide to altered hydration and renal (e.g., polyuria, hematuria) and liver (biliverdinuria) function. Alterations in these organs can affect drug elimination and metabolic homeostasis.

Diseases associated with increased anesthetic risk occur more often in some species. For example, Grey parrots (*Psittacus erithacus*) may have altered calcium hemostasis[5]; for this reason, measurement of ionized calcium is recommended (see Chapter 13). Alternatively, some clinicians preemptively give calcium supplementation to this species before anesthesia. Hypomagnesemia has also been postulated as a cause of hypocalcemia-associated seizures in this species.[5]

Physical examination may reveal problems requiring further diagnostics and stabilization before induction. Owners are usually very receptive to rescheduling based on clinical concerns related to anesthetic safety.

Minimizing Anesthetic Time

Many of the factors causing morbidity and mortality during anesthesia are time dependent. One way the clinician can reduce these problems is by minimizing time under anesthesia. This involves adequate preparation before induction and awareness of time once the animal is anesthetized. This does not mean, as mentioned previously, avoiding the use of sedatives, analgesics, and anxiolytics to hasten recovery.

Importance of a Dedicated Anesthetist

Besides minimizing the length of time a bird is under anesthesia, it is also essential to employ a dedicated anesthetist. This does not necessarily mean a specialist but does require someone who is trained to monitor the process and can react to identified problems. In most birds the window of time for successful resuscitation is very small (< 30 seconds) because of their high metabolic rate. Having someone dedicated to watching the patient will detect problems early, allowing correction before catastrophic physiologic failure. This person should also make the clinician aware of anesthetic and procedural time.

Emergency Drugs and Vascular Access

Resuscitation drug dosages should be calculated before induction to reduce reaction time in an emergency. For most patients it is also inexpensive to draw up and label the drugs; they can be discarded when they are hopefully not used. Similarly, for anything except the shortest procedures there should be intravascular access, whether it is an IV or intraosseous (IO) catheter (Figure 19-3 in Box 19-1). This should be established before induction or soon after.

Fasting

Standardized recommendations for preanesthetic withdrawal of food are difficult to make because of species differences and potential for underlying disease. The main aim is to reduce the potential for regurgitation or passive reflux that may then be aspirated. This risk must be balanced against the potential for hypoglycemia due to anorexia and a high metabolic rate. A full gastrointestinal tract is unlikely to affect ventilation, especially in those birds in which it is assisted. Certain species are more likely to regurgitate or vomit in the perianesthetic period; these especially include carnivores (e.g., raptors, corvids), piscivores (e.g., wading birds, cormorants), and frugivores (e.g., toucans, mynahs). Birds with full crops can be fasted to reduce their volume. Fledging parrots are particularly problematic because, in addition to their crops, large volumes of liquid food may be stored in the proventriculus and ventriculus. It is virtually impossible and undesirable to completely empty the upper gastrointestinal tract in these birds; doing so predisposes to the development of hypoglycemia. This author avoids anesthetizing birds of this age or empties the crop by gavage, keeps the bird as upright as possible, and minimizes anesthesia time. In birds predisposed to reflux, gauze swabs connected to tape extending from the mouth can be packed in the back of the pharynx.

LOCAL AND REGIONAL ANESTHESIA

Local Anesthetic Infiltration

Local anesthetics can be used in avian species. Care must be taken, however, to ensure accurate calculation and administration to prevent intoxication. There are two main groups of local anesthetics: short acting (e.g., lidocaine and mepivacaine) and long acting (e.g., bupivacaine). In general, long-acting local anesthetics have a lower therapeutic index and longer onset of action and duration of effect. Intrathecal injection of local anesthetics for spinal cord blockade and analgesia is not feasible due to the presence of large vessels.

Birds are not more sensitive to the adverse effects of local anesthetics than mammals. In broiler chickens anesthetized with isoflurane, lidocaine at 6 mg/kg IV produced no adverse cardiovascular effects.[6] The pharmacokinetics of lidocaine was also shown in chickens to be similar to that of mammals.[7] This author usually uses 10 mg/kg as the upper limit for lidocaine and mepivacaine use. For bupivacaine, calculated dosages are kept at 2 mg/kg or less. The local anesthetics are either infiltrated into an area or placed proximally to block a nerve(s) supplying the distal portion of a limb. Care should be taken when using topical and local anesthetic sprays formulated at concentrations for humans; the potential for frank overdosage is high.

Brachial Plexus Blockade

Brachial plexus blockade offers the potential to provide long-term anesthesia and analgesia for wing surgery. This technique has been evaluated in chickens[8,9] and ducks[10] with variable success. Figueiredo[9] determined landmarks for catheter placement using dissected chicken cadavers. Midazolam (1 mg/kg) and butorphanol (1 mg/kg) IM were used to restrain hens with their heads covered in lateral recumbency. The wing was abducted 90 degrees to the thorax and the apex

BOX 19-1 TECHNIQUE FOR PLACEMENT OF INTEROSSEOUS CATHETERS (TIBIOTARSUS, ULNA)

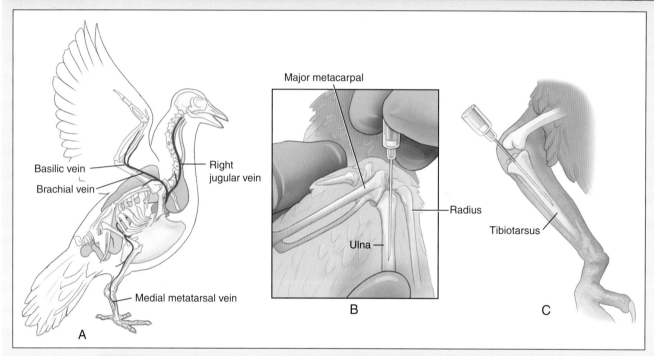

FIGURE 19-3 **A, Diagram of a bird showing potential vascular access sites during anesthesia.** The right jugular vein, basilic and brachial veins, and the medial metatarsal veins are depicted.

B, Diagram showing placement of IO catheter in distal ulna. Palpate the styloid process of the distal ulna at the dorsal side of the wing, proximal carpus. Pluck the feathers over this area and aseptically prepare it for better visualization of the landmark. Grasp the distal ulna between the fingers of one hand. With the other hand, the spinal needle is positioned over the distal ulna and aimed retrograde between the fingers holding the ulna. Apply a small amount of pressure as you rotate the point of the needle with your fingers, allowing it to cut through the cortex of the bone and enter the medullary cavity. Once the cortex has been entered, slowly advance the needle into the medullary cavity until the needle is seated in the ulna. Test the patency of the catheter by using an appropriate-sized syringe and a small amount of heparinized saline flush. The basilic vein should blanch as the fluid is injected. The intraosseous space is not elastic (as compared to a vein), and some resistance is expected. This resistance can be minimized by using small-volume syringes or by giving fluids by constant rate infusion. When you are sure the catheter is in place, attach a male adapter plug that has been flushed with heparinized saline. The catheter can be secured into the ulna by placing a small piece of tape at the hub in a "butterfly" fashion and suturing this tape to the skin. The catheter is then incorporated into a figure-eight wing bandage to minimize movement of the wing that can increase potential for fluid leakage from the catheter insertion site.

C, Diagram showing placement of IO catheter in proximal tibiotarsus. Palpate the cnemial crest at the proximal anterior surface of the tibiotarsus, just distal to the knee joint. Extend the leg at the coxofemoral joint, and flex the leg at the stifle, further exposing access to the femoral-tibiotarsal articulation. Pluck and aseptically prepare the area. The needle is inserted at the cnemial crest at, or to either side of, the insertion of the patellar tendon. As with the placement of the ulnar catheter, the cortex is penetrated by applying gentle pressure and concurrently rotating the needle point with the fingers of the driving hand. Once medullary cavity is entered, continue to drive the needle normograde until it is firmly seated in the cortex. Patency of the catheter can be checked by aspirating and seeing bone marrow, followed by the injection of a small amount of heparinized saline flush. Again, resistance should be expected in the small space of the medullary cavity. This resistance can be minimized by using small-volume syringes or by giving fluids by constant rate infusion. The catheter may be secured by placing a small piece of tape at the needle hub and suturing the tape to the skin.

of the axilla (proximal humeral condyle, coracoid, and scapula) palpated. A 20-SWG 50-mm Teflon-coated catheter electrode (Braun Melsungen AG, Melsungen, Germany) was attached to a peripheral nerve stimulator (2 to 5 Hz, 0.12 mA; S48 stimulator; Grass, Warwick, R.I., U.S.). The catheter extension was filled and connected to a 3-mL syringe containing either lidocaine (20 mg/mL, 1 mL/kg) with epinephrine or bupivacaine (5 mg/mL, 1 mL/kg). The catheter was inserted at a 45-degree angle to the skin just below the axillary apex. It was advanced through the pectoral muscle and fascia toward the chest wall to the area of the first rib. The appropriate muscle response and brachial plexus proximity were assessed as to when the strongest flexion of the wing occurred. The local anesthetic was then injected in 0.5-mL aliquots into the plexus sheath over 60 seconds. Onset of sensory denervation was 3 to 5 minutes, and duration of blockade was 60 to 90 minutes. The researchers, however, observed a relatively high failure rate of 33%. Cardoza[8] had more success using the long-acting local anesthetic ropivacaine (0.75%, 1 mL/kg). The onset and duration of effect were approximately 15 and 115 minutes, respectively. The effectiveness of brachial plexus blockade was also variable in ducks.[10]

DRUG ADMINISTRATION

Routes of drug administration include IM, subcutaneous (SC), IV (see Figure 19-3 and Box 19-1), IO, intranasal (IN), oral (PO), and cloacal. For anesthesia the most practical are IM, IV, and IN. PO administration has been used for the capture of wild birds using chloral hydrate (e.g., sandhill cranes,[11] *Grus canadensis*; rock doves,[12] *Columba livia*; Canada geese,[13] *Branta canadensis*) and tiletamine/zolazepam (e.g., common buzzard,[14] *Buteo buteo*). Uptake and dosing are variable, sometimes resulting in mortality. Cloacal administration offers the potential for rapid absorption but is impractical in the clinical setting.

Intravascular

For induction the author uses the dorsal metatarsal vein for administration of the parenteral anesthetics propofol, alfaxalone, or ketamine. The following technique is used to facilitate injection in a medium to large bird: The restrainer holds the patient in lateral recumbency and presents its back to the clinician. The lower leg is then pulled dorsally to expose the vein and allow an injection using a needle and syringe, or a butterfly or over-the-needle catheter. Alternatively, in parrots the patient is held upright with its ventrum toward the anesthetist. The lower right leg is held with the left hand, which simultaneously holds off the dorsal metatarsal vein. The parenteral anesthetic is then slowly injected into the vessel using a 25-gauge needle and 1-mL syringe. Grasp the syringe and leg in your left hand during injection to prevent the bird from moving and disengaging the needle. IO catheters can also be used for vascular access, for example, propofol injection in pigeons.[15]

Intramuscular

IM injections are usually given into the pectoral muscles from either side of the keel. This route must be carefully considered because of the potential for muscle damage that may render a bird flightless. Ketamine HCl, for example, will cause pain and damage due to its acidic pH. Conversely, alfaxalone has relatively neutral pH but can cause injury when given in large volumes.

Intranasal

IN administration is technically easy, and uptake is rapid due to a large vascular absorptive surface. Depending on the drug, it may be associated with nasal mucosal irritation.

PREMEDICATION

Premedication is regaining acceptance; drugs are used to facilitate handling, reduce anxiety, improve muscle relaxation, enhance analgesia, reduce inhalant anesthetic requirement, and perhaps avert some of the adverse physiologic effects of inhalation anesthesia.[1] The author does not use or recommend, however, the routine use of parasympatholytics (i.e., atropine, glycopyrrolate) except as indicated (e.g., for reducing bradyarrhythmias associated with butorphanol).

Benzodiazepines

Benzodiazepines include diazepam, midazolam, and zolazepam. The latter is combined with tiletamine in several commercial preparations (e.g., Telazol, Zoletil). Compared with diazepam, midazolam is water soluble, moderately more potent, and better absorbed from a parenteral injection. Water solubility allows combination with ketamine HCl or butorphanol for a single injection.

Benzodiazepines have minimal cardiopulmonary effects and are often combined with dissociative anesthetics to improve muscle relaxation. They are not, however, analgesics. Benzodiazepines produce dysphoria, making some birds difficult to work with and can cause flapping during recovery. The author has also observed midazolam exacerbate self-mutilation in some birds during recovery. Although benzodiazepines produce amnesia in humans, it is unknown whether this occurs in birds in the perianesthetic period. Flumazenil can be used to partially or completely reverse the effects of diazepam or midazolam. Repeat dosing may be required, however, due to its shorter half-life.

In zebra finches[16] (*Taeniopygia guttata*), diazepam (10 mg/kg IM) induced deep sedation and dorsal recumbency within minutes that lasted for several hours. Sedation was adequate to permit minimally invasive procedures. Flumazenil (0.3 mg/kg) provided complete rapid recovery. In Canada geese[17] (*Branta canadensis*) midazolam HCl (2.0 mg/kg IM) induced moderate sedation at 15 to 20 minutes adequate for positioning for radiography with minimal cardiopulmonary changes.

The addition of the mixed agonist-antagonist opioid butorphanol to a benzodiazepine can produce a more profound immobilization. For example, in great white pelicans[18] (*Pelecanus onocrotalus*) a combination of midazolam (1 mg/kg IM) and butorphanol (0.5 mg/kg IM) provided good sedation. As early as 10 minutes after injection, 43% of birds were less aggressive, and 29% exhibited a flaccid neck posture and closed eyes. The pelicans were completely recovered at 5 hours.

Both diazepam and midazolam, alone or in combination with ketamine or butorphanol, can be administered IN. In parrots, the author uses midazolam (0.5 to 2.0 mg/kg IN) to facilitate beak trimming and minor noninvasive procedures. Flumazenil (0.1 mg/mL, 0.03 to 0.05 mg/kg IN or IM) is used for reversal. For greater immobilization, butorphanol (0.3 to 0.5 mg/kg IN or IM) can be added. In Hispaniolan amazon parrots[19] (*Amazona ventralis*) midazolam (2.0 mg/kg IN) produced sedation within 3 minutes. The birds had reduced response to restraint, moderate bradypnea, and recovered within 10 minutes of flumazenil (0.05 mg/kg IN) administration.[19] In blue-fronted and vinaceous-breasted amazon parrots[20] (*A. aestiva, A. vinacea*), a combination of midazolam (1 mg/kg IN) and ketamine (15 mg/kg IN) administered by pipette provided good sedation. The same dosages IM had a slower onset and longer duration of effect. In budgerigars[21] (*Melopsittacus undulatus*), midazolam (13 mg/kg IN) produced a more rapid onset and shorter duration of effect (72 minutes) than diazepam (26 mg/kg IN). In ring-necked parakeets[22] (*Psittacula krameri*), midazolam (7.3 mg/kg IN) caused adequate sedation within a few minutes. Combinations of midazolam (3.65 mg/kg IN) and xylazine (10 mg/kg IN) with ketamine (40 to 50 mg/kg IN) also achieved sedation.[22] Flumazenil (0.13 mg/kg IN) hastened recovery from midazolam.

In canaries[23] (*Serinus canaria domestica*) IN diazepam (5 mg/μL, 25 mL per nostril) or midazolam (5 mg/mL, 25 μL) induced sedation within one to two minutes; birds did not move when placed in dorsal recumbency. The duration of recumbency was significantly longer with diazepam (38 minutes) than midazolam (17 minutes). Flumazenil (2.5 μg per nostril) significantly reduced recumbency time.

In pigeons[24] midazolam (5 mg/kg IN) alone had minimal cardiopulmonary effects, but inadequate restraint. In combination with dexmedetomidine (80 μg/kg IN), it produced effective immobilization 20 to 30 minutes after administration.[24] Atipamezole reversed the mild cardiopulmonary effects of this combination but did not produce complete recovery due to the presumed residual effects of the midazolam.

Alpha-2 Adrenergic Agonists

The alpha-2 adrenergic receptor agonists include xylazine, detomidine, medetomidine, and dexmedetomidine. Medetomidine and dexmedetomidine, its dextro-isomer, are more potent and selectively bound to the receptor than either xylazine or detomidine. Although marketed as twice as potent as medetomidine, in practice dexmedetomidine is around 1.6 times as potent as medetomidine.

Although alpha-2 adrenergic agonists produce analgesia and reduce inhalant anesthetic requirement, they can cause marked cardiopulmonary depression. These drugs are combined with ketamine to improve muscle relaxation, lower dosage, and provide longer immobilization. In mammals dexmedetomidine and medetomidine appear to have a larger therapeutic index than xylazine. All of these drugs can be reversed by atipamezole. It is recommended, however, that it be given IM or SC for reversal because with IV it can produce marked hypotension and negative inotropy. Absorption from IM injection is rapid.

Birds are relatively resistant to alpha-2-adrenergic agonists. For example, in pigeons xylazine[25] (16 mg/kg IM) or detomidine[26] (1.4 mg/kg IM) produced only minor to moderate sedation adequate for handling and sample collection. Similarly, in pigeons[27,28] and amazon parrots,[28] medetomidine (0.08 to 2.0 mg/kg IM) produced inadequate sedation for handling, as well as moderate bradypnea and bradycardia. At the lower dosages it only induced ataxia to sternal recumbency with retention of the righting reflex.[27] In rock partridges[29] (*Alectoris graeca*), xylazine (10 mg/kg IM), medetomidine (0.15 mg/kg IM) or detomidine (0.3 mg/kg IM) produced only variable sedation adequate for handling and radiography. Duration of effect and time to recovery were prolonged especially for detomidine. Xylazine produced the greatest sedation, but as would be expected, it produced profound respiratory depression. All drugs were associated with time-dependent hypothermia.

Similar to benzodiazepines, alpha-2 adrenergic agonists can be used IN, but immobilization appears poor. For example, in pigeons[30] xylazine (30 mg/kg IN) did not produce dorsal recumbency, and sedation was prolonged. In budgerigars[21] xylazine (26 mg/kg IN) produced prolonged sedation, but restraint was insufficient for even minor clinical procedures. In ring-necked parrots[22] detomidine (12 mg/kg IN) produced good sedation within 3.5 minutes. A combination of xylazine (10 mg/kg IN) with ketamine (40 to 50 mg/kg IN) also achieved adequate sedation.[22] Compared with detomidine, duration of dorsal recumbency was significantly longer with midazolam. Intranasal administration of yohimbine or atipamezole significantly decreased the duration of sedation induced by xylazine or detomidine, respectively.[22] In canaries,[23] xylazine (20 mg/mL, 12 μL per nostril) or detomidine (10 mg/mL, 12 μL per nostril) produced heavy sedation and sternal, but not dorsal, recumbency. Higher dosages of either xylazine (0.5 mg per nostril) or detomidine (0.25 mg per nostril) prolonged sedation but did not produce dorsal recumbency.[23] Yohimbine (120 μg per nostril) effectively antagonized xylazine and detomidine.[23]

Perianesthetic Analgesia

Analgesia is covered in Chapter 20. An analgesic plan should be part of any anesthetic regimen regardless of whether a procedure is predicted to be painful or not. The inhalant anesthetics isoflurane and sevoflurane, along with propofol, alfaxalone, and benzodiazepines, are not analgesic. Most birds appear to be kappa opioid receptor predominant; unfortunately, the short-acting mixed agonist/antagonist opioid butorphanol is the only commercially available kappa agonist. It can be combined with benzodiazepines IM or IN for more profound sedation and immobilization. Interestingly, in red-tailed hawks[31] (*Buteo jamaicensis*) fentanyl infusions produced a dose-dependent decrease in isoflurane requirement with minimal effects on measured cardiovascular variables. This suggests there is some species variation in response to κ and μ opioids.

Analgesia in the perianesthetic period will usually take a multimodal approach combining butorphanol with an NSAID, perhaps local analgesic blockade, and the use of tramadol postoperatively. This is also one area where ketamine is now becoming more in use because of its beneficial analgesic effects. Anesthetic drug groups are compared regarding their analgesic properties and side effects in Table 19-1, for a quick visual overview.

TABLE 19-1

Comparison of Anesthetic Groups, Routes of Administration, Analgesic Effects, Side Effects, and Potential for Reversal

Drug Group	Examples	Route of Administration	Analgesia?	Side Effects: Cardiopulmonary (0-+++)	Side Effects: Dysphoria (0-+++)	Reversal?
Benzodiazepines	Diazepam	IV, IM, IO, IN	No	+	++	Flumazenil*
	Midazolam	IV, IM, IO, IN				Flumazenil*
	Zolazepam	IV, IM, IO				?
Alpha-2 adrener-gic agonists	Xylazine	SC, IM, IV, IO, IN	Yes	+++	+	Atipamezole
	Detomidine					Atipamezole
	Medetomidine					Atipamezole
	Dexmedetomidine					Atipamezole
Dissociative anesthetics	Ketamine	IM, IV, IO	Yes	+	?	No
	Tiletamine	IM, PO			Recovery associated with incoordi-nation and struggling in the absence of other drugs.	
Propofol	Rapinovet	IV	No	++; dose and adminis-tration rate dependent	+	No
	PropoFlo					
	Diprivan					
Alfaxalone	Alfaxan	IM, IV	No	++	0	No
Inhalants	Isoflurane	Inhalant	No	++; dose dependent	0	No
	Sevoflurane					
	Desflurane					

IV, Intravenous; IM, intramuscular; IO, intraosseous; IN, intranasal.
*Flumazenil has shorter duration of effect than diazepam or midazolam.

INDUCTION

Parenteral

Dissociative Anesthetics

Available dissociative anesthetics include the relatively short-acting ketamine and the more potent long acting tiletamine. The latter is combined with the potent benzodiazepine zolazepam in several commercial preparations (i.e., Telazol and Zoletil). An advantage of these drug combinations is that they come as powders that can be concentrated for PO or remote IM administration in large birds. For example, tiletamine/zolazepam (80 mg/kg PO) (Zoletil) was used to immobilize common buzzards[14] (*Buteo buteo*). Birds receiving the drug combination in powder form were induced faster (30 minutes) than with the liquid (60 minutes). The effectiveness of immobilization was significantly decreased if the powder was combined with bait and stored for 7 to 14 hours or longer. Full recovery in some birds took up to 8 hours.

In Japanese quail[32] (*Cortunix cortunix japonica*) tiletamine/zolazepam (10 to 100 mg/kg IM) alone or in combination with xylazine or levomepromazine produced dose-dependent hypnosis but no anesthesia. A dosage of 30 mg/kg IM was recommended for noninvasive and minimally painful procedures

requiring restraint and recumbency. Histopathologic examination of the drug injection sites also showed focal discrete areas of myositis.

Telazol (10 mg/kg IM) provided rapid satisfactory immobilization for approximately 30 minutes in great horned (*Bubo virginianus*) and screech (*Otus asio*) owls, but not red-tailed hawks (*Buteo jamaicensis*) at any dosage (10 to 40 mg/kg IM).[33] Complete recoveries in all species required several hours or more. Additionally, recovery in the hawks was characterized by catalepsy, opisthotonos, and ataxia.

In adult king penguins[34] (*Aptenodytes patagonicus*) tiletamine/zolazepam (5 mg/kg IM) provided immobilization for about an hour after an induction time of 5 minutes or less. Dorsally recumbent birds without thermal insulation remained immobilized longer than those in ventral. In chicks, tiletamine/zolazepam (4 mg/kg IM) induced immobilization for 80 minutes. Penguins responded similarly to repeated injections and recovered without complications.

Ketamine HCl, the most commonly used dissociative anesthetic, is administered IV or IM. Dissociative anesthetics produce immobilization, but poor muscle relaxation. Consequently, it is usually combined with either a benzodiazepine or alpha-2 adrenergic agonist.[1] It does produce analgesia through its effects on NMDA receptors in the spinal cord.[35]

Consequently, in human anesthesia it may be added to propofol and used as an adjunct to opioids or local anesthetics to improve analgesia for minor painful procedures. Dissociative anesthetics produce complex effects on the circulatory system. In general, they increase sympathetic tone, with associated increase in arterial blood pressure. They do, however, produce a direct depressant effect on the myocardium; this may be "unmasked" in animals that are in shock.

Propofol

The short-acting anesthetic propofol is used IV for induction and maintenance. As described above, it is not analgesic and must be used with other drugs for painful procedures. Propofol has been evaluated in a variety of species including but not limited to pigeons,[15,36] wild turkeys[37] (Meleagris gallopavo), chickens,[38] waterfowl,[39-41] and amazon parrots.[42]

In turkeys,[37] propofol (5 mg/kg IV) administered over 20 seconds produced rapid induction but was associated with a short period of apnea, then bradypnea, hypercarbia, hypoxemia, and hypotension. Anesthesia was successfully maintained with a constant rate infusion of 0.5 mg/kg/min. Recovery was rapid and smooth once the infusion was discontinued. In pigeons,[36] propofol (14 mg/kg IV) also produced smooth, rapid induction and good muscle relaxation. The duration of effect was 2 to 7 minutes and was associated with marked respiratory depression. The safety margin was very narrow when ventilation was unassisted. In chickens,[38] propofol (4.5 to 9.7 mg/kg IV), followed by a constant rate infusion (0.5 to 1.5 mg/kg/min) for 20 minutes, produced rapid induction and general anesthesia. As in other species, sometimes marked cardiopulmonary depression was observed. Single or multiple runs of premature ventricular complexes were also observed in many birds. One required lidocaine (0.5 mg/kg IV) for ventricular tachycardia. Propofol at three times the induction dosage was fatal in all birds, indicating a low therapeutic index.[38]

In Hispaniolan amazon parrots[42] (Amazona ventralis), propofol (5 mg/kg IV) was used for induction, then for maintenance of anesthesia for 30 minutes using a constant rate infusion (1 mg/kg per min IV). The induction times with propofol were similar to those using isoflurane. Although both drugs produced respiratory depression (bradypnea, hypercapnia, hypoxemia), it was greater after induction with propofol. Propofol recovery times were prolonged compared to those with isoflurane, and several birds had agitated recoveries. The propofol constant rate infusion produced only light anesthesia in most birds.

Propofol facilitates induction to anesthesia of large birds when the use of a mask is impractical. For example, mute swans[41] (Cygnus olor) were induced with propofol (8 mg/kg IV) and then were maintained with either boluses (approximately 3 mg/kg every 1 to 8 minutes) or a continuous rate infusion (0.8 to 0.9 mg/kg/min) for 35 minutes of anesthesia. All swans recovered within 40 minutes, but in half, transient signs of central nervous system excitement occurred. Bolus dosing was unsatisfactory for general anesthesia because of sudden awakening. Hypoxemia was also noted in most birds.

Since propofol sometimes produces severe respiratory depression or apnea, supplemental oxygen and assisted ventilation are recommended. It can also produce profound hypotension. Since the cardiopulmonary effects are dependent on dose and rate of administration, it should be administered slowly in incremental boluses to effect.

Alfaxalone

The steroidal anesthetic alfaxalone was originally combined with alfadalone in the preparation Saffan and solubilized using cremophor EL. Saffan was discontinued due to side effects associated with the release of endogenous histamine. Alfaxalone has recently been remarketed in Australia and Europe, and now North America, as a 10-mg/mL water-soluble anesthetic (Alfaxan) for use in cats and dogs. Water solubility was achieved by binding alfaxalone to a cyclodextrine molecule. It does not cause histamine release and is rapidly metabolized by the liver in mammals. Its anesthetic effect is due to binding to GABA receptors. Alfaxalone is almost identical to propofol in its dosing and physiologic effects, including onset of action and duration of effect. Its main advantage is IM absorption suitable for anesthetic induction. Unfortunately, in large birds, a large injection volume is a major impediment to IM injection.

In wild rose flamingos[43] (Phoenicopterus roseus), alfaxalone (2 mg/kg IV) was used for induction for orthopedic surgery using isoflurane anesthesia. Its induction time was shorter, its induction quality smoother, and its recovery similar compared with mask induction with isoflurane. Flamingos given alfaxalone induction also required lower isoflurane concentrations for maintenance. Alfaxalone produced moderate cardiorespiratory depression.

Inhalant

The rapid uptake and induction with modern inhalant anesthetics make mask induction a common and feasible mechanism of induction. The mask must be placed over the patent nares at the base of the bill (Figure 19-4, A). This makes birds with elongated beaks a challenge; masks can be fashioned from either plastic bottles or bags (see Figure 19-4, B), or a small mask can be placed directly over the nares (see Figure 19-4, C). Isoflurane should be administered with a precision vaporizer or risk achieving fatal concentrations due to its high vapor pressure. Direct contact of liquid inhalant anesthetic with the eyes and mucous membranes may also cause irritation and injury. Table 19-1 provides a visual comparison of the above-mentioned anesthetic drug categories, their routes of administration, analgesic properties, and side effects.

INHALATION ANESTHESIA

Inhalant Anesthetic Choice

Inhalant anesthetics include desflurane, sevoflurane, and isoflurane; halothane and methoxyflurane are no longer available. Isoflurane and sevoflurane are the most commonly used inhalant anesthetics in clinical practice. Although uptake and elimination of desflurane is as fast as, or faster than, the other two, it has a low vapor pressure and potency necessitating purchase of an expensive, purpose-built heated vaporizer. Consequently, desflurane is unpopular and unlikely to become a major inhalant anesthetic in veterinary medicine. Differences in vapor pressures mean that there is need for purpose-built sevoflurane and isoflurane vaporizers, and these cannot be interchanged and used for the other inhalant

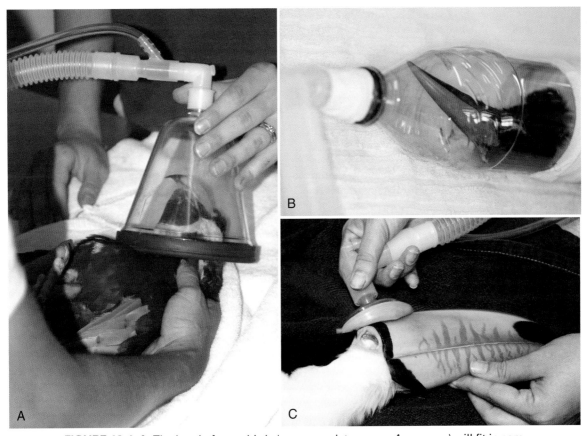

FIGURE 19-4 **A,** The head of most birds (e.g., a scarlet macaw, *Ara macao*) will fit in commercial small animal masks. The mask must cover the nares at the base of the beak. The patency of the nares should be assessed before mask induction. **B,** Long-billed birds require the manufacture of masks, if an inhalant anesthetic is to be used. A clear plastic water bottle has been modified to fit on a nonrebreathing system for delivery of the inhalant anesthetic. A latex glove has been added to form a seal around the face. **C,** A soft human pediatric mask is being used to form a seal over the nares of a toco toucan *(Ramphastos toco).*

anesthetic. If isoflurane is used in a sevoflurane vaporizer, it is theoretically possible to produce a very high, and potentially lethal, concentration.

Inhalant anesthetic potency (minimum anesthetic concentration, [MAC]; minimum anesthetic dosage, [MAD]) is similar for birds (isoflurane approximately 1.3% to 1.5%, sevoflurane 2.5%) as mammals.[44-49] Isoflurane MAC, however, appears to be lower for thick-billed parrots[50] *(Rhynchopsitta pachyrhyncha)* (1.07%) and cinereous vultures[51] *(Aegypius monachus)* (1.06%) than for other bird species.

Premedicants can reduce inhalant anesthetic requirement.[1] For example, in blue-fronted amazon parrots *(Amazona aestiva)* ketamine alone (10 mg/kg IM) or a combination of ketamine (10 mg/kg IM) and diazepam (0.5 mg/kg IM) decreased sevoflurane MAD from approximately 2.4% to 1.7% and 1.3%, respectively.[1] Ketamine alone or in combination with diazepam improved handling, reduced overt signs of stress in the parrots, and was associated with higher blood pressure than with sevoflurane alone.[1] In chickens,[52] both the mu opioid receptor agonist morphine and the kappa agonist U50488H decreased isoflurane MAC in a dose-dependent (1 to 3 mg/kg IV) manner without significant effects on heart rate and blood pressure.

In comparison with isoflurane, induction and recovery with sevoflurane are more rapid because of its lower blood solubility. For example, in red-tailed hawks[53] *(Buteo jamaicensis)* sevoflurane and desflurane produced more rapid return to function after anesthesia than isoflurane. Induction times and cardiopulmonary depressant effects were quantitatively the same.[53]

Both sevoflurane and isoflurane produce a similar dose-dependent cardiopulmonary depression.[44,51,53-56] Both induce hypotension by peripheral vasodilation and myocardial depression at higher settings. They also produce dose-dependent respiratory depression leading to hypercapnia and potentially hypoxemia. In rose-breasted cockatoos[57] *(Eolophus roseicapillus)*, hypothermia, hypercapnia, and arrhythmias were more marked with halothane than isoflurane. Compared with halothane or pentobarbital, isoflurane anesthesia resulted in a significantly lower threshold for electrical fibrillation of the chicken heart.[58] In bald eagles *(Haliaeetus leucocephalus)*, isoflurane anesthesia alone was associated with arrhythmias in 75% of birds, primarily during induction and recovery.[59] Another study of the same species[60] showed that isoflurane resulted in tachycardia, hypertension, and more arrhythmias compared with sevoflurane. Second-degree heart block was the arrhythmia most frequently observed, but it occurred at a low frequency.[60] Isoflurane and sevoflurane, however, both produced smooth, rapid induction and recovery, as in other species.

Intubation and Tracheal Stenosis

Intubation in most birds is usually simple, and the glottis is readily identified at the base of the tongue. The author uses a cotton-tipped applicator to pull the tongue forward in small birds. To prevent the tube being bitten off in parrots and in other hard-bills, a soft mouth gag can be constructed from gauze and tape. As mentioned above, penguins have a septum that comes close to the glottis. The jaws of flamingos prevent visualization of the glottis.

Postintubation stenosis is a potential adverse effect of endotracheal tubes. It is often due to trauma-induced mucosal and subcutaneous inflammation (see Figure 19-1). The birds usually present 1 to 3 weeks after an anesthetic event. Clinical signs are as expected for a partial tracheal obstruction and include respiratory noise, tachypnea, increased respiratory effort, and altered mentation.

The lesions usually correspond to the position of the end of the endotracheal tube. The tracheal rings of birds are complete; hence the recommendation not to inflate the cuff since there is no room for expansion and the mucosa would be damaged by compression. Tracheal trauma can still occur even if a cuff is not inflated. It is likely that this trauma results either from the movement of the endotracheal tube against the mucosa or from the end of the tube being jammed too tightly into the trachea. The trachea of birds narrows from the larynx to the middle of the external trachea. Other possibilities for trauma include rough intubation, chemical burns, and underlying disease. A stenotic lesion can be surgically removed.

Air Sac Cannulation

The unique aspects of avian respiration make it possible to bypass the upper system by inserting air sac cannulas for the purposes of ventilation, oxygenation, and inhalation anesthesia.[61] This technique can be used when there is partial or complete obstruction and surgery of the airway above the lungs. Air sac cannulas can even be used in very small birds. For example, this method has been used to deliver isoflurane to zebra finches for neurosurgery.[62]

Air sac cannulation requires tube placement in either the caudal thoracic or abdominal air sacs. Clavicular air sac administration was not successful in providing ventilation or maintaining anesthesia in isoflurane-anesthetized sulphur-crested cockatoos *(Cacatua galerita)*.[61] The author usually places the cannula through the left flank (paralumbar) into the caudal thoracic air sac. Alternatively, the cannula can be placed into the abdominal air sac behind the last rib and back of the leg. The paralumbar approach may make it easier to maintain and stabilize the cannula in birds that are awake, in the author's experience. When possible, use a commercially available cuffed endotracheal tube, shortened to length. A commercial tube is clear, allowing easy detection of mucus and other potential debris. It can also attach to an endotracheal tube adapter for inhalation anesthesia and ventilation. The inhalant concentrations and tidal volume may be higher due to gas escaping the upper airway. In an emergency, an over-the-needle cannula can be placed directly into the air sac and connected to an oxygen line to allow gas to flow past the lungs and out through a partial obstruction.

Effect of Body Position

In anesthetized red-tailed hawks, positioning in sternal recumbency resulted in the greatest lung and air sac volumes and lowest lung density, compared with positioning in right lateral and dorsal recumbency.[63] In a further study of red-tailed hawks,[64] it was shown that dorsal recumbency, the most common position for surgery and diagnostic procedures, did not compromise cardiopulmonary function any more than lateral recumbency. Birds hypoventilated in either lateral or dorsal recumbency. Differences in tidal volume with similar minute ventilation suggested that red-tailed hawks in dorsal recumbency might have lower dead space ventilation. Despite similar minute ventilation in both positions, birds in dorsal recumbency hypoventilated more yet maintained higher arterial oxygenation, suggesting parabronchial ventilatory or pulmonary blood flow distribution changes with position.

Breathing Systems

Most birds in clinical practice are less than 1 kg in body weight. Consequently, nonrebreathing systems are recommended. The smaller the birds, the more important mechanical dead space and resistance to air flow become. Minimum gas flow can be calculated from three times minute ventilation (tidal volume × respiration rate) or, alternatively, 220 mL/kg can be used as an estimate. The aim is to have a high enough gas flow to prevent rebreathing of exhaled carbon dioxide. Most precision vaporizers are not calibrated to work at very low flow rates, so the minimum flow is usually 500 mL. There are many commercially available nonrebreathing systems. Lightweight T-pieces can be constructed from tubing, and party balloons can be used as reservoir bags. Larger birds (i.e., over 5 kg) such as bald eagles and cranes can be maintained on circle or rebreathing systems designed for pediatric human or feline patients. Circle systems are less wasteful and provide warmed, humidified gases.

Muscle Relaxants

Although not an anesthetic or analgesic, the nondepolarizing, short-acting muscle relaxant atracurium besylate (0.15 to 0.45 mg/kg IV) can be used as an adjunct to inhalation anesthesia.[65] Muscle relaxation is monitored with a nerve stimulator and reversed with edrophonium (0.5 mg/kg IV). In chickens, the effective dosage of atracurium to result in 95% twitch depression in 50% of birds was 0.25 mg/kg, whereas the dosage to result in 95% twitch depression in 95% of birds was 0.46 mg/kg.[65]

The duration of effect at 0.25 mg/kg was approximately 35 minutes; at the highest dosage (0.45 mg/kg), 50 minutes. The cardiopulmonary effects of atracurium and edrophonium were clinically insignificant.

MONITORING

It is valuable when monitoring to have redundancy when possible. For example, when using a Doppler flow probe, have an esophageal stethoscope or electrocardiogram (ECG) also available. If the Doppler should stop, it is possible to quickly check the other monitors. If they confirm cardiac arrest, begin immediate chest compressions. When performing surgery, clear plastic drapes will also allow visualization of the patient, facilitating monitoring.

Allometric Scaling

Birds vary in size from the hummingbird to ostrich. Many of the variables monitored under anesthesia are related indirectly to size, a relationship that can be described in an allometric equation. Schmidt-Nielsen describes the concept of allometric scaling for many physiologic variables, including those of birds. An example of a useful equation for anesthesia is heart rate (bpm) = $155.8 \times$ body mass $(kg)^{-0.23}$.[66] Measured values over 20% outside the calculated weight are suggestive of abnormality, especially if they persist.

Anesthetic Depth

Anesthetic depth is determined using basic reflexes and responses, such as muscle and cloacal tone, pupil size, palpebral and corneal response, toe pinch, response to surgical incision, feather plucking, and heart rate. Interestingly, birds appear more likely to respond to feather plucking than a skin incision. This may be related to the clustering of nociceptors and mechanoreceptors around the feather follicles. Palpebral response is usually absent at light surgical planes of anesthesia. Sudden pilo-erection under anesthesia may reflect cardiac arrest rather than decreased anesthetic depth. The bispectral index has been successfully used and validated to monitor brain electrical activity and level of unconsciousness in chickens during isoflurane anesthesia.[67]

Pulse Oximetry

The use of pulse oximetry in birds is controversial. Pulse oximetry relies on differential absorption of two light wavelengths by saturated and unsaturated hemoglobin. This relationship was used to validate and describe an algorithm based on human hemoglobin. When using commercially available pulse oximeters, whether in mammals or birds, we make the assumption that the absorption pattern is the same. Spectral photometric analyses revealed a different photometric behavior of avian and human hemoglobin, which is expected to result in an underestimation of the actual saturation value in birds.[68] In pigeons and parrots, two commercially available pulse oximeters did not correlate well with arterial saturation values derived from blood gas analyses and calculation.[68] Pulse and heart rates, however, correlated well in both pulse oximeters tested.

Capnography

The end-tidal carbon dioxide concentration ($ETCO_2$) is an indirect measure of arterial carbon dioxide concentration (P_aCO_2). The latter is used to determine appropriate ventilation in the anesthetized patient. The two types of sampling methods are side-stream and in-line (Figure 19-5). The side-stream technique takes a continuous gas sample. This is minimally 300 to 500 mL/min, even in the best of pediatric monitors. This volume often exceeds the minute ventilation of small patients. This causes outside air to be entrained into a nonrebreathing system, causing the values to be lowered. The in-line capnographs have a sensor in the breathing system. This requires no gas sampling but does increase mechanical dead

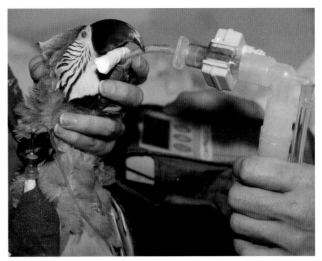

FIGURE 19-5 A blue gold macaw recovering from anesthesia. The bird is intubated with an uncuffed endotracheal tube connected to an in-line capnograph and nonrebreathing system. An intraosseous catheter has been secured into the distal ulna for fluid administration using a syringe pump. A mouth gag constructed from tape and gauze is present in the mouth to prevent the bird from biting the tube.

space, and the sensors tend to accumulate water and fail during prolonged usage. The capnograph wave is useful for assessing adequacy of ventilation. If the wave fails to fall to baseline, it indicates rebreathing of carbon dioxide. A dropping of the wave to zero can indicate decreased blood flow to the lungs, suggesting a failing heart before arrest.

The accuracy of capnography in birds is variable and related, in part, to the size and type of ventilation. In mechanically ventilated pigeons, $ETCO_2$ overestimated P_aCO_2.[69] In chickens ventilated using air sac cannulation, $ETCO_2$ was also not accurate in predicting P_aCO_2.[70] In isoflurane-anesthetized raptors, a sidestream capnograph provided a relatively good estimation of P_aCO_2 for birds weighing more than 400 g and receiving manual positive ventilation with a Bain system.[71] In isoflurane-anesthetized Grey parrots receiving intermittent positive pressure ventilation, there was a strong correlation between side-stream $ETCO_2$ and P_aCO_2.[72] The capnograph, however, consistently overestimated P_aCO_2 by approximately 5 mm Hg.

Doppler Flow Probe

Heart rate is monitored by palpation or placement of a Doppler flow probe on a peripheral artery (metatarsal, ulna), by auscultation of the heart (stethoscope including esophageal), or by pulse oximeter or electrocardiography. Positional maintenance of the Doppler flow probe is sometimes difficult. A soft clamp can be constructed from two tongue depressors and used to keep the probe in place over the ulna artery. Alternatively in large birds, the flow probe can be placed in the oropharynx or esophagus and directed at the major arteries ventral to the neck vertebra.

Electrocardiography

An avian ECG differs from an ECG for a domestic mammal. Attaching ECG leads and maintaining a good signal are sometimes difficult. An ECG should accurately monitor the rapid heart rates of small avian patients. There also should be a freeze function that allows the clinician to review an ECG while it continues to monitor. An electronic recording of the ECG throughout a procedure is now feasible and of value for retrospective review. Abnormal heart rates and auscultated arrhythmias should be investigated with an ECG before anesthesia.

Esophageal Stethoscopes

In addition to a good-quality regular stethoscope, an esophageal stethoscope with attached microphone is a simple and quickly placed method of monitoring heart rate (Figure 19-6). The complex crops of parrots and pigeons, and the presence of food, can make it difficult to place through the thoracic inlet. Another problem is the potential for passive reflux of fluid or active regurgitation and vomiting in response to the tube.

Blood Pressure

Direct Measurement

Direct arterial blood pressure measurement is usually not practical in a clinical setting. It requires placement of an indwelling catheter into a peripheral artery, which is then connected to a transducer that converts the pressure wave into an electrical signal. The systolic pressures of birds are usually much higher than those of mammals.[2] This is because the pressure wave is different due to the decreased elasticity of the arterial walls and the shape of the peripheral circulatory tree. Potential arterial catheter sites include the ulna and metatarsal arteries. In birds less than 2 kg, small catheters can be placed, but these small diameters will affect the pressure wave form, and they are more prone to clot formation. Concerns also exist about catheterization of major arteries to peripheral sites that may cause ischemic necrosis. These catheters cannot be maintained in awake birds because of the potential for catastrophic failure.

Indirect Measurement

Indirect blood pressure measurement is usually inaccurate at either low or high blood pressures.[73] For measurement, a Doppler cuff is placed on the distal humerus or femur.[74] A probe is then positioned on the medial surface of the proximal ulna or tibiotarsus, respectively. Doppler gel is used to enhance contact between the probe and skin. The cuff bladder is then inflated to a suprasystemic pressure that extinguishes the Doppler signal. As the cuff is slowly deflated, the first sound heard denotes the systolic pressure. The normal systolic blood pressure for psittacines under isoflurane or sevoflurane anesthesia is 90 to 150 mm Hg, and the same measurement for conscious psittacines is 90 to 180 mm Hg.[74]

Blood Gas and Clinical Chemistry Analysis

Blood gas analysis in the perianesthetic period is now feasible with the advent of small, portable analyzers that require only small amounts of blood. Additionally, some of these analyzers will give results for lactate and electrolytes. Several of the rapid blood glucose analyzers used in human medicine work for avian patients. Arterial blood samples can be collected from either the ulna or metatarsal arteries.

Temperature

Anesthetized birds rapidly lose heat, and continuous body temperature measurement is essential.[75] Birds have a higher body temperature than mammalian species. Cold climate birds can quickly become hyperthermic during the induction period due to struggling. Some aquatic birds have the ability to shunt blood away from the periphery to preserve heat. This feature may make cloacal temperature measurement inaccurate relative to core body temperature. An esophageal thermometer is recommended to measure core body temperature (see Figure 19-6). Conversely, in ringed turtle doves (*Streptopelia risoria*) anesthetized with isoflurane in oxygen, changes

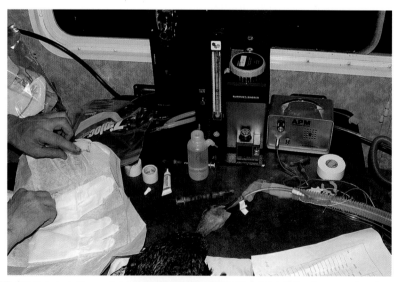

FIGURE 19-6 Inhalation of a mottled duck *(Anas fulvigula)* for intracoelomic surgical placement of a radiotransmitter. The bird is being monitored using an esophageal stethoscope and thermometer, and a Doppler flow probe on the medial metatarsal artery. The bird is also ventilated manually during the procedure.

in cloacal temperatures closely approximated changes in core body temperatures.[75]

SUPPORTIVE CARE

Ventilation

All birds, regardless of whether they appear to be breathing, hypoventilate under anesthesia. The author always prefers to provide supportive ventilation to birds under anesthesia. This becomes more critical in birds with decreased intracoelomic volume due to fat, fluid, or coelomic mass effects. The author will usually hand ventilate about six breaths per minute. Mechanical ventilators can also be used in birds.[72] For clinical practice, you want a ventilator with a wide range of rates that can deal with small tidal volumes and low pressures. For practical uses, a mechanical ventilator should have a long-life rechargeable battery and allow transportation of the patient. It should also be relatively lightweight and be easily understood by all. In isoflurane-anesthetized pigeons, controlled ventilation delivered by a pressure-limited device was not associated with clinically important adverse cardiopulmonary changes, but may be associated with respiratory alkalemia and cardiovascular depression when air sac integrity has been disrupted.[69]

Fluid Administration

Vascular access is essential for anesthetized patients. IO and IV catheter sites are summarized in Figure 19-3 and Box 19-1. For anesthesia, the author prefers to use the dorsal metatarsal vein for medium to large birds, and the jugular vein or ulna intraosseous (see Figure 19-5) in small birds. Once a catheter is placed, a syringe pump can accurately deliver small volumes over time. Although expensive, the author considers them an essential component of care in the perianesthetic period. Fluid rates during surgery will vary during a procedure from 5 to 10 mL/kg/h to even higher rates, depending on vascular status and blood loss.

Thermoregulation

For several reasons, birds will lose heat rapidly under anesthesia. These include large surface area to volume, large respiratory surface area, high minute ventilation, the use of cold, dry anesthetic gases, the impairment of central thermoregulation, the use of surgical prep liquids such as alcohol, and cold operating rooms.

In ringed turtle doves anesthetized with isoflurane in oxygen, a 680-W radiant heat source (poultry brooder) placed 27 cm above the birds maintained induction core body temperature for 120 minutes.[75] In comparison, neither a circulating 40° C warm-water blanket nor a gas warmer-humidifier, inserted in the fresh gas flow between the vaporizer and the nonrebreathing system, had any effect on maintenance of body temperature.[75]

In Hispaniolan amazon parrots anesthetized with isoflurane in oxygen, traditional heating devices, such as circulating-water blankets and 60-W infrared heat emitters positioned at a distance of 62.5 cm from the patient, helped attenuate decreases in body temperature during general anesthesia.[76] Forced-air warming, however, was the superior heating modality.[76] Forced-air warming is also advantageous because heat can be directed more specifically on the patient, it is less obstructive for the surgeon, and commercial units have a controllable thermostat.

Why Do Birds Not Recover or Die?

The recovery period is a critical period in the perianesthetic period, and deaths are not uncommon. Possible causes for prolonged recovery and mortality include extended elimination of drugs, hypoglycemia, hypothermia, hypercapnia, hypoxemia, electrolyte disturbances, hypotension, hypovolemia, and increased intracranial pressure.

Orthostatic hypotension, in the author's opinion, is an underappreciated cause of death in compromised patients during recovery. It refers to the pooling of blood due to the effects of gravity. This can result in temporary decreased return of blood to the heart and cardiac arrest. This can occur when the bird is moved rapidly during recovery and may explain a bird's death after a surgery during transport to recovery. This effect is exacerbated by hypovolemia, peripheral vasodilation, and the depressant effects of anesthetic drugs on the normal circulatory reflexes. During recovery from hypothermia, peripheral vessels that had been vasoconstricted will dilate, exacerbating hypovolemia and hypotension. Similarly, metabolic rate will increase, fueling the demand for glucose and exacerbating any marginal hypoglycemia.

CONCLUSION

Although avian anesthesia is more demanding of the clinician, several techniques and precautions should reduce potential morbidity and mortality. These include having an anesthetic and analgesic plan, minimizing anesthetic time, assessing the animal before anesthesia and correcting health-related issues, having a dedicated anesthetist, having vascular access for moderate to prolonged procedures, providing redundancy in monitoring, precalculating emergency drugs, and preventing hypothermia and taking care during recovery to ensure a smooth transition to normal homeostasis.

REFERENCES

1. Paula VV, Otsuki DA, Auler JOC, et al: The effect of premedication with ketamine, alone or with diazepam, on anaesthesia with sevoflurane in parrots (*Amazona aestiva*), *BMC Vet Res* 9:142–151, 2013.
2. Whittow GC, editor: *Sturkie's avian anatomy*, ed 5, San Diego, 2000, Academic Press.
3. Baumel JJ, King AS, Breazile JE, et al, editors: *Handbook of avian anatomy: nomina anatomica avium*, ed 2, Cambridge, 1993, Nuttall Ornithological Club.
4. Goldstein DL, Skadhauge E: Renal and extrarenal regulation of body fluid composition. In Whittow GC, editor: *Sturkie's avian physiology*, ed 5, San Diego, 2000, Academic Press, pp 265–297.
5. Kirchgessner MS, Tully TN Jr, Nevarez J, et al: Magnesium therapy in a hypocalcemic African grey parrot (*Psittacus erithacus*), *J Avian Med Surg* 26:17–21, 2012.
6. Brandão J, da Cunha AF, Pypendop B, et al: Cardiovascular tolerance of intravenous lidocaine in broiler chickens (*Gallus gallus domesticus*) anesthetized with isoflurane, *Vet Anaesth Analg* 42(4):442–448, 2015.
7. Da Cunha AF, Messenger KM, Stout RW, et al: Pharmacokinetics of lidocaine and its active metabolite monoethylglycinexylide after a single intravenous administration in chickens (*Gallus domesticus*) anesthetized with isoflurane, *J Vet Pharmacol Ther* 35:604–607, 2012.

8. Cardoza LB, Almeida RM, Flúza LC, et al: Brachial plexus block in chickens with 0.75% ropivacaine, *Vet Anaesth Analg* 36:396–400, 2009.

9. Figueiredo JP, Cruz ML, Mendes GM, et al: Assessment of brachial plexus blockade in chickens by an axillary approach, *Vet Anaesth Analg* 35:511–518, 2008.

10. Brenner DJ, Larsen RS, Dickinson PJ, et al: Development of an avian brachial plexus block technique for perioperative analgesia in mallard ducks (*Anas platyrhynchos*), *J Avian Med Surg* 24:24–34, 2010.

11. Hartup BK, Schneider L, Engels JM, et al: Capture of sandhill cranes using alpha-chloralose: a 10-year follow-up, *J Wildl Dis* 50:143–145, 2014.

12. Belant JL, Seamans TW: Alpha-chloralose immobilization of rock doves in Ohio, *J Wildl Dis* 35:239–242, 1999.

13. Belant JL, Seamans TW: Comparison of three formulations of alpha-chloralose for immobilization of Canada geese, *J Wildl Dis* 33:606–610, 1997.

14. Janovsky M, Ruf T, Zenker W: Oral administration of tiletamine/zolazepam for the immobilization of the common buzzard (*Buteo buteo*), *J Raptor Res* 36:188–193, 2002.

15. Guimarães LD, Natalini CC, Flores FN, et al: Evaluation of two intraosseous constant rate infusions of propofol in domestic pigeons, *Acta Scient Veterin* 34:325–329, 2006.

16. Prather JF: Rapid and reliable sedation induced by diazepam and antagonized by flumazenil in zebra finches (*Taeniopygia guttata*), *J Avian Med Surg* 26:76–84, 2012.

17. Valverde A, Honeyman VL, Dyson DH, et al: Determination of a sedative dose and influence of midazolam on cardiopulmonary function in Canada geese, *Am J Vet Res* 51:1071–1074, 1990.

18. Horowitz IH, Vaadia G, Landau S, et al: Butorphanol-midazolam combination injection for sedation of great white pelicans (*Pelecanus onocrotalus*), *Israel J Vet Med* 69:35–39, 2014.

19. Mans C, Guzman DS-M, Lahner LL, et al: Sedation and physiologic response to manual restraint after intranasal administration of midazolam in Hispaniolan amazon parrots (*Amazona ventralis*), *J Avian Med Surg* 26:130–139, 2012.

20. Bitencourt EH, Padilha VS, de Lima MPA, et al: Sedative effects of the association ketamine and midazolam administered intranasally or intramuscular in parrots (*Amazona aestiva* and *Amazona vinacea*), *Pesq Vet Bras* 33, 2013.

21. Sadegh AB: Comparison of intranasal administration of xylazine, diazepam, and midazolam in budgerigars (*Melopsittacus undulatus*): clinical evaluation, *J Zoo Wildl Med* 44:241–244, 2013.

22. Vesal N, Eskandari MH: Sedative effects of midazolam and xylazine with or without ketamine and detomidine alone following intranasal administration in ring-necked parakeets, *J Am Vet Med Assoc* 228:383–388, 2006.

23. Vesal N, Zare P: Clinical evaluation of intranasal benzodiazepines, alpha-agonists and their antagonists in canaries, *Vet Anaesth Analg* 33:143–148, 2006.

24. Hornak S, Liptak T, Ledecky V, et al: A preliminary trial of the sedation induced by intranasal administration of midazolam alone or in combination with dexmedetomidine and reversal by atipamezole for a short-term immobilization in pigeons, *Vet Anaesth Analg* 42(2):192–196, 2015.

25. Durrani UF, Ashraf M, Khan MA: A comparison of the clinical effects associated with xylazine, ketamine, and a xylazine-ketamine cocktail in pigeons (*Columba livia*), *Turkish J Vet Anim Sci* 33:413–417, 2009.

26. Durrani UF, Khan MA, Ahmad S: Comparative efficacy (sedative and anaesthetic) of detomidine, ketamine and detomidine-ketamine cocktail in pigeons (*Columba livia*), *Pakistan Vet J* 28:115–118, 2008.

27. Pollock CG, Schumacher J, Orosz SE, et al: Sedative effects of medetomidine in pigeons (*Columba livia*), *J Avian Med Surg* 15:95–100, 2001.

28. Sandmeier P: Evaluation of medetomidine for short-term immobilization of domestic pigeons (*Columba livia*) and amazon parrots (*Amazona* species), *J Avian Med Surg* 14:8–14, 2000.

29. Uzun M, Onder F, Atalan G, et al: Effects of xylazine, medetomidine, detomidine, and diazepam on sedation, heart and respiratory rates, and cloacal temperature in rock partridges (*Alectoris graeca*), *J Zoo Wildl Med* 37:135–140, 2006.

30. Moghadam AZ, Sadegh AB, Sharifi S, et al: Comparison of intranasal administration of diazepam, midazolam and xylazine in pigeons: clinical evaluation, *Iranian J Vet Sci Technol* 1:19–26, 2009.

31. Pavez JC, Hawkins MG, Pascoe PJ, et al: Effect of fentanyl target-controlled infusions on isoflurane minimum anaesthetic concentration and cardiovascular function in red-tailed hawks (*Buteo jamaicensis*), *Vet Anaesth Analg* 38:344–351, 2011.

32. Nicolau AA, De Souza Spinoza H, Maiorka PC, et al: Evaluation of tiletamine-zolazepam as an anesthetic in quail (*Cortunix cortunix japonica*), *J Am Assoc Lab Anim Sci* 38:73–75, 1999.

33. Kreeger TJ, Degernes LA, Kreeger JS, et al: Immobilization of raptors with tiletamine and zolazepam (*Telazol*). In Redig PT, Cooper JE, Remple D, et al, editors: *Raptor biomedicine*, Minneapolis, 1993, University of Minnesota Press, pp 141–144.

34. Thil MA, Groscolas R: Field immobilization of king penguins with tiletamine-zolazepam, *J Field Ornith* 73:308–317, 2002.

35. Schmid RL, Sandler AN, Katz J: Use and efficacy of low-dose ketamine in the management of acute postoperative pain: a review of current techniques and outcomes, *Pain* 82:111–125, 1999.

36. Fitzgerald G, Cooper JE: Preliminary studies on the use of propofol in the domestic pigeon (*Columba livia*), *Res Vet Sci* 49:334–338, 1990.

37. Schumacher J, Citino SB, Hernandez K, et al: Cardiopulmonary and anesthetic effects of propofol in wild turkeys, *Am J Vet Res* 58:1014–1017, 1997.

38. Lukasik VM, Gentz EJ, Erb HN, et al: Cardiopulmonary effects of propofol anesthesia in chickens (*Gallus gallus domesticus*), *J Avian Med Surg* 11:93–97, 1997.

39. Machin KL, Caulkett NA: Cardiopulmonary effects of propofol and a medetomidine-midazolam-ketamine combination in mallard ducks, *Am J Vet Res* 59:598–602, 1998.

40. Machin KL, Caulkett NA: Cardiopulmonary effects of propofol infusion in canvasback ducks (*Aythya valisineria*), *J Avian Med Surg* 13:167–172, 1999.

41. Müller K, Holzapfel J, Brunnberg L: Total intravenous anaesthesia by boluses or by continuous rate infusion of propofol in mute swans (*Cygnus olor*), *Vet Anaesth Analg* 38:286–291, 2011.

42. Langlois I, Harvey RC, Jones MP, et al: Cardiopulmonary and anesthetic effects of isoflurane and propofol in Hispaniolan amazon parrots (*Amazona ventralis*), *J Avian Med Surg* 17:4–10, 2003.

43. Villaverde-Morcillo S, Benito J, García-Sánchez R, et al: Comparison of isoflurane and alfaxalone (Alfaxan) for the induction of anesthesia in flamingos (*Phoenicopterus roseus*) undergoing orthopedic surgery, *J Zoo Wildl Med* 45(2):361–366, 2014.

44. Naganobu K, Fujisawa Y, Ohde H, et al: Determination of the minimum anesthetic concentration and cardiovascular dose response for sevoflurane in chickens during controlled ventilation, *Vet Surg* 29:102–105, 2000.

45. Phair KA, Larsen RS, Wack RF, et al: Determination of the minimum anesthetic concentration of sevoflurane in thick-billed parrots (*Rhynchopsitta pachyrhyncha*), *Am J Vet Res* 73:1350–1355, 2012.

46. Goelz MF, Hahn AW, Kelley ST: Effects of halothane and isoflurane on mean arterial blood pressure, heart rate, and respiratory rate in adult Pekin ducks, *Am J Vet Res* 51:458–460, 1990.

47. Curro TG, Brunson DB, Paul-Murphy J: Determination of the ED50 of isoflurane and evaluation of the isoflurane-sparing effect of butorphanol in cockatoos (*Cacatua spp.*), *Vet Surg* 23:429–433, 1994.

48. Ludders JW, Mitchell GS, Rode J: Minimal anesthetic concentration and cardiopulmonary dose response of isoflurane in ducks, *Vet Surg* 19:304–307, 1990.

49. Ludders JW, Rode J, Mitchell GS: Isoflurane anesthesia in sandhill cranes (*Grus canadensis*): minimal anesthetic concentration and cardiopulmonary dose-response during spontaneous and controlled breathing, *Anesth Analg* 68:511–516, 1989.

50. Mercado JA, Larsen RS, Wack RF, et al: Minimum anesthetic concentration of isoflurane in captive thick-billed parrots (*Rhynchopsitta pachyrhyncha*), *Am Vet Res* 69:189–194, 2008.

51. Kim YK, Lee SS, Suh EH, et al: Minimum anesthetic concentration and cardiovascular dose–response relationship of isoflurane in cinereous vultures (*Aegypius monachus*), *J Zoo Wildl* 42:499–503, 2011.

52. Concannon KT, Dodam JR, Hellyer PW: Influence of a mu- and kappa-opioid agonist on isoflurane minimal anesthetic concentration in chickens, *Am J Vet Res* 56:806–811, 1995.

53. Granone TD, de Francisco ON, Killos MB, et al: Comparison of three different inhalant anesthetic agents (isoflurane, sevoflurane, desflurane) in red-tailed hawks (*Buteo jamaicensis*), *Vet Anaesth Analg* 39:29–37, 2012.

54. Escobar A, Thiesen R, Vitaliano SN, et al: Some cardiopulmonary effects of sevoflurane in crested caracara (*Caracara plancus*), *Vet Anaesth Analg* 36:436–441, 2009.

55. Naganobu K, Ise K, Miyamoto T, et al: Sevoflurane anaesthesia in chickens during spontaneous and controlled ventilation, *Vet Rec* 152:45–48, 2003.

56. Naganobu K, Fujisawa Y, Ohde H, et al: Determination of the minimum anesthetic concentration and cardiovascular dose response for sevoflurane in chickens during controlled ventilation, *Vet Surg* 29:102–105, 2000.

57. Jaensch SM, Cullen L, Raidal SR: Comparative cardiopulmonary effects of halothane and isoflurane in galahs (*Eolophus roseicapillus*), *J Avian Med Surg* 13:15–22, 1999.

58. Greenlees KJ, Clutton RE, Larsen CT, et al: Effect of halothane, isoflurane, and pentobarbital anesthesia on myocardial irritability in chickens, *Am J Vet Res* 51:757–758, 1990.

59. Aguilar RF, Smith VE, Ogburn P, et al: Arrhythmias associated with isoflurane anesthesia in bald eagles (*Haliaeetus leucocephalus*), *J Zoo Wildl Med* 26:508–516, 1995.

60. Joyner PH, Jones MP, Ward D, et al: Induction and recovery characteristics and cardiopulmonary effects of sevoflurane and isoflurane in bald eagles, *Am J Vet Res* 69:13–22, 2008.

61. Jaensch SM, Cullen L, Raidal SR: Comparison of endotracheal, caudal thoracic air sac, and clavicular air sac administration of isoflurane in sulphur-crested cockatoos (*Cacatua galerita*), *J Avian Med Surg* 15:170–177, 2001.

62. Nilsona PC, Teramitsub I, White SA: Caudal thoracic air sac cannulation in zebra finches for isoflurane anesthesia, *J Neurosci Meth* 143:107–115, 2005.

63. Malka S, Hawkins MG, Jones JH, et al: Effect of body position on respiratory system volumes in anesthetized red-tailed hawks (*Buteo jamaicensis*) as measured via computed tomography, *Am J Vet Res* 70:1155–1160, 2009.

64. Hawkins MG, Malka S, Pascoe PJ, et al: Evaluation of the effects of dorsal versus lateral recumbency on the cardiopulmonary system during anesthesia with isoflurane in red-tailed hawks (*Buteo jamaicensis*), *Am J Vet Res* 74:136–143, 2013.

65. Nicholson A, Ilkiw JE: Neuromuscular and cardiovascular effects of atracurium in isoflurane-anesthetized chickens, *Am J Vet Res* 53:2337–2342, 1992.

66. Schmidt-Nielsen K: *Scaling. Why is animal size so important?* Cambridge, 1984, Cambridge University Press.

67. Martin-Jurado O, Vogt R, Kutter AP, et al: Effect of inhalation of isoflurane at end-tidal concentrations greater than, equal to, and less than the minimum anesthetic concentration on bispectral index in chickens, *Am J Vet Res* 69:1254–1261, 2008.

68. Schmitt PM, Göbel T, Trautvetter E: Evaluation of pulse oximetry as a monitoring method in avian anesthesia, *J Avian Med Surg* 12:91–99, 1998.

69. Touzot-Jourde G, Hernandez-Divers SJ, Trim CM: Cardiopulmonary effects of controlled versus spontaneous ventilation in pigeons anesthetized for coelioscopy, *J Am Vet Med Assoc* 227:1424–1428, 2005.

70. Paré M, Ludders JW, Erb HN: Association of partial pressure of carbon dioxide in expired gas and arterial blood at three different ventilation states in apneic chickens (*Gallus domesticus*) during air sac insufflation anesthesia, *Vet Anaesth Analg* 40:245–256, 2013.

71. Desmarchelier M, Rondenay Y, Fitzgerald G, et al: Monitoring of the ventilatory status of anesthetized birds of prey by using end-tidal carbon dioxide measured with a microstream capnometer, *J Zoo Wildl Med* 38:1–6, 2007.

72. Edling TM, Degernes LA, Flammer K, et al: Capnographic monitoring of anesthetized African grey parrots receiving intermittent positive pressure ventilation, *J Am Vet Med Assoc* 219:1714–1718, 2001.

73. Lichtenberger M, Orcutt C, Debehnke D, et al: Mortality and response to fluid resuscitation after blood loss in mallard ducks (*Anas platyrhynchos*), *Proc Assoc Avian Vet* 65–70, 2002.

74. Lichtenberger M: Determination of indirect blood pressure in the companion bird, *Sem Avian Exot Pet* 14:149–152, 2005.

75. Phalen DN, Mitchell ME, Cavazos-Martinez ML: Evaluation of three heat sources for their ability to maintain core body temperature in the anesthetized patient, *J Avian Med Surg* 10:174–178, 1996.

76. Rembert MS, Smith JA, Hosgood G, et al: Comparison of traditional thermal support devices with the forced-air warmer system in anesthetized Hispaniolan amazon parrots (*Amazona ventralis*), *J Avian Med Surg* 15:187–193, 2001.

Recognition, Assessment, and Management of Pain in Birds

Michelle G. Hawkins • Joanne Paul-Murphy • David Sanchez-Migallon Guzman

RECOGNITION AND ASSESSMENT OF PAIN

Pain is defined as the sensory and emotional experience associated with actual or potential tissue damage. Pain affects the animal's physiology and behavior to reduce or avoid the damage, to reduce the likelihood of recurrence and to promote recovery. Pain is subjective and the emotional component is difficult for us to translate because avian species lack facial expression and do not share verbal language with humans. In humans we accept that pain is what the patient says it is, but with birds, people's perceptions of the bird's behavior determines what is recognized as pain. Nociception is the transduction, conduction, and central nervous system (CNS) processing of signals generated by the stimulation of nociceptors. It is the physiologic process that, when completed, results in the conscious perception of pain.

Behavioral changes associated with pain in birds can be very obscure and subtle, but are often the earliest signs of pain detected by animal care staff or owners. Behavioral changes do not manifest uniformly among different species of birds; observers must become familiar with the full range of normal behaviors for the species as well as the individual. It is important to observe birds' behaviors at appropriate times for each species, for example, observing nocturnal species at night. Without knowing the range of normal behaviors, an observer will find it extremely difficult to detect abnormal behaviors, especially in prey species, which often only demonstrate quiet and subtle changes.

Birds tend to respond to noxious stimuli with a fight-or-flight response (i.e., escape reactions, vocalization, excessive movement) and/or conservation–withdrawal responses (i.e., no escape attempts or minimal vocalization and immobility). In domestic chickens (*Gallus gallus domesticus*), removal of feathers caused a progression of behavioral changes from an alert agitated response following the initial removal of feathers to periods of crouching immobility following successive feather removal.[1] In red-tailed hawks (*Buteo jamaicensis*) hospitalized with recent orthopedic injuries movement, head motions, and beak clacks were all significantly reduced when compared with birds without recent orthopedic injuries.[2] Studies using chickens with experimentally induced arthritis demonstrated that shifting their attention can reduce painful behaviors.[3]

Pain can change a bird's social interactions, especially in species with complex social systems. This may be an obvious change, such as perching away from the flock, or might be subtle, such as a reduction in social grooming. When birds are housed as single pets, their social interactions with the owner may be reduced or the bird may permit interactions that it would not otherwise allow. Birds in pain may display guarding behavior to protect a painful area, which may manifest as antisocial behaviors. Some forms of aggression have been linked to painful conditions in birds; anecdotal reports have suggested aggressive behaviors are sometimes reduced or dissipate following treatment of the painful condition.

Feather grooming is an avian behavior that runs the full spectrum of behavioral changes associated with pain, both acute and chronic. Grooming activity may decrease when a bird is in pain, but conversely overgrooming and feather-destructive behaviors have been associated with chronic pain, which may include neuropathic pain. In a social species housed within a group, a bird in pain frequently isolates itself from others, it may sleep apart from the rest of the flock, and mutual grooming is often decreased.[4] Increased self-grooming activities or preening other birds can be an intentional distraction.

Pain scales and score sheets are tools that are increasingly used to assess pain in animals, especially when specifically designed for a given species under well-defined conditions. Using pain scales requires an understanding of normal and pain-related behaviors for the species and individual. Pain score sheets can help maximize the efficacy of pain scoring using behavioral analysis. Score-sheet descriptions of behavior must be refined, and terms must be clearly defined to reduce observer bias and interobserver variability. In lieu of species-specific pain score sheets, there is tremendous value in using a generic visual analog pain scale of 1 to 10 to evaluate a bird's pain and the response to treatment and recovery from a painful condition. In a study completed by one of the authors, pigeons following orthopedic surgery were evaluated using a detailed numeric rating scale plus a simple 1 to 10 pain scale, and there was significant correlation between both methods.[5] Effective analgesia is expected to show a marked, easily discernable change in posture or behaviors that will effect a reliable change in the subjective pain score. If no change in pain score occurs, then the drugs, dosage, or frequency of administration should be re-evaluated for that patient.

PAIN MANAGEMENT

General Approaches to the Treatment of Pain

Surgical incision and other painful procedures in humans induce prolonged nervous system changes that later contribute to postoperative pain. This noxious stimulus-induced sensitization can be prevented or "pre-empted" by administration of analgesic agents prior to tissue injury. Pre-emptive analgesia with opiates, nonsteroidal antiinflammatory drugs (NSAIDs), and/or local anesthetics can block sensory noxious stimuli from onward transmission to the CNS, thus reducing the overall potential for inflammation and pain and improving the patient's short- and long-term recovery. Combinations of drugs in a multimodal protocol with opiates, NSAIDs, local anesthetics, and/or other drugs acting at different points in the nociceptive system provide a greater effect and potentially less toxicity than individual drugs given alone, which is especially important in avian species for which few analgesic data are available.

Opioids

Opioids are used for moderate to severe pain, such as traumatic or surgical pain. Opioids reversibly bind to specific receptors in the central and peripheral nervous system. These drugs are categorized as agonists, partial agonists, mixed agonist/antagonists, or antagonists based on their ability to induce an analgesic response once bound to a specific receptor. The action of opioid drugs on these receptors activates G-proteins, leading to a reduction in transmission of nerve impulses and inhibition of neurotransmitter release.[6] Agonist drugs have a linear dose–response curve that may be titrated to reach the desired effect, whereas the agonist/antagonist drugs may reach a ceiling effect after which increasing the dose does not appear to provide additional analgesia. During anesthesia, opioids are used to provide perioperative analgesia that may reduce the concentrations of volatile anesthetics (i.e., gas anesthesia-sparing

effects). The most common adverse effects reported with opioids are cardiac and/or respiratory depression. In many cases, these drugs may be reversed with antagonists, which will also terminate analgesia. The application and dosages of several opioid formulations have been scientifically evaluated and clinically applied in birds (Table 20-1).

Few studies have been conducted regarding the distribution, quantity, and function of each opioid receptor type in birds, and although marked species variability is assumed, further studies are necessary. In pigeons, the regional distributions of μ, κ, and δ receptors in the forebrain and midbrain were similar to mammals but the κ and δ receptors were more prominent in the pigeon forebrain and midbrain than μ receptors, and 76% of opioid receptors in the forebrain were determined to be κ type.[7] In day-old chicks, marked dissimilarities to this distribution suggest either age- or species-related differences.[8] Some of these dissimilarities might account for the varying responses to different opioid drugs identified between bird species.

Morphine is a μ-receptor agonist that has been infrequently used in avian medicine because some of the early studies with this drug in domestic fowl yielded conflicting results and suggested that very high dosages were required to reduce response to the toe pinch[9] or a noxious electrical stimulation.[10] Further investigations that involved the use of noxious thermal stimulation revealed strain-dependent effects in two lines of White Leghorns and a cross of Rhode Island Red X Light Sussex requiring dosages of 15, 30, and 100 mg/kg, respectively, to induce analgesia,[11] while in a different study 30 mg/kg resulted in analgesia in Rhode Island Red crossbreds

TABLE 20-1

Opioid and Opioid-Like Analgesics Evaluated in Avian Species by Either Pharmacokinetic or Pharmacodynamic Studies

Drug	Dosage (mg/kg)	Route	Frequency (q/h)	Species	Comments	Type of Study	References
Buprenorphine	0.6, 1.2, 1.8	IM, IV	Single dose	Cockatiels	Failed to increase thermal nociception thresholds. Some birds experience mild sedation at the highest dosages.	PK/PD	41
	0.1, 0.3, 0.6	IM, IV	Single dose	American kestrels	Increased withdrawal thresholds to thermal noxious stimulus for 0.5-6 hours.	PK/PD	39,40
	0.1	IM	Single dose	Grey parrots	No change in withdrawal response to noxious stimulus. May not achieve effective plasma concentrations at this dose.	PK/PD	24,37
	0.25, 0.5	IM	Single dose	Domestic pigeons	Increased latency withdrawal from a noxious electrical stimulus of 2 hours at 0.25 mg/kg and for 5 hours for 0.5 mg/kg.	PD	38
	0.05-1.0	Intra-articular	Single dose	Chickens	No significant effect on induced arthritis.	PD	14
Buprenorphine sustained-release formulation	1.8	IM, SC	Single dose	American kestrels	Increased thermal threshold for almost 24 hours.	PK/PD	Guzman, personal communication

CRI, Constant rate infusion; IM, intramuscular; IV, intravenous; PD, pharmacodynamic; PK, pharmacokinetic; PO, orally; q/h, every hour; $t_{(1/2)}$, half-life.

Continued

TABLE 20-1

Opioid and Opioid-Like Analgesics Evaluated in Avian Species by Either Pharmacokinetic or Pharmacodynamic Studies—cont'd

Drug	Dosage (mg/kg)	Route	Frequency (q/h)	Species	Comments	Type of Study	References
Butorphanol	1.0, 3.0, 6.0	IM	Single dose	American kestrel	Failed to increase foot withdrawal thermal thresholds, but instead caused hyperesthesia or hyperalgesia and agitation in males receiving 6 mg/kg; do not recommend in American kestrels.	PK, PD	100
	2.0, 4.0	IV	Single dose	Guineafowl	4 mg/kg resulted in arrhythmias and hypotension; one bird died.	PD	101
	2.0	IV	Single dose	Domestic chickens	Remained above minimum effective concentration for analgesia in mammals for approximately 2 hours.	PK	102
	5.0	PO	Single dose	Hispaniolan Amazon parrots	Oral bioavailability <10%; do not recommend PO administration.	PK	29
	2.0	IM	Single dose	Hispaniolan Amazon parrots	Safe and effective pre-emptive analgesia with sevoflurane anesthesia for endoscopy.	PD	26
	2.0-5.0	IM	Single dose	Hispaniolan Amazon parrots	Low mean plasma concentrations at 2 hours after 5 mg/kg IM. Withdrawal thresholds to noxious stimuli did not significantly change after 2 mg/kg IM.	PK, PD	30
	1.0	IM	Single dose	Cockatoos Grey parrots Blue-fronted Amazon parrots	Isoflurane-sparing study showed significant reduction in MAC in the cockatoos and Greys, but not Amazon parrots.	PD	22,103
	1.0–2.0	IM	Single dose	Grey parrots	Electrical stimuli to assess withdrawal thresholds—a more significant reduction of withdrawal response at 2 mg/kg.	PD	24
Fentanyl	Targeted controlled infusions	IV	CRI	Hispaniolan Amazon parrot	Reduced isoflurane MAC% in a dose-related manner, with significant effects on heart rate and blood pressure.	PD	21
	Targeted controlled infusions 10 to 30 µg/kg/min	IV	CRI	Red-tailed hawks	Reduced isoflurane MAC 31%–55% in a dose-related manner, without significant effects on heart rate, blood pressure, $PaCO_2$, or PaO_2.	PD	99
	0.02, 0.2	IM, SC	Single dose	White cockatoos	Rapid absorption and elimination. Withdrawal thresholds to electrical and thermal stimuli. 0.02 mg/kg did not affect either threshold; 0.2 mg/kg did affect both withdrawal thresholds but only some birds; hyperactivity in first 15–30 minutes.	PK/PD	19
	0.05–1.0	Intra-articular	Single dose	Chickens	No significant effect on induced arthritis.	PD	14

TABLE 20-1

Opioid and Opioid-Like Analgesics Evaluated in Avian Species by Either Pharmacokinetic or Pharmacodynamic Studies—cont'd

Drug	Dosage (mg/kg)	Route	Frequency (q/h)	Species	Comments	Type of Study	References
Hydromor-phone	0.1, 0.3, 0.6	IM, IV	Single dose	Cockatiels	Failed to increase thermal nociception thresholds. Some birds experience mild seda-tion at the highest dosages.	PK/PD	18
	0.1, 0.3, 0.6	IM, IV	Single dose	American kestrels	Increased the thermal nocicep-tion threshold for 3–6 hours. Some birds experience mod-erate sedation at the highest dosages.	PK/PD	16,17
Nalbuphine	12.5, 25, 50	IM	Single dose	Hispaniolan Amazon parrots	$t_{(1/2)}$ IM and IV less than 0.35 hour. Excellent IM bioavailability. 12.5 mg/kg produced 3 hours analgesia; higher doses did not increase analgesic time.	PK/PD	33,34
Nalbuphine sustained-release formulation	33.7, 37.5	IM, IV	Single dose	Hispaniolan Amazon parrots	37.5 mg/kg IV maintained plasma human therapeutic concentrations for 24 hours. 33.7 mg/kg produced 12 hours analgesia.	PK/PD	35,36
Tramadol	10.0	PO	Single dose	Penguin	Dose once daily appears adequate.	PK	43
	5.0, 15.0, 30.0	PO	Single dose	American kestrel	5 mg/kg significantly increased thermal nociception thresh-olds; higher doses resulted in less pronounced antinocicep-tive effects.	PD	49
	10.0, 20.0, 30.0	PO	Single and multiple dose	Hispaniolan Amazon parrots	30.0 mg/kg maintained target plasma therapeutic concen-trations for approximately 8 hours. Reduced thermal withdrawal response for approximately 6 hours.	PK, PD	44,48,104
	11.0	PO	Single dose	Red-tailed hawks	Maintained human plasma therapeutic concentrations for approximately 4 hours (but only three birds in study).	PK	45
	7.5	PO	Single dose	Indian peafowl	Maintained plasma human therapeutic concentrations for 12–24 hours.	PK	46
	11.0	PO	Single dose	American bald eagles	PO bioavailability high, 5 mg/kg PO every 12 hours suggested based on study; sedation with multiple dosing.	PK	47

and hyperalgesia in White Leghorns and Cal-White strains.[12] A more recent study of adult chickens that involved the use of the isoflurane-sparing technique found that increasing doses of morphine (0.1, 1, and 3 mg/kg) caused a significant decrease in the isoflurane minimum anesthetic concentration (MAC).[13] A study evaluating intra-articular injection of 1 to 3 mg mor-phine in a domestic fowl arthritis model identified no signifi-cant antinociceptive effects, but it is unclear whether synovial fluid pH differences may have affected the activity of the drug.[14] The pharmacokinetics of morphine at 2 mg/kg intra-venously (IV) also have been recently evaluated in the domes-tic chicken.[15] At this dose, chickens cleared morphine at a higher rate than man or cats. Plasma morphine analgesic con-centrations were similar to humans for approximately 2 hours.

Hydromorphone is a semisynthetic μ-opioid receptor ago-nist with a potency approximately three to four times that of morphine. Hydromorphone hydrochloride has shown a dose-responsive thermal antinociceptive effect when administered at 0.1, 0.3, and 0.6 mg/kg intramuscularly (IM) to American kestrels (*Falco sparverius*), suggesting that it may produce analgesia in this species for up to 6 hours (see Table 20-1).[16] The estimated relative potency of hydromorphone to morphine is 5–7:1.[16a] Severe sedation was detected in four birds when administered 0.6 mg/kg hydromorphone, and when the sedated birds were handled, they appeared agitated for a few seconds but then resumed a sedated behavior. The pharmacokinetics of hydromorphone following intramuscular and intravenous administration in American kestrels found a high intramuscular bioavailability (75%) and rapid elimination, with a short terminal half-life and a rapid plasma clearance.[17] A similar thermal nociception study in cockatiels (*Nymphicus hollandicus*) that were administered 0.1, 0.3, and 0.6 mg/kg IM hydromorphone and saline treatment showed no significant effect on the thermal threshold, and the highest dosages resulted in only a mild sedative effect.[18] More work evaluating other species is necessary before making recommendations on dosing and dosing frequency of this opioid agonist in other species.

Fentanyl is a short-acting μ-receptor agonist that is not commonly used in avian medicine because of the historical findings that μ-receptor agonists may not be useful for avian analgesia. Fentanyl administered at 0.02 mg/kg IM did not affect the withdrawal thresholds to electrical or thermal stimuli of white cockatoos[19]; however, a 10-fold increase in the dosage (0.2 mg/kg) administered subcutaneously (SC) did produce an antinociceptive response, but some birds were hyperactive for the first 15 to 30 min after receiving the high dose.[19] Fentanyl had rapid absorption and elimination in cockatoos (*Cacatua spp.*), with a terminal half-life of 1.15 hours.[19] Administered as an intravenous constant rate infusion (CRI) in red-tailed hawks, fentanyl reduced the minimum anesthetic concentration of isoflurane 31% to 55% in a dose-related manner, without significant effects on heart rate, blood pressure, PaCO$_2$, or PaO$_2$ (see Table 20-1).[20] In a similar study with Hispaniolan Amazon parrots (*Amazona ventralis*), fentanyl administered as an intravenous CRI reduced isoflurane MAC similarly to the red-tailed hawks; however, approximately 20 times higher dosing was necessary to achieve the same effects (M.G. Hawkins, Personal communication, June 28, 2015). Significant effects were detected in heart rate and blood pressure suggesting that while this can also be an effective opioid in these birds, close monitoring is recommended.[21]

Butorphanol is a mixed κ-opioid receptor agonist and μ-opioid receptor antagonist opioid drug. This opioid has historically been one of the most commonly used opioid analgesics in birds, despite many studies suggesting it requires very frequent dosing. Earlier isoflurane-sparing studies using 1 mg/kg IM butorphanol in three psittacine species showed a significant MAC reduction in cockatoos and Grey parrots (*Psittacus erithacus erithacus*), but not in blue-fronted Amazon parrots (*A. aestiva*), indicating species variability either in response to the drug itself or to the dose administered.[22,23] In a study using withdrawal thresholds to electrical stimuli in conscious Grey parrots, butorphanol at 1 mg/kg showed antinociceptive properties.[24] In a thermal antinociceptive study in which butorphanol dosages of 3 and 6 mg/kg IM were evaluated in Hispaniolan Amazon parrots, both dosages similarly increased thermal withdrawal thresholds (J Paul-Murphy, Personal communication, June 26, 2015). Based on these

studies, dosages of 1 to 4 mg/kg have been recommended in psittacines (see Table 20-1). In contrast American kestrels[25] administered butorphanol tartrate at 1, 3, and 6 mg/kg IM showed no significant increase in foot withdrawal thermal threshold values and no sedative effects were observed. Instead hyperesthesia or hyperalgesia and agitation were noted in males receiving 6 mg/kg. Because of these findings, butorphanol is not recommended in kestrels for pain management until further evidence of its analgesic properties is available. There is some evidence to suggest that butorphanol does not produce dose-related respiratory depression in contrast to μ-receptor agonists. Preoperative butorphanol administration (2 mg/kg IM) did not show significant anesthetic (including time to intubation and extubation) or cardiopulmonary changes in Hispaniolan Amazon parrots anesthetized with sevoflurane.[26] In a similar study in guineafowl (*Numida meleagris*),[27] administration of 4 mg/kg IV butorphanol did not significantly reduce MAC of sevoflurane but was associated with arrhythmias in all birds, significant decreases in heart rates and arterial blood pressures, and one bird died. Butorphanol pharmacokinetic (PK) studies have been published in several species of birds. One study evaluating the PK of 0.5 mg/kg butorphanol in red-tailed hawks and great-horned owls (*Bubo virginianus*) found terminal half-lives of 0.93 and 1.78 hours, respectively, when given intravenously and 0.94 and 1.84 hours, respectively, when given intramuscularly, suggesting the drug requires very frequent dosing in these species.[28] Likewise, when a dose of 2 mg/kg butorphanol was administered intravenously to domestic chickens, its terminal half-life was shorter in chickens than in humans, dogs, cattle, rabbits, and owls but longer than the red-tailed hawks.[15] In a PK study in Hispaniolan Amazon parrots,[29] mean target plasma concentrations greater than 100 ng/mL were maintained for 1.5 to 2 hours and 2 to 3 hours after intravenous and intramuscular administration, respectively. The terminal half-life also was very short (0.49 hours and 0.51 hours for intravenous and intramuscular administration, respectively). The calculated oral bioavailability of butorphanol was only 5.9%. This extraordinarily low oral bioavailability limits the use of this administration route for clinical purposes. Based on results in Hispaniolan Amazon parrots, butorphanol tartrate administered at 5 mg/kg IV or IM would have to be administered every 2 and 3 hours, respectively, to achieve target plasma concentrations determined in pharmacodynamic (PD) studies.[30] In American kestrels butorphanol tartrate administered at 6 mg/kg IM attained high plasma concentrations, which decreased rapidly over time.[25] All of these data confirm that frequent dosing of butorphanol is necessary in birds. This may be impractical because of lack of personnel to provide frequent dosing and the stress of frequent handling on the patient. Further research evaluating CRIs of butorphanol is needed to identify whether this is a good drug for use in balanced anesthesia/analgesia protocols. An experimental liposome-encapsulated, long-acting form of butorphanol tartrate was shown to be safe and effective in Hispaniolan Amazon parrots[30,31] and in green-cheeked conures (*Pyrrhura molinae*)[32] with induced arthritis for up to 5 days following subcutaneous administration but, unfortunately, this formulation is not commercially available.

Nalbuphine hydrochloride is a κ-opioid receptor agonist and μ-opioid receptor antagonist with a mechanism of action similar to butorphanol. It is used as an analgesic in the treatment of moderate to severe pain in humans and has a relatively lower incidence of respiratory depression that does not increase with additional dosing. Nalbuphine was rapidly cleared after 12.5 mg/kg IM and IV in Hispaniolan Amazon parrots and had excellent bioavailability following intramuscular administration, with little sedation and no adverse effects (see Table 20-1).[33] The same dosage increased thermal foot withdrawal threshold values in this species for up to 3 hours; higher dosages (25 and 50 mg/kg IM) did not significantly increase thermal foot withdrawal threshold values above those of the 12.5 mg/kg dosage.[34] While this opioid is promising for some species, frequent administration as with butorphanol is of concern. Nalbuphine decanoate, a slow-release nalbuphine experimental formulation, was administered at 33.7 mg/kg IM to Hispaniolan Amazon parrots and thermal withdrawal threshold values were increased for up to 12 hours, four times longer than the standard formulation.[35] Nalbuphine decanoate resulted in prolonged plasma concentrations after intramuscular administration in Hispaniolan Amazon parrots as well. When compared with previous studies with nalbuphine HCl, plasma concentrations that could be associated with antinociception were maintained for up to 24 hours when administered at 37.5 mg/kg.[36] Unfortunately, as with the liposome-encapsulated butorphanol, nalbuphine decanoate is not currently commercially available. Based on its potential for minor to few side effects, nalbuphine may show promise as an additional analgesic in pain-management protocols in avian patients.

Buprenorphine hydrochloride has a slow onset of action with longer duration than other opioid drugs and a unique and complex pharmacological profile. Buprenorphine is thought to act as a partial μ agonist but its κ-receptor activities are less well defined. Several studies suggest that buprenorphine demonstrates κ-receptor agonist effects but other evidence in mammals and pigeons (Columba livia) suggests that it also displays some κ-antagonistic activities. Buprenorphine has unusual receptor binding characteristics that appear to be the result of slow drug dissociation from opioid receptors. Doses from 0.05 to 1.0 mg buprenorphine administered intra-articularly in a domestic fowl arthritis model found no significant antinociceptive effects, but it is unclear whether synovial fluid pH differences may have affected the activity of the drug.[14] Buprenorphine at 0.1 mg/kg IM in Grey parrots did not demonstrate an antinociceptive effect when tested by noxious electrical stimulus, and PK analysis suggests this dose may not achieve effective plasma concentrations determined for mammals.[37] Pigeons administered 0.25 and 0.5 mg/kg IM buprenorphine had an increased withdrawal threshold from a noxious electrical stimulus for 2 and 5 hours, respectively, suggesting in different species this drug may have some effect at relatively low doses.[38] In American kestrels,[39] buprenorphine did cause a significant dose-dependent thermal antinociceptive response at 0.1, 0.3, and 0.6 mg/kg IM for 6 hours compared with control treatment. At 0.6 mg/kg, a mild sedative effect was appreciated. The PK of 0.6 mg/kg IM and IV buprenorphine was also evaluated in kestrels and high bioavailability (94.8%) after intramuscular dosing and a longer elimination rate than other opioids was identified.[40] In a similar study, a commercially available slow-release formulation of buprenorphine resulted in thermal antinociception in American kestrels for almost 24 hours following 1.8 mg/kg IM administration (D. Guzman, personal communication, June 26, 2015). In contrast, studies using cockatiels showed no significant difference in thermal withdrawal threshold using the same dosages of buprenorphine hydrochloride as in the kestrel studies, and no sedative effects were observed at any dosage.[41] Additional studies to evaluate other species are definitely warranted with this long-acting commercially available preparation.

Tramadol hydrochloride is an analgesic drug that has become popular recently despite minimal evidence of its efficacy. It is active at opioid, α-adrenergic, and serotonergic receptors.[42] Tramadol is a weak μ agonist but the O-desmethyl metabolite (M1) is a much more potent agonist in mammals. Other metabolites including M2 to M5 have also been described but their analgesic properties, if any, are not yet known. The conversion to the M1 metabolite is variable among species, but it is produced in the bird species studied thus far.[43-47] In humans, less respiratory depression and constipation are seen with tramadol than with μ-agonist opioids, but there are no data on these potential adverse effects in other species. PK profiles have been reported for American bald eagles (*Haliaeetus leucocephalus*),[47] Hispaniolan Amazon parrots,[44] red-tailed hawks,[45] African penguins (*Spheniscus demersus*),[43] Indian peafowl (*Pavo cristatus*),[46] and important differences exist with PK parameters between species. Oral bioavailability of tramadol was higher (97.94%) for American bald eagles than humans and dogs, suggesting this as a useful route of administration in this species. Tramadol 11 mg/kg orally (PO) achieved concentrations in the human analgesic range for 10 hours in 5 of 6 bald eagles; M1 plasma concentrations reached the human therapeutic range only in two eagles at much earlier time points.[47] The terminal half-life of tramadol in American bald eagles after oral dosing was two times that reported in dogs, but half as long as in humans. In Indian peafowl administered 7.5 mg/kg PO, plasma M1 concentrations remained at or near the human therapeutic range for 12 to 24 hours (see Table 20-1).[46] In Hispaniolan Amazon parrots, a much lower oral bioavailability (23.48%) and rapid clearance of a compounded oral suspension of tramadol leads to a requirement of a higher dose for oral administration to achieve similar plasma concentrations reported for other species.[44] Tramadol at a dose of 30 mg/kg PO induced thermal antinociception in Hispaniolan Amazon parrots for up to 6 hours, while lower dosages of 10 and 20 mg/kg did not have a significant effect.[48] In American kestrels, tramadol at 5 mg/kg PO significantly increased thermal thresholds for 1.5 hours when compared with the same birds given oral saline and for 9 hours when compared with baseline thresholds, while 15 and 30 mg/kg PO resulted in less antinociceptive effects (see Table 20-1).[49]

Nonsteroidal Antiinflammatory Drugs

NSAIDs are used to relieve musculoskeletal and visceral pain, acute pain, and chronic pain such as in osteoarthritis. The pharmacological activity of NSAIDs has been reviewed elsewhere and the mechanism of action is similar when administered to birds.[50,51] A broad tissue distribution of cyclooxygenase (COX) has been demonstrated in chickens.[52] The relative expression of COX-1 and COX-2 enzymes varies between species and both enzymes are important in avian

TABLE 20-2

NSAIDs Evaluated in Avian Species by Pharmacokinetic, Pharmacodynamic Evaluations, Toxicologic, or Clinical Studies

Drug	Dosage (mg/kg)	Route	Frequency (q/h)	Species	Comments	Type of Study	References
Carprofen	30.0	IM	Single dose	Chickens	Arthritis painful behaviors reduced 1 hour after treatment.	PD	72
	3.0	IM	12	Hispaniolan Amazon parrots,	Arthritis pain partially reduced, effect <12 hours.	PD	31
	1.0	IM	Single dose	Chickens	Improved locomotion of lame birds 1 hour after treatment.	PD	71
Flunixin meglumine	5.0	IV	Single dose	Budgerigars and Patagonian conures			75a
	5.0	IM	Single dose	Mallard ducks	12-hour activity, but muscle necrosis at the injection site.	PD	106
	5.5	IM	24 for 7 days	Budgerigars	Severe renal lesions.	TOX	63
	1.1	IV	Single dose	Chickens, ostrich, ducks, turkeys, pigeons	Chickens had long half-life but 10 minutes $t_{(1/2)}$ in ostrich.	PK	55
	3.0	IM	Single dose	Chickens	Arthritis painful behaviors reduced 1 hour after treatment.	PD	72
Ketoprofen	2.0	IV, IM, PO	Single dose	Quail	Low bioavailability IM, PO. Short IV $t_{(1/2)}$.	PK	73
	12.0	IM	Single dose	Chickens	Arthritis painful behaviors reduced 1 hour after treatment.	PD	72
	2.5	IM	24 for 7 days	Budgerigars	Tubular necrosis.	TOX	63
	5.0	IM	Single dose	Mallard Ducks	12-hour activity.	PD	105
	2.0, 5.0	PO, IM, IV	12-24	Eiders	Mortality associated with male eiders.	CS	75

CS, Care report or case series; IV, intravenous; PD, pharmacodynamic; PK, pharmacokinetic; PO, orally; q/h, every hour; TOX, toxicity; $t_{(1/2)}$, half life.

pain and inflammation. The application and dosages of NSAID formulations continues to be scientifically evaluated and clinically applied in birds (Table 20-2). The intention of recently developed NSAIDs has been to spare COX-1 and emphasize COX-2 inhibition with the goal of providing analgesia and suppressing inflammation without inhibiting physiologically important prostaglandins. The common NSAIDs used in avian medicine include meloxicam, carprofen, ketoprofen, celecoxib, and piroxicam, each with a distinct COX-1/COX-2 ratio and differing reports of effectiveness and toxicity in birds.

The most common adverse effects of NSAIDs include effects on the gastrointestinal system, renal system, and coagulation. NSAIDs have been recently implicated in humans and mammals with an increased risk of myocardial infarction and delays in bone healing,[53,54] but these effects have not been substantiated in birds. However, it is prudent to be aware that these adverse effects are often dose dependent and associated with chronic administration. The kidney uses both COX-1 and COX-2 for prostaglandin synthesis and injury occurs when renal prostaglandin synthesis is inhibited. Originally it was hypothesized that the adverse renal effects of NSAIDs

were linked primarily to COX-1 inhibition but COX-2 metabolites have been implicated in maintenance of renal blood flow, mediation of renin release, and regulation of sodium excretion. Therefore, in conditions of relative intravascular volume depletion and/or renal hypoperfusion such as dehydration, hemorrhage, hemodynamic compromise, heart failure, and renal disease, interference with COX-2 activity can have significant deleterious effects on renal blood flow and glomerular filtration rate.

Meloxicam is a COX-2-selective NSAID that has become the most widely used antiinflammatory medication in avian practice (see Table 20-2). Meloxicam is currently available as oral tablets, oral suspension, and an injectable formulation. Studies investigating the pharmacokinetics of meloxicam in chickens,[55] ostriches (Struthio camelus),[55] ducks,[55] turkeys (Meleagris spp.),[55] pigeons,[55] vultures,[56] ring-necked parakeets (Psittacula krameri),[57] Hispaniolan Amazon parrots,[58] Grey parrots,[59] red-tailed hawks, and great-horned owls[60] have been published. The terminal half-life and bioavailability of meloxicam in Hispaniolan Amazon parrots following 1 mg/kg PO administration were determined to be 15.8 ± 8.6 hours, and 49% to 75%, respectively.[58] A PD study in Hispaniolan

CHAPTER 20 • *Recognition, Assessment, and Management of Pain in Birds* **623**

TABLE 20-2

NSAIDs Evaluated in Avian Species by Pharmacokinetic, Pharmacodynamic Evaluations, Toxicologic, or Clinical Studies—cont'd

Drug	Dosage (mg/kg)	Route	Frequency (q/h)	Species	Comments	Type of Study	References
Meloxicam	0.5	IV, PO	Single dose	Red-tailed hawks and great-horned owls		PK	60
	2.0	IM	Multiple dose	Japanese quail	2 mg/kg IM q12h for 14d did not cause significant lesions but resulted in muscle necrosis.	TOX	65
	0.5, 2.0	IM-PO	Multiple dose	Pigeon	2 mg/kg was needed for significant analgesia in orthopedic pain.	PD	62
	1.0, 0.5	IM, IV, PO	Single and multiple dose (24 and 24)	Grey parrots	1 mg/kg IM would maintain target plasma concentrations for 24 hours; 0.5 mg/kg IM q12h did not cause renal lesion based on endoscopic biopsies.	PK/TOX	59,64
	1.0	IM, IV, PO	Single dose	Hispaniolan Amazon parrots	Improved weight bearing on arthritic limb.	PK, PD	58,61
	2.0	IM, PO	Single dose	Cape Griffon vultures	Short $t_{(1/2)}$; <45 min.	PK	56
	0.1	IM	24 for 7 days	Budgerigars	Glomerular congestion.	TOX	63
		IM	Single dose	Ring-necked parakeets		PK	57
	0.5	IV	Single dose	Chickens, ostrich, ducks, turkeys, pigeons	Variable distribution, slow clearance except ostrich.	PK	55
Piroxicam	0.5-0.8	PO	12	Whooping cranes	Used for acute myopathy and chronic arthritis.	CS	77
	0.5	PO	Single dose	Brolga cranes		PK	78

Amazon parrots with experimentally induced arthritis concluded that 1 mg/kg meloxicam IM every 12 hours significantly improved weight bearing but 0.5 mg/kg did not.[61] In pigeons,[62] meloxicam at 2 mg/kg PO every 12 hours provided quantifiable postoperative analgesia for orthopedic pain associated with experimental femoral osteotomy, but 0.5 mg/kg was ineffective. In addition, several studies have evaluated the adverse effects of meloxicam in budgerigars *(Melopsittacus undulates)*[63] (0.1 mg/kg IM), Grey parrots[64] (0.5 mg/kg IM), domestic pigeons[62] (2 mg/kg IM), Japanese quail *(Coturnix japonica)*[65] (2 mg/kg IM), and Hispaniolan Amazon parrots (1.6 mg/kg PO). In these studies, there were no significant renal, gastrointestinal, or hemostatic adverse effects reported at the dosages evaluated. A survey to determine NSAID toxicity in captive birds treated in zoos reported zero fatalities when meloxicam was administered to over 700 birds from 60 species.[66] The renal effects of NSAIDs have been of particular concern in the Asian vultures *(Gyps bengalensis, G. indicus,* and *G. tenuirostris).*[67,68] These species are more sensitive to the adverse renal effects of several NSAIDs, with the exception of meloxicam.[69] Despite meloxicam's large therapeutic range and relative safety compared with other NSAIDs,

species-specific potential adverse effects should continue to be evaluated.

Carprofen is considered a weak COX inhibitor at therapeutic doses yet exhibits good antiinflammatory activity. This weak inhibition of both COX isoforms may explain its apparent wide margin of safety and it may achieve its therapeutic effects partially through other pathways.[70] Carprofen given subcutaneously significantly improved the speed and walking ability of lame chickens in a dose-dependent manner.[71] An extremely high carprofen dose when compared with mammalian doses of 30 mg/kg IM was needed for analgesia in chickens with experimental arthritis[69]; this dose is 6 to 10 times higher than standard mammal doses.[72] An analgesic study utilizing Hispaniolan Amazon parrots with experimental arthritis noted that 3 mg/kg IM carprofen administered every 12 hours markedly improved the lameness in the short term. Longer term, treatment with carprofen alone caused a slight but nonsignificant improvement in weight-bearing load on the arthritic limb compared with the control treatment over the full 30-hour study period.[31] Much work is needed to determine appropriate dosages, dosing routes, and dosing frequency of carprofen in birds.

Ketoprofen is a potent nonselective COX-1 inhibitor that has been used extensively in small animal medicine. The excellent oral ketoprofen bioavailability in mammals makes this drug attractive for oral dosing. However, ketoprofen is most commonly used parenterally in birds because of limited oral PK data and difficulty in accurately dosing the oral formulation in small species. PK studies evaluating a single dose of 2 mg/kg ketoprofen given orally, intramuscularly, and intravenously in Japanese quail showed very low oral (24%) and intramuscular (54%) bioavailability of the drug and the shortest half-life reported for this NSAID in any species (see Table 20-2).[73] While it is possible that drug formulation could account for the low bioavailability of the drug in this study, additional studies are needed to determine whether drug formulations or physiological differences between species could account for these differences. PD studies of 5mg/kg IM ketoprofen in mallard ducks (*Anas platyrhynchos*) found an overall decrease in the inflammatory mediator thromboxane (TBX) for approximately 12 hours after administration.[74] This suggests that the duration of antiinflammatory effect in the mallards may parallel that of some mammals studied; further studies in additional species are necessary to evaluate the duration of effect and bioavailability of ketoprofen in birds. When ketoprofen 2 to 5 mg/kg IM was administered to free-ranging spectacled eiders (*Somateria fischeri*) and king eiders (*S. spectabilis*), 4 of 10 male spectacled eiders and 5 of 6 male king eiders died within 1 to 4 days after surgery.[75] The histological findings included severe renal tubular necrosis, acute rhabdomyolysis, and mild visceral gout. Male behaviors during mating season may have predisposed these birds to dehydration and the adverse effects of COX inhibition.[75]

Flunixin meglumine is a nonselective COX inhibitor. It was effective in reducing a model of arthritic pain in chickens when administered at 3.0 mg/kg IM.[72] A dose of 5 mg/kg IM suppressed plasma TBX activity, a surrogate indicator of pain, in mallard ducks for approximately 12 hours, suggesting that its physiologic action may be that long.[74] PK studies of flunixin have been performed in budgerigars and Patagonian conures[75a] (*Cyanoliseus patagonus*), ducks,[55] turkeys,[55] pigeons,[55] ostriches,[55] and chickens.[55] Northern bobwhite quail (*Colinus virginianus*) were treated for 7 days with a range of flunixin meglumine dosages and even the lowest dose (0.1 mg/kg) caused glomerular lesions.[76] Plasma uric acid and protein levels did not change in budgerigars treated with 5.5 mg/kg IM flunixin meglumine for 3 or 7 days, but a low frequency of glomerular congestion, degeneration, and dilation of tubules occurred with increased mesangial matrix synthesis.[63]

Piroxicam is a nonselective NSAID used for is antiinflammatory properties and its value as a chemopreventative and antitumor agent. It has a much higher potency against COX-1 than COX-2. Despite the high incidence of negative side effects of piroxicam used in humans, there are no reports of its toxicity in birds. It has been used clinically for long-term treatment of chronic arthritis in cranes.[77] A PK study in brolga cranes (*Grus rubicunda*) evaluated a dosage of 0.5 mg/kg PO, finding that daily administration might be appropriate for this species based on plasma concentrations (see Table 20-2).[78]

Diclofenac (DF) has been linked to the massive mortalities reported in multiple vulture species on the Asian subcontinent, leading to banning of DF on the Indian subcontinent. Common findings of diffuse visceral gout and proximal convoluted tubular damage indicated that the site of toxicosis was the kidneys or the renal supportive vascular system.[67,79-81] The association of DF with vulture mortalities led to several investigations to establish the mechanism of toxicity for DF and other NSAIDs in several avian species. The effect of DF on inhibition of renal prostaglandins and subsequent renal portal valve closure was proposed to cause the severe renal ischemia and nephrotoxicity,[80] but additional studies determined that vulture susceptibility to DF results from a combination of increases in reactive oxygen molecules (such as oxygen ions and peroxide), interference with uric acid transport, and duration of exposure.[78,79] Both DF and meloxicam were toxic to renal tubular epithelial cells following 12 hours of cell culture exposure, but meloxicam showed no toxicity in cultures incubated for only 2 hours.[78,79] DF decreased the transport of uric acid by interfering with the p-aminohippuric acid channel. Additionally, the terminal half-life of DF in vultures (14 hours) is much longer than in chickens (2 hours), exposing vultures to toxic effects of DF for prolonged periods whereas the rapid half-life of meloxicam in vultures intramuscularly (0.42 hour) or orally (0.41 hour) suggests it is unlikely this drug will accumulate.[56]

Local Anesthetics

Local anesthetics reversibly bind to Na^+ channels and block impulse conduction. Local anesthetics will be absorbed by the vasculature in the region blocked. Systemic uptake of the local anesthetics can be rapid in birds, and metabolism may be prolonged, increasing the potential for toxic reactions. The duration of action depends on the molecular properties and lipid solubility of the drug. Dosage recommendations have been lower for birds than mammals because anecdotal evidence has suggested that birds may be more sensitive to the adverse effects of these drugs. Toxic effects reported in birds include fine tremors, ataxia, recumbency, seizures, stupor, cardiovascular effects, and death. No adverse cardiovascular effects were identified in a recent study in chickens under isoflurane anesthesia when lidocaine was administered at 6 mg/kg IV.[82]

Lidocaine is available as a commercial preparation of 2% (20 mg/mL) and the "without epinephrine" formulation is recommended. Based on empirical use, the recommended dosage is 2 to 3 mg/kg, although 15 mg/kg with epinephrine had no adverse effects when used for brachial plexus block in mallard ducks.[83] For small birds, the commercial preparation may need to be diluted 1:10 or more to achieve an effective volume for the block, but it is unknown whether dilution allows either appropriate tissue drug concentrations for analgesia or the expected duration of analgesia to occur. The pharmacokinetics of lidocaine following 2.5 mg/kg IV administration in anesthetized chickens showed a rapid half-life and appears to share similar mechanisms of metabolism and elimination to mammalian species reported (Table 20-3).[84]

Bupivacaine is the most clinically useful perioperative local anesthetic in mammals because it is a long-acting local anesthetic. The commercial preparations of bupivacaine available are 0.25, 0.5, and 0.75% solutions (2.5, 5, and 7.5 mg/mL, respectively), and the lower concentration may not need dilution for birds. It has been used conservatively in birds because of concerns that toxic effects may take longer to resolve because of this drug's longer duration of effect.

TABLE 20-3

Local Anesthetic Evaluated in Avian Species by Either Pharmacokinetic or Pharmacodynamic Evaluations

Drug	Dosage (mg/kg)	Route	Frequency (q/h)	Species	Comments	Type of Study	References
Bupivacaine	2.0, 8.0	PN	Single dose	Mallard ducks	Ineffective in producing local analgesia.	PD	83
	5.0	PN	Single dose	Chickens	High failure rate.	PD	89
	2.0	SC	Single dose	Mallard ducks		PK	85
	3.0	IA	Single dose	Chickens	Effective in treating arthritic pain.	PD	86
Lidocaine	6.0	IV	Single dose	Chicken	6 mg/kg did not cause clinically relevant effects on HR or MAP.	PD	82
	2.5	IV	Single dose	Chicken		PK	
	2.0	PN	Single dose	Hispaniolan Amazon parrot	No effect on motor function, muscle relaxation or wing droop was observed.	PD	90
	15.0	PN	Single dose	Mallard ducks	Ineffective in producing local analgesia.	PD	83
	20.0	PN	Single dose	Chickens	High failure rate.	PD	89

HR, Heart rate; IA, intra-articular administration; IV, intravenous; MAP, mean arterial pressure; PD, pharmacodynamic; PK, pharmacokinetic; PN, perineural; q/h, every hour; SC, subcutaneous.

The recommended maximum dosage of bupivacaine for mammals is 2 mg/kg. Results from a study where mallard ducks were administered bupivacaine 2 mg/kg SC suggested the drug is shorter acting than in mammals, and potential for delayed toxicity was suggested by increased plasma concentrations at 6 and 12 hours.[85] Intra-articular bupivacaine (3 mg in 0.3 mL saline) was effective for treating arthritic pain in chickens.[86] A 1:1 mixture of bupivacaine and dimethyl sulfoxide was applied to amputated chicken beaks immediately after amputation, and feed intake improved.[87]

Local line or splash blocks are the most common methods of regional infiltration used in birds. The subcutaneous space in most avian species is very thin so a small gauge needle is recommended to make several subcutaneous injections into the operative area. Brachial plexus blockade has been described in a variety of avian species (see Table 20-3), but neither bupivacaine (2 and 8 mg/kg) or lidocaine (15 mg/kg) with epinephrine perineurally effectively blocked nerve transmission in the brachial plexus of mallard ducks.[88] Similar findings were reported in chickens with lidocaine (20 mg/kg) or bupivacaine (5 mg/kg) with epinephrine for brachial plexus blockade using a nerve locator.[89] In Hispaniolan Amazon parrots, neither palpation- or ultrasound-guided brachial plexus blockade was found to result in an effective block using lidocaine at 2 mg/kg perineurally.[90] Ischiatic-femoral nerve block has also been described in peregrine falcons (*Falco peregrinus*), and was considered a feasible technique applying lidocaine at 2 mg/kg perineurally with the aid of a nerve locator (see Table 20-3).[91] The safe use of transdermal patches and creams, epidural infusions, spinal blocks, and intravenous blocks have not yet been reported in birds.

Other Drugs

Gabapentin, a GABA analog, has been used to treat neuropathic pain in humans. Its exact mechanism of action is unknown, but its therapeutic action on neuropathic pain is thought to involve voltage-gated N-type calcium ion channels. As in humans and other mammals gabapentin is generally considered synergistic with other drugs and may not obtain the effect expected as a sole agent.[92,93] There are limited reports of use of gabapentin as part of a multimodal therapeutic plan for suspected neuropathic pain in birds. Recently, a pharmacokinetic study in Hispaniolan Amazon parrots[94] has suggested 10 mg/kg PO every 12 hours, and suggested that increasing dosages might be necessary as increasing dosing stepwise is generally necessary in other species.

Dietary Supplements

Omega-3 polyunsaturated fatty acids like eicosapentaenoic acid (EPA) and docosahexaenoic acid (DHA) have antiinflammatory effects that might reduce the pain associated with osteoarthritis (see Chapter 4, the section on Navigating the Nutraceutical Industry: A Guide to Help Veterinarians Make Informed Clinical Decisions). The total EPA and DHA dosages are the primary factors to consider, and the omega-3 to omega-6 fatty acid ratio are considered less important. Other omega-3 fatty acids (e.g., plant-based omega-3 fatty acid, α-linoleic acid) do not have similar effects.[95] There have been no studies in birds evaluating the effects and optimal dosage of EPA and DHA in osteoarthritic pain.

Glucosamine, methylsulfonylmethane, and chondroitin sulfate may be beneficial in the treatment of osteoarthritis through their antiinflammatory effects, but there are no studies in birds evaluating dosages and potential adverse effects (see Chapter 4, the section on Navigating the Nutraceutical Industry: A Guide to Help Veterinarians Make Informed Clinical Decisions). Polysulfated glycosaminoglycans (PSGAGs) have also been used anecdotally in the management of degenerative joint disease in birds, but fatal coagulopathies in different avian species (one Coraciiforme, two raptors, and one psittacine) following intramuscular administration have been reported.[96]

Physical Therapy

Treatment for pain in humans and companion mammal species may include physical modalities, manual therapy, and therapeutic exercise. The application of adjunctive therapy should be considered for acute and chronic pain in birds, although evidence-based information is not yet available. Therapeutic exercises, such as static weight bearing, can generally be utilized in the acute phase of injury with gradual progression of difficulty as healing occurs. Physical modalities such as thermotherapy and laser are used to diminish pain. Thermotherapy can have analgesic effects after the inflammatory effect has subsided. Low-level laser therapy (660 nm, 9 J/cm^2) has been shown to decrease indicators of neuropathic pain. Manual physical therapeutic techniques for joint mobilization can decrease pain but trigger-point pressure techniques might induce central sensitization.[97] There are a number of anecdotal reports of the use of acupuncture in pain management protocols for birds; however, no objective studies have been published.

Nursing and Supporting Care

The environmental effect on pain, stress, and anxiety can have a modulatory effect. The bird should be in an environment where it is as emotionally and physically comfortable as possible. Human presence or absence, decreasing light and noise, and separating other animals from the bird can reduce stress and anxiety during the painful period. When handling and moving an animal, avoid painful areas (e.g., surgical/trauma site, osteoarthritic joints), even when the animal is anaesthetized or sedated, to avoid inflicting a noxious stimulus, which can begin a new pain cascade.[97]

Cold compress during acute injury can reduce swelling and provide analgesia. Cold compress generally needs to be in place for 15 to 20 minutes to be effective. Warm compress is generally more comfortable after the acute phase has passed, but can aid tissue relaxation and act as a precursor to massage or stretching. Warm compress generally needs to be in place for 10 to 15 minutes.[96,97]

PAIN MANAGEMENT FOR SPECIFIC CONDITIONS AND PROCEDURES

Orthopedic Surgery

Orthopedic surgery can result in moderate to severe postoperative pain. Preventive and multimodal analgesic techniques should be used for all procedures. The balance between preoperative, intraoperative, and postoperative analgesia will depend on the severity of the preoperative condition and the location and magnitude of surgical trauma.[97]

Preoperative: Combinations of an opioid and an NSAID are often administered to birds when initially presenting for orthopedic trauma. General anesthesia can cause hypotension and reduce renal perfusion, thus it is still recommended to avoid NSAID administration in the immediate preoperative and perioperative periods. Opioids coupled with benzodiazepines administered intramuscularly are frequently recommended for the immediate pre-anesthetic period and may assist in reducing the amount of inhalation anesthetic needed for induction and maintenance of anesthesia.

Intraoperative: CRI using opioids has been used as an adjunct to inhalation anesthesia for orthopedic pain. An effective local anesthetic block at the surgical site and splash blocks of nerves in the surgical area of the fracture can decrease sensitization and windup that might occur during tissue handling.

Immediate postoperative (24 hours): Assuming the patient is well hydrated, a combination of an NSAID and continued opioid CRI, or parenteral opioid administration with gradual reduction in doses during the 24- to 48-hour postoperative period are recommended. Adjunctive protocols including physical therapy and cold or warm thermal therapy may be included as needed. Cold therapy will help reduce swelling whereas warm therapy may stimulate blood flow to specific areas.

Later postoperative period: Opioid administration with titration to effect and gradual discontinuation. NSAIDs or oral tramadol may be utilized when the patient returns to home care. Cold therapy of the affected regions should be continued for a minimum of 3 days, at which point it can be alternated with heat therapy prior to stretching and gentle weight bearing (with icing following these therapies).

Soft Tissue Surgery

Soft tissue surgery may cause mild, moderate, or severe postoperative pain. Preventive and multimodal analgesic techniques should be used and local anesthetic techniques included whenever possible. The balance between preoperative, intraoperative, and postoperative analgesia as described previously (see Orthopedic Surgery) will depend on the severity of the preoperative condition and the location and magnitude of surgical trauma. When postoperative pain is not successfully controlled with NSAIDs, alternative or additional analgesics or analgesic techniques should be used. Major soft tissue surgery may lead to chronic pain and may develop a neuropathic component. No veterinary studies have been performed assessing the benefit of adding gabapentin to the perioperative anesthetic and analgesic protocol in surgical situations where there is significant nerve damage. However, based on its use in human medicine, there may be potential value for use in the prevention of neuropathic pain.[97,98]

Minor soft tissue surgery

Preoperative and intraoperative: Combination of an opioid and local anesthetic techniques.

Postoperative analgesia: NSAIDs ± opioid and/or nondrug therapies such as physical therapy and cold or warm thermal therapy based on desired outcome.

Major soft tissue surgery

Preoperative: Same as for minor soft tissue surgery.

Intraoperative: CRI or parenteral opioids, local anesthetic blocks as needed.

Immediate and later postoperative (24 hours): NSAIDs if the patient is well hydrated and blood pressures are within the normal range, continuous infusions or boluses of drugs used intraoperatively as needed ± other adjunctive drugs and nondrug therapies such as physical therapy and cold or warm thermal therapy based on desired outcome.

Visceral Pain

Coelomic visceral pain occurs in conditions associated with distension and/or inflammation of hollow organs, ischemia, pulmonary thrombosis, acute enlargement of solid organs resulting in stretching of the capsule, and inflammation of any organ (e.g., pancreatitis, acute kidney injury, pneumonia/pleuritis). Visceral pain tends to be diffuse in nature; however, pain can be localized to an area within the cavity when pressure is applied externally.[97]

Mild pain

Use NSAID of choice (where indicated) and/or tramadol are recommended.

Moderate pain

Use buprenorphine (e.g., raptor) or butorphanol/nalbuphine (psittacines) or μ-agonist opioid (e.g., hydromorphone in raptor), depending on species. Add an NSAID when hemodynamically stable and no contraindications are identified.

Severe pain

Use μ-agonist opioid (e.g., hydromorphone in raptor) and titrate to effect, or opioid CRI. Add an NSAID when hemodynamically stable and no contraindications are identified.

Osteoarthritic Pain

Osteoarthritis is one of the most common causes of chronic pain in birds, and can be caused by trauma, infection, immune-mediated diseases, or developmental malformations. Pain develops secondary to joint dysfunction, muscle atrophy, and limb disuse, and the severity varies.

Mild pain

Weight loss, implementation of an appropriate exercise regimen, use of dietary supplements (e.g., glucosamine or chondroitin sulfate), and occasional NSAIDs during intermittent flare-ups are recommended.

Moderate pain

Same as above, but NSAIDs administered daily titrating down to the animal's minimal effective dose.

Severe pain

Same as above with increasing dosages of NSAIDs, adding other drugs (tramadol and gabapentin) as needed; arthrodesis may be necessary to minimize the pain of severe osteoarthritis.

Cancer-Related Pain

Cancer pain has varying degrees of severity dependent on duration, location, and type of cancer. Pain may originate from inflammation from tumor necrosis or direct pressure from muscle spasms in the area of the lesions, or from tissue that has been infiltrated. Most patients with cancer suffer pain to some degree, and the best documented is bone pain. A multimodal drug approach to control of cancer pain is recommended. NSAIDs are widely used to minimize cancer pain and even cancer growth in many mammalian species. They are recommended with the addition of opioids and tramadol as needed. Other modalities that can prove beneficial to reduce pain are surgery, chemotherapy, and radiotherapy and should be used concurrently.[97]

REFERENCES

1. Gentle MJ, Hunter LN: Physiological and behavioural responses associated with feather removal in *Gallus gallus* var *domesticus*, *Res Vet Sci* 50:95–101, 1991.
2. Mazor-Thomas JE, Mann PE, Karas AZ, et al: Pain-suppressed behaviors in the red-tailed hawk, *Appl Anim Behav Sci* 152:83–91, 2014.
3. Gentle MJ, Tilston VL: Reduction in peripheral inflammation by changes in attention, *Physiol Behav* 66:289–292, 1999.
4. Le Maho Y, Karmann H, Briot D, et al: Stress in birds due to routine handling and a technique to avoid it, *Am J Physiol* 263:775–781, 1992.
5. Desmarchelier M, Troncy E, Beauchamp G, et al: Evaluation of a fracture pain model in domestic pigeons (*Columba livia*), *Am J Vet Res* 73:353–360, 2012.
6. Bovill JG: Mechanisms of actions of opioids and non-steroidal anti-inflammatory drugs, *Eur J Anaesthesiol Suppl* 15:9–15, 1997.
7. Mansour A, Khachaturian H, Lewis ME, et al: Anatomy of CNS opioid receptors, *Trends Neurosci* 11:308–314, 1988.
8. Csillag A, Bourne RC, Stewart MG: Distribution of mu, delta, and kappa opioid receptor binding sites in the brain of the one-day-old domestic chick (*Gallus domesticus*): an in vitro quantitative autoradiographic study, *J Comp Neurol* 302:543–551, 1990.
9. Schneider C: Effects of morphine-like drugs in chicks, *Nature* 191:607–608, 1961.
10. Bardo MT, Hughes RA: Brief communication. Shock-elicited flight response in chickens as an index of morphine analgesia, *Pharmacol Biochem Behav* 9:147–149, 1978.
11. Fan S, Shutt AJ, Vogt M: The importance of 5-hydroxytryptamine turnover for the analgesic effect of morphine in the chicken, *Neuroscience* 6:2223–2227, 1981.
12. Hughes RA: Strain-dependent morphine-induced analgesic and hyperalgesic effects on thermal nociception in domestic fowl (*Gallus gallus*), *Behav Neurosci* 104:619–624, 1990.
13. Concannon KT, Dodam JR, Hellyer PW: Influence of a mu- and kappa-opioid agonist on isoflurane minimal anesthetic concentration in chickens, *Am J Vet Res* 56:806–811, 1995.
14. Gentle MJ, Hocking PM, Bernard R, et al: Evaluation of intraarticular opioid analgesia for the relief of articular pain in the domestic fowl, *Pharmacol Biochem Behav* 63:339–343, 1999.
15. Singh PM, Johnson C, Gartrell B, et al: Pharmacokinetics of morphine after intravenous administration in broiler chickens, *J Vet Pharmacol Ther* 33:515–518, 2010.
16. Guzman DS, Drazenovich TL, Olsen GH, et al: Evaluation of thermal antinociceptive effects after intramuscular administration of hydromorphone hydrochloride to American kestrels (*Falco sparverius*), *Am J Vet Res* 74:817–822, 2013.
16a. Dunbar PJ, Chapman CR, Buckley FP, et al: Clinical analgesic equivalence for morphine and hydromorphone with prolonged PCA, *Pain* 68:265–270, 1996.
17. Guzman DS, KuKanich B, Drazenovich TL, et al: Pharmacokinetics of hydromorphone hydrochloride after intravenous and intramuscular administration of a single dose to American kestrels (*Falco sparverius*), *Am J Vet Res* 75:527–531, 2014.
18. Sanchez Migallon-Guzman D, Houck E, Beaufrere H, et al: Evaluation of the thermal antinociceptive effects of hydromorphone hydrochloride in cockatiels (*Nymphicus hollandicus*). In *Proceedings of the Association of Avian Veterinarians*, 2014, pp 23–24.
19. Hoppes S, Flammer K, Hoersch K, et al: Disposition and analgesic effects of fentanyl in white cockatoos (*Cacatua alba*), *J Avian Med Surg* 17:124–130, 2003.

20. Pavez JC, Hawkins MG, Pascoe PJ, et al: Effect of fentanyl target-controlled infusions on isoflurane minimum anaesthetic concentration and cardiovascular function in red-tailed hawks (*Buteo jamaicensis*), *Vet Anaesth Analg* 38:344–351, 2011.

21. Hawkins MG, Pascoe PJ, DiMaio Knych HK, et al: Effect of fentanyl citrate target-controlled-infusions on isoflurane MAC and cardiovascular function in Hispaniolan Amazon parrots (*Amazona ventralis*). In *Proceedings of the Annual Conference of the Association of Avian Veterinarians*, 2014, pp 15–16.

22. Curro TG: Evaluation of the isoflurane-sparing effects of butorphanol and flunixin in psittaciformes. In *Proceedings of Association of Avian Veterinarians*,1994, pp 17–19.

23. Curro TG, Brunson DB, Paul-Murphy J: Determination of the ED50 of isoflurane and evaluation of the isoflurane-sparing effect of butorphanol in cockatoos (*Cacatua* spp.), *Vet Surg* 23:429–433, 1994.

24. Paul-Murphy J, Brunson DB, Miletic V: Analgesic effects of butorphanol and buprenorphine in conscious African grey parrots (*Psittacus erithacus erithacus* and *Psittacus erithacus timneh*), *Am J Vet Res* 60:1218–1221, 1999.

25. Guzman DS, Drazenovich TL, KuKanich B, et al: Evaluation of thermal antinociceptive effects and pharmacokinetics after intramuscular administration of butorphanol tartrate to American kestrels (*Falco sparverius*), *Am J Vet Res* 75:11–18, 2014.

26. Klaphake E, Schumacher J, Greenacre C, et al: Comparative anesthetic and cardiopulmonary effects of pre- versus postoperative butorphanol administration in Hispaniolan amazon parrots (*Amazona ventralis*) anesthetized with sevoflurane, *J Avian Med Surg* 20:2–7, 2006.

27. Escobar A, Valadão CA, Brosnan RJ, et al: Cardiopulmonary effects of butorphanol in sevoflurane-anesthetized guineafowl (*Numida meleagris*), *Vet Anaesth Analg* 41:284–289, 2014.

28. Riggs SM, Hawkins MG, Craigmill AL, et al: Pharmacokinetics of butorphanol tartrate in red-tailed hawks (*Buteo jamaicensis*) and great horned owls (*Bubo virginianus*), *Am J Vet Res* 69:596–603, 2008.

29. Guzman DS, Flammer K, Paul-Murphy JR, et al: Pharmacokinetics of butorphanol after intravenous, intramuscular, and oral administration in Hispaniolan Amazon parrots (*Amazona ventralis*), *J Avian Med Surg* 25:185–191, 2011.

30. Sladky K, Krugner-Higby L, Meek-Walker E, et al: Serum concentrations and analgesic effects of liposome-encapsulated and standard butorphanol tartrate in parrots, *Am J Vet Res* 67:775–781, 2006.

31. Paul-Murphy JR, Sladky KK, Krugner-Higby LA, et al: Analgesic effects of carprofen and liposome-encapsulated butorphanol tartrate in Hispaniolan parrots (*Amazona ventralis*) with experimentally induced arthritis, *Am J Vet Res* 70:1201–1210, 2009.

32. Paul-Murphy JR, Krugner-Higby LA, Tourdot RL, et al: Evaluation of liposome-encapsulated butorphanol tartrate for alleviation of experimentally induced arthritic pain in green-cheeked conures (*Pyrrhura molinae*), *Am J Vet Res* 70:1211–1219, 2009.

33. Keller DL, Sanchez-Migallon Guzman D, Klauer JM, et al: Pharmacokinetics of nalbuphine hydrochloride after intravenous and intramuscular administration to Hispaniolan Amazon parrots (*Amazona ventralis*), *Am J Vet Res* 72:741–745, 2011.

34. Sanchez-Migallon Guzman D, KuKanich B, Keuler NS, et al: Antinociceptive effects of nalbuphine hydrochloride in Hispaniolan Amazon parrots (*Amazona ventralis*), *Am J Vet Res* 72:736–740, 2011.

35. Sanchez-Migallon Guzman D, Braun JM, Steagall PV, et al: Antinociceptive effects of long-acting nalbuphine decanoate after intramuscular administration to Hispaniolan Amazon parrots (*Amazona ventralis*), *Am J Vet Res* 74:196–200, 2013.

36. Sanchez-Migallon Guzman D, KuKanich B, Heath TD, et al: Pharmacokinetics of long-acting nalbuphine decanoate after intramuscular administration to Hispaniolan Amazon parrots (*Amazona ventralis*), *Am J Vet Res* 74:191–195, 2013.

37. Paul-Murphy J, Hess J, Fialkowski JP: Pharmokinetic properties of a single intramuscular dose of buprenorphine in African grey parrots (*Psittacus erithacus erithacus*), *J Avian Med Surg* 18:224–228, 2004.

38. Gaggermeier B, Henke J, Schatzmann U. Investigations on analgesia in domestic pigeons (*C. livia*, Gmel., 1789, var. dom.) using buprenorphine and butorphanol. In *Proceedings of the European Association of Avian Veterinarians*, 2003, pp 70–73.

39. Ceulemans SM, Guzman DS, Olsen GH, et al: Evaluation of thermal antinociceptive effects after intramuscular administration of buprenorphine hydrochloride to American kestrels (*Falco sparverius*), *Am J Vet Res* 75:705–710, 2014.

40. Gustavsen KA, Guzman DS, Knych HK, et al: Pharmacokinetics of buprenorphine hydrochloride following intramuscular and intravenous administration to American kestrels (*Falco sparverius*), *Am J Vet Res* 75:711–715, 2014.

41. Sanchez Migallon-Guzman D, Houck E, Beaufrere H, et al: Evaluation of the thermal antinociceptive effects of buprenorphine hydrochloride in cockatiels (*Nymphicus hollandicus*). In *Proceedings of the Association of American Association of Zoo Veterinarians*, 2014.

42. Scott LJ, Perry CM: Tramadol: a review of its use in perioperative pain. *Drugs* 60:139–176, 2000.

43. Kilburn JJ, Cox SK, Kottyan J, et al: Pharmacokinetics of tramadol and its primary metabolite O-desmethyltramadol in African penguins (*Spheniscus demersus*), *J Zoo Wildl Med* 45:93–99, 2014.

44. Souza MJ, Sanchez-Migallon Guzman D, Paul-Murphy JR, et al: Pharmacokinetics after oral and intravenous administration of a single dose of tramadol hydrochloride to Hispaniolan Amazon parrots (*Amazona ventralis*), *Am J Vet Res* 73:1142–1147, 2012.

45. Souza MJ, Martin-Jimenez T, Jones MP, et al: Pharmacokinetics of oral tramadol in red-tailed hawks (*Buteo jamaicensis*), *J Vet Pharmacol Ther* 34:86–88, 2011.

46. Black PA, Cox SK, Macek M, et al: Pharmacokinetics of tramadol hydrochloride and its metabolite O-desmethyltramadol in peafowl (*Pavo cristatus*), *J Zoo Wildl Med* 41:671–676, 2010.

47. Souza MJ, Martin-Jimenez T, Jones MP, et al: Pharmacokinetics of intravenous and oral tramadol in the bald eagle (*Haliaeetus leucocephalus*), *J Avian Med Surg* 23:247–252, 2009.

48. Sanchez-Migallon Guzman D, Souza MJ, Braun JM, et al: Antinociceptive effects after oral administration of tramadol hydrochloride in Hispaniolan Amazon parrots (*Amazona ventralis*), *Am J Vet Res* 73:1148–1152, 2012.

49. Guzman DS, Drazenovich TL, Olsen GH, et al: Evaluation of thermal antinociceptive effects after oral administration of tramadol hydrochloride to American kestrels (*Falco sparverius*), *Am J Vet Res* 75:117–123, 2014.

50. Papich MG: An update on nonsteroidal anti-inflammatory drugs (NSAIDs) in small animals, *Vet Clin North Am Small Anim Pract* 38:1243–1266, vi, 2008.

51. Bergh MS, Budsberg SC: The coxib NSAIDs: potential clinical and pharmacologic importance in veterinary medicine, *J Vet Intern Med* 19:633–643, 2005.

52. Mathonnet M, Lalloue F, Danty E, et al: Cyclo-oxygenase 2 tissue distribution and developmental pattern of expression in the chicken, *Clin Exp Pharmacol Physiol* 28:425–432, 2001.

53. Dajani EZ, Islam K: Cardiovascular and gastrointestinal toxicity of selective cyclo-oxygenase-2 inhibitors in man, *J Physiol Pharmacol* 59(Suppl 2):117 133, 2008.

54. Gerstenfeld LC, Thiede M, Seibert K, et al: Differential inhibition of fracture healing by non-selective and cyclooxygenase-2 selective non-steroidal anti-inflammatory drugs, *J Orthop Res* 21:670–675, 2003.

55. Baert K, De Backer P: Comparative pharmacokinetics of three non-steroidal anti-inflammatory drugs in five bird species, *Comp Biochem Physiol Part C Toxicol Pharmacol* 134:25–33, 2003.

56. Naidoo V, Wolter K, Cromarty AD, et al: The pharmacokinetics of meloxicam in vultures, *J Vet Pharmacol Ther* 31:128–134, 2008.

57. Wilson G, Hernandez-Divers S, Budsberg S, et al: Pharmacokinetics and use of meloxican in psittacine birds. In *Proceedings of the Association of Avian Veterinarians*, 2004, pp 7–9.

58. Molter CM, Court MH, Cole GA, et al: Pharmacokinetics of meloxicam after intravenous, intramuscular, and oral administration of a single dose to Hispaniolan Amazon parrots (*Amazona ventralis*), *Am J Vet Res* 74:375–380, 2013.

59. Montesinos A, Ardiaca M, Diez-Delgado I, et al: Pharmacokinetics of parenteral and oral meloxicam in African grey parrots (*Psittacus erithacus erithacus*). In *Proceedings of the European Association of Avian Veterinarians Conference*, 2011, pp 129–134.

60. Lacasse C, Gamble KC, Boothe DM: Pharmacokinetics of a single dose of intravenous and oral meloxicam in red-tailed hawks (*Buteo jamaicensis*) and great horned owls (*Bubo virginianus*), *J Avian Med Surg* 27:204–210, 2013.

61. Cole GA, Paul-Murphy J, Krugner-Higby L, et al: Analgesic effects of intramuscular administration of meloxicam in Hispaniolan parrots (*Amazona ventralis*) with experimentally induced arthritis, *Am J Vet Res* 70:1471–1476, 2009.

62. Desmarchelier M, Troncy E, Fitzgerald G, et al: Analgesic effects of meloxicam administration on postoperative orthopedic pain in domestic pigeons (*Columba livia*), *Am J Vet Res* 73:361–367, 2012.

63. Pereira M, Werther K: Evaluation of the renal effects of flunixin meglumine, ketoprofen and meloxicam in budgerigars (*Melopsittacus undulatus*), *Vet Rec* 160:844–846, 2007.

64. Montesinos A, Ardiaca M, Juan-Selles C, et al: Evaluation of the renal effects of meloxicam in African grey parrots (*Psittacus erithacus erithacus*). In *Proceedings of the European Association of Avian Veterinarians Conference*, 2009, pp 171–176.

65. Sinclair KM, Church ME, Farver TB, et al: Effects of meloxicam on hematologic and plasma biochemical analysis variables and results of histologic examination of tissue specimens of Japanese quail (*Coturnix japonica*), *Am J Vet Res* 73:1720–727, 2012.

66. Cuthbert R, Parry-Jones J, Green RE, et al: NSAIDs and scavenging birds: potential impacts beyond Asia's critically endangered vultures, *Biol Lett* 3:90–93, 2007.

67. Oaks JL, Gilbert M, Virani MZ, et al: Diclofenac residues as the cause of vulture population decline in Pakistan, *Nature* 427:630–633, 2004.

68. Naidoo V, Wolter K, Cromarty D, et al: Toxicity of non-steroidal anti-inflammatory drugs to Gyps vultures: a new threat from ketoprofen, *Biol Lett* 6:339–341, 2010.

69. Swarup D, Patra RC, Prakash V, et al: Safety of meloxicam to critically endangered Gyps vultures and other scavenging birds in India, *Anim Conserv* 10:192–198, 2007.

70. Lees P, Landoni MF: Pharmacodynamics and enantioselective pharmacokinetics of racemic carprofen in the horse, *J Vet Pharmacol Ther* 25:433–448, 2002.

71. McGeowen D, Danbury TC, Waterman-Pearson AE, et al: Effect of carprofen on lameness in broiler chickens, *Vet Rec* 144:668–671, 1999.

72. Hocking PM, Robertson GW, Gentle MJ: Effects of non-steroidal anti-inflammatory drugs on pain-related behaviour in a model of articular pain in the domestic fowl, *Res Vet Sci* 78:69–75, 2005.

73. Graham JE, Kollias-Baker C, Craigmill AL, et al: Pharmacokinetics of ketoprofen in Japanese quail (*Coturnix japonica*), *J Vet Pharmacol Ther* 28:399–402, 2005.

74. Machin KL, Tellier LA, Lair S, et al: Pharmacodynamics of flunixin and ketoprofen in mallard ducks (*Anas platyrhynchos*), *J Zoo Wildl Med* 32:222–229, 2001.

75. Mulcahy DM, Tuomi P, Larsen RS: Differential mortality of male spectacled eiders (*Somateria fischeri*) and king eiders (*Somateria spectabilis*) subsequent to anesthesia with propofol, bupivacaine, and ketoprofen, *J Avian Med Surg* 17:117–123, 2013.

75a. Musser JM, Heatley JJ, Phalen DN: Pharmacokinetics after intravenous administration of flunixin meglumine in budgerigars (*Melopsittacus undulatus*) and Patagonian conures (*Cyanoliseus patagonus*), *J Am Vet Med Assoc* 242:205–208, 2013.

76. Klein PN, Charmatz K, Langenberg J: The effect of flunixin meglumine (banamine) on the renal function of northern bobwhite quail (*Colinus virginianus*): an avian model. In *Proceedings of the American Association of Zoo Veterinarians*, 1994, pp 128–131.

77. Hanley CS, Thomas NJ, Paul-Murphy J, et al: Exertional myopathy in whooping cranes (*Grus americana*) with prognostic guidelines, *J Zoo Wildl Med* 36:489–497, 2005.

78. Keiper NL, Hartup BK: Pharmacokinetics of piroxicam in brolgas. In *Proceedings of the Annual Conference of the Association of Avian Veterinarians*, 2014, p 291.

79. Naidoo V, Swan GE: Diclofenac toxicity in Gyps vulture is associated with decreased uric acid excretion and not renal portal vasoconstriction, *Comp Biochem Physiol Part C Toxicol Pharmacol*, 149:269–274, 2009.

80. Meteyer CU, Rideout BA, Gilbert M, et al: Pathology and proposed pathophysiology of diclofenac poisoning in free-living and experimentally exposed oriental white-backed vultures (*Gyps bengalensis*), *J Wildl Dis* 41:707–716, 2005.

81. Swan GE, Cuthbert R, Quevedo M, et al: Toxicity of diclofenac to Gyps vultures, *Biol Lett* 2:279–282, 2006.

82. Brandão J, da Cunha AF, Pypendop B, et al: Cardiovascular tolerance of intravenous lidocaine in broiler chickens (*Gallus gallus domesticus*) anesthetized with isoflurane, *Vet Anaesth Analg* 42:442–448, 2014.

83. Brenner DJ, Larsen RS, Dickinson PJ, et al: Development of an avian brachial plexus nerve block technique for perioperative analgesia in mallard ducks (*Anas platyrhynchos*), *J Avian Med Surg* 24:24–34, 2010.

84. Da Cunha AF, Messenger KM, Stout RW, et al: Pharmacokinetics of lidocaine and its active metabolite monoethylglycinexylidide after a single intravenous administration in chickens (*Gallus domesticus*) anesthetized with isoflurane, *J Vet Pharmacol Ther* 35:604–607, 2012.

85. Machin KL, Livingston A: Plasma bupivacaine levels in mallard ducks (*Anas platyrhynchos*) following a single subcutaneous dose. In *Proceedings of the American Association of Zoo Veterinarians*, 2001, pp 159–163.

86. Hocking PM, Gentle MJ, Bernard R, et al: Evaluation of a protocol for determining the effectiveness of pretreatment with local analgesics for reducing experimentally induced articular pain in domestic fowl, *Res Vet Sci* 63:263–267, 1997.

87. Glatz PC, Murphy LB, Preston AP: Analgesic therapy of beak-trimmed chickens, *Aust Vet J* 69:18, 1992.

88. Brenner DJ, Larsen RS, Dickinson PJ, et al: Development of an avian brachial plexus nerve block technique for perioperative analgesia in mallard ducks (*Anas platyrhynchos*), *J Avian Med Surg* 24:24–34, 2010.

89. Figueiredo JP, Cruz ML, Mendes GM, et al: Assessment of brachial plexus blockade in chickens by an axillary approach, *Vet Anaesth Analg* 35:511–518, 2008.

90. da Cunha AF, Strain GM, Rademacher N, et al: Palpation- and ultrasound-guided brachial plexus blockade in Hispaniolan Amazon parrots (*Amazona ventralis*), *Vet Anaesth Analg* 40:96–102, 2013.

91. d'Ovidio D, Noviello E, Adami C: Nerve stimulator-guided sciatic-femoral nerve block in raptors undergoing surgical treatment of pododermatitis, *Vet Anaesth Analg* 42:449–453, 2014.

92. Shaver SL, Robinson NG, Wright BD, et al: A multimodal approach to management of suspected neuropathic pain in a prairie falcon (*Falco mexicanus*), *J Avian Med Surg* 23:209–213, 2009.

93. Doneley B: The use of gabapentin to treat presumed neuralgia in a little corella (*Cacatua sanguinea*). In *Proceedings of Australian Association of Avian Veterinarians*, 2007, pp 169–172.

94. Baine K, Jones M, Cox S, et al: Pharmacokinetics of gabapentin in Hispaniolan Amazon parrots (*Amazona ventralis*). In *Proceedings of the Annual Conference of the Association of Avian Veterinarians*, 2013, pp 19–20.

95. Heinze CR, Hawkins MG, Gillies LA, et al: Effect of dietary omega-3 fatty acids on red blood cell lipid composition and plasma

metabolites in the cockatiel, *Nymphicus hollandicus*, *J Anim Sci* 90:3068–3079, 2012.

96. Anderson K, Garner MM, Reed HH, et al: Hemorrhagic diathesis in avian species following intramuscular administration of polysulfated glycosaminoglycan, *J Zoo Wildl Med* 44:93–99, 2013.

97. Mathews K, Kronen PW, Lascelles D, et al: Guidelines for recognition, assessment and treatment of pain: WSAVA Global Pain Council members and co-authors of this document, *J Small Anim Pract* 55:E10–E68, 2014.

98. Dworkin RH, O'Connor AB, Backonja M, et al: Pharmacologic management of neuropathic pain: evidence-based recommendations, *Pain* 132:237–251, 2007.

99. Pavez JC, Hawkins MG, Pascoe PJ, et al: Effect of fentanyl target-controlled infusions on isoflurane minimum anaesthetic concentration and cardiovascular function in red-tailed hawks (*Buteo jamaicensis*), *Vet Anaesth Analg* 38:344–351, 2011.

100. Guzman DS-M, Drazenovich T, KuKanich B, et al: Evaluation of the thermal antinociceptive effects and pharmacokinetics after intramuscular administration of butorphanol tartrate to American kestrels (*Falco sparverius*), *Am J Vet Res* 75:11–18, 2013.

101. Escobar A, Valadao CA, Brosnan RJ, et al: Effects of butorphanol on the minimum anesthetic concentration for sevoflurane in guineafowl (*Numida meleagris*), *Am J Vet Res* 73:183–188, 2012.

102. Singh PM, Johnson C, Gartrell B, et al: Pharmacokinetics of butorphanol in broiler chickens, *Vet Rec* 168:588, 2011.

103. Curro T, Brunson D, Paul-Murphy J: Determination of the ED50 of isoflurane and evaluation of the analgesic properties of butorphanol in cockatoos (*Cacatua* spp.), *Vet Surg* 23:429–433, 1994.

104. Souza MJ, Gerhardt L, Cox S: Pharmacokinetics of repeated oral administration of tramadol hydrochloride in Hispaniolan Amazon parrots (*Amazona ventralis*), *Am J Vet Res* 74:957–962, 2013.

105. Machin KL, Livingston A: Assessment of the analgesic effects of ketoprofen in ducks anesthetized with isoflurane, *Am J Vet Res* 63:821–826, 2002.

106. Machin KL, Tellier LA, Lair S, et al: Pharmacodynamics of flunixin and ketoprofen in mallard ducks (*Anas platyrhynchos*), *J Zoo Wildl Med* 32:222–229, 2001.

CHAPTER 21

Surgery

Jacob A. Rubin • Jeffrey J. Runge • Michael Mison • Steve Mehler • Michael Scott Echols • Nathaniel K.Y. Lam • Brian L. Speer • R. Avery Bennett • Julia B. Ponder • Patrick Redig

PRINCIPLES OF MICROSURGERY

Jacob A. Rubin, Jeffrey J. Runge

HISTORY

Over the last 25 years, there has been tremendous advancement in the development of both instrumentation and surgical materials within veterinary surgery as would be applied in avian species.[1-3] These developments have improved the precision with which surgery is performed. These advances have enabled clinicians to perform operations in birds that were once considered extremely difficult or nearly impossible. A turning point in modern-day microsurgery was the introduction and widespread adoption of high-power magnification through either the operating microscope or surgical loupes. Today these modalities are routinely used in both human and veterinary surgery alike.

Microsurgery is commonly defined as a surgical technique utilizing fine-tipped instruments to perform delicate operations with the help of optical magnification.[4] Microsurgical techniques are considered mainstream for human medical applications including plastic, transplantation, orthopedic, neurologic, and cardiothoracic surgery and have been around for the last half-century.[5-7,8a,9-12] While initial experimental studies utilized animal models for training purposes,[13,14] it is only over the last 20 years that microsurgical techniques have translated into mainstream veterinary surgery.[4,15-17] While most commonly used in small-animal medicine, the size of the patient and critical nature of many of the procedures make microsurgery and the use of the operating microscope or surgical loupes natural adjuncts for avian surgery.

OVERVIEW OF MICROSURGICAL TECHNIQUES

To accomplish some of the microsurgical procedures, one must become familiar with the technical knowledge and instrumentation and develop some expertise in the area. While most procedures used in macroscopic surgery can be adapted to microsurgical practice, a few key changes must be made to achieve excellence in microsurgery. Although in a macroscopic (normal, unmagnified) surgery some surgeons may exhibit little to no grossly applicable tremors associated with their hand movements, once the field is magnified, all hand movements are exaggerated tremendously, and an inherent hand tremor is present in all surgeons. To minimize hand tremors, a few basic concepts should be followed. There will be an inherent amount of stress and frustration when starting the learning curve of microsurgery. Minimizing controllable external factors will allow for more rapid skill acquisition. Surgeons should strive to get a full eight hours of sleep before commencing any microsurgical procedure, especially in their early training. Studies have shown that a lack of sleep will increase the inherent tremors of the novice microsurgeon.[18] Many other factors, including strenuous physical exercise, irritation or anxiety, and nicotine, caffeine, and other drugs, have all been shown to increase one's baseline tremors.[19] Although caffeine has been shown to increase one's inherent physiologic tremors, those individuals who are habitual in their caffeine intake will likely suffer from withdrawal if acutely stopped. The effects from caffeine withdrawal include headaches, muscle aches, and agitation and will likely make the tremors and the microsurgical experience worse.[20] As such, the authors recommend limiting caffeine intake to the minimal possible level to limit tremors and the negative aspects of withdrawal.

DIFFERENCES FROM MACROSCOPIC SURGERY

As previously discussed, there are some fundamental differences between microscopic and macroscopic (traditional open, nonmagnified) surgery. Although tremors are inherent in both techniques, the magnification of the microscope makes the tremors more apparent. The smallest width of some of the tissues being sutured and dissected is approximately 10 to 20 μm, which is considered extremely delicate.[21] As such, slow, deliberate motions are necessary. The goal of any procedure is to eliminate any wasted motions and to minimize the trauma to the tissue. Another striking difference observed between microsurgery and macrosurgery is that operative time differs dramatically, with microsurgery often requiring longer procedure times. Most anesthetized patients require the surgeon to perform a procedure with both operative time and overall anesthesia time at a minimum; it should be noted, however, that the surgical pace involved with utilizing magnification is slower than without magnification. One should plan accordingly when preparing the anesthetic protocol.[22,23]

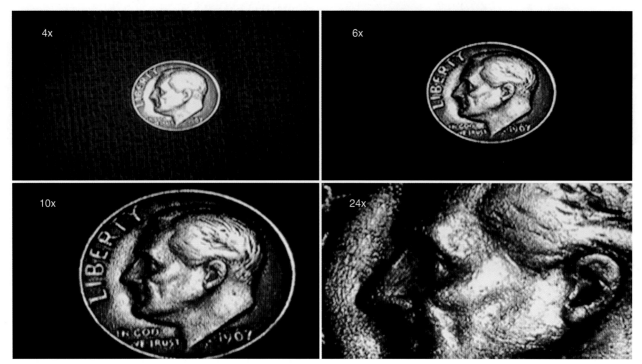

FIGURE 21-1 A dime imaged under an operating microscope. Note the difference in clarity and the loss of peripheral vision with increasing magnification.

The use of magnification (Figure 21-1), while greatly adding to the visualization of the direct surgical field, will limit the ability of the wearer to visualize the peripheral field. This makes an assistant necessary when utilizing the operating microscope and helpful when utilizing magnifying loupes. The assistant will help minimize the need to turn away from the surgical field to reach additional instruments and will limit unnecessary movement of the hands. This will be discussed in more detail later in this chapter.

INSTRUMENTATION AND SUTURE MATERIAL

To transition from a macroscopic area to a microscopic one, specifically designed equipment and instruments are required. Broadly speaking, these tools can be divided into three categories:
1. Fine operating instruments
2. Fine suturing material
3. Operative magnifying capabilities, including either loupes or an operative microscope

Standard surgical instruments and suture used under magnification can be difficult to work with, as they will appear very large and will likely traumatize the fine tissues. It is the opinion of this section's authors that these instruments are unsuitable for microsurgical procedures.

Instrumentation

The instruments required for most microsurgical techniques are microneedle driver, jeweler's forceps, and microscissors. Instruments intended for microsurgery are designed for minimal movement with the use of spring-loaded jaws, which allow these instruments to be used without changing hand

position. In addition to these basic instruments, a microsurgical irrigation device is also recommended.

Needle holder

Microsurgical needle holders should have a fine tip that meets along its entire surface when the instrument platform is closed (Figure 21-2). The apposition can be confirmed by

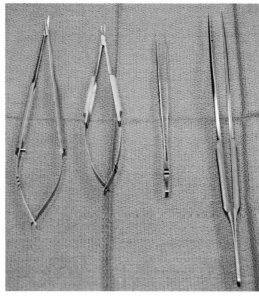

FIGURE 21-2 This figure shows each of the following from left to right: adventitia scissors, Barraquer microneedle holder, jeweler's Pierse forceps, and Spetzler neurovascular forceps.

closing the instrument gently under direct observation with magnification at the closing space between the jaws. There should be no gap between the jaws along the entire closed platform surface. Needle holders come with either straight or curved jaws, and use of each is operator preference dependent. Unlike macrosurgical instruments, they should not have any locking capabilities, as the action of locking and unlocking will transmit unwanted movements to the instrument tip. Ideally the microneedle holder will rest in the web space between the thumb and the index finger. As such the handles should be rounded for easier rotation in the fingertips. For microsurgical repairs in which the needle diameter is 100 μm or smaller, jeweler's forceps can be substituted for needle holders, as they have finer tips, but caution must be taken due to the delicate nature of the tips.[24,25]

Jeweler's forceps

One of the primary instruments among a surgeon's microsurgical armament is the jeweler's forceps. This instrument is manufactured in a variety of sizes and materials. Most are manufactured straight along their entire length, although variations have been developed that include angled and curved tips. The numbering system for jeweler's forceps indicates tip size and overall design.[24] The numbers for straight forceps range from 2 to 5, with the No. 2 designated as the coarsest tip and No. 5 the finest tip. The No. 3 straight forceps are the most commonly used forceps in microvascular surgery. All jeweler's forceps have a closing tension that tends to vary with the instrument type, manufacturer, instrument length, and history of use.[26] The tension for closing should allow the instrument to be held easily without falling from the grasp while the tips are still open at least 1 to 2 mm. On the other extreme, the force required to close the tips should be gentle enough so that hand fatigue does not develop, resulting in increased tremor. The tips of the forceps should be accurately aligned with minimal discrepancies on the sides or at the extreme tip. This instrument has by far the greatest versatility, as it can be used to perform blunt dissection and retraction. It is also a critical component of suturing and knot placement. Modifications of the jeweler's forceps include specialized tips of these thumb forceps, including ring tips, platform tips, and toothed forceps (Figure 21-3). Each of these is unique and allows for delicate dissection of avian tissues, with the ring tip allowing for a slightly more evenly distributed pressure on tissue. Additionally, the rounded tips are not likely to cause the puncture damage that jeweler's forceps can. The toothed forceps should be reserved for slightly tougher tissue, and neurovascular bundles should be avoided when utilizing these forceps.

Adventitia and suture scissors

Within veterinary surgery the two most useful types of microscissors are dissection and adventitia scissors, both of which are spring-handled with relatively short cutting tips. Dissection microscissors usually have curved blades and rounded tips. The curved blade allows dissectional approaches without awkward hand positioning, while the blunt tips permit fine dissection with a reduced risk of puncture damage. These are the microsurgical equivalent of Metzenbaum scissors. Adventitia scissors are used in microvascular surgery for trimming the adventitia from the end of the vessels to better appose the ends to prevent thrombus formation. A separate set of suture scissors, usually an older dedicated pair of dissection microscissors, should be used to prevent dulling of the blades of the primary microscissors used for tissue dissection.

Irrigation device

Irrigation of the field is necessary to prevent tissues from desiccating and sticking to the instruments. There are many commercially available irrigation tips that can be used. The authors prefer the use of a 3-cc syringe fitted with a 25-gauge needle that is bent at an approximately 45-degree angle. Alternatively, an ophthalmic bulb syringe with a nasolacrimal duct cannula works well for tissue irrigation during microsurgery.

Bipolar cautery

A bipolar coagulator is an important addition to any microsurgery setting. Good bipolar forceps have fine, undamaged tips similar in size to the jeweler's forceps with a variable control for the current setting.

Suture material choices

The appropriate selection of suture material for the procedure is a function of many factors, including (1) the anatomic features of the tissue, (2) the tensile strength of the tissue, (3) the duration that the suture needs to remain in place for tissue healing, and (4) the type of suture pattern that is to be used. The ideal suture for microsurgery should have excellent knot-holding capabilities and ease of handling, and should stimulate minimal inflammatory reaction (Figure 21-4). The suture material commonly used in microvascular surgery

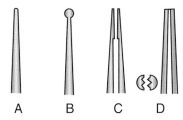

FIGURE 21-3 Microsurgical thumb forceps' tips. **A,** Smooth. **B,** Ring. **C,** Platform. **D,** 1 × 2 Toothed.

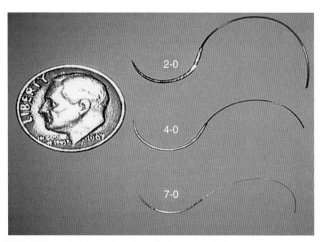

FIGURE 21-4 Note the size difference of Prolene suture materials compared with a representative dime.

ranges in size from 6-0 to 11-0, depending on the tissue being sutured. The diameters of 8-0, 9-0, 10-0, and 11-0 sutures range from 40 to 49, 30 to 39, 20 to 29, and 10 to 19 µM, respectively.[24]

The needle should likely be a taper needle to minimize trauma. Monofilament suture such as nylon or polypropylene is generally preferred in microsurgery because of its greater strength and durability and its decreased tissue reactivity, although braided multifilament sutures have excellent knot-holding capabilities. If using a braided multifilament, one can pass the suture through bone wax to minimize drag as it passes through the tissues. The use of absorbable monofilament material smaller than 6-0 is limited in veterinary medicine due to the difficulty of handling and the lack of commercially available materials in very small sizes. The most popular needles are curved with diameters of 70 to 140 µm.[15] There are two styles of tips for the microsurgical needles that are currently on the market: a standard tip that has a taper end, and the micro-edge taper (M.E.T., Angiotech, Vancouver, British Columbia, Canada) needle, which has a three-faced, pyramidal cutting tip that passes through the tissue planes with more ease.

Magnification

There are certainly limits to the unaided human eye in surgery. Although clinicians have routinely strived for close apposition of structures, the resolving power of the unaided human eye is only approximately 0.2 mm.[8a] Most surgeons who view two points closer than 0.2 mm will see only one point. Optical aids (e.g., loupes, operating microscopes, surgical headlamps, and fiber-optic handpiece lights) can improve resolution by many orders of magnitude. For example, a common operating microscope can raise the resolving limit from 0.2 to 0.006 mm (6 µm), which is a dramatic improvement compared with other magnification devices. The key to microsurgery is using the appropriate magnification for the specific operative technique. The primary goal of magnification is to improve the detail of the affected tissue to execute the most accurate operative procedure. Magnifying loupes were developed to address the problem of proximity, decreased depth of field, and eyestrain occasioned by moving closer to the subject.

Loupes are classified by the optical method by which they produce magnification. There are three types of binocular magnifying loupes: (1) a diopter, flat-plane, single-lens loupe, (2) a surgical telescope with a Galilean system configuration (two-lens system), and (3) a surgical telescope with a Keplerian system configuration (prism roof design that folds the path of light) (Figure 21-5).

The diopter system (see Figure 21-5, *A*) relies on a simple magnifying lens, and the degree of magnification is measured in diopters. One diopter (D) means that a ray of light that would be focused at infinity would now be focused at 1 meter. A lens with 2-D designation would focus light at 50 cm. The only advantage of the single-lens system is that it is relatively inexpensive, but it is less desirable because the plastic lenses that it uses are not always optically correct, and one must continuously move one's head to maintain the operating field in focus. Given these limitations, single-lens systems have limited use in the operating room but can be useful in examining patients in a nonsterile setting. The surgical telescope of either the Galilean or the Keplerian design produces an enlarged viewing image with a multiple-lens system (see Figure 21-5, *B* and *C*). The Galilean system provides a magnification range from 2× to 4.5× and is a small, light, and compact system. The prism loupes (Keplerian system) use refractive prisms and are actually telescopes with complicated light paths that provide magnifications up to 8×. Both systems produce superior magnification, correct spherical and chromatic aberrations, and have an excellent depth of field, thereby reducing eyestrain and head and neck fatigue.[15,16] These loupes offer significant advantages over simple magnification eyeglasses. The disadvantage of loupes is that the practical maximum magnification is only about 4.5×. Loupes with higher magnification are available, but they are heavy and unwieldy with a limited field of view. Such loupes require a constrained physical posture and cannot be worn for long periods of time without producing significant head, neck, and back strain.

In addition to magnification, the use of a surgical headlamp is often necessary to improve the overall visualization. Headlamps can be incorporated into the loupes themselves or used as stand-alone devices. The operating microscope (Figure 21-6) is the most robust form of magnification. It is often a costly investment, but it can usually be shared and utilized in cases from other specialties (surgery, ophthalmology, neurology). The operating microscope should provide a binocular, stereoscopic

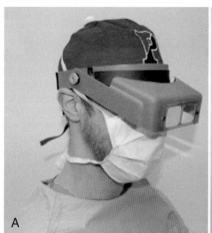 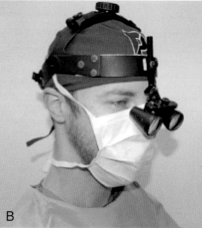 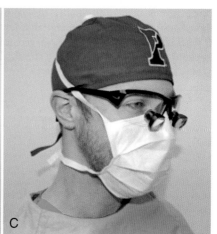

FIGURE 21-5 Three different surgical loupes. **A,** Diopter lenses. **B,** Over-the-head Galilean-style loupes. **C,** Through-the-lens Galilean-style loupes.

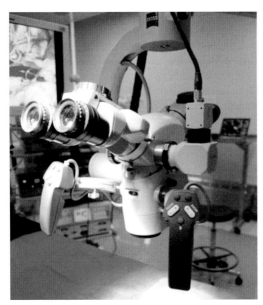

FIGURE 21-6 Operating microscope.

view of the surgical field at magnifications ranging from 8× to 25× (see Figure 21-1). Most systems will actually provide a wider range than this with the use of interchangeable lenses. While some operating microscopes have a single head, the ideal microscope has a dual head that allows an assistant to view the surgical field and assist with the operative techniques. (Figure 21-7) The optics of each head should converge, so that the same field of view is observed by each surgeon.[5,6,8b,24]

Most microscopes come on portable floor stands or table-mounted stands with the latter used primarily for research laboratories. There are two main features for intraoperative control of any operating microscope: the focus control and the magnification controls. These are controlled by either foot pedals or hand controls. The focus should have a smooth, nondrifting control, while the magnification can either be continuous or a turret magnification changer. Some microscopes also allow for *X*- and *Y*-coordinate changes with a built-in joystick mechanism on the foot pedal, although this is not necessary for the entry-level microsurgeon. Along with

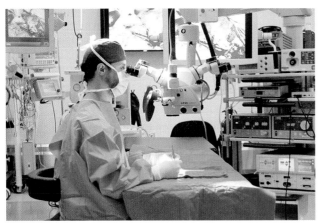

FIGURE 21-7 Note the operator's posture with an upright seated position, straight back, and forearms resting on the operative surface. This will help to minimize back strain and subsequent fatigue.

moving the microscope head in three dimensions, there should also be a means to rotate and tilt the microscope head for repositioning the optical path and visualization of different structures.

Some of the advantages of the microscope are the increased levels of magnification, the ability to change magnification levels, and the optics resulting in great visualization. Also, after one has gained experience with the microscope, the comfort level when using the scope will put less strain on the neck and back during longer procedures as compared with optical loupes.

The primary disadvantage of an operating microscope is associated with the cost. While a brand-new, state-of-the-art operating microscope can cost upward of $100k, many used older systems can be purchased for use in veterinary medicine by contacting human hospitals that are currently upgrading to newer systems. In addition, some older basic systems such as the Vasconcellos may be an option for a starting microsurgeon (see Figure 21-7). When purchasing an operating microscope for veterinary use, one should strive to find one that can be used in conjunction with other specialties to help defray some of the initial startup costs.[27]

Basic Microsuturing Techniques

Posture

Before starting a procedure with magnification, the surgeon must be ergonomically comfortable to achieve success. For the most part, surgical procedures should be performed in a sitting position to facilitate a fixed working distance and to minimize eyestrain (see Figure 21-7). There are two commonly used sitting postures in microsurgery. The first is a relaxed posture, resting against the backrest of the chair with virtually no weight placed on the feet. The other posture is created by shifting forward on the seat, not using the backrest, keeping a very straight back and neck, and placing even weight distribution on both feet. This is the authors' preferred position.

The position of one's hands is the next crucial step to be a successful microsurgeon. One should rest both arms comfortably on the workbench/operating table without supporting one's body weight on the arms (see Figure 21-7). This will both reduce the inherent tremors of the forearms, as well as reduce strain on the upper back and shoulders. Unlike macroscopic surgery, where instruments are grasped in a variety of positions, microsurgical instruments are always grasped in a normal "writing" grip similar to how one grasps a pencil (Figure 21-8). The thumb, index finger, and ring finger should grasp the instruments approximately 3 cm from the tip, with the butt end of the instrument positioned over the web of the thumb and index finger for support.[25]

The main goal of these initial steps is to maintain a comfortable position, yet to minimize unwanted and unnecessary motions, particularly of the upper arm and wrist. The instruments are controlled with the thumb and index fingers and with primarily only the fingertips in very slight motion. With round-handled instruments, most importantly the needle holder, the instrument is rolled between the thumb and index finger to manipulate the tip—for example, to pass a curved needle through the tissue. Once one becomes comfortable with the basics of handling the instruments, variations in hand position can be developed.

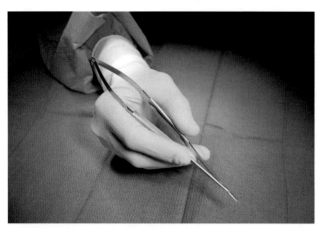

FIGURE 21-8 The needle holder is grasped in a "pencil grip" with the butt end of the instrument supported with the web of the thumb and index finger.

Focusing the microscope

For most microsurgical procedures in birds, high magnification is not necessary. However, when discrete structures must be visualized, higher magnification is very important. At higher magnifications, however, it is paramount that the surgeon be accustomed to compensating for the narrow depth of field, a limiting factor at high magnifications, by making frequent fine-focus adjustments. Once a surgeon is in a comfortable posture and has the patient situated, focusing the microscope on the area of interest is important. Most modern operating microscopes are equipped with parfocal lenses, which will keep the focus approximately the same when changing magnification. For optimal visualization, focusing the image under highest magnification first will lead to the best results. Unfortunately, the use of the microscope will limit the movement of the patient. Any movement of the operating field, such as when the patient's location is changed or the surgeon is operating at a different depth, will cause loss of focus. To limit the effects of this, it is often recommended that one magnify only to the level that is needed for the current technique, minimizing overmagnification.

Needle handling

The most appropriate region to grasp a microsurgical needle is midway down the needle shaft (approximately in the middle). Since micropoint needles are extremely delicate, they can be easily bent if grasped too close to the swage. Grasping the needle too close to the tip can both dull the tip and limit the depth of tissue penetration. Because of its small size, suture used in microsurgery can easily be damaged if grasped forcefully with needle holders. To prevent suture damage, the suture should first be grasped with jeweler's forceps. Because the tips are easily damaged, jeweler's forceps should not be used routinely to grasp needles; instead, the suture is grasped 5 to 10 mm from the swage of the needle. With a dangling type of maneuver, the needle can be adequately immobilized by the surrounding tissue while it is grasped in the correct position with the needle holder.

Needle driving

The accurate placement of a microsurgical needle requires that the tissue be firmly stabilized while the needle is passed. This requires that the tissue be firmly grasped with forceps adjacent to the intended point of needle insertion. As the near margin is stabilized with forceps, the needle is positioned nearly perpendicular and inserted. As the needle reaches the desired tissue depth, the needle holder is rolled between the thumb and index fingertips. The needle should come out completely between the two sides of the tissue being sutured. The far tissue is then grasped identically, and the tip of the needle is positioned parallel at a depth corresponding to the first bite. When the needle has just penetrated the deep tissue, the needle holder is again rolled, causing the needle to exit the surface. The needle is then grasped, and the arc of the needle is continued out of the tissue. It is imperative that the needle be rolled through the tissue, as the arc of the needle can be easily damaged, causing increased trauma to the tissue. With experience, the microsurgeon develops the skills to preferentially use the forceps for counterpressure, as opposed to grasping the tissue directly. With this method, the open forceps are inserted into the tissue gap; then the needle is pushed through the tissue, exiting between the open tips of the forceps.

Knot tying

There appears to be little consensus on the most ideal method to tie microsurgical suture. In general, because the holding power of the knot depends on the friction between suture strands, smooth suture materials are considered to require more throws than braided suture material.[28] Nonetheless, in one study the standard three-throw square knot was found to provide optimal results for all suture materials.[28] Surgeon's knots also are commonly used to increase the security of the tension on the first throw.[25] When using surgeon's knots, however, remember that the addition of the second throw may result in increased tightness of the suture loop, particularly if stiff monofilament is used. Deliberately leaving the first throw loose accommodates this effect. The technique for knot tying will vary with individual preference and the particular team approach used in microsurgery at any given institution. A single technique described in this text is the preferred method of the authors (Figure 21-9). This common technique uses the same pattern of throwing suture as is done in macroscopic surgery: The jeweler's forceps are held in the surgeon's nondominant hand while the needle holder is placed in the surgeon's dominant hand. The jeweler's forceps then grasp the needle end of the suture and wrap it upon the needle holders for all throws of knot formation. The jeweler's forceps initially grasp the suture in an overhand technique. The needle holders are placed between the jeweler's forceps and the free end of the suture material. Once the surgeon is comfortable, he makes a lazy horseshoe with the needle end of the suture over the needle holder. With the needle holder tips closed, the forceps tips are moved around the needle holder tip to create the loops of the first throw. This is easiest if the circles are kept small and the tips of the instruments are kept in close proximity. If performing a surgeon's throw, this initial step is repeated to get two loops on the first throw. The tips of the needle holders are then opened slowly so that the short end of the suture may be grasped. Finally, the instruments are moved apart so that the knot can be cinched down. The second throw must be done in the opposite direction to the first throw to create a square knot rather than a granny knot. Additional throws can be completed at the discretion of the primary surgeon. Once the knot is complete, the ends of the suture are cut short.

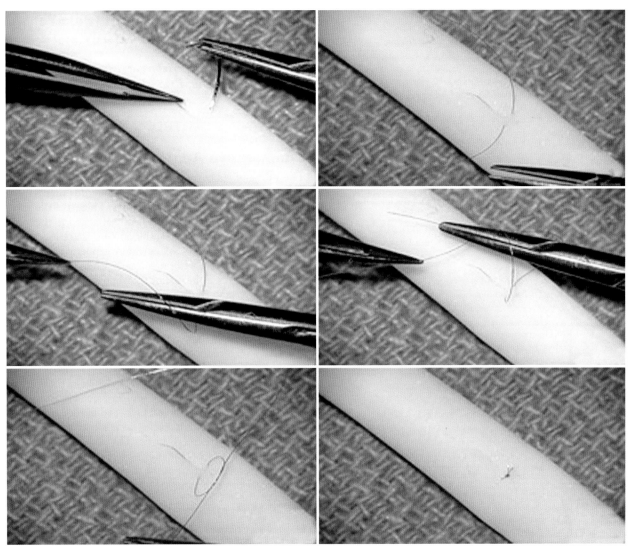

FIGURE 21-9 Knot tying in microsurgery.

ASSISTING IN MICROSURGERY

While not essential, having an assistant who is comfortable with the microsurgical instrumentation, the surgical table, and magnification can help to expedite the surgery as well as the learning process. If the individuals are using surgical loupes, it may be necessary for the assistant to pass instruments and to guide the primary surgeon's instruments into the surgical field because the surgeon's peripheral vision is limited. If surgeries are taking place under the operating microscope, the previous statement holds true, but also the assistant may play a more intricate role within the surgery itself. This may involve cutting suture, retracting tissue, and running the instrument table. Typically an assistant will utilize the microscope at the same time as the primary surgeon and, as such, the microscope should be fitted with dual heads. The preferred microscope in veterinary surgery would have a binocular view of the surgical field and coaxial with the optical path of the primary viewer, although other configurations exist. For the assistant's view to be coaxial, it is necessary for the assistant to share the same image as the surgeon, which requires a beam splitter to split the light in the primary optical pathway into both the surgeon's and assistant's oculars.[6] This usually requires the assistant and primary surgeon to sit across the table from each other.

Additional Training

While the novice microsurgeon can gain a lot of insight with some of the techniques discussed here, the initial learning curve is relatively steep. Practicing both suturing and operating under the microscope on models is strongly recommended before scheduling the first clinical case. There are also a number of microsurgery courses that allow for hands-on practice on both models and cadaveric/live tissue. With the increase in the interest in microsurgery in veterinary medicine, there are a few courses that specialize in training veterinarians (e.g., Columbia University Microvascular Course).

REFERENCES

1. Altman RB: General surgical considerations. In Altman RB, Clubb SL, Dorrestein GM, et al, editors: *Avian medicine and surgery*, Philadelphia, 1997, WB Saunders.

2. Bennett RA, Harrison GJ: Soft tissue surgery. In Ritchie RW, Harrison GJ, Harrison LR, editors: *Avian medicine: principles and application*, Lake Worth, Fla, 1994, Wingers Publishing.

3. Hernandez-Divers SJ: Minimally invasive endoscopic surgery of birds, *J Avian Med Surg* 19(2):107–120, 2005.

4. Doyle JE: Introduction to microsurgery. In Harrison JG, Harrison LR, editors: *Clinical avian medicine and surgery including aviculture*, Philadelphia, 1986, WB Saunders.

5. Barraquer JI: The history of the microscope in ocular surgery, *J Microsurg* 1:288, 1980.

6. Feldman MD, Wifnicki HJ: Use of the operating microscope, *J Reconstr Microsurg* 5:399, 1989.

7. Harms H, Mackensen G: *Ocular surgery under the microscope*, Chicago, 1967, Year Book Medical.

8a. Horenz P: The operating microscope. I. Optical principles, illumination systems, and support systems, *J Microsurg* 1:364, 1980.

8b. Horenz P: The operating microscope. II. Individual parts, handling, assembling, focusing, and balancing, *J Microsurg* 1:419, 1980.

9. Murray JW: The operating microscope, *Plast Surg Nurs* 6:65, 1986.

10. Nylen CO: The microscope in aural surgery, its first use and later development, *Acta Otolaryngol Suppl* 11:226, 1954.

11. Dale WA: The beginnings of vascular surgery, *Surgery* 76:849–866, 1974.

12. Rutherford RB: Diagnostic evaluations of arteriovenous fistulas and vascular anomalies. In Rutherford RB, editor: *Vascular surgery*, ed 6, Philadelphia, 2005, Elsevier Saunders, p 1602.

13. Goldwyn RM, Lamb DL, White WL: An experimental study of island flaps in dogs, *Plast Reconstr Surg* 31:528–536, 1963.

14. Goldwyn RM, Beach M, Feldman D, et al: Canine limb homotransplantation, *Plast Reconstr Surg* 37:184–195, 1966.

15. Nasisse MP: Principles of microsurgery, *Vet Clin North Am Small Anim Pract* 27(5):987–1010, 1997.

16. Sackman J: Principles of vascular surgery. In Slatter D, editor: *Textbook of small animal surgery*, ed 3, Philadelphia, 2002, Saunders, p 996.

17. van Ee RT, Nasisse MP, Helman G, et al: Effects of nylon and polyglactin 910 suture material on perilimbal corneal wound healing in the dog, *Vet Surg* 15:435, 1986.

18. Reznick RM, Folse JR: Effect of sleep deprivation on the performance of surgical residents, *Am J Surg* 154(5):520–525, 1987.

19. Wesensten NJ, Killgore WDS, Balkin TJ: Performance and alertness effects of caffeine, dextroamphetamine, and modafinil during sleep deprivation, *J Sleep Res* 14:255–266, 2005.

20. Silverman K, Evans SM, Strain EC, et al: Withdrawal syndrome after the double-blind cessation of caffeine consumption, *New Engl J Med* 327(16):1109–1114, 1992.

21. Rutherford RB: Basic vascular techniques. In Rutherford RB, editor: *Atlas of vascular surgery: basic techniques and exposures*, Philadelphia, 1993, Saunders.

22. Collins BK, Gross ME, Moore CP, et al: Physiologic, pharmacologic, and practical considerations for anesthesia of domestic animals with eye disease, *J Am Vet Med Assoc* 207:220–230, 1995.

23. Sullivan TC, Hellyer PW, Lee DO, et al: Low-dose pancuronium neuromuscular blockade during intraocular surgery: evaluation of efficacy in inducing extraocular muscle paralysis and effects on respiratory function, *Trans Am Coll Vet Ophthalmol* 29, 1996.

24. Chacha PB: Operating microscopes, microsurgical instruments and microsutures, *Ann Acad Med Singapore* 8:371, 1979.

25. Cooley BC: *A laboratory manual for microvascular and microtubal surgery*, Reading, PA, 2001, Surgical Specialties Corp.

26. Rhoton AL: Operative techniques and instrumentation for neurosurgery, *Neurosurgery* 53(4):907–934, 2003.

27. McGrouther DA: The operating microscope: a necessity or a luxury, *Br J Ophthalmol* 33:453, 1980.

28. Brouwers JE, Oosting H, deHaas O, et al: Dynamic loading of surgical knots, *Surg Gynecol Obstet* 173:443, 1991.

APPROACHES TO THE COELOM AND SELECTED PROCEDURES

Michael Mison, Steve Mehler, Michael Scott Echols, Nathaniel K.Y. Lam, Brian L. Speer, R. Avery Bennett

GETTING STARTED

Comparative Anatomy

The skin and subcutaneous tissues of birds differ from those of mammals. Birds have a very thin epidermis that is diffusely supplied by capillaries in the dermis.[1] There is little subcutaneous tissue, and the dermis is firmly attached to the underlying muscle fascia. Most avian blood vessels are less protected by surrounding tissues, leaving more potential for hemorrhage as compared with mammals, where the tissues surrounding the vessel heat slightly when traumatized and help to seal the vessel. This becomes more important when performing surgery in small birds with little total blood volume. Body feathers are easily plucked in the direction of their growth; however, flight feathers are difficult and painful to remove, and oftentimes the removal of primary remiges is avoided. Some bird species may have particularly thin skin, predisposing them to iatrogenic tears while feathers are being plucked. Plucked feathers are replaced quickly from undamaged contour feather follicles. Cut feathers are replaced only during the normal molt cycle, which may take as long as 2 years in some species of birds. The abdominal muscles are the same as those in the mammal, but species variation exists with regard to the extent of the midventral body wall muscles and their relative thicknesses.[2]

Patient Preparation

Halsted's principles of surgery should be followed when performing surgery in any species (Box 21-1). These principles are oftentimes forgotten when performing surgery in the avian patient, or may be dismissed in the interest of procedural speed or risk of problems during surgery. The overall goal of a short operative time is best achieved by having all of the necessary equipment ready and accessible.[3]

The patient is usually placed in lateral or dorsal recumbency when a coeliotomy is performed. The surgical site is generally plucked, not clipped, under general anesthesia (Figure 21-10). Plucking feathers is a painful procedure. Minimal feather plucking is performed, especially for wild birds intended for release. Feathers should be plucked

BOX 21-1 HALSTED'S PRINCIPLES OF SURGERY

Gentle handling of tissue
Meticulous hemostasis
Preservation of blood supply
Strict aseptic technique
Minimum tension on tissues
Accurate tissue apposition
Obliteration of dead space

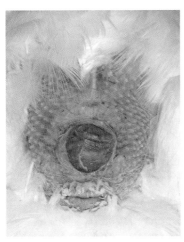

FIGURE 21-10 This pigeon has been placed in dorsal recumbency and plucked for a midventral coeliotomy and surgical repair of the visible hernia. There was concurrent septic salpingitis, egg retention, and oviductal impaction, necessitating salpingohysterectomy.

generally to a distance of 2 to 3 cm around the surgical site. In areas where the skin has been damaged or torn, the feathers may be cut to avoid further damage to the skin. Water-soluble gel, masking tape, and stockinette may be used to keep down and contour feathers under control. The skin is then aseptically prepared with chlorhexidine solution. Although povidone iodine solution can also be used, chlorhexidine is generally preferred due to its broader spectrum of activity, its residual antimicrobial effects, and the fact that it is not inactivated by organic matter. Scrub solutions may be too irritating for avian skin and should not always be used. The final prep is performed by wiping the surgical site gently with alcohol. Keep in mind that patient preparation with excessive amounts of saline or alcohol can predispose the patient to hypothermia. Draping the patient as quickly as possible with clear plastic drapes instead of cloth ones seems to help retain heat better. Clear, transparent plastic drapes also allow respiration to be monitored during the procedure (Figure 21-11).

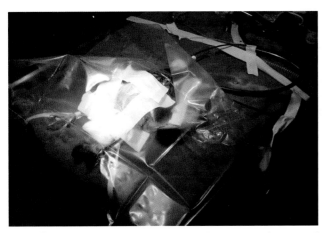

FIGURE 21-11 Clear surgical drapes facilitate patient monitoring and maintenance of a clear surgical field. This Bantam chicken hen is being prepared for ventral coelomotomy to address septic yolk coelomitis and oviductal impaction.

Plastic drapes with varying-size adhesive centers, fenestrations, and overall sizes are available from Veterinary Specialty Products, Inc. (VSP, Boca Raton, FL). This drape is placed over the patient, and a table drape is placed over that. A large fenestration is then cut into the paper drape over the plastic drape. This allows the surgeon to maintain a sterile field over the entire table and still be able to visually monitor the patient. Loss of body heat must be minimized during anesthesia. This is especially true for the smaller avian patients. Some form of supplemental heat (for example, warm water bottles, circulating warm water blankets, heat lamps, and forced warm air) should be provided to the patient.

Instrumentation

Magnification and microsurgery was covered in the previous chapter, and both are highly important in coelomic surgery. With the small size and blood volume of avian patients, close attention to hemostasis is required to minimize blood loss. Radiofrequency electrosurgery is useful in minimizing hemorrhage. It is important to know that when a fine-tip electrode is used to cut the relatively dry skin of birds, a higher setting is required compared with that for mammalian skin. When vessels are encountered at these high settings, they are cut and not coagulated, resulting in hemorrhage. Bipolar forceps have a broader surface area to disperse the current and may be used at a lower setting. They contain both electrodes, so there is no need for a ground plate, and their use seems to provide better hemostasis (Figure 21-12). These forceps can make skin incisions, coagulate before blade incision, and coagulate individual vessels. One of the best techniques for skin incision involves the use of the Harrison modified ophthalmic bipolar electrode. Fine, delicate instruments are very useful, if not essential, in avian surgery (this is discussed earlier in this section). Gauze pads (2 × 2) can be cut from the standard 4 × 4 sponges, or can be specifically purchased. The basic surgery pack, in addition to the standard set of instruments, should include three instruments for magnification surgery: a microneedle holder, micro tissue holding forceps, and microscissors. Once surgeon skill and experience advance, other instruments and equipment can be added. Sterile cotton-tipped applicators should also be available. They are very useful for gentle tissue retraction and for absorbing blood and fluid. Surgical Spears are small, wedge-shaped synthetic sponges attached to the end of a stick that are

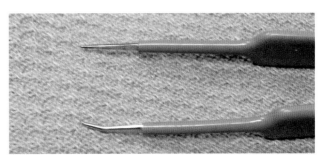

FIGURE 21-12 An excellent method for skin incisions, coagulation before blade incision, and coagulation of individual vessels is the use of the Ellman modified ophthalmic bipolar electrode, pictured here.

very absorbent (Weck-Cell Surgical Spears, Beaver-Visitec International, Inc., Waltham, MA). Absorbable gelatin sponges (Gelfoam, Pfizer, Inc., New York, NY) are also valuable for controlling hemorrhage. Hemostatic clips are also very useful (Ligaclip- or Hemoclip-Weck,). Right-angled appliers are also available for special applications in deep cavities (Figure 21-13). Hemoclips are available in at least five sizes, with small and medium most applicable for most avian surgery. No. 15 and No. 11 scalpel blades are most appropriate for surgery in birds. Heiss blunt retractors, Alm retractors, and ring retractors are suitable for use in medium to smaller species. The Lone Star Ring Retractor is another excellent instrument that provides excellent visualization of the surgical field (Cooper Surgical, Trumbull, CT; 203-601-5202).

The Skin Incision Using the Harrison Bipolar Forceps

A location should be chosen that has minimal effect on feathers and feather tracts, and that avoids the blood supply to major feathers. The skin is lifted with atraumatic forceps, creating a fold of skin at the center and perpendicular to the proposed incision. The tips of the electrodes are lightly closed on this fold, and current is activated. This will create the beginning of the incision. A very light touch is needed. If the forceps close too tightly on the skin, the current will not have an effect on the tissue. If there is no effect on the tissue, try lightening the grip on the tissue. The indifferent pole is then inserted into this slit subcutaneously to the extent of the proposed incision in one direction. The tips are closed, the current is activated, and the forceps withdrawn. The process is repeated in the other direction. This will create a skin incision and provide hemostasis for the majority of the blood vessels. If a longer incision is needed than the length of the forceps can create, the initial incision is made as described, and then additional length is achieved by inserting the indifferent electrode farther subcutaneously and the process repeated. This can be done on both ends of the incision to extend it to the needed length. This technique may also be utilized to incise abdominal wall or other structures where precision and hemostasis are critical.

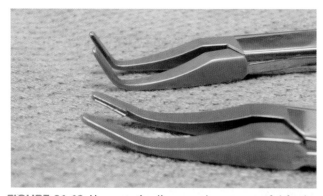

FIGURE 21-13 Hemostatic clips are also very useful for hemostasis in avian surgery. Regular applicators *(pictured below)* are more commonly used, but right-angled applicators *(pictured above)* can facilitate applications in deep body cavities.

Managing Blood Loss

Relatively small amounts of hemorrhage can be disastrous in small surgical patients. It is best if blood from a conspecific is available for transfusion if required. Blood is collected and cross-matched before surgery in case a transfusion is required. Strict attention to hemostasis is vital. The average cotton-tipped applicator holds approximately 0.1 cc of blood. Loss of 10% of the total blood volume is usually viewed as safe (approximately 1% of body weight), assuming the patient is not anemic at the start of the procedure. Intravascular fluid volume should always be maintained with the aid of colloid or crystalloid fluids during general anesthesia and surgery. If intravenous access cannot be established then an intraosseous catheter is placed. Monopolar electrosurgery or radiofrequency electrosurgery is employed for hemostasis and tissue dissection but should not be used on the gastric tissue or other tissues that might be negatively affected by the collateral heat produced. It has been well documented that radiofrequency electrosurgery causes less collateral heat damage than a CO_2 laser or electrosurgery at other frequencies. The Surgitron radiofrequency electrosurgical unit (Ellman International, Inc., Hewlett, NY) uses radiofrequency current that is received by the indifferent electrode acting as an antenna. As such, the indifferent electrode or ground plate does not even have to be touching the patient, eliminating the concern of burning the patient at the exit site of the ground plate contact. Bipolar electrosurgical forceps have a broader surface to disperse the current and, therefore, can be used at a lower setting. They contain both electrodes in the forceps, negating the need for a ground plate. They are most useful for aiding in hemostasis within body cavities, as the current passes between the tips of the electrodes, rather than through the patient to the ground plate as occurs with monopolar electrosurgery.

Suture Materials

In surgery of typical companion bird species, suture sizes of 4-0 to 6-0 are most commonly used, considering the 30- to 1500-gram range of those species. Keep in mind that variation in bird size is significant, so the choice of suture sizes will also vary with patient size. Though psittacine species can potentially remove suture materials easily, they generally preen the suture tails carefully but do not pull them out. Because of this, it is quite acceptable to use continuous patterns in the skin of avian patients, and the routine use of restraint collars or other mechanical restraint devices is much less common than in mammals.

When selecting an appropriate suture material, the tissue reaction to the material should be considered. In a study to evaluate the tissue reaction to suture materials in birds, five materials were evaluated (medium chromic catgut, polyglactin 910, polydioxanone, monofilament nylon, and monofilament stainless steel).[4] Catgut is absorbed in mammals by the action of proteolytic enzymes released from monocytes. In birds, catgut caused a marked granulocytic inflammatory response. The material was still present at the conclusion of the study (120 days). Polyglactin 910 is absorbed by hydrolysis, but in this study it produced the most intense inflammatory reaction of the materials evaluated; however, it was completely absorbed by 60 days. Polyglactin 910 is rapidly absorbed and soft, almost feather-like when the ends unravel, encouraging birds to preen them. Monofilament sutures are stiff and poke the adjacent skin, often causing irritation and getting the attention of the bird. Polydioxanone is absorbed by hydrolysis also. It caused minimal tissue reaction and was in the process of being degraded at the close of the study. Both nylon and steel caused minimal tissue reaction, but these stiffer, nonabsorbable materials were more likely to cause seromas, hematomas, and caseogranulomas. Newer, more rapidly absorbed monofilament materials should be evaluated in birds and likely have a place in avian surgery when a monofilament, rapidly absorbed material is indicated. When selecting suture materials, a variety of factors should be considered. Tissue reaction and absorbability should be taken into account. For body wall closure, a strong, slowly absorbable material that causes minimal tissue reaction is needed. In the skin, a rapidly absorbed material may be chosen, as it might eliminate the need for suture removal.

BRIEF COMMENT ON ANATOMY TERMINOLOGY

Birds have vastly different anatomy from that of mammals. Birds lack a distinct diaphragm and as such do not have a true abdominal or thoracic cavity. Rather, birds have a number of unique cavities within the coelom. Current nomenclature often lists terms with mammalian origins such as the "abdominal" and "thoracic" air sacs. Many of these terms do not accurately fit with avian anatomy but are commonplace in the literature. Until a generally recognized publication redefines some of these "mammalian themed" avian anatomic features, the nomenclature herein will reflect the current literature.

THE COELIOTOMY

Although endoscopy is a commonly used diagnostic and even therapeutic instrument to visually examine, obtain biopsies, and endosurgically debride, resect, and treat disease processes of many internal organs, it is not always the most appropriate choice for a particular patient and clinical circumstance.[5] If endoscopy is not to be used, a coeliotomy will provide access to the coelomic cavities. Direct access to the intestinal peritoneal cavity is accomplished via a ventral (midline or transverse) approach. Alternately, a left (or right) lateral flank approach may be used to access the intestinal peritoneal cavity by first entering the subpulmonary cavity, then incising the caudal thoracic and abdominal air sac walls. The specific approach is dependent on the nature of the problem and degree of access required, surgeon preference, individual bird anatomy and size, and relevant patient physical conditions. Each entry method has distinct advantages and disadvantages. Approaches commonly made include a ventral midline approach, a midline-L approach, a midline-T approach, and left and right lateral approaches that may or may not include L flaps (Figure 21-14). These surgical approaches generally require the bird to be in dorsal or lateral recumbency. If ascites or significant organomegaly is present, elevating the cranial half of the body may help reduce pressure on the heart, lungs, and more cranial air sacs, improving ventilation.

Ventral Coeliotomy

A ventral midline, transverse, or combination coeliotomy is used to expose the middle and/or both sides of the intestinal peritoneal cavity. This approach is used for surgical access to small and large intestines, pancreas, kidneys, ureters, cloaca, and the oviduct. The testes and ovary can also be accessed via a ventral approach, although in most cases, a lateral approach may be more effective for access to the gonads. The liver can be accessed from a cranial ventral coeliotomy, but the ventral hepatic peritoneal cavities must be entered. The bird is placed in dorsal recumbency, and the legs are pulled caudally. The skin is initially incised on the ventral midline. The midventral body wall is tented to hold it away from the underlying viscera and incised cranially to the caudal sternum and caudally to the interpubic space. This initial incision should preferably be performed with the aid of bipolar radiofrequency electrosurgery to minimize hemorrhage. If more exposure is needed, the incision can be extended by creating flaps (partial or full). This is done by making lateral (transverse) incisions parallel to the caudal edge of the sternum (parasternal) and/or parallel to the cranial edge of the pubis (parapubic). These additional incisions or others can be used to make an "L" pattern, a "T" pattern, and an "inverted T" pattern and are used only if improved exposure is required (see Figure 21-14, *B*). The supraduodenal loop (ileum) lies relatively ventral along the midline of the caudal coelom in Psittaciformes and can be easily transected if the surgeon is not careful. The presence of adhesions, yolk, and inflammatory debris can further complicate visualization of the supraduodenal loop of intestine. For this reason, the midline incision should, in general, be initially made as cranial as possible, unless the caudal ventral (coelom) portion must be explored, as with some cloacal surgeries. In general, the air sacs are preserved using ventral approaches, unless the nature of the pathology present necessitates their entry. The approach chosen should minimize the tissue exposure necessary to accomplish the task; it should also limit the compromise to the blood supply and the disruption of air sacs. It may be more difficult to maintain anesthesia with large abdominal approaches and procedures that result in disruption of multiple air sacs, and adjustments to anesthetic techniques may be necessary (Figure 21-15). Holding the incision closed or covering it with saline-moistened sponges for several breaths, along with increasing the percent of inspired anesthetic gas, will often help maintain the anesthesia level. The midventral body wall and muscles that have been transected, should flap incisions be used, are closed in a simple interrupted pattern. In some circumstances, a cruciate pattern may be used where the body wall is thin or overly distended. In larger bird species, the subcutaneous tissue may need to be closed, and a simple continuous pattern or mattress pattern is commonly used. The skin is closed in a simple interrupted, mattress, or Ford interlocking continuous pattern.

Transverse Coeliotomy

A transverse approach to the intestinal peritoneal cavity offers good exposure to a large portion of the abdomen. With the bird in dorsal recumbency, a transverse incision is made midway between the vent and the caudal extent of the sternum. Make sure to leave enough tissue along the caudal margin of the sternum to allow for closure. As the body wall is lifted and incised, be careful to protect underlying structures, as mentioned above in the midventral approaches. The duodenal loop containing pancreas lies immediately under the body wall in this location and the supraduodenal loop more caudally. Using this approach, the ventriculus and small intestine are most accessible (see Figure 21-14, *B*). If there is hepatomegaly, the caudal extent of the liver, usually the larger right lobe, may also be accessible by making an incision in the hepatic peritoneal cavity. The ventriculus is found in the left

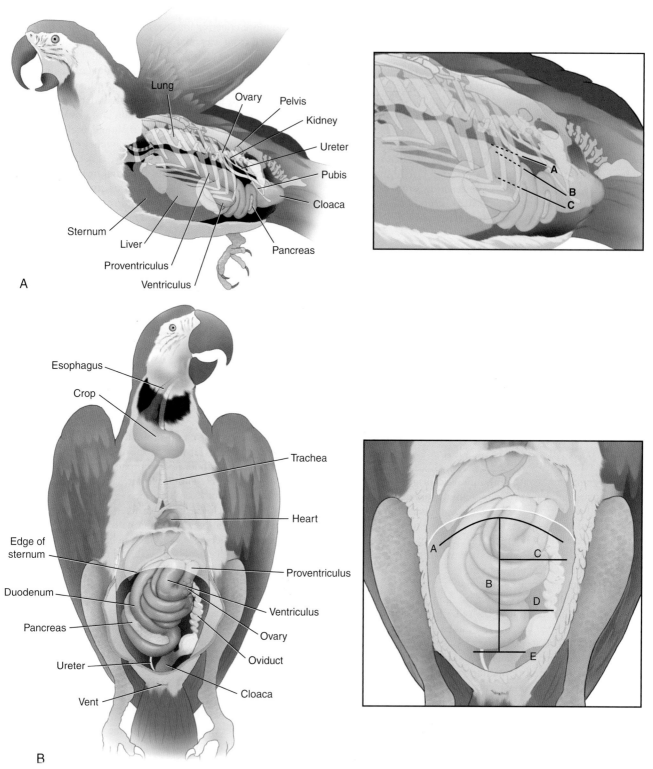

FIGURE 21-14 A, Line drawing of a macaw in right lateral recumbency, left leg forward and abducted, and right leg caudally extended, with viscera depicted. Incisions are depicted in *A* to *C.* The dashed portions of the lines represent where the incisions could be extended through the caudal two ribs and the additional exposure obtained. The more dorsal incisions (*A* and *B*) offer easier access to the ovary and reproductive tract, whereas the more ventral incision facilitates greater access to the gastrointestinal system. Modifying ventral flap incisions may be used for additional exposure for any of these incisions. **B,** Patient is placed in dorsal recumbency, with viscera depicted. Incisions shown are: ventral midline approach *(B),* a midline-L approach (*B* plus *C, D,* or *E*), a midline-T approach (*B* plus *A*), and an inverted T incision (*B* plus *E*). Combinations of these incisions may be used to greatly enhance the basic incisions (*A* or *B*), to facilitate access to specific areas of need.

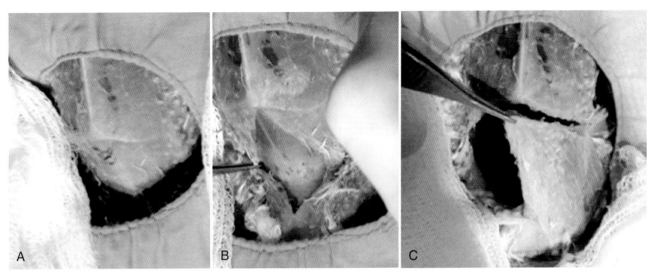

FIGURE 21-15 A, The bird is positioned in dorsal recumbency for a ventral midline coeliotomy. The wings are taped down in an extended position. The legs are retracted caudally and taped down. The feathers along both sides of the bird are plucked because this incision limits what can be performed in the coelomic cavity, and flaps may need to be created to increase exposure. **B,** The skin incision is made from the caudal apex of the sternum to the area of the vent along ventral midline between pubic bones. Once the skin incision is complete, an almost transparent fibrous tissue is identified on ventral midline. This is the linea alba, and it is incised by being elevated with jeweler's forceps and being nicked with bipolar forceps. The incision in the linea is continued cranially and caudally the length of the skin incision. The duodenum and pancreas are immediately dorsal to the linea, so great care is taken not to incise these structures. **C,** Adding a flap to the ventral midline approach allows for better visualization of the stomach. The approach combines a ventral midline coeliotomy with a parasternal or parapubic incision, or a combination. Flap incisions can be made on one or both sides of the sternum or pubic bones. The author most commonly uses a Y-shaped parasternal flap approach. It is important to leave a few millimeters of parasternal muscle to suture the body wall closed. As much as possible, the approach should limit hemorrhage and compromise to blood supply, and minimize tissue exposure and the disruption of multiple air sacs. It may be difficult to maintain body temperature and anesthesia with large abdominal approaches that disrupt multiple air sacs. If the bird is difficult to maintain under general anesthesia during these approaches, it may be necessary to pack off the opened air sacs with gauze for a few minutes, allowing inhalant anesthesia to resume. (Photos courtesy Steve Mehler.)

portion of the intestinal peritoneal cavity. The viscera may be reflected to expose the middle and caudal lobes of the kidneys, the cranial cloaca, and the lower reproductive tract (shell gland of females and vas deferentia of males). The body wall incision is closed in a simple interrupted pattern. The skin is closed in a simple interrupted, mattress, or Ford interlocking continuous pattern.

Left Lateral Coeliotomy

A left lateral approach provides exposure to the proventriculus, ventriculus, spleen, colon, left male and female reproductive tracts, left hepatic lobe, lung, heart apex, kidney, and ureter[6] (see Figure 21-14, *A*). The bird is positioned in right lateral recumbency with the wings pulled dorsally, and the right and left legs caudally. In some cases, the left leg is best pulled cranially, especially when a more cranial approach to the lateral coelom is not required. The thoracic and pelvic limbs are taped in place with masking tape, Durapore (3M, St Paul, MN), or any other tape that is easily removed (Figure 21-16). A tape stirrup can be fashioned for the left leg, which can allow for an assistant to move the leg from under the drape as needed when the leg is freed up, or if it needs to be moved for any reason during surgery. The skin incision is made from the proximal end of the pubis to the

last rib dorsal to the uncinate process (Figure 21-17, *A* and *B*) After the skin is incised, the left leg can be retracted farther caudally to provide improved exposure. A branch of the femoral artery is located within the body wall, coursing toward midline from the area of the coxofemoral joint. This vessel must be coagulated, ligated, or clipped before the abdominal musculature is incised. The skin incision is initiated with bipolar radiofrequency electrosurgery forceps as described above to create a small nick in the skin of the web. Using jeweler's forceps in one hand and bipolar electrosurgery in the other, the incision is extended as previously described. Using this technique, the incision is extended craniodorsal to the second to the last rib and caudally (making sure you are parallel to midline) to the pubic bone. After the skin incision is completed, the left leg can be abducted farther by an assistant using tape stirrups, as mentioned earlier. This is an important step and will greatly increase exposure and visualization.

The last two ribs are visualized at this time. This initially large incision is often necessary to accomplish most procedures performed through this lateral approach, especially when a bird has a dilated proventriculus or when dealing with a mass associated with the paired stomach system. If these steps are not taken, considerable procedural time can be

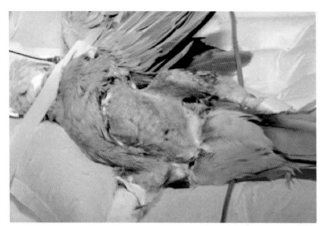

FIGURE 21-16 Shown is a male adult Amazon parrot under anesthesia positioned correctly in right lateral recumbency for a left lateral coeliotomy. The head is pointing away from the surgeon. The wings are pulled dorsally over the back. The down leg (right leg) is pulled at a 90-degree angle to the spine. The left leg is pulled caudal and dorsal (externally rotated at the hip or abducted) and secured in place. The skin incision should extend from the sixth rib to the pubic bone on the left side. The seventh and eighth ribs will be transected for most procedures performed through this approach. (Photo courtesy Steve Mehler.)

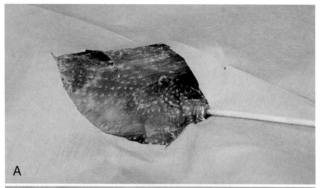

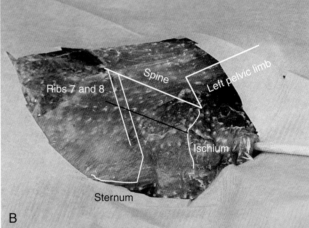

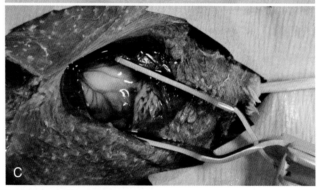

FIGURE 21-17 A, The patient is draped, and the skin has been appropriately prepared for surgery. **B,** The landmarks for palpation and the length and direction of the skin incision *(dark line)* are marked. **C,** The left lateral coeliotomy is completed by incising the skin as outlined in image **B** and by incising the muscular body wall paralleling the skin incision. A Heiss retractor is used in this case to increase exposure of the coelomic cavity, specifically the intestinal peritoneal cavity. The ventriculus is readily identified using this approach. A Lone Star ring retractor could also be used for body wall retraction. (Photos courtesy Steve Mehler.)

consumed while struggling to visualize the viscera, and risk of traumatizing tissues may be increased.

The superficial branch of the medial femoral artery and vein will need to be coagulated before entering the subpulmonary cavity. This is done by grasping the vessel between the tips of the bipolar electrosurgery forceps and activating the current in two places so the body wall can be cut between the locations where the vessels were coagulated. Then one tip of the cautery can be inserted superficially into the body wall, while the other is left external so that when the tips are apposed and the current activated, the body wall can be transected, creating an opening into the coelom. Alternatively, small vascular clips may be placed on these and other vessels before cutting them during the surgical approach. These techniques will greatly decrease hemorrhage. The body wall incision is continued using the technique described, extending caudally to the pubis and cranially to the border of the last rib. Alternatively, the surgeon can bluntly dissect through the lateral (coelomic) muscles of the body wall, including the external oblique, internal oblique, and transversus abdominus. It is best to dissect the muscles in the direction of their fibers to reduce excessive tearing. This muscle layer-by-layer approach is termed the grid approach, and it can carry the risk of ultimately yielding a reduced field of exposure unless the progressive lengths of these incisions are adequate. After the body wall is incised, the caudal thoracic air sacs and possibly the abdominal air sacs are visible dorsally. To reach the gonad(s) and proventriculus in most procedures, these air sacs must ultimately be incised.

The intercostal vessels need to be cauterized where they run cranially to the rib, before the last two ribs are cut. Follow the ribs from dorsal to ventral, and you should notice that there is a sharp bend in the ribs where the sternal and vertebral components of each rib meet. The intercostal vessels should be coagulated just cranial to the ribs and dorsal to the sharp bend. This is done by inserting the bipolar forceps under the rib, gently opposing the tips cranial to the rib, and activating the electrodes. The body wall incision may extend from the caudal aspect of the sixth rib to the pubic bone. Variation can be seen between species: In some species, up to three ribs may need to be cut to facilitate exposure to the gonad(s). The abdominal air sac is often opened during this approach, so flushing of the coelomic cavity should not be performed during these procedures. Once this is done, the eighth and seventh ribs can be transected just dorsal to the bend with heavy scissors. A Heiss retractor is inserted between the cut ends of the ribs with the handle pointing caudally (see Figure 21-17). Alternatively, a Lone Star ring retractor can be used to maintain exposure to the coelomic cavity. Once the procedure is complete, the retractor is removed, and the body wall is closed. Absorbable monofilament suture is used in a continuous, cruciate, or simple interrupted pattern. The left leg will need to be released to achieve a tension-free closure. No attempt is made to oppose the ribs or to close the abdominal air sac. Before commencing skin closure, consider having your anesthetist bag and inflate the respiratory tract, allowing you to see any air leakage through the body wall. The skin is then closed with a Ford interlocking or simple continuous pattern using an absorbable or nonabsorbable monofilament suture. Postoperatively, monitor for subcutaneous emphysema and air leakage through the skin incision. If noted, the skin incision can be opened to allow the air to leak out; most body wall incisions seal quickly. Persistent subcutaneous air leakage may require a repeat surgical exploration of the area and efforts to more effectively close the body wall.

Right Lateral Coeliotomy

A right lateral approach to the intestinal peritoneal cavity provides good exposure to the duodenum and pancreas and right male and female (if present) reproductive tracts, lung, heart apex, kidney, ureter, and right hepatic lobe. This approach is far less commonly performed given the more frequent need to access the ventriculus and female reproductive tract via a left lateral coeliotomy. The approach is otherwise reversed from a left lateral coeliotomy, and closure is routine, as previously described.

SELECTED COELOMIC SURGICAL PROCEDURES

Michael Mison, Steve Mehler, Michael Scott Echols, Nathaniel K.Y. Lam, Brian L. Speer, R. Avery Bennett

SURGERY OF THE PROVENTRICULUS AND VENTRICULUS

Relevant Surgical Anatomy and Physiology

The functional stomach of birds consists of the proventriculus, the intermediate zone or isthmus, the ventriculus, and the pylorus. The proventriculus includes the glandular compartment, which functions similarly to the mammalian stomach. The proventriculus varies in size and shape amongst species, being relatively small in granivorous species and relatively large in carnivorous and piscivorous species.[7-11] The mucosal surface of the proventriculus lacks the longitudinal folds observed in the esophagus and is lined by mucous secreting cells and multiple pit-like glands that secrete hydrochloric acid and pepsin. The intermediate zone or isthmus is the aglandular junction between the proventriculus and the ventriculus. Myenteric nerves cover the entire surface of the ventricular muscles and isthmus. Studies in domestic fowl have shown that for proper gastroduodenal motility to occur, the myenteric plexus associated with the

isthmus must remain intact. It is also suspected that initiation and regulation of the thick muscles also act via the nerves covering the isthmus. Specifically, isthmus denervation reduces the frequency of duodenal and muscular stomach contractions by 50% and abolishes glandular stomach contractions (in turkeys).[12] The nerves encircling the isthmus do not appear important in regulating thin muscle contractions.[13]

The ventriculus, also known as the gizzard, is the muscular compartment of the paired stomach system, which has no equivalent in the mammalian gastrointestinal tract. There are two distinct anatomic forms of the ventriculus in birds, which impact the surgical options for ventriculotomy between species. In general, ratite species have a large, thin-walled proventriculus that passes dorsal to the ventriculus and empties into the ventriculus at its caudal aspect.[7,8,11] This makes the caudal ventral ventriculotomy approach in these species difficult, but the opening between the proventriculus and ventriculus is large, making removal of some ventricular foreign bodies easier in this species using endoscopic techniques. In those species that feed on relatively soft food (carnivores and piscivores), the gizzard is more of a rounded, uniformly thin muscled structure that may be indistinguishable in appearance from the proventriculus.[14] In bird species that feed predominately on harder items that may require more functional grinding and mixing for digestion (insectivores, herbivores, and granivores), the gizzard is thickened and biconvex.[14-16] This anatomic feature, where the isthmus empties into the ventriculus opposite the caudal ventral ventricular sac, makes the caudal-ventral ventriculotomy feasible and preferable for some surgeons.

Grit in the ventriculus functions normally to provide additional abrasive action for those species that may require it (Columbiformes, Galliformes, most Psittaciformes, and ratites). The presence of grit may make surgery more difficult and can provide a constant source of coelomic contamination during ventriculotomy. It is important to be proactive when performing ventriculotomy and to prevent contamination of the coelom by isolating the stomach with multiple layers of moistened gauze sponges. The proventriculus and ventriculus act as a unit, propelling the ingesta back and forth between the two components to optimize mechanical and enzymatic digestion.[10,11,17-20] The proventriculus and ventriculus do not represent a major site for absorption of nutrients, most of which are absorbed in the small and large bowel.[11,17] The pylorus, Latin for "gatekeeper," arises from the right face of the ventriculus and connects the ventriculus to the duodenum. The pylorus regulates the rate of passage of food between the stomach and duodenum. It is a simple but effective muscular slit in Psittaciformes, Columbiformes, and Galliformes, in which it regulates the passage of triturated ingesta based upon particle size. The pylorus forms a distinct chamber in aquatic species.

Indications for surgery of avian paired stomach system

There are a limited number of conditions of the avian stomach that justify surgical intervention. The most common indications are to obtain diagnostic biopsy and other samples, the presence of a clinically significant gastric foreign body, complete or partial gastric outflow obstruction, or excision of gastric neoplasms or ulcerative and infiltrative intramural lesions. Surgically obtained biopsy or diagnostic samples are typically reserved for a disease process that is judged less likely to be diagnosed and/or concurrently managed with endoscopic methods.

Biopsy

Full-thickness or partial-thickness biopsies of the proventriculus and ventriculus can be used for obtaining appropriate samples for histopathology, microbiology, and molecular diagnostic testing. Diagnosis of many intramural and/or invasive mucosal disease processes (infectious, neoplastic, toxic, degenerative, parasitic and neuropathic) can be greatly facilitated by direct visualization of these organs and appropriate sample collection. Physical examination findings, clinical history, and supportive diagnostic testing are important to ascertain whether there is clear surgical indication for biopsy, and to target a specific location for sample collection.

Gastric foreign body and outflow obstruction

Most of the reported cases involve gastrointestinal impactions in ostriches, but impactions have also been described in kiwis (*Apteryx australis*), umbrella cockatoos (*Cacatua alba*), Micronesian kingfishers (*Halcyon cinnamomina cinnamomina*), sarus cranes (*Grus antigone*), bustards, and waterfowl.[14,21-25] Clinical signs associated with the presence of a gastric foreign body are often nonspecific.[26,27] Medical management is frequently recommended and used as a first line in therapy of treatment of birds with known or suspected partial obstructions due to the presence of gastric foreign material; birds with signs of complete obstruction of the gastric outflow tract should be stabilized and taken to surgery immediately.

Gastric neoplasms or ulcerative and infiltrative intramural lesions

Neoplasms of the proventriculus are often located at the isthmus. Carcinoma, squamous cell carcinoma, adenocarcinoma, adenoma, lymphoma, rhabdosarcoma, and leiomyosarcoma have been described.[28-35] Gastric carcinomas and adenocarcinomas are more often described in *Brotogeris* species, budgerigars, lovebirds, and cockatiels, as well as in smaller numbers of conures, Amazon parrots, cockatoos, African Greys, macaws, and Eclectus.[36] The more prevalent nonneoplastic lesions of the proventriculus and ventriculus of companion bird species include those associated with macrorhabdosis (budgerigars, cockatiels, parrotlets, finches), ulcerative proventriculitis, mineralization (cockatiels, budgerigars, lories and lorikeets, macaws), proventricular dilation disease (many species), and cryptosporidiosis (cockatiels, lovebirds, parrotlets, finches). Less frequent proventricular and ventricular lesions that may be amenable to surgical biopsy include fatty degeneration of the ventricular muscular tunics, transmural fungal ventriculitis, hypertrophy or atrophy of the ventricular muscular tunics, hypertrophy or atrophy of the proventricular mucosa, koilin fragmentation, mucosal papillomas, proventricular and ventricular mucosal granulomas, squamous metaplasia of the proventricular mucosa, proventricular or ventricular candidiasis, and xanthoma.[36]

Clinical signs and diagnostic methods of neoplastic diseases are similar to those described for foreign material and gastric obstruction. Surgical treatments primarily involve excision or resection of these lesions. Surgical excision may be palliative or with curative intent. Palliative surgical excision is performed with the goal of controlling hemorrhage from a bleeding lesion, or of alleviating a cancerous obstruction with debulking methods, without the ability to achieve a clean surgical margin. Curative-intent surgery involves tumor resection and an acceptable margin of healthy tissue surrounding the tumor to obtain a clean surgical margin. A clean surgical margin does not mean the patient has been cured. It refers to local disease control and does not imply resolution of metastatic lesions or multicentric disease processes. For these reasons, before, during, and after diagnosis and surgical procedures, considerations regarding the staging of these types of disease processes can offer help in economic strategies, prognostic implication, and welfare and quality-of-life informed consent discussions with owners.

Surgical Approaches and Patient Preparation

The left lateral approach transverse coeliotomy and the ventral midline with flap coeliotomy are used to access the proventriculus, isthmus, and ventriculus. For adult birds undergoing proventriculotomy or ventriculotomy, food is withheld from the patient for roughly 6 to 12 hours to allow for gastric emptying. This timeline is in part dependent on case and species-specific details and can vary. Grit will likely still be present in the ventriculus. If possible, the use of hand feeding formula 1 to 2 days before surgery will decrease the amount of residue in the ventriculus. Formula feedings should be discontinued 6 to 12 hours before surgery for many species.

Proventriculotomy and ventriculotomy

Once the ventriculus is identified, the suspensory ligaments (extension of the left portion of the posthepatic septum to oblique septum) associated with the ventriculus are bluntly dissected, and stay sutures are placed in the white tendinous portion of the ventriculus (Figure 21-18, *A*).[4] Monofilament suture on a taper needle is used for the stay sutures.[37] The stay sutures elevate the ventriculus and isthmus into the surgical field. Do not place stay sutures in the proventriculus or in the muscular parts of the ventriculus. Neither of these areas is strong enough to hold stay sutures, and tearing of the delicate tissue will occur with traction on the stay sutures. The proventriculus and ventriculus are isolated from the rest of coelom with sterile laparotomy sponges or moistened gauze to collect any spilled contents (see Figure 21-18, *B*). The isthmus, the anatomic region between the proventriculus and the ventriculus, is identified. A No. 11 scalpel blade is used to make a stab incision in the near wall of a relatively avascular portion of the isthmus. Electrosurgery, radiofrequency electrosurgery, and lasers should not be used to create an incision in the stomach or isthmus because of the potential for lateral heat damage, leading to incisional dehiscence in the immediate postoperative period. The incision can then be extended orad for a proventriculotomy or aborad for a ventriculotomy using a No. 11 blade or fine Metzenbaum, microscissors, or iris scissors (Figure 21-19). The use of a scalpel blade is the preferred technique for extending the incision because the technique creates no crushing or shearing injury to the tissues during cutting. Scissors, even fine, sharp scissors, shear and crush the tissue, leading to more inflammation and a greater chance of dehiscence. Manipulation of the tissues is performed with great care and precision. Many surgeons manipulate

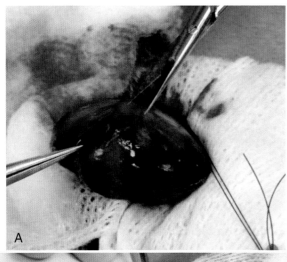

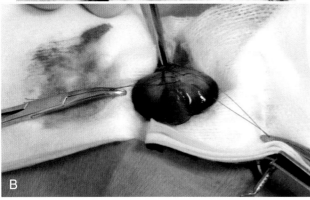

FIGURE 21-18 **A,** Once the ventriculus is identified, the suspensory ligaments associated with ventriculus are bluntly dissected, and the ventriculus is well isolated with moistened laparotomy sponges or gauze squares. **B,** Stay sutures are placed in the white tendinous portion of the ventriculus. For the stay sutures, 4-0 or 5-0 monofilament suture on a taper needle is used. The stay sutures are used to elevate the ventriculus and isthmus into the surgical field. Do not place stay sutures in the proventriculus or in the muscular parts of the ventriculus. Both of these areas are not strong enough to hold stay sutures, and tearing of the delicate tissue will occur with retraction of the stay sutures. (Photos courtesy Steve Mehler.)

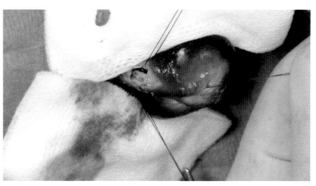

FIGURE 21-19 The isthmus, the anatomic region between the proventriculus and the ventriculus, is identified. A No. 11 blade on a bard Parker scalpel handle is used to make a stab incision in the ventral wall of an avascular portion of the isthmus. It is best to use carefully placed stay sutures for manipulation of the stomach and the edges of the incision during surgery and during closure of the isthmus, proventriculotomy, or ventriculotomy incision to prevent crushing injury to the edges of the incision. (Photo courtesy Steve Mehler.)

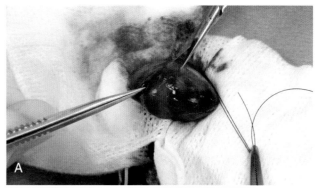

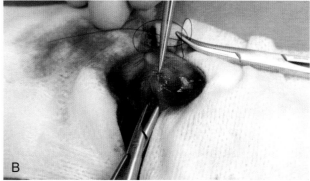

FIGURE 21-20 **A,** Depending on the location of the foreign body or region of interest, a caudal ventral ventriculotomy can be performed instead of entering the ventriculus via the isthmus. The thinner caudoventral region of the ventriculus may be approached by way of the caudoventral sac. This approach requires a meticulous closing technique incorporating a closely placed simple interrupted or simple continuous suture pattern because a second overlaying inverting pattern is not possible in this area of the ventriculus. This is performed on the caudal ventral surface of the ventriculus away from the isthmus. The isthmus is not incised using this technique. **B,** The caudal ventral sac has been incised, and access to the ventriculus is achieved. This approach is best used for lesions or foreign body retrieval close to the pyloric outflow tract. (Photos courtesy Steve Mehler.)

gastrointestinal structures with thumb forceps held in the nondominant hand. Most of us have poor control with our nondominant hand, and the tissues are often held too tightly and crushed in the tips of the thumb forceps. If the forceps are used for counterpressure as described in the microsurgery section earlier, they will not traumatize the tissue and will make it easier for surgeons to place the sutures. Rigid endoscopy can be used intraoperatively to reduce tissue trauma and to facilitate foreign body removal, in some circumstances.[21] It is best to use carefully placed stay sutures for manipulation of the stomach during surgery and during closure of the isthmus, proventriculotomy, or ventriculotomy incision (see Figures 21-18 and 21-19).

Some surgeons prefer a caudoventral ventriculotomy instead of entering the ventriculus via the isthmus. The isthmus is not incised using this technique. The ventriculus has two blind sacs (craniodorsal and caudoventral) covered with relatively thin muscles (Figure 21-20, *A*). An incision through

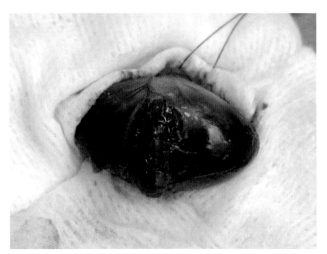

FIGURE 21-21 The incision is closed with a simple interrupted or continuous pattern with a fine absorbable monofilament material on a small taper needle. The author prefers 5-0 or 6-0 PDS on an RB-1 taper needle. No attempt is made at repairing the suspensory ligaments. (Photo courtesy Steve Mehler.)

their overlying thin muscle fibers allows relatively easy entry into the ventricular lumen[37,38] (see Figure 21-20, *B*). Again, use meticulous closure. This tissue does not invert, so use interrupted sutures placed close together (Figure 21-21).

The proventriculotomy or isthmus incision in most common companion bird species is closed with a fine 4-0 to 6-0 monofilament absorbable material on a small atraumatic taper needle using a simple continuous oversewn pattern. The specific choice of suture size, of course, is dependent on patient size and the integrity and characteristics of the tissues involved. For a ventriculotomy, the incision is closed with a simple interrupted or continuous pattern with a fine, absorbable monofilament material on a small taper needle (see Figure 21-21). In a study of Coturnix quail undergoing caudoventral sac ventriculotomy, ventricular mucosal healing was

not complete until 21 days postsurgery.[38] No attempt is made at repairing the suspensory ligaments. In general, there is a greater potential for incisional leaking of gastric content from a ventriculotomy incision as compared with one in the proventriculus or isthmus. A serosal patch of the incision can be performed to help prevent dehiscence and coelomitis. The liver lobe closest to the incision is gently manipulated over the incision (Figure 21-22). Using 5-0 or 6-0 monofilament absorbable suture on a taper needle, two to three simple interrupted sutures are placed between the seromuscular layers of the gastric incision to the capsule of the caudal edge of the liver lobe. Each suture is placed at least 5 mm lateral to the gastric incision and tightened such that the liver lobe covers the entire incision.

Resection and anastomosis of the isthmus

In cases of isthmus neoplasia or severe compromise or perforation of the isthmus secondary to a foreign body obstruction or other infiltrative disease process, a resection and anastomosis may be indicated and can be performed. The surgical approach is preferably a left lateral one; however, in some species and in individual patient circumstances, a midventral incisional approach may be acceptable. It is imperative that all soft tissue attachments and suspensory structures to the ventriculus be manually broken down before this procedure is attempted. Any residual tension along the anastomosis incision will lead to dehiscence. Once the proventriculus, isthmus, and ventriculus are identified and thoroughly isolated from the rest of the coelom with moistened gauze squares or laparotomy sponges, stay sutures are placed in the white tendinous portion of the ventriculus for manipulation during the anastomosis. The isthmus is transected off of the ventriculus with a No. 11 blade, leaving a 2- to 5-mm cuff of tissue at its junction with the proventriculus. This rim of tissue will be used to create the anastomosis. Hemorrhage is controlled with ligatures or Microhemoclips. Neither radiofrequency electrosurgery, electrosurgery, nor a CO_2 laser is used on the stomach at any time. Any visible grit or food is carefully removed from the opening

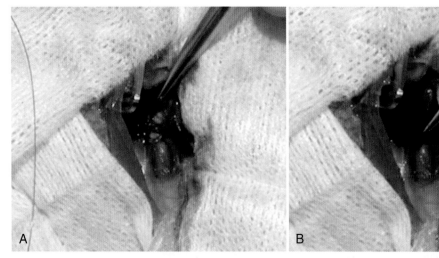

FIGURE 21-22 A serosal patch of an isthmus and proventriculotomy incision is being performed. **A,** Demonstrates the suture in the closed incision and the relationship of the incision to the caudal edge of the liver. **B,** The caudal aspect of the liver lobe is gently manipulated over the incision in the isthmus and proventriculus. (Photos courtesy Steve Mehler.)

to the ventriculus, and the ventriculus is wrapped in sterile moistened gauze or a laparotomy sponge. The opening into the ventriculus is sutured closed with 6-0 to 4-0 monofilament absorbable or similar monofilament absorbable suture, on a taper needle, preferably a small, fine-tipped taper needle, in a simple interrupted pattern. Once the ventriculus is sutured close, the caudal ventral sac is identified. The tissue of this blind-ended sac is thinner and holds suture better than other locations of the ventriculus. The sac is opened as is described above for ventriculotomy. The isthmus is sutured to the opening in the caudal ventral sac with a suture similar to the monofilament absorbable suture above on a taper needle in a simple interrupted pattern. There is no good way to leak test the incision, so the sutures must be placed close together and with meticulous effort. If after releasing all of the suspensory structures of the ventriculus there is still tension on the anastomosis, tension-relieving sutures can be placed between the proventriculus and ventriculus. Two to three interrupted monofilament sutures on a taper needle are placed between the proventriculus and the white tendinous portion of the ventriculus. Care is taken when tightening these sutures that they do not tear through the stomach and that tightening them does not create a kink or bend at the anastomosis site. Saline-soaked sponges or cotton-tipped applicators are used to wipe any contaminants off of the stomach or bowel before placing the organ back into the coelom.

Surgery of the Male Reproductive Tract
Relevant surgical anatomy and physiology
The key components of the reproductive anatomy of most male birds include the testes, epididymides, and ductus deferentes.[39] Some bird species also have a phallus. The paired testes are located ventral to the left and right cranial renal division. The mesorchium connects the testes to the dorsal body wall and provides suspensory support. The left testicle is typically larger than the right in most birds. During breeding activity, the testicular size may increase dramatically within normal physiologic parameters. The color of the testes varies in appearance from white to yellow or black, depending on the species. The epididymides are located at the testicular hilus at the dorsomedial aspect of the testes. The ductus deferentes continue from the epididymides as highly convoluted tubes (in adults) and parallel the ureters, terminating at the ureteral ostium in the urodeum. The testicular artery arises from the cranial renal artery. This vessel provides most of the arterial blood supply to the testes in most birds. An accessory testicular artery may also be present, arising directly from the aorta caudal to the cranial renal artery. Testicular venous blood returns directly to the caudal vena cava or via a common stem with the adrenal veins. Two testicular veins empty directly into the caudal vena cava of Pekin drakes (*Anas platyrhynchos*).[40] Given the diversity within the class Aves, it is likely that multiple variations of the testicular vasculature exist.

Orchidectomy (castration)
Clinical need for orchidectomy in birds is less frequent than the need for ovarian and oviductal surgical procedures in hens. Routine or prophylactic castration in companion bird species is rarely performed. As such, there is little information regarding the longer-term effects of castration in pet bird

species. Castration, as a sole maneuver for the purpose of elimination problem behaviors in male birds, is not recommended, due to the potential for the presence of previously learned "problem" behaviors in male birds and the possible lack of dependency on testosterone for those behaviors to be maintained. The effects of castration on aggressive Psittacine behaviors remains uncertain, although in other species, more variable effects have been seen following castration. In one study of ring-necked doves, castration reduced or eliminated courtship behavior and some aggressive behaviors.[40a] Castrated Gambel's (*Callipepla gambelii*) and scaled (*C. Squamata*) quail showed reduced or eliminated courtship behaviors and lower rates of male-male threats. Their gender-specific plumage remained unchanged, and the castrated male birds continued to exhibit overt aggression.[41] European starlings (*Sturnus vulgaris*) castrated at 1 year of age when nonreproductively active were more aggressive than noncastrated controls.[42] In that study, the authors concluded that nonreproductive aggression in yearling male starlings was independent of gonadal sex steroids and suggested that it even increased following castration. In addition to questions about the effects of castration on undesired aggressive male behavior, there is concern that remaining testicular tissue or an appendix epididymis that may continue to secrete androgens remains after castration. Castration is more medically indicated as a treatment for testicular neoplasia, orchitis, and other conditions that may not respond to medical management alone.

Caponization (castration) is commonly performed in commercial poultry, typically between 1 and 2 weeks of age. Caponized chickens have increased coelomic fat weight, total hepatic lipid content, and saturated fatty acid percentage as compared with intact birds.[43] The longer-term medical consequences of these changes are not known. There are several methods that have been described for surgical castration in avian species. These include simple extraction (caponization), endosurgical methods, and open surgical removal. Endoscopic castration methods are discussed in Chapter 12. With all of these procedures, there remains the potential for incomplete removal of all testicular tissue and partial regrowth or hypertrophy of the remaining testicular tissues.

Caponization
Caponization is performed in young male chickens to improve meat quality.[44] Heavy chicken breeds are caponized at 2 to 4 weeks, while slow-growing meat-type birds are caponized after 6 weeks old. Caponization becomes more difficult with age, due to progressive firmness of the tunica albuginea. In many lay personnel settings and parts of the world, the caponization procedure is typically done without anesthesia, with the bird held or strapped to a table. It is not necessary to emphasize further that appropriate anesthesia and pain management are ethically and medically indicated for such a procedure. The appropriate side is prepared for aseptic surgery, and an incision is made through the lateral body wall between the last two ribs, which are then separated with a tissue retractor. Specialized caponizing forceps are used to enter the incision, to delicately hold the entire testes, and to pull with a twisting motion until the testicle is free and removed. The wound is disinfected and left to close by second intention, or may be surgically closed. Incompletely caponized birds may hypertrophy the remaining testicular tissues, and those birds

tend to develop secondary sex characteristics unlike those of true capons.[44,45]

Open surgical castration

The surgical approach for open surgical castration is either a cranial left lateral approach or ventral midline incision with transverse flap to provide surgical access to the testes. The right testis may be exposed through the left lateral approach by dissecting through the dorsal mesentery, or the procedure may be repeated using a right lateral approach to remove the right testis. A left-handed surgeon may be best suited to attempting bilateral orchidectomy from a right lateral incision, whereas a right-handed surgeon typically is more comfortable with the left lateral approach. Unless the testicle is approached via a ventral midline coeliotomy with the left abdominal air sac reflected dorsally, an air sac wall will lay over the testis. This should be incised. Using gentle traction, pull the testis ventrally and apply at least one hemostatic clip. to the dorsal testicular blood supply. If two or three can be placed, incise distal to two. The testicle is removed either in one piece or is sometimes transected into more than one piece to facilitate removal. Radiofrequency electrosurgery or a diode laser can be used to free the testis from its soft tissue attachments and the remnants of the vascular cord. When radiofrequency electrosurgery or an intraoperative diode laser is used, care must be taken not to damage the adjacent blood vessels, kidney, or adrenal gland. Reported complications of open surgical castration include hemorrhage and hypertrophy of residual testicular tissues.

Castration has been described in ostriches and is typically performed through a lateral incision through the costal notch and lumbar fossa on each side.[46] A gloved hand is introduced, and the testicle can simply be palpated, grasped, and twisted to tear its attachments. Reported complications include subcutaneous emphysema and incisional dehiscence.

In juvenile birds or where the testicular blood supply is not well developed, a small, fine-tipped hemostat can be temporarily used in place of a Hemoclip and the testis pulled free. Leave the hemostat on the vascular stump for 1 to 2 minutes before release. Take care not to inadvertently jar the hemostat, as this can result in tissue trauma and augmented risk of hemorrhage. Use direct pressure hemostasis as needed. Diode laser excision can also be used to cut the testis from its attachments and may be performed without a hemostat. A topical hemostatic agent may be applied over these areas before closure to help ensure that continued hemorrhage does not reoccur during recovery.

Vasectomy

Endoscopic and external vasectomy methods are described in Chapter 12. Open coeliotomy surgical techniques for vasectomy are useful primarily as an aid in population control, particularly where normal courtship and pair bonding behaviors are desired in the absence of fertility.

A left lateral approach, sometimes paired with a right lateral approach, is used. The ductus deferens can be identified where they course lateral to the ureters. The overlying air sac is incised, and the ductus are lifted and transected, removing a large enough portion of the duct to minimize the risk of recanalization. Application of hemostatic clips to these severed ends of the ductus may also aid in prevention of recanalization. Care is required to avoid damage to the ureter. Vasectomized roosters ceased producing viable semen within 5 to 7 days.[47] Vasectomy does not stop courtship and copulation behaviors.[48] Hypothesized complications of open vasectomy procedures include reconnecting of the severed ends of the ductus and recanalization, leading to return of fertility. Reported complications include anesthetic-associated mortalities and inadvertent laceration of the adjacent ureter.

Surgery of the Female Reproductive Tract
Relevant anatomy and physiology

The anatomy and function of the female reproductive tract seem to be very consistent in the majority of bird species.[49] A right and left ovary and oviduct are present in the embryologic stages of all birds, but the right side regresses due to the action of Mullerian inhibiting substance before hatch.[49] In the majority of birds, only the organs on the left side (ovary and oviduct) are functional, although rudiments of the right gonad and oviduct can persist.[50] Two fully developed ovaries are known to occur in some birds of prey and the brown Kiwi (*Apteryx mantelli*), but right and left ovaries have been observed in at least 16 taxonomic orders that typically are seen with only one.

The ovary is attached to the cranial renal division and dorsal body wall by the mesovarian ligament. The blood supply to the ovary comes from the ovarian artery, which originates from the left cranial renal artery or comes directly off the aorta.[51] Accessory ovarian arteries may also arise from other adjacent arteries (see Chapter 6).[52] Multiple left ovarian veins may exist and drain into the cranial oviductal vein, which then enters the common iliac vein and finally the caudal vena cava (see Chapter 6).[52] These vascular anatomic variations, in part, contribute to the complexity of ovariectomy in adult birds, as there is rarely a single artery and vein to ligate. The oviduct is suspended within the intestinal peritoneal cavity via a dorsal and ventral ligament, and is supplied by five arteries. The cranial oviductal artery originates from the left cranial renal artery, supplying the infundibulum and magnum. The accessory cranial oviductal artery arises from the left external iliac artery and supplies the magnum. The middle oviductal artery arises from the left ischiadic artery and supplies the magnum and uterus. The caudal oviductal artery arises from the pudendal branch of the internal iliac artery and supplies the uterus. The vaginal artery also arises from the pudendal artery. The cranial and accessory arteries vary among species. The ovarian and oviductal arteries are greatly enlarged during periods of egg laying. The common iliac vein drains the cranial parts of the oviduct, and the internal iliac vein drains the caudal portions of the oviduct and the cloaca.[51]

The right mesonephros and mesonephric duct persist in many normal adult females, adjoining the cloaca.[49,53] Larger cystic right oviducts are not uncommon, and these are typically equivalent to the magnum or infundibulum, but not the uterus or vagina.[49] These cystic structures can be benign or can be associated with health problems including egg binding[54] and coelomic space-occupying effects.[49] After removal of the left ovary, these ducts can enlarge and become associated with the right gonad to form an epididymis and ductus deferens, potentially creating a fully functional male system.[49] In psittacine species, the prevalence of a cystic right oviduct was 90% in hens that had their left oviduct previously removed, but that maintained persistent estrogenic activity. In contrast, an overall prevalence at the time of coelomic surgery was 40%, and in birds with left ovarian or left oviductal disease processes, the prevalence was 70%.[55]

Surgery of the Ovary

Partial and complete ovariectomy

Indications for ovariectomy, either partial or complete, include the presence of ovarian disease processes including neoplasia, chronic recurring cysts, oophoritis, and other diseases that cannot be managed medically and that are life-threatening without further treatment. Clinical signs of ovarian disease are nonspecific and include coelomic swelling, dyspnea, ascites, poor or altered reproductive performance, and lethargy. If an ovarian mass-effect compresses the overlying lumbar or sacral nerve plexus, neurologic lameness (usually left-sided) may be seen. Diagnosis can be further supported using radiography, ultrasonography, computed tomography (CT), magnetic resonance imagery (MRI), exploratory coeliotomy, endoscopy, and biopsy. Although the cause is often unknown, cystic ovarian disease has been reported in numerous bird species.[56,57] Cystic ovaries are not uncommon and are sometimes secondary to neoplasia.[56,57] Ovarian infections (bacterial oophoritis) can be life-threatening and are often associated with septicemia and hematogenous delivery to the ovary. Granulosa cell tumors and ovarian adenocarcinomas are most frequently reported, but carcinomas, leiomyosarcomas, leiomyomas, adenomas, teratomas, dysgerminomas, fibrosarcomas, lipomas, and lymphomatosis have all been identified in bird ovaries.[53,56,58,59] Steroidogenic and morphologically distinctive granulosa cell tumors originating from follicles in atrophic ovaries represent another common ovarian tumor type.[58] Polyostotic (medullary) hyperostosis may also occur as a result of estradiol production or paraneoplastic syndrome with functional ovarian and oviductal neoplasms.[59,60] At least one study found that hyperestrogenism did not cause polyostotic hyperostosis in several species of birds with various neoplastic and nonneoplastic reproductive tract diseases.[61]

A true complete ovariectomy is very difficult to achieve in adult birds. Although ovariectomy has been described as a challenging and oftentimes high-risk procedure, it is also mentioned as a viable procedure in the literature, predominately in poultry species.[62-66] Most described ovariectomies are partial, with the more realistic goals of debulking abnormal tissue. The ovary can dramatically change in size and vascularity with reproductive activity. In circumstances where immediate surgery is not required, the bird is ideally conditioned to help reduce the degree of ovarian vascularity. Some diseases requiring ovariectomy do not allow clinicians time to "condition" the avian patient before surgery. Conditioning maneuvers may include the use of environmental, nutritional, and behavioral intervention, as well as GnRH agonists, depending on case specifics (see Chapters 5 and 12).

The surgical approach for ovariectomy is most often a left lateral approach but can, in some circumstances, include a cranial midventral approach. Once entry into the coelom has been accomplished, fluid and debris are cleared to enable visualization of the ovary and its associated vasculature. In some circumstances, removal of a diseased oviduct will be required to facilitate optimal surgical exposure of the ovary.

The first step of ovariectomy, particularly when there is a mature and active or diseased ovary, is to debulk its mass. The goal of debulking is to enable visualization of the ovarian attachments to the overlying common iliac vein and any other vessels that may be present. Large preovulatory follicles are removed using a twirling method. Using cotton-tipped applicators, rotate the follicle in one direction continuously 15 to 30 rotations until it separates from its pedicle. Alternatively, two cotton-tipped applicators can be used to apply gentle but progressive force to cause rupture of the follicle at its stigma, releasing the ovum. Once free, simply remove the follicle from the body cavity. Large cystic follicles that are present are aspirated, which in turn enables their removal using hemostatic clips where appropriate. Neoplastic growths of the ovary can also be segmentally debulked using hemostatic clips, a diode laser, or other means. Once there has been adequate debulking, the second aspect of ovariectomy can commence. The body of the ovary is progressively clamped along its dorsal attachments to the mesovarian ligament and ovarian arteries and veins using hemostatic clips. Often working from caudal to cranial at the ovarian base seems to be most efficient. Using an angled clip applicator allows placement of the clips parallel to the spine, avoiding trauma to underlying structures. When using surgical vascular instruments for this process, angled Debakey neonatal vascular clamps are atraumatic, can be positioned to rest in the surgical site without obstructing the view, and seem to provide some degree of hemostasis to the mass of the ovary. Once a section of the ventrocaudal portion of the ovary is clipped or clamped, it is surgically excised or electrocoagulated and removed. The surgical site is reassessed, and the vascular clamps are moved, or new Hemoclips are placed closer to the ovarian base, repeating the excision process. This process is repeated until the surrounding vasculature is identified and the underlying common iliac vein can be seen, deep to or dorsal to the ovary. Radiofrequency electrosurgical or laser ablation can be used, as indicated, for removal of any remaining ovarian tissue. Closure is in at least two layers and is routine. Potential complications include potentially fatal hemorrhage, leakage of air subcutaneously, and hypertrophy of remaining ovarian tissue.

Surgery of the Oviduct

Disorders of the oviduct may be incidental findings or may be clinically relevant, requiring surgical attention. Indications for oviductal surgery include ectopic ovulation and yolk coelomitis, oviductal impaction or binding, oviductal rupture and torsion, neoplasia, cystic hyperplasia of the oviduct, oviductal prolapse, salpingitis, and metritis.[67] Ectopic ovulations are, at times, comparatively innocuous and do not require surgical treatment and also can be a component of other, more significant peritoneal concerns. Severe sterile and life-threatening septic egg yolk peritonitis may result from ectopic ovulation or eggs and may be the result of systemic sepsis and oophoritis or ascending oviductal infections. Clinical signs may include significant depression, anorexia, respiratory distress, or death. Coliforms such as *Escherichia coli*, *Yersinia pseudotuberculosis*, *Salmonella* spp. and *Staphylococcus* spp. have been identified in septic yolk coelomitis.[68] Many yolk peritonitis cases are sterile and have no bacterial component involved. Depending on the degree of inflammation associated with egg yolk peritonitis,

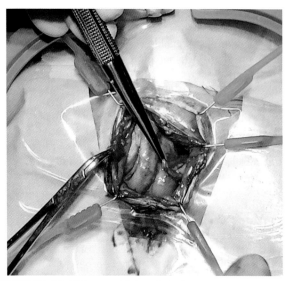

FIGURE 21-23 This pet chicken is being explored surgically, and visible peritonitis, serositis, and yolk material can be seen. One of the particular challenges at surgery is to safely identify anatomy, break down adhesions, and provide a view of the primary problem in order to address it. In this case, there was a septic salpingitis *(Escherichia coli)*, oviductal impaction, yolk peritonitis, multiple serosal adhesions, and free inspissated yolk material in the peritoneal cavity. (Photo courtesy Nathaniel Kane.)

adhesions may result and be found during coeliotomy days to more than a year after the episode (Figure 21-23).

Birds with oviductal disease may present with nonspecific clinical signs. The most commonly recognized signs are related to the resultant space-occupying mass-effect of oviductal enlargement, causing compression of the surrounding organs, peritoneal distension, peritonitis, and ascites. Peritoneal distension, however, is not always a characteristic of oviductal disease. Affected birds may show persistent "broodiness" with recent cessation of egg laying. Definitive diagnosis is typically made at coeliotomy; however, physical examination findings, ultrasound imaging, and radiographic imaging can aid in making the diagnosis.[69]

Salpingohysterectomy

Salpingohysterectomy is the surgical removal of the oviduct, infundibulum to uterus, and is primarily indicated for treatment of oviductal disease that cannot be medically managed.[70] Surgical approaches to the left oviduct can include the left flank coeliotomy (most common) or midventral approaches. When there is reason to suspect the presence of clinically significant right oviductal disease, a midventral approach will provide better access than a left flank coeliotomy. Once the intestinal peritoneal cavity has been entered, as with ovariectomy, fluid and debris are cleared to enable visualization of the oviduct. The oviduct is located along the dorsal aspect of the intestinal peritoneal cavity.[71] Incise through the left abdominal air sac. The ovary and oviduct are readily visible. When performing a ventral midline coeliotomy, the air sacs do not need to be breached. In reproductively active hens or when oviductal disease is present, these structures will be enlarged and potentially adhered to other viscera, and the

anatomy often is less straightforward. In some circumstances, a salpingotomy may be required to remove retained egg(s) or material to facilitate exposure of the oviductal suspensory ligaments and vasculature. Carefully elevate and dissect the oviduct away from the caudal vena cava. Inadvertent trauma to this vessel will lead to fatal hemorrhage. The ventral oviductal ligament is relatively avascular and can be dissected to allow the reproductive tract to be extended linearly. The oviduct can be removed moving from cranial to caudal, caudal to cranial, or in portions and segments as best fits the clinical circumstances. Presuming you are starting craniad, elevate the fimbria of the infundibulum located caudal to the ovary, exposing the dorsal attachments to the infundibulum. The dorsal ligament at the base of the infundibulum suspends the uterus and a branch of the ovarian artery that can be seen coursing from the ovary through the infundibulum. Apply a hemostatic clip or coagulate this vessel carefully at its location in the dorsal ligament to avoid hemorrhage from this vessel, which is difficult to control after it has been transected and retracts. Should hemorrhage be encountered, place gel foam and apply gentle pressure. When hemostasis has been accomplished, continue dissecting caudally and go back after completion and make sure there is no further hemorrhage. The remainder of the dorsal ligament may be dissected using bipolar cautery forceps or with Hemoclips or blunt dissection, where appropriate. Dissection may be more straightforward if efforts remain as close to the oviduct as possible. In general, the deeper and closer vessels are to the caudal vena cava, the larger they are. Those closer to the oviduct are smaller and oftentimes do not require clips or ligation. After the infundibulum is completely freed, retract the oviduct ventrally and caudally to expose the dorsal suspensory ligament. Clip or coagulate branches of the ovarian artery that lie perpendicular to the oviduct. Continue dissection caudally toward the cloaca, taking care to avoid the ureter. Clip or ligate the uterus at the uterovaginal junction by placing 1 to 2 hemostatic clips or an encircling suture a short distance from the cloaca, or at the cloaca if the vaginal tissues have been damaged. In larger birds, transfixation ligatures may be used at the amputation site of the distal oviduct. Closure is in 2 to 3 layers and is routine.

Salpingotomy

Salpingotomy is indicated in some cases of egg binding or dystocia where medical management has been judged to be ineffective.[68] This procedure may be required as part of a complete salpingohysterectomy, or may be carried out with the intent to spare the bird's reproductive capabilities if there is an otherwise normal or minimally diseased oviduct. The surgical approach to the oviduct is, in part, dependent on the location of the egg and can be either a caudal left lateral or ventral midline approach. The oviduct is incised directly over the bound egg and away from prominent blood vessels. The oviductal tissue is typically friable, and the incision should be made large enough to enable removal of the egg and material without stretching that causes tears in the tissue. Atraumatic microsurgical technique is important. Closure of the oviduct is in a single layer using a simple interrupted or continuous pattern with fine monofilament absorbable suture material. Closure of the body wall and skin is in 2 to 3 layers. Complications of salpingotomy may include dehiscence and oviductal rupture, or strictures and secondary oviductal impaction.

Surgery of the Intestinal Tract

Enterotomy, intestinal resection, and anastomosis

Enterotomy for the purpose of foreign body removal is described in various bird species.[72,73] Intestinal resection and anastomosis procedures are described but remain infrequently represented in the literature.[22,73] Nonmetallic lower gastrointestinal foreign bodies are most frequently linear and occasionally perforate, leading to abscessation and leaving a functional nidus of infection or lead to enterolith formation. Resection and anastomosis can be considered for localized intestinal neoplasms. Radiographs, with or without barium or iodine, and ultrasound may aid in obtaining a diagnosis, as can other imaging options, including, but not limited to, contrast fluoroscopy or advanced imaging modalities.

Based on the location of the intestinal lesion, a midline or transverse coeliotomy can be utilized to provide access to the surgical target. Intestinal surgery in general, including resection, repair, and anastomosis, is a delicate procedure in birds. As such, magnification and microsurgical techniques are recommended and generally required. The procedures themselves are no different from those described in mammalian species. Following enterotomy or resection and anastomosis of intestines in typical companion bird species, 6-0 to 10-0 suture is used in a simple appositional pattern.[3] The typical intestinal anastomosis usually requires 6 to 8 sutures for end-to-end anastomosis; however, in many cases side-to-side anastomosis is an acceptable technique that is less challenging to perform, especially in smaller birds. The movement of intestinal content can be stopped using sterilized bobby pins, or atraumatic vascular clamps or vessel approximators.

Duodenal feeding tube placement

In patients with severe gastrointestinal disease, bypassing a compromised or dysfunctional segment of the gastrointestinal tract may be necessary to facilitate provision of adequate nutrition in hyporexic or anorectic patients while allowing the surgical site to heal. Conditions that may require enteric feeding include those with upper gastrointestinal tract infections, dysfunction, obstructions, or severe injury. Maintaining a positive energy balance in these patients is critical to maximizing the potential for successful healing and recovery.

The surgical approach to the duodenum is either a ventral midline or ventral transverse coeliotomy. After identification of the ascending and descending duodenal loops by their attachments to the pancreas, a "through the needle" indwelling venous catheter of sufficient gauge (less than half the diameter of the intestine) is passed through the left body wall and then into a loop of descending duodenum.[3,74] The catheter is advanced over the needle approximately 4 to 6 cm through the descending and ascending loops of duodenum, and the needle is withdrawn. An enteropexy is performed to create permanent adhesions between the body wall and the enteric ostomy site by placing one to two absorbable monofilament sutures between the left body wall and the duodenum at the catheter entry site. After routine closure of the coeliotomy, the catheter should be secured to the outer abdominal wall using a finger trap with 3-0 or 4-0 nonabsorbable suture. The needle should be contained within the included snap guard, and the snap

guard should be sutured to the skin and conformed to the bird's body. The catheter is routed behind the leg and under the wing, and is sutured to the lateral and dorsal body wall (2 sutures). This functionally secures it in an unobtrusive position and prevents it from dislodgement. The catheter should be flushed with warm saline or water to ensure patency, and its hub should be sealed with an injection cap.

After calculation of the caloric needs, feedings should be divided into 4 to 6 equal volumes at regular intervals and injected at a rate of 1 mL/15 s (4 mL/min). The catheter should be flushed (1 to 2 mL of warm water or lactated Ringer's solution) before and after enteric feeding to maintain patency within the lumen. To prevent complications from leakage of intestinal contents, the enterostomy tube should remain in place for a minimum of 5 days to allow a seal to form between the intestine and body wall at the ostomy site. A cervical restraint collar or Elizabethan collar may be required in some circumstances to prevent patients from chewing or dislodging the enterostomy tube. Once the catheter is no longer needed, the securing sutures are cut, and the indwelling portion of the catheter is removed. In healthy pigeons, experimental placement of duodenostomy tubes sustained only minor weight loss, even after total enteral nutrition for 14 days.[74]

Surgery of the Cloaca

The cloaca of birds consists of three main compartments (from orad to aborad): the coprodeum, the urodeum, and proctodeum. The distal colon enters the coprodeum, which is separated from the urodeum by the coprourodeal fold. The ureters enter the urodeum through a sphincter muscle and an opening that is covered by transitional epithelium preventing ureteral reflux.[75] Further, the urodeum is separated from the proctodeum by the uroproctodeal fold. Feces combined with urine and urates form the complete dropping, which is eliminated through the proctodeum and out the external vent.

Indications for open surgery of the cloaca include prolapse of the entire cloaca, severe cloacal atony, recurrence of prolapse after closed reduction, failure of temporary percutaneous ventplasty or cloacopexy procedures, surgical management of cloacolithiasis, and for the purpose of visual assessment and biopsy/resection of chronic inflammatory or neoplastic lesions. The goal of most cloacal surgery is to facilitate obtaining a diagnosis and to restore as much of the normal anatomy and function as possible. Anatomy, form, and function of the cloaca have been discussed in detail in Chapter 7. Specific procedures include cloacotomy, cloacal resection, cloacopexy, and ventplasty.

Cloacotomy

Indications for cloacotomy include resection of inflammatory or neoplastic lesions, removal of cloacoliths, as a component of an open cloacopexy procedure or of open reduction of cloacal prolapse. Cloacotomy is generally reserved for access to lesions that cannot be diagnosed or managed endoscopically or medically, including, but not limited to, resection of neoplastic or traumatic lesions and removal of cloacoliths.[76,77] The basic surgical approach to the ventral cloaca is a ventral midline coeliotomy. As described with cloacopexy below, use a cotton-tipped applicator or other inserted instrument through the vent to identify the ventral cloacal wall. The cloacal incision is midventral, so care must be taken to avoid causing tears or further damage to these tissues. Following the procedure, closure is accomplished using appropriate monofilament suture. Potential complications following cloacotomy include dehiscence, entrapment of intestine, stricture formation, or inadvertent trauma to the ureteral, oviductal, or ductus deferentes juncture of the urodeum.

Cloacopexy

Several techniques for cloacopexy are described, and often these are used in combination with ventplasty to reduce cloacal prolapse, to maintain the position of the cloaca within the coelom, and to constrain the size of the vent opening. Cloacopexy procedures may include open cloacotomy methods or closed procedures.[78] The purpose of open cloacopexy is to create permanent adhesions from the cloaca to the body wall to anchor the organ in a reduced position. As with cloacotomy, a ventral midline coeliotomy is performed with extension of the incision parasternal bilaterally to provide access to the last ribs. The serosal surface of the cloaca is isolated, and any fat or other connective tissue is dissected from the ventral surface to prevent interference with adhesion formation between the serosa and body wall. Using a cotton-tipped applicator or other instrument inserted through the vent, the cloaca is distended, and its limits are visually defined. The cloacal serosal surface is located midventrally, and care must be taken to avoid causing tears or further damage to these tissues. Following the procedure, closure is routine, using appropriate monofilament suture. Cloacopexy can be performed circumcostally if there is minimal tension present when the cranial limits of the cloaca are moved cranially toward their potential attachment sites at the last rib. Alternatively or in combination, the cloaca can be sutured to the ventral body wall if the subserosal surfaces of the cloaca and peritoneal surface of the body wall are exposed and apposed. For circumcostal cloacopexy, two sutures are preplaced around the last rib on each side at the junction of the sternal and vertebral portions of the rib and full thickness through the cloaca. For sternal cloacopexy, if the cloaca cannot be advanced cranially to the ribs, two sutures are passed through the cartilaginous border of the sternum before placement through the cloaca. For subserosal cloacopexy, a 2- to 5-mm incision is made in the serosa to the level of the submucosa of the coprodeum parallel to its length approximately 5 to 10 mm from the midline. An incision of similar length is made on the opposite side paramedian at a point that will maintain the cloaca in a position that results in slight inversion of the vent. Preplace 3 to 4 sutures, and examine the position of the cloaca. Once all sutures are preplaced and in position, they are tied to form temporary adhesions. Eventually these sutures will stretch, break, or degrade; thus permanent adhesions must be created by the procedure to prevent recurrence. Following placement of the sutures, an incorporating cloacopexy can be performed. Incise or scarify the ventral aspect of the cloaca, and during closure of the ventral midline coeliotomy, the suture should be passed through one side of the body wall incision, full thickness through the cloaca, and through the other side of the body wall. Incisional colopexy has also been described to treat chronic cloacal prolapse through a U-shaped coeliotomy.[78a] After incision through the seromuscular layer, the colon was sutured to the left abdominal wall in a sulphur-crested cockatoo with long-term success. Complications of cloacopexy may include dehiscence of the pexy, failure of permanent adhesion resulting in reprolapse, hypertrophy of the cloaca leading to reprolapse, penetration of the cloaca and subsequent peritonitis, or colonic entrapment.[79]

Ventplasty

Since ventplasty is often paired with cloacopexy, this procedure is described here even though it alone does not require coeliotomy. Ventplasty is most often reserved as a portion of surgical treatment of chronic cloacal prolapse. Additional indications for ventplasty may include the resection of known or suspect neoplastic lesions or traumatic injuries of the vent. The goal of ventplasty is to reduce the vent size to a more normal size such that cloacal prolapse is less likely to recur. As with cloacopexy, ventplasty will likely fail as a sole form of treatment for chronic cloacal prolapse unless underlying cause(s) of the prolapse is not resolved and the bird continues to strain postoperatively.

The extent to which the vent sphincter is enlarged will determine how much tissue must be resected. For mild to moderate distension of the vent sphincter, usually one section of the vent is resected. For more severe distension, two areas of vent resection may be required. The basic incision is the same, but the choice to use one or two areas for resection is in large part based on surgeon preference and his assessment of what the need(s) are in a specific patient. Before making the incision(s), estimate how much tissue needs to be resected to make a normal vent diameter. Triangular incisions work best with the "base" of the triangle on the leading edge of the vent and the "point" away from the vent (Figures 21-24 and 25). A single incision works best over the cranioventral side of the vent, while two opposing incisions can be performed at the right and left lateral sides. Once the resection site(s) is(are) determined, excise the desired triangular area(s), taking

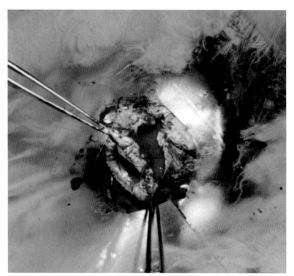

FIGURE 21-24 A triangular incision is being made for the purpose of a combined ventral abdominal wall cloacopexy and ventplasty in this cockatoo with a history of chronic cloacal prolapse. This procedure was strategically timed to follow careful integration of behavior change and dietary modification and concurrent medical management of secondary cloacitis.

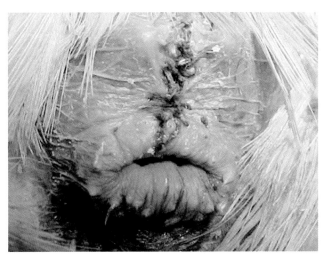

FIGURE 21-25 The same cockatoo from Figure 21-24 postoperatively. The prior locations of the two paired vent sutures are visible, which were used to help manage the prolapse condition while the patient was being prepared and conditioned for surgery. Approximately half of the ventral wall of the sphincter was removed and reanastomosed during the ventplasty procedure.

epidermis and dermis. If the sphincter and transverse cloacal muscles are visible, spare these muscles. The dermis can usually be bluntly dissected from the underlying muscular and submucosal tissue layers. When apposed, the new epidermal edges should form the desired vent diameter. If needed, more epidermal/dermal tissue is removed. With the appropriate "new" vent margins, the surgery site is closed. First the submucosa is closed with the dermis. Simple interrupted absorbable sutures are placed medial (which represents the new vent wall) to lateral for all tissue layers. The sphincter muscle itself is then closed, using a mattress suture in the muscle from cranial to caudal on each side. Next, the dermis is closed in the same fashion. Finally, the overlying epidermis is closed. The caudal cloacal mucosa should extend caudally to the vent epithelial margins without additional measures. If not, the mucosa is sutured in place as needed. The end result should be one suture line extending cranially (single vent resection) or one suture line extending laterally on the left and right sides of the vent (double vent resection). The new vent diameter should be just large enough to allow passage of droppings. Use lubricated cotton-tipped applicators to test the patency of the vent.

REFERENCES

1. King AS, McLelland J: Integument. In King AS, McLelland J, editors: *Birds: their structure and function*, Philadelphia, 1984, Bailliere-Tindall, pp 23–26.
2. King AS, McLelland J: Skeletomuscular system. In King AS, McLelland J, editors: *Birds: their structure and function*, Philadelphia, 1984, Bailliere-Tindall, pp 43–49.
3. Bowles HL, et al: Surgical resolution of soft tissue disorders. In Harrison GJ, Lightfoot TL, editors: *Clinical avian medicine*, vol 2, Palm Beach, Fla, 2006, Spix Publishing, pp 775–829.
4. Bennett RA, Yaeger MJ, Trapp A, et al: Histologic evaluation of the tissue reaction to five suture materials in the body wall of rock doves (*Columba livia*), *J Avian Med Surg* 11:175–182, 1997.
5. Divers SJ: Avian endosurgery, *Vet Clin North Am Exot Anim Pract* 13:203–216, 2010.
6. Dennis PM, Bennett RA: Ureterolithiasis in a double-yellow headed Amazon parrot (*Amazona ochrocephala*), *Proceedings of the Association of Avian Veterinarians* 161–162, 1999.
7. Lumeij JT: Gastroenterology. In Ritchie BW, Harrison GJ, Harrison LR, editors: *Avian medicine: principles and application*, Lake Worth, Fla, 1994, Wingers Publishing, pp 482–521.
8. Hoefer HL: Diseases of the gastrointestinal tract. In Altman RB, Clubb SL, Dorrestein GM, et al, editors: *Avian medicine and surgery*, Philadelphia, 1997, WB Saunders, pp 419–453.
9. Girling S: Diseases of the digestive tract of psittacine birds, *In Pract* 26:146–153, 2004.
10. Archambault AL, Timm KI: Treatment of acute lead ingestion in a juvenile macaw, *J Am Vet Med Assoc* 205:852–854, 1994.
11. Fowler ME: Comparative clinical anatomy of ratites, *J Zoo Wildl Med* 22:204–227, 1991.
12. Chaplin SB, Duke GE: Effect of denervation of the myenteric plexus on gastroduodenal motility in turkeys, *Am J Physiol* 259:G481–G489, 1990.
13. Hall AJ, Duke GE: Effect of selective gastric intrinsic denervation on gastric motility in turkeys, *Poult Sci* 79:240–244, 2000.
14. Degernes LA, Wolf KN, Zombeck DJ, et al: Ventricular diverticula formation in captive parakeet auklets (*Aethia psittacula*) secondary to foreign body ingestion, *J Zoo Wildl Med* 43:889–897, 2012.
15. King AS, McLelland J: External anatomy. In King AS, McLelland J, editors: *Birds: their structure and function*, Philadelphia, 1984, Bailliere-Tindall, p 97.
16. Hall AJ, Duke GE: Effect of selective gastric intrinsic denervation on gastric motility in turkeys, *Poult Sci* 79:240–244, 2000.
17. Duke GE: Alimentary canal: anatomy, regulation of feeding and motility. In Sturkie PD, editor: *Avian physiology*, ed 4, New York, 1986, Springer-Verlag, pp 269–301.
18. Tully TN, Hoefer H, Vansant F, et al: Heavy metal toxicosis, *J Avian Med Surg* 11:115–118, 1997.
19. Denver MC, Tell LA, Galey FD, et al: Comparison of two heavy metal chelators for treatment of lead toxicosis in cockatiels, *Am J Vet Res* 61:935–940, 2000.
20. Hoogesteijn AL, Raphael BL, Calle P, et al: Oral treatment of avian lead intoxication with meso-2,3-dimercaptosuccinic acid, *J Zoo Wildl Med* 34:82–87, 2003.
21. Speer BL: Chronic partial proventricular obstruction caused by multiple gastrointestinal foreign bodies in a juvenile umbrella cockatoo (*Cacatua alba*), *J Avian Med Surg* 12:271–275, 1998.
22. Honnas CM, Blue-McLendon A, Zamos DT, et al: Proventriculotomy in ostriches: 18 cases (1990–1992), *J Am Vet Med Assoc* 202:1989–1992, 1993.
23. Honnas CM, Jensen J, Cornick JL, et al: Proventriculotomy to relieve foreign body impaction in ostriches, *J Am Vet Med Assoc* 199:461–465, 1991.
24. Kinsel MJ, Briggs MB, Crang RFE, et al: Ventricular phytobezoar impaction in three Micronesian kingfishers (*Halcyon cinnamomina cinnamomina*), *J Zoo Wildl Med* 35:525–529, 2004.
25. Bailey TA, Kinne J, Naldo J, et al: Two cases of ventricular foreign bodies in the kori bustard (*Ardeotis kori*), *Vet Rec* 149:187–188, 2001.
26. Morrisey JK: Gastrointestinal diseases of psittacine birds, *Semin Avian Exotic Pet Med* 8:66–74, 1999.
27. Rupley AE: Diagnostic techniques for gastrointestinal diseases of psittacines, *Semin Avian Exotic Pet Med* 8:51–65, 1999.
28. Snyder JM, Treuting PM: Pathology in practice. Adenocarcinoma of the proventriculus with liver metastasis and marked, diffuse chronic-active proventriculitis and ventriculitis with moderate *M. ornithogaster* infection in a budgerigar, *J Am Vet Med Assoc* 244:667–669, 2014.
29. Yonemaru K, Sakai H, Asaoka Y, et al: Proventricular adenocarcinoma in a Humboldt penguin (*Spheniscus humboldti*) and a great horned owl (*Bubo virginianus*); identification of origin by mucin histochemistry, *Avian Pathol* 33:77–81, 2004.

30. Leach W, Paul-Murphy J, Lowenstine LJ: Three cases of gastric neoplasia in psittacines, *Avian Dis* 33:204–210, 1989.

31. János G, Marosán M, Kozma A, et al: Solitary adenoma in the proventriculus of a budgerigar *(Melopsittacus undulatus)* diagnosed by immunochemistry—short communication, *Acta Vet Hung* 59:439–444, 2011.

32. Schmidt RE, Dustin LR, Slevin RW: Proventricular adenocarcinoma in a budgerigar *(Melopsittacus undulatus)* and a grey-cheeked parakeet *(Brotogeris pyrrhopterus)*, *AAV Today* 2:140–142, 1988.

33. Schmidt V, Philipp HC, Thielebein J, et al: Malignant lymphoma of T-cell origin in a Humboldt penguin *(Spheniscus humboldti)* and a pink-backed pelican *(Pelecanus rufescens)*, *J Avian Med Surg* 26:101–106, 2012.

34. Gibbons PM, Busch MD, Tell LA, et al: Internal papillomatosis with intrahepatic cholangiocarcinoma and gastrointestinal adenocarcinoma in a peach-fronted conure *(Aratinga aurea)*, *Avian Dis* 46:1062–1069, 2002.

35. Maluenda ACH, Casagrande RA, Kanamura CT, et al: Rhabdomyosarcoma in a yellow-headed caracara *(Milvago chimachima)*, *Avian Dis* 54:951–954, 2010.

36. Reavill DR, Schmidt RE: Lesions of the proventriculus/ventriculus of pet birds: 1640 cases, *Proceedings of the Association of Avian Veterinarians* 89–93, 2007.

37. Bennett RA: Techniques in avian thoracoabdominal surgery, *Proceedings of the Association of Avian Veterinarians Core Seminar* 45–57, 1994.

38. Ferrell S, Werner J, Kyles A, et al: Evaluation of a collage patch as a method of enhancing ventriculotomy healing in Japanese quail *(Coturnix coturnix japonica)*, *Vet Surg* 32:103–112, 2003.

39. King AS, McLelland J: Male reproductive system. In King AS, McLelland J, editors: *Birds: their structure and function*, Philadelphia, 1984, Bailliere-Tindall, pp 166–174.

40. Kremer VA, Budras KD: The blood vascular system in the testis of Peking drakes *(Anas platyrhynchos)*: Macroscopic, light microscopic, and scanning electron microscopic investigations, *Anat Anz* 171:73–87, 1990.

40a. Adkins-Regan: Effects of sex steroids on reproductive behavior of castrated male ring doves, *Physiol Behavior* 26(4):561–565, 1981.

41. Hagelin JC: Castration in Gambel's and scaled quail: ornate plumage and dominance persist, but courtship and threat behaviors do not, *Horm Behav* 39:1–10, 2001.

42. Pinxten R, DeRidder E, DeCock M, et al: Castration does not decrease nonreproductive aggression in yearling male European starlings *(Sturnus vulgaris)*, *Horm Behav* 43:394–401, 2003.

43. Chen KL, Lee TY, Chen TW, et al: Effect of caponization and different exogenous androgen on hepatic lipid and β-oxidase of male chickens, *Poult Sci* 88:1033–1039, 2009.

44. Rikimaru K, Takahashi H, Nichols MA: An efficient method of early caponization in slow-growing meat-type chickens, *Poult Sci* 90:1852–1857, 2011.

45. Friedlander RC, Olson LD, McCune EL: Histologic pattern of testicular regrowths in caponized tom turkeys, *Avian Dis* 36:101–107, 1992.

46. Sikarski JG: Ostrich castration for behavioral control, *Proceedings of the First International Conf of Zoo and Avian Medicine* 416, 1987.

47. Janssen SJ, Kirby JD, Hess RA: Identification of epididymal stones in diverse rooster population, *Poult Sci* 79:568–574, 2000.

48. Samour J: Vasectomy in birds: a review, *J Avian Med Surg* 24:169–173, 2010.

49. King AS, McLelland, J: Female reproductive system. In King AS, McLelland J, editors: *Birds: their structure and function*, Philadelphia, 1984, Bailliere-Tindall, pp 145–165.

50. Johnson AL: Reproduction in the female. In Whittow GC, editor: *Sturkie's avian physiology*, ed 5, San Diego, 2000, Academic Press, pp 569–596.

51. King AS, McLelland J: Cardiovascular system. In King AS, McLelland J, editors: *Birds: their structure and function*, Philadelphia, 1984, Bailliere Tindall, pp 214–228.

52. Baumel JL: Systema cardiovasculare. In Baumal JL, King AS, Breazile JE, editors: *Handbook of avian anatomy: nomina anatomica avium*, ed 2, Cambridge, Mass, 1993, Nuttall Ornithological Club, pp 407–475.

53. Joyner KL: Theriogenology. In Ritchie BW, Harrison GJ, Harrison LR, editors: *Avian medicine: principles and application*, Lake Worth, Fla, 1994, Wingers Publishing, pp 748–804.

54. Hochleitner M, Lechner C: Egg binding in a budgerigar *(Melopsittacus undulatus)* caused by a cyst of the right oviduct, *AAV Today* 2:136–138, 1988.

55. Nemetz L: Clinical pathology of a persistent right oviduct in psittacine birds, *Proceedings of the Association of Avian Veterinarians*, 73–77, 2010.

56. Speer BL: Diseases of the urogenital system. In Altman RB, Clubb SL, Dorrestein GM, et al, editors: *Avian medicine and surgery*, Philadelphia, 1997, WB Saunders, pp 625–644.

57. Vegad JL, Kolte GN: An ovarian condition with multiple cystic follicles in a hen, *Vet Rec* 105:446, 1979.

58. Fredrickson TN: Ovarian tumors of the hen, *Environ Health Perspect* 73:35–51, 1987.

59. Latimer KS: Oncology. In Ritchie BW, Harrison GJ, Harrison LR, editors: *Avian medicine: principles and application*, Lake Worth, Fla, 1994, Wingers Publishing, pp 640–672.

60. Stauber E, Papageorges M, Sande R: Polyostotic hyperostosis associated with oviductal tumor in a cockatiel, *J Am Vet Med Assoc* 196:939–940, 1990.

61. Baumgartner R, Hatt J-M, Dobeli M, et al: Endocrinologic and pathologic findings in birds with polyostotic hyperostosis, *J Avian Med Surg* 9:251–254, 1995.

62. Lea RW, Richard-Yris MA, Sharp PJ: The effect of ovariectomy on concentrations of plasma prolactin and LH and parental behavior in the domestic fowl, *Gen Comp Endocrinol* 101:115–121, 1996.

63. Petrowski ML, Wong EA, Ishii S: Influence of ovariectomy and photostimulation on luteinizing hormone in the domestic turkey: evidence for differential regulation of gene expression and hormone secretion, *Biol Reprod* 49:295–299, 1993.

64. Proudman JA, Opel H: Daily changes in plasma prolactin, corticosterone, and luteinizing hormone in the unrestrained, ovariectomized hen, *Poult Sci* 68:177–184, 1989.

65. Terada O, Shimada K, Saito N: Effect of oestradiol replacement in ovariectomized chickens on pituitary LH concentrations and concentrations of mRNAs encoding LH β and α subunits, *J Reprod Fertil* 111:59–64, 1997.

66. Zadworny D, Etches RJ: Effects of ovariectomy or force feeding on the plasma concentrations of prolactin and luteinizing hormone in incubating turkey hens, *Biol Reprod* 36:81–88, 1987.

67. Martin HD: Avian reproductive emergencies: surgical management, *Vet Med Rep* 2:250–255, 1990.

68. Romagnano A: Avian obstetrics, *Semin Avian Exotic Pet Med* 5:180–188, 1996.

69. Honnas CM, Jensen JM, Blue-McLendon A: Surgical treatment of egg retention in emus, *J Am Vet Med Assoc* 203:1445–1447, 1993.

70. Harcourt-Brown N: Torsion and displacement of the oviduct as a cause of egg-binding in four psittacine birds, *J Avian Med Surg* 10:262–267, 1996.

71. Gorham SL, Akins M, Carter B: Ectopic egg yolk in the abdominal cavity of a cockatiel, *Avian Dis* 36:816–817, 1992.

72. Jenkins JR: Surgery of the avian reproductive and gastrointestinal systems, *Vet Clin North Am Exot Anim Pract* 3:673–692, 2000.

73. Wagner WM: Small intestinal foreign body in an adult Eclectus parrot *(Eclectus roratus)*, *J S Afr Vet Assoc* 76:46–48, 2005.

74. Goring RL, Goldman A, Kaufman KJ, et al: Needle catheter duodenostomy: a technique for duodenal alimentation of birds, *J Am Vet Med Assoc* 189:1017–1019, 1986.

75. Gumus E: The relationship between uretero-cloacal structure in birds and sigmoidalrectal pouch surgery in humans, *Aktuelle Urol* 35:228–232, 2004.

76. Beaufrere H, Nevarez J, Tully TN: Cloacolith in a blue-fronted amazon parrot (*Amazona aestiva*), *J Avian Med Surg* 24:142–145, 2010.

77. Mehler SJ, Briscoe JA, Hendrick MJ, et al: Infiltrative lipoma in a blue-crowned conure (*Aratinga acuticaudata*), *J Avian Med Surg* 21:146–149, 2007.

78. Avergis S, Rigg D: Cloacopexy in a sulphur-crested cockatoo, *J Am Anim Hosp Assoc* 24:407–410, 1988.

78a. Van Zeeland YRA, Schoemaker NJ, Van Sluijs FJ: Incisional colopexy for treatment of chronic, recurrent colocloacal prolapse in a sulphur-crested cockatoo (*Cacatua galerita*), *Vet Surg* 43(7):882–887, 2014.

79. Radlinsky MG, Carpenter JW, Mison MB, et al: Colonic entrapment after cloacopexy in two psittacine birds, *J Avian Med Surg* 18:175–182, 2004.

ORTHOPEDICS

Julia B. Ponder, Patrick Redig

Successful fracture management in the avian patient will be enhanced with an understanding of orthopedic principles, an appreciation of the unique characteristics of birds, and clear objectives for patient outcome, whether release back to the wild or pain-free life in captivity. The best treatment outcomes will be achieved through adherence to basic orthopedic principles that are consistent across species. While much can be extrapolated from mammalian medicine, the avian patient will be best served by an approach that is adapted to meet the tremendous variation among avian species, as well as the unique anatomy and physiology inherent in a body designed for flight. Depending on the environment a bird must function in after healing, the outcome goals may vary among patients. A wild bird undergoing rehabilitation for release back to the wild must have total restoration of musculoskeletal function before returning to its native habitat. While the physical demands for a captive bird's lifestyle are less rigorous, the ideal goal is still restoration of full function. When this is not possible, however, it may be appropriate to set a goal of returning to a comfortable and pain-free life.

From the very beginning of treatment, the clinician must make every effort to reduce morbidity by applying sound treatment techniques. The goals in fracture management include establishing early and rigid stability of the bone fragments while maintaining normal longitudinal and axial alignment of the bone. Whether using a surgically applied fixation device or external coaptation, the preservation of soft tissues is paramount for maintaining bone integrity. Where possible, fixation devices should promote load sharing with the bone, which results in quicker fracture healing when done appropriately. The use of fixation that will allow return of the limb to normal function and range of motion as soon as possible will shorten healing times and minimize secondary complications. It will also promote patient mobility and comfort.

While the objectives of orthopedic management in the avian patient are similar to those for mammalian patients, bird anatomy presents some unique characteristics and challenges. The cortices of the long bones of birds are thin and brittle. Although they are quite strong when intact, avian bones tend to shatter when they break, often resulting in severely comminuted fractures. With their centralized musculature, thin skin, and minimal subdermal tissues, birds have less soft tissue covering and protecting their bones. Fractures in free-ranging bird species are often open with bone fragments exteriorized and at risk of devitalization. Most birds have a strong ability to incorporate bone fragments into a healing fracture if soft tissue connections to fragments are maintained. There is a high risk of sequestrum formation when bone fragments become separated from their soft tissue attachments.

In general, bone healing times in birds are rapid. A simple humeral fracture with good fixation and vascular integrity will heal in as little as 3 weeks. Healing times are longer in fractures of more distally located bones on a given limb, as well as in cases with comminuted or open fractures, more distal diaphyseal fractures, infections, or poor nutritional status. Psittacine birds maintained in captivity, in particular, are prone to poor bone quality owing to long-term inadequate nutrition, and this can be a negative factor in the outcome of an attempt at fracture repair.

The decision whether to use surgical or nonsurgical fracture management techniques in any given case is based on the ability to meet orthopedic objectives, as well as on the resources and expertise available. The type of definitive fixation chosen for a case depends on the characteristics of the fracture, as well as on external factors such as owner consent and financial considerations. In wild birds, where the ultimate goal is complete restoration of full function, decisions are driven by an understanding of fracture elements, clinician experience, and available resources, as well as on comorbidities, age of the bird, and likelihood of repatriation if released. In companion birds, full function is still desirable, but may be less crucial. Since companion birds often have their food supplied daily with minimal physical demands, the primary consideration becomes comfort and lack of pain. Too often, though, the adaptability of companion birds is used as an excuse for less than optimal treatment of fracture. This can lead to prolonged recoveries, increased morbidity, less than ideal resolutions, and long-term problems. Approaching decision making in a fracture case with an understanding of orthopedic principles and how they apply to specific situations will improve clinical outcomes and result in better patient care.

EVALUATION OF THE FRACTURE PATIENT

Many of the decisions made during the initial presentation of a patient with a fracture have an impact on the case's eventual outcome. A holistic approach to the patient and good initial triage will result in more successful outcomes. Whether the patient is a wild bird or a captive bird, the goal is to capitalize on the body's healing potential while minimizing secondary morbidity. While early stabilization of the fracture and preservation of soft tissues are high priorities, the clinician must first and foremost address the critical care needs of the traumatized patient. Initial fracture stabilization, usually addressed on presentation of the patient, is very dependent on the patient's overall condition. Definitive fracture repair should be delayed until the patient is stable.

Patient Assessment

Upon presentation, the patient should be evaluated completely, including signalment, history, and physical and orthopedic examinations. Patient assessment, which is done concurrently with emergency stabilization, may require a staged approach if the bird's condition is too delicate to withstand the required handling. In total, assessment should include a complete physical exam, minimum database (including hematology, serum chemistries, and radiology), and fracture assessment. If possible, the physical exam should include hands-off observation, allowing the patient time to unmask clinical signs and the clinician the opportunity to evaluate mentation, posture, respiration, and general appearance. Indications of respiratory distress may include a tail bob in rhythm with breathing pattern or excessive movement of the ventral and lateral abdominal musculature. The use of anesthesia or sedation during physical exam and treatment should be considered, as it is often beneficial (see Chapter 17). While a fracture may be the most obvious problem a bird has on initial presentation, it is important to recognize the potential that the traumatic injuries might be far more extensive than just one bone. Traumatic incidents often result in eye, head, or intracoelomic trauma. An ophthalmologic exam is particularly important in the traumatized wild patient, as ocular impairment is common and may influence decisions regarding the ability of the bird to be released back to the wild. In addition to experiencing trauma, the patient may have underlying health issues such as poor nutrition, poor body condition, or chronic disease. Malnutrition and associated poor bone condition are common in companion birds. Deficits in nutrients such as vitamin K, calcium, and vitamin D can adversely impact surgical success as well as healing. Besides imaging fractures, radiographs may reveal evidence of internal trauma, or show sources of respiratory compromise.

Clinical signs of fractures may include wing droop, local swelling, apparent loss of limb function, localized pain, and/or altered limb positioning. Shoulder girdle fractures (coracoid, furcula, or scapula) are often more subtle, showing just a slight wing droop. One key clinical finding in a patient with a coracoid fracture or luxation is the inability to elevate the wing above the horizontal plane.

Fracture Assessment

When evaluating a fracture, the patient's treatment options, and prognosis, it is helpful to understand the factors that contributed to the breaking of the bone, as well as the characteristics of the fracture itself. Important considerations are the type of fracture, bone integrity, soft tissue compromise (open or closed fracture, additional soft tissue trauma), and the degree of fracture displacement.[1]

Poor bone integrity can be both a contributing factor to fractures and a consideration for fracture management. It is particularly relevant in captive birds. Many of these patients have poor bone quality as a result of malnutrition and/or lack of exercise. Diets with inadequate calcium are common, as is a lack of exposure to sunlight for vitamin D production.[2] Loss of bone mass associated with inactivity also contributes to poor bone quality in caged birds, as exercise is a key component of normal bone physiology. Load-bearing exercise contributes to the formation and maintenance of healthy bone. Reproduction is another physiologic process that has impact on bone integrity, as hens mobilize large amounts of calcium from medullary bone during egg-laying. In situations of excessive egg laying, this can be a factor in predisposing to fractures.[3] Less commonly, underlying bone disease such as neoplasia or osteomyelitis (e.g., mycobacterial infection) can predispose a patient to a fracture or impede attempts to repair.

The characteristics of the fracture are important to consider when determining treatment. Because of the minimal amount of soft tissue covering, avian fractures are very often open. In open fractures, the exposed bone is readily separated from its blood supply at the time of fracture or during improper handling afterward.[4] Exteriorized bone is often nonviable, an important consideration during initial triage. Open fractures also have a higher risk of bone infection. Strict attention to wound management and soft tissue preservation throughout triage and treatment will help prevent loss of bone viability and improve the long-term prognosis. Protecting protruding or uncovered bone is crucial to avoid devitalization from exposure.

Long bone fractures can be transverse, oblique, spiral, segmental, or comminuted.[1] Although it has high strength, avian cortical bone is quite thin. The forces that cause fractures can be high or low energy. A high-energy force (e.g., projectile) is more likely to shatter a bone, resulting in a comminuted fracture, while a low-energy force (e.g., collision with a stationary object) often results in a simple transverse or oblique fracture. High-energy fractures are also more likely to have significant soft tissue damage associated with them.[1] In general, lower energy force–induced fractures tend to be more commonly seen in companion bird species as compared to free-living wildlife, and as a result, there is comparatively less soft tissue damage, less comminution, and fewer open fractures encountered in companion birds.

These various fracture configurations have different abilities to accept load sharing with fixation. In a transverse fracture where the ends can be solidly opposed and can buttress each other, and where the muscles and mechanical forces assist in holding the fractured bone segments in place, healing will be facilitated, and the fixation device does not need to bear all the stresses. In comminuted fractures, the fixation device must be constructed more robustly, as the fractured bone cannot contribute to load sharing. This is particularly important in pelvic limb fractures. Understanding these mechanical forces will influence the clinician's choice of treatment.

FRACTURE MANAGEMENT OPTIONS

Three options exist for fracture management in birds: confinement/cage rest, coaptation, and application of a fixation device. Instances occur where all three are used simultaneously or successively in an individual patient. Regardless of the method of stabilization used, fractures require active management to ensure the optimal outcome. Benign neglect or a "set it and forget it" mentality are not usually associated with success.

Confinement and Cage Rest

Cage rest is suitable in a very small number of situations, typically those involving very small birds (finches, canaries) and/or injuries that are not amenable to bandaging or surgery (pelvic fractures) in other birds. Careful consideration must be given to the housing that is provided, and it generally matches that which is used for early postsurgical care of orthopedic patients (See section on convalescent care). Small patients can be easily confined in a smooth-sided container such as an aquarium; a cardboard box will suffice short-term in a pinch. Use of cage rest in any other situation will be accompanied by an overall reduction in rate of success, and clinicians are advised to consider the use of active management modalities as detailed below.

Nonsurgical Fracture Management: Coaptation[5]

Coaptation is most commonly used for initial or temporary fracture immobilization, providing short-term immobilization of wings and stabilization of leg fractures distal to the midpoint of the tibiotarsus as a temporary measure before surgical fixation. It can also be the preferred definitive (final) management technique in select cases such as very small birds or birds that are not good surgical candidates and do not require full flight (Table 21-1). Specific fractures for which it is considered the preferred management method include shoulder girdle fractures, metacarpal fractures, and tarsometatarsal fractures of small birds.[5-7] A variety of coaptive methods have been used to manage fractures in avian patients. Many of these methods, such as the Robert Jones bandage, Schroeder-Thomas splints, and spica splints, are modifications from mammalian techniques that have been applied to birds. Others, such as the figure-of-8 wrap, body wrap, and Altman tape splint, are unique to birds. In addition, a wide variety of products have been used to create splints, including syringe cases, moldable thermoplastic, and moldable padded aluminum strips.[8]

The major goals of applying any bandage are to provide protection and support for the injured area. Bandages can also provide prophylactic covering of vulnerable anatomy and be an integral part of the treatment in traumatic fractures with associated soft tissue trauma. Additional advantages of coaptation are that the required materials are relatively inexpensive and that most bandages are easily applied, requiring minimal effort to learn proper technique.

The use of coaptation alone for fracture management is often accompanied by poorer outcomes and difficult complications. In most avian fracture cases, the chances of achieving and maintaining functional alignment are poor when managed with coaptation. Certain applications of coaptation are to be avoided. These include, for instance, attempts to stabilize a

femoral fracture or a fracture in the proximal third of the tibiotarsus with a variation of a Robert Jones splint. These splints do not achieve the necessary joint immobilization of either the hip or the stifle. As a result, this violates the basic bandaging tenet of immobilizing the joints proximal and distal to a fracture, and will result in an exaggerated application of bending and torsional forces to the fracture site. In such cases, a hip-spica splint made from moldable materials is the better option. The figure-of-8 bandage applied to the wing can lead to compression, contraction, and dysfunction of the patagium, the leading edge of the wing between the shoulder and the carpus, if wrapped too tightly or not removed every 2 to 3 days for physical therapy of the patagium. Lastly, fractures of the radius and/or ulna that are managed with coaptation have a much higher likelihood of radioulnar synostosis (a bony bridge between the two bones adjacent to the fracture site that forms as a result of inadequate alignment of bone fragments or movement of the bones during healing) than those managed with surgical fixation.[9] A final challenge when using coaptation to stabilize a fracture is that it complicates the use of physical therapy. Stabilizing bandages prohibit normal range of motion and must be removed to perform physical therapy exercises such as passive range of motion. The following section, excerpted from an article on tips for raptor bandaging, highlights bandages that are commonly used in avian fracture management.[5]

Body wrap
A body wrap is used for simple stabilization of the wing and consists of a band of adhesive tape applied directly to the torso of the bird and incorporating the affected wing. Proper application entails holding the wing in its normal at-rest position and extending the hip joints so that the stifles are not unintentionally bound. Placement of the tape should begin mid-keel, with the tape direction moving away from the fractured wing and wrapping once around the torso, and then incorporating the injured wing into the wrap on the second pass around the bird. The direction of the wrapping is important, as crossing the wing in a dorsal to ventral progression effectively folds the wing to the body form. The final tape placement should cross the affected wing at the midpoint between the shoulder and the elbow joint and be centered at the mid-keel level. Care must be taken to ensure sufficient latitude for respiratory movements while remaining snug enough to still hold the wing in place (Figure 21-26). A body wrap can be used alone or in conjunction with a figure-of-8 bandage, and is indicated for temporary stabilization of wing fractures. It may be combined with a figure-of-8 bandage for definitive stabilization of a radius *or* ulna fracture, recognizing the increased risk of synostosis and nonunion relative to surgical repair, and with a metacarpal splint for treatment of distal wing fractures. The authors also have extensive experience with the use of a body wrap and physical therapy for successful management of coracoid and other shoulder girdle fractures (Figure 21-27).

Figure-of-8 bandage
The figure-of-8 bandage encompasses the wing from elbow to carpus and immobilizes the distal wing. It is used to stabilize fractures and support soft tissues of the wing distal to the elbow, and may also be used with reduced elbow luxations

TABLE 21-1
Recommended Methods of Fixation

Bone	Preferred Fixation	Alternative Fixations
Coracoid	Coaptation	
Humerus	ESF-IM Tie-in	IM Pin, Type I ESF
Ulna	ESF-IM Tie-in	IM Pin, Type I ESF
Radius	IM pin	
Metacarpus	Type I fixator	Curved-edge splint
Femur	ESF-IM Tie-in	IM Pin
Tibiotarsus	ESF-IM Tie-in, T	Type II fixator
Metatarsus	Splint	Type III fixator

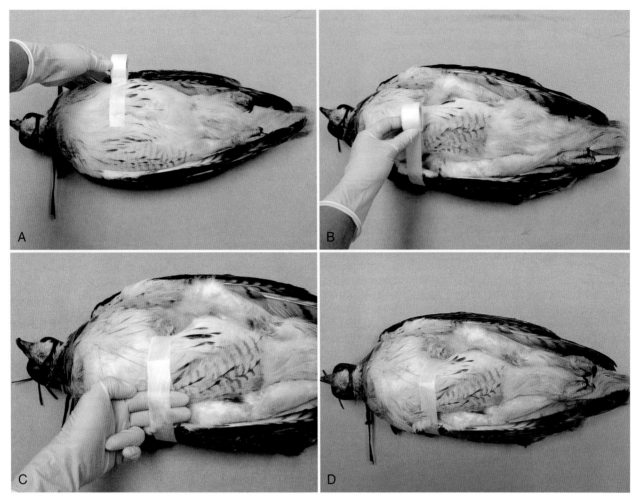

FIGURE 21-26 Application of a body wrap: Beginning mid-keel **(A)**, the tape is passed away from the injured wing **(B)** and wrapped once around the body with the second wrap incorporating the injured wing **(C)**. Final wrap should be snug, but not tight **(D)**.

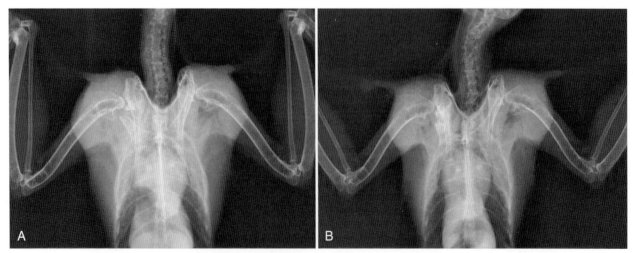

FIGURE 21-27 Radiographs of a merlin with a right coracoid fracture at admission **(A)** and prerelease **(B)**.

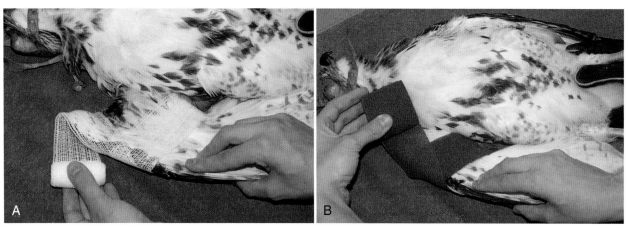

FIGURE 21-28 Application of figure-of-8 bandage to the right wing of a hawk, beginning with a gauze layer **(A)** and following with self-adherent wrap in the same pattern **(B)**.

(Figure 21-28). It is not recommended for humeral fractures due to the distraction pressure it applies to the bone fragments. The bandage is applied in two layers, except in very small birds (<200 g), where only one layer is used to avoid excessive bulk. The first layer is rolled conforming gauze, followed by a second layer of self-adherent bandage material. Beginning with the gauze, the wrap is loosely applied beginning on the body of the wing and unrolling toward the bird's body, crossing the dorsal aspect of the proximal metacarpus. The bandage material should be placed as proximal as possible on the humerus, into the axilla, and should not extend distal to the elbow. After two wraps around the body of the wing, the bandage material is passed across the dorsal wing and looped around the carpus loosely. This establishes the figure-of-8 pattern around the body of the wing and the carpus, which is continued for several wraps using gauze, then repeated with a layer of self-adherent bandage. It is important to note that the wing is immobilized by the bulk of bandaging layers, not the only tightness of the bandage. Complications in the use of the figure-of-8 bandage arise from (1) extended use of the bandage longer than 7 to 10 days, (2) too long an interval between bandage changes (e.g., no more than 2 to 3 days), (3) hyperflexion of the carpus that leads to reduced range of motion, (4) distortion of the patagium that occurs when the bandage is improperly applied so as to compress the leading edge of the wing, (5) overall application of the bandage too tightly, and (6) excessive bulk in very small birds (<100 g).

Curved edge splint

A curved edge splint is used in conjunction with a body wrap to align and stabilize metacarpal fractures (Figure 21-29). A strip of moldable thermoplastic that extends the length from the carpus to the distal phalanx is conformed to the ventral aspect of the metacarpus and folded over the leading edge of the bone. It is important to note that the lateral edge of the splint is bent upward at 90 degrees and does not extend above the plane of the dorsal surface of the wing (i.e., it does not wrap around the carpus). The splint is sandwiched in place with tape covering the distal wing and a body wrap applied. This may be a temporary technique before surgical

stabilization or a definitive repair in cases with minimal displacement. It is important to monitor soft tissue swelling and to adjust the fit as needed.

Modified Robert Jones bandage

This heavily padded bandage is used for temporary stabilization of tibiotarsus and tarsometatarsal fractures in medium to large birds. It is important to stabilize the joint proximal and distal to the fracture, as well as to monitor toes for swelling or coolness. This should be used only for very short-term coaptation. Adequate immobilization requires full extension of the stifle, which is not a normal anatomical positioning in a bird. With the leg fully extended, tape stirrups are applied medially and laterally, extending beyond the foot. The length of the fractured bone and adjoining joints may be wrapped in layers of cotton batting to provide good padding. The leg is then wrapped in rolled gauze with each sequential layer used to tighten the bandage evenly. The tape stirrups are reflected back along the bandage before a final wrap of self-adherent bandage material is applied. Complications resulting from excessive or uneven tightness of the bandage include swelling of the distal limb and impairment of circulation. For fractures in locations where the joints above and below the fracture site cannot be immobilized with this bandage, such as femoral fractures, cage rest in a deep bedding of shredded paper may be a more suitable option.

Tape splint

A tape splint may be used to stabilize tibiotarsus and metatarsus fractures in small birds (<300 g) (Figure 21-30). It is not acceptable for femoral fractures. After reducing the fracture, the tape splint is applied with joints flexed in normal perching position. Strips of porous adhesive tape are overlapped and layered horizontally to create two sheets of tape, which are applied to the medial and lateral aspect of the bird's leg, sandwiching the distal limb. The tape sheets are pinched together as close to the leg as possible, using a hemostat to tighten the tape. Once the tape splint is formed tightly to the leg, the excess tape is trimmed and the completed splint coated in cyanoacrylate such as Vetbond (3M, St Paul, MN) to harden it.

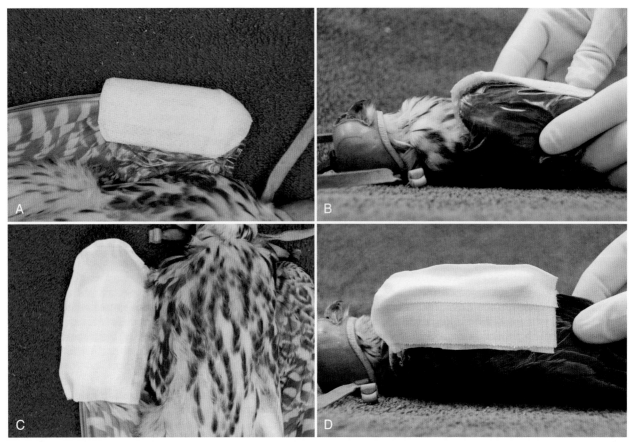

FIGURE 21-29 Curved-edge splint made from moldable thermoplastic. A piece of thermoplastic is cut to the length of the metacarpus and molded to the ventral aspect of the bone **(A)** with a right-angle bend covering the leading edge of the bone **(B)**. The splint is sandwiched in place using overlapping pieces of adhesive tape applied ventrally **(C)** and dorsally **(D)**.

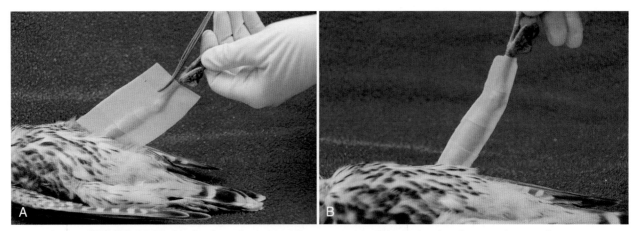

FIGURE 21-30 Application of a tape splint to a tarsometatarsus, showing two layers of tape sandwiching the injured leg **(A)**. Final splint after trimming and hardening with cyanoacrylate **(B)**.

Surgical Fracture Management

To achieve the goal of returning a bird to normal function in the shortest amount of time and with the greatest certainty of outcome, surgical management is the treatment of choice for most avian fractures. A well-constructed fixation device should be rigid, lightweight, versatile, and removable Ideally, the device should stabilize the forces that apply tension, torsion, shearing, and bending movements to bone, and also provide load sharing with the fracture, where possible, or assume entire load-bearing where not. Application of fixation should follow the principle of minimally invasive surgery, thereby preserving soft tissues. The surgeon should strive for spatial alignment of the main bone fragments with components of the fixation, preferably engaging the bone away from the fracture site. Bone fragments that have no soft tissue attachments should be removed to prevent sequestrum formation, while those with attachments should be left in place to function similarly to a vascularized graft. Finally, an ideal device will not restrict range of motion of the limb and will allow passive physical therapy and limited return to function. Three basic surgical fixation techniques and their applications in avian orthopedics are presented here.

Intramedullary pin

An intramedullary pin provides excellent opposition to the bending forces of a long bone and is applied relatively easily. Because of its inability to resist torsional, compressive, and tensile forces, the IM pin is typically used with coaptation. While this provides additional stabilization, coaptation also inhibits normal range of motion and access for physical therapy during the healing process. There is also risk of the pin falling out or being pulled out by the patient if it is not secured in some manner. The most common use of a single intramedullary pin in an avian long bone fracture is in the radius, and it is a key element in the hybrid fixator (see below). Capitalizing on the curved anatomy of most avian long bones, the intramedullary pin is typically inserted in such a way as to avoid joint involvement, and is passed normograde where possible to reduce soft tissue disruption at the fracture site. An intramedullary pin can be inserted retrograde (humerus, femur) so long as it exits at the proximal end or normograde (humerus, ulna, tibiotarsus); when done in a closed fashion, normograde insertion can significantly reduce the amount of overall morbidity necessarily associated with open reduction surgery. Retrograde insertion into the proximal ulna or the distal humerus where the pin exits at the elbow joint is strictly contraindicated. Insertion into the tibiotarsus requires lateral displacement of the patellar tendon. Penetration of the stifle joint, while unavoidable, has not proven detrimental. Lastly, experience has shown that use of cerclage to align fragments in oblique fractures is also contraindicated in avian orthopedics, as it frequently leads to loss of bone viability and sequestrum formation in the author's experience. A more successful outcome will be achieved by leaving bone fragments with soft tissue attachments in place and using a more robust fixator apparatus to achieve rigid stabilization.

External skeletal fixator

Type I, II, and III external skeletal fixators (ESF) can be used in birds. In general, they are very good at resisting rotational movement as well as compressive or tensile forces, and have moderate capacity to oppose bending if sufficiently robust. A partially threaded, positive-profile ESF half-pin (IMEX Veterinary Inc., Texas, USA), designed for birds, provides good cortical anchoring. A critical objective in building the fixator is to ensure that the threaded end of each ESF pin engages both bone cortices. These pins also have a central roughened area on the shaft designed to provide a good bonding surface for acrylic materials, which are used for the connecting system in place of stainless steel bar and clamps to reduce fixator weight. If these are not available, a conventionally threaded K-wire may be substituted; preferably, the use of a non-threaded pin should be avoided.

External skeletal fixators are used in situations where a hybrid fixator (see below) cannot be used due to inability to insert an intramedullary pin without joint impingement in bones lacking an intramedullary cavity (e.g., tarsometatarsus), or where fractures are highly comminuted with significant soft tissue compromise. Metacarpal fractures are very amenable to a Type I ESF, as are some ulna fractures. A Type II fixator can be used for metatarsal fractures in raptors and other large birds. Application of a Type II to the tibiotarsus (a type I is not adequately robust) requires modification on the medial side to avoid conflict with the body wall. For definitive fixation with an ESF, a minimum of two ESF pins must be placed in each fracture segment to assure fixator integrity. Transarticular configurations may be used to stabilize periarticular fractures of the proximal ulna, distal humerus, distal femur, and proximal tibiotarsus.[10] For transarticular fixations, the pins should span the length of the bone. If they do not, they can create a stress riser, and the bone can fracture through a fixation pin track. This is especially a problem in long-legged birds. One pin should be close to each end of the bone, and the other pin should be as close to the fracture as possible for the best fracture stabilization.

A variant of the external skeletal fixator, a ring fixator, was used effectively to repair a long-standing nonunion tibiotarsal fracture with substantial bone loss in a yellow-naped Amazon parrot.[11] In this case, the device allowed periodic lengthening of the limb as new bone formed in a process referred to as bone transport osteogenesis. Transport osteogenesis has also been used to re-establish limb length in two raptor cases in the absence of bone graft options.[12]

The hybrid fixator

The most versatile and effective system for long-bone fixation in birds is a hybrid system known as the external skeletal fixator-intramedullary (ESF-IM) pin tie-in (Figure 21-31).[4,13] This system is inexpensive, easily learned, lightweight, adaptable, and very effective in most cases. The fixator construction consists of an intramedullary pin, two ESF pins, and an external connecting bar that joins these components. The technique for the insertion of the intramedullary pin component of the ESF-IM tie-in is as described above to avoid joint impairment. Where possible, the pin is inserted in a normograde fashion. Once the fracture is reduced and the IM pin inserted, the two ESF pins are placed in the proximal and distal segments of the bone; care must be taken that each ESF pin engages both cortices. The ESF-IM tie-in is completed by bending the IM pin 90 degrees and aligning it with the

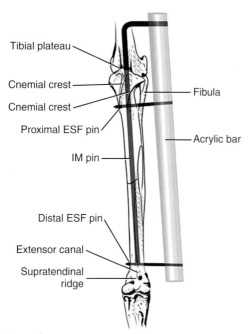

Tibial plateau

Cnemial crest

Cnemial crest

Proximal ESF pin

IM pin

Fibula

Acrylic bar

Distal ESF pin

Extensor canal

Supratendinal ridge

FIGURE 21-31 Diagram of an external skeletal fixator/intramedullary pin tie-in (ESF-IM tie-in) applied to a tibiotarsus.

ESF pins. With a Penrose drain as a mold, an acrylic connecting bar is created, connecting all three pins. Various available materials are suitable for the acrylic bar, including horsehoof repair acrylic (Technovit, Jorvet; Acrylix, IMEX, Dallas). Once completed, this construct has incredible strength and integrity, resisting all forces on the bone.[14] Additional ESF

pins can be added to the structure in cases where additional load-bearing needs to be handled by the fixation. As healing progresses, sequential dismantling of the fixator allows transfer of load sharing to the bone, promoting bone healing[15] (Figure 21-32).

The ESF-IM tie-in is effective for most diaphyseal long-bone fractures in birds, as described, and can be adapted for more proximal or distal fractures using cross-pinning techniques. A commercially available form of a hybrid fixator marketed as the Fixateur Externe du Service de Santé des Armées (FESSA) system, or tubular system, is available from United States (Jorgensen Labs, Loveland, CO) and European suppliers. In place of an acrylic bar is a stainless steel tube drilled with holes for the ESF pins and orthogonally drilled holes that contain locking set-screws. Its utility in repair of tibiotarsal fractures in falcons and across a number of avian species and cases has been demonstrated.[16,17]

Plates and nails

Plates have been used with varying degrees of success in repairing avian fractures. Available information derives predominately from individual case reports. The novel use of an externally applied locking compression plate as an ESF connector bar, and its associated cortical screws, was reported successful in managing a tarsometatarsal fracture in an eagle.[18] An interlocking nail was used successfully to repair a tibiotarsal fracture in a bald eagle.[19] Controlled studies to evaluate the utility of various miniplate systems for fracture management in pigeons (Columba livia) are increasingly defining important aspects unique and important to utilization of plates, but must be currently regarded as a work in progress.[20,21] Limitations include lack of suitably sized plates and nails to accommodate the wide range of bone sizes

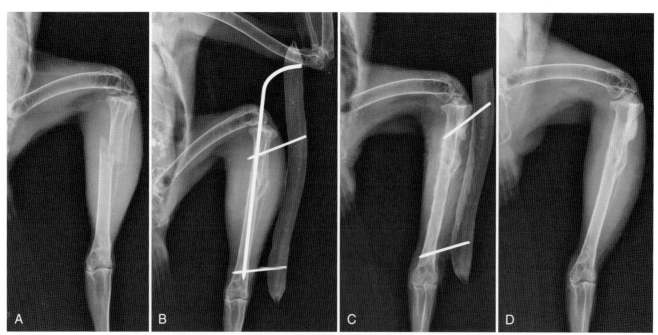

FIGURE 21-32 Radiographs showing progression of a tibiotarsal fracture in a red-tailed hawk. Admission radiograph **(A)**, fracture fixation with an ESF-IM tie-in apparatus **(B)**, deconstruction of the fixation by removal of IM pin **(C)**, and final resolution **(D)**.

encountered across the spectrum of avian species, lack of strength of the small plates to accommodate applied forces, morbidity associated with their placement, including ischemic necrosis of the skin pulled over the plate at closure, and also the expense.

CONVALESCENT CARE OF THE FRACTURE PATIENT

Pain Management

Recommendations for pain management in different bird species are changing rapidly in the field of avian medicine as new research increases our knowledge of pharmacokinetics and effectiveness. Multimodal therapy is recognized to have greater efficacy on pain management with less chance of negative side effects or toxicity (see Chapter 20). Opioids are indicated for moderate or severe pain in birds, especially in initial management and perioperatively in surgical cases (see Chapter 20). Although fairly short-acting, butorphanol[22] is commonly used in birds. Buprenorphine, which has a slower onset and longer duration, is increasingly being used, particularly in birds of prey. Nonsteroidal antiinflammatory drugs (NSAIDs) have both antiinflammatory and analgesic effects with substantially longer duration than opioids. NSAIDs used routinely in avian medicine include meloxicam[22] and carprofen.[22] Several studies have demonstrated extensive species variability in metabolism of all of these drugs. As pain management in avian species is an area of active research with new information routinely being published, the reader is encouraged to refer to recent literature in this area (see Chapter 20).[23]

Patient Management

Prevention of new trauma is a key concern immediately postoperatively. Patients should be adequately restrained during anesthetic recovery and not returned to a cage until fully able to balance and control their activity. The recovery cage should be prepared by removing or lowering any perching and providing a padded cage bottom. Many birds are less anxious when able to perch, yet are too unsteady to safely climb and perch postoperatively. A rolled-up towel or wooden dowel covered in self-adherent wrap on the bottom of the cage floor can be used to allow safe perching. Climbing should be prevented by using a solid-sided cage, which should be placed in a low-stress environment away from dogs, cats, humans, and any other predators. The use of low light and limited visibility will also encourage quiet recovery. Many patients will benefit from supplemental heat. A quiet, warm (85° to 90° F) environment with easy access for observation is ideal. In raptors, attention should be paid to preservation of flight feathers; it is routine to use a tail protector to prevent breakage of the rectrices during convalescence in most species (Figure 21-33).

Surgical patients should be re-evaluated 24 hours postoperatively for wound care and fixator integrity. Pin tracts should be cleaned of dried exudate. In the case of surgically repaired wing fractures, a body wrap should be kept in place for several days postoperatively until the bird can support the wing itself. With adequate fixation, it is usually possible to remove the body wrap within a week and allow the patient to

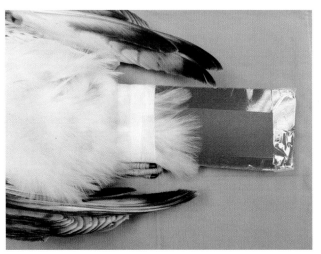

FIGURE 21-33 A tail protector made from a plastic file folder is fashioned to fit the tail. The retrices are inserted between two layers that have been taped together to form a pocket. The completed tail protector is taped to the covert feathers ventrally and dorsally.

return to normal range of motion on its own. Physical therapy in the form of passive range of motion should be initiated at the first postoperative check (see next section).

As with any patient, nutritional support is critical. Many avian patients are nutritionally compromised when presented for treatment. Wild birds may have been down and unable to eat for several days or weeks before presentation, and captive birds, while well fed, are often likely to be on nutritionally inadequate diets. Calcium and vitamins A and D_3 may be marginal or deficient in companion birds that eat only seeds and may need to be supplemented.

Diets designed for critical care are important initially, but getting the patient to self-feed on species-appropriate food items reduces stress in the long term. The immediate postoperative phase is not the time to do long-term diet correction in a companion bird. Also, consideration must be given to the patient's ability to access food, grasp and manipulate it, and eat. For example, raptor patients with leg fractures require cut-up food, especially if protective bandaging is applied to the contralateral foot to prevent bumblefoot. Some wild species such as osprey are notorious for not eating in captivity unless coaxed using operant learning methods. The clinician should work closely with a knowledgeable rehabilitator on nutritional support of wild birds.

Physical Therapy

Physical therapy includes a variety of noninvasive treatment modalities that encourage normal physiological function when applied appropriately. The goals of physical therapy are to promote mobility and joint range of motion, improve circulation to injured limb, maintain soft tissue integrity, and reduce the recovery time required after surgery or trauma. Although the need to treat soft tissue wounds and other concurrent issues may require a more frequent treatment schedule, the orthopedic patient should be examined a minimum of twice weekly during the first 2 weeks; during these sessions, it

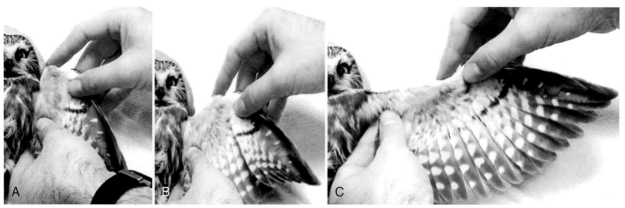

FIGURE 21-34 A northern saw-whet owl undergoing physiotherapy of the left wing. While the metacarpus and elbow are held, the wing is flexed **(A)** and moved through its range of motion **(B)** to complete extension **(C)**.

should also receive gentle passive physical therapy to maintain or increase range of motion of the affected limb.

As soon as possible, coaptation such as body and wing wraps should be removed, allowing the limb to return to normal function. These can normally be removed a few days after surgery, except in the case of metacarpal fractures, where additional support is required due to the weight of fixation at the end of the wing. If fixation allows for normal use of the limb with no coaptation, the requirement for physiotherapy is greatly reduced. Physiotherapy is often carried out under inhalant gas anesthesia with the addition of an analgesic to reduce responses to pain and to avoid unwanted movement. The limb is extended and held in a gentle stretch several times over a 5-minute period (Figure 21-34). Each joint is evaluated for range of motion relative to the normal limb. Soft tissues such as the patagium are stretched and massaged to prevent contraction of their elastic fibers; any portions showing signs of fibrotic condensation should be gently stretched to break down the fibrotic fibers. Initially, range of motion may be limited, but over a period of about 3 weeks with twice-a-week therapy, it can be restored, in most instances.

Monitoring of Healing and Dynamic Destabilization

As healing progresses, the ability to sequentially dismantle the surgical device (dynamic destabilization) allows load sharing to be increasingly shifted to the bone, promoting bone healing. Radiographs should be taken at 10 to 14 days and 20 to 24 days postoperatively, and biweekly thereafter until fracture is healed. Staged deconstruction should begin when early signs of callus formation at the fracture site are seen radiographically. Both ESF and ESF-IM tie-in fixators have the potential for sequential deconstruction. Type II ESF fixators can be changed to Type I fixators by the removal of one external bar, effectively reducing the rigidity of the construction. Continued deconstruction can occur with reduction of the number of ESF pins several days later. Any pins showing signs of loosening should be the first to be removed. With an ESF-IM tie-in apparatus, dismantling of the fixator construction can start with cutting the linkage between the IM pin and the external bar. Subsequent steps can include removal of the IM pin, reduction of the number of ESF pins, and removal of the ESF.

ORTHOPEDIC COMPLICATIONS

Regular evaluation of the orthopedic patient during healing will facilitate early detection of orthopedic complications, enable quicker interventions, and increase potential for successful outcomes. In the experience of the authors, the most common orthopedic complications seen in avian patients are loose fixator pins, radioulnar synostosis, sequestration of dead bone, and osteomyelitis.

During rechecks, the fixation apparatus should be monitored for loosening of pins or exudate around pin tracts/surgical sites. The presence of a radiolucent halo at the intersection of a fixation pin and bone is a good indication of pin loosening. Loose pins should be removed promptly, followed by rebuilding the fixation if resulting rigidity is inadequate for the phase of fracture healing, or by beginning the fixator deconstruction if more appropriate.

As noted previously, there is a high probability of synostosis formation between the distal radius and ulna fractures, especially if the radius is not stabilized. The development of synostosis will limit rotation at the radius/ulna and extension of the wing. The bony bridge formed can be relatively easily removed using rongeurs or an osteotome. Placement of bone wax or a fat pad (harvested from the subcutaneous tissue in the abdominal area) between the radius and ulna after the removal of the bony bridge will deter recurrence.[9]

In comminuted fractures, bony fragments that have lost their soft tissue connections will frequently develop into sequestra. Bone that has been externalized will often become dry, dirty, and devitalized. It can be difficult to determine the viability of these ends of long bones. Radiographic evidence of a sequestrum can be seen around 3 weeks into the healing process and will present as a radiolucent area around a bone fragment or segment of bone. Oftentimes, new callus formation can be seen trying to bridge around the sequestrum. This new bone formation is often of poor integrity. The presence of a sequestrum will delay or impair fracture healing and may be the cause of a draining tract. Surgical removal is recommended as soon as the extent of the sequestrum is clear. After debridement of all devitalized bone and tissue, bone edges should be freshened and fixation adjusted as required for stability.

The presence of exudate around pins or signs of inflammation are indications of potential secondary infection and should be pursued diagnostically, including culture and sensitivity, as well as therapeutically. A sample for culture can be collected by fine-needle aspiration if indicated from the area of infection. Besides indications of osteomyelitis on radiological exam, the patient may have an elevated white blood cell count and present nonspecific clinical signs such as anorexia or wing droop. Oftentimes, poor wound or bone healing will be present and, in some cases, a draining tract may occur. Broad-spectrum antibiotics that achieve high concentration in bone, such as clindamycin (50 mg/kg q12h, PO, or 100 mg/kg q24h, PO), should be used if osteomyelitis is suspected. Removal of surgically embedded fixation such as an IM pin may be necessary to control the infection. If so, culture and sensitivity of the removed pin will allow more strategic antimicrobial choice. Depending on the stage of healing, external fixation or coaptation may need to be added when internal fixation is removed.

SUMMARY

Managing fractures in the avian patient is based on the same principles as mammalian orthopedics, with some adjustments made to meet the unique characteristics of birds. The best outcomes will be achieved when close attention is paid to soft tissue preservation, when there is early and rigid stabilization of the fracture, and when the fixation maximizes opportunity for the patient to maintain range of motion and use of the limb. The clinician has the option of using cage rest, coaptation, or surgical fixation, depending on the characteristics of the individual situation and the desired outcome.

REFERENCES

1. Piermattei DL, Flo GL, DeCamp CE: *Brinker, Piermattei, and Flo's handbook of small animal orthopedics and fracture repair,* ed 4, St. Louis, 2006, Saunders/Elsevier.
2. de Matos R: Calcium metabolism in birds, *Vet Clin North Am Exot Anim Pract* 11(1):59–82, 2008.
3. Tully TN: Basic avian bone growth and healing, *Vet Clin North Am Exot Anim Pract* 5:23–30, 2002.
4. Redig PT, Cruz L: The avian skeleton and fracture management, a sub-section in trauma-related medical conditions. In Samour J, editor: *Avian medicine,* ed 2, London, 2008, Elsevier, pp 215–248.
5. Bueno-Padilla I, Arent LR, Ponder JB: Tips for raptor bandaging, *Exotic DVM* 12(3):29–47, 2011.
6. Redig PT, Nicolas Francisco O, Froembling M, et al: Coracoid fracture management in raptors: assessment of conservative approach. In *Proceedings. 30th Annu Meet Assoc Avian Vet* 351–352, 2009.
7. Murray M: Management of metacarpal fractures in free-living raptors. In *Proceedings. 33rd Annu Meet Assoc Avian Vet* 283–284, 2012.
8. Redig PT: Evaluation and non-surgical management of avian fractures. In Harrison JG, Harrison LR, editors: *Clinical avian medicine and surgery,* Philadelphia, 1986, Saunders, pp 380–394.
9. Beaufrere H, Ammersbach M, Nevarez J, et al: Successful treatment of a radioulnar synostosis in a Mississippi kite (*Ictinia mississippiensis*), *J Avian Med Surg* 26(2):94–100, 2012.
10. Rosenthal K, Hillyer E, Matheissen D: Stifle luxation in a Moluccan cockatoo and a barn owl, *J Avian Med Surg* 8(4):173–178, 1994.
11. Johnston MS, Thode HO, Ehrhart NP: Bone transport osteogenesis for reconstruction of a bone defect in the tibiotarsus of a yellow-naped Amazon parrot (*Amazona ochrocephala auropalliata*), *J Avian Med Surg* 22(1):47–56, 2008.
12. Ponder JB, Anderson GM, Bueno-Padilla IB: Distraction osteogenesis in two wild raptor species. In *Proceedings. 33rd Annu Meet Assoc Avian Vet* 43–44, 2012.
13. Redig PT: The use of an external skeletal fixator-intramedullary pin tie-in fixator for treatment of long bone fractures in raptors. In Lumeij JT, Poffers J, editors: *Raptor biomedicine III,* Lake Worth, Fla, 2000, Zoological Education Network, pp 239–254.
14. Van Wettere AJ, Redig PT, Wallace LJ, et al: Mechanical evaluation of external skeletal fixator-intramedullary pin tie-in configurations applied to cadaveral humeri from red-tailed hawks (*Buteo jamaicensis*), *J Avian Med Surg* 23(4):277–285, 2009.
15. Egger EL: External skeletal fixation – general principles. In Slatter DH, editor: *Textbook of small animal surgery,* ed 2, Philadelphia, 1993, WB Saunders, pp 1641–1656.
16. Hatt JM, Christen C, Sandmeier P: Clinical application of an external fixator in the repair of bone fractures in 28 birds, *Vet Rec* 160:188–194, 2007.
17. Muller M, Nafeez JM: Use of the FixEx Tubulaire Type F.E.S.S.A System for tibiotarsal fractures in falcons, *Falco* 29:25–29, 2007.
18. Montgomery RD, Crandall E, Bellah JR: Use of a locking compression plate as an external fixator for repair of a tarsometatarsal fracture in a bald eagle (*Haliaeetus leucocephalus*), *J Avian Med Surg* 25:119–125, 2011.
19. Hollamby S, Dejardin LM, Sikarskie JG, et al: Tibiotarsal fracture repair in a bald eagle (*Haliaeetus leucocephalus*) using an interlocking nail, *J Zoo Wildl Med* 35(1):77–81, 2004.
20. Christen C, Fischer I, von Rechenberg B, et al: Evaluation of a maxillofacial miniplate 1.0 for stabilization of the ulna in experimentally induced ulnar and radial fractures in pigeons (*Columba livia*), *J Avian Med Surg* 19(3):185–190, 2005.
21. Gull JM, Saveraid TC, Szabo D, et al: Evaluation of three miniplate systems for fracture stabilization in pigeons (*Columba livia*), *J Avian Med Surg* 26(4):203–212, 2012.
22. Hawkins MG, Barron HW, Speer BL, et al: Birds. In Carpenter JW, Marion CJ, editors: *Exotic animal formulary,* ed 4, St. Louis, 2013, Elsevier Saunders, pp 183–437.
23. Paul-Murphy J: Pain management. In Harrison GJ, Lightfoot TL, editors: *Clinical avian medicine,* Palm Beach, Fla, 2006, Spix Publishing, pp 233–240.

CHAPTER 22

Advancements in Management of the Welfare of Avian Species

Joanne Paul-Murphy • V. Wensley Koch • Jeleen A. Briscoe • Claudia M. Vinke
• Nico J. Schoemaker • Franck L.B. Meijboom • Yvonne R.A. van Zeeland
• Nienke Endenburg • Cheryl B. Greenacre

FOUNDATIONS IN AVIAN WELFARE

Joanne Paul-Murphy

WHAT IS AVIAN WELFARE?

Veterinarians in many countries take an oath to ensure or protect animal health and welfare, including the welfare of birds. This oath extends to companion birds; birds in captive environments such as farms, zoos, breeding facilities, sanctuaries, and research institutions; and free-ranging birds. It is often stated that the fundamental goals of avian veterinary medicine overlap with avian welfare concerns, but not everyone is familiar with what is involved in the protection of avian welfare. Avian clinicians are very familiar with methods to determine the health and wellness of a bird, which is certainly a very important component of a bird's welfare; however, the ability to assess welfare is something veterinarians are recognizing as an important aspect of their stewardship. Veterinarians have a responsibility to their avian patients and, as advocates for birds, to work toward maximizing their welfare. In the larger perspective, each person has an effect on avian welfare, from how we treat birds under our care, to the organizations we support for avian conservation, or even the choices we make when we purchase bird food.

Societies' concern for animal welfare includes an expectation for avian veterinarians to be able to consider concepts and standards that are determined for all animals and apply these specifically to birds. Knowledge of the veterinary commitment to welfare includes familiarity with the American Veterinary Medical Association's Animal Welfare Principles developed in 2006 (https://www.avma.org/KB/Policies/Pages/AVMA-Animal-Welfare-Principles.aspx). In addition, awareness of contributions made by veterinary specialty

organizations to animal welfare in several countries, including the European College of Animal Welfare and Behavior Management (http://www.ecawbm.org/), the American College of Animal Welfare (www.acaw.org), and The Australian and New Zealand College of Veterinary Scientists Animal Welfare Chapter (http://www.anzcvs.org.au/info/chapters/#4), is necessary.

Animal welfare has many definitions that have evolved as the science of animal welfare has advanced. If the term *animal* is exchanged for the single order of vertebrates called *avian*, the definition of welfare remains constant. The American College of Animal Welfare had the following definition adopted in 2010: "Animal welfare refers to the state of the animal. An assessment of welfare includes consideration of the animal's health, behavior, and biological function" (http://www.acaw.org/animal_welfare_principles.html). The World Organization for Animal Health (OIE) defines an animal as having good welfare if it is "healthy, comfortable, well nourished, safe, able to express innate behavior, and if it is not suffering from unpleasant states such as pain, fear and distress. Good animal welfare requires disease prevention and veterinary treatment, appropriate shelter, management, nutrition, humane handling and humane slaughter/killing" (OIE, 2010; Terrestrial Animal Health Code 2012 Volume 1, Article 7.1.1, http://www.oie.int/doc/ged/D7597.PDF). Avian veterinarians are well trained in addressing most of the physical aspects of avian welfare as defined by the OIE; however, the definition of welfare includes the bird's psychological well-being, which requires advanced training and experience to evaluate.

At the heart of welfare definitions is the understanding that the welfare of a bird belongs to the bird. Welfare refers to a characteristic of the individual animal rather than something given to the animal by people.[1] It is about the subjective state of the bird, including what is and is not good in the bird's life (see section on "As Free as a Bird on the Wing: Some Welfare and Ethical Considerations on Flight Restraint Methods in Birds"). Because welfare belongs to the individual bird, it may differ between different animals, even when provided the exact same conditions, and the welfare of the same bird may change as the bird ages. Avian welfare considers both physical and mental wellness of the bird. The welfare of a species can result in different conclusions dependent on the goal of keeping an animal. An animal that stays in zoos its whole life requires different skills from an animal that is kept for reintroduction into the natural environment for conservation.[2]

Avian welfare is *not* about what humans think is right and wrong for birds or society's view of what is acceptable for birds—those are ethical issues. Disagreements about avian welfare are often generated when people confuse scientific questions about the welfare of birds with ethical questions about how we think we *should* treat and care for birds. It is difficult to define animal welfare in a purely scientific manner, because much of the development of animal welfare science has grown out of a response to public concerns regarding the ethical treatment of animals. Humans are using animals for their own purposes, including companionship. Therefore it is an ethical decision to accept the responsibility to care for animals, including an obligation to ensure that the welfare of the animals is the best that can be provided. Humans have tremendous influence on avian welfare and often our conviction to ensure welfare for birds, either captive or free ranging, can invoke ethical dilemmas where conflicting responsibilities must be considered for decisions affecting the care and use of birds.

Veterinarians often assume the role as the birds' advocate, but may also have obligations to the client, caregivers, peers within the profession, society, and themselves. Ethical challenges may arise when these commitments conflict. As an avian veterinarian, it helps to be mindful that it is an ethical decision to prevent poor welfare and to promote good welfare of birds. Different stakeholders will place importance on different aspects of a bird's welfare. Welfare for the captive or wild bird is always a compromise among several factors, and there is not a single combination of variables that can claim to be the perfect model for the best avian welfare. The critical issue is to prevent the preventable, and every individual

BOX 22-1 THE FIVE FREEDOMS

1. Freedom from thirst, hunger, and malnutrition—by ready access to fresh water and a diet to maintain full health and vigor.
2. Freedom from discomfort—by providing an appropriate environment including shelter and a comfortable resting area.
3. Freedom from pain, injury, and disease—by prevention or rapid diagnosis and treatment.
4. Freedom to express normal behavior—by providing sufficient space, proper facilities, and company of the animal's own kind.
5. Freedom from fear and distress—by ensuring conditions and treatment that avoid mental suffering.

Adapted from Council FAW: *Farm animal welfare in Great Britain: past, present and future*, London, 2009.[8]

BOX 22-2 RE-INTERPRETATION AND ADAPTATION OF THE FIVE FREEDOMS BY THE UNITED KINGDOM'S ANIMAL WELFARE ACT OF 2006

1. Need for a suitable environment
2. Need for a suitable diet
3. Need to be able to exhibit normal behavior patterns
4. Need for the company of, or to be apart from, other animals
5. Need to be protected against pain, suffering, injury, and disease

From Animal Welfare Act of 2006.

who interacts with animals—which is most of us—needs to understand and accept his responsibility in delivering animal welfare, whether it is a laboratory animal, pet animal, farm animal, or wild animal.[3]

Many welfare definitions refer to an explanation put forth by the Farm Animal Welfare Council in 1979 as the Five Freedoms (Box 22-1). This definition was originally developed for agricultural animals, but now underlies the legislation and standards guiding not only farm and laboratory operations, but also zoological institutions.[4-7]

Avian welfare principles are consistent with the internationally recognized Five Freedoms; birds must be provided food, water, proper handling, health care, and environments appropriate to their species and use, and should be cared for in ways that prevent and minimize fear, pain, distress, and suffering. Current attitudes have transformed the Five Freedoms into a focus on satisfying needs, leading to lists of what aspects are crucial to the animal's welfare rather than identifying the negative. It seems more sensible to have a discussion of "providing food" than of "preventing malnutrition" or "hunger." In this way the provision of stimulation and freedom from boredom can be part of the same discussion.[9]

To view animal welfare as interacting domains, the Five Freedoms have been reinterpreted and adapted by the United Kingdom's Animal Welfare Act of 2006 (Box 22-2).[10] The Animal Welfare Act also places an extra imperative on training veterinarians and places a legal duty of care on animal owners. This means that those with responsibility for animals are legally bound to provide for their needs.[11]

Good welfare is not just the absence of negative experiences such as pain, fear, or disease but also depends on the bird having positive experiences, and the absence of positive experiences may compromise a bird's welfare. Minimizing the negative components addressed in the Five Freedoms can provide opportunities for a bird. Welfare is a continuum, and the bird's overall welfare status is affected by the bird's subjective experiences, although these are difficult to assess. Good welfare may include the animal's ability to experience vitality, companionship, contentment, satiety, happiness, curiosity, exploration, foraging, and play.[12] This last statement tries to account for the subjective feelings of animals, with freedom from the unpleasant subjective feelings of suffering and pain, using qualitative approaches to evaluate animal behavior.

ANIMAL WELFARE SCIENCE

Animal welfare as a science is recognized and supported by international peer-reviewed journals, numerous books, organizations, research departments, academic courses, and degree programs specific to the science of animal welfare. Animal welfare courses have been incorporated into the core curriculum of many veterinary schools. Inclusion of scientific information about animal welfare in university and training courses changes attitudes and practices, generally resulting in improved welfare for animals, which hopefully translates into improving avian welfare.

Animal welfare science applies rigorous scientific methods using a variety of behavioral or physiological measures as indicators of animal welfare for the purpose of providing objective data. The goal of animal welfare science is to develop methods for assessing and improving the welfare of animals in a variety of settings including laboratories, zoos, farms, shelters, and private homes. A clearly defined concept of welfare is needed for use in precise scientific measurements, in legal documents, and in public statements or discussion.[13] However, in the scientific literature, an explicit definition of welfare is difficult to identify. In most cases, a feeling of consensus is assumed about what welfare means, which is unfortunate because significant differences between the definitions results in differences in the selection and use of welfare indicators.[2] For example, in many zoo animal investigations, use of a naturalistic definition of animal welfare is preferred for the following reasons: the performance of species-typical behavior is emphasized in zoos, comparative research that examines species both in the wild and in captivity provides important insights into this definition, the definition is intuitively appealing to the public, and captive animals often fail to adapt to the zoo environment.[14]

The recognition of animal welfare science has resulted in a multidisciplinary approach, distinguishing animal welfare from animal health. The scientific assessment of animal welfare, including animal physical and mental health, has developed rapidly in recent years and the sophistication of these assessments will continue to evolve. Like any science, welfare information is continuously advanced, debated by newer investigations, and refined as it progresses. Emerging research in the area of what constitutes good animal welfare rather than identification of what needs to be avoided may yield constructive information to design best practices.[15]

Assessment measurements are intended to be independent of ethical considerations; however, culture influences how animals are used in a society, which also affects what questions are asked and which welfare issues are engaged in scientific inquiry.[16] The science can influence decisions about ethics, philosophy, sociology, economics, law, and politics. The earliest studies were concerned with assessment of welfare of agricultural animals, which provided general principles applicable to animals in a variety of other situations. Animal scientists and veterinarians have been exploring welfare issues for poultry, which has led to important advancements for the commercial poultry industry. However, the science of animal welfare as it relates to nonpoultry captive and wild birds is an emerging field with contributions from veterinarians, avian biologists, behaviorists, and others for understanding how birds' health, biological functions, behavior, and ability to cope and stabilize during change can be assessed.

BIRDS ARE SENTIENT BEINGS

Public concern about the welfare of animals is increasing rapidly. This has occurred, in part, because of new information and investigations about animal cognitive abilities and a more inclusive approach to the concept of which individuals are sentient. The definition of sentient includes (1) responsiveness to or consciousness of sense impressions (http://www.merriam-webster.com/dictionary/sentient) and (2) the ability to perceive or feel things (http://www.oxforddictionaries.com/us/definition/american_english/sentient).

Human opinion as to which species are sentient has generally changed over time in well-educated societies to encompass first all humans, instead of just a subset of humans, and then certain mammals that were kept as companions; animals that seemed most similar to humans such as monkeys; the larger mammals; all mammals; all warm-blooded animals; then all vertebrates; and now some invertebrates.[17] In general, veterinarians do not need to be convinced that animals, including birds, are sentient beings because they work so closely with them. Avian veterinarians witness how the individual bird responds to sensation, and great advances have been made in understanding the avian sensation of pain and response to relief of pain.[18] The ability of birds to experience pleasure, the opposite of pain, is more challenging to identify; however, feelings and emotions are included in the capacity of a sentient being.

The previous reluctance of science to attribute complex abilities and feelings to nonhumans slowed the gain of knowledge regarding the highly developed brain function in other groups of animals, including birds. Previously, researchers had been unwilling to carry out studies in the area of cognition and sentience because, if they used words such as awareness, feeling, emotion and mood, they risked the scorn of other scientists, which might have created difficulties in obtaining future research funding and in getting papers published.[19]

Training in animal welfare science in addition to avian medicine can provide veterinarians with tools to understand the needs of birds, as viewed from the birds' perspective. Birds may have their basic health needs met and yet still be experiencing significant welfare compromises because of issues such as frustration, boredom, loneliness, and anxiety. Studies to understand and objectively measure emotions and cognition of birds are fraught with challenges. Current understandings of the avian brain organization, homologies, evolution, and function have facilitated a better assimilation of scientific insights into the study of avian brain function.[20] Although the gross structure of avian and mammalian brains is radically different, there are connectional similarities in the brains of these two taxa, which may explain their similar behavior and cognition.[21]

ASSESSMENT OF AVIAN WELFARE

There is a growing interest in developing and implementing animal welfare assessment schemes for farms, zoos, aquaria, laboratories, and even for wild populations.[22] Veterinarians have a responsibility to improve the welfare of birds under their care, which might include birds owned by clients; birds arriving at a shelter, a sanctuary, or a wildlife rehabilitation center; or resident captive birds in aviaries, zoological institutions, rehabilitation centers, sanctuaries, rescue facilities, and foster care. The welfare assessment involves identification of both problems and attributes and application of a system to evaluate the issues, followed by a re-evaluation of the welfare when changes have been made. Welfare assessments are tools that can provide information, which can then help improve health and wellness of the birds plus increase engagement of the caregiver and strengthen the veterinarian's relationships with clients and caregivers.

Welfare assessment of nonpoultry species of birds has not been well established, although advances are being made to assess welfare of collections that include birds. In the zoo literature there is an emphasis on evaluation of animal behavior indicators and indexes, with a stated purpose to start a science-based "dialogue" between the zoo animal and human caretakers, resulting in the creation and maintenance of transparent, quality care and an optimal environment for the zoo animal.[2] Laboratory animal welfare assessments have also included development of guidelines for psittacine birds used in research, addressing welfare concerns related to captive containment, and indications of distress and compromised welfare.[23] Monitoring companion animal welfare is difficult since the population size and demography is unknown and the conditions in which companion animals are kept lack specificity and stability.[24] Frameworks are being developed for assessing welfare of companion animals, primarily horses, dogs, and cats, which may provide a foundation for future assessment for companion birds. Hopefully, efforts will be increased to develop and apply practices for welfare assessment of companion birds.

There are concerns that most veterinarians' skills are focused on evaluation of husbandry and physical attributes of their patients, and additional training may be needed to evaluate animals' behavioral well-being for a thorough welfare assessment. It was recently stated that there is a need for companion animal welfare assessments in a veterinary context, and development of proper instruments for this assessment have become more apparent.[25] While illness can have a negative impact on welfare, the absence of illness does not necessarily mean that welfare is good and emphasizing physical health and ignoring behavioral and mental aspects in the welfare assessment puts the veterinary assessment at risk of being incomplete.[25,26] Veterinary professionals therefore need to become familiar with additional methods and apply a problem-solving approach to convert scientific information into animal welfare assessments and decisions. This inevitably—and beneficially—involves using both emotional processing and logical, comprehensive, and critical reasoning.[27] For example, a veterinary assessment of the severity of an animal's disease can often be based on a set of physical measures with a set of normal ranges, in contrast to the assessment of an animal's welfare, which is based on a wide range of elements to be evaluated, and many of these have no "normal ranges" for reference because an animal's breed, temperament, or "individuality" is so variable. However, the veterinary specialist working with zoological species,

birds, reptiles, amphibians, or fish has developed skills for resource seeking and problem solving and is accustomed to using extrapolation of reference intervals across species. These veterinarians often need to make evaluations using knowledge of species behaviors, in addition to physical findings. These are skills developed by many veterinary professionals; however, in the realm of avian behavior and mental well-being, veterinary specialists with experience working with birds may be the most comfortable and competent.

General Principles of Avian Welfare Assessment

When developing an avian welfare assessment, there are several overreaching principles that have been established that can be applied.

1. A team approach allows input from people with different perspectives of the bird's situation. Identification of who is involved with a team will vary depending on whether it is a companion animal or a collection of birds being assessed. An assessment often receives input from several different individuals and it works best when people in the team are prepared to work together. It is beneficial when all members of the team are familiar with normal behavior for the species of bird(s) and are able to recognize the abnormal.
   - *Caregiver*: This may be an owner or the care staff at an institution—these are the people who observe the bird(s) in the bird's home environment. This is often the person who has daily interactions with the bird and could notice subtle changes in activity, behavior, or food intake. The caregiver can often describe behaviors that the bird may not exhibit to the veterinarian.
   - *Veterinarian*: This is a person with special training to observe and examine the bird's health parameters and should also be familiar with physical attributes specific to the species of bird(s).
   - *Facilities manager*: Managers and curators are people trained to observe a variety of animal species in a facility with an awareness of requirements or compliance with guidelines or protocols. These people are often able to offer advice on improving or avoiding adverse effects on the bird's welfare.
   - *Research investigator*: When the birds are involved in any type of study, the investigators may be collecting specific information that changes over time relative to the birds' welfare. For birds engaged in studies it is often necessary to have an institutional animal care and use protocol reviewed by a committee that can initiate a welfare assessment protocol early in the planning of a project.

2. Consistency between observers, or at least between the veterinarian professionals participating in a welfare assessment of the same individual bird or facility, makes for better follow through and re-evaluation. There is predictable variation between observers; therefore, having the same people observing the birds is helpful. In addition, birds may be able to differentiate between the observers and display different behaviors depending on the level of familiarity with the person making observations. Good communication and records of the observations can aid in reducing the range of variability. Regarding birds involved

in studies or research projects, it is important that all team members understand the purpose of the study and the scientific objectives.

3. Identification of which indicators are to be monitored can be challenging for birds, including which behavioral and physiological parameters can be used as indicators of welfare. It is important to define and monitor the right types and number of indicators. Common errors include having too many parameters, which prolongs the process and makes it less effective, whereas too few may lead to inaccuracies. Setting the baseline is often the most challenging part of a welfare assessment because it involves agreement as to what may be considered the hypothetical "ideal." These concepts will be further developed in the next section.

4. The veterinarian often selects the record system for the welfare information based on what is appropriate for the practice, institution, or facility being evaluated. There are several systems available for recording welfare assessments in other animal facilities, particularly food or laboratory animal facilities, but few are developed for companion animals' welfare assessments. Record systems have predetermined lists of factors to be evaluated. These may be set up to answer with simple binary yes/no responses or may incorporate numerical or ranking scales from good to bad. Numerical scoring systems provide structure to evaluate clinical signs, physical indicators, and behavioral parameters; however, this system requires a subjective value judgment by each assessor.

5. Frequency and timing of welfare assessments are often determined by the degree of deviation from good welfare. Assessments for the companion bird will vary depending on each situation, whereas for large collections of birds the timing and frequency is often established by the number of birds involved and the allocation of resources to provide effective monitoring. Indicators of poor welfare should be determined first and addressed immediately. After specific thresholds are determined, indicators of good welfare can then be used for monitoring. Signs of poor welfare may be more challenging to detect in some species of birds, which could lead to more frequent assessments in hopes of identifying problems early. The age or condition of illness of a companion bird will also affect how frequently health and welfare assessments will be beneficial. With regard to birds involved in a study, often the experimental design affects the frequency and timing of observations. Signs of illness and pain are important initial considerations that would prompt an immediate corrective action if such signs were unexpected, or unrelated to the research.[28,29]

To advance the standards of avian welfare, changes in the animals' welfare state must be assessed and feedback provided, from those working daily with the animals to those responsible for management decisions, allowing completion of the "refinement loop."[3,30] This requires engagement of all stakeholders, at all levels, to allow discussion of the feedback and consideration of further modifications. It is the final step of the refinement loop—implementation—that really matters, yet in many environments, despite all the data collection, monitoring, and evaluation, it simply does not happen, or happens only slowly.[3]

What Is Included in a Welfare Assessment?

The aspect of scoring each aspect of the welfare assessment of a bird or a group of birds seems logical and attractive; however, no single measurement of overall welfare has yet been determined and is not likely to be easily quantified. Even the notion that an assortment of factors can be scored and combined is too simplistic because a bird's welfare is linked to its internal, subjective experience, which is challenging to quantify. In avian welfare, for which no gold standard exists, no set of specific measurements, and for which there are different definitions, the validity must be investigated thoroughly before the instrument can be accepted for general use.

Welfare assessment techniques used for certification, legislation, management, and research applications have broadly been based on assessments of inputs (provisions, resources, and engineering-based criteria) and outcomes (animal-based measures and performance-based criteria).[9,31] Because of the broad acceptance of the tenets of the Five Freedoms, they have come to be used as stand-alone assessment criteria. At a minimum, elements of each of the freedoms are incorporated into checklists for a welfare assessment. However, an assessment tool should allow for when variations from each of the freedoms are acceptable based on health, welfare, and protocol requirements.[28] Perhaps the fundamental questions used in the process of developing laboratory animal assessments (Box 22-3) can be used as a guide for future avian welfare assessments.

Welfare assessments for zoo animals share similar concerns as avian welfare assessments for both individual animals and populations of animals, regardless of the species. Some zoo studies have a common approach, which might be useful for the development of avian welfare assessments.[6] The key features to include in an avian welfare assessment are as follows:

1. Assessment of resources
2. Measures of the physical state of individual birds
3. Measures of the bird's behavioral state
4. Assessment of the bird's mental state

Assessment of Resources

Resource-based reviews are the most commonly applied evaluation of an animal's welfare assessment. This portion of an assessment considers the biological and physical needs of a bird, although evaluation of the environment, husbandry, and management practices has been considered an indirect

---

BOX 22-3 QUESTIONS FOR DEVELOPING A NEW ASSESSMENT[28]

1. What assessment practices for animal care and for animal environments should be used?
2. Should these assessments be qualitative or quantitative, performance-based, or input-based?
3. How important are metrics based on behavioral tendencies, such as affective states, natural behaviors, telos, or choices?
4. Is it appropriate to compare the selectively bred animal with either its domestic or wild counterpart?

measure of an animal's welfare by some evaluation processes. However, it is often the housing and management conditions for groups of animals maintained by an institution such as a sanctuary or laboratory that are scrutinized by the public, perhaps because of the inherent "unnaturalness." The resources and environmental parameters regarded as necessary to provide the potential for good welfare need to be identified first and then quantified for evaluation. These are often the inputs that can provide consistent and objective measures. Basic resource recommendations may be available for some species of common companion birds, common species of birds used in research, or birds common to zoological collections through documents such as the Association of Zoos and Aquariums Animal Care Manuals (https://www.aza.org/animal-care-manuals/).[32] These manuals are developed to identify the general biological and physical needs of zoo animals and often include husbandry templates and focus on describing the resources, and the environmental and social parameters, assumed to promote good welfare. These documents are often developed with a lack of scientific data for a given species; however, these are often the only sources of information for husbandry practices and environmental recommendations (e.g., shelter, space, nutrition).[15] Some welfare measures of resources are either positive or negative, such as providing the correct thermal zone (positive) or being outside of that thermal zone (negative), whereas other parameters are evaluated on a continuum. For example, sufficient food may be provided and the birds are not hungry; however, the diet may not be providing the correct nutritional balance, placing the birds in a malnourished or over-nutrition state. Owners of companion birds will often include in their husbandry description their interpretation of what their bird likes or wants, which can provide information for the category of assessment of the mental state.[9]

Assessment of the Physical State

Components included in the assessment of a bird's physical state will vary depending on the individual bird. Aspects of the physical state may require closer monitoring depending on the bird's age, sex, and current and previous health issues, or if this is a new bird being purchased or birds entering an established collection through quarantine. Evaluation of the physical state is most likely the area of greatest comfort for the veterinarian because it addresses the health of the bird. The physical state assessment includes information gathered in the history and is often information provided by the owner or caretaker such as food and water consumption, feces and urate production, level of activity, and what the bird actually eats versus what food is provided. Evaluation includes the objective measurements of a physical examination such as weight, heart rate, respiratory rate, and recovery time after handling. Additional information to assess the physical state of a bird often includes diagnostic evaluations such as the complete blood count, plasma biochemistry values, and parasitic examination of the feces. Radiographic or additional imaging studies may be included to assess aspects of the bird's health not accessible by the physical examination. Physical assessments also include several subjectively scored parameters such as the bird's degree of responsiveness, body condition score, posture, and feather condition.

Physical parameters are most often used to determine whether a bird is healthy or ill, but many animal welfare studies examine subclinical physiological changes to determine whether an animal is "stressed." Distress has been defined as when the stress response shifts sufficient resources to impair other biological functions.[32] Avian corticosterone has been used as an indication of avian adrenal function and the stress response. Chronically elevated concentrations in birds have been associated with poor welfare sequelae such as compromised cellular and humoral immunity, growth, reproduction, and cognitive ability.[33,34] However, interpretation of cortisol concentrations requires caution because it is affected by a long list of variables, not necessarily stressful or distressing, such as diurnal or seasonal rhythms, reproduction, vocalization, and eating. Despite the many factors that affect the assessment of corticosterone concentration, it is still accepted as a supportive measure of physiological stress when correlated with other indices. For example, fecal corticoid concentrations were monitored in young whooping cranes (*Grus americana*) undergoing reintroduction, and shipment of the cranes to the field training site was correlated with an 8- to 34-fold increase in fecal corticoid concentrations, which returned to baseline levels within 1 week, whereas other aspects in the reintroduction process did not have this degree of change.[35]

For companion birds as well as birds in a collection at an institution such as a sanctuary, research facility, zoological collection, or breeding facility, welfare assessments include information from flock management such as life spans, history of disease, reproduction, care of the chicks, growth rate of offspring, incidents of trauma, and special evaluations for social separation of birds would be included in this portion of the welfare assessment.

Assessment of the Behavioral State

Behavioral assessment includes information about the birds' behavioral repertoire and activity budgets (see Chapter 5). An activity budget is a tool used by behavior scientists and ethologists to determine how much time an animal spends in various activities such as sleeping, resting, foraging, eating, grooming, playing, social interactions, vocalizations, flying, and moving. These categories can be subdivided even further into social play, object play, sexual play, locomotor play, and play fighting. However, it is rare for a companion bird or birds in a collection to have their activity budgets determined, and even rarer to have a standard for what those activity budgets might be like in good welfare versus bad welfare. Behavioral assessments can help to evaluate if the bird is engaging in species-typical activities and not expressing maladaptive behaviors that result in injury or illness.

In most behavior assessments, the caretaker or owner provides information in addition to the veterinarian's observations and assessment of the presence of abnormal behaviors in terms of excessive or lack of activity, abnormal vocalizations, excessive grooming or self-mutilation, or even the development of a stereotypy.[28] Changes in a bird's behavior as well as physiological responses are used for clinical assessment of pain (see Chapter 20). Pain is a significant welfare concern and can be associated with inappropriate housing, husbandry, response to injury, surgery, or a disease process. Behavioral signs of pain will vary between avian species, but some are easily recognized regardless of species such as lameness, imbalances in weight bearing, wing droop, or blepharospasm. Alternatively it may not be a behavior developed specific to pain, but a change or decrease in the presentation of a normal behavior. A study observing red-tailed hawks following orthopedic trauma noticed a marked decrease in normal maintenance behaviors, specifically a decrease in head movements, as a sensitive measure of an affective state in hawks with painful injuries.[36] The study concluded that these behaviors can be scored humanely and with minimal expense, and should be considered for further research on pain and analgesia in avian species.

Abnormal repetitive behaviors without an obvious function are called stereotypes and are often behaviors used to assess welfare. Stereotypical behavior has been theorized to be the response of an animal to the presence of abnormal stimuli or lack of stimuli in the captive environment, or may involve an abnormality within the captive animal itself.[37] A survey of the literature by Mason and Latham found that across species and environments where data were provided, almost 68% of the situations that caused or increased stereotypes also decreased welfare, but also warned that stereotypes were linked to good or neutral welfare nearly as often as poor, and therefore should not be used as a sole index of welfare.[38] In some situations a high level of abnormal behavior in an animal is associated with better individual coping abilities. Feather-damaging behaviors (FDBs), when a bird removes its own feathers, is widely recognized as a common stereotypical behavior of some captive psittacine species and has been a point of concern for keeping parrots as companion birds.[39,40] The study of Grey parrots and cockatoos explored the association between risk factors and FDBs and found that many frequently hypothesized risk factors were not significantly associated with FDBs. Increasing hours of sleep and length of ownership were significantly associated with FDBs in Grey parrots, whereas pet shop origin, cage location against a wall, and annual vacations taken by owners were associated with FDBs in cockatoos, highlighting the importance of future investigations to explore these relationships.[40]

The possibility that captive birds cannot perform behaviors that they would normally perform in a more natural environment is an enduring welfare concern. Given that people want to have birds for companionship, some forms of restriction are accepted. Rather than focus on re-creating a natural environment, the behavior assessment can try to determine whether the bird is able to show natural behaviors. Not all natural behavior is desirable, but there is strong sentiment expressed that while freedom to perform the whole repertoire of natural behavior is not crucial for an animal's welfare, providing opportunities to perform natural behavior may be an effective way to improve welfare in practice.[22]

Assessment of the Mental State

Evaluation of the mental state of a bird is the most abstract and subjective part of the overall welfare assessment because it involves judgments concerning the animals' demeanor or emotion. An emphasis on affective states (emotions and feelings) of the animal has led to assessment methods based on indicators of pain, fear, distress, frustration, hunger, thirst, and similar experiences. This aspect of an assessment relates back to the Five Freedoms that address freedom from hunger and thirst; pain, injury, and disease; and fear and distress. Early welfare scientists indicated that it is the animal's awareness of what is happening that is crucial for its welfare, and

investigations into welfare should be striving for measures (albeit indirect measures) that give some indication of how positive or negative the animal feels.[41,42] Some welfare assessments focus on behavior as the most useful indicator of mental welfare,[28] but it is important to consider the overall effects of all parameters on the mental health of the bird. For example, physical parameters can be used to determine whether a bird has a specific illness, but there is also the bird's subjective experience of feeling ill or in pain that reduces the bird's welfare.

Assessment of mental welfare has also been referred to as an indication of the subjective state of the animal. How to evaluate a bird's subjective state has not been well studied historically, and still relies on a great deal of anecdotal evidence. Objective criteria for behavioral evaluation of an individual bird are discussed in depth in Chapter 5. Several animal welfare researchers and veterinarians have suggested that the best way to evaluate well-being may be for the person most familiar with an animal's temperament, preferences, behavior, and routine to be "the voice" for that individual.[25,43-51] Alternatively, a technique called free-choice profiling or qualitative behavioral assessment was developed by Wemelsfelder[52] to evaluate animals' subjective state. Free-choice profiling uses descriptive terms independently generated by multiple observers to score animals, either by direct observation or by watching video. Analysis of observer agreement has shown a high degree of inter-rater reliability, even when observers have no previous experience with the species being assessed.

Multiple factors such as appropriate husbandry and environment allow for the expression of natural behaviors and satisfactory mental well-being. Enrichment programs can provide animals opportunities for expressing behaviors driven by the positive emotional systems of seeking, play, and caring, and decrease activation of the fear, rage, or panic systems.[53,54] Preference and motivation tests have been used to study what conditions birds prefer in a captive environment. These types of studies are based on the premise that if an animal is willing to "work" for food or a resource by using a natural behavior, there is likely a positive preference to use those species-specific behaviors. Foraging behavior is highly motivated for many species of birds. Studies have been designed to show that many birds choose to spend time interacting with foraging devices even when identical food is freely available; this phenomenon is called *contrafreeloading* and has been reported in a number of bird species.[55] Using a feeder apparatus that required lifting a weighted lid to gain access to pellets, orange-winged Amazon parrots (*Amazona amazonica*) were motivated to work by lifting more than their own body weight to access a large-sized food pellet when regular-sized pellets were freely available, suggesting motivation to access food forms that enable podomandibulation, a naturalistic foraging and feeding behavior.[56,57]

When birds play with toys in their environment or talk with an owner, what can be used to determine whether the bird is experiencing a positive emotion? It is much more challenging to determine when positive effects are beneficial to an animal rather than just neutral.[58] Studies in mammals have tried to identify which activities are more likely to be performed when animals are in positive affective states. In mammals, indications of a positive affective state may include facial expressions, paw licks, tongue protrusions, and vocalizations such as purring in cats or chirping in rats[9]; unfortunately these are not markers that can be extrapolated across species to birds.

WHAT ARE THE CURRENT AVIAN WELFARE ISSUES?

Avian welfare could be greatly improved if more studies were developed to address how best to promote good welfare for birds in captivity. Since avian welfare is an emerging focus of welfare science, a logical approach to determine what welfare issues are most urgent would be useful. Methods to try to assess which issues cause the greatest impairment to animal welfare have been reviewed.[59] A consensus approach bringing together stakeholders from different fields of expertise to collate information on potential welfare concerns has been used for laboratory animals.[60,61] A recent study was undertaken to aid in prioritization of welfare issues of companion dogs. A consensus view was sought from experts in welfare and behavior sciences, veterinary science, epidemiology, and zoology disciplines to try to gather more robust information on which to base decisions regarding prioritization of welfare issues for British companion dogs.[62] Issues that were identified by this process included inappropriate husbandry, lack of owner knowledge, undesirable behaviors, inherited disease, inappropriate socialization and habituation, and conformation-related disorders. Other welfare issues, such as obese and overweight dogs, were judged as being important for welfare but not strategic priorities, because of the expert-perceived difficulties in their management and resolution.[62] Analogous welfare issues affect the companion bird (see Chapter 25). Acknowledging that minimal funds are available for avian welfare research, a similar approach to prioritize welfare issues for avian welfare would require experts to gather information, providing an opportunity to reach consensus by discussion and help determine which issues need to be tackled. J. Webster[63] introduced a paper on implementation of animal welfare with the following call to action: if science is to be of practical service to animal welfare, we must do more than just study it; we must take it out of the confines of the laboratory and into the world where these animals actually live.

REFERENCES

1. Duncan IJH: Animal Rights—Animal welfare: a scientist's assessment, *Poul Sci* 60:489, 1981.
2. Koene P: Behavioral ecology of captive species: using behavioral adaptations to assess and enhance welfare of nonhuman zoo animals, *J Appl Anim Welfare Sci* 16:360, 2013.
3. Wolfensohn S, Honess P: Laboratory animal, pet animal, farm animal, wild animal: which gets the best deal? *Anim Welfare* 16:117, 2007.
4. Barber J, Lewis D, Agoramoorthy G, et al: Setting standards for evaluation of captive facilities. In Kleiman DG, Thompson KV, Kirk Baer C, editors: *Wild mammals in captivity: principles and techniques for zoo management*, ed 2, Chicago IL, 2010, University of Chicago Press, pp 22–34.
5. Knierim U, Pajor EA, Jackson WT, et al: Incentives and enforcement. In Appleby MC, Mench JA, Olsson IAS, Hughes BO, editors: *Animal welfare*, ed 2, Cambridge, UK, 2011, CABI Publishing, pp 291–303.
6. Whitham JC, Wielebnowski N: New directions for zoo animal welfare science, *Appl Anim Behav Sci* 147:247, 2013.
7. Webster AJ: Farm animal welfare: the five freedoms and the free market, *Vet J* 161:229, 2001.
8. Council FAW: *Farm animal welfare in Great Britain: past, present and future*, London, 2009.
9. Yeates JW, Main DC: Assessment of positive welfare: a review, *Vet J* 175:293, 2008.
10. Yeates J: *Patients. Animal welfare in veterinary practice*, Ames, IA, 2013, Wiley-Blackwell, pp 1–32.
11. Wensley SP: Animal welfare and the human-animal bond: considerations for veterinary faculty, students, and practitioners, *J Vet Med Educ* 35:532, 2008.
12. Fraser D, Duncan IJH: Pleasures, pains and animal welfare: toward a natural history of affect, *Anim Welfare* 7:383, 1998.
13. Broom DM: Advances in studies of behavior and welfare in relation to animal production, *R Bras Zootec* 40:15, 2011.
14. Mason GJ: Species differences in responses to captivity: stress, welfare and the comparative method, *Trends Ecol Evol* 25:713, 2010.
15. Melfi VA: There are big gaps in our knowledge, and thus approach, to zoo animal welfare: a case for evidence-based zoo animal management, *Zoo Biol* 28:574, 2009.
16. Fraser D: *Understanding animal welfare: the science in its cultural context*, Ames, IA, 2008, Wiley-Blackwell.
17. Broom DM: *Sentience and animal welfare*, Boston, MA, 2014, CABI, pp 1–7.
18. Paul-Murphy J, Hawkins M: Avian analgesia. In Miller E, Fowler M, editors: *Fowler's zoo and wild animal medicine: current therapy*, St Louis, MO, 2011, Elsevier Saunders, pp 312–323.
19. Broom DM: Needs, freedoms and the assessment of welfare, *Appl Anim Behav Sci* 19:384, 1988.
20. Jarvis ED, Gunturkun O, Bruce L, et al: Avian brains and a new understanding of vertebrate brain evolution, *Nat Rev Neurosci* 6:151, 2005.
21. Emery NJ: Cognitive ornithology: the evolution of avian intelligence, *Philos Trans R Soc Lond B Biol Sci* 361:23, 2006.
22. Eadie EN: *Understanding animal welfare: an integrated approach*, New York, 2012, Springer.
23. Kalmar ID, Janssens GP, Moons CP: Guidelines and ethical considerations for housing and management of psittacine birds used in research, *ILAR J* 51:409, 2010.
24. McGreevy PD, Bennett PC: Challenges and paradoxes in the companion-animal niche, *Anim Welfare* 19:11, 2010.
25. Wojciechowska JI, Hewson CJ: Quality-of-life assessment in pet dogs, *J Am Vet Assoc* 226:722, 2005.
26. Wojciechowska JI, Hewson CJ, Stryhn H, et al: Evaluation of a questionnaire regarding nonphysical aspects of quality of life in sick and healthy dogs, *Am J Vet Res* 66:1461, 2005.
27. Yeates J: *Animal welfare in veterinary practice*, Ames, IA, 2013, Wiley-Blackwell.
28. Beaver BV, Bayne K: Animal welfare assessment considerations. In Turner KBV, editor: *Laboratory animal welfare*, Boston, MA, 2014, Academic Press, pp 29–38.
29. Cockram MS, Hughes BO: Health and disease. In Appleby MC, Mench JA, Olsson IAS, Hughes BO, editors: *Animal welfare*, ed 2, Cambridge, MA, 2011, CABI, pp 120–137.
30. Hartley P, Lloyd M, Burton N: Obstacles to the refinement of scientific procedures using living animals, *Anim Welfare* S242, 2004.
31. Main DCJ, Kent JP, Wemelsfelder F, et al: Applications for methods of on-farm welfare assessment, *Anim Welfare* 12:523, 2003.
32. Moberg GP: Biological response to stress: implications for animal welfare. In Moberg GP, Mench JA, editors: *The biology of animal stress: basic principles and implications for animal welfare*, New York, 2000, CABI, pp 1–21.
33. Carsia RV, Harvey S: Adrenals. In Whittow GC, editor: *Sturkie's avian physiology*, ed 5, San Diego, 2000, Academic Press, pp 489–537.
34. Sapolsky RM, Romero LM, Munck AU: How do glucocorticoids influence stress responses? Integrating permissive, suppressive, stimulatory, and preparative actions, *Endocr Rev* 21:55, 2000.
35. Hartup BK, Olsen GH, Czekala NM: Fecal corticoid monitoring in whooping cranes (*Grus americana*) undergoing reintroduction, *Zoo Biol* 24:15, 2005.

36. Mazor-Thomas JE, Mann PE, Karas AZ, et al: Pain-suppressed behaviors in the red-tailed hawk 1 (*Buteo jamaicensis*), *Appl Anim Behav Sci* 152:83, 2014.

37. Garner JP, Meehan CL, Mench JA: Stereotypies in caged parrots, schizophrenia and autism: evidence for a common mechanism, *Behav Brain Res* 145:125, 2003.

38. Mason GJ, Latham NR: Can't stop, won't stop: is stereotypy a reliable animal welfare indicator? *Anim Welfare* 13:57, 2004.

39. Engebretson M: The welfare and suitability of parrots as companion animals: a review, *Anim Welfare* 15: 263, 2006.

40. Jayson SL, Williams DL, Wood JLN: Prevalence and risk factors of feather plucking in African Grey parrots (*Psittacus erithacus erithacus* and *Psittacus erithacus timneh*) and cockatoos (*Cacatua* spp.), *J Exot Pet Med* 23:250, 2014.

41. Dawkins MS: *Through our eyes only? The search for animal consciousness*, New York, 1998, Oxford University Press.

42. Duncan IJH:The changing concept of animal sentience, *Appl Anim Behav Sci* 100:11, 2006.

43. McMillan FD: Maximizing quality of life in ill animals, *J Am Anim Hosp Assoc* 39:227, 2003.

44. Morton DB: A hypothetical strategy for the objective evaluation of animal well-being and quality of life using a dog model, *Anim Welfare* 16:75, 2007.

45. Whitham JC, Wielebnowski N: Animal-based welfare monitoring: using keeper ratings as an assessment tool, *Zoo Biol* 28:545, 2009.

46. Hsu Y, Serpell JA: Development and validation of a questionnaire for measuring behavior and temperament traits in pet dogs, *J Am Vet Med Assoc* 223:1293, 2003.

47. Wojciechowska JI, Hewson CJ, Stryhn H, et al: Development of a discriminative questionnaire to assess nonphysical aspects of quality of life of dogs, *Am J Vet Res* 66:1453, 2005.

48. Wiseman-Orr ML, Scott EM, Reid J, et al: Validation of a structured questionnaire as an instrument to measure chronic pain in dogs on the basis of effects on health-related quality of life, *Am J Vet Res* 67:1826, 2006.

49. Taylor KD, Mills DS: Is quality of life a useful concept for companion animals? *Anim Welfare* 16:55, 2007.

50. Timmins RP, Cliff KD, Day CT, et al: Enhancing quality of life for dogs and cats in confined situations, *Anim Welfare* 16:83, 2007.

51. Meagher RK: Observer ratings: validity and value as a tool for animal welfare research, *Appl Anim Behav Sci* 119:1, 2009.

52. Wemelsfelder F: How animals communicate quality of life: the qualitative assessment of behaviour, *Anim Welfare* 16:25, 2007.

53. Grandin T, Johnson C: *Animals make us human: creating the best life for animals*, New York, 2009, Houghton-Mifflin Harcourt.

54. Morris CL, Grandin T, Irlbeck NA: Companion animals symposium: environmental enrichment for companion, exotic, and laboratory animals, *J Anim Sci* 89:4227, 2011.

55. Inglis IR, Forkman B, Lazarus J: Free food or earned food? A review and fuzzy model of contrafreeloading, *Anim Behav* 53:1171, 1997.

56. Rozek JC, Danner LM, Stucky PA, et al: Over-sized pellets naturalize foraging time of captive orange-winged Amazon parrots (*Amazona amazonica*), *Appl Anim Behav Sci* 125:80, 2010.

57. Rozek JC, Millam JR: Preference and motivation for different diet forms and their effect on motivation for a foraging enrichment in captive orange-winged Amazon parrots (*Amazona amazonica*), *Appl Anim Behav Sci* 129:153, 2011.

58. Phillips C: Animal welfare: a construct of positive and negative affect? *Vet J* 175:291, 2008.

59. Scott EM, Fitzpatrick JL, Nolan AM, et al: Evaluation of welfare state based on interpretation of multiple indices, *Anim Welfare* 12:457, 2003.

60. Leach MC, Thornton PD, Main DCJ: Identification of appropriate measures for the assessment of laboratory mouse welfare, *Anim Welfare* 17:161, 2008.

61. Whaytt HR, Main DCJ, Greent LE, et al: Animal-based measures for the assessment of welfare state of dairy cattle, pigs and laying hens: consensus of expert opinion, *Anim Welfare* 12:205, 2003.

62. Buckland E, Corr S, Abeyesinghe S, et al: Prioritization of companion dog welfare issues using expert consensus, *Anim Welfare* 23:39, 2014.

63. Webster J: The assessment and implementation of animal welfare: theory into practice, *Rev Sci Tech* 24:723, 2005.

ANIMAL WELFARE LEGISLATION AND ITS INFLUENCE ON AVIAN WELFARE

V. Wensley Koch, Jeleen A. Briscoe[a]

Does animal welfare legislation influence avian welfare? Does it influence avian veterinarians? Do avian veterinarians need to know about such legislation? Is avian welfare even relevant to avian veterinarians?

The answers to the first three questions depend on the legislation and its enforcement, of course, but in general terms, the answer to all three questions is "yes." Most of the legislation addressing avian welfare consists of broad anticruelty laws covering all animals, and in some cases veterinarians are required to report animal cruelty. The American Veterinary Medical Association (AVMA) "considers it the responsibility of the veterinarian to report such cases to appropriate authorities, whether or not reporting is mandated by law."[1] Therefore, avian veterinarians should at least know whether their local anticruelty laws cover birds. Most such laws do, so avian welfare can, at a minimum, be influenced by reporting cases of cruelty to the appropriate authorities.

The answer to the fourth question is also "yes." Most veterinarians enter the profession because of their love for animals, so from that aspect alone, the welfare of birds is relevant to avian veterinarians. In addition, welfare and health are inextricably intertwined, and avian veterinarians should also be interested in avian welfare from a health standpoint. Because ensuring the welfare of clients' birds may help in resolving and/or preventing health problems, most veterinarians understand that discussing avian husbandry with their clients is equally as important as providing for the birds' immediate health requirements. Although animal welfare legislation specifically addressing the needs of birds is rare, the legislation that does exist can help veterinarians in initiating these husbandry discussions. Finally, avian welfare is relevant to avian veterinarians because the public considers veterinarians to be animal welfare experts, and animal welfare experts should be knowledgeable about all facets of animal welfare, including the legislative aspects.

In the United States the only legislation that affects avian welfare is at the state or local level. The Federal Animal Welfare Act (AWA)[2] was amended in 2002 to cover birds (except those bred for use in research), but standards for regulating birds have not yet been published. Federal regulation will begin whenever standards are finally published, and it should have a significant effect on both the birds regulated under the AWA and the avian veterinarians who care for them.

[a]Note: The views expressed in this subpart are those of the authors and do not represent the views of Animal and Plant Inspection Service (APHIS), the United States Department of Agriculture (USDA), or the United States government.

Consider the example of laboratory animals and laboratory animal veterinarians. In 1985, the AWA[2] was amended to add detailed requirements for the regulation of animals used in research, including mandating the involvement of veterinarians in the oversight of such research. This requirement likely influenced an increasing demand for laboratory animal veterinarians and an increasing interest in specialization in that field. In 1985, the American College of Laboratory Animal Medicine (ACLAM) had 33 candidates for certification as diplomates. That number was similar to the number of candidates applying each year for the last 15 years. In 1990, the ACLAM had 62 candidates for certification, and the numbers were even higher for the rest of the 1990s. In 2003, the number dropped to 40 (still higher than the number of candidates in the years from 1971 to 1985), but then it began increasing again, reaching 80 candidates in 2007. Was the change in the law responsible for this increase in the number of candidates interested in certification as diplomates in laboratory animal medicine? There is no way to know for certain, but the timing is certainly suggestive of this. The authors of the report[3] from which these numbers came also noted that "(f)rom 2000–2007, the emphasis was on recruitment and training. There were too few qualified laboratory animal veterinarians for the number of open positions."

Prior to 1985, government oversight of research facilities was minimally effective because of limited inspection authority. When the regulations implementing the new law went into effect and detailed inspections of research facilities began, the welfare of laboratory animals was noticeably improved. Such improvements continue to evolve as a result of the research community's dedication to animal welfare, but the implementation of effective government oversight was a major player in speeding up that evolution. Therefore, the animal welfare legislation of 1985 benefited laboratory animals not only indirectly (by increasing the number of laboratory animal veterinarians trained to care for them), but also directly (by improving government oversight of their care).

Another example of how animal welfare can be improved through legislation has to do with environmental enrichment. The U.S. AWA[2] amendments of 1985 also added a requirement for "a physical environment adequate to promote the psychological well-being of primates." The regulations[2] implementing that requirement mandated environmental enrichment as the means of promoting primate psychological well-being. The nation's zoos rightfully felt that the need for psychological well-being was not limited to primates, and they initiated environmental enrichment for all of their animals. Just as measures to improve the welfare of laboratory animals began evolving rapidly when effective government oversight was initiated, the use of environmental enrichment also began evolving rapidly as zoos became more experienced in providing such enrichment. The movement is now beginning to spread to other venues, including the homes of pet owners. So what began as a requirement for psychological well-being for regulated primates has evolved into a push for environmental enrichment for all animals. Psittacine species, in particular, have been considered the avian equivalents of primates in their need for measures to ensure their psychological well-being, so an increasing emphasis on enriching the environments of birds should be of special benefit to them.

Environmental enrichment itself has also improved, from the ineffective practice of just giving an animal a toy or two (ineffective because toys quickly become boring to the animal), to a recognition of the importance of companions for social animals, the utility of foraging activities in decreasing boredom, the need to enrich all five senses (visual, auditory, tactile, olfactory, and gustatory enrichment), the value of regular positive reinforcement training in providing cognitive enrichment as well as encouraging voluntary medical and husbandry behaviors (e.g., voluntary blood draws or toenail trimming). These indirect effects of the AWA on fostering and enhancing enrichment techniques for all species has already improved avian welfare, and the effects should increase whenever standards for birds are published and enforcement of those standards begins. Government oversight of bird dealers and exhibitors could serve to spread enrichment "best practices" to those businesses and thus improve the welfare of the birds they raise, sell, and exhibit.

THE UNITED STATES ANIMAL WELFARE ACT AND THE ATTENDING VETERINARIAN

Whenever standards for birds under the U.S. AWA are published and enforcement of those standards begins, the demand for U.S. veterinarians familiar with avian health and husbandry will likely increase, as the demand for laboratory animal veterinarians increased in 1985. The concern that there will not be enough experienced veterinarians to fill that demand is a serious one, because retaining a knowledgeable attending veterinarian will be mandatory to meet regulatory requirements, as it currently is for mammals regulated under the AWA. A 2013 article[4] in the *Journal of the American Veterinary Association* indicated that the "AVMA's 2012 U.S. Pet Ownership and Demographic Sourcebook estimated the size of the nation's pet bird population to be 8.3 million animals at year end 2011." A 2014 article by Kelly, McCarthy, Menzel, and Engebretson[5] reported that the 2013–2014 American Pet Product Association National Pet Owners Survey estimated there were 20.6 million birds in 6.9 million U.S. households. Whatever the actual number of pet birds might be, a search for U.S. veterinarians listed on the Association of Avian Veterinarians (AAV) website[6] indicated that, as of October, 2014, there were only 958 AAV member veterinarians in the United States to serve the nation's pet bird population. It would appear that the United States is already experiencing a shortage of veterinarians knowledgeable about avian medicine (and comfortable with its practice), and when birds become regulated under the AWA and licensed bird facilities are required to employ attending veterinarians, that shortage is likely to become even more noticeable. However, there are presently no hard data available on either the number of bird breeders and exhibitors or the number of avian veterinarians in the United States, so for now, we can only speculate on how the enforcement of regulatory welfare standards for bird industries will affect veterinary oversight of regulated and unregulated birds.

The role of the attending veterinarian is an important one under the AWA regulations,[2] which currently require all facilities regulated under the Act to ensure veterinary oversight of their programs by retaining an attending veterinarian to provide veterinary care and husbandry advice for the regulated animals. The attending veterinarian must have "training and/or experience in the care and management of the species being attended." It should be emphasized that the attending veterinarian is responsible for all aspects of animal care at regulated facilities, not just for veterinary care. The regulations require the attending veterinarian to make "regularly scheduled visits to the premises" so that he or she can "oversee the adequacy of other aspects of animal care and use," as well as ensuring the provision of adequate veterinary care.

When clinical veterinarians are asked by clients to become attending veterinarians for animals regulated under the AWA, they often do not understand the scope of the duties they are accepting, but when they do understand and exercise their authority, they can be a significant force in improving the welfare of the animals they serve. The same influence can also be exercised by veterinarians caring for unregulated birds. Avian veterinarians might not wish to make visits to the homes of their clients, but discussions of husbandry practices may be helpful in resolving and/or preventing clinical problems in their patients. Most clients should want to provide appropriate care for their birds, but even with reluctant clients, cost-benefit discussions can often make it clear that good husbandry practices are well worth the effort (and it is probably difficult enough to find a good avian veterinarian whose advice clients will be motivated to follow and whose expertise they respect).

The anticipated scarcity of veterinarians experienced enough to serve as attending veterinarians for avian facilities regulated under the AWA could be handled by federal regulators in the same way as it is currently handled for exotic animal facilities when they experience difficulty in finding a suitable veterinarian. Such facilities may be approved to retain a local veterinarian with little knowledge of the species attended on the condition that the local veterinarian will consult with a species specialist as needed. Over time, it is hoped that the supply of veterinarians will increase to meet the increased demand. For example, a heightened demand for avian veterinarians might improve the availability of specialist training, as it apparently did for the specialty of laboratory animal medicine. Also, in coordination with current avian veterinarians and avian veterinary associations (national and local chapters), federal regulators could develop a consultant network, model veterinary care plans, and veterinary training materials to help inexperienced attending veterinarians gain the knowledge and skills needed to provide appropriate care for the birds under their supervision. This on-the-job training would help increase the numbers of veterinarians qualified to provide veterinary care for birds, and as more veterinarians become knowledgeable in avian medicine and begin providing care to more birds, the welfare of all birds will be improved.

CURRENT LEGISLATION IN THE UNITED STATES AND OTHER COUNTRIES

Although birds are not yet regulated under the U.S. AWA,[2] the Act itself has existed since 1966, when it was first passed as the Laboratory Animal Welfare Act. At that time, the law only regulated dog and cat dealers and laboratories that used dogs, cats, hamsters, guinea pigs, rabbits, or nonhuman primates in research. It was adopted as a result of public outcry

in response to media stories about dealers stealing pet dogs for sale to research and the poor care provided to the dogs by such dealers. In 1970, the name was changed to the Animal Welfare Act and oversight was expanded to other warm-blooded animals used in research, exhibition, or the wholesale pet trade. In 1976, regulation of commercial transportation of animals was added and most animal fighting ventures were prohibited. As mentioned above, a 1985 amendment imposed additional requirements for the use of animals in research, as well as requirements covering psychological well-being for primates and exercise for dogs. However, birds were excluded from coverage, by regulation, until an amendment in 2002 added birds not bred for use in research to those animals specifically required by law to be regulated.[7] Standards for birds have not yet been published, so the actual regulation of birds has not yet begun.

To understand the current situation regarding federal regulation of birds in the United States, one must understand a few facts about how the U.S. system of federal regulation works. When Congress passes a law describing its intent for certain activities to be regulated, it designates the part of the government it wishes to be responsible for undertaking that regulation. The responsibility for regulating animal welfare was delegated to the U.S. Department of Agriculture (USDA). Within the USDA, an agency called the Animal and Plant Health Inspection Service (APHIS) was assigned the animal welfare responsibilities, and it formed a division called Animal Care to handle the assignment. Animal Care, then, is required to write the detailed regulations and standards needed to implement the intent of Congress as expressed in the AWA. Those regulations and standards must go through a process specified within the Executive Branch of the government to be published as official requirements enforceable by law. As a part of that process, proposed regulations and standards must obtain the approval of various agencies of the Executive Branch before they are published to allow comment by the public (including interested experts). Public comments must then be considered by the implementing agency before a final version of the regulations and standards may be published.

In 2002, Congress amended the definition of *animal* in the AWA to exclude birds, rats of the genus *Rattus*, and mice of the genus *Mus*, bred for use in research. Although the definition of animal in the regulations previously promulgated under the AWA had always excluded rats of the genus *Rattus* and mice of the genus *Mus* bred for use in research, that definition had also excluded all birds, not just birds bred for use in research. In essence, then, this 2002 amendment of the AWA added birds not bred for use in research to those animal species specifically required by law to be regulated. However, Animal Care has not yet been able to publish regulations and standards for birds, so enforcement of the AWA regarding birds has not been pursued.

Any standards for birds published under the AWA, though, are likely to reflect the existing standards for mammals. Currently, Animal Care has published specific standards[2] for dogs and cats, guinea pigs and hamsters, rabbits, nonhuman primates, and marine mammals, as well as general standards for all other mammals. These standards cover requirements for humane handling, care, treatment, and transportation of regulated animals. For the most part, they are performance standards rather than engineering standards; that is, they simply require that the species-specific needs of animals be met, rather than specifying particular techniques or quantitative parameters for doing so. They address facilities (e.g., construction, availability of water and electricity, lighting, ventilation, temperature and humidity, drainage, storage, waste disposal, space), care (e.g., feeding, watering, housekeeping, sanitation, pest control, group compatibility, employee numbers and training), and transportation of live animals (e.g., required documents, terminal facilities, conveyances, enclosures, handling, observation, feeding and watering, group compatibility). For marine mammals, they address the water quality of pools. Regulations that apply to all animals address such things as veterinary care, identification, records, and handling. Minimum age requirements for transporting dogs and cats are also included.

Standards for birds will probably be similar to the general standards for mammals, with a few changes to reflect the unique characteristics of birds (e.g., requirements for perches or the provision of nesting materials). Aquatic birds will require additional provisions similar to those for marine mammals. Regulations on methods of identification may address such things as the banding of birds, and minimum age requirements for transporting some birds may be included. For the most part, however, general performance standards for mammals also address many of the welfare needs of birds, so the U.S. standards for birds can be anticipated to be similar to those currently in place for mammals. Based on the breadth of avian species anticipated to be regulated under the U.S. AWA, it would be difficult to maintain species-specific standards for all the different types of birds (as is currently done for different types of mammals), but species-specific requirements for birds can be met by alluding to them within the more general guidelines and using performance-based standards. Regulations based on performance standards, rather than engineering standards, provide the necessary flexibility to address a wide range of species and situations.

It should be emphasized, however, that any standards promulgated under the AWA will apply only to the birds regulated under the Act; that is, to some birds at dealer, exhibitor, and research facilities and some birds during transportation. The U.S. standards specifically addressing birds will probably be unique in that they will apply only one single guideline to all types of birds in many different settings. That guideline will have to be broad enough to apply to the parrot at a dealer's facility and the penguin at a zoo, but many birds will still not be protected under the AWA. Consistent with the AWA regulations for mammals, birds at traditional pet shops and birds in sanctuaries will generally not be protected. Bird dealers will only be regulated if they sell birds wholesale or through Internet sales and birds in sanctuaries will not be regulated unless the sanctuary is exhibiting its animals. However, the existence of minimum standards for those birds that are eventually regulated under the Act could provide avian veterinarians with a reference for initiating husbandry discussions with the owners of pet birds brought to veterinary clinics.

Although there are no federal standards for avian welfare in the United States, most birds in the United States are protected by state anticruelty laws. These laws may or may not clearly cover birds (i.e., specifically define *animal* to include birds) and may or may not be adequately enforced, so the

actual level of protection varies from state to state. The laws are very general, prohibiting abuse and usually including some basic husbandry requirements but rarely addressing any unique requirements for birds. The authors are aware of only four states that have laws or regulations specifically addressing any of the unique welfare needs of birds. California has a law prohibiting the sale of unweaned psittacine birds by pet stores.[8] Massachusetts has a pet shop regulation requiring that birds be able "to fly, hop or otherwise move about, individually spread their wings and simultaneously and freely from obstruction perch in a normal position."[9] Colorado regulates breeders and dealers of pets, including birds. The bird-specific requirements include a statement that at least "two perches, one at each end of the cage, must be provided for all species that prefer flying or jumping rather than climbing."[10] Minnesota is unique in having a law covering the care of birds kept as pets, which requires that perches "or other space must be provided to allow the bird to roost without physical harassment from other birds." The rest of that law has requirements similar to those for mammalian husbandry, including a requirement for sufficient room for the bird "to obtain exercise."[11] Avian veterinarians in Minnesota, then, can actually refer to state law in husbandry discussions with their clients. In other states, veterinarians could use the California, Colorado, and Massachusetts requirements to begin such husbandry discussions, or they could use international laws as a basis for their conversations.

Internationally, the situation is similar to that which exists in the various states of the United States. Avian welfare is primarily addressed only in general animal welfare statutes that consist, in essence, of anticruelty legislation, that is, laws prohibiting abuse and usually including some basic husbandry requirements but rarely addressing any unique requirements for birds. A wide variety of countries, from Austria to Zimbabwe, have such laws, but the laws may or may not clearly cover birds (i.e., specifically define *animal* to include birds) and may or may not be adequately enforced, so the actual level of protection varies from country to country. In addition to the laws of individual countries, Europe also has the European Convention for the Protection of Pet Animals, although this legislation is yet another general anticruelty law that does not address the unique welfare needs of birds.[12]

As with the states of the United States, however, some countries do have laws or regulations specifically addressing birds. Legislation in the Netherlands prohibits the separation of psittacines from their parents prior to a minimum age calculated to prevent disturbing their well-being (unless separation is required for the well-being of the parents or chicks).[13] Germany has two sets of guidelines specific to caged birds: one for psittacines[14] and one for small birds such as larks, finches, and sparrows.[15] The guidelines address such things as perches spaced for flying and opportunities for bathing, but they do not address the sale of unweaned birds. They do not have the force of law but can be used as expert advice in court when an enforcement action is brought under the anticruelty law. Germany also recently began requiring that animal dealers provide customers with written information on caring for the animals they buy, and a private organization (the *Bundesverband für fachgerechten Natur-, Tier- und Artenschutz e.V.*) has worked with experts to summarize the bird guidelines in flyers that dealers can use to meet this requirement (T. Richter,

Personal communication, October 6, 2014). Six of the eight states of Australia (all except Tasmania and Western Australia)[16-21] have codes of practice specific to caged birds, addressing such things as perches, nesting, toenail and beak trimming, and bird-specific feeding requirements. Most mention opportunities for bathing and specifically require the freedom to fly. Some prohibit flight restriction methods (wing clipping, pinioning, and tethering), some make allowances for restriction, and some fail to address the issue. Some allow the sale of unweaned birds (to knowledgeable buyers) and some do not. These Australian states also have codes for pet shops and exhibited animals (zoos, circuses, films, and/or television), with varying degrees of bird-specific requirements. Most codes do not have the force of law and would only be used as guidelines in court when an enforcement action was brought under the state anticruelty law, but the South Australia code specifically states that "(f)ailure to abide by this code may result in prosecution under the Prevention of Cruelty to Animals Act, 1985."[20]

Almost all of the Australian states have requirements for poultry and farmed emus and/or ostriches and require permitting for the possession of wild animals, including birds. Such laws are also common internationally. Farm animal welfare is a worldwide concern, so many countries, and the Office International des Epizooties or World Organization for Animal Health, have standards for poultry welfare, as well as for animal transportation (usually aimed primarily at farm animal transportation). Many countries also have laws regarding the import, export, marketing, and possession of wild animals, including birds. Several countries have specific legislation regarding raptors (falconry). In the United States, some states require licenses or permits to market psittacines as a control measure for psittacosis. Some countries have laws regulating pet shops and exhibited animals (usually zoos and/or circuses), with varying degrees of bird-specific requirements. Many countries ban cock fighting, but many also allow it. In countries that ban it enforcement may be problematic. These types of bird-related laws are not addressed in detail in this section, which focuses on animal welfare legislation affecting the husbandry of pet birds, but they are mentioned here for the sake of completeness. Such laws are also avian welfare laws, although their effects on pet birds are minimal at best.

ANIMAL WELFARE ISSUES AND THEIR INFLUENCE ON LEGISLATION

Most animal welfare laws are passed as a result of public pressure on legislators. For example, the law in the Netherlands regarding the hand rearing of psittacines resulted from such activity (W. Weinbeck, Personal communication, October 3, 2014). In response to public concerns, the government requested the Wageningen University and Research Centre (WUR) to review existing legislation in the Netherlands prohibiting the separation of immature mammals from their parents and to include parrots in this research. The center then produced the WUR Livestock Research Report 428, "Weaning of animals,"[22] which described the welfare problems that can be caused by the separation of young animals from their parents, detailed which species were currently at risk, and proposed criteria for preventing problems caused by such separation. Based upon the report, the government

proposed draft legislation in 2011 and, after receiving public comments, issued final legislation in 2014.

In contrast, the law and regulations regarding pet animal facilities in Colorado were initiated by the pet animal industry itself. Prior to passage of the law, regulation of the industry was managed by the Department of Public Health and Environment, and industry members felt that oversight by the veterinarians in the Department of Agriculture would be more appropriate (K. Anderson, Personal communication, September 23, 2014). Having more specific guidelines than just anticruelty legislation is helpful to both industry and government inspectors to clarify what is expected of animal facility owners. Involvement of the industry in the writing of the regulations also helps ensure industry acceptance. Pet animal industry members did participate in the drafting of the Colorado law and regulations, and the law became final in 1995 (K. Anderson, Personal communication, September 23, 2014).

Enforcement of the Colorado law has indeed been effective at improving the welfare of birds. Initially, many substandard facilities were forced to improve or cease operating, and inspectors still identify and work to upgrade or eliminate deficient facilities (K. Anderson, Personal communication, September 23, 2014). The parent–chick separation law in the Netherlands is also likely to be enforced and should improve avian welfare by preventing hand feeding by inexperienced owners and allowing proper socialization of psittacines, hopefully decreasing the behavioral problems often seen in these birds (W. Weinbeck, Personal communication, October 3, 2014). However, as was mentioned regarding anticruelty laws, the efficacy of bird-specific laws in improving avian welfare depends upon enforcement of those laws. Also, although the bird-specific codes and/or guidelines that are written to help enforce general animal welfare laws can be used as educational tools to help improve avian welfare overall, such education is possible only if their availability is widely known. Obscure codes and guidelines are no more effective than unenforced laws, so enforcement of laws and dissemination of guidelines is critical to improving avian welfare through legislative avenues. Avian veterinarians can help in spreading the expert advice found in legal guidelines, but sometimes they may need to search out such information. For the sake of improving avian welfare, it is worth the effort to discover what guidelines are available to help ensure at least minimally adequate husbandry for pet birds.

Controversial issues in animal welfare may or may not be addressed legislatively. Regulations and guidelines tend to maintain the status quo regarding such issues, so if controversial issues are addressed, they are usually addressed by new laws, most commonly in response to social pressures. The sale of unweaned psittacines is an example of such an issue regarding avian welfare. Public pressure has resulted in laws addressing this practice in California and the Netherlands, but the matter has not been tackled in most jurisdictions. In Australia, some states allow the sale of unweaned birds (to knowledgeable buyers) and some do not. Whether or not bans on such sales become more common will depend on the politics of public pressure and industry resistance as played out on the worldwide scene.

Another example of a controversial issue regarding avian welfare is the topic of flying and flight restriction. The animal welfare community generally holds that animals should be provided with the freedom to express normal behavior, and flying is certainly normal behavior for most birds. However, flying is restricted in many ways for many captive birds. Perhaps the most common form of restriction is by keeping birds in enclosures too small to allow them to fly. Tethering is a customary restriction imposed on raptors. Pinioning and wing clipping are other conventional methods of flight restriction. Wing clipping is rarely banned but may be restricted to being performed by a veterinarian or experienced bird keeper. Pinioning is usually performed on water birds and game birds, so banning it in pet birds is not typically an issue. However, banning it in zoos, for example, would indeed be controversial in the jurisdictions where it still exists as a common and accepted practice. Pinioning without anesthesia raises questions of cruelty, but pinioning with anesthesia is still a welfare issue for those who believe that captive birds should be allowed to fly. In addition, less common means of flight restriction may become more widespread if pinioning is banned. Therefore, simply banning pinioning would not fully address the issue of flight restriction in bird species now commonly pinioned. As with other controversial issues, whether or not legislation addressing the ability of captive birds to fly becomes more common will depend on the politics of public pressure and industry resistance as played out on the global stage.

Not all avian welfare problems lend themselves to legislative solutions. For example, a high rate of abandonment of parrots and an overburdened rescue system trying to deal with the unwanted birds are problems unlikely to be resolved by laws or regulations. Dealing with dog and cat overpopulation challenges requires public education, and dealing with the parrot relinquishment and sanctuary needs will require the same. Federal and state legislation can bring bird dealer and rescue facilities under government oversight and potentially improve bird living conditions, but it cannot solve the problem of people abandoning unwanted pets. (As noted above, the U.S. AWA regulates some dealers, but sanctuaries are regulated only if they exhibit their animals. Therefore, regulation of birds under the U.S. AWA would still not provide most birds at rescue facilities with legislative protection beyond the local anticruelty laws.)

Avian veterinarians should ensure their understanding of avian welfare issues is current, so that they can counsel bird owners on the scientific aspects of such issues. Laws and regulations are political and thus may or may not be based on current scientific knowledge, but veterinarians should recognize both the science and the politics behind legislative initiatives so that they can provide science-based advice to their clients whenever possible. They should also understand what animal welfare legislation can and cannot do to move avian welfare forward, so that they can knowledgeably discuss controversial issues with their clients. As noted at the beginning of this section, good husbandry can help resolve and/or prevent health problems, so veterinarians should be well informed about the current science of avian husbandry and welfare for that reason alone, but veterinarians are also seen by the public as animal welfare experts, and animal welfare experts should be knowledgeable about all facets of animal welfare, including the legislative aspects. Hopefully, the information in this chapter will provide a good start in obtaining that knowledge.

REFERENCES

1. American Veterinary Medical Association: *Animal abuse and animal neglect.* https://www.avma.org/KB/Policies/Pages/Animal-Abuse-and-Animal-Neglect.aspx. Accessed October 16, 2014.
2. Animal and Plant Health Inspection Service: *Animal Welfare Act and animal welfare regulations,* 2013. http://www.aphis.usda.gov/animal_welfare/downloads/Animal%20Care%20Blue%20Book%20-%202013%20-%20FINAL.pdf. Accessed October 16, 2014.
3. American College of Laboratory Animal Medicine: *The history of the American College Of Laboratory Animal Medicine,* the first fifty years 1957–2007. Compiled by Middleton, C; edited by La Regina, M. http://www.aclam.org/Content/files/files/Public/Active/ACLAMHistoryComplete-02.pdf. Accessed October 16, 2014.
4. Nolen RS: Birds of a feather, *J Am Vet Med Assoc* 245(6):734–738, 2013. https://www.avma.org/News/JAVMANews/Pages/130915a.aspx. Accessed October 16, 2014.
5. Kelly D, McCarthy E, Menzel K, et al: *Avian welfare issues: an overview; avian welfare coalition,* 2014. http://www.avianwelfare.org/issues/overview.htm. Accessed October 16, 2014.
6. Association of Avian Veterinarians: *Find a vet form.* http://aav.site-ym.com/search/custom.asp?id=1803. Accessed October 16, 2014.
7. Adams B, Larson J: *Legislative history of the Animal Welfare Act, introduction,* National Agricultural Library. http://www.nal.usda.gov/awic/pubs/AWA2007/intro.shtml. Accessed October 16, 2014.
8. California legislative information: *Health and safety code, division 105 communicable disease prevention and control, part 6 veterinary public health and safety, chapter 6 sale of birds.* http://leginfo.legislature.ca.gov/faces/codes_displayText.xhtml?lawCode=HSC&division=105.&title=&part=6.&chapter=6.&article. Accessed October 16, 2014.
9. Massachusetts Energy and Environmental Affairs: *330 Code of Massachusetts Regulations (CMR): Department of Food & Agriculture, 12.00: licensing and operation of pet shops.* http://www.mass.gov/eea/docs/agr/legal/regs/330-cmr-12-00.pdf. Accessed October 16, 2014.
10. Colorado Secretary of State: *Department of Agriculture, Animal Industry Division, Rules and Regulations Pertaining to the Administration and Enforcement of the Pet Animal Care and Facilities Act, 8 Code of Colorado Regulations (CCR) 1201-11.* http://www.sos.state.co.us/CCR/GenerateRulePdf.do?ruleVersionId=5825. Accessed October 16, 2014.
11. Minnesota Office of the Revisor of Statutes: *Minnesota Statutes 346.40 Pet Birds,* 2014. https://www.revisor.mn.gov/statutes/?id=346.40. Accessed October 16, 2014.
12. Council of Europe's Treaty Office: *European Convention for the Protection of Pet Animals,* 1987. http://conventions.coe.int/Treaty/en/Treaties/Html/125.htm. Accessed October 16, 2014.
13. Netherlands Government: *Besluit houders van dieren, Geldend op 25-09-2014, Bijlage I. als bedoeld in artikel 1.20 van het Besluit houders van dieren.* http://wetten.overheid.nl/BWBR0035217/volledig/geldigheidsdatum_25-09-2014#BijlageI. Accessed October 16, 2014.
14. Brücher H, van den Elzen R, Fergenbauer-Kimmel A, et al: *Bundesministeriums für Ernährung und Landwirtschaft. Sachverständigengruppe Gutachten über die tierschutzgerechte Haltung von Vögeln, Mindestanforderungen an die Haltung von Papageien,* 1995. http://www.bmel.de/SharedDocs/Downloads/Landwirtschaft/Tier/Tierschutz/GutachtenLeitlinien/HaltungPapageien.pdf?__blob=publicationFile. Accessed October 16, 2014.
15. Tierschutzgutachten / Tierschutzleitlinien, Haltung von Kleinvögeln, Gutachten der Sachverständigengruppe über die tierschutzgerechte Haltung von Vögeln, Brücher H, van den Elzen R, Pagel T, et al: *Bundesministeriums für Ernährung und Landwirtschaft,* 1996. http://www.bmel.de/DE/Tier/1_Tierschutz/Tierschutzgutachten/_texte/GutachtenDossier.html?notFirst=true&docId=377432. Accessed October 16, 2014.
16. Australian Capital Territory (ACT) Government: *Animal Welfare (Welfare of Captive Birds Code of Practice) Approval 1995,* 1995. http://

www.legislation.act.gov.au/di/1995-129/default.asp. Accessed October 16, 2014.

17. New South Wales (NSW) Department of Primary Industries: *NSW Code of Practice No 4 - Keeping and Trading of Birds*, 1996. http://www.dpi.nsw.gov.au/agriculture/livestock/animal-welfare/codes/aw-code-4. Accessed October 16, 2014.

18. Northern Territory Government Department of Primary Industry and Fisheries: *Northern Territory Animal Welfare Advisory Committee Guidelines for the Care and Welfare of Caged Birds.* http://www.animalwelfare.nt.gov.au/__data/assets/pdf_file/0011/47990/Guidelines_Caged_Birds.pdf. Accessed October 16, 2014.

19. Queensland Government Department of Environment and Heritage Protection: *Code of Practice Aviculture.* http://www.ehp.qld.gov.au/register/p00055aa.pdf. Accessed October 16, 2014.

20. Government of South Australia Department of Environment, Water and Natural Resources: *Code of practice for the husbandry of captive birds.* http://www.environment.sa.gov.au/managing-natural-resources/plants-and-animals/Animal_welfare/Codes_of_practice/Animal_welfare_codes_of_practice. Accessed October 16, 2014.

21. State Government of Victoria Department of Environment and Primary Industries: *Code of Practice for the Housing of Caged Birds.* http://www.depi.vic.gov.au/pets/other-pets/birds/code-of-practice-for-the-housing-of-caged-birds. Accessed October 16, 2014.

22. Wageningen UR, van Dixhoorn IDE, van Dierendonck M, van Eerdenburg F, et al. *Wageningen UR Livestock Research Rapport 428 Scheiden van dieren*, 2011, http://edepot.wur.nl/165114. Accessed October 16, 2014.

AS FREE AS A BIRD ON THE WING: SOME WELFARE AND ETHICAL CONSIDERATIONS ON FLIGHT RESTRAINT METHODS IN BIRDS

Claudia M. Vinke, Yvonne R.A. van Zeeland, Nico J. Schoemaker, Franck L.B. Meijboom

As free as a bird on the wing—this saying alone may invite you to question what type of welfare implications might be involved if we want to prevent our pet and aviary birds from flying. Procedures like wing trimming and permanent deflighting procedures are among the most controversial topics on an international scale; yet deflighting is one of the most routinely performed procedures in veterinary practice. That this topic is surrounded by so much controversy raises these questions: Is wing trimming a basic service that an owner can and may expect when consulting a veterinarian for a routine checkup, or does the procedure warrant a more careful approach and critical analysis prior to deciding whether to temporarily or permanently deflight the bird? What are the *best* methods (i.e., least intrusive, least painful, and most effective) and to what purpose?

To answer these questions, some fundamental ethical and welfare aspects have to be addressed. These include discussions on whether flying is an essential behavioral needed for a bird, and whether a bird's welfare will be impaired when it is not able to fly. These issues are complex by nature, because deflighting a bird does not automatically imply reduced welfare. Paradoxically, it seems that some deflighting techniques may actually increase the bird's opportunities to express other biologically relevant behaviors, which they would otherwise miss out on if they had unclipped wings but were housed in a more restrictive enclosure. Other questions that are raised when discussing the topic of deflighting a bird concern the purposes for which we deflight our pet birds, pros and cons of deflighting, the techniques used to deflight a bird, and whether performing such a procedure is morally acceptable. In this chapter, the various techniques to deflight a bird will be discussed, including their pros and cons from a welfare and ethical perspective.

WHY DECISIONS TO DEFLIGHT A BIRD SHOULD NOT BE TAKEN LIGHTLY: THE GROWING ISSUE OF ANIMAL WELFARE

Throughout the decades, animal welfare has received growing attention in both public and academic realms. To understand this development, one could point to our improved knowledge of the biology and physiology of animals, including birds. However, this can only partly explain why one should pay attention to welfare issues related to trimming and deflighting procedures. Another argument that may explain the attention to bird welfare is the broadly shared idea that humans should not harm animals. This argument has a long tradition[1]; however, concern for cruelty was not always primarily related to animals. For instance, John Locke (1632–1704)[2] argued that children should be educated in a way that teaches them not to be cruel to animals. He nonetheless justified this by stressing the potential link between cruelty against animals in childhood and against humans in later life. The current attention to the welfare of birds is no longer justified merely by its impact on humans, but truly focuses on the welfare of the animal itself. This increased awareness of animal welfare often starts with the acknowledgment that birds have the capacity to experience pain and pleasure, and may even possess higher cognitive capacities, such as goal-directed behaviors. Consequently, birds may have interests and preferences that can be frustrated by human actions, emphasizing that humans have duties to prevent such frustrations and take animal welfare seriously. The aforementioned link further stresses the interplay between ethics and science: whereas the assessment of a bird's cognitive capacities as morally relevant involves normative assumptions, it also implies the need for scientific evidence to assess whether and to what level birds indeed possess such capacities and whether and which welfare issues may arise from human interventions such as deflighting a bird.

The welfare assessments of the various deflighting methods discussed in this chapter will start from the normative assumption that birds are morally considered for their own sake and not only because of the instrumental value they may have for humans. At the same time, physiology and behavioral science are used to address the question of whether and to what extent birds are harmed by deflighting.

THE PURPOSE AND INCIDENCE OF DEFLIGHTING

Before raising the welfare discussion on deflighting techniques, the purposes for which birds are deflighted and the biological and ethical issues and implications associated with

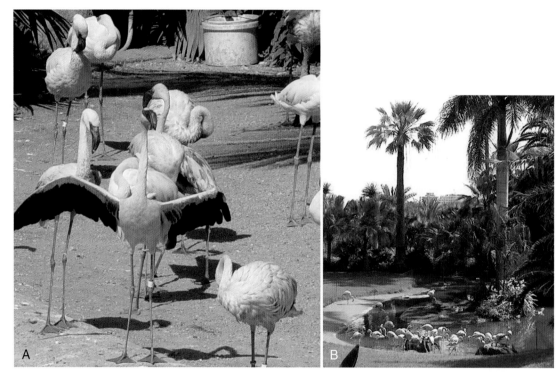

FIGURE 22-1 Permanent deflighting methods can offer distinct benefits for some zoo-logically displayed species, such as these flamingos. **A,** The pinioned left wing of the lead bird is clearly visible with its wings extended. **B,** A collection of pinioned birds on exhibit in a zoological park, with only light, almost transparent, fencing required for containment. (Photos courtesy Brian Speer.)

this procedure need to be addressed. Along with medical reasons, which necessitate wing amputation (e.g., tumors, trauma, wing tip necrosis, xanthomas, chronic inflammation), the most common indications for deflighting include the temporary or permanent removal of flight, the temporary limitation of flight, or the modification of flight capability.[3] These procedures are widely applied in various settings including the commercial poultry industry, laboratories, zoos, avicultural parks, and private homes.[4] For decades, deflighting procedures such as pinioning have been commonplace in waterfowl and large zoo birds, such as ducks, geese, swans, pelicans, and cranes, traditionally housed in open enclosures for public display and in private collections.[5] Despite deflighting procedures being commonly and routinely applied all over the world, there is no central registration keeping track of the numbers of birds that are deflighted on a yearly basis. Therefore, it is impossible to give exact insight into the total number of birds that are trimmed or deflighted (either using a temporary or permanent technique).

Although deflighting deprives birds of their ability to fly, the procedure also provides the bird with new opportunities to express alternative behavioral patterns that it would not have been able to express when confined to a conventional cage.[4] Because of the inability of the bird to fly away or escape, it is often allowed a greater range of motion, either by housing it in a large, open outdoor enclosure (e.g., in case of zoo birds or waterfowl; Figure 22-1) or because it is allowed to roam freely around the house and/or may be taken outside (in case of pet birds).

In addition, the deflighting may be beneficial at least temporarily when dealing with a bird that is displaying signs of aggression and/or biting toward humans or other animals, creating a safer environment for people to interact with the bird while trying to modify this behavior. Alternatively, it may also be an important tool to aid in training and socializing birds, especially those that are fearful and/or those that are untamed. In the proper situation, a temporary deflighting procedure can

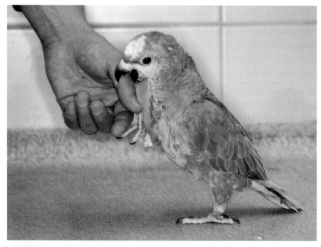

FIGURE 22-2 After trimming its wing feathers, this orange-winged Amazon parrot *(Amazona amazonica)* quickly gained trust in the owner and was willing to step up on the hand.

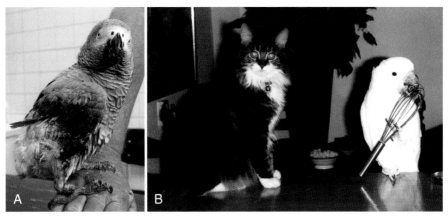

FIGURE 22-3 **A,** This Grey parrot *(Psittacus e. erithacus)* was attacked by a dog and unable to flee because its wings were trimmed. **B,** Some birds seem to live very harmoniously together with predators, such as cats. This cat and cockatoo are fully comfortable together, although the owner will never keep these animals together without supervision.

be used to render the bird more dependent on its caretaker (e.g., to be transported to a different location), increasing the chance of establishing a reinforced trustworthy relationship[6] (Figure 22-2). It should, however, be taken into consideration that this approach is a more forceful, intrusive, and possibly coercive intervention strategy compared with other alternatives for addressing aggressive and other behavioral problems. Therefore, it is recommended that other less intrusive strategies should always be considered prior to or concurrently with the contemplated deflighting procedure (see Chapter 5).

On the downside of deflighting pet birds, it should be realized that the inability of the bird to take off also prevents the bird from escaping potential danger, (e.g., when it is under attack from a dog, cat, or another bird) (Figure 22-3). Prior to deciding whether or not to deflight a bird, the bird's living conditions and its interaction with family members and other pets should always be considered while carefully weighing the potential benefits and disadvantages of the deflighting procedure.

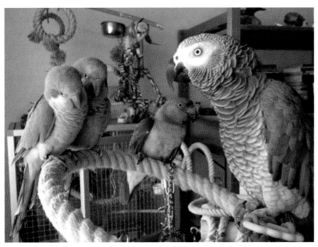

FIGURE 22-4 Trimming the wing feathers of birds allows them to come outside of the cage and be placed on a play stand. (Photo courtesy Ellen Uittenbogaard.)

Reasonably, today's pet bird owners want to see and engender more species-specific behavior from their animals. These desires lead to searches for alternatives to the traditional cage, housing them in less restrictive aviary housings or indoors on play stands, trees, and/or gyms, or even in rooms specifically designated for the bird (Figure 22-4). Similarly, public opinion warrants the choice for natural, open enclosures in a zoo instead of the unsightly, wire-mesh aviaries that were previously seen.[7] Parallel to this trend, more caged birds may be expected to be trimmed in the future to prevent them from flying away from their residence. Alternatively, for those who feel strongly about not clipping their bird's wings because of ethical, welfare, or cosmetic concerns, but do want to take their bird outside, the use of specially designed harnesses and/or flight training may be taken into consideration.

WHAT DOES FLIGHT MEAN FOR A BIRD?

Welfare may include physical, medical, and behavioral aspects. Some physical and medical implications of flight restraint and the meaning of behavioral needs or priorities are discussed below.

Physical and Medical Implications

The complex muscle architecture of the wing enables a bird to produce the aerodynamic power that is essential for lifting it into the air and advance and maneuver itself during flight[8] (Figure 22-5). Aside from flying, the wings of a bird have a substantial role in balance during sitting, walking, and running.[7,9] The inability of the bird to balance itself as a result of a deflighting procedure may cause serious injuries as the bird can fall and harm itself.[3]

Wing flapping is reported to increase the tibia strength (in hens[10]) while flying improves flight musculature[11] and provides cardiovascular exercise.[12] It has been proposed that flight deprivation may be a predisposing factor for avian atherosclerosis[13] because this disease is seen in flight-restrained species.[7] Just as in many other species, restricted exercise in birds may also result in obesity[14] and weight gain-related medical problems such as lipomas.[7] Deflighting procedures

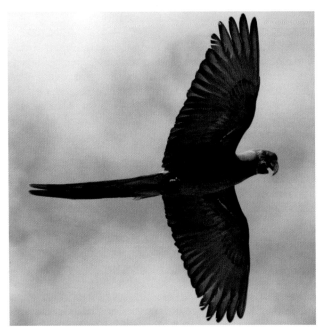

FIGURE 22-5 The primary role of the wings and flight feathers is for flight as demonstrated by this military macaw *(Ara militaris).*

may therefore pose a risk for the development of these medical problems.

Behavioral Implications

For biologists, the ultimate questions to be answered are *what does a captive bird want, and what does the captive bird miss*? Behavioral needs, or what the animal considers indispensable, have been described in various ways in the literature of animal welfare and welfare assessment. One approach is to reflect on the wild or the natural environment and suggests that all elements that are denied to animals in captivity can be described as either lacking or deprived.[15,16] This approach has been largely rejected by many animal welfare scientists citing the organism's behavioral plasticity and the effects of domestication and humans' selective breeding programs.[17-20] Therefore, the term *behavioral priority* is preferably used instead of behavioral needs. Behavioral priority takes into account a hierarchy of requirements in line with different motivations, whereby the need to satisfy these particular motivations depends on internal and external circumstances and previous experiences and current circumstances (context); it also takes into account the motivational and emotional state of the particular individual.[21] Despite many publications on this topic, it is not possible to give precise standards on the timing, duration, and frequency that a particular "indispensable" behavioral pattern should be performed by an individual member of that species, allowed to be labeled as "good" or "enough."[21,22] An animal's welfare status therefore may best be represented by the adaptive value of the individual's interaction with a given environmental setting (e.g., getting food, handling and restraint, social interaction)—a dynamic concept.[23] This adaptive value is dependent on the individual's life history, including emotional, behavioral, morphological, and physiological consequences, and the result of a variable mix of factors, e.g., genetic make-up, prenatal (stress) situations, early

life experiences (such as mother–child interactions, weaning age, imprinting and socialization), social relationships and status, diverse learning experiences, and traumatic experiences. Hence, an intermingled complex of genetic, species-specific and individual traits, ontogenetic development, and (later) learning processes occur as a result of specific environmental conditions and experiences.[24,25] Animal welfare assessment can best be seen in light of this dynamic complex whereby the animal's welfare is compromised "if the impact of adverse internal or external factors (or their interaction) challenges the animal's adaptability, such that the animal cannot adapt to the demands of the prevailing environmental circumstances to enable it to reach a state which it perceives as positive."[23,25a]

The first aspect to address is the wing and its basic function, which can be different in each separate bird species dependent on the evolutionary optimization that enables the bird to interact with and adapt to its natural habitat(s) and environment(s). Flying is the most well-known function of a bird's wing, although not in all species. Wings can be anatomically and morphologically adapted to serve in a specific function in the natural environment, which may vary from, for example, efficient foraging (the herons' "umbrella" to attract fish) and attracting sexual partners in courtship[9] to balancing on a partner during copulation[5] (Figure 22-6; for other functions of the wing see Figure 22-7). The type of function is often clearly visible in the feather structure, feather density, wing structure, and feather coloration and decoration, with great differences present between the species, for example, ostrich versus swallow.

In addition to the basic wing function, we can determine which basic ethological motivation is underlying flight. For many flighted bird species, flying is the preferred and the most efficient way of locomotion to fulfill several basic motivations enabling them to cope with the environment in an adequate way (e.g., escape from predators, search for sexual

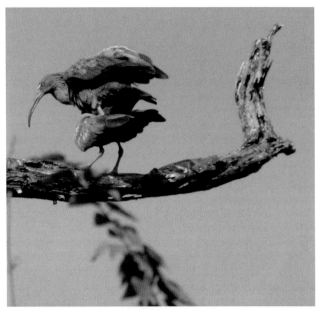

FIGURE 22-6 The wings of this male plumbeous ibis *(Theristicus caerulescens)* are used to balance on top of his female during copulation.

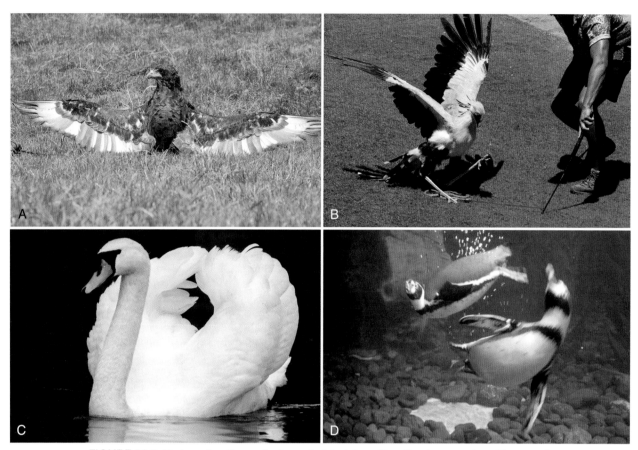

FIGURE 22-7 Various functions of wings. **A,** A bateleur *(Terathopius ecaudatus)* is spreading its wings during sunbathing to catch as much sun as possible. **B,** A secretary bird *(Sagittarius serpentarius)* uses its wings to balance while catching a fake snake during a demonstration. **C,** A male mute swan *(Cygnus olor)* using its wings for display. **D,** These black-footed penguins *(Spheniscus demersus)* use their wings to "fly" under water.

partners, reaching essential foraging or nesting sites). Generally, the inability to fulfill these kinds of basic motivations because of anatomical restriction, housing conditions, or management procedures may result in stress and the development of abnormal behaviors such as stereotypies, compulsive disorders, and automutilation.[12,26-30]

Based on the above, wings should be considered multifunctional extremities for a bird that may serve many basic functions and satisfy the motivations behind these functions. Especially the species-specific functions and basic motivations *beyond the wing* should carefully be considered in the decision-making process of whether or not to deflight a bird. Evidence-based answers on the indispensability of wings to perform certain behavioral patterns are scarce and open for future research. The impossibility of fulfilling essential basic motivations may, however, result in acute and/or chronic stress. With stress in captive birds considered as one of the most important predisposing causes of disease,[7,31] the potential stress induced by deflighting may negatively affect both the bird's health and welfare.

Although flight is one of the best-known functions of a bird wing, research on the consequences of flight restriction on the bird's welfare is scarce. In 2013, Peng et al[32] evaluated the pathological, ethological, and physiological consequences of deflighting in five wild caught, pinioned great mynahs

(Acridotheres grandis). In two birds that were evaluated for presence of neuroma formation, no abnormalities were detected at the site of amputation. In two other birds, space preference, as measured by entree frequency through a one-way door construction, was evaluated whereby the pinioned birds were found to have a preference for bigger cages or those with increased vertical space. In the fifth bird, electromyography of the pectoral muscle revealed diminished muscular strength. Based on these results, the authors concluded that the captive birds were still highly inclined to use flight as a means of transportation and deflighting resulted in marked physiologic changes in the flight musculature, which can be expected following a deflighting procedure. Although the scientific merit of this study should be considered low due to the limited number of birds evaluated, it is the only study performed regarding the effects of flight restriction in birds.

ETHICAL CONSIDERATIONS: WELFARE AND BEYOND

From the previous analysis it is clear that there are no easy answers to the welfare problems related to deflighting birds. Each technique requires its own welfare assessment. However, from an ethical perspective, the discussion already starts before choosing a specific technique. If we consider animals, including birds, to be morally relevant for their own sake we owe them respect. This attitude of respect should not only be translated in terms of attention to animal welfare, but also includes a referral to the notion of animal integrity. Respect for the integrity of the animal implies that we have a responsibility to take into account the wholeness and completeness of the animal, the species-specific balance of the creature, and the animal's capacity to maintain itself independently in an environment suitable to the species.[33] This responsibility cannot be reduced in terms of welfare alone. Even if an infringement of the bird's completeness or capacity to maintain itself independently would not result in pain or other discomfort, deflighting would still require an ethical justification if the performed procedure is not directly in the best interest of the animal. This not only applies to the permanent methods of deflighting involving surgical procedures, but also to the less invasive, temporary techniques of wing trimming. Although these methods may genuinely differ in terms of their impact on welfare, both alter the animal significantly and limit the bird in its capacities, at least in large part because of human interests.

The argument of animal integrity does not automatically rule out the option of deflighting, but does stress that deflighting a bird is never a neutral act. In practice, this ethical debate implies that it is imperative to first evaluate whether alternatives to deflighting or trimming a bird are available. Only when no true alternatives are found or when these alternatives are associated with other, genuine ethical problems, can the decision be made to deflight a bird and consider the various options that are available. In this decision-making process the discussion should focus on the possibilities to improve welfare by using the least intrusive method that is likely to result in a favorable outcome. The topic, however, necessitates another ethical debate, one regarding the aim of trimming or deflighting, which is closely related to the reasons for which we keep birds and the value attributed to bird keeping as a whole, based on which we justify our interventions. This discussion is rather fundamental and goes beyond the scope of this chapter. Nonetheless, it is important to be aware of such fundamental views on the values that underlie the claimed need to trim or deflight, because these directly influence the assessment and acceptability of the welfare issues related to the various methods and techniques.

COMMON DEFLIGHTING TECHNIQUES

Considering the abovementioned aspects, the decision might be made to deflight the bird. In this case, various types of deflighting techniques may be used. These techniques may either be reversible (temporary) or irreversible (permanent) and can be performed unilaterally or bilaterally, resulting in a partial or total removal of the wing's ability to lift. In practice, permanent methods are used if birds are planned to be kept uncaged long term; in other situations, temporary deflighting procedures may be opted. In 1996, Ellis and Dein[34] described nine methods of flight restraint: (1) limited amputation (removal of a portion of the wing; most common form is pinioning, which involves removal at the carpus), (2) tenotomy (severing the extensors of the carpus), (3) tenectomy (removal of a portion of the extensors of the carpus), (4) patagiectomy (removal of the patagial membrane and apposition of the

radius and the humerus), (5 and 6) wing (feather) clipping (cutting the distal functional ankyloses [fusion of the joint(s) of the wing], portions of the primary and secondary feathers), (7) brailing (binding one wing), (8) vane trimming, and (9) confinements under nets. Throughout the literature, the consensus is presented regarding the time at which the procedure is performed (i.e., deflighting should not be performed during the molting period or when growing primaries are present).[4]

A summary of the techniques that have thus far been described to (temporary or permanently) deflight a bird can be found in Tables 22-2 and 22-3 and the subsequent sections.

Temporary Deflighting Techniques

The most commonly used technique to temporarily limit the ability of a pet bird to fly is to trim the wing feathers (*remiges*; for an overview of the anatomy and nomenclature of the wing and feather see Figure 22-8). When performed in bilateral symmetry, the trim prevents the bird from generating sufficient speed and thrust to take off, directly reducing flight capacity while still allowing the bird to slowly descend in a gliding flight. Unilateral or asymmetric trimming, in contrast, frustrates flight by severely unbalancing the bird, only allowing the bird to spiral down in an uncontrolled flight, increasing the risk for injury or trauma from an inability to properly land.[4] For this reason, unilateral and asymmetric wing trims are strongly discouraged.

When clipping the wing feathers it is important to remove the least amount of feathers as possible. When the bird is still able to lift, more of the feather can be removed. If too many feathers are removed, however, the bird may crash land, potentially leading to serious injury. When performing a wing clip, clipping of the secondary feathers (as shown in Figure 22-9) should be avoided, as these feathers are important for landing and decreasing speed during landing. Clipping them removes the bird's ability to glide down.

The bilateral wing trim may be performed in various ways. The choice on how to cut the feathers is often based on personal preference, in which the cosmetic and esthetic effect as well as the support of neighboring feathers may be important factors to consider,[3,4] Three different methods of bilateral wing clipping are described in the following list.

Method 1: The primary feathers are clipped in a curved pattern whereby the outer primary (P10) is cut the shortest and the most inner primary (P1) is kept the longest (Figure 22-10). If performed in this way, a nice cosmetic result is achieved whereby, during a molt, the new primaries receive support during the development by their neighboring feathers. This method is preferred by the authors.

Method 2: The outer five to eight primaries are cut 5 to 25 mm distal to the coverts (Figure 22-11). The cut primaries should still have enough length to provide support for newly developing feathers during molt. With this method a less cosmetic effect is achieved compared with method 1.

Method 3 (often referred to as "show clip")[3]: The outer two to three primaries remain untouched, while the next five to eight primaries may be cut very short (up to or below the level of the coverts; Figure 22-12). Many perceive this method to be the most cosmetic, as the outer primaries are the ones that cross over the tail in a nonclipped bird. With

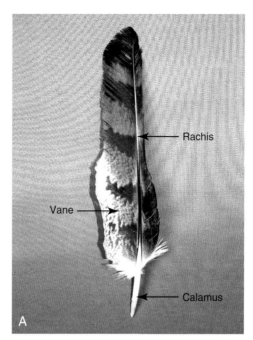

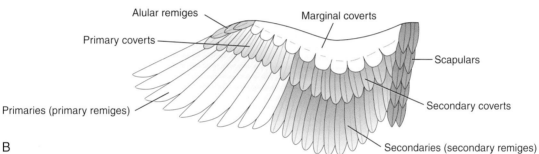

FIGURE 22-8 Anatomy and terminology of the wing feathers. The main shaft of the feather is the scapus and is divided into the vexillum (vaned portion) and calamus (unvaned portion). The vane is the majority of the feather extending perpendicular to the shaft. The scapus is the central axis of a feather composed of the calamus (unvaned) and the rachis (vaned). (From Miller RE, Fowler ME: *Fowler's zoo and wild animal medicine*, vol 8, St Louis, MO, 2015, Elsevier.)

this method, there is also potentially less risk of feather damage as the outer feathers do not have sharp edges that may irritate the bird. This method, however, does have several disadvantages:

- When the outer primaries are left untouched, the bird may be able to achieve enough lift to fly away and/or crash because of impaired flight capabilities. This is especially the case in the lighter built species (e.g., cockatiels).
- In the more heavily built species (e.g., Grey parrots, Amazon parrots) too much wing support may have been lost by removing the more inner placed feathers. As a result these birds may injure themselves during landing.
- The outer primaries have become more vulnerable to damage and during molt as there is insufficient support for the newly developing feathers. Since the latter feathers are heavily innervated, molting may become a painful event, which may result in self-inflicted damage to these new feathers.

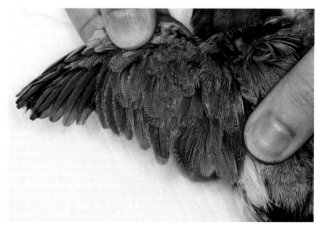

FIGURE 22-9 All primary and secondary wing feathers have been clipped in this lovebird. As a result, the wing does not have its weight-bearing capability anymore, which may easily lead to trauma during a fall or landing.

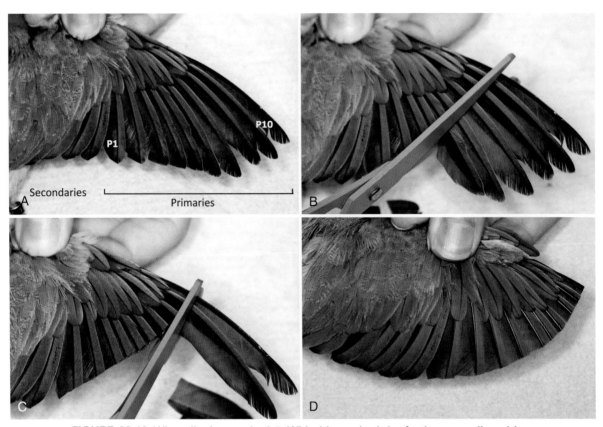

FIGURE 22-10 Wing clipping method 1. With this method the feathers are clipped in a curved pattern where primary 1 is kept the longest and primary 10 the shortest. **A,** Fully feathered spread wing of a lovebird. **B** and **C,** Demonstration of the direction in which the primary feathers are clipped. **D,** End result after clipping. In larger, heavily bodied birds typically fewer feathers are clipped because of problems with excessive alteration of lift.

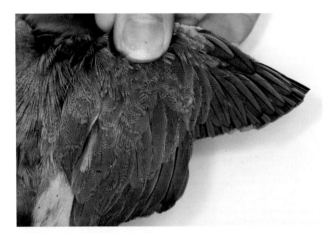

FIGURE 22-11 Wing clipping method 2. With this method a different cosmetic effect is achieved compared with method 1. All 10 of the primary flight feathers have been trimmed slightly longer than the level of the dorsal wing coverts. As mentioned in Figure 22-10, in larger, heavily bodied birds typically fewer feathers are clipped because of problems with excessive alteration of lift.

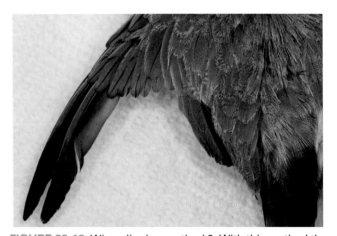

FIGURE 22-12 Wing clipping method 3. With this method the outer two to three primaries are left unclipped. When this wing is folded next to the body, it is not visible that the wings have been clipped, which is perceived by some as a more cosmetic option of wing clipping. Primaries 8-1 have been clipped, underneath the dorsal wing coverts. Fewer feathers are typically clipped in larger bird species.

TABLE 22-1

Recommended Wing Clip Patterns for Different Types of Psittacines

Body Type	Species	Wing Clip Pattern
Small, experienced flyers	Budgerigars and other parakeets	Frequently all 10 primaries need to be clipped
Light weight, strong, swift flyers	Cockatiels, small macaw species, lories	Frequently, up to a maximum of the outer seven primaries need to be clipped
Slower, heavy built birds	Grey parrots, Amazon parrots, *Poicephalus* spp.	Frequently, clipping of the outer four to six primaries or fewer is sufficient

From Speer BL: The clinical consequences of routine grooming, *Proceedings of the Association of Avian Veterinarians*, Orlando, Florida, 2001, pp 109–115.

The amount of feathers, and the extent to how far the feathers are cut, is dependent on the build of the bird involved. In heavy birds (e.g., Grey parrots) perhaps only five feathers are cut, while in light birds (e.g., cockatiels and macaws) more feathers are cut (Table 22-1). In addition, the age of the bird and its flight experience should also be taken into consideration when performing a wing trim. Especially young and unexperienced birds can be clumsy and are more prone to falling and injury.[35] Therefore, it is frequently recommended to delay wing clipping until the bird is a bit more confident and has learned to fly, and more important, land. Only once the young bird is able to fly and safely land on a perch may a wing trim be performed, with a gradual increase in the number and/or length of the feathers that are clipped to ensure a gradual reduction in the bird's flying capabilities, allowing it to become accustomed to the loss of flight ability and limiting the risk of injury (Figure 22-13). Interestingly, on the topic of gradual loss and prior experience, recent animal welfare discussions were launched addressing the topic of prior experience and its influence on the level of motivation for the resource or performing a specific behavior: *Can you miss what you never have experienced?* So far, the outcomes of this discussion are so unclear that it is impossible to assess the consequences of a bird's prior flight experiences on its motivation to flight, and more research should be done for sound conclusions.

In addition to the wing clip, other temporary deflighting techniques have been described. An overview of these other techniques, including a short description of the procedure, the handling procedures and post-operative recovery, and the potential risks for side effects and complications involved in these procedures are summarized in Table 22-2.

Permanent Deflighting Techniques

All permanent methods of deflighting involve surgery of the bone and/or soft tissue (for an overview of the patagia and osseous anatomy of the wing, see Figure 22-14), which generally necessitates the use of anesthesia and analgesia. The exception to this "rule" is pinioning of 2- to 3-day-old chicks, whereby the wings are cut with regular scissors without the use of anesthesia and analgesia (Figure 22-15). In these young animals hardly any blood loss is seen. Pinioning in adult birds, however, requires anesthesia and the use of a tourniquet, hemostatic agents, and sutures to minimize bleeding.[36] The most commonly applied pinioning technique is to cut the metacarpals just below the alula, which should preferably be performed at the time that the chick's bones are not yet

hardened, but at an age that the risk for hemorrhage is minimal.[4] The alular bone must remain intact to protect the stub. Alternatively, the wing may be amputated at the level of the carpometacarpal joint[37] (Figure 22-16) or ulna.[4,38]

Two other techniques that may be performed as alternatives to pinioning include patagiectomy and tenonectomy. During a tenonectomy a portion of the extensor tendons of

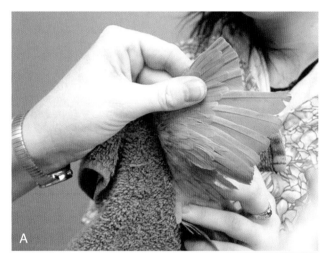

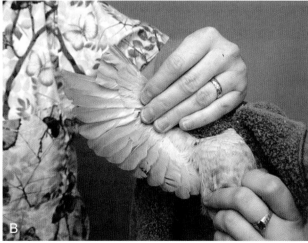

FIGURE 22-13 In this young green-cheeked conure *(Pyrrhura molinae)* only the outermost primaries (10-7) are bilaterally clipped to reduce thrust and lightly modify flight capabilities to facilitate a training plan. **A,** Dorsal view. **B,** Ventral view. (Photos courtesy Brian Speer.)

TABLE 22-2

Overview of Different Temporary Deflighting Techniques

Name	Procedure Description	Handling Aspects and Postoperative Recovery	Potential Risks and Complications	References
Wing/feather clipping	Clipping of the primaries using scissors. Various patterns may be used, with the extent of a wing clip varying from cutting a part of the primaries to all the primaries and most or all of the distal secondaries (unilaterally or bilaterally). Unilateral clips or clipping of the secondaries should be avoided because of increased risks of injury and stress to the birds.	Preferably two persons: one clipping and one holding the animals and positioning and stretching the wing. Repeated treatment necessary following a subsequent molt.	Splintering the calamus or tear the follicle (risk by using blunt instruments) → risk for irritation. Cutting too short → risk for severing the blood vessels. Cutting too long → risk for (handicapped) flight, thus higher risk for injuries. Cutting in growth stage: especially for feathers in development, hemorrhages can occur as the feathers are highly vascular at this moment. Indirect: unbalance by the unilateral clip → risk for injuries; insufficient support for newly developing feathers.	Speer, 2001[3]; Hesterman et al, 2001[4]; Ellis and Dein, 1996[34]; AZA Avian Scientific Advisory Group, 2013[65]
Brailing	Wing strapping in flexed position. Leather or plastic strap is fitted around the primaries and patagium. Brail is inserted between the bases of the third- and fourth-most distal primaries. Applied for temporary restraint, e.g., in young birds for transport.	Preferably two persons handling: one strapping and one immobilizing the bird and stretching the wing. Repeated treatment. For long-term use, a change to the opposite wing is necessary every 2 weeks.	No longer than 3 weeks, otherwise it may interfere with the growth of the wing. Must fit properly, otherwise blood circulation restrictions or skin lesions. Risk for damaging growing blood feathers. Stiffness after immobilizing (2 weeks change advised to prevent stiffness of the immobilized wing).	Hesterman et al, 2001[4]; Zhang et al, 2011[5]; Ellis and Dein, 1996[34]; AZA Avian Scientific Advisory Group, 2013[65]
Vane trimming	Applied when feathers are growing. Vanes usually trimmed when birds are 60–70 days old (comment from authors: young birds soon after their first flight experiences). A portion of the vanes of the primaries and the distal three secondaries of one wing are trimmed with scissors.	Preferably two persons handling: one clipping and one holding the animals and positioning and stretching the wing. Repeated treatment necessary as soon as the feathers are fully grown (see wing/feather clipping).	Not reported in the literature, but probably comparable to wing clipping.	Ellis and Dein, 1996[34]; AZA Avian Scientific Advisory Group, 2013[65]
Geometric changes of the barbs	Longitudinal removal of the ventral margin of barbs from the primaries using a scalpel, changing the aerodynamics and stiffness of the feather.	Preferably two persons handling: one treating the barbs and one immobilizing the bird and stretching the wing.	No bleeding, no inflammation, and no pain or other side effects reported.	Zhang et al,[5] 2011

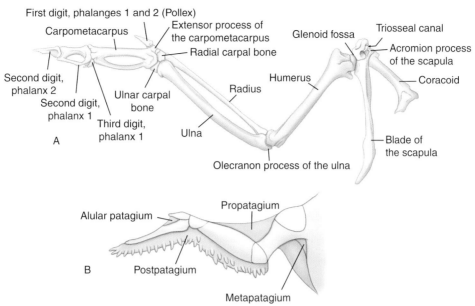

FIGURE 22-14 Anatomy of the wing. **A,** The osseous anatomy of the wing. (Diagram courtesy Dr. Stefan Harsch.) **B,** The four patagia of the wing include the propatagium, where the wing and the neck join the thorax; the postpatagium, which is located at the caudal angle of the carpus; the metapatagium at the caudal junction of the thorax and the wing; and the alular patagium between the alula and the carpometacarpus. (From Miller RE, Fowler ME: *Fowler's zoo and wild animal medicine*, vol 8, St Louis, MO, 2015, Elsevier.)

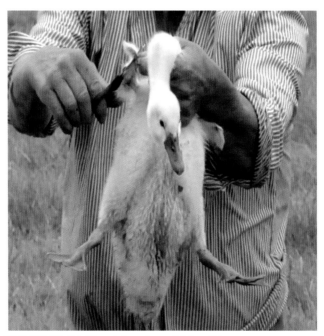

FIGURE 22-15 The right wing of this wild, young mute swan *(Cygnus olor)* is being illegally pinioned as this bird is certainly older than 3 days.

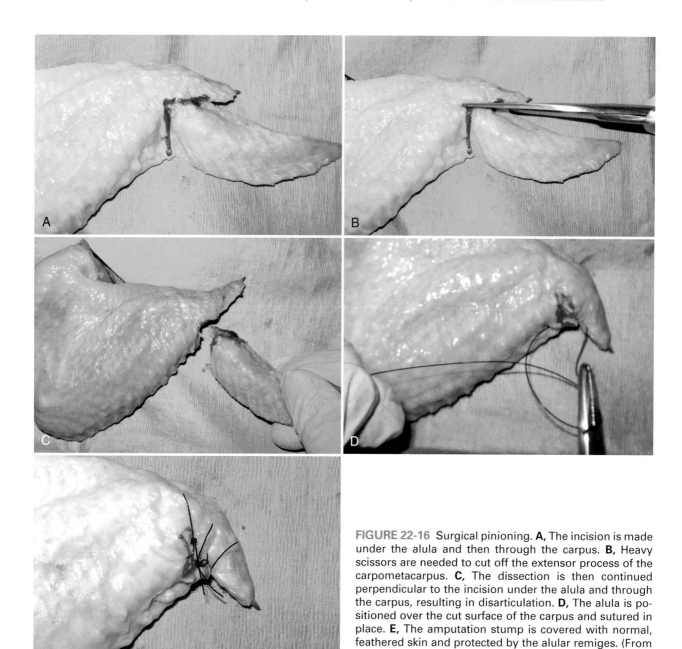

FIGURE 22-16 Surgical pinioning. **A,** The incision is made under the alula and then through the carpus. **B,** Heavy scissors are needed to cut off the extensor process of the carpometacarpus. **C,** The dissection is then continued perpendicular to the incision under the alula and through the carpus, resulting in disarticulation. **D,** The alula is positioned over the cut surface of the carpus and sutured in place. **E,** The amputation stump is covered with normal, feathered skin and protected by the alular remiges. (From Miller RE, Fowler ME: *Fowler's zoo and wild animal medicine,* vol 8, St Louis, MO, 2015, Elsevier.)

the manus is removed, followed by a 3-week period of taping to promote ankyloses of the carpal joint. In case of patagiectomy, the propatagium is removed followed by suturing of the skin and juxtaposing of the humerus and radius bones.[4] Several other techniques have been reported for permanent deflighting of birds, and an overview of these techniques can be found in Table 22-3 and seen in Figures 22-17 and 22-18.

In many countries (e.g., Great Britain, Austria, the Netherlands) most invasive permanent deflighting techniques are legally restricted by national animal protection or animal welfare and livestock regulations, unless performed by a

licensed veterinarian. An exception to this rule is made for poultry chicks (i.e., chickens, turkeys) and goslings, which may be pinioned by laymen in the first few days following hatching. Since all other permanent deflighting methods are considered more invasive and painful, anesthesia (general or local) and use of analgesics is required. Unfortunately, some laymen do pinion birds themselves at an older age by placing a ligature around the wing at the level of the proximal metacarpus leading to avascular necrosis. This technique not only results in considerable pain but will also predispose a bird for complications such as osteomyelitis, necrosis, and chronic wounds (Figure 22-19).

TABLE 22-3

Overview of Different Permanent Deflighting Techniques

Name	Procedure Description	Handling Aspects and Postoperative Recovery	Potential Risks and Complications	References
Patagiectomy	Removal of propatagium (patagial membrane) and subsequent juxtaposing of the humerus and radius bones by suturing the skin together. Should be performed under general anesthesia, with additional use of analgesics.	Operation performed under general anesthesia. Comment from authors: postoperative recovery period estimated at 1–2 weeks.	None reported, but expected to be similar to any surgical procedure.	Hesterman et al, 2001[4]; Ellis and Dein, 1996[34]; AZA Avian Scientific Advisory Group, 2013[65]; Robinson, 1975b[70]
Pinioning (see Figures 22-16 and 22-17)	Preferably performed 2–3 days after hatching. Amputation is generally performed at the level of the metacarpals (preferably leaving the alula intact). Alternatively amputation may be performed at level of metacarpus or ulna. To cut the bone hemostatic clips and/or sharp scissors (small birds) or surgical saw (larger-sized species) may be used. Tourniquet may be applied to temporarily occlude circulation. Should be performed under general anesthesia, with additional use of analgesics, except when pinioning 2–3-day-old chicks.	Operation performed under general anesthesia. Pinioning of 2–3-day-old chicks is generally performed using scissors and without anesthesia. Postoperative recovery period is 8–10 days.	Pinioning of large birds can be more complex and is therefore more often associated with complications than pinioning in smaller or younger birds. When performed during the growth of feathers, hemorrhage may occur from (accidental) trauma to the feathers. Hemorrhage resulting from trauma to other tissues may also occur. Insufficient skin to cover the bone may pose a risk for pressure necrosis. Skin trauma. Infection (preventive antibiosis may be considered). Bone splintering.	Hesterman et al, 2001[4]; Ellis and Dein, 1996[34]; Olsen, 1997[40]; D'Agustino et al, 2006[42]; AZA Avian Scientific Advisory Group, 2013[65]; Robinson, 1975a[69]; Fletcher and Miller,1980[71]
Tenectomy of the main wing tendons or extensor carpi radialis	Removal of a portion of the extensor tendons of the manus. Immobilized for 3 weeks in flexed position to allow for ankyloses of the carpal joint. Should be performed under general anesthesia, with additional use of analgesics warranted.	Operation under general anesthesia. Postoperative recovery period of 3 weeks necessary to allow for ankyloses of the carpal joint.	None reported, but expected to be similar to any surgical procedure.	Hesterman et al, 2001[4]; Ellis and Dein, 1996[34]; AZA Avian Scientific Advisory Group, 2013[65]; Miller, 1973[72]
Tenectomy of the musculus supracoracoideus	Transection of the tendon of the musculus supracoracoideus at its insertion on the proximal humerus. May be performed unilaterally or bilaterally. Should be performed under general anesthesia, with additional use of analgesics recommended.	Operation under general anesthesia. Transparent adhesive dressing applied for 3 days. Postoperative recovery period of 3–6 weeks (as some subjects start to fly).	None reported, but expected to be similar to any surgical procedure. Lack of efficacy reported in cockatiels and pigeons, rendering the technique ineffective for deflighting in these species.	Degernes and Feduccia, 2001[41]

Continued

TABLE 22-3

Overview of Different Permanent Deflighting Techniques—cont'd

Name	Procedure Description	Handling Aspects and Postoperative Recovery	Potential Risks and Complications	References
Tenotomy, notching, and dewinging	Severing the extensors of the manus with a thermocautery instrument. Cutting and cauterization of the main wing tendon: a small segment of the tendon of the musculus extensor metacarpi radialis is removed. Wing should be immobilized for 3 weeks in flexed position to promote ankyloses of the carpal joint. Alternatively, cut and removal of a section of the superficial pectoral muscle and propatagial tendon. Local anesthesia and analgesia.	Handling and restraint throughout the procedure (if local anesthesia is applied). Alternatively procedure may be performed under general anesthesia. Postoperative recovery period is 3 weeks (to allow sufficient ankylosis of the carpal joint).	Postoperative bleeding may occur in case of insufficient immobilization. Limited flight possible in some birds, warranting an additional wing trim.	Hesterman et al, 2001[4]; Ellis and Dein, 1996[34]; Olsen, 1997[40]; AZA Avian Scientific Advisory Group, 2013[65]; Fletcher, 1989[71]; Miller, 1973[72];
Functional ankylosis of the carpal joint	Fixing the ulna, carpal, and metacarpal bones in a bent position. Requires general anesthesia, with additional use of analgesics recommended.	Operation under general anesthesia. Postoperative recovery period not reported, but comparable to tenectomy (3–6 weeks).	None reported, but similar to any orthopedic surgery (e.g., osteomyelitis).	Ellis and Dein, 1996[34]; AZA Avian Scientific Advisory Group, 2013[65]
Radial neurectomy	Surgical removal of about 8–10 mm of the radial nerve. Requires general anesthesia, with additional use of analgesics recommended.	Operation under general anesthesia.	None reported, but expected to be similar to any surgical procedure. Reported ineffective at preventing flight.	Hesterman et al, 2001[4]
Feather follicle ablation/extirpation (see Figure 22-18)	Ablation of primary feather follicles through surgery, or using a diode laser or cryoprobe (freezing). Should be performed under general anesthesia, with additional use of analgesics recommended.	Operation under general anesthesia. Cryoprobe use: 5 seconds, three cycles. Diode laser use: 10 W, 2 seconds. Postoperative recovery period: all side effects were reported to resolve within 12 weeks.	D'Agustino reported diode laser (10 W) to be faster (2 seconds), easier to perform, and causing minimal tissue damage compared with a cryoprobe (20–30 seconds). Necrosis reported when using a cryoprobe. Other reported side effects include swelling, ulceration, hyperemia, edema, and serosanguineous discharge. Procedure does not appear successful for deflighting in all bird species.	D'Agustino, et al, 2006[42]; Krawinkel, 2011[73]; Shaw et al, 2012[74]

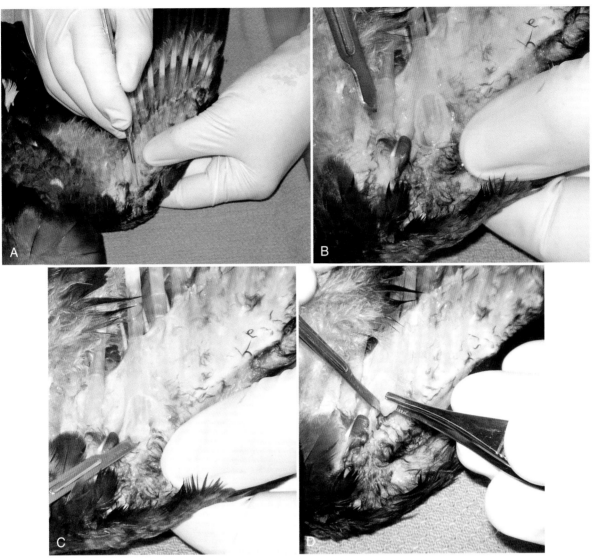

FIGURE 22-17 Feather follicle excision. For remige follicle excision in a large bird, make an incision parallel to the calamus from the insertion on the carpometacarpus about 1 cm long **(A)**. Expose the follicle and about 1 cm of calamus **(B)**. Elevate the follicle from its attachments **(C)**. Expose 5 to 10 mm of the calamus **(D)**. *Continued*

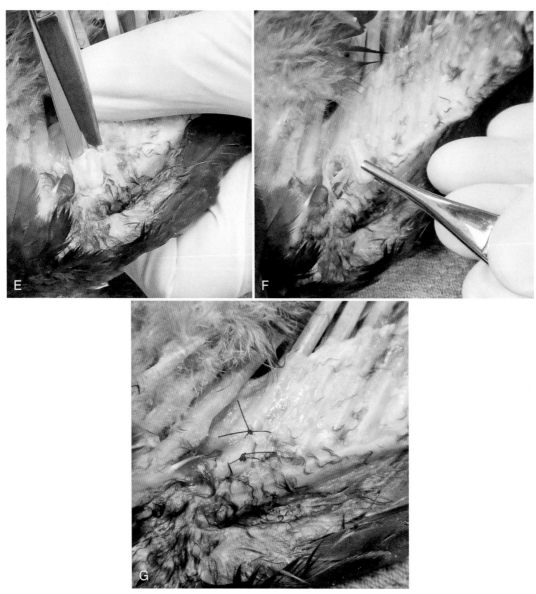

FIGURE 22-17, cont'd Cut the calamus proximal to the skin with heavy scissors **(E)**. Discard the piece of calamus with the follicle **(F)**. Place one or two sutures in the skin **(G)**. (From Miller RE, Fowler ME: *Fowler's zoo and wild animal medicine*, vol 8, St Louis, MO, 2015, Elsevier.)

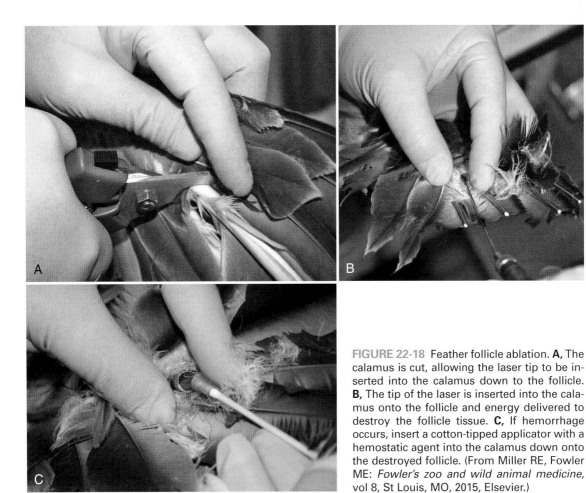

FIGURE 22-18 Feather follicle ablation. **A,** The calamus is cut, allowing the laser tip to be inserted into the calamus down to the follicle. **B,** The tip of the laser is inserted into the calamus onto the follicle and energy delivered to destroy the follicle tissue. **C,** If hemorrhage occurs, insert a cotton-tipped applicator with a hemostatic agent into the calamus down onto the destroyed follicle. (From Miller RE, Fowler ME: *Fowler's zoo and wild animal medicine,* vol 8, St Louis, MO, 2015, Elsevier.)

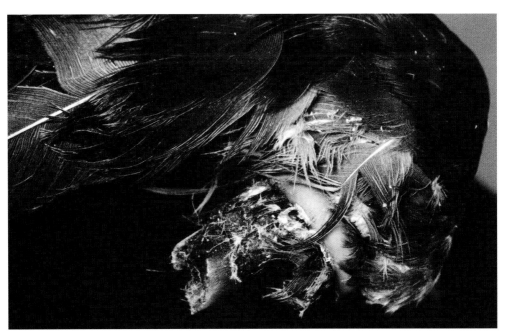

FIGURE 22-19 This black swan *(Cygnus atratus)* presented for a postpurchase examination. The right wing was found to be illegally pinioned by placing a rubber band around the metacarpal area of the right wing. This resulted in an avascular necrosis of the distal part of the wing, following which the distal part of the metacarpus was broken off, leaving an unprotected part of the metacarpus visible.

DIRECT WELFARE CONSEQUENCES AS A RESULT OF DEFLIGHTING PROCEDURES

Direct welfare consequences for the bird as a result of deflighting include direct or indirect medical and behavioral complications, pain, and stress related to handling and restraint. The specifically selected deflighting procedure, including its associated potential complications and side effects, could factually be categorized as mere technical implications. It should, however, be emphasized that the experience of pain and stress depends on the experiences early on in life and are perceived and experienced differently by each individual. For example, a wild-caught bird will likely experience a "routine" handling procedure as more stressful compared with a captive-bred bird, unless the captive bird has had an experience with forceful and stress-evoking restraint methods. Regular positive experiences with handling and restraint (e.g., in a training setup) may, however, help reduce the level of stress experienced during future restraint to a more acceptable level. These individual variations emphasize the importance of carefully assessing each individual case in its own context, taking the individual bird's behaviors and the purpose for which the procedure is performed into account.

Medical and Behavioral Complications of Deflighting Procedures

Various medical and behavioral complications may arise after a wing clip or other deflighting procedure. The various complications reported in literature are summarized in Table 22-4 and will be further illustrated below.

Hemorrhage

Even with the relative simple and noninvasive techniques of clipping, severe hemorrhage may occur, e.g., as a result of accidental clipping of blood feathers (Figure 22-20). Factors that may predispose the bird to extensive bleeding may include (1) the delicacy of the bird's skin, which makes it susceptible to tearing; (2) its loose attachment to underlying tissues, limiting the ability to control bleeding; and (3) relatively higher systemic blood pressure.[4] Control of bleeding is considered the most important factor to consider when deflighting a bird. Hemorrhage control may consist of compression, astringent

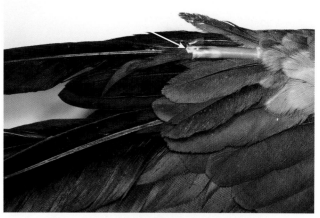

FIGURE 22-20 When trimming the wing feathers attention must be paid to new developing feathers *(arrow)*, also referred to as blood feathers, as the blood vessel present in the shaft may bleed profusely when cut.

hemostatic agents, careful placement of ligatures, and the use of electrocautery and/or suturing. Furthermore, risks of hemorrhage can be minimized by proper timing regarding the feather development stage and performing the procedure at lower ambient temperatures[4,34,39,40] (Table 22-4).

Trauma

Other frequently mentioned (indirect) complications that may occur during or after both invasive and noninvasive deflighting procedures are traumatic injuries.[3,4,11,35,41] These injuries may include injuries to the keel (Figure 22-21), beak (Figure 22-22), or tail (Figure 22-23) and fractured wings and/or legs, which in severe cases may even lead to death. Most of these injuries result directly from the lack of balance or loss of gliding ability caused by excessive trimming or unilaterally performed deflighting techniques.[3]

Other medical complications

Reported side effects directly resulting from surgical procedures include osteomyelitis (Figure 22-24), myiasis, sepsis, and death.[5,41] D'Agustino et al[42] mentioned the risk of mature birds traumatizing the pinioning site, eventually leading to

TABLE 22-4

Potential Complications That May Occur in Relation to Deflighting Procedures

Medical Complications	Behavioral Complications
• Bleeding of cut blood feathers or at the surgery site (see Figure 22-20) • Trauma to the keel (split keel; see Figure 22-21), the wings and legs (including fractures), or beak (see Figure 22-22) • Avulsion of the base of the tail (split tail injury; see Figure 22-23) • Osteomyelitis of cut bone (see Figure 22-24) • Chronic wounds (see Figure 22-25) • Development of feather follicle cysts (see Figure 22-26) • Ingrown or abnormal feathers (see Figure 22-27) • Myiasis at surgery site • Sepsis and potentially death	• Development of learned fear or anxiety disorders • Risk of developing feather damaging behavior or automutilation (see Figure 22-28)

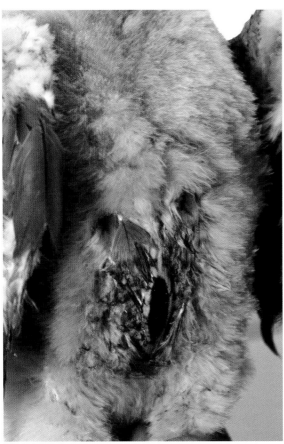

FIGURE 22-21 When the primary and secondary feathers are too short to break a fall to the ground, as in this Grey parrot *(Psittacus erithacus)*, the bird may land/fall on its chest, whereby the skin covering the keel is split. This is called a "split keel."

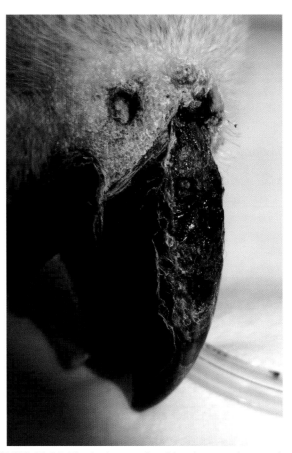

FIGURE 22-22 The lesion on the rhinotheca and upper beak structures of this Grey parrot *(Psittacus erithacus)* was the result of repeated trauma from falling onto a hard surface because of its inability to fly away when startled by unexpected sounds or movements.

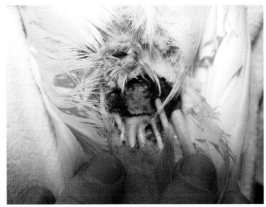

FIGURE 22-23 A split to the ventral skin of the pygostyle can be seen in this Goffin's cockatoo *(Cacatua goffiniana)*, which appeared to be the result of an uncontrolled fall. (Photo courtesy Brian Speer.)

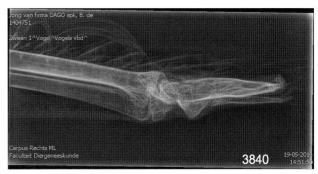

FIGURE 22-24 Posterior–anterior radiograph of a pinioned wing of a mute swan *(Cygnus olor)*. The distal end of the metacarpus shows an active periosteal reaction that may be due to continued trauma of the wing. (Photo courtesy the Division of Diagnostic Imaging, Faculty of Veterinary Medicine, Utrecht University, the Netherlands.)

chronic wounds (Figure 22-25). Furthermore, the risk of abnormal feather growth, including development of feather follicle cysts and ingrown feathers (Figures 22-26 and 22-27), is frequently mentioned in the literature. Often this is the result of trauma to the follicle or growing feather during or after the procedure.[41] Additionally, Hesterman et al[4] mentioned infection and neuroma formation as potential complications of surgical deflighting techniques.

Behavioral complications

Excessive grooming, potentially leading to feather-damaging behavior and/or automutilation, may occur if the remaining feather stumps irritate the skin (e.g., a wing clip at improper length or ragged stump resulting from the use of blunt scissors) (Figure 22-28). Alternative to the explanation of mechanical irritation, the observed excessive grooming activities may also reflect a redirected or displacement activity caused by frustration or stress from the sudden loss of wing function, following which the bird directs this frustration toward the cut ends of feathers. Although the end result is the same, the approach to these two hypothesized causations differs significantly. Whereas in the former feathers are clipped more extensively to remove the frayed ends (removing the source of mechanical irritation, but also potentially resulting in further

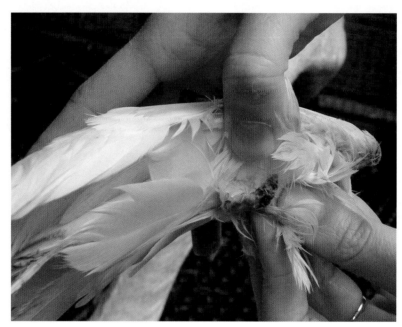

FIGURE 22-25 This mute swan *(Cygnus olor)* kept bumping the end of its wing against objects, resulting in a chronic wound on the lateral side of the pinioned wing.

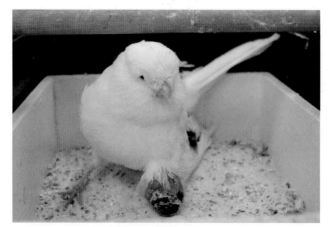

FIGURE 22-26 Feather cyst in a Norwich canary *(Serinus canaria domestica)*. Although the feather cyst in this bird is from a genetic condition, feather cysts may also develop as a result of a deflighting technique in which the feather follicle is damaged.

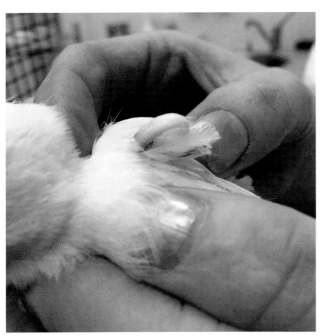

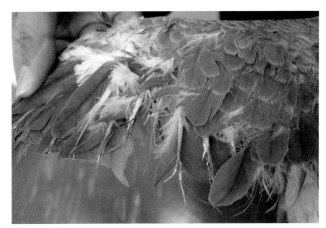

FIGURE 22-28 After clipping of the primary feathers, this Grey parrot *(Psittacus e. erithacus)* started to chew its feathers. Two divergent hypotheses for this behavior include redirected behavior from frustration/stress and mechanical irritation from the stumps.

FIGURE 22-27 Abnormal formed feather in a canary *(Serinus canaria domestica)*. Such feathers may result from incorrectly performed deflighting techniques or pulling of feathers, causing (permanent) damage to the feather follicle or growing feathers.

loss of lifting ability), the latter requires imping of the feathers or adjustment of the environment to minimize stress while simultaneously counterconditioning and desensitizing the bird to the known or theorized problems.

Additionally, when the feathers are clipped too rigorously and the bird is not able to glide to the ground and/or loses its ability to balance it may also become insecure and anxious. In some individuals, a fall may result in so much fear that it can at least, in theory, be classified as a phobia: a marked fear or anxiety related to a specific object or situation (human[42a]; dogs and cats[43]). Because of this intensely negative experience, some birds may generalize their response to its associated antecedents to other contexts, locations, or persons. The latter is highly undesirable for both the bird's welfare and the human–animal bond. This cascade of events is not limited to injuries resulting from falling, and can be initiated by the handling and restraint experience and other components and consequences of the entire procedure. In individuals that are believed to be susceptible to developing anxiety disorders (e.g., Grey parrots), it is recommended to decrease flight ability gradually to allow the bird to learn to cope with its restricted flight capabilities. In addition, positive reinforcement training techniques[44] may be useful for counterconditioning already negatively associated stimuli and situations to more positive ones.

Other long-term side effects of deflighting procedures are generally considered rare. However, no scientifically valuable statistics are available in the literature on this issue to make any definite conclusions regarding the overall negative outcomes in the long term.

Pain

Pain is an aversive sensory and emotional experience,[45] with freedom of pain considered as an important criterion for addressing welfare, as demonstrated by its inclusion in the Five Freedoms of the Brambell Committee (1965),[46] which are used to evaluate animal welfare.

As pain changes the animal's behavior and physiology, the ultimate goal is to try and avoid further damage and to promote recovery.[45] With respect to birds, pain issues are mostly discussed in relation to procedures such as beak trimming, feather pecking, and slaughter shackling in commercially kept poultry,[47-50] with behavioral indices developed in these species to assess welfare.[51] However, to the best of our knowledge, the effects of pain and irritation involved with invasive and noninvasive methods of deflighting have thus far not been systematically reported in the literature. Gentle and Hunter[52] did perform an experiment whereby feathers were artificially removed from hens (pulled out in *one pull*) to mimic feather pecking behavior in hens. They subsequently observed *agitated* birds showing wing flapping, vocalizing, increased heart rate, elevated blood pressure, and electroencephalographic arousal, based on which they concluded that feather removal is likely to be painful to the bird. The pulling method used here, however, is different from the deflighting methods described above, limiting extrapolation of their findings to the deflighting techniques used in practice. In addition, challenges are encountered while trying to assess pain in birds. For example, some birds may vocalize and become restless, aggressive, or try to escape, whereas others become more quiet and sedentary and respond with tonic immobility, especially when being handled.[53-55] Therefore, it is essential to be aware of the normal behavior of the individual bird and recognize any behavioral changes that may occur as a result of pain.

Aside from pain directly associated with the procedure, postamputation pains and postsurgical neuromas, which in humans have been associated with severe pain,[56] may also arise. Although Hesterman et al[4] concluded that neuromas are likely to occur after pinioning, thus far no evidence exists that this actually is the case. Pain, irritation, and injuries may, however, be the start of self-injurious behavior such as auto-mutilation in other species (dogs and cats[43,57]). Behavioral problems have also been observed after deflighting procedures. This self-injurious behavior may not occur only after invasive deflighting techniques, but also after a wing trim, and might be initiated either by a mechanically induced irritation and/or displacement behavior resulting from the sudden loss of wing function. Thus far, however, no clear evidence is available on the causality of self-directed and self-injurious behavior after wing trimming, thus emphasizing the need to investigate this link further.

Stress During Handling and Restraint

Deflighting procedures automatically imply moments of handling and restraint that may vary from repetitive (molt-dependent) procedures to one single intervention. Often, the

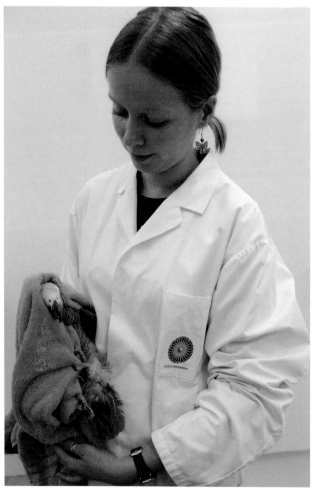

FIGURE 22-29 Training birds to accept being toweled using positive reinforcement strategies limits the amount of stress when having to be handled during procedures such as wing trimming.

help of an assistant is needed to restrain the bird if performing the procedure in a fully awake animal.[5] Although generally considered a routine procedure, these capture, handling, and restraint techniques can have a significant impact on the bird's health and welfare. For example, birds may easily develop hyperthermia following capture and restraint, especially when ambient temperatures are high.[58,59] Thus, chasing a bird should preferably be avoided. Other medical issues that may arise following capture, handling, and restraint include bone fractures, especially the fragile legs of long-legged species of birds.[4] Aside from medical issues, restraint may also result in stress. The duration and level of stress not only depends on the procedure used to *capture and restrain* the bird, but also on the use of analgesia, sedation, or anesthesia. The perceived levels of stress furthermore vary greatly between individuals, resulting in shorter or longer periods of physical and mental recovery. Accepted as *just a part of the game*, handling and restraint are often an underestimated factor of stress in veterinary practice.[59,60] This especially holds true for animals that have not been (or have only partially been) socialized to humans (e.g., wild-caught birds) and/or have no (or only limited) training and preparation for human handling procedures. Understandably, most veterinary practitioners have remained primarily focused on the medical problems and associated procedures, without uniformly taking into account the individual's prior experiences (e.g., socialization to humans, previous handling experiences, and training), which significantly influence the level of stress experienced by the individual bird. Moreover, veterinarians have seldom considered these previous experiences or the stress inflicted by their interventions as a criterion for choosing the most appropriate method to handle a particular individual. From a welfare point of view, however, criteria such as the degree and nature of socialization with humans, prior handling experiences, and training are of the utmost importance to create an *all-in* best practice and should, therefore, be embedded in the decision-making process regarding the method used for handling and restraint of the bird when performing a deflighting procedure.

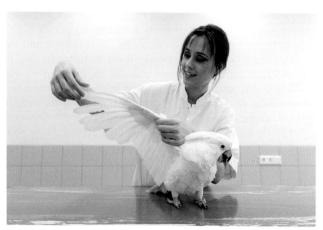

FIGURE 22-30 A well-trained bird will allow its wings to be spread and cut, minimizing the amount of stress involved in such a procedure.

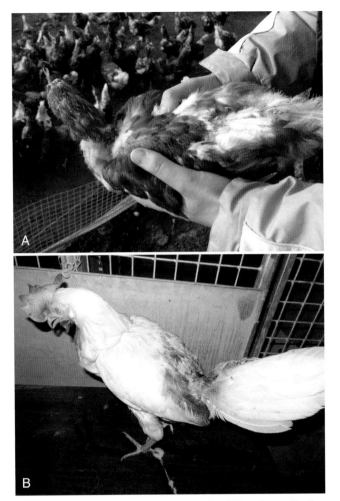

FIGURE 22-31 Excessive feather pecking **(A)** and cannibalism **(B)** are commonly seen in poultry because of overcrowding. Similar injuries may also occur in other avian species when returning a recently deflighted individual back into the flock. (Photos courtesy Bas Rodenburg **[A]** and Elske de Haas **[B]**.)

Handling and restraint are skills that should always be performed by trained personnel. Poor restraint techniques can easily produce fear and rapidly learned behavioral patterns of resistance[3] with subsequent consequences for future handling procedures and the stress level of the bird. Methods for stress reduction during catching, handling, and restraint in birds might be found in habituation and *teaching cooperative behavior* (training): by using operant condition techniques with positive reinforcement (see LeBlanc et al[61] for training artificial insemination procedures in macaws), feather-trimming sessions can be made less fearful for the bird. (See further reading on stress reduction in human–animal interactions [e.g., *handling and gentling*].[62-64]). Owners may, for example, get their birds accustomed to toweling and/or learn to trim their birds' feathers themselves by first teaching their birds to spread their wings followed by clipping the feathers (Figures 22-29 and 22-30). Although no studies appear available on training for deflighting

techniques specifically, general bird training information to optimize handling procedures might be helpful for owners when attempting to habituate their bird to toweling or wing trimming.[44] In some specific circumstances, the use of conscious sedation or even general anesthesia may facilitate stress reduction in some restraint situations. These types of procedures, however, should not be viewed as substitutes for skilled handling and restraint.

Aside from the technique used to handle and restrain the bird, the frequency with which the handling needs to be performed should also be taken into consideration. Nonpermanent methods of deflighting necessitate repeated treatment in relation to the species-specific molting seasons, necessitating multiple handling and restraint moments. The permanent, more invasive deflighting methods, in contrast, generally require fewer handling sessions, with no further handling or restraint needed after the last postoperative control.[65] Dependent on the bird species and the manner in which it is kept, this may pose as a valid argument in the decision-making process of the deflighting method used.

In group-housed birds, reintroduction in the group after intervention should always be carefully monitored: the introduced animal may look different, smell different, or may behave different following the procedure. Since many bird species are socially housed, the return of a bird into the group may cause stress for the returned individual as well as its group members, even if it is a well-known group member and/or even if the moment of isolation was short. Especially when the feathers look different or the skin or bandage material is visible, pecking behavior and aggression can be evoked, which may result in excessive pecking behavior and cannibalism, as described in some poultry species[66-68] (Figure 22-31).

CONCLUSIONS

Several noninvasive and invasive deflighting techniques may be considered by the veterinarian when confronted with the request and decision-making process to deflight a bird. The decision to deflight and the choice for a specific technique may, however, have several health and welfare implications, which may be more or less severe, dependent on the individual bird, its previous life experiences, and current living conditions. A decision *whether or not* and *how* to deflight a bird should not be taken lightly, but should follow a standardized process involving the precise formulations of the intended goals, the species' biology (including species-specific behaviors and social organization), the individual's previous life experiences (origin, imprinting and socialization, training, possible traumatic experiences, learned responses to handling, and restraint-associated stimuli) and current living environment (e.g., presence of potential predators and other hazards, social structure), and the short- and long-term costs and benefits regarding the bird's health and welfare. Taking all of the abovementioned factors into consideration allows for a balanced decision on whether or not to deflight the bird and, if so, which technique would be optimal for this specific bird in this particular situation (Figure 22-32).

STEP 1. Start to collect background information of the bird.

Checklist of Questions	ANSWER YES More risks for stress	ANSWER NO Less risks for stress
SPECIES' BIOLOGY		
• Wings are used for flying?		
• Wings are used for flight?		
• Wings are used for fight?		
• Wings are used for balance?		
• Wings are used for foraging?		
• Migration species?		
• Wings are used in the balts?		
• Wings are used during mating?		
•		
•		
INDIVIDUAL PAST		
• Weaned too early?		
• No socialization on humans?		
• No prior training for handling and restraint?		
• Had traumatic experiences with handling or restraint?		
• Had traumatic experiences in general?		
•		
•		
If prior history is unknown: is the bird frightened in the presence of known and unknown persons?		
HOUSING AND MANAGEMENT SITUATIONS		
• Predator environment? (dog/cat/bird household, neighboring cats, etc.)		
• No stable social structure in the group?		
• No stable/trustful relationship with owner/caretaker?		
• Unpredictable management procedures?		
• Uncontrollable management procedures?		
TOTAL		

FIGURE 22-32 Decision tree for deflighting procedures in birds. Deflighting procedures are interventions, either less or more invasive, with short-term or long-term effects. Every decision needs an individual approach to start with the precise formulations of the intended goals (for both the bird and human), the species' biology, the individual's previous life experiences (origin, imprinting and socialization, training, possible traumatic experiences) and current living environment (e.g., presence of potential predators and other hazards, social structure), and the short-term as well as long-term costs and benefits with regard to the bird's health and welfare.

STEP 2. The purpose for eventually applying deflighting techniques.

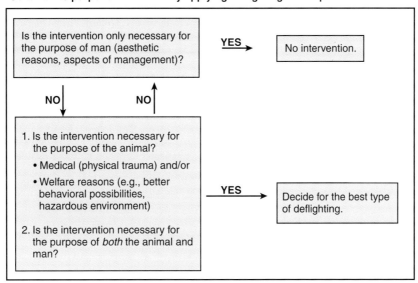

STEP 3. Decide the best deflighting technique

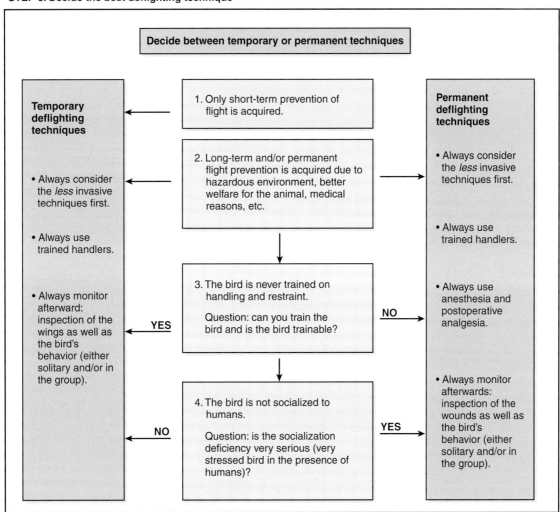

FIGURE 22-32, cont'd For legend see opposite page.

REFERENCES

1. Rollin BE: Animal agriculture and emerging social ethics for animals, *J Anim Sci* 82:955–964, 2004.
2. Locke J: *[1693]*. Some thoughts concerning education. In Grant RW, Tarcov N, editors: Indianapolis, IN, 1996, Hackett.
3. Speer BL: *The clinical consequences of routine grooming, Proceedings of the Association of Avian Veterinarians,* Orlando, Florida, 2001, pp 109–115.
4. Hesterman H, Gregory NG, Boardman WSJ: Deflighting procedures and their welfare implications in captive birds, *Anim Welfare* 10:405–419, 2001.
5. Zhang SL, Yang SH, Li B, et al: An alternate and reversible method for flight restraint of cranes. Technical report, *Zoo Biol* 30:342–348, 2011.
6. Wilson L, Luescher AU: Parrots and fear. In Luescher AU, editor: *Manual of parrot behavior,* Oxford, UK, 2006, Blackwell Publishing, pp 225–231.
7. Bračko A, King CE: Advantages of aviaries and the aviary database project: a new approach to an old option for birds. In Fisken FA (Managing Editor), Field D, Lees C, Leus K, Miller RE, Pullen K, Rübel A, editors: *International zoo yearbook,* London, 2014, The Zoological Society of London, p 48. Wiley Online Library, ISSN: 1748-1090/. DOI: 10.111/izy.12035.
8. Biewener AA: Muscle function in avian flight: achieving power and control, *Philos Trans R Soc Lond B Biol Sci* 366(1570):1496–1506, 2011, (abstract).
9. Kuslan JA: *The terminology of courtship, nesting, feeding and maintenance in herons,* 2011. http://www.HeronConservation.org. [online. non-peer-reviewed publication].
10. Hughes BO, Appelby MC: Increase in bone strength of spent laying hens housed in modified cages with perches, *Vet Rec* 124:483–484, 1989, (abstract).
11. Fair J, Paul E, Jones J, editors: *Guidelines to the use of wild birds in research,* ed 3, Washington, DC, 2010, Ornithological Council, p 215.
12. Engebretson M: The welfare and suitability of parrots as companion animals: a review, *Anim Welfare* 15:263–276, 2006.
13. St Leger A: Avian atherosclerosis. In: Miller RE, Fowler ME, editors: *Fowler's zoo and wild animal medicine: current therapy 6,* St Louis, MO, 2008, Elsevier Saunders, pp 200–205.
14. Tully TN, Dorrestein GM, Jones AK, editors: *Handbook of avian medicine,* ed 2, St Louis, MO, 2009, Elsevier Saunders.
15. Thorpe WH: The assessment of pain and distress in animals. In *Report of the technical committee to enquire into the welfare of animals kept under intensive livestock systems, Command paper 2836,* London, 1965, HMSO, pp 125–134.
16. Martin G: Zur Käfighaltung von Legehennen. Eine Stellungnahme aus der Sicht der Verhaltenswissenschaft. In Yeutsch GM, von Loeper E, Martin G, Müller J, editors: *Intensivhaltung von Nutztieren aus ethischer, rechtlicher und ethologischer Sicht,* Basel, 1979, Birkhäuser, pp 101–112.
17. Dawkins MS: Battery hens name their price: consumer demand theory and the measurement of ethological "needs", *Anim Behav* 31:1195–1205, 1983.
18. Poole TB: The nature and evolution of behavioural needs in mammals, *Anim Welfare* 1:203–220, 1992.
19. Veasey JS, Waran NK, Young RJ: On comparing the behaviour of zoo housed animals with wild conspecifics as a welfare indicator, *Anim Welfare* 5:13–24, 1996.
20. Price EO: Behavioural development in animals undergoing domestication, *Appl Anim Behav Sci* 65:245–271, 1999.
21. Cooper JJ, Albertosa MJ: Behavioural priorities of laying hens, *Avian and Poult Biol Rev* 14(3):127–149, 2003.
22. Jensen P, Toates FM: Who needs "behavioural needs"? Motivational aspects of the needs of animals, *Appl Anim Behav Sci* 37:161–181, 1993.
23. Ohl F, van der Staay FJ: Animal welfare: at the interface between science and society, *Vet J* 192(1):13–19, 2012.
24. Barash DP: In search of behavioural individuality, *Hum Nat* 8:153–169. 1997.
25. Piersma T, Drent J: Phenotypic flexibility and the evolution of organismal design, *Trends Ecol Evol* 18:228–233, 2003.
25a. Ohl F, Hellebrekers LJ: Animal welfare: the veterinary concept, *Tijdschrift voor Diergeneeskunde* 15:754–755, 2009.
26. Duncan IJH, Wood-Gush DGM: Thwarting of feeding behaviour in the domestic fowl, *Anim Behav* 20:444–451, 1972.
27. Cronin GM, Wiepkema PR: An analysis of stereotyped behaviour in tethered sows, *Annals de Recherches Veterinaires* 15(2):263–270, 1984.
28. Broom DM, Johnson KG: *Stress and animal welfare, Animal Behaviour Series, London,* London, 1993, Chapman and Hall.
29. Clubb R, Mason G: Captivity effects on wide-ranging carnivores, *Nature* 425:473–474, 2003.
30. van Zeeland YRA, Spruijt BM, Rodenburg TB: Feather damaging behaviour in parrots: a review with consideration of comparative aspects, *Appl Anim Behav Sci* 121:75–95, 2009.
31. Cooper J, Cooper M: *Captive birds in health and disease: game birds, raptors, parrots, waterfowl, and other species,* Surrey, BC, 2004, Hancock House Publishers.
32. Peng SJ, Chang F, Sheng-Ting J: Welfare assessment of flight-restrained captive birds: effects of inhibition of locomotion, *Thai J Vet Med* 43(2):235–241, 2013.
33. Rutgers B, Heeger R: Inherent worth and respect for animal integrity. In: Dol M, Fentener van Vlissingen M, Kasanmoentalib S, Visser T, Zwart H, editors: *Recognizing the intrinsic value of nature,* Assen, the Netherlands, 1999, Van Gorcum, pp 41–53.
34. Ellis DH, Dein FJ: Flight restraint. In Ellis DH, Gee GF, Mirande CM, editors: *Cranes: their biology, husbandry, and conservation,* Washington, DC and International Crane Foundation, Baraboo, WI, 1996, National Biological Service, pp 241–244.
35. Forbes NA, Glendell G: Wing clipping in psittacine birds, *Vet Rec* 144:299, 1999.
36. Gibbens N: Pinioning non-agricultural birds, *Vet Rec* 173:53, 2013, doi: 10.1136/vr.f4440.
37. Acharjyo LN, Ojha SC: Pinioning of wild birds in captivity: a clinical study, *Indian Vet J* 49:720–724, 1972.
38. Wallach JD: Surgical techniques for cage birds, *Vet Clin North Am* 3:231–237, 1987.
39. Fletcher KC, Miller BW: A technique for cosmetic pinioning of adult birds, *Vet Med Small Anim Clin* 75(12):1898–1904, 1980, (abstract).
40. Olsen JH: Anseriformes. In Ritchie BW, Harrison GJ, Harrison LR editors: *Avian medicine, principles and application,* Lake Worth, FL, 1997, Wingers Publishing, pp 694–719.
41. Degernes LA, Feduccia A: Tenectomy of the supracoracoideus muscle to deflight pigeons (*Columba livia*) and cockatiels (*Nymphicus hollandicus*), *J Avian Med Surg* 15(1):10–16, 2001.
42. D'Agustino JJ, Snider T, Hoover J, et al: Use of laser ablation and cryosurgery to prevent primary feather growth in a pigeon (*Columba livia*) model, *J Avian Med Surg* 20(4):219–224, 2006.
42a. Anonymous: *DSM-5 Diagnostics and statistical manual of mental disorders,* ed 5, Washington, DC, 2013, American Psychiatric Association.
43. Landsberg G, Hunthausen W, Ackerman L: *Behaviour problems of the dog & cat,* ed 3, St Louis, MO, 2013, Saunders Elsevier.
44. Heidenreich B: An introduction to positive reinforcement training and its benefits, *J Exot Pet Med* 16(1):19–22, 2007.
45. Molony V, Kent JF: Assessment of acute pain in farm animals using behavioural and physiological measurements, *J Anim Sci* 75:266–272, 1997.
46. Brambell Committee: *Report of the technical committee to enquire into the welfare of animals kept under intensive livestock husbandry systems, The Brambell Report,* London, 1965, HMSO, ISBN 0 10 850286 4.
47. Gentl MJ, Tilston VL: Nociceptors in the legs of poultry: implications for potential pain in pre-slaughter shackling, *Anim Welfare* 9:227–236, 2000.

48. Gentle MJ: Pain issues in poultry, *Appl Anim Behav Sci* 135:252–258, 2011.
49. Nasr MAF, Nicol CJ, Murrell JC: Do laying hens with keel bone fractures experience pain. *PLoS One* 7(8):1–6, 2012.
50. Prunier A, Mounier L, Le Neindre P, et al: Identifying and monitoring pain in farm animals: a review, *Animal* 7(6):998–1010, 2013.
51. Gentle MJ, Waddington D, Hunter LN, et al: Behavioural evidence for persistent pain following partial beak amputation in chickens, *Appl Anim Behav Sci* 27:149–157, 1990.
52. Gentle MJ, Hunter LN: Physiological and behavioural responses associated with feather removal in Gallus gallus var domesticus, *Res Vet Sci* 50:95–101, 1990.
53. Sanford J, Ewbank R, Molony V, et al: Guidelines for the recognition and assessment of pain in animals, *Vet Rec* 118:334, 1986.
54. Fraser AR, Quine JP: Veterinary examination of suffering as a behaviour-linked condition, *Appl Anim Behav Sci* 23:235–264, 1989.
55. Gentle MJ: Pain in birds, *Anim Welfare* 1:235–247, 1992.
56. Hsu E, Cohen SP: Postamputation pain: epidemiology, mechanisms, and treatment, *J Pain Res* 6:121–136, 2013.
57. Bowen J, Heath S: *Behaviour problems in small animals. Practical advice for the veterinary team*, St Louis, MO, 2005, Elsevier Saunders.
58. Fowler ME: *Restraint and handling of wild and domestic animals*, Ames, IA, 2008, Wiley Blackwell.
59. Greenacre CB, Lusby AL: Physiological responses of Amazon parrots (*Amazona* species) to manual restraint, *J Avian Med Surg* 18(1):19–22, 2004.
60. Straub J, Forbes N, Pees M, et al: Effect of handling-induced stress on the results of spectral Doppler echocardiography in falcons, *Res Vet Sci* 74:119–122, 2003.
61. Leblanc F, Pothet G, Jalme MS, et al: Training large macaws for artificial insemination procedures, *J Appl Anim Welfare Sci* 14:187–210, 2011.
62. Hemsworth PH, Barnett JL: Relationship between fear of humans, productivity and cage position of laying hens, *Br Poult Sci* 30:505–518, 1989, (abstract).
63. Barnett JL, Hemsworth PH, Hennessy TH, et al: The effects of modifying the amount of human contact on behavioural, physiological and production responses of laying hens, *Appl Anim Behav Sci* 41:87–100, 1994.
64. Zulkifli I: Review of human-animal interactions and their impact on animal productivity and welfare, *J Anim Sci Biotechnol* 4:25, 2013, 7P [Open Access].
65. Anonymous: *Recommendations for developing an institutional flight restriction policy*, developed by the Association of Zoos & Aquariums Avian Scientific Advisory Group, 2P, 2013.
66. Savory CJ: Feather pecking and cannibalism, *World's Poult Sci J* 51:215–219, 1995.
67. McAdie TM, Keeling LJ: Effect of manipulating feathers of laying hens on the incidence of feather pecking and cannibalism, *Appl Anim Behav Sci* 68:215–229, 2000.
68. Dixon LM: Feather pecking behaviour and associated welfare issues in laying hens, *Avian Biol Res* 1(2):73–87, 2008.
69. Robinson PT: Pinioning young birds with hemostatic clips (*a photographic essay*), *Vet Med Small Anim Clin* 70(12):1415–1417, 1975a.
70. Robinson PT: Unilateral patagiectomy: a technique for deflighting large birds, *Vet Med Small Anim Clin* 70(2):143–145, 1975b.
71. Fletcher KC: *Surgical deflighting of cranes without altering the normal osteology of the wing, Proceedings of the 44th Annual Conference of the International Union of Directors of Zoological Gardens*, Washington DC, 1989, National Zoological Park Library, Smithsonian Institution, pp 118–119.
72. Miller JC: The importance of immobilizing wings after tenectomy and tenotomy, *Vet Med Small Anim Clin* 68:35–38, 1973.
73. Krawinkel P: Feather follicle extirpation: operative techniques to prevent zoo birds from flying. In Miller RE, Fowler M, editors: *Fowler's zoo and wild animal medicine: current therapy*, vol 7, St Louis, MO, 2011, Elsevier, pp 275–280.
74. Shaw SN, D'Agostino JJ, Davis MR, et al: Primary feather follicle ablation in common pintails (*Anas anas acuta*) and a white faced whistling duck (*Dendrocygna viduata*), *J Zoo Wildl Med* 43(2):342–346, 2012.

THE HUMAN–AVIAN BOND

Nienke Endenburg

The bond between humans and pets is an ancient one[1] and is one of the world's most unique and enduring bonds. Pets are increasingly considered as "one of the family" and live in the home, rather than outside. People see their pets as important members of their families—they are friends, playmates, and protectors, providing their owners with love, security, and joy.[2] Pets have evolved to be true companion animals and most pet owners are emotionally attached to their pets.[3] In return for companionship, it is the owners' responsibility to take care of their pets, providing them with loving, safe, and happy homes; good health care and nutrition; and proper training and socialization. Ideally, the owner–pet relationship is beneficial to both parties.

While most human–companion animal research has focused on dogs and cats, birds are also kept as pets. The human–avian bond, however, has not been extensively investigated, which is puzzling because birds are the third most popular household pet.[4] The companionship quality of birds is often underestimated, possibly because people have little or no actual experience with birds or have had a poor relationship with birds as a result of poor socialization, miscommunication, and misunderstanding.[4] Unlike dogs, birds have not been bred and reared in captivity for thousands of years and as such cannot be considered truly domesticated. Some may consider canaries and budgerigars as domesticated, but parrots are wild animals, whether bred in captivity or not. This means that owners should be aware of the specific needs of these birds.

People buy parrots for a number of reasons: they are attractive with their glossy, brightly colored feathers; some are able to talk; and they are exotic, different from cats and dogs. Unfortunately, not all future parrot owners are knowledgeable about the needs of their pet in terms of food, exercise, attention, and housing, which could compromise the parrot's welfare. People often buy companion animals and also parrots on impulse, not knowing the commitment required.[5] They are messy, noisy animals but often very intelligent—it has been estimated that parrots have the intelligence of a 5-year-old child.[6] Like children who need to learn limits to their behavior, parrots can develop behavior problems if they are not raised correctly; problems that are difficult for the inexperienced owner to modify or reverse. Especially when they reach adolescence, out-of-control parrots may be a nightmare to live with and often a reason for owners to bring the parrot to a shelter or to have it euthanized.[7,8]

Different aspects of the human–avian bond are discussed in this chapter. First, the notion of attachment is discussed and how the different attachment styles of owners can influence the bond that owners develop with their birds. Second, the advantages and disadvantages of anthropomorphization to both owners and birds are explained. While the bird provides its owner with social support (how this occurs is discussed later), anthropomorphization can compromise the bird's welfare. The notion of animal welfare in relation to the owner–bird relationship is discussed, as is how the owner copes with the death of his bird and the role of the veterinarian in this loss.

ATTACHMENT

If genetically healthy and provided with competent avian veterinary medical support, even small birds like canaries and budgerigars can live longer than most dogs. Larger species, such as parrots, potentially live as long as humans.[5] This long life span has positive and negative aspects. People can become very attached to their bird, which "accompanies" them throughout life's ups and downs.[9] The bird is nonjudgmental and always "listens" to its owner, so that he does not feel alone.

In the wild, parrots live in flocks, meaning that potentially there will be a strong bond between owner and parrot. Owners that develop a strong bond with their pets spend more time with them and interact with them for longer periods of time. Lue et al[10] showed that these owners are also more likely to seek higher levels of veterinary care; are less sensitive to the price of veterinary care; and, crucially in relation to compliance, are more willing to follow the recommendations of the veterinarian.

Bird ownership not only involves considerable commitment and time on the part of the owner but also brings with it a financial commitment. The price of buying a bird is typically a minor aspect of the total cost of ownership. Think of food, the cage (which has to be much larger than owners think and, therefore, much more expensive), toys, and other necessities and enrichments. Veterinary care, because it can require an avian specialist, is probably more expensive than for dogs and cats. Parrot owners in particular need to invest a lot of time and money to keep their pets healthy, given the long life span of these birds. These factors tend to reinforce owner–bird attachment.

Attachment is a concept that comes from human developmental psychology. The attachment between children and their caretakers, primary attachment, is extremely important for a child's development. Fogany and Target[11] found that without secure attachment a child may develop a personality disorder, characterized by enduring maladaptive patterns of behavior, cognition, and inner experience, exhibited across many contexts and deviating markedly from those accepted by the individual's culture. These patterns develop early, are inflexible, and are associated with significant distress or disability.[12] The type of attachment formed (secure, preoccupied, dismissing, or fearful[13]) may influence the type of interpersonal relationships a person develops later in life (Figure 22-33). For instance, people with a preoccupied attachment style need to stay in close contact with their partner. They may find it difficult when a partner goes to work, because they feel insecure. The type of attachment formed depends, among other factors, on the relationship a child has with its primary caregiver. If that caregiver is not responsive, for instance, because of (postpartum) depression or not available because of family circumstances, an insecure attachment can develop. Early

MODEL OF OTHER (avoidance) \ MODEL OF SELF (Dependence)	POSITIVE (low)	NEGATIVE (high)
POSITIVE (low)	CELL I SECURE Comfortable with intimacy and autonomy	CELL II PREOCCUPIED Preoccupied with relationships
NEGATIVE (high)	CELL IV DISMISSING Dismissing of intimacy Counterdependent	CELL III FEARFUL Fearful of intimacy Socially avoidant

FIGURE 22-33 Attachment style categories and model of self and others. (Redrawn from Bartholomew K: Avoidance of intimacy: an attachment perspective, *J Soc Personal Relationsh* 7:147–178, 1990.)

attachment experiences are apparently represented and carried forward, setting conditions for seeking, interpreting, and reacting to later experiences.

The relationship between a person and an animal could also be called attachment.[14] However, the human–animal bond cannot be explained in terms of primary attachment[15] but in terms of other forms of attachment, such as adult attachment.[16] People describe their feelings for companion animals in very similar, if not the same, terms that they use to describe their attachment to relatives and partners or spouses.[15] The desire to be close or to keep close to the attachment figure is a measure of attachment that is often used to assess the strength of the human–animal bond.[17]

Children develop an internal working model with attachment figures.[18] This internal working model makes it possible to predict the behavior of the attachment figure and can later influence how children think of themselves. For example, if a primary caregiver is not available or is insufficiently available, a child might feel that he is not worth being looked after and cared for. If this feeling is elicited often enough, it will have a strong influence on the rest of that child's life and how he develops. It is possible that children who grow up with animals develop an internal working model with a certain type of animal, for instance, a bird.[19] If human caregivers are not always available, for whatever reason, children may form a secure attachment with a pet, which forms a protective factor during the child's development. On the basis of Bartholomew's model, it is also possible that a person, even a child, who is socially avoidant could develop a very strong bond or even become overattached to a bird. Research has shown that children who grow up with a certain animal are more likely to own that type of animal in adulthood.[20] However, as mentioned previously, the cost and commitment of keeping a bird for a long time may ultimately disrupt the owner–bird bond, to the detriment of the bird's welfare.

ANTHROPOMORPHIZATION

People anthropomorphize companion animals[21] and say that they get unconditional love from them. Anthropomorphism is "the attribution of human mental states (thoughts, feelings, motivations and beliefs) to nonhuman animals."[22] It is an almost universal trait among companion animal owners. They see their pets as members of their family, speak to and with them, think they understand what they are saying, and celebrate their birthdays.[19,20] People imbue animals with humanlike intelligence, desires, beliefs, and intentions, such as pride and guilt.[21] This inability to see the pet as an animal and inability to realize that the pet perceives the world through senses different to their own may cause owners to ignore or be ignorant of the specific needs of their pet. These deficits, in turn, can lead to behavior problems and compromise the pet's welfare.

SOCIAL SUPPORT

Serpell[21] expounded on the reasons why people own pets and concluded that ownership provides humans with social support. Cobb[23] defined social support as "information leading the subject to believe that he is cared for and loved, esteemed, and a member of a network of mutual obligation." The importance of social support to human well-being has long been recognized, with extensive medical literature confirming a strong, positive link between social support and improved human physical health and survival. Social support has been shown to protect against cardiovascular disease and strokes, rheumatic fever, diabetes, nephritis, pneumonia, and most forms of cancer, and depression and suicide.[21,24] The perception that family and friends would provide effective help during times of stress (i.e., perceived support) has been consistently linked to good mental health.[25]

Likewise, if there is a strong bond between an owner and bird, the owner feels that he gets support from the bird (Figure 22-34). People need a few ongoing personal relationships to maintain their emotional well-being, and one of these relationships could be with a bird. Rook[26] found companionship to be closely linked to well-being, and bird owners say they receive companionship from their pets.[27]

Animal Welfare

Many owners form close, emotionally rewarding relationships with their pets. However, the tendency to anthropomorphize pets may make it difficult for owners to disentangle their pets' real needs from their own emotional projections.[28]

Interest in animal welfare and welfare management has increased substantially in recent years,[29] as has research into companion animal welfare.[30] Despite the increasing number of studies into welfare-associated issues in captive parrots, much remains to be learned.[31] One problem is the lack of consensus on how to measure the welfare of an animal objectively. Moreover, every definition of animal welfare is influenced by the moral or ethical standards of society.[32] That said, progress has generated new concepts of animal welfare that are more dynamic than the original Five Freedoms of Brambell.[33] One of these concepts is that "an individual is in a positive welfare state when it has the freedom to react adequately to

◆ Hunger, thirst, or incorrect food;
◆ Thermal and physical discomfort;
◆ Injuries or diseases;
◆ Fear and chronic stress, and thus,
◆ The freedom to display normal behavioral patterns that allow the animal to adapt to the demands of the prevailing environmental circumstances and enable it to reach a state that it perceives as positive."[32]

This refers to the animal's ability to perceive negative states or conditions and to operate on its environment to adapt to them. An animal's welfare might best be represented by the adaptive value of that animal's interaction with a given environmental setting, but this dynamic welfare concept has significant implications for assessing welfare.[32] But if it is difficult for scientists and veterinarians to define and judge animal welfare, it is even more so for owners, who often lack specific knowledge of the requirements of their pet. For example, birds with inadequate environmental stimuli may develop problem behaviors, such as feather damaging, biting, and screaming, all of which are signs of a compromised welfare.[31] It is a veterinarian's job to educate owners and help them to adequately take care of their bird's welfare (Figure 22-35).

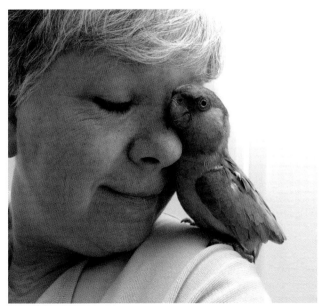

FIGURE 22-34 Owners can be very attached to their birds. (Photo courtesy Ellen Uittenbogaard, the Netherlands.)

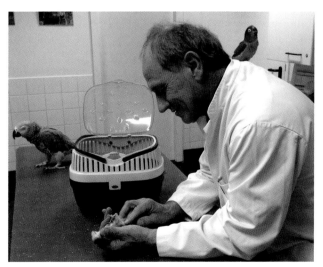

FIGURE 22-35 Veterinarians are animal welfare consultants. (Photo courtesy Ellen Uittenbogaard, the Netherlands.)

WHEN THE BOND IS BROKEN

Many parrot owners become deeply attached to their birds, in part because of their relative longevity.[27] This means that owners share a lot of life events, for example, the death of a cherished person, a child leaving home, and divorce, with their birds. The fact that bird owners experience unconditional love and social support from their bird ensures that the bond is strong.[34] This is an anthropomorphic presumption that many owners experience, and social support has, as stated before, a lot of positive influences on human mental and physical health.

Even though birds have a relatively long life, most owners will experience the death of their bird. This can be devastating to owners, who will go through a grieving process.[27] More than 85% of people report symptoms of grief after the death of a much-loved pet and over one third still grieve after 6 months.[35] The death of a pet is often the first loss that children experience and offers parents the opportunity to help them learn about loss and to express their grief.[36] However, too often, grief at the loss of a pet is unacknowledged, trivialized, or pathologized, which complicates mourning.[37,38] This is the case with dogs and cats, but even more so with birds.[36] Friends and relatives may not understand the importance of the pet to the owner—that the pet is not just "an animal." Complicated mourning may lead to depression and even to an inability to work. Factors that can complicate grieving include other recent losses, little or no support from friends or family, or not viewing the body of the bird after its death.

As pet birds age, their owners become aware that at some stage the animal will die or have to be euthanized. They will prepare mentally for this, and a part of the grieving process takes place while the bird is still alive, so-called anticipatory grief.[34] This is an important period because people can take pictures, think and talk about events that happened during the bird's lifetime, and say how much they love him and value him. However, for some owners this thought alone can be rather distressing—they feel that they cannot live without their pet, that the bird was the only thing they can trust, and even that they no longer have a reason to live. This problem is particularly acute when it comes to making the decision to euthanize the bird.[36] Owners often hope that the animal will die naturally, so they do not have to decide between life and death. It is the veterinarian's role to tell owners, gently but firmly, that the animal's welfare is compromised and that it is best to prevent suffering by allowing the bird to die.[39] In the end, most owners feel that this is the best decision. If they wait too long they will feel guilty that they let their beloved pet suffer, because they were not ready to let it be euthanized. Because owners get used to a certain behavior or how the bird looks, they do not always appreciate that their pet is ill or how ill it truly is. Moreover, what they consider acceptable regarding the health and welfare of their pet tends to change, especially as the bird ages, leaving it up to the veterinarian to explain to the owner that the bird is ill and suffering and that it is time to euthanize. Even so, many owners experience intense guilt and ruminate about the timing of euthanasia.[37] Owners who had their pet euthanized by a veterinarian reported significantly less grief than owners who lost their pets due to natural causes.[40] The grieving process is made easier if the owner is present when the bird is euthanized.[34,36] The veterinarian should explain the procedure, so that the owner knows what to expect, which in turn helps the owner to cope with the idea of euthanasia.

It is a different case when the bird dies unexpectedly, especially if it is a young bird.[34] Owners think it "unfair" that their pet has died because they thought it would live for years.[34] The grieving process is often difficult because there was no time to say goodbye. It may help if owners write a letter to the pet to say goodbye, make a scrapbook of the pet's memorabilia, or plant a tree. Sometimes it helps owners to do a postmortem examination because there is a chance to understand the cause(s) of the death, which can free them of guilt and helps to provide closure. But not all owners are willing to give the veterinarian permission to do this.

After euthanasia of their pet, many owners are in a state of shock.[41] They hardly can believe that their pet is dead and that it will not be back. They may blame themselves that the bird had to be euthanized.[41] If they had gone to the veterinarian earlier, would their pet still be alive? It is difficult to answer this question. Most owners go to their veterinarian when they think something is wrong, but sometimes this is not possible because of financial reasons, family problems, or other reasons. In most cases, it will not help if owners are told they should have come earlier, but they could be told about the appropriate time to come in the future.

Social support is very important during the mourning period. Owners have to be able to tell their story and explain that they are very sad and miss the presence of their pet (the sounds it made, talking and greeting the owner when he or she came home). The adjustment process for the loss of a pet bird may be hindered by a lack of social support and opportunities for healthy confiding in others.[42] Owners might find it upsetting if friends and family, who normally give social support, react with "it was only a bird, buy a new one." The bond between a bird and owner has taken time to develop and cannot be replaced by another bird: every bird has its own personality and character. Individuals who might have had an adequate social support network following the death of a human significant other may not fare as well when a pet dies.[43,44]

Most owners expect their veterinarian to give support and to understand that the loss of this special bird is a very sad experience.[42] However, not all veterinarians are adequately trained in how to comfort grieving clients[42] and may resort to "icy professionalism,"[42] although they care deeply about their clients. Veterinarians who support their owners will have clients forever (Figure 22-36). Giving support to grieving clients means listening to their nonmedical concerns, usually about whether the decision they made was the right one or feelings of guilt about the death of the animal.[41] Veterinarians should "wear their compassion on their sleeve, where all can see it, and balance compassion with scientific and medical skill and knowledge" (B. Speer, Personal communication, September 1, 2014). Supporting clients also means normalizing loss, allowing them to express thoughts and emotions, and listening to painful and pleasant memories. Veterinarians often feel they cannot be of help unless they know the "right" thing to say or the "right" thing to do, but most owners prefer someone who is really listening to them and not necessarily giving them good advice.[34] If the veterinarian fails to be understanding and show compassion, in most cases owners will go to another veterinarian if they have a new pet. Civil complaints and regulatory accusations against the veterinarian will more

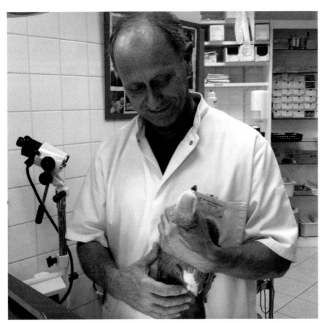

FIGURE 22-36 Veterinarians can play an important role for owners who have lost their birds. (Photo courtesy Ellen Uittenbogaard, the Netherlands.)

easily be started if there is a lack of trust and healthy communication between client and veterinarian during or after the process of medical care for their bird that has passed away.

While people grieve in their own way, at some stage many owners will ask the veterinarian when they should get a new bird. No general statements can be made, for one person that will be within a couple of days, for another after a couple of months or even years.[34] To prevent disappointment, it should be made clear to owners that even if the new bird looks like their old pet, it will have its own personality.

Veterinarians can also provide advice or suggestions to their clients when they are considering buying a new bird, specifically where to find the higher quality retailers, breeders, or rescue facilities in their area. Regardless, owners must have the freedom to decide for themselves when the time has come to get a new bird and from what sources it should come.

CONCLUSIONS

In many ways, the human–avian bond is different from other human–companion animal bonds. The longer life span of the bird means that the bond is probably stronger and more enduring; however, the longer life span also means that there is a longer commitment to the bird, which may hinder the development of a strong bond, especially in "impulse" owners without sufficient knowledge of the bird's needs. It is the task of veterinarians to monitor the welfare of the bird and to tell owners about the bird's specific needs—needs that might not be met, despite the owner's best intentions, if there is a tendency to anthropomorphize the bird. They also have a role in supporting grieving owners whose pets die, whether naturally or by euthanasia. Owners who feel supported by the veterinary practice staff will become loyal clients and practice staff will have the satisfaction of having done their job well.

REFERENCES

1. Serpell JA: Historical and cultural perspectives on human-pet interactions. In McCardle P, McCune S, Esposito L, Freund L, editors: *Animals in our lives: human–animal interaction in family, community, & therapeutic settings*, Baltimore MD, 2011, Paul H. Brooks, pp 11–22.
2. Walsh F: The human-animal bonds I: the relational significance of companion animals, *Fam Proc* 48:462–480, 2009a.
3. Friedmann E, Son H: The human-companion animal bond: how humans benefit, *Vet Clin Small Anim* 39:293–326, 2009.
4. Anderson PK: A bird in the house: an anthropological perspective on companion parrots, *Soc Anim* 11(4):394–418, 2003.
5. Wilson L: The appropriate bird for the appropriate owner, *Semin Avian Exot Pet Med* 8(4):165–173, 1999.
6. Pepperberg I: *The Alex studies: cognitive and communicative abilities of Grey parrots*, Cambridge, MA, 1999, Harvard University Press.
7. Gaskins LA, Bergman L: Surveys of avian practitioners and pet owners regarding common behavior problems in psittacine birds, *J Avian Med Surg* 25(2):111–118, 2011.
8. Meehan C, Mench J: Captive parrot welfare. In Luescher AU, editor: *Manual of parrot behavior*, Ames, IA, 2006, Blackwell Publishing, pp 301–318.
9. Beck L, Madresh EA: Romantic partners and four-legged friends: an extension of attachment theory to relationships with pets, *Anthrozoös* 21(1):43–56, 2008.
10. Lue TW, Pantenburg DP, Crawford PM: Impact of the owner-pet and client-veterinarian bond on the care that pets receive, *JAVMA* 232(4):531–540, 2008.
11. Fogany P, Target M: Attachment and reflective function: their role in self-organisation, *Dev Psychopathol* 9:679–700, 1997.
12. American Psychiatric Association: *Diagnostic and statistical manual of mental disorders*, ed 5, Arlington, VA, 2013, American Psychiatric Publishing.
13. Bartholomew K: Avoidance of intimacy: an attachment perspective, *J Soc Personal Relationsh* 7:147–178, 1991.
14. Gewirtz JL, Boyd EF: The infant conditions, the mother. In Alloway T, Pliner P, Krames L,editors: *Advances in the study of communication and affect, attachment behavior*, New York, 1977, Plenum Press, pp 109–143.
15. Colby PM, Sherman A: Attachment styles impact on pet visitation effectiveness, *Anthrozoös* 2:150–165, 2002.
16. Berman WH, Sperling MB: The structure and function of attachment. In Sperling MB, Berman WH, editors: *Attachment in adulthood: clinical and developmental perspectives*, New York, 1996, The Guilford Press, pp 3–28.
17. Cairns RB: Attachment behaviour in mammals, *Psychol Rev* 73:409–429, 1966.
18. Macfie J, Mcewain NL, Houts RM: Intergenerational transmission of role reversal between parent and child: dyadic and family systems internal working models, *Attachment Hum Dev* 7(1):51–65, 2005.
19. Endenburg N: The attachment of people to companion animals, *Anthrozoös* 8(2):83–89, 1995.
20. Endenburg N: Animals as companions. Demographic, motivational and ethical aspects of companion animal ownership, Thesis, 1991, University of Amsterdam.
21. Serpell JA: Anthropomorphism and anthropomorphic selection—beyond the "cute response," *Soc Anim* 10(4):437–454, 2003.
22. Lehman H: Anthropomorphism and scientific evidence for animal mental states. In Mitchell RW, Thompson NS, Miles HL, editors: *Anthropomorphism, anecdotes and animals*, Albany, NY, 1997, SUNY Press, pp 104–115.
23. Cobb S: Social support as a moderator of life stress, *Psychosomat Med* 38:300–314, 1976.
24. Uchino BN: Social support and health: a review of physiological processes potentially underlying links to disease outcomes, *J Behav Med* 29(4):377–387, 2006.

25. Lakey B, Orehek E: Relational regulation theory: a new approach to explain the link between perceived social support and mental health, *Psychol Rev* 118(3):482–495, 2011.

26. Rook KS: Social support versus companionship: effects on life stress, loneliness, and evaluation of others, *J Pers Soc Psychol* 52:1132–1147, 1987.

27. Lennox AM, Harrison GJ: The companion bird. In Harrison GJ, Lightfoot TL, editors: *Avian medicine: principles and application*, Lake Worth, 2006, Wingers Publishing, pp 26–44.

28. Bradshaw JWS, Casey RA: Anthropomorphism and anthropocentrism as influences in the quality of life of companion animals, *Anim Welfare* 16(Suppl 1):149–154, 2007.

29. Bayvel ACD, Cross N: Animal welfare: a complex domestic and international public-policy issue—who are the key players. *J Vet Med Educ* 37:3–12, 2010.

30. Odendaal JSJ: Science-based assessment of animal welfare: companion animals, *Rev Sci Tech* 24:493–502, 2005.

31. van Zeeland YRA: *The feather damaging Grey parrot: an analysis of its behavior and needs*, PhD thesis, The Netherlands, 2013, Utrecht University.

32. Ohl F, van der Staay FJ: Animal welfare: at the interface between science and society, *Vet J* 192:13–19, 2012.

33. Brambell Committee (Report): *Report of the technical committee to enquire into the welfare of animals kept under intensive livestock husbandry systems*, *The Brambell Report*, London, 1965, HMSO.

34. Lagoni L, Butler C, Hetts S: Responding to the human-animal bond: how veterinarians help clients. In *The human-animal bond and grief*, Philadelphia, PA, 1994, WB Saunders, pp 53–78.

35. Wrobel TA, Dye AL: Grieving pet death: normative, gender, and attachment issues, *Omega* 47:385–393, 2003.

36. Walsh F: The human-animal bonds II: the role of pets in family systems and family therapy, *Fam Proc* 48:481–499, 2009.

37. Meyers B: Disenfranchised grief and the loss of an animal companion. In Doka KJ, editor: *Disenfranchised grief: new directions, challenges, and strategies for practice*, Champaign, IL, 2002, Research Press, pp 251–264.

38. Werner-Lin A, Moro T: Unacknowledged and stigmatized losses. In Walsh F, McGoldrick M, editors: *Living beyond loss: death in the family*, ed 2, New York, 2004, Norton, pp 247–272.

39. Rollin BE: Euthanasia and quality of life, *JAVMA* 228(7):1014–1016, 2006.

40. McCutcheon KA, Fleming SJ: Grief resulting from euthanasia and natural death of companion animals, *Omega* 44(2):169–188, 2002.

41. Butler C, Short DeGraff P: Helping during pet loss and bereavement, *Vet Q* 18(1):58–60, 1996.

42. Pilgram MD: Communicating social support to grieving clients: the veterinarians' view, *Death Stud* 34:699–714, 2010.

43. Hall MJ, Ng A, Ursano RJ, et al: Psychological impact of the animal-human bond in disaster preparedness and response, *J Psychiatr Pract* 10:368–374, 2004.

44. Gerwolls MK, Labott SM: Adjustment to the death of a companion animal, *Anthrozoös* 7(3):172–187, 1994.

EUTHANASIA

Cheryl B. Greenacre

Clients and society in general are increasingly concerned about respectful and humane treatment of animals including all aspects of euthanasia. According to the American Veterinary Medical Association (AVMA) *Guidelines for the Euthanasia of Animals: 2013 Edition*, the term *euthanasia* "is usually used to describe ending the life of an individual animal in a way that minimizes or eliminates pain and distress."[1] This new, expanded version, hereafter referred to as the "AVMA Guidelines," is 102 pages long and includes sections on species that were not addressed in earlier versions, a section on how to handle animals before and during euthanasia, disposal of carcasses, and the human perspective of animal euthanasia including ethics. It also includes an avian section pertaining to pet birds; aviary birds; and birds used in falconry, racing, zoos, and educational facilities. There are separate sections in the AVMA Guidelines for wild birds under the "Captive and Free-ranging Nondomestic Animal" section and for birds raised for food under the "Animals Farmed for Food and Fiber" section.

The new AVMA Guidelines emphasize evidence-based medicine and research, but unfortunately in the area of euthanasia of birds, there is little, if any, research or evidence-based medicine published compared with what is present for mammals. What scientific literature is available pertains to chickens in a commercial environment in the form of peer-reviewed reports regarding euthanasia of individual or small groups of birds.[2-10] The majority of the information available on euthanasia of pet birds consists of anecdotal reports in book chapters, guidelines from various associations, journal roundtable discussions, and editorials.[11-21] The method of euthanasia depends on species, size, anatomic and physiologic characteristics, environment, degree of domestication, clinical state, and anticipated and actual response to restraint. People performing euthanasia should be knowledgeable in the method chosen and understand normal behavior for a bird, compared with what is considered a stressed or fearful bird, so that the bird can be handled appropriately to reduce stress before and during euthanasia.

An overview of acceptable, acceptable with conditions, and unacceptable methods of euthanasia are summarized in Table 22-5 and explained in depth below.

ACCEPTABLE METHODS FOR BIRDS

According to the AVMA Guidelines, acceptable methods of euthanasia for birds include intravenous injection of a sodium pentobarbital euthanasia solution with or without the bird being unconscious or under anesthesia.

Intravenous injection with an injectable euthanasia agent (such as sodium pentobarbital) is the quickest and most reliable means of euthanizing birds when it can be performed without causing undue stress. Most birds experience stress with handling and restraint, and many veterinarians prefer to gently restrain them in a towel while mask inducing with isoflurane or sevoflurane with or without prior sedation with midazolam given intramuscularly or intranasally at least 15 minutes prior to induction. Other sedatives can be used. Intravenous pentobarbital is the best option when combined with anesthesia since it is quick and reliable. A disadvantage of this method is the degree of potential stress from handling and restraint until the bird is rendered unconscious and that this method requires access to the venous system. If the bird is anesthetized, then there is less need to ensure venous access since an unconscious bird can also be given an intracardiac injection. A disadvantage is the disturbance of some tissues, such as cardiac tissue, from the euthanasia solution.[13]

TABLE 22-5

Acceptable, Conditionally Acceptable, and Unacceptable Methods of Euthanasia of Birds According to the American Veterinary Medical Association *Guidelines for the Euthanasia of Animals: 2013 Edition*

Method	Acceptable	Conditionally Acceptable	Unacceptable
Pentobarbital IV with prior sedation or anesthesia	Yes		
Pentobarbital IV without prior sedation or anesthesia	Yes		
Pentobarbital ICa or IC		If unconscious	
Inhalant agents alone		If performed appropriately	
Carbon dioxide		If necessary and performed appropriately	
Carbon monoxide		If necessary and performed appropriately	
Nitrogen		If necessary and performed appropriately	
Argon		If necessary and performed appropriately	
Cervical dislocation		If necessary and performed appropriately	
Decapitation		If necessary and performed appropriately	
Gunshot		If necessary and performed appropriately	
Potassium chloride			Unless unconscious
Exsanguination			Unless unconscious
Thoracic compression			Unless unconscious

IV, Intravenous; ICa, intracardiac; IC, intracoelomic.

ACCEPTABLE WITH CONDITIONS METHODS FOR BIRDS

The AVMA Guidelines make it very clear that "methods acceptable with conditions are equivalent to acceptable methods when all criteria for application of a method can be met."[1] According to the AVMA Guidelines, methods of euthanasia for birds that are acceptable with conditions include intraosseous, intracardiac, or intracoelomic injection of a sodium pentobarbital euthanasia solution; inhalant anesthetic overdose of carbon dioxide, carbon monoxide, nitrogen, or argon; cervical dislocation; decapitation; and gunshot. Euthanasia via injection with potassium chloride or exsanguination is only considered as secondary adjunctive methods if administered to an unconscious bird, such as a bird under general anesthesia. Each of these methods will be described individually below.

Pentobarbital via Route Other Than Intravenously

Administering pentobarbital by a route other than intravenously must be when the bird is unconscious under general anesthesia. Do not administer pentobarbital intramuscularly. Barbiturate salts are alkaline and therefore very irritating and painful if given intramuscularly or by an intracardiac or intracoelomic route, particularly if these injections inadvertently are delivered into an air sac. Although intermuscular administration of barbiturate euthanasia solutions is somewhat commonly used in birds by a number of veterinarians (Cheryl Greenacre, group discussion ICARE 2015), the argument remains that there is likely considerable pain induced *before* rendering the bird unconscious. For this reason, veterinarians are advised to devise euthanasia methods that cohere to the current AVMA and product label guidelines. Per AVMA guidelines, "With the exceptions of IM delivery of ultrapotent opioids (i.e., etorphine and carfentanil) and IM delivery of select injectable anesthetics, IM, SC, intrathoracic, intrapulmonary, intrathecal, and other nonvascular injections are not acceptable routes of administration for injectable euthanasia agents in awake animals."[21a] Intraosseous injections should be given under anesthesia because of the pain of the needle going through the periosteum and should not be given in pneumatic bones, such as the femur or humerus, because these are lined with respiratory epithelium and connect to the respiratory tract. An injection of pentobarbital euthanasia solution can be given into the occipital sinus if the bird is under general anesthesia.

Inhaled Anesthetics

Acceptable methods of euthanasia for birds with conditions include inhalant anesthetics such as isoflurane, sevoflurane, and halothane with or without nitrous oxide at high concentrations. Birds given high concentrations of inhaled gas anesthetics lose consciousness rapidly and death occurs after they are rendered unconscious, although the entire procedure may take a long time. An important consideration is that a high concentration of gas can be used and there may be minimal to no physical restraint and stress involved as a result. Advantages of this method are that it renders the bird unconscious before death, it is readily available in most practices, and it induces minimal tissue damage for later necropsy. Disadvantages are the possible exposure of personnel to these volatile gasses, the initial handling and restraint may be stressful, and possible aversion to the smell or delivery method of the volatile agent.

Carbon Dioxide

Birds require comparatively high (greater than 40%) concentrations of carbon dioxide to induce anesthesia prior to loss of consciousness. There is considerable scientific literature available on the use of carbon dioxide for euthanizing chickens, ducks, and turkeys.[2-5] It is important that the application rate of carbon dioxide is appropriate so that the increase in carbon dioxide is rapid enough to have a short time to the loss of posture and unconsciousness, but slow enough that there is less aversion or reaction to the gas. Even though birds are unconscious, they tend to flap with carbon dioxide and this can damage tissue if needed for necropsy.[13] Advantages of carbon dioxide are that it renders the bird unconscious prior to death and it has been extensively studied in chickens, turkeys, and ducks. The disadvantages are that unconscious motor activity such as flapping of wings may damage tissues for necropsy and may be disconcerting to the observer.

Carbon Monoxide

Carbon monoxide is not generally used in clinical settings because of the risk to personnel, but if used safely and levels are increased appropriately, carbon monoxide results in rapid unconsciousness prior to death.

Argon and Nitrogen

Inhaled nitrogen and argon are not generally used in clinical settings due to lack of ready availability, but they are used in commercial settings. If used safely and appropriately, these result in rapid unconsciousness prior to death. In fact, it was found that chickens had less of an aversion to argon than nitrogen or carbon dioxide, unlike rats.[2]

Cervical Dislocation

If other acceptable methods are available in the clinical setting, then those should be chosen, but sometimes cervical dislocation is the only feasible method available in a field situation, for example, an emergency at an aviary or in a field research setting. Cervical dislocation is typically performed in birds that are less than 200 g, but has been described in birds as large as 2.3 kg.[7,8] Cervical dislocation is a method that is acceptable with the condition that the person performing the cervical dislocation is experienced in performing the procedure. Practice is recommended on fresh cadavers, but learning from an experienced mentor is best. It should be performed as cranial as possible, ideally between the skull and the first cervical vertebra or between the first and second cervical vertebrae. An advantage of cervical dislocation is that no chemicals or special instrumentation is necessary. Disadvantages of cervical dislocation are that it is restricted to small birds (less than 200 g), it can be disconcerting to observers, the individuals performing the cervical dislocation must be skilled, and this method may not cause immediate unconsciousness.

Decapitation

If other acceptable methods are available in the clinical setting, then those should be chosen, but sometimes decapitation is needed in a field situation; for example, an emergency at an aviary, field research setting, or as assurance that cervical dislocation was complete may at times necessitate decapitation. Decapitation is typically performed in birds that are less than 200 g, but has been described in birds as large as 3.5 kg. This method is acceptable with the condition that the person performing the decapitation is experienced in performing the procedure and the device used is very sharp and kept in good working order. Decapitation should be performed as cranial as possible, ideally between the skull and the first cervical vertebra. One study in chickens showed that visual evoked responses were present up to 30 seconds after decapitation. Advantages of decapitation are that no chemical is necessary and it provides clear evidence of a successful procedure. Disadvantages of decapitation are that it is restricted to small birds (less than 200 g), it can be disconcerting to observers, individuals performing the euthanasia must be skilled, the equipment must be kept sharp and in good working order, and this procedure may not cause immediate unconsciousness.

Gunshot

This method is not used in a clinical setting because of obvious dangers to personnel and because there are better methods available. This method is used if necessary in field conditions with the condition that personnel are adequately trained and it is used in a manner safe to people. Gunshot to the head or neck is optimal.

UNACCEPTABLE METHODS FOR BIRDS

In the conscious bird it is unacceptable to perform thoracic compression, exsanguinate, or administer potassium chloride. Thoracic compression is the application of digital pressure to the heart and sternum of the bird to prevent respiratory and cardiac movement. The AVMA Guidelines cite concerns over lack of standardization or characterization of this technique and a lack of information regarding time of death and exact cause of death.[1,14,15,19] Adjunctive methods are those methods that can be used only if the bird is unconscious or anesthetized prior to their use, and include intravenous or intracardiac potassium chloride or exsanguination. If thoracic compression is performed in an unconscious bird then it is considered conditionally acceptable. These adjunctive methods are unacceptable if performed in a conscious bird, but if the bird is anesthetized then they are acceptable with this condition. Exsanguination is useful if the blood is needed for further testing in the bird. It is also unacceptable to inject solutions that are not euthanasia agents, such as cleaning products, in an attempt to euthanize.

EGG EUTHANASIA

Some research states that the neural tube of the bird embryo is completely formed and able to feel pain by 50% incubation.[19,20] Other literature states that there are no consistent electroencephalographic (EEG) readings in bird embryos until about 80% incubation (Day 17 for a chicken embryo), and even then the EEG waves are indicative of a sleeplike state until hatching.[21] The AVMA Euthanasia Guidelines cite these two conflicting findings, one in the poultry section, the other in avian section, leaving a discrepancy prompting an addendum to be written in the near future for clarification. In the meantime, companion bird species embryos that are greater than 50% through incubation should be euthanized by the above acceptable methods or acceptable with conditions methods including anesthetic overdose, decapitation, or prolonged (greater than 20 minutes) exposure to carbon dioxide. Eggs that are less than 50% through incubation can be destroyed by prolonged (greater than 20 minutes) exposure to carbon dioxide, cooling (less than 4° C for 4 hours), freezing, or egg addling.

DISPOSAL OF CARCASSES

No matter which euthanasia method is chosen proper disposal of the carcass must be taken into consideration and must adhere to local and state laws. Choices for disposal include burial, thermal or chemical cremation, or rendering. If pentobarbital solution is used, the carcass must be disposed in a manner so that wildlife such as raptors, carnivores, and other scavengers will not be exposed to it. If veterinarians fail to properly dispose of animal remains or fail to inform their clients of how to provide proper disposal of animal remains then the Migratory Bird Treaty Act, the Endangered Species Act, and the Bald and Golden Eagle Protection Act may be used and they carry civil penalties up to $25,000 and criminal penalties up to $500,000 and 2 years in jail. Cases of suspected wildlife death from animal remains containing pentobarbital are investigated by the regional U.S. Fish and Wildlife Service law enforcement office.[1,22-24]

To prevent secondary poisoning from pentobarbital-type euthanasia solutions by scavenger consumption of the carcasses, the U.S. Fish and Wildlife Service makes clear recommendations. These include incineration or cremation, immediate deep burial according to local laws and regulations, and securely storing animal remains until such time as deep burial is practical. Burial should follow local landfill practices to prevent access by scavengers to legally disposed animal remains. Animal remains should be properly tagged, and the outer bags or containers should display prominent poison tags.[1,22-24] Clients must be educated about proper disposal methods as a part of their signed euthanasia consent form.

HUMAN PERSPECTIVE

The human perspective of euthanasia includes the owners making a very difficult decision regarding their bird and the veterinarian and staff performing the euthanasia. Euthanasia should be handled with professionalism, respect, and compassion by all animal care staff. Communication is key to helping owners make end-of-life decisions regarding their pets. Various approaches can be used to make the setting of the euthanasia as comfortable as possible for owners, especially if they wish to be present for the euthanasia. A recent study found that over 75% of owners who recently experienced death of a pet reported a positive correlation between support from the veterinarian and staff and their ability to handle the grief associated with their pet's death.[25] Good communication includes preparing owners for what to expect during the euthanasia process including the method used and the potential for agonal movements (agonal breaths, muscle twitches, failure of the eyelids to close, and elimination from the cloaca). Some practices offer at-home euthanasia, some offer grief counseling, and others send sympathy cards and paw print impressions made with the pet's foot pressed into clay (Figure 22-37). Stress of performing euthanasia can adversely affect the animal

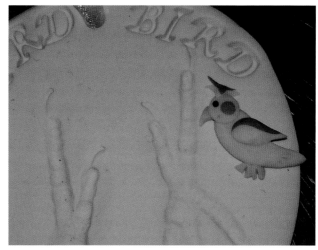

FIGURE 22-37 Picture of a paw imprint given to an owner in remembrance of their pet bird.

care staff. One potential solution to prevent or minimize such adverse effects is to attend mindful-based stress reduction classes that are available almost everywhere and can help with compassion fatigue.

REFERENCES

1. *AVMA Guidelines for the euthanasia of animals: 2013 edition*, Schaumburg, IL, 2013, American Veterinary Medical Association.
2. Raj ABM: Aversive reactions to argon, carbon dioxide and a mixture of carbon dioxide and argon, *Vet Rec* 138(24):592–593, 1996.
3. Blackshaw JK, Fenwick DC, Beattie AW, et al: The behavior of chickens, mice and rats during euthanasia with chloroform, carbon dioxide and ether, *Lab Anim* 22(1):67–75, 1998.
4. Close B, Banister K, Baumans V, et al: Recommendations for euthanasia of experimental animals: part 1, *Lab Anim* 30:293–316, 1996.
5. Close B, Banister K, Baumans V, et al: Recommendations for euthanasia of experimental animals: part 2, *Lab Anim* 31:1–32, 1997.
6. Coenen AML, Lankhaar J, Lowe JC, et al: Remote monitoring of electroencephalogram, electrocardiogram, and behavior during controlled atmosphere stunning in broilers: implications for welfare, *Poult Sci* 88(1):10–19, 2009.
7. Erasmus MA, Lawlis P, Duncan IJ, et al: Using time to insensibility and estimated time of death to evaluate a nonpenetrating captive bolt, cervical dislocation, and blunt trauma for on-farm killing of turkeys, *Poult Sci* 89(7):1345–1354, 2010.
8. Gregory NG, Wotton SB: Comparison of neck dislocation and percussion of the head on visual evoked responses in the chicken's brain, *Vet Rec* 126(23):570–572, 1990.
9. Mason C, Spence J, Bilbe L, et al: Methods for dispatching backyard poultry, *Vet Rec* 164(7):220, 2009.
10. Raj ABM: Recent developments in stunning and slaughter of poultry, *Worlds Poult Sci J* 62:462–484, 2006.
11. Miller EA, editor: Euthanasia of nonconventional species: zoo, wild, aquatic, and ectothermic animals. In Miller EA, editor: *Minimum standards for wildlife rehabilitation*, ed 3, St Cloud, MN, 2000, National Wildlife Rehabilitators Association, p 77, (Sec.7.3).
12. Franson JC: Euthanasia. In Friend M, Franson JC, editors: *Field manual of wildlife diseases. General field procedures and diseases of birds*, BRD Information and Technology Report, Washington, DC, 1999, U.S. Geological Survey, Biological Resources Division, pp 49–51.

13. Latimer KS, Rakich PM: Necropsy examination. In Ritchie BW, Harrison GJ, Harrison LR, editors: *Avian medicine: principles and application*, Lake Worth, FL, 1994, Wingers Publishing, pp 355–379.

14. Bennett RA: Association disagrees with euthanasia method for avian species (lett), *J Am Vet Med Assoc* 218:1262, 2001.

15. Ludders JW: Another reader opposing thoracic compression for avian euthanasia (lett), *J Am Vet Med Assoc* 218:1721, 2001.

16. Rae M: Necropsy. In *Clinical avian medicine*, vol 2, Palm Beach, FL, 2006, Spix Publishing, pp 661–678.

17. Hess L: Euthanasia techniques in birds—roundtable discussion, *J Avian Med Surg* 19:242–245, 2005.

18. Gaunt AS, Oring LW: *Guidelines to the use of wild birds in research*, Washington, DC, 1997, The Ornithological Council, pp 3–10.

19. Orosz S: Birds. In *Guidelines for euthanasia of nondomestic animals*, 2006, American Association of Zoo Veterinarians, pp 46–49.

20. Mellor DJ, Diesch TJ: Birth and hatching: key events in the onset of awareness in the lamb and chick, *N Z Vet J* 55(2):51–60, 2007.

21. Reilly JS, editor: Euthanasia of animals used for scientific purposes. In *Australia and New Zealand council for the care of animals in research and teaching*, Adelaide, Southern Australian, 2001, Adelaide University, pp 37–92.

21a. *AVMA Guidelines for the euthanasia of animals: 2013 edition*, Schaumburg, IL, 2013, American Veterinary Medical Association.

22. Krueger BW, Krueger KA: *U.S. Fish and Wildlife Service fact sheet: secondary pentobarbital poisoning in wildlife.* http://cpharm.vetmed.vt.edu/USFWS/. Accessed Mar 7, 2011.

23. O'Rourke K: Euthanatized animals can poison wildlife: veterinarians receive fines, *J Am Vet Med Assoc* 220:146–147, 2002.

24. Otten DR: Advisory on proper disposal of euthanatized animals, *J Am Vet Med Assoc* 219:1677–1678, 2001.

25. Adams CL, Bonnett BN, Meek AH: Predictors of owner response to companion animal death in 177 clients from 14 practices in Ontario, *J Am Vet Med Assoc* 217:1303–1309, 2000.

CHAPTER 23

Conservation of Avian Species

Glenn H. Olsen • Lorenzo Crosta • Brett D. Gartrell • Philip M. Marsh • Cynthia E. Stringfield

CONSERVATION MEDICINE

Glenn H. Olsen

Health of humans, animals, plants, and ecosystems are intertwined. Disturbance tips the balance in favor of weedy species, vectors, and disease agents. Biodiversity is important to prevent imbalance in nature. However, more scholarship is needed, and there is still much more to study, understand, and manage than we currently know.

As global warming changes species ranges, new species mixtures develop, with new hosts for old pathogens (or new pathogens finding old hosts). Conservation medicine focuses on pathogens in ecosystems. The examples in this chapter focus on ecosystem restoration or the restoration of biodiversity, and conservation plays an important part in these restoration projects. Restoration projects attempt to restore some biodiversity and to save ecosystems and maybe the planet. Are we becoming "plant doctors," as one author claims?[1]

Human-induced habitat alteration—often termed *habitat destruction*—and species loss lead to the disruption of ecosystems. This is followed by changes in disease transmission patterns, invasions of alien species and pathogens, and deposition of toxic pollutants. It is interesting that many "emerging" diseases are coming from areas where human-altered ecosystems first developed multimillennia ago. We see many types of pathogenic avian influenza coming from the Yangtze River and surrounding areas where ancient Chinese civilization developed. Middle Eastern respiratory disease is emerging from the ancient civilizations of the Tigris-Euphrates/Fertile Crescent areas of the Middle East, so even long-altered, long-disturbed human ecosystems can change, leading to new disease emergence factors.

We humans are still fumbling about trying to understand the health impacts generated by changing ecosystems. We need professionals with transdisciplinary skills to link ecosystems with animal and human health issues.[2] The link between ecosystems and health is partly addressed in the One Health, One Medicine concept that seeks to link the health of humans, animals, and the environment. Conservation medicine seeks to bring together the disciplines of health and ecology in a new transdisciplinary design.[2] Conservation medicine can address the effects of disease on threatened and endangered species, on reintroduction efforts for these species, and on ecosystem health. Conservation medicine can look at changes in species diversity as it impacts disease transmission and reservoirs of diseases. The transmission of Lyme disease, for example, is reduced by increased biodiversity in the environment.[3]

How will conservation medicine work in the future? Wildlife biologists recognize disease risks, but more biomedical research and diagnostic resources are needed to develop new, noninvasive health monitoring techniques. Already we are using fecal corticosteroids to monitor stress levels in sandhill and whooping cranes,[4,5] with the samples collected from the ground after the cranes walk by an area.

Disease risk analysis is one tool of conservation medicine. Covello and Merkhofer[6] developed a three-part risk analysis framework that is applied to conservation medicine and reintroduction programs.[7] Risk analysis or risk management is the overarching framework and has three sections or elements: hazard identification, risk assessment, and risk evaluation. Hazard identification is the component for identifying risk agents and the conditions where these agents produce harmful effects. Risk assessment is describing and then quantifying these risks. Risk evaluation involves comparing risks and evaluating the significance of each risk.

The Office International des Epizooties (OIE), also referred to as the World Organization for Animal Health, has used risk analysis for assessing disease risks for the importation of domestic animals.[8] However, this methodology is not as well developed for wild animal reintroductions because we do not have the same epidemiological knowledge base for infectious diseases in wildlife. Risk analysis is underutilized in wildlife, as reintroductions and wildlife populations are much more complicated, involving an ecosystem, not a barnyard environment under human control.[7]

Two authors[9,10] have looked at disease risk analysis in endangered species programs. Their analysis includes (1) disease/hazard list, (2) tools for ranking or prioritizing diseases and hazards, (3) how to collect information on diseases and hazards, and (4) qualitative disease risk analysis and is based on Covello and Merkhofer.[6]

Quantitative disease risk analysis appears to be a more difficult undertaking. Ballou[11] recognized the need for a quantitative approach to disease risk analysis and suggested using a population viability analysis to determine risk to the population. There is an epidemiological modeling package called OUTBREAK that is linked to the population viability analysis in a package called VORTEX, but one author[7] claims this quantified approach using OUTBREAK has never been used in a published example of disease risk analysis. One major hurdle is our poor understanding of infections and parasitic diseases in wildlife compared with what we know in domestic animal medicine and human medicine.

REINTRODUCTION BIOLOGY

What is reintroduction biology? One author[12] describes it as "the science and practice of restoring populations of animals and plants through translocations." Humankind has been doing this for decades, if not centuries. At first, reintroductions were done accidentally, such as the release of rats and mice into various habitats, often islands that were devoid of these species before the arrival of the first humans on ocean-going vessels. Later, reintroductions were done much more purposefully, such as the release of mongoose on various Caribbean and Pacific islands to combat, usually unsuccessfully, rats, which were, as often as not, accidental reintroductions themselves.

Avian reintroductions usually fall into the latter category of purposeful reintroductions, rather than accidental reintroductions. One exception to this may be the accidental escape of falcons from the armies of Genghis Khan that crossbred with native falcons in the Altay Mountains, producing a hybrid species.[13] Other accidental reintroductions in recent years have involved the escape or release of various species of pet birds, usually psittacines, into a habitat that proves suitable for the species to thrive and reproduce.

Purposeful reintroductions have included such programs as the barn owl *(Tyto alba)* releases in Hawaii, again to try to combat reintroduced rats and mice. A host of game bird releases such as the ring-necked pheasant *(Phasianus colchicus)* have been somewhat successful in various habitats around the world. Aesthetic releases to "improve" the environment, such as the release of starlings in North America to give the people some of the birds described in Shakespeare's works, have sometimes been exceedingly successful. Many passerine species were introduced to Hawaii by an organization dedicated to raising funds for the introduction of birds from around the world to improve the Hawaiian ecosystem. As late as 1965, Act 203 passed by the state of Hawaii legislature provided funds for importing more nongame bird species.[14]

Today purposeful reintroductions, such as the examples in this chapter, are often utilized as a tool to save a threatened or endangered species from extinction in the wild or to bolster low populations of a species. The whooping crane *(Grus americana)* example describes a technique using ultralight aircraft to reintroduce a migratory bird to a migration pathway where no members of the species remain. The California condor *(Gymnogyps californianus)* reintroductions started a few years after the political/biological decision was made in 1987 to remove the last of the species from the wild. As a result of improved captive propagation techniques, California condors were released again to the wild 5 years after the last one had been removed.

The Spix's macaw *(Cyanopsitta spixii)* recovery program is still in its infancy compared with the programs for the other species discussed in this chapter. No releases are currently being undertaken, and only one female bird has been released in the history of the program. There is a strong veterinary medical program that is attempting to identify important diseases, such as that caused by avian bornavirus (ABV), or proventricular dilation disease (PDD) (see Chapter 2), and to develop preventative medical programs. However, there is no overall cohesive organization or plan to implement the sustained reintroduction program that is required to restore this species to the wild.

The takahe *(Porphyrio hochstetteri)* reintroduction program is an interesting case study. One small remnant population of takahe, originally thought to be extinct, was located by a persistent biologist. Even this did not guarantee success, as political battles ensued between those who favored minimal or no intervention with this remnant population and those who favored more aggressive approaches. As the remnant population continued to drop, the more aggressive approach won. A captive breeding population was established and releases planned.

Unfortunately, much of the South Island of New Zealand is no longer appropriate habitat for the takahe because of introduced mammalian predators. Isolated islands that were free of introduced predators were the sites for five release programs. In addition, birds from the captive breeding center have been used to bolster the remnant population. In this example, a strong captive breeding center with an evolving veterinary program of successful intervention has helped the species to continue to make a recovery from near extinction.

TRACKING REINTRODUCED BIRDS

Although the species preservation efforts discussed in this chapter only briefly, if at all, mention the use of radiotelemetry devices to track birds, these units can be a very important part of any reintroduction program. Without radiotelemetry devices, dead, sick, or injured birds can be nearly impossible to locate, yet these are the birds that can help improve the veterinary care program for all the birds. Even though telemetry devices allow biologists and veterinarians to track the

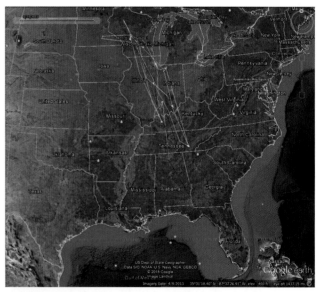

FIGURE 23-1 An example of tracking data for parent-reared whooping cranes released in Wisconsin. Tracks represent 5 young whooping cranes, 2 reintroduced in September 2013 and 3 reintroduced in September 2014. (Tracking data compiled by Kathleen M. Mcgrew, USGS/PWRC, on Google Earth map.)

daily movements of reintroduced birds, the devices and attachment methods need veterinary input, as pointed out in the section about the takahe reintroductions, where improper wing harness attachment was leading to soft tissue injuries and even fractures.

The advent of satellite telemetry using the Argos system with the launch of the NOAA-6 satellite in 1979 has been a major advance in our ability to track wildlife over remote and rugged terrain. The first satellite transmitters weighed 11.3 kg and were used to track large mammals only. By the early 1990s, transmitter weight was down to 450 g, and deployment was possible on larger birds such as bald eagles *(Haliaeetus leucocephalus)* and sandhill cranes *(Grus canadensis)*. By 2014, transmitter weight was down to 5 g for solar rechargeable backpack transmitters. Between 2010 and 2014, as the size and weight of transmitters shrank, the numbers of avian species tracked went from 30% to 39% of the total number of animals being tracked by satellite (Figure 23-1).

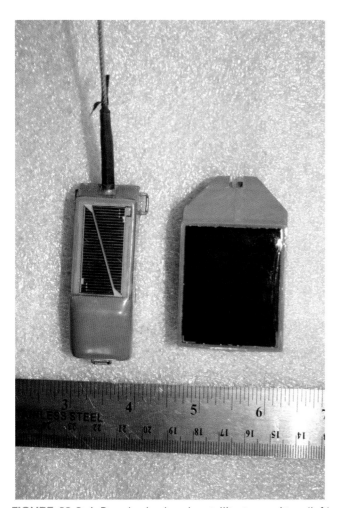

FIGURE 23-2 A Doppler backpack satellite transmitter *(left)* compared with a cellular backpack transmitter *(right)*. The cellular backpack transmitter has a larger solar panel array *(black areas)* than the Doppler backpack satellite transmitter. This can be an advantage in some species because feathers will not be groomed over the top of the solar panels, but in other species the larger size can pose physical problems for the bird.

Cellular telephone technology has contributed to this ability to track wild birds. The demand for smaller, more powerful cell phones with more functions has led to battery research and the development of smaller, more powerful batteries. Batteries are the major weight factor in transmitters, and even solar-powered transmitters have small rechargeable batteries that store the trickle charge from the solar panels and release the larger amount of energy needed for each transmission.

The widespread use of cellular telephones has led to another application for wildlife studies. Several companies are currently marketing backpack transmitters for avian species that communicate with cell phone towers instead of satellites. The units have GPS capability, store locations at set intervals, and then download the data through the cell phone towers as the bird passes near one. The birds are literally "phoning home." The advantage of this system is the lowered cost and more finely tuned locations of GPS versus the Doppler locations from satellite telemetry (although the satellite telemetry units can now also use GPS for locations). Currently cell phone backpack units are slightly heavier than the satellite units and have a larger solar panel array (Figure 23-2), but as the weight and size of the transmitters come down, the application will be used on more wild avian species. The one other disadvantage of the cellular telephone system is its dependence on cell towers to download data periodically. The bird carrying such a unit must pass within a few kilometers of a cell phone tower periodically. For tracking avian species that inhabit remote locations such as the Amazon rain forest or the Arctic, or for oceanic species, satellite telemetry continues to be the best option.

REFERENCES

1. Lovejoy TE: Forward: plant doctors. In Aguirre AA, Ostfeld RS, Daszak P, editors: *New directions in conservation medicine*, New York, 2012, Oxford University Press.
2. Aguirre AA, Tabor GM, Ostfeld RS: Conservation medicine: ontogeny of emerging discipline. In Aguirre AA, Ostfeld RS, Daszak P, editors: *New directions in conservation medicine*, New York, 2012, Oxford University Press, pp 3–16.
3. Schmidt KA, Ostfeld S: Biodiversity and the dilution effect in disease ecology, *Ecology* 82:609–619, 2001.
4. Hartup BK, Olsen GH, Czekala NM, et al: Levels of fecal corticosterone in sandhill cranes during a human-led migration, *J Wildlife Dis* 40(2):267–272, 2004.
5. Hartup BK, Olsen GH, Czekala NM: Fecal corticoid monitoring in whooping cranes (*Grus Americana*) undergoing reintroduction, *Zoo Biol* 24:15–28, 2005.
6. Covello BT, Merkhofer MW: *Risk assessment methods: approaches for assessing health and environment risks*, New York, 1993, Plenum Press.
7. Sainsbury AW, Armstrong DP, Ewen JG: Methods of disease risk analysis for reintroduction programs. In Ewen JG, Armstrong DP, Parker KA, et al, editors: *Reintroduction biology: integrating science and management*, West Sussex, UK, 2012, Blackwell Publishing.
8. Bruckner G, MacDiarmid S, Murray N: *Handbook on import risk analysis for animals and animal products*, Paris, France, 2010, Office International des Epizooties.
9. Armstrong D, Jakob-Hoff R, Seal US: *Animal movements and disease risk: a workshop*, Apple Valley, Minnesota, 2003, Conservation Breeding Specialist Group (SSC/IUCN).
10. Miller PS: Tools and techniques for disease risk assessment and threatened wildlife conservation programs, *International Zoo Yearbook* 41:38–51, 2007.

11. Ballou JD: Assessing the risk of infectious disease in captive breeding and reintroduction programs, *J Zoo Wildlife Med* 24:327–335, 1993.
12. Seddon PJ, Armstrong DP, Parker KA, et al: Summary: Chapter 14. In Ewen JG, Armstrong DP, Parker KA, et al, editors: *Reintroduction biology: integrating science and management*, West Sussex, UK, 2012, Blackwell Publishing.
13. Ellis DH: What is Falco altaicus Menzbier? *J Raptor Res*, 29(1): 15–25, 1995.
14. Berger AJ: Introduced birds. In *Hawaiian birdlife*, ed 2, Honolulu, Hawaii, 1981, University of Hawaii Press.

THE CONSERVATION PROJECT OF THE RAREST PARROT: THE SPIX'S MACAW (*CYANOPSITTA SPIXII*)

Lorenzo Crosta

The Spix's macaw (*Cyanopsitta spixii*) is extinct in the wild: The last free-ranging specimen, a male, paired with a female Illiger's macaw (*Primolius maracana*), disappeared in October 2000.[1-11]

BIOLOGICAL NOTES

The Spix's macaw is a medium-sized parrot weighing about 300 g and measuring around 60 cm in length. A typical feature of the species is the blue color, which changes its shade over the different body parts. In fact, it is lighter on the head, where it switches into a grayish-blue, while it is darker on the wings and back.

The naked facial patches, typical of most macaws, are light gray in the young specimens and dark gray in the mature birds. Furthermore, young birds will show a light horn-colored stripe along the curve of the upper bill, while this stripe will disappear in the adult Spix's macaws (Figures 23-3 and 23-4).

Even if there was some discussion about the fact that female Spix's macaws might show some white feathers scattered around the head, this has never been proven, at least not to a point to be used as a means to determine the gender of Spix's macaws. In other words, we can state there is no valid information about a defined sexual dimorphism in this species, so far.

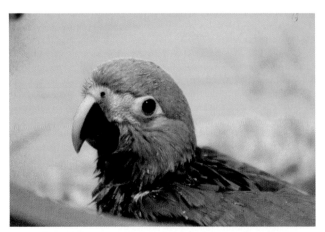

FIGURE 23-3 Spix's macaw chick, 70 days old.

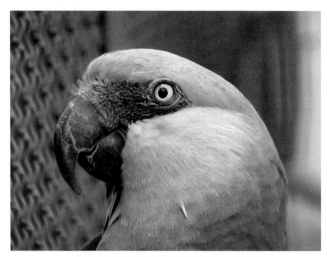

FIGURE 23-4 Adult Spix's macaw.

The Spix's macaw has traditionally been included with the group of blue macaws, which consists of four species divided in two genera:

- *Anodorhynchus*, including three species:
  - Hyacinth, or hyacinthine macaw (*Anodorhynchus hyacinthinus*)
  - Lear's, or indigo macaw (*Anodorhynchus leari*)
  - Glaucous macaw (*Anodorhynchus glaucus*)
- *Cyanopsitta*, a monospecific genus, including only the Spix's macaw (*Cyanopsitta spixii*).

The idea to include the Spix's within the other blue macaws was historically carried forward on the simple basis of their similar appearance, such as the blue color of the feathers. Nowadays, according to the latest genetic discoveries, we know that the Spix's macaw is more closely related to the medium-sized macaws of the genus *Orthopsittaca* and *Primolius*, including the Illiger's macaw, the blue-headed macaw, and the red-bellied macaw, and the large macaws belonging to the genus *Ara*. On the other hand, the other blue macaws (genus *Anodorhynchus*) are more related to the golden (or Queen of Bavaria) conure (*Guaruba guarouba*). For this reason, we would not be wrong defining the golden conure as the "real fourth Blue macaw."

The genus name *Cyanopsitta* means blue parrot, while *spixii* is named for Johann Baptist von Spix, a German physician and naturalist sent to Brazil to describe the local fauna and to eventually bring back some specimens. This is literally what von Spix did: In 1819 he shot a blue macaw and brought it back to Germany as a stuffed specimen. That bird was captured in a region that now belongs to the Pernambuco state, not too far from Bahia, where the last wild Spix's were known to live. In 1832 the species was described again by Johann Wagler, a well-known German zoologist, but afterward, the species remained a sort of mystery for about 150 years, until it was again seen in Brazil and described by Paul Roth, a Swiss ornithologist, in 1986.

It has been speculated that the natural range of the Spix's macaw has never been too large, and thus it is possible that the species population has never been very large, as well. However, it is thought that the original range included a vast portion of the Gerais area, in Bahia state, Brazil. The last known range of the Spix's macaw in the wild included an area called Caatinga, located in northeastern Brazil. The Caatinga is a very dry area, characterized by a low vegetation that evolved to stand periods of extremely hot climate and no rain. (Rainfall can be absent for months, sometimes years.) The species was supposedly thriving in woodland galleries that grew along the main local rivers, formed by "Caraibeiras" *(Tabebuia aurea)*. The natural habitat was very specific, and birds did depend on the trees for the most important aspects of their lives, such as nesting, feeding, and roosting. The Spix's macaw fed primarily on seeds and nuts of Caraibeira and shrubs of different Euphorbiaceae.

HOW MANY SPIX'S MACAWS STILL EXIST?

After a preliminary meeting, held in 1987 at the Loro Parque, in Tenerife (Canary Islands, Spain), 17 captive Spix's macaws were identified. In 1991, when the International Studbook was in the process of being officially recognized, the information about the real number of Spix's macaws in captivity became cloudier, with reports of captive numbers ranging from 11 to 17 birds. However, when the International Studbook was formally started, 15 captive birds were officially known to exist in the world. Of those, 11 were founders, or better "wild caught birds, with no known genetic relationship." Four of the starting 15 birds were captively bred and reared (Figure 23-5).

After the Brazilian government released an international amnesty for the species, declaring that no birds in the hands of the Permanent Committee for the Recovery of Spix's Macaw (CPRAA) members would be confiscated, Joseph Hämmerli, a private Swiss holder, joined the CPRAA, increasing the number to 18 birds, of which 12 were founders.

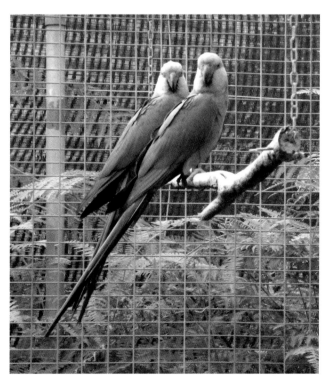

FIGURE 23-5 A pair of Spix's macaws, Loro Parque Tenerife.

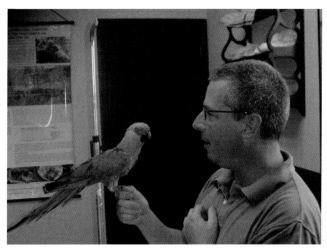

FIGURE 23-6 One of the last photos of Presley, the bird that inspired the movie "Rio."

Over the years, Spix's macaws have been bred successfully in different institutions, as outlined below:
- Birds International, Philippines (since 1999, hen birds were moved to Qatar)
- Private owners, Switzerland (birds moved to Germany and Qatar)
- Loro Parque, Tenerife, Spain (1992, 2004, and following years)
- AWWP, Qatar (2004–on)
- ACTP, Germany (2006–on)
- NEST, Brazil (2014)

Despite the number of Spix's macaws bred and raised in 2014, the year was not good for the species, since two important birds died. One was female #26, and the other was Presley, the bird originally repatriated from the United States, which inspired the cartoon movie "Rio" (Figure 23-6). The exact number of Spix's macaws in captivity is often debated both officially and nonofficially for the following reasons:

1. Some holders were not members of the previous CPRAA, and they were not obliged to declare the number of birds in their hands.
2. There are strong clues about some more Spix's macaws, likely in countries not adhering to the Convention on International Trade in Endangered Species of Wild Fauna and Flora (CITES), but no confirmed data are officially available.
3. Still, there is the hope that some unknown holders might show up and join the conservation program, increasing the number of the breeding population in captivity.

As of January 2015, 92 birds are officially registered, all of which are being maintained in captivity in three locations. Their numbers and locations are depicted in Table 23-1.

The Efforts for the Conservation of the Spix's Macaw

In 1990 (3 years after the meeting held in 1987 at the Loro Parque in Tenerife), the Brazilian Institute of Environment and Renewable Natural Resources (Instituto Brasileiro do Meio Ambiente e dos Recursos Naturais Renováveis [IBAMA]) started the CPRAA, with the purpose of conserving the Spix's macaws. In 2000, the last known wild Spix's macaw suddenly

TABLE 23-1

Current Known World Population of the Spix's Macaw, January 2015

Location	Male	Female	Unknown Gender
ACTP (Association for the Conservation of Threatened Parrots, Germany)	5	4	3
NEST (Criadouro Científico para a Conservação Estância, Brazil)	2	7	2
AWWP (Al Wabra Wildlife Preservation, Qatar)	30	40	0
TOTAL	37	51	5

disappeared. There were and still are almost never-ending disputes about possible responsibilities, faults, and what really happened to the bird (Was it dead? Had it been killed by any sort of predator? Had it been smuggled somewhere?). The author had the chance to speak with people working in the area, where a man claimed that he talked to a local farmer, who found the bird dead, just below high power lines. The farmer claimed to have buried the body because he was worried the confirmation of death would lead to termination of monies for the local project. This information is not corroborated or confirmed. The only simple fact was that the Spix's macaw was not flying free anymore. This was a tragedy for the CPRAA, whose members in the previous 10 years had been putting a lot of energy, effort, and money toward setting up a conservation program and, if possible, a reintroduction project.

There were widely used techniques of advertising and methods of increasing the awareness and pride of local people where that last Spix's macaw was living. Lectures about the birds in the schools of the local countryside were used and efforts were made to make people aware that such an emblematic bird would bring tourism and money into that remote area. Two projects, which had been carried over, were particularly intriguing, at least in the author's eyes. The first, original plan foresaw the introduction of a female Spix's macaw in the hope that she would mate with the last wild male. Actually, there was a good start for the project, and female stdb #7 was brought into the Caatinga region in August 1994. This female was illegally caught from the wild in 1987, discovered, and confiscated. Further, there was a very good chance that she was the original mate of the last wild male. This posed the best opportunity for the birds to rebuild a pair relationship that had already existed.

After almost 1 year of adaptation and preliminary work, female #7 was released in March 1995. In the beginning female #7 was just following the mixed couple (Spix's male × Illiger's female), but by June of the same year, she was already pairing with the male, while the Illiger's female was following behind. By that time, they were forming a triad, but the apparent rank of the Spix's female was constantly growing. Sadly, around the end of July 1995, female #7 disappeared.

Considering the high level of monitoring, smuggling was unlikely, and it was supposed that she died. Potential causes of death were hypothesized to include predation or an accident following collision with high power lines. At that point, another action was suggested: to release in the wild Spix's macaw chicks coming from captivity. In a few words, the plan contemplated three steps:
1. To transfer some breeding (proven fertile) Illiger's macaw *(Primolius maracana)* pairs in Caatinga, where the last Spix's macaw was flying free, and manage them on-site.
2. To try to put fertile Illiger's eggs into the nest of the mixed pair (Spix's × Illiger's), which in the meantime had bonded again. The idea was to verify whether the mixed pair was able to incubate and successfully raise a clutch of chicks from the same species of at least one of the two species in the pair.
3. In case the trial was successful, a similar approach would be attempted, but using fertile Spix's macaw eggs from captive pairs.

Although the plan had a good start, it crashed after the last wild bird disappeared in October 2000. This fact, together with other discouraging technical and political news, led to the dissolution of the CPRAA in the year 2002. Soon after, a new "Working Group" (WG) was started, whose members included Conservation International do Brasil, Cemave-Proaves, Fundãçao Parque Zoológico de São Paulo, and Loro Parque Fundación.

The newly founded WG first acted under the supervision of IBAMA, and some consulting experts for the different fields were selected. Those were as follows: Roberto Aceredo (bird breeder), Carlos Bianchi (biologist), Lorenzo Crosta (veterinarian), Yara de Melo Barros (biologist), and Cristina Miyaki (molecular geneticist). In 2007, the WG passed under the supervision of the Instituto Chico Mendes de Conservação da Biodiversidade (Chico Mendes Institute for the Conservation of Biodiversity [ICMBio]), a newly formed branch of IBAMA. At that point, the new WG concentrated on two primary actions: (1) setting up new breeding centers in Brazil (captive birds in Brazil had not bred successfully yet) and (2) setting up more breeding centers in other countries (for two main reasons: first, some institutions had been breeding the Spix's macaws successfully, and there was no reason to stop them; second, with such a limited number of birds, it was considered too risky to keep all birds in one or a few places in the same country). With more holding institutions, the chances that an accident or an infectious disease could put an end to the species were considered lower, and by implementing specific training for the staff working in the recovery centers, it was hoped that risk would be even lower.

Besides those major points, the WG members started setting the bases for a project to release the birds in the wild. This could take place only when the total number of birds in captivity and the local situation in the area chosen for the release showed that a reintroduction of Spix's macaws was safe (Figure 23-7). A minimum number of 200 birds in captivity was suggested as the safe background from which releases could be started.

With the understandable complexity of a program involving leading institutions from different countries, but kept together by the hope of seeing the Spix's macaw flying free

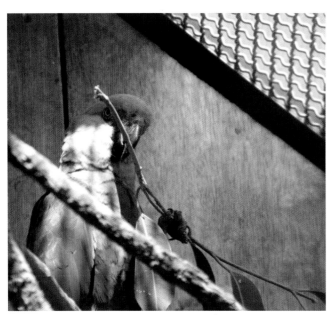

FIGURE 23-7 Adult Spix's macaw in a breeding aviary in Brazil.

again, the WG worked until 2012. In that year, as a result of different points of view and general disagreements between the holders, the Loro Parque Foundation (Tenerife, Spain) and the San Paulo Zoo (Brazil) eventually left the program. At that point the program kept on, with the name Brazilian National Action Plan for the Recovery of the Spix's Macaw. This new working group includes the following holders: Association for the Conservation of Threatened Parrots (ACTP, Germany), Al Wabra Wildlife Preservation (AWWP, Qatar), and Criadouro Científico para a Conservação Estância (Nest, Brazil). The Lymington Foundation, originally included within the holders, remained as a consulting institution after Presley passed away in 2014. The working group includes people with different profiles who are involved at different levels. Those are as follows:

1. Camile Lugarini and Patricia Serafini (CEMAVE), captive program coordinator and national center representative
2. Cromwell Purchase (AWWP), studbook keeper and genealogic consultant
3. Lorenzo Crosta and Marcus Vinícius Romero Marques, veterinary medicine
4. Cristina Yumi Miyaki, genetics
5. Ricardo Pereira, reproduction
6. João Luiz Xavier do Nascimento (CEMAVE/ICMBio)
7. Mark Stafford (Parrots International)
8. Ricardo Pereira (FMVZ-USP)
9. Tomas White (U.S. Fish and Wildlife Service)
10. Vanessa Kanaan (Instituto Espaço Silvestre), ethology and prerelease training.
11. Pedro Develey (SAVE Brasil)
12. Kilma Manso (ECO)

It must be pointed out that well before the last Spix's macaw disappeared from the wild, a recovery program was already in existence. The basis for a general management strategy had already been settled, and all that followed used the previous suggestions, goals, and mistakes as their guideline.

But . . . What is a Recovery Program? What is a Veterinarian's Role in this Story?

As a community, avian veterinarians are often called on to take part in "recovery programs," but often it is unclear what that request specifically means. What level of involvement is required? What are we expected to do, or not to do? "Recovery program" has too wide a definition, as it may range from a group of very committed people monitoring the nesting sites of an endangered species in a given area, to a very complex program involving people with different professional profiles and even government institutions. One possible definition is: A multidisciplinary program involving people with different experiences and skills, with the aim to reach a specific goal: the protection of a species.

In the spirit of teamwork, the best way to have different people work together is to seek to exploit the specialty of each member of the team, appreciating the skills of all. In fact, one of the most difficult tasks, especially when a very emblematic species is involved, is to work in a smooth way, understand the opinions of the different professionals involved, and try to pick up the best from each member of the team. The role of each professional depends on his or her previous experiences. For example, in the recovery program of the Spix's macaw, people with very different professional profiles have been involved. At some points, areas of expertise have ranged from genetics and field biology to international law. (Think about how difficult it may be to transfer a bird from Asia to Brazil and vice versa.) Addressing specifically the veterinary efforts involved, the veterinarians in the program have been asked to:

- Assess the general health of the specimens in the program
- Perform endoscopic examinations to evaluate health and maturity of the reproductive systems
- Write the guidelines for the health management of the birds. (This last task is particularly challenging, as it involves actions and efforts of other people, such as keepers, curators, and nutritionists.)
- Devise, implement, and refine prophylaxis and quarantine plans
- Define rules for the translocation of the birds from place to place

On a broader perspective, veterinary involvement in conservation medicine requires a broad skill set. Experience in avian medicine and surgery, captive breeding, fertility evaluation and assessment of infertility, and behavioral and environmental enrichment are all essential. There is also a strong need for the ability to cooperate with local veterinarians in each affiliated institution.

PROPHYLAXIS

The best approach to safeguarding the health of captive Spix's macaws is prophylaxis. Its main objective is to prevent the introduction and spread of pathogens and to diagnose, control, and eliminate them before they have a negative effect on the birds. In particular it is imperative to preclude entry and spread of the most dangerous infectious parrot diseases, from among those known to date. It is important to limit the risk of introducing and spreading diseases to other animal species (birds, mammals, reptiles, and man) through a careful and complete health examination, especially when birds are repatriated from countries in which the health situation and the common diseases are very different from the local ones in Brazil.

QUARANTINE

Every bird that enters a given breeding facility and/or is newly integrated in the Spix's recovery program must undergo a defined period of at least 50 days of strict isolated quarantine to help preclude the spread of diseases to the rest of the population/birds on site.

The quarantined birds must be tested for the aforementioned infectious diseases before they have been transferred and not before 3 to 5 days after their arrival to the quarantine. Birds are not allowed to leave the quarantine premises before the test results have arrived and the official veterinarian of the program has been consulted. It is important that the attending veterinarians critically assemble and standardize their recommended testing procedures, based on valid science, and best practices using current sensitivity and specificity of the tests being applied.

Considering the limited number of Spix's macaws still existing, the rules must be very strict. On the other hand, for the same reason, keepers and curators will know each bird personally, which makes monitoring the animals an easier task to perform on a day-to-day basis. The most common events that require medical treatment (and therefore prevention) are bacterial infections and parasitic infestations of the gastrointestinal and respiratory tracts. Most of these problems are sensitive to good hygiene measures and common-sense aviary management procedures. Thus it is important that routine health controls are carried out on a daily basis. These include daily rounds during which the birds are closely inspected, and collection of samples to be evaluated later on in the laboratory, when needed (Figure 23-8). Specific observational controls are based on the following:

1. Behavior
2. Physical appearance and posture
3. Plumage
4. Eyes

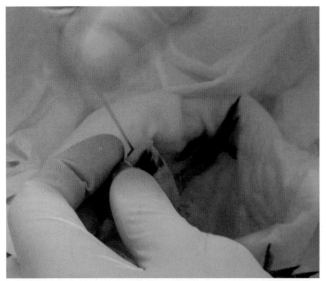

FIGURE 23-8 Sampling an 18-day-old Spix's chick.

5. Feces
6. Food and water intake
7. Visible presence of nasal, ocular, cloacal discharges
8. Visible abnormalities of the bill and toes
9. Visible presence of leg bands in the absence of problems attributable to them

SPECIFIC MEDICAL PROBLEMS

Apart from those routine preventative measures to help avoid what can be foreseen and predictable, the Spix's macaw captive population has been challenged with one particular infectious disease problem and the need to develop one new procedure. These include, respectively, PDD, ABV, and the use of artificial insemination to enhance reproductive success.

Proventricular Dilation Disease

Proventricular dilation disease (PDD) was first diagnosed in 2003 in the population kept in Qatar, well before the ABV–PDD connection was made. Fortunately, the problem was limited to a group of birds that, although participating in the international program, was isolated from the rest of the population for several reasons including geographical ones. The whole flock was subjected to several different tests, including screening crop biopsies and isolation of specific PMV-1 strains (at the time thought to be involved in the disease process). In 2008, a clear connection was made between ABV and PDD (see Chapter 2). This advancement in our understanding of the disease provided the opportunity to screen the whole Spix's macaw population kept in Qatar using a combination of methods rather than polymerase chain reaction (PCR) alone, and manage the flock accordingly. The ability to identify and isolate the sick subpopulations with disease and to identify and isolate ABV-infected but asymptomatic birds facilitated an upgrade in population management for the species. More importantly, we were able to identify and maintain our population of noninfected and healthy macaws. At this point ABV/PDD does not seem to be a major problem for the Spix's, or at least the disease is well managed and likely will not cause problems to the rest of the population. However, this success is a clear example of how careful we have to be when managing very rare species and that even a minor drop in our attention may lead to critical failure.

Use of Artificial Insemination

One of the reasons artificial insemination was first attempted in this species is that there has been a chronic lack of good breeding males in the Spix's macaw program (Figure 23-9). Even if this is not a problem in a specific location, where for example the sex ratio is good enough, it may occur in other breeding facilities where there are too many spare females or where the males that are forming good pairs and are actively stimulating their mate to lay eggs are infertile. These are the typical scenarios in which artificial insemination may be of greatest value. For example, in one location there may be two well-bonded pairs, one in which the male is a good and established breeder, while in the other the male is infertile. When the laying season is approaching, the first male can be used to artificially inseminate the female of the second pair. This

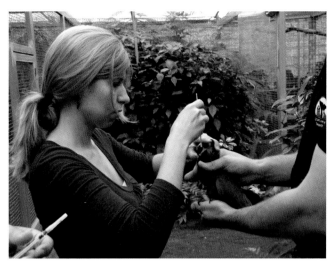

FIGURE 23-9 Sampling a blue-headed macaw *(Primolius couloni)* used as a cage mate for spare Spix's macaws. Monitoring the health of any bird that is allowed contact with the species is as important as monitoring the Spix's macaws themselves.

could be done without breaking the established bonded but infertile pair, and thereby avoiding the risks and logistical challenges of efforts to form new pairs. Another potential merit of artificial insemination in this program could be to use a given male to fertilize a female for specific genetic purposes. In summary, although the use of artificial insemination in this species' breeding program remains a newer developed and implemented technique, its potential positive impact on the number of Spix's macaws produced (and other Psittacine species) and their genetics is undeniable. To date, three Spix's macaw chicks have been produced by artificial insemination (see Chapter 12). The true impact of AI will remain to be proven over time in the effort to preserve the Spix's macaw.

ACKNOWLEDGMENTS

The author is particularly thankful to the following companies:
- Loro Parque Fundación, for funding the travel of the official veterinarian, as long as the LPF remained in the program.
- Abaxis Europe, in the person of Mrs. Bärbel Köhler, for providing all the Vetscan rotors to run the blood chemistry panels on the birds.
- Karl Storz Endoscopy and Strattner Brazil (representing Storz in Brazil), for providing, year after year, a full video endoscopy equipment to be used for the program.

REFERENCES

1. Bampi MI, Da-ré M: Recovery programme for the Spix's macaw *(Cyanopsitta spixii)*: conservation in the wild and reintroduction programme. In *Proceedings of the III International Parrot Convention*, Loro Parque, Tenerife, 1994, pp 188–194.

2. Crosta L: A journey to Brazil for the Spix's macaw, *AAV Newsletter & Clinical Forum* March-May:3–6, 2004.
3. Crosta L, Timossi L: The recovery program of the Spix's macaw *(Cyanopsitta spixii)*, four years of veterinary monitoring of the most endangered psittacine species. In *9th European AAV Conference*, Zurich, Switzerland, 2007, pp 67–71.
4. de Melo Barros Y, De Soye Y, Watson R, et al: *Plano de ação para a conservação da ararinha-azul (Cyanopsitta spixii) (Action plan for the conservation of the Spix's macaw)*, Brasilia, Brazil, 2012, Instituto Chico Mendes, de conservação de Biodiversidade.
5. Juniper T, Yamashita C: The habitat and status of the Spix's macaw *Cyanopsitta spixii*, *Bird Conserv Int* 1(1):1–9, 1991.
6. Juniper T, Parr M: *Parrots: a guide to parrots of the world*. England, 1998, Pica Press, pp 142–143, 419–420.
7. Juniper T: The Spix's macaw recovery program—a review. In *Proceedings of the V International Parrot Convention*, Loro Parque, Tenerife, 2002, pp 101–118.
8. Juniper T: *Spix's macaw: the race to save the world's rarest bird*, London, 2002, Fourth Estate Publishing.
9. Joshua S: *Cyanopsitta spixii*: DNA and fingerprinting. In *Proceedings of the III International Parrot Convention*, Loro Parque, Tenerife, 1994, pp 79–84.
10. Tavares FS, Baker AJ, Pereira SL, et al: Phylogenetic relationships and historical biogeography of neotropical parrots *(Psittaciformes: Psittacidae: Arini)* inferred from mitochondrial and nuclear DNA sequences, *Syst Biol* 55(3):454–470, 2006.
11. Watson R: Managing the world's largest population of Spix's macaws. In *33rd Annual Convention of the American Federation of Aviculture (AFA)*, Los Angeles, 2007.

VETERINARY INVOLVEMENT IN THE TAKAHE RECOVERY PROGRAM

Brett D. Gartrell, Philip M. Marsh

The takahe *(Porphyrio hochstetteri)* is a large flightless rail that is endemic to New Zealand (Figure 23-10). The decline of the takahe coincides with both Maori and European colonization

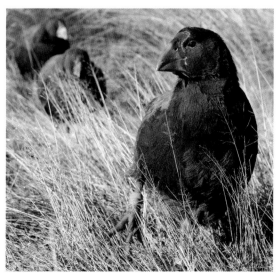

FIGURE 23-10 Takahe *(Porphyrio hochstetteri)*. (Photo courtesy Helen Dodson.)

of New Zealand. At these times, there were both deliberate and accidental introductions of a suite of mammalian predators, including rats, ferrets, stoats, cats, pigs, and dogs. These invasions into an island ecosystem that had previously been devoid of mammalian predators resulted in the extinction of much of New Zealand's endemic fauna.[1]

DECLINE AND CONSERVATION OF THE TAKAHE

Archaeological evidence shows that takahe were once present across both the North Island and South Islands of New Zealand (Figure 23-11). The North Island takahe *(Porphyrio mantelli)*

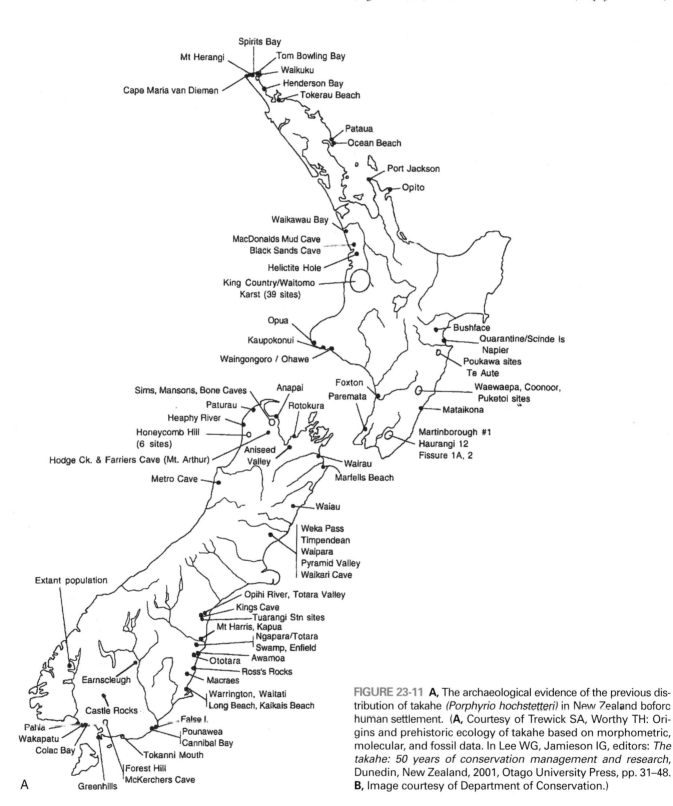

FIGURE 23-11 A, The archaeological evidence of the previous distribution of takahe *(Porphyrio hochstetteri)* in New Zealand before human settlement. **(A,** Courtesy of Trewick SA, Worthy TH: Origins and prehistoric ecology of takahe based on morphometric, molecular, and fossil data. In Lee WG, Jamieson IG, editors: *The takahe: 50 years of conservation management and research,* Dunedin, New Zealand, 2001, Otago University Press, pp. 31–48. **B,** Image courtesy of Department of Conservation.)

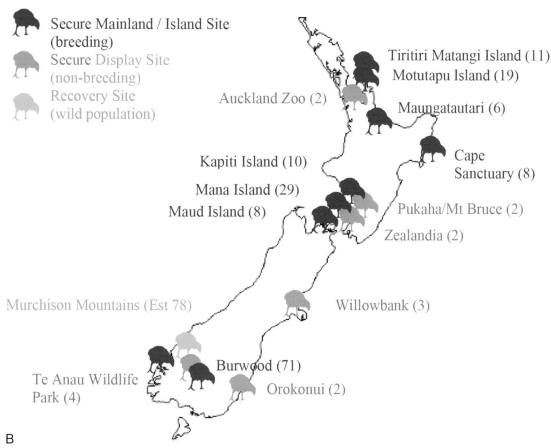

Secure Mainland / Island Site
(breeding)
Secure Display Site
(non-breeding)
Recovery Site
(wild population)

Auckland Zoo (2)

Tiritiri Matangi Island (11)
Motutapu Island (19)

Maungatautari (6)

Kapiti Island (10)

Cape
Sanctuary (8)

Mana Island (29)

Maud Island (8)

Pukaha/Mt Bruce (2)

Zealandia (2)

Murchison Mountains (Est 78)

Willowbank (3)

Burwood (71)

Te Anau Wildlife
Park (4)

Orokonui (2)

B

FIGURE 23-11, cont'd **B,** The current geographical distribution of takahe *(Porphyrio hochstetteri)* in New Zealand. One population from a private island has been excluded for privacy concerns.

was a separate species and is thought to have become extinct in the 1800s, although much of its decline has been attributed to habitat changes and earlier Maori hunting. The South Island takahe was also thought to have gone extinct in the late 1890s because of the combined effects of habitat change and destruction, hunting, and introduced predators.[2,3] However, a remnant population of takahe was discovered in 1948 in a remote mountainous region of Fiordland in the South Island called the Murchison Mountains. The steep-sided glacial valleys had slowed the invasion of the introduced predators long enough for about 250 birds of this once widespread species to survive. Initially, the takahe were not intensively managed, and the population continued to decline because of the habitat destruction caused by introduced red deer and mammalian predation, primarily by stoats. The population reached a low of 112 birds in 1981.[1,4,5]

Since that time, takahe have been intensively managed by the Department of Conservation, a branch of the New Zealand government. The conservation is carried out in partnership with Ngai Tahu, the Maori people of the South Island. As well as the protection of the Murchison Mountain population, subpopulations of the birds have been established on pest-free offshore islands and on predatorproof mainland sanctuaries. A captive breeding center has been established that initially pioneered techniques in artificial incubation of eggs and the hand-rearing of chicks, but it now exclusively focuses on producing parent-reared birds, who have been shown to have a much improved reproductive success rate on release.[6] These efforts have resulted in a slow recovery of the population number to an estimated 220 adult birds. The population is listed as Nationally Critical under the New Zealand Threat Classification System.[1,4,6,7]

The main aim of the current Takahe Recovery Plan is to increase the population by 25%. This will be achieved by maintaining and expanding the Murchison Mountain population using intensive control of predators and replenishing wild stocks of takahe with captive-bred and island-bred birds.[1] The proposed security aims to achieve by 2020 are to (1) manage for 125 breeding aged pairs at appropriately managed secure sites, (2) have at least two large and managed Recovery Sites with capacity for at least 30 breeding pairs each, one of which is the Murchison Mountains, and (3) have the value of takahe as a conservation icon and "taonga" (a Maori term that is simplistically translated as "sacred treasure") recognized and have their story widely known and understood (P. Marsh, personal communication, August 2014).

Veterinary Support for Takahe Conservation

Veterinary support for takahe conservation management has changed as the program has developed. Initially, veterinary support was limited to necropsy of dead birds, with the results being used to guide both the captive management and inform the program of causes of death in the wild population. More recently, medical and surgical care of individual takahe has been made available through private veterinary clinics, zoos, and university hospitals. Veterinary research is also being used to inform both wild and captive management of the birds as new health issues emerge as a result of intensive conservation management practices. Finally, disease ecology studies are emerging that are investigating the effects of population-level management of the microflora that takahe carry and are exposed to in the altered habitats that have become vital for their conservation.

PATHOLOGY

Takahe have been submitted to a variety of veterinary diagnostic laboratories for necropsy. McLelland et al[8] summarized 199 necropsy reports on takahe carried out during the period from 1992 to 2007. The reports comprised 56 eggs, 51 chicks up to 6 months of age, 13 subadults 6 to 18 months old, 74 adults, and five birds where age was not recorded. There were many cases where a cause of death could not be determined, which was caused by advanced decomposition of many carcasses, the freezing of some birds before pathological investigation, long delays between recovery and submission for postmortem examination, and variation in the extent of postmortem examination and ancillary diagnostic testing.[8]

Birds from the Murchison Mountains often die in winter, and their bodies are not recovered until snowmelt the following spring. Not surprisingly, for most of these birds a cause of death was not established, but signs of trauma and predation are sometimes still detected. Avalanches are known to kill several birds annually. For island populations, the most common cause of death in adult birds was either trauma; infectious or inflammatory disease, including septicemia caused by *Erysipelothrix rhusiopathiae* in 7% (5/74) of adult birds that died; and a range of visceral and articular infections. Mortality of captive birds over this period was very low with only six birds dying from a variety of causes.[8]

There has been a high reported incidence of developmental and congenital disorders in takahe chicks, especially relating to yolk sac disorders and limb malformations. Rotational limb deformity was common in early efforts at hand-rearing takahe, with a reported 13 of 135 chicks (10%) raised between 1985 and 1994 being affected. The condition reduced in incidence following the addition of potassium permanganate to the diet, implying an underlying manganese deficiency. Despite adjustments to the captive rearing diet, a low prevalence of angular limb deformities persisted until the captive breeding program switched exclusively to parent rearing of chicks. Limb deformities in parent-reared chicks are extremely rare.[8]

MEDICAL AND SURGICAL CARE OF INDIVIDUAL BIRDS

The medical and surgical care of individual birds is important in the conservation of takahe not only because they are a critically endangered species, but also because they are a long-lived, slowly reproducing species. For example in areas of Fiordland where stoat trapping is carried out, adult survival has been estimated at 82%.[9] In life history theory, these characteristics are typical of K-selected species and are associated with high net reproductive worth of individual animals. In veterinary terms, it means that there is considerable value in returning an adult takahe to the breeding population. Using these stark criteria, conservation managers often triage care and effort of breeding individuals over older animals or those considered of less value to the breeding population, for example animals whose genetics are already overrepresented in a limited population gene pool.

It is worth noting, however, a school of thought called compassionate conservation, where animal welfare is ranked as an important factor to consider in the conservation management of a species.[10,11] Where resources are available, a sound argument can be made for bringing best practice veterinary medical and surgical care to all animals of a threatened or endangered species, regardless of perceived breeding value. Conservation managers, however, are often operating in a resource-limited environment and must make difficult decisions regarding how to triage these resources. Veterinarians involved in conservation projects must provide conservation managers with the information to make informed decisions, and must be ready to advocate for the welfare of their patients. However, if they are to be successfully integrated within the conservation team, they must accept that individual patient decision making is sometimes influenced by factors outside of the veterinary sphere of expertise. Similarly, conservation managers need to be aware that animal welfare is not a luxury, that individual birds have a value beyond their potential contribution to the breeding population, and that the welfare of individual birds will become more important as conservation in New Zealand is increasingly being run by public partnerships with community groups.

Hospital care of takahe was initially limited by a lack of suitable husbandry and care protocols. This particularly related to nutritional support, as takahe that were anorexic would invariably lose weight despite tube feeding with a variety of liquid diets. With birds in catabolism, little could be done to address complicated medical or surgical problems, and the survival of birds in hospital situations was low. By trial and error, a liquid diet was developed comprising a 2:1 mix of a human critical care solution (Jevity, Abbott Nutrition, Auckland, New Zealand) and a parrot mash (High Potency Mash, Harrison's Bird Foods, Trentwood, TN). Takahe are difficult to tube feed, as they have a narrow gape and a very powerful bill. The use of a robust beak gag and a large bore feeding tube is recommended to minimize the chances of inadvertent tracheal intubation. Takahe from managed populations are familiar with a pelleted diet and usually begin self-feeding in hospital within a few days, at which time tube feeding is withdrawn. Birds from less intensively managed areas, such as the Murchison Mountains,

TABLE 23-2

Primary Diagnosis for 32 Takahe *(Porphyrio hochstetteri)* Admitted to Wildbase Hospital, Massey University, New Zealand, from 1999 to 2014

Diagnosis Classification	Frequency	Comments
Infection/inflammation	10	Arthritis, tenosynovitis, pododermatitis, enteritis
Trauma/misadventure	8	Fractures and injuries
Congenital/developmental	4	Rotational limb deformities and a pericloacal cyst
Iatrogenic	2	Aspiration pneumonia and nutritional deficiency
Myopathy	2	Unknown etiology
Neoplasia	2	Uterine adenocarcinoma and vertebral sarcoma
Undiagnosed	2	Severe central neuropathies that resolved with generic care
Parasitic	1	Severe coccidiosis
Toxicity	1	Lead toxicosis

often require supplementary feeding throughout the period of their hospitalization.

The takahe seem to have no specific thermal requirements in hospital and are routinely kept at temperatures of 18° to 25° C (65° to 77° F). While no definitive thermal tolerances have been established, anecdotally birds that have moved from a hospital environment back into a winter alpine habitat have died from exposure and hypothermia. The current protocol is to ensure that a period of habituation to colder temperatures occurs in a managed environment before birds are released in winter.

In behavioral terms, there is much variation in the expression of a stress response in hospitalized takahe. Some birds will show stereotypical pacing or "fence running" in small enclosures, whereas others appear to cope with hospitalization without overt signs of stress. Regardless, all birds are hospitalized in a screened-off room, and attempts are made to limit disturbance of the birds as much as is possible in a hospital setting. Potted native grasses and cut browse are used to provide hides, which dramatically reduces stereotypical pacing. The flooring used for the birds is usually rubberized matting, over which are laid towels that are changed every day. In the later stages of hospitalization, cut turf is often laid down within the hospital room for browse and environmental enrichment.

The territorial nature of takahe means that on the rare occasions when we have had multiple birds in hospital, they have been kept in separate enclosures, well separated to prevent intraspecific aggression. However, we were able to introduce a chick with limb deformities to an older hen, which was in hospital also for a musculoskeletal disorder. The goal of this introduction was to prevent imprinting in the chick, and the protocols for the introduction were discussed with and approved by experienced conservation managers. The older bird was seen to discipline the overenthusiastic greetings of the chick with a few hard whacks of her beak, but otherwise the shared hospitalization of these birds went well.

Anesthesia, analgesia, and surgical protocols, and medication doses for takahe have all been extrapolated from standard avian medical information on other species. To date, there have been no identified idiosyncrasies of takahe with regard to medical care; however, pharmacokinetic studies to validate the current medicinal doses used are entirely lacking.

Takahe have been presented for veterinary care for a variety of conditions (Table 23-2), most commonly for infections, inflammation, and musculoskeletal trauma, especially of the legs and feet.

VETERINARY RESEARCH INTO HEALTH ISSUES

Individual necropsies and clinical cases have been used to inform more extensive research into health issues affecting takahe and to inform the conservation management of the species. A significant example of this was the identification of injuries associated with the harness system used for radio tracking takahe. Radio transmitters are used for long periods in takahe with a double wing-loop style backpack harness. The use of radio transmitters is essential to manage the birds in often harsh and remote environments, especially the Murchison Mountain population. We identified two clinical cases of wing fractures through birds admitted to the Wildbase Hospital. We suspected that these injuries were associated with the radio transmitter harness system. We retrospectively examined 26 birds at necropsy by gross examination, radiography, and computed tomography to assess damage from the backpack harness. Ten birds that had never worn a harness had no evidence of wing injury. Of the 16 birds that had worn a harness, 10 (63%) had superficial soft tissue injury to skin or patagium or more severe injury, such as remodeling of the distal humerus at the harness cord-wing interface, or pathologic fractures[12] (Figure 23-12). Previously, radio transmitter harnesses were associated with a loss of fitness in takahe,[13] but these more severe injuries are hypothesized to be associated with discomfort, increased risk of infection or fracture, and occasionally death. In response to this research, the use of leg-mounted transmitters is being phased in.

Other health issues have been identified as requiring more study in takahe but have yet to be developed into full research projects. There is an increasing incidence of coccidiosis in captive-reared takahe as the captive management of the takahe becomes more focused on parent rearing in outdoor pens. An increased incidence of parasitic disease, including coccidiosis, has been seen in kiwi (*Apteryx* spp.) under intensive conservation management,[14,15] and we anticipate that takahe will be similarly affected. Species-specific research into

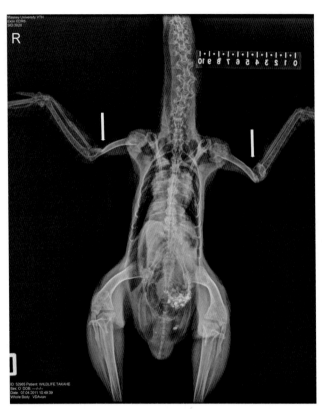

FIGURE 23-12 Ventrodorsal radiograph of a takahe *(Porphyrio hochstetteri)* showing patagial erosion and humeral remodeling and fracture *(white arrows)* at the site of load bearing of the radio transmitter harness. (Image courtesy Massey University.)

disease control in these conditions is essential to ensure the success of captive rearing programs.

Another issue that requires more research is the occasional incidence of erysipelas that occurs in adult takahe in the island populations. An inactivated vaccine (Eryvac, Pfizer, West Ryde, Australia) is used to good effect to minimize deaths from this pathogen, but research into the epidemiology of *Erysipelothrix rhusiopathiae* is needed. Previous research in another critically endangered New Zealand species, the kakapo *(Strigops habroptilus)*, has shown seabirds to be the most likely reservoir for erysipelas in offshore island refuges,[16] but more information is needed to accurately identify the risks to the takahe population.

Disease Ecology Research

The movement of individual takahe between the subpopulations has been common in order to manage the remaining genetic diversity of the species and to replenish the wild population in the Murchison Mountains.[1,7,17,18] The translocation of the animals between the subpopulations exposes the remnant animals to increased risk of the introduction of an infectious disease.[19] The disease risk to the subpopulations is currently managed by pretranslocation disease screening and limited use of quarantine. To more fully explore the risks of

disease transmission, we carried out a social network analysis of the takahe translocation network using individual movements of birds recorded between 2008 and 2011 (Figure 23-13). The networks changed over time and increased in size throughout the time frame considered. The network had some small-world characteristics, which means that most sites are not neighbors of one another but can be reached from every other by a small number of hops or steps. The sites with the highest cumulative tie weights connecting them were the captive breeding center, the Murchison Mountains, and two offshore islands. The key player fluctuated between the captive breeding center and the Murchison Mountains. Every year the cumulative networks identified the captive breeding center as the hub until the final network in 2011. Likewise, the wild Murchison Mountains population was consistently the sink of the network. Other nodes, such as the offshore islands and the wildlife hospital, varied in importance over time. The social network analysis was useful in identifying key sites for disease surveillance, the most critical sites for infectious disease control (hubs), and the sites most at risk from infectious disease (sinks).[20]

Following on from this work, a disease ecology study is in progress examining the movement within the takahe network of *Campylobacter* and *Salmonella* species and strains using a combination of culture, PCR, and whole-genome analysis of the pathogens. The initial results indicate that the conservation management of the animals and the locations of the host affect the epidemiology of these organisms. The results suggest that maintaining the biosecurity of subpopulations through disease screening, quarantine, and isolation of sick individuals is important to reduce the risk of infectious disease outbreaks.

SUMMARY

The takahe recovery program has successfully staved off extinction for the species, and the establishment of subpopulations and captive breeding has reduced the risk of a single stochastic event wiping out the population. Replenishment of the wild population has also been achieved. However, the challenges faced by takahe in their natural habitat remain, and intensive management of the species is necessary for the foreseeable future. Veterinary support should assist the conservation of the species. Basic veterinary services like pathology and clinical care of sick and injured animals are vital; however, extending our biomedical knowledge of the species and the epidemiology of its pathogens is also needed to ensure the continuation of this unique and endemic bird.

REFERENCES

1. Wickes C, Crouchley D, Maxwell JM: Takahe *(Porphyrio hochstetteri)* recovery plan 2007–2012, Wellington, New Zealand, 2009, Department of Conservation.
2. Mills JA, Lavers RB, Lee WG: The takahe–a relict of the Pleistocene grassland avifauna of New Zealand, *New Zeal J Ecol* 7:57–70, 1984.
3. Worthy TH, Swabey SEJ: Avifaunal changes revealed in quaternary deposits near Waitomo Caves, North Island, New Zealand, *J Roy Soc New Zeal* 32(2):293–325, 2002.

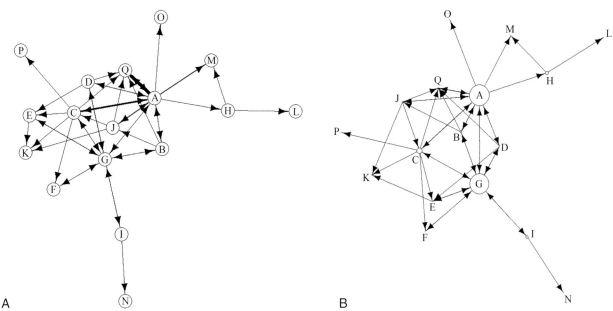

A   B

FIGURE 23-13 Node *(circles)* and tie *(lines)* networks of cumulative takahe translocations from 2007 to 2011: **(A)** tie weight between locations (the thicker the line, the more translocations between two directly connected locations) and **(B)** weighted betweenness for individual locations (i.e., measure of centrality determining the likelihood of a node connecting two random nodes via the shortest path while accounting for node strength [sum of node weights] of an individual node). Nodes are isolated geographic locations that are used for takahe conservation. Lines with either uni- or bidirectional arrows show the direction of human-mediated takahe translocations between locations. Size of the circle illustrates extent of centrality; the larger the node, the more central the location in the network. *A,* Burwood Bush breeding center; *B,* Kapiti Island; *C,* Mana Island; *D,* Maud Island; *E,* Maungatautari reserve; *F,* Pukaha Mount Bruce; *G,* Wildbase Hospital; *H,* Private island; *I,* Te Anau wildlife reserve; *J,* Tiritiri Matangi Island; *K,* Motutapu Island; *L,* Peacock Springs wildlife park; *M,* Secretary Island; *N,* Wellington Zoo; *O,* Willowbank reserve; *P,* Zealandia/Karori Sanctuary; *Q,* Murchison Mountains. (Figure from Grange Z, van Andel M, French NP, et al: Network analysis of translocated takahe populations to identify disease surveillance targets, *Conserv Biol* 28(2):518–528, 2014.)

4. Hegg D, Greaves G, Maxwell JM, et al: Demography of takahe *(Porphyrio hochstetteri)* in Fiordland: environmental factors and management affect survival and breeding success, *New Zeal J Ecol* 36(1):75–89, 2012.

5. Moore PD: Red deer or takahe? *Nature* 271(5645):507, 1978.

6. Maxwell JM, Jamieson IG: Survival and recruitment of captive-reared and wild-reared takahe in Fiordland, New Zealand, *Conserv Biol* 11(3):683–691, 1997.

7. Grueber CE, Maxwell JM, Jamieson IG: Are introduced takahe populations on offshore islands at carrying capacity? Implications for genetic management, *New Zeal J Ecol* 36(2):223–227, 2012.

8. McLelland JM, Gartrell BD, Roe WD: A retrospective study of post-mortem examination findings in takahe *(Porphyrio hochstetteri)*, *New Zeal Vet J* 59(4):160–165, 2011.

9. Jamieson IG, Ryan CJ: Increased egg infertility associated with translocating inbred takahe *(Porphyrio hochstetteri)* to island refuges in New Zealand, *Biol Conserv* 94(1):107–114, 2000.

10. Cattet MRL: Falling through the cracks: shortcomings in the collaboration between biologists and veterinarians and their consequences for wildlife, *ILAR J* 54(1):33–40, 2013.

11. Draper C, Bekoff M: Animal welfare and the importance of compassionate conservation - a comment on McMahon et al. (2012), *Biol Conserv* 158:422–423, 2013.

12. Michael S, Gartrell B, Hunter S: Humeral remodeling and soft tissue injury of the wings caused by backpack harnesses for radio transmitters in New Zealand Takahē *(Porphyrio hochstetteri)*, *J Wildlife Dis* 49(3):552–559, 2013.

13. Godfrey JD, Bryant DM, Williams MJ: Radio-telemetry increases free-living energy costs in the endangered Takahe *Porphyrio mantelli*, *Biol Conserv* 114(1):35–38, 2003.

14. Morgan KJ, Alley MR, Pomroy WE, et al: Enteric coccidiosis in the brown kiwi *(Apteryx mantelli)*, *Parasitol Res* 111(4):1689–1699, 2012.

15. Morgan KJ, Alley MR, Pomroy WE, et al: Extra-intestinal coccidiosis in the kiwi *(Apteryx spp.)*, *Avian Pathol* 42(2):137–146, 2013.

16. Gartrell BD, Alley MR, Mack H, et al: Erysipelas in the critically endangered kakapo *(Strigops habroptilus)*, *Avian Pathol* 34(5):383–387, 2005.

17. Grueber CE, Jamieson IG: Low genetic diversity and small population size of Takahe *Porphyrio hochstetteri* on European arrival in New Zealand, *Ibis* 153(2):384–394, 2011.

18. Grueber CE, Laws RJ, Nakagawa S, et al: Inbreeding depression accumulation across life-history stages of the endangered takahe, *Conserv Biol* 24(6):1617–1625, 2010.

19. Cunningham AA: Disease risks of wildlife translocations, *Conserv Biol* 10(2):349–353, 1996.

20. Grange ZL, Van Andel M, French NP, et al: Network analysis of translocated takahe populations to identify disease surveillance targets, *Conserv Biol* 28(2):518–528, 2014.

VETERINARY CONTRIBUTIONS TO THE RECOVERY OF THE CALIFORNIA CONDOR

Cynthia E. Stringfield

"The California Condor has long been symbolic of avian conservation in the U.S. Following their extirpation from the wild in 1987, many questioned whether they could ever be returned to the natural environment. Yet the California Condor Recovery Program has achieved success beyond what many imagined possible . . . But the birds survive in nature only through constant and costly human assistance and intervention." AOU report, 2010

Veterinary "human assistance and intervention" has been a crucial part of bringing the California condor back from the brink of extinction. However, if the saying "It takes a village" was ever true, it has been for the California condor program. While this chapter focuses on the veterinary contributions to the California condor program, successfully battling all the veterinary issues would have been impossible without the tremendous dedication of condor biologists and volunteers, researchers, and zoo condor staffs. This intervention started in the 1940s and continues today, and a chronologic look reveals many important lessons learned during one of America's oldest and most complex efforts to recover an endangered species.

THE LATE 1940s TO 1950s: NO LUCK

In 1949, after decades of decline, the California condor population was estimated to be about 150 birds. After success during the 1940s in breeding Andean condors in captivity, in 1949 the San Diego Zoological Society (SDZS) approached the California Department of Fish and Game requesting a permit to bring a pair of condors into captivity to serve as a source of birds to release to the wild to bolster the population. This permit was approved; however, it did not allow release of progeny into the wild for fear of disease transmission. Numerous wildlife biologists protested the permit, and they eventually succeeded in blocking any trapping by lobbying the California legislature, which in 1954 prohibited any taking of wild condors. This was the beginning of continual ongoing debates about how "hands on," or aggressive, management of wild birds should be. Thirty years after this decision, when many fewer birds remained, the SDZS, along with the Los Angeles Zoo (LAZ), would be left holding the responsibility for saving this species.

THE 1960s TO 1970s: THE BEGINNING

Twenty years later, in 1974, a Recovery Plan for the continued dwindling population of California condors was developed by the California Condor Recovery Team (CCRT). This Recovery Team was an advisory body to the U.S. Fish and Wildlife Service (USFWS), created in 1973 after passage of the federal Endangered Species Act. The California Condor Recovery Plan was the first such plan developed for any endangered species. This first step was followed by a 1978 report by a joint panel of scientists outside the program from the American Ornithologists' Union (AOU) and the National Audubon Society (NAS). The report urged a much more intensive program, including captive breeding, and was endorsed by the USFWS. By late 1979 the NAS successfully lobbied Congress to establish a greatly expanded effort to conserve the species.

THE 1980s: KNOWLEDGE AND ACTION

Opposition continued, but in 1980 a permit was requested to trap, examine, take samples, and place radio transmitters on 10 birds, and to trap an immature female to bring into captivity as a mate for a lone captive male ("Topa Topa," who had lived at the LAZ since 1967, when he was found as a starving fledgling). The permit was granted, but did not allow blood sampling or the use of yet-untested cannon nets. Unfortunately, a chick died during the stress of handling by a lone biologist in the middle of that year, and Noel Snyder, who accepted the ultimate responsibility in his book, *The California Condor*, stated that "actual handling should not have been attempted by one person alone, a veterinarian should have been present."[1] The consequences of the loss of this chick resulted in an immediate revocation of the permit, and this was an enormous step backward.

Subsequently, a project in Peru on Andean condors for the PhD of wildlife biologist Mike Wallace gave handlers much more experience, and patagial transmitters were also perfected. Phil Ensley, a veterinarian from the SDZS who had experience with Andean condors in captivity, was part of the team to capture, sex, sample, and handle these birds. Additionally, an expedition to South Africa to attempt trapping of vultures taught researchers that the cannon net was the best method to trap California condors. Work with black and turkey vultures in Florida in 1979 also allowed biologists to improve their methods. Permits were reinstated with additional safeguards, including a requirement that a veterinarian be present anytime a condor was handled. Zoo veterinarians were now a part of the capture team.[2,3]

1982 was a very big year for the California condor. The first chick ("Xol xol") was brought into captivity in the late summer of 1982; emergency permission had been given to capture this nestling condor, whose father had disappeared. This was the first chick handling done since the mortality of the chick in 1980 and, per Snyder, "All aspects of the operation proceeded smoothly, with Phil Ensley doing most of the handling. Here at last was a concrete demonstration that not all intensive activities might be lethal for the species."[1] The captive flock was established in two ways from 1982 to 1987. Between 1982 and 1986, eggs and nestlings were removed from wild nests, and eggs were hatched at the San Diego Wild Animal Park (SDWAP). In 1982 it was observed that condors would re-lay if they lost their egg, and a program of replacement clutching of wild pairs started in 1983. By 1986, 16 eggs were taken from wild nests, resulting in 13 surviving chicks. More young condors were also brought in. The first comprehensive condor census via photo census (because the telemetry permit had been denied) was also completed in 1982. This census showed only 21 birds remaining: 14 adults and 7 immatures. On the heels of this, permits were granted again, and the first wild condor ("IC1") was trapped and radiotagged in October with Phil Ensley again involved

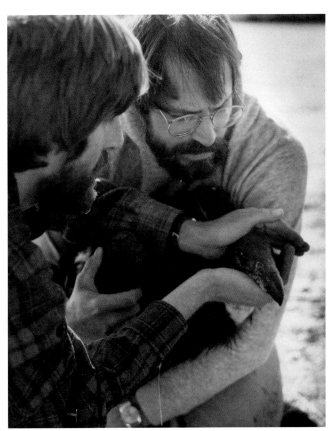

FIGURE 23-14 First California condor captured in 1982, IC1. (Photo courtesy Helen Snyder.)

(Figure 23-14). As a result of this success, a second bird ("AC2") was allowed and successfully tagged. A free-flying bird ("PAX") was trapped as a potential mate for "Topa Topa." He turned out to be a male but had health problems, and the veterinarians at the zoos appealed to the Fish and Game Commission (FGC) that he be made part of the captive flock. The FGC agreed that he fit the description of what had been requested from the USFWS, and he was allowed to stay in captivity."[1] Nine birds total were handled with the assistance of LAZ and SDZS veterinarians in the next five years with no further problems. Snyder again stated, "Without the efforts of both of these institutions, the prospects for ultimate success of the program would have been minimal."[1]

Only after having the first census in 1982 was mortality data able to be discovered. Before this, assumed causes for the population decline included shooting, ritual sacrifice by Indian tribes, collision with power lines, and birds becoming mired in oil seeps. Having some birds outfitted with radiotelemetry greatly assisted in the gathering of pathology data. Between 1982 and 1986, the condor population plummeted by about 25%: By the summer of 1983, 19 birds remained; in 1984, only 15. After a catastrophic excessive mortality event during the winter of 1984 to 1985 that claimed 40% of the population in just a few months, only nine wild birds and only one breeding pair remained. Despite attempts at preserving them in the wild, it was not enough to reverse the decline, and in fact, the decline had accelerated. Out of the first four recovered wild birds that died in the winter of 1984 to 1985, three died of lead poisoning. The other, and first mortality,

was likely caused by cyanide used for trapping coyotes. A new important category was now added to condor mortality causes: poisoning. These four cases are historically very important and relied heavily on veterinary intervention, data, and evaluation. This was the beginning of the SDZS pathology department's critical role in performing postmortem evaluations. The lead poisoning deaths included the second mortality: "IC1," the first bird captured in 1982, was found dead after his telemetry signal stopped moving. A bullet fragment was found in his digestive tract, and he also became the first documented lead-poisoned bird. The third mortality occurred a year later. Ben Gonzales, LAZ veterinarian, went to assist a 7-year-old bird that had just had his first breeding attempt, but the bird died soon after discovery. The fourth mortality was a bird found severely ill, and with crop stasis, in November of 1985. Despite veterinary intervention at the San Diego Zoo (SDZ), this bird died in January 1986. These cases were published in a historically important article, "Lead Poisoning in Free-Ranging California Condors," in *JAVMA* by Don Janssen et al.[4] Additionally, out of 14 condors that were sampled between 1982 and 1986, five birds had increased lead levels: Two of those birds were two of the cases above, and one of the birds later disappeared.

Because of the drastic decline in numbers, in 1985 it was decided that captive breeding and removal of all wild birds were the only hope for the species. This "taking of captives" (as it was called) was very controversial and contentious, and a lawsuit was filed by the NAS resulting in a tremendous battle finally won by USFWS. Using cannon net and pit trapping, three birds were trapped in the summer of 1985. The previously mentioned lead-poisoned bird died at the SDZ in January of 1986, and the remaining five birds were trapped by 1987. The last wild condor ("AC9") was brought into captivity on Easter Day in 1987, and California condors were extinct in the wild. These birds had their gender and family lines determined by the genetics department at the SDZS and were arranged in pairs to maximize outbreeding. They were placed off exhibit at SDWAP and LAZ in large aviary breeding facilities similar to successful captive breeding facilities used for Andean condors.

This was the beginning of what was to be an extremely successful captive breeding program, starting with these 27 birds in captivity (the eight trapped birds, "Topa Topa," "PAX," and the 17 chicks that never flew in the wild). The condors readily adapted to life in the zoo, and zoo incubation experts were able to double or even triple clutch birds by removing the first (and more rarely a second) egg for artificial incubation. The first captive chick was hatched in 1988 at the SDWAP. Zoo veterinarians at the LAZ and SDWAP treated these eggs just like live patients, and hatching assistance, radiographing for malpositions, antibiotic treatment while still in the shell, and breakout techniques were worked out, and chicks were saved who otherwise would have died before hatch.[5,6]

THE 1990s: GROWTH AND RELEASE

Only 4 years after the first captive hatch, there had been 25 chicks fledged in captivity, and it was time for the first release of California condors back into the wild. On January 14, 1992, two captive reared fledgling California condors and two

Andean condors were released in the Sespe wilderness. Mike Wallace, now a curator at the LAZ, was running the releases because of his experience with Andeans in Peru. (The details had been worked out with just Andean condors in the several years before.) The first California condors were pulled back in and then rereleased because of behavioral problems, which were worked on at a special workshop on release methods in 1994. Released birds were perching on power poles and had no fear of people, and these issues were mediated by prerelease exposure of birds to fake power poles that delivered a shock when they perched on them, and a "hazing" program (people posing as hikers who capture birds). By 1994, there were 14 free-flying birds when I took over the responsibilities of veterinary coordinator. Zoo veterinarians at the LAZ and SDWAP had the responsibility for the veterinary care of the captive birds, and because of proximity and Mike Wallace's involvement, the LAZ had the responsibility for the veterinary care for the released birds. The responsibility for field birds rested with the veterinary coordinator,[3] a position previously held by Ben Gonzales and subsequently Michele Miller. In 1993, Pat Redig of the University of Minnesota's Raptor Center was appointed to the Recovery Team as the only veterinarian on the team.

Thankfully, the founders were extremely healthy; however, physical exams and lab work were performed on them every year from a preventive medicine approach. One year on routine annual lab work, after running electrophoresis testing to get normal values, I noticed what appeared to be a previously unseen abnormal electrophoretic pattern on two females. The birds were captured again and radiographed. They both had eggs in their coelomic cavities, but it was not laying season. They both went to surgery, and our LAZ veterinary surgeon, Steve Klause, who was to become the most experienced California condor surgeon, found egg yolk peritonitis in both. We warned that this was a guarded prognosis for survival and certainly for the birds' reproductive abilities. Both birds never looked back and reproduced successfully that same season, with one even triple clutching. Another case in a wild bird taught us the species resilience again. A field bird was brought in with a severe necrotic, infected old open comminuted leg fracture—he was difficult to catch, and it took biologists a while to capture him. Again, Steve Klause performed the surgery, and we pushed the boundaries in aftercare. We had to manage this bird (nicknamed "Bad Boy" because he was so challenging to catch and restrain), with an external fixator, restraining and doing wound management on him every couple of days for weeks (Figures 23-15 and 23-16). Again, we warned that this might end badly, but again, the bird prevailed and completely healed. These were just two of the many teaching lessons to come about how tough this species is when it comes to medical problems. During this early time we also struggled with biologists' concerns about behavior problems and fear of imprinting, which led to many discussions about how often and how we could handle birds for treatment. The gunshot bird's attitude helped teach us that a young wild bird would not become habituated to people as a result of veterinary treatment.

Meanwhile, in 1993, a new captive flock was created at the Peregrine Fund's World Center for Birds of Prey in Boise, Idaho. A local veterinarian was utilized for emergent care, but the Peregrine Fund management then did not agree with

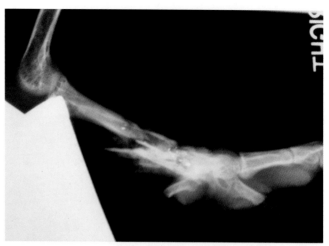

FIGURE 23-15 Tarsometatarsal fracture of free-ranging condor.

doing annual physicals or egg interventions as we did at LAZ and SDWAP, so their veterinary program was minimal. This was a different, more "hands off" management veterinary philosophy that the Peregrine Fund brought to the program. A new release site, also run by the Peregrine Fund, at the Grand Canyon in Arizona was added to the program in 1996, and we brought condors by helicopter to the edge of the Vermilion Cliffs. Kathy Orr, veterinarian at the Phoenix Zoo and later Liberty Wildlife, was and continues to be the site veterinarian for these wild birds. This started a program of having a local veterinarian providing care while the veterinary coordinator consulted, and we tried, but struggled, to keep care standardized. Also in 1996, Phil Ensley came to visit the LAZ to review records and ask many detailed questions as he prepared the first veterinary chapter on California condors. This extremely thorough chapter included information through March of 1997 and was published in 1999.[6]

In 1997, another new release site, managed by the Ventana Wildlife Society, was added in the Big Sur area of California. Field veterinary care was initially provided by Mike Murray, then Amy Wells, out of a local private practice, and on a volunteer basis. This same year, I also received a phone call from Kathy Orr, who was concerned she had a botulism case at a prerelease pen in Arizona. There was not much data in the

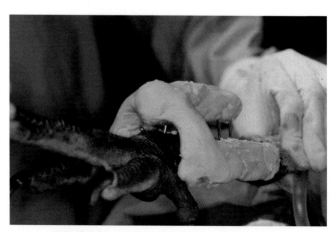

FIGURE 23-16 External fixator after surgery.

literature about this, and it was initially hard to believe that a condor could get botulism. SDWAP veterinarian Jeff Zuba assisted by shipping antitoxin, and Kathy pulled this bird through.[7] This was another learning experience about putting hand-reared chicks that had only been fed clean food into a prerelease pen where they were not disturbed and so were eating rotting food. Some literature suggested that vultures that are "immune" to botulism actually build a tolerance to it, much like a vaccination program.[8] This was another team effort; a change in this management ensued, and we have not seen any more botulism cases. Also in 1997 LAZ veterinarians taught other zoo veterinarians egg intervention techniques at an egg workshop Susie Kasielke created for the American Association of Zoo Veterinarians conference.

It was now September of 1997, five years after the first California releases, when lead reared its ugly head again. Our battle with lead had begun, and life for all of us managing these birds changed forever. Field biologists reported that older birds, with younger birds following, had begun to forage for food on their own instead of eating food left for them by biologists. Two birds were observed feeding on a dead deer during hunting season, and biologists brought in our first two cases of lead poisoning postrelease. The first case was "W5," a 3-year-old dominant bird showing no symptoms but with metal in his gizzard on x-rays and a 1.6-ppm blood lead level. After consultation with experts in this field, including Pat Redig, Mike Murray, and Charles Sedgwick, and research into treatment protocols, the bird was treated for 10 days and passed the metal. His blood levels decreased, and he was rereleased. The second bird was similar but with lower blood levels and no metal in his digestive tract. Eight months later, "W5" was back in the hospital, but in much worse shape. His legs and digestive tract were paralyzed, and he had crop stasis and a crop full of rotten food.[9] Another consultation with Pat Redig yielded a grave prognosis. He reported that if it were an eagle, they would euthanize him because they do not come back from that level of severity of clinical signs, but it was a condor, and no one was giving up. LAZ veterinarians Janna Wynne, Charles Sedgwick, and I pioneered the use of a feeding tube and continuous feeding machine, along with chelation.[10] Mike Wallace was immediately at the health center when this bird arrived and was instrumental in helping us figure out how to manage him from a behavioral standpoint. As we looked around the treatment room after placing the feeding tube, a technician came up with the idea of modifying a plastic water pitcher as an Elizabethan collar (Figure 23-17). After a 3½-month recovery, numerous consultations with the condor team, and the first-ever discussions about euthanizing a wild California condor, the bird finally regained use of his crop, made a full recovery, and was rereleased. Soon after, I received a phone call from a field biologist reporting how "W5" had regained his dominance in the flock and had just fought with a golden eagle at a carcass. Both birds went over the edge of a cliff while grappling, with only "W5" coming back victorious. This was the first of many more cases that taught us how incredibly tough and resilient condors are in the face of lead poisoning, and that they have an amazing threshold and tolerance for lead. This was a different conclusion than that reported in 2006 based on a study from Patuxent of captive Andean condors who were experimentally poisoned with lead.[11]

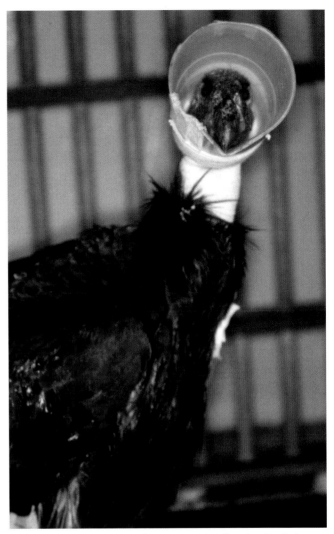

FIGURE 23-17 Makeshift collar made of a plastic pitcher.

Sadly, "W5" disappeared on July 30, 2000, and the other bird that first came in with him had disappeared December 29, 1999. Unfortunately, this was the beginning of what was to come: Many more lead poisoning cases and mortalities and birds routinely coming into the LAZ for treatment. As veterinary coordinator, I worked with biologists to adopt a program of routine lead screening in California, pioneering the use of the handheld human LeadCare analyzer for field testing. As we so often had to do in medicine of species where no data exist, literature was reviewed, and treatment cutoff values and treatment and rerelease protocols created.[12] They appeared to work well; however, years later I reviewed all the cases and double-checked that no birds had "slipped through the cracks" with the treatment cutoff values protocol; it was a relief to see that it had withstood the test of time. One treatment protocol was discontinued in 2007 after many successful cases but several visceral gout mortalities: This was the practice of using both calcium ethylenediaminetetraacetic acid (EDTA) and meso-2,3-dimercaptosuccinic acid (DMSA) together. This protocol initially seemed promising[13] and was attempted to decrease handling and injections to once a day instead of twice a day with solely calcium EDTA.[14]

It was not long before the first phone call came from Chris Parish, the field supervisor in Arizona, describing a sick wild bird. Arizona had now started seeing lead poisoning as well, and they adopted that same first protocol, except because of the remote nature of their birds, they utilize their field biologists much more to do the treatment in the field, and only bring clinically sick birds in from the field to the veterinarian.[15]

THE 2000s: ADDING WNV AND CHICKS TO THE MIX

After West Nile Virus (WNV) hit New York in 1999, USFWS California condor program manager Jesse Grantham phoned, and after discussing many other things, he asked what we were going to do about WNV. That was a very good question that still required a plan. Mike Mace, bird curator at the SDWAP, had relayed information about two zoo Andean condors who had become very ill with WNV in New York, and all the data coming in suggested that condors would be "sitting ducks" to be wiped out by this virus. The Centers for Disease Control (CDC) was testing a new vaccine, and after researching it, with nothing to lose, the author gave lead researcher (and veterinarian) Jeff Chang a call. This phone conversation between two veterinarians led to an enormous cooperative effort by avian veterinarians, virologists, conservationists, the CDC, and a private corporation, Aldevron. This undertaking, using a new DNA recombinant vaccine that had never been used outside of a research setting, was our best chance. Although there were some unnerving moments pioneering this in a critically endangered species, we really had no choice. The early data on the only other available WNV vaccine at the time, a killed equine product, was not encouraging for protecting birds. After many conference calls to discuss the plan, and with complete and total support by the condor team, we embarked on our WNV vaccination program. We decided to test the vaccine on Andeans first, and in October of 2002, the first Andean condor was vaccinated. After good results, we moved on to some of the "least valuable" birds (genetically) and then, with no additional funding or manpower, managed to get the entire captive and wild population vaccinated in time. It was a Herculean team effort by all involved, as it included hundreds of restraints and procedures and could not be done during the reproductive season. We did not have one problem, either from restraint or vaccination (Figure 23-18). After continually reviewing serology data with Jeff Chang, we felt ready as WNV came our way. In July 2004, thanks to excellent surveillance by the City of Los Angeles Public Health WNV surveillance team, we knew the actual day WNV arrived at the condor facility at the LAZ. We saw zero morbidity. Serology results after this time showed birds that had definitely been exposed as their serologic titers had increased: A huge bullet was dodged. This program is detailed in several publications[16-18] and was run by LAZ: All data and vaccines came through this source to avoid overloading the CDC, who was doing us such a huge favor. Christine Lutz, our LAZ laboratory veterinary technician, was a master of organization and a critical part of this program. Unfortunately, high-level management at the Peregrine Fund decided to leave the vaccination program after starting with it and then suffered a serious WNV mortality event in 2006, losing four birds over 10 days. After numerous

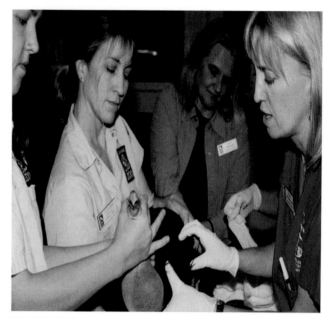

FIGURE 23-18 West Nile vaccination at the Los Angeles Zoo.

emergency phone calls, we expedited vaccine to them to vaccinate in the face of this outbreak, but they lost two more chicks and a juvenile that had been transferred to Arizona for release. Jeff Chang then agreed to what the Peregrine Fund wanted, to be allowed to run their own vaccination program independently, and they commenced vaccinating again. Pat Redig had also started testing this vaccine at the Raptor Center in an attempt to get it licensed and available for use in birds, but unfortunately, this has not yet occurred.[19]

In 2001 the veterinary coordinator was asked to become a member of the CCRT. It was becoming very obvious that the health issues for the birds required this. It was an honor and a privilege to be a part of this group and to be the only veterinarian actually working with condors on the team. Working with Pat Redig and other team scientists, we eventually created a subset group we called the Scientific Advisory Committee.

Finally, the time we had been all hoping for was here: Eggs and chicks also started happening in the wild in 2001. Excitement led to sadness as we realized we had what would become a very big new intensive veterinary problem: garbage impaction in chicks. An obstructed chick with zinc toxicosis died in the nest in 2002, and again discussion commenced about hands off and letting nature take its course vs. hands on and more aggressive intervention. Biologist concerns included that pairs would not learn to change their behavior if we intervened. In 2003, a chick was helicoptered out and landed in the parking lot of the LAZ, and though we tried to save it from trash impaction and a perforation, we had to euthanize it because of secondary aspergillosis (Figures 23-19 and 23-20). Thankfully in Arizona, the first successful wild chick fledged in 2003. In 2004, two more severe trash impaction cases died in southern California, and finally one chick fledged. There were two more cases in 2005: One survived surgery at the LAZ, and one died during nest removal. Mike Clark, LAZ condor keeper and an integral member of the field team, and I were doing the nest visit for the chick that died with a new

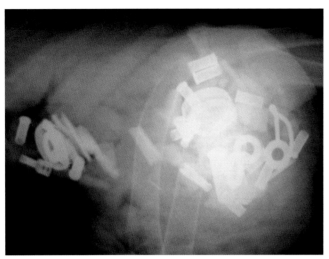

FIGURE 23-19 Lateral radiographic image of trash impaction in a condor chick. (Courtesy Mike Clark and the Los Angeles Zoo.)

USFWS biologist, Joseph Brandt; the nest entry culminated in bringing a dead chick back in a bag. Joseph went on to create a detailed, expertly organized, and aggressive nest entry program that formally started in 2007.[12] Thankfully, he was an expert climber and could teach others those skills. In 2006 Janna Wynne, Steve Klause, and the condor crew pushed the envelope again by surgically removing trash from a chick and returning it to the nest the very next day. We knew how tough the birds were but wondered if a chick could really be that tough. That chick went on to recover fully in a wild nest with no aftercare one day after major surgery. These early chick interventions and the trash (termed junk, then microtrash) ingestion problem were detailed in a publication in 2007 by Allan Mee with SDZS pathologist Bruce Rideout as a coauthor.[20] In the new nest monitoring program, nestling feather

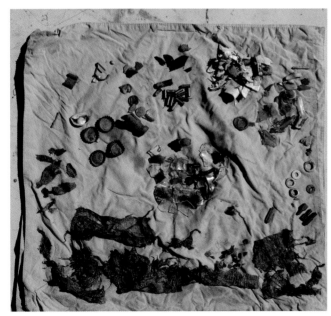

FIGURE 23-20 Foreign material removed from an impacted condor chick during ventriculotomy. (Courtesy Mike Clark.)

growth and development were carefully monitored because stunting had been noted when these wild chicks were compared with zoo chicks. During nest visits, veterinarians examined nestlings, vaccinated for WNV, and checked lab parameters.[12,21] Trash was removed from the nest cavity and bone fragments provided instead.[20] During the 2007 breeding season, all six breeding attempts were successful. The nest program continues on, with the important assistance of the Santa Barbara Zoo joining the program and focusing on monitoring nests and helping with veterinary nest visits, and with LAZ veterinary and condor staff providing an enormous effort as they continue to assist with interventions for the next several years. The hikes and climbs could be brutal, and helicopter rides were routine because of the remote nature of some of the nests. In the Big Sur area, Amy Wells assists with nests, while Kathy Orr helps with medical care for Arizona birds (Figure 23-21).

Mike Wallace created a new international release site in Baja, Mexico, with the SDZ and Jeff Zuba working with Mexican veterinarians and handling the care for these wild birds, but initially all the birds were to come from the LAZ. The permits and testing and their timing, and quarantine with testing that was required to bring birds into Mexico were huge veterinary challenges and could never have occurred successfully without Mike Wallace's persistence and bilingual skills.[22] In 2002, we made the small plane trip, almost having birds held at customs. Again, with smooth talking in fluent Spanish by Mike Wallace, we passed customs and brought birds to a pine forest (where it snows in winter) in Sierra de San Pedro Martir National Park (SDSP). This was another major accomplishment in the expansion of the recovery program.[9]

In 2003, another new release site was started with the U.S. Geological Service at Pinnacles National Monument, and the

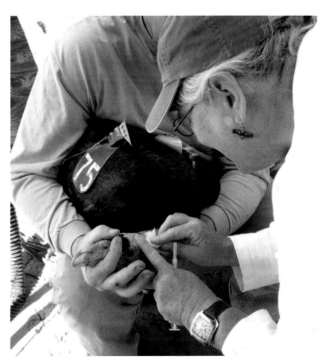

FIGURE 23-21 Dr. Kathy Orr examines and treats a condor in Arizona. It has been through the contributions on-site by local veterinarians that the expansion of this project has been strengthened.

Oregon Zoo received captive condors and started a fourth breeding colony. Also in 2003 Pat Redig was named chair of the Lead Mitigation subcommittee for the CCRT. He was invited by the USFWS to head up an initiative to mitigate lead poisoning in California condors in southern California and Arizona. In addition to the CCRT, project partners included several gun lobbying organizations such as the National Rifle Association and Safari Club. This was an attempt to work with, instead of against, these groups that were steadfast in their denial that lead in ammunition was a problem; however, this attempt was unsuccessful.

In 2003, with data and collaboration with Bruce Rideout, I initiated a formal mortality review. Previous concerns had instigated behavioral training for power line aversion that had been successful in decreasing mortalities. Trauma and lead poisoning were the current concerns, with lead poisoning being the most serious.[23] In 2005 hematology normal values were published as veterinarians continued to add to the knowledge of this species.[24] Occasional trauma cases continued, and in 2006 a fracture repair on a bird from Arizona was done by Pat Redig at the University of Minnesota's Raptor Center, and the bird was rereleased.

In this decade as well, the poultry industry in Southern California experienced an outbreak of avian influenza (H6N2), creating concern for zoos with valuable captive bird collections, including our captive California condors. Don Janssen of the SDWAP took the lead in extending the detailed plan for their facility to the condors. Thankfully, this outbreak was controlled, and preventive measures to keep it from entering our facilities were successful.

While at the LAZ, we had been carefully collecting samples for a researcher, Molly Church, working with Don Smith at UC Santa Cruz. Little did we know how important this lab would be to the science of lead poisoning. In 2006, along with Bruce Rideout, they reported their findings. They measured lead concentrations and isotope ratios in blood from 18 condors living in the wild in central California, in eight prerelease birds, and in diet and ammunition samples to determine the importance of ammunition as a source of exposure. Blood lead levels in prerelease condors were low and isotopically similar to dietary and background environmental lead in California. In contrast, blood lead levels in free-flying condors were substantially higher (almost 10 times higher) with lead isotopic compositions that approached or matched those of the lead ammunition. They also looked at a lead-poisoned condor in Arizona and found that the lead in tissues and in a serially sampled growing feather recovered postmortem was from an isotopically distinct lead source. They concluded: "Together, these data indicate that incidental ingestion of ammunition in carcasses of animals killed by hunters is the principal source of elevated lead exposure that threatens the recovery in the wild of this endangered species."[25]

In February of 2007, veterinarians at the Wildlife Health Center at UC Davis created a report titled "Lead Exposure in California Condors and Sentinel Species in California." In this report, they began an important veterinary involvement by an outside agency, UC Davis, regarding the lead issue.[26]

In August of 2007, as California continued to cite a lack of scientific evidence to support implementation of a lead ammunition ban, I was asked to testify in front of the Fish and Wildlife Commission as its members yet again considered a ban of lead ammunition in condor territory. This presentation told the commissioners individual stories (with pictures) of lead poisoning. They learned that programwide, the overall mortality rate for released birds was 33% through 2003 (the first 10 years of the program), that it currently was 36%, and that California's rate was 39%. They learned how the conservative conclusion was reached that a minimum of 8% to 24% of California's deaths were caused by lead poisoning (4 to 12 birds out of 51), and how without treatment, the rate would be at minimum 14% to 45% (15 to 23 birds out of 51). They also learned about lead poisoning in human adults and children (that very low levels affect development, intellect, and behavior), that treatment was not a substitute for removing the lead from the environment, and that condors too were smart, social, and long-lived. The commissioners seemed friendly, grateful, and interested. They were attentive and asked intelligent questions, and afterwards, one of them said that the report "was the best presentation putting things together the commission had heard over the four years it had been considering the issue."[21,27] Don Smith followed, presenting the data from UC Santa Cruz on isotope work. The commissioners passed the ban that year, and not only that, but then the governor, Arnold Schwarzenegger, signed an even more restrictive bill.

Lead debates in 2006 started focusing on not just the immediate health of the bird, but also the longer-term effect of low lead levels in birds with no symptoms. We discussed the reality that birds would constantly be out of the wild if all of them with subclinical levels were treated. It was a trade-off between having wild behavior and birds in the field versus birds constantly in captivity for treatment. This difficult balancing act continues.

Meanwhile, the AOU and NAS had been investigating the condor program again, and in 2008, 30 years after their last report, they published their assessment. The veterinary recommendations were as follows: "We recommend continuing the existing veterinary coordinator position to facilitate information transfer on topics such as vaccines and procedures. The Field Working Group meetings have assisted greatly in this information exchange and should be continued as well, reformed as the Recovery Implementation Team. Addition of a research and monitoring coordinator and data manager to the program will make the veterinary coordinator more effective. We also recommend that the veterinary coordinator oversee development of general health protocols for the program. These should be carefully reviewed by participating veterinary representatives and updated appropriately."[28] Writing protocols had definitely taken a backseat to stomping out and preventing fires, and many written protocols were dated or short and minimal.

2010 TO JULY 2014

On the heels of the AOU report, the Recovery Team was disbanded in March of 2010. I finished a condor chapter covering the medicine of condors from March of 1997 (where Phil Ensley's chapter left off) to March of 2010, and this was published in 2012.[12] These two chapters form a complete clinical reference through that time. Also in 2010, two important publications came out from veterinarians Terra Kelly and Christine Kreuder-Johnson at the Wildlife Health Center at the University of California—Davis. They had been studying lead in turkey vultures before the lead ban, and then in golden eagles and turkey vultures after the lead ban took effect in condor range. The first study showed that blood lead concentration in turkey vultures was significantly higher during the deer hunting season compared with the off-season, and blood lead concentration also increased with increasing intensity of wild pig hunting at study sites.[29] The second study found that lead exposure in both golden eagles and turkey vultures declined significantly in the first year after the 2008 ban of lead ammunition within condor range was implemented.[30]

In 2011, Don Janssen, who had continued his stalwart support of condors since the beginning of the program, arranged for a special field team meeting in San Diego. In facilitated groups, we prioritized what the field needed. Everyone came to the conclusion that the veterinary coordinator position had grown so large and complicated, and was such an integral part of the recovery of the species, that it needed dedicated and funded time. This was something that I had been requesting for many years but had not had success in achieving. After leaving the LAZ and moving on to Moorpark College's Exotic Animal Training and Management program in 2004, all condor veterinary coordinator efforts had become purely volunteer. The conclusion of this meeting was that while this position needed to be funded, there was no funding for it, so the LAZ and SDZS would alternate in hosting this position. The initial idea at this meeting of creating a formal medical team to work on protocols and scientific publications has not yet come to fruition, but frontline veterinarians continue to labor hard, often with minimal monetary support, caring for the ever-increasing numbers of birds: (1) Amy Wells volunteering her time for the Ventana birds; (2) condor keeper staff taking over lead-poisoned bird treatments at LAZ because of high veterinary staff turnover, budget cuts, and caseload increases (and a decrease in veterinarians in the field to assess chicks); (3) Kathy Orr and Liberty Wildlife volunteering their services to work with the Peregrine Fund biologists to maintain the high level of care for the Arizona and Utah birds; and (4) the SDSP continuing its support and veterinary program for Mexico. Thankfully, the Oakland Zoo started helping LAZ with the lead-poisoned California condors in 2012. In 2013, SDZS turned over condor pathology services to the USFWS Forensics Laboratory in Ashland, Oregon, where previously only suspected criminal cases had been submitted.

Publications from 2012 included an article about ingluviotomy feeding tube case studies in lead-poisoned birds from the Phoenix Zoo[31] and the long-awaited, hugely time-intensive "Patterns of Mortality in Free-ranging California Condors," a gigantic undertaking by Bruce Rideout and 19 coauthors from 10 different agencies. This article details and documents the mortality data from 17 years and 135 deaths, illustrating a 38% mortality level. Seventy percent of cases where a cause of death could be determined were from anthropogenic causes, of which lead remained the most important mortality cause affecting the sustainability of the wild condor population.[32] This paper was followed in July of 2012 by another important paper from the UC Santa Cruz lab, entitled "Lead Poisoning

and the Deceptive Recovery of the Critically Endangered California Condor,"[33] and in March of 2013 by a statement titled "Health Risks from Lead-Based Ammunition in the Environment: A Consensus Statement of Scientists," signed by 30 experts in the field, including six veterinarians.[34] This statement was rapidly followed in June of 2013 by Johnson, Kelly, and Rideout with the article "Lead in Ammunition: A Persistent Threat to Health and Conservation,"[35] and then another declaration titled "Health Risks from Lead-based Ammunition in the Environment," authored by 15 scientists, including Bruce Rideout and Pat Redig.[36] On October 11, 2013, California became the first state to ban lead ammunition for hunting when the governor signed A.B. 711. The ban is to be implemented gradually and will not take effect until 2019, so the California team will have years more of morbidities and mortalities, but at least there is more hope on the horizon. Governor Jerry Brown noted that hunters and anglers are "the original conservationists" and that switching to nontoxic ammunition "will allow them to continue the conservation heritage of California." He also added, "Lead poses a danger to wildlife. This danger has been known for a long time."[37] Arizona continues to work with the public in a different way: through an enormous education and voluntary compliance effort, and the number of California condors treated for lead exposure in Utah and Arizona recently dropped to its lowest level since 2005.

LOOKING BACK, AND THE FUTURE

The California condor is currently classified as Critically Endangered on the IUCN Red List. The California Condor Recovery Plan, written by the California Condor Recovery Team, states that before reclassification to threatened status can occur, three disjunct populations of California condors are needed, numbering at least 150 birds each: two in the wild and one in captivity, and each population should have approximately 15 breeding pairs and have a positive rate of increase. At this writing (data from the end of August 2014), 232 birds currently fly in the wild: 130 in California; 29 in Baja, California; and 73 in Arizona/Utah. In addition, 202 birds are in captivity, and the populations continue to increase, now with second-generation wild birds fledging.

This program taught me the definition of success through teamwork and true scientific collaboration. As the program grew because of success, it also became extremely complex, with debates among individuals and organizations commonplace. The veterinary problems this species has suffered have been extreme, and without conquering them, recovery could not have occurred. Many determined and dedicated people have fought as hard as the condors themselves, not giving up when others said it was impossible or too expensive. We wondered how we could give up when our species caused the decline of this magnificent creature that has been here since the Pleistocene, and who is certainly not giving up. The people of this incredible program will continue to stand on the shoulders of our predecessors, just as the birds alive now stand on the wings of the dead condors before them. As the veterinary part of this effort, we continue to soldier on to bring the California condor to a place of full recovery where our drastic interventions are no longer needed.

REFERENCES

1. Snyder N, Snyder H: *The California condor*, San Diego, 2000, Academic Press.
2. Oosterhuis J: Veterinary involvement in the California condor recovery program. In *Proceedings of the American Association of Zoo Veterinarians*, Chicago, 1986, p 93.
3. Shima AL, Gonzales B: Veterinary involvement in the California and Andean condor recovery and release projects. In *Proceedings of the American Association of Zoo Veterinarians*, Calgary, Alberta, Canada, pp 90–97, 1991.
4. Janssen DL, Oosterhuis JE, Allen JL, et al: Lead poisoning in free-ranging California condors, *J Am Vet Med Assoc* 189(9):1115–1117, 1986.
5. Ensley PK, Rideout BA, Sterner DJ: Radiographic imaging to evaluate chick position in California condor eggs. In *Proceedings of the American Association of Zoo Veterinarians*, Pittsburgh, 1994, pp 132–133.
6. Ensley PK: Medical management of the California condor. In Fowler ME, Miller, RE, editors: *Zoo and wild animal medicine, current therapy*, vol 4, Philadelphia, 1999, Saunders, pp 272–292.
7. Orr K: Botulism in a California condor. In *Proceedings of the American Association of Zoo Veterinarians*, Milwaukee, 2002, pp 101–103.
8. Rocke TE, Bollinger TK: Avian botulism. In Thomas NJ, Hunter B, Atkinson CT, editors: *Infectious diseases of wild birds*, ed 1, 2008, Wiley, p 405.
9. Stringfield CE: Medical management of the free-ranging California condor. In *Proceedings of the American Association of Zoo Veterinarians*, Omaha, 1998, pp 423–424.
10. Wynne J, Stringfield CE: Treatment of lead toxicity and crop stasis in a California condor, *J Zoo Wildlife Med* 38(4):588–590, 2007.
11. Pattee OH, Carpenter JW, Fritts SH, et al: Lead poisoning in captive Andean condors, *J Wildlife Dis* 42(4):772–229, 2006.
12. Stringfield CE: The California condor veterinary program: 1997–2010. In Fowler ME, Miller RE editors: *Zoo and wild animal medicine, current therapy*, vol 7, St. Louis, 2011, Elsevier, pp 286–296.
13. Denver MC, Tell LA, Galey FD, et al: Comparison of two heavy metal chelators for treatment of lead toxicosis in cockatiels, *Am J Vet Res* 61(8):935–940, 2000.
14. Simeone C, Zuba J, Rideout B, et al: Visceral gout and death of a California condor under dual chelation treatment for lead toxicity. In *Proceedings of the American Association of Zoo Veterinarians*, Kansas City, 2011, p 58.
15. Hunt WG, Parish CN, Orr K, et al: Lead poisoning and the reintroduction of the California condor in northern Arizona, *J Avian Med Surg* 23(2):145–150, 2009.
16. Chang GJ, Davis BS, Stringfield C, et al: Prospective immunization of the endangered California condors protects this species from lethal West Nile virus infection, *Vaccine* 25(12):2325–2330, 2007.
17. Stringfield CE, Davis BS, Chang GJ: Vaccination of Andean condors and California condors with a West Nile virus DNA vaccine. In *Proceedings of the American Association of Zoo Veterinarians*, Minneapolis, pp 193–194, 2003.
18. Stringfield CE, Davis BS, Chang GJ: Vaccination of Andean condors and California condors with a West Nile Virus DNA vaccine. In *Proceedings of the American Avian Veterinarians*, 2003.
19. Redig PT, Tully TN, Ritchie BW, et al: Effect of West Nile virus DNA-plasmid vaccination on response to live virus challenge in red-tailed hawks, *Am J Vet Res* 72(8):1065–1070, 2011.
20. Mee A, Rideout BA, Hamber JA, et al: Junk ingestion and nestling mortality in a reintroduced population of California condors, *Bird Conserv Int* 17(2):119–130, 2007.
21. Stringfield, CE: SSP veterinary update: California condor. In *Proceedings of the American Association of Zoo Veterinarians*, Los Angeles, 2008, p 190.
22. Mercado JA, Zuba JR, Fernandez FS, et al: California condor conservation in Baja California: successes and challenges across the border. In *Proceedings of the American Association of Zoo Veterinarians*, Milwaukee, 2002, pp 101–103.
23. Stringfield, CE, Wong A, Wallace M, et al: Causes of death in released California condors from 1992–2002. In *Proceedings of the American Association of Zoo Veterinarians*, San Diego, 2004, pp 85–86.
24. Dujowich M, Mazet JK, Zuba JR: Hematologic and biochemical reference ranges for captive California condors, *J Zoo Wildlife Med* 36:590–597, 2005.
25. Church ME, Gwiazda R, Risebrough RW, et al: Ammunition is the principal source of lead accumulated by California condors reintroduced to the wild, *Environ Sci Technol* 40(19):6143–6150, 2006.
26. Johnson CK, Vodovoz T, Boyce WM, et al: Lead exposure in California condors and sentinel species in California. www.researchgate.net/publication/252987498.
27. Herdt T: Commissioners near bullet ban. The Ventura County Star, 8/28/2007. http://www.vcstar.com/news/commissioners-near-bullet-ban.
28. Walters JR, Derrickson SR, Fry DM, et al: Status of the California condor and efforts to achieve its recovery, pp 70–72. http://www.aou.org/committees/conservation/docs/AOU_Condor_Report.pdf.
29. Kelly TR, Johnson CK: Lead exposure in free-flying turkey vultures is associated with big game hunting in California, *PLoS One* 6(4):e15350, 2011.
30. Kelly TR, Bloom PH, Torres SG, et al: Impact of the California lead ammunition ban on reducing lead exposure in golden eagles and turkey vultures, *PLoS One* 6(4):e17656, 2011.
31. Aguilar RF, Yoshicedo JN, Parish CN: Ingluviotomy tube placement for lead-induced crop stasis in the California condor, *J Avian Med Surg* 26(3):176–181, 2012.
32. Rideout BA, Stalis I, Papendick R, et al: Patterns of mortality in free-ranging California condors, *J Wildlife Dis* 48(1):95–112, 2012.
33. Finkelstein ME, Doak DF, George D, et al: Lead poisoning and the deceptive recovery of the critically endangered California condor, *Proc Natl Acad Sci USA* 109(28):11449–11454, 2012.
34. Bellinger DC, Bradman A, Burger J: Health risks from lead-based ammunition in the environment: a consensus statement of scientists. https://escholarship.org/uc/item/6dq3h64x#page-1.
35. Johnson CK, Kelly TR, Rideout BA: Lead in ammunition: a persistent threat to health and conservation, *EcoHealth* 10:455–456, 2013.
36. Bellinger DC, Burger J, Cade TY, et al: Health risks from lead-based ammunition in the environment, *Environ Health Perspect* 121:A178–A179, 2013.
37. Brown J: Signing Message, Oct 11, 2013. http://gov.ca.gov/docs/AB_711_2013_Signing_Message.pdf.

THE WHOOPING CRANE RECOVERY PROJECT

Glenn H. Olsen

Among the 15 species of cranes in the world, Whooping cranes (*Grus americana*) (Figure 23-22) are the most endangered, numbering as few as 22 birds several times during the period between 1937 to 1944. The location of the last remaining migratory flock's wintering area was known and protected in Aransas National Wildlife Refuge (NWR) on the Texas Gulf Coast in 1937, but the breeding grounds were not known until accidently discovered in 1954 by a pilot flying in support of a fire-fighting effort in a remote area in northwestern Alberta, Canada. Fortunately, this area had already been protected as part of a vast tract included in Wood Buffalo National Park (Figure 23-23).

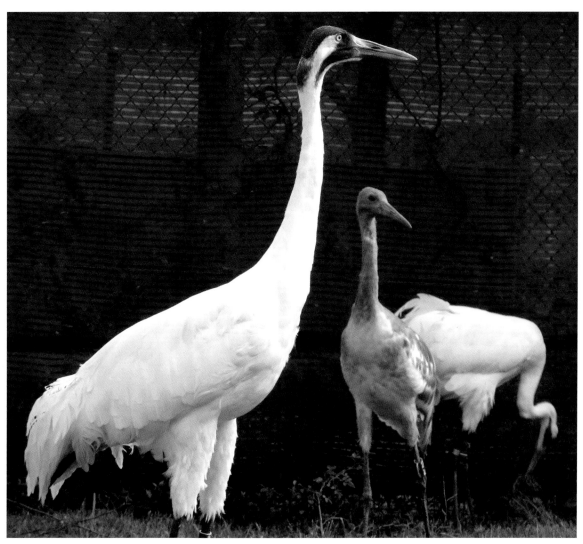

FIGURE 23-22 Adult whooping cranes stand 5 feet (1.7 m) high and can have a wingspan of 9 to 10 feet (3 m). Primary feathers are black, while all other body feathers are white. The red color on the head is skin. Adult whooping cranes weigh 5.5 to 7.5 kg. Young whooping cranes under 1 year of age have a mixture of white and cinnamon-colored body feathers, black primaries, and no red-colored skin on the top of the head.

The estimated population numbers of whooping cranes during the period of pre-European settlement of North America range up to 10,000 birds, meaning that they were never very abundant. The first scientific description of the species is attributed to the English artist-naturalist Mark Catesby after he was given a dead whooping crane by a group of Iroquois Native Americans.[1] Samuel Hearn, while exploring the Great Slave Lake area of Canada in 1770, saw whooping crane pairs in the area that almost 200 years later would prove to be their breeding grounds. Lewis and Clark in 1805 sighted migrating whooping cranes over the Little Missouri River mouth.[1]

Subsistence hunting by settlers in the United States and Canada, plus drainage of wetlands required by whooping cranes, led to declines in number to an estimated 1000 birds by 1870. Draining wetlands was an especially critical blow across the recognized breeding range from northern Illinois and southern Wisconsin through Iowa, Minnesota, eastern

South and North Dakota, and the southern Canadian Prairie provinces of Manitoba, Saskatchewan, and Alberta. The last known whooping crane nest on the prairies was found in western Saskatchewan in 1922.

Even though the numbers of whooping cranes were low, 22 total (16 migratory whooping cranes, plus 6 nonmigratory whooping cranes in a flock in Louisiana) when Aransas NWR was established in 1937, further efforts to study and protect whooping cranes were sidetracked by a combination of the ongoing depression and the descent into the global conflict of World War II. Following the war, the National Audubon Society and the USFWS established the Cooperative Whooping Crane Project in 1946. Robert Porter Allen, a National Audubon Society wildlife biologist, began studying these birds. Additionally, a campaign was begun to educate hunters and farmers about whooping cranes and the fact that these magnificent birds were protected under law in both the United States and Canada by a joint Migratory Bird Treaty

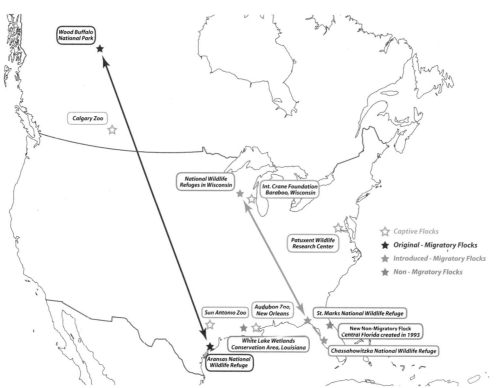

FIGURE 23-23 Wintering areas, breeding grounds, and migration routes of the remaining wild flocks of whooping cranes. The flock from Texas to Alberta and the reintroduced flock from Wisconsin to Florida are depicted. Captive breeding centers participating in the reintroduction programs are identified by a star. (Map courtesy of the USGS/PWRC.)

Act of 1918. This campaign effectively stopped illegal shooting of whooping cranes for almost five decades, but in the past decade there has been an alarming increase in shooting incidents. Most of the recent incidents have been attributed not to hunters but to teenagers with guns shooting at targets of opportunity in any season. The newly established reintroduction efforts have been especially hard hit by this vandalism.

The low number of whooping cranes in North America was one driving force leading to the enactment of the Endangered Species Act in the United States (1966, amended 1973). The first captive propagation efforts were begun by the Audubon Zoo in New Orleans in the 1950s after the capture of the last wild nonmigratory whooping crane in the state in 1950. The program had some success in breeding birds in captivity, but numbers were never sustainable, even within the captive population. In 1966 Ray Erickson with the USFWS initiated a captive breeding program at the USFWS Patuxent Wildlife Research Center (Patuxent) (see Figure 23-23). The first whooping crane located there was named Canus for *Can*ada and *U*nited *S*tates; indeed, all whooping cranes are considered jointly owned by the two countries. During the following decades, starting in the 1980s, Patuxent produced hundreds of eggs and chicks for various release programs.

The first effort at establishing a new wild flock took place at Grays Lake NWR in Idaho. Whooping crane eggs from Patuxent and the wild whooping crane flock at Wood Buffalo National Park were removed from nests and flown to Idaho, where the eggs were placed in the nests of greater sandhill cranes (*Grus canadensis tabida*). The sandhill cranes hatched the eggs, raised the whooping crane chicks, and taught the

chicks the migration route in the fall. However, as the whooping crane chicks matured into colts and young adults, it was found that the now adult birds would not mate with other white cranes. Because of imprinting, which we now know occurs within a few days to weeks after hatching, these new whooping cranes were imprinted on their sandhill crane parents. The project ended in 1989, but the whooping cranes that were released persisted in the western states well into the 1990s.

DISEASE ISSUES AND THE ESTABLISHMENT OF SEVERAL BREEDING FLOCKS

In 1984 at Patuxent, there was an epizootic of an unknown disease that at the time killed 7 adult whooping cranes, including 5 breeding-age females. This was a big setback for a program that only numbered 45 birds. The causative agent was identified as eastern equine encephalitis virus (EEE), and a vaccination program was developed, first using a human EEE vaccine (Salk Institute), then later an equine product (Fort Dodge, now Pfizer Encephalomyelitis West Nile Virus Vaccine).[2,3]

In the fall of 1987, another epizootic claimed 15 cranes at Patuxent: 12 sandhill and 3 whooping cranes. This time the causative agents were two mycotoxins (T-2 and DON) associated with mold on corn and in pelleted feed.[4] A program to test all incoming feed was established and proved worthwhile.

However, because of these two epizootics, and because the highly endangered whooping cranes existed in only two places in the world—between Texas and Alberta as a wild flock, and as a captive flock in Maryland—it was decided to split the captive flock among several institutions. Whooping crane adults and eggs from Patuxent and eggs from the wild flock nesting in Alberta were sent to the International Crane Foundation in Baraboo, Wisconsin; to the Calgary Zoo's Devonian Breeding Center, in Alberta; and to the Audubon Zoo's Species Conservation Center in New Orleans, Louisiana. Between 1989 and 1993, no reintroductions occurred, with all efforts going to establishing these new captive breeding flocks.

Continued Reintroductions 1994 to Present

Reintroduction efforts started again in 1994 in Florida. To avoid imprinting whooping cranes on people, caregivers dressed in costumes (Figure 23-24) reared whooping cranes from the captive facilities, and these birds were soft released into various locations in central Florida around Kissimmee. Initially a few eggs were brought in from the wild flock at Wood Buffalo National Park, but after 1996 no further reintroduction efforts using eggs from this source occurred. The new method developed for this reintroduction and all subsequent reintroductions is for the crane chicks to be reared by costumed caregivers. The costumes and puppet heads (Figure 23-25) are used to prevent the chicks from imprinting on the human form. To avoid the young crane chicks from imprinting solely on the costumed humans, the chicks are always in view of adult whooping cranes in adjacent pens. All four of the captive facilities contributed eggs and chicks toward this Florida nonmigratory reintroduction for 12 years, but a population viability analysis in 2005 showed that the chance of this reintroduction succeeding was less than 1%. Severe drought, land use changes (urbanization), and low reproductive performance were the reasons for the dire predictions, so the reintroduction effort was discontinued, although there is still a remnant population of whooping cranes in central Florida in 2015.

Starting in 2001, a new reintroduction effort was begun in Wisconsin. Whooping crane chicks were again costume-reared, but these chicks were also taught to fly with their

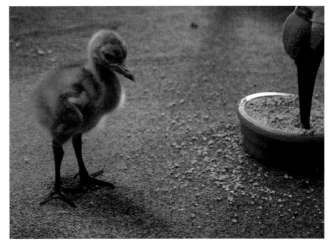

FIGURE 23-25 Young whooping crane chick being taught to eat a commercial crane diet by using a puppet head to point out the food.

costumed caregivers when the caregivers flew off in an ultralight aircraft (Figure 23-26). The first attempt to teach a migration route to whooping crane chicks involved seven chicks reared at Patuxent in partnership with Operation Migration. The chicks were led on a 2000-km (1240 mile) migration from Necedah NWR in central Wisconsin to Chassahowitzka NWR on the Florida Gulf Coast (Figure 23-27).

Some birds innately know to migrate; others—most notably swans, geese and cranes—learn a migration route by following parents south in the first autumn and afterward refining this migratory ability by accompanying older, more experienced birds on subsequent migrations.[5] Because no whooping cranes were left in eastern North America, and because we did not want to have our released whooping cranes imprinted on and following sandhill cranes, we needed to develop methods to teach the young cranes migratory routes. This effort involved both whooping cranes, sandhill

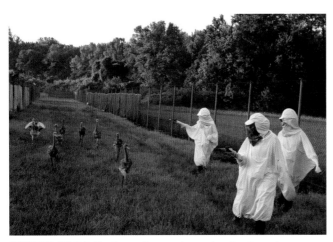

FIGURE 23-24 Costumed caregivers lead whooping crane chicks on a walk at USGS Patuxent Wildlife Research Center, Laurel, Maryland. Costumes are used to avoid imprinting whooping crane chicks on humans.

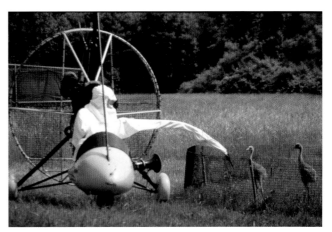

FIGURE 23-26 Early ultralight training of whooping crane chicks begins as soon as they are old enough to follow the costumed caregiver carrying the crane puppet head. This early training is called circle pen training, as the chicks are confined to a circular pen and encouraged to follow the ultralight by being offered periodic rewards of mealworms.

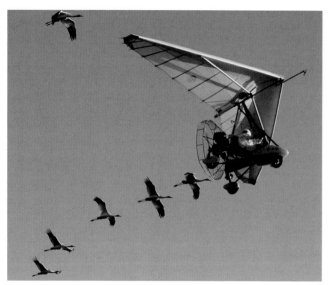

FIGURE 23-27 Whooping cranes following an ultralight aircraft, flown by pilots from Operation Migration, on a migration route from Wisconsin to Florida.

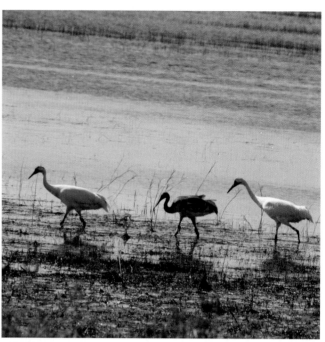

FIGURE 23-28 Whooping crane colt with alloparents, a few days after release in September at Necedah National Wildlife Refuge, Wisconsin.

cranes (as surrogate species), and trumpeter swans over a decade and used land-based vehicles,[6] hot air balloons, and various ultralight aircraft designs.[7]

Starting in 2005, a new introduction method was developed at the International Crane Foundation in Baraboo, Wisconsin.[8] This new method relied upon the proven methodology of costume rearing by human caregivers dressed in the crane costumes (see Figure 23-24) but without involvement of ultralight aircraft. Instead, cranes are released in groups in autumn and follow adult whooping cranes or sandhill cranes to learn their migration route. Therefore, this method is referred to as the direct autumn release. Other than a slightly higher mortality rate in the first year, this method has been highly successful in the reintroduction of whooping cranes at Necedah NWR and Horicon NWR.

In 2013 for the first time, a third reintroduction method was tested. Because of some possible issues with reproductive behavior, especially incubation and nest defense, research staff was concerned about what whooping crane chicks might be missing by being costume-reared, not parent-reared. So four whooping crane chicks in both 2013 and 2014 have been reared by captive parent birds at Patuxent and soft released in central Wisconsin, where alloparents were present to lead the chicks on migration (Figure 23-28).

Louisiana Reintroduction

Starting in early 2011, a new reintroduction program began in south Louisiana at White Lake Marsh, the same area that a nonmigratory whooping crane flock occupied until 1950. There were two reintroductions the first year (2011): one in late winter and one the following fall, with one reintroduction each subsequent year. All crane chicks used for this reintroduction are costume-reared, with soft releases following the successful direct autumn release pattern used in Wisconsin. In 2014, a pair of these new whooping cranes built a nest and laid two eggs. The eggs were infertile, not unusual for first-time nesting cranes.

Health Issues with Reintroductions

The reintroduction program to establish the Eastern migratory population of whooping cranes has been successful in initiating a migratory population between Wisconsin and Florida. Birds are intensively monitored with both VHF transmitters and satellite transmitters attached to leg bands. Therefore, any disease or mortality issues after release are easily documented by recovering the carcasses and performing a full necropsy. Necropsies have been done at the Department of Infectious Diseases and Pathology, College of Veterinary Medicine, University of Florida, Gainesville; at the USGS National Wildlife Health Center, Madison, Wisconsin; and at the USFWS National Wildlife Forensic Laboratory, Ashland, Oregon. In 2009 postmortem summary results about this population were published.[9] The authors found causes of mortality to include predation (47%, n = 8), trauma (12%, n = 2), and degenerative disease (6%, n = 1), while the cause of mortality was undetermined in 35% (n = 6) of the cases. Predation was commonly caused by bobcats (*Lynx rufus*). The one case of degenerative disease was associated with exertional myopathy following a capture and translocation of a crane that had wandered far off course. In addition, 5 nonfatal traumatic injuries were reported, including gunshot (n = 1), utility line collision (n = 3), and impact trauma (n = 1). No infectious diseases were found in this reintroduced population.[9]

During the Florida releases, similar mortality events were documented.[9] Predation, primarily bobcat, accounted for 58% of mortality (n = 108/186). Traumatic injuries accounted for 7.5% (14/186), and undetermined 27% (50/186). However, infectious diseases caused 7.5% (14/186) of mortality in the Florida population versus 0% in the Eastern migratory population. Infectious disease mortality in the Florida population was caused by EEE, disseminated visceral coccidiosis, aspergillosis, and a wasting syndrome associated with an infectious bursal disease-like virus.[10]

General Health Issues of Captive Crane Populations

Because of the effort put forth to learn how to rear and reproduce whooping cranes, sandhill cranes, and other cranes in captivity, a number of book chapters summarizing the health care issues have been published over the past three decades. The largest captive populations of cranes in North America are at the USGS Patuxent Wildlife Research Center in Laurel, Maryland, and the International Crane Foundation in Baraboo, Wisconsin, with smaller populations at some zoos, notably the Calgary Zoo in Calgary, Alberta, and the Audubon Zoo in New Orleans.

The first summary chapter on crane medicine was published in 1978,[11] though the chapter also included Sphenisciformes (penguins), Ciconiiformes (storks and herons), and Phoenicopteriformes (flamingos) in addition to Gruiformes. The chapter included only the two sentences under the heading of "disease description" for Gruiformes: "There are no unique diseases in this group of birds. They are subject to trauma of limbs, aspergillosis, and other general avian infections and parasitic disease."

The second edition of Fowler's *Zoo and Wild Animal Medicine* had an 11-page chapter devoted solely to cranes.[12] Ten years later, an entire book devoted to captive crane husbandry was published, including chapters on adult and juvenile crane diseases and medicine.[13,14] Recent avian medicine books have included chapters on crane diseases.[15,16]

Several major health issues exist for captive husbandry and reintroduced cranes. The first of these is a herpes virus infection caused by the aptly named inclusion body disease of cranes virus (IBDC). This virus caused some morbidity and mortality among captive cranes at the International Crane Foundation in 1978. The disease is thought to have arrived in some cranes imported from Europe, as the virus does not occur in wild North American cranes. The outbreak was confined to this one institution and, through the judicious use of testing and quarantine, was eliminated from the institution and never spread to other institutions. However, testing of captive flocks and especially of all captive cranes for release continues to this day. The USGS National Wildlife Health Center is the only laboratory in North America to do the testing (antibody titer).

IBDC is characterized by lethargy and loss of appetite for 48 hours, followed by diarrhea and death.[17] Mortality occurred in sandhill cranes, red-crowned cranes (*Grus japonensis*), blue cranes (*Anthropoides paradise*), and hooded cranes (*Grus monacha*). All were captive birds at the International Crane Foundation, and only the sandhill cranes are native to North America.[17] Pathologic lesions include enlargement of the liver and spleen with small (about 1-mm diameter) yellow-white sessions, plus hemorrhage in the thymus and intestines. There are characteristic intranuclear inclusion bodies in liver and splenic tissue.[17]

IBDC is an important disease from a conservation standpoint. It does not occur in wild crane flocks in North America but has occurred in captive crane collections. Because whooping cranes and endangered Mississippi sandhill cranes (*Grus*

canadensis pulla) are bred and reared for release programs at some zoological institutions that also house old-world cranes, increased diligence must be maintained to ensure that all release cranes are free from this disease.

EEE has proven deadly to whooping cranes at Patuxent in 1984[2] and Mississippi sandhill cranes.[18] Most cranes show no clinical signs or only brief neurological signs such as ataxia before death. Unlike IBDC, EEE is a disease of North America, with native passerine birds acting as reservoir hosts. The virus is spread among the passerine birds and to cranes, horses, and humans by a mosquito (*Culiseta melanura*). Therefore the release programs for cranes concentrate on preexposure immunization using killed equine vaccines.[19] Several vaccines have been used over a period of years, with Vetera EWT (Boehringer Ingelheim Vetmedica, Inc., St. Joseph, MO; mention of trade name does not imply U.S. Government endorsement) currently being used to protect the young cranes before release. No challenge studies have been done to date, but the vaccination program has proven efficacious based on retrospective studies examining incidence of carrier mosquitos and antibody titer in sentinel quail and sandhill cranes.[3]

EEE is under control for the present time through the use of a vaccination program to protect captive and released whooping cranes. EEE is known to occur on occasion in Wisconsin, Louisiana, and other southeastern states where we are releasing whooping cranes and hope to establish breeding and migrating populations. EEE has the potential to impact these efforts but not in the immediate future, as all wild-hatched chicks are eventually captured around fledging age to receive a leg band radio transmitter and metal Bird Banding Laboratory band. They receive a health evaluation and can be vaccinated at that time, also. However, when the re-introduction programs become self-sustaining and large numbers of wild whooping crane chicks are fledged into the population, and the banding program is discontinued, EEE may become one of the mortality factors affecting these populations (Figure 23-29).

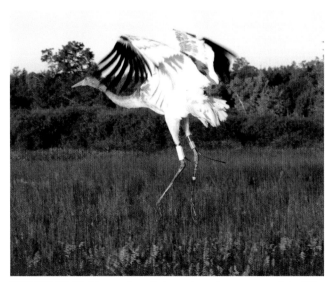

FIGURE 23-29 Young, free-flying whooping crane colt in Wisconsin, showing colored leg bands with radio transmitters (0.6 ounces, 18 grams) that allow biologists and veterinarians to closely monitor these endangered birds after reintroduction.

West Nile Virus first occurred in North America in 1999. The disease has occurred in Africa, Europe, and the Middle East and was first described from Africa in the 1930s. During the 80+ years since the disease was first recognized, mortality has been reported in some species of birds, but not cranes. After the arrival of WNV in North America and its spread from New York City to Maryland (about 300 km), one adult greater sandhill crane and two 3-month-old Florida sandhill cranes *(G. c. pratensis)* died from the disease. Therefore, a vaccination research program was developed to test and challenge Florida sandhill crane adults and chicks.[20,21] WNV-vaccinated sandhill cranes developed a less severe infectious response and suffered no mortalities among chicks or adults as compared with unvaccinated challenged cranes. This information was then used to protect captive and released whooping cranes, and no WNV mortalities have been documented among the protected whooping crane populations.

For a species that once only numbered 22 individuals, the whooping crane has come a long way back on the road to recovery, but there are several more hurdles to cross to establish viable populations in several locations in North America. Introducing healthy birds by maintaining vigilant preventive medicine programs in the captive flocks used for this reintroduction effort is one important step. Another step is to remain vigilant for exotic diseases such as IBDC and WNV that could have negative impacts on captive breeding and reintroduction efforts.

REFERENCES

1. Sakrison D: *Chasing the ghost birds: saving swans and cranes from extinction*, Baraboo, Wisconsin, 2007, International Crane Foundation.
2. Dein FJ, Carpenter JW, Clark JW, et al: Mortality of captive whooping cranes caused by eastern equine encephalitis virus, *J Am Vet Med A* 189:1006–1010, 1986.
3. Olsen GH, Turell MH, Pagac BB: Efficacy of eastern equine encephalitis immunization in whooping cranes, *J Wildlife Dis* 33:312–315, 1997.
4. Olsen GH, Carpenter JW, Gee GF, et al: Mycotoxin-induced disease in captive whooping cranes (*Grus americana*) and sandhill cranes (*Grus canadensis*), *J Zoo Wildlife Med* 26:569–576, 1995.
5. Mueller T, O'Hara RB, Converse SJ, et al: Social learning of migratory performance, *Science* 341(6149):999–1002, 2013.
6. Ellis DH. Wings across the desert: the incredible motorized crane migration, Surrey, B.C., 2001, Hancock House.
7. Ellis DH, Sladen WJL, Lishman WA, et al: Motorized migrations: the future or mere fantasy? *BioScience* 53(3):260–264, 2003.
8. Wellington MM, Urbanek RP: The direct autumn release of whooping cranes into the eastern migratory population:a summary of the first three years. In *Proceedings of the North American Crane Workshop*, 11:215, 2010.
9. Cole GA, Thomas NJ, Spalding M, et al: Postmortem evaluation of reintroduced migratory whooping cranes in Eastern North America, *J Wildlife Dis* 45(1):29–40, 2009.
10. Spalding MG, Sellers HS, Hartup BK, et al: Infectious bursal disease virus associated with a wasting syndrome in released whooping cranes in Florida. In *Proceeding of the American Association of Zoo Veterinarians, American Association of Wildlife Veterinarians, Wildlife Disease Association Joint Conference*, San Diego, CA, 2004, p 73.
11. Fowler ME: Penguins, cranes, storks, and flamingos (Sphenisciformes, Gruiformes, Ciconiiformes, and Phoenicopteriformes). In Fowler ME, editor: *Zoo and wild animal medicine*, Philadelphia, 1978, WB Saunders Company.
12. Carpenter JW: Cranes. In Fowler ME, editor: *Zoo and animal medicine*, ed 2, Philadelphia, 1986, WB Saunders and Company.
13. Olsen GH, Carpenter JW, Langenberg JA: Medicine and surgery. In Ellis DH, Gee GF, Mirande CM, editors: *Cranes, their biology, husbandry and conservation*. Washington, D.C., 1996, U.S. Department of Interior, pp 137–174.
14. Olsen GH, Langenberg JA: Veterinary techniques for rearing crane chicks. In Ellis DH, Gee GF, Mirande CM, editors: *Cranes, their biology, husbandry and conservation*. Washington, D.C., 1996, U.S. Department of Interior, pp 95–104.
15. Olsen GH, Carpenter JW: Cranes. In Altman RB, Clubb SL, Dorrestein GM, et al, editors: *Avian medicine and surgery*, Philadelphia, 1997, WB Saunders and Company.
16. Olsen GH: Cranes. In Tully TN Jr., Dorrenstein GM, Jones AK, editors: *Avian medicine*, ed 2, Edinburgh, UK, 2009, Saunders Elsevier.
17. Docherty DE: Inclusion body disease of cranes. In Friend M, editor: *Field guide to wildlife diseases*, Washington, D.C., 1987, U.S. Department of Interior, Fish and Wildlife Service.
18. Young LA, Citino SB, Seccareccia V, et al: Eastern equine encephalitis in an exotic avian collection. In LaBonde J, editor: *Proceedings of the Association of Avian Veterinarians*, 1996, pp 163–165.
19. Clark GC, Dein FJ, Crabbs CL, et al: Antibody response of sandhill and whooping cranes to an eastern equine encephalitis virus vaccine, *J Wildlife Dis* 23:539–544, 1987.
20. Olsen GH, Miller KJ, Docherty D, et al: West Nile virus vaccination and challenge in sandhill cranes (*Grus canadensis*). In *Proceedings of the Association of Avian Veterinarians*, 2003, pp 123–124.
21. Olsen GH, Miller KJ, Docherty DE, et al: Pathogenicity of West Nile virus and response to vaccination in sandhill cranes (*Grus canadensis*) using a killed vaccine, *J Zoo Wildlife Med* 40(2):263–271, 2009.

CHAPTER 24

Practice Management and Risk Management

Thomas E. Catanzaro • Brian L. Speer • Charlotte Lacroix • Robert E. Schmidt

PRACTICE MANAGEMENT

Thomas E. Catanzaro, Brian L. Speer

This chapter explores some of the concepts and managerial logistics associated with the development and maintenance of a successful avian practice, and the business aspects of seeing avian patients and integrating them into this practice. Good medical practice, delivered optimally, promotes good business. Concurrently, good business management skills are essential for the continual delivery of excellent medical services and require their continued development and refinement. Both of these are important for success when combined and fit to your own passion and interest in avian practice.

There are between 10 and 20 million birds kept as pets in the United States alone. These numbers vary based on the individual survey involved and include a large number of pet birds. Birds are the third most popular companion pet behind dogs and cats in the United States. In many other countries, keeping birds often is believed to be even more popular. Excluding aquarium or pond fish, the caged bird is the fourth most popular pet in the United Kingdom, with combined caged birds and pet domestic fowl in 2.8% of households, behind dogs (25%), cats (19%), and rabbits (3%).[1] There are estimated to be more than 25 million pets in Australia (2013 data), with nearly 5 million of Australia's 7.6 million households having pets. At 63%, Australia has one of the highest rates of pet ownership in the world; there are about 5 million companion birds, with a 20% household penetration. Data provided by the American Veterinary Medical Association (AVMA) show a similar percentage of households owning birds as seen in the United Kingdom. From the AVMA data, it is also apparent that there are considerably fewer veterinary visits per year per household compared with dogs, cats, and horses and a lower veterinary expenditure per household and lower veterinary expenditure per animal (Table 24-1).

Although there are approximately 8800 to 9000 species of birds, comparatively few of these are commonly maintained as pets or companions. The more commonly kept pet bird species as companion and aviary birds vary depending on the region of the world, but in many regions the top 10 most commonly seen pet species probably account for greater than 50% of most pet bird veterinary patient accessions. A positive impact can likely be achieved pertinent to the health care of these species with solidly managed veterinary health care systems that adjust to more current methods of management, husbandry, and health care delivery. An integral requirement for attaining the most effective medical efforts is sound practice management, which is explored in this chapter.

PRACTICE PRINCIPLES IN MANAGEMENT

There is no real debate that the practice doctors and staff need to function as a team to provide the level of health care needed. The debate is over how a practice functions as a team or a business.[2-4] In this light, the business of a well-managed practice is not an accident and requires focus, structure, and a shared goal among all the staff. In true "team-based" health care delivery, the income that those

---

TABLE 24-1

2012 American Veterinary Medical Association U.S. Pet Ownership Data

	Dogs	Cats	Birds	Horses
Percent of households owning	36.5%	30.4%	3.1%	1.5%
Number of households owning	43,346,000	36,117,000	3,671,000	1,780,000
Average number owned per household	1.6	2.1	2.3	2.7
Total number in United States	69,926,000	74,059,000	8,300,000	4,856,000
Veterinary visits per household per year (mean)	2.6	1.6	0.3	1.9
Veterinary expenditure per household per year (mean)	$378	$191	$33	$373
Veterinary expenditure per animal (mean)	$227	$90	$14	$133

Source: 2012 AVMA U.S. Pet Ownership and Demographics Source Book. https://www.avma.org/KB/Resources/Statistics/Pages/Market-research-statistics-US-Pet-Ownership-Demographics-Sourcebook.aspx

practices generate is the outcome and product of a shared, concerned, and compassionate vision of a high standard of patient care. The entire practice remains grounded by the cornerstones of its stability: consistent clinical case management philosophy and uniformity in patient advocacy by all doctors in case management. In comparison, when there is inconsistent management, core values, and philosophy, there will be internal stress, disruption, and impairment of the goal to do the best job possible. These in turn can easily lead to an eventual erosion of the client-centered practice management philosophy and economic detriment to the practice's well-being. It is true that practice management philosophy is not the same as case management, and that individual doctors can deliver excellent case management in a variety of management philosophical settings. It is also true that the consistency of case management, across the board between all doctors and staff, is often a clear reflection of a practice philosophy focused on the client, rather than its doctors.

The typical routine for an avian veterinarian (in companion or zoological collection practice) includes performing physical examinations, diagnosing illnesses, drawing blood and collecting other diagnostic samples, outlining treatment plans for individual patients or groups of birds, prescribing medications, making dietary recommendations, setting fractures, performing surgeries, and completing follow-up evaluations. This is unfortunately a self-limiting approach to companion bird practice, but follows the paradigms of typical veterinary education to focus on the "broken animals." In reality, 70% of a companion animal practice's front door swing rate is driven by pet stewards who want to keep their pets healthy compared with those who perceive that their animals are ill and require treatment. This demand for "wellness care" is often inconsistently met and is inconsistently applied through typical practice management methods and philosophies. Internal promotion of a practice, resulting in greatly enhanced practice stability and overall success, relies on the establishment of a practice culture that solidly embraces this demand for preventative health care or wellness care services (Box 24-1).

There is an interesting paradigm in veterinary practice, which is not exclusively limited to birds. In this paradigm the shared goal to enhance and extend quality of life is focused on procedures, tests, and treatments in the search for disease, and success is often proclaimed by negative test results—the

absence of documentable disease. This approach contrasts starkly with an approach that combines a focused effort to add in positive impact wellness components, such as training, behavioral guidance, enrichment, and educational discussions regarding welfare and empowerment of the stewards of these animals to facilitate favorable changes. Once a practice accepts that wellness is much more than a diagnostic quest, the sooner the caseload becomes balanced and the practice begins to truly stand proud and succeed.

Savvy practitioners know that their next steps are to understand their organizational behaviors and skills, to establish a practice culture, and to empower their practice team to be true veterinary service extenders. Some of the best ideas are often discarded by management, since they did not think of them, or they use the old adage: "We tried it once, it will never work." Different times, different staff, and different clients all provide new ideas, each having some value. As a veterinary practice owner, how you handle your fear and stress regarding changes in your practice sends ripple effects throughout your practice team.

Below are steps you can take to keep practice operations on an even keel:

1. Ensure that you have "trained to trust" during the first 90 days of employment, then macromanage and understeer. This approach empowers staff and lessens their anxiety.
2. Increase communications (the getting and giving of information). You can encourage positive storytelling and prevent rumors among staff about the practice's leadership initiatives and operational upgrades.
3. Be approachable. You will increase the chance that direct reports will provide ideas and feedback without fear.
4. Use strategic thinking centered on the big picture. Strategic assessment is an immediate call for strategic action (usually with new metrics); this leaves staff with good direction, a positive attitude, and faith that you have the practice moving in the right direction.
5. Provide resources so staff members have the knowledge, skills, tools, and the capacity and time to serve the clients and care for the patients.
6. Keep things professional both ethically and bioethically and in alignment with the practice's core values and mission focus. This professional balance causes staff to take action instead of placing blame.
7. Be encouraging. Faultfinding only generates more blame, paranoia, and political gamesmanship within the practice team.
8. Take care of yourself with proper diet, sleep, and exercise. Dress for success, but within the practice's dress code.

DOCTOR-CENTERED VERSUS CLIENT-CENTERED PRACTICE STYLE

The above eight points assume an understanding of client-centered versus doctor-centered practice style. In essence and summary, the *doctor-centered* style looks at internal quality factors, the doctor's schedule, and pride in procedures; it keeps the doctor in the spotlight. *Client-centered* style seeks client satisfaction, fear-free services for the patient, and speaks of the health care plan (rather than the "estimate").

BOX 24-1 EXAMPLES OF GENERAL CATEGORIES OF INTERNAL PROMOTION OF AVIAN PRACTICE

Wellness health care services
Lifestyle enrichment
Integration of behavioral medicine with patient care
Dietary programs and nutritional diversity enhancement
Recurring laboratory screening tests
Recurring care services (grooming and training)

*The following is an **overall practice comparison** of functions and focus in a doctor-centered versus client-centered practice philosophy:*

Doctor-centered	Client-centered
Staff works to support the needs and goals of the individual doctors	Doctor(s) function as a part of a team with their practice staff
Doctors work individually to provide patient care and client service as best they can	Constant focus on the client by the entire practice team
Focus is on supporting the doctor(s) who maintain their focus primarily on the client	Patient advocacy is a team-based concern, and when shared with a client, they listen and try to understand

First noted by Lau-Tzu in the fifth century BC, this concept is an application of Servant Leadership. Most veterinary practices (private and institutional) are predominately doctor centered in their manner of operation. Although both the doctor-centered and the client-centered practice operate with shared goals of patient care and client service, the client-centered practice offers a clearer vision that is easiest to maintain by the entire practice team. There are key and recognizable differences between these conceptual operational modes. In a doctor-centered practice, the staff typically waits to do the next "duty as assigned." As the doctors move from the outpatient consultation rooms to the inpatient treatment area, a sizable number of the staff tends to follow those doctors. The staff that does not follow often shifts to a lower productivity mode of work when the doctor is not present in their work zone. Also, in the doctor-centered practice, the doctors more often can be found performing the nursing rounds of inpatients, doing the daily treatments themselves, and in some cases using well-qualified nursing staff as animal holders only so they can do the nursing work themselves. Veterinarians in a doctor-centered practice typically do not effectively delegate to their staff, and they do not encourage or schedule regular client nursing appointments. In summary, in a doctor-centered practice, the staff works to support the needs and goals of the individual doctors, who in turn strive individually to provide patient care and client service as they best can.

*The following is a comparison of veterinary **staff functions and focus** in a doctor-centered versus client-centered practice:*

Doctor-centered	Client-centered
Staff waits to do the next "duty as assigned"	There is a large staff role in most forms of client communications; support staff is empowered
Staff tends to follow doctors as they move about practice zones	Outpatient staff: keeps the doctor on schedule
Remaining staff drops productivity when doctor is not present	Inpatient nurse keeps the surgeon/inpatient doctor on schedule

In the client-centered practice, the staff has a much larger role in most forms of client communications, and they are empowered to do so by the practice ownership and management. When the doctor moves from outpatient consultation rooms to the inpatient treatment area, the outpatient nurses revert to nursing appointments and client telephone outreach activities and never leave their outpatient zone of responsibility. Concurrently, the inpatient nursing staff meets with the doctor and both review the priorities for the inpatient demands and detailed planning for in-patient procedures and/or surgery. The outpatient nursing staff works to keep the doctor on schedule in the consultation rooms and oversees and augments client and patient service. The inpatient nurse keeps the surgeon/inpatient doctor on schedule within their zone of responsibility.

*The following is a comparison of **doctor functions and focus** in a doctor-centered versus client-centered practice:*

Doctor-centered	Client-centered
Do not effectively delegate to their staff	Keep on schedule in both inpatient and outpatient zones of operation
Do not typically encourage or schedule regular client nursing appointments	Work with staff in the appropriate zone, maintaining focus on client and patient
Doctors perform more of the nursing rounds of inpatients	Assume role of client follow-up for adherence to prescribed actions
Do the daily treatments themselves	Do rounds before the veterinarian arrives, and prioritize per practice protocols
May use well-qualified nursing staff as animal holders only	Independent action for Risk Level 1 animals after adequate training

In summary, in a client-centered practice, the doctor(s) work more with their practice staff as a functional part of a team that has a constant focus on the client, as opposed to a practice team that focuses on supporting the doctor(s) who maintain their focus primarily on the client. The differences between these two operations-management philosophies become more apparent as the practice grows in size and number of clients, patients, doctors, and staff. These same differences can also dramatically influence the ability of a practice to consistently deliver optimal patient care and client service.

How does this relate to avian medical practice and adding or augmenting these species in your practice? None of the above points are clearly unique to avian practice. These core aspects of practice management philosophy apply across the board in all aspects of veterinary health care. Consistency, the hallmark of client-focused operations management, can become more challenging to deliver the more "unique" the species group our patients represent. As a practice's vision focuses on avian species, the potential volume of available clients and patients is reduced, and the need for maintaining a superior niche in marketing to and maintaining a growing client base becomes increasingly important. For these practices to grow and flourish outside of the mold of a single doctor practice, client-centered practice operations are essential not only for growth, but likely for their own economic survival.

SHARING LEADERSHIP AND PARTICIPATIVE MANAGEMENT

Shared leadership is an important key to effective practice leadership because it overtly promotes the distribution of the functions of the doctors among the health care delivery team. This aspect of management (shared problem solving and decision making) is an increasingly prevalent aspect of human health care management worldwide. Traditional "competitive" styles of leadership are less and less responsive to the complex, multigenerational society we find in most health care settings today. Participative or cooperative styles of interaction are the key to successful veterinary practice operations, whereas case management remains doctor centered and the medical record is maintained and documented for others to follow.

An individual's style of interaction with others is an outward sign of the substance within their leadership style. With experience, we can tell a lot about a manager's or doctor's capabilities by observing them in operational situations, but it is better to watch them in health care delivery action. How does a good leader behave when the group is confronted with the need for decision? Situational leadership describes a method of leadership in relation to the needs of the members; in health care delivery, these are usually operational issues of the workplace rather than urgent patient care situations. There are a number of models for participative management or leadership advocated by different authors. One of these is *situational leadership* as described by Dr. Paul Hersey.[5]

Situational leadership basically implies that there is no one best way to lead in every situation. It suggests that effective leadership varies with the maturity levels involved—that is, members' willingness and ability to lead or follow—within a group, as well as the issues at hand. In other publications, this author has described these styles of leadership as directive, persuasion, coaching, delegation, mentoring, consulting, and finally joining. Sharing leadership in veterinary health care delivery is a style of participative management. Participative management concepts have been around for many years as listed below:

- *Situational Leadership*, as originally defined by Hersey and Blanchard, identifies four leadership styles—directing, coaching, supporting, delegating—for leading groups that range from high to low membership maturity.[6,7]
- *Managerial Grid*: This model, the so-called "Nine-Nine" model of leadership, is described in *Facilitating Group Behavior*.[8] The Nine-Nine model was formalized and popularized by behavioral scientists R.R. Blake and J.S. Mouton. For more information, see *Managerial Grid* (1964).[7] An example of how this grid may be applied to veterinary practice management and client service is illustrated in Figure 24-1.
- *Theory X and theory Y*: Both of these theories conceptualized by McGregor are about human motivation.[9] In theory X, management assumes employees are inherently lazy and will avoid work if they can and that they inherently dislike work. As a result, management believes that workers need

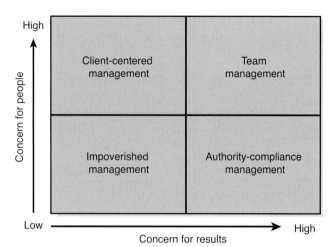

FIGURE 24-1 An example of the Blake Mouton Managerial Grid as may be applied to veterinary practice management and client service. This grid, when applied to practice management operations, can facilitate your ability to identify your current leadership style, to identify areas of desired improvement or development in leadership style, and keep the grid in situational context. Team management and leadership is not always the best approach to all situations.

to be closely supervised and comprehensive systems of control developed. In theory Y, management assumes that employees are ambitious, self-motivated, and exercise self-control. As a result, managers believe that employees will learn to seek out and accept responsibility and will exercise self-control and direction in accomplishing goals to which they are committed. These two theories were not viewed by McGregor as representatives of different ends of the same continuum, but more as different continua entirely.

- *Four-Model System*: Likert articulated the "Four-Model System."[10] This system was used to assist organizations in moving away from bureaucratic model (system 1) management toward system 4 management or to determine the extent that organizations exist along this spectrum.
  - Exploitative–Authoritative
  - Benevolent–Authoritative
  - Consultative–Democratic
  - Participative–Democratic

One of the key concepts in all these models is that empowered individuals on the team will feel better about their contributions and be more productive. The other key factor is now being called "Servant Leadership" (first coined by Robert K. Greenleaf in "The Servant as Leader," an essay that he first published in 1977.[11]) The reciprocal is that each team member must be willing to accept accountability for improved outcomes within their sphere of practice influence, on a continual basis (Continual Quality Improvement [CQI]). These styles of leadership are appropriate depending on the task, the situation, and the group (Figure 24-1).

The last decade of the past century saw a great revolution in the science of veterinary practice management. The historical patterns of just adding gimmicks was replaced by integrated programs of fiscal management, effective use of human resources, and client-centered service to deliver quality health care. The veterinary practices that opted to overhaul their old habits and establish a new practice environment are commonly found with the ones that survived and flourished during recessionary times. This millennium saw many systems modified to better meet Generation-Y needs as an example of an evolved and adaptive management focus.

EVOLUTION AND REVOLUTION IN VETERINARY PRACTICE MANAGEMENT

There are periods of time that are evolutionary in each practice, and there are times that require a revolutionary phase. The recessionary economic times noted over the recent decade have made this a mandate for most all veterinary practices. Since change is needed in this new era of abundant veterinary services, revolution is causing parabolic changes unlike the linear changes seen with past practice management evolution.

In today's health care market, where the consumer has become well informed through the media and client education, needs for change are expected to be processed quickly and effectively. Veterinary practices must become lean and mean in an effort to meet the challenges that can be controlled, particularly in the current environment of waste control; controlled substance enforcement; chemical hazards; veterinarian/client/patient relationships; drug surveillance; practice marketing review of ethics as restraint of trade; and a host of provincial, state, and local restrictions and rules. The veterinary practices that want to change are dissatisfied with what was, are led by veterinarians not interested in preserving the past, and are usually looking for a prime competitive advantage within their community. The problem in the United States, the United Kingdom, New Zealand, or Australia today is that the real prime competitive edge always ends up as the human resources within our own sphere of influence. In fact, *Fortune* magazine recently stated: "The most successful corporations of the new millennium will be something called a learning organization." Arie DeGeus of Royal Dutch/Shell stated: "The ability to learn faster than your competition may be the only sustainable competitive advantage."

Counterfeit programs have abounded in recent years, claiming to bring the desired changes in practice management. Guest relations, fancy job descriptions, standards of performance, smile training, cost center controls, profit center marketing, price schedules, and even the paper chase caused by computers are only symptomatic treatments that cannot cure the disorder. If we look to the leaders in service, and veterinary medicine is a service industry, one item becomes evident: the secret to success lies within our own walls. McDonalds, Marriott, SAS Airlines, Federal Express, and Disney are all examples of real service success stories. They treat their own people the way they want their customers/clients/guests to be treated. They have reduced the hierarchy and shared simplified corporate expectations for quality, unity, excellence, empathy, and/or teamwork. McDonalds even has a vice president in charge of fun. They also have eliminated "employee" and "subordinate" from everyone's vocabulary; they all speak of "associates," except for Disney, which considers everyone as a member of the "cast"—always on display. Without those types of basic mind-set changes, the "team" cannot be elevated into empowered positions.

THE IMPORTANCE OF CLIENT PERCEPTION: COMMON COURTESY

In the business of veterinary health care, taking the time to be courteous is an absolute must. Considering that a comparatively smaller number of clients and patients are available compared with the typical canine/feline practice, communication skills and common courtesy may be even more important for client retention in an avian practice. When people bring their birds to your office they are most often stressed. When compared with their domestic companion mammalian counterparts, a larger proportion of birds still are presented to veterinary offices with the client perception that they are ill. They are worried about their animal's health, about how their bird may be handled, and about the potential size of the ultimate invoice when services are completed. Many clients in this "crisis" mode do not want to make uninformed choices; they want answers and specific statements of what is needed to be done and why. They want some degree of control over what is done and to have an active role in the informed consent established during their consultation with you. They want to be informed, but not coerced, forced, or preached at. As such, when veterinarians consult with these clients, discussions focused on what is needed for their bird as opposed to what your recommendations are become extremely important. This principle is important when there is a physical disease known or suspected to be present, but it is equally (if not more) important when considering routine preventative health or wellness management of avian patients. Offering gold-, silver-, and bronze-level options for wellness care to your clients and then recommending that they make their choice is not an effective way to establish the needed working relationship between yourself and the clients. People want to feel good about their decision to come to your practice, as well as the "correctness" of their decisions after the examination. Through the extension of common courtesy, many of these concerns can be addressed. By merely being nice to people, you are more capable of listening to (and hearing) their frustrations, worries, or concerns. A good listener and communicator is capable of building rapport with his or her clients, while at the same time educating them and maintaining focus on the patient's health and welfare.

A common component of staff courtesy training is the use of "pedestal words" during client communication. These are brief words or phrases that function to raise the client to a level above the ordinary, and they make clients feel that they have been put onto a pedestal. Examples of pedestal words or phrases may include the following:

1. "May I?" (asking permission implies authority)
2. "I'd like your advice," or "What do you think?" (suggests superior wisdom)
3. "I'd sure appreciate it if" (there is an implication here that the client has the power to refuse or grant a favor)
4. "You are so right," or providing a "high five" (a pat on the back)
5. "As you know" (implies an understanding and professional skill)
6. "Please" (always a great lubricator in human relations)

Whether the doctors and staff of your practice use a caring approach (body language; thoughtful, listening, interested, and compassionate), pedestal words, or a combination of techniques, client confidence in your practice will be re-inforced and grow. The birds and your clients will have a greater chance of becoming less of a target for rigid medical and wellness protocols in your clinical mind's eye. More importantly, individuals (clients and patients) that you come to know at this level become a part of a greater picture of a tailored delivery of wellness health care.

EIGHT MANAGEMENT STARTING POINTS

Medicine

Medical and surgical knowledge and skills must remain the cornerstone of a quality health care marketing program. In today's marketplace, we can never overpromise and underde-liver; we must be current with the state of the art. In today's practice, that means wellness care must be "front and center" in staff training programs and client education; staff members as veterinary extenders show a higher level of pride. From this expertise comes the pride that is required to do the rest.

Money

This is based on health care delivery commitments and starts with the use of an annual cash budget, with paired income and expense centers, monitored monthly with an internal opera-tional accounting system. It is supported by a staff-monitored and staff-operated expense control program that keeps in-come statement expenses (less rent, veterinarian monies, and return on investment [ROI]) below 50% of the revenues ev-ery month. More interestingly, staff members can be client-bonding assets and primary care providers for husbandry and well care services; in some practices, empowered (trained and supported) staff drive up to 30% of the primary care income generated.

Mission Focus

This starts with a practice philosophy and an inviolate set of core values, which state the belief and vision of the ownership. This makes the practice team *focus* the core values on the mis-sion of quality health care delivery. As an example, these are extended into a written Standards of Care (SOCs) for Risk Level 1 animals (the *what* and *why*); staff then produces the protocols with the *who* and *how*. To be most effective, the *when* is then developed in joint session (leadership and zone teams) and includes milestones and specific new measure-ments for identifying success. This effort becomes the basis for key terms of behavior, employment, and expectations to exceed, not just meet.

Method

This starts with changing the practice's traditional standard operational format of input→process→output. It adds a fourth element to the operational format: input→process →output→outcome. The practice tasks to the outcome, not the process or output. A sick patient (input) is treated (pro-cess) and made well (output) but the progressive veterinary practice of the new millennium aims at client satisfaction (outcome), staff harmony (outcome), and a concurrent net income for the practice (outcome). As is seen in behavioral

medicine and applied behavior analysis, the consequence (outcome) of a behavior (or in this case, process) functions to either reinforce or punish the behavior.

Marketing

Persuasive marketing is based on developing the client's "needs" awareness, not just sales of products. It is a form of internal promotion of needed services and/or products. This begins with stating the pet's needs (patient advocacy) and the practice's needs in each case, then giving the client two op-tions to say "yes." In health care, the terms *should, recommend, you could,* and *we could* leave questions of need in the client's mind and obscures the decision to do the right thing. A com-mon adage comparing mere practice protocol and sound pa-tient advocacy might be the difference between "doing the right things" versus "doing things right."

Manpower

This starts with a progressive practice orientation program at the point of hire and continues with regular training toward excellence. The competency standard is excellence and has no compromise. Pride is sought and achieved by helping staff members exceed the practice expectations and standards. When pride is the staff input, quality will be the perception of the clients.

Minutes

This starts with increasing the doctor's time with patients and clients, which requires veterinarians to let go of routine treat-ments and basic client education so the staff may deliver it more economically, as well as the banking, scheduling, drug ordering, and other administrative tasks. Using the staff to leverage the doctor's time is working smarter, not harder. This is called training and tasking to the accountability for the desired outcome.

Morale

This starts with hiring people first and foremost for their at-titude; skills can be taught. It is demonstrated in the practice culture maintained by the leadership. Attitude is what is nurtured and promoted on a daily basis with recognition and a sense of belonging. This concept is summarized by Dr. Michael LeBoeuf in *The Greatest Management Principle in the World.*[12]

The above eight items seem easy at first glance, but em-bracing each, on a daily basis, without reverting to the old habits is a process that takes months to learn. Team-based health care delivery systems can be built, maintained, and integrated into the practice style and philosophy best fitting for a practice. These items cannot be used as either/or choices. The three key business factors for any product, manufacturing, or service industry are market opportunity, capital availability, and people power (human resources). The human resources of a practice are the key factor when seeking CQI. They are the most important, the highest cost, and the key to business and competitive success. The veterinary prac-tice of tomorrow will build to fit what works for people—both our clients and our employees. The elements of successful management are used, as each of the eight starting points below are placed into action in your management plans.

The Elements of Successful Management

1. Build the management machine. Build wide participation, share expectations, and depend on client feedback.
2. Look to bank only excellence (forsake old comparisons). Find only the most successful companies and practices to emulate.
3. Move to value-centered management, freeing up the control of changes by veterinarians only to leadership.
4. Power up frontline managers and let them take over the day-to-day duties.
5. Build a solid "ballpark" of standardized management expectations—the core values. Do not violate these values, and set the example at all times.
6. Redesign the measurements and rewards. Avoid reinforcement for the nonperformers; feed the players and magnify the strong points of the human resources.
7. Make the client king. If the client is perceived as interfering with someone's time, that staff person does not really understand his or her real job, which is client service.
8. Use innovation and streamline the system. Give small teams 30 days to solve problems for the good of the whole.

Organizational change efforts do not always work; in fact, they are often the hardest task to successfully accomplish. There have been three key reasons for failures to organize change in practice:

1. The agent for change—the consultant. A veterinary consultant can underestimate the immediate requirements of maintaining an ongoing business while demolishing the old system. Consultants do not always meet the client's need for an integrated approach that fits with an individual practice's philosophy. A cookbook approach is often offered as a "cure all" solution, or there may be an erroneous downplay of the need for management walkarounds and reassessments. These all can result in the promotion of a downwardly cascading system of program accountability.
2. The practice owner may have too low a desire to change, may have a lack of commitment to the plan, may have a lack of follow-up enforcement, or may not take timely action to remove problem people from the practice formula.
3. Many middle managers may think the fad for motivation to change will pass, and as a result do not support increased discussion and empowerment, lack a consistent discipline to apply to new behaviors that are desired, or may embrace a cycle of pain from the past too strongly to let go and move forward.

ATTRIBUTES OF PEAK PERFORMERS AND SUCCESSFUL BUSINESS LEADERS

For 18 years, Charles Garfield studied high achievers to determine what it takes to lead a discipline while performing at peak levels. He studied everyone from Tom Landry to Victor Kiam but eventually identified six basic attributes common to people who achieve peak performance in his book, *Peak Performers: The New Heroes of American Business*.[13]

1. *A commitment to mission*: This is the source of peak performance. Peak performers decide what they really care about and what they want to do.
2. *Results in real time*: Peak performers work to achieve goals that move them closer to fulfilling their missions.
3. *Self-management through self-mastery*: Peak performers not only turn a critical eye on past behavior, but also know how to mentally rehearse for new behavior (*accepting* the blame and *giving* credit).
4. *Team building and team playing*: Team builders know how to stretch the abilities of others and encourage risk taking. Believers in team health care systems do not just lead the teams they build, they join them.
5. *Course correction*: Peak performers know how to introduce change by learning from mistakes and applying the *vision* of the future.
6. *Change management*: Peak performers know how to anticipate and deal with external changes from new technology or new opportunities and then construct alternative futures. When we apply these six basic attributes to the veterinary practices that are progressive, growing, and still having fun, we see two more attributes in the peak performers:
7. The ability to differentiate between output and outcomes.
8. The ability to align programs to meet the desired outcomes that are expected.

To reach desired outcomes, we need to use detailed planning. In simplistic terms, output is the recovered pet or, in some practices, a paid bill. Veterinary practice needs to be more than this output; it needs to be centered on an outcome. The outcome is the client's perception that they have improved their enjoyable relationship with a healthy and happy family companion, and it is the practice's wish for the client to refer a neighbor because of their high satisfaction level. There is a significant difference between output- and outcome-orientated practices, and our practice philosophies can be adjusted to do either, but not both, efficiently.

The bottom line in what motivates peak performers to fulfill their own best talents is their values. These values, the real tangible qualities that make up the character of a person or an organization, are the internal drives to excel and put an operation onto a fast track to success. In veterinary medicine, the core values of the staff center on caring for people and their animals, not dollars and cents. The uncommon leader of a veterinary practice understands this as fact and converts all goals and objectives to issues of caring, continuity of care, and the quality of care offered as patient advocates. The doctor who centers his or her focus on common figures such as the average client transaction (ACT) will be seen as a money-oriented task master (the staff produces net, not gross), and will not get the same staff support as a patient advocate who desires wellness and better health care for each patient.

Patricia Aburdene, co-author of *Re-Inventing the Corporation*, summarized that tomorrow's successful business leaders must create an environment that nourishes personal growth and satisfaction. Intuition, she explained, will be highly valued, and the principles of both quality service and quality of life will emerge as part of the new work ethic. Part of leadership is the ability to master change. Rosabeth Kanter, author of *The Change Masters* and *Men and Women of the Corporation*, has stated that the renaissance of American business will come through innovation, entrepreneurship, and participative management. She also believes that motivating people to innovate can transform any traditional health care delivery system to meet the changing tomorrows. Harvard's

Dr. Harry Levinson, best-selling author of *CEO: Corporate Leadership in Action*, claims that leaders are servants, teachers, and facilitators.[14] These people establish purpose, support values, and know how and when to say good-bye. The ultimate definition of a high-achieving leader will be clarified in the practices across the United States, the United Kingdom, New Zealand, Australia, and other countries. The answer is up to each veterinarian. It depends on who you are and what you want to contribute to the profession and the veterinary health care delivery system.

Change will not occur unless there is a fire that will not be put out. If you listen only to your accountant, remember that most of them count beans behind the bow wave of the system. They are not known to be leaders of the future, only counters of what has been past. The samurai management style, the dedication to the end result, must be an element of pride, not apology. Samuel Johnson said it well: "Nothing will ever be attempted if all possible objections must first be overcome." Change is not for the weak of heart or those with marginal dreams. It is for those that dare to dream of what could be and are willing to sacrifice to make it happen. You need to believe that it must be completed within 3 years and not delay in attacking the underlying causes. Whether you think you can or you think you cannot, you will be the one who makes your thoughts right.

The trick to building a great veterinary practice, surviving and thriving in these turbulent times, is to be true to yourself. Go back to your roots; remember why you joined the veterinary profession, not the logic that has occurred since that time. Your own dreams can create your own reality, in this regard. The way to be special in the minds of your clients is to be distinctly yourself. Be a personality, think of yourself as a product (since that is all the traditional veterinarian is comfortable in "selling" to clients).

RULES TO HELP TRANSFORM DREAMS TO REALITY

Know What Is Important

Always remember why you entered the profession, and establish clarity to your reason(s). Remember what you dreamed *before* the education and school of hard knocks altered your vision. Listen to your heart. Define this dream into solid parameters that can be monitored and measured while the implementation and accomplishment efforts are conducted.

Build a Prototype

Try a model that can be tested, tasted, felt, seen, smelled, or touched. It does not have to be pretty, and it does not have to be 110% accurate. Take baseline laboratory databases (complete blood counts [CBCs] and/or chemistries); start with the higher risk birds you see (e.g., older, higher historical risk factors such as poor diet) and discuss and offer every client the opportunity to let you establish the baseline you need in the medical records for later when problems occur. Remember what you were taught in veterinary school: sequential blood chemistries and hemograms are far more meaningful than single tests.

Take Responsibility

Stop blaming others, or the economy, or the community—if you look internally, the alternatives and solutions are within your reach. If you blame others, you are abdicating accountability for your role in changing the outcome. Leadership is dangerous (the buck stops with you), it is scary (followers will do what you tell them), lonely (fault lies with those atop the pyramid), fun (you can define the success milestones as well as the celebrations of the attempts), and exhilarating (seeing others learn to stretch and innovate, in a safe environment, requires an uncommon leader).

Keep It Simple—Make It Fun

Managers are most often concerned with style and process, while leaders concentrate on substance and creativity of the outcomes. Managers fear chaos because they often must become aggressive, while leaders love the aggression required to make dreams reality. The clear and distinct identification of the end point (and alternative outcomes possible) allows chaos to become simplified—process belongs to the followers and there are very few rules that are critical. First and foremost, make it fun. Clients like to buy from people who are not selling. They like to buy from practices that offer good encounters with friendly and fun people. This does not mean euthanasia must be fun (remember the motive, proper time, and proper place), but it does mean that our personal stress must stay out of sight, waiting to be scrubbed away and flushed down the drain. And almost always, there will be at least one individual on your staff who will probably not want to let go of his or her baggage.

Review the Motives

Fighting the windmills of competition is far easier than fighting the windmills of your own dreams. Leaders must be motivated at all times; fatigue makes you a lemming, looking for the sea. You must want to make a difference for someone or something else, and the purity of this "cause" comes from knowing you are doing the right thing, at the right time, for the right reasons. If your goal is pure and selfless, fame and fortune will find you; it need not be a pursuit with its own reward.

Inspire Excellence

Anyone can be average, and today's excellence is tomorrow's average. Excellence in health care is a mandate—an undeniable common goal that we all share, but not all achieve. Togetherness and support of the team in the quest for excellence helps develop pride and pride comes when expectations are exceeded. Clients want to believe their veterinarian is special. It is human nature. If the expectation is excellence, and you help fend off the negative thoughts that poison daily activities, clients will perceive a level of pride that will differentiate the practice in the community.

Require Continual Improvement

Know your strengths and know your areas where you must use others to "make it happen." Know when to ask for help and know when to release control. Good leaders inspire others to perform above their abilities, and provide training so the initial leap of faith is just a long stretching step rather than a leap into the unknown. The expectation to continually improve must overwhelm the safety concerns of "no risk" operations.

Rapid Response

Whatever time of response is average, make it twice as fast. Clients are busy, and they often do not want to be in your practice more than 30 minutes, much less have an appointment and not be seen on time. In physics, we know that momentum is a function of mass and velocity. If you want to improve the momentum, regardless of how big the challenge, just increase the velocity.

The most effective change programs are usually an interactive set of staff training programs, step by baby step. In the United States, New Zealand, and Australia, approximately 65% of veterinary staff represents "status quo" behavior styles, which means they move slowly into change mode. They must be trained to a level of being trusted, and then have small projects to demonstrate they have the respect of the leadership. After the initial project successes, they can then move into new programs. Effective practice leaders ensure that all new programs have new metrics, since experienced leaders know that old metrics cause reversion to the old systems.

KEY MANAGEMENT METRICS FROM WHICH TO WORK

The journals and seminar speakers love to speak of average client transaction and gross sales as indicators of success and often provide the national averages as benchmarks. A benchmark is what the top 15% are doing, but they need to be of similar size, similar to operational format, and similar outcome expectations to really be a "benchmark." To be at the national average, you must be seeking to be "the best of the worse" or "the worse of the best"; using the average as a benchmark is nothing more than striving for mediocrity. For a bird or other specialty practice, a goal of being 10% better in a program of interest, or specifically aiming to be better than last year in the same period, is a form of benchmark specific to the practice. If you do not measure it, you cannot manage it.

Program Procedures Per 100 Patients Seen

It is amazing why veterinarians equate dollars with program procedures. Depending on epidemiology and circumstances, pet or aviary birds may deserve a number of procedures, including hematology, fecal assays, pathogen-specific screening tests, routine grooming procedures, and vaccines. A question that often is not considered but should be is, *How many program procedures are being done per 100 birds seen?*

Cases Referred to Nursing or Technical Staff for Follow-Up

Feeding and enrichment plans, observation of patient progress for inpatients and outpatients, telephone follow-up review of progress and status following outpatient or inpatient visits, or training and furthering enrichment plans for the home setting are all at least in part nurse and technical staff

functions. These functions require that the staff is trained to a level of trust to effect the desired outcome.

Diagnostic Ratios

The simplest ratio is "pharmacy sales:diagnostic sales"; we expect about 1:1 in a general practice, maybe 4:1 in a mobile production practice, and about 1:2 or 1:3 in a bird practice. The ratio will vary by provider (caseload dependent), but the practice will have an average that can be used as a "rough yardstick."

Number of Positive Recognitions Per Day

Larry was a traditional veterinarian who had been in practice "forever." He expected competency and had been through it all. He seldom recognized good work, and was perceived to "not be happy" with staff performance. We had him write each staff member's name on the back of his business card every morning, and check off the name when he provided positive feedback . . . the goal was to have every name checked off before going home for the night. At the 90-day follow-up visit, he had special cards printed with everyone's name; the system had changed the practice's culture to one of harmony, with an amazing upbeat performance.

Update Frequency of Written Standards of Care

The written SOCs are for well care initially, and as such, require 110% compliance by all providers. When the bird is showing signs of illness, clinical freedom within protocols is expected. The *compliance* to SOCs is internal to the practice team, while the *adherence* is what the client does with what the respective practice providers have told the client. Internal compliance to the SOCs will reinforce the "safe haven" for the staff, but reduces the "owner's" variances, since he or she must set the example 24 hours a day, 7 days a week, 365 days per year. As a means of implementing an update of segments of a practice's SOCs, many practices will update or add to their written SOCs following every continuing educational event attended.

Husbandry Hints Revised/Updated

Too many practices use a copy of a copy of older handouts, and their clients can see the apathy. Client handouts deserve the quality of practice-specific information, and staff members are more than able to keep them current and contemporary.

Trained Locums/Relief Veterinarians

Mark spent 2 years looking for an associate who knew birds, or was willing to learn about birds; he did not want to spend the time training multiple new relief vets on a recurring basis. Finally, he was convinced to build a team of two or three part-time associates/locums/relief veterinarians, and when he did, he found the secret formula for gaining family time. Interestingly, as one of the part-time veterinarians moved away, the remaining two found a replacement and trained that person to the practice standards. In fact, Mark posted his schedule, and gave the trio the opportunity to schedule themselves into duty slots per their own needs. His family time became part of his weekly schedule, which spouse and kids really appreciated (and the burnout threat was minimized).

Catchment Area Assessment

Take the time to assess the details of your new clients coming to your practice. Why did they pick you? How did they hear about you? We know we should have over 50% of a practice's new clients referred by satisfied clients. Use this type of information to send personal thank you acknowledgments to those who have referred new clients to you.

FINANCIAL MANAGEMENT

Generally good financial planning is boring. If you find it exciting, stressful, regretful, depressing, combative, or any other state of high emotion, you are probably doing something wrong. Here are eight boring financial rules to live by to live a happier financial life (in no particular order).

Live Within Your Means

Simply stated, if you cannot live within your means, you are doomed and the rest of your life is made miserable as a byproduct. Credit is not a valid method for supporting a family. You know how it is said that finances are the major cause of relationship difficulties? This first point is a major culprit. If you are already in trouble, start living within your income today. Sketch out a common-sense budget, cut your expenses, make a plan to pay off the debt, and start an automatic savings deposit at some minimal level. When cutting expenses, remember that every expense falls into one of two categories: an absolute requirement or a desire, want, or luxury. When the debt is paid off, bulk up the automatic savings and investment amounts and live off what is left after savings and investments.

Make a Plan for Your Future

Without a plan, you are walking through a totally dark doorway with no idea what is on the other side. Do not blame someone else when you end up somewhere undesirable. Your plan should be pretty simple. Starting today, make your goal a small financial footprint as you go into retirement. By financial footprint, we are referring to your living expenses. Ideally and relatively speaking, a small financial footprint either requires less retirement income or allows you to live a larger life on the income you created. Veterinary students are wise to start immediately with their first pay check after graduation. Many veterinary graduates have rarely had this large a recurring income, so putting 10% to 15% away before anything else with every pay check is a worthy discipline to allow money to compound over time (use a savings account until there is adequate money for a longer term CD, which then lends to an investment portfolio, e.g., real estate trust).

Protect Your Family, Practice, and Staff

If death or major disability takes away your family's living income or your practice earning potential, you must have alternative sources of funds available for them to continue to live at a reasonable standard of living. Role play your own or your spouse's death (or lack of earning potential) and see what happens. Where will the survivors turn? How much will they need? How long will they need it? How will they manage their funds? Who will help manage the funds? Consider all these questions at different ages because your needs will change over time. Also, consider home, auto, health, disability, long-term care, and liability protection for worst-case scenarios.

You Must Invest

Investment does not have to be complicated. Simply, you should be contributing to your employer plan (401K, TSP) or an Individual Retirement Account, or both. Keep your investment expenses low. Contribute out of every pay check. Have the right allocation of funds in your account and rebalance to your original allocation of funds annually.

All of these concepts have probably been discussed and described by your financial planner or by your accountant or both. It does not have to be complicated, and most veterinarians can do this easily. It does take some reading and understanding on your own part, or you may be vulnerable to some of the poor judgments and expensive mistakes people can make. Stop and think about liquidity and cash flow rather than gross turnover and average client transaction.

Have a Savings Account

Although this is a basic point to bring forward, you always must have access to quick and stable value money. Why? So you do not go into hock or debt for any one thing that may arise requiring immediate funds. You occasionally need money for emergencies, large purchases, expenses after a job loss, and a splurge every once in a while (you have to live a bit sometimes). Remember, credit is not a valid way to pay for life. Have money available at all times.

Consolidate Accounts and Eliminate Where Possible

Too many accounts complicate your life. If you were a juggler, you could juggle only so many balls in the air. You take on too many, and balls start falling to the ground. Fewer accounts, better control, easier management, and missions accomplished. Accounts to consolidate or eliminate should include credit, loans, retirement, savings, investments, and others.

Pay Your Bills on Time

Paying on time (and when possible more than required) positively affects your credit rating. The better your credit rating, the lower future borrowing rates can become. A good credit rating allows for better or more financing options for you should you need credit in the future. Creditors prefer to do business with people they can trust and that have a record to prove it.

Get You and Your Spouse (and Practice Manager) on the Same Page

You cannot be working against each other. Take the time to schedule and follow through in discussions of these key personnel. These actions are the basic building blocks to financial success—like the foundation of a home. To disagree or disregard these actions is risking ruin. Here are a few starter questions for your discussions:

- The practice's written SOCs are used at every quarterly budget review; how are we tracking individual provider commitment to the SOC agreements? *Note: failure to "make budget" is just a lack of discipline by individuals to do what they have committed to do in the previous budget review.*

- What's the difference between "risk" and "risky?" *Example: a new program is often a risk, but to start it without adequate training-to-trust of staff is risky.*
- How can risk be managed to minimize it while investing in stock funds that ensure long-term wealth creation? *A qualified SEC financial planner may be needed to explain this factor.*
- Most people think *the stock market going down is the risk,* but why must the stock market go down for you to build wealth?
- How can you use your recurring and one-time fund allocations (at home and in the practice) to manage risk?

Take a little time to become familiar with financial basics (including understanding your balance sheet) and these questions will be easy. Once you do these things, you will be on the road to happiness because you will have your financial house in order.

Management Accounting versus Tax Accounting

Every practice needs to track line items, especially cost of drugs, since it is often such a large line item. The "paired" line items have been categorized in the American Animal Hospital Association Chart of Accounts (income item versus expense for the item). Some vendors will even give you an end of month (EOM) breakdown by major category. The major expense categories are best summarized to match the major income categories shown by your veterinary software. This is usually done by using QuickBooks, My Money, Xero (in the cloud), or other user-friendly bookkeeping software. The basic business formula, "Income − Expense = Profit," is important to use, and yet most veterinary practice management software systems cannot compute this basic business number. When you use the previously mentioned software or another user-friendly bookkeeping system, you will have the EOM data in real time. If you use your accountant, this is usually delayed by weeks or months and comes back in a tax-friendly format (no paired line items).

Program-Based Budget Planning

Budgeting should not be viewed as an accountant's exercise. Tax accounting is differentiated from managerial accounting. The cash budget is only a series of clinical programs to which we have historical data on the income or expense impact on any practice. A good leader promotes income development activities and allows his team to increase net by controlling expenses and extending the health care delivery programs beyond the professional diagnostician. Therefore, the annual budget cycle includes an annual marketing plan and the communication/training plan for the team and a continually refreshed commitment to higher levels of quality health care delivery.

Programs = Net Income

More veterinary practice owners are learning that a focus on the front door is good business; they know when their procedures are down. A good program-based budget provides the needed measurements for growth: how many procedures are we doing and what the relationships to each other are. These measurements are essential to make success happen. In *Building*

the Successful Veterinary Practice: Programs and Procedures (Volume 2), examples are provided that most practices can follow to build a monthly cash budget, establish effective income statements, and build on an established Chart of Accounts.[15] Mechanically, the income statements of a practice should reflect the major income categories produced by the practice's veterinary software at EOM, and those major categories are then used for the top left-hand column of the budget instead of "sales," and the income history of the last 3 years can be used to determine the average earning power of each month (percent of annual income). The chart is not the planning process, and the planning and projections are what are needed to make it happen.

Controlling Cash Flow

The traditional approach to restrict expenses and inch the prices upward is adequate to maintain average growth to defend against inflation, but it does not promote expansion. The cost of professional services continually rises as do the fixed and variable costs associated with a practice. It is one thing to project an increased income for next year, but it is far more difficult to make it happen. The secret to obtaining those extra degrees of expansion (practice growth) is based on the increasing horizontal (adding services) and vertical (expanding existing services) levels of income available to the practice. Income production (new or expanded services and products) is the major variable in controlling liquidity, which is also called "cash flow."

To control (or monitor) income levels, fees must be projected and cash must be received (and bad debt must be minimized). We will assume the practice has a clear set of values and core competencies, a future-based vision, and a consistent practice philosophy in place (an accepted core platform of services and products). This is started with a cash budget, with paired income and expense centers where possible, projected by month, for the coming fiscal year. In program-based budgeting:

1. The historical income (percentage of the annual income earned per month) must be established, either by historical records or experience factors. This will help decide the percentage of cost allocation per specific month for variable and semifixed expenses.
2. Ancillary income sources must be assessed as opportunities to the available practice team (space and equipment, client acceptance, and human resources). Using historical expenses will be helpful and must be assessed, expanded, and allocated to specific months based on the horizontal and vertical diversification planned for the upcoming year.
3. A flexible model must be established built on zero-based budgeting. Start with the assumed profit level required to make the practice grow at the desired rate in the upcoming year, then look at the current and possible income potentials.
4. The practice plan (vision of the practitioner) outlines the 1-, 3-, and 5-year hospital director's health care delivery plan, marketing plan, business plan, and staff utilization plan (names vary by practice).

Controlling the cash flow means knowing what is expected then measuring the accomplishment of that performance level. The program-based budget must be compared with actual performance on a monthly basis and adjustments need to be made in the remaining monthly targets if the year-end goals are to be met. This is often done in dollars, but when variances occur, you must look at procedure counts or you are just fooling yourself.

The Front Door Must Swing

It is commonly understood that if there is no client flow through your doors then it is hard to deliver health care or earn a living. The secret is what makes *your* practice front door swing. Every practice has a different formula, but there are common components, and they are called programs (as in program-based budgeting). Examples of programs that can reinforce client return visits and their resulting revenues and practice growth include strategically designed wellness services aimed at using some of the biological data traditionally collected as a component of lifestyle enrichment, behavioral intervention and enrichment programs, inpatient as well as outpatient integration of behavioral medicine with every patient and client interaction, strategic dietary management and implementation, and recurring care services including but not limited to grooming of nails and wings (if needed). Examples of program diagnostic centers that may be in need of evaluation for their roles in avian practice are seen in the following sections.

Baseline screening or diagnostic databases

This includes but is not limited to CBCs, serum biochemistries, and cytology and some appropriate pathogen-specific screening assays. These, chosen and applied well, have shown great value in the management of risk factors pertinent to individual bird health as well as populations. Many of these tests can be performed in a standardized manner in-house. Although in many practices these types of tests are used, there are still many more available, and which may have particular proactive preventative health management value in some settings (see Chapters 1, 2, and 13).

Anesthesia and surgery

This includes intravenous or intraosseous fluid support, Doppler pulse monitoring and indirect blood pressure, current and bimodal if not even trimodal analgesia, microsurgical instrumentation, and magnifying loupes and operating or surgical microscopy. All, if used with skill and expertise, can elevate the standard of care, case management outcome, and client perception of value (see Chapters 19 to 21).

Diagnostic imaging

Imaging modalities and their documented diagnostic value have expanded greatly beyond plain radiographic film images in avian medicine. With training, ultrasonography can significantly enhance the diagnosis and management of cardiovascular and coelomic disease processes in birds. Fluoroscopy can provide real-time diagnostic abilities at comparatively low used machine outlay costs, and computed tomography and magnetic resonance imaging are increasingly more available and directly applicable in avian medical practice (see Chapter 14). If you are not aware of their potential benefits for a case and its management, it is hard, if not impossible, to discuss with their owners the real need for their use, and these modalities may not be even considered as a result.

The front door swings because we believe in our health care programs and share that conviction with clients. If you do not medically believe it is needed, do not do it. In this light, program centers are client-oriented services, not designed as income centers or profit centers. These same program centers, if not designed, kept current, and challenged for continual evidence of solid medical and scientific merit, could of course be used as profit or income centers under the guise of real programs. We can mistakenly try to save our clients' money by avoiding the implementation of good medical programs, and we can also mistakenly use medical programs for the generation of practice revenue instead of carefully assessed outcome, which is accomplished through critical thinking and scientific methodologies.

The ability to believe in good medicine is the cornerstone of a successful practice. The ability to convey this need to clients is the cornerstone of a profitable practice. The overhead of a veterinary practice is pretty fixed (in well-managed practices, less than 50% of the gross income is spent on monthly profit and loss expenses, not counting rent, doctor monies, and ROI benefits [quarterly rate stays below 48%]). So, it is the delivery of services and products within existing staff and facility capabilities that can make the net income difference.

Every year, newer and recurrent continuing education courses mean you have the opportunity to enhance practice programs. The continuing education experience that does not add one new program was a wasted expense. That new program is designed to provide better care, and there is a value associated with that client benefit. That value, as assessed to clients, should be reflected in your program-based budget for the year. The cash flow reports from that computer in your office only reflect the "belief level" of the providers in the new program(s) offered. The choice is yours, and we are here to help, but the belief starts in your gut and ascends to your heart. When your heart believes in the program, the clients will accept the care as needed and essential. It is your choice—lower the net each year or provide better health care delivery programs.

Protocols Are Not Necessarily the Same as Programs

In the client-centered practice, the team functions to be consistent, and the doctors are a component of this team. For consistency to be most effectively delivered, some basic and clearly understood methods of operation (internal standards of care) are integral for success to be achieved. On the other hand, these same standards, or protocols, can pose potential hazards to health care delivery and ultimately the long-term health of the practice itself. In avian health care, the mixture of species that a practice sees is considerably broader and more complex than seen in a canine/feline practice. Those practices that work with additional species groups such as reptiles and amphibians, exotic small mammals, fish, wildlife, and other zoological species have an even greater species differential with which to develop in-depth familiarity. There is a clear need for more uniform and in-depth knowledge and training with these species by the entire practice team. This level of familiarity is essential to avoid a practice approach that is founded on mere standard protocols adopted from outside sources compared with tailored wellness health care delivery. Lack of knowledge and species familiarity can result in an internal management that either drifts with no standards of operation when these patients are seen or that applies sweeping standardized protocols across species and epidemiologic lines that probably should not be crossed. Wellness screening protocols and procedures are only as valuable for patient care as the total of their relative strength and accuracy as reliable tools for screening common true health risk factors. The assessment of the tests that are used requires critical scientific challenge regarding their sensitivity and specificity and economic merit, and remains a primary responsibility of practice management and the health care delivery team. These internal SOCs need to be critically balanced with detailed knowledge and expertise, and must be based on careful assessment of their true merit, rather than the income that they generate or the mere (but unsubstantiated) belief that they have merit. As an example of a shift in internal SOCs away from simple protocol (output) toward a more effective outcome, one could look at a common grooming procedure—the beak trim. A practice management philosophy and SOCs may be altered to acknowledge that "beak trims" are no longer accepted as a standardized and simple procedure or protocol (e.g., wing-, beak-, and nail-trimming appointments). Instead of this simple protocol driving to a simple procedure and simple output, a change of internal standards can be made. A concerted team effort should be made, via telephone and at examination, to ensure that these types of procedures be accompanied by a well-defined individual clinical need (examination and diagnosis). With this more focused level of diagnosis, appropriate client-informed awareness of what may be best for their bird and their issue of concern can be achieved. Normal beaks do not typically overgrow, and they typically do not require trimming. Some beak-trimming procedures simply are not needed at all. Often, there can be problems with the functional anatomy, nutrition, or general health of these birds that can lead to these changes.

By applying the behavioral principles of the Law of Effect, the business aspects of the use of standardized wellness testing protocols can be evaluated from the client's perspective of their desire to return to your practice. The Law of Effect simply states that behavior (in this case, client return visits to your practice) is a function of its consequences. In other words, the frequency of a client's return visits is influenced by

the consequences that followed their earlier visits (see Chapter 5). The Law of Effect is applied with two basic procedures: reinforcement and punishment. Reinforcement increases the frequency of behavior and punishment decreases the frequency of behavior. Reinforcement (both positive and negative) refers to an event that occurs in conjunction with a behavior and increases the likelihood that a behavior will occur again. A positive reinforcer is a stimulus that is sought and added to the environment that the client finds "pleasant." A negative reinforcer is a stimulus that is avoided and that the client in this case finds "unpleasant," leading the client to avoid this aversive stimulus by repeating their visits to your practice. Both positive and negative reinforcers function to increase the frequency of the target behavior, but by very different means. Punishment (both positive and negative) refers to an event that occurs in conjunction with a behavior and decreases the likelihood that a behavior (client return visits) will occur again. A positive punisher in this case would be a stimulus that occurs in conjunction with the client visit, is added to the environment or experience, and that functions to decrease the probability of the client's return. A negative punisher would be a stimulus that occurs in conjunction with the client visit, is removed from the environment, and functions to decrease the probability of the client's return. The proof of their classification lies strictly in the assessed rate or predicted future rate of the client's return visit frequency. If your client's return visit rate is not increasing, it is being punished, regardless of your practice management intentions (Table 24-2).

The probability of return client visits to your practice can suffer the consequences of negative punishment (clients lose money and return visits decrease) and positive punishment (clients receive suboptimal care and recognize it and return visits decrease). Client return rate can be increased through positive reinforcement (clients are pleased with their experience and feel that they take home something of value) and negative reinforcement (tests performed either confirm the absence of problem or identify a problem, enabling treatment—both leading to a desirable outcome of relief). A common deficit in many wellness protocols used in avian practice is the belief that negative reinforcement can function as a key drive for return visits—the marketing of peace of mind. In this system, it is argued that clients increase their probability of return visits as a result of the use of protocols

TABLE 24-2

Skinner's Paradigms Applied to Client Return Visits

	Positive (Addition of a Stimulus as a Result of the Visit)	Negative (Subtraction of a Stimulus as a Result of the Visit)
Reinforcement (increased rate of return to the practice)	Perceived value Direct benefit to wellness and strength of the human–animal bond	"Peace of mind" Relief from the perception of disease Removal of visible or suspected disease
Punishment (decreased rate of return to the practice)	Suboptimal health care Lack of common courtesy (perceived discourtesy) Stress or injury to the birds	Loss of money Inconvenience to client

Client-centered veterinary health care providers will always strive to make sure that both outpatient and inpatient visits result in client-perceived substance in that upper left hand box: positive reinforcement. These differences highlight the important comparison between the *output* of what we do compared with the *outcome* (client perception) of those actions (see Chapter 5).

for routine documentation of the absence of disease. This type of a management system can be contrasted to those that are focused on positive reinforcement (client return visits are increased by their perception of increased value at the time of the visit). In general, bird owners state that their perceived value of veterinary service is based on things that directly influence the quality of their relationship with their bird at home. Although a sense of relief because of the absence of disease does have value, the direct infusion of fun, knowledge, and improved home relationships with companion birds should be viewed as a more probable strong drive for those return visits. In this light, some standardized testing protocols can be counterproductive to the development of a growing clientele if the practice philosophy is not client centered. Positive reinforcement for regular returns in wellness management (clients receive valued and desired service and increase their probability of returns) should be viewed as the ideally structured, most ethical, and strongest driving factor for their return visits. This may be clearly contrasted with a practice that emphasizes a negative reinforcement system for encouraging client return (clients receive the "good" news that their bird is not diseased at the moment and return regularly for this peace of mind).

The Practice Budget Team

The control of the cash flow from programs that match the core values of the practice is a team responsibility and, as such, the plan must be a team effort. The practice budget team should include the practice owners, bookkeeper, office manager, lead technician(s), lead receptionist(s), and an outside mentor. The technician and receptionist should be involved in those areas where they have a firsthand interest and impact but need not be involved in all parts of the team planning. The outside mentor, to be most effective, must be detached from the practice's patient health care plan.

Key financial and operational relationships need to be discussed to determine indicators that management can observe to easily monitor trends on a monthly basis. Examples would include, but should not be limited to, the following:

Cost of drugs and medical supplies	12%–15%
Paraprofessional salaries	17%–21%
Total W-2 compensation, doctors clinical and staff	<43%
Percent of transactions that are new clients	Target 10%
Number of new clients by referral	>60%
Percent gross from consultations/surgery/anesthesia	Individual practice data points, and less so standard targets of performance
Percent of gross for mailing	>0.6%
Number of transactions per veterinarian	Individual practice data points to monitor
Percent "net" given away (adjustments/discounts by veterinarian)	Individual practice data points to monitor

Aging rate of accounts receivable (30, 60, or 90 days)	Individual practice data points to monitor
Rate of follow-up scheduling by doctor	Individual practice data points to define and monitor
Diagnostic ratio (pharmacy sales:diagnostic sales)	Individual practice and doctor data points to monitor

Some of these ratios, like the pharmacy sales:diagnostic sales by veterinarian, are very individual ratios, but center the doctor's attention on what they can do for the quality of care provided by the practice. Many of these ratios can be graphed for more clarity when evaluating trends. These ratios are indicators to watch, positioning you to know when to look deeper into the operational trends or fiscal management of the practice.

Beware of the easy factors so often published without "the rest of the story," such as the ACT, which is often counterproductive because it centers attention on the wrong thing: What is the "computer's definition" of a transaction? Is the ACT reported by veterinarian or by hospital? What is the over-the-counter sales impact? What is the income per inpatient visit versus outpatient visit? What are the payroll hours per transaction? What is the return rate per year (client or patient)? Some consultants demand that the square footage of the practice be used to compute cost centers, but the allocations of circulating space makes potentially profitable areas appear worthless. Evaluate services within the resources available to the practice and maximize income from each cost center. The bottom line of fee structuring is simply if you are within about 10% of the community high, variances from national norms are not significant for the clients who seek quality veterinary health care services.

The veterinary computer systems of today are designed to give abundant data. Unfortunately, this most often is minimally true information for management decision making. A good practice manager must be able to take the information available and process it into knowledge that can be used for the good of the practice. In any practice, less than 30 factors are needed to reveal the monthly trends. In the area of laboratory services, expenses should be tracked by in-house versus commercial and income should be tracked by preventative, presurgical, and medical support functions. The examination/office call (better called "doctor's consultation") should be tracked by rechecks and normal and extended consultations. In a healthy mature practice, monthly operational expenses, *without the major variables of rent, DVM salaries, or ROI*, would be expected to be between 45% and 48% of the gross. Quicken and QuickBooks (from Intuit) are excellent software systems for expense summaries and accounts payable needed to support the Chart of Accounts.

Comparisons could include outpatient drugs and medical supplies versus inpatient drugs and medical supplies, hospitalization income, imaging income compared with expenses, over-the-counter sales, boarding fill rate, or others. Other expected ratios include rent at 1% per month of the fair market value (triple net lease), DVM wages (owner(s), et al) at 18% to 23%, CPA and legal fees at 0.8% to 2%, office supplies at 1.4% to 2.2%, or maintenance costs of 0.5% to 1.5%.

Using the practice team to keep the budget plan on track will be enhanced when the accurate data are shared in a timely manner by using a format that is user friendly. Remember, the staff knows how much a practice takes in each day (they close out the computer), they just do not know what the costs are in most cases. The team used to keep the budget on track will provide feedback that will show the benefit of the time taken to make the information readable. The practice management methodologies required to make the budget plan happen include the following principles: accurate data, timeliness of data availability, user friendliness, controlled cost of capturing data, and keeping on track monthly.

REFERENCES

1. <http://www.pfma.org.uk/pet-population/#>.
2. Catanzaro T: *Building the successful veterinary practice* (vols 1–3), Hoboken, NJ, 1997–1998, Wiley Blackwell.
3. Catanzaro T: *The practice success prescription: team-based veterinary healthcare delivery*, VIN Library. <www.vin.com>.
4. Catanzaro T: *Fundamental money management for the veterinary practice*, 2009, VCI Signature Series Monographs.
5. Hersey P: *The situational leader*, ed 4, 1985, Warner Books.
6. Hersey P, Blanchard KH: Life cycle theory of leadership, *Training and Development Journal* 23(5):26–34, 1969.
7. Blake R, Mouton J: *The managerial grid: the key to leadership excellence*, Houston, 1964, Gulf Publishing.
8. Blake R, Mouton J: *The managerial grid III: the key to leadership excellence*, Houston, 1985, Gulf Publishing.
9. McGregor D: *The human side of enterprise*, New York, 1960, McGraw-Hill.
10. Likert R, Likert JG: *New ways of managing conflict*, New York, 1976, McGraw-Hill.
11. Greenleaf RK: *Servant leadership: a journey into the nature of legitimate power and greatness*, 1977, Paulist Press.
12. LeBoeuf M: *The greatest management principle in the world*, 1985, Putnam.
13. Garfield C: *Peak performers: the new heroes of American business*, 1987, William Morrow.
14. Levinson H, Rosenthal S: *CEO: corporate leadership in action*, 1985, BasicBooks.
15. Catanzaro TE: *Building the successful veterinary practice. Vol 2: programs and procedures*, 1998, Wiley-Blackwell.

MANAGING RISK IN AVIAN PRACTICE

Charlotte Lacroix

In the law of professional negligence, the standard of care is the benchmark by which others assess a veterinarian's competence. To be within the standard of care, veterinarians must perform their duties with an average degree of skill, care, and diligence exercised by colleagues practicing under the same or similar circumstances. Unfortunately, this is a general rule and not always helpful when a veterinarian is trying to determine whether or not to do something in a given situation. For example, when is it necessary or not necessary to refer a patient?

In general, compared with other professionals, veterinarians are minimally regulated. Aside from the state board of examiners, Drug Enforcement Agency and Occupational Safety and Health Administration, few governmental agencies have oversight on how veterinary medicine is practiced. This is a good thing, because veterinarians can still exercise independent judgment with minimal anxiety of having Big Brother watch over them. The downside, however, is that it is unclear as to what is and what is not the standard of practice. For this reason, it is important that veterinary professionals keep the conversation going as to what does or does not constitute the standard of care, for it is better that such standards are articulated and shared within and for the industry versus waiting around and having the lawyers and courts determine the standards, one by one, each at the expense of a veterinarian's career.

There are two primary areas of law that regulate the conduct of veterinarians and help ensure that veterinarians act prudently and reasonably in their dealings with clients and their animals. The first is the civil court system, which adjudicates claims made by clients who allege that their veterinarians have acted carelessly. The second is the state board of examiners, which is an administrative office of the state in which the veterinarian is licensed. It is charged with enforcing a state's veterinary practice act, which sets forth laws with which veterinarians must comply to obtain and maintain their veterinary licenses. In performing their daily clinical duties, veterinarians need to be cognizant of these two areas of law, since they represent the two principal avenues by which clients may have complaints addressed.

Receiving letters from the state board of examiners and/or an accusatory client's attorney can be stressful, causing veterinarians to respond impulsively and not always in their best interests. This is especially the case with veterinarians who have been practicing for only a few years, since they are not likely to have been previously named in a lawsuit or reprimanded by a regulatory agency. It is important for veterinarians to realize that how they initially respond to such allegations can have a significant impact on the outcome. For this reason, it behooves us to become knowledgeable about the processes by which state boards and the courts adjudicate such allegations. The following scenario illustrates how these procedures work in real life.

CRACKERS' CASE HISTORY

Dr. Snape has been in practice for 6 years and has a small animal practice on Main Street in the center of town. He prides himself on keeping current on the standards of care and continually investing in his professional development. He has very recently developed an interest in exotics and has joined several associations, including the Association of Exotic Mammal Veterinarians. Dr. Snape has a loyal following and is beginning to get known in the neighborhood as the modern James Harriot because there is nothing he cannot treat.

Mr. Smith brings in Crackers, an adult yellow-naped Amazon, to be examined by Dr. Snape, and explains that Crackers has not been eating well lately and has lost some weight. He recently noticed discharge from Crackers' eyes and nose, as well. Mr. Smith does not know much about birds and adopted Crackers about 6 months ago from a friend who moved abroad. Dr. Snape performs a physical examination and concludes that Crackers probably has an infection and prescribes a 2-week course of enrofloxacin. While Crackers' symptoms improve, they persist enough that Dr. Snape prescribes an additional 4 weeks of antibiotic therapy.

Two years later, Crackers has a relapse and, this time, both Mr. and Mrs. Smith bring Crackers to Dr. Snape. They came together because Mr. Smith had flu-like symptoms and did not think he could manage bringing Crackers for this visit by himself. In Crackers' relapse, he once again exhibited reduced appetite and weight loss, plus the Smiths noticed that Crackers' droppings were loose with bright yellow urine. They also informed the doctor that Crackers had recently laid eggs.

Dr. Snape's physical examination revealed a distended abdomen and a palpable coelomic mass effect. He diagnosed egg binding, a common condition in both birds and reptiles. Then, without advising the Smiths of his limited experience with birds or offering a referral to a more experienced colleague, he recommended surgery. Dr. Snape obtained verbal consent and informed the Smiths that he felt comfortable performing the surgery since he had done several similar procedures on reptiles. During the surgery, even though no egg was identified, Dr. Snape also performed a salpingohysterectomy as a precautionary measure. Crackers recovered from surgery, and was sent home on antibiotics.

Within a couple of days, Crackers again had a distended abdomen. Losing faith in Dr. Snape, the Smiths sought a second opinion from Dr. Owlson, another veterinarian, whom their neighbor had told them specialized in bird medicine. The Smiths had no idea that such specialists existed. The Smiths requested that Dr. Snape transfer Crackers' medical records to Dr. Owlson and made an appointment. The entries in the medical record were as follows:

> September 16th exam: Adult yellow-naped Amazon, not doing well. Dx: Upper respiratory infection. Rx: Enrofloxacin.
> September 29th: Client called. Crackers improving but still not acting normally. Rx: 4-week refill.
> June 1st exam: Have not seen client for 2 years. Loose feces, distended abdomen. Dx: Egg binding. Tx: No egg identified at surgery; uneventful prophylactic spay performed.

Since Mr. Smith was still not feeling well, Mrs. Smith brought in Crackers. Dr. Owlson's examination and preliminary diagnostics led to a differential diagnosis including liver disease and the probability of reproductive tract disease. Surgical exploration was discussed and recommended for the purpose of obtaining the most expedient diagnosis and determining treatment options. During surgery, Dr. Owlson obtained biopsies of what was a visibly enlarged liver and removed the left oviduct, which had not been entirely removed by Dr. Snape and was impacted with retained egg and yolk debris. Histologic evaluation of the liver biopsies confirmed the presence of liver disease, specifically chlamydiosis and aseptic salpingitis with impaction. Crackers was treated successfully over the next several months and fully recovered.

During the same time, and in addition, Mr. Smith was confirmed to have the disease by his physician after having become very seriously ill, and was treated successfully after a protracted course of hospitalization and nursing care.

Six months later, Dr. Snape receives two letters: one from the state veterinary board of examiners and another from the Smiths' attorney. The state board letter requests that Dr. Snape respond to the Smiths' accusations that Dr. Snape was negligent in (1) failing to inform Mr. Smith that he had limited experience in treating birds; (2) failing to offer a referral to a veterinarian who was qualified and experienced in treating birds; (3) misdiagnosing Crackers' condition; (4) performing a surgical procedure below the standard of care; (5) failing to warn Mr. Smith of the zoonotic potential of chlamydiosis; and (6) failure to maintain appropriate medical records, including a complete surgical report. The correspondence from the attorney includes a copy of a complaint filed with the state court, alleging malpractice and seeking: (1) $65,000 for Mr. Smith's lost wages, (2) $115,000 for emotional distress, and (3) $3700.00 for veterinary expenses and the $4500.00 value of Crackers' lost breeding potential.

What should Dr. Snape do?

Responding to Allegations of Professional Malpractice

How veterinarians address such accusations will in part depend on whether the allegations are in the form of a lawsuit, state board complaint, or both. Regardless of the form in which the allegation is made, the first step veterinarians should take is to carefully read the complaint and determine what is being requested of them and in what time frame. Once this information has been ascertained, they should gather the pertinent medical records and any other documentation relating to the services in question and write down in chronological order their recollection of the events. This should also include obtaining statements from staff members that were involved.

In this case, the complaints allege that Dr. Snape performed a procedure for which he was not qualified or experienced, failed to refer the case, failed to identify a zoonotic potential risk to his client, and had poor medical records. The facts indicate that Dr. Snape examined Crackers, made a diagnosis, and performed a surgical procedure to treat the egg binding. Dr. Snape should carefully review the medical records to corroborate his recollection of the events. Unfortunately, in this case, because the documentation is poor, it will be a scenario of Dr. Snape's word against the Smiths' word. For example, it will be difficult for Dr. Snape to claim that he informed the client of the differential diagnoses and options, including a referral, as there are no such notations in the records. Since Dr. Snape has a legal obligation to maintain medical records, the fact that he has not will imply that he also was careless with his medicine. As he reviews the records, Dr. Snape should write down the events that led to the complaint and ask his staff to do the same. Most veterinarians will find this helpful since it will refresh their memories, help them develop a consistent "story" about what happened, and provide a draft from which to develop a written response.

To not compromise his defense in the lawsuit or state board action, Dr. Snape should immediately contact his professional liability insurance carrier and ask for advice. However, if Dr. Snape suspected earlier that the Smiths might pursue legal action, he should have contacted his insurance carrier at that time. It certainly was a red flag when the Smiths requested that the medical records be transferred to a recognized specialist in avian medicine. Insurance carriers may differ in how they handle negligence actions, but usually require the defendant to fill out a claims form in which the veterinarian describes the circumstances that led to the claim. A claims representative then reviews the facts, makes a recommendation as to a course of action, and may assign an attorney to the case if the complaint cannot be settled quickly. If the Smiths are offered a settlement and reject it, it is likely that an attorney would be assigned to defend Dr. Snape, since in this case, it appears that Dr. Snape's care was substandard in several respects.

In dealing with the letter from the state board, Dr. Snape should be aware that he will most likely be defending his conduct at his own expense, since professional liability insurance carriers generally do not provide coverage for state board actions (exception: AVMA-PLIT offers a limited policy insuring against state board actions). While Dr. Snape may respond on his own, it is usually advisable to obtain legal advice as to how to respond to the allegation(s) and, at the very least, have an attorney review his letter. In drafting his response, Dr. Snape should not underestimate the time and effort it will take to address all the issues in the complaint in an organized and articulate manner. Responses that are disorganized, incomplete, inflammatory, and/or difficult to follow often lead to further investigation by the board as opposed to an early dismissal of the charges. Additionally, Dr. Snape may find it helpful to consult with other veterinarians to see what they think about his set of circumstances and how they would have responded. This will assist Dr. Snape in determining whether he acted within the standard of care and provide an indication as to his liability.

Negligence

The burning issues for Dr. Snape, of course, are whether he was negligent in (1) failing to make the correct diagnosis, (2) performing an unnecessary surgery, (3) failing to refer Crackers to an avian specialist or someone with experience in treating birds, and (4) failing to maintain proper medical records. Our courts and juries decide negligence on a case-by-case basis in light of the specific facts and circumstances of each situation, but veterinarians should be aware of a few general principles. First and foremost, it is important to note that a veterinarian can be found negligent even if he did not intend to cause harm. Simply put, "I didn't mean to" is no defense to "You should have known better." A simple mistake can lead to liability.

Secondly, veterinarians can be found negligent even if the rest of their colleagues would have acted in the exact same way. Judges can determine that the entire industry is at fault if it is in the public's interest. A famous judge, Leonard Hand, once wrote in his opinion that "[c]ourts must in the end say what is required; there are precautions so imperative that even their universal disregard will not excuse their omission."[1] Hence, it is a false security to rely solely on what the rest of your colleagues are doing.

To recover damages from a veterinarian based on negligence, a client must prove four elements by a preponderance of the evidence, meaning it is more likely than not that the veterinarian acted below the standard of care:

Duty of care

Clients must show that their veterinarians "owed" them a duty of care to provide veterinary services of a certain standard. This element is easy to prove because courts almost always find that, once a veterinarian has agreed to provide veterinary services, the veterinarian has also assumed the legal duty to take reasonable care in providing such services. In this scenario, Dr. Snape clearly owed the Smiths a duty to take reasonable care in providing veterinary services to Crackers.

Breach of standard of care

A duty to provide services within the standard of care is breached when veterinarians fail to meet the standard of care as established by the veterinary profession, that is, when they fail to act with the level of skill and learning commonly possessed by members of the profession in good standing. The Smiths will probably be able to prove breach of duty if their attorney can show one or more of the following: (1) veterinarians competent in avian medicine would have made the correct diagnosis and not performed an unnecessary surgery, (2) Mr. Smith would have been warned of the zoonotic potential of the disease (chlamydiosis), and (3) records were not SOAPed (subjective, objective, assessment, and plan methodology of documentation).

Conversely, Dr. Snape will attempt to establish that he did not breach his duty of care by showing that most general practitioners competent in avian medicine (like himself) would have missed the diagnosis and certainly not alarmed Mr. Smith about a zoonotic potential that had no evidence to support its existence. He also would argue that his medical records are consistent with recordkeeping practices of his colleagues. It is at this stage that expert witnesses are hired to testify as to what the standard is in the case.

Proximate cause

Clients must also prove that the veterinarian's failure to provide services within the standard of care "proximately" or "closely" caused the harm suffered by the clients. If the harm suffered by the client is not a result of the veterinarian's actions or omissions, it would be unfair to hold the veterinarian responsible. In our case, it is clear that Dr. Snape's unnecessary salpingohysterectomy and the delay in correct diagnosis caused the additional veterinary expenses and Mr. Smith's lost wages. Suppose, however, that Mr. Smith had lost time at work because of a reason that was unrelated to Crackers' condition (i.e., seasonal downsizing of his employer's workforce). Even though the warning of zoonosis still should have been given, the fact that it was not is not the direct cause of Mr. Smith's lost wages. It would therefore be a lot harder to prove that Mr. Smith's lost wages resulted from *anything* Dr. Snape did or failed to do.

Damages

Even after they have proved negligence, clients must also establish that they suffered harm resulting from such negligence. Since animals are considered to be property under the law and most state courts do not recognize loss of companionship, this harm is usually in the form of an economic loss. As a result, veterinary malpractice awards are usually much lower than in human malpractice cases and clients usually only recover the fair market value of the animal, costs incurred for veterinary care, and the loss of income or profits in cases where the use of the animal is lost. In this case, the Smiths will attempt to collect damages for the veterinary fees and lost value in Crackers, since Crackers can no longer be used for breeding, a purpose that they claimed was their intent. They will also want to be compensated for Mr. Smith's lost wages, as well as emotional distress.

Avoiding Client Complaints

Veterinarians can often avoid receiving letters from clients' attorneys and state boards by addressing client complaints long before client dissatisfaction leads to legal recourse. Clients often resort to litigation and/or state board action when they believe their veterinarian either acted negligently or failed to respond appropriately to their concerns. When faced with a client complaint, veterinarians should consider the following:

1. Listen to the client.
   a. Clients who have complaints are often angry and need the opportunity to vent.
   b. Veterinarians should show their clients that they are taking the matter seriously by listening carefully to what they say and taking notes of the conversation.
   c. Do not interrupt the clients since this will only anger them further and likely interfere with a clear understanding of the facts.
2. Remain calm and objective.
   a. Avoid becoming defensive and/or emotional, since this may inadvertently reinforce the client's belief that the veterinarian acted inappropriately with respect to the care of the client's pet.
   b. A client's criticism of a veterinarian's actions, even when fully justified, does not necessarily mean that any negligence occurred. Veterinary medicine is an imperfect science and veterinarians are not omnipotent.
3. Communicate, communicate, communicate.
   a. Many lawsuits are filed because veterinarians fail to adequately communicate with their clients. Often the client does not fully understand the diagnosis and/or proposed treatment and has unrealistic expectations as to the veterinarian's services and the respective outcome.
   b. Veterinarians can enhance communication and reduce potential misunderstandings by (1) obtaining informed consents, (2) providing fee estimates, (3) encouraging questions, and (4) providing handouts explaining the contemplated services.
   c. Veterinarians should use plain English when communicating to clients since medical jargon may not only confuse clients but also intimidate them, making them reluctant to ask important questions.
4. Show sympathy and concern.
   a. Clients whose pets have died are often emotionally distraught and, under certain circumstances, may seek to blame someone (sometimes their veterinarian) for their pet's death. Veterinarians who are compassionate and attempt to comfort their clients are more likely to diffuse their client's perception that the veterinarian should be held accountable for their pet's death.
   b. Veterinarians should not hesitate to recommend grief counseling for clients who appear to have difficulty coping with the loss of their pet. Several veterinary schools have such hotlines, including the University of California at Davis, University of Florida, and Colorado State University.
5. Coach the staff.
   a. Staff members can help diffuse client complaints and should be coached in what to do and say, if anything, when a client complains.
   b. The staff should remain professional at all times and avoid offensive/defensive discussions with clients who may be less intimidated by staff members and therefore more hostile to the staff compared with the veterinarian.
6. When a mistake may have been made:
   a. Veterinarians should always express empathy and compassion for unfortunate outcomes. Apologetic statements and admissions of fault should be avoided and only be made when the veterinarian is certain of the facts and is sure that a mistake was made. These statements should be made only after coaching from a legal advisor in conjunction with the malpractice insurance carrier and in a controlled setting. This will avoid inflaming a situation that is already riddled with potential misunderstandings. Veterinarians with only a few years of experience should ensure that they have all the facts, as they are more likely to feel guilty and accountable for bad outcomes, even though there was no negligence. Remember that feeling guilty is *not* the same thing as being guilty.
   b. Veterinarians should not offer to settle a malpractice charge or agree to any settlement offered by the client without first contacting their insurance carrier and attorney, since it may be interpreted as an admission of fault, thereby prejudicing their case. Under certain circumstances, it may be appropriate to reduce the client's bill as a gesture of goodwill, in an attempt to amicably and expeditiously resolve a dispute without admitting liability.
7. Do not throw your colleague under the bus.
   a. Veterinarians should exercise caution any time a client or someone else makes disparaging comments about a colleague. Clients who feel they have been wronged will seek reaffirmation by attempting to "color" their story to persuade their new veterinarian that the prior veterinarian made an obvious mistake.
   b. Veterinarians should avoid jumping to conclusions, because circumstances are often not as they appear. You may wonder why a certain test was not performed or a particular recommendation was not made. All too often the recommendation was not made—and a test not performed—because the patient was not yet sick enough and/or the client declined because of financial or other reasons.
   c. If there is a question about the way a case was handled, a veterinarian should contact the colleague and get an

explanation before making any judgments about the set of circumstances. Treat your colleagues as you would like to be treated by giving them the benefit of the doubt.

Just as an ounce of prevention is worth a pound of cure, the best practice to avoid being dragged into a lawsuit or state board investigation is to take measures to avoid client complaints. Even if successful, Dr. Snape will spend a lot of time, effort, and money defending himself in court and before the state board. In retrospect, it would have been far less costly and burdensome if Dr. Snape had informed Mr. Smith that he had limited experience with birds and offered a referral to a veterinarian with experience in treating birds; at a minimum, Dr. Snape should have done his research before arriving at a diagnosis.

Veterinarians will save themselves a lot of grief if they periodically evaluate their practices to identify areas where preventive measures and procedures will help avoid complaints before they start. Additionally, veterinarians should regularly consult with the staff, their colleagues, and perhaps even their insurance carrier to ensure that they are aware of the latest preventive measures adopted by other practitioners. Keeping abreast of developments in the legal liability field should be an integral part of any veterinarian's continuing professional education. Because people are people, there is no way to prevent client complaints entirely. But, in this area like in many others, ignorance is dangerous and a preventive attitude is the best approach.

IMPORTANCE OF SOAPED MEDICAL RECORDS

The importance of medical records in general, and what they should encompass, cannot be overemphasized. The proper and complete documentation of patients' medical information and client communications is by far the best way veterinarians can limit their potential liability. The large majority of sanctions imposed by veterinary state boards, for example, are a result of a veterinarian's failure to maintain complete and accurate medical records.[2]

The medical record is an evidentiary document generated for the main purpose of communicating to others what was done and why it was done, or, if not done, why it was not done. The information within medical records must explain and substantiate a veterinarian's actions or omissions. The shortcoming of most medical records is that they do not contain sufficient information to describe the veterinarian's actions or inactions, and/or the information is not presented in a way that the reader can follow the cognitive reasoning of the veterinarian. Additionally, rarely do veterinarians record clients' refusals to follow their recommendations or clients' noncompliance with important treatments and follow-ups. And, even if some of this information is documented, it is far too frequently rendered meaningless because it is illegible.

Medical records typically encompass the patient records of individual pets, but also include the business and legal documents of the hospital, such as estimates, invoices, hospital handouts, financial records, and all logs. The amount and types of information recorded should be consistent with the

level and complexity of the services rendered. The first place to look for what is required is your state's practice act. Another good comprehensive resource is the American Animal Hospital Association (AAHA) guidelines for an accredited hospital, which are found on the AAHA website.

State practice acts vary but, as a general rule, they require:
1. Separate records for each patient
2. Accuracy: The vet is responsible for this, even if using dictation
3. Complete: Normals, abnormals, *and* not examined
4. Legible: Can dictate; does not have to be your handwriting
5. Unalterable: Set a lock-up time and do not alter the original afterward
6. Easily accessible/retrievable
7. Retained for 3 to 5 years

Generally, the most common information veterinarians fail to include in the medical record is communications with clients, staff, and colleagues regarding the care of the patient. This is likely because, when the communication occurs, the medical record is nowhere to be found and most practices are just not sufficiently well organized to make locating the record any easier than finding a needle in a haystack. Fortunately, advances in computer and intercom technology are helping to reduce this administrative nightmare. As to information that should not be recorded, under no circumstances should medical records include derogatory statements about clients, patients, or colleagues, as such comments come back to crush the credibility of the author.

CONFIDENTIAL CLIENT INFORMATION

Protecting personal information of clients is an ethical duty for all veterinarians, and a legal duty in about half of the states. For example, Illinois Practice Act, 225 ILCS 115/25.17 stipulates: "No veterinarian shall be required to disclose any information concerning the veterinarian's care of any animal except on written authorization or other waiver by the veterinarian's client or an appropriate court order or subpoena . . . When communicable disease laws, cruelty to animals laws, or laws providing for public health or safety are involved, this privilege is waived."

The American Veterinary Medical Association (AVMA) Principles of Veterinary Medical Ethics under Principle II (L) states, "*Veterinarians and their associates should protect the personal privacy of patients and clients.* Veterinarians should not reveal confidences unless required to by law or unless it becomes necessary to protect the health and welfare of other individuals or animals." Even in those states that do not have explicit prohibitions on divulging client confidential information, veterinarians should still exercise caution before revealing client information to a third party. Always attempt to obtain client consent and, in cases of emergency, such as when the health of a person or pet is at risk, be sure there is a paper trail that justifies the disclosure of the confidential information.

To maintain confidentiality of medical records, veterinarians must establish specific procedures for the release of information and adhere to them. Generally, it is preferable to send copies of medical records directly to follow-up veterinarians.

The use of a release form simplifies this process and could look like the following:

> To: [Insert practice name and address of sender]
> I, the owner of or agent for the animal(s) named [insert pet(s) name(s)], hereby request that copies or summaries of the medical records of these animals be released to [Insert recipient practice name, doctor name, address, telephone and fax]
> Owner's signature: _____ Date: _____
> Payment of $ _____ is provided/enclosed for you to photocopy and mail this information as directed.

Necessity of Informed Consent

Consent forms are evidentiary documents that serve to prove that clients agreed to professional services after having been informed of the medical procedure, its risks, and probable outcomes. Veterinarians use these forms to defend themselves against actions in negligence suits brought by dissatisfied clients and to collect unpaid fees from clients who claim that the services were not authorized. Consent forms help to ensure that clients understand the contemplated medical procedure and agree to have it performed on their animals.

Veterinarians and their staff must do more than just present consent forms to their clients to sign. It is not enough for clients to agree to have their animals undergo a medical or surgical procedure; they must also understand the consent they are giving. "Informed" means the clients acknowledge that they have been apprised of feasible alternatives and the possible adverse effects that might arise from the procedure. Veterinarians may be responsible for damages in cases where clients convince judges that they have signed consent forms without understanding their ramifications.

While it is not necessary for veterinarians to provide their clients with mini courses in veterinary medicine, they are required to provide enough information about the risks that would materially affect a "reasonable person's decision" to have his or her pet undergo the contemplated procedure.[a] Furthermore, veterinarians need not disclose risks that are already known to clients or risks that are unknown to the veterinary community. In deciding whether they have provided their clients with enough information about the proposed procedure, practitioners should ask themselves: "Have we discussed this to the point that a reasonable client would be able to make an informed decision?"

The following are elements that should be present in all consent forms to ensure their enforceability[3]:

- Identification of the hospital, veterinarians performing the procedures, the pet/animal owners or agents, and the pets/animals receiving the treatments
- A brief description of the recommended procedures and their associated complications
- Clients' acknowledgment that the procedures have been explained and they understand the procedures and their risks and benefits
- Clients' acknowledgment that they have had an opportunity to ask questions and have received satisfactory responses
- Recorded lists of specific recommended procedures that clients refuse
- Blocks for client signatures and dates

When are consent forms unenforceable?

Even when veterinarians have explained everything that a reasonable client would need to know before agreeing to a procedure and have been successful in getting a signed informed consent, there are certain circumstances when the consent is likely to be unenforceable. Such is the case when clients have based their consents on false, misleading, or incomplete information. Courts are also reluctant to enforce consents signed by clients who are mentally incompetent, under duress, under age, or under the influence of drugs or alcohol. This last condition is often seen in emergency settings where clinicians are faced with clients who have returned from an evening out and are not capable of making informed decisions.

Finally, consent forms that are drafted too broadly, allowing veterinarians to undertake any and all medical and surgical procedures or giving permission for any and all treatments in the future, are usually unenforceable. In the interest of practicality, clients are asked to sign such consents when they first bring their pets to their veterinarians with the intent that they will serve as consents for subsequent visits. Although such consents are valid for the performance of routine procedures and for a reasonable time, veterinarians must realize that, generally, consents are ineffective unless they specifically pertain to procedures they plan to perform.

Problems with obtaining informed consents

There are several reasons why many veterinarians are reluctant to use consent forms in their practices. Obtaining informed consents is time-consuming for staff members and veterinarians because it may require lengthy explanations and generates additional paperwork and paper storage. Additionally, veterinarians fear that, if the procedure is "too clearly" explained, their clients will be overwhelmed by the information, refuse to provide a signature, or overreact, leaving their pets untreated or incompletely treated.

While these are all valid concerns, they must be weighed against the financial, emotional, and clerical burdens of collecting unpaid fees and defending lawsuits. Veterinarians should recognize that signing consent forms is normal in the human health care industry and clients have accepted this as essential to their receipt of medical care. Implementing consent forms as part of the practice's policies may seem daunting initially but will become quite routine with time and practice, and undoubtedly will facilitate the delivery of professional services.

CONCLUSION

Being accused of malpractice can be a disconcerting experience for any veterinarian, but especially for associates who have been in practice for only a few years. These allegations can come in the form of a civil lawsuit or state board action, and require veterinarians' immediate attention so as not to

---

[a]This standard is extrapolated from that which is required of physicians in New Jersey; see *Largey v. Rothman*, 110 N.J. 204 (1988). Readers should note that states differ on what standard is used to determine whether physicians provided their patients with enough information about the risks associated with the contemplated procedure.

compromise their defense. Preparing a defense against such allegations is facilitated by having knowledge of the law of negligence and an understanding of the adjudicatory process. Nonetheless, the best defense lies in addressing client complaints when they first arise by using honed listening and communication skills, keeping abreast of the standard of care within the industry, and adopting preventative measures.

REFERENCES

1. Hooper TJ: [60 F.2d 737 (2d Cir. 1932)].
2. Babcock SL, Doehne JR, Carlin EP: Special report, *JAVMA*, 244(12):1397–1402, 2014.
3. Flemming D: The informed consent doctrine: what you should tell your clients, *Calif Vet* 13, 1997.

FORENSIC NECROPSY

Robert E. Schmidt

Forensic medicine is a relatively new concept in veterinary medicine.[1] Much of what has been written is concerned primarily with animal abuse.[2] The dictionary definition of *forensic* is of, relating to, or denoting the application of scientific methods and techniques to the investigation of crime. This definition has been expanded to imply detailed collection of evidence whether or not there is/was a specific legal case.[3] In avian medicine, forensic cases have involved litigation over environmental, nutritional, and medical hazards, particularly allegations of malpractice and animal abuse. The avian practitioner can become involved in such cases as a referral source or as one directly involved in a particular case. Cases involving wildlife are less likely to be encountered as any that appear to involve federal laws are sent to the U.S. Fish and Wildlife Service Forensics Laboratory. Because there is a potential for monetary and reputational damage when such cases occur, the avian practitioner should have a clear picture of all the steps necessary to achieve a satisfactory result, including a thorough and proper necropsy. This discussion is a part of an overall chapter covering practice management and risk management topics and will cover the avian necropsy, including necessary documentation and sample collection.

Although this discussion is designed to give the avian practitioner guidance in performing a forensic necropsy, it is recommended that, if possible, the necropsy be referred to a board-certified pathologist with avian experience. This is because there may be court proceedings, and there could be challenges to the information gleaned from the necropsy based on the practitioner's appropriate credentials. Ideally, in any legal case, the practitioner would be working complementarily with the pathologist to evaluate all aspects of the case. In reality, however, in most instances the avian practitioner will be responsible for the necropsy portion of the postmortem examination. There are several reviews of avian necropsy procedures available.[4-7]

To obtain the maximum value from a necropsy, consultation with a pathologist with training and experience in avian disease and histopathology is necessary. Although pathologists that primarily see mammalian tissues may be able to make morphologic diagnoses, in some cases interpretation of the lesions requires knowledge of avian diseases and the ability to discuss what the findings mean for the particular species in question. Not only are there species-specific diseases, but the same disease can have different morphologic presentations in different avian species. Remember that you are the pathologist's client, and as such have a professional relationship similar to the one your clients have with you. This implies that there are ethical considerations to be adhered to regarding information exchange and release. For any given case, the pathologist cannot discuss findings with third parties unless your permission is given.

In many cases the bird is presented dead with a request for a necropsy. In these cases as detailed a history as possible should be obtained. In other situations you may be called to the place where the dead bird was found. Again, a detailed history is important, but a careful examination of the environment must be made. Anything that does not seem "normal" should be noted and photographically documented. This includes alterations in size, shape, and color of organs; excessive fluid accumulation; and anything that appears to be traumatically induced.

Since any given case may end up in legal proceedings and possibly a trial, accurate and thorough documentation is necessary. This requires that the prosecutor or an assistant take complete notes and photographs. Photographs should begin with the unopened body and be taken at each stage of the necropsy. They should include all organ systems even if no gross change is apparent. Save the leg band and/or any other identifying material, record the microchip number if present, and always be sure to obtain signed written permission for the necropsy. This is especially important when there is potential legal action.

Necropsy of most birds (except the very large) can be done with a minimum of equipment. Poultry shears, scissors, scalpel, and thumb forceps are all that is required. Appropriate safety precautions must be observed. At the minimum, an apron or protective coat and gloves should be worn. If there is any possibility of a zoonotic disease, a mask and possibly more extensive protection would be advised (Figures 24-2 and 24-3).

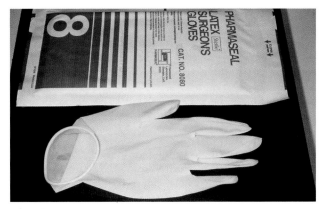

FIGURE 24-2 Example of gloves used in necropsy. Examination gloves are also acceptable.

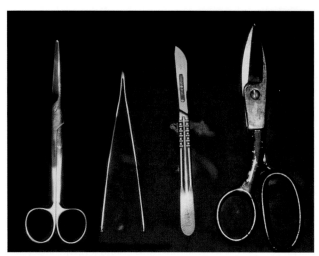

FIGURE 24-3 Minimal set of instruments for an avian necropsy. All birds except very large species can be necropsied using these instruments.

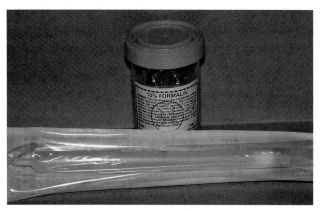

FIGURE 24-4 Formalin for collecting tissue and sterile swab used to collect samples for bacteriology.

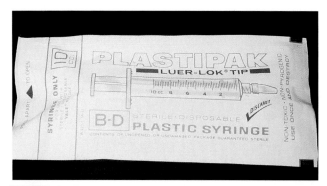

FIGURE 24-5 Sterile syringe needed to collect fluids when microbiologic examination is necessary.

To obtain appropriate samples for immediate examination or submission to the laboratory, clean glass slides, paper towels, sterile swabs, and a container with fixative should be available. The best routine fixative is 10% neutral buffered formalin. Supplies can usually be obtained from a commercial laboratory or local medical laboratories. Sterile syringes may be needed to collect fluids for culture and are useful for

cytology so there is no confusion as to the source of microorganisms on the slide. Containers for tissue to be frozen should also be available. Frozen tissue will be needed for toxicology if indicated and for polymerase chain reaction or DNA analysis if needed (Figures 24-4 and 24-5).

ORGANIZATION AND METHODOLOGY

The keys to gaining the maximum information from the gross necropsy are thoroughness and consistency. The actual approach is less important than conducting the necropsy the same way each time. Each organ and tissue should be evaluated and described to ensure that nothing is overlooked. All changes should be documented with a description, not a diagnosis. Use terms that include size, shape, color, consistency, and smell that the prosecutor should quantitate when possible. Avoid redundancies such as "brown in color." Samples for toxicology and microbiology should be taken as soon as possible. Samples for microbiology in particular should be obtained before there is much carcass manipulation. A representative sample of all tissues should be saved, and in forensic cases a duplicate set is advisable in case there is any problem, particularly with shipping to the laboratory.

If the necropsy is done in the clinic certain guidelines should be observed. Do not allow the owner to view the necropsy. In almost all cases the owner is not capable of interpreting what is seen and done. Always be sure the owner is aware of what a necropsy entails, and that unless it was a *cosmetic* necropsy, remains returned for home burial or other disposition should not be viewed by family members.

Return the body to the owner or agency requesting the necropsy or obtain signed written permission to keep/dispose of it. It probably should be kept frozen until the case is finalized. Remember to document the chain of custody for all material sent to any laboratory/pathologist. It is also a good idea to always have a third party present during all discussions of problems or disputes with the owner of the bird, if applicable. In many cases the bird is presented dead with a history of "sudden death." This history should be evaluated in light of the gross changes.

General Considerations in Interpreting Gross Lesions

A relative lack or excess of blood contributes to the size, color, and consistency of any organ. Color changes may occur before or after death. The differences will be noted with experience. The consistency of any organ may be affected by both antemortem conditions including cell infiltration and connective tissue proliferation, and by the amount of time postmortem that lapses before the necropsy is done. Tissue loss may lead to symmetrical or asymmetrical changes in organ size and weight. Loss can indicate necrosis or atrophy and excess tissue may be from hypertrophy, hyperplasia, or neoplasia.

Necropsy Procedure and Systematic Review

Weights and measurement of the carcass and organs may be of benefit if there are published normals for the species.

After carefully examining the carcass, the bird should be placed on its back (Figure 24-6).

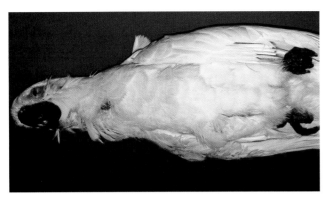

FIGURE 24-6 Placing the carcass on its back to begin the necropsy procedure.

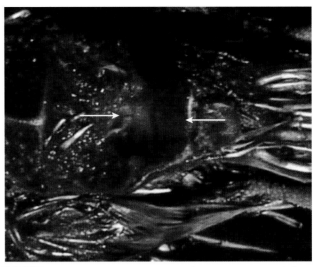

FIGURE 24-8 Green discoloration of the skin *(arrows)* from postmortem degeneration.

A. *Integument.* Feathers should be removed from the jaw to the cloaca (Figure 24-7). Feathers grow in tracts with areas of nonfeathered skin between. The shape and general appearance are similar across most avian species. With increasing time postmortem, feathers become easier to remove. If the skin rips when removing feathers, it is usually a sign of advanced autolysis. With autolysis the skin will be green-black (Figure 24-8). Check for signs of trauma such as bruises and lacerations. Also check for "stress" marks in feathers. Examine for lumps and areas of thickening.

If there is poor feathering and loss of feathers, review specific conditions.

B. Musculoskeletal system. Normal color of muscle in most pet species is red-brown. Pale areas and streaks can indicate degeneration and/or inflammation; the size and shape of pectoral muscles are indicators of general condition and nutritional status (Figure 24-9). In young birds, malformations of leg, wing, or beak are probably from congenital problems of skeletal development, and soft bones that bend but do not break indicate osteopenia or osteodystrophy. Specific disease syndromes include:
   a. *Polyomavirus infection.* May lead to muscle hemorrhage.
   b. *Sarcocystis infection.* Can lead to foci of necrosis and some hemorrhage, as well as white foci representing areas of sarcocyst formation in some species.

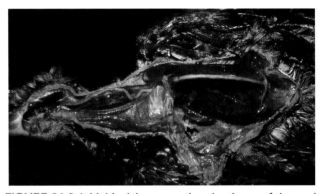

FIGURE 24-9 Initial incision, exposing the tissue of the neck and the pectoral muscles.

   c. *Vitamin E deficiency.* Common cause of muscle pallor, which can be seen as streaks or large pale areas.
   d. *Parasitism.* Includes sarcosporidiosis and migrating metazoans.
   e. *Rickets and osteomalacia.* Lead to bones that may bend under pressure.
   f. *Trauma.* There should be a careful examination for penetrating wounds and fractures.
   g. *Neoplasia.* Unusual in the muscle of typical pet species; however, bone tumors are not uncommon.
After examining the skin, skeletal muscle, and bone, the abdominal cavity should be opened (Figure 24-10). If there is an effusion, samples can be taken for cytology and microbiology. The incision should then be continued through the ribs and up the neck to the jaw. The angle of the jaw should be transected to expose the oral cavity and pharynx (Figure 24-11). All organs should then be examined in situ before removing.

C. *Cardiovascular system.* The pericardial sac should be translucent, with minimal pericardial fluid. The shape of the heart is roughly conical. The left atrioventricular (A-V) valve is membranous but the right A-V valve is a muscular flap. Color changes include pallor (degeneration

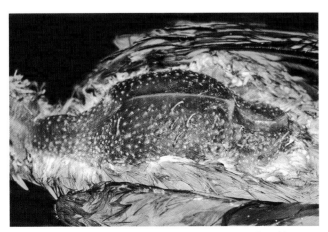

FIGURE 24-7 Plucking feathers to expose the skin.

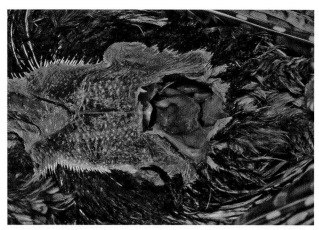

FIGURE 24-10 Opening the peritoneal cavity for initial inspection.

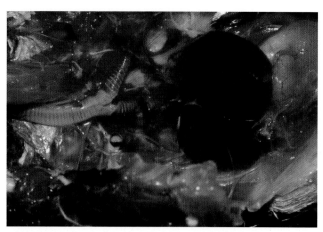

FIGURE 24-12 Visualizing the lungs and liver after removing the heart.

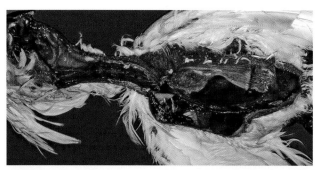

FIGURE 24-11 Extending the incision to open the entire peritoneal cavity.

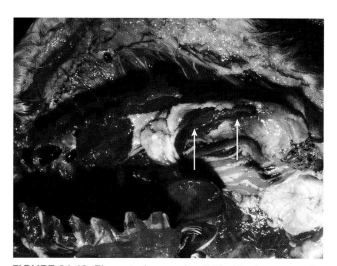

FIGURE 24-13 Elongated normal gall bladder in a penguin.

or inflammation), reddening (hemorrhage), and yellowing (often associated with atherosclerosis). In atherosclerosis the blood vessels of the heart may be more rigid than normal. Open the heart in the path of the blood flow if possible. Complete hemisection is often done in small birds. Open major blood vessels and check for atherosclerotic plaques either visually or by touch. Do not mistake fat for lesions. Specific disease syndromes include:

a. *Viral infections.* Gross lesions include hemorrhage and pale streaks and foci.
b. *Localization of other systemic infections.* Include bacterial infections and systemic protozoal infections such as *Sarcocystis* sp.
c. *Nutritional myopathy.* Usually presents as areas of pale streaking in the myocardium. No exudate should be seen.
d. *Metabolic lesions*
   1. *Gout.* Gross changes associated with visceral gout will include the deposition of white material in/on the pericardium and epicardium.
   2. *Atherosclerosis.* Presents grossly as yellow foci or streaks that usually are associated with medium or large intramural arteries.
e. *Traumatic lesions are usually obvious.* If there appears to be trauma foreign objects should be looked for.

D. *Alimentary system including liver and pancreas.* Examine the liver and entire alimentary tract in situ, including tongue, oral cavity, and cloaca, and remember species variations in size and shape of the crop and ventriculus particularly. Some species have cecae, but there is considerable variability. In many herons and bitterns, only one cecum is present, and in the secretary bird there are two pairs of ceca.[8] In general, herbivorous birds have larger ceca than either omnivores or carnivores. Remove and examine the liver. Normal liver is red-purple and has smooth margins (Figure 24-12). Many species have small or essentially no gall bladder, but some can be large (Figure 24-13). The liver is involved in many systemic processes and may be uniformly enlarged, contain variably sized focal or multifocal lesions, or be discolored. There are a number of specific diseases of liver with gross changes that are similar and cannot be distinguished on gross examination. Autolysis must be differentiated from antemortem lesions, which may necessitate histopathology.

In the intestinal tract, color changes may be due to postmortem autolysis. Do not overdiagnose gastrointestinal

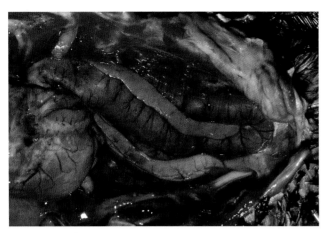

FIGURE 24-14 Normal avian pancreas.

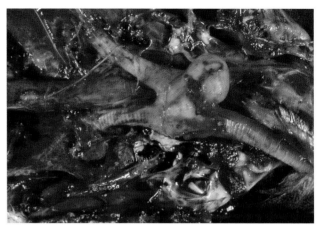

FIGURE 24-15 Normal syrinx in a male duck. This could be diagnosed as an abnormality if species differences are not known.

disease. The intestinal contents become progressively more bile stained in the distal position of the tract. Differentiate hemorrhage from severe congestion if possible. Open all segments. Check for abnormal contents (e.g., parasites). Save gastrointestinal contents for toxicology.

Specific intestinal diseases include bacterial, mycotic, and parasitic infections; viral infections; and neoplasia. A common tumor is proventricular carcinoma, usually seen at the junction with the ventriculus. It may be flat and difficult to see grossly. The pancreas should fill duodenal loop and is usually cream colored or slightly pink (Figure 24-14). Nodularity or a granular appearance is abnormal. Acute pancreatic necrosis is most common in Quaker parakeets, but may also be seen in other psittacines. Grossly there is hemorrhage and discoloration.

After removal of the gastrointestinal tract and pancreas, other organ systems can be examined and appropriate tissues taken for histologic examination.

E. *Respiratory system*. There are species differences in size and shape of the trachea and syrinx (Figure 24-15). Do not mistake syringeal muscles for the thyroids (Figure 24-16). The lower respiratory system should be examined first. Foreign material or excess secretion may accumulate in airways. The lungs should be removed and all surfaces examined (Figure 24-17). The air sacs should be translucent, but will opacify with age. The avian respiratory system is very sensitive to irritation and birds will have problems in environments that do not obviously affect mammals. Numerous inhaled irritants/toxins can cause respiratory difficulty and sudden death. The common gross appearance is a red wet lung. Remember that the pneumatized air spaces in the bones communicate with the respiratory system. Pneumatized bones include cervical and anterior thoracic vertebrae, the posterior thoracic vertebrae, synsacrum and hind limb and the sternum, sternal ribs, coracoid, clavicle, scapula, and forelimb.

The upper respiratory system—nasal passages and sinuses—can be accessed after the brain has been removed. The head can be transected longitudinally. Infections can lead to accumulation of exudate, and neoplasia may present as solid, space-occupying masses in nasal passages or sinuses.

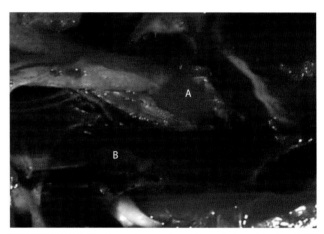

FIGURE 24-16 Syringeal muscles *(A)* and thyroid gland *(B)*. Note proximity and similar shape and color. Syringeal muscles can be mistaken for the thyroid gland.

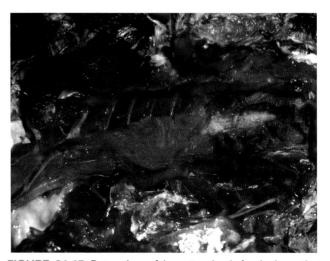

FIGURE 24-17 Retraction of lung to check for lesions that may only be visible on the dorsal surface.

F. *Urinary system.* The kidneys have three main divisions and are usually red-brown or yellow-brown. The cranial division of the kidney is usually the largest and is often mistakenly considered abnormal grossly, although there is no lesion and the kidneys are histologically normal.

In young birds, the kidney is often actively hematopoietic, which can lead to gross mottling (Figure 24-18). Color and consistency changes can be antemortem or postmortem.

Specific diseases include viral infections, such as polyomavirus, herpesvirus, and adenovirus, and bacterial infections. Renal *Coccidia* is seen in some species, particularly waterfowl. Other types of protozoa may also affect the kidney, such as toxoplasma and cryptosporidia.

Nutritional and metabolic disorders may affect the kidney. The common gross appearance with any of these conditions is paleness of the renal parenchyma and multiple yellow-white foci or streaks

G. *Hematopoietic and lymphoid tissue.* In young birds hematopoiesis can be seen in kidney, liver, spleen, and bone marrow. In parenchymal organs it may present as multifocal to confluent red foci in the liver and kidney.

Primary lymphoid organs are the thymus and bursa of Fabricius. Thymic tissue is present in the neck, from the angle of the mandible to the thoracic inlet, in young psittacines (Figure 24-19). The bursa of Fabricius is in the dorsal portion of the cloacal wall (proctodeum), slightly to the left of midline in most psittacine birds. It is round to oval (Figure 24-20). In ratites the bursa is comprised of papillary structures and is more difficult to see grossly. The bursa will involute with age, and knowing the age of the bird to be necropsied is important in assessing the appearance and condition of the bursa. In young birds, stress of any sort can lead to premature bursal atrophy.

Long bones can be broken and marrow placed in formalin for histology. Marrow smears can also be made at this time. The spleen is a sensitive indicator of primary and secondary disease in birds.

Specific diseases include infectious diseases that can affect all hematopoietic tissue. Viral infections may destroy the bursa and/or thymus in young birds. Lymphoid and myeloid neoplasms will present as enlargement of the affected organ.

Metabolic diseases ("fatty" spleen) may result in enlargement and discoloration of affected tissue.

H. *Endocrine system.* The pituitary gland is present at the base of the brain and may become neoplastic, particularly in budgerigars, leading to distortion/displacement of the brain. The thyroid glands and parathyroid glands are cranial to the thoracic inlet, associated with the carotid arteries. The syringeal muscle is almost the same color as the thyroid glands and is often mistaken for the thyroid. The thyroid and associated parathyroid glands will be slightly more cranial and lateral in the neck. The adrenal glands are at the cranial division of the kidney. Any enlargement in this area must be carefully located to see if it originates in the cranial kidney, the gonad, or the adrenal gland.

Specific disease conditions include atrophy, degeneration or hyperplasia of any endocrine organ, inflammation that can lead to gross swelling and reddening, and neoplasia. Adrenal degeneration is most common in Grey parrots, and may be a cause of sudden death.

I. *Reproductive system.* In females the right ovary and oviduct are vestigial and the gonads in some species may be pigmented. In seasonal breeders, the testicles may be greatly

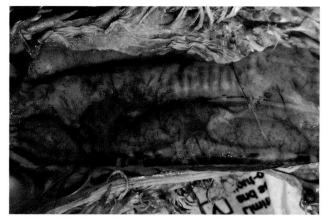

FIGURE 24-19 Normal thymus in a young bird. The tissue can be extensive and occur anywhere in the neck.

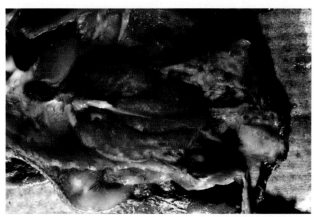

FIGURE 24-18 Renal discoloration in a young bird from extramedullary hematopoiesis; this is normal for many species.

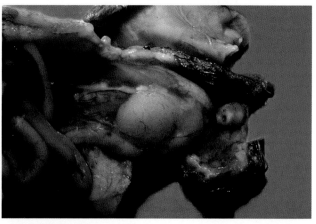

FIGURE 24-20 Normal bursa in a young psittacine bird.

enlarged. In females the oviduct is flat when inactive, but enlarges and becomes tortuous after ovulation. If no ova are in transit, enlargement and dilatation can indicate inflammation.

Specific diseases include oophoritis from any cause. Grossly the ovary may be enlarged and discolored. Salpingitis cases may have exudate in the oviduct, and if the oviduct is perforated there may be associated peritonitis. Egg binding/dystocia will be obvious when an egg or portion of an egg is present in the oviduct/uterus associated with discoloration, hemorrhage, and/or necrosis of a portion of the oviduct.

Neoplasia may be of ovarian or oviductal origin in females. When extensive, it may be difficult to determine the exact origin, as proliferative lesions can be present throughout the peritoneal cavity. In males testicular neoplasia must be differentiated from adrenal gland and cranial renal tumors. Common testicular tumors include seminoma, Sertoli cell tumor, and interstitial cell adenoma. Grossly they cannot be differentiated.

J. *Central and peripheral nervous systems.* In larger birds the brain can be removed after the cranial cap is removed. In smaller birds the entire head can be hemisected and the brain removed (Figure 24-21). Traumatic injury must be differentiated from other conditions that cause clinical central nervous system (CNS) signs. In young birds congenital malformations and hydrocephalus may be causes of neurologic signs. Specific diseases may be viral including paramyxovirus, polyomavirus, adenovirus, and bornavirus (proventricular dilatation disease). Bacterial meningoencephalitis will usually lead to gross exudate in the meninges, particularly on the basilar surface of the brain.

Toxicities usually have no gross change. Neoplasia can be central or peripheral but this is uncommon. Inflammation of ganglia and peripheral nerves is seen histologically in proventricular dilatation disease, but gross changes are limited to the affected viscera.

K. *Special senses:*
a. *Eye.* If the bird is blind or has an obvious ocular lesion, the eye should be removed and examined histologically. All extraneous tissue and extraocular muscles should be removed prior to fixing. Specific ocular diseases may be viral; particularly poxvirus may cause proliferative lesions on the eyelids. Viruses that can cause CNS lesions can potentially cause retinitis. A variety of bacterial organisms can cause inflammation of all or part of the eye. Chronic granulomatous inflammation may be associated with generalized mycobacterial infections. Aspergillus is a common cause of severe keratitis or conjunctivitis and some protozoal infections can include keratitis. Nematodes may be present in the conjunctival sac or be intraocular. Primary tumors of the eye include medulloepithelioma, lymphosarcoma, and melanoma. With the exception of possible pigmentation in melanomas, a specific diagnosis cannot be made grossly.
b. *Ear.* Otitis externa may be grossly obvious, but the inner ear is rarely examined. With vestibular signs, the middle and inner ears should be examined histologically as paramyxovirus infection can cause otitis interna, particularly in finches and *Neophema* sp. Bacterial or fungal infections are usually a cause of otitis externa and cause obvious signs of inflammation including redness and exudation. Carcinoma of the glands of the ear canal is occasionally seen.

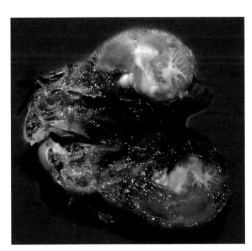

FIGURE 24-21 Longitudinal section of the head exposing the nasal cavity, sinuses, and brain.

REFERENCES

1. Munro R, Munro HMC: Some challenges in forensic veterinary pathology: a review, *J Comp Pathol* 149:57–73, 2013.
2. Merck MD: Veterinary forensics: animal cruelty investigations, Ames, IA, 2007, Blackwell Publishing.
3. Cooper JE, Cooper ME: Forensic veterinary medicine: a rapidly evolving discipline, *Forens Sci Med Pathol* 4:75–82, 2008.
4. Williams BH: Ten steps to better pathology results, *Vet Pract News* 14(6):32–35, 2002.
5. Schmidt RE: Necropsy. In Olsen GH and Orosz SE, editors: *Manual of avian medicine*, St. Louis, MO, 2000, Mosby, pp 542–552.
6. Latimer KS, Rakich PM: Necropsy examination. In Ritchie BW, Harrison GJ, Harrison LR editors: *Avian medicine: principles and application*, Lake Worth, FL, 1994, Wingers Publishing, pp 355–379.
7. Munger LL, McGavin MD: Sequential postmortem changes in chicken kidney at 4, 20, or 37C, *Avian Dis* 16:606–621, 1972.
8. McLelland J: Anatomy of the avian cecum, *J Exp Zool Suppl* 3:2–9, 1989.

CHAPTER 25

Common Conditions of Commonly Held Companion Birds in Multiple Parts of the World

Brian L. Speer • Geoffrey P. Olsen • Robert Doneley • Deborah Monks • Frank Verstappen • Enrique Yarto-Jaramillo • Dorianne Elliott • Maggie Weston • Jorge Rivero • Anne McDonald

Although a large number of avian species are kept as companion animals, the more prevalent species likely constitute the majority of what most veterinarians will statistically be seeing in practice. As an example, in one surveyed North American avian species-specific practice, 51.7% of all patient accessions over a surveyed 5-year period were represented by 10 single species, and 70.6% of all patient accessions were represented by their respective genus categories.

The distribution of what particular species or taxonomic groups may be more common in different parts of the world and the nature of their presenting medical and behavioral problems should be expected to vary regionally. This chapter takes a different approach to the scope of companion avian practice and is regionally oriented, comparing data by region to facilitate comparisons of what species practitioners may be more likely to expect to see, depending on their geographic location, and what kinds of issues and problems may be more prevalent among those species. In these times when there is a continual need to devote limited time and revenues toward continuing education and improvement of clinical skills, awareness of expected needs and their probabilities should have value.

To guide part of this chapter, practitioners were recruited to participate and provide data from various parts of the world. Regions represented in this survey include North America (Canada), North America (the United States), Mexico and Central America, South America, Africa (South Africa), Northern Europe (Netherlands), and Australasia (Australia). Where possible, computer record-keeping databases were searched to provide as much objective data as possible. Where digital databases were less available, contributors were asked to confer with as many colleagues as possible to assemble the most complete, albeit subjective, input possible. Participating veterinarians were asked to fill out the spreadsheets provided to answer the questions described in Box 25-1.

BOX 25-1 SURVEY QUESTIONS

1. What are the 10 most common pet bird species that are seen?
2. What are the most common medical problems that are seen in each of these species?
3. What are the most common behavioral problems that are seen in each of these species?
4. What are the most common signalment and history for these problems?
5. What are the most common physical examination findings associated with those problems?
6. How was the diagnosis most commonly supported or confirmed?
7. What treatment(s) are available and more common for these problems?
8. What is the expected outcome?

Variations in the species or groups being identified were noted, where appropriate.

The types of problems reported were categorized and grouped empirically by metabolic/nutritional, infectious/inflammatory, behavior, trauma/toxic, neoplasia, anomalous, and degenerative/developmental. There was some degree of understandable overlap between some of these categories (e.g., gout was characterized as metabolic/nutritional, but it could be the result of toxic or even a neoplastic disease condition). Portions of these data are presented here for the reader's benefit.

FINDINGS

Selected portions of the data obtained are displayed in the Tables at the end of the chapter.

DISCUSSION

Many of the medical conditions seen in companion birds around the world have direct or indirect origins in nutrition, husbandry, and lack of owner knowledge. These issues are similar to those that have been cited as pertinent to canine welfare (see Chapter 22).[1] In addition, multiple chronic diseases or conditions were identified, often overlapping and/or concurrently present in avian patients. The greatest variation by region was noted in commonly seen species and most commonly presented problems. Means of diagnosis varied to a lesser degree, and there was less variation in treatment and outcome expectations.

These findings correspond closely in many ways to similar human data: As many as half of all adults, approximately 117 million people in the United States, have one or more chronic health conditions. One of four adults has two or more chronic health conditions.[2] Obesity, cancer, arthritis, heart disease, stroke, and diabetes are included in 7 of the top 10 causes of death in 2010.[3-7] Lack of exercise or physical activity, poor nutrition, tobacco use, and excessive alcohol consumption combine to cause much of the illness, suffering, and early deaths of Americans related to chronic diseases and conditions. Tobacco use continues to be the leading cause of preventable disease and death in the United States.[8]

Intervention at the primary health care level, for example, can have a great impact on reducing relative risk through the consistent delivery of information at the individual patient level in both medical and veterinary medical practices, but its delivery can be inconsistent. As an example, the Centers for Disease Control and Prevention (CDC) reviewed office-based physician visits by patients 11 to 21 years of age that were accompanied by documentation of screening for tobacco use and tobacco cessation counseling, including the provision of medications.[8] Overall, 69.5% of the patients seen were screened for tobacco use. Of those that screened affirmative for tobacco use, only 19.8% received any cessation assistance. Perhaps not surprisingly, cessation assistance was more likely to be delivered during visits in which preventative care was the major reason for the visit (28.9%) than during visits for other reasons (16.7%). Obviously, tobacco use is not nearly as significant in companion bird health, but other aspects of lifestyle, specifically screening for nutritional, husbandry, behavioral, and enrichment factors, likely offer somewhat similar correlates. In the tobacco use survey, noted barriers to assessment and treatment of smokers included lack of knowledge of effective intervention strategies, lack of time, inadequate payment for treatment, and lack of institutional support for routine assessment and treatment of tobacco use. Additionally, physicians specifically cited similar and additional barriers, including (1) large patient caseloads, resulting in limited time per patient; (2) competing health care demands during preventive visits; (3) inadequate training; (4) lack of information on how to access referral and treatment resources; (5) lack of dissemination of research to physicians that supports positive treatment outcomes and prevents negative effects from failing to intervene; (6) fear of alienating patients and their families; and (7) inadequate reimbursement. Promising approaches for increasing delivery of tobacco preventative services were noted to be a variety of provider and client reminder systems and increased provider training. These noted barriers and potential approaches to reduction of risk

factors have many almost identical correlates in primary and secondary prevention methods of avian health care. In primary prevention, methods are used before the patient becomes diseased, with the goal of preventing the disease from occurring. Secondary prevention is used after the disease has developed but before the patient is profoundly affected by the condition, with the goals being diagnosis and early treatment.

It is highly probable that similar barriers exist in the delivery of avian health care. Identification of inappropriate dietary management or early clinical signs of illness with caged and companion bird species can likely offer proactive intervention opportunities similar to screening and cessation counseling for the risk behavior of cigarette smoking for age groups 11 to 21, as noted above. As with cigarette smoking, in which only 19.8% of cigarette smokers were provided cessation advice, there is likely to be weak discussion, advice, and counseling about diet change for birds during typical veterinary consultations. The barriers cited by physicians in regard to tobacco use screening and cessation guidance probably have similar correlates in avian health care.

Improved screening and interventions likely can have great preventative value for issues pertinent to nutrition, husbandry, behavior, and welfare of companion bird species. Standardized history collection and record-keeping methods, leveraging empowered staff as part of client-centered practice methods to facilitate screening and interventions, and good communication skills are essential for effectiveness. These details are balanced with a regionally specific and sound understanding of risk factors and their associations with health and welfare issues. Executed well, these maneuvers should enable veterinarians to reduce the number of nutritional and metabolic health–associated problems that so commonly afflict companion birds on a worldwide basis, as well as improve the quality of their lives. There are, however, additional challenges for veterinarians in their efforts to deliver preventative health care for birds, above and beyond issues of need for improved screening and proactive, evidence-based preventative intervention. These challenges are slightly varied, depending on region of the world, but are largely affected by details of the nature of the pet trade itself, along with cultural, economic, and ethnic variables. The perspective provided from South America highlights some of these issues, and potential areas where veterinary involvement can favorably influence the health and welfare of companion birds are described below.

THE PERSPECTIVE ON AVIAN MEDICINE IN SOUTH AMERICA

Jorge Rivero, Maggie Weston

South America, comprising 12 individual countries, is the planet's fourth largest continent. This continent is highly diverse in a multitude of ways. The continent is dominated by the Andes Mountains in the west, while the east contains highland regions, large river basins, and the Amazon rainforest. The geographical diversity of South America is second only to the diversity seen among its people. South America is host to cultures originating from the traditions of indigenous people, combined with those of European, African, and Asian immigrants. Because of the wide variety of cultural, ethnic, and economic backgrounds, how the people of this continent view birds, both in the wild and in captivity, can vary significantly. South America is home to over 3000 different bird species, comprising over one third of the world's total. Many of the continent's wild bird species are involved in illegal pet trafficking, most of these of the family Psittacidae; these species are the most popular in the trade, with the number one reason being that people buy parrots in the belief that they will get a "talking" bird.[9]

The illegal parrot trade is rampant in all South American countries.[10,11] Although the majority of countries have legislation in place against this practice, most of this legislation is poorly enforced.[11-13] Parrot species commonly seen in the trade, including multiple *Amazona*, *Ara*, and *Aratinga* species, vary according to the region involved.[14] These birds taken from the wild eventually end up in big city markets, where they can be purchased and kept as pets.[10,12] Other avian species commonly kept as pets include canaries, budgerigars, cockatiels, and lovebirds, all of which are domestically bred. Few bird owners understand the proper diet and husbandry for the birds that they keep, and even fewer seek veterinary care.

The majority of the diseases most commonly seen by avian veterinarians in South America are directly related to improper husbandry and diet.[10] Most birds are kept in cages far too small for their size with limited enrichment opportunities. This is a result of a widespread misunderstanding of how a bird should be properly kept, and of economic factors. This can lead to a variety of behavioral conditions such as feather-destructive behavior (FDB). In addition, most pet birds are fed sunflower seed–based diets, occasionally supplemented with corn or fruit and sometimes leftovers from the family dinner. A contributing factor to this problem is the sheer lack of commercially made formulated diets in many South American countries. Limited availability of formulated diets can pose difficult challenges to efforts to adequately balance a bird's diet. For those few countries that do have access to either imported or domestically produced diets, cost can be a significant inhibiting, if not prohibiting, factor for many bird owners. Improper nutritional conditions can predispose birds to the development of hypovitaminosis A, hypocalcemia and metabolic bone disease, egg laying difficulties, and gastrointestinal infections, and they can increase the risk for developing respiratory infections such as aspergillosis and chlamydiosis.[10,15] Improper nutrition combined with an inadequate captive environment can also contribute to feather-destructive behavior. The same nutritional problems are seen in the smaller pet birds (e.g., canaries, budgerigars, and cockatiels). These species are commonly fed only canary seed or a general small parrot–designated seed mixture. The scope and breadth of the problem of improper nutrition are a mixture of cultural, economic, and educational issues all too common in South America. This situation, in the authors' opinion, is the one that can be most influenced by the avian veterinarian.

Several other problems exist for the avian veterinarian in regard to parrot trafficking. One is the depopulation of wild species, resulting in risk for endangerment and extinction. Through education, avian veterinarians can directly influence conservation efforts. Existing laws must be better enforced, and the general population must be educated not to buy birds from markets dealing with illegally trafficked birds. Veterinarians can educate potential bird owners about what type of bird would best suit their household, and direct these people to the proper channels for acquiring a bird. Veterinarians can also educate people about the illegal parrot trade so that the general public can understand the poor conditions in which birds are often housed and sold. Public health is also a concern. Transporting ill birds across regional and country borders and selling these birds in crowded conditions can increase the risk that people will contract psittacosis, avian influenza, and other diseases.[16,17]

Providing medical and surgical care for birds in South America can be a challenge. Most avian veterinarians have to make do with medications that are typically designed and formulated in strengths for humans. Compounding pharmacies are not as widely available in most South American countries as they are in the United States. Fortunately, most medications designed for dogs and cats can also be typically found and their use extrapolated when treating a bird. As in North America, both name brands and generics for drugs can be found. The most commonly used medications prescribed by South American avian veterinarians include enrofloxacin; ivermectin; doxycycline; metronidazole; meloxicam; vitamin A, D, E, B complex; fipronil; and amoxicillin with clavulanic acid.

Many South American veterinarians have difficulty gaining access to advanced diagnostic and therapeutic medical equipment. In addition, many veterinarians do not have access to ultrasound, radiography, endoscopy, gas anesthesia, or lab machines for blood work. Some can contract out to a lab or university veterinary clinic for needed diagnostics. However, in regard to performing blood work, many diagnostic labs require an excess of blood or are simply unable to run avian blood hematologic and biochemical evaluations. In regard to running a complete blood count (CBC), this problem can be corrected by having more veterinarians learn how to perform a CBC in-house. Microscopes are readily available to veterinarians in most veterinary practices. The cost of diagnosing and treating a bird is also challenging. Many bird owners simply cannot afford veterinary care, and most veterinarians are forced to treat a bird based on history and physical examination findings alone.

The veterinary profession can influence much of how birds are treated in South America. Veterinarians interested in treating birds should strive to gain more opportunities for continuing education in the form of books, publications, online groups, and membership in the Association of Avian Veterinarians (AAV). The type of continuing education brought to South American veterinarians should also be practical according to the individual conditions and limitations of the region and should not just reflect what can be done in the "ivory tower" of avian medicine. Veterinarians can encourage pet food companies to gain affordable access to pelleted bird diets in all South American countries and then educate the bird owner on proper diet and diet conversion. In cases where the bird owner will not feed a pelleted diet, the veterinarian can provide a list of appropriate foods that can be fed that would achieve a more balanced diet. The owners of pet birds should also be informed about how to recognize signs of illness in their bird in order to be more proactive and to reduce or eliminate pain and suffering. Veterinarians can offer public education courses to bird owners in regard to proper husbandry, nutrition, and behavior. In general, economic stability is improving throughout much of South America. In time, it is likely that many veterinarians will have better access to advanced diagnostics and therapeutics, and with proper bird owner education, the need for these things can be recognized. More veterinary schools in South America are starting to offer courses on avian and wildlife medicine. Many veterinarians are also working with wildlife biologists on conservation efforts and on public education to discourage the illegal parrot trade. To encourage domestic bird ownership, veterinarians can work with bird breeders to establish a domestically bred pet bird population. In the authors' opinion, it would be highly beneficial if Latin American avian veterinarians could create an association that represents each country, and that is capable of holding an annual avian conference in Spanish and Portuguese for these veterinarians, enabling a current reality-based education that still keeps an eye on long-term needs for improvement and development in Latin America.

ACKNOWLEDGMENTS

The authors would like to acknowledge the following veterinarians who were interviewed for this chapter: J Rivero (Peru); R. Valderrama (Chile); F. Baschetto (Argentina); R. Mattiello (Argentina); D. Di Nucci (Argentina); F. Pedrosa (Argentina); S. Ierino (Argentina); L. Piparo (Argentina); I. Rodriguez (Bolivia); D. Wehdeking (Colombia); J. Lugo (Colombia); J. Pena (Colombia); A. Castro (Colombia); A. Ortega (Ecuador); A. Coppola (Paraguay); A. Simoza (Venezuela); G. Gonzales (Venezuela); C. Tosta (Venezuela); N. Boede (Venezuela); E. Couto (Brazil); A. Grespan (Brazil); C. Niemeyer (Brazil); R. Prazeres (Brazil).

ADDITIONAL PERSPECTIVES FROM MEXICO AND CENTRAL AMERICA

Enrique Yarto-Jaramillo

The above South American perspectives are in large part reflected in Mexico and Central America, as seen in similar survey information obtained from veterinarians. As in South America, in both of the surveyed geographical regions there are excellent clinicians and surgeons (many specifically from the small animal medicine field) who offer a high-quality service and who have been additionally trained either in general exotic pet medicine, in zoo medicine, or with a solid basis in small animal medicine and surgery. To this author's knowledge, there is not one recognized resident specialist serving in the private or zoo practice settings in Mexico or in Central America, including the American Board of Veterinary Practitioners (ABVP), the American College of Zoological Medicine (ACZM), the European College of Zoological Medicine (ECZM), or Fellow, Australian and New Zealand College of Veterinary Scientists (FANZCVS). The AAV was established in 1980 and is currently the most recognized avian veterinary professional organization in the United States, Europe, and Australia, and presumably has several members from other parts of the world as well. At the present time, no avian species group veterinary association has been formed in Mexico,

Central America, South America, or Africa in conjunction with the AAV, as is seen in Australasia and Europe. Continued communications with the International Committee of the AAV shows promise for improved involvement and participation of our colleagues and students from these parts of the world in the AAV and other professional organizations involved with the field of avian medicine and surgery. The Mexican Association of Zoo, Exotic Pets and Wildlife Veterinarians (AMMVEZOO, AC) was established in 2010, giving rise to different networking possibilities and training programs focused on exotic birds and other taxonomic species groups. AMMVEZOO has promoted and supported the establishment of ALVEFAS (Latin Association of Wildlife Veterinarians), which includes zoo, wildlife, and exotic pet veterinarians, and whose legal formation is taking place at the time of the writing of this chapter (January 2015). The National Autonomous University of Mexico (UNAM) recently launched a specialty program in zoo and wildlife medicine and surgery. This program has been very appealing for students and veterinarians from Mexico, Central America, and South America. It does not, however, provide targeted training of candidates for credentialing for currently recognized specialties with avian species included.

Birds (parrots and canaries) remain among the top three most popular nondomestic animal groups in Mexico, along with reptiles and small mammals, apparently not related to income but to culture. However, as is seen in South America, we know that many birds are still purchased from vendors in the illegal pet trade. Mesoamerican cultures had a fundamental relationship with nature, especially birds. These animals have represented concepts, special meaning, and religious values, as well as serving to form an essential part in their rituals and cosmogony. Continual increases of new information, treatment, and surgical procedures have provided opportunities for avian veterinarians to practice at very high levels.[18] These developments, although they position veterinarians to deliver more science and evidence-based medicine, stand opposite to the historical trends of veterinary health care delivery. In the past, a lack of trained avian veterinary health care professionals was typical (and remains so in some regions); pseudoscientific and non–veterinary-trained health care remains common. An excellent quote summarizes the reality of this to date in many parts of Mexico, Central America, South America, and Africa: "Bird dealers and store owners were a logical resource because of their apparent practical experience with small animals and animal diseases. Pet shops distributed proprietary bottled medications, dispensed written advice, and even performed procedures on sick or injured pets when the need arose."[19] These trends are changing, predominately in the more populated areas of Mexico and Central America. Changes have been most notable in the past few years and should be expected to continue in the future. With improved veterinary contact, a higher level of trained health care, and communication, the future and the changes that it shall bring look bright.

ACKNOWLEDGMENTS

I (EYJ) would like to deeply acknowledge the invaluable support and willingness of my colleagues who took the time to review their extensive files, respond to our questionnaire, and produce tabulated data: Miroslava Alonso Estrada (Mexico); Itzcóatl Maldonado and Aline Ixtab Morales Estrada (Mexico); and Julio C. Reyes (Panama). Other names of contributors are not included at their request.

REFERENCES

1. Buckland E, Corr S, Abeyesinghe S,et al: Prioritization of companion dog welfare issues using expert consensus, *Anim Welfare* 23:39, 2014.
2. Ward BW, Schiller JS, Goodman RA: Multiple chronic conditions among US adults: a 2012 update, *Prev Chronic Dis*: (serial online). http://dx.doi.org/10.5888/pcd11.130389.
3. Centers for Disease Control and Prevention: *Death and mortality*. http://www.cdc.gov/nchs/fastats/deaths.htm. Accessed December 20, 2013.
4. Centers for Disease Control and Prevention: *NCHS data on obesity*. http://www.cdc.gov/nchs/data/factsheets/factsheet_obesity.htm. Accessed December 20, 2013.
5. Hootman JM, Brault MW, Helmick CG, et al: Prevalence and most common causes of disability among adults—United States, 2005, *MMWR Morb Mortal Wkly Rep* 58(16):421–426, 2009. http://www.cdc.gov/mmwr/preview/mmwrhtml/mm5816a2.htm?s_cid=mm5816a2_e. Accessed December 23, 2013.
6. Barbour KE, Helmick CG, Theis KA, et al: Prevalence of doctor-diagnosed arthritis and arthritis-attributable activity limitation—United States, 2010-2012, *MMWR Morb Mortal Wkly Rep* 62(14):869–873, 2013. http://www.cdc.gov/mmwr/preview/mmwrhtml/mm6244a1.htm. Accessed March 13, 2014.
7. Centers for Disease Control and Prevention: *National diabetes fact sheet*, 2011. http://www.cdc.gov/diabetes/pubs/pdf/ndfs_2011.pdf. Accessed December 20, 2013.
8. Jamal A, Dube SR, Babb SD, et al: Tobacco use screening and cessation assistance during physician office visits among persons aged 11–21 years—National Ambulatory Medical Care Survey, United States, 2004–2010, *MMWR Surveill Summ* 63:71–79, 2014.
9. Doest O: Abducted from the wild: illegal pet, illegal vet? *Proc AAV* 361–366, 2007.
10. Weston MK, Memon MA: The illegal parrot trade in Latin America and its consequences to parrot nutrition, health, and conservation, *Bird Populations* 9:76–83, 2009.
11. Juniper NJ, et al: Dimensions and causes of the parrot conservation crisis. In Beissinger SR, Snyder N, editors: *New world parrots in crisis*, Washington, DC, 1992, Smithsonian Institution, pp 1–24.
12. Gonzalez JA: Harvesting, local trade, and conservation of parrots in the Northeastern Peruvian Amazon, *Biol Conserv* 114:437–446, 2003.
13. Guzman JC, Sanchez Saldana ME, Grosselet M, et al: *The illegal parrot trade in Mexico: a comprehensive assessment*, Washington, DC, 2007, The Defenders of Wildlife.
14. Snyder N, McGowan P, Gilardi J, et al: *Parrots: status survey and conservation action plan 2000–2004*, *Gland*, Switzerland, and Cambridge, UK, 2000, IUCN.
15. McDonald D: Nutritional considerations. In Harrison G, Lightfoot T, editors: *Clinical avian medicine*, vol 1, Palm Beach, 2006, Spix Publishing, pp 86–140.
16. Freitas Raso T, Godoy SN, Milanelo L: An outbreak of chlamydiosis in captive blue-fronted amazon parrots *(Amazona aestiva)* in Brazil, *J Zoo Wildlife Med* 35:94–96, 2004.
17. Godoy SN, Matushima ER: A survey of diseases in Passeriform birds obtained from illegal wildlife trade in São Paulo City, Brazil, *J Avian Med Surg* 24(3):199–209, 2010.
18. Lennox AM, Harrison GJ: The companion bird. In Harrison G, Lightfoot T, editors: *Clinical avian medicine*, vol 1, Palm Beach, 2006, Spix Publishing, pp 29–44.
19. Pollock CG: Companion birds in early America, *J Avian Med Surg* 27(2):148–151, 2013.

TABLE 25-1

Common Pet Bird Species by Region

Most Common Species by Region and Order of Prevalence	North America (Western Canada)	North America (Western US)	Central America and Mexico
1	Budgerigar (*Melopsittacus undulatus*)	Cockatiel (*Nymphicus hollandicus*)	Red-lored Amazon (*Amazona autumnalis*)
2	Peach-faced lovebird (*Agapornis roseicollis*)	Grey parrot (*Psittacus erithacus*)	Orange-fronted parakeet (*Eupsittula canicularis*)
3	Cockatiel (*Nymphicus hollandicus*)	Umbrella cockatoo (*Cacatua alba*)	Canary (*Serinus canaria domestica*)
4	Grey parrot (*Psittacus erithacus*)	Budgerigar (*Melopsittacus undulatus*)	Budgerigar (*Melopsittacus undulatus*)
5	Pacific parrotlet (*Forpus coelestis*)	Blue and gold macaw (*Ara ararauna*)	*Ara* spp. macaws
6	Pyrrhura Conure sp	Peach-faced lovebird (*Agapornis roseicollis*)	Feral pigeon (*Columba livia domestica*)
7	Blue-fronted Amazon (*Amazona aestiva*)	Moluccan cockatoo (*Cacatua moluccensis*)	Domestic duck
8	Ring-necked parakeet (*Psittacula krameri*)	Yellow-naped Amazon (*Amazona auropalliata*)	Cockatoo group (*Eolophus/Cacatua* spp.)
9	Citron-crested cockatoo (*Cacatua sulphurea citrinocristata*)	Green-cheeked conure (*Pyrrhura molinae*)	Owls
10	Moluccan cockatoo (*Cacatua moluccensis*)	Chicken (*Gallus gallus domesticus*)	Chicken (*Gallus gallus domesticus*)
11			Moluccan cockatoo (*Cacatua moluccensis*)

South America (Peru)	Northern Europe (Netherlands)	Africa (South Africa)	Australia (Eastern)
Orange-winged Amazon (*Amazona amazonica*)	Grey parrot (*Psittacus erithacus*)	Grey parrot (*Psittacus erithacus*)	Cockatiel (*Nymphicus hollandicus*)
Aratinga conure sp. (*Aratinga* spp)	Budgerigar (*Melopsittacus undulatus*)	Ring-necked parakeet (*Psittacula krameri*)	Budgerigar (*Melopsittacus undulatus*)
Brotogeris sp.	Peach-faced lovebird (*Agapornis roseicollis*)	Cockatiel (*Nymphicus hollandicus*)	Chicken (*Gallus gallus domesticus*)
Canary (*Serinus canaria domestica*)	Cockatiel (*Nymphicus hollandicus*)	Eclectus parrot (*Eclectus roratus*)	Pyrrhura conure sp
Budgerigar (*Melopsittacus undulatus*)	Chicken (*Gallus gallus domesticus*)	Budgerigar (*Melopsittacus undulatus*)	Lorikeets (tribe Loriini)
Pigeons and doves (Order: Columbiformes, Family: Columbidae)	Amazon sp (*Amazona* spp)	Blue and gold macaw (*Ara ararauna*)	Ring-necked parakeet (*Psittacula krameri*)
Mealy Amazon (*Amazona farinosa*)	Senegal parrot (*Poicephalus senegalus*)	Umbrella cockatoo (*Cacatua alba*)	Rose-breasted cockatoo (*Eolophus roseicapilla*)
Festive Amazon (*Amazona festiva*)	Eclectus parrot (*Eclectus roratus*)	Sun conure (*Aratinga solstitialis*)	Eclectus parrot (*Eclectus roratus*)
Yellow-crowned Amazon (*Amazona ochrocephala*)	Rose-breasted cockatoo (*Eolophus roseicapilla*)	Blue-fronted Amazon (*Amazona aestiva*)	Alexandrine parakeet (*Psittacula eupatria*)
Blue-headed pionus (*Pionus menstruus*)	Green-cheeked conure (*Pyrrhura molinae*)	Peach-faced lovebird (*Agapornis roseicollis*)	Sulfur-crested cockatoo (*Cacatua galerita*)
	Blue and gold macaw (*Ara ararauna*)		Blue and gold macaw (*Ara ararauna*)

TABLE 25-2

Commonly Encountered Problems in the Budgerigar *(Melopsittacus undulatus)*

Problem	North America (Western Canada)	North America (Western US)	Central America and Mexico	South America (Peru)	Northern Europe (Netherlands)	Africa (South Africa)	Australia (Eastern)
METABOLIC/NUTRITIONAL							
Obesity	X	X	X	X	X	X	
Malabsorption/maldigestion	X						
Hypovitaminosis A		X	X	X			
Reproductive tract disease (female and male)	X	X	X	X	X		
Noninfectious hepatopathies	X		X				
Chronic egg laying			X	X			X
Egg binding		X	X	X		X	X
Gout	X			X			
INFECTIOUS/INFLAMMATORY							
Sinusitis	X		X	X		X	
Conjunctivitis			X	X			X
Avian polyoma virus				X		X	
Trichomoniasis				X			X
Ectoparasitism			X	X			
Giardiasis				X			
Knemidokoptes sp.			X	X		X	X
Macrorhabdosis		X		X	X	X	X
Coccidiosis				X			X
Bacterial Enteritis			X	X		X	
BEHAVIOR							
Generalized/learned fear							X
TRAUMA/TOXIC							
Lead toxicosis	X						
Trauma		X	X	X	X		
NEOPLASIA							
Neoplasia, nonspecified			X	X			X
Gastrointestinal neoplasia		X					
Renal neoplasia		X		X			
Pituitary tumors	X	X					
Gonadal neoplasia	X	X	X	X	X	X	
Squamous cell carcinoma of uropygial gland		X		X			
ANOMALOUS							
Abdominal Hernia				X		X	
Ingested foreign material/nonspecific gastroenteritis		X			X		
DEGENERATIVE/DEVELOPMENTAL							
Arthritis	X	X					
Renal pathology					X		
Pododermatitis		X		X			
Arthritis/articular gout				X	X		

TABLE 25-3

Commonly Encountered Problems in the Cockatiel (*Nymphicus hollandicus*)

Problem	North America (Western Canada)	North America (Western US)	Central America and Mexico	South America (Peru)	Northern Europe (Netherlands)	Africa (South Africa)	Australia (Eastern)
METABOLIC/NUTRITIONAL							
Malnutrition	X		*	*			
Hypovitaminosis A		X	*	*		X	
Obesity		X	*	*	X		
Xanthoma		X	*	*	X		
Noninfectious hepatopathies	X		*	*		X	
Female reproductive disorders	X		*	*	X		X
Chronic egg laying	X		*	*		X	X
Egg binding	X		*	*		X	X
Gout	X		*	*			
INFECTIOUS/INFLAMMATORY							
Chlamydiosis			*	*		X	
Macrorhabdosis		X	*	*			X
Sinusitis	X	X	*	*	X		
Conjunctivitis			*	*			X
Dermatitis/self-mutilation	X		*	*			
BEHAVIOR							
Male aggressive behavior	X		*	*			
Feather damaging behavior		X	*	*	X	X	X
TRAUMA/TOXIC							
Trauma	X	X	*	*	X	X	X
Heavy metal toxicosis			*	*		X	
NEOPLASIA							
Reproductive neoplasms		X	*	*			
ANOMALOUS							
Ingested foreign material/nonspecific gastroenteritis		X	*	*	X		
Tracheal occlusion		X	*	*	X		
DEGENERATIVE/DEVELOPMENTAL							
Arthritis		X	*	*			
Renal disease		X	*	*	X		X
Neonatal ingluvitis			*	*		X	

*Not reported in this surveyed species group for this region.

TABLE 25-4

Commonly Encountered Problems in *Amazona* sp.

Problem	North America (Western Canada)	North America (Western US)	Central America and Mexico	South America (Peru)	Northern Europe (Netherlands)	Africa (South Africa)	Australia (Eastern)
METABOLIC/NUTRITIONAL							
Malnutrition	X	X	X	X	X	X	*
Hypovitaminosis A				X			*
Obesity		X		X	X	X	*
Noninfectious hepatopathies	X	X		X	X	X	*
Female reproductive disorders						X	*
Cardiovascular disease	X	X			X		*
INFECTIOUS/INFLAMMATORY							
Sinusitis	X	X			X	X	*
Candidiasis				X			*
Ectoparasitism				X			*
Lower respiratory/fungal respiratory disease/aspergillosis	X			X		X	*
Mycobacteriosis		X					*
Papillomatous disease	X						*
Chlamydiosis						X	*
Bacterial enteritis			X	X			*
BEHAVIOR							
Learned aggression		X			X	X	*
Inappropriate pair bonding				X		X	*
Feather damaging behavior		X	X	X			*
TRAUMA/TOXIC							
Trauma	X	X	X	X			*
Heavy metal toxicosis						X	*
NEOPLASIA							
Gastrointestinal neoplasms		X					*
Neoplasia, nonspecific	X		X				*
ANOMALOUS							
Cataracts	X						*
DEGENERATIVE/DEVELOPMENTAL							
Arthritis	X	X	X		X		*
Pododermatitis				X			*

*Not reported in this surveyed species group for this region.

TABLE 25-5

Commonly Encountered Problems in the Grey Parrot *(Psittacus erithacus)*

Problem	North America (Western Canada)	North America (Western US)	Central America and Mexico	South America (Peru)	Northern Europe (Netherlands)	Africa (South Africa)	Australia (Eastern)
METABOLIC/NUTRITIONAL							
Seizures resulting from hypocalcemia			✕	*		✕	
Rhinolithiasis	✕			*			
Cardiovascular disease	✕	✕		*	✕		
Malnutrition		✕	✕	*	✕		
Hypovitaminosis A			✕	*		✕	
Noninfectious hepatopathies	✕			*			
INFECTIOUS/INFLAMMATORY							
Psittacine beak and feather disease	✕			*	✕	✕	
PDD	✕			*	✕	✕	
Fungal respiratory disease/Aspergillosis	✕	✕		*	✕	✕	
Chlamydiosis				*		✕	
Sinusitis				*	✕		
BEHAVIOR							
Generalized/learned fear	✕	✕		*	✕	✕	
Biting behaviors		✕		*			
Feather damaging behavior		✕	✕	*	✕	✕	✕
TRAUMA/TOXIC							
Ingluvial burns				*		✕	
Trauma		✕		*	✕	✕	✕
Heavy metal toxicosis			✕	*		✕	
NEOPLASIA							
Squamous carcinoma of uropygial gland	✕			*			
ANOMALOUS							
Trauma secondary to inappropriate wing trim	✕			*			✕
Ingested foreign material/nonspecific gastroenteritis			✕	*			
DEGENERATIVE/DEVELOPMENTAL							
Arthritis			✕	*			
Renal pathology				*	✕		
Skeleton growth abnormalities				*	✕		

*Not reported in this surveyed species group for this region.

TABLE 25-6

International Patterns of Common Problems and Common Means of Diagnosis*

Problem	North America (Western Canada)	North America (Western USA)	Central America and Mexico
Obesity	Physical examination Radiographs +/− barium Assessment for fatty liver	Physical examination	Physical examination, history, hematology, serum chemistry, tumor excision, and biopsy
Malnutrition	Physical examination, complete blood count, serum biochemistry panel, radiographs, ultrasound	History and signalment, physical examination findings; Diagnostic workup for secondary or tertiary-associated diseases	History (seed-only diets), physical examination, complete blood count, serum biochemistry panel, and radiographs
Cardiovascular disease	Ultrasound Serum biochemistry panel, radiographs	Physical examination, signalment and history, radiographs, ultrasonography	NA
Arthritis	Physical examination, radiographs	Physical examination, radiographs	Clinical history, physical examination, radiographs, and cytology of synovial fluids
Noninfectious hepatopathies	Physical examination, complete blood count, serum biochemistry panel, ultrasonography, radiographs	Physical examination, elevated serum bile acids and sometimes GGT, radiographs (increased or reduced hepatic silhouette); definitive diagnosis via hepatic biopsy	Clinical history, physical examination, radiographs, lipemic blood, serum biochemistry, elevated cholesterol, elevated bile acids.
Egg binding	Physical examination, complete blood count, serum biochemistry panel to include bile acids Ultrasound Radiographs	NA	History and physical examination, radiographs, coelomic ultrasound
Female reproductive disorders	Physical examination, ultrasound, +/− radiographs, +/− coelomocentesis	Clinical history, physical examination, ultrasound, fluoroscopic and/or plain radiographic imaging, surgically obtained biopsy and histopathology	Clinical history, physical examination, radiographs, ultrasound
Sinusitis	Physical examination, complete blood count, serum biochemistry panel, sinus aspirate for cytology and culture, deep nasal Gram stain with culture Skull and whole body radiographs, CT scan imaging	Physical examination findings, cytology of nasal discharge, PCR, aerobic culture	Clinical history, physical examination, radiographs, complete blood count, culture and cytology of exudates
Conjunctivitis	Maybe complicated by MRSA, recommend extended bacterial sensitivity if MRSA present with fungal elements, repeat CBCs to monitor systemic effects	NA	NA
Ectoparasitism	NA	Physical examination	Skin irritation, partial baldness, crusty lesions on legs

CBC, Complete blood count; GGT, γ-glutamyltransferase; NA, not available from data obtained in this survey; PCR, polymerase chain reaction.
*Common problems seen internationally and common means of diagnosis across all surveyed species.

South America (Peru)	Northern Europe (Netherlands)	Africa (South Africa)	Australia (Eastern)
Physical examination, fat deposit over the body, pododermatitis	Physical examination and observation	Compare body weight to average, body condition score.	Physical examination
History and physical examination	History and signalment, physical examination	History of poor diet, typical presenting complaints	NA
NA	Physical examination, radiographs, ultrasound, electrocardiography, serum biochemistry panel	NA	NA
Physical examination, clinical history, radiographs	Physical examination, radiographs	NA	Physical examination, radiographs
Physical examination, clinical history, radiographs	Physical examination, elevated serum bile acids and sometimes GGT, radiographs (increased or reduced hepatic silhouette); definitive diagnosis via hepatic biopsy (hepatic fibrosis most common finding)	Complete blood count, lipemia, raised bile acids, hepatic biopsy for definitive diagnosis	Clinical history, physical examination, radiographs, serum biochemistry with bile acids and cholesterol
Physical examination, clinical history, radiographs	History and physical examination, radiographs, coelomocentesis.	Physical examination and radiographs	Physical examination and radiographs
Physical examination, clinical history, radiographs	Clinical history, physical examination, coelomic ultrasound or plain radiographic imaging, coelomocentesis	Physical examination, Triglyceride and Cholesterol levels on serum chemistry panel, presence of hormonal activity such as aggression or nesting behavior.	Clinical history, physical examination, serum biochemistry to include cholesterol and triglycerides, radiographs
Physical examination, referral for radiographs; blood can be sent to an outside private lab for complete blood count and serum biochemistry panel	Physical examination	Physical examination, culture of exudates	NA
Physical examination, clinical history	NA	NA	Examination, conjunctival cytology, chlamydia diagnostics
Physical examination, feather examination under microscope	Physical examination	NA	NA

Continued

TABLE 25-6

International Patterns of Common Problems and Common Means of Diagnosis—cont'd

Problem	North America (Western Canada)	North America (Western USA)	Central America and Mexico
Bacterial enteritis	GI culture in enteropathic medium, in-house Gram stain/cytology, radiographs with possibly barium contrast, serum biochemistry panel, coelomic ultrasound if GI perforation is suspected	Fecal cytology, aerobic culture and sensitivity, radiographic and fluoroscopic imaging with contrast, ultrasonography	History, clinical, and physical assessments, direct fecal examination, fecal cytology, complete blood count
Chlamydiosis	NA	NA	NA
Psittacine beak and feather disease (PBFD)	Complete blood count PBFDV PCR of feather pulp	Physical examination, whole blood PCR, skin and feather follicle biopsy	NA
PDD/Bornavirus infection	Bornavirus PCR Rarely biopsy crop Clinical history Radiographs Ultrasound for evaluation of gastrointestinal motility	History and clinical signs, physical examination, rule-outs of other differential diagnoses, plain radiographic and contrast imaging (with fluoroscopy) of the gastrointestinal tract, biopsy of diseased organ system with diagnostic lesions provides definitive diagnosis	NA
Macrorhabdosis	NA	Fecal direct wet mount, PCR	
Fungal respiratory disease/ Aspergillosis	Complete blood cell count, electrophoresis, BP/BA/EPH-often substantial ele WBC, globulin level elevation and low-grade anemia if chronic, radiographs, tracheal endoscopy and cytology Aspergillosis Panel— antibody and galactomannan. Coelomic endoscopy and topical painting of lesions with Amphotericin B. Biopsy for cytology, fungal culture and PCR testing for concurrent Mycobacterium.	Physical examination and history, supportive hematology data, radiography, endoscopy; PCR, aerobic culture or cytology of endoscopy-derived samples	NA
Self-Mutilation	Physical examination, culture and sensitivity of wounds	Physical examination, clinical history, signalment	NA
Learned aggression	Clinical history	Clinical history, physical examination; behavioral evaluation, observation	NA
Inappropriate pair bonding	Clinical history and physical examination	Clinical history and physical examination	Clinical history and physical examination

BA, Bile acids; BP, blood pressure; EPH, serum electrophoresis; GI, gastrointestinal; PBFDV, Psittacine beak and feather disease virus; WBC, white blood cell count.

South America (Peru)	Northern Europe (Netherlands)	Africa (South Africa)	Australia (Eastern)
Fecal cytology and Gram stain, radiographs, complete blood count, serum biochemistry panel	NA	Clinical examination, direct fecal examination and Gram stain, fecal culture	NA
NA	NA	Complete blood count. Antigen PCR on blood and feces, antibody ELISA on blood.	NA
NA	Clinical history, physical examination, complete blood count, serum biochemistry panel, PBFDV PCR and ELISA, sometimes in severe cases necropsy results	Clinical examination and PBFDV PCR	Physical examination, circovirus PCR, hemagglutination assay/hemagglutination inhibition
NA	Clinical history, physical examination; complete blood count with serum biochemistry panel, PCR and ELISA, sometimes in severe cases necropsy results	Radiographs, complete blood cell count, bornavirus PCR on blood/feces, histopathology of crop or proventricular biopsy, necropsy	NA
History and physical examination, fecal Gram stain, fecal direct wet mount	Fecal direct wet mount and hemacolor, culture for bacteria	Fecal direct wet mount	Physical examination, fecal direct wet mount
NA	Physical examination and history, complete blood count, radiographs, endoscopy; PCR, aerobic culture or cytology of endoscopy-derived samples	Complete blood count, serum biochemistry panel, radiographs and endoscopy	NA
Behavioral and husbandry history	NA	Physical examination and history of self-mutilation.	Physical examination, complete blood count, serum biochemistry panel, radiographs
NA	Clinical history, physical examination; behavioral evaluation, observation	History of agonistic behavior, demonstration of aggression.	Behavior assessment
Behavioral and husbandry history	Clinical history and physical examination	Clinical history and physical examination	NA

ELISA, Enzyme-linked immunosorbent assay.

Continued

TABLE 25-6

International Patterns of Common Problems and Common Means of Diagnosis—cont'd

Problem	North America (Western Canada)	North America (Western USA)	Central America and Mexico
Generalized/ learned fear	Rule out underlying health issues. Behavior training Confidence building	Careful behavioral evaluation; medical management of significant concurrent or traumatic injuries	NA
Feather damaging behavior	Complete blood count with serum biochemistry panel, radiographs, skin culture for yeast organisms as an initial data base, skin biopsy, PBFDV PCR and Bornavirus PCR	Physical examination, clinical history, behavioral evaluation, foundational diagnostic database for physical health assessment	Clinical history, physical examination, complete blood count, serum biochemistry panel, PBFDV and polyoma PCR, skin cytology, skin biopsy
Trauma	Physical examination, assess for blood loss and lesions of oral cavity, skull and neck	Clinical history, physical examination, radiographic imaging if indicated	Clinical history, physical examination, and radiographs
Heavy metal toxicosis	Clinical history, radiographs, lead check sticks, blood lead	Clinical history, physical examination findings, radiography/ fluoroscopy, blood lead levels, response to treatment	NA
Gonadal neoplasms	Physical examination, ultrasound, radiographs, +/− barium contrast	Physical examination, coelomic ultrasound, radiographic imaging, surgical, endoscopic or necropsy-derived biopsy for confirmed diagnosis	NA
Ingested foreign material/ Nonspecific gastroenteritis	Radiographs, barium contrast, endoscopy	Clinical history, radiographic or fluoroscopic imaging, gastric endoscopy	Physical examination, clinical history, radiographs, endoscopy, exploratory laparotomy

South America (Peru)	Northern Europe (Netherlands)	Africa (South Africa)	Australia (Eastern)
NA	Behavioral evaluation; history and partially per exclusion	Clinical history, no abnormalities on complete blood count and serum biochemistry panel or radiographs	NA
Behavioral history and husbandry history	Physical examination, clinical history, behavioral evaluation, per exclusion for viral etiologies	Radiographs, complete blood count with serum biochemistry panel, cytology of feathers and feather pulp, and behavioral evaluation	Physical examination, clinical history, skin biopsy
Physical examination findings, radiographic imaging if indicated	Physical examination findings, radiographic imaging if indicated	Clinical examination, palpation and radiographs	Physical examination findings, radiographic imaging if indicated
NA	NA	Radiographs, blood lead and blood zinc concentrations	Clinical signs, hyperuricemia; clinical history
Physical examination, clinical history, radiographs	Physical examination findings, coelomic ultrasound, radiographic imaging, surgical and endoscopic evaluation	Physical examination, radiographs, and ultrasound	NA
Physical examination, clinical history, radiographs	Clinical history, radiographs, complete blood count with serum biochemistry panel per exclusion.	Physical examination, radiography, endoscopy	Physical examination, radiographs

Appendices

APPENDIX 1

Table of Common Drugs and Approximate Doses

James W. Carpenter • *Michelle G. Hawkins* • *Heather Barron**

TABLE 1

Antibacterial Agents

Agent	Dosage	Species/Comments
Amikacin	7–20 mg/kg SC, IM, IV q8–12h	Most species; may cause myositis with IM injection; least nephrotoxic of the aminoglycosides, but renal toxicosis has been demonstrated in some species at 10 mg/kg after 11 days; uric acid levels may be abnormal for up to 7 days after cessation; maintain hydration during use
	15 mg/kg IM q12h, IV q8h	Blue-fronted Amazon parrots/PD
	15–20 mg/kg IM q8–12h	Cockatiels/PD
	528 mg/L water	Ratites/egg dip
	3 g/40 packet bone cement	PMMA bead formation (1:14 ratio); same dose for all aminoglycoside beads
Amoxicillin/clavulanate (Clavamox, Pfizer)	125–250 mg/kg PO q8–12h	Most species, including pigeons, psittacines, and raptors
	500 mg/L drinking water	Chickens/PD
Amoxicillin sodium	50–250 mg/kg IM, IV q8–12h	Most species, including bustards, pigeons, passerines, soft bills, and gram-positive and gram-negative bacteria
Amoxicillin trihydrate	55–200 mg/kg PO, SC, IM, IV, q4–12h	Most species/broad-spectrum bactericidal penicillin antibiotic; minimal activity for common gram-negative infections of birds; relatively low availability after oral administration
	150 mg/kg SC, IM q24h × 5 days (administer q48h with long-acting preparation)	Pigeons
	200–1500 mg/L drinking water	Pigeons, canaries, waterfowl
	1500–4500 mg/L drinking water	Psittacines
	300–600 mg/kg soft feed	Canaries, psittacines

IM, Intramuscular; IV, intravenous; PD, pharmacodynamic; PMMA, polymethyl methacrylate; PO, oral; SC, subcutaneous.

Continued

---

*Although the authors attempted to verify dosages contained in this formulary, errors in the original sources or in the preparation of this chapter may have occurred. All users of this reference, therefore, should empirically evaluate all dosages to determine that they are reasonable before use. The publisher assumes no responsibility and makes no warranty with respect to results obtained from the uses or dosages listed, for any misstatement or error, negligent, or otherwise, contained in this chapter. In addition, the authors do not necessarily endorse specific products or dosages reported in this formulary. Also, the listing of a drug or commercial product in this chapter does not indicate approval by the Food and Drug Administration or the manufacturer for use in exotic animals.

Most of the avian formulary information has been modified with permission from: Carpenter JW, editor: Exotic animal formulary, ed 4,.St. Louis, 2013, Saunders.

Drug dosages are listed in ascending order; feed and water dosages are listed last.

TABLE 1

Antibacterial Agents—cont'd

Agent	Dosage	Species/Comments
Ampicillin sodium	50–150 mg/kg IM q6–12h	Most species/PD
	150–200 mg/kg PO q8–12h	Amazon parrots/PD; therapeutic levels not achieved in one species at this dosage
	528 mg/L drinking water	Pigeons/PD; *Streptococcus bovis*
Ampicillin trihydrate	15–25 mg/kg SC, IM q12h	Ratites, cranes, raptors/PD
	100 mg/kg PO, IM q4–12h	Most species
	1000–2000 mg/L drinking water	Galliformes, canaries/flock use
	2000–3000 mg/kg soft feed	Canaries/aviary use
Ampicillin/sulbactam (Unasyn, Pfizer)	200–300 mg/kg IM, IV q8h[9,10]	Poultry/PD
Azithromycin (Zithromax, Pfizer)	10–40 PO q24–48h	Most species/PD in cockatiels and macaws; found to be effective in eliminating *Chlamydophila psittaci* infections after 21 days
Carbenicillin (Geocillin, Roerig; Pyopen, Smith-Kline Beecham)	100–200 mg PO, IM, IV q6–12h	Most species
Cefadroxil	100 mg/kg PO q12h	Most species
Cefazolin	25–75 mg/kg PO, IM, IV q12h	Most species
Cefotaxime (Claforan, Hoechst-Roussel)	50–100 mg/kg IM, IV q 8–12h	Most species
Cefovecin (Convenia, Pfizer)	10 mg/kg SC, IM, IV q1h	Pigeons, chickens/PD; not recommended for use in birds due to short half-life; cannot be used q14d as in dogs and cats
Cefoxitin	50–100 mg/kg IM, IV q6–12h	Most species
Ceftazidime	50–100 mg/kg IM, IV q4–8h	Most species
Ceftiofur (Naxcel, Pfizer or the extended-release formulation, Excede, Pfizer)	10–20 mg/kg IM q3–5 days (Excede)[17,28,34]	Red-tailed hawks/PD; American black ducks/PD; helmeted guineafowl/PD
	10–50 mg/kg IM q4–12h (Naxcel)	Most species/PD in cockatiels and one species of Amazon parrot
Ceftriaxone	75–100 mg/kg IM q4–8h	Most species/PD in chickens
Cephalexin	50–125 mg/kg IM, PO q6–12h	Most species/PD mostly in poultry
Cephalothin	100 mg/kg IM, IV q6–8h	Most species/PD in poultry
Chloramphenicol palmitate (oral suspension)	25–50 mg/kg PO q8h	Most species
Chloramphenicol succinate	22 mg/kg IM, IV q3h	Ducks (PD), raptors
	50 mg/kg IM q6–12h	Most species; PD in macaws, conures, peafowl, eagles, geese
	200 mg/kg IM q12h × 5 days	Budgerigars/PD
Chlortetracycline (Aureomycin Soluble Powder, Cyanamid)	15–20 mg/kg PO q8h	Pigeons/PD
	100 mg/kg PO q6h	Raptors
	0.5–1% pellets × 30–45 days	Psittacines/*Chlamydophila*; reduce calcium in diet to 0.7%
	5000 mg/kg soft feed × 45 days	Chickens, turkeys/PD; medication of feed and water required to reach therapeutic level
	2500 mg/L drinking water	Most species
Ciprofloxacin (Cipro, Bayer)	15–40 mg/kg PO, IM, IV q12h	Most species
	50 mg/kg PO q12h	Raptors/PD
	80 mg/kg PO q24h	Most species/*Mycobacterium*; use in combination with other agents
Clarithromycin (Biaxin, Abbott)	10–85 mg/kg PO q24h	Most species/*Mycobacterium*; allometrically scaled
Clindamycin	25–50 mg/kg PO q8–12h	Most species
	100 mg/kg PO q6h[20]	Pigeons/PD
	100–150 mg/kg PO q12h	Raptors; osteomyelitis
Clofazimine (Lamprene, Novartis)	1–12 mg/kg PO q12–24h	Most species/*Mycobacterium*; use in combination with other agents
Cloxacillin	100–250 mg/kg PO, IM q12–24h	Most species, including raptors; recommended for treating pododermatitis
Danofloxacin mesylate (A180, Pfizer)	5 mg/kg PO, IM, IV	Most species

TABLE 1

Antibacterial Agents—cont'd

Agent	Dosage	Species/Comments
Doxycycline (Vibramycin, Pfizer)	25–50 mg/kg PO q12–24h	Cockatiels/PD; *Chlamydophila*; treatment for 21 and 45 days both effective; may cause regurgitation; use low end of dose range for macaws and cockatoos
	400–800 mg/L drinking water (make fresh daily)	Waterfowl, budgerigars (PD); treatment for 21 days in cockatiels with spiral bacteria
	300 mg/kg diet (wet weight) × 42 days[11]	Cockatiels/PD; doxycycline was added to soybean oil and then mixed with a pelleted diet formulated with reduced calcium (to reduce doxycycline chelation) and a low fat content
	1000 mg/kg feed	Large psittacines on dehulled seed (PD), macaws on corn (PD), canaries, large psittacines on soft feed (10 mg/mL syrup mixed into 29% kidney beans, 29% canned corn, 29% cooked rice, and 13% dry oatmeal cereal)
Doxycycline (Vibravenös, Pfizer)	50–100 mg/kg SC, IM q5–7d × 5–7 doses	Most species; PD in pigeons and houbara bustards
Doxycycline hyclate (Vibramycin injection, Pfizer)	25–50 mg/kg slow bolus IV q24h × 3 days	Psittacines (cardiovascular collapse associated with the propylene glycol carrier can occur after rapid IV injection)
	75–100 mg/kg SC, IM q5–7 days	Pigeons/PD
Doxycycline (Doxirobe gel, Pharmacia)	Topical	Most species/apply to beak or pododermatitis lesions; use in conjunction with debridement; antibiotic is released for 28 days
Enrofloxacin	—	Injectable formulation is highly alkaline and may cause tissue necrosis and pain; repeated IM injections are not recommended; no detectable effect on cartilage in day-old chicks; appears stable when compounded and stored at room temperature[25]; may be administered in some food items[31]
	7.5–9.5 mg/kg IM, IV q24h[32]	Crested caracaras/PD
	10–15 mg/kg PO, SC, IM q12h	Most species/PD
	15 mg/kg PO, IM, IV q12h	Raptors/PD; IV administration in owls may result in weakness, tachycardia, and vasoconstriction
	15–30 mg/kg PO, SC, IM q12–24h	Most species/PD for pulse dosing in some species
	50 mg/L drinking water	Chickens, turkeys/PD
	100–200 mg/L drinking water	Psittacines, pigeons/PD
	200–750 mg/mL drinking water	Psittacines/PD
	250–1000 mg/kg feed	Passerines; psittacines/PD
	50 mg/kg via nebulization × 4 h (Day 1, AM), then 25 mg/kg × 4 h/day × 4 days	Muscovy, Pekin ducklings/*Riemerella* (*Pasteurella*)
	0.2 mg/mL saline, flush q24h × 10 days	Raptors/nasal flush
Erythromycin	10–20 PO, IM q12–24h	Most species; IM injection can cause muscle necrosis
	100 mg/kg PO	Pigeons/PD
	100–1500 mg/L drinking water	Most species; pigeons/PD
Ethambutol (Myambutol, Lederle)	10–30 mg/kg PO q12–24h	Most species/*Mycobacterium*; use in combination with other agents
Gentamicin	2.5–5 mg/kg IM q8–12h	Most species; nephrotoxic; should be well hydrated; caution at higher doses
	5–10 mg/kg IM q8–12h	Cockatiels/PD
	5–10 mg/kg IM q4–6h	Pigeons, quail/PD
	2–3 drops ophthalmic solution intranasal q8h	Most species
Isoniazid	5–30 mg/kg PO q12–24h	Most species/*Mycobacterium;* should be used in combination with other drugs
Kanamycin (Kantrim, Fort Dodge)	10–20 mg/kg IM q12h	Most species
	13–65 mg/L drinking water	Most species; make fresh daily
Lincomycin	0.25–0.5 mL intra-articular q24h	Raptors
	25–50 mg/kg PO q12h	Most species
	50–100 mg/kg PO, IM q12–24h	Psittacines, raptors

Continued

TABLE 1

Antibacterial Agents—cont'd

Agent	Dosage	Species/Comments
Lincomycin/spectinomycin (LS-50 Water Soluble, Upjohn; Linco-Spectin 100 Soluble Powder, Upjohn)	50 mg/kg PO q24h 528 mg/L drinking water 750 mg/L drinking water × 3–7 days	Most species Turkey poults/PD; *Mycoplasma* airsacculitis Waterfowl
Marbofloxacin (Zeniquin, Pfizer)	2–2.5 mg/kg PO q24h[14,35] 2.5–5 mg/kg PO q24h 2–3 mg/kg IV, IO q24h 3–12 mg/kg PO q24h 5 mg/kg IM, IV 10–15 mg/kg IV q24h[12] 10–15 mg/kg PO, IM q12–24h	Broiler chickens and muscovy ducks/PD Blue and gold macaws/PD Raptors/PD Turkeys/PD Ostriches/PD Ducks/PD Raptors, bustards/PD
Meropenem (Merrem, Abbott)	175 mg/kg IM q24h	Pigeons/PD; broad-spectrum carbapenem antibiotic, penetrates most tissues and fluids
Metronidazole	10–50 mg/kg PO q 12–24h	Most species
Minocycline	10–15 mg/kg PO q12h 5000 mg/kg feed	Penguins, raptors Parakeets/use as antibiotic impregnated millet
Neomycin	Topical q6–12h 10 mg/kg PO q8–12h 80–264 mg/L drinking water 70–220 mg/kg feed × 14–21 days	Use is generally limited to topical formulations for skin, eyes, and ears, and, occasionally, oral treatment of enteric infections; not absorbed from GI tract Most species Waterfowl, galliformes Waterfowl, galliformes/*Clostridium*, necrotizing enteritis
Norfloxacin (Noroxin, Merck; Vetriflox 20% Oral Solution, Lavet Ltd., Budapest)	— 8 mg/kg PO q24h 10 mg/kg PO q24h 10 mg/kg PO q6–8h 15 mg/kg in water over 2–4 hr 100 mg/L drinking water × 5 days	Fluoroquinolone; not approved for use in food-producing birds in the United States; administration of the total daily dose to chickens over 2–4 h (pulse dosing) has been recommended Chickens/PD Chickens, geese/PD Turkeys/PD Turkeys/PD Chickens/PD
Novobiocin sodium	15–30 mg/kg PO q24h 220–385 mg/kg feed	Poultry/effective against some gram-positive cocci Poultry, waterfowl
Orbifloxacin (Orbax, Schering-Plough)	15–20 mg/kg PO q24h[16]	Japanese quail/PD
Ormetoprim-sulfadimethoxine (Primor, Pfizer)	60 mg/kg PO q12h 475–951 mg/L drinking water × 7–10 days 200–800 mg/kg feed	Pigeons Pigeons Waterfowl/colibacillosis
Oxytetracycline	— 2 mg/mL nebulization q4–6h 5 mg/kg SC, IM q12–24h 16 mg/kg IM q24h 23 mg/kg IV q6–8h or 43 mg/kg IM q24h 50–100 mg/kg SC, IM q2–3d 58 mg/kg IM q24h 2500 mg/L drinking water and 2500 mg/kg feed 300 mg/kg soft feed	IM administration may cause muscle irritation or necrosis; may be useful in treating *Chlamydophila*, fowl cholera; products or foods containing Al, Ca, Mg, Fe reduce or alter absorption; outdated tetracycline is nephrotoxic Parakeets/requires ultrasonic nebulizer; therapeutic concentrations of antibiotic were present in lung and trachea Chicken chicks/PD Great horned owls/PD Pheasants/PD Cockatoos (PD), passerines Amazon parrots/PD Chickens (PD), turkeys (PD), waterfowl/simultaneous medication of feed and water required to reach therapeutic level Psittacines
Penicillin	50,000 IU/kg IM 8 g/40 g packet bone cement	Waterfowl/*Erysipelas*, new duck disease PMMA beads (ratio 1:5)
Penicillin benzathine/procaine	200 mg/kg IM q24h	Most species; anecdotal reports suggest should not be used in birds <1 kg BW because of possible toxic effects
Penicillin G	6 mg/kg IV	Ostriches, emus/PD; rapidly eliminated; small volume of distribution

BW, Body weight; GI, gastrointestinal.

TABLE 1

Antibacterial Agents—cont'd

Agent	Dosage	Species/Comments
Piperacillin sodium	—	Extended-spectrum penicillin; not available as a veterinary product in the United States; see piperacillin/tazobactam
	100 mg/kg IM q4–6h	Red-tailed hawks, great horned owls/PD
	200 mg/kg IM q8h	Budgerigars (PD), raptors
	0.02 mL (4 mg) in macaw eggs; 0.01 mL (2 mg) in small eggs	Eggs/inject 200 mg/mL solution into air cell on Days 14, 18, and 22
Piperacillin(P)/ tazobactam(t) (Zosyn, Tazocin, Wyeth)	(P) 87 mg/kg + (t) 11 mg/kg IM q3–4h[3]	Amazon parrots/PD
Rifabutin (Mycobutin, Pharmacia)	15–45 mg/kg PO q24h	Most species including passerines/*Mycobacterium*; use in combination with other agents
Rifampin	10–20 mg/kg PO 12–24h 45 mg/kg PO q24h	Most species/*Mycobacterium*; use with other agents; may cause/be associated with hepatitis, CNS signs, depression, and vomiting;
Silver sulfadiazine	Topical q12–24h	Most species/burns, ulcers; Amazon foot necrosis; bandage application preferred
Streptomycin (Strepto- mycin Sulfate, Roerig)	—	May be nephrotoxic or neurotoxic; not recommended; consider amikacin as an alternative; *Mycobacterium*; use in combination with other agents
Sulfadimethoxine (Albon, Pfizer)	20–50 mg/kg PO, IM q12–24h	Most species; chickens/PD
	25–55 mg/kg PO q24h × 3–7 days	Raptors; loading dose at higher end × 1 day
	50 mg/kg PO q24h	Cranes
	330–400 mg/L drinking water on Day 1 followed by 200–265 mg/L × 4 days	Pigeons
Tetracycline	50 mg/kg PO q8h	Most species, including passerines
	200–250 mg/kg PO q12–24h	Most species/gavage
	40–200 mg/L drinking water	Most species, including game birds
	100–600 mg/kg feed	Game birds
Tiamulin (Denagard, Novartis)	12.5 mg/kg PO × 3 days	Poultry/intestinal spirochetosis
	25–50 mg/kg PO q24h	Most species; bacteriostatic antibiotic; effective against *Mycoplasma*
Ticarcillin/clavulanate (Ti- mentin, SmithKline Beecham)	100–200 mg/kg IM, IV q12h	Most species; extended-spectrum penicillin; very poor absorption if injectable given orally
Tilmicosin (Micotil 300 In- jection, Provitil-powder and Pulmotil AC-liquid, Elanco)	30 mg/kg PO q24h	Poultry/PD
	100–500 mg/L drinking water × 5 days	Poultry chicks/*Mycoplasma*; macrolide; handle with caution; potentially fatal to humans
Tobramycin	0.25–0.5 mL intra-articular flush q24h × 7–10 days	Raptors/septic arthritis
	2.5–5 mg/kg IM q8–12h	Most species; neurotoxicity or nephrotoxicity may develop
Trimethoprim-sulfadiazine (Tribrissen, Schering- Plough; Septra, Monarch)	12–60 mg/kg PO q12h	Raptors/useful for sensitive infections in neonates
	20 mg/kg SC, IM q12h	Psittacines
	30 mg/kg PO, IM, IV q12h	Ostriches/PD
	30 mg/kg PO q8h	Psittacines; combine with pyrimethamine for treatment of sarcocystosis
	107 mg/L drinking water	Galliformes
Trimethoprim/sulfa- methoxazole (Bactrim, Roche; Septra, Bur- roughs Wellcome)	48 mg/kg PO, IM q12h	Raptors
	60 mg/kg PO q24h	Pigeons
	100 mg/kg PO q12h	Most species, including psittacines; reduce dose if regurgitation occurs
	360–400 mg/L drinking water	Most species, including pigeons
	400 mg/kg feed	Geese
Tylosin (Tylan, Elanco)	15–30 mg/kg IM q6–12h	Most species; effective against gram-positive bacteria, *Mycoplasma*, *Chlamydophila*, *Pasteurella*; very irritating to muscles when administered IM
	50 mg/kg PO q24h	Passerines, pigeons
	50 mg/L drinking water	Most species
	250–1000 mg/L drinking water	Most species/*Mycoplasma*

CNS, Central nervous system.

TABLE 2

Antifungal Agents

Agent	Dosage	Species/Comments
Amphotericin B	—	Fungicidal; lipid-based amphotericin B products are now available that have less toxicity than conventional desoxycholate form; *Macrorhabdus ornithogaster* (avian gastric yeast); preferred IV agent for aspergillosis; intratracheal administration for syringeal aspergilloma may cause tracheitis; potentially nephrotoxic; resistance may develop
	1.5 mg/kg IV q8h × 3–7 days	Most species
	1 mg/kg intratracheal q8–12h, dilute to 1 mL with sterile water	Psittacines, raptors/aspergillosis
	1 mg/kg intratracheal q12h × 12 days, then q48h × 5 weeks	Raptors/syringeal aspergilloma
	100–109 mg/kg PO by gavage q12h × 10–30 days	Budgerigars/avian gastric yeast; compound in simple syrup
	0.05 mg/mL sterile water	Most species/nasal flush
	0.2 mL PO q12h × 10 days	Budgerigars/avian gastric yeast; use IV formulation (5 mg/mL)
	0.25–1 mL PO q24h × 4–5 days	Raptor neonates/candidiasis; not absorbed from alimentary tract
	1000 mg/L drinking water × 10 days	Budgerigars/avian gastric yeast
	Topical	Apply 10% solution to oropharynx
	7 mg/mL saline q12h	Most species/nebulization × 15 min
Amphotericin B (3% cream)	Topical to affected area q12h	Most species/mycoses
Amphotericin B (A)/proteolytic nasal flush (P)	Nasal flush (A) 1 mg/kg + (P) 0.2–0.4 mL diluted in 20 mL saline q24h	Uses a commercial neomycin-chymotrypsin-trypsin-hydrocortisone ointment (Kymar, Schering-Plough); 10 mL per naris (flushed vigorously in small amounts)
Clotrimazole	—	Broad-spectrum antifungal agent; inhibits the growth of pathogenic yeasts such as *Candida albicans*; used commonly as adjunctive therapy for aspergillosis; administer via air sac, intratracheally, nebulization, or topically
	2 mg/kg intratracheal q24h × 5 days	Psittacines/syringeal aspergilloma; apply with catheter or endoscope directly into syrinx during anesthesia
	10 mg/mL saline flush	Most species/effective against *Aspergillus* at sites that can be flushed
	1% solution	Nebulization × 30–60 min
Enilconazole emulsion	6 mg/kg PO q12h	Eclectus parrots/glossal candidiasis
	1 mg (0.5 mL)/kg intratracheal of a 1:10 dilution q24h	Falcons/aspergillosis
	200 mg/L drinking water	Canaries/cutaneous dermatophytosis
	Topical 1:10 dilution q12h	Raptors/cutaneous aspergillosis, candidiasis
	Topical or intratracheal 1:10–1:100 dilution	Psittacines/aspergillosis, candidiasis
	0.1 mL/kg in 5 mL sterile water, nebulize × 30 min, 5 days on, 2 off, up to 3 months	Raptors/aspergillosis
Fluconazole (Diflucan, Pfizer)	—	Fungistatic; penetrates well into brain, cerebrospinal fluids, and eyes; *Candida;* only indicated if topical treatment (i.e., nystatin) is not feasible; water-soluble; safest therapeutic index of the azoles; may be ineffective against aspergillosis; death observed in budgerigars at 10 mg/kg PO q12h (this dose was also ineffective against avian gastric yeast with *Macrorhabdus*); compounded oral suspension stable for 14 days when refrigerated
	2–6 mg/kg PO q12–24h	Most species
	5 mg/kg PO q24h, 10 mg/kg PO q48h[27]	Cockatiels/PD
	5–15 mg/kg PO q12h × 14–60 days	Most species
	8 mg/kg PO q24h × 30 days	Psittacines/cryptococcosis
	20 mg/kg PO q48h	Psittacines/PD; mucosal, systemic yeast infections
	100 mg/L in drinking water[27]	Cockatiels/PD
	100 mg/kg soft food	Gouldian finches/candidiasis

IV, Intravenous; PD, pharmacodynamic; PO, oral.

TABLE 2

Antifungal Agents—cont'd

Agent	Dosage	Species/Comments
Flucytosine (Ancobon, Roche)	—	Fungistatic agent; penetrates well into CNS; used prophylactically in raptors (especially falcons) and waterfowl to prevent aspergillosis; may be administered as adjunctive treatment; about 50% of *Aspergillus* strains are resistant; toxicity is low, however adverse effects may include gastrointestinal effects, hepatotoxicity, and bone marrow depression
	20–75 mg/kg PO q6–12h	Most species/generalized yeast or fungal infections
	75 mg/kg q12h × 5–7 days, then q24h × 14 days	Raptors/prophylaxis for prevention of aspergillosis
	75–120 mg/kg PO q6–12h	Most species/aspergillosis
	50–250 mg/kg feed	Psittacines, mynah birds
Griseofulvin	10 mg/kg PO q12h	Pigeons/dermatophytosis; gavage
	30–50 mg/kg q24h in drinking water	Ostriches/mycotic dermatitis
Itraconazole (Sporanox, Janssen)	—	Most species/systemic mycoses, superficial candidiasis, dermatophytosis; fungistatic; maximal oral bioavailability when taken with a full meal; commercially available suspension is recommended as a first choice; do not use compounded formulations because bulk drug is not bioavailable or stable
	2.5–5 mg/kg PO q24h	Grey parrots/anorexia, depression, and toxicity reported at higher doses in this species
	5–10 mg/kg PO q24h	Blue-fronted Amazon parrots/PD; aspergillosis; 10 mg/kg is required to achieve therapeutic concentrations in poorly perfused tissues
	5–10 mg/kg PO q12–24h × 10–14 days, then q48h	Raptors/aspergillosis prophylaxis
	5–10 mg/kg PO q12h	Passerines, waterfowl
	20 mg/kg PO q24h	Penguins/PD
	26 mg/kg PO q12h	Pigeons/PD; fungicidal levels achieved in respiratory tissue; further toxicologic studies required
	200 mg/kg feed up to 100 days	Gouldian finches/PD; dermatomycoses; beads from capsules were mixed with small amount of oil and seed
Ketoconazole (Nizoral, Janssen)	—	Most species/systemic mycoses (e.g., aspergillosis), candidiasis; fungistatic; less toxic than amphotericin B; more toxic than itraconazole; may be associated with potentially fatal hepatotoxicity; 20 mg/kg may cause regurgitation (discontinue for 1–2 days, then restart)
	30 mg/kg PO q12h × 7–14 days	Amazon parrots/PD
	30 mg/kg PO q12h × 7–30 days	Pigeons (PD), raptors/prophylactic in raptors for aspergillosis
	60 mg/kg PO q12h	Raptors/PD (common buzzard); aspergillosis
	200 mg/L drinking water, nectar, or soft feed × 7–14 days	Canaries, hummingbirds, Gouldian finches/dissolve crushed tablet in ½–1 tsp vinegar
Miconazole	—	Fungistatic; inhibits the growth of *Candida albicans*, Malassezia, and dermatophytes; injectable miconazole is not available in the United States
	5 mg/kg intratracheal q12h	Psittacines/10 mg/mL solution diluted with saline; syringeal mycoses
	10–20 mg/kg IM, IV q8–24h	Raptors, psittacines
	Topical to affected areas q12h	Cutaneous fungal infections; used in conjunction with oral itraconazole

IM, Intramuscular.

Continued

TABLE 2		
Antifungal Agents—cont'd		
Agent	**Dosage**	**Species/Comments**
Nystatin	—	Drug of choice for treatment of candidiasis; not systemically absorbed across intact gastrointestinal tract; oral lesions must be treated by direct contact with medication; when treating neonates, administer separately from formula to maximize concentration and contact time
	20,000–100,000 U PO q12–24h	Raptors, pigeons
	300,000–600,000 U/kg PO q8–12h	Most species
	Topical q6h	Hummingbirds/candidiasis; direct application using a cotton swab
	100,000 U/L drinking water	Canaries, finches
Pimaricin (Natamycin, Alcon)	1 drop in affected eye q8h	Lovebirds/macrolide antifungal; keratomycosis
Silver sulfadiazine	Topical to affected areas q12–24h	Most species/bandage application preferred
Terbinafine	—	Fungicidal; questionable therapeutic potential for the treatment of aspergillosis in avian species; higher dose or use in combination with itraconazole may be more effective
	10–30 mg/kg PO q12–24h	Most species
	15 mg/kg PO q24h	Penguins/PD
	22 mg/kg PO q24h	Raptors/PD
	60 mg/kg PO q24h[7]	Amazon parrots/PD
	1 mg/mL solution via nebulization[6]	Amazon parrots/PD; may need higher concentration, frequent administration, or nebulization times more than 15 min to achieve therapeutic levels
Voriconazole (Vfend, Pfizer)	—	Most active drug against aspergillosis; some strains resistant; dose extrapolation difficult between species; PO and IV solutions available; may need to adjust dose for long-term treatment to maintain therapeutic concentrations; compounded suspensions stable up to 30 days at room temperature
	10 mg/kg PO, IV q12h	Chickens/PD
	10 mg/kg PO q12h or 20 mg/kg q24h	Pigeons/PD
	10 mg/kg PO q8h[13]	Hawks/PD; more frequent dosing (e.g., up to q8h) may be necessary to maintain target concentrations during prolonged therapy
	12–18 mg/kg PO q12h	Grey parrots/PD
	18 mg/kg PO q8h	Amazons/PD
	40 mg/kg PO q24h	Quail/PD
	20 mg/kg IV, PO q8–12h[19]	Ducks/PD

TABLE 3

Antiviral and Immunomodulating Agents

Agent	Dosage	Species/Comments
Acemannan (CarraVet, Carrington Laboratories)	—	Has been demonstrated in poultry to induce macrophages to secrete interferon, tumor necrosis factor-α, and interleukins and thus may have immunostimulant, antiviral, antineoplastic, and gastrointestinal properties; used as adjuvant in some avian vaccines
	1–2 mg/kg SC or intralesional q7d	Chemotherapeutic adjunct therapy
Acyclovir (Zovirax, Burroughs Wellcome)	—	Antiviral agent; active against herpesviruses and cytomegalovirus; IM injection of the water-soluble sodium salt (IV formulation) may cause severe muscle necrosis; phlebitis and neurologic signs may occur with IV administration; most effective when administered before clinical signs begin; birds should be treated for a minimum of 7 days; the reconstituted solution is unstable and should be divided into aliquots and frozen
	10 mg/kg IM q24h × 5–14 days	Chickens/Marek's disease
	20–40 mg/kg IM q12h	Psittacines/psittacine herpesvirus
	29 mg/bird PO q8h × 7 days	Pigeons/herpesvirus
	80 mg/kg PO q8h × 7 days	Quaker parakeets/PD; psittacine herpesvirus prophylaxis or treatment
	120 mg/kg PO q12h	Tragopans/PD
	330 mg/kg PO q12h × 4–7 days	Psittacine neonates/psittacine herpesvirus
	330 mg/kg PO q12h	Raptors/falcon and owl herpesvirus; may cause vomiting
	1000 mg/L drinking water	Quaker parakeets/herpesvirus; gavage
Amantadine (Symmetrel, Endo Labs)	—	Antiviral agent; inhibits replication of influenza A viruses
	1 mg/kg PO q24h × 3 weeks	Grey parrots/no effect on avian bornavirus infection
	10 mg/kg PO × 3 days pre- and 18 days postexposure	Turkeys/influenza viruses; must be administered before and during virus exposure
	25 mg/kg PO × 10 days following infection	Chickens
	100 mg/L drinking water	Chickens/can use simultaneously with killed influenza vaccine
Entecavir (Baraclude, Bristol-Myers Squibb)	—	Oral antiviral drug used in the treatment of hepatitis viruses
	1 mg/kg PO q24h × 14 days[8]	Ducklings/PD; antiviral agent; duck hepatitis B; given with duck hepatitis B virus (DHBV) deoxyribonucleic acid vaccines
Famciclovir (Famvir, Novartis)	25 mg/kg PO q12h	Ducklings/PD; antiviral agent; duck hepatitis; toxic effects were not reported
Imiquimod cream (Aldara, 3M)	Topical application	Psittacines/cloacal papillomatosis; thought to boost host cell-mediated immunity; masses decreased in size in one report, but not in another; complete remission did not occur in either
Interferon α2a	—	Glycoprotein with immunomodulating and antiproliferative capabilities as well as antiviral activity
	30 U q24h × 5 days, 30 U 2X/week × 2 weeks, then 30 U q7d × 2 weeks	Most species
	60–240 U/kg SC, IM q12h or 300–1200 U/kg PO q12h	Most species/stock solution: mix 1 mL (3,000,000 U/mL) with 100 mL sterile water (30,000 U/mL); can freeze as 2 mL vials up to 1 year; mix 2 mL of stock into 1 L LRS (60 U/mL); refrigerate up to 3 months
Levamisole	—	Anthelmintic with immunostimulation properties; low therapeutic index (toxic reactions and deaths reported)
	1.25–2.5 mg/kg PO, IM, SC q7–14d	Most species

IM, Intramuscular; IV, intravenous; LRS, lactated Ringer's solution; PO, oral; SC, subcutaneous.

Continued

TABLE 3

Antiviral and Immunomodulating Agents—cont'd

Agent	Dosage	Species/Comments
Oseltamivir	—	Neuraminidase inhibitor used for treatment of avian influenza
	0.5 mg/kg PO q12h × 5 days[5]	Duck, chickens/PD; administered prophylactically to healthy animals in the event of an outbreak in valuable zoological collections
Penciclovir (Denavir, Novartis)	10 mg/kg IP q24h × 12–24 weeks	Ducks/PD; antiviral agent active against herpesviruses; DHBV; viral levels were significantly reduced; no toxic effects observed; dissolve in 2 mL of 1% DMSO
Rimantadine (Flumadine, Forest)	100 mg/L drinking water	Chickens/influenza viruses; must be used before and during exposure

DMSO, Dimethyl sulfoxide.

TABLE 4

Antiparasitic Drugs

Agent	Dosage	Species/Comments
Albendazole	5–50 mg/kg PO	Broad-spectrum anthelmintic; may be toxic in keas, some Columbiformes at 50–100 mg/kg
Amprolium	13–30 mg/kg PO	Pyrimidine derivative coccidiostat; most species
Carnidazole	5–50 mg/kg PO	Treatment for *Trichomonas, Giardia*, Hexamita, *Histomonas*, most species
Chloroquine phosphate	5–25 mg/kg PO	Generally used with primaquine for *Plasmodium, Haemoproteus*, and *Leucocytozoon*; overdose can result in death
Clazuril	3–7 mg/kg PO	Most species; drug detected in eggs after multiple dosing
Diclazuril	5–10 mg/L drinking water	Some *Eimeria* resistance in poultry documented recently; rotate for long-term prevention
Fenbendazole	10–50 mg/kg PO	Most species/anthelmintic effective against cestodes, nematodes, trematodes, *Giardia*, and acanthocephalans; toxicity documented in pigeons and doves; may be toxic to other species, including raptors, vultures, lories, storks, and pelicans
Fipronil	7.5 mg/kg; spray on skin once, repeat in 30 days prn	Apply via pad to base of neck, tail base, and under each wing; avoid plumage during application; alcohol may create dry, brittle feathers; do not soak bird; do not exceed 7.5 mg/kg
Imidocarb dipropionate	5–7 mg/kg IM once, repeat in 7 days	Raptors/*Babesia*; some cases require a total of three treatments
Ivermectin	0.2–0.4 mg/kg PO, SC, IM, topical once, can repeat in 10–14 days	Dilute with water or saline for immediate use; dilute with propylene glycol for extended use; parenteral ivermectin may be toxic to finches and budgerigars
Metronidazole	10–30 mg/kg PO q12	Most species/antiprotozoal, including alimentary tract protozoa (especially flagellates such as *Giardia, Histomonas, Spironucleus*, and *Trichomonas*)
	30–50 mg/kg PO q24h	Most species
	100 mg/L drinking water or soft food	Canaries
	200 mg/L drinking water × 7 days	Passerines
Milbemycin oxime	2 mg/kg PO, repeat in 28 days	Galliformes
Ponazuril	10–20 mg/kg PO repeat in 10–14 days	Most species including pigeons, waterfowl
	25 mg/kg PO, IM, repeat in 10–14 days	Bali mynahs/cestodes
Primaquine	—	Hematozoa (i.e., *Plasmodium, Haemoproteus*, and *Leucocytozoon*); use in conjunction with chloroquine; dosage based on amount of active base rather than total tablet weight
	0.3 mg/kg PO (at 24 h following the initial chloroquine dose) q24h × 7–10 days	Penguins and raptors/use with chloroquine (10 mg/kg at 0 h, then 5 mg/kg at 6, 24, and 48 h)
	0.75–1 mg/kg PO once	Most species, including raptors/*Plasmodium*; use with chloroquine (25 mg/kg at 0 h, then 15 mg/kg at 12, 24, and 48 h); palliative therapy
	1 mg/kg PO q7d	Use with chloroquine (10 mg/kg q7d) as a preventative regimen for birds recovering from *Plasmodium* infection
	1 mg/kg PO q24h × 2 days, repeat q7d × 3–5 treatments to prevent relapse	Raptors/*Plasmodium*; use with chloroquine (20 mg/kg IV initially, followed by 10 mg/kg PO at 6, 18, and 24 h)

IM, Intramuscular; IV, intravenous; PO, oral; prn, as needed; SC, subcutaneous.

Continued

TABLE 4		
Antiparasitic Drugs—cont'd		
Agent	**Dosage**	**Species/Comments**
Pyrimethamine (Fansidar, Roche)	—	Most species/*Atoxoplasma, Plasmodium;* chloroquine and primaquine are preferred; overdosage may cause hepatoxicity; *Toxoplasma, Atoxoplasma, Sarcocystis;* may be effective for *Leucocytozoon;* supplement with folic acid
	0.25–0.5 mg/kg PO q12h × 30 days	Raptors, waterfowl/*Sarcocystis, Toxoplasma*
	0.5 mg/kg PO q12h × 14–28 days	Most species/use for 28 days for *Leucocytozoon* in raptors
	0.5 mg/kg PO q12h × 30 days	Waterfowl/*Sarcocystis*
	0.5–1 mg/kg PO q12h × 30 days	Eclectus, Amazon parrots/use with trimethoprim-sulfadiazine (30 mg/kg)
	1 mg/kg feed	Game birds
	100 mg/kg feed	Most species
Quinacrine HCl (Atabrine, Sanofi)	—	Most species/*Atoxoplasma, Plasmodium;* chloroquine and primaquine preferred; overdosage may cause hepatoxicity
	5–10 mg/kg PO q24h × 7–10 days	Most species/use higher doses for *Atoxoplasma, Lankesterella, Plasmodium*
	26–79 mg/L drinking water × 10–21 days	Pigeons
Ronidazole	2.5 mg/kg PO × 6 days	Pigeons
	6–10 mg/kg PO q24h × 6–10 days	Most species
	10–20 mg/kg PO q24h × 7 days	Pigeons
Selamectin	—	No adverse effects, including neurological signs, were seen in healthy zebra finches with doses up to 92 mg/kg
	23 mg/kg topically, repeat in 3–4 weeks	Budgerigars/*Knemidokoptes* improvement 13/14 birds at 4 weeks, no neurological signs identified but monitor for weight loss
Sulfachloropyrazine	1 g of 30% powder/L of drinking water × 5 days, off 3 days, on 5 days, then repeat cycle 4×; administer treatment 3× annually	Bali mynahs/*Atoxoplasma;* significantly reduced or totally cleared oocyst shedding for extended time; it is uncertain if the drug is safe to use when parents are feeding chicks; supplement with vitamin B$_6$. No adverse effects, including neurological signs, were seen in healthy zebra finches with doses up to 92 mg/kg
Sulfachloropyridazine	150–300 mg/L drinking water; 5 days/week × 2–3 weeks	Passerines, including canaries/may need to treat for months for systemic coccidiosis
	300 mg/L drinking water × 5 days, off 3 days, on 5 days, then repeat cycle 4×; administer treatment 3× annually	Passerines, including Bali mynahs/*Atoxoplasma*
	300 mg/L drinking water × 7–10 days	Pigeons
	300–1000 mg/L drinking water × 3 days, off 2 days, then repeat course	Pigeons
	400–500 mg/L drinking water × 5 days, off 2 days, on 5 days	Most species
Sulfadimethoxine	25 mg/kg PO q12h × 5 days	Raptors
	25–50 mg/kg PO q24h × 3 days	Raptors
	25–50 mg/kg PO q24h × 3 days, off 2 days, then q24h × 3 days	Raptors/*Eimeria, Sarcocystis*
	25–55 mg/kg PO q24h × 3–7 days	Raptors
	50 mg/kg PO once, followed by 25 mg/kg PO q24h × 7–10 days	Psittacines
	50 mg/kg PO q24h × 5 days, off 3 days, on 5 days	Pigeons/close to toxic levels
	250 mg/L drinking water × 5 days	Turkeys
	330–400 mg/L drinking water × 1 day then 200 mg/L × 4 days	Pigeons/supplement with vitamin B for 5 days
	500 mg/L drinking water × 6 days	Chickens

TABLE 4

Antiparasitic Drugs—cont'd

Agent	Dosage	Species/Comments
Sulfaquinoxaline	—	Contraindicated with dehydration, liver disease, or bone marrow suppression; gastrointestinal upset, regurgitation are common, especially in macaws; use for longer than 2 weeks may require vitamin B (folic acid) supplementation
	250 mg/L drinking water × 6 days, off 2 days, on 6 days	Turkeys
	400 mg/L (1.4 mL/L) drinking water × 6 days, off 2 days, on 6 days	Chickens
	500 mg/L (1.8 mL/L) drinking water × 6 days, off 2 days, on 6 days	Pigeons
	225 mg/kg feed continuously	Turkeys
	450 mg/kg feed continuously	Chickens
Thiabendazole	40–100 mg/kg PO q24h × 7 days	Most species
	50 mg/kg PO, repeat in 14 days	Ostriches
	100 mg/kg PO once, repeat in 10–14 days	Raptors
	100–200 mg/kg PO q12h × 10 days	Raptors/nematodes; may interfere with egg laying
	100–500 mg/kg PO once	Most species
	250–500 mg/kg PO, repeat in 10–14 days	Most species, including psittacines
	425 mg/kg feed × 14 days	Pheasants, cranes
Toltrazuril (Baycox, Bayer)	—	Has been successful in reducing mortality from *Atoxoplasma* in passerines and may affect systemic stages of the disease; not very effective against *Atoxoplasma* when given in water; bitter taste, mixing with soft drink (i.e., cola) increases palatability; 2.5% solution is very alkaline and should not be gavaged directly into the crop
	7 mg/kg PO q24h × 2–3 days	Budgerigars, raptors
	10 mg/kg PO q24h × 2 days	Raptors/preferred treatment for *Caryospora*
	10 mg/kg PO q48h × 3 treatments	Raptors/treatment of choice for coccidiosis in falcons
	12.5 mg/kg PO q24h × 14 days	Bali mynahs/*Atoxoplasma*; dosage is based on a limited number of clinical cases
	15–25 mg/kg PO q24h × 2 days	Raptors
	25 mg/kg PO q7d × 3 treatments	Raptors
	50 mg/kg PO once	Most species/*Giardia, Trichomonas, Entamoeba*
	2 mg/L drinking water × 2 consecutive days/week	Psittacines
	5 mg/L drinking water × 2 days, repeat in 14–21 days	Lories/10 mg/L administered during second course of treatment
	12.5 mg/L drinking water × 2 days	Waterfowl
	20 mg/kg in drinking water × 2 days	Pigeons
	25 mg/L drinking water × 2 days	Chickens
	25 mg/L drinking water × 2 days, repeat in 14–21 days	Cockatiels, passerines (including goldfinches, manikins, siskins)
	75 mg/L drinking water × 2 days/week × 4 weeks	Passerines
	125 mg/L drinking water × 5 days	Pigeons
	200-400 mg/kg feed	Chickens/Histomonas; depressed weight gain on higher dosage
Trimethoprim-sulfadiazine	5 mg/kg IM q12h	Companion birds/*Sarcocystis*; use in conjunction with pyrimethamine (0.5–1 mg/kg PO q12h × 2 days, then 0.25 mg/kg PO q12h × 30 days)
	30 mg/kg PO q8–12h	Most species, including psittacines, raptors/*Sarcocystis* (treat for at least 6 weeks); coccidia
	60 mg/kg PO, SC q12h × 3 days, off 2 days, on 3 days	Raptors, waterfowl/coccidia
	80 mg/mL drinking water (trimethoprim)/40 mg/mL water (sulfadiazine)	Canaries/*Toxoplasma gondii*
Trimethoprim-sulfamethoxazole	25 mg/kg PO q24h	Toucans, mynahs/coccidia
	30 mg/kg PO q12–24h	Passerines/antiprotozoal
	320–525 mg/L drinking water	Poultry/coccidia
	480 mg/L drinking water q24h	Pigeons/antiprotozoal; See sulfonamides

TABLE 5

Chemical Restraint/Anesthetic/Analgesic Agents[a]

Agent	Dosage	Species/Comments
Acepromazine	0.1–0.2 mg/kg IV 0.25–0.5 mg/kg IM	Ratites/most commonly used in combination with other anesthetics; rarely used in other species
Atipamezole	2.5–5× α2 adrenergic agonist dose IM, IV	α2 adrenergic antagonist; 1:1 volume reversal of dexmedetomidine and medetomidine is general rule; can be divided ½ IM and ½ SC
Atropine sulfate	0.01–0.02 mg/kg SC, IM, IV	Most species/premedication
	0.04–0.1 mg/kg SC, IM, IV, IO, IT	Most species/bradycardia; higher doses with CPR
Bupivacaine HCl	—	May be shorter acting in some birds; minimize dose to limit potential toxic effects
	2 mg/kg infused SC	Mallard ducks/PD; high plasma levels at 6 and 12 h post-administration so possible for delayed toxicity
	2–8 mg/kg perineurally	Mallard ducks/variable effectiveness for brachial plexus nerve block
Butorphanol tartrate	—	PO bioavailability <10% in Hispaniolan Amazon parrots; do not recommend in American kestrels
	0.05–0.25 mg/kg IV	Ratites
	0.5–5 mg/kg IM, IV q1–4h	Most species, including psittacines
	3 mg/kg (premedication) + 75 μg/kg/min IV CRI (maintenance)	Psittacines; significantly reduced isoflurane MAC
Dexmedetomidine HCl	25 μg/kg IM	Common buzzards/adequate restraint to prevent reaction to handling but did not allow for intubation; no arrhythmias, excitement, or major adverse effects noted; complete reversal with atipamezole
	75 μg/kg	Common kestrels/adequate restraint to prevent reaction to handling but did not allow for intubation
Diazepam	0.05–0.5 mg/kg IV	Most species
	0.25–0.5 mg/kg IM, IV q24h × 2–3 days	Raptors/appetite stimulant
	5 mg/kg PO, IV	Ratites/sedation
	12–15 mg/kg intranasally	Ring-necked parakeets, canaries/ dose divided into each nare and given slowly; intranasal flumazenil significantly reduced recumbency time
Dobutamine	15 μg/kg/min IV[30]	β1-adrenergic agonist used to treat anesthetic-induced hypotension
Dopamine HCl	7–10 μg/kg/min IV[30]	Inotropic vasopressor used to treat anesthetic-induced hypotension
Fentanyl citrate	0.2 mg/kg loading dose + 10–30 μg/kg/min IV CRI	Reduced isoflurane MAC 31%–55% in a dose-related manner in red-tailed hawks; significant effects on heart rate/blood pressure in Hispaniolan Amazon parrots
Flumazenil	0.02–0.05 mg/kg IM, IV	Most species
	0.05–0.25 mg/kg intranasally[21]	Canaries, mallard ducks, Hispaniolan Amazon parrots, ring-necked parakeets/dose divided evenly between nares and given slowly, significantly reduced recumbency time
Gabapentin	—	Neuropathic pain (chronic pain; often associated with traumatic and self-induced injuries); analgesic
	10 mg/kg PO q12h	Little corella/long-term analgesia (>90 days); sole analgesic for self-mutilation; no adverse effects noted
	11 mg/kg PO q12h	Prairie falcon/long-term (>90 days) analgesic adjunct to multimodal therapy for self-mutilation
	30 mg/kg PO[1]	Hispaniolan Amazon parrots/PD; additional studies are needed
Glycopyrrolate	0.01–0.02 mg/kg IM, IV	Most species/preanesthetic

CPR, Cardiopulmonary resuscitation; CRI, Constant rate infusion; IM, intramuscular; IO, intraosseous; IT, intratracheal; IV, intravenous; MAC, minimum alveolar concentration; PD, pharmacodynamic; PO, oral; SC, subcutaneous.
[a]All opioid agonists and agonist-antagonists may cause respiratory depression; profound bradypnea may occur with potent opioid agonists.

TABLE 5

Chemical Restraint/Anesthetic/Analgesic Agents—cont'd

Agent	Dosage	Species/Comments
Ketamine HCl	—	Seldom used as sole agent because of poor muscle relaxation and prolonged, violent recoveries; may produce excitation or convulsions; may fail to produce general anesthesia in some species including raptors and waterfowl
	5–50 mg/kg SC, IM, IV	Smaller species require a higher dose; large birds tend to recover more slowly
	50 mg/kg IO	Pigeons/provided effective anesthesia
Ketamine (K)/diazepam (D)	(K) 2–5 mg/kg IV + (D) 0.25 mg/kg IV	Ostriches/ketamine may be given 15–30 min after diazepam
	(K) 3–8 mg/kg + (D) 0.5–1 mg/kg IM	Eagles, vultures
	(K) 8–15 mg/kg + (D) 0.5–1 mg/kg IM	Falcons
	(K) 10–40 mg/kg IV + (D) 1–1.5 mg/kg IM, IV	Raptors, pigeons, waterfowl/rapid bolus may produce apnea, arrhythmia, and increased risk of death
	(K) 20 mg/kg + (D) 1 mg/kg IV	Toucans/short procedures (15–20 min)
	(K) 75 mg/kg IM + (D) 2.5 mg/kg IV	White leghorn cockerels/ diazepam administered 5 min before ketamine for typhlectomy; some limb contracture, hypothermia, hypoxia, hypercapnia
Ketamine (K)/midazolam (Mi)	(K) 10–40 mg/kg + (Mi) 0.2–2 mg/kg SC, IM	Most species, including psittacines
	(K) 40–50 mg/kg + (Mi) 3.65 mg/kg intranasally	Ring-necked parakeets/dose divided into each nare and given slowly; onset of action less than 3 min, dorsal recumbency for 70.7 ± 46.7 min, recovery times reduced with flumazenil intranasally
Ketamine (K)/midazolam (Mi)/butorphanol (B)	(Mi) 0.2 mg/kg + (B) 0.4 mg/kg IM followed by (K) 8.7 +/– 0.5 mg/kg IV	Ostriches/induction; followed by intubation and isoflurane anesthesia
Lidocaine	—	Toxic effects have been documented in birds at overall lower total doses (2.7–3.3 mg/kg) than dogs; may need to dilute 1:10 in small birds
	1–3 mg/kg	Most species
	15 mg/kg + 3.8 μg/kg lidocaine perineurally	Mallard ducks/variable effectiveness for brachial plexus nerve block
Midazolam HCl	0.1–2 mg/kg IM, IV	Most species/premedication at lower doses, onset approximately 15 min when administered IM
	0.15 mg/kg IV	Ostriches/rapid sternal recumbency in adults
	2 mg/kg intranasally	Hispaniolan Amazon parrots/ mild-to-moderate sedation in 3 min; reduced vocalizations, struggling and defensive behaviors for 15 min; reversed with intranasal flumazenil
	2–6 mg/kg IM	Quail/PD; mild-to-heavy sedation
	5 mg/kg IV	Turkeys, chickens, ring-necked pheasants, bobwhite quail
	7.3–8.8 mg/kg intranasally	Ring-necked parakeets, canaries/dose divided into each nare and given slowly; time to onset, 3 min; dorsal recumbency, 57.7 ± 24.4 min; flumazenil administered intranasally significantly reduced recovery time
	12.5–15.6 mg/kg intranasally	Canaries/dose divided into each nare and given slowly; time to onset, less than 3 min; dorsal recumbency, 17.1 ± 5 min; flumazenil intranasally significantly reduced recovery time
Nalbuphine HCl	12.5 mg/kg IM q2–3h	Opioid partial κ-agonist and partial μ-antagonist; Hispaniolan Amazon parrots/PK, PD; excellent bioavailability, little sedation; rapidly cleared after IM dosing; higher dosages (25 and 50 mg/kg IM) did not significantly increase withdrawal values
Naloxone HCl	0.01 mg/kg IV	Ostriches
	2 mg IV q4–12h	Most species, including psittacines

PK, Pharmacokinetic.

TABLE 5

Chemical Restraint/Anesthetic/Analgesic Agents—cont'd

Agent	Dosage	Species/Comments
Naltrexone HCl	300–330 mg IM, IV	Ostriches
Propofol	—	IV sedative-hypnotic agent; give slowly for induction to minimize apnea; intubation and IPPV required
	1–5 mg/kg IV	Most species/induction
	3 mg/kg IV (induction); 0.2 mg/kg/min IV (maintenance)	Ostriches/PD; anesthesia
	4 mg/kg IV (induction); 0.5 mg/kg/min IV (maintenance)	Barn owl/anesthesia
	5 mg/kg IV (induction); 1 mg/kg/min IV (maintenance)	Hispaniolan Amazon parrots/PD; recovery times (15.4 ± 15.2 min) were prolonged when compared with isoflurane; 6 of 10 birds had agitated recoveries; light anesthetic plane in 8 of 10 birds
Tolazoline HCl	1 mg/kg IV	Ostriches
	15 mg/kg IV	Raptors, including vultures
Tramadol HCl	5 mg/kg PO, IV q12h	Bald eagles/similar plasma concentrations to humans for analgesia (but analgesia not evaluated); PO bioavailability in bald eagles higher than in humans and dogs; monitor for sedation and reduce dose and/or frequency prn
	7.5 mg/kg PO	Peafowl/2 of 6 birds reached human tramadol analgesic concentrations
	8–11 mg/kg PO q12h	Red-tailed hawks/15 mg/kg PO q12h data model suggested more frequent dosing to achieve human analgesic plasma tramadol concentrations; monitor for sedation and reduce dose and/or frequency prn
	30 mg/kg PO q6h	Hispaniolan Amazon parrots/similar plasma concentrations to humans for analgesia

IPPV, Intermittent positive pressure ventilation; prn, as needed.

TABLE 6

Nonsteroidal Antiinflammatory Agents[a,b]

Agent	Dosage	Species/Comments
Carprofen	2–10 mg/kg SC, IM	Most species; caution should be used when administering to *Gyps* vultures; Hispaniolan Amazon parrots may need more frequent dosing recommended than q12h
	30 mg/kg IM	Chickens/PD; arthritis painful behaviors reduced 1 h post-treatment only with this high dose
Celecoxib (Celebrex, Pfizer)	10 mg/kg PO q24h × 6–24 weeks	Psittacines/clinical proventricular dilatation disease; clinical improvement may be seen within 14 days
Ibuprofen	5–10 mg/kg PO q8–12h	Psittacines/use pediatric suspension for small birds; avoid in *Gyps* vultures
Ketoprofen	1–5 mg/kg IM q12h	Avoid in *Gyps* vultures; raptors, waterfowl
	2.5 mg/kg IM q24h × 3 or 7 days	Budgerigars/low frequency of glomerular congestion, degeneration/dilation of tubules occurred at 3–7 days treatment
	5–10 mg/kg IM, IV	Waterfowl; caution in eider ducks/high mortality may be owing to high bupivacaine dose, or cumulative toxicity of bupivacaine and ketoprofen
Meloxicam	—	No reported mortalities including *Gyps* vultures, few studies evaluating renal effects of higher doses
	1 mg/kg PO, IM, IV q12h[23]	Hispaniolan Amazon parrots/ improved weight-bearing on arthritic limb compared with lower doses; PO lower bioavailability than parenteral; concentrations similar to humans for analgesia for IM, IV for only 6 h
	2 mg/kg IM q12h × 14 days	Japanese quail/unremarkable histological and minimal biochemical changes
	2 mg/kg IM, PO	Cape Griffon vultures/rapid metabolism and short elimination t½ suggests low potential for drug accumulation
Piroxicam	—	Has been used to treat pain associated with chronic degenerative joint disease in cranes and other species
	0.5 mg/kg q12h	Psittacines
	0.5–0.8 mg/kg PO q12h[c]	Whooping cranes/used for acute myopathy, chronic degenerative joint disease

IM, Intramuscular; IV, intravenous; PD, pharmacodynamic; PO, oral; SC, subcutaneous.

[a]Unless otherwise noted, drugs provide analgesic, antipyretic, and antiinflammatory effects.

[b]Nonsteroidal antiinflammatory agents may potentially cause gastrointestinal upset and hemorrhage as well as adverse renal effects ranging from fluid retention to renal failure.

[c]Paul-Murphy J. Personal communication. 2011.

TABLE 7

Hormones and Steroids

Agent	Dosage	Species/Comments
Human chorionic gonadotropin	500–1000 U/kg IM on Day 1, 3, 7 q3–6wk prn	Inhibits egg laying; administer on Days 3 and 7 if hen lays eggs after Day 1
Deslorelin acetate	—	Synthetic long-acting GnRH agonist; used to treat reproductive tract disorders or conditions exacerbated by circulating concentrations of reproductive hormones; reported to suppress ovarian carcinoma in a cockatiel[24]
	4.7 mg long-acting implant IM[4]	Pigeons/effective for controlling egg laying in females for at least 49 days
	4.7 mg or 9.4 mg implant placed SC intrascapularly[4,22,26]	GnRH agonist available as long-term implant; no adverse reports with use till date
Dexamethasone[a]	0.2–1 mg/kg IM, IV once or q12–24h × 2–7 days, then q48h × 5 days	Most species, including raptors/antiinflammatory
	2–4 mg/kg IM, IV q12–24h	Most species, including ratites/shock, trauma
Dexamethasone sodium phosphate[a]	2–4 mg/kg SC, IM, IV q6h–24h	Most species/head trauma, shock, hyperthermia; higher dose for shock, head trauma, endotoxemia
Insulin	0.002 U/bird IM q12–48h	Budgerigars/NPH insulin
	0.01–0.1 U/bird IM q12–48h	Amazon parrots/NPH insulin
	0.5–3 U/kg IM	Psittacines/NPH insulin
	1.4 U/kg IM q12–24h	Cockatiels, toco toucans/NPH insulin
	2 U/bird IM	Toco toucans/ultralente or PZI; adjust dose or frequency based on glucose curves
Leuprolide acetate	—	Administration before onset of egg laying may be more successful than treatment during breeding; 1 month depot formulation generally requires q4wk treatment
	(Number of days for desired effect) × (52 or 156 μg/kg) = dosage IM	Cockatiels
	200–1000 μg/kg IM q2–6wk	Most species
	1250 μg/kg IM once	Penguins/induced molt in 1 of 2 birds dosed

GnRH, Gonadotropin-releasing hormone; IM, intramuscular; IV, intravenous; NPH, neutral protamine Hagedorn; prn, as needed; PZI, protamine zinc insulin; SC, subcutaneous.

[a]Steroid administration may predispose birds to aspergillosis and other mycoses; administration may also be associated with the development of polyuria/polydipsia/polyphagia, increased protein catabolism, glycosuria, and diabetes mellitus; toxic levels may be attained even with topical application; administration should ideally not exceed 5 days; rapid onset, shorter-acting drugs are generally less likely to cause serious adverse effects.

TABLE 7
Hormones and Steroids—cont'd

Agent	Dosage	Species/Comments
Levothyroxine (L-thyroxine)	1–200 μg/kg PO q12h × 4 weeks	Psittacines, raptors
Methylprednisolone acetate[a]	200 mg/bird IM	Ratites (adults)
Oxytocin	0.5–10 U/kg IM	Most species; should be preceded by calcium administration for egg binding; contraindicated unless uterovaginal sphincter is well dilated and uterus is free of adhesions; used alone to stop uterine bleeding; may need to repeat injection
Prednisolone[a]	0.5–1 mg/kg IM, IV once	Most species
	1–1.25 mg/kg PO q48h	Ratites
	2 mg/kg PO q12h	Psittacines/inflammation
	2–4 mg/kg IM, IV	Raptors/shock
Prednisolone sodium succinate[a]	0.5–1 mg/kg IM, IV	Psittacines/antiinflammatory
	1.5–2 mg/kg IM q12h	Ratites/immunosuppression
	2–4 mg/kg IM, IV once	Psittacines/shock; trauma; endotoxemia; immunosuppression
	5–8.5 mg/kg IV q1h	Ratites/shock
Prednisone[a]	—	See prednisolone
Prostaglandin E2	0.02–0.1 mg/kg applied topically to the uterovaginal sphincter	Relaxes uterovaginal sphincter; lower dosage may be effective; freeze into aliquots
Prostaglandin F2α	0.02–0.1 mg/kg IM, intracloacal once	Dystocia; may be helpful when the egg is located distally and the uterovaginal sphincter is dilated; can result in uterine rupture, bronchoconstriction, hypertension, and death
Thyroid-stimulating hormone (TSH)	0.1 U IM	Cockatiels
	0.2 U/kg IM	Macaws/PD; T_4 doubled in 6 of 11 birds 4 h after receiving TSH
	1 U/kg IM	T_4 doubled in Hispaniolan and blue-fronted Amazon parrots 6 h after receiving TSH
	1–2 U/kg IM	Psittacines/obtain blood at 0 h, then 4–6 h after TSH stimulation

PD, Pharmacodynamic; PO, oral.

TABLE 8

Nebulization Agents[a]

Agent	Dosage	Species/Comments
N-acetyl-L-cysteine 10%–20% (Mucomyst, Bristol)	22 mg/mL sterile water until dissipated	Most species/mucolytic agent; tracheal irritation and reflex bronchoconstriction reported in mammals; use is preceded by bronchodilators in mammals; see amikacin, gentamicin, terbinafine for combinations
Amikacin	5–6 mg/mL sterile water or saline × 15 min q8–12h	Most species/discontinue if polyuria develops
	6 mg/mL sterile water and 1 mL acetyl-cysteine (20%) until dissipated q8h	Most species
Aminophylline	3 mg/mL sterile water or saline × 15 min	Most species/bronchial and pulmonary vasculature smooth muscle relaxation; incompatible with amikacin, cephalothin, clindamycin, erythromycin, oxytetracycline, methylprednisone, penicillin G, tetracycline; consult with specialized references for more information
Amphotericin B (Fungizone, Squibb)	—	May lead to hypokalemia; corticosteroids may exacerbate this effect; minor systemic absorption with aerosol administration; can be nebulized long term
	0.3–1 mg/mL × 15 min q6–12h	Most species
	7–10 mg/mL saline	Most species
Carbenicillin (Geocillin, Roerig)	20 mg/mL saline × 15 min q12h	Psittacines/Pseudomonas pneumonia; use in combination with parenteral aminoglycosides
Cefotaxime	10 mg/mL saline × 10–30 min q6–12h	Most species
Ceftriaxone	40 mg/mL sterile water	Poultry/PD
	40 mg/mL sterile water and DMSO	Poultry/PD; 1 g ceftriaxone in 10 mL sterile water, plus 15 mL DMSO
	200 mg/mL sterile water and DMSO	Poultry/PD; 4 g ceftriaxone in 10 mL sterile water, plus 10 mL DMSO
Clotrimazole (1%)	10 mg/mL propylene glycol or polyethylene glycol × 30–60 min q24h × 3 days, off 2 days, repeat prn for up to 4 months	Most species/treatment of aspergillosis for stable patients without respiratory distress; can be toxic to psittacines at this dose; may use in combination with systemic amphotericin B, flucytosine, and itraconazole
	10% clotrimazole in propylene glycol with 5% DMSO	Raptors
Doxycycline hyclate	13 mg/mL saline	Psittacines
Enilconazole	0.2 mg/5 mL saline q12h × 21 days	Most species, including raptors, psittacines
	10 mg/mL sterile saline or water	Most species/antifungal (e.g., aspergillosis)
Enrofloxacin	10 mg/mL saline	Most species
Gentamicin	3–6 mg/mL saline or sterile water and 1–2 mL acetylcysteine (20%) × 20 min q8h	Most species
	5 mg/mL saline × 15 min q8h	Most species
Lincomycin	250 mg/mL water	Most species
Miconazole	Nebulize 15 min q8h × 10 days	Raptors/aspergillosis
Oxytetracycline	2 mg/mL × 60 min q4–6h	Parakeets/PD
Piperacillin	10 mg/mL saline × 10–30 min q6–12h	Most species
Sodium chloride	—	Viscosity of respiratory secretions may be decreased by hydration
Spectinomycin	13 mg/mL saline	Most species
Sterile water	—	Viscosity of respiratory secretions may be decreased by hydration
Sulfadimethoxine	13 mg/ml saline	Most species
Terbinafine	500 mg and 1 mL acetyl-L-cysteine and 500 mL distilled water	Psittacines/aspergillosis
Terbutaline	0.01 mg/kg with 9 mL saline	Psittacines/bronchodilation
Tylosin	10 mg/mL saline × 10–60 min q12h	Most species
	20 mg/mL DMSO or distilled water × 1 h	Pigeons, quail (PD), most species
	20 mg/mL DMSO and 0.5 mL saline	Psittacines

DMSO, Dimethyl sulfoxide; PD, pharmacodynamic; prn, as needed.
[a]Nebulization is an adjunctive therapy indicated for rhinitis, sinusitis, tracheitis, pneumonia, airsacculitis, and syringeal aspergilloma, where there is air movement occurring in the patient's disease state; optimal particle size for deposition in the trachea is 2–10 μm; optimal particle size for peripheral airways is 0.5–5 μm; treatments of 30–45 min repeated q4–12h are recommended; caution: do not overhydrate airways.

TABLE 9

Agents Used in the Treatment of Toxigenic Conditions

Agent	Dosage	Species/Comments
Bismuth subsalicylate	2–5 mg/kg PO once	Adsorbent; gavage; alternatively, can use activated charcoal
Calcium EDTA (edetate calcium disodium)	—	Preferred initial chelator for lead and zinc toxicosis; may cause renal tubular necrosis in mammals; maintain hydration and monitor patient for polyuria/polydipsia; SC, IM absorbed well
	10–50 mg/kg IM q12h × 5–10 days or longer	Raptors
	20–70 mg/kg IV	Most species/empirical diagnosis; signs should resolve for up to 48 h; diluted 1:4 in saline
	25–50 mg/kg IV q12h	Geese
	30–35 mg/kg IM, IV q8–12h × 3–5 days, off 3–4 days, repeat prn	Most species
	40 mg/kg IM q12h	Cockatiels/PD; reduces lead levels when used alone or with DMSA
Charcoal, activated	—	Adsorbs toxins from the intestinal tract; may be mixed with hemicellulose to act as a bulk laxative to aid in the passage of ingested toxins; administration before cathartic use may help bind small particles of heavy metal; see magnesium hydroxide for combination
	52 mg/kg PO once	A component of oiled bird treatment; alternatively, may use bismuth
	2000–8000 mg/kg PO	Most species
Charcoal, activated/electrolyte slurry (ToxiBan, Vet-A-Mix)	—	Orally administered adsorbent for GI tract toxins
	50 mL/kg by gavage	Three bottles of charcoal slurry (3.75 g/kg) added to 250 mL of electrolyte solution; use in treatment of oiled birds
Detergent (Dawn, Procter & Gamble)	1%–5% bath	Submerse bird up to mid-neck region; rinse with water; use water at 103–105°F (39–41°C) and 40–60 psi; use in treatment of oiled birds
Dimercaptosuccinic acid	—	Oral chelator for lead or zinc; may be effective for mercury toxicity
	25–35 mg/kg PO q12h × 5 days/week × 3–5 weeks	Most species, including raptors/lead toxicosis
	25–35 mg/kg PO q24h × 10 days	Psittacines, raptors/lead and zinc toxicosis
	40 mg/kg PO q12h × 21 days	Cockatiels/PD; lead toxicosis; reduces lead levels when used alone or in combination with CaEDTA; 80 mg/kg resulted in death in >60% of cockatiels
Fluid therapy	—	Dehydration, shock, nutritional support, etc.
Magnesium hydroxide (M) (Milk of Magnesia, Roxane)/activated charcoal (C)	(M) 10–12 mL + (C) 1 tsp powder	Most species/cathartic[a]; adsorbent
Oral electrolyte solutions (Pedialyte; Ross Labs)	30 mL/kg by gavage	Most species/at field stabilization site
Penicillamine	—	Preferred chelator for copper toxicosis; may be used for lead, zinc, and mercury toxicosis
	30 mg/kg PO q12h × ≥7 days	Most species/initially supplemented with CaEDTA once in severe neurological disease
	30–55 mg/kg PO q12h × 7–14 days	Most species, including raptors, waterfowl
	50–55 mg/kg PO q24h × 1–6 weeks	Most species, including psittacines, raptors/use in combination with CaEDTA for several days followed by penicillamine × 3–6 weeks
Vitamin K[1]	0.2–2.2 mg/kg IM q4–8h until stable, then q24h PO, IM × 14–28 days	Most species, including raptors/rodenticide anticoagulant toxicosis

DMSA, Dimercaptosuccinic acid; EDTA, ethylenediaminetetraacetic acid; GI, gastrointestinal; IM, intramuscular; IV, intravenous; PD, pharmacodynamic; PO, oral; prn, as needed; SC, subcutaneous.

[a]Cathartics increase gastrointestinal motility and are used to evacuate the gut and prevent absorption of toxins.

TABLE 10

Psychotropic Agents[a]

Agent	Dosage	Species/Comments
Amitriptyline	—	Tricyclic antidepressant; antihistaminergic action; used in the treatment of pruritic conditions (including feather damaging behavior), anxiety disorders, and/or depression
	1–5 mg/kg q12–24h; PO	Most species/feather damaging behavior; obsessive compulsive disorders; phobias
	2 mg/kg q24h; PO	Psittacines/minimum of 30 days
Buspirone	0.5 mg/kg q12h; PO	Anxiolytic drug, used in the treatment of anxiety disorders
Carbamazepine	3–10 mg/kg q24h; PO	Anticonvulsant; treatment of seizure disorders; may also be beneficial to treat feather damaging behavior and anxiety- or frustration-related aggression
	166 mg/L drinking water	Most species/anticonvulsant; analgesic; may cause bone marrow suppression; combination with chlorpromazine or haloperidol recommended for the initial 2 weeks of the treatment
Chlorpromazine	—	Phenothiazine derivative; antipsychotic drug; dopamine antagonist (less specific than haloperidol); main effect is sedation, but may be useful for feather damaging behavior as well
	0.1–0.2 mg/kg once (tranquilizer)	Cockatoos, Ring-necked parakeets/use with carbamazepine after the removal of Elizabethan collar; mild sedation and decreases obsessive behaviors
	1 mL stock solution[b]/120 mL drinking water	Most species/mild sedation
	0.2–1 mL stock solution/kg q12–24h	Most species/mild sedation
Clomipramine	—	Tricyclic antidepressant; antihistamine; used for example in the treatment of impulsive and obsessive-compulsive disorders (ICD/OCD), depression and/or anxiety disorders
	0.5–1 mg/kg q12–24h; PO	Psittacines/feather damaging behavior; automutilation; start with low dose and gradually increase over 4–5 days
	3–5 mg/kg q12–24h; PO	Psittacines/compulsive feather damaging behavior or impulse control disorder; anxiety
	4–9.5 mg/kg q12h; PO	Grey parrots/behavior interpreted as paradoxical anxiety; combine with anxiolytic therapy (buspirone)
Diazepam	—	Benzodiazepine sedative; anxiolytic/stress-associated feather picking; useful as sole agent or in combination with phenobarbital for seizure control
	0.25–0.5 mg/kg IM, IV q24h × 2–3 days	Raptors/appetite stimulant
	0.5 mg/kg PO	Passerines/calm fractious species
	0.5–0.6 mg/kg IM	Most species/facilitates acceptance of Elizabethan collar
	0.5–1(–1.5) mg/kg PO, IM, IV q8–12h	Most species/control of seizures
	2.5–4 mg/kg PO q6–8h	Psittacines/sedation
	10–20 mg/L drinking water	Most species
Diphenhydramine	—	Antihistamine; mild hypnotic effects; suspected allergic feather picking
	2–4 mg/kg PO q12h	Most species
	2 mg/L drinking water	Most species
Doxepin	—	Tricyclic antidepressant; antihistaminergic action; used in the treatment of pruritic conditions (including feather damaging behavior), anxiety disorders, and/or depression
	0.5–1 mg/kg q12h; PO	Most species/feather damaging behavior
	1–2 mg/kg q12h; PO	Psittacines/anxiety; pruritus
	1–5 mg/kg q24h; PO	Psittacines/feather damaging behavior

IM, Intramuscular; IV, intravenous; PO, oral.

[a]The use of psychotropic agents in birds is controversial because safety, efficacy, and pharmacologic effects are poorly documented; anxiolytics or tricyclic antidepressants may be useful for stereotypic behaviors or mutilation; selective serotonin reuptake inhibitors may prove helpful for explosive behaviors; consider metabolic scaling when calculating dosages; these treatments should be used as components of a structured behavior change strategy. Note: most of the dosages mentioned in this table have been derived from case reports and/or anecdotal evidence. As information on pharmacokinetics, pharmacodynamics, efficacy, and toxicity is currently lacking for most of these drugs, no specific recommendations can be made at this stage.

[b]Stock solution: 125 mg chlorpromazine in 31 mL simple syrup.

TABLE 10

Psychotropic Agents—cont'd

Agent	Dosage	Species/Comments
Fluoxetine	—	Selective serotonin re-uptake inhibitor; antidepressant; adjunctive treatment for depression-induced feather picking
	0.4–4 mg/kg PO q24h	Psittacines/compulsive feather picking
	2–3 mg/kg PO q12–24h	Most species, including psittacines
	1 mg/kg q24h; PO	Psittacines
	1–5 mg/kg q24h; PO	Psittacines
Haloperidol	—	Butyrophenone derivative; dopamine antagonist, antipsychotic drug
	0.1–0.2 mg/kg q12h; PO	Psittacines/automutilation; feather damaging behavior
	0.2–0.9 mg/kg q24h; PO	Most species/stereotypic preening behavior
	1–2 mg/kg q14–21d; IM	Most species, including psittacines
Hydroxyzine	—	Antihistamine; treatment of allergic responses, pruritus and pruritus-associated behavioral disorders
	2 mg/kg q8–12h; PO	Most species/pruritus
	30–40 mg/L drinking water	Most species
Levetiracetam	50 mg/kg PO q8h or 100 mg/kg PO q12h[29]	Hispaniolan Amazon parrots/antiepileptic; potential use in long-term anticonvulsive treatment; drug levels should be monitored
Lorazepam	—	Benzodiazepine, tranquilizer/sedative; used in macaws with feather picking or aggression (may be used concurrently with haloperidol)
	0.1 mg/kg q12h; PO	Macaws/aggression; feather damaging behavior; use alone or with haloperidol
Naloxone	—	Opiate receptor antagonist, used in the acute treatment of stereotypies, compulsive, and self-injurious behaviors or addictions
	2 mg/kg; IV	Psittacines/may be used to determine the response of stereotypic behavior to antagonist therapy; reduction of behavior should be observed within 20 min
Naltrexone	—	Opiate receptor antagonist, used in the acute treatment of stereotypies, compulsive and self-injurious behaviors or addictions
	1.5 mg/kg q8–12h; PO	Most species/feather damaging behavior; automutilation; contraindicated in patients with liver disease; may need to increase dosage 2–6× to be effective; dissolve tablet in 10 mL sterile water; preservative does not go into solution
Nortriptyline	—	Tricyclic antidepressant; may be beneficial for treating feather damaging behavior, anxiety and/or depression. Hyperactivity commonly noted as side effect
	16 mg/L drinking water	Most species/feather damaging behavior; seldom used; decrease dose or discontinue if hyperactivity develops; taper dose to discontinue
Paroxetine	—	Selective serotonin reuptake inhibitor, antidepressant, used in the treatment of depression, post-traumatic stress and panic disorders and ICD/OCD
	1–2 mg/kg q12–24h; PO	Macaws, ibis/feather damaging behavior; automutilation; generally requires long-term therapy
	3 mg/kg q12h; PO	Pigeons/reduce compulsive behavior
	4 mg/kg q12h; PO	Grey parrots
Phenobarbital sodium	—	Barbiturate anticonvulsant; mild sedative effect; long-term seizure management; adjust dosage based on blood levels; may cause deep sedation and inability to perch
	1–5 mg/kg IV bolus	Most species/status epilepticus; begin at low end of dosage range and increase for refractory seizures
	2–7 mg/kg PO q8–12h	Most species/feather picking; seizures; self-mutilation
	50–80 mg/L drinking water	Most species, including Amazon parrots/idiopathic epilepsy
Potassium bromide	—	Long-term seizure management; use as sole agent or in conjunction with phenobarbital; monitor blood levels that may take up to 90 days to establish steady state; not available in approved dosage forms in North America; may be obtained from chemical companies or compounding pharmacies; for a concentration of 250 mg/mL, add distilled water as needed to 25 g of potassium bromide for a final volume of 100 mL
	25 mg/kg PO q24h	Most species
	50–80 mg/kg PO q24h	Pigeons
	75 mg/kg PO	Psittacines

TABLE 11

Nutritional/Mineral Support

Agent	Dosage	Species/Comments
Calcium	—	Recommended dietary levels[a]
	3–10 mg/kg feed (0.3%–1%)	Laying parrots
	4–8 mg/kg feed (0.4%–0.8%)	Growing Muscovy ducks
	8 mg/kg feed (0.8%)	Growing Japanese quail
	8–10 mg/kg feed (0.8%–1%)	Growing chickens
	18.8–32.5 mg/kg feed (1.88%–3.25%)	Laying chickens/3.25% recommended for hens that lay eggs daily
	22.5 mg/kg feed (2.25%)	Laying turkeys
Calcium borogluconate (10%)	50–100 mg/kg IM, IV	Psittacines/20% solution
	100–500 mg/kg SC, IV (slow) once	Raptors/hypocalcemic
Calcium glubionate	25–150 mg/kg PO q12h	Most species/hypocalcemia, calcium supplementation
Calcium gluconate (10%)	—	Hypocalcemia; dilute 1:1 with saline or sterile water for IM or IV injections
	5–10 mg/kg SC, IM, IV (slow) q12h prn	Psittacines/hypocalcemic tetany
	10–100 mg/kg IM	Psittacines/acute presentation of hypocalcemia
	25–50 mg/kg SC, IV (slow)	Pigeons
	50–100 mg/kg IM (diluted), IV (slow)	Most species, including psittacines, pigeons, raptors
	1 mL/30 mL (3300 mg/L) drinking water	Psittacines/calcium supplementation
Calcium lactate/calcium glycerophosphate	5–10 mg/kg IM q7d prn	Most species, including raptors/hypocalcemia
	50–100 mg/kg IV (slow bolus) once	Grey parrots
Dextrose (50%)	50–100 mg/kg IV (slow bolus) to effect	Psittacines/hypoglycemia; can dilute with fluids
	500–1000 mg/kg IV (slow bolus)	Hypoglycemia; can dilute with fluids
Hemicellulose (Metamucil, Searle)	Small amount on food daily	Most species/for bulk in diet; facilitates defecation in bowel deficit disorders and other conditions
	0.5 tsp/60 mL hand-feeding formula or baby food gruel	Psittacines/bulk diet to delay absorption of an ingested toxin
Iodine (Lugol's iodine)	0.2 mL/L drinking water daily	Most species/thyroid hyperplasia
	2 parts iodine + 28 parts water; 3 drops into 100 mL drinking water	Budgerigars/thyroid hyperplasia
Iron	20–40 mg/kg feed	Toucans/levels recommended for a low-iron diet
Iron dextran	10 mg/kg IM, repeat in 7–10 days prn	Most species/iron deficiency anemia; use cautiously in species in which iron storage disease is common
Lactobacillus (Bene-Bac, Pet-Ag)	1 pinch/day/bird	Psittacines/stimulation of normal gastrointestinal flora regrowth
	1 tsp/L hand-feeding formula	Most species
Pancreatic enzyme powder (Viokase-V Powder, Fort Dodge)	—	Most species/exocrine pancreatic insufficiency; maldigestion; mix with food and let stand 30 min
	2–5 g/kg	Most species
	⅛ tsp/kg feed	Most species
	⅛ tsp/60–120 g lightly oil-coated seed	Most species
	⅛ tsp/30–120 mL hand-feeding formula prn	Psittacine neonates
Selenium (Se)	0.05–0.1 mg Se/kg IM q3–14d	Most species/neuromuscular diseases (capture myopathy, white muscle disease, some cardiomyopathies); may be useful in some cockatiels with jaw, eyelid, and tongue paralysis
Vitamin A	200 U/kg IM	Raptor juveniles/ supplemental therapy for pox infection
	2000 U/kg PO, IM	Psittacines/adjunctive therapy for pox infection
	5000 U/kg IM q24h × 14 days, then 250–1000 IU/kg q24h PO	Psittacines/adjunctive therapy for respiratory or epithelial disease
	20,000–33,000 U/kg IM q7d	Most species/hypovitaminosis A; maximum dose; improves skin healing

IM, Intramuscular; IV, intravenous; PO, oral; prn, as needed; SC, subcutaneous.
[a]Grains and seeds commonly fed to parrots contain calcium levels of approximately 0.02–0.1% dry matter (DM).
[b]Food items known to contain appreciable amounts of thiaminase include clams, herring, smelt, and mackerel.

TABLE 11

Nutritional/Mineral Support—cont'd

Agent	Dosage	Species/Comments
Vitamin B_1 (thiamine)	—	Thiamine deficiency; requirements may be higher if thiaminase is present in diet[b]
	1–2 mg/kg PO q24h	Raptors, penguins, cranes/daily supplement
	1–2 mg/kg IM q24h	Vultures, raptors, cranes, penguins/CNS signs
	1–3 mg/kg IM q7d	Most species, including raptors
	1–50 mg/kg PO q24h × 7 days or indefinitely	Raptors
	3–30 mg/kg IM q7d	Raptors/stimulates appetite, hematopoiesis; neuromuscular disease; liver disease; supportive therapy; adjunct to sulfa therapy
	25–30 mg/kg feed or fish	Piscivorous species/recommended level of supplementation
	2850 mg/L drinking water q7d	Pigeons
Vitamin B_{12} (cyanocobalamin)	0.25–0.5 mg/kg IM q7d	Most species/anemia
	2–5 mg/bird SC	Pigeons/vitamin B_{12} deficiency
Vitamin B complex	—	Usually dosed based on thiamine (see vitamin B_1)
Vitamin D_3	3300 U/kg IM q7d prn	Most species/hypovitaminosis D_3; hypervitaminosis D may occur with excessive use
	6600 U/kg IM once	Most species
	11–30 min of direct sunlight/day	Chickens/sufficient for endogenous synthesis of vitamin D
Vitamin E	0.06 mg/kg IM q7d	Psittacines/hypovitaminosis E
	0.06 mg/kg IM	Ratites/prevention or treatment of capture myopathy
	15 mg/kg PO once	Raptors/PD; administer without food
	200–400 mg/bird PO q24h	Great blue herons
	100 mg/kg fish (wet basis)	Piscivorous species/recommended level of supplementation
Vitamin K_1 (phytonadione)	0.025–2.5 mg/kg IM q12h	Most species
	0.2–2.2 mg/kg IM q4–8h until stable, then q24h × 14 days	Most species/rodenticide toxicity
	2.5 mg/kg IM q24h until hemostasis, then q7d prn	Psittacines/vitamin K responsive disorders; hematochezia; coagulopathy
	10–20 mg/kg IM q12–24h	Psittacines
	0.1 mg/kg feed	Turkeys/PD; as effective as 1–2 mg/kg in reducing plasma prothrombin time

CNS, Central nervous system; PD, pharmacodynamic.

TABLE 12

Ophthalmologic Agents

Agent	Dosage	Species/Comments
Bacitracin/neomycin/polymyxin B sulfate	Small bead topical	Most species/antibiotic; corneal ulcers, conjunctivitis
Chloramphenicol ophthalmic drops	1 drop topical q6–8h	Most species, antibiotic
Ciprofloxacin HCl	1 drop topical q4–8h	Most species/antibiotic; corneal ulcers, conjunctivitis (e.g., *Chlamydophila*, *Mycoplasma*)
	One drop topical q12h; use in conjunction with tylosin 1 mg/mL drinking water × 21–77 days	House finches/*Mycoplasma gallisepticum* conjunctivitis
Flurbiprofen ophthalmic solution	Topical as indicated[33]	NSAID used in the eye to treat or prevent inflammation (i.e., uveitis, conjunctivitis)
Neomycin/polymyxin B/gramicidin	1 drop topical q2–8h	Most species/antibiotic; corneal ulcers; conjunctivitis
Oxytetracycline/polymyxin B	Small bead topical	Most species/antibiotic; conjunctivitis
Prednisolone acetate (1%)	1 drop q4–8h	Raptors/traumatic anterior uveitis without corneal ulceration
Proparacaine (0.5%)	Topical	Topical anesthesia
Rocuronium bromide	—	Neuromuscular blocking agent
	0.12 mg topical in each eye[2]	European kestrels/mydriatic agent; maximal mydriasis was achieved in 90 min
Tetracaine (6%)	Topical	Topical anesthetic

NSAID, Nonsteroidal antiinflammatory drugs.

TABLE 13

Agents Used in Emergencies

Agent	Dosage	Species/Comments
Atropine sulfate	0.2–0.5 mg/kg IM, IV, IO	Bradycardia; CPR
Aminophylline	4 mg/kg PO q6–12h	Can give orally after initial response
	10 mg/kg IV q3h	Use for pulmonary edema
Calcium gluconate	50–100 mg/kg IM, IV (slow bolus)	Hypocalcemia; dilute 50 mg/mL; hyperkalemia
Dexamethasone Na phosphate	2–6 mg/kg IM, IV q12–24h	Head trauma (until signs abate); shock (one dose); hyperthermia (until stable); use in these conditions is controversial
Dextrose (50%)	50–100 mg/kg IV (slow bolus to effect)	Hypoglycemia; can dilute with fluids
	500–1000 mg/kg IV (slow bolus)	Hypoglycemia; can dilute with fluids
Dextran 70	10–20 mL/kg	Most species/hypovolemic shock
Diazepam	0.5–1 mg/kg IM, IV prn	Seizures
Doxapram	5–20 mg/kg IM, IV, IO	Most species/respiratory depression or arrest; CPR
Epinephrine (1:1000)	0.5–1 mL/kg IM, IV, IO, intratracheal	CPR; bradycardia
Fluids	10–25 mL/kg IV, IO	Bolus over 5–7 min
	50–90 mL/kg fluids SC,[a] IV, IO	Most species
Hetastarch	10–15 mL/kg IV (slow) q8h × 1–4 treatments	Most species, including raptors/hypoproteinemia; hypovolemia
Mannitol	0.2–2 mg/kg IV (slow) q24h	Raptors/cerebral edema; anuric renal failure; contraindicated in intracranial bleeding
Magnesium sulfate	20 mg/kg IM once[18]	African Grey parrot/treatment for seizure activity associated with hypomagnesemia (associated with hypocalcemia that is not responsive to calcium therapy)
Prednisolone Na succinate	10–20 mg/kg IM, IV q15min prn	Historically it has been used for head trauma and CPR; use in these conditions is controversial; no longer appears to be a treatment for traumatic brain injury, and may actually exacerbate mortality.
	15–30 mg/kg IV	Raptors/see comment above
Sodium bicarbonate	1 mEq/kg q15–30min to maximum of 4 mEq/kg total dose	Metabolic acidosis
	5 mEq/kg IV, IO once	CPR
Terbutaline	0.01 mg/kg PO, IM q6h	Psittacines/α2-selective smooth muscle bronchodilator
	0.1 mg/kg PO q12–24h	Macaws, Amazon parrots/bronchodilator; obstructive pulmonary disease, pneumonitis

CPR, Cardiopulmonary resuscitation; IM, intramuscular; IO, intraosseous; IV, intravenous; PO, oral; prn, as needed; SC, subcutaneous.
[a]Because of the presence of peripheral vasoconstriction, subcutaneous administration is not adequate for patients in shock.

TABLE 14

Miscellaneous Agents

Agent	Dosage	Species/Comments
Aminophylline	4–5 mg/kg PO, IM, IV q6–12h	Most species/bronchodilator; need to prepare as a suspension daily
	8–10 mg/kg PO, IM, IV q6–8h	Raptors, ratites
	10 mg/kg IV q3h, then PO after initial response	Most species
	10 mg/kg IM, IV q8–12h	Most species/for IV use, dilute in 10–20 mL saline or 5% dextrose in water and inject slowly
Anticoagulant citrate dextrose (A-C-D Solution, Sanofi)	0.15 mL/1 mL whole blood	Anticoagulant for transfusions; not effective for extended storage of whole blood; heparin can be substituted if A-C-D is not available
Armor All Protectant (Armor All Protectant Corp.)	Topical to affected plumage	Most species/softens sticky trap glue-covered plumage; use detergent (Dawn) to remove Armor All
Bismuth subsalicylate (Pepto Bismol, Procter & Gamble)	1–2 mL/kg PO q12h	Most species/weak adsorbent, demulcent
	2–5 mL/kg PO once	Most species/a component of oiled bird treatment; alternatively can use activated charcoal
Chlorhexidine (0.05%–0.1% solution)	Topical	Presurgical skin cleaner; antiseptic
Cimetidine	—	Prototype histamine-2 blocker used to reduce gastrointestinal (GI) acid production
	3–10 mg/kg PO, IM, IV q8–12h	Ratites
	5 mg/kg PO, IM q8–12h	Psittacines/proventriculitis; gastric ulceration
Cisapride	0.5–1.5 mg/kg PO q8h	Most species/GI prokinetic agent, stimulates motility; not commercially available in United States; can be compounded
Citrate phosphate dextrose adenine solution (CPDA)	1 part CPDA:5 parts whole blood	Most species/anticoagulant for blood collection for transfusion; not for extended storage of whole blood
Dextran 70	10–20 mL/kg IV	Most species/hypovolemic shock; colloid with a t½ shorter than hetastarch
Digoxin	—	Congestive heart disease; toxic reactions include depression, ataxia, vomiting, diarrhea; contraindicated with renal or liver disease; monitoring of serum digoxin, potassium, magnesium, calcium, and ECG is recommended; induced arrhythmias in pigeons at 0.2 mg/kg/day
	0.0035 mg/kg IV q24h	Turkeys
	0.0049 mg/kg IV q12h	Poultry
	0.01 mg/kg PO q24h × 6 weeks	Chickens/ascites syndrome; reduced ascites; no apparent toxicity
	0.01–0.02 mg/kg PO q12h	Psittacines, passerines, raptors/congestive heart disease
	0.02 mg/kg PO q24h × 5 days	Parakeets, sparrows (PD)/this dose led to signs of toxicity in a mynah
	0.05 mg/kg PO q24h	Quaker parakeets/PD; congestive heart failure; cardiomyopathy
	0.13 mg/L drinking water	Psittacines, passerines, raptors/congestive heart disease
Diphenhydramine	1–4 mg/kg PO q8–12h	Psittacines/allergic rhinitis, hypersensitivity, pruritus
	2 mg/kg IV, IO once	Cockatoos/used before chemotherapy
	2–4 mg/kg PO, IM, IV q12h	Most species/has calming effect in some anxious birds; may cause hypotension
	20–40 mg/L drinking water	Most species

ECG, Electrocardiogram; IM, intramuscular; IO, intraosseous; IV, intravenous; PD, pharmacodynamic; PO, oral.

TABLE 14

Miscellaneous Agents—cont'd

Agent	Dosage	Species/Comments
Enalapril	0.25–0.5 mg/kg PO q24–48h	Most species/dilated cardiomyopathy; monitor uric acid levels; reduce dose or discontinue if concurrent renal disease
	1.25 mg/kg PO q8–12h	Pigeons, Amazon parrots/PK
	2.5–5 mg/kg PO q12h	Amazon parrot/right-sided heart failure; long-term therapy
Ferric subsulfate	Topical	Most species/hemostasis of bleeding nail or beak tip; will cause necrosis if used on open skin lesions
Fluids	PO, SC, IV as needed	Fluid requirement for most birds is 50 mL/kg/day
Furosemide	—	Diuretic; overdose can cause dehydration and electrolyte abnormalities; toxicity characterized by neurologic signs and death
	0.1–2 mg/kg PO, SC, IM, IV q6–24h	Most species, including psittacines, raptors/lories are extremely sensitive
	0.15 mg/kg IM q8h	Mynahs/ascites, hemochromatosis
	0.5–2.2 mg/kg PO, IM q12–24h	Most species/cardiac disease, ascites
	2–5 mg/kg PO, IM q12–24h	Raptors/cardiac disease, pulmonary congestion
	2.5–10 mg/kg PO q12h × 7–14 days	Cockatiels, budgerigars/ascites
	40 mg/L drinking water	Most species/congestive heart failure; can be used with digoxin and ACE inhibitors
Gadopentetate dimeglumine (Magnevist, Berlex)	0.25 mmol/kg IV	Contrast agent for magnetic resonance imaging
Glipizide	—	Sulfonylurea antidiabetic; contraindicated in ketotic patients; patients should be maintained at trace glycosuria to prevent hypoglycemia
	0.5 mg/kg PO q12h	Cockatiels/diabetes mellitus
	1.25 mg/kg PO q24h	Most species/diabetes mellitus
Heparin	2 U/mL whole blood	Anticoagulant for blood transfusions
Hetastarch (Hespan, DuPont)	—	Colloid with a t½ of 25 h; use with caution in patients suffering from congestive heart failure or renal failure
	10–15 mL/kg IV q8h × 1–4 treatments	Most species/chronic hypoproteinemia; decrease fluid treatment to ⅓–½ maintenance fluid dose
Hydroxyzine (Atarax, Roerig)	2–2.2 mg/kg PO q8h	Allergic pruritus; feather picking; self-mutilation
	34–40 mg/L drinking water	Most species/respiratory allergy; feather picking
Iohexol (Omnipaque, Sanofi Winthrop)	25–30 mL/kg PO	Cockatoos, Amazon parrots/gavage; radiographic GI iodinated contrast media; 1:1 dilution with water can also be used
	50 mL/kg PO	Quaker parakeets, budgerigars
Kaolin/pectin	2 mL/kg PO q6–12h	Psittacine neonates/intestinal protectant, antidiarrheal
	≤15 mL/kg PO, repeat prn	Raptors
Lactulose	—	Reduces blood ammonia levels; does not treat liver disease
	150–650 mg/kg (0.2–1 mL/kg) PO q8–12h	Most species, including psittacines/hepatic encephalopathy
	200 mg/kg (0.3 mL/kg) PO q8–12h	Psittacine neonates
Magnesium hydroxide (M)/activated charcoal (C)	(M) 10–12 mL + (C) 1 tsp powder	Most species/cathartic; adsorbent
Magnesium sulfate (Epsom salts)	0.25–1 g/kg PO q24h × 1–2 days	Most species/purgative, cathartic; may cause lethargy; see peanut butter for combination
Mannitol	0.25–2 mg/kg q24h IV (slow bolus)	Most species/osmotic diuretic used to treat cerebral edema, especially after head trauma; may be used with furosemide

ACE, Angiotensin-converting-enzyme; prn, as needed; PK, pharmacokinetic; SC, subcutaneous.

TABLE 14

Miscellaneous Agents—cont'd

Agent	Dosage	Species/Comments
Metoclopramide	—	GI motility disorders; regurgitation; slow crop motility; no alterations in motility observed after a single dose of 1 mg/kg IM
	0.3 mg/kg PO, IM, IV	Most species
	0.5 mg/kg PO, IM, IV q8–12h	Most species, including psittacines/GI ileus; regurgitation
	2 mg/kg IM, IV q8–12h	Raptors, waterfowl/crop stasis; ileus
	12.5 mg/kg PO	Ratites/GI disorders
Mineral oil	5–10 mL/kg PO via gavage	Most species/cathartic; used to aid passage of grit and other foreign bodies; administer directly into the crop because oral administration may result in aspiration pneumonia; see peanut butter for combination
Peanut butter	Peanut butter and mineral oil (2:1)	Most species/add to diet; cathartic
	Dilute peanut butter and magnesium sulfate	Most species/add to diet; cathartic; dilute with water
Pentobarbital sodium	0.2–1 mL/kg IV, ICe	Most species/birds may react unpredictably with IV administration; ICe administration is smooth, quiet
Pimobendan (Vetmedin, Boehringer-Ingelheim)	—	Phosphodiesterase-inhibitor and calcium sensitizer used in treatment of congestive heart failure
	10 mg/kg PO[15]	Hispaniolan Amazon parrots/use tablet suspension; safety and efficacy are unknown; potential use in other birds is unknown
Povidone iodine	Topical, wash off within 5 min	Raptors/wound cleansing; antiseptic; but is infrequently used in avian dermatology owing to its drying, irritating, and staining effects
Propranolol	0.04 mg/kg IV (slow)	Most species/supraventricular arrhythmia, atrial flutter, fibrillation
	0.2 mg/kg IM	
Psyllium (Metamucil, Procter & Gamble)	0.5 tsp/60 mL hand-feeding formula	Most species/bulk diet; can use mineral oil as alternative or in addition to psyllium
Silymarin (milk thistle)	50–75 mg/kg PO q12h	Most species/hepatic antioxidant; use in patients with liver disease and as ancillary to chemotherapy; use a low-alcohol or alcohol-free liquid formulation
Skin-So-Soft (Avon)	Topical to affected plumage	Most species/softens and removes sticky trap glue from plumage; use Dawn dish detergent to remove Skin-So-Soft product[a]
Sucralfate	25 mg/kg PO q8h	Most species/oral, esophageal, gastric, duodenal ulcers; give 1 h before food or other drugs
Terbutaline	0.01 mg/kg PO, IM q6h	Psittacines/α2-selective smooth muscle bronchodilator
	0.1 mg/kg PO q12–24h	Macaws, Amazon parrots/bronchodilator; obstructive pulmonary disease; pneumonitis
Theophylline	2 mg/kg PO q12h	Severe macaws/bronchodilation
Tincture of iodine	Topical	Most species, raptors/wounds
Trypsin-balsam of Peru-castor oil (Granulex, Pfizer)	Topical	Most species/digests necrotic tissue (may have debriding action); may have analgesic effects; may cause local inflammation and pyogenic reaction; do not use for long-term management[a]
Urate oxidase (Uricozyme, Sanofi Winthrop)	100–200 U/kg IM q24h	Red-tailed hawks, pigeons/PD; significantly lowered plasma uric acid, including postprandial plasma uric acid
Yeast cell derivatives (Preparation H, WhiteHall)	Topical q24h	Most species/pododermatitis; stimulation of epithelialization

ICe, Intracoelomic.
[a]Many topical agents contain oils that adhere to plumage. These agents should be used sparingly and generally in non-feathered regions to prevent losing the insulative properties of the plumage.

REFERENCES

1. Baine K, Jones MP, Cox S, Martin-Jimènez T: Pharmacokinetics of gabapentin in Hispaniolan Amazon parrots (*Amazona ventralis*), *Proc Annu Conf Assoc Avian Vet* 19–20, 2013.

2. Barsotti G, Briganti A, Spratte JR, et al: Safety and efficacy of bilateral topical application of rocuronium bromide for mydriasis in European kestrels (*Falco tinnunculus*), *J Avian Med Surg* 26:1–5, 2012.

3. Carpenter JW, Tully TN Jr, Gehring R, Guzman DS-M: Single-dose pharmacokinetics of piperacillin/tazobactam in the Hispaniolan Amazon parrot (*Amazona ventralis*). In press.

4. Cowan ML, Martin GB, Monks DJ, et al: Inhibition of the reproductive system by deslorelin in male and female pigeons (*Columba livia*), *J Avian Med Surg* 28:102–108, 2014.

5. Dong-Hun L, Yu-Na L, Jae-keun P, et al: Antiviral efficacy of oseltamivir against avian influenza virus in avian species, *Avian Dis* 55:677–679, 2011.

6. Emery LC, Cox SK, Souza MJ: Pharmacokinetics of nebulized terbinafine in Hispaniolan Amazon parrots (*Amazona ventralis*), *J Avian Med Surg* 26:161–166, 2012.

7. Evans EE, Emery LC, Cox SK, et al: Pharmacokinetics of terbinafine after oral administration of a single dose to Hispaniolan Amazon parrots (*Amazona ventralis*), *Am J Vet Res* 74:835–838, 2013.

8. Feng F, Teoh CQ, Qiao Q, et al: The development of persistent duck hepatitis B virus infection can be prevented using antiviral therapy combined with DNA or recombinant fowl poxvirus vaccines, *Vaccine* 28:7436–7443, 2010.

9. Fernández-Varón E, Carceles C, Espuny A, et al: Pharmacokinetics of a combination preparation of ampicillin and sulbactam in turkeys, *Am J Vet Res* 65:1658–1663, 2004.

10. Fernández-Varón E, Carceles C, Espuny A, et al: Pharmacokinetics of an ampicillin–sulbactam (2:1) combination after intravenous and intramuscular administration to chickens, *Vet Res Commun* 30:285–291, 2006.

11. Flammer K, Massey JG, Roudybush T, Meek C: Doxycycline-medicated pelleted diet in cockatiels, *Proc Annu Conf Assoc Avian Vet* 15, 2011.

12. Garcia-Montijano M, de Lucas JJ, Rodriguez C: Marbofloxacin disposition after intravenous administration of a single dose in wild mallard ducks (*Anas platyrhynchos*), *J Avian Med Surg* 26:6–10, 2012.

13. Gentry J, Montgerard C, Crandall E, et al: Voriconazole disposition after single and multiple, oral doses in healthy, adult red-tailed hawks (*Buteo jamaicensis*), *J Avian Med Surg* 28(3):201–208, 2014.

14. Goudah A, Hasabelnaby S: The disposition of marbofloxacin after single dose intravenous, intramuscular and oral administration to Muscovy ducks, *J Vet Pharmcol Ther* 34:197–201, 2011.

15. Guzman DS-M, Beaufrère H, Kukanich B, et al: Pharmacokinetics of single dose oral pimobendan in Hispaniolan Amazon parrots (*Amazon ventralis*), *J Avian Med Surg* 28:95–101, 2014.

16. Hawkins MG, Taylor IT, Byrne BA, et al: Pharmacokinetic-pharmacodynamic integration of orbifloxacin in Japanese quail (*Coturnix japonica*) following oral and intravenous administration, *J Vet Pharmacol Ther* 34:350–358, 2011.

17. Hope KL, Tell LA, Byrne BA, et al: Pharmacokinetics of a single intramuscular injection of ceftiofur crystalline-free acid in American black ducks (*Anas rubripes*), *Am J Vet Res* 73:620–627, 2012.

18. Kirchgessner MS, Tully TN Jr, Naverez J, et al: Magnesium therapy in a hypocalcemic African grey parrot (*Psittacus erithacus*), *J Avian Med Surg* 26:17–21, 2012.

19. Kline Y, Clemons KV, Woods L, et al: Pharmacokinetics of voriconazole in adult mallard ducks (*Anas platyrhynchos*), *Med Mycol* 49:500–512, 2011.

20. Lenarduzzi T, Langston C, Ross MK: Pharmacokinetics of clindamycin administered orally to pigeons, *J Avian Med Surg* 25:259–265, 2011.

21. Mans C, Guzman DS-M, Lahner LL, et al: Sedation and physiologic response to manual restraint after intranasal administration of midazolam in Hispaniolan Amazon parrots (*Amazona ventralis*), *J Avian Med Surg* 26:130–139, 2012.

22. Mans C, Pilny A: Use of GnRH-agonists for medical management of reproductive disorders in birds, *Vet Clin North Am Exot Anim Pract* 17:22–33, 2014.

23. Molter CM, Court MH, Cole GA, et al: Pharmacokinetics of meloxicam after intravenous, intramuscular, and oral administration of a single dose to Hispaniolan Amazon parrots (*Amazona ventralis*), *Am J Vet Res* 74:375–380, 2013.

24. Nemetz L: Deslorelin acetate long-term suppression of ovarian carcinoma in a cockatiel (*Nymphicus hollandicus*), *Proc Annu Conf Assoc Avian Vet* 37–42, 2012.

25. Petritz OA, Guzman DS-M, Wiebe VJ, et al: Stability of three commonly compounded extemporaneous enrofloxacin suspensions for oral administration to exotic animals, *J Am Vet Med Assoc* 243:85–90, 2013.

26. Petritz OA, Guzman DS-M, Paul-Murphy J, et al: Evaluation of the efficacy and safety of single administration of 4.7-mg deslorelin acetate implants on egg production and plasma sex hormones in Japanese quail (*Coturnix coturnix japonica*), *Am J Vet Res* 74:316–323, 2013.

27. Ratzlaff K, Papich MG, Flammer K: Plasma concentrations of fluconazole after a single oral dose and administration in drinking water in cockatiels (*Nymphicus hollandicus*), *J Avian Med Surg* 25:23–31, 2011.

28. Sadar MJ, Hawkins MG, Drzenovich T, et al: Pharmacokinetic-pharmacodynamic integration of an extended-release ceftiofur formulation administered to red-tailed hawks (*Buteo jamaicensis*), *Proc Annu Conf Assoc Avian Vet* 11, 2014.

29. Schnellbacher R, Beaufrère H, Arnold RD, et al: Pharmacokinetics of levetiracetam in healthy Hispaniolan Amazon parrots (*Amazona ventralis*) after oral administration of a single dose, *J Avian Med Surg* 28:193–200, 2014.

30. Schnellbacher RW, da Cunha AF, Beaufrère H, et al: Effects of dopamine and dobutamine on isoflurane-induced hypotension in Hispaniolan Amazon parrots (*Amazona ventralis*), *Am J Vet Res* 73:952–958, 2012.

31. Wack AN, KuKanich B, Bronson E, et al: Pharmacokinetics of enrofloxacin after single dose oral and intravenous administration in the African penguin (*Spheniscus demersus*), *J Zoo Wildl Med* 43:309–316, 2012.

32. Waxman S, Prados AP, de Lucas J, et al: Pharmacokinetic and pharmacodynamic properties of enrofloxacin in Southern crested caracaras (*Caracara plancus*), *J Avian Med Surg* 27:180–186, 2013.

33. Williams DL: *The avian eye: Ophthalmology of Exotic Pets*, West Sussex, UK, 2012, John Wiley & Sons, pp 119–158.

34. Wojick KB, Langan JN, Adkesson MJ, et al: Pharmacokinetics of long-acting ceftiofur crystalline-free acid in helmeted guineafowl (*Numida meleagris*) after a single intramuscular injection, *Am J Vet Res* 72:1514–1518, 2011.

35. Yuan LG, Wang R, Sun LH, et al: Pharmacokinetics of marbofloxacin in muscovy ducks (*Cairina moschata*), *J Vet Pharmacol Ther* 34:82–85, 2011.

Normal Clinical Pathologic Data

Alan M. Fudge • *Brian L. Speer*

TABLE 1

Hematology: Laboratory Reference Ranges for Selected Species*

Species Common Name (Common name synonyms) Scientific Name	N[†]	Units	Packed Cell Volume (%)		White Blood Cell Count C Units: ×10⁹/L S.I.: ×10³/mcL (%)		Heterophils C Units: ×10⁹/L S.I.: ×10³/mcL (%)	
			Mean	Range	Mean	Range	Mean	Range
Grey parrot (African Grey) genus *Psittacus* sp.	5571	Conventional			10.3	6–13	6.0667	4.635–7.519
		S.I.			10.3	6–13	6.0667	4.635–7.519
		%	48.2	45–53			58.9	45–73
Grey parrot (African Grey, Congo) *Psittacus erithacus*	495	Conventional			12.0	8–15	7.236	5.520–8.880
		S.I.			12.0	8–15	7.236	5.520–8.880
		%	46.1	42–52			60.3	46–74
Timneh parrot (African Grey, timneh) *P. timneh*	219	Conventional			11.3	9–13	6.486	5.085–7.91
		S.I.			11.3	9–13	6.486	5.085–7.91
		%	47.8	45–50			57.4	45–70
Amazon genus *Amazona* sp.	8375	Conventional			12.3	5–17	6.273	3.813–8.733
		S.I.			12.3	5–17	6.273	3.813–8.733
		%	47.6	41–53			51	31–71
Amazon, blue-fronted *Amazona aestiva*	828	Conventional			10.4	6–13	5.4808	3.432–7.488
		S.I.			10.4	6–13	5.4808	3.432–7.488
		%	47.7	42–53			52.7	33–72
Amazon, double yellow-headed *A. oratrix*	565	Conventional			10.4	6–13	5.5224	3.952–7.384
		S.I.			10.4	6–13	5.5224	3.952–7.384
		%	47.5	40–53			53.1	38–71
Amazon, lilac crown *A. finschi*	57	Conventional			11.0	7–13	5.566	3.19–8.03
		S.I.			11.0	7–13	5.566	3.19–8.03
		%	47.2	44–52			50.6	29–73
Amazon, mealy *A. farinosa*	54	Conventional			13.2	9–16	7.4844	5.016–10.032
		S.I.			13.2	9–16	7.4844	5.016–10.032
		%	49.7	42–55			56.7	38–76
Amazon, green-cheeked (Mexican red head) *A. viridigenalis*	206	Conventional			11.8	6–16	6.0652	3.894–8.26
		S.I.			11.8	6–16	6.0652	3.894–8.26
		%	46.5	40–51			51.4	33–70
Amazon, orange wing *A. amazonica*	240	Conventional			12.2	7–16	6.3806	3.782–8.906
		S.I.			12.2	7–16	6.3806	3.782–8.906
		%	47.1	40–52			52.3	31–73
Amazon, panama *A. ochrocephala panamensis*	67	Conventional			11.7	8–16	6.7158	3.51–9.009
		S.I.			11.7	8–16	6.7158	3.51–9.009
		%	49.4	46–54			57.4	30–77
Amazon, red-lored *A. autumnalis*	299	Conventional			12.3	6–16	6.2484	4.059–8.979
		S.I.			12.3	6–16	6.2484	4.059–8.979
		%	48.1	42–55			50.8	33–73
Amazon, yellow nape *A. auropalliata*	1074	Conventional			12.4	6–17	6.4852	3.844–9.052
		S.I.			12.4	6–17	6.4852	3.844–9.052
		%	48.4	42–55			52.3	31–73

C Units, Conventional units.
*Methodology: WBC estimated from smear; manual cell differential count.
[†]Sample size number.

Lymphocytes C Units: $\times 10^9$/L S.I.: $\times 10^3$/mcL (%)		Monocytes C Units: $\times 10^9$/L S.I.: $\times 10^3$/mcL (%)		Eosinophils C Units: $\times 10^9$/L S.I.: $\times 10^3$/mcL (%)		Basophils C Units: $\times 10^9$/L S.I.: $\times 10^3$/mcL (%)	
Mean	Range	Mean	Range	Mean	Range	Mean	Range
3.914	1.957–5.150	0.0309	0–0.206	0.0257	0–0.103	0.0824	0–0.103
3.914	1.957–5.150	0.0309	0–0.206	0.0257	0–0.103	0.0824	0–0.103
38	19–50	0.03	0–2	0.24	0–1	0.08	0–1
4.392	2.400–6.480	0.192	0.120–0.360	0.1608	0.120–0.240	0.0852	0–0.120
4.392	2.400–6.480	0.192	1–3	1.34	1–2	0.71	0–1
36.6	20–54	1.6	1–3	1.34	1–2	0.71	0–1
3.819	2.147–5.424	0.00452	0–0.113	0.07119	0–1.226	0.00791	0–0.113
3.819	2.147–5.424	0.00452	0–0.113	0.07119	0–1.226	0.00791	0–0.113
33.8	19–48	0.04	0–1	0.63	0–2	0.07	0–1
5.387	2.460–8.241	0.00615	0–0.246	0	0–0	0.0578	0–0.246
5.387	2.460–8.241	0.00615	0–0.246	0	0–0	0.0578	0–0.246
43.8	20–67	0.05	0–2	0	0–0	0.47	0–2
4.524	2.288–6.67	0.00208	0–0.104	0.00416	0–0.104	0.02808	0–0.104
4.524	2.288–6.67	0.00208	0–0.104	0.00416	0–0.104	0.02808	0–0.104
43.5	22–65	0.02	0–1	0.04	0–1	0.27	0–1
4.6072	2.08–6.76	0.03432	0–0.104	0.0052	0–0.104	0.0364	0–0.104
4.6072	2.08–6.76	0.03432	0–0.104	0.0052	0–0.104	0.0364	0–0.104
44.3	20–65	0.33	0–1	0.05	0–1	0.35	0–1
4.686	2.09–7.37	0.0033	0–0.11	0.0044	0–0.11	0.0319	0–0.11
4.686	2.09–7.37	0.0033	0–0.11	0.0044	0–0.11	0.0319	0–0.11
42.6	19–67	0.03	0–1	0.04	0–1	0.29	0–1
5.94	3.036–8.58	0.00264	0–0.132	0	0–0	0.01584	0–0.132
5.94	3.036–8.58	0.00264	0–0.132	0	0–0	0.01584	0–0.132
45	23–65	0.02	0–1	0	0–0	0.12	0–1
4.8852	2.478–7.67	0.00708	0–0.118	0	0–0	0.07788	0–0.236
4.8852	2.478–7.67	0.00708	0–0.118	0	0–0	0.07788	0–0.236
41.4	21–65	0.06	0–1	0	0–0	0.66	0–2
5.2582	2.44–7.808	0.00244	0–0.122	0	0–0	0.003584	0–0.224
5.2582	2.44–7.808	0.00244	0–0.122	0	0–0	0.003584	0–0.224
43.1	20–64	0.02	0–1	0	0–0	0.32	0–2
5.0193	2.691–8.19	0	0–0.117	0	0–0.117	0.01053	0–0.117
5.0193	2.691–8.19	0	0–0.117	0	0–0.117	0.01053	0–0.117
42.9	23–70	0	0–1	0	0–1	0.09	0–1
5.6949	2.706–8.118	0.00369	0–0.123	0	0–0	0.05289	0–0.246
5.6949	2.706–8.118	0.00369	0–0.123	0	0–0	0.05289	0–0.246
46.3	22–66	0.03	0–1	0	0–0	0.43	0–2
5.4684	2.48–8.308	0.00248	0–0.124	0	0–0	0.05084	0–0.248
5.4684	2.48–8.308	0.00248	0–0.124	0	0–0	0.05084	0–0.248
44.1	20–67	0.02	0–1	0	0–0	0.41	0–2

Continued

TABLE 1

Hematology: Laboratory Reference Ranges for Selected Species—cont'd

Species Common Name (Common name synonyms) Scientific Name	N†	Units	Packed Cell Volume (%)		White Blood Cell Count C Units: ×10⁹/L S.I.: ×10³/mcL (%)		Heterophils C Units: ×10⁹/L S.I.: ×10³/mcL (%)	
			Mean	Range	Mean	Range	Mean	Range
Amazon, yellow-crowned *A. ochrocephala*	36	Conventional			12.7	8–15	6.4389	4.699–8.763
		S.I.			12.7	8–15	6.4389	4.699–8.763
		%	47.8	42–55			50.7	37–69
Budgerigar *Melopsittacus undulatus*	1542	Conventional			6.7	3–10	3.7989	2.68–4.556
		S.I.			6.7	3–10	3.7989	2.68–4.556
		%	51.5	44–58			56.7	40–68
Caique *Pionites* sp.	30	Conventional			12	8–15	6.768	4.68–8.64
		S.I.			12	8–15	6.768	4.68–8.64
		%	50.8	47–55			56.4	39–72
Canary *Serinus canaria forma domestica*	300	Conventional			7.0	3–10	2.576	1.47–4.2
		S.I.			7.0	3–10	2.576	1.47–4.2
		%	49.9	45–56			36.8	21–60
Cockatiel *Nymphicus hollandicus*	9267	Conventional			8.0	5–11	4.752	3.68–5.76
		S.I.			8.0	5–11	4.752	3.68–5.76
		%	51.2	43–57			59.4	46–72
Cockatoo group family *Cacatuidae*	5928	Conventional			10.4	5–13	6.2	4.68–7.49
		S.I.			10.4	5–13	6.2	4.68–7.49
		%	45.4	40–54			59.6	45–72
Cockatoo, bare eye (Little corella) *C. sanguinea*	30	Conventional			10.6	6–14	6.4978	4.346–8.162
		S.I.			10.6	6–14	6.4978	4.346–8.162
		%	48.3	43–55			61.3	41–77
Cockatoo, Goffin's (Tanimbar corella) *C. goffiniana*	298	Conventional			10.8	7–13	6.372	4.86–7.776
		S.I.			10.8	7–13	6.372	4.86–7.776
		%	47.3	42–55			59	45–72
Cockatoo, lesser sulfur-crested *C. sulphurea*	17	Conventional			12.3	15	8.364	5.412–9.717
		S.I.			12.3	15	8.364	5.412–9.717
		%	49.3	45–56			68	44–79
Cockatoo, Major Mitchell (Leadbeater's cockatoo, Pink cockatoo) *Lophochroa leadbeateri*	14	Conventional			10.0		6.03	3.7–7.8
		S.I.			10.0	6–13	6.03	3.7–7.8
		%	47.9	42–53			60.3	37–78
Cockatoo, Moluccan (Salmon-crested cockatoo) *Cacatua moluccensis*	772	Conventional			10.6	8–12	6.201	4.664–7.526
		S.I.			10.6	8–12	6.201	4.664–7.526
		%	45.3	41–54			58.5	44–71
Cockatoo, rose-breasted (Galah, Roseate cockatoo, Pink and grey cockatoo) *Eolophus roseicapilla*	92	Conventional			12.3	8–15	7.4538	5.289–9.102
		S.I.			12.3	8–15	7.4538	5.289–9.102
		%	48.8	40–55			60.6	43–74
Cockatoo, triton *Cacatua galerita triton*	544	Conventional			14.6	12–16	8.7892	6.424–10.95
		S.I.			14.6	12–16	8.7892	6.424–10.95
		%	45.5	42–50			60.2	44–75

Lymphocytes C Units: ×10⁹/L S.I.: ×10³/mcL (%)		Monocytes C Units: ×10⁹/L S.I.: ×10³/mcL (%)		Eosinophils C Units: ×10⁹/L S.I.: ×10³/mcL (%)		Basophils C Units: ×10⁹/L S.I.: ×10³/mcL (%)	
Mean	**Range**	**Mean**	**Range**	**Mean**	**Range**	**Mean**	**Range**
5.5372	2.286–8.001	0	0–0.127	0	0–0.127	0.03429	0–0.127
5.5372	2.286–8.001	0	0–0.127	0	0–0.127	0.03429	0–0.127
43.6	18–63	0	0–1	0	0–1	0.27	0–1
2.5259	1.474–4.02	0.00737	0–0.134	0	0–0	0.03216	0–0.134
2.5259	1.474–4.02	0.00737	0–0.134	0	0–0	0.03216	0–0.134
37.7	22–60	0.11	0–2	0	0–0	0.48	0–2
4.176	2.4–7.32	0	0–0.24	0	1–0.12	0	1–0.12
4.176	2.4–7.32	0	0–0.24	0	1–0.12	0	1–0.12
34.8	20–61	0	0–2	0	0–1	0	0–1
3.031	1.4–4.55	0.0028	0–0.07	0.0028	1–0.07	0.0056	0–0.07
3.031	1.4–4.55	0.0028	0–0.07	0.0028	1–0.07	0.0056	0–0.07
43.3	20–65	0.04	0–1	0.04	0–1	0.08	0–1
3.392	2.08–4.8	0.004	0–0.08	0.0488	0–0.16	0.0096	0–0.08
3.392	2.08–4.8	0.004	0–0.08	0.0488	0–0.16	0.0096	0–0.08
42.4	26–60	0.05	0–1	0.61	0–2	0.12	0–1
3.56	2.08–5.20	0.003	0–0.2	0.033	0–0.2	0	0–0.1
3.56	2.08–5.20	0.003	0–0.2	0.033	0–0.2	0	0–0.1
34.2	20–50	0.03	0–2	0.33	0–2	0	0–1
4.0492	2.332–6.042	0	0–0.212	0.00954	0–0.106	0	0–0.106
4.0492	2.332–6.042	0	0–0.212	0.00954	0–0.106	0	0–0.106
38.2	22–57	0	0–2	0.09	0–1	0	0–1
3.8556	2.376–5.508	0.00324	0–0.108	0.0378	0–0.216	0	0–0.108
3.8556	2.376–5.508	0.00324	0–0.108	0.0378	0–0.216	0	0–0.108
35.7	22–51	0.03	0–1	0.35	0–2	0	0–1
3.936	2.583–6.888		0–0.246		0–0.246		0–0.123
3.936	2.583–6.888		0–0.246		0–0.246		0–0.123
32	21–56		0–2		0–2		0–1
3.74	2–6.2	0	0–0.02	0	0–0.01	0	0–0.01
3.74	2–6.2	0	0–0.02	0	0–0.01	0	0–0.01
37.4	20–62	0	0–2	0	0–1	0	0–1
3.6252	2.014–5.3	0.00212	0–0.106	0.02968	0–0.212	0	0–0.106
3.6252	2.014–5.3	0.00212	0–0.106	0.02968	0–0.212	0	0–0.106
34.2	19–50	0.02	0–1	0.28	0–2	0	0–1
4.2312	2.46–6.396	0	0–0.246	0.02952	0–0.123	0	0–0.123
4.2312	2.46–6.396	0	0–0.246	0.02952	0–0.123	0	0–0.123
34.3	20–52	0	0–2	0.24	0–1	0	0–1
5.5626	3.212–8.176	0	0–0.292	0	0–0.146	0	0–0.146
5.5626	3.212–8.176	0	0–0.292	0	0–0.146	0	0–0.146
38.1	22–56	0	0–2	0	0–1	0	0–1

Continued

TABLE 1

Hematology: Laboratory Reference Ranges for Selected Species—cont'd

Species Common Name (Common name synonyms) Scientific Name	N†	Units	Packed Cell Volume (%)		White Blood Cell Count C Units: ×10⁹/L S.I.: ×10³/mcL (%)		Heterophils C Units: ×10⁹/L S.I.: ×10³/mcL (%)	
			Mean	Range	Mean	Range	Mean	Range
Cockatoo, umbrella	951	Conventional			12.8	8–16	7.616	5.76–9.088
C. alba		S.I.			12.8	8–16	7.616	5.76–9.088
		%	44.8	40–50			59.5	45–71
Conure group *Aratinga* and *Pyrrhura* sp.	2911	Conventional			9.6	5–13	5.6064	4.224–6.912
		S.I.			9.6	5–13	5.6064	4.224–6.912
		%	49.2	42–54			58.4	44–72
Conure, blue-crowned	93	Conventional			7.8	14	4.6644	3.354–5.772
Aratinga acuticaudata		S.I.			7.8	14	4.6644	3.354–5.772
		%	49.2	40–53			59.8	43–74
Conure, cherry-headed (Red masked parakeet)	66	Conventional			8.0	5–10	4.808	3.84–5.84
		S.I.			8.0	5–10	4.808	3.84–5.84
A. erythrogenys		%	49.9	43–56			60.1	48–73
Conure, dusky (Dusky-headed parakeet, Weddell's	29	Conventional			9.9	5–13	5.7618	4.257
parakeet)		S.I.			9.9	5–13	5.7618	4.257
A. weddellii		%	49.3	41–55			58.2	43–70
Conure, gold-capped	36	Conventional			10.1	6–13	5.7065	4.444–6.969
A. auricapillus		S.I.			10.1	6–13	5.7065	4.444–6.969
		%	52.6	50–55			56.5	44–69
Conure, green-cheeked	41	Conventional			7.7	5–10	4.3736	3.542–5.467
Pyrrhura molinae		S.I.			7.7	5–10	4.3736	3.542–5.467
		%	50.9	42–55			56.8	46–71
Conure, half moon (Orange-fronted parakeet)	29	Conventional			8.2	6–10	5.2808	4.1–5.986
		S.I.			8.2	6–10	5.2808	4.1–5.986
Eupsittula canicularis		%	49.1	42–54			64.4	50–73
Conure, jenday	55	Conventional			8.1	6–10	4.60	3.726–5.751
Aratinga jandaya		S.I.			8.1	6–10	4.60	3.726–5.751
		%	50.6	42–55			56.8	46–71
Conure, maroon bellied (Red bellied conure, Brown eared	28	Conventional			10.4	7–13	5.751	4.576–7.384
conure)		S.I.			10.4	7–13	5.751	4.576–7.384
Pyrrhura frontalis		%	50.7	46–55			55.3	44–71
Conure, mitred	74	Conventional			8.1	5–11	4.795	3.564–5.832
Psittacara mitrata		S.I.			8.1	5–11	4.795	3.564–5.832
		%	47.1	40–52			59.2	44–72
Conure, nanday	179	Conventional			8.7	5–11	5.203	4.176–6.177
Aratinga nenday		S.I.			8.7	5–11	5.203	4.170–0.177
		%	50.1	40–55			59.8	48–71
Conure, Patagonian	57	Conventional			8.8	6–11	5.262	3.872–6.336
Cyanoliseus patagonus		S.I.			8.8	6–11	5.262	3.872–6.336
		%	48.4	42–55			59.8	44–72

Lymphocytes C Units: ×10⁹/L S.I.: ×10³/mcL (%)		Monocytes C Units: ×10⁹/L S.I.: ×10³/mcL (%)		Eosinophils C Units: ×10⁹/L S.I.: ×10³/mcL (%)		Basophils C Units: ×10⁹/L S.I.: ×10³/mcL (%)	
Mean	**Range**	**Mean**	**Range**	**Mean**	**Range**	**Mean**	**Range**
4.416	2.56–6.528	0.00384	0–0.256	0.04864	0–0.256	0	0–0.128
4.416	2.56–6.528	0.00384	0–0.256	0.04864	0–0.256	0	0–0.128
34.5	20–51	0.03	0–2	0.38	0–2	0	0–1
3.4656	2.112–4.896	0.00384	0–0.096	0.00768	0–0.096	0.01536	0–0.096
3.4656	2.112–4.896	0.00384	0–0.096	0.00768	0–0.096	0.01536	0–0.096
36.1	22–51	0.04	0–1	0.08	0–1	0.16	0–1
2.8002	1.794–3.9	0	0–0.078	0.01326	0–0.078	0.01638	0–0.156
2.8002	1.794–3.9	0	0–0.078	0.01326	0–0.078	0.01638	0–0.156
35.9	23–50	0	0–1	0.17	0–1	0.21	0–2
2.888	1.84–4	0	0–0.16	0	0–0.08	0	0–0.08
2.888	1.84–4	0	0–0.16	0	0–0.08	0	0–0.08
36.1	23–50	0	0–2	0	0–1	0	0–1
3.6531	1.98–5.148	0	0–0.198	0	0–0.099	0	0–0.099
3.6531	1.98–5.148	0	0–0.198	0	0–0.099	0	0–0.099
36.9	20–52	0	0–2	0	0–1	0	0–1
3.8481	2.626–4.949	0	0–0.101	0	0–0.101	0.03333	0–0.202
3.8481	2.626–4.949	0	0–0.101	0	0–0.101	0.03333	0–0.202
38.1	26–49	0	0–1	0	0–1	0.33	0–2
3.0492	1.694–4.081	0	0–0.154	0	0–0.077	0	0–0.077
3.0492	1.694–4.081	0	0–0.154	0	0–0.077	0	0–0.077
39.6	22–53	0	0–2	0	0–1	0	0–1
2.7306	1.64–5.002	0	0–0.164	0	0–0.082	0	0–0.082
2.7306	1.64–5.002	0	0–0.164	0	0–0.082	0	0–0.082
33.3	20–51	0	0–2	0	0–1	0	0–1
3.305	1.782–4.374	0	0–0.162	0	0–0.104	0	0–0.32
3.305	1.782–4.374	0	0–0.162	0	0–0.104	0	0–0.32
40.8	22–54	0	0–2	0	0–1	0	0–4
4.222	2.496–5.824	0	0–0.028	0	0–0.081	0	0–0.104
4.222	2.496–5.824	0	0–0.028	0	0–0.081	0	0–0.104
40.6	24–56	0	0–2	0	0–1	0	0–1
2.900	1.863–4.05	0	0–0.162	0	0–0.081	0	0–0.081
2.900	1.863–4.05	0	0–0.162	0	0–0.081	0	0–0.081
35.8	23–50	0	0–2	0	0–1	0	0–1
3.036	2.088–4.089	0	0–0.087	0.096	0–0.087	0.053	0–0.174
3.036	2.088–4.089	0	0–0.087	0.096	0–0.087	0.053	0–0.174
34.9	24–47	0	0–1	0.11	0–1	0.61	0–2
2.939	1.848–4.576	0	0–0.088	0	0–0.088	0.021	0–0.088
2.939	1.848–4.576	0	0–0.088	0	0–0.088	0.021	0–0.088
33.4	21–52	0	0–1	0	0–1	0.24	0–1

Continued

TABLE 1

Hematology: Laboratory Reference Ranges for Selected Species—cont'd

Species Common Name (Common name synonyms) Scientific Name	N[†]	Units	Packed Cell Volume (%)		White Blood Cell Count C Units: ×10⁹/L S.I.: ×10³/mcL (%)		Heterophils C Units: ×10⁹/L S.I.: ×10³/mcL (%)	
			Mean	Range	Mean	Range	Mean	Range
Conure, sun	286	Conventional			9.0	6–11	4.797	3.96–6.48
Aratinga solstitialis		S.I.			9.0	6–11	4.797	3.96–6.48
		%	49.7	42–55			53.3	44–72
Dove	45	Conventional			11.0	9–13	5.951	4.73–6.93
Streptopelia risoria and *Geopelia*		S.I.			11.0	9–13	5.951	4.73–6.93
cuneata		%	47.3	92			54.1	43–63
Duck domestic	73	Conventional			18.1	14–24	11.132	9.593–12.489
Anas platyrhynchos domestica		S.I.			18.1	14–24	11.132	9.593–12.489
		%	43.4	35–50			61.5	53–69
Combined Eagle species	18	Conventional			16.9	12–21	11.762	8.788–13.52
Bald eagle		S.I.			16.9	12–21	11.762	8.788–13.52
Haliaeetus leucocephalus		%	41.9	37–48			69.6	52–80
Golden eagle								
Aquila chrysaetos								
Eclectus parrot	415	Conventional			12.5	9–15	7.25	5.75–8.75
Eclectus roratus		S.I.			12.5	9–15	7.25	5.75–8.75
		%	49.5	45–55			58	46–70
Emu	98	Conventional			14.9	8–21	11.7412	8.046–13.112
Dromaius novaehollandiae		S.I.			14.9	8–21	11.7412	8.046–13.112
		%	47.4	39–57			78.8	54–88
Grey-cheeked parakeet	449	Conventional			8.3	4–12	4.6729	3.735–5.644
(Fire-winged parakeet)		S.I.			8.3	4–12	4.6729	3.735–5.644
Brotogeris pyrrhoptera		%	50.2	45–56			56.3	45–68
Hawk, red-tailed	13	Conventional			19.5	15–24	9.7305	6.825–12.87
Buteo jamaicensis		S.I.			19.5	15–24	9.7305	6.825–12.87
		%	45.1	38–52			49.9	35–66
Lory (11 genera, 53 species)	130	Conventional			10.8	8–13	5.4216	4.212–6.48
		S.I.			10.8	8–13	5.4216	4.212–6.48
		%	50.6	47–55			50.2	39–60
Lovebird	650	Conventional			11.7	7–16	5.6511	11.232
Agapornis sp.		S.I.			11.7	7–16	5.6511	11.232
		%	50.5	44–55			48.3	96
Macaw group	5338	Conventional			15.2	10–20	9.5912	7.6–11.4
mostly *Ara* and some *Anodorhynchus*		S.I.			15.2	10–20	9.5912	7.6–11.4
		%	48.5	42–56			63.1	50–75
Macaw, blue and gold	1367	Conventional			12.8	8–16	7.7568	6.272 0.000
(Blue and yellow macaw)		S.I.			12.8	8–16	7.7568	6.272–9.088
Ara ararauna		%	48.7	44–55			60.6	49–71
Macaw, green-winged	347	Conventional			14.2	11–16	8.9602	6.958–10.366
(Red and green macaw)		S.I.			14.2	11–16	8.9602	6.958–10.366
A. chloroptera		%	47.2	42–54			63.1	49–73

Lymphocytes C Units: ×10⁹/L S.I.: ×10³/mcL (%)		Monocytes C Units: ×10⁹/L S.I.: ×10³/mcL (%)		Eosinophils C Units: ×10⁹/L S.I.: ×10³/mcL (%)		Basophils C Units: ×10⁹/L S.I.: ×10³/mcL (%)	
Mean	**Range**	**Mean**	**Range**	**Mean**	**Range**	**Mean**	**Range**
3.141	1.8–4.41	0.0054	0–0.09	0	0–0	0.0684	0–0.18
3.141	1.8–4.41	0.0054	0–0.09	0	0–0	0.0684	0–0.18
34.9	20–49	0.06	0–1	0	0–0	0.76	0–2
5.709	4.62–6.71	0.0011	0–0.22	0	0–0.22	0	0–0.22
5.709	4.62–6.71	0.0011	0–0.22	0	0–0.22	0	0–0.22
51.9	42–61	0.1	0–2	0	0–2	0	0–2
6.588	4.887–9.05	0	0–0.362	0.0468	0–0.181	0	0–0.181
6.588	4.887–9.05	0	0–0.362	0.0468	0–0.181	0	0–0.181
36.4	27–50	0	0–2	0.26	0–1	0	0–1
4.039	3.042–5.746	0	0–0.507	0.197	0–0.676	0	0–0.338
4.039	3.042–5.746	0	0–0.507	0.197	0–0.676	0	0–0.338
23.9	18–34	0	0–3	1.17	0–4	0	0–2
5.05	2.875–7.125	0	0–0.125	0.0175	0–0.125	0.01	0–0.125
5.05	2.875–7.125	0	0–0.125	0.0175	0–0.125	0.01	0–0.125
40.4	23–57	0	0–1	0.14	0–1	0.08	0–1
2.9502	1.49–6.556	0.00149	0–0.149	0.447	0–0.894	0.0298	0–0.149
2.9502	1.49–6.556	0.00149	0–0.149	0.447	0–0.894	0.0298	0–0.149
19.8	10–44	0.1	0–1	3	0–6	0.2	0–1
2.9382	1.826–3.984	0.00415	0–0.083	0.00581	0–0.083	0.00415	0–0.083
2.9382	1.826–3.984	0.00415	0–0.083	0.00581	0–0.083	0.00415	0–0.083
35.4	22–48	0.05	0–1	0.07	0–1	0.05	0–1
6.6495	3.705–9.75	0	0–0.585	0	0–78	0	0–0.39
6.6495	3.705–9.75	0	0–0.585	0	0–78	0	0–0.39
34.1	19–50	0	0–3	0	0–4	0	0–2
4.7196	2.376–7.452	0	0–0.216	0	0–0.108	0	0–0.108
4.7196	2.376–7.452	0	0–0.216	0	0–0.108	0	0–0.108
43.7	22–69	0	0–2	0	0–1	0	0–1
4.212	2.34–6.201	0.00468	0–0.117	0.03159	0–0.234	0.02691	0–0.234
4.212	2.34–6.201	0.00468	0–0.117	0.03159	0–0.234	0.02691	0–0.234
36	20–53	0.04	0–1	0.27	0–2	0.23	0–2
5.624	3.496–8.056	0.00456	0–0.152	0	0–0	0.01064	0–0.152
5.624	3.496–8.056	0.00456	0–0.152	0	0–0	0.01064	0–0.152
37	23–53	0.03	0–1	0	0–0	0.07	0–1
4.4416	2.304–6.784	0.00512	0–0.256			0.00512	0–0.128
4.4416	2.304–6.784	0.00512	0–0.256			0.00512	0–0.128
34.7	18–53	0.04	0–2			0.04	0–1
5.1972	3.124–8.52		0–0.284		0–0.284	0.01704	0–0.142
5.1972	3.124–8.52		0–0.284		0–0.284	0.01704	0–0.142
36.6	22–60		0–2		0–2	0.12	0–1

Continued

TABLE 1

Hematology: Laboratory Reference Ranges for Selected Species—cont'd

Species Common Name (Common name synonyms) Scientific Name	N†	Units	Packed Cell Volume (%)		White Blood Cell Count C Units: ×10⁹/L S.I.: ×10³/mcL (%)		Heterophils C Units: ×10⁹/L S.I.: ×10³/mcL (%)	
			Mean	Range	Mean	Range	Mean	Range
Macaw, Hahn's (Red-shouldered macaw) *Diopsittaca nobilis nobilis*	51	Conventional			14.1	10–18	7.5999	5.781–10.152
		S.I.			14.1	10–18	7.5999	5.781–10.152
		%	51.3	47–55			53.9	41–72
Macaw, hyacinth *Anodorhynchus hyacinthinus*	149	Conventional			13.4	11–16	9.2862	7.504–10.72
		S.I.			13.4	11–16	9.2862	7.504–10.72
		%	50.1	45–55			69.3	56–80
Macaw, military *Ara militaris*	88	Conventional			16.5	12–20	11.8305	9.57–14.025
		S.I.			16.5	12–20	11.8305	9.57–14.025
		%	46.8	44–51			71.7	58–85
Macaw, noble (Red-shouldered macaw) *Diopsittaca nobilis cumanensis*	22	Conventional			14.6	8–22	7.2708	4.964–9.198
		S.I.			14.6	8–22	7.2708	4.964–9.198
		%	52.3	48–56			49.8	34–63
Macaw, scarlet (Red and yellow macaw) *Ara macao*	146	Conventional			12.5	10–14	7.525	6–9.125
		S.I.			12.5	10–14	7.525	6–9.125
		%	49.1	45–55			60.2	48–73
Macaw, severe (Chestnut-fronted macaw) *A. severus*	104	Conventional			12.1	9–14	7.3931	5.445–9.68
		S.I.			12.1	9–14	7.3931	5.445–9.68
		%	49.1	45–55			61.1	45–80
Macaw, yellow collared (Golden-collared macaw) *Primolius auricollis*	70	Conventional			13.6	10–16	8.6904	7.344–10.064
		S.I.			13.6	10–16	8.6904	7.344–10.064
		%	50.9	42–55			63.9	54–74
Moustache parakeet (Rose-breasted parakeet) *Psittacula alexandri*	26	Conventional			11.6	8–15	7.6676	5.8–9.164
		S.I.			11.6	8–15	7.6676	5.8–9.164
		%	46.1	42–51			66.1	50–79
Mynah species, mostly *Acridotheres tristis*	44	Conventional			9.9	8–12	5.4945	4.455–6.336
		S.I.			9.9	8–12	5.4945	4.455–6.336
		%	47.7	38–50			55.5	45–64
Ostrich *Struthio camelus*	140	Conventional			18.7	10–24	5.2173	10.846–16.643
		S.I.			18.7	10–24	5.2173	10.846–16.643
		%	45	41–57			27.9	58–89
Owl, great-horned *Bubo virginianus*	18	Conventional			17.0	10–25	11.764	9.52–13.43
		S.I.			17.0	10–25	11.764	9.52–13.43
		%	38.1	30–50			69.2	56–79
Parakeet, Alexandrine *Psittacula eupatria*	18	Conventional			14.3	10–16	8.923	7.293–10.439
		S.I.			14.3	10–16	8.923	7.293–10.439
		%	47.4	45–54			62.4	51–73
Parakeet, ringneck (Rose-ringed parakeet) *Psittacula krameri*	16	Conventional			11.2	8–14	6.0144	4.48–7.616
		S.I.			11.2	8–14	6.0144	4.48–7.616
		%	49.5	45–54			53.7	40–68
Parrot, Meyers *Poicephalus meyeri*	39	Conventional			11.2	8–14	6.9328	5.376–8.4
		S.I.			11.2	8–14	6.9328	5.376–8.4
		%	49.9	98			61.9	48–75

Lymphocytes C Units: ×10⁹/L S.I.: ×10³/mcL (%)		Monocytes C Units: ×10⁹/L S.I.: ×10³/mcL (%)		Eosinophils C Units: ×10⁹/L S.I.: ×10³/mcL (%)		Basophils C Units: ×10⁹/L S.I.: ×10³/mcL (%)	
Mean	**Range**	**Mean**	**Range**	**Mean**	**Range**	**Mean**	**Range**
7.191	3.807–10.011		0–0.282		0–0.141	0	0–0.141
7.191	3.807–10.011		0–0.282		0–0.141	0	0–0.141
51	27–71		0–2		0–1	0	0–1
4.355	2.412–8.308		0–0.268		0–0.268	0.01206	0–0.134
4.355	2.412–8.308		0–0.268		0–0.268	0.01206	0–0.134
32.5	18–62		0–2		0–2	0.09	0–1
5.28	4.125–6.6		0–0.33		0–0.165		0–0.165
5.28	4.125–6.6		0–0.33		0–0.165		0–0.165
32	25–40		0–2		0–1		0–1
7.0226	4.672–9.636	0	0–0.146	0	0–0.146	0	0–0.146
7.0226	4.672–9.636	0	0–0.146	0	0–0.146	0	0–0.146
48.1	32–66	0	0–1	0	0–1	0	0–1
4.55	2.875–6.25	0	0–0.25	0	0–0.125	0.0175	0–0.125
4.55	2.875–6.25	0	0–0.25	0	0–0.125	0.0175	0–0.125
36.4	23–50	0	0–2	0	0–1	0.14	0–1
4.3681	3.025–5.687	0	0–0.242	0	0–0.121	0.05203	0–0.242
4.3681	3.025–5.687	0	0–0.242	0	0–0.121	0.05203	0–0.242
36.1	25–47	0	0–2	0	0–1	0.43	0–2
5.1952	3.4–7.072	0	0–0.136	0	0–0.136	0	0–0.136
5.1952	3.4–7.072	0	0–0.136	0	0–0.136	0	0–0.136
38.2	25–52	0	0–1	0	0–1	0	0–1
4.3384	2.436–6.38	0	0–0.116	0	0–0.116	0	0–0.116
4.3384	2.436–6.38	0	0–0.116	0	0–0.116	0	0–0.116
37.4	21–55	0	0–1	0	0–1	0	0–1
4.0095	2.079–5.445	0	0–0.099	0.07128	0–0.396	0	0–0.099
4.0095	2.079–5.445	0	0–0.099	0.07128	0–0.396	0	0–0.099
40.5	21–55	0	0–1	0.72	0–4	0	0–1
4.5254	2.244–7.667	0.49368	0–0.748	0.00748	0–0.374	0.0374	0–0.374
4.5254	2.244–7.667	0.49368	0–0.748	0.00748	0–0.374	0.0374	0–0.374
24.2	12–41	2.64	0–4	0.04	0–2	0.2	0–2
4.76	3.4–8.16		0–0.34	0.7888	0–1.87		0–0.17
4.76	3.4–8.16		0–0.34	0.7888	0–1.87		0–0.17
28	20–48		0–2	4.64	0–11		0–1
5.22	3.861–7.007	0	0–0.143	0	0–0.143	0	0–0.143
5.22	3.861–7.007	0	0–0.143	0	0–0.143	0	0–0.143
36.5	27–49	0	0–1	0	0–1	0	0–1
4.9392	3.584–6.272	0	0–0.112	0	0–0.112	0	0–0.112
4.9392	3.584–6.272	0	0–0.112	0	0–0.112	0	0–0.112
44.1	32–56	0	0–1	0	0–1	0	0–1
3.8304	2.576–5.264	0	0–0.224	0	0–0.112	0	0–0.112
3.8304	2.576–5.264	0	0–0.224	0	0–0.112	0	0–0.112
34.2	23–47	0	0–2	0	0–1	0	0–1

Continued

TABLE 1

Hematology: Laboratory Reference Ranges for Selected Species—cont'd

Species Common Name (Common name synonyms) Scientific Name	N[†]	Units	Packed Cell Volume (%)		White Blood Cell Count C Units: $\times 10^9$/L S.I.: $\times 10^3$/mcL (%)		Heterophils C Units: $\times 10^9$/L S.I.: $\times 10^3$/mcL (%)	
			Mean	Range	Mean	Range	Mean	Range
Parrot, red-bellied *Poicephalus rufiventris*	14	Conventional			12.6	9–16	7.5474	7.056–8.442
		S.I.			12.6	9–16	7.5474	7.056–8.442
		%	48.3	45–51			59.9	56–67
Parrot, thick-billed *Rhynchopsitta pachyrhyncha*	10	Conventional			12.3	8–21	6.1623	3.936–8.364
		S.I.			12.3	8–21	6.1623	3.936–8.364
		%	39.3	33–43			50.1	32–68
Parrotlet species Genus *Forpus* sp.	29	Conventional			8.8	6–13	5.6496	4.84–6.512
		S.I.			8.8	6–13	5.6496	4.84–6.512
		%	50.8	48–55			64.2	55–74
Pionus species group Genus *Pionus* sp.	431	Conventional			9.6	5–13	6.3168	0.48–7.104
		S.I.			9.6	5–13	6.3168	0.48–7.104
		%	49.8	45–54			65.8	5–74
Pionus, blue-headed *Pionus menstruus*	26	Conventional			12.6	10–16	7.4844	5.544–9.702
		S.I.			12.6	10–16	7.4844	5.544–9.702
		%	48.1	40–53			59.4	44–77
Pionus, white-capped *P. senilis*	49	Conventional			8.8	5–11	5.3504	4.136–6.512
		S.I.			8.8	5–11	5.3504	4.136–6.512
		%	50.6	47–55			60.8	47–74
Quaker parrot (Monk parakeet) *Myiopsitta monachus*	210	Conventional			12.2	8–17	7.442	5.734–8.54
		S.I.			12.2	8–17	7.442	5.734–8.54
		%	49.7	45–58			61	47–70
Rosella, Genus *Platycercus* sp.	21	Conventional			11.8	9–15	6.7142	5.428–8.142
		S.I.			11.8	9–15	6.7142	5.428–8.142
		%	51	45–60			56.9	46–69
Parrot, Senegal *Poicephalus senegalus*	244	Conventional			10.7	6–14	6.2702	4.708–7.811
		S.I.			10.7	6–14	6.2702	4.708–7.811
		%	50.6	45–60			58.6	44–73
Swan *Cygnus* sp.	36	Conventional			13.4	11–16	7.1288	4.556–8.978
		S.I.			13.4	11–16	7.1288	4.556–8.978
		%	45.6	42–50			53.2	34–67
Toucan *Ramphastos* sp.	86	Conventional			13.5	8–18	7.0065	5.535–8.37
		S.I.			13.5	8–18	7.0065	5.535–8.37
		%	49.8	42–60			51.9	41–62

Lymphocytes C Units: ×10⁹/L S.I.: ×10³/mcL (%)		Monocytes C Units: ×10⁹/L S.I.: ×10³/mcL (%)		Eosinophils C Units: ×10⁹/L S.I.: ×10³/mcL (%)		Basophils C Units: ×10⁹/L S.I.: ×10³/mcL (%)	
Mean	**Range**	**Mean**	**Range**	**Mean**	**Range**	**Mean**	**Range**
5.922	4.158–9.072	0	0–0.252	0	0–0.252	0	0–0.126
5.922	4.158–9.072	0	0–0.252	0	0–0.252	0	0–0.126
47	33–72	0	0–2	0	0–2	0	0–1
4.797	2.46–6.888		0–0.123		0–0.123		0–0.123
4.797	2.46–6.888		0–0.123		0–0.123		0–0.123
39	20–56		0–1		0–1		0–1
3.1328	2.112–4.4	0	0–0.088	0	0–0.088	0	0–0.088
3.1328	2.112–4.4	0	0–0.088	0	0–0.088	0	0–0.088
35.6	24–50	0	0–1	0	0–1	0	0–1
3.9936	1.824–6.72	0	0–0.096	0	0–0.096	0.0144	0–0.096
3.9936	1.824–6.72	0	0–0.096	0	0–0.096	0.0144	0–0.096
41.6	19–70	0	0–1	0	0–1	0.15	0–1
4.5108	2.394–6.552	0	0–0.126	0	0–0.126	0	0–0.252
4.5108	2.394–6.552	0	0–0.126	0	0–0.126	0	0–0.252
35.8	19–52	0	0–1	0	0–1	0	0–2
3.7488	1.76–6.16	0	0–0.088	0	0–0.088	0	0–0.176
3.7488	1.76–6.16	0	0–0.088	0	0–0.088	0	0–0.176
42.6	20–70	0	0–1	0	0–1	0	0–2
4.209	2.44–7.686	0.04758	0–0.488			0.07686	0–0.366
4.209	2.44–7.686	0.04758	0–0.488			0.07686	0–0.366
34.5	20–63	0.39	0–4			0.63	0–3
5.3454	2.95–7.552	0	0–0.236	0	0–0.118	0	0–0.236
5.3454	2.95–7.552	0	0–0.236	0	0–0.118	0	0–0.236
45.3	25–64	0	0–2	0	0–1	0	0–2
4.9541	2.354–7.49	0	0–0.107	0.02675	0–0.214	0.00749	0–0.107
4.9541	2.354–7.49	0	0–0.107	0.02675	0–0.214	0.00749	0–0.107
46.3	22–70	0	0–1	0.25	0–2	0.07	0–1
5.494	3.082–8.844	0	0–0.268	0	0–0.134	0	0–0.134
5.494	3.082–8.844	0	0–0.268	0	0–0.134	0	0–0.134
41	23–66	0	0–2	0	0–1	0	0–1
6.8175	4.725–9.45	0	0–0.27	0.09045	0–0.405	0	0–0.135
6.8175	4.725–9.45	0	0–0.27	0.09045	0–0.405	0	0–0.135
50.5	35–70	0	0–2	0.67	0–3	0	0–1

TABLE 2

Erythrocytic Parameters[a]

Species Common Name (Common name synonyms) Scientific Name	Units	Red Blood Cell Count (RBC) Conventional: ×10⁶/μL S.I.: ×10¹²/L Mean	Range	Packed Cell Volume (PCV), (%) Mean	Range
Grey parrot (African Grey) genus *Psittacus* sp.	Conventional	3.27	2.84–3.62		
	S.I.	3.27	2.84–3.62		
	%			48.96	41.1–53.5
Amazon genus *Amazona* sp.	Conventional	2.82	2.45–3.18		
	S.I.	2.82	2.45–3.18		
	%			47.83	41.96–52.5
Budgerigar *Melopsittacus undulatus*	Conventional	4.32	3.77–4.6		
	S.I.	4.32	3.77–4.6		
	%			51.45	43.4–56.1
Cockatiel *Nymphicus hollandicus*	Conventional	3.93	3.1–4.4		
	S.I.	3.93	3.1–4.4		
	%			52.63	41.4–58.9
Cockatoo group family Cacatuidae	Conventional	2.84	2.44–3.34		
	S.I.	2.84	2.44–3.34		
	%			47.1	40.2–55.12
Duck domestic *Anas platyrhynchos domestica*	Conventional	3.61	3.2–4.01		
	S.I.	3.61	3.2–4.01		
	%			52.06	42.3–57.7
Eclectus parrot *Eclectus roratus*	Conventional	2.98	2.5–3.7		
	S.I.	2.98	2.5–3.7		
	%			47.51	42.4–53.7
Emu *Dromaius novaehollandiae*	Conventional	2.93	2.38–3.33		
	S.I.	2.93	2.38–3.33		
	%			49.38	42.2–54.6
Lory (11 genera, 53 species)	Conventional	1.85	1.72–2.1		
	S.I.	1.85	1.72–2.1		
	%			47.4	39–57
Lovebird *Agapornis* sp.	Conventional	3.79	3.25–3.95		
	S.I.	3.79	3.25–3.95		
	%			48.3	41.5–55.4
Macaw group mostly *Ara* and some *Anodorhynchus*	Conventional	3.82	3.45–4.04		
	S.I.	3.82	3.45–4.04		
	%			50.7	44.6–55.3
Ostrich *Struthio camelus*	Conventional	3.11	2.63–3.49		
	S.I.	3.11	2.63–3.49		
	%			48.87	41.7–53.9
Parrot, Senegal *Poicephalus senegalus*	Conventional	1.8	1.70–2.17		
	S.I.	1.8	1.70–2.17		
	%			45	41–57

[a]Methodology: PCV: Centrifugation. All other parameters: Cell-Dyn 3500, Abbott Laboratories, Abbott Park, IL.

Hemoglobin (Hb) Conventional: g/dL S.I.: g/L		Mean Corpuscular Volume (MCV) = PCV/RBC Conventional: μm^3/cell S.I.: fl/cell		Mean Corpuscular Hemoglobin (MCH) = Hb/RBC Conventional: pg/cell S.I.: pg/cell		Mean Corpuscular Hemoglobin Concentration = MCH/MCV Conventional: g/dL S.I.: g/L	
Mean	Range	Mean	Range	Mean	Range	Mean	Range
13.81	12.7–15.9	150	144–155	41	36.4–43.9	27.36	25.38–28.1
138.1	127–159	150	144–155	41	36.4–43.9	273.6	253.8–281
14.46	12.2–15.89	168	160–175	51.7	47.2–56.8	30.53	29.07–31.89
144.6	122–158.9	168	160–175	51.7	47.2–56.8	305.3	290.7–318.9
14.7	12.42–16.89	121.5	116–127	26.1	23.1–30.89	21.79	19.8–23.9
147	124.2–168.9	121.5	116–127	26.1	23.1–30.89	217.9	198–239
12.15	10.2–14.7	135.9	126–142	31	26.4–35.8	22.68	20.45–25.2
121.5	102–147	135.9	126–142	31	26.4–35.8	226.8	204.5–252
13.61	11.1–16.0	166.3	158–175	47.7	40.45–53.7	28.85	25.8–31.5
136.1	111–160	166.3	158–175	47.7	40.45–53.7	288.5	258–315
13.06	10.9–15.98	145.9	136–156	35.8	31.8–39.4	24.46	21.9–26.1
130.6	109–159.8	145.9	136–156	35.8	31.8–39.4	244.6	219–261
12.36	11.1–13.99	164.3	157–170	42	37.5–44.6	25.53	22.69–27.53
123.6	111–139.9	164.3	157–170	42	37.5–44.6	255.3	226.9–275.3
14.35	11.8–16.31	167.1	159–173	48.1	44.96–53.08	28.87	26.79–31.4
143.5	118–163.1	167.1	159–173	48.1	44.96–53.08	288.7	267.9–314
16.04	13.6–17.0	219	206–220	86.5	78.2–89.0	39.37	35.2–43.3
160.4	136–170	219	206–220	86.5	78.2–89.0	393.7	352–433
11.82	10.8–14.76	135.1	128–140	29.3	27.5–31.4	21.51	20.29–23.14
118.2	108–147.6	135.1	128–140	29.3	27.5–31.4	215.1	202.9–231.4
11.4	10.1–13.82	130.4	125–138	29	27.5–31.4	21.51	20.29–23.14
114	101–138.2	130.4	125–138	29	27.5–31.4	215.1	202.9–231.4
13.7	11.3–16.04	161.1	149–173	43.5	27.3–31.3	22.08	20.58–22.94
137	113–160.4	161.1	149–173	43.5	27.3–31.3	220.8	205.8–229.4
16.92	14–17.2	212	205–218	82.2	76.4–88.4	37.65	34.7–41.2
169.2	140–172	212	205–218	82.2	76.4–88.4	376.5	347–412

TABLE 3

Enzymes: Laboratory Reference Ranges for Selected Species

Species Common Name (Common name synonyms) Scientific Name	N*	Lactate Dehydrogenase (U/L)		Creatine Kinase (U/L)	
		Mean	Range	Mean	Range
Grey parrot (African Grey) genus *Psittacus* sp.	5571	248.2	154–378	303	140–411
Grey parrot (African Grey, Congo) *Psittacus erithacus*	495	243.1	144–390	306.1	135–410
Timneh parrot (African Grey, timneh) *P. timneh*	219	238.5	144–402	286.3	126–420
Amazon genus *Amazona* sp.	8375	230.4	160–368	257.1	117–425
Amazon, blue-fronted *Amazona aestiva*	828	228.3	158–366	22.5	130–417
Amazon, double yellow-headed *A. oratrix*	565	233.3	160–354	260.9	128–420
Amazon, lilac crown *A. finschi*	57	225.7	160–332	248.3	153–376
Amazon, mealy *A. farinosa*	54	228.8	159–381	278.5	208–348
Amazon, green-cheeked (Mexican red head) *A. viridigenalis*	206	246.1	145–388	2435.4	123–429
Amazon, orange wing *A. amazonica*	240	251.6	148–451	278.2	120–455
Amazon, panama *A. ochrocephala panamensis*	67	233.5	160–387	318.6	157–458
Amazon, red-lored *A. autumnalis*	299	229.2	150–412	262.5	136–420
Amazon, yellow nape *A. auropalliata*	1074	228.5	160–360	252.5	132–402
Amazon, yellow crowned *A. ochrocephala*	36	197.6	171–265	391.8	260–490
Budgerigar *Melopsittacus undulatus*	1542	251.7	156–384	235	117–368
Caique *Pionites* sp.	30	192.3	147–270	249.3	124–384
Canary *Serinus canaria forma domestica*	300				
Cockatiel *Nymphicus hollandicus*	9267	255	122–378	269.1	160–420
Cockatoo group family Cacatuidae	5928	302.8	208–414	266.4	147–418
Cockatoo, bare eye (Little corella) *Cacatua sanguinea*	30	314.2	256–415	279.7	155–420
Cockatoo, Goffin's (Tanimbar corella) *C. goffiniana*	298	329.9	198–452	281.8	144–439
Cockatoo, lesser sulfur crested *C. sulphurea*	17	285.6	173–398	281.1	157–408

*Number of normal animals in the data set.

Aspartate Aminotransferase (U/L)		Alkaline Phosphatase (U/L)		Amylase (U/L)		Bile Acids (μmol/L)	
Mean	Range	Mean	Range	Mean	Range	Mean	Range
173.8	110–340	33.9	12–92	510.9	415–626	55.8	12–96
161.1	81–369	40.2	14–64	283.3	200–384	53	12–96
191.4	120–342	39.8	12–125	304.5	170–436	60.8	23–97
221	150–344	52	8–100	330.1	184–478	89	33–154
231.5	146–408	57.8	20–108			87	34–140
210.4	152–400	73.4	50–100	410.3	327–474	86.5	32–148
227.5	150–382	46.3	11–75			84.1	33–144
225.8	138–377			305	36–574	68	31–145
210.6	150–328	53.8	18–92			88.2	36–154
205.8	114–389	35	20–64	0	0–0	93.6	29–157
208.7	154–394	42.8	14–64	381	200–645	90.2	31–148
224.3	150–408	53.5	26–101	346.7	156–472	68.7	24–120
218.8	150–390	52.7	20–96	336.2	187–546	85.1	36–144
214.2	150–380					119	59–188
262.3	156–375	68.3	24–96	437.3	302–560	81.1	32–117
222.5	118–364			267	244–290	67.4	12–112
224.4	132–351						
244.6	128–396	51.1	12–100	360.7	113–870	75.8	44–108
204.4	140–360	58.9	24–104	557.9	228–876	70	34–112
219	130–340	17.5	4–28			55	26–96
210.8	140–350	43.6	20–92	370.3	273–536	56	15–96
191.4	134–276	65	21–100	414.3	236–750	59.3	24–95

Continued

TABLE 3

Enzymes: Laboratory Reference Ranges for Selected Species—cont'd

Species Common Name (Common name synonyms) Scientific Name	N*	Lactate Dehydrogenase (U/L)		Creatine Kinase (U/L)	
		Mean	Range	Mean	Range
Cockatoo, Major Mitchell (Leadbeater's cockatoo, Pink cockatoo) *Lophochroa leadbeateri*	14	303.7	240–390	247.8	132–376
Cockatoo, Moluccan (Salmon-crested cockatoo) *C. moluccensis*	772	304.6	192–456	272.1	148–404
Cockatoo, rose breasted (Galah, Roseate cockatoo, Pink and grey cockatoo) *Eolophus roseicapilla*	92	320.5	161–395	228.9	120–395
Cockatoo, triton *C. galerita triton*	44	269.6	118–374	296.3	164–396
Cockatoo, umbrella *C. alba*	951	296.4	208–405	269.8	152–444
Conure group Aratinga and *Pyrrhura* sp.	2911	292.1	216–408	262.4	153–408
Conure, blue crowned *Aratinga acuticaudata*	93	221.6	148–380	256.3	120–344
Conure, cherry headed (Red-masked parakeet) *Aratinga erythrogenys*	66	249.4	180–441	253.1	146–396
Conure, dusky (Dusky-headed parakeet, Wed- dell's parakeet) *Aratinga weddellii*	29	220.1	114–328	202.6	108–375
Conure, gold-capped *Aratinga auricapillus*	36	250.1	175–387	284.9	200–384
Conure, green-cheeked *Pyrrhura molinae*	41	251.5	168–370	207.6	144–276
Conure, half moon (Orange-fronted parakeet) *Eupsittula canicularis*	29	222.2	104–368		
Conure, jenday *Aratinga jandaya*	55	279.7	224–354	276.8	167–388
Conure, maroon-bellied (Red-bellied conure, Brown- eared conure) *Pyrrhura frontalis*	28	281	204–372	201.5	111–491
Conure, mitred *Psittacara mitrata*	74	212	140–360	193.2	136–311
Conure, nanday *Aratinga nenday*	179	285.8	204–396	251.7	135–400
Conure, orange-fronted *Eupsittula canicularis*	13				
Conure, Patagonian *Cyanoliseus patagonus*	13			305.7	221–387
Conure, sun *Aratinga solstitialis*	57	257.7	188–392	280.1	153–372
Dove *Streptopelia risoria* *Geopelia cuneata*	45	263.1	150–388	260.2	180–388

Aspartate Aminotransferase (U/L)		Alkaline Phosphatase (U/L)		Amylase (U/L)		Bile Acids (μmol/L)	
Mean	Range	Mean	Range	Mean	Range	Mean	Range
182.2	165–210	54	50–60			166	142–189
189.3	136–366	60.2	21–104	542.9	228–780	66.9	30–110
264.8	150–344	65	48–82			128	101–148
162.4	120–208	75.3	54–100			67.5	24–98
204.1	140–376	68.5	38–106	632	264–876	74.5	38–114
229.5	147–378	54.6	24–104	441.1	192–954	65.7	32–105
201.4	140–354					68	24–105
215.9	132–385					59	32–94
257.2	162–356					17	16–18
232.8	147–363					20.7	9–32
204	138–270					53.2	10–93
207.2	120–324					64.2	28–138
233.7	140–312					71	20–114
224.2	136–378						
189	118–342	40.4	12–78			51.7	12–96
238.8	147–378	41	28–64			69.1	16–129
178	120–360					47.2	15–93
238.6	138–355					51.5	12–92
217.7	111–372					71.8	40–106

Continued

TABLE 3

Enzymes: Laboratory Reference Ranges for Selected Species—cont'd

Species Common Name (Common name synonyms) Scientific Name	N*	Lactate Dehydrogenase (U/L)		Creatine Kinase (U/L)	
		Mean	Range	Mean	Range
Duck domestic *Anas platyrhynchos domestica*	73	193.8	120–246	266.1	165–378
Combined Bald eagle *Haliaeetus leucocephalus* Golden eagle *Aquila chrysaetos*	18	289.4	252–340	334.6	234–485
Eclectus parrot *Eclectus roratus*	415	275.3	198–386	264.3	132–410
Emu *Dromaius novaehollandiae*	98	778.1	318–1243	428.8	70–818
Grey-cheeked parakeet (Fire-winged parakeet) *Brotogeris pyrrhoptera*	449	262.7	154–356	278.8	164–378
Hawk, red-tailed *Buteo jamaicensis*	13	339.8	230–398		
Lory (11 genera, 53 species)	130	194.6	124–302	295.6	178–396
Lovebird *Agapornis* sp.	650	277.1	225–354	250.7	160–392
Macaw group mostly *Ara* and some *Anodorhynchus*	5338	135.3	70–220	214.7	88–361
Macaw, blue and gold (Blue and yellow macaw) *Ara ararauna*	1367	133.7	69–220	219.4	92–380
Macaw, green-winged (Red and green macaw) *Ara chloroptera*	347	139.9	72–224	220.9	96–368
Macaw, Hahn's (Red-shouldered macaw) *Diopsittaca nobilis nobilis*	51	184.8	132–260	292.8	242–380
Macaw, hyacinth *Anodorhynchus hyacinthinus*	149	136.3	90–208	280.2	138–369
Macaw, military *Ara militaris*	88	134.8	72–216	219.7	126–321
Macaw, noble (Red shouldered macaw) *Diopsittaca nobilis cumanensis*	22				
Macaw, scarlet (Red and yellow macaw) *Ara macao*	146	122.2	60–210	240.1	98–366
Macaw, severe (Chestnut fronted macaw) *Ara severus*	104	128.9	66–210	225.7	123–356
Macaw, yellow-collared (Golden-collared macaw) *Primolius auricollis*	70	152	96–213	291.1	210–361
Moustache parakeet (Rose-breasted parakeet) *Psittacula alexandri*	26	300	208–360		
Mynah species, mostly *Acridotheres tristis*	44			336.6	250–414

Aspartate Aminotransferase (U/L)		Alkaline Phosphatase (U/L)		Amylase (U/L)		Bile Acids (μmol/L)	
Mean	Range	Mean	Range	Mean	Range	Mean	Range
33.9	12–73					54.9	22–82
231.3	134–339						
219.9	144–339	72.2	32–111	622.2	562–684	70.7	30–110
227.2	80–380					18	2–34
324.6	189–388					53.7	81
242	110–392						
257.5	141–369					57.3	20–97
214.5	130–360					56	12–90
121.5	65–168	50.3	12–100	421.2	239–564	48.9	7–100
118.9	64–168	60.2	32–100	407.8	239–516	52.8	27–86
116.9	62–168	59.9	30–106			44.5	15–78
184.1	133–216						
143.2	110–174	41.8	15–84			50.5	13–91
123.3	76–166	41.9	17–88			66.2	24–130
176.7	126–215						
120.1	74–177	30.1	16–58			68.3	21–100
129	72–170	41.7	12–76			54.3	25–82
129.4	104–150					57.9	21–93
266.7	143–380						
284.4	200–352					58.2	30–96

Continued

TABLE 3

Enzymes: Laboratory Reference Ranges for Selected Species—cont'd

Species Common Name (Common name synonyms) Scientific Name	N*	Lactate Dehydrogenase (U/L)		Creatine Kinase (U/L)	
		Mean	Range	Mean	Range
Ostrich *Struthio camelus*	140	970	408–1236	3702	800–6508
Owl, great-horned *Bubo virginianus*	18	282.8	142–383	286.7	252–376
Parakeet, Alexandrine *Psittacula eupatria*	18				
Parakeet, ringneck (Rose-ringed parakeet) *Psittacula krameri*	46	213.9	150–318		
Parrot, Meyers *Poicephalus meyeri*	39				
Parrot, red-bellied *Poicephalus rufiventris*	14				
Parrot, Senegal *Poicephalus senegalus*	244	254.1	153–396	288	151–396
Parrot, thick-billed *Rhynchopsitta pachyrhyncha*	10	173	158–202	251.6	200–344
Parrotlet species Genus *Forpus* sp.	29				
Pionus species group Genus *Pionus* sp.	431	248.5	179–384	276.2	116–408
Pionus, blue-headed *Pionus menstruus*	26	225.3	138–384		
Pionus, white capped *Pionus senilis*	49	228.5	157–354	219.6	106–365
Quaker parrot (Monk parakeet) *Myiopsitta monachus*	210	243	138–360	318.8	192–402
Rosella, Genus *Platycercus* sp.	21	223.9	121–348		
Swan *Cygnus* sp.	36	244.2	150–352	246.9	130–389
Toucan *Ramphastos* sp.	86	257.6	180–319		

Aspartate Aminotransferase (U/L)		Alkaline Phosphatase (U/L)		Amylase (U/L)		Bile Acids (μmol/L)	
Mean	Range	Mean	Range	Mean	Range	Mean	Range
447.9	226–547					21	2–30
196.7	104–344	39	8–102			23.5	8–54
252.7	159–303						
178	120–360						
229.8	156–352						
245.8	176–316						
202.8	120–330					587	20–94
186.5	143–280	81.5	70–93			55	22–98
173.7	110–224						
222.3	135–358					47	15–92
241.8	148–342						
213.5	120–346						
248.6	130–380					55.3	21–90
176.3	116–258						
52.3	10–108	66.7	48–92			38.9	18–85
243.3	141–340	43.3	14–88			54.4	16–86

TABLE 4

Metabolic: Laboratory Reference Ranges for Selected Species*

Species Common Name (Common name synonyms) Scientific Name	N[†]	Units	Uric Acid Conventional: (mg/dL) S.I.: (μmol/L) Mean	Range
Grey parrot (African Grey) genus *Psittacus* sp.	5571	Conventional	5.55	2.0–11
		S.I.	330.1	117.8–648.3
Grey parrot (African Grey, Congo) *Psittacus erithacus*	495	Conventional	5.65	2.5–10
		S.I.	336.1	146.9–593.6
Timneh parrot (African Grey, Timneh) *P. timneh*	219	Conventional	5.5	1.7–10
		S.I.	327.1	103.5–604.9
Amazon genus *Amazona* sp.	8375	Conventional	5.1	2.2–10
		S.I.	303.3	132.0–618.0
Amazon, blue-fronted *Amazona aestiva*	828	Conventional	5.03	2.3–10
		S.I.	299.2	137.4–604.3
Amazon, double yellow-headed *A. oratrix*	565	Conventional	4.88	2.3–9.9
		S.I.	290.3	136.8–585.9
Amazon, lilac crown *A. finschi*	57	Conventional	5.65	2.6–10
		S.I.	336.1	155.2–612.6
Amazon, mealy *A. farinosa*	54	Conventional	5.27	2.3–12
		S.I.	313.5	138.6–699.5
Amazon, green-cheeked (Mexican red head) *A. viridigenalis*	206	Conventional	5.51	2.2–11
		S.I.	327.7	130.9–625.1
Amazon, orange wing *A. amazonica*	240	Conventional	5.32	2.3–11
		S.I.	316.4	136.8–624.5
Amazon, panama *A. ochrocephala panamensis*	67	Conventional	5.58	2.8–10
		S.I.	331.9	164.8–606.1
Amazon, red-lored *A. autumnalis*	299	Conventional	5.23	2.2–9.9
		S.I.	311.1	130.9–587.1
Amazon, yellow nape *A. auropalliata*	1074	Conventional	5.07	2.3–11
		S.I.	301.6	137.4–636.4
Amazon, yellow-crowned *A. ochrocephala*	36	Conventional	5.37	2.3–11
		S.I.	319.4	134.4–624.5
Budgerigar *Melopsittacus undulatus*	1542	Conventional	8.61	4.8–13
		S.I.	512.1	285.5–764.9
Caique *Pionites* sp.	30	Conventional	5.13	2.5–11
		S.I.	305.1	149.9–631.7
Canary *Serinus canaria forma domestica*	300	Conventional	8.68	4.1–13
		S.I.	516.3	246.2–750.0
Cockatiel *Nymphicus hollandicus*	9267	Conventional	7.05	3.4–11
		S.I.	419.3	202.2–648.3
Cockatoo group family Cacatuidae	5928	Conventional	7.05	3.4–11
		S.I.	397.9	226.0–654.3
Cockatoo, bare eye (Little corella) *C. sanguinea*	30	Conventional	5.95	3.0–11
		S.I.	353.9	176.1–638.2

*Data from the California Avian Laboratory, Citrus Heights, CA.
[†]Number of normal animals in the data set.

Glucose Conventional: (mg/dL) S.I.: (mmol/L)		Cholesterol Conventional: (mg/dL) S.I.: (mmol/L)		Total Protein Conventional: (g/dL) S.I.: (g/L)		Total Calcium Conventional: (mg/dL) S.I.: (mmol/L)	
Mean	**Range**	**Mean**	**Range**	**Mean**	**Range**	**Mean**	**Range**
281.1	256–360	193.2	100–250	3.5	2.7–4.4	9.29	8.0–14
15.6	14.21–19.98	5	2.59–6.47	35.1	27–44	2.32	2.00–3.49
281.1	256–360	193.2	100–250	3.3	2.8–3.7	9.29	8.0–14
15.5	13.99–19.15	5.72	3.59–6.83	33	28–37	2.27	1
295.6	274–372	203.9	96–268	3.5	2.4–4.4	9.15	7.5–14.4
16.41	15.21–20.65	5.27	2.48–6.93	34.5	24–44	2.28	1.87–3.59
286.6	246–378	190.6	148–228	3.7	2.6–4.5	9.83	8.0–13.9
15.91	13.66–20.98	4.93	3.83–5.9	36.8	26–45	2.45	2.00–3.46
287.5	246–389	200	100–270	4.5	3.5–6.5	9.9	8.2–13.8
15.96	13.66–21.59	5.17	2.59–6.98	45	35–64.8	2.47	2.05–3.44
279.6	248–369	194.2	100–252	3.7	2.4–4.4	9.76	8.4–13.1
15.52	13.77–20.48	5.02	2.59–6.52	36.6	24–43.7	2.44	1
292.1	245–353	201.4	160–232	3.5	2.6–4.4	9.63	8.4–12.9
16.21	13.60–19.60	5.21	4.14–6.00	34.7	26–44	2.4	2.10–3.21
264	201–337	184.4	111–239	3.5	2.4–4.2	10.3	8.6–12.9
14.65	11.16–18.71	4.77	2.87–6.44	34.7	24–42	2.58	2.15–3.22
286.6	248–370	188.5	144–230	3.4	2.1–4.4	9.77	8.3–15
15.91	13.77–20.54	4.88	3.72–5.95	34.2	21–44	2.44	2.07–3.74
295.3	249–482	215.2	180–254	3.8	2.7–4.9	9.52	8.0–14.5
16.39	13.82–26.76	5.57	4.65–6.57	38.1	27–49	2.38	2.00–3.62
272.4	248–330	203.3	178–237	3.6	2.9–4.6	8.97	8.0–12
15.12	13.77–18.32	5.26	4.60–6.13	36.2	29–46	2.24	2.00–2.99
285.9	250–388	201.1	150–228	3.9	2.3–4.4	9.51	8.0–13.2
15.87	13.88–21.54	5.2	3.88–5.90	39	23–44.4	2.37	2.00–3.29
284.1	249–377	188.8	100–256	3.8	2.8–4.7	985	8.4–13.2
15.77	13.82–20.93	4.88	2.59–6.62	37.6	28–47	2.46	2.10–3.29
255.4	170–316	211.9	125–246	4	3.2–4.6	9.97	8.6–11.7
14.18	9.44–17.54	5.48	3.23–6.36	40.4	32–46	2.49	2.15–2.91
329.8	216–456	181.1	120–230	2.8	2.1–4.3	9.27	8.0–11.2
18.31	11.99–25.31	4.68	3.10–5.95	28.3	21–43	2.31	2.00–2.80
267.2	170–372	174	126–220	3.1	2.5–3.5	9.25	8.3–11.1
14.83	9.44–20.65	4.5	3.26–5.69	30.8	25–35	2.31	2.07–2.77
297	160–360						
16.49	8.88–19.98						
326.1	228–440	151.7	90–200	2.9	2.1–4.8	9.2	8.2–10.9
18.1	12.66–24.42	3.92	2.33–5.17	29	21–47.9	2.3	2.05–2.71
326.1	228–440	151.7	90–200	3.6	2.6–4.8	9.2	8.2–10.9
14.87	11.44–23.2	4.28	2.48–5.48	36.2	26–48.3	2.35	2.05–2.86
265.5	220–378	195.2	174–223	3.1	2.6–3.8	9.78	8.1–11.9
14.74	12.21–20.98	5.05	4.50–5.77	30.5	26–38	2.44	2.02–2.96

Continued

TABLE 4

Metabolic: Laboratory Reference Ranges for Selected Species—cont'd

Species Common Name (Common name synonyms) Scientific Name	N†	Units	Uric Acid Conventional: (mg/dL) S.I.: (μmol/L)	
			Mean	Range
Cockatoo, Goffin's (Tanimbar corella) C. goffiniana	298	Conventional	6.85	3.5–11
		S.I.	407.4	208.2–639.4
Cockatoo, lesser sulfur-crested C. sulphurea	17	Conventional	6.76	2.1–11
		S.I.	402.1	123.7–638.2
Cockatoo, Major Mitchell (Leadbeater's cockatoo, Pink cockatoo) Lophochroa leadbeateri	14	Conventional	7.4	2.2–11
		S.I.	440.2	130.9–672.1
Cockatoo, Moluccan (Salmon crested cockatoo) C. moluccensis	772	Conventional	6.05	3.2–11
		S.I.	359.9	190.3–632.9
Cockatoo, rose breasted (Galah, Roseate cockatoo, Pink and grey cockatoo) Eolophus roseicapilla	92	Conventional	6.92	3.9–11
		S.I.	411.6	231.4–635.2
Cockatoo, triton Cacatua galerita triton	44	Conventional	5.55	2.2–11
		S.I.	330.1	127.9–654.9
Cockatoo, umbrella C. alba	951	Conventional	6.67	3.5–11
		S.I.	396.7	208.2–648.3
Conure group Aratinga and Pyrrhura sp.	2911	Conventional	6.58	3.0–11
		S.I.	391.4	178.4–665.0
Conure, blue-crowned Aratinga acuticaudata	93	Conventional	5.31	2.3–11
		S.I.	315.8	137.4–638.2
Conure, cherry-headed (Red-masked parakeet) A. erythrogenys	66	Conventional	5.8	2.1–11
		S.I.	345	124.9–678.7
Conure, dusky (Dusky-headed parakeet, Weddell's parakeet) A. weddellii	29	Conventional	7.52	3.1–11
		S.I.	447.3	186.2–644.2
Conure, gold-capped A. auricapillus	36	Conventional	6.2	2.5–11
		S.I.	368.8	124.9–666.2
Conure, green-cheeked Pyrrhura molinae	41	Conventional	8.11	3.2–12
		S.I.	482.4	189.7–742.3
Conure, half moon (Orange-fronted parakeet) Eupsittula canicularis	29	Conventional	7.17	3.1–11
		S.I.	426.5	182.0–666.8
Conure, jenday Aratinga jandaya	55	Conventional	6.32	2.1–11
		S.I.	375.9	122.5–673.9
Conure, maroon-bellied (Red-bellied conure, Brown-eared conure) Pyrrhura frontalis	28	Conventional	6.16	3.0–12
		S.I.	366.4	178.4–738.7
Conure, mitred Psittacara mitrata	74	Conventional	5.94	2.2–13
		S.I.	353.3	130.9–772.1
Conure, nanday Aratinga nenday	179	Conventional	6.48	2.3–11
		S.I.	385.4	137.4–660.2

Glucose Conventional: (mg/dL) S.I.: (mmol/L)		Cholesterol Conventional: (mg/dL) S.I.: (mmol/L)		Total Protein Conventional: (g/dL) S.I.: (g/L)		Total Calcium Conventional: (mg/dL) S.I.: (mmol/L)	
Mean	Range	Mean	Range	Mean	Range	Mean	Range
274.2	220–412	169.9	114–214	3.4	2.4–4.3	9.07	8.0–11.4
15.22	12.21–22.87	4.39	2.95–5.53	34	24–43	2.26	2.00–2.84
245.2	138–304	138.8	113–206	3.5	2.8–4.6	9.16	8.1–10.3
13.61	7.66–16.88	3.59	2.92–5.33	34.8	28–46	2.29	2.02–2.57
301.9	242–392	202	152–252	3.5	3–3.9	9.26	8.4–11.6
16.76	13.43–21.76	5.22	3.93–6.52	34.8	30–39	2.31	2.10–2.89
259	198–424	171.9	104–224	3.6	2.5–4.8	9.39	8.0–11.7
14.38	10.99–23.54	4.45	2.69–5.79	36.1	25–48	2.34	2.00–2.92
300	198–376	185	146–224	3.2	2.4–4.5	8.62	8.4–9.1
16.65	10.99–20.87	4.78	3.78–5.79	31.6	24–45	2.15	2.10–2.27
270.3	200–345	198.6	146–248	4	2.4–4.8	9.49	8.0–12
15	11.10–19.15	5.14	3.78–6.41	39.5	24–48	2.37	2.00–2.99
269.4	214–426	162.4	96–212	3.6	2.3–6.1	9.33	8.1–11
14.95	11.88–23.65	4.2	2.48–5.48	36	23–61	2.33	2.02–2.74
291	216–418	174.4	144–202	3.4	2.4–4.9	9.38	8.1–11.7
16.15	11.99–23.20	4.51	3.72–5.22	33.9	24–49	2.34	2.02–2.91
292.3	228–377	187.2	162–227	3.8	2.4–4.9	9.45	8.3–12
16.23	12.66–20.93	4.84	4.19–5.87	37.5	24–49	2.36	2.07–2.99
290.8	220–384	162.1	96–245	3.3	2.8–4.9	9.57	8.1–11
16.14	12.21–21.32	4.19	2.48–6.34	33.2	28–49	2.39	2.02–2.73
273.5	213–350	142.8	120–163			9.77	8.1–11.7
15.18	11.82–19.43	3.69	3.10–4.22			2.44	2.02–292
280.3	202–366	215.7	170–246	3.4	2.7–3.9	9.44	8.0–11.1
15.56	11.21–20.32	5.58	4.40–6.36	33.8	27–39	2.36	2.00–2.77
288.6	215–395	165	96–220	4.1	3.4–4.8	9.28	8.0–12.5
16.02	11.93–21.93	4.27	2.48–5.69	41	34–48	2.32	2.00–3.2
281.3	189–388	165.8	120–237			9.5	8.4–12.6
15.61	10.49–21.54	4.29	3.10–6.13			2.37	2.10–3.14
277.5	192–346	190.1	102–258			9.97	8.6–11.7
15.4	10.66–19.21	4.92	2.64–6.67			2.49	2.15–2.92
300.6	261–340	182.6	104–207			9.38	8.1–11.4
16.69	14.49–18.87	4.72	2.69–5.35			2.34	2.02–2.84
292.6	228–370	193.1	123–240	3	2.5–3.7	9.17	8.4–10.9
16.24	12.66–20.54	4.99	3.18–6.21	30.4	25–37.3	2.29	2.10–2.72
290.8	231–393	180.6	117–248	3	1.9–3.7	9.2	8.0–11
16.14	12.82–21.82	4.67	3.03–6.41	30.4	19–37	2.28	2.00–2.73

Continued

TABLE 4

Metabolic: Laboratory Reference Ranges for Selected Species—cont'd

Species Common Name (Common name synonyms) Scientific Name	N[†]	Units	Uric Acid Conventional: (mg/dL) S.I.: (μmol/L)	
			Mean	Range
Conure, orange-fronted *Eupsittula canicularis*	13	Conventional	6.6	3.6–11
		S.I.	392.6	213.5–647.1
Conure, Patagonian *Cyanoliseus patagonus*	13	Conventional	5.53	2.3–11
		S.I.	328.9	133.8–678.1
Conure, sun *Aratinga solstitialis*	57	Conventional	6.66	2.2–12
		S.I.	396.1	131.5–688.8
Dove *Streptopelia risoria, Geopelia cuneata*	45	Conventional	7.25	2.5–12
		S.I.	431.2	146.9–710.2
Duck domestic *Anas platyrhynchos domestica*	73	Conventional	6.39	2.0–12
		S.I.	380.1	119.0–701.3
Combined Eagle species Bald eagle *Haliaeetus leucocephalus* Golden eagle *Aquila chrysaetos*	18	Conventional	6.17	2.1–13
		S.I.	367	121.9–761.3
Eclectus parrot *Eclectus roratus*	415	Conventional	5.45	2.0–11
		S.I.	324.2	120.1–645.4
Emu *Dromaius novaehollandiae*	98	Conventional	6.3	1.0–14
		S.I.	374.7	59.5–832.7
Grey-cheeked parakeet (Fire-winged parakeet) *Brotogeris pyrrhoptera*	449	Conventional	6.29	0.3–12
		S.I.	374.1	19.6–706.6
Hawk, red tailed *Buteo jamaicensis*	13	Conventional	11.1	6.3–18
		S.I.	658.4	375.9–1068.9
Lory (11 genera, 53 species)	130	Conventional	6.23	2.0–12
		S.I.	370.6	119.6–703.1
Lovebird *Agapornis* sp.	650	Conventional	7.44	3.3–11
		S.I.	442.5	193.9–634.1
Macaw group mostly *Ara* and some *Anodorhynchus*	5338	Conventional	5.57	1.8–12
		S.I.	331.3	107.1–701.3
Macaw, blue and gold (Blue and yellow macaw) *Ara ararauna*	1367	Conventional	5.32	1.9–11
		S.I.	316.4	113.0–655.5
Macaw, green winged (Red and green macaw) *A. chloroptera*	347	Conventional	5.31	1.5–11
		S.I.	315.8	90.4–659.6
Macaw, Hahn's (Red-shouldered macaw) *Diopsittaca nobilis nobilis*	51	Conventional	7.26	3.9–11
		S.I.	431.8	230.8–645.4
Macaw, hyacinth *Anodorhynchus hyacinthinus*	149	Conventional	6.79	1.5–12
		S.I.	403.9	91.0–734.0
Macaw, military *Ara militaris*	88	Conventional	5.14	2.0–11
		S.I.	305.7	121.3–653.7
Macaw, noble (Red-shouldered macaw) *Diopsittaca nobilis cumanensis*	22	Conventional	6.38	2.2–10
		S.I.	379.5	129.7–622.2

Glucose Conventional: (mg/dL) S.I.: (mmol/L)		Cholesterol Conventional: (mg/dL) S.I.: (mmol/L)		Total Protein Conventional: (g/dL) S.I.: (g/L)		Total Calcium Conventional: (mg/dL) S.I.: (mmol/L)	
Mean	**Range**	**Mean**	**Range**	**Mean**	**Range**	**Mean**	**Range**
310.7	236–389	189.4	94–255	3	2.2–3.8	9.06	8.2–10.4
17.25	13.10–21.59	4.9	2.43–6.59	29.8	22–38	2.26	2.05–2.59
273.4	167–380	175.6	112–255	3.4	2.4–4.5	9.22	8.0–11.2
15.17	9.27–21.09	4.54	2.90–6.590	34.2	24–45	2.3	2.00–2.80
299.9	164–386	219.6	124–257	2.9	2.1–3.7	9.41	8.0–12.6
16.65	9.10–21.43	5.68	3.21–6.65	28.6	21–37	2.35	2.00–3.14
206.5	127–319	170.2	104–244	4.5	3.5–5.5	10	8.7–12.7
11.46	7.05–17.71	4.4	2.69–6.31	44.7	35–55	2.5	2.17–3.18
325.6	253–389	205.4	134–268			10.8	8.9–13.5
18.08	14.04–21.59	5.31	3.47–6.93			2.68	2.22–3.37
265.7	216–396	198.6	100–261	3.7	3.2–4.3	9.31	8.1–11.9
14.8	11.99–21.98	5.13	2.59–6.75	36.6	32–42.8	2.32	2.02–2.98
134.1	101–243	122	68–170	3.9	3.4–4.4	11.1	8.8–12.5
7.4	5.61–13.49	3.15	1.76–4.40	39	34–44	2.77	2.20–3.12
289.3	210–385	185.1	96–249			9.16	8.0–11.6
16.1	11.66–21.37	4.79	2.48–6.44			2.29	2.00–2.89
310.8	222–388					10.6	8.4–13.8
17.3	12.32–21.54					2.65	2.10–3.43
287.2	192–388	197.5	100–257	3.1	1.9–4.1	9.08	8.0–11.5
15.9	10.66–21.54	5.11	2.59–6.65	30.9	19–41	2.27	2.00–2.87
305.7	220–390	163.8	100–228	2.7	1.8–3.7	9.5	8.4–11.7
17	12.21–21.65	4.24	2.59–5.90	27.1	18–37	2.37	2.10–2.92
277.2	210–360	167.8	96–264	3.4	2.4–4.4	9.66	8.4–11.9
15.4	11.66–19.98	4.34	2.48–6.83	34.2	24–43.9	2.41	2.10–2.96
279.7	210–368	160.7	96–249	3.5	2.5–4.2	9.73	8.4–11.8
15.5	11.66–20.43	4.16	2.48–6.44	34.7	25–42	2.43	2.10–2.94
275.7	210–360	163.3	108–256	3.5	2.7–4.2	9.65	8.4–11.8
15.3	11.66–19.98	4.22	2.79–6.62	34.8	27–42	2.41	2.10–2.94
265.9	190–322	156.9	96–238			9.08	8.1–10.4
14.8	10.55–17.87	4.06	2.48–6.15			2.27	2.02–2.59
271.1	216–352	132.9	96–216	3	2.6–3.4	9.37	8.2–11.4
15.1	11.99–19.54	3.44	2.48–5.59	30.5	26–34	2.34	2.05–2.84
274.1	214–340	167.5	110–237	3.5	3–3.9	9.27	8.4–10.9
15.2	11.88–18.87	4.33	2.84–6.13	34.5	30–39	2.31	2.10–2.72
270.8	231–300						
15	12.82–16.65						

Continued

TABLE 4

Metabolic: Laboratory Reference Ranges for Selected Species—cont'd

Species Common Name (Common name synonyms) Scientific Name	N†	Units	Uric Acid Conventional: (mg/dL) S.I.: (μmol/L)	
			Mean	Range
Macaw, scarlet (Red and yellow macaw) *Ara macao*	146	Conventional	5.15	2.1–11
		S.I.	306.3	121.9–642.4
Macaw, severe (Chestnut-fronted macaw) *A. severus*	104	Conventional	6.51	2.2–12
		S.I.	387.2	129.7–701.9
Macaw, yellow-collared (Golden-collared macaw) *Primolius auricollis*	70	Conventional	7.44	3.4–12
		S.I.	442.5	204.0–702.5
Moustache parakeet (Rose-breasted parakeet) *Psittacula alexandri*	26	Conventional	6.81	3.1–11
		S.I.	405.1	185.0–624.5
Mynah species, mostly *Acridotheres tristis*	44	Conventional	7.57	2.3–12
		S.I.	450.3	134.4–713.2
Ostrich *Struthio camelus*	140	Conventional	8.62	1.0–15
		S.I.	512.7	59.5–892.2
Owl, great-horned *Bubo virginianus*	18	Conventional	8.52	3.1–12
		S.I.	506.8	183.2–703.6
Parakeet, Alexandrine *Psittacula eupatria*	18	Conventional	7.16	4.3–11
		S.I.	425.9	257.5–640.0
Parakeet, ringneck (Rose-ringed parakeet) *Psittacula krameri*	46	Conventional	6.7	3.3–12
		S.I.	398.5	193.9–700.7
Parrot, Meyers *Poicephalus meyeri*	39	Conventional	5.72	2.1–11
		S.I.	340.2	26.1–672.1
Parrot, red-bellied *Poicephalus rufiventris*	14	Conventional	6.55	3.0–9.5
		S.I.	389.6	178.4–562.7
Parrot, Senegal *Poicephalus senegalus*	244	Conventional	5.95	2.3–12
		S.I.	353.9	134.4–707.8
Parrot, thick-billed *Rhynchopsitta pachyrhyncha*	10	Conventional	6.47	3.4–11
		S.I.	384.8	202.2–683.4
Parrotlet species Genus *Forpus* sp.	29	Conventional	8.23	4.1–12
		S.I.	489.5	244.5–694.1
Pionus species group Genus *Pionus* sp.	431	Conventional	5.91	2.0–12
		S.I.	351.5	120.7–685.2
Pionus, blue-headed *Pionus menstruus*	26	Conventional	6.11	3.1–12
		S.I.	363.4	184.4–710.8
Pionus, white-capped *P. senilis*	49	Conventional	5.62	2.1–11
		S.I.	334.3	126.7–662.0
Quaker parrot (Monk parakeet) *Myiopsitta monachus*	210	Conventional	6.8	2.2–12
		S.I.	404.5	133.2–712.6
Rosella, Genus *Platycercus* sp.	21	Conventional	7.22	3.4–11
		S.I.	429.4	201.6–634.7
Swan *Cygnus* sp.	36	Conventional	6.82	2.1–11
		S.I.	405.7	126.1–654.3
Toucan *Ramphastos* sp.	86	Conventional	7.93	2.4–14
		S.I.	471.7	144.5–832.7

Glucose Conventional: (mg/dL) S.I.: (mmol/L)		Cholesterol Conventional: (mg/dL) S.I.: (mmol/L)		Total Protein Conventional: (g/dL) S.I.: (g/L)		Total Calcium Conventional: (mg/dL) S.I.: (mmol/L)	
Mean	**Range**	**Mean**	**Range**	**Mean**	**Range**	**Mean**	**Range**
265.7	210–333	183.2	12–247	3.2	2.4–3.8	9.38	8.4–10.9
14.8	11.66–18.48	4.74	3.10–6.39	32.3	24–37.7	2.34	2.10–2.72
278.5	220–366	180.6	100–252	3.3	2.3–3.9	9.4	8.4–10.8
15.5	12.21–20.32	4.67	2.59–6.52	32.9	23–39	2.35	2.10–2.69
278.6	126–363	181.7	108–240	3.7	3.2–4.4	10.1	8.8–11.7
15.5	6.99–20.15	4.7	2.79–6.21	36.9	32–44	2.52	2.20–2.92
284.6	225–348					9.3	8.3–10.8
15.8	12.49–19.32					2.32	2.07–2.69
318.5	228–372	204.1	126–244	3.6	3–4.3	9.41	8.2–10.8
17.7	12.66–20.65	5.28	3.26–6.31	35.6	30–43	2.35	2.05–2.69
217	164–330	103	39–172	3.9	2.4–5.3	10.7	8.0–13.6
12.1	9.10–18.32			39	24–53	2.67	2.00–3.39
319.1	237–390	191.4	114–261	4	3.3–4.6	10.2	8.8–12.4
17.7	13.16–21.65	4.95	2.95–6.75	39.5	33–45.9	2.6	2.20–3.09
254.3	192–308					9.13	8.0–10.9
14.1	10.66–17.10					2.28	2.00–2.73
294.4	220–354					9.21	8.4–10.4
16.34	12.21–19.65					2.3	2.10–2.59
255.5	212–294					9.34	8.2–10.4
14.2	11.7–16.32					2.33	2.05–2.59
275.1	232–326						
15.27	12.88–18.10						
288.7	256–354	193.8	114–250	3.4	2.9–4.1	9.24	8.4–10.8
16.02	14.21–19.65	5.01	2.95–6.47	34.2	29–41.2	2.31	2.10–2.69
295	246–350	159.8	102–214	3	2.8–3.6	9.11	8.0–10.5
16.38	13.66–19.43	4.13	2.64–5.53	30.3	28–36	2.27	2.00–2.62
308.7	252–384						
17.13	13.99–21.32						
279.5	212–368	229	176–258	3.4	2.3–4.3	9.23	8.2–10.4
15.51	11.77–20.43	5.92	4.55–6.67	34.1	23–43	2.3	2.05–2.59
276.4	200–348					8.93	8.0–10
15.34	11.10–19.32					2.23	2.00–2.50
282.5	221–348					8.94	8.2–10
15.68	12.27–19.32					2.23	2.05–2.50
287.9	210–395	219.1	100–262	3.1	2.5–3.7	9.23	8.4–10.8
15.98	11.66–21.93	5.67	2.59–6.78	31.2	25–37	2.3	2.10–2.69
337.6	281–396					9.27	8.0–10.9
18.74	15.60–21.98					2.31	2.00–2.72
187.9	132–360	164.6	92–250	3.4	2.3–4.4	10.9	8.2–13.4
10.43	7.33–19.98	4.26	2.38–6.47	33.6	23–44	2.72	2.05–3.34
297.9	222–363	175.1	104–254	3.5	2.8–4.4	10.2	8.8–11.8
16.53	12.32–20.15	4.53	2.69–6.57	34.9	28–44.2	2.55	2.20–295

Normal Biological Data

Christal Pollock • James W. Carpenter

TABLE 1

Classification of Selected Avian Species Groups

FALCONIFORMES

American kestrel	*Falco sparverius*
Bald eagle	*Haliaeetus leucocephalus*
Black vulture	*Coragyps atratus*
Common kestrel	*Falco tinnunculus*
Cooper's hawk	*Accipiter cooperii*
Eurasian buzzard	*Buteo buteo*
Eurasian (northern) sparrowhawk	*Accipiter nisus*
Gyrfalcon	*Falco rusticolus*
Harris hawk	*Parabuteo unicinctus*
Merlin	*Falco columbarius*
Northern goshawk	*Accipiter gentilis*
Golden eagle	*Aquila chrysaetos*
Osprey	*Pandion haliaetus*
Peregrine falcon	*Falco peregrinus*
Prairie falcon	*Falco mexicanus*
Red-tailed hawk	*Buteo jamaicensis*
Sharp-shinned hawk	*Accipiter striatus*
Turkey vulture	*Cathartes aura*

STRIGIFORMES

Barn owl	*Tyto alba*
Barred owl	*Strix varia*
Eurasian eagle owl	*Bubo bubo*
Great horned owl	*Bubo virginianus*
Screech owl, eastern	*Megascops asio*
Screech owl, western	*Megascops kennicottii*
Snowy owl	*Bubo scandiacus*

RATITES

Emu	*Dromaius novaehollandiae*
Ostrich	*Struthio camelus*
Rhea	*Rhea americana*

PICIFORMES (RAMPHASTIDAE)

Channel-billed toucan	*Ramphastos vitellinus*
Toco toucan	*Ramphastos toco*

CICONIIFORMES

American (Caribbean) flamingo	*Phoenicopterus ruber*
Great blue heron	*Ardea herodias*

GRUIFORMES

Houbara bustard	*Chlamydotis undulata*
Sandhill crane	*Grus canadensis*

CORACIIFORMES

Rufous hornbill	*Buceros hydrocorax*

TABLE 2

Biologic and Physiologic Values of Selected Psittacine Birds[1-5]

| Species | Body Weight (kg) | Lifespan (yr) | | Temp °C (°F)[a] |
		Range	Maximum Reported	
Amazon parrot (*Amazona* spp.)	—	>50	80	—
Amazon, blue-crowned (Mealy) (*Amazona farinosa guatemalae*)	540–700	4–8	—	—
Amazon, blue-fronted (*Amazona aestiva*)	361–485 (432)	—	—	—
Amazon, double yellow-headed (*A. oratrix*)	463–694 (568)	1.5 wild	19.3 wild	—
Amazon, green-cheeked (Mexican red head) (*A. viridigenalis*)	343–377 (360)	4–8 (6)	35	—
Amazon, yellow-crowned (yellow-fronted) (*Amazona ochrocephala*)	—	—	—	—
Amazon, yellow-naped (*A. auropalliata*)	476–795 (596)	—	—	—
Amazon, white-fronted (spectacled) (*A. albifrons*)	—	—	—	—
Bourke's parakeet (*Neopsephotus bourkii*)	35–50 (40)	—	—	—
Brotogeris spp.	—	—	—	—
Budgerigar (*Melopsittacus undulatus*)	26–35	Median: 5	18	—
Cockatiel (*Nymphicus hollandicus*)	80–100	Median: 10–12	36	—
Cockatoo (*Cacatua* spp.)	—	—	—	—
Cockatoo, medium	—	—	—	—
Cockatoo, large	—	—	—	—
Cockatoo, bare-eyed (little corella) (*C. sanguinea*)	331	—	—	—
Cockatoo, citron-crested (*C. sulphurea citrinocristata*)	—	—	—	—
Cockatoo, galah (rose-breasted) (*Eolophus roseicapilla*)	299	40–60	—	—
Cockatoo, greater sulphur-crested (*Cacatua galerita*)	806	—	—	—
Cockatoo, Leadbeater's (Major Mitchell) (*Lophochroa leadbeateri*)	381–474 (423)	—	—	—
Cockatoo, lesser sulphur-crested (*Cacatua sulphurea*)	303	—	—	—
Cockatoo, Moluccan (salmon-crested) (*C. moluccensis*)	808	—	—	—
Cockatoo, palm (*Probosciger aterrimus*)	—	—	—	—
Cockatoo, triton (*Cacatua galerita triton*)	559	—	—	—
Cockatoo, umbrella (*C. alba*)	552	—	—	—
Conure	80–100	—	—	—
Conure, small	—	—	—	—
Conure, large	—	—	—	—
Conure, blue-crowned (*Thectocercus acuticaudatus*)	—	—	—	—
Conure, golden (Queen of Bavaria) (*Guaruba guarouba*)	252–276 (262)	—	—	—

bpm, Beats per minute.
[a]Body temperature is not routinely measured during physical examination.
[b]Restraint can increase respiratory rate 1.5–2-fold.

Heart Rate (bpm)	Respiratory Rate (bpm)[b]	Clutch Size	Incubation Period (d)	Hatching Weight (g)	Fledging Age (d)		Weaning Age (days)	Sexual Maturity
					Parent-Raised	Hand-Raised		
—	15–45	—	24–29	—	45–60	90–120	75–90	4–6 yr
—	—	—	—	—	—	—	—	—
—	—	—	26	—	—	—	—	—
—	—	—	28–29	—	—	—	—	—
—	—	—	26	—	—	—	—	—
—	—	—	28–29	—	—	—	—	—
—	—	—	28–29	—	—	—	—	—
—	—	—	24	—	—	—	—	—
—	—	—	—	—	—	—	—	—
—	—	—	22	—	—	—	—	—
—	60–75	4–6	16–18	—	22–26	30–40	30	6–9 mo
—	40–50	4–5	18–20	—	32–38	47–52	42–49	6–12 mo
—	15–40	—	—	—	—	—	—	—
—	—	—	—	—	45–60	90–120	75–100	3–4 yr
—	—	—	—	—	60–80	120–150	95–120	5–6 yr
—	—	—	23–24	—	—	—	—	—
—	—	—	25–26	—	—	—	—	—
—	—	—	22–24	—	45–55	90–120	89–90	12 mo
—	—	—	24–25	—	—	—	—	—
—	—	—	—	—	—	—	—	—
—	—	—	—	—	—	—	—	—
—	—	—	28–29	—	—	—	—	—
—	—	—	28–30	—	—	—	—	—
—	—	—	27–28	—	—	—	—	—
—	—	—	28	—	—	—	—	—
—	—	—	—	—	35–40	45–70	60	2–3 yr
—	40–50	—	—	—	—	—	—	—
—	30–45	—	—	—	—	—	—	—
—	—	—	23–24	—	—	—	—	—
—	—	—	—	—	—	—	—	—

Continued

TABLE 2

Biologic and Physiologic Values of Selected Psittacine Birds—cont'd

Species	Body Weight (kg)	Lifespan (yr) Range	Maximum Reported	Temp °C (°F)[a]
Conure, Nanday (Black-hooded) (*Aratinga nenday*)	—	—	—	—
Conure, orange-fronted (*Eupsittula canicularis*)	—	—	—	—
Conure, Patagonian (burrowing parrot) (*Cyanoliseus patagonus*)	—	—	—	—
Conure, sun (*Aratinga solstitialis*)	120–130	Median: 19	30	—
Eclectus parrot (*Eclectus roratus*)	347–512 (432)	20–40	80	—
Grey parrot (*Psittacus erithacus*)	370–534 (407–454)	40–60 45 captivity 22.7 wild	48–60	41 (105.8)
Lory/lorikeet	—	20–30	—	—
Lorikeet, rainbow (*Trichoglossus haematodus*)	75–157	Median: 7	38	—
Lovebird	42–48	15–30	—	—
Lovebird, Fischer's (*Agapornis fischeri*)	42–58	Median: 8	32	—
Lovebird, masked (yellow-collared) (*A. personatus*)	43–47	Median: 6	24	—
Macaw	—	—	—	—
Macaw, large	—	75–100	—	—
Macaw, small	—	50–80	—	—
Macaw, blue and gold (blue and yellow) (*Ara ararauna*)	1021 995–1380 (1021)	21	48	—
Macaw, green-winged (red and green) (*A. chloroptera*)	1050–1708 (1179)	19	63	—
Macaw, hyacinth (*Anodorhynchus hyacinthinus*)	1197–1695 (1355)	22	54	—
Macaw, military (*Ara militaris*)	788–1134	Median: 20	54	—
Macaw, red-fronted (*A. rubrogenys*)	458	—	—	—
Macaw, scarlet (*A. macao*)	900–1490 (1103)	Median: 21	48	—
Pionus parrot (*Pionus* spp.)	—	—	—	—
Princess of Wales parakeet (*Polytelis alexandrae*)	100–129 (108)	—	—	—
Quaker (monk) parakeet (*Myiopsitta monachus*)	—	—	—	—
Red-crowned parakeet (*Cyanoramphus novaezelandiae*)	95–100	—	—	—
Red-rumped parakeet (*Psephotus haematonotus*)	60–69 (65)	—	—	—
Ring-neck parakeet (*Psittacula krameri*)	115	18–25	—	—
Senegal parrot (*Poicephalus senegalus*)	—	—	—	—

Heart Rate (bpm)	Respiratory Rate (bpm)[b]	Clutch Size	Incubation Period (d)	Hatching Weight (g)	Fledging Age (d)		Weaning Age (days)	Sexual Maturity
					Parent-Raised	Hand-Raised		
—	—	—	21–23	—	—	—	—	—
—	—	—	30	—	—	—	—	—
—	—	—	24–25	—	—	—	—	—
—	—	4–5	23–28	—	49–56	—	—	2–3 yr
—	—	—	26–28	—	72–80	120–150	100–110	4 yr
340–600	24–45	2–5	26–30 Congo: 28 Timneh: 26	—	77–94	100–120	75–90	3–6 yr
—	—	—	21–27	—	42–50	62–70	50–60	2 yr
—	—	1–3	24–25	—	49–56	—	—	1 yr
—	50–60	—	18–24	—	30–35	45–55	40–55	6–12 mo
—	—	3–8	20–22	—	28–35	—	—	—
—	—	3–8	20–22	—	28–35	—	—	—
	20–25	—	—	—	—	—	—	—
—	—	—	26–28	—	70–80	120–150	95–120	5–7 yr
—	—	—	23–26	—	45–60	90–120	75–90	4–6 yr
—	—	1–3	25–27	—	84–98	—	—	3–4 yr
—	—	2–3	26–28	—	84–98	—	—	4–5 yr
—	—	2–3	29	31.6	98–112 (108)	—	—	5–6 yr
—	—	2–4	28	—	91	—	—	3–4 yr
—	—	—	—	—	—	—	—	—
—	—	1–4	28	—	84–91	—	—	4–6 yr
—	—	—	25–26	—	—	—	—	—
—	—	—	—	—	—	—	—	—
—	—	—	23	—	—	—	—	—
—	—	—	—	—	—	—	—	—
—	—	—	—	—	—	—	—	—
—	—	—	22–23	—	40–45	55–65		3 yr
—	—	—	24–25	—	—	—	—	—

TABLE 3

Biologic and Physiologic Values of Selected Passerine Birds[1,6-38]

Family	Species	Body Weight (g)	Lifespan (yr) Range	Max reported	Temp °C (°F)[a]
Bombycillidae	Cedar waxwing (*Bombycilla cedrorum*)	30–32	—	8	40–41.3 (104–106.3)
Cardinalidae	Northern cardinal (*Cardinalis cardinalis*)	33.6–64 (42–48) Males are slightly larger than females	Annual survival rates for adults have been estimated at 60%–65%	15	40–41.3 (104–106.3)
Corvidae	—	—	—	—	40–41.3 (104–106.3)
	American crow (*Corvus brachyrhynchos*)	316–620 (438–458) Males are slightly larger		16 wild 59 captive	—
	Blue jay (*Cyanocitta cristata*)	64.1–109 (85)	7 wild	17 wild 26.25 captive	—
Estrildidae	—	—	—	—	40–41.3 (104–106.3)
	Bengalese finch (Society or Japanese Mövchen) (*Lonchura striata domestica*)	7.5–16	4–7	—	—
	Common waxbill (*Estrilda astrild*)	7.5–16 (8.9)	4 wild	—	—
	Gouldian finch (*Erythrura gouldiae*)	7.5–35	—	—	—
	Java sparrow (*Padda oryzivora*)	7.5–35 (24–30)	—	—	—
	Zebra finch (*Taeniopygia guttata*)	7.5–16 (12)	4–7	—	—
Fringillidae	—	—	—	—	40–41.3 (104–106.3)
	American goldfinch (*Carduelis tristis*)	8.6–20.7 (12.6)	—	10	—
	Common canary (Island or Atlantic) (*Serinus canaria*)	12–30	5–15	20–25	—
	House finch (*Carpodacus mexicanus*)	16–27 (21)	—	11	—
	Purple finch (*C. purpureus*)	18–32 (25)	2 wild	14	—
Hirundinidae	Tree swallow (*Tachycineta bicolor*)	16–25 (20)	8–11 (2.7)	12	40–41.3 (104–106.3)
Mimidae	Northern mockingbird (*Mimus polyglottos*)	36.2–58 (43–49)		20 captivity	40–41.3 (104–106.3)
Paridae	Black-capped chickadee (*Parus atricapillus*)	8.2–14 (10.8)	2.5 wild	12	40–41.3 (104–106.3)
Passeridae	House sparrow (*Passer domesticus*)	20.1–34.5 (27.4–28)	—	13	40–41.3 (104–106.3)
Sturnidae	—	—	—	—	40–41.3 (104–106.3)
	European starling (Common) (*Sturnus vulgaris*)	64–100	—	—	—
	Golden-breasted starling (*Cosmopsarus regius*)	80	—	—	—
	Hill Mynah (myna) (*Gracula religiosa*)	180–270 (205)	12	20	—
Timaliidae	Pekin robin (red-billed leiothrix) (*Leiothrix lutea*)	26	—	—	40–41.3 (104–106.3)
Turdidae	American robin (*Turdus migratorius*)	64.8–85 (77)	2 (wild) Only 25% of fledged young survive to November	14	40–41.3 (104–106.3)[c]

bpm, Beats per minute.
[a]Potential diurnal variation of 2–3° C.
[b]Pip-to-hatch interval is usually 24 hr or less.[33]
[c]Less than or equal to 38° C (100.4° F) considered slightly hypothermic in the American robin.[37]

Heart Rate (bpm)	Respiratory Rate (bpm)	Clutch Size	Incubation Period (d)[b]	Hatching Weight (g)	Eyes Open (d)	Fledging Age (d)	Weaning Age (d)	Sexual Maturity
—	—	2–6 (4–5)	10–17	—	Eyes remain closed in the first week	14–18 (15) fledging weight of 30 g	—	1 yr
—	—	1–5 (3)	11–14	3.5		9–15	—	1 yr
—	—	—	—	—	—	—	—	—
—	—	2–9	16–22	15.6–70	10–15 (110–210 g)	20–45	—	—
—	—	2–8	16–22	—	—	20–45	—	1 yr
—	—	—	—	—	—	—	—	—
—	—	4–8	12–16	—	—	18–20	25–28	9–10 mo
—	—	4–6	11–12	—	—	17–28	33–44	6–12 mo
—	—	—	—	—	—	19–28	33–44	—
—	—	4–8	14–14	—	—	26–28 captivity 19–28 wild	33–44	—
—	—	4–6	12–16	—	—	14–28	33–44 25–28	9–10 mo captivity 2.5–3 mo wild
—	—	—	—	—	—	—	—	—
—	—	2–7	12–14	<1–2	—	12–18	2–7	12–14 mo
265–325 resting	60–80 resting	3–5	12–14	—	—	11–17 (14)	21	<1 yr
—	—	2–6 (4–5)	13–14	<1–2	—	12–19 (14)	—	<1 yr
—	—	2–7	12–13	—	—	14–17	—	—
—	—	4–7	11–20 (14.5)	—	—	20–25	—	1 yr
—	—	2–6 (4–5)	10–17	3.5–18	—	11–13 fledging weight of 32g	—	1 yr
—	—	1–13 (6–8)	12–13	—	—	14–18	—	6 mo
—	—	2–5	12–14	<1–2		13–17	—	—
—	—	—	—	—	—	—	—	—
—	92 resting 180 flight	4–5	10–17	5.5–30	—	20–23	—	—
—	—	—	—	—	—	—	—	—
—	—	2	14–15	—	—	30	60	2–3 yr
—	—	—	—	—	—	—	—	—
—	—	3–5 (3.5)	10–17	5–35	—	13–15 fledging weight of 48–50 g	—	1 yr

TABLE 4

Biologic and Physiologic Values of Selected Raptors[1,39-47]

Order	Species	Body Weight (kg)		Longevity (yr)
		Male	**Female**	
Falconiformes	American kestrel *(Falco sparverius)*	0.1–0.12	0.13–0.17	2–7
	Bald eagle *(Haliaeetus leucocephalus)*	4.1–4.3	5.6–6.3	20–30 wild, 47 captivity
	Black vulture *(Coragyps atratus)*	2.0–2.7		25
	Cooper's hawk *(Accipiter cooperii)*	0.28–0.35	0.44–0.57	12 (20)
	Eurasian buzzard *(Buteo buteo)*	0.55–0.86	0.7–1.2	25
	Eurasian (northern) sparrowhawk *(Accipiter nisus)*	0.15–0.2	0.19–0.3	15
	Golden eagle *(Aquila chrysaetos)*	2.5–4.0	3.25–6.35	>38
	Gyrfalcon *(Falco rusticolus)*	0.8–1.3	1.4–2.1	—
	Harris's hawk *(Parabuteo unicinctus)*	0.7–1.0		20–30
	Kestrel *(Falco tinnunculus)*	0.14–0.25	0.15–0.31	—
	Merlin *(F. columbarius)*	0.15–0.21	0.19–0.26	10–14
	Northern goshawk *(Accipiter gentilis)*	0.6–1.1	0.8–1.4	15–19
	Osprey *(Pandion haliaetus)*	1.0–1.7	1.1–1.9	—
	Peregrine falcon *(Falco peregrinus)*	0.56–0.85	1.1–1.5	15–20
	Prairie falcon *(F. mexicanus)*	0.50–0.65	0.70–0.98	10–15
	Red-tailed hawk *(Buteo jamaicensis)*	0.69–1.15	1.0–1.35	21
	Sharp-shinned hawk *(Accipiter striatus)*	0.08–0.13	0.14–0.21	10
	Turkey vulture *(Cathartes aura)*	0.85–2.0		16
Strigiformes	Barn owl *(Tyto alba)*	0.44–0.47	0.49–0.57	>15
	Barred owl *(Strix varia)*	0.63	0.8	18
	Eurasian eagle owl *(Bubo bubo)*	1.5–2.8	1.8–4.2	50–60
	Great-horned owl *(B. virginianus)*	1.3	1.7	20
	Screech owl, eastern *(Megascops asio)*	0.16–0.18	0.18–0.22	>14
	Screech owl, western *(M. kennicottii)*	0.13–0.21	0.16–0.25	>13
	Snowy owl *(Bubo scandiacus)*	1.4–2.5	1.6–2.9	28

bpm, Beats per minute.

Heart Rate (bpm)	Respiratory Rate (bpm)	Clutch Size	Incubation Period (d)	Interval Between Eggs (d)	Fledging (d)	Sexual Maturity (yr)
—	—	3–7	29–31	2–3	30–31	1
—	—	1–3	34–36	—	70–98	4–5
—	—	1–3	37–48	—	80–94	3
—	—	3–6	32–36	—	27–34	2
—	18	2–4	36–38	3	49–56	2–3
—	—	2–4	32–43	—	24–30	1–2
—	—	1–3	43–45	3–5	70	>5
—	—	3–5	34–36	—	49–56	—
—	—	2–5	32	2–3	43–49	>3
—	—	3–6	27–29	1–2	27–30	1
—	—	2–7	28–32	2	30–35	2
—	—	4–6	35	2–3	35–42	>3
—	—	3–4	29–32	2–3	48–59	3
—	—	2–7	29–33	—	35–42	>3
—	—	3–4	29–31	—	35–42	1–2
—	—	2–4	28–35	—	42–46	2
—	—	3–9+	30–33	2–3	24–27	—
—	9.2	1–3	30–40	—	66–88	—
—	—	2–9	30–31	2–3	70–75	1
—	—	2–4	28–33	—	42	—
—	—	2–4	34–36	2–3	90	2–3
—	—	1–4	30–37	—	42–63	1–3
—	—	2–6	21–30	—	—	—
—	—	3–8	32–35	—	28	—
—	—	1–3 (11)	38–41	—	16	2

TABLE 5

Biologic and Physiologic Values of Selected Galliformes[1,48-59]

Family	Species	Body Weight (kg)		Lifespan (yr)	
		Males	Females	Average	Maximum Reported
Cracidae	Curassow			24 Great curassow	—
	Red-billed (southeast) curassow	3.5		—	—
	(*Crax blumenbachii*)				
Meleagrididae	Turkey, wild	6.8–11	3.6–5.4	—	—
	(*Meleagris gallopavo*)				
Numididae	Guineafowl	—		—	—
	(*Acryllium* spp.)				
Phasianidae	Chicken, Greater prairie	—		—	—
	(*Tympanuchus cupido*)				
	Jungle fowl, red	2.58		30 captivity	—
	(*Gallus gallus*)				
	Domestic chicken	2–12		25	—
	(*G. gallus*)				
	Francolin, Erckel's	—		—	—
	(*Francolinus erckelii*)				
	Francolin, black	—		—	—
	(*Francolinus francolinus*)				
	Peafowl, Indian	2.7–6 (4)		10–25 (16–18)	25 wild
	(*Pavo cristatus*)				23.2 captivity
	Pheasant, Blood	—		—	—
	(*Ithaginis cruentus*)				
	Pheasant, ring-necked or common	1.263		10–18	—
	(*Phasianus colchicus*)				
	Quail, common	0.070–0.155		11	—
	(*Coturnix coturnix*)				
	Quail, Japanese	0.090–0.115		6	—
	(*Coturnix japonica*)				
	Quail, northern bobwhite	0.140–0.170		6	—
	(*Colinus virginianus*)				
	Tragopan	—		—	—
	(*Tragopan* spp.)				
Opisthocomidae	Hoatzin				
	(*Opisthocomus hoazin*)				
Tetraonidae	Grouse				

bpm, Beats per minute.
[a]Best layers average between 250–280 eggs per year.

Clutch Size	Incubation Period (d)	Fledging (d)	Sexual Maturity (yr)
2	28–32	—	—
2 rarely 3	30.5	—	2–3 yr
4–17 (8–15)	25–31 (28)	—	10 mo–1 yr
6–20	26–28	—	—
12	23–26	—	—
5–10 (4–6)	21	—	—
12–16[a]	—	—	12–20 weeks for most, 26 weeks in Jersey Giants
5–10	21–23	—	—
8–12	18–19	—	—
2–8 (max 12)	27–29	7–14	1–3 yr
5–12	27–29	—	—
7–15 (10)	23–28 (24)	7–12	1 yr
6–13	17–20	11	—
7–14	19–20 (17)	—	Male: 52 d Female: 63 d
—	23	14	1 yr
2–6	28	—	—
2–3			
2	28–32		

TABLE 6

Biologic and Physiologic Values of Selected Waterfowl[1,60-77]

Family, Subfamily	Species	Body Weight (kg, mean)		Lifespan	
		Male	Female	Range	Maximum Reported
Anatinae	American black duck (*Anas rubripes*)	(1080)		—	—
	American wigeon (*A. americana*)	538–649 (594)		—	—
	Blue-winged teal (*A. discors*)	314–387 (335–352)		—	—
	Cinnamon teal (*A. cyanoptera*)	310–355 (333)		—	—
	Eurasian teal (common) (*A. crecca*)	280		—	—
	Eurasian wigeon (*A. penelope*)	990–1160	700–800	10–15	35
	Gadwall (*A. strepera*)	587–697 (642)		—	—
	Mallard (*A. platyrhynchos*)	837–1047 (901–982)		10–15	—
	Mandarin duck (*Aix galericulata*)	428–693		10–15	
	Mottled duck (*Anas fulvigula*)	734–860 (797)		—	—
	Muscovy duck (*Cairina moschata*)	2000–4000	1100–1500	10–15	—
	Mute swan (*Cygnus olor*)	12.2	8.9	25–30	—
	Northern pintail (*Anas acuta*)	454–1362 (612)	454–1135	—	—
	Northern shoveler (*A. clypeata*)	466–569 (518)		—	—
	Ringed teal[a] (*Callonetta leucophrys*)	360		—	—
	Wood duck (*Aix sponsa*)	548–610 (579–582)		—	—
Anhimidae	Screamers	3500–5000		—	—
Anserinae	Bar-headed goose (*Anser indicus*)	2000–3000 (2600)		15–20	
	Black-necked swan (*Cygnus melancoryphus*)	7000		—	—
	Barnacle goose (*Branta leucopsis*)	1454–2020 (1737–2100) Body mass ↓ by ~25% during molt		—	—
	Canada goose (*B. canadensis*)	—		—	—
	B. c. canadensis	3554–4628 (4091)		—	—
	B. c. occidentalis	2495–3206 (2851)		—	—
	B. c. minima	1095–1387 (1241)		—	—
	B. c. moffitti	3137–4305 (3721)		—	—
	Emperor goose (*Anser canagicus*)	1770–2233 (2002)		—	—
	Greater white-fronted goose (*A. albifrons*)	2661		—	—
	Greylag goose (*A. anser*)	2500–4100		—	—
	Hawaiian (nēnē) goose (*Branta sandvicensis*)	2200 1800–2300	1900	15–20	28 wild 42 captivity
	Pink-footed goose (*Anser brachyrhynchus*)	2600	2350	15–20	—
	Red-breasted goose (*Branta ruficollis*)	1300–1600	1150	15–20	—
	Snow goose (*Anser c. caerulescens*)	1710–2530 (2120)		—	—
	Trumpeter swan (*Cygnus buccinators*)	(9639)		—	—
	Tundra swan (*C. columbianus*)	(6300)		—	—
	Whooper swan (*C. cygnus*)	(8100)		—	—
Aythyinae	Canvasback (*Aythya valisineria*)	1001–1157 (1079)		—	—
	Common pochard (*A. ferina*)	—		—	—
	Lesser scaup (*A. affinis*)	629 (559–698)		—	—
	Redhead (*A. americana*)	852–1044 (948)		—	—
	Ring-necked duck (*A. collaris*)	594–666 (630)		—	—
	Tufted duck (*A. fuligula*)	589–740 (665)		10–15	
Dendrocygninae	Black-bellied whistling duck (*Dendrocygna autumnalis*)	716	705–756 (731)	—	—

bpm, Beats per minute.
[a]Sometimes placed in subfamily Tadorninae.

Heart Rate (bpm)	Respiratory Rate (bpm)	Clutch Size	Incubation Period (d)	Mean Body Weight of 1-day-old (g)	Fledging (d)	Sexual Maturity (yr)
—	—	3–7	29–31	2–3	30–31	1
—	—	—	25	—	37–48	1
—	—	—	23	—	—	—
—	—	—	23	—	—	—
—	—	—	—	16.8	—	—
180–230	30–95	7–11	23–25	26.4	40–45	1
—	—	—	26	—	—	—
180–230	30–95	8–12	23–29	28.8	42–60	1
180–230	30–95	9–12	28–30	—	41–46	1–2
—	—	—	26	—	—	—
180–230	30–95	8–15	35	—	—	1
80–150	13–40	4–8	35–40	—	—	5
—	—	7–9	22–24	—	46–47	0.5–1
—	—	—	23	—	—	—
—	—	—	—	—	—	—
—	—	—	—	30	—	—
—	—	—	—	—	—	—
80–150 (104 ± 7)	13–40	4–6	27–30	—	55–60	2–3
—	—	—	—	—	—	—
113 ± 11	—	—	24	—	—	—
—	—	4–10	25–30	—	40–73	2–3
—	—	—	28	—	—	—
—	—	—	27	—	—	—
—	—	—	26	—	—	—
—	—	—	28	—	—	—
—	—	—	25	—	—	—
—	—	—	—	—	—	—
—	—	3–12 (4–6)	27–28	—	—	2–3
80–150	13–40	1–5 (3)	29–31	—	3 mo	2–3
80–150	13–40	3–5	26–27	—	—	2
80–150	13–40	3–7	23–25	—	—	2
—	—	—	23	—	—	—
—	—	—	—	—	—	—
—	—	—	—	—	—	—
—	—	—	24	—	—	—
—	—	—	—	40.1	—	—
—	—	—	—	—	—	—
—	—	—	26	—	—	—
—	—	—	26	—	—	—
180–230	30–95	6–14	23–25	34.1	—	1
—	—	—	31	—	—	—

Continued

TABLE 6

Biologic and Physiologic Values of Selected Waterfowl—cont'd

Family, Subfamily	Species	Body Weight (kg, mean)		Lifespan	
		Male	Female	Range	Maximum Reported
Merginae	Common eider *(Somateria mollissima)*	2250 850–3025 (1800)	2120	10–15	
	Common golden eye *(Bucephala clangula americana)*	645–687 (666)		10–15	
	Common merganser *(Mergus merganser)*	—	1076	—	—
	Hooded merganser *(M. cucullatus)*	521–536 (529)		—	—
	Red-breasted merganser *(M. serrator)*	—		—	—
	Velvet scoter *(Melanitta fusca fusca)*	—	1316	—	—
	White-winged scoter *(M. f. deglandi)*	1091–1440 (1204–1326)		—	—
Oxyurinae	Maccoa duck *(Oxyura maccoa)*	673–761 (717)		—	—
	Ruddy duck *(O. Jamaicensis)*	508–619 (564)		—	—
Tadorninae	Common shelduck *(Tadorna tadorna)*	—	960	—	—
	Egyptian goose *(Alopochen aegyptiaca)*	1500–2250		—	—

Heart Rate (bpm)	Respiratory Rate (bpm)	Clutch Size	Incubation Period (d)	Mean Body Weight of 1-day-old (g)	Fledging (d)	Sexual Maturity (yr)
180–230	30–95	3–6	25–30 (26)	61.4	60–75	1–2
180–230	30–95	9–11	27–32 (31)	32.4	—	1
—	—	—	—	46.2	—	—
—	—	—	—	—	—	—
—	—	—	—	46.2	—	—
—	—	—	—	54.7	—	—
—	—	—	28	—	—	—
—	—	—	25	—	—	—
—	—	—	24	—	—	—
—	—	—	—	—	—	—
—	—	5–12	28–30	—	70	2

TABLE 7

Biologic and Physiologic Values of Selected Pigeons and Doves[78-81]

Species	Body Weight (g)		Lifespan (yr)		Clutch Size	Incubation Period (d)	Fledging (d)	Sexual Maturity
	Males	Females	Average	Maximum Reported				
African collared dove (*Streptopelia roseogrisea*)	150–160		—	—	—	—	—	—
Common ground dove (*Columbina passerina*)	30		4–8	—	—	12 to >14	18	1 yr
European turtle dove (*Streptopelia turtur*)	85–186		—	—	1–2	13–14	20	—
Mourning dove (*Zenaida macroura*)	96–170 (120)		1.5 wild	19.3 wild	2	13–15	12–15	85 d
Pigeon (rock dove) (*Columba livia*)	240–300 (358.7)		4–8 (6)	35	2	16–19	28–35	—
Pink pigeon (*C. mayeri*)	240–410	213–369	—	—	—	—	—	—
Southern crowned pigeon (*Goura scheepmakeri*)	2250		—	—	1	—	—	—
Spotted dove (*Streptopelia chinensis*)	146–198		—	—	2 (rarely 3)	14–16	14–15	—

TABLE 8

Biologic and Physiologic Values of Other Selected Species[1,31,40,82-101]

Taxonomic Group	Species	Body Weight (kg)		Longevity (yr)		Body Temp, °C (°F)
		Male	Female	Reported	Maximum	
Apodiformes Subfamily						
Apodidae	Alpine swift (Tachymarptis melba)	—		—	26	—
	Chimney swift (Chaetura pelagica)	0.017–0.030 (0.023)		—	14	40–41 (104–105.8), potential diurnal variation of 2–3° C
	Common swift (Apus apus)	—		—	21	—
Tribe Chaeturini	Spinetails					
Trochilidae	Most hummingbirds	0.003–0.007		5–12 (5–8)	17 captivity	39–45 (102.2–113) As low as 14 (57.2) during torpor
	Reddish hermits (Phaethornis ruber)	<0.002		—	—	—
	Bee hummingbirds (Mellisuga helenae)	<0.002		—	—	—
	Giant hummingbirds (Patagonia gigas)	0.019–0.021		—	—	—
Ciconiiformes	American flamingo (Caribbean) (Phoenicopterus ruber)	2.8	2.2	—	>60 captivity	—
	Great-blue heron (Ardea herodias)	2.1–2.5		15	24	—
Coraciiformes	Rufous hornbill (Buceros hydrocorax)	—	0.75	—	—	—
Gruiformes	Houbara bustard (Chlamydotis undulata)	2.2	1.2	10–15	—	—
	Sandhill crane (Grus canadensis)	2.7–5.4		20–30	—	—
Pelecaniformes						
Anhingidae	Anhinga (Anhinga anhinga)	1.08–1.35		11.9 wild	16.4 wild	—
Fregatidae	Frigatebird, magnificent (Fregata magnificens)	1.2–1.815		20–30 estimated	—	—
Phalacrocoracidae	Cormorants	—		—	—	—
	Cormorant, double-crested (Phalacrocorax auritus)	1.2–2.5 (2.0), Males slightly larger		—	—	—
	Cormorant, Guanay (P. bougainvillii)	1.55–3.2		—	—	—
Pelecanidae	Pelicans	Up to 15		—	—	—
	Pelican, American white (Pelecanus erythrorhynchos)	6.18–8.0 4.54–9.0	4.21–8.0	—	26.4 wild	—
	Pelican, Australian (P. conspicillatus)	4.4–6.8		15–25	50 captivity	—
	Pelican, brown (P. occidentalis)	2.05–5		27.83	43 wild	—
	Pelican, pink-backed (P. rufescens)	3.86–5.55	3.42–4.57	—	—	—
Phaethontidae	Tropicbirds	—		—	—	—
	Tropicbird, red-tailed (Phaethon rubricauda)	0.64–1.1		—	—	—

bpm, Beats per minute.
[a]48-hr interval between egg laying.

Heart Rate (bpm)	Respiratory Rate (bpm)	Clutch Size[a]	Incubation Period (d)	Birth Weight (g)	Weaning Age	Fledging Age (d)	Sexual Maturity (yr)
			14–32				
		1–7 (2–3)					
—	—	—	—	—	—	—	—
—	—	2–7	16–21	1.0–1.5	—	28–30	—
—	—	1	—	—	—	—	—
		4–5	—		—	—	—
500–600 resting	13–40 resting	2	13–19	—	—	20–35	—
>1000 active	30–95 active						
<50, down to							
30 torpor							
—	—	—	—	—	—	—	—
—	—	—	—	—	—	—	—
—	—	—	—	—	—	—	—
—	—	3–5 (2–7)	27–31	—	28–42 d	63–91	3–5
—	—	2	27–29	—	—	56–60	1.8
—	—	2–3	—	—	—	119–136	—
—	—	2–3	21–22	—	—	35–40	1–3
—	—	2 (1–3)	28–31	—	Precocial	67–75	3–6 (wild)
—	—	—	—	—	—	—	—
—	—	1–7 (3)	25–28	—	—	21–28	2
—	—	2-4	24-31	—	—	—	—
—	—	2	41	—	—	—	—
—	—	—	—	—	—	—	—
—	—	2–4	28–35	—	—	—	3–4
—	—	2	30	—	—	70–77	3
—	—	1-3 (2)	32–35 (32)	—	—	60	3–4
—	—	2-3 (3)	29–30	—	—	77	Male: 2–4 yr; Female: 3–4 yr
—	—	—	—	—	—	—	—
—	—	1	40–46	—	—	—	4
—	—	—	—	—	—	—	—

Continued

TABLE 8

Biologic and Physiologic Values of Other Selected Species—cont'd

Taxonomic Group	Species	Body Weight (kg)		Longevity (yr)		Body Temp, °C (°F)
		Male	Female	Reported	Maximum	
Sulidae	Boobies	—		—	—	—
	Booby, blue-footed (*Sula nebouxii*)	1.53		18 captivity	—	—
	Booby, red-footed (*S. sula*)	0.85–1.0		—	—	—
	Gannet, northern (*Morus bassanus*)	2.932 / 2.2–3.6	3.067	—	21 wild	—
Piciformes (Ramphastidae)	Channel-billed toucan (*Ramphastos vitellinus*)	0.6–0.7		20	—	—
	Toco toucan (*Ramphastos toco*)	0.59–0.76		18–20	—	—
Ratites	Emu (*Dromaius novaehollandiae*)	30–55		19	30	—
	Ostrich (*Struthio camelus*)	120–160		50	—	—
	Rhea (*Rhea americana*)	25		—	—	—

bUnder isoflurane anesthesia.

Heart Rate (bpm)	Respiratory Rate (bpm)	Clutch Size[a]	Incubation Period (d)	Birth Weight (g)	Weaning Age	Fledging Age (d)	Sexual Maturity (yr)
—	—	1–3	40–45	—	—	—	1–6
—	—	2–6 (4)	25–30	—	—	42	—
—	—	—	—	—	—	—	—
—	—	1	42–50	—	—	120–200	3
—	—	2–4 (5)	15–16	—	—	—	1
—	—	2–4	15–18	—	—	42–56	3–4
42–76 hr[b]	4–17 hr[b]	5–15	50–56	—	Precocial	—	3–5
60–72 hr[b]	6–12	10 (20)	41–43	—	Precocial	—	4
—	8.5	—	36–41	—	Precocial	—	1.5–2

TABLE 9

Values Reported for Selected Ophthalmic Diagnostic Tests in Avian Species[1,102-110]

| Species | Ultrasound (mm ± STD)[a] | Intraocular Pressure (mm Hg) | | Schirmer Tear Test (mm/min) | Phenol Red Thread Test (mm/15 s ± STD) |
		Applanation Tonometry	Rebound Tonometry		
American flamingo *(Phoenicopterus ruber)*	—	16.1 ± 4.2	9.5 ± 1.7	12.3 ± 4.5	24.2 ± 4.4
Axial globe length	13.8 ± 0.16	—	—	—	—
Anterior chamber depth	1.75 ± 0.05	—	—	—	—
Lens thickness	4.6 ± 0.06	—	—	—	—
Vitreous body depth	6.95 ± 0.1	—	—	—	—
Pecten dimensions	5.1 ± 0.38 length 2.2 ± 0.14 width	—	—	—	—
Bald eagle *(Haliaeetus leucocephalus)*	—	20.6 ± 2	—	14 ± 2	—
Barn owl *(Tyto alba)*	—	—	10.8 ± 3.8	—	—
Blue-fronted Amazon[b] *(Amazona aestiva)*	—	—	—	—	—
D1	1.7 ± 0.3	—	—	—	—
D2	3.5 ± 0.2	—	—	—	—
D3	7.3 ± 0.4	—	—	—	—
Axial length	12.6 ± 0.6	—	—	—	—
Common buzzard *(Buteo buteo)*	—	—	26.9 ± 7.0	—	—
Chicken, 3-week-old	—	—	17.5 ± 0.1	—	—
Golden eagle *(Aquila chrysaetos)*	—	21.5 ± 3	—	—	—
Great-horned owl *(Bubo virginianus)*	—	10.8 ± 3.6	—	—	—
Eurasian eagle owl *(Bubo bubo)*	—	—	10.5 ± 1.6	—	—
Eurasian sparrowhawk *(Accipiter nisus)*	—	—	15.5 ± 2.5	—	—
Kestrel *(Falco tinnunculus)*	—	—	9.8 ± 2.5	—	—
Large psittacines[c]	—	—	—	—	19.1 ± 3.3–25.5 ± 6.3 (OS) 19.8 ± 4.3–28.2 ± 6.3 (OD)
Long-eared owl *(Asio otus)*	—	—	7.8 ± 3.2	—	—
Northern goshawk *(Accipiter gentilis)*	—	—	18.3 ± 3.8	—	—
Peregrine falcon *(Falco peregrinus)*	—	—	12.7 ± 5.8	—	—
Red kite *(Milvus milvus)*	—	—	13.0 ± 5.5	—	—
Red-tailed hawk *(Buteo jamaicensis)*	—	20.6 ± 3.4	—	—	—
Swainson's hawk *(Buteo swainsoni)*	—	20.8 ± 2.3	—	—	—
Tawny owl *(Strix aluco)*	—	—	9.4 ± 4.1	—	—
Juvenile	—	—	8.7 ± 4.9	7.2	—
Adult	—	9.4 ± 1.8	11.1 ± 3.1	4.3	—
White-tailed sea eagle *(Haliaeetus albicilla)*	—	—	26.9 ± 5.8	—	—

STD, Standard deviation; OD, right eye; OS, left eye.

[a]Mean values reported.

[b]Transpalpebral ocular ultrasound examinations were performed on 32 blue-fronted Amazon parrots with no history of ocular disease; measurements were taken in sagittal planes using a 10-MHz linear probe without a standoff pad; D1 is the distance between the cornea and the anterior lens capsule; D2 is the distance between the anterior and posterior lens capsule; D3 is the distance between the posterior lens capsule and the optic papilla.

[c]Group of large parrots including 22 macaws, 17 cockatoos, 10 Amazon parrots, 1 Grey parrot, 1 eclectus, and 1 pionus.

TABLE 10

Approximate Resting Respiratory Rates of Selected Avian Species and by Weight[111-113]

Species	Respiratory Rate (breaths/min)[a]
Finch	90–110
Canary	60–80
Budgerigar	60–75
Lovebird	50–60
Cockatiel	40–50
Small conure	40–50
Large conure	30–45
Toucan	15–45
Amazon parrot	15–45
Cockatoo	15–40
Macaw	20–25
Mallard	30–95
Raptor	10–20
Mute swan	13–40

Weight (g)	Respiratory Rate (breaths/min)[a]
100	40–52
200	35–50
300	30–45
400	25–30
500	20–30
1000	15–20

[a]Restraint can increase respiratory rate by 1.5–2× resting rate.

REFERENCES

1. Carpenter JW, Marion CJ, editors: *Exotic animal formulary*, ed 4, St. Louis, 2013, Elsevier.
2. Heatley JJ, Cornejo J: Psittaciformes. In Miller RE, Fowler ME, editors: *Fowler's zoo and wild animal medicine*, Vol 8, St. Louis, 2015, Saunders, p 173.
3. Holman R: *Psittacus erithacus*, 2008. http://animaldiversity.ummz.umich.edu/accounts/Psittacus_erithacus/. Accessed July 18, 2014.
4. Robaldo Guedes NM, Scherer PN: The large macaws. In Fowler ME, Cubas ZS, editors: *Biology, medicine, and surgery of South American wild animals*, Ames, 2001, Iowa State University Press, pp 150–152.
5. Sholty K: *Amazona farinosa*, 2006. http://animaldiversity.ummz.umich.edu/accounts/Amazona_farinosa/. Accessed August, 25, 2014.
6. Backues K, Carmel B, Coke R, et al: Mynah (Family Sturnidae), *Exotic DVM* 8:31, 2007.
7. Ballard B, Cheek R: *Exotic animal medicine for the veterinary technician*, ed 2, Ames, 2010, Blackwell Publishing, p 484.
8. BirdLife International Species factsheet—multiple species: 2014. http://www.birdlife.org. Accessed August 12, 2014.
9. Bowers V: Passerines: swallows, bushtits, and wrens. In Gage LJ, Duerr RS, editors: *Hand-rearing birds*, Ames, 2007, Blackwell Publishing, pp 403–413.
10. Breitmeyer E: *Mimus polyglottos*, 2004. http://animaldiversity.ummz.umich.edu/accounts/Mimus_polyglottos/. Accessed August 23, 2014.
11. Burton M, Burton R: *The wildlife encyclopedia*, Tarrtown, 2002, Marshall Cavendish Corporation.
12. Coles BH, editor: *Essentials of avian medicine and surgery*, ed 3, Ames, 2007, Blackwell Publishing, p 397.
13. The Cornell Lab of Ornithology: *Bird Guide—Multiple Species*, 2014. http://www.allaboutbirds.org. Accessed August 11, 2014.
14. Dewey T: *Cardinalis cardinalis*, 2011. http://animaldiversity.ummz.umich.edu/accounts/Cardinalis_cardinalis/. Accessed August 23, 2014.
15. Doneley B: *Avian medicine and surgery in practice: companion and aviary birds*, London, 2010, Manson Publishing, p 336.
16. Duerr R, Purdin G: Passerines: house finches, goldfinches, and house sparrows. In Gage LJ, Duerr RS, editors: *Hand-rearing birds*, Ames, 2007, Blackwell Publishing, pp 381–392.
17. Eng ML, Williams TD, Letcher RJ, et al: Assessment of concentrations and effects of organohalogen contaminants in a terrestrial passerine, the European starling, *Sci Total Environ* 473–474:589–596, 2014.
18. Friedman E: Corvids. In Gage LJ, Duerr RS, editors: *Hand-rearing birds*, Ames, 2007, Blackwell Publishing, pp 361–375.
19. Frysinger J: *Cyanocitta cristata*, 2001. http://animaldiversity.ummz.umich.edu/accounts/Cyanocitta_cristata/. Accessed August 23, 2014.
20. Harms CA, Harms, RV: Venous blood gas and lactate values of Mourning doves (*Zenaida macroura*), Boat-tailed grackles (*Quiscalus major*), and House sparrows (*Passer domesticus*) after capture by mist net, banding, and venipuncture, *J Zoo Wildl Med* 43(1):77–84, 2012.
21. Heatley JJ, Cary J, Russell KE, et al: Clinicopathologic analysis of Passeriform venous blood reflects transitions in elevation and habitat, *Vet Med Res Rep* 4:21–29, 2013.
22. Howard J: Passerines: American robins, mockingbirds, thrashers, waxwings, and bluebirds. In Gage LJ, Duerr RS, editors: *Hand-rearing birds*, Ames, 2007, Blackwell Publishing, pp 393–401.
23. Huntington S: Passerines: exotic finches. In Gage LJ, Duerr RS, editors: *Hand-rearing birds*, Ames, 2007, Blackwell Publishing, pp 415–420.
24. Johnson S: American crow (*Corvus brachyrhynchos*), *Exotic DVM* 10:13–14, 2008.
25. Johnson-Delaney CA: *Exotic companion medicine handbook for veterinarians*, Lake Worth, 2008, Zoological Education Network.
26. Klein L: *Bombycilla cedrorum*, 2003. http://animaldiversity.ummz.umich.edu/accounts/Bombycilla_cedrorum/. Accessed August 23, 2014.
27. Payevsky VA: Phylogeny and classification of passerine birds, Passeriformes, *Biol Bull Rev* 4(2):143–156, 2014.
28. Purdin G: Chick identification. In Gage LJ, Duerr RS, editors: *Hand-rearing birds*, Ames, 2007, Blackwell Publishing, pp 15–37.
29. Roof J: *Parus atricapillus*, 2011. http://animaldiversity.ummz.umich.edu/accounts/Parus_atricapillus/. Accessed August 23, 2014.
30. Roof J, Harris M: *Tachycineta bicolor*, 2001. http://animaldiversity.ummz.umich.edu/accounts/Tachycineta_bicolor/. Accessed August 23, 2014.
31. Sibley DA: *The Sibley guide to birds*, ed 2, New York, 2014, Alfred A. Knopf, p 598.
32. Sims K: *Gracula religiosa*, 2000. http://animaldiversity.ummz.umich.edu/accounts/Gracula_religiosa/. Accessed August 23, 2014.
33. Smith JA: Passeriformes (songbirds, perching birds). In Miller RE, Fowler ME, editors: *Fowler's zoo and wild animal medicine*, Vol 8, St. Louis, 2015, Saunders, p 245.
34. Sterling R: *Carpodacus purpureus*, 2011. http://animaldiversity.ummz.umich.edu/accounts/Carpodacus_purpureus/. Accessed August 23, 2014.
35. Sung W: Passerines. In Tynes VV, editor: *Behavior of exotic pets*, Ames, 2010, Wiley Blackwell, pp 12–20.
36. Tarr L: *Estrilda astrild*, 2011. http://animaldiversity.ummz.umich.edu/accounts/Estrilda_astrild/. Accessed August 23, 2014.
37. Wagner DN, Mineo PM, Sgueo C, et al: Does low daily energy expenditure drive low metabolic capacity in the tropical robin, Turdus grayi? *J Comp Physiol B* 183:833–841, 2013.
38. White R: *Taeniopygia guttata*, 2007. http://animaldiversity.ummz.umich.edu/accounts/Taeniopygia_guttata/. Accessed August 23, 2014.
39. Best R: Breeding problems. In Beynon PH, Forbes NA, Lawton MPC, editors: *BSAVA manual of raptors, pigeons and waterfowl*, Ames, 1996, Iowa State University Press, pp 202–215.

40. Carey JR, Judge DS: *Longevity records: life spans of mammals, birds, amphibians, reptiles, and fish*, Denmark, 2002, Odense University Press.

41. Chitty J: Birds of prey. In Meredith A, Redrobe S, editors: *BSAVA manual of exotic pets*, Gloucester, 2002, British Small Animal Veterinary Association, pp 179–192.

42. Erlich PR, Dobkin DS, Wheye D: *The birder's handbook: a field guide to the natural history of north american birds*, New York, 1988, Simon & Schuster.

43. Forbes NA, Richardson T: Husbandry and nutrition. In Beynon PH, Forbes NA, Harcourt-Brown NH, editors: *BSAVA manual of raptors, pigeons and waterfowl*, Ames, 1996, Iowa State University Press, pp 289–298.

44. Hardey J, Crick H, Wernham C, et al: *Raptors: a field guide to survey and monitoring*, Edinburgh, 2006, Scottish Natural Heritage.

45. Samour J: Management of raptors. In Harrison GJ, Lightfoot TL, editors: *Clinical avian medicine*, Vol II, Palm Beach, 2006, Spix Publishing, pp 948–954.

46. Samour J: *Avian medicine*, London, 2000, Harcourt Publishers, pp 309–377.

47. Tully Jr TN, Dorrestein GM, Jones AK: *Handbook of avian medicine*, ed 2, Philadelphia, 2009, Saunders.

48. Chumchal M: *Colinus virginianus*, 2000. http://animaldiversity.ummz.umich.edu/accounts/Colinus_virginianus/. Accessed July 18, 2014.

49. Damerow G: *Storey's guide to raising chickens*, North Adams, 2010, Storey Publishing.

50. de Avelar Azeredo RM, Simpson JGP, Barros LP: Order Galliformes, Family Cracidae. In Fowler ME, Cubas ZS, editors: *Biology, medicine, and surgery of South American wild animals*, Ames, 2001, Iowa State University Press, p 136.

51. Fowler E: *Pavo cristatus*, 2011. http://animaldiversity.ummz.umich.edu/accounts/Pavo_cristatus/. Accessed July 18, 2014.

52. Gautier Z: *Gallus gallus*, 2002. http://animaldiversity.ummz.umich.edu/accounts/Gallus_gallus/. Accessed July 18, 2014.

53. Howard L: *Cracidae*, 2004. http://animaldiversity.ummz.umich.edu/accounts/Cracidae/. Accessed August 25, 2014.

54. Jackson CE: *Peacock*, London, 2006, Reaktion Books Ltd.

55. McCullough J: *Meleagris gallopavo*, 2001. http://animaldiversity.ummz.umich.edu/accounts/Meleagris_gallopavo/. Accessed July 18, 2014.

56. Morishita TY: Galliformes. In Miller RE, Fowler ME, editors: *Fowler's zoo and wild animal medicine*, Vol 8, St. Louis, 2015, Saunders, p 153.

57. Pappas J: *Coturnix japonica*, 2002. http://animaldiversity.ummz.umich.edu/accounts/Coturnix_japonica/. Accessed July 18, 2014.

58. Pappas J: *Coturnix coturnix*, 2002. http://animaldiversity.ummz.umich.edu/accounts/Coturnix_coturnix/.Appendix-9781455746712.doc Accessed July 18, 2014.

59. Switzer C: *Phasianus colchicus*, 2011. http://animaldiversity.ummz.umich.edu/accounts/Phasianus_colchicus/. Accessed July 18, 2014.

60. Batouli A: *Branta sandvicensis*, 2007. http://animaldiversity.ummz.umich.edu/accounts/Branta_sandvicensis/. Accessed July 18, 2014.

61. Batt BDJ, Afton AD, Anderson MG, et al, editors: *Ecology and management of breeding waterfowl*, Minneapolis, 1992, University of Minnesota Press.

62. de Magalhaes J, Costa J: A database of vertebrate longevity records and their relation to other life-history traits, *J Evol Biol* 22:1770–1774, 2009.

63. Fransson T, Kolehmainen T, Kroon C, et al: *European longevity records*, 2001. http://www.euring.org/data_and_codes/longevity-voous.htm. Accessed July 18, 2014.

64. Harris M: *Aix galericulata*, 1999. http://animaldiversity.ummz.umich.edu/accounts/Aix_galericulata/. Accessed July 18, 2014.

65. Hohman WL, Taylor TS, Weller MW: Annual body weight change in ring-necked ducks (*Aytha collaris*). In Weller MW, editor: *Waterfowl in Winter*, Minneapolis, 1988, University of Minnesota Press, p 260.

66. Pope A: *Aix sponsa*, 2004. http://animaldiversity.ummz.umich.edu/accounts/Aix_sponsa/. Accessed July 18, 2014.

67. Portugal SJ, Green JA, Butler PJ: Annual changes in body mass and resting metabolism in captive barnacle geese (*Branta leucopsis*): the importance of wing moult, *J Exp Biol* 210(Pt 8):1391–1397, 2007.

68. Robinson J: *Anas acuta*, 2002. http://animaldiversity.ummz.umich.edu/accounts/Anas_acuta/. Accessed July 18, 2014.

69. Rogers C: *Somateria mollissima*, 2002. http://animaldiversity.ummz.umich.edu/accounts/Somateria_mollissima/. Accessed August 18, 2014.

70. Silveira LF, Fowler ME: Order Anseriformes (ducks, geese, swans). In Fowler ME, Cubas ZS, editors: *Biology, medicine, and surgery of South American wild animals*, Ames, 2001, Iowa State University Press, pp 103–104.

71. Takekawa J, Heath S, Douglas D, et al: Geographic variation in bar-headed geese Anser indicus: connectivity of wintering areas and breeding grounds across a broad front, *Wildfowl* 59:100–123, 2009.

72. Tattan A: *Alopochen aegyptiaca*, 2004. http://animaldiversity.ummz.umich.edu/accounts/Alopochen_aegyptiaca/. Accessed July 18, 2014.

73. Taylor S: *Anas Americana*, 2002. http://animaldiversity.ummz.umich.edu/accounts/Anas_americana/. Accessed July 18, 2014.

74. Tromberg C: *Anas Penelope*, 2014. http://animaldiversity.ummz.umich.edu/accounts/Anas_penelope/. Accessed July 18, 2014.

75. Vargas S: *Anser anser*, 2002. http://animaldiversity.ummz.umich.edu/accounts/Anser_anser/. Accessed July 18, 2014.

76. Ward S, Bishop C, Woakes A, Butler P: Heart rate and the rate of oxygen consumption of flying and walking barnacle geese (*branta leucopsis*) and bar-headed geese (*Anser indicus*), *J Exp Biol* 205:3347–3356, 2002.

77. Yarza F: *Branta Canadensis*, 2014. http://animaldiversity.ummz.umich.edu/accounts/Branta_canadensis/. Accessed July 18, 2014.

78. Emiley A, Dewey T: *Zenaida macroura*, 2014. http://animaldiversity.ummz.umich.edu/accounts/Zenaida_macroura/.Appendix-9781455746712.doc. Accessed July 18, 2014.

79. Gibbs D, Barnes E, Cox J: *Pigeons and doves: a guide to the pigeons and doves of the world*, Sussex, 2001, Pica Press.

80. Gyimesi ZS: Columbiformes. In Miller RE, Fowler ME, editors: *Fowler's zoo and wild animal medicine*, Vol 8, St. Louis, 2015, Saunders, p 168.

81. Roof J: *Columba livia*, 2001. http://animaldiversity.ummz.umich.edu/accounts/Columba_livia/. Accessed July 18, 2014.

82. BirdLife International Species Factsheet—Multiple Species: 2014. http://www.birdlife.org. Accessed August 12, 2014.

83. Camfield A: *Apodidae*, 2004. http://animaldiversity.ummz.umich.edu/accounts/Apodidae/. Accessed July 18, 2014.

84. Camfield A: *Trochilidae*, 2004. http://animaldiversity.ummz.umich.edu/accounts/Trochilidae/. Accessed July 18, 2014.

85. Chantler P, Driessens G: *Swifts: a guide to the swifts and treeswifts of the world*, ed 2, Sussex, 2000, Pica Press.

86. Collins C: Swifts. In: Elphick C, Dunning J, Sibley D, editors: *The Sibley guide to bird life and behavior*, New York, 2001, Alfred A. Knopf, pp 353–356.

87. The Cornell Lab of Ornithology Bird Guide—Multiple Species: 2014. http://www.allaboutbirds.org. Accessed August 11, 2014.

88. Kyle P, Kyle G: Swifts. In Gage LJ, Duerr RS, editors: *Hand-rearing birds*, Ames, 2007, Blackwell Publishing, pp 311–322.

89. Orr KA, Fowler ME: Order Trochiliformes (*Hummingbirds*). In Fowler ME, Cubas ZS, editors: *Biology, medicine, and surgery of South American wild animals*, Ames, 2001, Iowa State University Press, pp 175–176.

90. Purdin G: Chick identification. In Gage LJ, Duerr RS, editors: *Hand-rearing birds*, Ames, 2007, Blackwell Publishing, pp 15–37.

91. Sargent R, Sargent M: Hummingbirds. In Elphick C, Dunning J, Sibley D, editors: *The Sibley guide to bird life and behavior*, New York, 2001, Alfred A. Knopf, pp 357–365.

92. Beletsky L: *Birds of the world*, New York, 2006, The Johns Hopkins University Press.

93. Christie J: Pelecaniformes *(Pelicans and cormorants).* In Jackson J, Bock W, Olendorf D, Hutchins M, editors: *Grzimek's animal life encyclopedia,* Vol. 8, New York, 2003, Thomson and Gale, pp 183–186.

94. Dewey T: *Pelecanus erythrorhynchos,* 2009. http://animaldiversity.ummz.umich.edu/accounts/Pelecanus_erythrorhynchos/. Accessed July 18, 2014.

95. Harris M: *Sula nebouxii,* 2001. http://animaldiversity.ummz.umich.edu/accounts/Sula_nebouxii/. Accessed July 18, 2014.

96. Kearns L: *Anhinga anhinga,* 2009. http://animaldiversity.ummz.umich.edu/accounts/Anhinga_anhinga/. Accessed July 18, 2014.

97. Poole E: *Pelecanus conspicillatus,* 2011. http://animaldiversity.ummz.umich.edu/accounts/Pelecanus_conspicillatus/. Accessed July 18, 2014.

98. Redrobe S: Pelecaniformes. In Miller RE, Fowler ME, editors: *Fowler's zoo and wild animal medicine,* Vol 8, St. Louis, MO, 2015, Saunders, p 99.

99. Scott V: *Pelecanus occidentalis,* 2012. http://animaldiversity.ummz.umich.edu/accounts/Pelecanus_occidentalis/. Accessed July 18, 2014.

100. Ward E: *Phalacrocorax auritus,* 2000. http://animaldiversity.ummz.umich.edu/accounts/Phalacrocorax_auritus/. Accessed July 18, 2014.

101. Tully TN, Shane SM: *Ratite: management, medicine, and surgery,* Malabar, 1996, Krieger Publishing Company, pp 47–60.

102. Cousquer G: Ophthalmological findings in free-living tawny owls *(Strix aluco)* examined at a wildlife veterinary hospital, *Vet Rec* 156:734–739, 2005.

103. Holt E, Rosenthal K, Shofer FS: The phenol red thread tear test in large Psittaciformes, *Vet Ophthalmol* 9:109–113, 2006.

104. Jeong MB, Kim YG, Yi NY, et al: Comparison of the rebound tonometer *(TonoVet)* with the applanation tonometer *(TonoPen XL)* in normal Eurasian eagle owls *(Bubo bubo),* *Vet Ophthalmol* 10:376–379, 2007.

105. Kuhn SE, Jones MP, Hendrix DVH, et al: Normal ocular parameters and characterization of ophthalmic lesions in a group of captive bald eagles *(Haliaeetus leucocephalus),* *J Avian Med Surg* 27:90–98, 2013.

106. Lehmkul RC, Almedia MF, Mamprim MJ, et al: B-mode ultrasonography biometry of the Amazon parrot *(Amazona aestiva)* eye, *Vet Ophthalmol* 13(Suppl):26–28, 2010.

107. Meekins JM, Stuckey JA, Carpenter JW, et al: Ophthalmic diagnostic tests and ocular findings in a flock of captive American flamingos *(Phoenicopterus ruber ruber),* *J Avian Med Surg* 29:95–571, 2015.

108. Prashar A, Guggenheim JA, Erichsen JT, et al: Measurement of intraocular pressure (IOP) in chickens using a rebound tonometer: quantitative evaluation of variance due to position inaccuracies, *Exp Eye Res* 85:563–571, 2007.

109. Reuter A, Müller K, Arndt G, Eule JC: Reference intervals for intraocular pressure measured by rebound tonometry in ten raptor species and factors affecting the intraocular pressure, *J Avian Med Surg* 25:165–172, 2011.

110. Stiles J, Buyukmihci NC, Farver TB: Tonometry of normal eyes in raptors, *Am J Vet Res* 55:477–479, 1994.

111. Cooper JE: Appendix IX. Medicines and other agents used in treatment, including emergency anaesthesia kit and avian resuscitation protocol. In Cooper JE, editor: *Birds of prey: health and disease,* ed 3, Ames, 2002, Blackwell Publishing, pp 271–277.

112. Forbes NA, Richardson T: Husbandry and nutrition. In Beynon PH, Forbes NA, Harcourt–Brown NH, editors: *BSAVA manual of raptors, pigeons and waterfowl,* Ames, 1996, Iowa State University Press, pp 289–298.

113. Rupley AE: Critical care of pet birds, *Vet Clin North Am Exot Anim Pract* 1:11–41, 1998.

Index

Artificial insemination, 437–443, 554–555
    on Spix's macaw, 726–727, 727f
Ascaridia sp., ovum of, 519f
Ascending aorta, of domestic fowl, 255f
Ascites, 355–356
    due to hepatic cirrhosis, 358f
    secondary to cardiomyopathy, 356–357
    secondary to pulmonary hypertension, 356–357
Aspergilloma
    air sac, 66f
    in cranial thoracic air sac, endoscopic view of, 68f
    of syrinx, 68f
Aspergillosis, 63–70
    clinical signs and lesions of, 66–67
        acute form, 66
        chronic form, 66
    diagnosis of, 67–69
        antibody and antigen detection, 67
        cytology, 68
        endoscopy, 68, 68f
        fungal culture, 69
        hematology and serum chemistry, 67
        histopathology, 68, 69f
        polymerase chain reaction (PCR), 68
        radiology, 67–68
    disease predisposition of, 64–65
    etiology of, 63–64, 64f
    host immune response to, 65–66
    infection, international patterns of, 788-792t
    localized, 66, 66f
    pathogenesis of, 65–66
    in poultry, 563
    prevention for, 70
    treatment of, 69–70, 69t
        allylamines, 70
        azoles, 70
        polyenes, 69–70
Aspergillus fumigatus, 63
    culture, 64f
    granuloma, 65f
    virulence factors, 66
Aspergillus-related toxins, immunosuppressive effects of, 422
Aspergillus spp., 274–275
Assessment
    of catchment area, in key management metrics, 758
    fertility, 459–460
Association for the Conservation of Threatened Parrots (ACTP), 724–725
Association of Avian Veterinarians (AAV), 7, 7f, 8b, 678, 779–780
Association of Zoos and Aquariums Animal Care Manuals, 673–674
ASVCP. *see* American Society for Veterinary Clinical Pathology (ASVCP)
Atenolol, for cardiovascular disease in birds, 312t
Atherosclerosis, 265–271, 266f, 268f, 288, 377
    Amazon parrot with severe, 288
    avian nutrition and, 146
    clinical signs of, 288
    columbiformes, 270–271
    etiology and development of, 266

Atherosclerosis *(Continued)*
    galliformes, 270
    impact of diet in, 269
    isoxsuprine for, 311–313
    lesion characterization of, 266–267, 266f
    lesion location of, 267, 267f, 268f
    myocardial infarction associated with, 270
    in other avian orders, 269–271
    pathophysiology of, 266
    prevalence and risk factors, 267–269, 269f, 270t
    prognosis of, 320
    in raptors, 270
    risk factors of, 271
    treatment of, 311
Atipamezole, 606
Atoxoplasma, 74–75
Atoxoplasmosis, 359, 359f
Atracurium besylate, 610
Atropine, for cardiovascular disease in birds, 312t
Attachment, human-avian bond and, 710
Attending veterinarian, animal welfare and, 678–679
Atypical antipsychotics, 222
Auricapillus (Conure, gold-caped)
    enzymatic laboratory reference ranges for, 840-847t
    hematologic laboratory reference ranges for, 826-837t
    metabolic laboratory reference ranges for, 848-855t
Auricle, 365f
Auropalliata (Amazon, yellow nape)
    enzymatic laboratory reference ranges for, 840-847t
    hematologic laboratory reference ranges for, 826-837t
    metabolic laboratory reference ranges for, 848-855t
Australaves, 20
Australian and New Zealand College of Veterinary Scientists (ANZCVS), 14
Autoimmune diseases, 413
Autoimmune hemolytic anemia, 415
Autoimmune skin disease, 415, 415f
Autoimmune thyroiditis, 415
Automated hematology analyzers, 468
Automutilation, 226–234, 227f, 228f
    diagnostic workup for, 203t, 226f, 230–231, 231f
    etiologic considerations, 228–230
    factors involved in onset and maintenance of, 206t
    prognosis and monitoring of, 233–234, 234b
    species, age, and gender predilections in, 227–228, 227f
    therapeutic considerations of, 217f, 231–233, 232f, 233f
Autonomic innervation, on cloaca, 329
Autumnalis (Amazon, red-lored)
    enzymatic laboratory reference ranges for, 840-847t
    hematologic laboratory reference ranges for, 826-837t
    metabolic laboratory reference ranges for, 848-855t

AV node, in cardiac conduction system and coronary arteries, 259f
AV (mitral) valve, left, 254, 259f
Avascular necrosis, pinioning and, 699f
Average client transaction (ACT), 755
Avian
    chemistry panels of, 487t
    clinical neuroanatomy of, 363–369, 364f
    clinical neurology of, 363–377
    hematology, monitoring and preparation of reagents in, 464
    medicine, reference intervals and their applications, 478–482
    neurologic examination of, 369–374, 374b
        cranial nerve examination, 369–371
        mentation for, 369
Avian acute inflammatory demyelinating polyneuropathy (AvIDP), 418–419
Avian behavioral history form, 198-200b
Avian bornavirus (ABV), 28–33, 417
    as cause of PDD, 30–31
    clinical disease of, 37–38
    diagnosis of, 33–39
    disease patterns of, 37–38
    flock clearance from, 41
    flock management for, 40f, 41–43, 42f
    isolation of, 34
    occurrence of, 31
    potential pathogenesis of, 32–33
    tests for detection of, 35-36t
    therapy for, 39–41
    transmission of, 31–32
    vaccination for, 43
Avian bornavirus (ABV) antigen, 34
Avian bornavirus-specific antibodies, detection of, 34–37
Avian cancer patients, support of, 133–137
    client support in, 137–138
    nutritional support for, 136–137
    pain management in, 136
    quality of life assessment tool for, 135t
Avian cardiomyocytes, 254
Avian chlamydiosis, 86
Avian clinical pathology
    examples for analytical errors in, 464
    general concepts and limitations, 478–480, 480f
Avian encephalomyelitis, 561
Avian heart, 252, 255f, 256f, 257f
    computed tomography and magnetic resonance imaging for, 308–309, 309f
Avian influenza, 561
Avian influenza viruses (AIVs), 421
    in birds, 61–62
    current HPAI dynamics, 62
    diagnosis of, 60–61
    ecology of, 59–60
    pathobiology of, 59–60
    reportable, 61
    type A, biology of, 59
    vaccination for, 62
    virology of, 59–60
    zoonotic potential of, 61
        pet bird species, 61–62
Avian medicine, 1–21
    critical thinking, of evidence-based, 16–21
    growth of, 3–4